Y0-EGI-687

SURGICAL INFECTIOUS DISEASES

SURGICAL INFECTIOUS DISEASES

edited by

Richard L. Simmons, M.D.
Professor of Surgery and Microbiology
University of Minnesota Health Sciences Center
Minneapolis, Minnesota

Richard J. Howard, M.D., PH.D.
Associate Professor of Surgery
University of Florida College of Medicine
Gainesville, Florida

with

Angela I. Henriksen, B.A.
Editor, Department of Surgery
University of Minnesota Health Sciences Center
Minneapolis, Minnesota

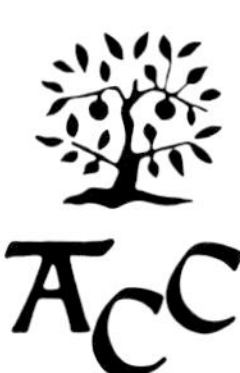

APPLETON-CENTURY-CROFTS/NEW YORK

82 83 84 85 86 / 10 9 8 7 6 5 4 3 2 1

Prentice-Hall International, Inc., London
Prentice-Hall of Australia, Pty. Ltd., Sydney
Prentice-Hall of India Private Limited, New Delhi
Prentice-Hall of Japan, Inc., Tokyo
Prentice-Hall of Southeast Asia (Pte.) Ltd., Singapore
Whitehall Books Ltd., Wellington, New Zealand

Library of Congress Cataloging in Publication Data
Main entry under title:

Surgical infectious diseases.

Bibliography: p.
Includes index.
1. Surgical wound infections. I. Simmons, Richard Lawrence, 1934– . II. Howard, Richard J. [DNLM: 1. Surgical wound infection. WO 185 S592s]
RD98.3.S953 617′.01 81–12739
ISBN 0–8385–8729–1 AACR2

NOTICE: Every effort has been made to ensure that the drug selection and dosage reported in this text include the recommendations and practice in use at the time of publication. We urge, however, that the package insert for each drug be consulted for recent changes in indications and dosage, and for added warnings and precautions. This is particularly important when the recommended agent is new or seldom used.

Design: Gloria J. Moyer

PRODUCTION: Lucinda C. Carbuto, Richard Horgan, John Morgan, Piedad Palencia, Jean M. Sabato, Judith Warm Steinig

PRINTED IN THE UNITED STATES OF AMERICA

DEDICATED TO

OWEN H. WANGENSTEEN
1898–1981
Chairman, Department of Surgery,
University of Minnesota, 1930–1967

AND

JOHN S. NAJARIAN
1927–
Chairman, Department of Surgery,
University of Minnesota, 1967–

Enthusiastic Teachers, Innovative Surgeons, and Leaders in American Surgery—For Establishing and Maintaining a Department of Surgery Devoted to Research, Scholarship, and Clinical Excellence

Contributors

George L. Adams, M.D.
Associate Professor, Department of Otolaryngology, University of Minnesota Medical School, Minneapolis, Minnesota

David H. Ahrenholz, M.D.
Medical Fellow, Department of Surgery, University of Minnesota Medical School, Minneapolis, Minnesota

J. Wesley Alexander, M.D., Sc.D.
Professor of Surgery; Director, Transplantation Division, University of Cincinnati; Director of Research, Shriners Burns Institute, Cincinnati, Ohio

Raymond A. Amoury, M.D.
Surgeon-in-Chief, The Children's Mercy Hospital, Kansas City, Missouri; Katharine Berry Richardson Professor of Pediatric Surgery, University of Missouri, Kansas City School of Medicine; Clinical Professor of Surgery, Creighton University School of Medicine, Omaha, Nebraska; Consultant in Surgery, Truman Medical Center and St. Luke's Hospital, Kansas City, Missouri

Robert W. Anderson, M.D.
Professor of Surgery; Director of Cardiovascular and Thoracic Surgery, University of Minnesota Medical School, Minneapolis, Minnesota

Louis H. Aulick, Ph.D., Lieutenant Colonel, MSC
Research Physiologist, US Army Institute of Surgical Research, Brooke Army Medical Center, Fort Sam Houston, Texas

Ian M. Baird, M.D.
Director of Infectious Diseases Section, Riverside Methodist Hospital, Columbus, Ohio

Henry H. Balfour, Jr., M.D.
Professor, Department of Laboratory Medicine and Pathology, and Pediatrics; Director, Division of Clinical Microbiology, University of Minnesota Medical School, Minneapolis, Minnesota

Donna J. Blazevic, M.P.H.
Professor, Department of Laboratory Medicine and Pathology, University of Minnesota Medical School, Minneapolis, Minnesota

John F. Burke, M.D.
Helen Andrus Benedict Professor of Surgery, Harvard Medical School; Chief, Trauma Services, Massachusetts General Hospital, Boston, Massachusetts

Daniel M. Canafax, Pharm.D.
Assistant Professor, Department and College of Pharmacy, University of Minnesota Medical School, Minneapolis, Minnesota

Michael E. Carey, M.D.
Professor, Department of Neurosurgery, Louisiana State University Medical School, New Orleans, Louisiana

Frank B. Cerra, M.D.
Associate Professor, Department of Surgery, State University of New York at Buffalo; Buffalo General Hospital, Buffalo, New York

A. Benedict Cosimi, M.D.
Chief, Clinical Transplant Surgery, Massachusetts General Hospital; Associate Professor, Department of Surgery, Harvard Medical School, Boston, Massachusetts

Robert E. Condon, M.D., M.S.
Professor and Chairman, Department of Surgery, The Medical College of Wisconsin; Chief of Surgical Services, Milwaukee County General Hospital, Wood Veterans Administration Hospital, and Froedtert Memorial Hospital; Consultant Surgeon, Columbia, Deaconess, Lutheran, Mt. Sinai, St. Joseph's, St. Luke's, and St. Mary's Hospitals, Milwaukee, Wisconsin

John H. Crandon, M.D.
Associate Clinical Professor, Department of Surgery, Tufts University Medical School, Boston, Massachusetts

Peter J.E. Cruse, M.D.
Professor and Chairman, Department of Surgery, University of South Alabama, Mobile, Alabama

P. William Curreri, M.D.
Johnson and Johnson Distinguished Professor of Surgery, Cornell Medical Center, New York, New York

Scott F. Davies, M.D.
Director, Section of Pulmonary Medicine, Department of Medicine, Hennepin County Medical Center, Minneapolis, Minnesota; Assistant Professor, Department of Medicine, University of Minnesota Medical School, Minneapolis, Minnesota

Gordon W. Douglas, M.D.
Professor and Chairman, Department of Obstetrics and Gynecology, New York University Medical Center, New York, New York

Thomas D. Dressel, M.D.
Medical Fellow, Department of Surgery, University of Minnesota Medical School, Minneapolis, Minnesota

Richard F. Edlich, M.D.
Professor of Plastic Surgery and Biomedical Engineering, Department of Plastic Surgery, University of Virginia Medical School, Charlottesville, Virginia

Thomas J. Enright, M.D., F.A.C.S.
Assistant Clinical Professor, Department of Surgery, Duke University School of Medicine, Durham, North Carolina; Assistant Chief, Surgical Service, Veterans Administration Medical Center, Asheville, North Carolina

Sydney M. Finegold, M.D.
Chief, Infectious Disease Section, Wadsworth Veterans Administration Medical Center; Professor, Department of Medicine, UCLA School of Medicine, Los Angeles, California

Michael P. Finn, M.D.
Instructor, Department of Surgery, University of Louisville School of Medicine, Louisville, Kentucky

Robert H. Fitzgerald, Jr., M.D.
Consultant and Assistant Professor, Department of Orthopedic Surgery, Mayo Clinic and Mayo Foundation, Rochester, Minnesota

Wesley Furste, M.D., F.A.C.S.
Clinical Professor, Department of Surgery, Ohio State University, Columbus, Ohio

Dale N. Gerding, M.D.
Chief, Infectious Disease Section, Veterans Administration Medical Center; Associate Professor, Department of Medicine, University of Minnesota Medical School, Minneapolis, Minnesota

Robert L. Goodale, Jr., M.D., Ph.D.
Associate Professor, Department of Surgery, University of Minnesota Medical School, Minneapolis, Minnesota

Patrick F. Hagihara, M.D.
Associate Professor, Department of Surgery, University of Kentucky College of Medicine, Lexington, Kentucky

Toni Hau, M.D.
Associate Professor, Department of Surgery, Case Western Reserve University, Cleveland, Ohio

David C. Hohn, M.D.
Assistant Professor, Department of Surgery, University of California Medical Center, San Francisco, California

Richard J. Howard, M.D., Ph.D.
Associate Professor, Department of Surgery, University of Florida College of Medicine, Gainesville, Florida

Thomas K. Hunt, M.D.
Professor, Department of Surgery and Ambulatory and Community Medicine, University of California San Francisco, San Francisco, California

Stephen C. Jacobs, M.D.
Assistant Professor, Department of Urology, Medical College of Wisconsin, Milwaukee County Medical Complex, Milwaukee, Wisconsin

Frank E. Jones, M.D.
Assistant Professor, Department of Surgery, Medical College of Wisconsin, Milwaukee County Medical Complex, Milwaukee, Wisconsin

Patrick J. Kelly, M.D.
Professor, Department of Orthopedic Surgery, Mayo Clinic and Mayo Foundation, Rochester, Minnesota

Charles F. Klinger, Ph.D.
Visiting Assistant Professor of History, University of Minnesota, Minneapolis, Minnesota

Harold Laufman, M.D., Ph.D., F.A.C.S.
Emeritus Professor, Department of Surgery, Albert Einstein College of Medicine; Emeritus Director, Institute for Surgical Studies, Montefiore Hospital and Medical Center, Bronx, New York

Russell K. Lawson, M.D.
Professor and Chairman, Department of Urology, Medical College of Wisconsin, Milwaukee County Medical Complex, Milwaukee, Wisconsin

Thom E. Lobe, M.D.
Clinical Instructor, Department of Surgery, Ohio State University Hospitals, Columbus, Ohio

James M. Malone, M.D.
Assistant Professor, Department of Surgery; Assistant Chief of Vascular Surgery, University of Arizona, Arizona Health Science Center, Tucson, Arizona

Stephen C. Marker, M.D.
Clinical Assistant Professor, Department of Laboratory Medicine and Pathology, and Pediatrics, University of Minnesota Medical School, Minneapolis, Minnesota

William J. Martin, Ph.D.
Head, Microbiology, Clinical Laboratories, UCLA Hospital and Clinics; Professor, Departments of Pathology, Microbiology and Immunology, UCLA School of Medicine, Los Angeles, California

Jonathan L. Meakins, M.D.
Associate Professor, Departments of Surgery and Microbiology, Royal Victoria Hospital and McGill University, Montreal, Quebec

Lee S. Monroe, M.D.
Clinical Professor, Department of Medicine, University of California, San Diego, California; Senior Consultant, Scripps Clinic and Research Foundation, LaJolla, California

Wesley S. Moore, M.D.
Professor, Department of Surgery, University of California Center for the Health Sciences, Los Angeles, California

Ronald Lee Nichols, M.D.
Henderson Professor of Surgery; Professor of Microbiology and Immunology, Tulane University Medical Center Hospital; and Attending Surgeon, Charity Hospital of Louisiana at New Orleans, Louisiana

Phillip K. Peterson, M.D.
Associate Professor, Department of Medicine, University of Minnesota Medical School, Minneapolis, Minnesota

Hiram C. Polk, Jr., M.D.
Professor and Chairman, Department of Surgery, University of Louisville School of Medicine, Louisville, Kentucky

Samuel R. Powers, Jr., M.D. (Deceased)
Professor and Chairman, Department of Surgery; Professor, Department of Physiology, Albany Medical College of Union University, Albany, New York

George T. Rodeheaver, Ph.D.
Research Associate Professor, Department of Plastic Surgery, University of Virginia Medical School, Charlottesville, Virginia

Robert H. Rubin, M.D.
Associate Professor, Department of Medicine, Harvard Medical School; Associate Physician, Infectious Disease and Transplant Units, Massachusetts General Hospital, Boston, Massachusetts

Thomas M. Saba, Ph.D.
Professor and Harold C. Wiggers Chairman, Department of Physiology, Albany Medical College of Union University, Albany, New York

Lee D. Sabath, M.D.
Professor, Department of Medicine, University of Minnesota Medical School, Minneapolis, Minnesota

George A. Sarosi, M.D.
Chief, Medical Service, Veterans Administration Medical Center; Professor and Vice-Chairman, Department of Medicine, University of Minnesota Medical School, Minneapolis, Minnesota

Stewart M. Scott, M.D.
Associate Chief of Staff for Research and Development, Veterans Administration Medical Center, Asheville, North Carolina; Associate Clinical Professor, Department of Surgery, Duke University Medical Center, Durham, North Carolina

Gordon F. Schwartz, M.D., F.A.C.S.
Professor, Department of Surgery, Jefferson Medical College, Philadelphia, Pennsylvania; Attending Physician (Surgery), Thomas Jefferson University Hospital, Philadelphia; Consultant Surgeon, Bryn Mawr Hospital, Bryn Mawr, Pennsylvania, Chestnut Hill Hospital, Philadelphia, and Veterans Administration Center, Wilmington, Delaware

Gulshan K. Sethi, M.D.
Chief, Cardiac Surgical Section, Veterans Administration Medical Center, Asheville, North Carolina; Associate Clinical Professor, Department of Surgery, Duke University School of Medicine, Durham, North Carolina

Herbert M. Sommers, M.D.
Professor, Department of Pathology, Northwestern University Medical School, Chicago, Illinois

J. Dwight Stinnett, Ph.D.
Associate Professor, Research Surgery and Microbiology, Department of Surgery, University of Cincinnati College of Medicine, Cincinnati, Ohio

Edward H. Storer, M.D.
Professor, Department of Surgery, Yale University; Chief Surgical Service, West Haven Veterans Administration Medical Center, West Haven, Connecticut

Timothy Takaro, M.D.
Chief, Surgical Service, Veterans Administration Medical Center, Asheville, North Carolina; Clinical Professor, Department of Surgery, Duke University School of Medicine, Durham, North Carolina

John G. Thacker, Ph.D.
Associate Professor, Department of Mechanical Engineering, University of Virginia, Charlottesville, Virginia

M. David Tilson, M.D.
Associate Professor, Department of Surgery, Yale University School of Medicine, New Haven, Connecticut

Marc S. Visner, M.D.
Fellow, Department of Surgery, University of Minnesota Medical School, Minneapolis, Minnesota

Stephen R. Waltman, M.D.
Professor, Department of Ophthalmology, Washington University School of Medicine, St. Louis, Missouri

Owen H. Wangensteen, M.D. (Deceased)
Chairman and Regents Professor Emeritus, Department of Surgery, University of Minnesota Medical School, Minneapolis, Minnesota

Sarah D. Wangensteen, B.A.
Senior Medical Historian Emeritus, Department of Medical History, University of Minnesota Medical School, Minneapolis, Minnesota

Vallee L. Willmann, M.D.
Professor, Department of Surgery, St. Louis University, St. Louis, Missouri

Douglas W. Wilmore, M.D.
Associate Professor, Department of Surgery, Harvard Medical School at the Brigham and Women's Hospital, Boston, Massachusetts

Lowell S. Young, M.D.
Professor, Division of Infectious Diseases, School of Medicine, University of California, Los Angeles, California

Contents

PART VIII. SPECIAL PROBLEMS IN SURGICAL INFECTIONS

Preface

INFECTION IS encountered by all surgeons and surgical specialists who, by the nature of their craft, invariably impair the first lines of host defense—the cutaneous or mucosal barrier—between the environmental microbe and the host's interior milieu. In the past surgeons made some of the most important contributions to the development of early antiseptic techniques and the environmental control of infection. With the standardization of these approaches and the advent of modern antibiotic therapy, however, surgeons as a group tended to lose interest in the study of infection. Progress in the understanding of its pathogenesis and treatment was given over to medical specialists in infectious diseases, who in turn tended to focus on systemic diseases caused by single organisms occurring in otherwise normal hosts.

For these reasons, there has not been a comprehensive textbook of surgical infections since Frank Meleney's *Clinical Aspects and Treatment of Surgical Infections,* published in 1949. Although there are several excellent medical reference-textbooks, their emphasis is on virology and single agent etiology. Surgeons tend to ignore these texts because surgical infections are regional infections caused by polymicrobial endogenous flora in hosts whose defenses are compromised.

This reference text is an attempt to gather together useful material on the pathogenesis, diagnosis, and treatment of infectious diseases for the library of both the mature surgeon and the surgeon in training. We hope that this compiled information will be used as a basis for further advances in the understanding of surgical infectious diseases.

We have divided this book into eight sections: history, surgical microbiology, host defenses, systemic response to infection, antimicrobial therapy, wound infections and their prevention, regional surgical infections, and special problems in surgical infection. The sections on surgical microbiology and antimicrobial therapy concentrate on those microorganisms that are most likely to cause infection in surgical patients.

We feel that the section on host defenses is particularly important because in the end it is the host's own defenses that rid the patient of infection. We predict that the field of host defenses, and how to improve them, will receive intensive investigation in the remaining years of this decade.

Because the surgeon is the physician who frequently deals with the septic patient, septic shock, and systemic organ failure in sepsis, we included a section on the physiologic and metabolic alterations occurring in the infection patient.

The final three sections deal with actual clinical problems. The section on wound infections discusses the epidemiology, causes, and prevention of wound infections. The section on regional surgical infection adopts the anatomic, regional approach because surgeons frequently think in these terms and clinically are usually presented with infections in a single region. This is not a how-to-do-it section.

Like all multi-authored books, style and clarity may vary from chapter to chapter, but we have exerted a strong editing hand in all chapters in an attempt to provide consistency. Therefore, any criticism should be reserved for us. We believe that the advantages of having experts write clearly about their areas of specialty far outweigh the potential consistency provided by a single-authored book.

This book could not have come into being without the help of several other individuals. We would like to thank Dr. John S. Najarian for his constant support and encouragement. We are especially grateful to Angela I. Henriksen for her creative editorial contribution during every stage of our book's development. We are also grateful to Carolyn M. Keene, Candy Swain, Carol A. Markwood (Gainesville), and Kathryn P. Anderson and Ann Marie Klapperich (Minneapolis) for typing the manuscripts.

R.L.S., R.J.H.

Surgical Infectious Diseases

PART I: HISTORY

CHAPTER 1
Surgical Infection and History

OWEN H. WANGENSTEEN, SARAH D. WANGENSTEEN, AND CHARLES F. KLINGER

THE mid-sixteenth century witnessed three significant events in the advance of medicine: Girolamo Fracastoro described the significance of direct contact in the propagation of infection (1546); Ambroise Paré demonstrated, conclusively, the superiority of instillation of turpentine, instead of burning-hot oil, into battle wounds (1545); and Andreas Vesalius' great and beautifully illustrated book, *On the Fabric of the Human Body*, appeared in print (1543). Perhaps never in medical history have three such important works appeared within so brief a period, and each was to leave an indelible imprint on medical progress.

For centuries before and more than three centuries after Fracastoro, the nature of infection remained an enigma. He conceived of seminaria (germs) as the provocative agents of infection. The microscope was more than a century away, as were the animalcules (bacteria) of Leeuwenhoek. The proof of the pathogenicity of bacteria awaited the methodology and the careful work of Robert Koch (1876–78). Robert Hooke's *Micrographia* (1665) marked the beginnings of microbiology, a science that has greatly enriched medicine in this romantic period, which witnessed a steady succession of contributions to medicine's advance. Jacob Henle (1840) directed notice to the role of bacteria in the origins of miasmas, and the imaginative research of the wide-ranging chemist Louis Pasteur, unhindered by the restrictive barriers of conventional scientific disciplines, helped solve the mysteries of many diseases of animals and man. The careful and systematic methodology of that greatest of microbiologists of the nineteenth century, Robert Koch, succeeded in separating and identifying bacteria by substituting use of solid culture media for broth. His demonstration of the life cycle of the anthrax bacillus was labeled by Cohnheim (April 1876) as the greatest discovery in microbiology up to that time. Koch's innovation of photographing bacteria rather than describing them also marked an important advance. Koch's postulates sketching the means of establishing the pathogenicity of bacteria as the causative agents of disease have found universal acceptance.

Samuel Johnson's *Dictionary of the English Language* (1755), consisting of two huge tomes that rapidly went through a second and third edition, contains the words contagion, contagious, infectious, infective, and infection. The contagious nature of many diseases had already been well established. Puerperal fever was believed to be contagious in nature until Ignacz Semmelweis (1847) demonstrated it was carried by the unclean hands of the accoucheur. Scrubbing the hands in warm soap and water with a nail brush, followed by a similar scrub in chlorine water (Dakin's solution of World War I), quickly decimated the mortality of that dreadful scourge. With general acceptance of the prophylactic surgical antisepsis of Semmelweis, puerperal fever has virtually disappeared. Bacteria is a post-Semmelweis word innovation of the mid-nineteenth century.

Semmelweis (March 1847) was led to his conclusion while studying the autopsy report on his friend Kolletschka, who died from sepsis after he had sustained a finger prick while performing an autopsy on a patient who had died of sepsis at Vienna's Allgemeines Krankenhaus. Semmelweis inferred that the lethal agents in puerperal fever were the unclean hands, instruments, and linen employed by accoucheurs. By mid-May 1847, Semmelweis had initiated a strict program at the Vienna hospital involving scrubbing of the hands in soap and warm water with a fingernail brush, followed by a similar scrub in Dakin's solution. Instruments to be employed in the delivery were also immersed in a solution of chlorine water. By June, Karl Haller, an adjunct director of the hospital, wrote: "A fresh breeze permeates the hospital atmosphere that augurs well for the future of obstetrics and surgery." Although Semmelweis, a direct and brusque man in dealing with associates, initially incurred the wrath and enmity of many professional colleagues, not many years after publication of his 1861 monograph, *Die Aetiologie, der Begriff und die Prophylaxis des Kindbettfiebers,* his antagonists capitulated to his views. Why the Vienna surgeons took no note of Semmelweis' significant innovation remains a mystery. Other than Haller, the first to take serious note thereof was Ferdinand von Hebra, who was originally intent on surgery but turned to dermatology. Actually, the first to employ Semmelweis' methods in elective abdominal surgery was the Freiburg gynecologist Alfred Hegar who, in 1876–77, reported 15 successive excisions of ovarian cysts without mortality, an operation that in the hands of well-known ovariotomists of that period commanded an operative mortality of 25 to 40 percent. Semmelweis' initial work (1847–49) antedated recognition and acceptance of the pathogenicity of bacteria by approximately four decades and the first publication of Lister (1867) by 20 years.

Placement of antiseptics into wounds is an ancient practice, featured in the parable of the Good Samaritan (Luke 10:34). Lister lent great impetus to surgery's advance by instilling varying concentrations of carbolic acid into the open wounds of compound fractures (1867), a practice he extended to other wounds and later to elective operations. Over great opposition in Britain and America, Listerian practices had found general adoption by the mid-1880s, to be supplanted shortly thereafter by the prophylactic surgical antisepsis of Semmelweis (1847). At the end of World War I, Alexander Fleming (1919) protested the placement of antiseptic agents into wounds, saying they did more harm to the tissues than to the bacteria. In later publications, Fleming described the bactericidal properties of lysozyme and of penicillium mold (1929), which led to the development of penicillin and other antibiotics.

Prior to the innovation of printing (ca 1450), the art and practice of surgery were taught to apprentices primarily by word of mouth and observation. Surgeons of that period were essentially an unlettered lot, disdained by physicians. Surgeons, despite their low status, did have the advantage of acquiring practical experience through their labors, while physicians in their teaching exercises devoted themselves solely to philosophic discussions of the disease they were called upon to treat, failing to employ patient demonstrations in their lectures to students. Jean Louis Petit (1710), an accomplished Paris surgeon, was among the first who declined to acknowledge the superiority of physicians.

Until the demonstration of the pathogenicity of bacteria by Koch (1876–78) and the acceptance of bacterial etiology of tissue infection, surgical management and avoidance of wound infection remained in a chaotic state. Erysipelas and "hospital gangrene" in wounds were commonplace. In the mid-1870s, Volkmann of Halle and Nussbaum of Munich informed university authorities that the frequency of these lethal complications was forcing them to close their surgical wards.

Methods of treating wounds were subjected to argument rather than trial. Very little note had been taken of the study of James Lind, the Haslar Hospital naval surgeon, who had taken 12 sailors with scurvy to sea (1747). They were divided into six groups, two in each, and fed a basic naval diet, with various additions for each group. At six days, the two sick sailors provided with two oranges and one lemon each day were already seaworthy. This was probably the first published, controlled, clinical study in medicine (1753).

Open wound management of amputations and "minute particulars" permitted a few surgeons to achieve results rarely excelled, even following the acceptance of prophylactic surgical antisepsis. Pouteau of Lyons (1760), in 120 instances of perineal lithotomy for the removal of vesical calculi, lost three patients, a hospital mortality of 2.5 percent. Pouteau stressed cleanliness and left the perineal wound open, permitting the urine to wash the wound.

Alexander Monro I of the Royal Infirmary in Edinburgh (1737, 1752) was able to report a hospital mortality for amputations of 8 percent; almost a century later (1843) in the same hospital the mortality was more than five times greater (49 percent), definitely suggesting that surgical cleanliness had deteriorated, giving way to speed in the performance of amputation, with neglect of "minute particulars."

SPONTANEOUS GENERATION

The belief in spontaneous generation was present throughout antiquity; Aristotle and Van Helmont firmly believed in it. The strongest advocate of the thesis of spontaneous generation in the eighteenth century was Needham (1713–81), and in the nineteenth, Pouchet (1800–72). The English neurologist Henry Bastian (1837–1915) entered the fray on their side in 1911. Spallanzani (1729–99) had, in the view of many scientists (1767, 1776), disproved the validity of the Needham thesis, but doubt persisted until Pasteur and Tyndall brought conclusive proof to bear on the invalidity of spontaneous generation.

PASTEUR'S IMPRINT

John Hughes Bennett (1868), fellow of the Royal Society of Edinburgh, professor of the Institutes of Medicine, and senior professor of clinical medicine at the University of Edinburgh, wrote a pamphlet entitled *On the Atmospheric Germ Theory and Origin of Infusoria.* The author challenged Pasteur's finding of the sterility of fluids subjected to boiling, including sealed bent tubes that precluded admission of air. In fact, Bennett was unable to confirm Pasteur's observations. He was apparently unaware of the work of Davaine on the multiplication and fission of bacteria (1860). Bennett's work also antedated the observations of Ferdinand Cohn (1876), who confirmed Davaine's earlier findings of the extraordinary rapidity of germination and propagation of bacteria.

John Farley (1977) critically analyzed the historic and philosophic background of spontaneous generation, and Aleksandr Oparin (1936) reviewed the history of the "Origin of Life" on the planet earth. Toncsik reviewed the entire history of experimentation on the theory of spontaneous generation from the time of Francesco Redi (1668) up through the work of Pasteur (1861), who, with the aid of Tyndall's studies on moteless air and discontinuous repetitive fractional sterilization (1877, 1881), dealt the death blow to the thesis of spontaneous generation.

Pasteur Vallery-Radot, a grandson of Pasteur, traced Pasteur's origins and successively enumerated his more important contributions. First came his work with crystals and their separation into tartrate and paratartrate. Pasteur's first work in the biologic field concerned fermentation; then spontaneous generation, in which area he made a very significant contribution; followed by studies of wine, vinegar, and beer; then silkworm disease. Pasteur was interested in the germ theory and its application to medicine and surgery, and began his research in 1873. In 1877, Pasteur addressed the problem of anthrax. He also studied cholera of chickens and prepared a vaccine for its prevention and treatment.

Louis Nicol (1974) stressed the role of Pasteur's keen interest in and knowledge of veterinary medicine in the progress of his work and discoveries. Nicol expanded on the role of Henri Bouley, the French apostle of veterinary medicine, and his relationship to Pasteur, whose contact with veterinary medicine over long years was intimate. Nicol's chatty monograph contains many letter exchanges between the principals, with considerable emphasis on rabies. The death of Bouley (1884) terminated the long collaboration between Pasteur and veterinary medicine, an influence extended by Nocard, a pupil of Bouley, and again through Nocard's friendship with Duclaux, Roux, and Chamberland.

Albert Delaunay summarized the growth and development of Pasteur's interest in microbiology. Casimir-Joseph Davaine (1812–82) was the first to recognize the pathogenicity of microbes. He wrote (1860) of the rapidity with which bacteria divide and reproduce themselves.

Delaunay described the birth of microbiology, tracing the development of knowledge of the pathogenicity of bacteria and viruses, natural and acquired immunity, the mechanisms of immunity, and the prevention and treatment of infectious diseases. Delaunay dealt at some length with Metchnikoff and phagocytosis.

The Dijon, Dole, and Arbois areas, the scenes of Pasteur's early life in the Jura section of eastern France, contain important memorabilia of Pasteur's development into a keen, mature, and creative scientist. A visit there can definitely be recommended to all students of Pasteur and his brilliant achievements. Pasteur spent the final years of a productive life at the Pasteur Institute in Paris in the company of many celebrated pupils including Roux, Duclaux, Chamberland, Metchnikoff, and others. A visit to the Pasteur Institute can be an experience that stirs the emotions and makes one appreciate Pasteur's durable contributions to human welfare.

THEORIES OF IMMUNITY

Élie Metchnikoff (1845–1916), a zoologist and embryologist by training, spent the final 25 years of his life at the Pasteur Institute. He is usually regarded as the founder of the phagocytic theory of immunity. He introduced a rose thorn into the transparent larvae of the starfish and noted hours later that the mobile cells of the larvae worked their way to the splinter. Metchnikoff noted that when the transparent crustacean daphnia was infected with a small parasitic fungus, a struggle ensued between the daphnia's mobile cells and the parasite. He observed also that in mammalian laboratory animals, white blood corpuscles engulfed bacteria. With the advice of Greek scholars, Metchnikoff called the phenomenon of engulfing and devouring organisms phagocytosis.

A long struggle ensued between proponents of the humoral theory and the proponents of Metchnikoff's cellular theory of immunity. Today, it is conceded that both have significant roles to play in immunity. Development of the cellular theory undoubtedly represents Metchnikoff's most important scientific contribution.

Metchnikoff expressed the belief and hope that man's useful life could be extended to 140 years. He thought that the absorptive capacity of the colon, which permits toxic substances to enter the blood, was the chief deterrent to the achievement of that objective. He entertained the idea that at some future date the colon could be safely removed by surgery to obviate this occurrence. Meanwhile, his attack on the problem was to alter the bacterial flora of the colon by the ingestion of lactic acid milk, of which yogurt is probably the current counterpart. Metchnikoff subsequently labeled intestinal microbes a significant cause of senility. He was an abstainer from alcohol and tobacco, which he regarded as important ancillary causes of arteriosclerosis and senility. Despite his long dietary reliance on lactic acid milk, Metchnikoff spent his final years as an invalid. He suffered almost daily from painful anginal and cardiac attacks, requiring narcotics for relief. He died at age 71, achieving only half the life expectancy of 140 years that he had projected for man. He quoted the Bible frequently in his writings but made no allusion to the admonition of verse 10 of Psalm 90: "The days of our years are threescore years and ten; and if by reason of strength they be fourscore years, yet is their strength labour and sorrow."

As related to freedom from taxation and other fiscal or religious obligations, immunity is a word of ancient origin. As applied to disease, it probably originated with Pasteur, who noted that there are some infections of man to which many laboratory animals are naturally immune. Acquired immunity and its mechanism of acquisition are not completely understood.

The original theory of the body's defense against bacterial invasion held to the humoral thesis that the blood plasma possessed great bactericidal qualities. Metchnikoff was primarily responsible for promulgating the cellular theory of immunity; allusion has already been made to his studies on phagocytosis in crustacean larvae. Denys and LeClef observed that removing the leukocytes from the blood resulted in a considerable reduction of the bactericidal property of the blood; the addition of leukocytes restored its antibacterial quality. They showed that washed leukocytes are deprived of their phagocytic activity. This activity is restored only when the leukocytes are again placed in blood serum or plasma, a circumstance indicating how interdependent the cellular and humoral theories of immunity are in action.

A succession of events characterized by chemotactic attraction of polymorphonuclear leukocytes, macrophages, and lymphocytes brings the bacteria to the leukocytes that have escaped by a process of diapedesis through the venules and capillary blood vessels in the area. The bacteria become adherent to the wall of the leukocytes, which then ingest and digest the offenders. Bordet has shown that some bacteria, notably streptococcus, exude a substance that inhibits this sequence of events, thus interfering with and delaying phagocytosis. It is this repellent action of streptococci upon leukocytes that permits rapid spread of the ensuing cellulitic infection.

Jenner (1749–1823), a pupil of John Hunter, securely established the protective effect of cowpox vaccination against smallpox, an accomplishment that military leaders like Napoleon I greatly appreciated. The Jennerian program of vaccination prevented the decimation of armies. H. J. Parish has suggested that "smallpox may have preserved Canada for the British Empire." General Washington failed to take Quebec in 1776 because his army under Generals Richard Montgomery and Benedict Arnold had not been vaccinated, and losses from smallpox were great. Today, prophylactic vaccination has apparently eliminated smallpox throughout the world.

The humoral thesis of immunity undoubtedly had its origin in Jenner's great accomplishment, but scientific proof of the validity of the humoral thesis of immunity awaited the work of Nuttall (1888) and of Buchner (1889–90), who demonstrated that a cell-free serum has bactericidal activity.

MANAGEMENT OF CONTAMINATED WOUNDS

OPEN MANAGEMENT

The thirteenth century surgeon Theodoric (1205–96) held that wounds could heal without suppuration, a thesis that Henri de Mondeville (1260–1329) also supported. The erudite surgeon Guy de Chauliac (1298–1368) of Avignon favored open management of contaminated wounds; many surgical historians believed he thereby retarded surgery's advance, as much as six centuries according to Garrison (1922). A few pre-Listerian surgeons, notably von Kern of Vienna (1826), Liston (1841) of London's University College Hospital, and the German surgeon Burow (1859), employed open-wound management in amputation, with mortalities considerably lower than that of surgeons primarily closing wounds.

DEBRIDEMENT

In March 1917, before American entry into World War I, the Inter-Allied Surgical Conference of English–French Military Surgeons convened in Paris and resolved that all contaminated wounds should be subjected to debridement with excision of all dead tissue and left open. On April 26, 1943, in World War II, Surgeon General Norman Kirk of the American Army Medical Corps mandated debridement for all contaminated wounds, with open-wound management. Circular amputations without skin flaps were also mandated, leaving such wounds open, to be closed secondarily. Guy's (1363) wound practices of almost six centuries earlier finally found universal adoption in military circles, and soon thereafter in civilian surgery.

SURGICAL ACCOUNTABILITY

Before the acceptance of prophylactic surgical antisepsis, surgeons were reluctant to publish their operative and hospital mortalities, and understandably so, because of the frequency of serious wound infections that proved lethal. Florence Nightingale, who emerged from the Crimean War (1854–56) as a legendary hero, and who devoted the remainder of her long life to improving nursing and hospitals, had repeatedly urged on hospital authorities and surgeons the need to publish their hospital and operative mortalities. Yet very few went along with the suggestion. As late as 1875, Lawson Tait, a well-known Birmingham gynecologist and surgeon, urged the board of a large municipal hospital to publish the hospital and operative mortalities. The hospital's board of supervisors advised Tait that they did not elect to do so. Tait threatened to publish their letter of refusal in a widely read medical journal if they did not provide the data. The board capitulated and, said Tait, with the elapsing of a few years, the operative mortality of that hospital decreased by 50 percent.

Sir James Paget of London's Guy's Hospital related in *Lancet* (1862) that Sir Astley Cooper had visited a prominent Paris surgeon (undoubtedly Dominique Larrey) and had made hospital rounds with him approximately 20 years previously. Larrey had declared to Cooper that he had no mortality from amputation at the shoulder joint. When they visited the dead house together, there lay upon the autopsy table a fresh body upon which a recent disarticulation at the shoulder joint had been performed, a favorite operation of Larrey's. Larrey remarked that the patient died of pneumonia, not from the operation. "We must beware of such dishonesty," wrote Paget. He added, "I have as yet scarcely lost a case in true consequence of hernia, tracheotomy, or trephining . . . yet nearly half of all that I have operated on for hernia had died, and more than half after tracheotomy and nearly all after trephining. But these were deaths after operations; not because of them."

HOSPITAL REFORMERS

England's first great hospital and prison reformer was John Howard (1727–90), who on a vacation-bound ship to Lisbon in 1756 underwent imprisonment in Brest, France, at the hands of a French privateer. The misery of the imprisonment left an enduring impression on Howard. He was shocked to discover in 1773 the health conditions in his small county jail, and sought comparison with nearby institutions. Howard then began an investigation and self-appointed mission that was to occupy the remainder of his life and entail 50,000 miles of travel. He particularly criticized the environmental conditions of hospitalization, as well as diets in lazarettos and hospitals in many countries. At Hôtel Dieu in Paris, he found as many as five to six patients in a single bed, some of them dying. Howard's last journey took him to St. Petersburg (Leningrad), Moscow, and Cherson (Sevastopol), where he died of an infectious fever characterized by convulsions; he became the hero and martyr to a great cause. The Russian government erected an impressive monument near the Black Sea to honor Howard's contribution to the health of the Russian people. Commented Edmund Burke, English statesman, "Howard's life was a voyage of discovery."

In Jacques Tenon (1724–1816), France had its first great sanitarian and hospital reformer. The eldest of 11 children of an impecunious surgeon in a village south of Paris, young Tenon went to Paris at age 17 to learn something of his father's profession. Witnessing surgery at Hôtel Dieu filled him with horror. He then joined the Danish anatomist, Jacques Winslow, at Jardin-du-Roi in Paris. When Winslow observed a heart preparation Tenon had made, he gave the young investigator a position on his staff. Quickly, Tenon learned to read Latin and Greek and received a degree in philosophy. After a tour as an army surgeon, he won the chair of surgery at the Paris Salpetrière. Later, he occupied the chair of pathology at the Royal Academy for many years. Tenon studied the conditions in hospitals in France and England, visiting hospitals in Oxford, Birmingham, Bristol, Plymouth, Exeter, Salisbury, Winchester, and Portsmouth, making a detailed inventory of the care of the sick, including diet, beds, attitude toward patients, hours and frequency of meals, and general care. He studied the water supply of hospitals, their amphitheaters, operating room suites, and hospital ventilation. His epochal report remains pertinent for hospital construction and bed assignments today. He studied hospital records and found that Hôtel Dieu in Paris had probably the highest mortality among hospitals. He recommended that surgical wards should not be near the postmortem rooms; that separate rooms be set aside for operations, for preparing patients for operations, and for postoperative care; he suggested too that obstetrical beds not be mingled with surgical beds in the wards.

THE IMPRINT OF A FEW PUBLIC SANITARIANS

Chadwick (1890), a young English attorney, abandoned the law to study systems of public health. He became a follower of Jeremy Bentham (1748–1832), the founder of utilitarianism—the greatest good to the greatest number—and an ardent champion of the cause of sanitation and betterment of public health. Chadwick was primarily responsible for passage of the act that established a board of public health in England (1848). His memorable *Report on the Sanitary Condition of the Labouring Population of Great Britain* was presented to the House of Lords in 1842. He found that the length of life was shorter among laborers than among the gentry and professional persons; he then made a serious plea to improve the living conditions of the poor. To this end, he spent the remainder of his long professional life attempting to reduce filth and the physical suffering of the poor, and to remedy the moral disorder prevalent among the lower classes of English society.

The year 1858 marked the period of the "Great Stink," owing to the pollution of the Thames by sewage, which was so bad that Parliament had to adjourn periodically; the unpleasant odor made work impossible. Ultimately, the sewage of London was dumped into the lower reaches of the Thames and washed out to sea.

John Simon (1816–1904), distinguished St. Thomas Hospital surgeon, abandoned the practice of surgery at age 32 to become the first medical officer of the city of London (1848). Simon had been broadly trained. He was the first in 1852 to do a successful ureterorectal anastomosis for urinary incontinence caused by congenital vesical ectopia. Simon regarded trial by jury, in court hearings in which professional experts from opposite sides vigorously supported their partisan interests, as "moral prostitution and subordination of science." Simon studied the medical literature for clues of the sources of hospital insalubrity, and he cited Semmelweis's contribution to the establishment of prophylactic surgical antisepsis; Lister's first publication on wound antisepsis (1867) was still 3 years away. It was obvious that Simon was more knowledgeable concerning the status of hospital sanitation than most men of his time.

The New York surgeon Stephen Smith (1823–1922), who remained active and healthy into his late nineties, devoted a good segment of his long professional life to questions of public health on a voluntary basis. With the help of William Cullen Bryant, editor of the *Evening News*, he threatened to expose an extensive and wealthy landowner, one of whose apartments was a fever nest and the source of an epidemic. The culprit immediately initiated corrective measures, which converted the long-neglected apartment complex into a safe place to live and also brought the owner high rents. Smith's stress on improving the public health brought about in legislative sessions the Metropolitan Health Bill (1865), which succeeded in ridding New York City of much of the filth in which many of its poor lived. In his story of his struggles to do away with rubbish heaps and filth, Smith alluded to the insistence of the Hebrew fathers on cleanliness in formulation of the Mosaic Sanitary Code.

SOME REGIONAL VARIETIES OF INFECTION

EMPYEMA

Toward the end of World War I and before the availability of the sulfonamides and penicillin, the pandemic of streptococcal pneumonia terminating in empyema commanded worldwide attention. The mortality was horrendous, reaching 90 percent according to some reports, owing in large measure to employment of early open drainage. The current practice then was to follow one of Hippocrates' rules concerning suppuration, that wherever collections of pus occur, they should be immediately evacuated. But physicians and surgeons continued to overlook the stricture that Hippocrates had advised and imposed upon suppuration in the pleural cavity: in the presence of serous exudation, open drainage, whether by an intercostal incision or a rib resection, should be delayed until the exudate, on aspiration, had become thickened by the presence of fibrin. It remained for the French surgeon C. E. Sédillot (1841) to recall the admonition of Hippocrates on this score. Yet despite Sédillot's advice, physicians and surgeons almost universally continued to establish early open drainage for all empyemas. Only in World War I did Evarts Graham and the chemist R. D. Bell redirect attention to the hazards of open drainage of the thoracic cavity in the presence of serous streptococcal empyemas. Fortunately, with the arrival of sulfanilamide (1935) and penicillin for army (1942) and civilian use (1944–45), empyema became rare.

SUBPHRENIC AND OTHER INTRAPERITONEAL ABSCESSES

Subphrenic abscesses occur as a consequence of a perforated tubular abdominal viscus, notably from perforation of a duodenal or gastric ulcer, the appendix, gallbladder, or colon; it may also occur as an iatrogenic complication following intra-abdominal surgery, in which a leak occurs as a sequel to imperfect techniques in operations upon the gastrointestinal tract. An infected hematoma from injury of the pancreas or spleen may also give rise to subphrenic abscess. An imperfect inversion of the duodenal stump attending Billroth II gastric resections has continued to be an occasional antecedent of subphrenic abscess.

A large pneumoperitoneum, attending perforation of a duodenal ulcer, indicates that the perforation is also large and leaking, a circumstance suggesting that digestion of the diaphragm with a resultant hole and extension of digestive juices into the thorax is a possibility. An accumulation of acid peptic juice immediately beneath the diaphragm can readily do this with the development of an empyema. Howard Beye reported that in a series of 337 patients with thoracic empyema, he had only once observed transversion of the diaphragm from above with resultant subphrenic abscess. To the contrary, in 31 patients with subphrenic abscess of abdominal origin, Beye noted thoracic complications in 23 instances (74 percent), usually empyema.

The Finnish surgeon Autio reported that in performing appendectomy he left 10 ml of an opaque sterile x-ray medium in the lateral gutter of the pericecal area. X-ray films were taken at intervals between 3 and 12 hours and again between 24 and 72 hours after the operation in a large number of patients. He noted wide dispersion of the opaque x-ray medium into the subhepatic and suprahepatic spaces, the pelvis, and even the left paracolic gutter.

Recognition of a left subphrenic abscess is relatively simple. With the patient in the steep Trendelenburg position on the x-ray table, a few ounces of swallowed barium will come to occupy the upper end of the gastric fundus. If there is a spatial separation of a centimeter or more between the diaphragm and the gastric fundus, a subphrenic collection of pus or blood is a possibility.

Recognition of a right subphrenic collection is not so easy; a high right diaphragm of limited mobility when viewed fluoroscopically, accompanied by fever and leukocytosis with a likely antecedent cause, points the way. Rarely is it possible to identify with certainty the presence of a subhepatic collection on the right side preoperatively. The important item in any abdominal collection of exudate is to detect its presence early and to provide dependent drainage. Antibiotics cannot reach or overcome an abscess; the only effective remedy is surgical drainage. The senior author (O. H. W.) was once partial to a technique of exploration of abscess-prone areas of the peritoneal cavity, using a long suction device patterned after a tonsillectomy sucker. The long handle is provided with a thumb release to interrupt suction during introduction of the instrument. A 4-cm incision is made beneath the lateral costal margin of that side of the abdomen where the collection is believed to be. The probing suction device is kept gently but firmly applied to the lateral abdominal wall, and in succession reaches the lateral gutter, the subhepatic and suprahepatic spaces, and finally the cul-de-sac. Dependent drainage through a short drainage tract, performed without risk of opening the pleural cavity, is the best technique in managing a subphrenic abscess. An inch of gravity drainage is the most effective force in evacuating an abscess. From the standpoint of dependent drainage, the classical posterior approach with paraspinal resection of a low-lying thoracic rib provides the most dependent drainage. The surgeon must be aware, however, that the parietal pleura descends to a level lower than the 12th rib. Before an incision is made in the diaphragm, it must be ascertained that the lung lying immediately below the pleura is not moving freely. In such an event, it is well to insert a gauze pack for a few days, extending out beyond the skin level, so that firm adhesions between the pleura and the lung will develop. When the diaphragm is incised a few days later, the pleural cavity itself will not be opened. The best assurance against opening the pleura is provided by the Nather-Ochsner approach; its shortcoming is the long tract, which often precludes dependent drainage.

Pelvic collections in the female are easily evacuated by a colpotomy incision. In the male, a dissection plane needs to be developed between the rectum and the bladder for evacuation of a pelvic collection. The paracolic gutters can be readily evacuated.

Hudspeth of the Bowman Gray School of Medicine has urged a more radical direct approach to intraperitoneal collections of exudate. In fact, he calls his operation "radical surgical debridement in the treatment of advanced generalized bacterial peritonitis"; he recorded a succession of 92 patients thus treated without hospital mortality, obviously a unique achievement, not readily duplicated without case selection. Effective evacuation of abscesses, with addition of appropriate antibiotics, is in the final analysis the critical measure of a successful surgical drainage procedure. How widely Hudspeth's success has been duplicated in the hands of other abdominal surgeons yet awaits confirmation. Halaz (1970) also favors the intraperitoneal approach and has provided some data to support this view.

A plea for early surgical intervention is definitely in order in cases of intraperitoneal infection. When the acutely obstructed appendix is excised before perforation, the risk to the patient is minimal. Over several years in the late 1930s, in the preantibiotic era, the mortality of perforated peptic ulcer in our University Hospitals was zero. All the physicians in Minnesota were then alert to the importance of early surgical intervention. Today, a sizable mortality is still being reported in many areas. Is the profession placing too much dependence on antibiotics? One may also ask, with justification, should there be a return to closed intestinal anastomoses? Before the availability of antibiotics, over a 2-year period (1941–43), the senior author (O. H. W.) and his residents performed a succession of 61 colon resections, the majority for malignancy, without clinically demonstrable leak. There was one death in the series. One patient was found, at operation, to have a fistula between the hepatic flexure and the duodenum in consequence of perforation of the cancer into the duodenum; he died 16 days after operation of a Mann-Williamson neostomal ulcer. The biliary-pancreatic ampulla had unwittingly been excised with the cancerous duodenal fistula.

In a recent report, Nealon and his associates reviewed the reported mortality of subphrenic abscess from seven medical centers. The overall operative mortality was nearly 33 percent; the mortality for the nonoperative treatment of wait and see was almost 90 percent, an occurrence that serves to emphasize the importance of early recognition and prompt surgical intervention.

In recent years, liver and lung scans employing radioactive agents have enhanced the ability of radiologists to recognize subphrenic abscess. There have been both false-positive and false-negative interpretations of such scans with this method in the detection of such abscesses. Continued pursuit of the method with technical advances will no doubt improve the performance. It was in the early recognition of right subphrenic abscess that the senior author (O. H. W.) found the tonsil sucker-probe, described previously, was helpful.

THE OBSTRUCTED APPENDIX

Reginald Fitz (1886) gave appendicitis its name, implying that it is an infection, a thesis that gained widespread support for a number of years. Clarence Dennis and one of us (O. H. W.) showed in the 1930s that perforation of the appendix in the rabbit, chimpanzee, and man was caused by the high secretory pressure within the appendix, which exceeded diastolic blood pressure when there was obstruction to the appendical outlet. In man, the usual cause of obstruction is the fecalith, whose origin still remains a mystery. Owing to its thin wall, the appendix of the rabbit will perforate 70 percent of the time within 10 hours of obstruction; in chimpanzee and man, within 24 to 36 hours. Measured secretory pressures in chimpanzee and man of the obstructed appendix are in the area of 100 mm Hg, approximating systolic blood pressure. In the mid-1930s, exteriorization operations for cancer of the colon were usual. We had no misgivings, when excising an exteriorized malignancy upon the abdominal wall, about placing an untied ligature around the base of the appendix, which was occluded 48 hours later when fibrin had sealed the base of the cecum to the parietal peritoneum. Only then were secretory pressure determinations made. This procedure was undertaken in 22 patients with malignancy of the colon. In seven, the appendix was atrophic and not susceptible to cannulation. In 15 patients whose ages ranged between 60 and 72, the appendix appeared normal (68 percent). In fact, the oldest patient in the group had a secretory pressure of 100 mm Hg. This pressure probably represents the highest secretory pressure of any tubular structure in man. (Carl Ludwig of Leipzig [1851] cannulated the canine submaxillary duct and described a secretory pressure of 250 mm Hg.) The role of generous deposits of lymphoid tissue in the appendix, probably greater than in the remainder of the colon, has long been recognized. It is of interest, however, that when the cecal area and the appendix of the rabbit were subjected to x-ray irradiation, destroying completely the lymphoid tissue of the appendix, the high secretory pressure remained in the presence of obstruction.

C. N. McBurney of the New York Roosevelt Hospital wrote in 1889 that when the "acute appendix" came to be routinely excised early, the mortality of appendicitis would disappear. There has, in fact, been a 99 percent decrease in the mortality of appendicitis in the United States since 1930, when approximately 16,000 appendicitis-associated deaths occurred annually. In 1973, there were only 1,066 deaths from appendicitis in the overall population of the United States, a laudable achievement over four decades. It is too late to change the name of appendicitis, but the profession has begun to recognize the serious threat of perforation in the presence of an obstructed appendix, reflected in the current accomplishment.

MANAGEMENT OF CELLULITIC INFECTIONS

Before the arrival of sulfanilamide (1935) and penicillin (1944), there was no effective treatment for cellulitic streptococcal infections. In the mid-1920s, the professor of ophthalmology at the University of Minnesota sustained a prick of his left thumb while performing a mastoidectomy. A severe cellulitis of the entire left forearm developed. Arthur Strachauer, chief of surgery, amputated the arm above the elbow, a procedure that failed to halt the cellulitic process. Shortly thereafter, a graduate student in anatomy, while working with a streptococcal culture, spilled a drop on her forearm. The rabbit she was about to inject with the culture scratched the spot, and within a few days the student was dead. Prior to the availability of sulfanilamide, the surgeon in his attack upon bacterial infection was delimited to evacuation of abscesses. Whenever he tried to do more, he usually did harm.

Some surgeons returning from World War I were imbued with the idea that implantation of an antiseptic into infected wounds would stop the ravages of cellulitis, following the thesis of Lister (1867) who implanted varying concentrations of carbolic acid into the wounds of compound (open) fractures. In World War I, Dakin (1915) devised a solution, a hypochlorite, an agent Semmelweis put to good use almost seven decades earlier at the Vienna Allgemeines Krankenhaus (1847) as a prophylaxis against puerperal fever.

In January 1934, a young schoolteacher at a one-room rural school in Minnesota was admitted to our University Hospitals with a septic phlegmon from a compound fracture of the left femur, accompanied by swelling of both thigh and leg. The accident resulted from an explosion in the wood-burning stove employed to heat the schoolroom. A lid of the stove struck the patient's left thigh in its midsection with great force, causing a compound fracture of the femur. On arrival at the hospital, the patient had a picket-fence fever varying from 101 to 104F. An immediate debridement of the open wound was done, but the cellulitic process accompanied by high fever persisted. An experienced World War I surgeon of the clinical staff recommended multiple incisions in the thigh and leg. Appreciating that drainage alone could not stop the cellulitic process, O. H. W. persuaded the military surgeon, who had a large experience with use of Dakin's solution, to undertake the procedure. Two operative sessions were necessary, during which long posterior and lateral incisions in the thigh and leg were made. Continuous irrigation of the resultant wounds with large quantities of Dakin's solution, employing the Carrel technique, did not restrain the infection. The senior orthopedic surgeon, also with World War I experience, was then consulted, and counseled amputation at the hip joint, which advice the patient rejected. O. H. W., having had a nodding acquaintance with the interesting book *On Rest and Pain* (1863), by John Hilton of London's Guy's Hospital, in which complete rest was stressed for all types of surgical infections, completely immobilized both lower extremities in a spica cast, extending from the toes up to both axillary folds. When the cast had thoroughly solidified, the patient could be turned freely, without her prior pain or distress. The effect on the fever was remarkable; within 2 days the patient was essentially afebrile. Her appetite returned, and she was obviously on the way to a dramatic recovery from what had appeared to be a hopeless situation.

For similar cellulitic infections, the sulfonamides and antibiotics have had a significant impact, but they were unavailable for approximately 2 years after this patient was admitted. Over the ensuing years, elevation and complete immobilization of the involved extremity were used in this clinic with very favorable responses.

GUNSHOT INJURIES

In World War I, Pierre Duval of Paris (1918) indicated that wounds of the chest had been considered trivial, since they were usually caused by small-caliber bullets. Only when a large blood vessel was injured was there grave danger. It was Duval's view that approximately one-quarter of missile wounds were caused by small-caliber bullets, with a resultant mortality of 2 percent; the mortality of injury from higher-caliber shells approximated 30 percent. Duval was of the opinion that surgery for thoracic bullet wounds was feasible and that the hazard of an open surgical pneumothorax was not great. He believed that a large proportion of patients so injured, if operated upon in good time, could be saved.

In the mid-1930s, O. H. W. observed four children, all under 10 years of age, who had been shot through the thorax with a 38-caliber revolver. All the children recovered without incident, responding well to intercostal suction drainage without recourse to open operation. Obviously, no large vessel had been injured.

GUNSHOT WOUNDS OF THE ABDOMEN

Following the death of James Garfield in September 1881, there was much discussion in the surgical literature of why the President had died. He had been shot in the back at a distance of 6 to 8 feet by an assassin with a small-caliber revolver. Unfortunately, the wound had been examined 17 times by "socially clean" but unsterile hands. The President died of a mycotic aneurysm of the splenic artery. Had a piece of adhesive tape been applied over the point of entry of the bullet, probably the President would have survived. The American gynecologist Marion Sims wrote a series of articles urging early operation for such wounds. X-rays were more than 15 years away, yet because of damage to the genitofemoral nerve to the scrotum, it was surmised that the tract of the bullet had perforated Garfield's lower thoracic vertebra, severing the adjacent nerve.

Charles T. Parkes (1884), a Chicago surgeon, fired shots into the abdomens of anesthetized dogs, which had been prepared antiseptically for operation. He observed that intestinal spillage was a consistent finding, and the operative mortality, despite immediate operation, was high.

Upon his return from the Boer War (1899–1900), the English surgeon George H. Makins wrote a monograph summarizing his experiences. The war was an itinerant type of warfare without established bases to permit emergency operations. It was Makins' conclusion that nonoperative management of bullet wounds was the wisest scheme, attended by a mortality of 33 percent. Nicholas Senn of Chicago, at the Siege of Santiago in the Spanish-American War (1900), came to the same conclusion. When President William McKinley was felled by an assassin's bullet in September 1901 at the Pan American Exposition in Buffalo, New York, he was on the operating table within 75 minutes of the shooting. Matthew Mann, local gynecologist who did the operation, noted perforation of both walls of the stomach by a bullet that penetrated into the pancreas, which neither Mann nor the goiter pathologist Harvey Gaylord could find after 7 hours of searching at postmortem.

At the outbreak of World War I, the London surgeon P. Lockhart-Mummery reaffirmed his stand that gunshot wounds involving the bowel are best treated by observation, even when proper operating facilities are available. In July 1915, Enderlen and Sauerbruch, German surgeons, observed in a controlled study that when bullet wounds of the intestine were treated conservatively, 94 percent died; the recovery rate of those submitted to early operation was 44.4 percent.

Frederick F. Cartwright, anesthesiologist of the London Hospital, pointed out that Princess Vera Gedroitz, a Russian surgeon in the Russo-Japanese War (1904–05), had brought to the front a well-equipped ambulance train. This permitted her to operate on battle casualties in good condition, within a relatively short time following the wounding, a policy she adopted for all penetrating wounds of the abdomen. Cartwright reported that the results were better than any yet attained—182 operations for various wounds had been done by the Princess.*

Gerald W. Shafton (1960) indicated that he had introduced a policy of observing patients with penetrating wounds of the abdomen, including stab wounds and small caliber bullet wounds. He concluded that in civil practice,

* Boris Petrovsky, minister of health in the U.S.S.R., personal communication.

patients so injured, if closely observed, could be treated conservatively with surprising success. In fact, he concluded that conservative management was at least as safe as operative intervention. In a consecutive series of 125 bullet-wound patients, the mortality in the group treated nonoperatively was less than 1 percent; for those operated on, it was 20 percent. In papers of 1966 and 1969, Shafton continued to endorse a conservative regimen. Under conditions of modern warfare with high velocity weapons, it may rightfully be inferred that Shafton's treatment could not compete with operative management.

SURGICAL STYLES OF OPERATING

Appreciation by surgeons of advances in knowledge of microbiology is reflected in successive styles of operating. Prior to demonstration of the pathogenicity of bacteria by Koch (1876–78), no accepted ritual or manner of dress by surgeons had been adopted. Robert Liston, a colorful and facile operator, performed a high amputation under ether anesthesia at London's University College Hospital on December 21, 1846, the first major operation under anesthesia in Britain. The extremity was amputated in 25 seconds. On occasion, Liston transferred the handle of the operating knife to his mouth to quicken such procedures. Like Kern (1826) of Vienna before him, Liston did not close the amputation wound primarily. He left it open, and his assistants periodically applied cold water gauze packs to the wound until a glaze appeared over the entire wound surface. At that time, a single percutaneous suture was placed, approximating the midsector of the wound, the edges of which were then brought together by several strips of adhesive tape. Omission of many percutaneous sutures and secondary wound closure were undoubtedly largely responsible for Liston's acceptable amputation mortality of approximately 11 percent, a mortality half that of Lister's in his first skirmishes with amputation for compound (open) fractures employing instillation of varying concentrations of carbolic. The usual Listerian dress and the carbolic acid spray which Lister adopted in 1871 were continued by surgeons in the best university surgical clinics until Neuber (1883) of Kiel introduced washed gowns and boiled instruments. Said Neuber, "For many years white linen operating gowns have been in use in the Kiel clinic. As soon as they are unclean, and after every operation, they are replaced with washed gowns. The entire operating personnel wears them, surgeons, assistants and nurses." Victor Hacker (1884), of Billroth's surgical clinic, wrote, "The operator and assistants wear washed linen coats during operative procedures." An American translation appeared in 1892. Actually, the first suggestion of sterilized gowns to appear in print in Germany came from the pen of the Berlin surgeon Curt Schimmelbusch in Bergmann's surgical clinic. Said Schimmelbusch, "At operations the surgeons and participants in the procedure wear sterilized white linen gowns."

In his famous speech of 1874 before a group of medical scientists, Pasteur urged upon surgeons the need to sterilize their instruments and operating material with heat, which suggestion the French surgeon Leon Tripier put into practice in 1883 and Paul Redard in 1886.* Pasteur's associate Charles Chamberland described his autoclave (1880) to sterilize his culture media for bacteria, which Koch described independently in 1881, demonstrating too the superiority of moist over dry heat.

Neuber's practice is nicely shown in Thomas Eakins' painting of Hayes Agnew operating at the University of Pennsylvania Hospital in 1889. A nurse too is present in the operating arena, a practice not yet adopted by Billroth (1890) or other German-speaking surgeons until near the turn of the century. Nurses began to participate actively in the surgical arena at New York's Bellevue Hospital in the early 1870s. Rubber gloves were first worn by Caroline Hamptom (1889), Halsted's operating scrub nurse (later to become Mrs. Halsted), whose hands were allergic to mercuric chloride, a hand dip used by the Halsted operating team. In February 1897, Bloodgood, an early trainee of Halsted, invoked use of rubber gloves by all participants in operative procedures. By 1904 all members of Halsted's operating team were wearing rubber gloves but no face masks, an innovation of Johann Mikulicz and the microbiologist Carl Flügge of Breslau (now Wroclaw) in 1897. The full ritual dress of operating personnel was depicted in Fowler's operative manual in 1906.

ADVANCES IN OTHER DISCIPLINES INFLUENCE SURGEON'S ROLE

Prophylaxis in the prevention of many infectious fevers has had a tremendous influence on human welfare throughout the world. The work of the Veterinary American Live-Stock Commission (1911–17) in eliminating bovine tuberculosis by pasteurization of milk and the killing of tuberculous cattle has affected the work role of the surgeon significantly. No longer is the surgeon called upon to deal with tuberculous cervical lymph nodes and similar lesions of bones and joints, which commanded much of his time in the 1920s. Similarly, the discovery of Enders and his associates (1949) in cultivating the poliomyelitis virus, along with the vaccination program of Sabin (1955) and Salk (1953) against poliomyelitis virus, have virtually eliminated the need for orthopedic surgeons to devote a major share of their activity to the repair of serious deformities occasioned by this paralytic and devastating disorder.

Streptomycin and other antibiotics and pharmacologic antituberculous agents have also had a profound effect on the control of pulmonary tuberculosis. Surgical wards devoted to patients with thoracoplasty have been eliminated, and bronchiectasis, which commanded much of the thoracic surgeon's time in the 1930s and 1940s, has disappeared. Prophylaxis directly affects the role of the surgeon in disease control.

WHAT OF TOMORROW?

Progress is a discontinuous process, with long periods of lull. Occasionally, a review of indications for operations can make a tremendous impact for the better. Well into

* See Wangensteen and Wangensteen: *The Rise of Surgery*, 1978, pp 7, 8, 491, 692, 706.

this century, cesarean section was often delayed for difficult labor in term pregnancies until the parturient had been in labor for several days, with resultant uterine mucosal necrosis and ensuing uterine sepsis, accompanied by an operative mortality of 40 to 60 percent. Over the past decade, a fetal position indicating a long and difficult labor has come to be looked on as an adequate indication for cesarean section before the onset of labor. In a few large university clinics, where this practice has been invoked regularly, large series of cesareans have been performed without maternal mortality.

If similar management was carried out consistently in such emergencies as acute appendicitis, before perforation of the obstructed appendix, McBurney's 1889 prediction of no mortality could be anticipated. Similar results might be obtained with perforated peptic ulcer. The availability of antibiotics has occasioned family physicians, who ordinarily see such patients first, to be less alert to the importance of early operative intervention. Sharper attention must be directed to the need to invoke the earliest possible surgical intervention.

BIBLIOGRAPHY

Wangensteen OH, Wangensteen SD: *The Rise of Surgery from Empiric Craft to Scientific Discipline*. Minneapolis, Univ. of Minnesota Press, 1978.

PART II: SURGICAL MICROBIOLOGY

CHAPTER 2 Microbes and Their Pathogenicity

RICHARD J. HOWARD

OF the myriad of microorganisms, only a small fraction cause disease in man, and only a few of these cause surgical infections—infections that appear to be a consequence of an operative procedure or infections for which surgical therapy may be required.

TYPES OF MICROORGANISMS

While the classification of microorganisms is not entirely satisfactory, they are conveniently placed into groups based on structural properties (Table 2-1). Microorganisms can be classified on the basis of increasing complexity: (1) viruses; (2) prokaryotes (primitive nucleus) lack a true nucleus and include bacteria, spirochetes, rickettsia, chlamydia, and mycoplasmas; and (3) eukaryocytes (true nucleus) have a nucleus bound by a nuclear membrane and include protozoans and fungi. Multicellular eukaryotic organisms—metazoans—such as platyhelminths (flatworms) and nematyhelminths (round worms) are not microorganisms but can cause infection (see Chapter 11).

VIRUSES

Viruses are the smallest (20–300 nm in diameter) infectious agents and have the simplest structure (Fig. 2-1). They were originally distinguished by their small size ("filtrable viruses") and because they are obligate intracellular parasites. Some small prokaryotes (chlamydia, rickettsia, and mycoplasma), however, also share these properties, so that the distinctive features of viruses lie in their simple structure and their unique mode of replication. Whereas bacteria and higher organisms reproduce by binary cell division, virus multiplication occurs by synthesis of the individual components within the host cell, followed by assembly of the components into complete virus particles.

A complete virus particle, a virion, has a central core of genetic material surrounded by a protein coat, which protects the nucleic acid from the environment and serves as a vehicle of transmission from one host to another. The nucleic acid accounts for only a small part of the total mass of the virion—approximately 1 percent in the case of influenza virus. All viruses have a central core containing either RNA or DNA, never both. The nucleic acid can be either single-stranded or double-stranded. Most DNA viruses of clinical importance have double-stranded DNA, while medically important RNA viruses have either single- or double-stranded RNA. Viruses have a limited genetic capacity (Table 2-1). For instance, the genome of poliovirus can code for only seven or eight polypeptides, while herpesviruses have sufficient genetic information to code for 150 polypeptides. Nevertheless, viruses are effective intracellular parasites and can cause substantial tissue damage.

The nucleic acid is surrounded by a protein coat, the capsid. The capsid is composed of individual polypeptide chains, termed protomeres. Protomeres aggregate in groups of five or six to form structural subunits, capsomeres (Fig. 2-1). The capsomeres then assemble to form the capsid. Capsid proteins are specified by the viral genome. Because of their limited genetic capacity, viruses cannot spare too many genes to determine capsid proteins. Hence, for the majority of viruses the capsid consists of many identical capsomeres. Viruses that have helical capsids (eg, influenza virus) usually have a single type of capsomere. Icosahedral viruses (ie, herpesviruses, poliovirus) can have capsids made of single protein subunits or several types of protein subunits. The capsid protects the nucleic acid from physical and chemical inactivation. The capsid may also play a role in attachment of the virus to sites on susceptible cells.

Some viruses have a second coat, the envelope. The envelopes of viruses consist of proteins (often linked to carbohydrates) and lipids. The proteins of the envelope are determined by the viral genome, but the lipid and carbohydrate come from the host cell. Viruses in which

TABLE 2-1. CLASSIFICATION OF MICROORGANISMS

	Mean Diameter (μm)	Genetic mass (daltons)	Number of genes
Viruses			
Poliovirus	0.02–0.03	2.5×10^6	7–8
Herpesviruses	0.10–0.20	6×10^7	150
Vaccinia	0.20–0.30	1.6×10^8	4×10^2
Prokaryotes			
Bacteria			
E. coli	0.6×2–3	3.9	6×10^3
B. anthracis	1.3×10		
Chlamydias	0.20–0.30	4×10^8	10^3
Mycoplasmas	0.20–0.30	5×10^8	10^3
Rickettsias	0.30–0.60	10^9	2×10^3
Spirochetes	0.1×5–20		
Eukaryocytes			
Fungi	2–4		
Protozoans			
Entamoeba histolytica	40		
Human cells	8–50	1.6×10^{12}	3×10^6

assembly takes place in the cell nucleus (ie, herpes simplex, cytomegalovirus) acquire much of the lipid from nuclear membrane as they "bud" from the nucleus—a process similar to reverse pinocytosis. Enveloped RNA viruses (eg, influenza virus), in which assembly occurs in the cytoplasm, bud from the plasma membrane and thus acquire their envelope lipids and carbohydrate from the cytoplasmic membrane. The presence of lipid in the envelope prevents formation of a rigid structure; hence, the outer surface of enveloped viruses makes the virus sensitive to organic solvents, such as ether. This lipoprotein envelope is an integral part of the virion and aids attachment and penetration of the virus into subsequent cellular hosts.

All viruses are obligate intracellular parasites because they contain no biosynthetic or energy-generating mechanisms. They are entirely dependent on host cells for energy generation and for biosynthesis. Many viruses are not completely devoid of enzymes—they may contain enzymes important in the replication of their nucleic acid.

PROKARYOTES

Bacteria

Bacteria are the smallest organisms that contain all the biosynthetic machinery and energy-generating mechanisms required for an independent existence and for self-replication. Bacteria are prokaryotic organisms because they lack a true nucleus surrounded by a nuclear membrane, chromosomes, and a mitotic apparatus (Figs. 2-2 and 2-3). The most obvious differences between bacterial and animal cells are size and simplicity of structure (Table 2-1). Bacteria have three general shapes: rods *(E. coli, Bacteroides fragilis)*, spheres *(Staphylococcus aureus, Streptococcus pyogenes)*, and spirals *(Treponema pallidum)*.

Several classification systems have been devised for bacteria, which suggests that none of them is completely satisfactory. Classification systems include bacterial shape, oxygen requirement, metabolic characteristics, genetic composition, staining properties, and computer systems that group bacteria on the basis of more than 100 taxonomic characteristics. *Bergey's Manual of Determinative Bacteriology*[1] attempts an exhaustive phylogenetic classification of bacteria, but major changes in its system have occurred in each of its eight editions, which suggests that it is not entirely satisfactory either.

Bacterial Structure

Nuclear Body. Although bacteria lack a true nucleus, a nuclear region consisting of DNA fibrils can be seen in electron micrographs (Fig. 2-2). Furthermore, discrete nuclear bodies can be recognized in bacteria by light microscopy using DNA-specific stains. The DNA exists as a single circular molecule, and bacteria are thus considered to have a single chromosome. The DNA of a typical bacterium *(E. coli)* weighs 3×10^9 daltons, compared to 2.5×10^6 daltons for poliovirus and 1.6×10^{12} daltons for a human somatic cell (Table 2-1). When unfolded, the DNA is approximately 1,000 times as long as the bacterium.

In addition to the large circular chromosome, bacteria occasionally contain small autonomously replicating DNA strands called plasmids. These plasmids may contain genes responsible for antibiotic resistance, and since they can be transferred between bacteria by conjugation, they have

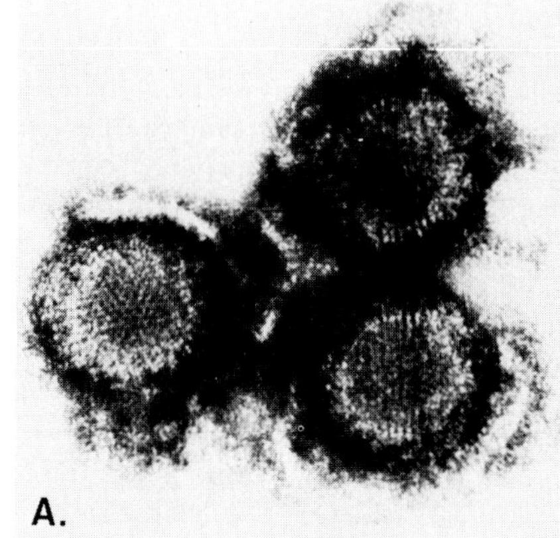

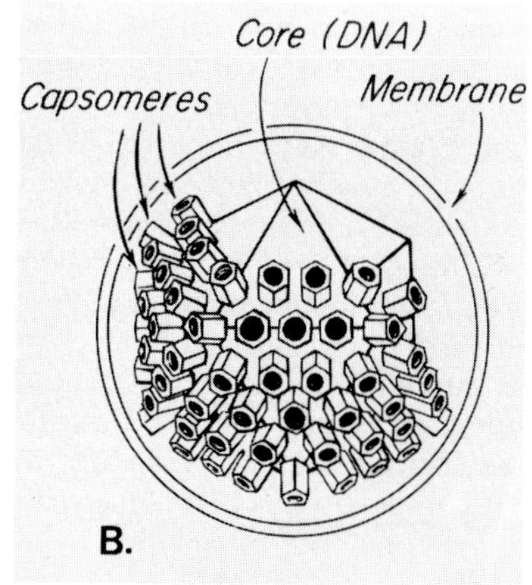

Fig. 2-1. **A. Cytomegalovirus negatively stained with uranyl acetate. The capsomeres and the irregularly shaped surrounding envelope are readily seen. (Courtesy Lee FK, Nahmias AJ, Stagno S: *N Eng J Med* 229:1266, 1978.) B. Diagrammatic drawing of a typical herpesvirus. The central core contains DNA. The core is surrounded by a layer of protein called the capsid, which is composed of individual units termed capsomeres. The capsid of herpesviruses is an icosahedron and has 162 capsomeres. Herpesviruses acquire a membrane coat (envelope) when they bud from the nuclear membrane of the host cell.**

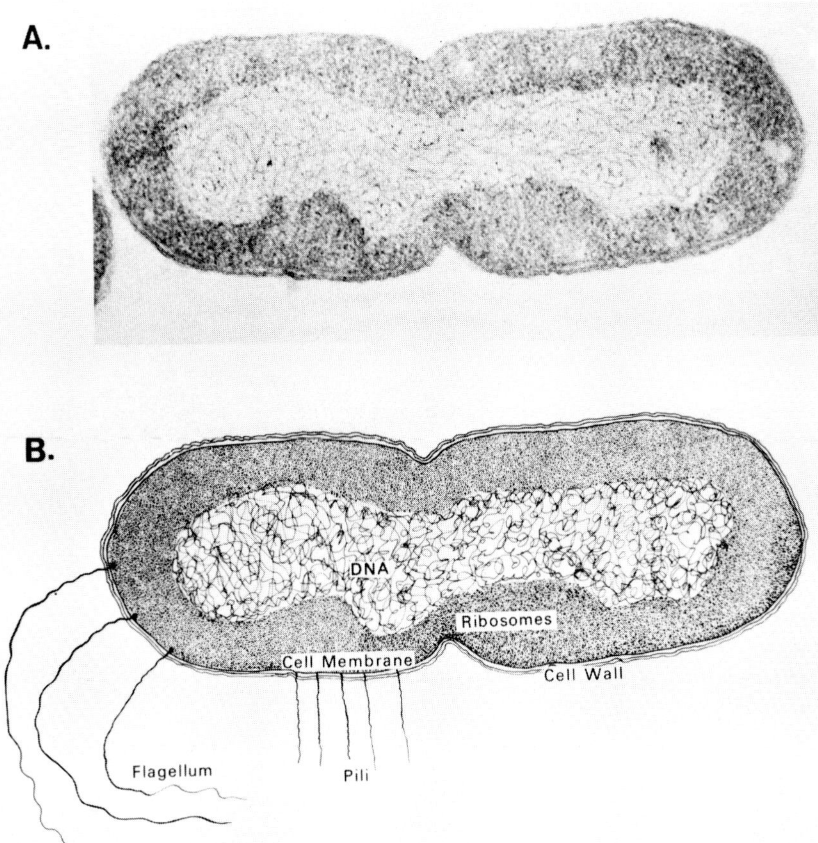

Fig. 2-2. A. ***Escherichia coli*** cell showing central nucleoid containing DNA fibers coagulated by the fixative osmium tetroxide. There is a lack of distinct nuclear membrane, a feature that differentiates prokaryotic cells from eukaryotic cells. A central constriction in the membrane can be seen indicating that cell division has begun. The dark area surrounding the nucleoid is filled with ribosomes. No flagellae or pili can be seen in this micrograph. (Courtesy Woldringh CL, de Jong MA, van den Berg W, Koppes L: *J Bacteriol* 131:270, 1977.) B. Diagrammatic drawing of an *E. coli* cell showing the essential structural features of a typical bacterium. The flagella and pili are located over the entire cell surface of the *E. coli.*

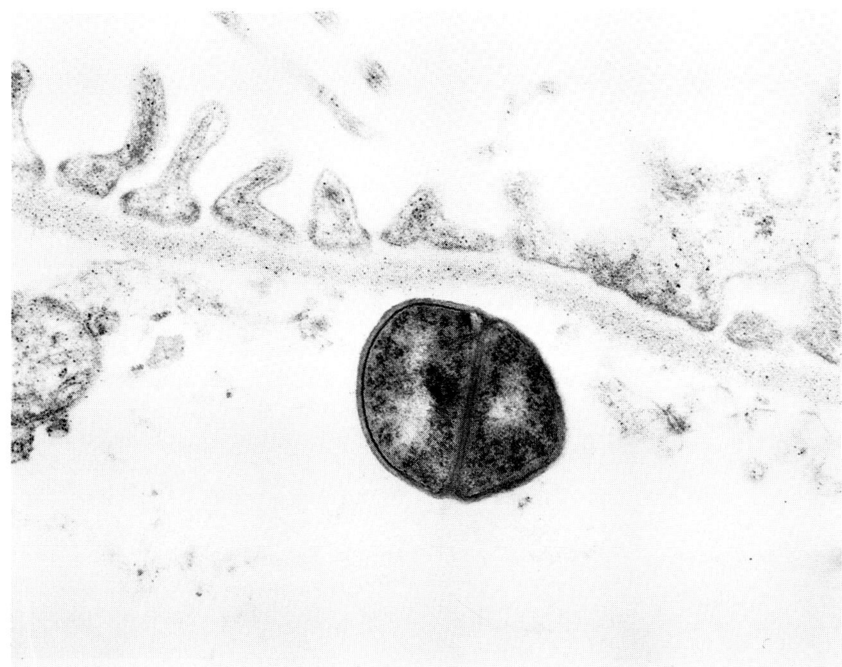

Fig. 2-3. ***Staphylococcus aureus.*** Note the light nucleoid regions surrounded by the dark cytoplasm containing abundant ribosomes. The cell membrane is surrounded by a thicker cell wall than is found in gram-negative bacteria. This cell has already divided with the vertical cell membranes separating the two cells. 35,400×. (Courtesy NL Staley.)

been called resistance transfer factors, or R factors. They are common in enteric bacteria such as *E. coli, Salmonella,* and *Shigella.* In 1959, strains of *Shigella* suddenly appeared which were resistant to four widely used antibiotics—sulfonamides, chloramphenicol, streptomycin, and tetracycline.[2] A plasmid had been introduced into these *Shigella,* which had genes for resistance to each of the four antibiotics.

Cytoplasmic Contents. Bacterial cytoplasm is thickly populated with ribosomes. Bacteria have 70S ribosomes composed of 50S and 30S subunits. Animal cells have larger 80S ribosomes. The ribosomes are the sites where synthesis of polypeptides from amino acids occurs. Many bacteria also have granular inclusions composed of cellular storage materials, eg, glycogen and lipid. Bacteria do not have mitochondria. Instead, enzymes and cytochromes involved in electron transport and oxidative phosphorylation are located on the plasma membrane.

Plasma Membrane. The cytoplasmic membrane is a typical three-layered "unit membrane," which appears as three dark-light-dark bands on electron micrographs (Fig. 2-2). The plasma membrane's major functions are: (1) selective permeability and transport of solutes into the cell, (2) electron transport and oxidative phosphorylation, (3) excretion of exoenzymes, and (4) serving as the site of enzymes responsible for synthesis of DNA, cell wall polymers, and membrane lipids.

Mesosomes are convoluted invaginations of the cytoplasmic membrane. Mesosomes serve as the attachment site of the bacterial chromosome to the cytoplasmic membrane. They are also involved in cell division. The extra membrane of the mesosome may facilitate separation of the segregating chromosomes and the initiation of a membrane bridge between two newly formed cells. Some mesosomes attached to nonseptal regions of the cell appear to function in secretion and electron transport.

Cell Wall. Gram-positive bacteria have a rigid, relatively thick (15–80 nm) electron-dense cell wall, external to the plasma membrane, that gives shape to the bacteria and enables the plasma membrane to resist bursting as a result of the high intracellular osmotic pressure (5 atmospheres for gram-negative bacteria and up to 20 atmospheres for gram-positive bacteria) (Fig. 2-3). In gram-negative bacteria, this electron-dense layer is only 2–3 nm thick. Gram-negative bacteria have an additional trilaminar outer membrane layer 6 to 18 nm thick (Fig. 2-4). Differences in cell wall structure determine whether bacteria are gram-positive or gram-negative.

The walls of gram-positive bacteria are relatively easy to purify. Their basic structure is peptidoglycan (also called murein, glycopeptide, or mucopeptide) (Fig. 2-5). Peptidoglycan consists of polysaccharide chains (the backbone) of alternating residues of N-acetylglucosamine and N-acetylmuramic acid. These polysaccharide chains are cross-linked by polypeptide chains (nine amino acids long in the case of *S. aureus*). Gram-positive bacteria may also have teichoic acids covalently bound to some N-acetylmuramic acid residues. Teichoic acids are polymers of either ribotal or glycerol residues and are major surface antigens. The cell walls of gram-negative bacteria are also composed of peptidoglycan, but there is much less of it than in gram-positive bacteria and there is no teichoic acid.

The outer membrane of gram-negative bacteria is a trilamellar structure that resembles the plasma membrane (Fig. 2-4). This outer membrane contains lipopolysaccharide and is also known as endotoxin because it is toxic and is firmly bound to the cells. Westphal and Lüderitz[3-5] determined the molecular structure of the endotoxin of *Salmonella minnesota.* Endotoxin is extracted from the bacteria by hot phenol and split by acid hydrolysis into lipid A (which has the toxicity of endotoxin) and polysaccharide, which is responsible for antigenicity. The structure of lipid A is constant, but the polysaccharide structure may vary, contributing to the numerous O antigens of the enteric bacteria.

The cell wall can be removed from gram-positive organisms by treatment with lysozyme. Usually the cell lyses, but if it is digested in an osmotically protected environment, the bacterium survives, surrounded only by the plasma membrane. This form is termed a protoplast. Similar treatment of gram-negative bacteria also yields an organism that must be in a protected osmotic environment and is called a spheroplast. Spheroplasts, however, retain an outer wall layer. L forms are morphologically similar to protoplasts or spheroplasts, but the term "L form" is limited to cells that can multiply.

Capsules. Capsules are loose, gel-like structures composed of polysaccharides or polypeptides, or both. They are most easily demonstrated by negative staining in India ink, where they form a clear layer between the ink and the darker bacterial cell. Capsules also impart a glistening mucoid appearance to colonies on agar gel. Capsules protect bacteria from phagocytosis, and their presence is usually correlated with virulence. Capsule formation is determined in part by the environment of the bacterium. Bacteria tend to form capsules in host tissues. When grown in vitro, however, bacteria tend not to make capsules unless specific nutrients are provided.

Flagella and Pili. Flagella and pili are hairlike structures on bacteria (Fig. 2-2). Flagella are responsible for motility of bacteria. They are long (30–200 nm) and thin (12–25 nm) structures composed mostly of protein. Bacteria may have a single flagellum at one end or a few flagella at one or both poles (polar flagellation). Alternatively, the flagella may be distributed over the entire cell surface (peritrichous flagellation). With the aid of an electron microscope, a base plate may be seen at the end of each flagellum, which anchors it to the plasma membrane. Pili are shorter (up to several nm) and thinner (7.5–10 nm) than flagella and are found only on gram-negative bacteria.

Spores. Spores are formed within some gram-positive bacteria when nutrition is inadequate (Fig. 2-6). Spores are much more resistant to the lethal effects of heat, drying, freezing, radiation, and toxic chemicals than are the vegetative bacteria. The spore wall and cortex contain peptidoglycan. The central core contains the complete genome of the vegetative cell. A variety of catabolic and biosynthetic enzymes are also present.

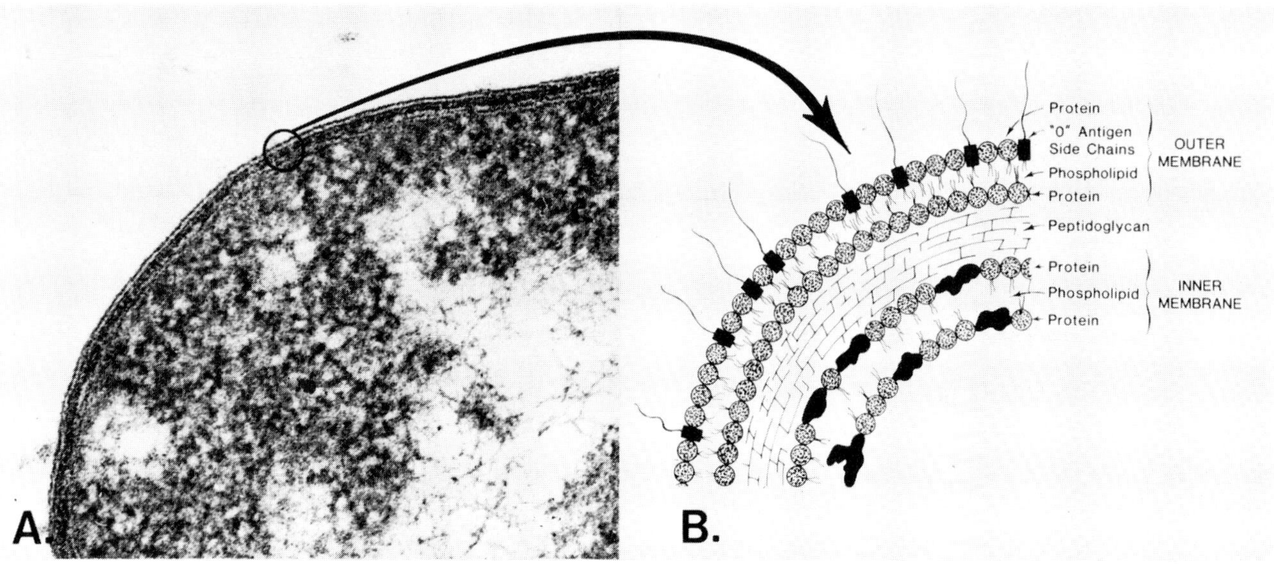

Fig. 2-4. A. *E. coli* showing the cell wall (200,000×). (Courtesy RGE Murray.) B. Diagrammatic drawing of the *E. coli* cell envelope.

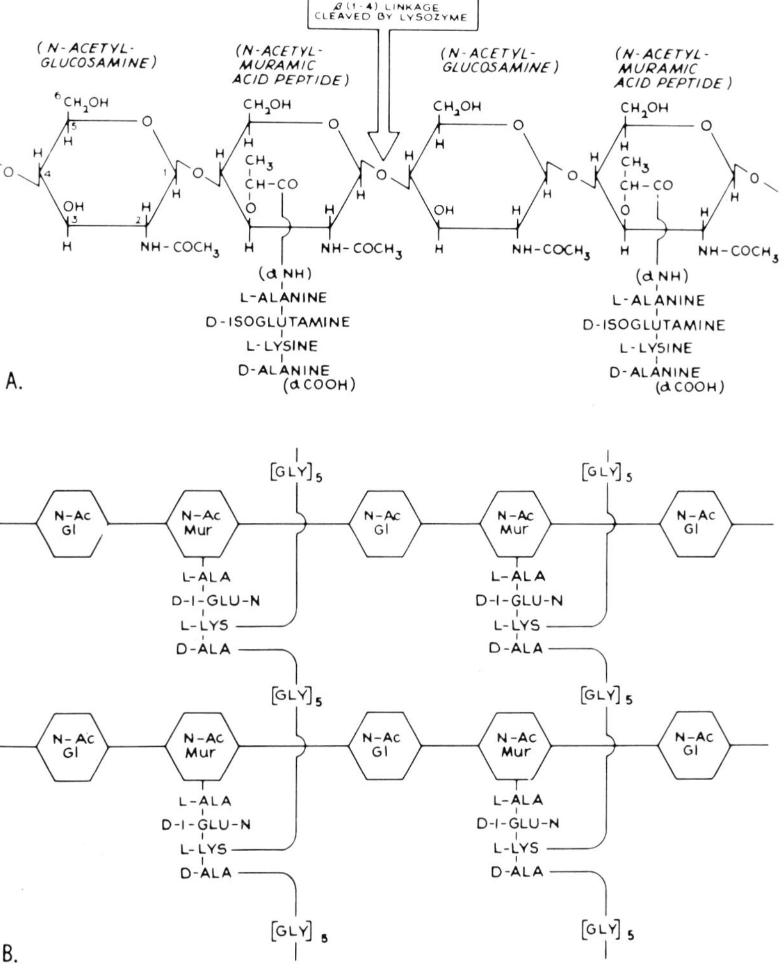

Fig. 2-5. A. A segment of the peptidoglycan of *Staphylococcus aureus.* The backbone of the polymer consists of alternating subunits of N-acetylglucosamine and N-acetylmuramic acid connected by β(1–4) linkages. The muramic acid residues are linked to short peptides, the composition of which varies from one bacterial species to another. In some species the L-lysine residues are replaced by diaminopimelic acid, an amino acid found in nature only in prokaryotic cell walls. The D-amino acids, which are also characteristic constituents of prokaryotic cell walls, are not found in eukaryotic cells. The peptide chains of the peptidoglycan are cross-linked between parallel polysaccharide backbones. B. Schematic representation of the peptidoglycan lattice which is formed by cross-linking. Bridges composed of pentaglycine peptide chains connect the α-carboxyl of the terminal D-alanine residue of one chain with the ϵ-amino group of the L-lysine residue of the next chain. The nature of the cross-linking bridge varies among different species. (Reproduced with permission from Jawetz E, Melnick JL, Adelberg EA: *Review of Medical Microbiology,* 13th ed., Los Altos, California, Lange Medical Publications, 1978.)

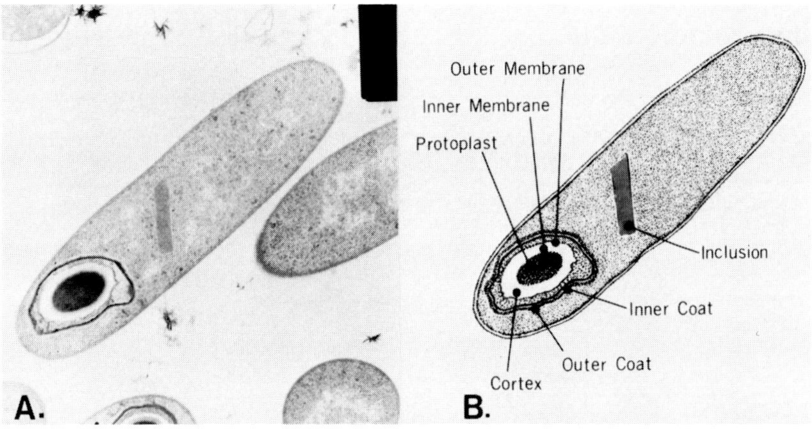

Fig. 2-6. **A. *Clostridium perfringens* cell containing a mature spore located at one end. The centrally located rod-shaped inclusion forms during sporulation. Its function is not known. (Courtesy Duncan CP, King GJ, Frieben WR: *J Bacteriol* 114:845, 1973.) B. Diagrammatic drawing of the *C. perfringens* cell showing the essential features of the spore. The protoplast contains the complete genome of the bacterial cell.**

Bacterial Growth

Bacteria have the ability to grow under a variety of environmental conditions. In general, bacteria require a suitable oxidation-reduction potential, an energy source, an appropriate hydrogen ion concentration, a suitable temperature, and nutrients.

The primary energy source for most bacteria is chemical energy, supplied by organic or inorganic compounds. Release of energy involves oxidation-reduction reactions. The energy source (eg, glucose) becomes oxidized (to CO_2 and H_2O), and another substance becomes reduced. Although many oxidation-reduction reactions involve oxygen, many do not. When oxygen is the electron receptor, aerobic respiration occurs. Some bacteria (anaerobes) can carry out respiration in the absence of oxygen as the electron acceptor. Bacteria that require oxygen for growth are obligate aerobes. Some bacteria *(Clostridium, Bacteroides)* cannot grow in the presence of oxygen and are obligate anaerobes, although the precise reason for their oxygen intolerance is uncertain. Still other bacteria (eg, *Streptococcus pyogenes*) may grow with or without oxygen but tend to grow better under one condition, and are termed facultative anaerobes or aerobes. Many facultative organisms can adjust their metabolism to aerobic and anaerobic conditions.

Bacteria also need a suitable hydrogen ion concentration and temperature for growth. For instance, most bacteria that make up the normal flora of the human gastrointestinal tract grow best in a slightly alkaline pH and at a temperature of 37C. There are bacteria, however, that grow in hot springs and some that grow at colder temperatures, although few grow below 29C. Most bacteria tolerate a pH range of 3–4 units. *E. coli* grows optimally at a pH between 4.5 and 8. Some bacteria can tolerate a pH of 0, and others thrive at a pH of up to 9. Each bacterium has a pH and temperature that provide optimal growth, which is related to the optimal conditions for its enzyme systems. Under suboptimal conditions, enzyme activity rapidly falls off and bacteria fail to grow—although they may survive and resume growth when conditions improve.

Bacteria also require minerals and vitamins plus other nutrients from which to generate energy and as building blocks for more complex macromolecules. The nutrients required vary widely, depending on the genetic capacity of the bacterium. Some bacteria can synthesize most sugars, amino acids, and vitamins, and thus need only minimal nutrients added to the growth medium. Other bacteria have limited capacity to synthesize their own nutrients and require enriched media.

Rickettsiae

The rickettsiae are small, nonmotile, obligate intracellular bacteria (Fig. 2-7). They appear as spherical forms 0.3 μm in diameter or as short rods 0.3 μm × 1.0 μm. Because of their small size and because they are obligate intracellular organisms, for years they were thought to constitute a separate phylum somewhere between viruses and bacteria on the phylogenetic scale. They are true bacteria: (1) they multiply by binary fission, (2) they contain both DNA and RNA, (3) they contain enzymes of the Krebs cycle and of electron transport, (4) at least one species contains muramic acid—a constituent found only in bacterial cell walls—and (5) their growth is inhibited by antibacterial agents. Rickettsiae are probably obligate intracellular parasites because their membranes are permeable to adenosine triphosphate, nicotinamide adenine dinucleotide, coenzyme A, and other essential cofactors. They must get these molecules from the host cell.

The survival of most rickettsiae requires that they be transmitted from one host to another in a manner that minimizes their exposure to the extracellular world. Most rickettsiae therefore usually have an arthropod vector. Rickettsial diseases are characterized by exanthematous rashes. They are the etiologic agents of typhus, Rocky Mountain spotted fever, and other exanthematous fevers. It is estimated that more human lives have been lost from rickettsial diseases than from any illness, except malaria.

Chlamydias

Chlamydias are small (0.2–0.3 μm in diameter) obligate intracellular bacteria (Fig. 2-8). Like bacteria: (1) they contain both DNA and RNA, (2) they divide by binary fission, (3) their cell walls contain peptidoglycan, (4) their ribosomes are similar to bacterial ribosomes, and (5) they are susceptible to antibiotics. Isolated chlamydias lack the ability to synthesize protein, DNA, and RNA, but within host cells they make their own macromolecules. They lack en-

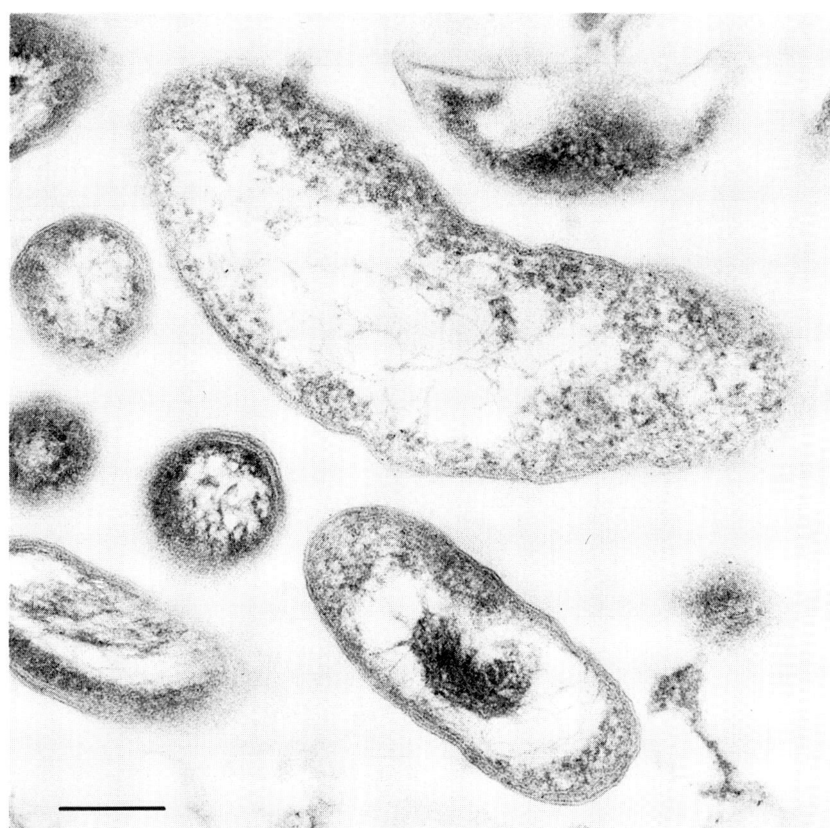

Fig. 2-7. Coxiella burnetii (a rickettsia) with light central nucleoid with coagulated DNA fibrils. The dark area contains ribosomes. The cell is surrounded by a trilamellar cell membrane and a cell wall containing peptidoglycan. Bar indicates 0.2 μm. 86,000×. (Courtesy Wiebe ME, Burton PH, Shankel DM: *J Bacteriol* 110:368, 1972.)

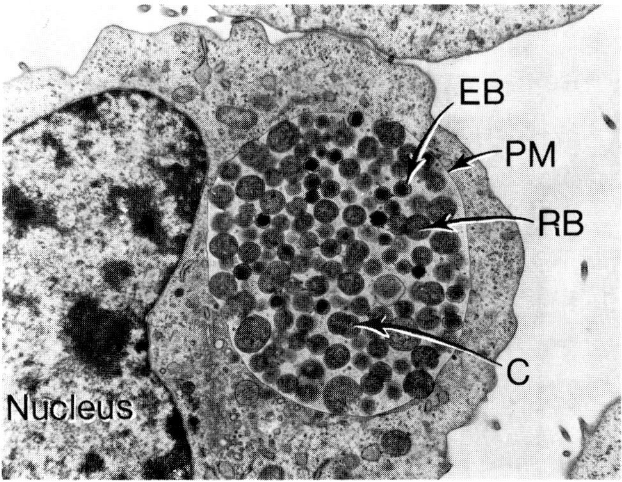

Fig. 2-8. Chlamydia psittaci in a phagosome of a human phagocytic cell. PM = phagosome membrane; EB = elementary body; RB = reticulate body; C = cell undergoing binary fission. 5,040×. (Courtesy GP Manire.)

ergy-producing enzyme systems and cannot synthesize adenosine triphosphate. Thus, they depend on host cells for generating metabolic energy. They produce typical cytoplasmic inclusions in infected cells, which are pathognomonic of chlamydia infections. Chlamydias are the etiologic agents of trachoma, inclusion conjunctivitis, lymphogranuloma venereum, ornithosis, nongonococcal urethritis, and neonatal pneumonia.

Mycoplasmas

Mycoplasmas are the smallest (150–300 nm in diameter) cells capable of independent extracellular existence (Fig. 2-9). They do not have cell walls and do not stain with Gram stain. They are not susceptible to antimicrobials which inhibit cell wall synthesis. Only one mycoplasma, *Mycoplasma pneumoniae*—the agent of primary atypical pneumonia—causes disease in humans.

EUKARYOTES

Fungi

Fungi are eukaryotic cells (Figs. 2-10 to 2-14). Their DNA is separated into chromosomes during cell division, and the nuclei are separated from the cytoplasm by a nuclear membrane. Their nuclei also contain nucleoli and histones, features lacking in bacteria. Unlike prokaryotic cells, the cytoplasm of fungi contains organelles such as mitochondria and endoplasmic reticulum. The plasma membrane of fungi contains sterols, a component absent from the plasma membranes of bacteria.

Fungi have a rigid cell wall, external to the plasma membrane, that serves to protect the cell from osmotic disruption. The cell wall of fungi does not contain peptidoglycan; instead it is composed almost entirely of polysaccharide. In many molds and yeasts, the principal structural material is chitin, which is a polymer of N-acetylglucosamine residues. Some yeasts also have a polysaccharide capsule surrounding the cell wall which, like bacterial capsules, inhibits phagocytosis (Fig. 2-10).

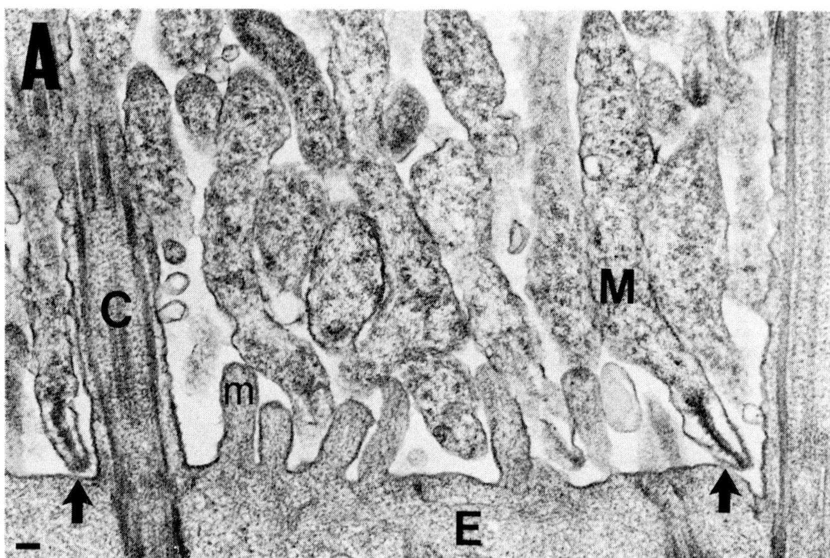

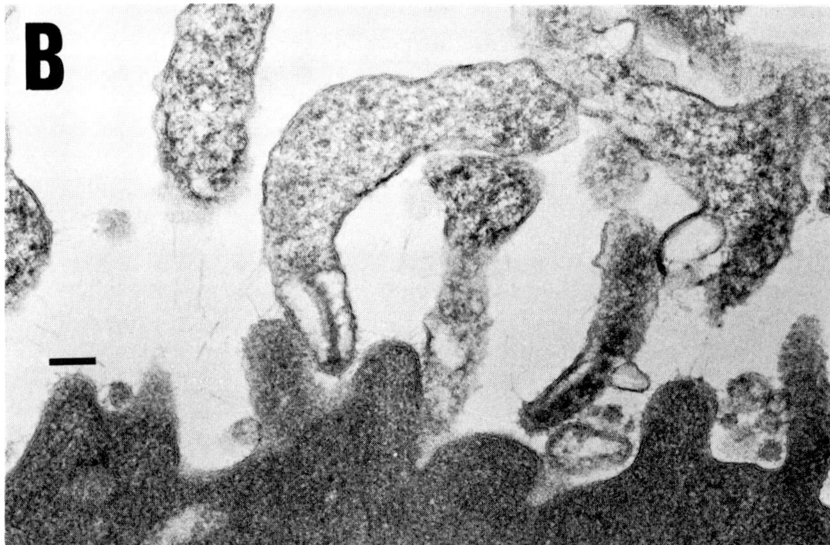

Fig. 2-9. A. *Mycoplasma pneumoniae* in tracheal ring organ culture for 72 hours. There is heavy parasitization of the cell with specialized tips for attachment to the tracheal cells (arrows) in close apposition to the bases of the cilia and microvilli. Bar indicates 0.1 μm. C = cilium; M = mycoplasma, m = microvillus; E = epithelium. B. *M. pneumoniae* = infected tracheal ring showing the classical filamentous structure of the organism, its tip touching a nonciliated cell. The encircling unit membrane, the body containing ribosomes and fibrils of nuclear material are all present. Bar indicated 0.1 μm. (Courtesy Wilson MH, Collier AM: *J Bacteriol* 125:332, 1976.)

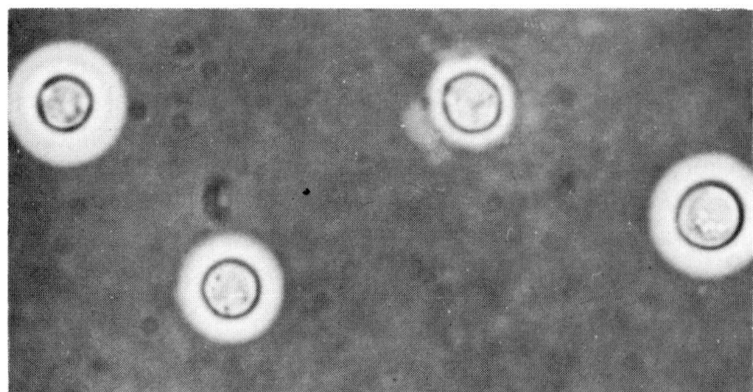

Fig. 2-10. India ink preparation of *Cryptococcus neoformans* from spinal fluid. The dark India ink background outlines the thick, clear capsule of the yeast cell.

Fungi grow either as single cells (yeasts) or as multicellular filamentous colonies (molds). Yeasts are unicellular, ovoid organisms 3–5 μm in diameter. The hyphae of molds are long septate chains, 2–10 μm in diameter.

Molds are characterized by tubular branching hyphae (Fig. 2-11), often divided into cells by transverse cell walls (septae). Spores (conidia) develop on specialized hyphae conidiophores of most fungi growing on solid medium and are primarily reproductive structures (Figs. 2-12–2-14). Of the estimated 80,000 species of fungi, only about 100 cause disease in man (mycoses). They are classified as systemic (deep) and superficial (cutaneous) mycoses. Systemic mycoses usually result in a granulomatous reaction in the host, with abscess formation. Fungi capable of causing infection include *Histoplasma capsulatum, Blastomyces dermatitides, Cryptococcus neoformans,* and *Coccidioides immitis.* Other fungi such as *Candida albicans, Aspergillus fumigatus,* and *Phycomycetes* are opportunists, and usually cause disease only in hosts with compromised defense mechanisms.

Cutaneous mycoses (dermatomycoses) are caused by fungi belonging to the genera *Trichophyton, Epidermophyton,* and *Microsporum.* They have a predilection for keratin-rich structures such as hair, nails, and epidermis.

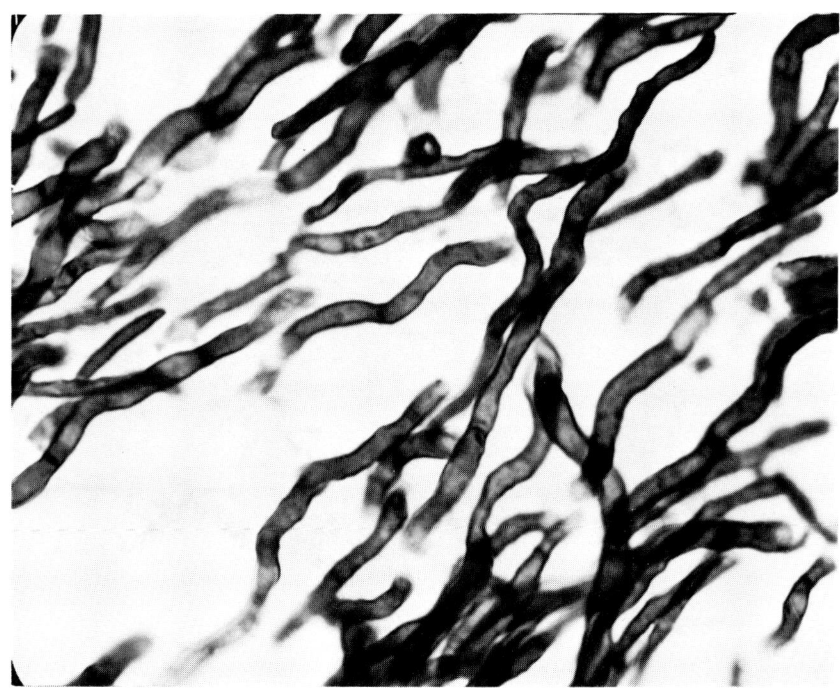

Fig. 2-11. Candida albicans nonseptate pseudohyphae in lung tissue (990×).

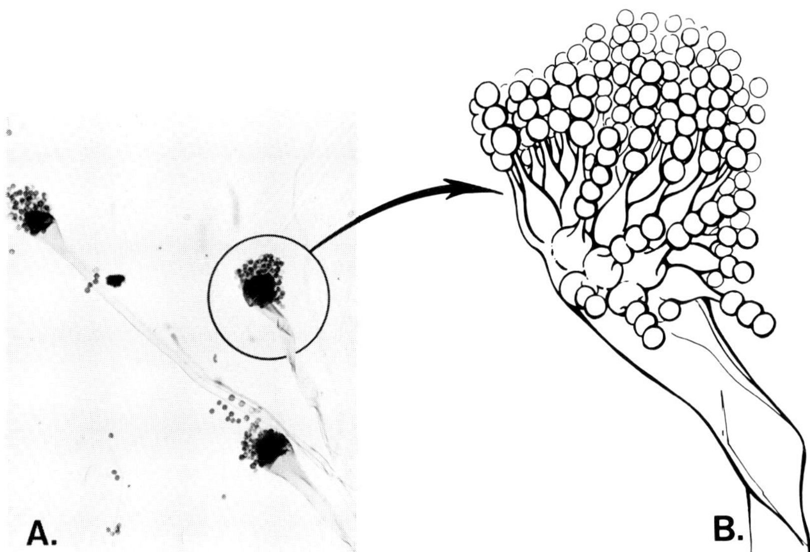

Fig. 2-12. A. *Aspergillus fumigatus.* The long conidiophores have long vesicle-like tips (× 472). B. The surface has flask-shaped sterigmata to which are attached chains of conida.

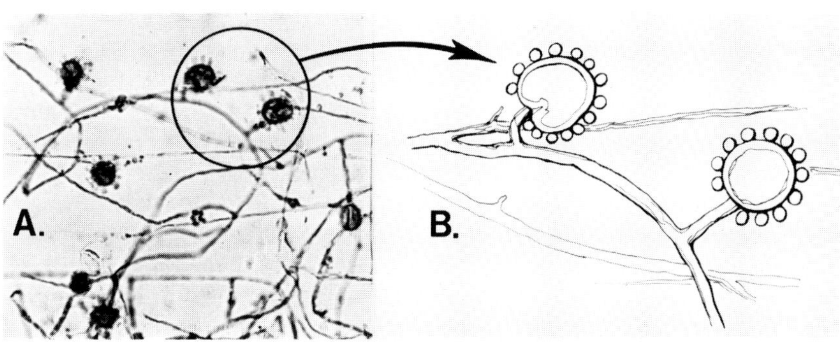

Fig. 2-13. Macroconidia (chlamydospores) of *Histoplasma capsulatum* (380×).

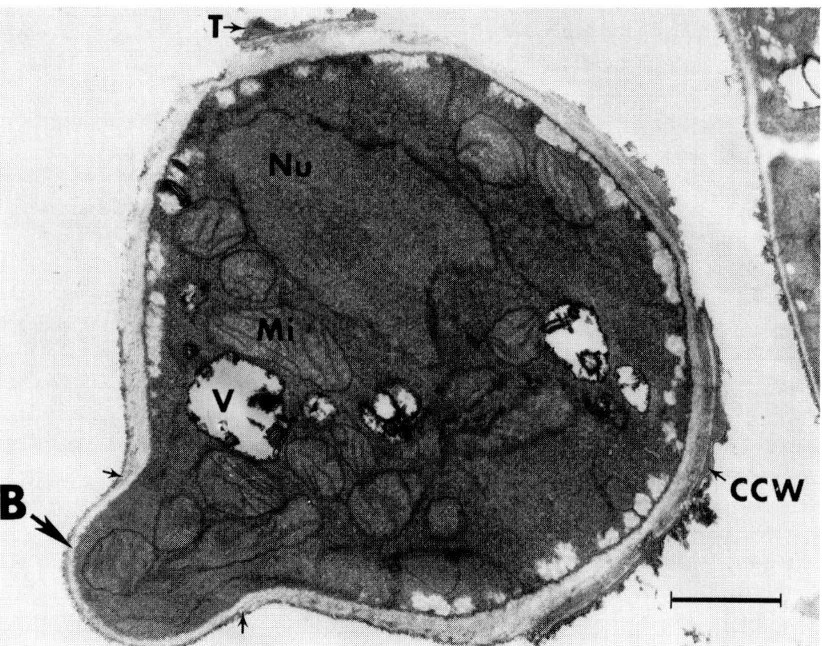

Fig. 2-14. Germinating microconidium of *H. capsulatum*. The remnants of the conidial cell wall (CCW), the presence of tubercles (T), and the origin of the cell wall of the budlike germ tube (B) are indicated by arrows. The cytoplasm contains a true, membrane-bound nucleus (Nu), mitochondria (Mi), and vacuoles (V), thus making it a eukaryotic cell. Bar indicates 0.5 μm (Courtesy Garrison RG, Boyd KS: *J Bacteriol* 133:345, 1978.)

Protozoa

Protozoa are unicellular, eukaryotic microorganisms. Their cellular structure has many characteristics in common with human cells. Like all eukaryotic cells, they have a true nucleus with a nuclear membrane, mitotic structures, histones, chromosomes, and a nucleolus. Their cytoplasm contains well-defined organelles such as mitochondria and endoplasmic reticulum. The plasma membrane is stabilized with sterols. There is no cell wall. The smaller protozoa, such as *Leishmania,* measure 2×4 μm, whereas the giant ameba, with a diameter of approximately 1 mm, is visible to the naked eye.

Medically important protozoa can be conveniently grouped according to the principal site of infection: intestine *(Entamoeba histolytica, Balantidium coli),* blood *(Plasmodium, Trypanosoma, Leishmania),* genital tract *(Trichomonas vaginalis),* and parenchymal cells *(Pneumocystis carinii, Toxoplasma gondii).*

HOST-MICROBIAL RELATIONSHIPS

Humans are constantly colonized with a variety of microorganisms. Vast numbers of bacteria live harmlessly in the human oral cavity, nasal cavity, intestine, female genital tract, eyes, and skin. Each site provides a variety of microenvironments suitable for different kinds of bacteria. It is also estimated that approximately 150 viruses infect people without causing detectable illness. This state, where neither host nor infecting agent harms the other, is called commensalism and may even be mutually beneficial (mutualism). The human host provides a suitable environment for intestinal bacteria, and the bacteria synthesize vitamin K or vitamin B_{12}, which are required by the human host. Only when the microorganisms cause pathologic changes in the host does disease occur. Pathogenic microorganisms can produce disease in the infected host.

Parasitism occurs when one organism lives at the expense of another. For successful parasitism, a microorganism cannot cause the death of the host, because the parasite will also die unless it finds another host. There is no sharp distinction between a parasite and a nonparasite (saprophyte). There is a steady gradation from microorganisms with almost no capacity to injure the host to those that injure the host with great regularity when they infect. For instance, *Lactobacillus* rarely, if ever, causes disease, whereas *Yersinia pestis* (plaque bacillus) regularly causes disease in the infected host. Poliovirus causes disease in only about 1 percent of the hosts who are infected. *E. coli* is part of the normal flora of the intestine, and most strains cause no disease when confined there; however, disease can result when it escapes the confines of the intestine. It may enter the bladder by passage of a catheter through the urethra, or it may ascend the short female urethra, without catheterization, and cause cystitis and pyelonephritis. *E. coli* can cause peritonitis or abdominal abscess when it gains entrance to the peritoneal cavity during intestinal operation, penetrating trauma to the intestine, or intestinal infarction. Microorganisms that cause disease only in a person with abnormal host defenses are referred to as opportunists.

Virulence is synonymous with pathogenicity, but is occasionally used to reflect the degree of pathogenicity. Most writers now prefer not to make this distinction and use the terms virulent and pathogenic interchangeably. Thus, if two strains of a bacterium can cause disease in a host but fewer organisms of one strain are required, the latter strain is said to be more pathogenic or virulent.

Traditionally, pathogens have been regarded as having some unique characteristics that allowed them to produce disease. Indeed, some bacteria do have special disease-producing characteristics. For instance, *Corynebacterium diphtheriae, S. dysenteriae, C. botulinum,* and *C. tetani* cause disease because they elaborate a specific toxin, which adversely alters the function of host cells. Such special disease-producing characteristics are the exception rather than the rule. We simply do not understand how most pathogens cause disease. Some bacteria have characteristics (eg, capsules) that allow them to escape host defenses and thus to multiply in tissues, but how they actually cause tissue or organ injury is unknown.

Some microbes can thrive only in host tissues outside phagocytic and other cells. Other microorganisms are found almost entirely in intracellular locations—usually in phagocytic cells. In general, extracellular parasites (*S. aureus, S. pneumoniae, Klebsiella pneumoniae, S. pyogenes,* and *Neisseria gonorrheae*) cause acute, rapidly progressive diseases. These types of bacteria are readily killed after they have been phagocytosed by neutrophils and macrophages. On the other hand, intracellular parasites such as the bacteria *Mycobacterium tuberculosis, M. leprae, Brucella abortis, Salmonella typhi,* and the fungi *Histoplasma capsulatum, Candida albicans, Coccidioides immitis* and *Blastomyces dermatitidis* are usually found in tissues inside phagocytic cells, but are capable of extracellular existence. They can resist intracellular digestion and killing by the lysosomal enzymes, but their means of survival are not well understood. They even grow and multiply within phagocytic cells. These types of intracellular bacteria and fungi commonly cause chronic, slowly progressive illnesses. Other microorganisms, such as chlamydias, rickettsiae, and viruses, are obliged to live inside the cells they invade because they lack the necessary metabolic machinery for an independent existence. They must use the host cell's metabolic and synthetic apparatus for growth and obtain necessary molecules from the host.

MICROBIAL PATHOGENICITY

The extent of an infection is determined by the interplay of the host's defense mechanisms and microbial virulence factors. Some failure in local or systemic host defenses must occur for a microbe to cause disease (Chapter 13). The ability to avoid or withstand host defenses is one of the most important microbial characteristics contributing to disease-producing capacity. When the host's defenses are compromised by burns, trauma, operation, drugs, and poor nutrition, microbes that normally have a low degree of pathogenicity are able to invade tissues and cause disease.

The factors that contribute to virulence have been studied more extensively for bacteria than for other microbes. Special characteristics by which bacteria, fungi, and other microbes resist host defenses and thus increase their disease-producing capacity are probably the exception. We do not understand the mechanisms by which many microorganisms resist host defenses, especially microbes of low pathogenicity.

ATTACHMENT TO EPITHELIAL SURFACES

Because most "naturally" occurring infections take place via the respiratory, gastrointestinal, or genitourinary tract, an important initial step in many infections is the ability of microbes to attach to an epithelial surface. This ability helps them escape local host defenses and compete successfully with the normal flora for nutrients and space. In fact, the normal flora can also attach to epithelial surfaces and may prevent colonization of more pathogenic microbes, in part, by covering up specific attachment sites required by pathogenic microorganisms.

Bacteria and viruses appear to attach to epithelial cells via pairs of complementary receptors on microbe and cell. Influenza virus attaches to respiratory epithelial cells, because the viral hemagglutinin reacts with neuraminic acid receptors on these cells. Other viruses (eg, poliovirus, adenovirus) attach to susceptible cells because there are specific receptors on these cells for viral capsid protein. *S. pyogenes* attaches to pharyngeal epithelium by means of the M protein on the cell surface—experimentally, anti-M protein IgA antibody can prevent this attachment. *Neissera gonorrheae* attaches to urethral epithelium via pili. In addition, attachment of *N. gonorrheae* is favored because this bacterium has an IgA protease which can inactivate IgA, which normally seems to mask bacterial receptors for urethral epithelium. Other bacteria also show specific attachment to host cell surfaces, but the mechanism is unknown: *E. coli, Salmonella typhi,* and *Vibrio cholerae* attach to intestinal epithelium; *Haemophilus influenzae* and *H. pertussis* attach to respiratory epithelium, and *Chlamydia trachomatis* specifically attaches to conjunctival epithelium.

Once attached, bacteria cause disease by tissue invasion, by elaboration of extracellular or cell surface toxins, and by immunologic means (ie, poststreptococcal glomerulonephritis and rheumatic valvular disease). *S. pneumoniae* produce disease solely by their ability to invade tissues and have no toxigenic capability. Dead pneumococci or cell-free filtrates of broth cultures of pneumococci do not cause illness or the inflammatory response characteristic of pneumococcal infection. At the other end of the spectrum is *Clostridium botulinum,* which lacks all ability to invade tissues and hardly elaborates its exotoxin at normal body temperatures. Toxin production occurs optimally when the bacteria are cultured at 25C to 30C. In fact, botulism is not an infection at all, it is an intoxication. In between these two bacteria are microorganisms that can both invade tissues and elaborate toxins or extracellular enzymes, such as *S. aureus, S. pyogenes, C. perfringens,* and *Corynebacterium diphtheriae.* With these bacteria, experimental illness similar to that caused by inoculation of live organisms can be produced by administration of killed organisms or of cell-free broth cultures. This ability to cause disease in the absence of live organisms implicates toxins and extracellular enzymes as having a part in the illness caused by the live organism. But most infections, and almost all surgical infections, require a microbe to invade tissues and multiply within the host. To do this, the microorganism must be able to escape local and systemic host defenses.

In the case of many surgically related infections, the surgeon disrupts the physical integrity of the skin, intestine, and other body surfaces that harbor bacteria, thus permitting them to become implanted in tissues. Microbes also escape local defenses when burns, trauma, intestinal ischemia, or gangrene render local defenses incompetent and permit direct tissue access.

MECHANISMS BY WHICH MICROBES ESCAPE HOST DEFENSES

In general, two mechanisms of resisting host defenses have been investigated: (1) some bacteria actually escape phagocytosis and intracellular killing, and (2) some bacteria elaborate toxins and extracellular enzymes that inhibit host defenses and facilitate tissue spread of bacteria. Exotoxins, of course, can also affect cells having nothing to do with host defenses. Exotoxins and bacterial extracellular enzymes are discussed together, because many toxins are enzymes and because both are extracellular macromolecules—usually proteins.

Mechanisms Whereby Microorganisms Escape Phagocytosis and Intracellular Killing

One way to avoid phagocytosis is to eliminate chemotaxis. Some streptococci secrete a streptolysin which inhibits PMN chemotaxis so that PMNs are less readily drawn toward the invading bacteria. The same streptolysin is also lethal for phagocytes.

Many bacteria *(S. pneumoniae, Haemophilus influenzae, Klebsiella pneumoniae, E. coli, Salmonella typhi)*, and fungi (ie, *Histoplasma capsulatum, Cryptococcus neoformans, C. albicans*) possess thick capsules, which seem to enable the microbe to resist phagocytosis. Perhaps the capsules prevent antibody or complement absorption to the subcapsular cell membrane. Alternatively, they may create a "slippery" surface, so the phagocyte cannot surround the organism and engulf it. Only if antibodies to the capsule itself are present is phagocytosis easily accomplished. Whatever the mechanism, the presence of capsules is correlated with virulence. For instance, as few as 10 encapsulated *S. pneumoniae* can kill a mouse when inoculated intraperitoneally, whereas 10,000 bacteria are required if the capsules are removed by hyaluronidase.[6] If the mouse is rendered incapable of forming antibodies (opsonins) against the capsule, a single bacterium is sufficient to cause death.

Like capsules, the M protein of *Streptococcus pyogenes* is associated with the ability to resist phagocytosis. Under the microscope it appears that streptococci do not absorb to the phagocyte and seem to "slither" off the surface of PMNs that are attempting to engulf them.[6] When the M protein is covered with antibody (opsonized), phagocytosis readily occurs.

Another mechanism that bacteria use to resist phagocytosis is exhibited by *S. aureus.* A component of the cell wall, protein A, inhibits the phagocytosis even of opsonized bacteria. Protein A acts by blocking the Fc portion of IgG antibody, preventing binding of the Fc portion to the receptors on the PMNs. Protein A is found only in highly pathogenic staphylococci and may thus be an important virulence factor. The complex of other virulence factors at work for the extensively investigated *S. aureus* are discussed in Chapter 4.

Bacteria have also evolved mechanisms of avoiding intracellular killing after they have been phagocytosed. Normally, the first step in intracellular killing is fusion of the lysosome with the phagosome, so that the microbe is rapidly exposed to the digestive enzymes. Virulent *Mycobacterium tuberculosis,* which is phagocytosed readily, somehow inhibits the lysosomes from fusing with the phagosome. However, lysosomal fusion readily occurs when strains of *M. tuberculosis* of low virulence are phagocytosed, and the organisms are killed. Lysosomal fusion also fails to occur when *Toxoplasma gondii* is phagocytosed by macrophages, when *Aspergillus flavus* is phagocytosed by alveolar macrophages of susceptible mouse strains, when chlamydia enter cells in tissue culture, and when *S. aureus* enters Küpffer cells of the in vitro perfused liver. Furthermore, *S. aureus* produces catalase, an enzyme that enables it to degrade hydrogen peroxide—potent bactericidal component of the PMN myeloperoxidase–hydrogen peroxide–halide system.

Other microbes successfully resist digestion by lysosomal enzymes in the phagolysosome. In fact, certain microbes regularly grow in macrophages. Microorganisms that can multiply in macrophages include viruses (herpesviruses), rickettsia, bacteria *(M. tuberculosis, Brucella abortis)*, fungi (*Cryptococcus neoformans)*, and protozoa *(Toxoplasma gondii)*. How these microorganisms resist intracellular killing is not known, but the mechanisms probably depend on structural properties of the outer surfaces of the microorganisms.

Exotoxins and Extracellular Enzymes

Many bacteria produce extracellular enzymes and toxins (exotoxins) that may facilitate their disease-producing capacity (Tables 2-2 and 2-3). For other microorganisms, exotoxins are the most important or even the sole factor contributing to the production of disease. Almost all exotoxins are proteins and are readily inactivated by heat, formaldehyde, and other chemical treatments. These inactive exotoxins, toxoids, sometimes retain their antigenic determinants, and can be used for immunization against the toxin.

TABLE 2-2. TOXICITY OF WELL-KNOWN POISONS AND BACTERIAL TOXINS

Poison or toxin	Toxicity for man (mg)*
Strychnine	100
Arsenic	100
Cyanide	50
Cobra venom	25
Endotoxin	100
Clostridium botulinum	
Botulinum A	0.00009
Botulinum D	0.00003
Clostridium tetani toxin	0.0001
Clostridium welchi E toxin	0.28
Clostridium novyi toxin	0.001
Shigella dysenteriae neurotoxin	0.00006
Corynebacterium diphtheriae toxin	0.02

* The numbers given here are approximations from animal data. Because animal species may vary in susceptibility to toxins, the figures will vary depending on which species the toxicity is based. Therefore these numbers must be regarded as rough approximations for a 70-kg man.

TABLE 2-3. EXOTOXINS PRODUCED BY THE PRINCIPAL TOXIGENIC BACTERIA

Bacterium	Disease	Toxin	Action
Streptococcus pyogenes	Pyogenic infections	Streptolysin O	Hemolytic
	Scarlet fever	Streptolysin S	Hemolytic
		Erythrogenic	Causes scarlet fever rash
		Streptokinase	Deoxyribonuclease
		Streptodornase	Fibrinolytic
		Streptococcal DPNase	Cardiotoxic, leukotoxic (?)
Staphylococcus aureus	Pyogenic infections	α-toxin	Necrotizing, hemolytic, leukocidic
		β-toxin	Hemolytic, lethal
		γ-toxin	hemolytic, necrotizing, lethal
		δ-toxin	Hemolytic, leukolytic
		ϵ-toxin	Hemolytic
		Enterotoxin	Emetic
		Leukocidin	Kills leukocytes
		Hyaluronidase	Spreading factor
		Coagulase	Coagulates plasma
Clostridium tetani	Tetanus	Tetanospasm	Muscle spasms
		Tetanolysin	Hemolytic cardiotoxin
Clostridium perfringens	Gas gangrene	α-toxin	Lecithinase: necrotizing, hemolytic
		β-toxin	Necrotizing, lethal
		γ-toxin	Lethality
		δ-toxin	Hemolysis
		ϵ-toxin	Necrotizing
		η-toxin	Lethality
		θ-toxin	Hemolytic cardiotoxin
		ι-toxin	Necrotizing
		κ-toxin	Collagenase
		λ-toxin	Protoclytic
		μ-toxin	Hyaluronidase, spreading factor
Clostridium novyi	Gas gangrene	α-toxin	Necrotizing
		β-toxin	Lecithinase: necrotizing, hemolytic
		γ-toxin	Lecithinase: necrotizing, hemolytic
		δ-toxin	Hemolytic
		ϵ-toxin	Lipase, hemolytic
		ζ-toxin	Hemolytic
Clostridium botulinum	Botulism	Neurotoxin (6 types)	Paralytic
Corynebacterium diphtheriae	Diphtheria	Diphtheritic toxin	Necrotizing
Shigella dysenteriae	Dysentery	Neurotoxin	Paralytic, hemorrhagic
Haemophilus pertussis	Whooping cough	Whooping cough toxin	Necrotizing

The precise role for many enzymes and exotoxins in bacterial pathogenicity is uncertain. Some of these exotoxins are produced only under appropriate in vitro culture conditions and may not be synthesized or released in vivo. One method of attempting to determine whether enzymes and exotoxins have a real role in the pathogenicity of a bacterium is to determine whether an acellular broth culture of the bacterium can reproduce any of the characteristics of an experimental infection with live bacteria. These bacterial enzymes and exotoxins cause hemolysis of red blood cells, death of white blood cells, necrosis of tissues, degradation of intercellular substances such as nucleic acid, hyaluronic acid, collagen and other proteins, and clotting of plasma. Many bacteria cause hemolysis of erythrocytes when grown on blood agar, but the importance of hemolysins in vivo is uncertain. Similarly, enzymes that cause degradation of intercellular substances such as collagen and hyaluronic acid may favor spread of bacteria through tissue planes, but there is no solid evidence to support this hypothesis. For instance, administering an antihyaluronidase antibody does not affect pathogenicity of bacteria that produce this toxin.

S. aureus produces a coagulase that causes clotting of plasma. While the ability to produce coagulase is correlated with virulence of *S. aureus*, there is no evidence that the coagulase itself is responsible for this virulence. It has been hypothesized that by converting fibrinogen to fibrin, coagulase contributes to pathogenicity by entrapping the bacteria in the clot, thus protecting them from phagocytes. Pathogenic strains of *S. aureus* which do not elaborate coagulase, however, produce similar tissue lesions and are no more readily phagocytosed. *S. aureus* when grown in broth also elaborates a necrotizing toxin that can cause necrosis of cells. Its role in actual infections is not known.

Streptolysin produced by *S. pyogenes* inhibits in vitro chemotaxis of PMNs, but its in vivo importance is not certain. Streptolysin O is cardiotoxic, causes hemolysis of red blood cells, and is lethal when administered to mice. Streptokinase causes fibrinolysis, and streptodornase degrades nucleic acids and may facilitate spread of the bacteria in tissue planes.

Clostridium perfringens produces at least ten separate exotoxins, including collagenase, a hyaluronidase, a lecithinase, proteolytic enzymes, necrotizing toxins, and hemolytic toxins (Table 2-3). These toxins are believed to be important in the pathogenesis of gas gangrene by causing tissue necrosis, thus lowering the oxidation-reduction potential and providing a favorable environment for anaerobic bacterial growth. The collagenase breaks down the framework of muscle and other tissues, facilitating the spread of these infections along tissue planes.

For some bacteria, such as *C. tetani*, *C. botulinum*, *Corynebacterium diphtheriae*, and *Shigella dysenteriae*, intoxication is the most prominent and in some case sole mechanism of disease. In addition, *S. aureus* produces a potent enterotoxin that is the cause of staphylococcal food poisoning. Some *E. coli* strains also produce an enterotoxin that results in a cholera-like illness in infants. These bacterial exotoxins are the most potent toxins known (Table 2-2). Diseases caused by toxigenic bacteria typically require many hours to a few days before symptoms become apparent.

Tetanus and botulinum toxin are potent neurotoxins. *C. botulinus* produces at least six separate protein exotoxins. Botulinum toxin attaches to preganglionic and postganglionic synapses of the peripheral autonomic system and to the nerve ends at the myoneural junction, where it blocks neural transmission at cholinergic synapses. At these sites, botulinum toxin prevents release of acetylcholine from cholinergic nerve fibers, which results in paralysis. Death usually occurs from suffocation after the respiratory muscles become paralyzed. *C. tetani* produces two exotoxins, tetanolysin and tetanospasm. Tetanolysin is cardiotoxic and causes hemolysis, but it is not thought to be of major clinical importance. Tetanospasm is responsible for the spasms and hyperreflexia of clinical tetanus. Tetanus exotoxin acts mainly on the anterior horn cells of the spinal cord and on the brain stem. At these sites, it leads to muscle spasms and hyperreflexia by blocking spinal inhibitory synapses. Its physiologic effects are similar to those of strychnine poisoning.

The neurotoxin of *Shigella dysenteriae* can lead to paralysis and death of the animal several days after injection. The exotoxin of *S. dysenteriae*, however, does not appear to be a neurotoxin. Rather, it affects the central nervous system primarily by its toxicity for the vascular endothelium of blood vessels in the brain and spinal cord, thus affecting the blood flow to central nervous tissue.

Of all the bacterial exotoxins, the mechanism of action of diphtheria toxin is best understood. In fact the toxin is not produced unless the bacterium itself is infected by a virus (bacteriophage) whose genome codes for the toxin. On a molecular basis, the toxin inhibits polypeptide chain elongation by catalyzing the inactivation of a translocation factor required for addition of amino acids to the growing polypeptide chain. Physiologically, this leads to death of cells of the mucous membrane, resulting in the diphtheritic pseudomembrane and favoring further bacterial growth. The heart and peripheral nerves are especially susceptible and, if recovery ensues, late neurologic and cardiac complications are relatively common.

The enterotoxin of *Vibrio cholerae* binds irreversibly to intestinal epithelium, activating adenyl cyclase and increasing intracellular cyclic AMP. The results are intestinal electrolyte and water loss, producing diarrhea, dehydration, and electrolyte depletion characteristic of clinical cholera. Cell-free filtrates of *V. cholerae* produce the disease in volunteers, implicating the exotoxin as a major etiologic factor in this disease.

While not all exotoxins play a role in bacterial virulence, the pathogenic properties of tetanus, botulinus, and diphtheria toxins, staphylococcal enterotoxin, and the erythrogenic toxin of *S. pyogenes* have been conclusively established. The evidence is also convincing that the exotoxin of *Bordetella pertussis* is responsible for the deep broncheal wall lesions in whooping cough. Similarly, there is decisive evidence that the neurotoxin of *S. dysenteriae*, the α-toxin of *S. aureus*, and the lethal toxin of *Bacillus anthracis* are important to the pathogenicity of these organisms. On the other hand, there is no conclusive evidence that any of the other exotoxins produced by gram-positive bacteria are active in vivo.

Endotoxins

Endotoxins form the outer layer of the cell wall of gram-negative bacteria. They are an integral part of the cell wall and are released only with death of the bacteria. They are less toxic than an equivalent weight of exotoxin and, unlike most exotoxins, they are heat stable and cannot be converted to toxoids. Table 2-4 compares the properties of exotoxins and endotoxins.

Endotoxins are macromolecular complexes of phospholipids, polysaccharide, and protein. Their toxic biologic

TABLE 2-4. COMPARISON OF EXOTOXINS AND ENDOTOXINS

Exotoxins	Endotoxins
Excreted by living cells; found in high concentrations in fluid medium	Integral part of microbial cell walls of gram-negative organisms liberated upon their disintegration
Polypeptides, molecular weight 10,000–900,000	Lipopolysaccharide complexes. Lipid A portion probably responsible for toxicity
Relatively unstable; toxicity often destroyed rapidly by heat over 60C	Relatively stable; withstand heat over 60C for hours without loss of toxicity
Highly antigenic; stimulate the formation of high-titer antitoxin. Antitoxin neutralizes toxin	Do not stimulate formation of antitoxin; stimulate formation of antibodies to polysaccharide moiety
Converted into antigenic, nontoxic toxoids by formalin, acid, heat, etc.	Not converted into toxoids
Highly toxic; fatal for laboratory animals in micrograms or less	Weakly toxic; fatal for laboratory animals in hundreds of micrograms
Do not produce fever in host	Often produce fever in host

Reproduced with permission from Jawetz E, Melnick JL, Adelberg EA: *Review of Medical Microbiology,* 12th ed. Los Altos, California, Lange Medical Publications, 1978, p 130.

properties are associated with the lipopolysaccharide (LPS) moiety. The lipopolysaccharide consists of a polysaccharide region covalently bound to a lipid region (lipid A) (Fig. 2-15). The polysaccharide region of the lipopolysaccharides molecule consists of a "core" polysaccharide and an "O antigen" polysaccharide. The O antigen is chemically unique for each type of organism and lipopolysaccharide. Neither polysaccharide is toxic when it has been disassociated from lipid A.

Lipid A is thought to be responsible for all endotoxin or lipopolysaccharide toxicity listed in Table 2-5. In small doses, endotoxin causes fever through the release of an endogenous pyrogen from PMNs and macrophages. The pyrogenic action of endotoxin is believed to be mediated through prostaglandin E. When administered in larger doses (approximately 1 mg per kg for most mammalian species), endotoxin causes irreversible shock and death within an hour or two. Thus, the lethal effects of endotoxin occur much faster than those of exotoxins, which usually require many hours to days before death occurs.

At less than lethal doses, endotoxin causes many systemic biologic effects (Table 2-5). It can activate the complement system in vitro by an alternate pathway through C3. This pathway spares the early complement components, C1, C4, C2, which are required for complement activation by antigen-antibody complexes. In fact, some authorities [7,8] assert that complement is the final common pathway for all the biologic effects of endotoxin. Endotoxin also causes rapid drop in complement when administered in vivo, and complement depletion can reduce the hypotension and lethality caused by administration, and the localized and generalized Schwartzman reaction as well.

Endotoxin can also activate the coagulation system directly through activation of Factor XII (Hageman factor) or indirectly through PMNs and monocytes, which release a tissue factor which then activates Factor VIII.[8] The ability of endotoxin to activate Hageman factor not only initiates the clotting sequence; Hageman factor also activates the entire kinin system, a system of vasoactive polypeptides. Endotoxin can thus produce tissue injury through initiation of intravascular coagulation.[8]

Endotoxin also causes thrombocytopenia, platelet aggregation, and release of serotonin in animals. The thrombocytopenia is abrogated by complement depletion. Aggregation of human platelets does not occur when they are exposed to endotoxin in vitro, but serotonin release from platelets does occur. Endotoxin also causes a prompt profound transient leukopenia followed by leukocytosis.[8] Macrophages release several substances in response to endotoxins—procoagulants, collagenase, pyrogens, prosta-

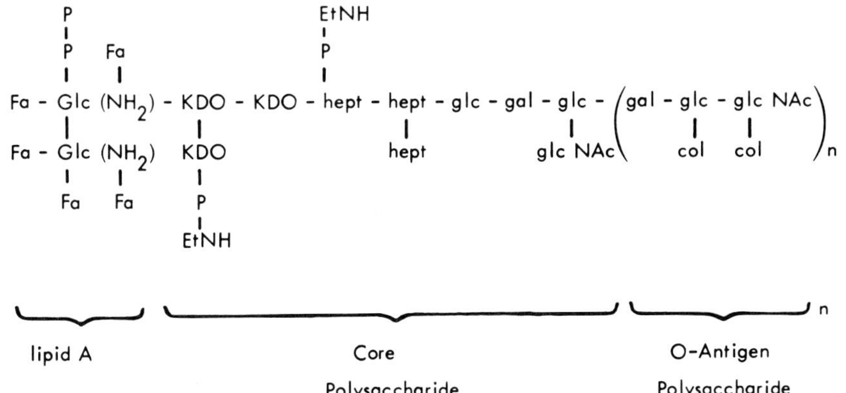

Fig. 2-15. Chemical structure of *E. coli* lipopolysaccharide (endotoxin). Abbreviations: Fa = fatty acid; P = phosphate; Glc (NH_2) = glycosamine; KDO = 2-keto 2-deoxy-octulosonate; EtNH = ethanolamine; hept = L-glycero-D-mannoheptose; glc = glucose; gal = galactose; glcNAc = N-acetyl-glucosamine; col = colitose. (Courtesy Morrison DC, Ulevitch RJ: *Am J Pathol* 93:525, 1978.)

TABLE 2-5. BIOLOGIC EFFECTS OF ENDOTOXIN

Site	Comment
Thermoregulatory center	Causes fever; releases pyrogens from neutrophils; directly affects thermoregulatory center in the hypothalamus
Blood	
Erythrocytes	Shifts erythropoiesis from bone marrow to spleen
Leukocytes	Leukopenia to 10 percent of normal occurs within minutes, maximal leukopenia at 2 hours; leukocyte count returns to normal 4–6 hours after injection; later leukocytosis. Increased phagocytosis and bacterial killing in vitro
Platelets	Thrombocytopenia; platelet aggregation; release of platelet constituents (ADP, vasoactive amines, histamine, serotonin, platelet factor 3)
Coagulation system	Extrinsic coagulation pathway: Causes release of platelet factor 3 which acts to form thromboplastin; releases tissue factor from macrophages
	Intrinsic coagulation pathway: activates factor XII (Hageman factor), the initial component of the intrinsic clotting system
	Causes disseminated intravascular coagulation
Complement	Activates complement via the alternative pathway (C3)
Vascular system	
Shock	Mechanism uncertain; causes decreased systemic pressure, decreased cardiac output, decreased venous return, increased peripheral resistance, pooling of blood
Vasoactive substances	Causes release or activation of histamine, serotonin, kinins
Endocrine system	Causes release of ACTH and growth hormone, increases plasma cortisol; no effect on TSH or LH
Immune system	
Endotoxin is an immunogen	Antibodies can be detected 7–10 days after endotoxin administration
Adjuvant	Endotoxin is an adjuvant for a variety of antigens
B cell mitogen	
Stimulates reticuloendothelial system	Increases processing of antigen
Metabolism	
Carbohydrate	Initial hyperglycemia followed by hypoglycemia with concomitant decrease in liver glycogen
Lipid	Hyperlipidemia; increased free fatty acids, serum cholesterol, serum phospholipids, and plasma triglycerides
Proteins	Stimulates liver protein synthesis; increases serum lactic acid dehydrogenase, isocitric dehydrogenase, transaminase, and creatine phosphokinase
Minerals	Decreases serum iron and iron binding capacity
Gastrointestinal system	Decreased thirst, appetite, and gastric emptying; diarrhea
Reticuloendothelial system	Enhanced blood clearance of colloidal carbon; releases mediators from macrophages (collagenase, pyrogens, prostaglandins, colony stimulating factor, and a tissue factor that promotes coagulation); stimulated macrophages to become cytotoxic
Schwartzman phenomenon	Localized and generalized Schwartzman phenomenon, mediated through coagulation system
Resistance to infection	Increases nonspecific resistance to bacteria, fungi, and viruses

glandin, and factors cytotoxic for tumor cells. Endotoxin also enhances the ability of macrophages to phagocytose bacteria and colloidal gold. Similar types of macrophage activation may be the mechanism of the increased resistance to infection in experimental animals treated with endotoxin.

Endotoxin also causes release of adrenocorticotropic and growth hormones from the pituitary gland, alteration of protein, carbohydrate, and lipid metabolism, abortion, hemorrhage into tumors, and the local and generalized Schwartzman reactions. In addition, endotoxin is an immunologic adjuvant, nonspecifically increasing the immune response to a variety of antigens.

Despite the hundreds of articles dealing with the chemistry and biologic effects of endotoxin, its role in the initiation of clinical infection is unknown—even though much circumstantial evidence supports its role in the complication of overwhelming gram-negative sepsis.

IMMUNOLOGIC INJURY AS A RESULT OF INFECTION

The immune response to infections may have evolved as protective devices, but these devices can themselves produce inflammation, cell infiltration, tissue destruction, and even ultimately lead to death. Indeed, Thomas[9] has observed that "our arsenals for fighting off bacteria are so powerful and involve so many different defense mechanisms, that we are in more danger from them than from the invaders."

There are many examples of immunopathology resulting from experimental infections in animals and a few human infections with clear-cut immunopathologic sequelae.[10] Perhaps the best known is rheumatic fever, which follows group A streptococcal infections. Streptococci have antigens that cross-react with heart muscle, and antibodies against these streptococcal antigens can react with heart muscle and valve tissue. The antigen-antibody complexes that result can activate the complement cascade and activate inflammatory changes, which lead to myocarditis and endocarditis. Because many strains of streptococci have these antigens, recurrent attacks of rheumatic fever can occur.

Antibodies to other microbes also form during the course of infection, and antigen-antibody complexes can themselves lead to disease. For example, immune complexes can become deposited on the basement membranes of the renal glomerulus and blood vessels. In these sites, immune complexes activate the complement system and produce inflammation and immune injury. This injury causes acute glomerulonephritis and vasculitis. Kidney deposits of immune complexes have been found in people with hepatitis B infection, infection with *S. pyogenes*, and malaria. These glomerulonephritides are usually acute. The antigen responsible for chronic glomerulonephritis has not been identified.

Immune complexes have been implicated in arthralgias and rashes caused by certain arboviruses. The dengue shock syndrome is thought to be an anaphylactic-type reaction to dengue virus infection.

Delayed-type hypersensitivity reactions to microbial antigens are responsible for some of the most prominent clinical manifestations of microbial disease. For example, dermatophytes grow in the stratum corneum of the skin. During the first 10 to 35 days of infection, the skin appears normal or only slightly inflamed. These fungi do not seem to produce any irritant or toxins that directly damage the skin; however, after 2 to 3 weeks the advancing border of the infection may become inflamed. This inflammation stems from the host immunity to the dermatophyte. This immunity then produces most of the pathology observed in clinical dermatophytoses. This host response to the fungus is an intense immune inflammatory reaction, which produces erythema and edema. The cell-mediated immune damage has some benefit to the host, however, because it prevents the spread or the lateral migration of the fungus within the skin. If cell-mediated immunity to dermatophyte antigen does not develop, the skin does not become inflamed and the infection is not eradicated. Consequently, in patients without the ability to express cell-mediated immunity, the infected skin is only minimally inflamed, but the fungus infection persists to produce scaling erythema, puritis, fissures, and cracks. The acute inflammatory type of skin infection usually heals spontaneously or responds well to treatment. The chronic or noninflammatory type of infection, however, associated with failure to express cell-mediated immunity to the fungus, is relapsing and responds poorly to treatment.

Another example of the immune response to an infection resulting in pathology is that seen with experimental lymphocytic choriomeningitis virus in mice. Infection of healthy, adult animals with this virus produces choroiditis and meningitis. A persistent carrier state ensues, however, if lymphocytic choriomeningitis virus is inoculated into immunologically incompetent neonatal mice within 24 hours of birth or into adult mice that have been immunosuppressed and are unable to mount an immune response against the virus. Both inoculated neonatal mice and adult immunosuppressed mice persistently carry the virus but do not develop meningitis or choroiditis. Histologically, lymphocytic infiltrates can be seen in the choroid plexus and meninges of animals that develop choriomeningitis. Thus, in these animals the immune response to the virus is responsible for the cerebral injury and subsequent death. Lymphocytic choriomeningitis virus can be detected by immunofluorescence in the cerebrum and cerebellum, liver, and other organs of mice inoculated at birth, despite lack of cellular destruction or pathologic or functional changes. If, however, immune lymphocytes are passively transferred to these animals, they rapidly die of diffuse tissue damage caused by a vigorous inflammatory infiltrate.

PATTERNS OF INFECTION

Microorganisms can cause infections that have different time courses—acute, chronic, persistent (latent), and slow. These divisions are for convenience, because microbes can cause more than one pattern of infection. Furthermore, acute infections can become chronic, latent, or develop into slow infections, and latent infections can become acute infections.

Acute infections have an abrupt onset and last for several days or several weeks. Most acute surgical infections are localized to one organ or body region, such as pneumonia, cellulitis, carbuncle, abscess, pyelonephritis, peritonitis, infection of an artificial valve, aortic graft.

Disseminated infections involve multiple tissues or organs and are spread via the bloodstream. Disseminated infections are rare in surgical patients but when they do occur they are frequently fatal. In addition, surgical patients with compromised host defenses are susceptible to opportunistic disseminated bacterial, fungal, and viral diseases.

Inapparent infections occur when the host has evidence of infection but there are no clinical manifestations and no disease occurs. Most infections with poliovirus and mumps virus are inapparent; patients manifest serum antibody to the virus but have never had clinical disease. Inapparent infection also occurs with *Histoplasma capsulatum, M. tuberculosis, Coccidioidis immitis, Treponema pallidum, S. pyogenes* (streptococcus carrier), *Salmonella typhi,* and others.

Chronic infections last from weeks to months and years and are particularly common with facultative intracellular parasites. Most surgical infections do not fall into this category, but the surgeon can encounter leprosy, syphilis, tuberculosis, anthrax, and osteomyelitis.

Persistent (latent) infections occur when the microbial parasite and host have reached an equilibrium so that the microbe does not cause disease but remains in the host—unaffected by host defenses. Viruses—especially members of the herpesvirus family—are the best examples of persistent infections. Varicella-zoster virus can persist in the dorsal root ganglia for years without causing disease, only to appear as an acute case of zoster when the appropriate stimulus reactivates it. Herpes simplex virus, the etiologic agent of fever blister, is also a latent virus that can be reactivated by stress, heat, actinic radiation, and illness. Most adults have been infected by another herpesvirus, cytomegalovirus (an inapparent infection). It can remain latent until reactivated by pregnancy, immunosuppression, or cancer chemotherapy. All latent herpes viruses can be reactivated by operation, immunosuppressive drugs, or cancer chemotherapy. Syphilis, tuberculosis, and other bacteria may exist as latent infection, and their reactivation may present with local (and therefore surgical) manifestations.

Slow viral infections refer to viral infections that may require several years to become clinically manifest. Virus replication is not slow, but the disease occurs over a prolonged period. Almost all slow virus disease primarily affects the central nervous system. Subacute sclerosing panencephalitis is caused by measles viruses. Other slow virus infections are Kuru and Kreutzfeld-Jacob disease.

BIBLIOGRAPHY

Ajl SJ, Kadis S, Montie TC, Weinbaum G, Ciegler A (eds): Microbial Toxins: A Comprehensive Treatise, Vols 1–8. New York, Academic, 1971.

Brock TD: Biology of Microorganisms. Englewood Cliffs, NJ, Prentice-Hall, 1970.

David BD, Dulbecco R, Eisen H, Ginsberg HS, Wood WB Jr, McCarty, M: Microbiology; Including Immunology and Molecular Genetics, 2nd ed. Hagerstown, MD, Harper and Row, 1973, p 1107.

Elsbach P: Degradation of microorganisms by phagocytic cells. Rev Infect Dis 2:106, 1980.

Luria SE, Darnell JE Jr, Baltimore D, Campbell A: General Virology, 3rd ed. New York, Wiley, 1978.

Mims CA: The Pathogenesis of Infectious Disease. New York, Grune and Stratton, 1976.

Morrison DC, Ulevitch RJ: The effect of bacterial endotoxins on host mediation systems. Am J Pathol 93:526, 1978.

REFERENCES

1. Buchanan RE, Gibbons NE (eds): Bergey's Manual of Determinative Bacteriology, 8th Ed. Baltimore, Williams and Wilkins, 1974.
2. Davis BD, Dulbecco R, Eisen H, Ginsberg HS, Wood WB, Jr, McCarty M: Microbiology: Including Immunology and Molecular Genetics, 2nd ed. Hagerstown, Maryland, Harper and Row, 1973, p 1107.
3. Lüderitz O, Staub AM, Westphal O: Immunochemistry of O and R antigens of *Salmonella* and related Enterobacteriaceae. Bacteriol Rev 30:192, 1966.
4. Rietschel ET, Gottert H, Lüderitz O, Westphal O: Nature and linkages of the fatty acids present in the lipid-A component of Salmonella lipopolysaccharides. Eur J Biochem 28:166, 1972.
5. Westphal O: Bacterial endotoxins: the second Carl Prausnitz Memorial Lecture. Int Allerg Appl Immunol 49:1, 1975.
6. Mims CA: The Pathogenesis of Infectious Disease. New York, Grune and Stratton, 1976, p 13.
7. Gewurz H, Mergenhagen SE, Nowotny A, Phillips EJK: Interactions of the complement system with native and chemically modified endotoxins. J Bacteriol 95:397, 1968.
8. Morrison DC, Ulevitch RJ: The effects of bacterial endotoxins on host mediation systems. A review. Am J Pathol 93:526, 1978.
9. Thomas LP: The Lives of a Cell; Notes of a Biology Watcher. New York, Viking, 1974, p 78.
10. Theofilopoulos AN, Dixon FJ: Immune complexes in human diseases: A review. Am J Pathol 100:531, 1980.

CHAPTER 3
Indigenous Microbiota in the Human

HERBERT M. SOMMERS

PATIENTS today are more at risk from members of their own indigenous flora than from exogenous infectious agents. Historically, epidemics of infectious disease were caused by organisms with unique virulence factors that gave them a selective edge over the indigenous microbiota. The organisms that caused plague, anthrax, tuberculosis, and cholera were capable of causing infection when introduced, even in small numbers, into healthy hosts. Control of infectious disease from highly contagious agents therefore depended on the isolation of patients to reduce person-to-person spread and the development of effective vaccines to selectively stimulate the patient's immune system. In contrast, the common infectious diseases found in hospitalized patients today are primarily the result of changes in host resistance factors and modification of the host's indigenous microbial flora.

Changes in the host's resistance to infection can occur under many conditions, including acute and chronic illness, nutritional deprivation, and acquired or congenital immunologic defects. Trauma, severe burns, irradiation for malignant disease, and the use of immunosuppressive or cytotoxic drugs can all cause changes in local and systemic defense mechanisms and predispose the patient to infection from microorganisms that might otherwise be considered nonpathogenic. Surgical infections result from the natural or iatrogenic inoculation of ambient flora into sites that are normally guarded by intact cutaneous or mucosal barriers.

Changes in the numbers and species of the host's indigenous microbiota can occur rapidly, along with the acquisition of new phage or serotypes of bacteria, which can replace less virulent strains. Under the pressure of antibiotic therapy, episomes that code for resistance to multiple antimicrobial agents can rapidly transfer between organisms of the same and differing species and even those of separate genera. It seems likely that other virulence factors may similarly be transferred between organisms, conferring certain advantages for invasion of, or attachment to, host epithelial cells and thereby augmenting their ability to cause infection. Because one lives in harmony with many indigenous microbiota, the concept of "non-pathogens" developed. We now know that with immunosuppression, variable amounts of necrosis associated with operation, the use of cytotoxic drugs, and possibly the acquisition of virulence factors, many of these "non-pathogens" develop the ability to invade the host and become "pathogens." For this reason, the terms "pathogen" and "non-pathogen" should be used with qualifying adjectives.

BACTERIAL NOMENCLATURE

One of the irritating problems facing the practicing surgeon is the continued reclassification and changing nomenclature of bacteria and other infectious agents. One such example is the organism that causes pneumococcal pneumonia. For many years, this organism was called *Diplococcus pneumoniae,* although taxonomists had known of similarities between the pneumococcus and members of the genus *Streptococcus.* In 1967, the name was changed from *Diplococcus pneumoniae* to *Streptococcus pneumoniae.* This change in nomenclature has caused confusion for generations of physicians who first learned the characteristics of the organism under its former name.

The reclassification and renaming of infectious agents usually follows information gained from determining metabolic characteristics, antibiotic susceptibility patterns, susceptibility to specific bacteriophages, deoxyribonucleic acid (DNA) relatedness, or computerized identification programs. The combined use of several of these methods has been called the polyphasic approach to taxonomy. Such programs are powerful aids in distinguishing among bacterial isolates that may vary only slightly from a typical pattern, and have provided a means for distinguishing among otherwise closely related and sometimes previously undescribed groups of bacteria. Examples of new and reclassified bacterial species in the Enterobacteriaceae are listed in Table 3-1. The previous species designations are given for comparison when applicable.

Often, the reasons for changing the names of microorganisms are not apparent and may not be relevant to the medical significance of the microorganism. To provide continuity in nomenclature during transition periods, it has been suggested that the new name be used with the

TABLE 3-1. CHANGES IN TAXONOMY AND NOMENCLATURE OF THE ENTEROBACTERIACEAE BY THE ENTERIC SECTION OF THE CENTER FOR DISEASE CONTROL IN 1977

New Designation	Previous Designation
Klebsiella oxytoca	*Klebsiella pneumoniae,* indole positive or indole positive and gelatin positive
Enterobacter sakazakii	*Enterobacter cloacae,* yellow pigment
E. gergoviae	
Hafnia alvei	*E. hafniae*
Citrobacter amalonaticus	*Citrobacter freundii,* malonate negative, H_2S negative, KCN negative, indole positive, adonitol positive; or *Levinea amalonatica*
Providencia stuartii, urea positive	*Proteus rettgeri,* Biogroup 5
P. stuartii, Biogroup 4	*Providencia alcalifaciens* Biogroup 4
P. rettgeri	*Proteus rettgeri,* Biogroups 1–4
Morganella morganii	*P. morganii*
Yersinia enterocolitica (typical)	*Y. enterocolitica*
Y. enterocolitica, sucrose negative	*Y. enterocolitica*
Y. enterocolitica, rhamnose positive	*Y. enterocolitica*
Y. enterocolitica, rhamnose and raffinose positive	*Y. enterocolitica*
Y. ruckeri	Red mouth bacterium

Adapted from Brenner DJ, Farmer JJ, Hickman FW, et al: *Taxonomic and Nomenclature Changes in Enterobacteriaceae.* HEW Publications No. (CDC) 78–8356. Atlanta, Center for Disease Control, 1978.

previous name in parenthesis, i.e., *Streptococcus (Diplococcus) pneumoniae* or *Acinetobacter calcoaceticus (Herellea vaginicola).* Although the reclassification of microbes can at times be confusing, we should all be able to recognize an old friend in new clothes.

One of the most obvious changes is in the taxonomy of the genus *Proteus* (Table 3-1). For many years, the tribe proteae in the family of Enterobacteriaceae consisted of *Proteus vulgaris, P. mirabilis, P. rettgeri,* and *P. morganii* and two species in the genus *Providencia, P. stuartii* and *P. alcalifaciens.* For the purpose of identification of most isolates, distinction between the members of the tribe proteae and other members of the Enterobacteriaceae was made by demonstrating the production of the enzyme phenylalanine deamidase by the organism. The members of the genus *Proteus* could be further separated from the *Providencia* by the presence of the enzyme urease. Recently, *P. rettgeri* has been found to be more closely related to the Providenciae than to the Proteae. Accordingly, it has been proposed that Biogroups 1 to 4 of this organism be called *P. rettgeri,* while Biogroup 5 has been reclassified as *P. stuartii,* urea-positive. Similarly, a more discriminating review of certain characteristics of *Proteus morganii* has shown this organism to have a significantly different content of guanidine plus cytosine than the remaining two species, and appears to be less related to the Proteae than to other bacteria in the Enterobacteriaceae such as *E. coli* and Salmonellae. It has therefore been proposed to make a completely new genus and species, *Morganella morganii,* to reflect this difference.

Table 3-2 lists the current names recommended for the members of the Enterobacteriaceae, a large group of gram-negative bacteria representing many of the most common organisms associated with infections in humans (Chapter 5, Tables 5-2, 5-3). Many of these organisms are members of our indigenous microbiota and are particularly important in infections that develop in hospitalized patients who commonly have some defect in host resistance factors or have factors predisposing to infection such as foreign bodies, eg, urinary or intravenous catheters.

TABLE 3-2. FAMILY ENTEROBACTERIACEAE*

Escherichia coli	*Enterobacter cloacae*
Shigella dysenteriae	*sakazakii*
flexneri	*aerogenes*
boydii	*gergoviae*
sonnei	*agglomerans*
Edwardsiella tarda	*Hafnia alvei*
Salmonella cholerasuis	*Serratia marcescens*
typhi	*liquefaciens*
enteritidis (2000 + varieties)	*rubidaea*
	Morganella morganii
Arizona hinshawii	*Proteus vulgaris*
Citrobacter freundii	*mirabilis*
diversus	*Providencia alcalifaciens*
amalonaticus	*stuartii,* Biogroup 4
Klebsiella pneumoniae	*stuartii,* urease positive
ozaenae	
rhinoscleromatis	*rettgeri*
oxytoca	

* See also Tables 5-2, 5-3

Modified from Edwards PR, Ewings WH: *Identification of Enterobacteriaceae,* 3rd ed. Minneapolis, Burgess, 1972, and Brenner DJ, Farmer JJ, Hickman FW, et al: *Taxonomic and Nomenclature Changes in Enterobacteraceae.* HEW Publication No. (CDC) 78-8356, Atlanta, Center for Disease Control, 1978.

TABLE 3-3. NONFERMENTATIVE GLUCOSE-OXIDIZING AND NONOXIDIZING BACTERIA

Glucose-oxidizing bacteria	Glucose-nonoxidizing bacteria
Pseudomonas aeruginosa	*Pseudomonas maltophilia*
cepacia	*denitrificans*
fluorescens	*diminuta*
pseudomallei	*alkaligenes*
stutzeri	*putrifaciens*
putida	*Alkaligenes faecalis*
vesicularae	*odorans*
Acinetobacter calcoaceticus	*denitrificans*
var. anitratus (Herellea vaginicola)	*Acinetobacter calcoaceticus var. lwoffi (Mima polymorpha)*
Flavobacterium meningosepticum species	
Moraxella kingii	

In addition to the members of Enterobacteriaceae, there is a large group of gram-negative bacteria that are occasionally associated with clinically significant infections. These organisms are distinguished from the Enterobacteriaceae by the inability to ferment glucose anaerobically. Many of these organisms are capable of utilizing glucose by oxidative enzymes, while others are unable to use carbohydrate at all. These organisms are frequently referred to in the laboratory by the terms glucose-oxidizing or glucose-nonoxidizing bacteria. The most significant organism in this group is *Pseudomonas aeruginosa,* but it also includes other species of the genera *Pseudomonas, Acinetobacter, Moraxella,* and *Flavobacter,* with organisms of the genus *Alkaligenes* seen less commonly. Representative, but not all, members of these two groups of organisms are listed in Table 3-3.

As clinical microbiology laboratories have become more sophisticated, increasing numbers of bacteria have been isolated from infections that are not easily identified. Many are found that do not fit existing taxonomic tables and are forwarded to reference laboratories, where similarities of metabolic and cultural characteristics and types of infection they cause are catalogued until the organism is given a name. Prior to that time, arbitrary designations are often used to refer to similar groups of organisms such as EF #1 (eugonic fermenter #1). Because many of these earlier designations have been used in publications prior to assigning a valid name to the organism, a series of such organsisms is listed in Table 3-4.

TABLE 3-4. PROVISIONAL AND APPROVED NAMES FOR UNCOMMON GRAM-NEGATIVE BACTERIA

CDC Letters and Numbers	Approved Names
EO-1	*Pseudomonas cepacia; Pseudomonas multivorans*
HB-1	*Eikenella corrodens*
HB-2	*Hemophilus aphrophilus*
HB-3 & 4	*Actinobacillus actinomycetemcomitans*
HB-5	None (Hemophilus-like)
M-1	*Moraxella kingii, Kingella kingae*
M-4	*M. urethralis*
I	*Pseudomonas maltophilia*
Ia	*P. diminuta*
Ib-1	*P. putrefaciens*
IIa	*Flavobacterium meningosepticum*
IIb	*Flavobacterium* species
IIc	None (saccharolytic flavobacterium)
IId	*Cardiobacterium hominis*
IIk-1	*Xanthomonas* species; *Pseudomonas paucimobilis*
IIk-2	*Xanthomonas* species
IIIa	*Achromobacter xylosoxidans*
IIIb	*A. xylosoxidans*
IVb	*Bordetella parapertussis*
Va-2	*Pseudomonas pickettii*
Vb-1	*P. stutzeri*
Vb-3	None
Vc	*Alcaligenes denitrificans*
Vd-1	*Achromobacter* species
Vd-2	*Achromobacter* species
Ve-1	*Chromobacterium typhiflavum*
Ve-2	*C. typhiflavum*
VI	*Alcaligenes faecalis*

STUDY OF THE INDIGENOUS MICROBIOTA

A knowledge of the indigenous microbiota in different locations of the body can be helpful in providing the clinician with a list of organisms that may be the cause of an infection that follows injury at one of these sites. It is also helpful in determining the source and significance of microorganisms isolated from unrelated sites of the body. For example, bacterial endocarditis from *Streptococcus faecalis* is more often associated with urinary tract infection in middle-aged males than with poor dental hygiene and tooth extraction. A knowledge of the indigenous microbiota is also helpful in determining the consequence of overgrowth of one microorganism by another. For example, *Candida* overgrowth within the gastrointestinal tract is frequent in patients given neomycin because neomycin effectively inhibits the bacteria of the family Enterobacteriaceae but has little effect on *Candida.* Similarly, clindamycin and other antimicrobial agents that suppress the intestinal bacteria select for the growth of *Clostridium difficile.* Uncontrolled proliferation of *C. difficile* can result in the elaboration of a potent enterotoxin that causes pseudomembranous enterocolitis.

INTERACTION AMONG DIFFERENT BACTERIAL SPECIES

The interaction among indigenous microbial organisms can serve two contrary functions. They can protect us from infection, and they can help determine the kind of infection that we develop. Unfortunately, relatively little is known of these complex relationships, but several examples illustrate the principle.

The microflora of the oropharynx are thought to perform an important protective function. Sanders[1] has shown that certain pharyngeal strains of alpha-hemolytic streptococci were capable of inhibiting the growth of *Staphylococcus aureus* and *Neisseria meningitidis.* In addition, only alpha-hemolytic streptococci, among organisms from several different genera, antagonized the growth of *Streptococcus pyogenes* (Lancefield group A) in vitro. Closer study showed this antagonism to be the result of more rapid use of growth metabolites by the alpha-hemolytic streptococci than *S. pyogenes.* Of interest was the observation that children not infected with Lancefield group A streptococci harbored alpha-hemolytic streptococci that were highly antagonistic to *S. pyogenes* in vitro and that the alpha-hemolytic streptococci from infected children lacked this property. Similarly, Johanson et al [2] have shown that 82 percent of pharyngeal cultures from normal individuals contain bacterial species (predominantly alpha-hemolytic streptococci) that will inhibit the growth of stock strains of pneumococci. Both of these studies suggest a protective effect by the alpha-hemolytic streptococci against colonization from organisms likely to be associated with clinical infection.

Another important interaction among bacteria is synergism between one or more organisms to cause infection. One example is a virulent, necrotizing infection of the mouth,[3] from which four separate bacteria can be cultured; *Bacteroides melaninogenicus,* a diphtheroid, and two other species of bacteroides. No one organism alone, or in combinations of two or three, will cause the infection in experimental animals. All four strains must be introduced at the same time for infection to occur. Although all the potential interactions between these organisms are not known, the diphtheroid secretes vitamin K, a growth factor needed by *B. melaninogenicus. B. melaninogenicus* in turn secretes proteolytic enzymes, which contribute to the extensive necrosis characteristic of this infection. The role of the other two organisms is not clear.

Indigenous microbiota can sometimes stimulate nonspecific immune responses, which provide protection from true pathogens. One example is the ability of pharyngeal *Neisseria lactamica* to stimulate protective antibodies to *N. meningitidis.*[4] This suggests that *N. lactamica* can stimulate cross-reacting, protective antibodies against certain capsular types of *N. meningitidis.* Cross-reactive bactericidal antibodies against *Haemophilus influenza* will also develop in experimental animals fed selected strains of *E. coli.* This fact has prompted a speculation that stimulation of cross-protective antibodies by this means may be more important in protecting young children from infection from *H. influenzae* than subclinical infection.[5,6]

Interactions among bacteria within the colon are complex and difficult to study. Many microorganisms can interfere with the function or proliferation of others by the production of bacteriocins, competition for nutrients, or the creation of unfriendly environments. An example is the inhibitory effect of volatile, short-chain, organic fatty acids produced by many anaerobic bacteria on the growth of *Salmonella typhimurium* as well as *Shigellae, Pseudomonas aeruginosa,* and *Klebsiella pneumoniae.*[7]

Intestinal motility also has a significant effect on the composition of the normal flora. Rapid peristalsis is of great value in maintaining low levels of indigenous flora in the small intestine. Obstruction in either the small or large intestine may result in bacterial overgrowth in the proximal segment. Similarly, intestinal bypass procedures for obesity can result in changes in the numbers and types of microorganisms at different levels in the intestine.[8]

INDIGENOUS MICROBIOTA BY ANATOMIC REGION

SKIN

The common members of the cutaneous microflora are listed in Table 3-5. Such a list does not take account of the fact that the indigenous microbiota of the skin will vary greatly, depending on different sites of the body and the characteristics of the skin at these sites. The anaerobic propionibacteria, for example, live preferentially in the lipid-secreting glands of the dermis of the face; most other species are found only on desquamating epithelial cells of the stratum corneum. Organisms that require living cells for hosts, like viruses, must invade cells of the basal epithelial layers where there is active cellular metabolism.

Because of their habitat deep in the sebaceous glands of the skin, the anaerobic, lipophilic bacteria, *Propionibacterium acnes* and species, are rarely affected by surface decontamination solutions. They can be found after 7 to 10 days of incubation as contaminants in blood and spinal fluid cultures or taken from deep sites where a transcutaneous needle puncture has been made to collect the specimen. Fortunately, this group of bacteria are seldom encountered in cutaneous wound infections.

The phenomenon of "bacterial interference" is well illustrated by skin microflora. This phenomenon depends on the attachment of one bacterial organism to an epithelial cell in preference to a second. The principle of bacterial interference was used prophylactically in the 1950s to prevent staphylococcal infections in newborn nurseries. In the early antibiotic era, it was noted that penicillin-resistant strains of *S. aureus* were associated with severe

TABLE 3-5. MICROORGANISMS FOUND IN THE SKIN

Microorganism	Range of Incidence (Percent)
Staphylococcus epidermidis (albus) (coagulase negative)	85–100
S. aureus (coagulase positive)	5–25
Streptococcus pyogenes (group A)	0–4
Clostridium perfringens (especially lower extremities)	2–60
Propionibacterium acne (anaerobic corynebacteria)	45–100
Anaerobic corynebacteria (diphtheroids)	55
Lactobacillus	55
Enterobacteriaceae	Uncommon
Acinetobacter calcoaceticus	25
Moraxella species	5–15
Mycobacteria	Uncommon
Candida albicans	Uncommon
Other *Candida* species, particularly *C. parapsilosis*	1–15
Dermatophytes (feet)	2–30

nursery infections of neonates. Prospective studies showed that colonization of the umbilical cord by virulent staphylococcal phage types could often be demonstrated prior to the onset of infection in the infant. In an attempt to reduce colonization by the virulent strain, and presumably avoid infection, a less virulent strain of the same species, *S. aureus*, strain 502A, was used to deliberately colonize the umbilical cord stump shortly after birth. This strain was considerably less virulent than organisms belonging to phage type 80/81 *S. aureus*, and in most infants it appeared to prevent colonization by the more virulent strains. The use of *S. aureus* 502A has been helpful in selected instances, although clinically significant infections from the 502A strain have also been reported.

Some important pathogens commonly found in skin are really transient residents, which contaminate the area around orifices. The best example is *S. aureus*, which is resident in the nostrils and perianal region but survives poorly elsewhere on the skin. *Clostridium perfringens* similarly, usually, contaminates only the perineum and thighs.[9] In this location, however, it can cause gas gangrene in as many as 1 percent of the patients undergoing above-knee amputations for diabetic vascular insufficiency. To control this threat, Drewett et al [9] have shown that iodophor compresses applied for 15 minutes before operation resulted in the failure to isolate the organism from 60 patients who had previously yielded *C. perfringens* on skin culture.

The skin of the normal host has a number of mechanisms to control overgrowth by bacterial species and prevent infection (Chapters 13 and 25). Sebaceous glands secrete complex lipids, which can be degraded by specific enzymes from certain gram-positive bacteria. Some of these lipids are changed to unsaturated fatty acids, which have a strong antimicrobial activity against many gram-negative bacteria and certain fungi. Among these lipids are unsaturated fatty acids, which are volatile and can be associated with a strong and offensive odor. To minimize these odors, deodorants were formulated that contained antibacterial substances directed against the gram-positive bacteria that split the lipids into the unsaturated acids. The use of antibacterial agents of this type can quickly result in a shift of the skin flora to a predominantly gram-negative population. Under these circumstances, the shift from a predominantly gram-positive to gram-negative bacterial population can result in an increased incidence of skin infections.[10]

NOSE AND NASOPHARYNX

Staphylococci, both *S. aureus* and *S. epidermidis*, compose the largest number of bacteria in the nasal passages (Table 3-6). In this location, the staphylococci are the most common indigenous microbiota and extend to the skin of the face, particularly at the nasal-labial fold. Most microorganisms known to be associated with significant infection in the nasopharynx are recovered primarily in the posterior portion of the nasal passages. It may be difficult to adequately sample the posterior nasal pharynx for culture without special swabs with fine tips of calcium alginate.

Diphtheroids are one of the frequently found group of organisms in the nasal passages. Diphtheroids are a large and poorly classified group of gram-positive bacilli, which are rarely associated with infection. These organisms are members of the genus *Corynebacteria* but, with the exception of *C. diphtheriae*, are rarely speciated.

TABLE 3-6. MICROORGANISMS FOUND IN THE NOSE AND NASOPHARYNX

Microorganism	Range of Incidence (Percent)
Staphylococcus aureus	20–85
S. epidermidis	90
Aerobic corynebacteria (diphtheroids)	5–80
Streptococcus pneumoniae	0–17
S. pyogenes (group A)	0.1–5
S. mitis	30–80
Alpha or nonhemolytic streptococci	30–70
Branhamella (Neisseria) *catarrhalis*	12–60
Haemophilus influenzae	12
H. parainfluenzae	35–65
Neisseria meningitidis	0–10
Enterobacteriaceae	20
Moraxella nonliquefaciens	5–10

Anaerobic bacteria frequently cause infection in the nasal sinuses, but systematic surveys to determine the incidence and species of different types of anaerobic bacteria in normal subjects have been difficult to obtain. For that reason, the normal anaerobic bacterial flora of the nasal passages, sinuses, and the nasopharynx is not well defined. Many of the anaerobic bacterial species found in the oropharynx and the upper respiratory passages are probably present within the nasal passages and the nasopharynx.

Although small numbers of *Streptococcus pneumoniae, Neisseria meningitidis,* and *Haemophilus influenzae* may be found in the nasopharynx, most are not encapsulated with the polysaccharides often associated with strains causing clinical infection. The significance of these organisms in the patient without infection is not clear, but most consultants agree that in the absence of classical virulence factors, such as specific polysaccharide capsules, no attempt should be made to eradicate such organisms by chemotherapy.

OROPHARYNX

The most important single group of microorganisms native to the oropharynx are the alpha-hemolytic streptococci (Table 3-7). For many years, these organisms have been called *S. viridans*, implying a single species. *S. viridans* is a general term, usually referring to several species of alpha-hemolytic streptococci. Perhaps a more appropriate term would be the viridans group of streptococci, which would include the species *S. mitis, S. milleri, S. sanguis, S. salivarius,* and several others. Although species identification of these organisms is routinely performed by dental microbiologists, there has not been the same need for identification of these organisms by medical microbiologists. With improved clinical laboratory capability and the need to identify the source of bacteria associated with subacute bacterial endocarditis, more laboratories are adopting procedures to speciate alpha-hemolytic streptococci.

TABLE 3-7. MICROORGANISMS FOUND IN THE OROPHARYNX

Microorganism	Incidence Range of (Percent)
Staphylococcus aureus	35–50
S. epidermidis	30–70
Streptococcus pyogenes (group A)	0–9
S. pneumoniae	0–50
Alpha and nonhemolytic streptococci	25–99
Lactobacilli	50–70
Aerobic corynebacteria (diphtheroids)	50–90
Branhamella (Neisseria) catarrhalis	10–97
Neisseria meningitidis	0–15
N. lactamica	0–20
Haemophilus influenzae	5–20
H. parainfluenzae	20–50
Gram-negative bacteria, eg, *Klebsiella pneumoniae*	18
Acinetobacter calcoaceticus	5–30
Anaerobic micrococci	Common
Anaerobic streptococci	Common
Bacteroides fragilis	Common
B. melaninogenicus	Common
B. oralis	Common
Fusobacterium necrophorum	Common
Campylobacter sputorum	5

Another large group of organisms native to the oropharynx are the gram-negative diplococci. One of the most common of these groups, *Branhamella* (Neisseria) *catarrhalis*, are small gram-negative cocci which are rarely the cause of serious infection, such as meningitis. As in the nasopharynx, small numbers of *N. meningitidis* can be found in the oropharynx. Similarly, *N. lactamica* can be recovered in 1 to 15 percent of children and adults and on rare occasions can cause meningitis.

The oropharynx contains large numbers of *S. aureus* and *S. epidermidis*. It should be emphasized that recovery of *S. aureus* from either a nose or a throat culture does not mean that the patient should be treated for staphylococcal infection. Previous concepts that the isolation of *S. aureus* from the throat indicated that the carrier was a threat to patients or attending medical personnel are now being reevaluated.

A few bacterial species are capable of causing acute pharyngitis, and Lancefield group A streptococci *(S. pyogenes)* and *N. gonorrhoeae* are clearly among them. Although *S. pneumoniae* and *H. influenzae* are occasionally recovered from patients complaining of acute pharyngitis, their contribution to the signs and symptoms of infection in these patients has not been established.

Anaerobic bacteria are present in large numbers in both the mouth and the oropharynx, particularly in patients with poor dental hygiene, caries, or periodontal disease. Anaerobic micrococci, streptococci, and *Veillonella* species can commonly be demonstrated on culture as well as species of *Bacteroides* and *Fusobacterium*. These organisms are a potential source of aspiration pneumonia in patients recovering from general anesthesia.

The normal oropharynx is seldom colonized by gram-negative Enterobacteriaceae. In contrast, hospitalized patients are heavily colonized. The exact reasons for this change in microflora is not known,[11-13] but the shift probably contributes to the high incidence of pneumonia caused by gram-negative bacteria in patients with severe illness.

THE MOUTH

The microbial flora of the mouth is dependent on the presence or absence of teeth, caries, or periodontal disease (Table 3-8). The recognition of selective colonization of certain streptococcal strains, *S. sanguis* and *S. mutans*, for tooth surface and *S. salivarius* for buccal and gingival epithelial surfaces have shown that highly specific factors are involved in bacterial attachment, colonization, and infection. These organisms in the presence of different types of food, particularly sucrose, can contribute to the formation of dental plaque and caries. Dental plaque, with large numbers of actively metabolizing bacteria, results in the production of a low oxidation-reduction potential (Eh) on the surface of, and in the crevices between, teeth. A reduced Eh permits the growth of anaerobic bacteria, such as *Bacteroides melaninogenicus*, *Veillonella*, and *Fusobacterium* species as well as many others. The presence of carious teeth with cavities usually results in a further increase of bacterial growth and decrease of the Eh. Therefore, uncontrolled dental caries predispose to the growth of large numbers of anaerobic bacteria and anaerobic oral treponemes. This group of patients is at special risk for incurring anaerobic pulmonary infections should they aspirate oropharyngeal secretions during or following general anesthesia. Removal of carious teeth significantly reduces the numbers of oral anaerobic bacteria and treponemes.

TABLE 3-8. MICROORGANISMS FOUND IN THE MOUTH (SALIVA, TOOTH SURFACES)

Microorganism	Range of Incidence (Percent)
Staphylococcus epidermidis (coagulase-negative)	75–100
S. aureus (coagulase-positive)	10–35
Anaerobic micrococci	100
Streptococcus mitis and other alpha-hemolytic streptococci	100
S. sanguis	100
S. salivarius	100
S. mutans	100
Enterococci	5–20
Peptostreptococci	Prominent
Veillonella alcalescens	100
Lactobacilli	95
Actinomyces israelii	Common
Enterobacteriaceae	65
Eikenella corrodens	0–5
Bacteroides fragilis	Common
B. melaninogenicus	Common
B. oralis	Common
Fusobacterium nucleatum	15–90
Mycobacteria	0–3
Candida albicans	6–50
Treponema denticola	Common
T. refringens	Common

TABLE 3-9. MICROORGANISMS FOUND IN THE STOMACH AND SMALL INTESTINE

Microorganism	Range of Incidence (Percent)
Stomach—usually sterile owing to gastric pH of 2–3	
Jejunum—gram-positive facultative bacteria (Enterococci, lactobacilli, diphtheroids) Strict anaerobic bacteria absent	Small numbers $<10^5$/ml
Ileum—distal portion may show small numbers of Enterobacteriaceae and increasing numbers of anaerobic gram-negative bacteria	
Candida albicans	40

STOMACH

The strongly acid pH of the normal stomach (2.0 to 3.0) plays a big part in reducing the microbial population in this organ (Table 3-9). Most bacteria die rapidly when exposed for even a short time to such a low pH, especially when the stomach is empty. The number of viable microorganisms that can be recovered from a stomach goes up with food ingestion. Food acts to buffer the low pH and increases the probability of more rapid transit through the stomach. Rapid gastric emptying results in a shorter exposure to an acid environment, and hence the total number of microorganisms that can be recovered from the stomach will drop with gastric emptying.

The microbial flora of the stomach can change rapidly with intestinal obstruction distal to the ampulla of Vater. This leads to an increase in the gastric pH following an influx of bile, pancreatic secretions, and alkaline duodenal and jejunal fluid into the stomach. Under these conditions, the bacterial content of the stomach begins to mirror the microbial flora of the oropharynx and will include both gram-negative aerobic and anaerobic bacteria (Table 3-9). Relatively few organisms withstand passage through the normal empty stomach, but several, including *M. tuberculosis* and several other mycobacterial species as well as some strains of *Candida albicans*, can survive short periods in the highly acid environment.

SMALL INTESTINE AND BILIARY TRACT

The upper portion of the small intestine contains few microorganisms because of the combined influence of a strongly acid environment in the stomach and the inhibitory action of bile on many microorganisms. Gram-positive cocci and bacilli make up most of the bacterial population in the upper jejunum, with *S. faecalis*, lactobacilli, and diphtheroids representing the types of organisms that best withstand the inhibitory characteristics of both bile and pancreatic secretions.

The indigenous microbiota of the biliary tract are not known; however, in the few patients without biliary disease who have been studied, the bile was sterile. It is likely that a number of different bacteria may be found in the bile ducts and gallbladder as the result of transphincteric reflux or of occasional invasion of the portal blood system from the intestinal tract and excretion by the liver. The antibacterial activity of bile tends to limit the types of bacteria that could survive. Examples of organisms that can tolerate increased concentrations of bile salts include the *Salmonella* species, especially *S. typhi, Streptococcus faecalis, C. perfringens*, and *Bacteroides fragilis*.[14,15] Conversely, susceptibility of pneumococci to the surface active action of bile makes infection from these organisms uncommon in the hepatobiliary tract.

C. albicans can be recovered by culture from the distal portion of the small intestine in 40 percent of healthy people. Although colonization with *C. albicans* is not a problem for the normal person, patients on immunosuppressive therapy or those with lymphomas or leukemias that involve lymphoid tissue in Peyer patches of the distal ileum are at special risk of developing either local or disseminated candidiasis. Antitumor chemotherapy can result in necrosis of the involved submucosal lymphoid tissue, providing a portal of entry for *Candida* in the ileum. Because many of these patients also have defects in their humoral and cellular immune systems, they are at high risk for candidemia and disseminated *Candida* infection.

Occasionally, the administration of antibiotics to patients in preparation for intestinal surgery results in the overgrowth of large numbers of yeast. This can result from suppression of the facultatively anaerobic Enterobacteriaceae with a source of neomycin-resistant *Candida* emptying from the small intestine into the colon.

In the distal portion of the small intestine, the indigenous flora begin to take on the characteristics of the colonic flora. Increasing numbers of anaerobic bacteria appear, along with Enterobacteriaceae and enterococci. Modification of the normal small intestinal motility pattern or anatomic relationships following surgical procedures for obstruction or intestinal bypass can result in bacterial overgrowth producing a number of clinical syndromes.[8,16]

LARGE INTESTINE

The colon contains the largest concentration of microorganisms in the body (Table 3-10). As much as 60 percent of the dry weight of the stool is bacterial mass. The anaerobic gram-negative non-spore-forming bacteria comprise the vast majority of the 10^{11} to 10^{12} organisms per gram that may be present. The ratio of anaerobic bacteria to the facultative bacteria varies from 300:1 to 1000:1. Although it was previously believed that the majority of the bacteria in the colon were members of the Enterobacteriaceae or related species, studies for the quantitative recovery and identification of the indigenous flora have indicated that less than 0.3 percent of all colonic bacteria belong to this family.[17]

Recently, there has been renewed interest in determining the number and identification of the bacteria present in the stool. This has followed the suggestion that changes in the indigenous flora of the colon may be one explanation for the wide variations in incidence of carcinoma of the colon among people in different countries[18,19] (Table 3-10). The validity of the methods used for isolation

TABLE 3-10. RELATIVE FREQUENCY OF BACTERIAL SPECIES IN FECAL FLORA

Rank	Percent	Organism(s)
1	12	*Bacteroides vulgatus*
2	7	*Fusobacterium prausnitzii*
3	6.5	*Bacteroides adolescentia*
4	6	*Eubacterium aerofaciens*
5	6	*Peptococcus productus II*
6	4.5	*Bacteroides thetaiotaomicron*
7	3.6	*Eubacterium eligens*
8	3.3	*Peptococcus productus I*
9	3.2	*Eubacterium biforme*
10	2.5	*E. aerofaciens III*
11	2.3	*Bacteroides distasonis*
28	0.7	*B. ovatus*
29	0.6	*B. fragilis*
59–75	0.13	*Streptococcus faecalis*
76–113	0.06	*Escherichia coli, Klebsiella pneumoniae,* and 37 other bacterial species

Adapted from Moore WEC, Holdeman LV. *Appl Microbiol* 27:916, 1974.

was established in part by determining counts of bacterial cells from dilutions of the stool and comparing these with the number of viable colony-forming units recovered by culture. Using this technique, 93 percent of the bacteria estimated to be present in the stool by direct Gram stain were recovered by culture.

More than 113 separate species of microorganisms were found in the stool specimens in this study, each representing at least 0.05 percent of the flora in the colon. Of the first ten most common species ranked, only *Bacteroides thetaiotaomicron* is seen with any frequency in cultures from patients with clinical anaerobic bacterial infections. By far the most common *Bacteroides* species that can be recovered from patients with clinical infection is *B. fragilis,* which makes up only 0.6 percent of all organisms in the stool.[17] *Streptococcus faecalis* is more common than the members of the Enterobacteriaceae, making up 0.13 percent of all fecal bacteria.

A review of the organisms isolated from patients with clinical infections from anaerobic bacteria at Northwestern Memorial Hospital in Chicago shows that *B. fragilis* is associated with a much higher incidence than might be expected when compared to its rank frequency in the colon (Table 3-11). Conversely, *B. vulgaris,* the organism ranked first in order of frequency of isolation, was recovered from patients with clinical infection in much smaller numbers. This discrepancy emphasizes the differences in virulence factors between species. Although not all the virulence factors associated with *B. fragilis* are known, it has a polysaccharide capsule, which provides protection from phagocytosis. Similarly, the frequency of recovery of *E. coli* and *Klebsiella pneumoniae* from postoperative or traumatic abdominal wounds occurs more often than their incidence in the stool would suggest. This indicates that these organisms also possess important virulence factors, which provide for a distinct pathogenic advantage over normal host defense mechanisms.

It is generally agreed that the source of *C. perfringens* on the skin and in the biliary tract results from organisms present in the colon. This organism, as well as other members of *Clostridia,* are available for growth and production of toxic enzymes whenever trauma or surgery involves the contents of the colon with a decrease in the local Eh. Similarly, the presence of *C. perfringens* within the biliary tract without evidence of gas-producing infection suggests the possibility that the organism is readily available but causes disease only under certain circumstances.[14,15] Table

TABLE 3-11. ANAEROBIC BACTERIAL ISOLATES, NORTHWESTERN MEMORIAL HOSPITAL

	Rank Frequency	Source of Isolates						
		Blood	*Blood Culture—Autopsy*	*G-I*	*TTA* PULM*	*G-U*	*Wounds*	*Abscess*
Bacteroides vulgatus	1	4	5	1	2	1	7	7
B. thetaiotaomicron	6	3	2	4	1	1	6	6
B. distasonis	11–12	1	0	2	0	2	6	2
B. ovatus	25–28	1	1	0	0	0	5	1
B. fragilis	29	28	4	9	3	3	32	13
B. melaninogenicus		0	0	1	3	3	10	21
Bacteroides species †		14	6	15	21	15	72	37
Fusobacterium nucleatum	113	0	0	5	2	1	5	8
Fusobacterium species		1	4	3	1	2	9	10
Clostridium perfringens	113	9	14	9	0	4	14	2
C. ramosum	50–58	2	2	0	0	0	4	3
Bifidobacterium adolescentis	3	0	2	0	2	5	1	2
Eubacterium species ‡		2	2	3	6	2	11	2
Peptococcus magnus	50–58	9	0	2	0	10	32	9
Peptostreptococcus species		8	3	3	2	15	24	20
Propionobacterium acnes	50–58	10	4	2	12	1	15	1

* Transtracheal aspiration

† To include *Bacteroides oralis, ruminicola ss brevis,* and *clostridiformis ss clostridiformis, capillosis, corrodens,* and *amylophilus.*

‡ Not further speciated.

TABLE 3-12. MICROORGANISMS FOUND IN THE LARGE INTESTINE

Microorganism	Range of Incidence (Percent)
Anaerobic bacteria—300 times as many anaerobic bacteria as facultative aerobic bacteria (eg, Enterobacteriaceae)	
Gram-negative bacilli *(non-spore-forming)*	100
Bacteroides distasonis	100
B. fragilis	100
B. melaninogenicus (3 subspecies)	100
B. oralis (2 subspecies)	100
B. thetaiotaomicron	100
B. vulgatus	100
Fusobacterium nucleatum	100
F. necrophorum	100
Gram-positive bacilli (with and without spores)	
Lactobacilli	20–60
Clostridium perfringens	25–35
C. difficile	1–4
C. innocuum	5–25
C. ramosum	5–25
C. septicum	30–70
C. tetani	30–70
Eubacterium limosum	30–70
Bifidobacterium bifidum	30–70
Gram-positive cocci	
Peptostreptococcus (anaerobic streptococci)	Common
Peptococcus (anaerobic staphylococci)	Moderate
Facultative aerobic and anaerobic bacteria	
Gram-positive cocci	
Staphylococcus aureus (associated with nasal carriage)	30–50
Enterococci (group D streptococcus)	100
Streptococcus pyogenes (groups B, C, E and G)	0–16
Escherichia coli	100
Shigella—groups A–D	0–1
Salmonella enteritidis (2200 serotypes)	3–7
S. typhi	0.0001
Klebsiella species	40–90
Enterobacter species	40–90
Proteus mirabilis and *vulgaris, Morganella morganii,* and *Providencia* species	5–55
Pseudomonas aeruginosa	3–11
Candida albicans	15–30

3-12 lists many of the more common microorganisms that can be isolated from the large intestine.

The recovery of certain species of bacteria from blood cultures can be associated with a previously inapparent, ulcerating malignant lesion of the colon. Examples include *C. septicum*[20] and *Streptococcus bovis,* a member of the Lancefield group D streptococci. With *S. bovis,* the patient may have subacute endocarditis, but a carcinoma of the colon is present in many cases.[21,22] The incidence of *S. bovis* in the colon is not clearly established, as most previous studies have not distinguished between *S. faecalis* and *S. bovis* but have considered both under the more general heading of enterococci.

GENITOURINARY TRACT

Normally the kidneys, ureters, and urinary bladder do not have an indigenous microbiota. In both the male and female, small numbers of organisms may be present in the distal portion of the urethra. The number of bacteria near the bladder sphincter is usually negligible.

In a woman, the vagina can have a complex microbial flora (Table 3-13). In the newborn infant, lactobacilli colonize the vagina shortly after birth, following the influence of the mother's hormonal stimulation. As the influence of maternal hormones wanes, lactobacilli (Döderlein's bacilli) are replaced with gram-positive cocci. With menarche and cyclic hormonal stimulation, the glycogen content of squamous epithelium again increases and is correlated with the return of lactobacilli. Lactobacilli metabolize glycogen, producing lactic acid, which in turn contributes to a low vaginal pH of 4.5 to 5.5 in the normal human adult female. The low pH will select for certain microorganisms, such as *C. albicans* and anaerobic bacteria, while inhibiting the growth of more fastidious bacteria, including the growth of certain Enterobacteriaceae.

Like the microbial flora of the oropharynx and colon, the vagina has many organisms that can interact with one another and influence their growth. One of the organisms associated with infection in the vagina is *N. gonorrhoeae.* Several groups of investigators[23,24] have shown an inhibi-

TABLE 3-13. MICROORGANISMS FOUND IN THE GENITOURINARY TRACT

Microorganism	Range of Incidence (Percent)
Kidney and urinary bladder normally sterile. Female and male urethra usually sterile except for short anterior segment	
Vagina and Uterine cervix	
Lactobacilli	70–80
Bacteroides species	60–80
Fusobacterium species	10–20
Clostridium species	15–30
C. perfringens	0–10
Peptostreptococcus	30–75
Bifidobacterium species	10–75
Eubacterium species	5–10
Actinomyces species	25–60
Aerobic corynebacteria (diphtheroids)	45–75
Staphylococcus aureus	5–15
S. epidermidis	35–80
Enterococci (group D Streptococcus)	30–80
Streptococcus pyogenes (usually group B, also C, F and G)	5–20
Streptococcus species (not group D)	20–50
Enterobacteriaceae	18–40
Haemophilus (Corynebacterium) vaginalis	10–40
Moraxella osloensis	5–15
Acinetobacter species	5–15
Candida albicans	30–50
Torulopsis glabrata	1–10
Trichomonas vaginalis	6–10
Mycoplasma species	15–20

tory relationship between lactobacilli and *N. gonorrhoeae*, where it was found that lactobacilli secreted substances that prevented the growth of *N. gonorrhoeae*. The lactobacilli secreting inhibitory substances were recovered less frequently from women infected with *N. gonorrhoeae* than from uninfected women. Similarly, among women having contact with an infected sexual partner, those subsequently developing gonorrhea were less likely to have inhibitory lactobacilli than those who did not become infected. Of interest was the observation that the recovery of inhibitory lactobacilli was highest during the 2 weeks following the onset of the menses, when the recovery of *N. gonorrhoeae* from infected patients was lowest. These observations suggest that a protective effect against infection from *N. gonorrhoeae* is present from certain strains of the indigenous lactobacilli and may be related to changes associated with the menstrual cycle.

Cyclic hormonal fluctuation may influence the microbial flora by several means. Progesterone tends to increase the content of glycogen in the epithelial cells and thereby increase the amount of carbohydrate available for microbial growth. More glycogen availability can also be associated with increased numbers of *C. albicans*. Use of the first birth control pills containing large amounts of progesterone was often associated with an increase in vaginal candidiasis, presumably by increasing vaginal epithelial glycogen.

The large numbers of both gram-positive and gram-negative anaerobic and facultative bacteria in the vagina and in the region of the endocervical os represent a potential threat of infection at the time of either spontaneous or induced abortion. The presence of small fragments of necrotic tissue in the endometrium or the vagina can offer a substrate for growth of clostridia, which can be ideal for toxin secretion.

BIBLIOGRAPHY

Rosebury T: Microorganisms Indigenous to Man. New York, McGraw-Hill, 1962.

Savage DC: Survival on mucosal epithelia, epithelial penetration and growth in tissues of pathogenic bacteria. In Smith H, Pearce JH (eds): Microbial Pathogenicity in Man and Animals (22nd Symposium of the Society for General Microbiology). New York, Cambridge Univ. Press, 1972, p 25.

Skinner FA, Carr JG (eds): The Normal Microbial Flora of Man. New York, Academic, 1974.

Youmans GP, Paterson PY, Sommers HM: The Biologic and Clinical Basis of Infectious Diseases. Philadelphia, Saunders, 1980.

REFERENCES

1. Sanders E: Bacterial interference. I. Its occurrence among the respiratory tract flora and characterization of inhibition of group A streptococci and viridans streptococci. J Infect Dis 120:698, 1969.
2. Johanson WG Jr, Blackstock R, Pierce AK, Sanford JP: The role of bacterial antagonism in pneumococcal colonization of the human pharynx. J Lab Clin Med 75:946, 1970.
3. Socransky SS, Gibbons RJ: Required role of *Bacteroides melaninogenicus* in mixed anaerobic infections. J Infect Dis 115:247, 1965.
4. Gold R, Goldschneider I, Lepow ML, Draper TF, Randolph M: Carriage of *Neisseria lactamica* in infants and children. J Infect Dis 137:112, 1978.
5. Myerowitz RL, Handzel ZT, Schneerson R, Robbins JB: Induction of *Haemophilus influenzae* type b capsular antibody in neonatal rabbits by gastrointestinal colonization with cross-reacting *Escherichia coli*. Infect Immun 7:137, 1973.
6. Robbins JB, Schneerson R, Argaman M, Handzel ZT: *Haemophilus influenzae* type b: disease and immunity in humans. Ann Intern Med 78:259, 1973.
7. Levison ME: Effect of colon flora and short-chain fatty acids on growth in vitro of *Pseudomonas aeruginosa* and Enterobacteriaceae. Infect Immun 8:30, 1973.
8. Corrodi P, Wideman PA, Sutter VL, Drenick EJ, Passaro E Jr, Finegold SM: Bacterial flora of the small bowel before and after bypass procedure for morbid obesity. J Infect Dis 137:1, 1978.
9. Drewett SE, Tuke W, Payne DJ, Verdon PE: Skin distribution of *Clostridium welchii:* use of iodophor as sporicidal agent. Lancet 1:1172, 1972.
10. Marples RR: Effects of soaps, germicides and disinfectants on the skin flora. In Skinner FA, Carr JG (eds): The Normal Microbial Flora of Man. New York, Academic, 1974, p 35.
11. Johanson WG, Pierce AK, Sanford JP: Changing pharyngeal bacterial flora of hospitalized patients. Emergence of gram-negative bacilli. N Engl J Med 281:1137, 1969.
12. Valenti WM, Trudell RG, Bentley DW: Factors predisposing to oropharyngeal colonization with gram-negative bacilli in the aged. N Engl J Med 298:1108, 1978.
13. Johanson WG Jr, Woods DE, Chauduri T: Association of respiratory tract colonization with adherence of gram-negative bacilli to epithelial cells. J Infect Dis 139:667, 1979.
14. England DM, Rosenblatt JE: Anaerobes in human biliary tracts. J Clin Microbiol 6:494, 1977.
15. Campbell ES, Kelly AG: Acute emphysematous cholecystitis due to *Clostridium perfringens*. Ala J Med Sci 15:234, 1978.
16. King CE, Toskes PP: Small intestine bacterial overgrowth. Gastroenterology 76:1035, 1979.
17. Moore WE, Holdeman LV: Human fecal flora: the normal flora of 20 Japanese-Hawaiians. Appl Microbiol 27:961, 1974.
18. Hill MJ, Drasar BS, Hawksworth G, Aries V, Crowther JS, Williams REO: Bacteria and aetiology of cancer of large bowel. Lancet 1:95, 1971.
19. Howell MA: Diet as an etiological factor in the development of cancers of the colon and rectum. J Chron Dis 28:67, 1975.
20. Alpern RJ, Dowell VR Jr: Nonhistotoxic clostridial bacteremia. Am J Clin Pathol 55:717, 1971.
21. Klein RS, Recco RA, Catalano MT, Edberg SC, Casey JI, Steigbigel NH: Association of *Streptococcus bovis* with carcinoma of the colon. N Engl J Med 297:800, 1977.
22. Brooks RJ, Ravreby WD, Keusch G, Bottone E: More on *Streptococcus bovis* endocarditis and bowel carcinoma. N Engl J Med 298:572, 1978.
23. Saigh JH, Sanders CC, Sanders WE Jr: Inhibition of *Neisseria gonorrhoeae* by aerobic and facultatively anaerobic components of the endocervical flora: evidence for a protective effect against infection. Infect Immun 19:704, 1978.
24. Kraus SJ, Geller RC, Perkins GH, Rhoden DL: Interference by *Neisseria gonorrhoeae* growth by other bacterial species. J Clin Microbiol 4:288, 1976.

CHAPTER 4
The Pyogenic Cocci

PHILLIP K. PETERSON

Therefore it is certain that the air, water, and earth are filled with innumerable small animals; and furthermore that they can be demonstrated.
Athanasius Kircher (1602–80)

ATHANASIUS KIRCHER was probably the first investigator to use the microscope in the study of disease and the first to espouse the theory that contagious disease was spread by animaliculae (small living animals invisible to the naked eye). Nearly two centuries after Kircher's death, Billroth and Ehrlich applied the term *Streptococcus* to a chain-forming coccus they saw in infected wounds. Within a year (1877), Koch observed staphylococci in pus, and in 1879 Neisser saw the gonococcus in pus cells of patients with gonorrhea. Thus, the bacterial etiology of suppuration, a process recognized since antiquity, was established.

Over the past century, the legacy of these great men has resulted in an explosive growth of knowledge about the pathogenesis of infections caused by these pyogenic cocci. A great deal has been learned about mechanisms of bacterial virulence and host defense and about the basis of the inflammatory process. The purpose of this chapter is to outline the pathogenesis of infections caused by these microbes, so that some feeling for the dynamic nature of investigation in this area will emerge.

STAPHYLOCOCCI

IDENTIFICATION AND CLASSIFICATION

The genus *Staphylococcus* is comprised of facultatively anaerobic gram-positive cocci, which ferment glucose, produce catalase, and tend to form irregular grape-like clusters. Staphylococci are members of the family Micrococcaceae, the other genus of this family being Micrococcus. Unlike staphylococci, micrococci are usually strict aerobes and do not ferment glucose. A variety of biochemical tests can be used to identify a number of staphylococcal species. The most widely recognized staphylococcal species are *Staphylococcus aureus, S. epidermidis,* and *S. saprophyticus. S. aureus* is the best characterized and also clearly the most pathogenic of these species.

S. aureus strains usually produce golden or pale yellow colonies on solid media, hence the name of the species and its distinction from the white colonies of *S. albus* (now called *S. epidermidis*). Pigment production is an unstable characteristic; some *S. aureus* strains produce only white colonies. *S. aureus* is more consistently, and most practically, identified by its production of coagulase.[1] Many laboratories define *S. aureus* as a coagulase-positive staphylococcus, whereas coagulase-negative staphylococci are referred to as *S. epidermidis*. However, there are rare strains of *S. aureus* that are coagulase-negative, and some laboratories define *S. aureus* as staphylococci that produce deoxyribonuclease (DNase), a characteristic that also correlates highly with this species. Unfortunately, a number of coagulase-negative, DNase-positive staphylococci belong to species other than *S. aureus*.[2] There is no totally acceptable, practical solution to the classification of staphylococci. Although both coagulase-negative staphylococci and micrococci can cause human disease under certain circumstances, the coagulase-positive staphylococci *(S. aureus)* are unquestionably the most pathogenic.

PATHOGENESIS

Source of Infection

The natural habitat of staphylococci is the body surface of many species of mammals and birds. Staphylococci are also found in the air and dust of occupied buildings and in milk, food, and sewage.[1] *S. aureus* is a commensal bacterium found on moist areas of skin and in the anterior nares of up to 40 percent of healthy persons.[3] *S. epidermidis* is an ubiquitous member of the flora of the skin and mucous membranes. Carriers of *S. aureus* can serve as a reservoir of this microorganism, and the skin often provides a vehicle for spread of staphylococci from person to person. The hospital environment is particularly favorable for transmission of *S. aureus* because of the intimate care of patients. Organisms can be transferred from patient to patient by the hands of attendants, and airborne transmission of staphylococci can be facilitated by improper room ventilation, as well as by the clothing of nurses and physicians.[4]

In addition, the use of antibiotics by those who are staphylococcal carriers can enhance the spread of antibiotic-resistant organisms.[5]

S. aureus is the most common pathogen isolated from operative wound infections.[6] In some surgical units, 10 percent of operative wounds are infected with staphylococci.[3] Such patients are a serious source for nosocomial staphylococcal infection, and some means of isolation should be practiced.

Intact skin and mucous membranes provide an effective barrier to staphylococci. When these barriers are breached, however, *S. aureus* is endowed with a number of characteristics that favor its survival within the invaded host. Given the frequency with which this barrier is violated and the environment that facilitates transmission of staphylococci within hospitals, it is not surprising that *S. aureus* is one of the most common causes of nosocomial infections. *S. epidermidis* infection is largely a product of modern medical and surgical technology. Although this staphylococcal species is not as pathogenic as *S. aureus*, it is particularly well suited for a tenacious existence in the presence of foreign bodies such as prosthetic heart valves and ventricular-atrial shunts.

Bacterial Factors

Although *S. aureus* is one of the principal bacterial pathogens that causes human infections, experimental infections can be produced only when high numbers of the bacteria are used. In a series of classic experiments, Elek [7] and Elek and Conen [8] demonstrated that it required a minimum of 7.5×10^6 cocci to produce a pustule when bacteria were injected intradermally, subcutaneously, or in full thickness wounds of volunteers. No differences were found in the virulence of strains obtained from clinical lesions, from healthy carriers, and from epidemic sources. When organisms were introduced by skin sutures left in situ, 500 times fewer bacteria produced severe local abscesses. In one volunteer, a suture containing only 100 cocci caused suppuration. To date, the mechanisms by which foreign bodies enhance pathogenicity remain largely unexplained.

Over the past several decades, an appreciation has been gained of the great diversity of staphylococcal pathogenicity factors.[9] A number of these factors are possessed by some *S. aureus* strains and not by others, and thus some strains are more virulent. It has also become clear that there is no single important staphylococcal virulence factor, but rather there is an array of mechanisms by which these bacteria can both evade host defenses and injure the host. Virulence factors of *S. aureus* can be divided into three general categories: (1) bacterial cell surface components, (2) extracellular products, and (3) genotypic and phenotypic variability (Fig. 4-1).

Bacterial Cell Surface Components

The cell wall of most *S. aureus* strains is composed of three major constituents—peptidoglycan, teichoic acid, and protein A. The peptidoglycan (mucopeptide) is a polysaccharide with extensively cross-linked peptide side chains (Fig. 2-5). Attached to the carboxyl group of each N-acetylmuramic acid is a short peptide, which is usually cross-linked by a pentaglycine bridge to a neighboring peptide unit. About 50 percent of the weight of the cell wall is contributed by peptidoglycan, which provides rigidity.[10] Cell wall teichoic acids, comprising about 40 percent of cell wall weight, are charged polymers of ribitol-phosphate with *N*-acetyl-D-glucosamine and D-alanine substituents. Protein A, contributing about 5 percent of the cell wall weight, is covalently linked to the peptidoglycan component.

Many strains of *S. aureus* possess a cell wall peptidoglycan which has been associated with pathogenicity.[11] When injected intradermally in animals, this cell wall "aggressin" inhibits edema production and migration of leukocytes, thus allowing bacteria to multiply and to produce necropurulent lesions. *S. aureus* peptidoglycan also possesses endotoxin-like properties,[12] and can activate both the classical and alternative pathways of the serum complement system, and elicit a cell-mediated immune response.

A role in the pathogenesis of *S. aureus* infections has not been defined for teichoic acid, although it appears that this cell wall component may contribute to complement activation.[13] Therefore, along with protein A and peptidoglycan, teichoic acid may contribute to the formation of pus, which is a major manifestation of staphylococcal infection. The teichoic acids are largely responsible for the serologic specificity of staphylococci, and high titers of antibodies have been found in patients with serious or deep-seated staphylococcal infections.[14] Testing for the development of teichoic acid antibodies may be of diagnostic value in certain clinical settings.

Protein A is present in the cell walls of virtually all *S. aureus* strains, and is found in only a small percentage

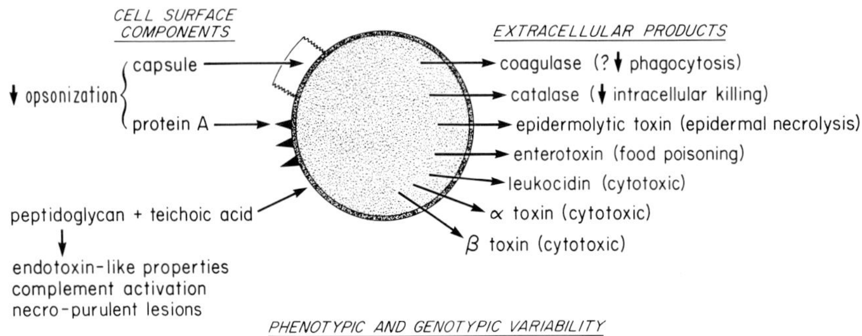

Fig. 4-1. **Virulence factors of *S. aureus* and their proposed biologic effects.**

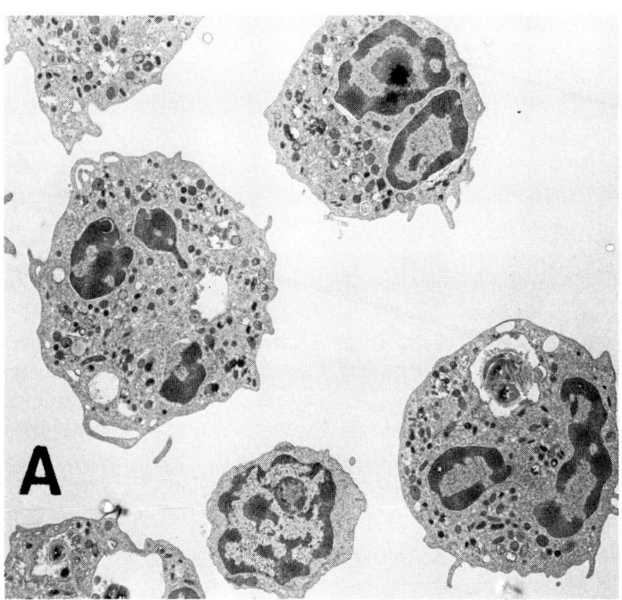

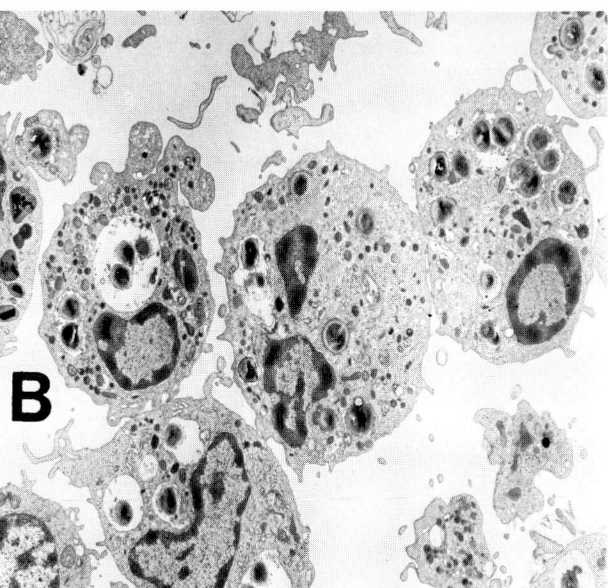

Fig. 4-2. Electronmicrograph of human polymorphonuclear leukocytes incubated with equal concentrations of (A) an encapsulated *S. aureus* strain, and (B) an unencapsulated variant. Bacteria were incubated in normal human serum before being added to the leukocytes. Note the paucity of ingested encapsulated bacteria in comparison to the unencapsulated organisms.

of *S. epidermidis* strains. In 1966, Forsgren and Sjöquist [15] reported that protein A reacted nonspecifically with the Fc fragment of immunoglobulin G (IgG) rather than with the Fab combining site, which would be the case in classical antigen-antibody reactions. This phenomenon was called a pseudoimmune reaction. Sjöquist and Stalenheim [16] demonstrated that protein A possessed anticomplementary properties as a result of the formation of protein A–IgG complexes, and that these complexes could activate both classical and alternative complement pathways. Although in vitro evidence suggests that both cell wall-associated and isolated protein A can interfere with opsonization of staphylococci,[17] and that this protein can thereby be regarded as being "antiphagocytic," there is no in vivo evidence of its function as a virulence factor.

The cell surface of some *S. aureus* strains contains a fourth component, a polysaccharide capsule. Although encapsulated *S. aureus* strains are rarely encountered in vitro, evidence suggests that they may be common in vivo. There is both in vitro and in vivo evidence to indicate that the capsule *can* serve as a significant virulence factor. Encapsulated staphylococci have been shown to "resist phagocytosis" in nonimmunized animals, a phenomenon that appears to be related to inhibition of opsonization of these strains by the serum complement system (Fig. 4-2).[18]

Extracellular Products

Many *S. aureus* strains produce a large number of extracellular, enzymatically active factors that are believed to be important in the pathogenesis of staphylococcal disease. The enzyme coagulase is used to differentiate the more pathogenic coagulase-positive staphylococcal species. Although early investigators suggested that coagulase protected staphylococci from phagocytosis, this concept has been disputed.[19] Recent studies have shown that coagulase-negative, DNase-positive variants of *S. aureus* are significantly less virulent than are related coagulase-positive, DNase-negative variants.[20] The mechanism by which coagulase acts as a virulence factor was not elucidated.

Mandell [21] has proposed that another staphylococcal enzyme, catalase, may protect bacteria from the lethal effects of hydrogen peroxide that is produced by phagocytic cells, and that catalase may thereby function as a virulence factor. This observation may in part explain the previously recognized ability of some staphylococci to survive within phagocytic cells.

About one-third of the clinical isolates of *S. aureus* produce a toxin capable of causing staphylococcal food poisoning,[22] which is characterized by vomiting and diarrhea 1 to 6 hours after ingestion of this enterotoxin. It is believed that enterotoxins enter the circulation in an unchanged state via the digestive tract and that their activity is mediated via the central nervous system.

Epidermolytic toxin can cause a variety of skin lesions, the most characteristic of which are the diffuse exfoliative bullae seen in children with staphylococcal scalded skin syndrome. Only certain staphylococcal strains (phage group II) are capable of producing this toxin, whose mode of action has been delineated. Although relatively uncommon in older patients, this disease has been reported with increasing frequency in adults with compromised immune defenses.[23]

Recently, Todd and Fishaut [24] have reported a clinical syndrome characterized by fever, conjuctival hyperemia, hypotension, renal failure, liver injury, and generalized erythroderma, which they postulate is caused by a distinct toxin (exfoliatin B) produced by phage group I staphylococci. In their series, this syndrome was seen primarily in older children. Another newly recognized staphylococcal toxic-shock syndrome, seen almost exclusively in menstruating women who use tampons,[24a,24b] shares many similarities to the syndrome described by Todd and Fishaut. This syndrome may be caused by a pyrogenic exotoxin produced by certain *S. aureus* strains (P. Schlievert, personal communication) that colonize the women at risk of this disease. The toxic shock syndrome, with a mortality of about 10 percent, is being seen in nearly epidemic proportions in Minnesota, Wisconsin, and Utah. It is speculated that a new toxic-producing strain of *S. aureus* has gained a foothold in these states. It should be pointed out that males can develop this syndrome, and that a few cases have been associated with skin infection.

Other extracellular products of *S. aureus* that appear to play a role in pathogenicity include the cytotoxic factors, leucocidin and alpha- and beta-hemolysins.[25]

Genotypic and Phenotypic Variability

Given the right environmental conditions, *S. aureus* is capable of changing its genotypic and phenotypic characteristics, and this adaptability can contribute to pathogenicity. The development of antibiotic resistance is an important example of staphylococcal adaptability. Genotypic changes occur through the processes of mutation, transformation, and transduction (a phenomenon by which extrachromosomal genetic material, such as a plasmid, is transported to a new bacterial cell by a bacteriophage). When a mutation occurs or the bacterial genotype changes by the acceptance of a plasmid, growth under the prevailing conditions of the host may be enhanced. For example, an enzyme may be produced which inactivates a therapeutic agent, or a change in antigenic structure may occur which allows the mutant to escape the host's existing immunologic defenses.

Staphylococci also have variable phenotypic characteristics. Park et al [26] have commented on the hidden potential of *S. aureus* to produce additional surface polysaccharides under certain environmental conditions. When cultured in hypertonic media or in the presence of cell wall inhibiting drugs such as penicillin, staphylococci may grow as L-forms, ie, small protoplasmic bodies without cell walls.[27] Although it has been suggested that the L-forms may function in the bacterial persistence that occurs during antibiotic therapy and may be responsible for relapse after therapy, the clinical importance of L-forms is unknown.

Many pathogenetic factors are not understood. Unlike many other bacterial species which appear to have a preference for only certain tissues (tropism), *S. aureus* has the capacity to establish infection and survive in a variety of sites including, as an important example, normal heart valves. Little is known about the factors that promote staphylococcal attachment or adherence to cells or about the factors that facilitate its long-term survival in certain areas, such as bone.

Host Factors

Host response to staphylococcal infections is characterized by an extraordinary interplay of factors which, on the one hand, are involved in defense against the bacterial cell and, on the other, contribute to many of the signs and symptoms of staphylococcal disease. Over the past several decades, the basis of host defense, the genesis of the inflammatory process, and the factors contributing to abscess formation have become more completely understood (Chapter 13). These concepts will be discussed as they relate to the host's immune response to *S. aureus* (Fig. 4-3).

The major means of defense of the invaded host against staphylococci is provided by phagocytic cells, including both wandering polymorphonuclear leukocytes and the mononuclear phagocyte system. Patients with quantitative or qualitative defects of these cells are predisposed to recurrent and severe staphylococcal diseases.[9] The invading staphylococci invoke the egress of phagocytic cells from the bone marrow, a process that appears to be mediated via various leukopoietic factors, perhaps monocyte products and certain components of the activated complement system.[28] Diapedesis of phagocytic cells from the vascular space and directed movement of these cells toward bacteria (leukotaxis) appear to depend on normal cell motility and on activation of serum complement with an attendant gradient of activated complement factors (probably involving at least C5a). A number of bacterial cell wall and extracellular products appear to be responsible for the generation of chemotactic factors. Patients with defective leukotactic responsiveness and deficiencies of certain components of the complement system have difficulty with recurrent *S. aureus* infections.[29]

An effective interaction of phagocytes with bacterial cells depends on the ability of the phagocyte to recognize its prey. In the case of *S. aureus*, this process of recognition is mediated by bacterial opsonization (the interaction of certain components of the complement system and of immunoglobulins with the bacterial cell surface that facilitates phagocytosis). The peptidoglycan component of the staphylococcal cell wall appears to initiate the process of opsonization.[30] Phagocytic cells function as though they possess receptors for an activated form of the third component of complement (C3b) and for the Fc portion of IgG.[31] Although antibodies are probably active in host defense against staphylococci, they are also capable of producing immune complexes that can result in certain complications of staphylococcal disease, such as immune complex glomerulonephritis.

Phagocytosis or ingestion of staphylococci is followed rapidly by intracellular killing, a process that depends at least in part on the generation of active oxygen radicals. The best defined, and probably most common, primary intracellular killing defect is found in patients with chronic granulomatous disease, a disease characterized by frequent and severe *S. aureus* infections, including abscesses of the skin, lungs, liver, lymph nodes, and bones. Phagocytic cells from these patients are unable to kill intracellular staphylococci, an abnormality related to the inability of these cells to mount a respiratory burst after ingesting staphylococci, presumably caused by a defect in the enzyme NADPH.[32]

Although T lymphocytes and macrophages are undoubtedly involved in host response to *S. aureus*, the exact role of cell-mediated immunity in host defense against staphylococci and the nature of the involvement of cell-mediated immunity in tissue damage are not clearly established.

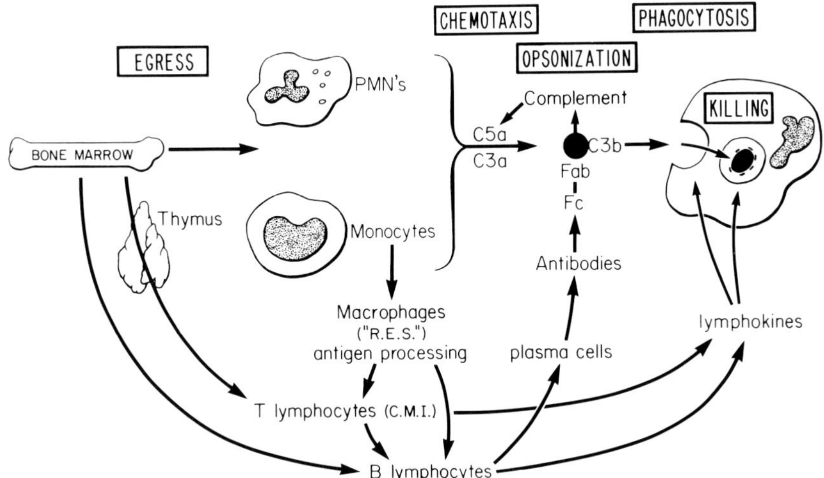

Fig. 4-3. **The immune response to *S. aureus.***

CLINICAL MANIFESTATION AND THERAPEUTIC CONSIDERATIONS

As discussed, the clinical manifestations of staphylococcal disease are largely the combined result of bacterial toxicity and host response to this organism. Specific disease entities involving staphylococci and their treatment are dealt with in subsequent chapters, so selected clinical problems will be mentioned here briefly. A review of staphylococcal diseases has been provided by Musher and McKenzie.[33]

As soon as *S. aureus* gains access to the circulation, the potential for serious disease is present, even in the host with normal immune defense mechanisms. *S. aureus* bacteremia is therefore regarded as a serious clinical problem because of its well-recognized pathogenicity, as witnessed by its ability to establish infection on normal heart valves and to localize in other deep foci, including bone, kidney, and brain. Although a primary skin focus is often implicated, the source of infection is sometimes obscure. There is recent, controversial evidence that *S. aureus* bacteremia that arises from a removable focus, such as an infected intravenous line, may not be as portentous as once considered.[34] Many authorities continue to recommend 4 to 6 weeks of parenteral antistaphylococcal therapy for all cases of *S. aureus* bacteremia. Monitoring a patient for the development of antistaphylococcal antibodies may help predict which patients are more likely to have deep-seated infection and would therefore benefit from such long-term therapy.[35]

In contrast to *S. aureus*, the isolation of coagulase-negative staphylococci from a blood culture usually signifies contamination of the culture from the skin. When multiple blood culture results are positive, however, infective endocarditis, an infected foreign body, or immunologic compromise must be considered. Because of the ubiquity of coagulase-negative staphylococci, their isolation from any site may indicate contamination; these organisms can also cause suppurative [36] and lower urinary tract infections.

An important aspect of the management of most staphylococcal abscesses is incision and drainage. For some infections, such as cutaneous abscesses or wound infections that are not recurrent or severe, or associated with systemic symptoms, incision and drainage is sufficient treatment and antibiotic therapy is not required. Abscesses that involve internal organs generally necessitate operative drainage, although occasionally antibiotic therapy alone can be curative. Foreign bodies or necrotic tissue must generally be removed or debrided for effective eradication of infection. Generally, because of the widespread emergence of penicillin resistance among staphylococci, a penicillinase-resistant antibiotic must be used. When parenteral therapy is indicated, drugs such as nafcillin or oxacillin can be used. Recent reports suggest that methicillin may be associated with a greater incidence of nephrotoxicity than either of these other semisynthetic penicillins. The dosage and duration of therapy, neither of which have been clearly established for any of the staphylococcal diseases, are generally decided by considerations related to the nature and severity of the disease being treated. A cephalosporin can be used in the penicillin-allergic patient who does not have a history of an immediate or accelerated type of hypersensitivity. Vancomycin also seems effective and is probably the best drug for methicillin-resistant staphylococcal strains. Although there are in vitro and animal studies indicating aminoglycosides may provide a synergistic effect when used in combination with penicillinase-resistant penicillins, the benefit of combination therapy has not been established in humans.

STREPTOCOCCI

IDENTIFICATION AND CLASSIFICATION

Bacteria belonging to the genus *Streptococcus* are gram-positive ovoid or spherical cells arranged in chains or pairs. Streptococci are nonsporing, usually nonmotile, and fail to reduce nitrate. They ferment cabohydrates with the production of acid, but never gas. Unlike staphylococci, streptococci are catalase-negative. Streptococci are similar to staphylococci in that they are facultatively anaerobic. The strictly anaerobic chain-forming cocci (anaerobic streptococci) differ so greatly in their metabolic characteristics from the streptococci that they are excluded from the genus *Streptococcus*, and therefore will not be discussed in this chapter. Although not of major surgical significance, the pneumococci are recognized as a separate and well-defined streptococcal species.

Three major characteristics are used for the classification of the streptococci; (1) changes induced by colonies of bacteria grown on sheep blood agar (β-hemolysis, ie, complete destruction of erythrocytes; α-hemolysis, ie, zones of greenish discoloration containing intact red cells; "γ-hemolysis," no hemolysis in the surrounding culture medium); (2) serologic reactions (Lancefield classification); and (3) biochemical and physiologic characteristics such as the production of specific enzymes and the ability to grow in the presence of various chemical substances. On the basis of these characteristics, many of the streptococci can be identified at a species level (Table 4-1). Although this method of classification is somewhat cumbersome, it is clinically relevant. When provided such information about a streptococcal isolate, the clinician (1) may have a better appreciation of the most likely source of infection, (2) may anticipate specific complications, eg, endocarditis, rheumatic fever, or suppurative foci, and (3) may make significant therapeutic decisions regarding choice of antibiotic and operative intervention. Some of the tests used to identify the streptococcal species that are the most pathogenic in man are listed in Table 4-1.

In 1933 Lancefield described a method for classifying β-hemolytic streptococci. She used a precipitin reaction and antigens extracted from these bacteria. Originally, five antigenic groups were identified (A, B, C, D, and E); there are now 19 groups (A through H and K through T). The Lancefield serologic classification is based on a heat- and acid-stable carbohydrate antigen located in the cell walls of organisms of all groups except groups D and N (which are identified on the basis of a lipoteichoic acid moiety). Although a number of clinical isolates are nongroupable,[37] serologic classification remains a valuable method.

Group A streptococci, the most common streptococcal pathogens of man, constitute a single species (*S. pyogenes*). Almost all group A streptococci are β-hemolytic and are extremely susceptible to bacitracin—two features that are commonly used in the presumptive identification of this species. The limitations of these and of other methods used in the classification of the streptococci have been reviewed by Facklam.[38] Group A streptococci can be subclassified according to their cell wall protein antigens (M and T). More than 60 M types are recognized.

Group B streptococci also comprise only one species, *S. agalactiae*. Group B streptococci are almost always β-hemolytic, and virtually all produce hippuricase, an enzyme that hydrolyzes hippuric acid. Most of the other β-hemolytic streptococci do not produce this enzyme; however, some strains of enterococci hydrolyze hippuric

TABLE 4-1. GENERAL CHARACTERISTICS OF STREPTOCOCCUS SPECIES COMMONLY PATHOGENIC FOR MAN

Species	Serologic Group	Hemolysis	Identifying Features	Common Infections	MICs, of Benzyl Penicillin (μg/ml) *
S. pyogenes	A	β †	Bacitracin susceptibility †	Skin, wound, respiratory tract (nonsuppurative complications)	0.005
S. agalactiae	B	β †	Hippurate hydrolysis, CAMP test	Neonatal meningitis, bacteremia, genitourinary tract	0.05
Enterococci *S. faecalis* *S. faecium* *S. durans*	D	α, β, γ	Bile-esculin hydrolysis, salt tolerant	Endocarditis, intra-abdominal and intrapelvic, urinary tract	2
Nonenterococci S. bovis S. equinus	D	α, β, γ	Bile-esculin hydrolysis, not salt tolerant	Endocarditis	0.06
Viridans streptococci *S. mutans* *S. mitior* *S. salivarius* *S. sanguis* *S. milleri*		α, γ		Endocarditis Abscesses	0.012
S. pneumoniae		α †	Bile solubility, optochin susceptibility	Pneumonia, otitis media, meningitis	0.01

* Concentrations given are approximate estimates of mean minimal inhibitory concentrations (MICs) taken from many sources.
† An occasional exception.

acid. Most enterococci are not β-hemolytic. The CAMP test is frequently used in the identification of group B streptococci.[38] Typing within the B group is based upon envelope carbohydrate rather than protein antigens, as in group A. Currently, there are five recognized serotypes of group B streptococci (Ia, Ib, Ic, II, III).

There are five streptococcal species within group D (Table 4-1). Three species, *S. faecalis*, *S. faecium*, and *S. durans*, are collectively referred to as enterococci. The two nonenterococcal species, *S. bovis* and *S. equinus*, share the group D antigen and also, like the enterococci, give a positive bile-esculin reaction. Tolerance to 6.5 percent NaCl broth is a major characteristic of the enterococci, a feature used in distinguishing them from the nonenterococcal species. The separation of these two groups is of major clinical significance, as the enterococci are much less susceptible to penicillin, and important therapeutic considerations are based on the identification of this group when endocarditis is diagnosed.

The viridans streptococci can also be classified into five different species (Table 4-1). All species are non-β-hemolytic and also by definition are not non-β-hemolytic members of group A, B, D, and N. Although many viridans streptococci cannot be grouped by the Lancefield classification, there are strains that do react with antisera to groups H, K, and O. These species of streptococci do not grow in broth containing 6.5 percent NaCl and do not give a positive bile-esculin reaction. Parker and Ball [39] have provided a detailed discussion of other tests used in classification of the viridans streptococci.

S. pneumoniae is an easily distinguishable α-hemolytic streptococcal species that might be considered as belonging to the viridans group, which shares a number of immunologic cross-reactions.[40] Pneumococci have a characteristic lanceolate morphology and are arranged in pairs or chains. Solubility in bile and susceptibility to optochin are two tests commonly used in the clinical laboratory to distinguish this species (Table 4-1). The pneumococci possess one of a series of antigenically specific capsular polysaccharides. Using antisera to these polysaccharides, 82 pneumococcal types can be identified; however, 14 types cause about 80 percent of all serious infections.[41] Polysaccharides from these 14 types are included as antigens in the current pneumococcal vaccine. When pneumococci react with homologous anticapsular serum, a capsular precipitin reaction (quellung reaction) occurs, and the capsule appears refractile under the microscope. The use of an omniserum containing antibodies to all 82 pneumococcal types can be used in identifying pneumococci. The quellung reaction produced by this omniserum may prove to be superior to a Gram stain in the rapid identification of this species in some clinical specimens.

PATHOGENESIS

Source of Infection

Group A streptococci that cause soft tissue infections are spread by direct contact of an injured area with the organisms in the environment; pharyngitis is spread by large airborne droplets. The spread of group A streptococci that causes pyoderma and impetigo is enhanced by crowding and poor hygiene. A recent study of an epidemic of operative wound infections caused by group A streptococci was traced to a nurse with streptococcal cellulitis of the finger, but later cases appeared to be caused by airborne or droplet spread of organisms from the vagina of the same nurse. Skin or wound infections and the respiratory tract are the most frequent sources for group A streptococcal bacteremia.[37]

The epidemiology of group B streptococcal infections indicates that the female genital tract is the primary reservoir of these organisms; the frequency of carriage has been variously reported from less than 5 to 25 percent.[42] The acquisition rate of group B streptococci is high in infants born of colonized mothers, but the risk of clinical disease is low. The portal of entry of group B streptococci that causes neonatal meningitis or bacteremia, respiratory distress, and pneumonia probably involves multiple body orifices. Group B streptococci can also be isolated from rectal swabs and from urethral cultures of asymptomatic males and females—these sites also may be important reservoirs.

Group D streptococci (enterococci) are normal residents of the bowel and vagina. Endogenous infection from one of these sites appears to be the major source of a diverse group of clinical diseases, including nosocomial enterococcal urinary tract infection, intra-abdominal or intrapelvic infection, bacteremia, and endocarditis. In surgical practice, they are most often found in mixed infections in wounds or intraperitoneal sepsis.

The viridans streptococci are found as part of the normal flora of many of the body's surfaces, including the mouth and bowel. They are the most prominent inhabitants of the oral cavity, an important portal of entry for infections such as endocarditis and brain abscess. The bowel may be an important source of *S. milleri*, occasionally found in intra-abdominal abscesses.[43]

Pneumococci colonize the upper respiratory tract in from 30 to 60 percent of healthy people. Recent epidemiologic evidence indicates that person-to-person spread of these organisms may be facilitated by viral infection of the upper respiratory tract. The portal of entry for many pneumococcal infections is presumably this site. Overwhelming pneumococcal infection is the principal late septic complication after splenectomy and is the principal cause of primary peritonitis in children.

Bacterial Factors of Group A Streptococci

Group A streptococci are the most pathogenic and most thoroughly studied of the streptococcal groups. This is the only streptococcal species associated with suppurative and nonsuppurative complications, ie, acute rheumatic fever and poststreptococcal glomerulonephritis. As was pointed out for *S. aureus*, both bacterial cell surface components and extracellular products play a role in pathogenesis (Table 4-2). Wannamaker [42] has reviewed these bacterial factors in detail.

Bacterial Cell Surface Components (Group A Streptococci)

The cell surface of the group A streptococcus is currently regarded as a mosaic network comprised of four major

TABLE 4-2. VIRULENCE FACTORS OF GROUP A STREPTOCOCCI

Bacterial Factors	Biologic Effects
Cell surface components	
M protein	Antiphagocytic (decreased opsonization)
Hyaluronic capsule	Antiphagocytic
Peptidoglycan	Endotoxin-like properties, necropurulent lesions
Lipoteichoic acid	Attachment to epithelial cells
Extracellular products	
Streptolysins O and S	Cytotoxic
Proteinase	Cytotoxic
Hyaluronidase, streptokinase	Promote spread of infection
Pyrogenic exotoxins	Endotoxin-like properties

constituents—hyaluronic acid, Lancefield group-specific carbohydrate, peptidoglycan, and surface proteins (M, T, and R antigens). Although there is evidence that the hyaluronic acid capsule is antiphagocytic, its role in pathogenicity in human infections is not established. The group-specific carbohydrate is a polysaccharide polymer of N-acetyl-D-glucosamine and L-rhamnose. This polymer has antigenic components that cross-react with glycoprotein from human cardiac valves, but its role in the pathogenesis of rheumatic carditis is unknown.

The M protein of group A streptococci, which is located in hairlike structures of fimbriae on the cell surface (Fig. 4-4), is a major virulence factor for this group of organisms.[44] Group A variant strains lacking M protein rarely cause human disease because they are readily phagocytized by human leukocytes. The exact mechanism by which M protein interferes with phagocytosis is unclear. Recent evidence, however, suggests that it may do so by inhibiting bacterial opsonization by masking the cell surface components that are responsible for activation of the alternative complement pathway.[45] Type-specific, anti-M protein antibodies are essential for promoting efficient phagocytosis of M protein-positive strains. The T and R proteins are not important for virulence and do not stimulate protective antibodies.

The peptidoglycan component of the streptococcal cell wall has a structure and significance similar to the staphylococcal peptidoglycan. It gives the cells its shape and rigidity, and it shares antigens. Such sharing may be involved in natural immunity to gram-positive bacteria. Streptococcal peptidoglycan, like staphylococcal peptidoglycan, produces fever and a local Schwartzman reaction in rabbits. Peptidoglycan also produces dermal necrosis with infiltration of polymorphonuclear leukocytes and can activate the alternative pathway of complement.[46] Thus, this cell wall constituent shares a number of characteristics of the endotoxins of gram-negative bacteria.

The initiation of infection in the upper respiratory tract requires that group A streptococci possess a mechanism for adhering to mucosal cells of the pharynx and tonsils. Adherence to epithelial cells appears to be a property of lipoteichoic acid, which is located in the surface fimbriae of group A streptococci along with M proteins.[47]

Extracellular Products (Group A Streptococci)

Group A streptococci release a large array of toxins and enzymes, some of which have been implicated in pathogenesis. Two distinct hemolysins, O and S, are produced by group A streptococci. Streptolysin S is responsible for the β-hemolysis that surrounds colonies on the surface of blood agar; subsurface hemolysis is caused by oxygen-labile, streptolysin O. Streptolysin O, a potent cardiotoxin,[48] can act on any sterol-containing membrane, including the cell membranes of polymorphonuclear leukocytes and platelets and of mammalian mitochondria. Measurement of antibodies to this hemolysin have been useful as a diagnostic test in recent group A streptococcal infection. Because streptolysin S, which also has leukotoxic properties, is nonantigenic, it has been suggested that it might be active during repeated streptococcal infections and in recurrences of rheumatic fever.[49] Streptococcal proteinase may be responsible for tissue invasion or tissue damage.

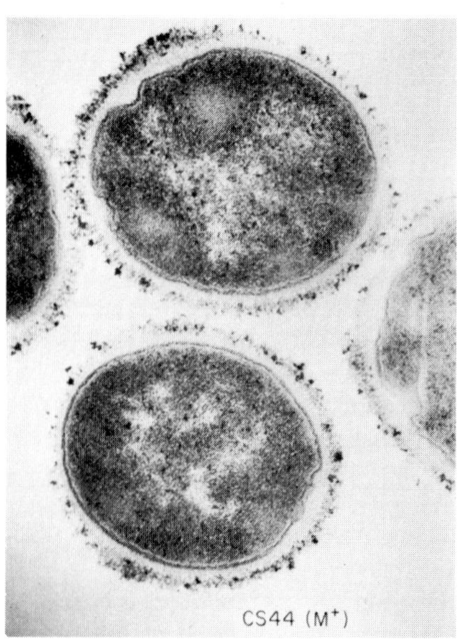

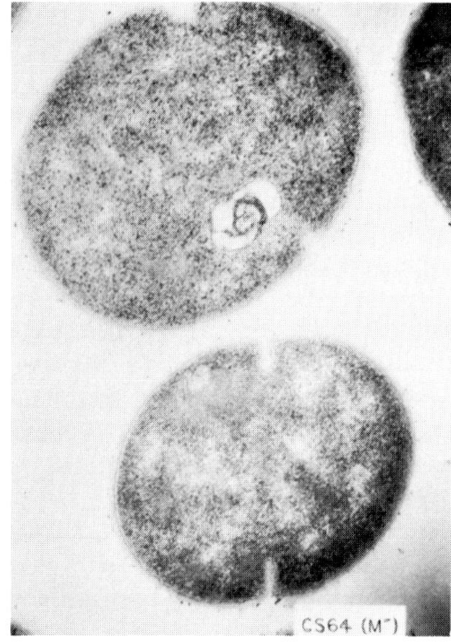

Fig. 4-4. **Electronmicrographs of an M protein-positive group A streptococcal strain, CS44 (M⁺), and an M protein-negative variant of this strain, CS64 (M⁻). The hairlike structures seen on the surface of CS44 contain M protein, a major streptococcal virulence factor. (Photomicrographs courtesy of P. P. Cleary)**

Pyrogenic exotoxins (erythrogenic toxins) and the enzymes hyaluronidase and streptokinase may all promote spread of infection. The pyrogenic exotoxins were originally thought to have only erythrogenic activity (scarlet fever); however, it is now clear that these toxins can produce fever and share many of the properties of endotoxin from gram-negative bacteria.[50]

Bacterial Factors in Other Streptococci

Bacterial factors involved in the pathogenicity of streptococcal infections caused by species other than group A are not as clearly understood. Although the factors responsible for virulence in group B streptococci are largely unknown, immunologic studies suggest that virulence may be related to the capsular antigen. Sialic acid, a major constituent of the polysaccharide capsules of group B streptococci, has been considered a possible virulence factor for invasion of neonatal meninges. The presence of sialic acid in all serotypes, however, does not explain the propensity of type III organisms for invasion of this site.[51] The function of extracellular products of group B streptococci in pathogenesis is obscure.[42]

The major virulence factor of *S. pneumoniae* appears to be its capsular polysaccharide. The antiphagocytic property of this cell surface component may be similar to that of the capsular polysaccharide found in some staphylococcal strains. This polysaccharide appears to mask cell wall peptidoglycan from the opsonic activity of certain serum factors, in particular the complement system.[52] Type-specific anticapsular antibodies promote phagocytosis of these organisms and are, in general, protective against serious infection—hence the renewed interest in capsular antigen vaccines for susceptible individuals.

A major factor involved in the pathogenesis of the most serious infection caused by both the viridans streptococci and by group D organisms, ie, endocarditis, is adherence of these organisms to damaged or abnormal heart valves. It is possible that glucan, a dextran frequently produced by endocarditis-associated species of streptococci, may contribute to the stickiness of these bacteria and may thus play a role in the initiation of this infection.[39,53] The ecologic or pathogenetic role of these organisms in mixed infections is unknown.

Host Factors

Mechanisms of host response to, and defense against, streptococci are in many respects similar to those seen with staphylococci (Fig. 4-2). An intact integument and mucous membrane barrier are of primary importance in defense against streptococci. Breaks in these barriers are essential for tissue invasion and the bacteremia seen with many of the streptococcal species. Purulent infections of the tonsils and pharynx by group A streptococci can occur without local trauma.

Many streptococci have a predilection for special hosts.[42] The majority of group B streptococcal infections occur in neonates or mothers in the postpartum period. In other adults, group B infections appear to be largely opportunistic, occurring with a high frequency in diabetics and in patients with underlying malignancy.[54] Another example of special host requirements for some streptococcal infections is the finding that the pharyngeal cells of patients with rheumatic heart disease have an increased avidity for adherence of rheumatic fever–associated group A streptococci, a phenomenon that may be important in the pathogenesis of rheumatic fever.[55] Group A streptococci can also behave as opportunistic organisms in immunologically compromised hosts, such as patients with leukemia, solid tumors, collagen-vascular diseases, and burns.[42] In patients with burns who have received skin grafts, infections with group A streptococci can lead to graft rejection. An important host factor to consider, when dealing with bacteremia or endocarditis caused by *S. bovis*, is the association of these problems with occult carcinoma of the colon.[56]

The factors responsible for the production of pus in streptococcal lesions are not clearly established. Increased chemotactic responsiveness of circulating polymorphonuclear leukocytes has been demonstrated in streptococcal skin infections.[57] Multiple cell wall and secretory products of streptococci can activate the serum complement system.[58] Presumably, a significant concentration of factors such as C5a and C3a is formed at the site of infection, and leukocytes may then follow a gradient of these factors into the site of infection. Although there is evidence that some streptococcal strains can be phagocytized without opsonization (surface phagocytosis), it appears that both antibodies [44] and the complement system [45] are necessary for effective opsonization and phagocytosis of most streptococci. Patients with quantitative defects of either immunoglobulins or certain complement components [29] have frequent streptococcal infections. For those strains with surface polymers that interfere with the process of opsonization, such as the encapsulated pneumococci and M protein–positive group A streptococci, type-specific antibodies appear to be essential for both effective phagocytosis and protection against serious sequelae of infection.

During infection, numerous antibodies also develop to a variety of extracellular bacterial products (enzymes and toxins). These antibodies may be active in neutralizing the potentially tissue-damaging effects of these products. Measurement of antibody levels to streptolysin O (ASO titer) and to DNase B is of diagnostic value. Anti-DNase B antibodies are more consistently elevated than are ASO antibodies in patients with streptococcal skin infection and glomerulonephritis.[59]

Streptococci are rapidly killed after being phagocytized. Because these organisms are catalase-negative they do not survive within phagocytes, even within phagocytes from patients with chronic granulomatous disease. After phagocytosis, endogenous pyrogen may be produced and released by phagocytic cells; pyrogens capable of acting on the central nervous system appear to be at least one mechanism responsible for the fever in streptococcal infection. After phagocytosis, group A streptococcal cell walls persist in macrophages and these cells can become cytotoxic. The persistence of indigestible residues of group A streptococci in mononuclear phagocytes may result in chronic release of acid hydrolases which lead to inflammation and tissue damage.[60]

The spleen has an especially important function in host defense against overwhelming pneumococcal infection. The reasons for the prominent role of the spleen in host defense against this streptococcal infection are not entirely clear. After splenectomy, certain humoral factors are reduced,[61] and the passive filtering effect of the spleen for encapsulated organisms is lost.

Cell-mediated immunity also appears to be involved in host defense against, and response to, certain streptococcal infections.[42]

As has already been mentioned, group A streptococci are the only members of the *Streptococcus* genus to be associated with nonsuppurative complications, namely, glomerulonephritis and acute rheumatic fever. The evidence indicates that poststreptococcal glomerulonephritis (which can be seen after both skin and pharyngeal infections) is a manifestation of an immune complex disease. The pathogenesis of rheumatic fever (which occurs only after pharyngeal infection) is unknown, although there are a number of attractive hypotheses, including cross-reacting antibodies and a cell-mediated immune response.[42]

CLINICAL MANIFESTATIONS AND THERAPEUTIC CONSIDERATIONS

Group A streptococci remain the most common cause of human streptococcal infections. These organisms can cause infections of almost any organ system, although infections of the skin, subcutaneous tissues and pharynx are by far the most frequently affected.[62] The pyogenic potential of these organisms is perhaps best demonstrated by the striking propensity for empyema formation after group A pneumonia. For unknown reasons, the nonsuppurative complications of group A streptococcal infection have become relatively uncommon in industrialized countries,[63] and in recent years group B streptococcal infections have become more common. In some hospitals, group B streptococci are now the principal streptococcal pathogens, especially in neonates (bacteremia, meningitis, acute respiratory distress) and postpartum patients. Group B infections have rarely received comment in the surgical literature.

Infections caused by group D streptococci are particularly important in hospitalized patients, a fact that is largely related to their existence as part of the normal flora of the genitourinary and gastrointestinal tracts. The insertion of instruments in the genitourinary tract can lead to urinary tract infection, bacteremia, and endocarditis. Perforation of the gastrointestinal tract or infection of the pelvic organs is a common association with the development of intra-abdominal or intrapelvic infection caused by a mixed bacterial flora, including group D streptococci. Operative intervention is usually mandatory. As has already been pointed out, the distinction between enterococcal and nonenterococcal group D species is important in guiding antibiotic therapy. Of all the streptococcal species, the enterococci are routinely resistant to penicillin (Table 4-1), so ampicillin is generally substituted. When enterococci are the cause of endocarditis, gentamicin should be added to the regimen because of its therapeutic synergy. Vancomycin should be used in the penicillin-allergic patient.

The viridans streptococci remain the most common cause of infective endocarditis. Although not generally regarded as pyogenic, recent investigations have shown that one species, *S. milleri*, is highly pyogenic, being found in abscesses in many sites such as the liver and brain.[43] The isolation of *S. milleri* from a blood culture should alert the physician to look for such a complication. This is one reason for the proposal that clinical microbiology laboratories should routinely speciate the viridans streptococci.

Penicillin is still the best drug for group A streptococcal infections. Fortunately, resistance to penicillin has not appeared among group A streptococci, although resistance to erythromycin and lincomycin may be increasing. Cephalosporins can be used as an alternative in patients with a history of penicillin allergy that is not of the immediate type. The dose and duration of antibiotic therapy are determined by the site (cephalothin and cefazolin should not be used for central nervous system infections) and severity of infection. Although penicillin is also the best drug for pneumococcal infections, the recent emergence of resistant strains in some countries is a cause of concern.[64] Penicillin, or an appropriate alternative drug, should also be used prophylactically in patients at high risk for rheumatic fever recurrences, infective endocarditis (congenital heart disease, valvular heart disease, and prosthetic grafts and valves), and overwhelming pneumococcal infection (anytime after splenectomy). Immunization with the newly released pneumococcal vaccine appears to be warranted in all patients who are functionally asplenic or who have undergone splenectomy.[65] Even vaccination will not prevent all pneumococcal sepsis in asplenic patients, and long term chemoprophylaxis may be necessary.

NEISSERIAE

IDENTIFICATION AND CLASSIFICATION

Although other members of this group of microorganisms can cause human disease, *Neisseria gonorrhoeae* and *N. meningitidis* are clearly the most pathogenic species for people. These bacteria are gram-negative spherical or ovoid cocci found in pairs with flattened adjacent sides. They do not produce spores, are nonmotile, and are strict aerobes. *Neisseriae* produce indophenol oxidase, and although not specific for this group, a positive oxidase reaction is used in the process of identification. Gonococci and meningococci are relatively fragile organisms with fastidious nutritional and growth requirements. This characteristic necessitates special care in the transport of clinical specimens, special culture media (chocolate agar or Thayer Martin medium), and the presence of carbon dioxide and humidity to assure growth. Differentiation between gonococci and meningococci is often based on their different means of breakdown of specific sugars with concomitant production of acid (gonococci degrade only glucose, meningococci degrade maltose and glucose, and neither species can degrade sucrose or lactose).

Immunofluorescence tests can be used to distinguish gonococci from other Neisseriae and for the subtyping of gonococci. Different gonococcal strains can also be identified by specific growth requirements *(auxotyping)* and by various outer membrane antigens.[66] Five distinct colony forms of gonococci have been recognized. In contrast to T3, T4, and T5 colony forms, T1 and T2 colonies contain organisms that are covered with pili and are more highly virulent.[67] The serogroups of meningococci (A, B, C, D, X, Y, and Z) are differentiated on the basis of specific polysaccharides found on the bacterial surface, all of which, except for serogroups B and D, are clearly capsular in nature.

PATHOGENESIS

Source of Infection

N. gonorrhoeae and *N. meningitidis* are both specifically human pathogens. Gonococci can infect epithelial cells of the urethra, endocervix, anal canal, pharynx, and conjunctiva. Gonococcal infection is transmitted from person to person by the apposition of these mucosal surfaces, usually during sexual contact. Infection is not necessarily accompanied by symptoms, and asymptomatic carriers are the primary reservoir for gonococcal infection. Contiguous spread of bacteria from the endocervix can result in endometritis, salpingitis, tubo-ovarian abscess, and peritonitis. Invasion from any infected mucosal surface into the bloodstream can result in the clinical syndrome of disseminated gonococcal infection. *N. meningitidis* can be found as a member of the normal flora of the pharynx (the carrier rate has been variously reported from 2 to 38 percent). Although the attack rate clearly increases with crowding (eg, among military recruits) and with exposure to patients with active infection, the relationship between colonization and the development of overt disease is not entirely clear. In the case of meningococcal meningitis, for example, the portal of entry is often covert. Surgically treatable metastatic abscesses are rare complications of meningococcemia.

Bacterial Factors

The cell surface of gonococci has several functions in pathogenesis (Table 4-3). The outer membrane of the gonococcal cell envelope contains several constituents that are important in this regard—outer membrane protein, lipopolysaccharide, and pili (hairlike structures traversing the cell wall). Endotoxin is one part of the lipopolysaccharide component. Pili appear to be important for the initial attachment to epithelial cells, and may also inhibit phagocytosis and bacterial killing.[67] Resistance to phagocytosis may also be correlated with the protein components of the outer layer of the cell surface.[68] Recent evidence indicates that the surface of some gonococci may be encapsulated and that encapsulated strains are resistant to non-antibody-mediated phagocytosis.[69] Most meningococcal strains are encapsulated, and the capsule is presumably an important bacterial defense factor.

The ability of some microorganisms to acquire iron within a host is an important determinant both of virulence and of the nature of the engendered infection.[70] Strains of *N. gonorrhoeae* isolated from patients with disseminated gonococcal infection have an enhanced ability to acquire iron in an experimental host, when compared to urogenital isolates from patients with uncomplicated infection. *N. meningitidis*, which can produce septicemia and disseminated infection, is also unaffected by reduced iron concentrations.[70]

IgA protease is an extracellular enzyme produced by both gonococci and meningococci. The only known substrate for this enzyme is human immunoglobulin of the IgA1 subclass, which is important in local mucosal immune defense. Mulks and Plaut [71] have shown that all clinical isolates of *N. gonorrhoeae* and *N. meningitidis* tested were IgA protease positive, in contrast to eight species of nonpathogenic Neisseriae that commonly colonize the normal human nasopharynx.

Host Factors

Inhibition of attachment of *N. gonorrhoeae* to epithelial cells is, at least in part, associated with the local production of antibody. Tramont [72] has shown that antibodies of the classes IgG and IgA (primarily secretory IgA) are capable of inhibiting such attachment. Other humoral factors and polymorphonuclear leukocytes appear to have a major role in the killing of gonococci and in preventing invasion and spread of infection.

Whereas serum by itself does not possess significant bactericidal activity for staphylococci or streptococci, serum is clearly bactericidal for a number of gonococcal strains. Both antibodies and the complement system are involved in the bactericidal action. Antibodies of the IgG and IgM classes are capable of initiating complement activation at the gonococcal surface, and the terminal components of complement seem to be essential for the lethal

TABLE 4-3. VIRULENCE FACTORS OF *N. GONORRHOEAE*

Bacterial Factors	Biologic Effects
Cell surface components	
Lipopolysaccharide (endotoxin)	Cytotoxic, pyrogenic
Pili	Attachment to epithelial cells, inhibit, phagocytosis, killing
Outer layer proteins	Inhibit phagocytosis
Capsule	Inhibits phagocytosis
Iron-binding ability	Promotes survival, dissemination
IgA protease	Degrades local IgA

event (bacterial lysis). Patients with isolated deficiencies of C6, C7, or C8 have suffered recurrent severe gonococcal or meningococcal infections.[73] It seems that several surface antigens can trigger the antibody-mediated, complement-dependent bactericidal reaction, and that occasional gonococcal strains are killed via the alternative complement pathway in the absence of antibody. Schoolnik et al.[74] have shown that gonococcal strains that disseminate from local sites are more serum-resistant than are strains isolated from patients with uncomplicated gonorrhea. Recently, Ingwer et al.[75] found that sera from patients with disseminated gonococcal infection or hypogammaglobulinemia do not have bactericidal activity for gonococci.

Within 2 or 3 days after infection of the urethra, polymorphonuclear leukocytes appear. Although the gonococcal and host factors responsible for leukotaxis have not been established, activation of complement by bacterial surface components, with the production of factors such as C3a and C5a, may be involved. Phagocytosis of gonococci is promoted by serum opsonins, presumably involving both antibodies and complement with fixation of C3b at the bacterial surface. Most of the ingested gonococci are killed, although it has been suggested that gonococci are capable of surviving and multiplying within polymorphonuclear leukocytes. Antibodies directed against the cell surface of meningococci, probably primarily anticapsular antibodies, promote efficient killing and phagocytosis of these bacteria.

Host factors that may promote the spread of gonococcal infections into the endometrial cavity and the fallopian tubes include menstruation and the implantation of an intrauterine device.

At least two important questions related to host defense against gonococci remain: Why is it that everyone exposed to gonococcal infection does not develop an infection, and why does there appear to be little or no lasting immunity after gonococcal infection? An effective meningococcal vaccine protective against serogroups A and C has been produced. There is concern, however, that infection with other serogroups may be increased by immunization with this vaccine.[76]

CLINICAL MANIFESTATIONS AND THERAPEUTIC CONSIDERATIONS

Gonococcal infection remains an extremely important social problem. In the United States, over one million cases of gonorrhea were reported in 1977. Gynecologists, urologists, orthopedic surgeons, and even general surgeons will encounter this disease in its local and systemic manifestations (eg, skin lesions, tenosynovitis, acute septic arthritis, pelvic peritonitis).[77] In contrast, most patients with meningococcal disease, ie, patients with meningitis, meningococcemia, or pneumonitis, will not be seen in surgical consultation.

About 20 percent of the exposed females who become infected with gonococci develop acute salpingitis (acute pelvic inflammatory disease). An estimated 500,000 cases of acute pelvic inflammatory disease occur in the United States each year, and about 50 percent of the cases are caused by gonococci alone or in combination with other flora indigenous to the genital tract. When complicated by the development of tubo-ovarian abscess, surgical intervention is generally warranted. Anorectal infection, seen primarily in females, neonates, and homosexual males, usually involves rectal bleeding. Anorectal infection can be complicated by pararectal abscess formation or fistula in ano. Spread of gonococci into the upper abdomen can result in gonococcal perihepatitis (Fitz-Hugh-Curtis syndrome). Patients with this disease have right upper quadrant or bilateral upper abdominal pain and tenderness. The clinical findings, plus mild liver function test abnormalities and associated nonvisualization of the gallbladder on oral cholecystography, can mimic acute cholecystitis. Epididymitis and prostatitis are seldom caused by gonococci, presumably because of early antibiotic therapy.

Although penicillin remains the best drug for gonococcal and meningococcal infection, the emergence of plasmid-mediated, penicillinase-producing strains of gonococci, first recognized in 1975, is a cause for great concern.[78] The total impact and final outcome of this alarming new development in gonococcal disease are unknown.

BIBLIOGRAPHY

Buchanan R, Gibbons NE (eds): Bergey's Manual of Determinative Bacteriology, 8th ed. Baltimore, Williams & Wilkins, 1974.

Feldman HA: Meningococcal infections. Adv Intern Med 18:177, 1972.

Jeljaszewicz J (ed): Proceedings of the 3rd International Symposium on Staphylococci and Staphylococcal Infections. New York, Springer-Verlag, 1976.

Parker MT (ed): The Pathogenic Streptococci. Reedbooks, Chertsey, Surrey, 1980.

Patterson MJ, Hafeez A: Group B streptococci in human disease. Bacteriol Rev 40:774, 1976.

Sparling PF, Lee TJ: Gonorrhea: New insights and problems. In Weinstein L, Field BN (eds): Seminars in Infectious Disease, Vol 1. New York, Stratton Intercontinental Medical Book Corporation, 1978, p 34.

REFERENCES

STAPHYLOCOCCI

1. Wilson GS, Miles A: Topley and Wilson's Principles of Bacteriology, Vol. 1, 6th ed., Virology and Immunity. Baltimore, Williams and Wilkins, 1975, p 764.
2. Gramoli JL, Wilkinson BJ: Characterization and identification of coagulase-negative, heat-stable deoxyribonuclease-positive staphylococci. J Gen Microbiol 105:275, 1978.
3. Williams REO, Blowers R, Garrod LP, Shooter RA: Hospital Infections, 2nd ed. London, Lloyd-Luke, 1966.
4. Lidwell OM, Brock B, Shooter RA, Cooke EM, Thomas GE: Airborne infection in a fully air-conditioned hospital. IV. Airborne dispersal of *Staphylococcus aureus* and its nasal acquisition by patients. J Hygiene 75:445, 1975.
5. Ehrenkranz NJ: Person-to-person transmission of *Staphylococcus aureus:* quantitative characterization of nasal carriers spreading infection. N Engl J Med 271:225, 1964.

6. National nosocomial infections study—United States, 1975–76. Morbid Mortal Weekly Rep 26:377, 1977.
7. Elek SD: Experimental staphylococcal infections in the skin of man. Ann NY Acad Sci 65:85, 1956.
8. Elek SD, Conen PE: The virulence of *Staphylococcus pyogenes* for man: a study of wound infection. Br J Exp Path 38:573, 1957.
9. Verhoef J, Peterson PK, Quie PG: Immunology of staphylococcal infection. In Nahmias AJ, O'Reilly R (eds): Immunology of Human Infections. New York, Plenum, 1980.
10. Ghuysen JM, Strominger JL, Tipper DJ: Bacterial cell walls. Compr Biochem 26:53, 1968.
11. Van der Vijver JCM, Van Es-Boon MM, Michel MF: A study of virulence factors with induced mutants of *Staphylococcus aureus.* J Med Microbiol 8:279, 1975.
12. Rotta J: Endotoxin-like properties of the peptidoglycan. Z Immunitaetsforsch 149:230, 1975.
13. Wilkinson, BJ, Kim Y, Peterson, PK, Quie PG, Michael AF: Activation of complement by cell surface components of *Staphylococcus aureus.* Infect Immun 20:338, 1978.
14. Crowder JG, White A: Teichoic acid antibodies in staphylococcal and nonstaphylococcal endocarditis. Ann Intern Med 77:87, 1972.
15. Forsgren A, Sjöquist J: "Protein A" from *S. aureus.* I. Pseudoimmune reaction with human γ-globulin. J Immunol 97:822, 1966.
16. Sjöquist J, Stolenheim G: Protein A from *Staphylococcus aureus* IX. Complement-fixing activity of protein A-IgG complexes. J Immunol 103:467, 1969.
17. Peterson PK, Verhoef J, Sabath LD, Quie PG: Effect of protein A on staphylococcal opsonization. Infect Immun 15:760, 1977.
18. Peterson PK, Wilkinson BJ, Kim Y, Schmeling D, Quie PG: Influence of encapsulation on staphylococcal opsonization and phagocytosis by human polymorphonuclear leukocytes. Infect Immun 19:943, 1978.
19. Cawdery M, Foster WD, Hawgood BC, Taylor C: The role of coagulase in the defense of *Staphylococcus aureus* against phagocytosis. Br J Exp Pathol 50:408, 1969.
20. Hasegawa N, San Clemente CL: Virulence and immunity of *Staphylococcus aureus* BB and certain deficient mutants. Infect Immun 22:473, 1978.
21. Mandell GL: Catalase, superoxide dismutase, and virulence of *Staphylococcus aureus.* In vitro and in vivo studies with emphasis on staphylococcal-leukocyte interaction. J Clin Invest 55:561, 1975.
22. Casman EP: Staphylococcal enterotoxin. Ann NY Acad Sci 128:124, 1965.
23. Peterson PK, Laverdiere M, Quie PG, Sabath LD: Abnormal neutrophil chemotaxis and T-lymphocyte function in staphylococcal scalded skin syndrome in an adult patient. Infection 5:128, 1977.
24. Todd J, Fishaut M: Toxic-shock syndrome associated with phage-group-I staphylocci. Lancet 2:1116, 1978.
24a. Follow-up on toxic shock syndrome. MMWR 29:441–445, 1980 (Sept. 19).
24b. Update on toxic shock syndrome. FDA Drug Bull. 10:17–19, 1980 (Nov.).
25. Cohen J (ed): The Staphylococci. New York, Wiley, 1972.
26. Park JT, Shaw DRD, Chatterjee AN, Mirelman D, Wu T: Mutants of staphylococci with altered cell walls. Ann NY Acad Sci 236:54, 1974.
27. Kagan BM: L-forms. In Cohen J (ed): The Staphylococci. New York, Wiley, 1972, p 65.
28. Cline MJ, Craddock CG, Gale RP, Golde DW, Lehrer RI: Granulocytes in human disease. Ann Intern Med 81:801, 1974.
29. Johnston RB, Stroud RM: Complement and host defense against infection. J Pediatr 90:169, 1977.
30. Peterson PK, Wilkinson BJ, Kim Y, Schmeling D, Douglas SD, Quie PG, Verhoef J: The key role of peptidoglycan in the opsonization of *Staphylococcus aureus.* J Clin Invest 61:597, 1978.
31. Verhoef J, Peterson PK, Quie PG: Human polymorphonuclear leukocyte receptors for staphylococcal opsonins. Immunology 33:231, 1977.
32. Quie PG, White JG, Holmes B, Good RA: In vitro bactericidal capacity of human polymorphonuclear leukocytes: diminished activity in chronic granulomatous disease of childhood. J Clin Invest 46:668, 1967.
33. Musher DM, McKenzie SO: Infections due to *Staphylococcus aureus.* Medicine (Baltimore) 56:383, 1977.
34. Iannini PB, Crossley K: Therapy of *Staphylococcus aureus* bacteremia associated with a removable focus of infection. Ann Intern Med 84:558, 1976.
35. Tuazon CU, Sheagren JN, Choa MS, Marcus D, Curtin JA: *Staphylococcus aureus* bacteremia: Relationship between formation of antibodies to teichoic acid and development of metastatic abscesses. J Infect Dis 137:57, 1978.
36. Polaczek-Kornecka B, Dziadur-Goldsztajn Z, Komorowski A: Coagulase-negative staphylococci in clinical surgery. In Jeljaszewicz J (ed): Staphylococci and Staphylococcal Diseases. Published as supplement 5 to Zentralblatt für Bakteriologie, Parasitenkunde, Intfektionskrankheiten und Hygiene. New York, Fischer Verlag, 1976, p 145.

STREPTOCOCCI

37. Duma RJ, Weinberg AN, Medrek TF, Kunz LJ: Streptococcal infections: A bacteriologic and clinical study of streptococcal bacteremia. Medicine (Baltimore) 48:87, 1969.
38. Facklam RR: A review of the microbiological techniques for the isolation and identification of streptococci. CRC Crit Rev Clin Lab Sci 6:287, 1976.
39. Parker MT, Ball LC: Streptococci and aerococci associated with systemic infection in man. J Med Microbiol 9:275, 1976.
40. Wannamaker LW, Matsen JM (eds): Streptococci and Streptococcal Diseases: Recognition, Understanding and Management. New York, Academic, 1972, p 355.
41. Kaiser AB, Schaffner W: Prospectus: the prevention of bacteremic pneumococcal pneumonia: a conservative appraisal of vaccine intervention. JAMA 230:404, 1974.
42. Wannamaker LW: Immunology of streptococci. In Nahmias AJ, O'Reilly R (eds): Immunology of Human Infections. New York, Plenum, 1980.
43. Parker MT, Ball LC: Streptococcus milleri as a pathogen for man. In Parker MT (ed): The Pathogenic Streptococci: Streptococcal Disease in Man and Animals. Chertsey, Surrey, Reedbooks, 1980.
44. Fox EN: M proteins of group A streptococci. Bacteriol Rev 38:57, 1974.
45. Peterson PK, Schmeling D, Cleary PP, Wilkinson BJ, Kim Y, Quie PG: Inhibition of alternative complement pathway opsonization by group A streptococcal M protein. J Infect Dis 139:575, 1979.
46. Greenblatt J, Boackle RJ, Schwab JH: Activation of the alternative complement pathway by peptidoglycan from streptococcal cell wall. Infect Immun 19:296,1978.
47. Beachey EH, Ofek I: Epithelial cell binding of group A streptococci by lipoteichoic acid on fimbriae denuded of M protein. J Exp Med 143:759, 1976.
48. Halbert SP: Streptolysin O. In Ajl SJ, Kadis S, Montie TC (eds): Microbial Toxins. Vol III. New York, Academic, 1970, p 69.
49. MacLeod CM: Hypersensitivity and disease. In Lawrence HS

(ed): Cellular and Humoral Aspects of the Hypersensitive States. New York: PB Hoeber, 1959, p 615.

50. Schlievert PM, Watson DW: Group A streptococcal pyrogenic exotoxin: pyrogenicity, alteration of blood-brain barrier, and separation of sites for pyrogenicity and enhancement of lethal endotoxin shock. Infect Immun 21:753, 1978.
51. Patterson MJ, Hafeez AEB: Group B streptococci in human disease. Bacteriol Rev 40:774, 1976.
52. Wilkinson BJ, Peterson PK, Quie PG: Cryptic peptidoglycan and the antiphagocytic effect of the *Staphylococcus aureus* capsule: model for the antiphagocytic effect of bacterial cell surface polymers. Infect Immun, 23:502, 1979.
53. Ramirez-Ronda CH: Adherence of glucan-positive and glucan-negative streptococcal strains to normal and damaged heart valves. J Clin Invest 62:805, 1978.
54. Lerner PI, Gopalakrishna KV, Wolinsky E, McHenry MC, Tan JS, Rosenthal M: Group B Streptococcus *(S. agalactiae)* bacteremia in adults: analysis of 32 cases and review of the literature. Med (Baltimore) 56:457, 1977.
55. Selinger DS, Julie N, Reed WP, Williams RC Jr: Adherence of group A streptococci to pharyngeal cells: a role in the pathogenesis of rheumatic fever. Science 201:455, 1978.
56. Murray HW, Roberts RB: *Streptococcus bovis* bacteremia and underlying gastrointestinal disease. Arch Intern Med 138:1097, 1978.
57. Hill HR, Kaplan EL, Dajani AD, Wannamaker LW, Quie PG: Leukotactic activity and reduction of nitroblue tetrazolium by neutrophil granulocytes from patients with streptococcal skin infection. J Infect Dis 129:322, 1974.
58. Gallis HA: Complement (C) and immunoglobulin (Ig) interactions of streptococci. In Parker MT (ed): The Pathogenic Streptococci. Chertsey, Surrey, Reedbooks, 1980.
59. Dilton HC Jr, Reeves MSA: Streptococcal immune responses in nephritis after skin infections. Am J Med 56:333, 1974.
60. Ginsburg I, Sela MN: The role of leukocytes and their hydrolases in the persistence, degradation and transport of bacterial constituents in tissues: relation to chronic inflammatory processes in staphylococcal, streptococcal, and mycobacterial infections, and in chronic periodontal disease. CRC Crit Rev Microbiol 4:249, 1976.
61. Krivit W: Overwhelming postsplenectomy infection. Am J Hematol 2:193, 1977.
62. Peter G, Smith AL: Group A streptococcal infections of the skin and pharynx (Part I, II). N Engl J Med 297:311, 365, 1977.
63. McCarty M: The streptococcus and human disease. Am J Med 65:717, 1978.

PNEUMOCOCCI

64. Editorial. Resistant pneumococci. Lancet 2:803, 1977.
65. Austrian R: The assessment of pneumococcal vaccine. N Eng J Med 303:578, 1980.

GONOCOCCI

66. Johnston KH, Holmes KK, Gotschlich EC: The serological classification of *Neisseria gonorrhoeae.* I. Isolation of the outer membrane complex responsible for serotype specificity. J Exp Med 143:741, 1976.
67. Ofek I, Beachey EH, Bisno AL: Resistance of Neisseria gonorrhoeae to phagocytosis: relationship to colonial morphology and surface pili. J Infect Dis 129:310, 1974.
68. King GJ, Swanson J: Studies on gonococcus infection XV. Identification of surface proteins of *Neisseria gonorrhoeae* correlated with leukocyte association. Infect Immun 21:575, 1978.
69. Richardson WP, Sadoff JC: Production of a capsule of *Neisseria gonorrhoeae.* Infect Immun 15:663, 1977.
70. Payne SM, Finkelstein RA: The critical role of iron in host-bacterial interactions. J Clin Invest 61:1428, 1978.
71. Mulks MH, Plaut AG: IgA protease production as a characteristic distinguishing pathogenic from harmless neisseriaceae. N Engl J Med 299:973, 1978.
72. Tramont EC: Inhibition of adherence of *Neisseria gonorrhoeae* by human genital secretions. J Clin Invest 59:117, 1977.
73. Lee TJ, Utsinger PD, Snyderman R, Yount WJ, Sparling PF: Familial deficiency of the seventh component of complement associated with recurrent bacteremic infections due to *Neisseria.* J Infect Dis 138:359, 1978.
74. Schoolnik GK, Buchanan TM, Holmes KK: Gonococci causing disseminated gonococcal infection are resistant to the bactericidal action of normal human sera. J Clin Invest 58:1163, 1976.
75. Ingwer I, Petersen BH, Brooks G: Serum bactericidal action and activation of the classic and alternate complement pathways by *Neisseri gonorrhoeae.* J Lab Clin Med 92:211, 1978.
76. Nikoskelainen J, Leino A, Lähtönen E, Kalliomäki JL, Toivanen A: Is group-specific meningococcal vaccination resulting in epidemics caused by groups of virulent meningococci? Lancet 2:403, 1978.
77. Holmes KK, Counts GW, Beaty HN: Disseminated gonococcal infection. Ann Intern Med 74:979, 1971.
78. Sparling PF, Holmes KK, Wiesner PJ, Puziss M: Summary of the conference on the problem of penicillin-resistant gonococci. J Infect Dis 135:865, 1977.

CHAPTER 5
Enteric Gram-Negative Bacteria and Pseudomonads

WILLIAM J. MARTIN AND LOWELL S. YOUNG

GRAM-NEGATIVE bacilli were once considered saprophytes of limited virulence. Over the past 40 years, however, they have replaced staphylococci as the principal etiologic agents in surgical infections.[1] In fact, gram-negative bacilli now comprise the single greatest infection hazard in hospitalized patients.[2-4] The principal reason for this shift has been the fact that debilitated individuals, who in another era would have been considered nonoperable, now qualify for a variety of surgical procedures. Gram-negative bacilli are true pathogens in such hosts.

Gram-negative bacilli have frequently been viewed as a single group of potential pathogens, but important differences exist, even among members of the family Enterobacteriaceae. Furthermore, it has commonly been assumed that many gram-negative organisms (eg, the pseudomonads) belong within this family. This is incorrect for taxonomic reasons.[5,6] Nonetheless, because of the frequent appearance of *Pseudomonas* and a variety of nonenteric bacilli in surgical infections, and their presence in "mixed infections" including enteric gram-negative organisms, it seems appropriate to discuss the bacteriology and basic clinical syndromes associated with these organisms.

Table 5-1 is an attempt to group aerobic or facultative gram-negative bacilli by their order of clinical importance. Some of these organisms of lesser surgical significance are discussed in Chapter 7.

MICROBIOLOGIC ASPECTS OF GRAM-NEGATIVE BACILLI

BASIC STRUCTURE OF THE GRAM-NEGATIVE BACILLARY ORGANISMS

Aerobic gram-negative bacilli of clinical importance are non-spore-forming organisms that fail to take the Gram stain, may or may not be motile, and have certain structural or cell wall constituents that underlie this tinctorial property. Bacterial nomenclature is a changing field (see Table 3-1), and recognition that organisms previously grouped on the basis of physical or taxonomic properties may in fact not be closely related has led to a systematic reevaluation of bacterial classification according to such factors as DNA homology. Both old and new associations must be borne in mind as various microbiology laboratories adapt to these new terms.

The basic cell wall structure of clinically significant gram-negative bacilli includes most of the components that are illustrated in Figure 5-1 (also see Chapter 2). Many organisms, such as *Klebsiella pneumoniae* and *Escherichia coli*, are encapsulated with a polysaccharide-containing material. Designation for this encapsulated material is K, or capsular antigen, but other synonymous terms have been the Vi antigen of *Salmonella typhi* and the serotype antigen of *K. pneumoniae*. The acidic, negatively charged, structural capsule may allow the organisms to resist phagocytosis and can be an important virulence factor. Penetrating through the outer capsule of motile organisms is a relatively large proteinaceous whiplike structure [5] called flagella(ae), which carries the H antigen. Motility may be an important microbial factor involved in pathogenesis of infections such as occur in the urinary tract, which are usually ascending infections. Localized surface structures called pili or fimbriae that protrude from the capsule or outer cell wall facilitate attachment of infecting microbes to the mucosa of alimentary, respiratory, or genitourinary tracts. Pili-mediated ability to attach to surfaces is probably important in the initial interaction between parasite and host.

Much attention has been focused on the somatic heat-stable cell wall antigens, the so-called O antigens of gram-negative bacilli. Other synonyms for these structures are lipopolysaccharide or endotoxin. Most gram-negative bacilli contain endotoxins, the material left (both structurally and in terms of biologic activity) after cell wall structures are boiled for 30 to 60 minutes. When injected, they elicit fever, leukopenia followed by leukocytosis, and if given in sufficient quantities, hemodynamic instability leading to shock and death (see Chapter 16).

The structure of bacterial endotoxins has been elucidated in the past 15 years (Chapter 2). Lipopolysaccharide derived from strains of organisms that are usually isolated from urinary tract infections or bloodstream invasion have three regions or layers:

TABLE 5-1. AEROBIC (OR FACULTATIVE) GRAM-NEGATIVE BACTERIA OF SURGICAL SIGNIFICANCE

Important	Occasionally Important	Rarely Significant
Enterobacteriaceae	Enterobacteriaceae	
E. coli	*Arizona*	*Achromobacter*
Enterobacter	*Citrobacter*	*Alcaligenes*
Klebsiella	*Edwardsiella*	*Flavobacterium*
Proteus	*Providencia*	*Moraxella*
Serratia	*Salmonella*	
	Shigella	
	Yersinia	
Pseudomonas aeruginosa	*Acinetobacter calcoaceticus (Herellea)*	
	Acinetobacter lwoffi (Mima)	
	Aeromonas	
	Legionella pneumophila	
	Pasteurella	
	Pseudomonas, not aeruginosa	
	Vibrio	

1. The *outer membrane* contains O-specific lipopolysaccharides, ie, repetitive units of specific sugars that convey the serologic specificity of an organism. Thus, the familiar O agglutination pattern reported from *Salmonella* and *E. coli* reflects the ability of specific antiserum to agglutinate these organisms in high dilution. The O-specific lipopolysaccharide in turn is linked to a core region, which consists of common repetitive sugars linked to an inner core comprised of ketodeoxyoctonate linked to lipid A. The structure of the core glycolipid is widely shared among gram-negative bacteria; antibodies to it are broadly cross-reactive. Since the lipid A appears to be responsible for all of the toxic biologic properties of lipopolysaccharide, it is possible that vaccines could be developed to protect against many types of gram-negative bacillary infections. One reservation about this approach, however, is that other determinants more peripheral to the cell wall membrane may obscure or protect the core so that antibodies directed against core regions may not have access to directly neutralize the toxic effects of lipopolysaccharides.

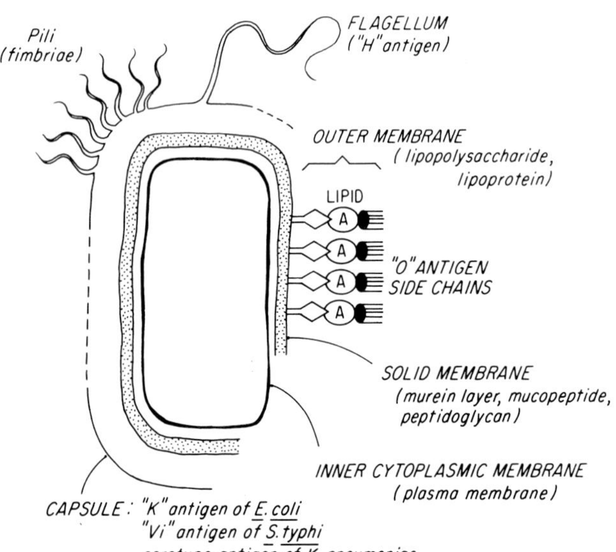

Fig. 5-1. **The major cell wall antigens of the gram-negative bacillus. Some are flagellated (H antigen) and may have capsules (K antigen). The O, or heat-stable somatic antigen, is part of the outer of three membranes and contains lipid A, which is responsible for endotoxicity. (Reproduced from Young et al., *Ann Intern Med* 86:456, 1977, with permission of the publishers.)**

O-antigenic structures and capsular antigens may further enhance resistance to phagocytosis as well as to the bactericidal activity of serum complement plus circulating antibodies. The so-called outer membrane portion of the gram-negative bacillary wall thus contains capsules (for encapsulated organisms), lipopolysaccharide, and protein constituents.

2. The *intermediate layer* is composed of murein or mucopeptide, and it is at this structure that beta lactam agents (penicillins, cephalosporins) exert their effect in disrupting cell wall synthesis.

3. The inner cell wall membrane, or *cytoplasmic membrane,* is the truly limiting structure in the presence of beta-lactam antibiotics; organisms exposed to penicillin-type agents tend to swell up and form spheroplasts that are osmotically fragile.

Cell wall structures of gram-negative bacilli appear to be related to some properties of invasiveness, but extracellular products such as tissue-destroying proteolytic enzymes and exoenzymes can also function as virulence factors.

For example, exotoxins from enteropathogenic *E. coli* are most responsible for the production of diarrhea in a manner analogous to cholera toxin. Most clinical isolates of *P. aeruginosa* produce both proteolytic enzymes and at least one exotoxin. Exotoxin A, the best characterized of these *Pseudomonas* toxins, is a potent inhibitor of protein synthesis, similar to diphtheria toxin. Just as antibodies directed against capsular and outer membrane components (O-specific lipopolysaccharide, core glycolipid) can protect against the sequelae of shock and death complicating bacteremic infections,[7-9] antibodies directed against toxins such as exotoxin A are also protective.[10]

TAXONOMY AND NOMENCLATURE

Family Enterobacteriaceae (Enteric Bacteria)

The best known and most easily recognized of the gram-negative facultative bacilli (that is, bacilli that grow aerobically and under conditions of increased CO_2) are the bacteria that currently make up the family Enterobacteriaceae. Members of this family are usually motile, although some species are nonmotile (genera *Shigella* and *Klebsiella*). The motile species possess peritrichous flagella, differing from members of the family Pseudomonadaceae, which have polar flagella. Several strains of *Salmonella, Shigella,*

Escherichia, Klebsiella, Enterobacter, and *Proteus* possess fimbriae or pili.

All species of enteric bacilli ferment glucose. Aerogenic (ie, gas-producing) and anaerogenic forms are found. The absence of gas in the fermentation of carbohydrates is characteristic of some genera. Nitrates are usually reduced to nitrites. Indophenol-oxidase is not produced.

The family is composed of a large and diverse group of organisms varying in antigenic structure and biochemical properties. The genera within the family have been established mainly on the basis of biochemical characteristics. Original species designations are still widely used and were established by both biochemical and ecologic criteria. The antigenic complexity of these bacteria has led to the development of antigenic schemes, patterned after the Kauffmann-White scheme for *Salmonella,* in which numerous serotypes based on O and H antigen typing were derived. Many of these serotypes are biochemically similar and can be distinguished only by serologic procedures.

After cultivation on laboratory media, enteric bacteria produce similar growth on blood agar, usually appearing as relatively large, shiny, gray colonies, which may or may not be hemolytic. Species that produce hydrogen sulfide show a definite greening around subsurface colonies in blood agar. On trypticase soy agar, nutrient agar, or meat infusion agar, the colonies vary in size, depending on the genus, but they are usually grayish white, translucent, and slightly convex. Some colonies are large and mucoid (*Klebsiella,* certain types of *Shigella,* and certain variants of *Salmonella,* especially *S. typhimurium*). Colony variation does occur, giving rise to smooth and rough forms. The terms smooth and rough are often used by microbiologists, but unfortunately they have several meanings. Although it may describe the morphologic appearance of colonies, roughness additionally indicates autoagglutinability in saline and susceptibility to the bacteriolytic activity of complement in fresh serum. Individual species or type colony characteristics are described under the respective genera.

Although the eighth edition of *Bergey's Manual of Determinative Bacteriology*[11] is widely used in the classification of the family Enterobacteriaceae, the classification system of Edwards and Ewing[6] has had the greatest impact on clinical microbiologists and infectious disease physicians. Table 5-2 summarizes both systems without intentional prejudice. The classification of Edwards and Ewing will be used in this chapter. More recent changes in taxonomy and nomenclature of these organisms as advocated by the Center for Disease Control are shown in Table 5-3.[12] These changes have been proposed on the basis of sophisticated biochemical and immunochemical patterns, particularly the use of DNA homology to establish the relatedness of bacterial species. Some designations made by clinical laboratories are in a state of flux; sometimes a seemingly new bacteriologic entity is simply an organism whose name has been changed.

Family Pseudomonadaceae

A member of the family Pseudomonadaceae, *P. aeruginosa,* is a polar monotrichous, gram-negative rod occurring singly, in pairs, or in short chains. On blood agar, the organism grows as a large, flat colony with a ground-glass appearance, and produces a zone of hemolysis. In patients with cystic fibrosis, mucoid strains are frequently isolated from the sputum. The colonies tend to spread and give off a characteristic grapelike odor. Most strains excrete pyocyanin and fluorescein (pyoverdin), giving the colony a characteristic blue-green color; approximately 4 percent are apyocyanogenic.

P. aeruginosa is oxidase-positive by Kovacs method[5] and utilizes glucose oxidatively in oxidation and fermentation (O-F) medium; gluconate is oxidized to ketogluconate (but not by other pseudomonads). *P. aeruginosa* is lysine and ornithine decarboxylase-negative and arginine dihydrolase-positive. Most strains grow at 42C on trypticase agar slants. They also grow on a selective agar medium containing cetyltrimethylamine bromide (Cetrimide). Most other members of the genus are inhibited on the latter medium.

IDENTIFICATION

Preliminary Identification of Cultures

Colonies of *Salmonellae* and *Shigellae* are recognized by their lactose-negative appearance on isolation plates. Suspected colonies of these two genera should be picked carefully with an inoculating needle and transferred to screening media such as triple sugar iron agar (TSI) or Kligler's iron agar (KIA).

Some colonies of *Proteus* species can be confused with *Salmonellae* and other lactose-negative enterobacteria on initial isolation; therefore, all TSI (or KIA) cultures should be further screened on urea agar or urea broth (weakly buffered). The reactions observed on TSI (or KIA) agar slants, together with the effect on urea, usually indicate the possible genus to which the isolate belongs. However, final identification depends on additional biochemical and serologic tests.

Because *P. aeruginosa* grows on EMB or MacConkey agar as a nonlactose-fermenting organism, it can be selected and transferred to TSI (or Kligler) agar as a suspicious colony from stool cultures and may be incorrectly identified.

Lactose-Fermenting Members of Enterobacteriaceae

A large number of organisms within the family Enterobacteriaceae ferment the carbohydrate lactose, and can be tentatively identified by the reactions shown in Figure 5-2 and Table 5-4. Some lactose-positive species ferment the sugar promptly, whereas others exhibit a delayed reaction, and the vast majority of the clinically important isolates fall into one of these categories. The lactose reaction can provide important information in the bacteriologic evaluation of a gram-negative rod. In fact, we feel certain that one of the most important sets of bacteriologic information on these bacilli that a clinician should know is that the lactose-positive organisms—*E. coli* and *Klebsiella*—tend to be more susceptible to antimicrobial agents like cephalosporins and chloramphenicol, whereas those or-

TABLE 5-2. CLASSIFICATION OF ENTEROBACTERIACEAE-TWO OF THE MAJOR SYSTEMS IN WIDESPREAD USE

Edwards and Ewing	Bergey's *Manual*
Family Enterobacteriaceae	Family Enterobacteriaceae
Tribe I Escherichieae	Genus I *Escherichia*
Genus I *Escherichia*	Species *E. coli*
Species *E. coli*	Genus II *Edwardsiella*
Genus II *Shigella*	Species *E. tarda*
Species *S. dysenteriae*	Genus III *Citrobacter*
S. flexneri	Species *C. freundii*
S. boydii	*C. intermedius*
S. sonnei	Genus IV *Salmonella*
Tribe II Edwardsielleae	Species *S. choleraesuis*
Genus I *Edwardsiella*	*S. typhi*
Species *E. tarda*	*S. enteritidis*
Tribe III Salmonelleae	Genus V *Shigella*
Genus I *Salmonella*	Species *S. dysenteriae*
Species *S. choleraesuis*	*S. flexneri*
S. typhi	*S. boydii*
S. enteritidis	*S. sonnei*
Genus II *Arizona*	Genus VI *Klebsiella*
Species *A. hinshawii*	Species *K. pneumoniae*
Genus III *Citrobacter*	*K. ozaenae*
Species *C. freundii*	*K. rhinoscleromatis*
C. diversus	Genus VII *Enterobacter*
Tribe IV Klebsielleae	Species *E. cloacae*
Genus I *Klebsiella*	*E. aerogenes*
Species *K. pneumoniae*	Genus VIII *Hafnia*
K. ozaenae	Species *H. alvei*
K. rhinoscleromatis	Genus IX *Serratia*
Genus II *Enterobacter*	Species *S. marcescens*
Species *E. cloacae*	Genus X *Proteus*
E. aerogenes	Species *P. vulgaris*
E. hafnia	*P. mirabilis*
E. agglomerans	*P. morganii*
Genus III *Serratia*	*P. rettgeri*
Species *S. marcescens*	*P. inconstans*
S. liquefaciens	Genus XI *Yersinia*
S. rubidaea	Species *Y. enterocoliticia*
Tribe V Proteeae	*Y. pseudotuberculosis*
Genus I *Proteus*	*Y. pestis*
Species *P. vulgaris*	Genus XII *Erwinia* (plant pathogens)
P. mirabilis	Species *E. herbicola* (has been considered a human pathogen)
P. morganii	
P. rettgeri	
Genus II *Providencia*	
Species *P. stuartii*	
P. alcalifaciens	
Tribe VI Yersineae	
Genus I *Yersinia*	
Species *Y. enterocolitica*	
Y. pseudotuberculosis	
Y. pestis	
Tribe VII Erwinieae (plant pathogens)	
Genus I *Erwinia*	
Genus II *Pectobacterium*	

ganisms that do not or slowly ferment lactose—*Pseudomonas, Serratia, Enterobacter,* indole-positive *Proteus*—often require therapy with potentially toxic agents like aminoglycosides (see Tables 5-7 and 5-8).

The IMViC (indole, methyl red, Voges-Proskauer, and citrate [the "i" is inserted for euphony]) reaction is used primarily to distinguish between the coliform bacteria, but may also be applied advantageously to other organisms in the family. Again, final identification must depend on an extended profile of biochemical tests.

Rapid procedures designed to reduce the amount of time for identifying members of the Enterobacteriaceae as well as other gram-negative bacilli have been developed commercially. All systems have been rated as good, with

TABLE 5-3. CURRENT CLASSIFICATION OF ENTEROBACTERIACEAE AS PROPOSED BY THE CENTER FOR DISEASE CONTROL

Tribe	Genus	Species	Changes	Additions
I. Escherichieae				
	Escherichia	*coli*		
	Shigella	*dysenteriae*		
		flexneri		
		boydii		
		sonnei		
II. Edwardsielleae				
	Edwardsiella	*tarda*		
III. Salmonelleae				
	Salmonella	*choleraesuis*		
		typhi		
		enteritidis		
	Arizona	*hinshawii*		
	Citrobacter	*freundii*		
		diversus		
				C. amalonaticus
IV. Klebsielleae				
	Klebsiella	*pneumoniae*		
		ozaenae		
		rhinoscleramatis		
				K. oxytoca
	Enterobacter	*aerogenes*		
		cloacae		
		agglomerans		
		hafniae	*Hafnia alvei*	
				E. sakazakii
				E. gergoviae
	Serratia	*marcescens*		
		liquifaciens		
		rubidaea		
V. Proteeae				
	Proteus	*mirabilis*		
		vulgaris		
		rettgeri		
		(biogroup 1–4)	*Providencia rettgeri*	
		(biogroup 5)	*P. stuartii*	
		morganii	*Morganella morganii*	
	Providencia	*alcalifaciens*		
		stuartii		
VI. Yersineae				
	Yersinia	*pestis*		
		pseudotuberculosis		
		enterocolitica		
				Y. intermedia
				Y. frederiksenii
				Y. ruckeri
VII. Erwinieae	├—Not human pathogens—┤			

Adapted from: Brenner DJ et al.[12]

an accuracy correlation ranging from 87 to 96 percent, or higher depending on the number and variety of cultures tested. A competent and well-trained technician is essential to achieve this degree of accuracy.

Basically, each system utilizes a battery of biochemical tests that can produce results from a single or several bacterial colonies in less than 24 hours. The tests and their manufacturers are listed in Table 5-5.

TABLE 5-4. REACTIONS OBSERVED IN TSI AGAR

Reactions	Explanation
Acid butt (yellow), alkaline slant (red)	Glucose fermented
Acid throughout medium, butt and slant yellow	Lactose or sucrose or both fermented
Gas bubbles in butt, medium sometimes split	Aerogenic culture
Blackening in the butt	Hydrogen sulfide produced
Alkaline slant and butt (medium entirely red)	None of the three sugars fermented

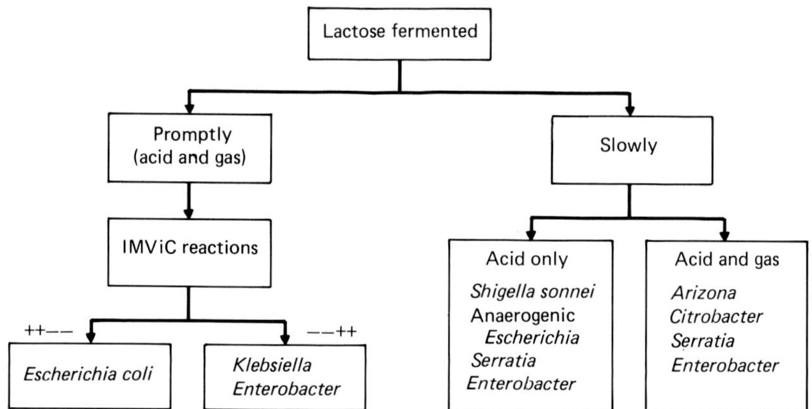

Fig. 5-2. **Immediate screening and tentative identification of Enterobacteriaceae by Lactose, IMViC, and TSI Reactions.**

IMMUNITY AGAINST GRAM-NEGATIVE BACILLI

Host defenses against infection are extensively covered in other chapters of this book (Chapter 13) and in recent reviews.[2,13,14] Only a brief summary will be made of the mechanisms that appear to prevent normal individuals from developing systemic enterobacillary infection.

Many individuals have circulating antibodies against disease-causing organisms without history of disease.[15] Natural antibodies probably result from gastrointestinal colonization or inapparent infection. Another possibility is that these antibodies developed after exposure to avirulent organisms which share antigens with disease-causing microbes. Cross-reactions between cell wall components of pneumococci and gram-negative organisms like *E. coli* and *Klebsiella* have been described.[2,16]

The obvious risk of gram-negative bacillary infection, particularly *P. aeruginosa* infection in the neutropenic patient, attests to the critical role of neutrophils in the defense against systemic invasion by gram-negative rods; monocytes appear to be less active and efficient phagocytes for encapsulated bacteria. In order for neutrophils to function optimally, opsonic support through the complement and antibody systems is required.[17] The antibodies are of the IgG and IgM class and are heat stable, but IgM requires complement in order to act as an opsonin. IgA is the primary antibody of the mucosal surfaces, and both IgA and IgG have been implicated in blocking the attachment of microbes to mucosal surfaces. Diseases such as acquired or native hypogammaglobulinemia are clearly associated with increased susceptibility to infection, and the prospect for survival from bacteremic gram-negative bacillary infections even in patients with normal levels of phagocytic cells but decreased antibody levels has been shown to be poor.[18] Thus, neither adequate antibody levels nor adequate numbers of circulating phagocytes (usually a neutrophil count in excess of 1,000) by itself is sufficient for adequate defenses against disease-causing pyogenic organisms.

From a therapeutic standpoint, however, granulocyte transfusions and supplemental immunoglobulin infusion may ultimately prove to be useful.[19]

Cell-mediated immunity does not appear to have a major role in defenses against gram-negative organisms, though some diseases characterized by depressed cell-mediated immunity have been associated with parallel deficiencies in humoral defenses and phagocytic cell function.

IMPORTANT ENTEROBACTERIACEAE

The epidemiology of infections with these organisms is of the utmost importance in current hospital practice.[20-23] Chapter 24 is devoted to nosocomial problems.

ESCHERICHIA COLI

E. coli is a motile, flagellated, usually piliated bacillus, whose biochemical characteristics have already been summarized. It is the most common facultative aerobic gram-negative bacillus in the gastrointestinal tract and in biliary and mixed intra-abdominal infections associated with perforations of the gastrointestinal tract. The ascending course

TABLE 5-5. COMMERCIAL BIOCHEMICAL TESTS FOR IDENTIFICATION OF GRAM-NEGATIVE BACILLI

Name	Manufacturer
API	Analytab Products, Inc. Plainview, NY
Enterotube System	Roche Diagnostics Division of Hoffmann, La Roche, Inc. Nutley, NJ
Entero-Set 20 (Inolex)	Fisher Diagnostics Orangeburg, NY
Minitek System	BBL, Division of Becton, Dickenson and Co. Cockeysville, MD
Micro-ID	General Diagnostic Division Warner-Lambert Co. Morris Plains, NJ
R/B System	Flow Laboratories, Inc. McLean, VA
N/F (nonfermenter) System	Flow Laboratories, Inc.

of these organisms from feces to urethra, ureter, kidney, and ultimately to blood is thought to account for their predominance as a cause of both urinary tract infections and bacteremia.

These organisms can also be an important cause of gram-negative pneumonia.[23,24] Wound infections, osteomyelitis, and meningitis appear to develop either as a result of direct extension of infection from a primarily infected site or on a bacteremic basis.

E. coli is also an important cause of diarrhea. Originally, the role of *E. coli* in diarrheal illness was obscured by its ubiquity in stool. It was far easier to focus on such obvious pathogens as *Salmonella* and *Shigella*. With more sophisticated techniques for epidemiologic "fingerprinting" of *E. coli* strains and the ability to evaluate diarrheageneic properties in vitro, the association has been made between *E. coli* and a number of well-studied epidemics.[7,8] Diarrhea-producing strains attach more readily (adhere) to gastrointestinal mucosal surfaces through their piliated surface structures. Once adherent, there appear to be several mechanisms for the pathogenesis of diarrhea: (1) local invasion (mucosal penetration) in a manner akin to invasiveness of *Shigella* species; (2) one of several heat-labile or heat-stable extracellular toxins triggers intestinal secretions in a manner analogous to cholera. The diarrhea-producing characteristics seem linked to a plasmid which contains chromosomal material coding for the production of the exotoxin. In prospective studies of diarrhea in tropical countries, as many as 75 percent of episodes of apparently infectious diarrhea can be traced to one or more of the enteropathogenic *E. coli*. Some debate exists as to whether the properties of enteropathogenicity are associated with specific serotypes. Presumptive identification of some enteropathogenic strains have been made on the basis of serotyping by agglutination or immunofluorescent methods, but the more specific diagnosis of diarrhea caused by extracellular products should probably rest upon the demonstration of toxin activity by a variety of sophisticated laboratory techniques.

Several methods are now available for epidemiologic studies of *E. coli* infections. These include tracing of biologic properties of the organism (enzyme production, utilization of certain substrates are the basis for so-called biotyping schema) and the more classic identification of cell wall surface structures by agglutination reactions. Flagellar serotyping is carried out with unheated cultures and thus allows the investigator to determine the H antigen of implicated strains. Somatic typing is carried out with heated or boiled cultures, and agglutination patterns are read after an appropriate incubation period with specific O antiserum. K typing is designed to identify the capsular material that surrounds the O type. Techniques such as electrophoresis, agglutination, and immunodiffusion have been used.[25]

Over 160 O groups and as many as 100 K or capsular types have been described for *E. coli* infections, but a small number, less than ten O and K types, probably account for the majority of serious systemic infections.[25] The ability to type *E. coli* by agglutination reactions or related methods may be of value in certain epidemiologic situations, such as an outbreak of nosocomial infections or the identification of the etiology of infectious diarrhea.

Fortunately, *E. coli* are usually sensitive to a wide variety of antimicrobial agents including the tetracyclines, chloramphenicol, the broad spectrum penicillins, cephalosporins, the aminoglycosides, and polymyxins. For uncomplicated urinary tract infections, sulfonamides will suffice, and the efficacy of bacteriostatic agents like tetracyclines and chloramphenicol is as good as with bactericidal agents if the organisms are susceptible in vitro. Chloramphenicol's superior distribution into fatty tissues and into the central nervous system places it at a singular advantage in infections occurring in the central nervous system and possibly in the lung. The latter infections, however, should be severe before this agent is used. For neutropenic patients the use of bactericidal agents is to be preferred, particularly the pairing of one of the beta-lactam (ampicillin or cephalosporin) agents with an aminoglycoside to achieve a bactericidal and possibly synergistic effect.[26]

KLEBSIELLA, ENTEROBACTER, SERRATIA

Organisms belonging to this group of enteric organisms are important causes of surgical infections associated with the biliary tree and the perforations of the gastrointestinal tract. Originally the serotypes described by Friedlander, *K. pneumoniae* A through F (now redesignated 1 through 6), were recognized as the etiologic agents of a life-threatening gram-negative pneumonia afflicting alcoholics. Today, we realize that this particular type of pneumonitis is not unique to the lower-numbered serotypes of *Klebsiella*. In fact *Klebsiella*, *Enterobacter*, and *Serratia* can all be important causes of pneumonia as well as urinary tract infections.

Klebsiella Species

Within the genus *Klebsiella,* three species have been recognized: *K. pneumoniae, K. ozaenae,* and *K. rhinoschleromatis.* A recent addition is the indole-positive species, *K. oxytoca.* These organisms are usually encapsulated and often produce large mucoid colonies on agar. Of the *Klebsiella* types, more than 75 have been identified by their specific agglutination patterns. Strains of *K. ozaenae* usually belong to type 4, 5, or 6, and strains of *K. rhinoschleromatis* to type 3.

Patients who develop community-acquired (ie, nonnosocomial) *Klebsiella* pneumonia are often afflicted with a disease such as alcoholism. In the classic radiologic description this infection was found to involve the upper lobes. Sputum has been described as both bloody and mucoid, and the consolidated parenchyma of the involved lobe may be "bowed" or bulging as the fissure is demarcated by x-ray. Nonetheless, these features are not a reliable basis for distinguishing *K. pneumoniae* infection from other bacterial or even fungal pneumonias. Histopathologically, *Klebsiella* pneumonitis is a necrotizing process characterized by destruction of alveolar septate linings and occasional caviation.

K. pneumoniae accounts for up to 10 percent of all hospital-acquired infections. Urinary tract infections are most common, followed by lower respiratory tract and wound infections. Increased risk of infection has been associated with Foley catheterization and endotracheal intubation. Multidrug-resistant strains of *Klebsiella* have become endemic in a number of institutions.

K. rhinoschleromatis is a cause of scleroma, a chronic granulomatous process of the nasal mucosa, paranasal sinuses, pharynx, larynx, middle ear, and the respiratory epithelium down to the bronchi.[27] Histologically, there is evidence of necrosis and fibrosis. Large foamy cells containing rod-shaped gram-negative organisms (Mikulicz cells) can be seen. This invasive growth, which can invade bone and result in the destruction of respiratory passages, has been mistaken for a neoplastic process or a mycobacterial disease. The disease is endemic in Eastern Europe (slavic leprosy), but the organism is actually of low infectivity and appears to spread by close and prolonged exposure between afflicted persons. Antimicrobial treatment of scleroma must be combined with surgical excision for optimum benefit.

K. ozaenae has been isolated from patients with a chronic atrophic rhinitis called ozaena. Histopathologically, there is loss of mucosal architecture, and clinically there is a chronic production of a foul-smelling discharge. In contrast to scleroma, ozaena is not believed to be a primary bacterial process and may have multiple etiologies with other gram-negative organisms acting as copathogens. *K. ozaenae* could also be an opportunistic secondary invader of damaged nasal mucosa. Many patients in technologically advanced societies have the isolates recovered from sputum or bronchoalveolar lavage. This organism is generally not a pathogen but can cause pneumonia or other deep-seated infection.

As a group, organisms belonging to the *Klebsiella* species are susceptible to cephalosporins, chloramphenicol, tetracyclines, the aminoglycosides, polymyxins, and trimethoprim–sulfamethoxazole. The important factor is that except for *K. ozaenae, Klebsiella* species are usually resistant to ampicillin, carbenicillin, and ticarcillin; when these drugs are used for the systemic therapy for *Pseudomonas* and *Serratia, Klebsiella* species which may coexist are not likely to be eradicated.

Enterobacter Species

The genus *Enterobacter* includes several distinct species: *E. aerogenes, E. cloacae,* and *E. agglomerans.* In contrast to *Klebsiella, Enterobacter* species rarely cause primary infection alone but are often isolated in combination with *E. coli* or *Klebsiella* from biliary or intraperitoneal infections and from the sputum, urine, or wound drainage from hospitalized patients. In intensive care units, *Enterobacter* and *Serratia* species have been a particularly vexing cause of cross-infection in patients who have indwelling urethral catheters, endotracheal tubes, or tracheostomies. Outbreaks of septicemia have also been implicated with contaminated parenteral fluids or with indwelling venous catheters.[22]

Serratia Species

Serratia species has been recognized as a significant human pathogen only within the last two decades.[28] These lactose-negative gram-negative organisms include *S. marcescens, S. liquefaciens,* and *S. rubidaea. Serratia* has been particularly implicated in the types of nosocomial infections; bacteremia linked to indwelling intravenous or intraperitoneal catheters or to instrumentation of the genitourinary tract, and pneumonia associated with contaminated inhalation therapy equipment. Both *Serratia* and *Pseudomonas aeruginosa* are often superinfecting pathogens that affect patients initially receiving broad spectrum antimicrobials like the cephalosporins, ampicillin, and the tetracyclines. Septic arthritis caused by *Serratia* organisms occasionally occurs and may be introduced into joints after aspiration or injection of medication or as a result of bacteremia. *Serratia* may be a common infecting organism in heroin addicts.

Serratia organisms tend to be highly resistant to cephalosporins, penicillins, and polymyxins. The agents of choice are aminoglycosides (gentamicin or amikacin), high concentrations of the extended-spectrum penicillins like carbenicillin or ticarcillin, and the combination of trimethoprim/sulfamethoxazole. Chloramphenicol may be active but should probably be considered after the other agents. A new cephalosporin-like antibiotic, cefoxitin, inhibits up to 50 percent of *Serratia* in vitro.

THE TRIBE PROTEEAE: *PROTEUS* AND *PROVIDENCIA*

The tribe Proteeae consists of two genera, *Proteus* and *Providencia.* These gram-negative organisms are motile, pleomorphic rods that are typically lactose-negative and are distinguished from other enteric bacilli by having the enzyme phenylalanine deaminase.

The Genus *Proteus*

Four species are traditionally assigned to the genus *Proteus*, of which the best known, *P. mirabilis*, does not ferment indole. In contrast, the indole-positive Proteeae are less common and include the species *P. vulgaris*, *P. rettgeri*, and *P. morganii (Morganella morganii)*. One of the most typical microbiologic properties of *P. mirabilis* and *P. vulgaris* is their ability to swarm on moist agar media. Discrete colonies are surrounded by a thin bluish-gray, confluent surface growth that occurs over a wide temperature range and complicates the isolation of other organisms present in mixed culture.

Proteus organisms are generally not carried in the stools of normal individuals but can be found in patients receiving oral antimicrobial therapy. The most common site of *Proteus* infections is the urinary tract, but it is a frequent isolate in mixed infections related to gastrointestinal perforations and has been implicated in bacteremic infections, wound infections, pulmonary infections, and brain abscesses.

P. mirabilis is the most common of the *Proteus* species encountered clinically and may cause 10 percent of all urinary tract infections. It often represents an even larger proportion of organisms causing hospital-acquired urinary tract infections. Several properties appear to underlie the pathogenicity of *Proteus* species for the urinary tract. Because many strains are urease producers, these organisms are able to split urea and form ammonium hydroxide. The shift in urinary pH to a markedly alkaline range potentiates the formation of stones. Stones may account for the chronicity or recurrence of *Proteus* urinary tract infections, because they act as a foreign body, and organisms remaining viable in the stony matrix could be protected from the effects of antimicrobial therapy. Other factors that contribute to the uropathogenicity of *Proteus* strains are the fact that many, if not all, of these organisms are piliated and can attach to urothelium.[29] The motility of *Proteus* species, particularly *P. mirabilis* and *P. vulgaris*, is a property conferred by the presence of many flagellae, and this may be an important factor in ascending infections.

One of the most noteworthy clinical-microbiologic aspects of *Proteus* infections is the differing antimicrobial susceptibility of the indole-positive versus indole-negative strains. The indole-negative species, *P. mirabilis*, are usually susceptible to high concentrations of penicillin G, although most clinicians tend to use ampicillin, amoxacillin, or a cephalosporin. This species is usually susceptible to other agents as well, including tetracyclines, chloramphenicol, and the aminoglycosides. On the other hand, indole-positive strains can be quite antibiotic-resistant and may be only inhibited by agents such as the aminoglycosides and trimethoprim-sulfamethoxazole. Some of the most resistant gram-negative organisms now encountered in the hospital, and of particular concern because some are aminoglycoside resistant, belong to *P. rettgeri* and *P. vulgaris* species.

TABLE 5-6. GRAM-NEGATIVE BACILLARY INFECTIONS WITH SYMPTOMS THAT CAN BE CONFUSED WITH ACUTE SURGICAL ABDOMEN

Enterobacteriaceae
Salmonella sp.
Shigella sp.
E. coli (enteropathogenic), invasive, toxigenic
Yersinia sp.
Campylobacter
Vibrio cholerae
Vibrio parahemolyticus
Rarely: *Arizona, Citrobacter, Edwardsiella, P. aeruginosa, Klebsiella, Aeromonas*

The Genus *Providencia*

Organisms belonging to this genus were previously grouped as the paracolon bacilli, a rather imprecise microbiologic designation representing a variety of organisms that could not be readily classified within other genera. Currently, the genus *Providencia* consists of three species, *alcalifaciens*, *rettgeri*, and *stuartii*. These organisms are readily identified on conventional media but may give biochemical reactions that could result in their being confused with *Salmonella* species. Of the three *Providencia* species, *P. stuartii* has received the most clinical attention. It has been implicated as a serious cause of complicated nosocomial urinary tract infections and in life-threatening infections occurring in burn units. *P. stuartii* is highly resistant to a number of conventionally used antimicrobial agents such as ampicillin, cephalosporins, and chloramphenicol, and it usually requires aminoglycoside therapy. However, even in this group a number of organisms are gentamicin-resistant and may require therapy with amikacin.

OCCASIONALLY IMPORTANT ENTERIC ORGANISMS

SALMONELLA AND *SHIGELLA*

Salmonella and *Shigella* are the classic gram-negative enteric pathogens associated with abdominal pain and diarrheal syndromes. Both groups of organisms contain many important species and serotypes, and the clinical manifestations can be protean. Perhaps of greatest concern to practicing surgeons is the likelihood that acute salmonellosis or shigellosis can mimic an acute surgical abdomen. Table 5-6 is an attempt to summarize some of the bacterial pathogens, including *Salmonella* and *Shigella*, which might cause a clinical picture leading to surgical intervention. It is not clear whether or not surgical intervention should be discouraged (see section on yersiniosis) and in fact might be encouraged even if the infection turns out to be amenable to antibiotic treatment alone.

Diarrhea is not a necessary clinical manifestation of either disease. In the early stages of classic typhoid, for instance, constipation or even intestinal obstruction may be the major clinical finding. This paradoxical observation has often been a stumbling block to the correct perception of the underlying diagnosis. Furthermore, *S. typhi* is classically associated with biliary tract disease and can on occasion mimic acute cholecystitis; chronic carriage of typhoid bacilli is more commonly associated with biliary stones and cure of typhoid carriers may require cholecystectomy.

Shigella

Shigellosis appears to cause a diarrheal syndrome either on the basis of local invasion of the gastrointestinal mucosa or the elaboration of a diarrhea-producing exotoxin. Its hallmark is a fairly short incubation period (average 2 days), fever, crampy abdominal pain, and a diarrheal product characterized by both blood and mucus. Abdominal tenderness is usually general, and the abdominal wall is not rigid. Sigmoidoscopy can reveal hyperemia, small bleeding sites, purulent mucus secretions, and Gram stain or methylene blue stain of feces reveals myriad fecal leukocytes (the latter being a helpful sign of intestinal shigellosis as opposed to other diarrheal entities).

Salmonella

Salmonellosis has innumerable animal reservoirs, and most people acquire the infection from environmental or foodborne sources. The mechanism of the diarrhea is unknown, and the disease is usually self-limited and requires only symptomatic treatment. Acute food poisoning, ie, *Salmonella* enterocolitis, is characterized by short incubation periods (18 to 72 hours), nausea, vomiting, colicky abdominal pain, and rapid onset of diarrhea. The finding of mucus and blood in the stool is less common than it is in shigellosis. Occasionally, severe abdominal tenderness even with rebound occurs, which can be confused with acute appendicitis or acute cholecystitis. Usually, however, the disease subsides within 5 days.

Of particular interest are the extraintestinal manifestations of salmonellosis. Although relatively few individuals are found to be bacteremic, organisms may cause arthritis, acute pericarditis, appendicitis, and have been found to colonize aortic aneurysms, causing primary peritonitis, pyelonephritis, and osteomyelitis. An increased susceptibility to *Salmonella* infections has been classically associated with asplenia such as occurs during the natural history of sickle cell anemia. There is a striking tendency of *Salmonella* species to be localized at sites of preexisting vascular disease, eg, aneurysms or vascular grafts.

Typhoid fever is on the decline in areas of improved sanitation. Immunization has had a questionable impact on its incidence. The overall mortality may reach 10 percent in certain series, with dangerous complications being intestinal hemorrhage and perforation of the bowel. The distinction between typhoid and other *Salmonella* enteric fevers (eg, paratyphoid) is difficult to make on clinical grounds alone.

While shigellosis should be treated with antimicrobial drugs, uncomplicated *Salmonella* diarrhea should not be treated. Good studies have shown that antibiotic treatment actually prolongs gastrointestinal carriage and selects for resistant fecal organisms. On the other hand, there is not much dispute about treating extraintestinal salmonellosis.

In many parts of the world, *Salmonella* and *Shigella* are often quite resistant to antimicrobials like tetracyclines, ampicillin, and sulfonamides. Chloramphenicol is the best agent for typhoid, though ampicillin is quite effective if given in adequate parenteral dose for susceptible organisms. Trimethoprim–sulfamethoxazole appears to be effective for both gastrointestinal and systemic *Salmonella* and *Shigella* infections.

THE GENUS *YERSINIA*

The genus *Yersinia* is a relatively recently created taxonomic entity now included in the family Enterobacteriaceae. These organisms were formerly classified among the genus *Pasteurella*. They are gram-negative coccobacillary forms of which three species are recognized as pathogenic for man: (1) *Y. pestis*, the agent of bubonic plague or the "black death," (2) *Y. pseudotuberculosis*, an occasional human pathogen known to cause tuberculous-like lesions in animals; and (3) *Y. enterocolitica*, by far the most important species because it is now recognized as an important cause of diarrhea and abdominal symptoms.

Yersinia Enterocolitica

Appreciation of the importance of *Y. enterocolitica* in human disease stems from investigations of both sporadic and epidemic cases of enterocolitis, often accompanying abdominal symptoms in a manner that has mimicked acute appendicitis. Usually, this organism produces a relatively mild and self-limited disease, which requires no treatment, but sometimes septicemias can occur. Severe diarrhea, often bloody, and temperatures in excess of 102F mimic disease caused by other intestinal pathogens such as *Shigella*, *Salmonella*, and enteropathogenic *E. coli*. Furthermore, mesenteric lymphadenitis due to *Y. enterocolitica* may occur with or without gastrointestinal symptoms and cause a syndrome indistinguishable from acute appendicitis. The appendix may be normal, but one study has demonstrated that approximately 5 percent of appendectomies will yield positive cultures of *Y. enterocolitica*.[30] For this reason, inflamed mesenteric nodes should be cultured when a normal appendix is discovered during operations for acute appendicitis. Recovery of *Y. enterocolitica* could alert the community to the possibility of an epidemic of pseudoappendicitis. Such epidemics have occasionally been traced to a common source such as contaminated food or water.[31]

An important epidemiologic observation is that outbreaks of *Yersinia* gastroenteritis seem to occur in the winter rather than in the summer. The organism has a peculiar preference for cold temperatures and flourishes in environmental sources. This special property has been utilized for recovery of the organism by the cold enrichment technique by placing fecal or other samples in an icebox where *Yersinia* multiplication still occurs. Patients who have yersiniosis should be isolated as for other enteric infections. Natural reservoirs of this infection have been poorly identified, but a small number of humans have been shown to be carriers and the organism has been found in other animal sources. Fecal transmission seems likely.

The only definitive means for diagnosing *Y. enterocolitica* infection is culture of stool or mesenteric nodes. Bacteremia is uncommon. Unfortunately, cultural recovery even with the best available techniques, such as cold enrichment, is slow, and appendectomy should not be deferred awaiting laboratory confirmation.

Most cases of mesenteric adenitis resolve spontaneously but there may be late complications of disease (such as infectious arthritis possibly on an autoimmune mechanism). Symptomatic treatment with fluids and bed rest is indicated in the milder cases, and there is no evidence that antimicrobial therapy shortens the course of the disease. Serious infections, on the other hand, particularly in the immunocompromised patient, require aggressive antimicrobial therapy with chloramphenicol, the aminoglycosides, or trimethoprim/sulfamethoxazole.

Yersinia Pestis

Y. pestis is the cause of all the clinical forms of plague. It is not an enteric organism.[32] The organisms are plump, gram-negative, nonmotile, lactose-negative pleomorphic bacilli whose bipolar (safety pin) appearance may not be evident on Gram stain. They grow on most bacteriologic media, although growth is slow at 35 to 37C. Rapid identification can be made using a fluorescent antibody technique, although cross-reactions with *Y. pseudotuberculosis* have been recorded.

The epidemiology of plague is complex, and foci occur throughout the world wherever wild rodents with fleas interact with people. It is endemic in the Rocky Mountain region of the United States. Ratborne plague is a far less serious problem in urban areas than previously, and now wild mammal transmission in the rural areas predominates (ie, ground squirrels, prairie dogs, and chipmunks). Human plague may result from pneumonic spread, human flea transmission, or contact with infected exudates.

Y. pestis in fleas develops into masses of organisms, which block the upper gut. Attempts to swallow blood lead to regurgitation of the organisms into the site of the bite. The human is an accidental victim of a bite by rat flea or by contact with infected tissue in carnivores or other wild rodents. The local tissues in the regional nodes become necrotic, infarcted, inflamed, hemorrhagic, and edematous, and progressive toxemia leads to death. The usual incubation period of bubonic plague is 2 to 6 days, and the severity at onset is variable. Initially, malaise, fever, pain, and tenderness occur in the area of the regional lymph nodes. Bubos (enlarged fluctuant nodes) most often appear in the inguinal or axillary regions, but any subcutaneous site is susceptible. Intermittent bacteremia is common. The progression of infection in bacteremia can be extremely rapid, and in some patients the onset of clinical toxicity is sudden and bubo formation can be delayed, making the diagnosis difficult.

The diagnosis depends on suspecting the disease, aspirating a bubo, and culturing the blood. A rapid tentative diagnosis can be made on smear if Giemsa stain is used. Gram stain preparations do not show the characteristic bipolarity. Fluorescent antibody tests on aspirated material will confirm the diagnosis. Bubos should not be excised or incised and drained for diagnostic purposes. Tularemia is a common incorrect diagnosis, and cultures of aspirates that are negative at 24 hours should increase the suspicion of plague or tularemia. Acute and convalescent sera are useful in epidemics.

Therapy should be started immediately. Streptomycin is the best drug, but other effective drugs include kanamycin, chloramphenicol, tetracyclines, and sulfadiazine. Quarantine of all patients and patient contacts should be carried out, and prophylactic chemotherapy should be instituted for contacts. Shock may require steroid administration.

A heat-killed vaccine is available which is reasonably effective in preventing disease. Booster injections are recommended every 6 months, but the principal protective method is environmental sanitation.

CITROBACTER

Organisms belonging to the genus *Citrobacter* are closely related to the *Salmonellae.* There are extensive cross-reactions between these organisms and other members of the family Enterobacteriaceae. *Citrobacter* are occasionally isolated from a variety of clinical sources and are most commonly implicated in urinary and respiratory tract infections. There have been reports of *Citrobacter* isolates as the cause of central nervous system infection in neonates. Cerebral abscesses, endocarditis, and sepsis secondary to contaminating intravenous fluids have been reported. The two most commonly encountered species of *Citrobacter* are *C. diversus* and *C. freundii. C. diversus* are found to be resistant to ampicillin and carbenicillin but susceptible to cephalothin, whereas strains of *C. freundii* are variably sensitive to all of these agents.

HAFNIA ALVEI

These organisms are related to the genera *Klebsiella, Enterobacter,* and *Serratia.* In some references the organism has been identified as *Enterobacter hafnia.* Clinical isolates have been mainly nosocomial in origin, and the types of infection include pneumonia, urinary tract infection, and surgical wounds. Most aminoglycosides, chloramphenicol, tetracyclines, and carbenicillin are active against this agent, but *Hafnia* species are resistant to ampicillin and cephalosporins.

EDWARDSIELLA TARDA

This group of organisms are similar to *Salmonella* in terms of the clinical disease produced, but the two genera are not closely related. The species name *tarda* refers to the relative slowness of this organism in fermenting various biochemical substrates. Most human isolates have been obtained from cases of acute gastroenteritis.[33] The syndrome involves intermittent watery diarrhea which persists for a few days but may last up to 2 weeks. Occasionally, low-grade fever and vomiting are present. Although the organism has been recovered from the stools of entirely asymptomatic individuals, *E. tarda* has been implicated as the source of bloodstream infection, liver abscess, meningitis, and soft-tissue infection. Most cases of gastroenteritis associated with this organism resolve without treatment. As with the management of *Salmonella* gastroenteritis, normal individuals should probably not receive antimicrobial therapy. For systemic infections, the organism is sensitive to a variety of common antimicrobials including ampicillin, cephalosporins, chloramphenicol, tetracyclines, and aminoglycosides.

ERWINIA

The genus *Erwinia* belongs within the family Enterobacteriaceae and has classically been associated with plant disease. Many strains previously belonging to the herbicola-lathryi group of *Erwinia* have now been reclassified as *Enterobacter agglomerans. Erwinia* of the herbicola-lathryi group have been isolated from cases of brain abscess, urinary tract infection, meningitis, pneumonia, empyema, and bacteremia caused by intrinsic contamination of intravenous fluid. The organisms have shown varying susceptibility to a variety of commonly used antimicrobial agents like cephalosporins, penicillins, and tetracyclines, but most are inhibited by nalidixic acid, aminoglycosides, and chloramphenicol.

FAMILY PSEUDOMONADACEAE

PSEUDOMONAS AERUGINOSA

As mentioned earlier in this chapter, *Pseudomonas aeruginosa (Bacillus pyocyaneus)* is an organism that technically does not belong within the family Enterobacteriaceae but is properly categorized within the family Pseudomonadaceae. In clinical practice, *P. aeruginosa* is probably the most important of the gram-negative rods that are referred to as nonfermenters. This term encompasses a taxonomically heterogeneous group of bacilli that have two important characteristics—they fail to ferment carbohydrates, and they are obligate aerobes. These two features are highly important in selection of laboratory techniques for the detection and identification of these microorganisms.

Because *P. aeruginosa* infections commonly occur in association with gastrointestinal disease, urinary tract abnormalities, burns, or other situations in which gram-negative enteric bacilli are often encountered, it is proper to consider *P. aeruginosa* when evaluating the enteric bacteria. The experience of many medical centers is that among the systemic and pulmonic gram-negative bacillary infections, those caused by *P. aeruginosa* rank highest in mortality.[8,34] This high mortality appears to be a reflection of the predilection of this organism for neutropenic subjects, subjects with thermal injury, and recipients of organ transplants.[21,35]

There is no consensus about the basis for the human virulence of *P. aeruginosa.* A number of interesting studies have investigated the ability of the organism to elaborate extracellular virulence factors such as exoenzymes and toxins,[10,36] the heat-stable cell wall structures that appear to convey resistance to phagocytosis,[17] and the physical properties of the microbe that allow it to survive in adverse environmental conditions.[20] Indeed, one of the most simplistic explanations for the opportunistic nature of *P. aeruginosa* is its saprophytic qualities, ie, it has minimal nutritional requirements and limited carbon sources will permit luxuriant growth. It survives readily in water, soil, and food products, and is so hardy that commonly used detergents and disinfectants have little effect on its viability. Since pseudomonads will survive in any moist environment, medical equipment using water is commonly contaminated.

Epidemiology

Attempts to colonize normal volunteers with *P. aeruginosa* have been unsuccessful unless concomitant antimicrobial agents like ampicillin have been given,[37] and this organism is not likely to be found in the gastrointestinal tract of normal individuals. Furthermore, leukocytes and serum from normal individuals show an excellent ability to phagocytose and kill strains of *P. aeruginosa* from a wide variety of sources.[17] The incidence of gastrointestinal carriage in hospitalized or clinically ill patients receiving special diets or antibiotics, however, may approach 50 percent. It seems, then, that the host is continually assaulted with strains of *P. aeruginosa* that abound in the environment and in ingested materials. Colonization occurs only with some debility of the host, and colonization usually precedes bacteremia, particularly in the neutropenic patient.[38]

A number of serologic typing systems have been used to study the epidemiology of *P. aeruginosa,*[39] and a number of cross-reactions have been noted. Agglutination tests have identified 10 to 15 O-antigenic serotypes, but Fisher et al.[40] have seven antisera which can adequately identify approximately 90 percent of clinically important strains. Other methods for epidemiologic study include phage typing and pyocin typing. All these techniques have been extremely useful in determining which nosocomial outbreaks of *P. aeruginosa* have a common source or an epidemic strain as opposed to multiple sources of infection.

Virulence Factors

Besides surface antigens, which are identified by agglutination reactions, the extracellular products of *P. aeruginosa* may be important virulence factors. Exotoxin A (of several exotoxins) is a potent inhibitor of protein synthesis, somewhat analogous to activity of diphtheria toxin.[10,36] Furthermore, most disease-causing *P. aeruginosa* elaborate potent proteolytic enzymes such as elastase and lecithinase.[36,41] At present, it is not possible to conclude which if any of these factors is most critical in the pathogenesis of *P. aeruginosa* infection. Proteases may be important in the initiation of tissue injury such as the early events following burn injury or inoculation of organisms into wounds. Exotoxins may be involved in the lethal events accompanying systemic *P. aeruginosa* infection.

Clinical Manifestations

Clinically, the onset of *Pseudomonas* bacteremia may be fulminant with a rapid progression to hypotension and shock. In a small percent of patients, bacteremia is accompanied by a striking necrotizing vasculitis.[42] The name *ecthyma gangrenosum* is the classic term for these lesions. Initially, the first indication of vasculitis is a vesicle or bulla surrounded by a slightly raised halo of erythema. Within a matter of hours, the central vesicle or bulla progresses to frank ulceration. The halo of erythema may become darkly ecchymotic (and might be mistaken for just subcutaneous bleeding in thrombocytopenic patients). Histopathologically, organisms are found invading the venular side of the vascular bed and appear to trigger thrombosis and infarction.[43] Some ecthyma gangrenosum skin lesions may be singular, while other patients may have showers of them. They appear on any surface of the body including the trunk, back, and extremities, but the area that should be carefully examined should be the perirectal area. Although some lesions have been attributed to a hypersensitivity phenomenon, the recovery of the organisms by aspiration or biopsy is readily achieved if the patient is not receiving systemic antimicrobial drugs. Thus, the finding of these lesions is prima facie evidence of bacteremia, and the patient should be treated.

The proclivity of *P. aeruginosa* to cause necrotizing vasculitis is one of the striking features of bacteremic disease syndromes, and these may also involve the gastrointestinal tract and the lungs. Indeed, the so-called shock lung syndrome may reflect the activation of complement, coagulation, and kinin systems, with the lung serving as one of several target organs. The rapid development of pulmonary infiltrates with evidence for increased alveolar capillary-arterial oxygen gradient may be a reflection of a diffuse intrapulmonary capillary leak triggered by bacterial products such as *Pseudomonas* endotoxins. The mortality in this complication is high, and aggressive antimicrobial therapy and maintenance of ventilatory function are imperative.

P. aeruginosa infections can involve all major organs and soft tissue sites. The organism can cause central nervous system infections, particularly meningitis and brain abscess, in patients with immunodeficiency or in individuals who have intracerebral catheters or shunts in place. External ear infections due to *P. aeruginosa* are quite common but may not necessarily call for the use of systemic antimicrobial therapy. Bone infections frequently represent a superinfection, ie, the onset of a *Pseudomonas* infection following an initial process caused by staphylococci. Caution must be exercised in interpreting the results of sinus tract cultures in diagnosing osteomyelitis. Biopsy of infected bone should be undertaken before committing the patient to a prolonged course of potentially toxic antipseudomonal therapy.

Pulmonary infections caused by *P. aeruginosa* are among the greatest therapeutic challenges that clinicians now face. Highly mucoid strains of *Pseudomonas* have caused life-threatening disease in children with cystic fibrosis. Mucoid strains of *P. aeruginosa* are rarely encountered in other types of *Pseudomonas* infection, but the nonmucoid strains are a particular problem in hospital-acquired aspiration pneumonia. These pneumonias tend to occur in intensive care units or burn units and in critically ill patients receiving assisted ventilation.

In the older literature, *P. aeruginosa* has been implicated as a cause of diarrheal illness (Shanghai fever), but this problem is seldom described in recent times. Intra-abdominal and urinary infections often present as superinfections after antimicrobial therapy for another infection has been initiated. Foreign bodies such as Foley catheters, intra-arterial and intravenular catheters, peritoneal lavage devices, and prostheses serve as the nidus of persistent infection. *Pseudomonas* arthritis and osteomyelitis develop on a bacteremic basis in heroin addicts, who also are prone to *Pseudomonas* endocarditis, a lethal complication that may require excision of infected cardiac valves.[44]

Treatment

There are three groups of antimicrobial drugs that can be used for *P. aeruginosa* infection; the aminoglycosides (gentamicin, tobramycin, amikacin), the antipseudomonal penicillins (carbenicillin and ticarcillin), and the polymyxins (polymyxin B and colistin). Historically, polymyxins were relatively ineffective, supposedly because of nephrotoxicity. No modern study, however, has compared these agents to the aminoglycosides and penicillins. The major advantage of the polymyxins has been the fact that isolates of *P. aeruginosa* have not developed resistance to this family of compounds. At present, the aminoglycosides appear to be the best agents, but some strains have already developed multidrug resistance. Amikacin is the most reliably effective of the aminoglycosides against *Pseudomonas* if evaluated on the basis of resistance to R-factor-mediated enzymatic inactivation. On a weight basis, tobramycin, factored for achievable blood levels, may be more potent against some strains but it is not as resistant to enzymatic attack as is amikacin. For systemic *Pseudomonas* infections, the use of at least two agents seems indicated, such as the pairing of the aminoglycoside with carbenicillin or ticarcillin. Some studies indicate that the use of such combinations is not only clinically beneficial but is paralleled by in vitro evidence of antibacterial synergy.[26]

Prevention

Prevention of *Pseudomonas* infections may be possible through the use of immunoprophylactic measures such as the administration of a vaccine or immunoglobulin, approaches that have been successfully demonstrated experimentally and in some clinical trials.[18,45] The use of granulocyte transfusions may be of benefit in neutropenic patients. Since the transfused white cells are short-lived, multiple daily transfusions are needed until the patients' own leukocytes return in sufficient numbers.[19]

NONAERUGINOSA PSEUDOMONAS SPECIES

Table 5-7 is a summary of nonaeruginosa pseudomonads of occasional medical and surgical importance. The three most important species listed are *P. cepacia, P. maltophilia,* and *P. pseudomallei.* All are found in soil and water and cause illnesses similar to those caused by *P. aeruginosa.* Unfortunately, their antibiotic sensitivity patterns are different.

P. cepacia is a recent appellation for organisms previously designated as *P. multivorans* or *P. kingii.* The organism has occasionally been encountered in wound and genitourinary tract infections. It colonizes foot ulcers or traumatized skin in a manner leading to the peculiar syndrome known as foot rot.[46] The most serious infections with *P. cepacia* are endocarditis (as in abusers of intravenous drugs), septicemia, and meningitis. *P. cepacia* appears to be a nosocomial pathogen of increasing importance which, like strains of *P. aeruginosa*, contaminates inhalation therapy equipment, water baths, and sinks. Also it has been isolated from outbreaks associated with contaminated blood products or infusion fluids.

P. pseudomallei is found in Southeast Asia. The syndrome of necrotizing pneumonia with occasional septicemia and metastatic spread of disease was recognized in United States troops in Vietnam.[47] Many years after leaving an endemic area, previously exposed individuals can develop necrotizing pulmonary infection by reactivation of latent disease.

P. maltophilia can occasionally cause nosocomial respiratory infections, wound infections, and granulomatous infections.[48,49]

Depending on the clinical circumstances, presumed infection by these organisms should be approached either cautiously or aggressively. Recovery of nonaeruginosa pseudomonads from skin or the oropharynx may represent new colonization. These organisms tend to overgrow during the selection pressure of antimicrobial therapy. On the other hand, the isolation of the organism in pure culture from a transtracheal aspirate, bone aspirate, carefully collected urine, or from blood unquestionably indicates infection that requires urgent treatment.

Table 5-8 is a summary of the antimicrobial susceptibility patterns of these organisms. Their susceptibility to aminoglycosides is variable. For instance, *P. cepacia* is usually resistant to aminoglycosides (with kanamycin perhaps being an exception) and variably susceptible to carbenicillin, so that the agents used for *P. aeruginosa* infections should not be assumed to be effective for *P. cepacia*. Further, *P. pseudomallei* is often resistant to those antimicrobials but susceptible to agents such as tetracyclines, the sulfonamides, or trimethoprim–sulfamethoxazole. The tetracyclines and chloramphenicol appear to be fairly effective against a large proportion of the nonaeruginosa pseudomonads, but polymyxins (colistin and polymyxin B) are often ineffective, as are most of the penicillins, like ampicillin and the cephalosporins.

TABLE 5-7. NONAERUGINOSA PSEUDOMONAS SPECIES OF OCCASIONAL MEDICAL AND SURGICAL IMPORTANCE

Species	Reference	Clinical Associations
cepacia *	46	Septicemia, "foot rot," endocarditis, wound infections, GU infections
fluorescens	50	Wounds, respiratory infections, catheter-associated bacteremia
maltophilia	48	Respiratory infections, ulcers, abscesses, wound infections, granulomas
stutzeri	49	Wounds, osteomyelitis, otitis
pseudomallei	47	Necrotizing pneumonia and metastatic disease
putida	50	Wounds, GU infections, catheter associated bacteriemia
putrefaciens	49	Wounds, abscesses, bacteriemia

* Also called *P. multivorans* or *P. kingii*

RECOMMENDATIONS FOR ANTIMICROBIAL CHEMOTHERAPY OF GRAM-NEGATIVE BACILLARY INFECTIONS

Individual recommendations for antimicrobial therapy have been made in the sections describing each pathogen. The differing antimicrobial susceptibility patterns of members of the genus *Pseudomonas* have been outlined in Table 5-8. Table 5-9 is a summary of recommended antimicrobial agents for gram-negative bacillary infections other than *Pseudomonas*, including many discussed in Chapter 7. These recommendations are made in general terms, and within each category of agents there are often several therapeutic alternatives. In vitro susceptibility patterns at a particular institution, local experience with one

TABLE 5-8. ANTIMICROBIAL SUSCEPTIBILITY OF PSEUDOMONAS SPECIES

Species	Aminoglycosides *	Carbenicillin †	Polymixins ‡	Tetracyclines	Chloramphenicol	Sulfa
aeruginosa	+	+	+	0	0	0
cepacia	0	±	0	0	±	+§
fluorescens	+	0	+	+	±	
maltophilia	0	±	+	±	±	± §
stutzeri	+	+	+	+	±	
pseudomallei	±	+	0	+	+	+
putida	+	0	+	±	0	

+, usually susceptible; ±, variable; 0, resistant

* Amikacin, gentamicin, tobramycin
† Or ticarcillin
‡ Polymixin B or colistin
§ Trimethoprim/sulfamethoxazole preferred

TABLE 5-9. RECOMMENDED ANTIMICROBIAL AGENTS FOR GRAM-NEGATIVE BACILLARY INFECTIONS

Organism	First Choice	Second Choice	Alternate	Comment
Enterobacteriaceae				
Citrobacter	Aminoglycoside	Chloramphenicol	Cephalosporins	Cephalosporin susceptibility varies
Enterobacter	Aminoglycoside	Carbenicillin *	Trimethoprim/sulfa	Some cephalosporins may be effective
E. coli	Aminoglycoside	Ampicillin	Cephalosporins	Often sensitive to wide variety of agents
Klebsiella	Aminoglycoside	Cephalosporins	Chloramphenicol	Often sensitive to wide variety of agents
Proteus	Aminoglycoside	Carbenicillin	Trimethoprim/sulfa	Ampicillin for *P. mirabilis*
Providencia	Aminoglycoside	Carbenicillin	Trimethoprim/sulfa	Some strains only inhibited by amikacin
Salmonella	Chloramphenicol	Ampicillin	Trimethoprim/sulfa	
Serratia	Aminoglycoside	Carbenicillin	Trimethoprim/sulfa	
Shigella	Ampicillin	Trimethoprim/sulfa	Chloramphenicol	Wide variations in susceptibility
Yersinia enterocolitica	Aminoglycoside	Chloramphenicol	Trimethoprim/sulfa	
Y. pseudotuberculosis	Streptomycin	Aminoglycoside	Tetracycline	
Y. pestis	Tetracycline	Streptomycin		
Acinetobacter	Aminoglycoside	Chloramphenicol	Tetracycline	
Aeromonas	Aminoglycoside	Carbenicillin	Chloramphenicol	
Legionella	Erythromycin	Rifampin	Trimethoprim/sulfa	
Pasteurella	Penicillin G	Tetracycline	Erythromycin	*P. multocida* only
Pseudomonas	See Table 5-8			
Vibrio	Tetracycline	Trimethoprim/sulfa	Aminoglycoside	

* Ticarcillin may be substituted for carbenicillin

preparation versus another, and the factors of cost and pharmacokinetics are often powerful determinants in placing individual agents in an order of preference (Chapter 18).

REFERENCES

1. McGowan JE, Barnes MW, Finland M: Bacteremia at Boston City Hospital: occurrence and mortality during 12 selected years (1935–1972), with special reference to hospital-acquired cases. J Infect Dis 132:316, 1975.
2. Young LS, Martin WJ, Meyer RD, Weinstein RJ, Anderson ET: Gram-negative rod bacteremia: microbiologic, immunologic, and therapeutic considerations, Ann Intern Med 86:456, 1977.
3. Bennett JV: Incidence and nature of endemic and epidemic nosocomial infections. In Bennett JV, Brachman PS (eds): Hospital Infections. Boston, Little, Brown, 1979, p 233.
4. Musher DM: Cutaneous and soft-tissue manifestations of sepsis due to gram-negative enteric bacilli. J Infect Dis 2:854, 1980.
5. Finegold SM, Martin WJ, Scott EG (eds): Bailey and Scott's Diagnostic Microbiology, 5th ed. St. Louis, Mosby, 1978.
6. Edwards PR, Ewing WH: Identification of Enterobacteriaceae, 3rd ed. Minneapolis, Burgess, 1972.
7. McCabe WR, Kreger BE, John M: Type-specific and cross-reactive antibodies in gram-negative bacteremia. N Engl J Med 287:261, 1972.
8. Young LS, Mandell GL, Douglas RG, Bennett JE: Principles and Practice of Infectious Diseases. New York, Wiley, 1979, p 571.
9. Zinner SH, McCabe WR: Effects of IgM and IgG antibody in patients with bacteremia due to gram-negative bacilli. J Infect Dis 133:35, 1976.
10. Pollack M, Young LS: Protective activity of antibodies to exotoxin A and lipopolysaccharide at the onset of *Pseudomonas aeruginosa* septicemia in man. J Clin Invest 63:276, 1979.
11. Buchanan RE, Gibbons NE (eds): Bergey's Manual of Determinative Bacteriology, 8th ed. Baltimore, William & Wilkins, 1974.
12. Brenner DJ, Farmer JJ III, Hickman FW, Ashbury MA, Steigerwalt AG: Taxonomic and Nomenclature Changes in *Enterobacteriaceae.* Atlanta, Center for Disease Control, 1977.
13. Stossel TP: Phagocytosis. N Engl J Med 290:717, 1974 (Part One); 290:774, 1974 (Part Two); 290:833, 1974 (Part Three).
14. Müller-Eberhard HJ: Complement. Ann Rev Biochem 44:697, 1975.
15. Young LS, Stevens P: Cross-protective immunity to gram-negative bacilli: Studies with core glycolipid of *Salmonella minnesota* and antigens to *Streptococcus pneumoniae.* J Infect Dis 136 (Suppl):S174, 1977.
16. Robbins JB, Myerowitz RL, Whisnant JK, Argaman M, Schneerson R, Handzel ZT, Gotschlich EC: Enteric bacteria cross-reactive with *Neisseria meningitidis* groups A and C and *Diplococcus pneumoniae* types I and III. Inf Immun 6:651, 1972.
17. Young LS, Armstrong D: Human immunity to *Pseudomonas aeruginosa.* I. In vitro interaction of bacteria, polymorphonuclear leukocytes, and serum factors. J Infect Dis 126:257, 1972.
18. Young LS, Meyer RD, Armstrong D: *Pseudomonas aeruginosa* vaccine in cancer patients. Ann Intern Med 79:518, 1973.
19. Berdischewsky MT, Young LS: Infectious complication of neoplastic disorders and their management. In Franklin EC (ed): Clinical Immunology Update. New York, Elsevier North Holland, 1979, p 307.
20. Young LS, Armstrong D: *Pseudomonas aeruginosa* infections. CRC Crit Rev Clin Lab Sci 3:291, 1972.
21. Brachman PS: Epidemiology of nosocomial infections. In Ben-

nett JV, Brachman PS (eds): Hospital Infections. Boston, Little, Brown, 1979, p 9.

22. Goldmann DA, Maki DG, Bennett JV: Intravenous infusion-associated infections, chap 26. In Bennett JV, Brachman PS (eds): Hospital Infections. Boston, Little, Brown, 1979, p 443.
23. Lorber B, Swenson RM: Bacteriology of aspiration pneumonia. A prospective study of community- and hospital-acquired cases. Ann Intern Med 81:329, 1974.

ENTEROBACTERIACEAE

24. Tillotson JR, Lerner AM: Characteristics of pneumonias caused by *Escherichia coli*. N Engl J Med 277:115, 1967.
25. Orskov I, Orskov F, Jann B, Jann K: Serology, chemistry and genetics of O and K antigens of *Escherichia coli*. Bact Rev 41:667, 1977.
26. Anderson ET, Young LS, Hewitt WL: Antimicrobial synergism in the therapy of gram-negative rod bacteremia. Chemotherapy 24:45, 1978.
27. Reyes E: Rhinoscleroma. Observations based on a study of two hundred cases. Arch Dermatol 54:531, 1946.
28. Wilfert JN, Barrett FF, Kass EH: Bacteremia due to *Serratia marcescens*. N Engl J Med 279:286, 1968.
29. Silverblatt FJ: Host parasite interactions in the rat renal pelvis. A possible role for pili in the pathogenesis of pyelonephritis. J Exp Med 140:1696, 1974.
30. Bottone EJ: *Yersinia enterocolitica:* a panoramic view of charismatic microorganism. CRC Crit Rev Microbiol 5:211, 1977.
31. Black RE, Jackson RJ, Tsai T, Medvesky M, Shayejani M, Feeley JC, McLeod KI, Wakelee AM: Epidemic *Yersinia enterocolitica* infection due to contaminated chocolate milk. N Engl J Med 298:76, 1978.
32. Poland JD: Plague. In Hoeprich PD (ed): Infectious Diseases: A Modern Treatise of Infectious Processes. Hagerstown, Harper & Row, 1977, p 1050.
32a. Lipsky BA, Hook EW III, Smith AA, Plorde JJ: Citrobacter infections in humans: Experience at the Seattle Veterans Administration Medical Center and a review of the literature. Rev Infect Dis 2:746, 1980.
33. Jordan GW, Hadley WK: Human infection with *Edwardsiella tarda*. Ann Intern Med 70:283, 1969.
34. Myerowitz RL, Medeiros AA, O'Brien TF: Recent experience with bacillemia due to gram-negative organisms. J Infect Dis 124:239, 1971.
35. Lau WK, Young LS, Black RE, Winston DJ, Linne SR, Weinstein RJ, Hewitt WL: Comparative efficacy and toxicity of amikacin/carbenicillin versus gentamicin/carbenicillin in leukopenic patients: a randomized prospective trial. Am J Med 62:959, 1977.

PSEUDOMONADS

36. Young LS: The role of exotoxins in the pathogenesis of *Pseudomonas aeruginosa* infections. J Infect Dis 142:626, 1980.
37. Buck AC, Cooke EM: The fate of ingested *Pseudomonas aeruginosa* in normal persons. J Med Microbiol 2:521, 1969.
38. Moody MR: Effect of acquisition on the incidence of *Pseudomonas aeruginosa* in hospitalized patients. In Young VM (ed): *Pseudomonas aeruginosa:* Ecological Aspects and Patient Colonization. New York, Raven, 1977, p 111.
39. Farmer JJ III, Herman LG: Epidemiological fingerprinting of *Pseudomonas aeruginosa* by the production of and sensitivity of pyocin and bacteriophage. Appl Microbiol 18:760, 1969.
40. Fisher MW, Devlin HB, Gnabasik FJ: New immunotype schema for *Pseudomonas aeruginosa* based on protective antigens. J Bacteriol 98:835, 1969.
41. Wretlind B, Mollby R, Wadstrom T: Separation of two hemolysins from *Aeromonas hydrophila* by isoelectric focusing. Infect Immun 4:503, 1971.
42. Forkner CE, Frei E III, Edgcomb JH, Utz JP: *Pseudomonas* septicemia. Observations on twenty-three cases. Am J Med 25:877, 1958.
43. Dorff GJ, Geimer NJ, Rosenthal DR, Rytel MW: *Pseudomonas* septicemia. Illustrated evolution of its skin lesion. Arch Intern Med 128:591, 1971.
44. Reyes MP, Palutke WA, Wylin RF, Lerner AM: *Pseudomonas* endocarditis in the Detroit Medical Center. Med 52:173, 1973.
45. Alexander JW, Fisher MW, MacMillan BG: Immunological control of *Pseudomonas* infection in burn patients: a clinical evaluation. Arch Surg 102:31, 1971.
46. Taplin D, Bassett DCJ, Mertz PM: Foot lesions associated with *Pseudomonas cepacia*. Lancet 2:568, 1971.
47. Spotnitz M, Rudnitzky J, Rambaud JJ: Melioidosis pneumonitis. Analysis of nine cases of a beginning form of melioidosis. JAMA 202:950, 1967.
48. Gilardi GL: *Pseudomonas maltophilia* infections in man. Am J Clin Pathol 51:58, 1969.
49. Gilardi GL: Infrequently encountered *Pseudomonas* species causing infection in humans. Ann Int Med 77:211, 1972.
50. Von Graevenitz A, Weinstein J: Pathogenic significance of *Pseudomonas fluorescens* and *Pseudomonas putida*. Yale J Biol Med 44:265, 1971.

CHAPTER 6
Anaerobic Bacteria

SYDNEY M. FINEGOLD

THERE is considerable disagreement as to how to define an anaerobe. A practical operational definition is that an anaerobe is a bacterium that requires reduced oxygen tension for growth; it cannot grow on the surface of solid media in 10 percent carbon dioxide in air (18 percent oxygen). Facultative organisms can grow in either the presence or the absence of air. The term microaerophilic is commonly used for organisms that grow poorly or not at all in air but that will grow distinctly better under 10 percent carbon dioxide in air (reduced oxygen content) or anaerobically. Aerotolerant organisms are anaerobes that tolerate oxygen well enough to grow to some extent on the surface of freshly prepared solid media.

CLASSIFICATION

Anaerobic bacteria are represented by all morphologic types. The most commonly encountered are the gram-negative anaerobic bacilli, which are seen in at least one-third of clinically significant anaerobic infections. Although there are a large number of gram-negative anaerobic cocci, the gram-positive anaerobic cocci are generally more important. The gram-positive spore-forming anaerobic rods are next to last in frequency of isolation from clinical infections, but they are important as potent toxin producers and can produce devastating disease. Finally, there are gram-positive non-spore-forming anaerobic bacilli, but only *Actinomyces* and *Arachnia* are of much clinical significance.

Table 6-1 is a simplified classification of the anaerobes that are of greatest clinical importance. Five organisms or groups taken together account for two-thirds of all clinically significant anaerobic infections. Included are the *Bacteroides fragilis* group, the *B. melaninogenicus–B. asaccharolyticus* group, *Fusobacterium nucleatum*, the anaerobic cocci, and *Clostridium perfringens*. A table is included on the common anaerobic pathogens in each of the chapters on regional infections.

GRAM-NEGATIVE BACILLI

Bacteroides and *Fusobacterium* are the pathogenic organisms of the gram-negative non-spore-forming rods. The others are of much less clinical significance. Because of their fastidious requirements for growth and the inability to form spores, *Bacteroides* and *Fusobacterium* are apparently commensal with people. They contribute to the normal flora of the mouth, the intestines, and the female genital tract and, as strict anaerobes, can produce foul odor and gas. Many grow slowly, taking a week or longer for identification, which delays the start of appropriate drug therapy for the patient.

Although most *Bacteroides* species are pleomorphic, *B. fragilis* is a nonpleomorphic, nonfilamentous organism, difficult to distinguish from *E. coli*. It is frequently associated with *E. coli*. *B. fragilis* is the most clinically significant of these bacilli. It is the most common anaerobic organism in clinical infections and septicemia.

B. melaninogenicus (group) is usually found mixed with other species of *Bacteroides*. Although it is difficult to maintain in pure culture, it grows well when mixed with other anaerobes. This organism is active in establishing synergistic infections: without the presence of *B. melaninogenicus*, mixed oral or intestinal anaerobic bacteria injected subcutaneously into animals do not cause infection.

Fusobacterium and *Bacteroides* have been implicated in many localized infections. The ear, nose, and throat regions were common sites of infection by anaerobes before the widespread use of penicillin and tetracycline for the treatment of undiagnosed acute pharyngitis. Other infections attributed to the gram-negative anaerobic organisms are abscesses of the abdominal cavity and pelvis, acute appendicitis, lung, liver, and brain abscesses, infections of the gallbladder, perirectal infections, and pilonidal and sebaceous cyst infections. *Bacteroides* infection often causes thrombophlebitis and secondary septic embolization to the liver, lungs, peritoneum, and joints. *Bacteroides* bacteremias are more frequently recognized now, with most cases originating from the gastrointestinal tract. Most of the *Fusobacterium* bacteremias originate from upper respiratory sites.

GRAM-POSITIVE COCCI
(*Peptococcus* and *Peptostreptococcus*)

Peptostreptococcus is the more significant pathogen and has been associated with anaerobic myositis, septic abortion, liver abscesses, and empyema as well as with *Bacteroides* in a variety of mixed infections. Both *Peptococcus* and *Peptostreptococcus* can produce a foul odor and gas. Both organisms occur normally in the vagina, mouth, and feces. Because *Peptostreptococcus* and *Bacteroides* have a similar commensal distribution, the anaerobic strepto-

TABLE 6-1 MAJOR ANAEROBES ENCOUNTERED CLINICALLY

Gram-negative bacilli
Bacteroides fragilis group
especially B. fragilis, B. thetaiotaomicron;
B. distasonis, B. ovatus, B. vulgatus
B. melaninogenicus
B. asaccharolyticus
B. ruminicola
B. oralis
B. bivius
B. disiens
Fusobacterium nucleatum
F. necrophorum
F. mortiferum
F. varium
Gram-positive cocci
Peptococcus
Especially *P. magnus, P. asaccharolyticus, P. prevotii*
Peptostreptococcus
Especially *P. anaerobius, P. intermedius* * *P. micros*
Microaerophilic streptococci *
Gram-positive spore-forming bacilli
Clostridium perfringens
C. ramosum
C. septicum
C. novyii
C. histolyticum
C. sporogenes
C. sordellii
C. bifermentans
C. fallax
C. difficile
C. inocuum
C. botulinum
C. tetani
Gram-positive non-spore-forming bacilli
Actinomyces (israelii, meyerii, naeslundii, odontolyticus, viscosus)
Arachnia propionica
Bifidobacterium eriksonii
Propionibacterium acnes

* Not true anaerobes

cocci and *Bacteroides* are frequently found together in infections.

Peptococcus has been shown to be a frequent cause of infected sebaceous cysts, breast abscesses, and joint and finger infections.

GRAM-POSITIVE SPORE-FORMING BACILLI

Clostridium

The characteristics, classification, and pathogenic properties of the clostridia are best understood of all the anaerobic bacilli. They are the only spore-forming anaerobic organisms, and their identification depends on the demonstration of spores, which can be difficult in the case of *C. perfringens* and *C. ramosum*. *C. perfringens,* the most common pathogenic species, does not produce spores in tissues. Although most of the clostridia are obligate anaerobes, two species, *C. tertium* and *C. histolyticum,* can grow aerobically, and C. *perfringens* is quite aerotolerant. Less than a dozen of the 100 species of clostridia are associated with human disease. Tetanus produced by *C. tetani* and botulism caused by *C. botulinum* are more properly described as intoxications rather than infections (Chapter 47). In addition to *C. perfringens,* the less common *C. novyi* and *C. septicum,* and the still rarer *C. histolyticum, C. bifermentans,* and *C. fallax* are all capable of causing myonecrosis (gas gangrene), anaerobic cellulitis, septic abortions, and operative wound infections. *C. difficile* causes pseudomembranous colitis. Clostridia are found as part of the normal bowel flora, in the soil, and irregularly in the mouth and female genital tract.

GRAM-POSITIVE NON-SPORE-FORMING BACILLI

Actinomyces

A. israelii and *A. naeslundii* have both been identified as a part of the normal flora of the mouth. *A. israelii* also occurs in the intestines of humans, but never exists as a saprophyte outside of the body. Most strains of *A. israelii* are obligate anaerobes and will not grow on Sabouraud medium, which typically supports fungal growth. Clinical infections by this organism are always endogenous, complex, and accompanied by anaerobic cocci, *B. melaninogenicus, Actinobacillus actinomycetemcomitans,* and staphylococci. These concomitant organisms are effective because they lower the oxidation-reduction potential and secrete enzymes that facilitate tissue invasion by disrupting the mechanical structure of the tissues. Sulfur granules can usually be detected in the purulent material obtained from *Actinomyces* infections. The gram-positive rods result from fragmentation of the short branching filaments and can often be confused with those of *Propionibacterium acnes,* but the catalase-positive activity of the latter will distinguish the two organisms. *A. viscosus,* however, is also catalase-positive.

Propionibacterium

The anaerobic diphtheroid *Corynebacterium acnes* has been reclassified as *Propionibacterium acnes.* This organism is significant because it is probably the most prominent bacterium of the normal skin flora and is often a contaminant in mixed cultures. It also occurs in the mouth and in the intestinal tract. *P. acnes* can be confused with *A. israelii.* In rare instances, *P. acnes* has been implicated as a primary pathogen in cases of sinusitis, infected prosthetic devices, and endocarditis either with or without rheumatic heart disease.

Other gram-negative non-spore-forming rods (*Eubacterium, Bifidobacterium,* and *Lactobacillus*) have seldom been associated with clinical infections.

GRAM-NEGATIVE COCCI

Veillonella

Veillonella is the most common gram-negative anaerobic cocci found in people. This strict anaerobe is found normally in the mouth, upper respiratory tract, vagina, and intestinal tract. Strains of *Veillonella* have been identified from abscesses, cysts, pleural fluid, and bronchial infections, usually in combination with other anaerobic or aerobic bacteria. Their role in infection is probably minor.

GROWTH CHARACTERISTICS

Certain characteristics of the anaerobes present problems in clinical identification.[1-3] For example, gram-positive anaerobic bacteria commonly destain and may therefore appear gram-negative. Occasionally, young gram-negative forms appear to be gram-positive or contain gram-positive granules. Certain short bacilli, *B. melaninogenicus–B. asaccharolyticus* group, commonly look like cocci. On occasion, cocci may be pleomorphic enough to appear to be short rods. Spores are often difficult to detect. This is especially true in the case of *C. perfringens*. Finally, some of the anaerobic organisms, particularly a number of clostridia, are aerotolerant and will grow to some extent on the surface of culture media. Thus, it can be difficult to decide whether or not a given organism is anaerobic, although experienced bacteriologists usually do not find these characteristics to be major problems. Table 6-2 lists certain microscopic characteristics and the morphologic features of colonies of the more common anaerobic bacteria.

The most simple and practical way to cultivate clinical anaerobic bacteria is in a GasPak jar. After appropriate plates are inoculated and placed into this jar, the anaerobic atmosphere is created by adding 10 ml of water to a commercially available gas-generating packet and then placing the lid on the jar. Hydrogen and carbon dioxide are liberated, and the hydrogen combines with oxygen in the jar, in the presence of catalysts incorporated in a basket on the underside of the jar lid to produce water and make conditions within the jar anaerobic. The procedure is so simple that house staff members, if provided with the jars and appropriate plate media, can set up the cultures themselves if necessary. However, specialized techniques are required to ensure that anaerobes growing on the plate do not die, to determine that a given colony represents a true anaerobe and not a facultative organism, and to identify the organisms accurately. Jars should not be opened until after 48 hours of incubation. The jars should only be opened by experienced bacteriologists to examine plates and to subculture. When results are needed as soon as possible, duplicate samples can be taken so one jar can be opened early, or a Bio-Bag can also be used. One or two petri dishes can be placed in a plastic Bio-Bag, which incorporates a gas-generating system that can be activated after the bag is sealed. The plates can be examined through the bag without exposing them to oxygen.

ANAEROBES AS NORMAL FLORA

Anaerobes are prevalent as normal flora throughout the body, and most surgical anaerobic infections arise from indigenous organisms that gain entrance to deeper or devitalized tissues.[4] If an infection occurs in relation to a given mucosal surface, the normal flora at that site can provide a guide to the specific organisms that should be encountered (Fig. 6-1). It is also important to recognize that anaerobes are prevalent as normal flora so that specimens for culture will be obtained in such a way as to preclude mixing in normal flora with organisms causing the infection.

Table 6-3 lists the normal anaerobic flora at various sites throughout the body. All mucosal surfaces are heavily populated with anaerobic as well as aerobic bacteria. Anaerobes always outnumber aerobic or facultative bacteria. In the mouth and upper respiratory tract, anaerobes outnumber aerobes 10 to 1. In the colon, anaerobes outnumber aerobes 1,000 to 1. Thus, *E. coli* makes up only one-tenth of one percent of the total colonic flora, and the *B. fragilis* group is numerically dominant. In addition to mucosal surfaces, the skin also has an indigenous flora which includes certain anaerobes, particularly *P. acnes* and anaerobic cocci.

The normal anaerobic flora can be modified by disease, impaired drainage, and antimicrobial therapy. Normally, the stomach contains less than 10^3 organisms per ml and obligate anaerobes are absent. The small bowel flora is also relatively simple, with total counts of 10^4 to 10^5 per ml, or less, except for the distal ileum, where counts range from 10^6 per ml to somewhat higher levels. High in the small bowel, the flora consists entirely of gram-positive facultative forms—streptococci, lactobacilli, and yeasts. The further one goes distally in the small bowel, the more the flora varies. In the terminal ileum, there are equal numbers of aerobes and anaerobes. The major anaerobes encountered are *Bacteroides* and *Bifidobacterium*, the latter usually nonpathogenic in the setting. In the presence of bleeding or obstructing duodenal ulcer or with gastric ulcer or carcinoma, the flora of the stomach and upper small bowel are usually more profuse and may include anaerobes, coliforms, and other organisms found in fecal flora. The impact of antimicrobial therapy will, of course, depend on levels of drug achieved and the susceptibility of the normal flora. Thus, a knowledge of the pharmacology and antibacterial spectrum of various antimicrobial drugs will permit one to anticipate which elements of the normal flora will be suppressed, and to what extent, and also to predict which resistant organisms are likely to colonize that area. Because the normal flora of the body constitutes one of the most important defense mechanisms, antimicrobial agents should be used only when specifically indicated.

INCIDENCE AND TYPES OF ANAEROBIC INFECTIONS

Anaerobic bacteria may participate in any type of infection caused by any type of bacterium.[5-14] No organ or tissue is immune. Well-documented data of the impressive incidence of anaerobic bacteria in major infections involving the lung and pleural space, intra-abdominal sites, and the female genital tract have been available for some time. Additional data continually accumulate to indicate that anaerobes are important in many other categories of infection throughout the body. Table 6-4 shows a number of types of surgical infections in which anaerobes are common. Table 6-5 correlates the specific anaerobic bacteria recovered with the type of infection.

TABLE 6-2. MICROSCOPIC CHARACTERISTICS AND MORPHOLOGY OF COLONIES OF COMMONLY ENCOUNTERED ANAEROBES

	Microscopic Morphology	Morphology of Colonies on Blood Agar
Bacteroides fragilis group	Gram-negative bacilli with rounded ends, pleomorphic, may be coccobacillary, may show vacuolation and bipolar staining	Convex, entire, white-gray, semitranslucent, may be mucoid, shiny
Bacteroides melaninogenicus–B. asaccharolyticus group	Gram-negative short bacilli with rounded ends, often coccobacillary	Convex, entire edge, glistening or dull, yellow-beige-brown to black depending on length of incubation, medium, etc.
Fusobacterium nucleatum	Gram-negative bacilli, slender, spindle-shaped with tapered ends, sometimes in pairs end to end	Convex, glistening with internal irridescent flecking or raised opaque "bread crumb" colonies. Greening of medium
Fusobacterium necrophorum, F. mortiferum, F. varium	Very pleomorphic, filamentous, irregularly staining, gram-negative bacilli. Swellings along filaments. Large, free round bodies.	Often "fried egg" colonies. Raised center; flat, irregular periphery. Center opaque, edge translucent
Peptococcus	Gram-positive spherical cocci, occurring singly, in pairs, short chains, and irregular clumps	Convex, gray to white, opaque, shiny, entire edge. Small
Peptostreptococcus	Gram-positive spherical or elongated cocci, occurring singly, in pairs, or in chains	Convex, gray to white, opaque, shiny or dull, entire edge. Small
Clostridium perfringens	Gram-positive bacilli, broad, relatively short, with blunt ends. Spores rare	Low convex, semiopaque, shiny, entire, with double zone of hemolysis: narrow zone of complete hemolysis surrounded by a larger zone of incomplete hemolysis
Other clostridia	Thin to broad gram-positive bacilli. May or may not show spores	
Gram-positive nonsporeforming bacilli		
Bifidobacterium	Pleomorphic; often have bifurcated ends, but may be club-shaped or coccobacillary	
Propionibacterium	Regular or club-shaped, palisading or "Chinese-letter" arrangement may be seen	
Actinomyces	Thin, filamentous, long, branching	
Arachnia	Thin, filamentous, long, branching	

SURGICAL EPIDEMIOLOGY

Almost all anaerobic infections are endogenous. In the case of *Clostridium*, an organism widely distributed in soil and nature, there may be occasional exogenous infections, particularly relating to trauma. Nevertheless, most cases of clostridial myonecrosis that follow war injury are of endogenous origin and are primarily related to difficulties in maintaining good personal hygiene under battle conditions. Also, clostridial myonecrosis after operation is probably caused by a patient's own fecal flora rather than by spores of clostridia in the operating suite (even though the latter have been found).

Anaerobic infection may be facilitated by diagnostic

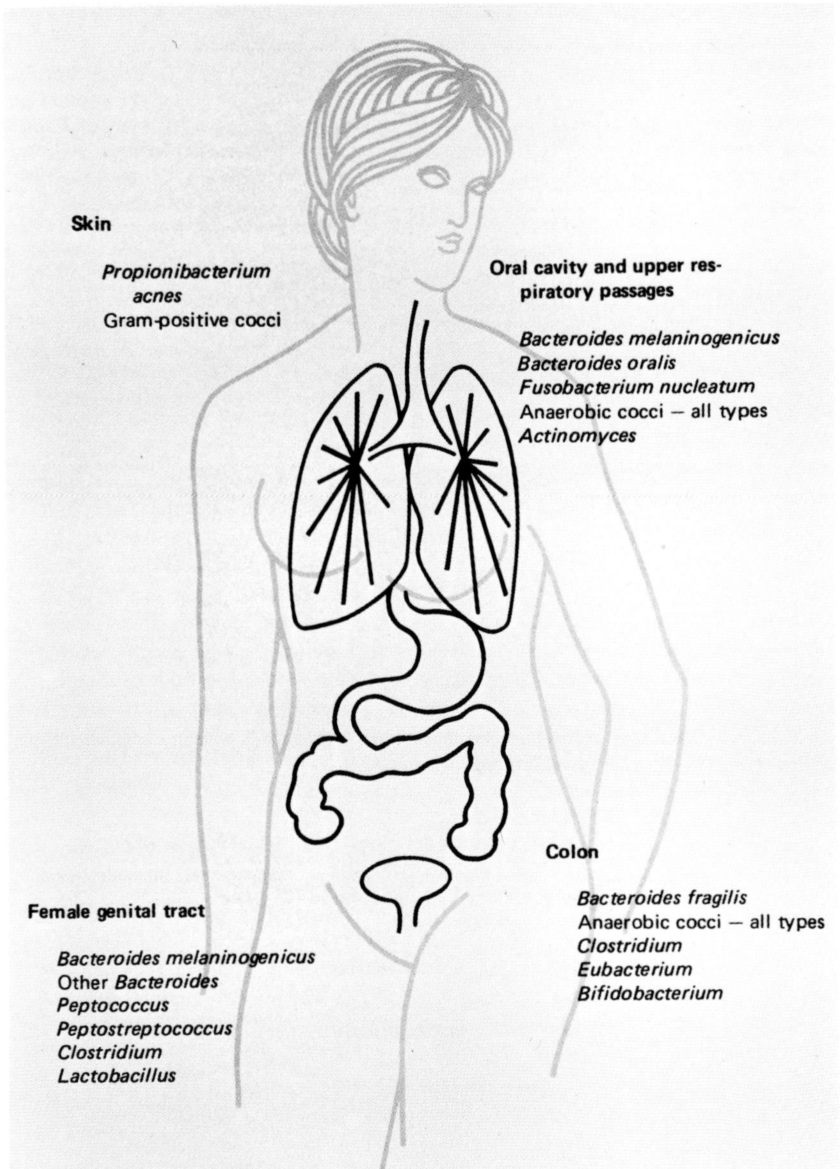

Fig. 6-1. Predominant anaerobes of the normal flora.

TABLE 6-3. INCIDENCE OF VARIOUS ANAEROBES AS NORMAL FLORA IN HUMANS

	Clostridium	*Actinomyces*	*Bifidobacterium*	*Eubacterium*	*Lacto Bacillus* †	*Propionibacterium*	*Bacteroides*	*Fusobacterium*	Cocci *Gram-positive*	*Gram-negative*
Skin	0	0	0	±	0	2	0	0	1	0
Upper respiratory tract *	0	1	0	±	0	1	1	1	1	1
Mouth	±	1	1	1	1	±	2	2	2	2
Intestine	2	±	2	2	1	±	2	1	2	1
External genitalia	0	0	0	U	0	U	1	1	1	0
Urethra	±	0	0	U	±	0	1	1	±	U
Vagina	±	0	1	±	2	1	1	±	1	1

U = Unknown; 0 = Not found or rare; ± = Irregular; 1 = Usually present; 2 = Usually present in large numbers

* Includes nasal passages, nasopharynx, oropharynx and tonsils

† Includes anaerobic, microaerophilic, and facultative strains

TABLE 6-4. SURGICAL INFECTIONS COMMONLY INVOLVING ANAEROBES

	Incidence (%)	Proportion of Cultures Positive for Anaerobes Yielding Only Anaerobes
Bacteremia	20	4/5
Central nervous system		
Brain abscess	89	1/2–2/3
Extradural or subdural empyema	10	
Head and neck		
Chronic sinusitis	52	4/5 *
Chronic otitis media	56	1/10
	33	0
Neck space infections	100	3/4
Wound infection following head and neck surgery	95	0
Dental, oral, facial		
Dental and oral		
Orofacial, of dental origin	94	4/10
Bite wounds	47	1/34
Thoracic		
Aspiration pneumonia	93	1/2 †
	62	1/3
	100	1/3
Lung abscess	93	1/2–2/3
	85	3/4
Bronchiectasis		
Empyema (nonsurgical)	76	1/3
	62	1/2
Abdominal		
Intra-abdominal infection (general)	86	1/10
	90	1/3
	81	1/3
	94	1/7
Appendicitis with peritonitis	96	1/100
Liver abscess	52	1/3
Other intra-abdominal infection (postsurgery)	93	1/6
Wound infection following bowel surgery	45	0
Biliary tract	41	2/117
Obstetric-gynecologic		
Miscellaneous types	100	1/3
	74	1/3
	72	
Pelvic abscess	88	1/2
Vulvovaginal abscess	75	1/4
Vaginal cuff abscess	98	1/30
Septic abortion, sepsis	67	
	63	
Pelvic inflammatory disease	25	1/14
	48	1/7
Soft tissue and miscellaneous		
Nonclostridial crepitant cellulitis	75	1/12
Pilonidal sinus	73+	
Diabetic foot ulcers	95	1/20
Soft tissue abscesses	60	1/4
Cutaneous abscesses	62	1/5
Decubitus ulcers with bacteremia	63	
Osteomyelitis	40	1/10
Gas gangrene (clostridial myonecrosis)		
Breast abscess		
Perirectal abscess		

* 23/28 cultures (82%) yielding heavy growth of one or more organisms had only anaerobes present

† Aspiration pneumonia occurring in the community, rather than in the hospital, involves anaerobes to the exclusion of aerobic or facultative forms two-thirds of the time

Modified from Sutter VL, Citron DM, Finegold SM [3]

and therapeutic modalities used in the hospital that lead to impaired blood supply, tissue necrosis, and breakdown of mucosal barriers, which create ideal conditions for invasion and multiplication of anaerobes from the normal flora. Radiation, cytotoxic drugs, and corticosteroids generally predispose to infection, anaerobic or otherwise. Antimicrobial therapy may select out resistant anaerobes, such as *B. fragilis*, which may then cause infection under appropriate conditions. Transmission of infection caused by anaerobes from animal to man has been rarely documented. Human-to-human transmission is even more rare, with the exception of certain venereal diseases. Infection following bites, animal or human, frequently involves anaerobic organisms. Administration of anesthetics or drugs that compromise consciousness, of course, may predispose to aspiration and subsequent pulmonary infection.

PATHOGENESIS OF ANAEROBIC INFECTIONS

PREDISPOSING CONDITIONS

Essentially all anaerobic infections arise indigenously. Under certain circumstances, anaerobes of the indigenous flora have an opportunity to penetrate tissues and to cause infection. Poor vascular supply and necrosis of tissue lower the oxidation-reduction potential, favoring their growth. The oxidation-reduction potential of the intestinal tract, necrotic tissue, and abscess cavities ranges from −150 to −250 mV. Accordingly, factors that predispose to anaerobic infection include vascular disease, epinephrine injection, cold, shock, edema, trauma, operation, foreign bodies, malignancy, and gas production by microorganisms. Prior infection with aerobic or facultative bacteria also makes conditions more favorable for anaerobic growth by lowering the potential. Under certain circumstances, such as aspiration pneumonia, the normal flora may be carried into another area normally free of bacteria and set up an infection.

As with infection involving aerobic or facultative bacteria, conditions that impair host defense mechanisms and prior antimicrobial therapy to which the infecting organisms are resistant (ie, aminoglycosides in the case of anaerobes) may pave the way for anaerobic infection.

AEROTOLERANCE

Certain elements of the normal flora which are sensitive to oxygen appear to be unable to participate in infections. In general, the pathogenic anaerobes are more aerotolerant—some surprisingly so. This feature, of course, permits these organisms to survive, after the normally protective mucosal barrier is broken, until conditions are satisfactory for their multiplication and further invasion. After the process has started, anaerobes can multiply rapidly and maintain their own reduced environment by virtue of excretion of end products of fermentative metabolism, including short-chain fatty acids, organic acids, and alcohols.

MIXED INFECTIONS

Two-thirds of the infections in which anaerobes participate are mixed, with both anaerobes and facultative or occasionally aerobic bacteria participating together.[7] Participation of the anaerobes in these mixed infections is often facilitated by the nonanaerobes. Lowering of the oxidation-reduction potential by growth of the nonanaerobes has already been mentioned. Other bacteria may also supply anaerobes with necessary growth factors. This has been demonstrated in mixed infections involving *B. melaninogenicus*, which often requires vitamin K or analogues and whose growth may be stimulated by hemin. In some cases, the mucosal barrier may have been penetrated early in the course of an infection by only facultative bacteria. Thus, acute otitis media and acute sinusitis typically involve only facultative bacteria, but chronic otitis media and chronic sinusitis often include anaerobes or are mixed. There are examples of specific synergy, such as postoperative bacterial synergistic gangrene, which requires the combination of a microaerophilic (or sometimes anaerobic) streptococcus and *Staphylococcus aureus* (or sometimes a gram-negative facultative bacillus) (Chapter 8).

Involvement of anaerobes in infections may depend on resistance of certain of these organisms to normal defense mechanism (Chapter 13). This may include resistance to normal bactericidal activity of serum and to phagocytosis. This will be discussed further.

ENZYMES

Superoxide dismutase has been found in a number of anaerobes, including members of the *B. fragilis* group. In general, there is a good correlation between superoxide dismutase activity and oxygen tolerance. Although catalase is found in some anaerobes, such as some members of the *B. fragilis* group, there is no relationship between catalase activity and oxygen tolerance. A number of anaerobes produce beta-lactamases which account for their resistance to cephalosporins and, to a lesser extent, to penicillins. Plasmids which code for resistance to several antimicrobial agents and for transferable resistance have been found in *Bacteroides* and in *Clostridium*. These points will be discussed in the treatment section.

EXOTOXINS

In the case of clostridia, the most virulent of all anaerobes, various exotoxins produced by these organisms are responsible for the nature of the local lesions and the systemic manifestations.[15,16] However, the modes of action of the toxins and the individual importance of each are complex and unclear. Lecithinases, such as those produced by *C. perfringens* (alpha toxin) and *C. novyi* (gamma toxin), can damage or destroy cell membranes. Capillaries are made freely permeable to fluid and protein, and the resulting extravasation of fluid can cause increased anoxia in tissues. Lysis of red blood cells by alpha toxin of *C. perfringens* is almost certainly the cause of the hemolytic anemia and hemoglobinuria seen in sepsis with this organism. The collagenases of *C. perfringens* and *C. histolyticum* destroy collagen barriers in the tissues and thus prevent localization of the infection. Destruction of reticulin around capillaries leads to hemorrhage and thrombosis, with further decrease in the oxidation-reduction potential. Proteolysis provides additional amino acids and peptides for bacterial growth. The hyaluronidase of *C. perfringens* greatly facilitates spread of the organism through the tissues. Other factors produced by pathogenic clostridia presumably are important in pathogenesis as well, but it is difficult to prove. Included would be deoxyribonucleases *(C. perfringens* and *C. septicum)*, lipases *(C. novyi)*, proteinases *(C. histolyticum)*, and fibrinolysins. Other toxins produced by clostridia include hemolysins, neuraminidase, phospholipase, lysolecithinase, elastase, and leukocidin. *C. perfringens* and *C. difficile* both produce an enterotoxin. *C. difficile*, the cause of pseudomembranous colitis related to antimicrobial therapy, also produces a toxin that causes a cytopathic effect on almost all tissue culture cell lines.

The gram-negative anaerobic rods also produce certain exotoxins.[15] *B. melaninogenicus* is one of the few organisms that produce collagenase. Certain *Bacteroides* produce neuraminidase. *B. fragilis* produces a heparinase which may contribute to intravascular clotting, and leads to a requirement for increased dosage of heparin in treating the septic thrombophlebitis which may be seen during the course of this infection. *B. asaccharolyticus* has extensive proteolytic activities, rendering it capable of hydrolysing gelatin, casein, coagulated protein, plasma protein, and azacol, as well as collagen. *F. necrophorum* produces a leukocidin. Most strains of *B. melaninogenicus*, ss. *intermedius*, produce a lipase. All species of the *B. fragilis* group, except for *B. vulgatus*, produce extracellular hyaluroni-

TABLE 6-5. INCIDENCE (PERCENT) OF SPECIFIC ANAEROBES IN VARIOUS INFECTIONS (WADSWORTH MEDICAL CENTER EXPERIENCE, 1973–1978)

	Specimen Source or Type of Infection					
Anaerobes	***Blood***	***Central Nervous System***	***Wound Infections Following Head and Neck Surgery***	***Dental***	***Human Bites***	***Animal Bites***
Number of Specimens Surveyed	(58)	(6)	(49)	(8)	(18)	(16)
B. fragilis	48*	0	0	0	0	0
B. thetaiotaomicron	10	0	0	0	0	0
Other bile resistant *Bacteroides* *	9	0	0	0	0	0
B. melaninogenicus ss *melaninogenicus*	2	0	45	13	28	0
B. melaninogenicus ss *intermedius*	0	17	53	13	50	13
B. melaninogenicus no subspecies	0	0	14	0	0	0
B. asaccharolyticus	0	0	4	0	0	13
Bile sensitive saccharolytic *Bacteroides* †	7	0	82	25	44	6
B. ureolyticus	0	0	4	0	6	0
Other *Bacteroides* sp ‡	7	17	49	13	22	13
F. nucleatum	3	50	47	0	22	19
F. necrophorum	7	0	2	25	0	0
F. mortiferum-varium grp	2	0	0	0	0	0
Other *Fusobacterium* sp §	2	0	4	13	0	75
Other gram-negative bacilli	2	0	2	0	0	6
Peptostreptococcus sp	2	0	43	50	33	6
Peptococcus sp	7	0	37	150	11	19
Veillonella sp	2	0	43	25	50	13
Other gram-negative cocci	0	0	6	0	0	0
C. perfringens	3	0	0	0	0	0
Other *Clostridium* sp	12	0	0	0	6	0
Actinomyces sp	0	67	2	50	0	0
Bifidobacterium sp	0	0	4	0	0	0
Lactobacillus sp	0	0	22	25	0	0
P. acnes	5	0	8	0	6	19
Other *Propionibacterium* sp	0	0	4	13	6	38
Eubacterium sp	3	0	27	13	6	13

* *B. Distasonis, B. vulgatus, B. ovatus, B. uniformis, B. splanchnicus, B. eggerthii.*
† *B. ruminicola* ss *brevis, B. ruminicola* ss *ruminicola, B. oralis, B. bivius, B. disiens.*
‡ Includes nonspeciable *Bacteroides* sp.
§ Includes nonspeciable *Fusobacterium* sp.

Modified from Sutter, Citron, Finegold[3]

Specimen Source or Type of Infection							
Transtracheal Aspirates; Pleural Fluid	*Miscellaneous Soft Tissue Infections Above the Waist*	*Intra-abdominal Infections*	*Peri-rectal abscess*	*Decubitus ulcers*	*Foot ulcers*	*Miscellaneous Soft Tissue Infections Below the Waist*	*Osteomyelitis*
(143)	(41)	(114)	(15)	(16)	(70)	(37)	(32)
4	5	54	73	56	39	24	6
1	0	32	53	25	11	8	6
3	0	33	33	31	10	10	0
20	0	8	13	0	6	3	6
31	22	12	0	19	13	11	3
4	5	4	0	25	6	0	13
3	10	9	13	13	13	5	3
47	34	17	20	25	19	14	13
9	10	5	7	0	7	3	13
36	70	29	27	31	19	14	31
22	20	14	13	6	3	5	6
3	5	4	0	0	1	0	3
0	0	5	7	0	1	3	0
13	2	8	7	0	1	3	0
3	2	0	7	0	0	0	0
13	22	29	13	44	24	41	38
22	29	27	20	69	81	46	106
30	12	6	7	6	3	5	0
0	0	3	0	0	0	0	0
4	5	21	13	6	4	8	0
6	0	51	93	63	11	3	3
12	10	0	0	13	4	14	9
6	0	2	0	0	0	5	6
18	12	17	7	13	9	3	3
4	2	4	0	0	6	3	19
2	7	1	0	0	1	5	0
21	15	47	20	6	14	16	19

dase and chondroitin sulfatase. Elastase is rarely found in *Bacteroides.* Other enzymes produced by certain members of the genus *Bacteroides* include fibrinolysin, lysozyme, lecithinase, deoxyribonuclease, phosphatase, protease, and lipase.

ENDOTOXINS

There have been a number of studies of the endotoxin of various gram-negative anaerobic rods.[15] In the case of the *Bacteroides fragilis* group, the endotoxin does not contain lipid A, 2-keto-deoxyoctanate, or heptose. It also lacks beta-hydroxymyristic acid. This endotoxin exhibits poor biologic activity in various test systems. *B. asaccharolyticus* also does not have any beta-hydroxymyristic acid and its endotoxin is biologically impotent. *B. melaninogenicus* endotoxin contains no 2-keto-deoxyoctanate or heptose, and it and the endotoxin of *B. oralis* show weak biologic activity. The endotoxins of *F. necrophorum* and *F. nucleatum* vary to some extent from strain to strain in terms of content of 2-keto-deoxyoctanate and sugars and in biologic activity, but many or most strains show strong biologic activity, comparable to that of *Salmonella enteritidis.*

HOST DEFENSE MECHANISMS AND IMMUNITY

The oxidation-reduction potential of healthy tissues is well above levels necessary for anaerobic growth. Thus, anaerobes cannot multiply in normal tissues. Atraumatic inoculation of guinea pigs with toxin-free spores of *Clostridium tetani* does not cause tetanus. Wounds, however, are by their very nature traumatic, and it is trauma that both initiates colonization by anaerobes and provides the atmosphere for their multiplication. Vascular damage or vascular insufficiency is probably the most important predisposing factor for anaerobic infection. Tissue damage results in a fall in both Eh and pH, and these changes, together with the breakdown of protein to produce amino acids, leads to conditions highly favorable to the growth of anaerobic bacteria. Postoperative gas gangrene following clean operations is most often encountered in patients with arterial insufficiency—patients with diabetes mellitus, atherosclerosis, and frostbite. Operations that require the use of tourniquets or bloodless field techniques favor growth of anaerobes introduced into the operative site. The same is true for procedures in which there is imperfect hemostasis, excessive heat coagulation of tissues, or prolonged and traumatic use of retractors. War wounds are the classic examples of wounds that contain large amounts of necrotic tissue, providing suitable conditions for anaerobic bacterial invasion. In addition, neither cellular nor humoral components of the host defense systems can reach the bacteria in an avascular microenvironment.

Both cell-mediated and humoral immunity may be important in protection against anaerobic infections. Certain anaerobes, such as *B. melaninogenicus,* may inhibit phagocytosis and the killing of other organisms that may be found together with *B. melaninogenicus* in mixed infection. The capsules of certain organisms, such as *B. fragilis, B. asaccharolyticus,* and *C. perfringens,* may be important factors in determining anaerobic infection. The mechanism by which the capsule facilitates infection with these organisms remains to be determined. There is no evidence that the capsule interferes with phagocytosis, but it is a possibility. It is interesting to note that *B. fragilis* strains adhere to rat peritoneal mesothelium better than unencapsulated species of *Bacteroides.*

Polymorphonuclear leukocytes have both oxygen-dependent and oxygen-independent microbicidal systems. Components of both of these systems might be important in phagocytic killing of anaerobes under conditions of varying oxygen tension. Studies performed to date have not provided a clear-cut picture of the situation. One study indicated normal killing of *B. fragilis* within polymorphonuclear leukocytes under anaerobic conditions, and another study noted normal killing of this organism under aerobic conditions. Neither random migration of polymorphonuclear leukocytes nor chemotaxis in response to factors generated by immune complexes in plasma differed significantly under aerobic or anaerobic conditions. However, chemotaxis in response to factors generated by bacteria in plasma was depressed under anaerobic conditions; one of the organisms used in this study was *B. fragilis.*

B. fragilis is more resistant to the normal bactericidal activity of serum than are other members of the *B. fragilis* group. *Fusobacterium mortiferum* is killed by serum alone or serum plus white blood cells under both aerobic and anaerobic conditions. *B. thetaiotaomicron* and *B. fragilis* are phagocytosed and killed intracellularly by human polymorphonuclear leukocytes in the presence of normal serum, but not by either leukocytes or serum alone, under anaerobic conditions. In an aerobic environment, similar results are obtained except that *B. fragilis* is phagocytosed and killed intracellularly to some extent in the absence of serum.

Immunoglobulin and components of the alternate complement pathway participate in opsonization of *B. fragilis* and *B. thetaiotaomicron.* Antibody to the capsular polysaccharide of *B. fragilis* can be induced in animals by infection with encapsulated strains or by implantation of the capsular material itself (along with outer membrane components which stimulate antibody response). This type of immunization confers significant protection in animals against subsequent abscess development caused by *B. fragilis.* Furthermore, a study of women with acute pelvic inflammatory disease demonstrated antibody to the capsular antigen of *B. fragilis* in those in whom *B. fragilis* was part of the infecting flora.[17]

Various techniques have been used to demonstrate antibodies in animals experimentally infected and in people undergoing natural infection. With some of the gram-negative anaerobic bacilli, there may be significant cross-reactions between species. Normal subjects can also show antibody to various gram-negative anaerobic bacilli.

Endotoxins of gram-negative anaerobic bacilli have been studied for their influence on blastic transformation of lymphocytes and on polymorphonuclear leukocyte migration. The reactions are proportionate to the potency of the endotoxin and therefore more impressive in the case of *Fusobacterium* than with *Bacteroides.*

TABLE 6-6. CLUES TO ANAEROBIC INFECTION

1. Four odor to specimen
2. Location of infection in proximity to a mucosal surface
3. Infections secondary to human or animal bite
4. Gas in specimen
5. Previous therapy with aminoglycoside antibiotics (such as neomycin, gentamicin, and amikacin)
6. Black discoloration of blood-containing exudates; these exudates may fluoresce red under ultraviolet light (*B. melaninogenicus, B. asaccharolyticus* infections)
7. Presence of "sulfur granules" in discharges (actinomycosis)
8. Unique morphology on Gram stain
9. Failure to grow, aerobically, organisms seen on Gram stain of original exudate
10. Growth in anaerobic zone of fluid media or of agar deeps
11. Growth anaerobically on media containing 75 to 100 μg/ml of kanamycin, neomycin, or paromomycin (or medium also containing 7.5 μg/ml of vancomycin, in the case of gram-negative anaerobic bacilli)
12. Characteristic colonies on agar plates anaerobically (eg, *F. nucleatum* and *C. perfringens*)
13. Young colonies of *B. melaninogenicus* and *B. asaccharolyticus* may fluoresce red under ultraviolet light (blood agar plate)

It is clear that *B. fragilis* is involved in infection more commonly than other members of the same group (such as *B. vulgatus* or *B. ovatus*), despite the fact that *B. fragilis* may be outnumbered by these other members in the normal colonic flora. This may be due to encapsulation of *B. fragilis* in contrast to the lack of a capsule in other members of the *B. fragilis* group. As suggested earlier, the capsule may interfere with host defense mechanisms. The same may apply to *B. asaccharolyticus*, which appears to be more important in infection than *B. melaninogenicus*, which is not encapsulated.

DIAGNOSTIC CONSIDERATIONS

A list of clues suggesting that a patient may have an anaerobic infection is given in Table 6-6. The only specific clue to anaerobic infection is foul or putrid odor to secretions. Only anaerobic infection produces this type of odor, although the absence of a foul odor does not exclude anaerobes from being involved in infection. Certain anaerobes, particularly some of the cocci, do not produce the end products of metabolism that have this characteristic odor. In other cases, there will not be communication between the infected site and the examiner's nose. The remainder of the clues are not specific but nonetheless are helpful, particularly when two or more are present together. Location of infection in proximity to a mucosal surface is, of course, a clue because this is a major location for indigenous anaerobic flora. Tissue necrosis and gas in tissues or discharges are nonspecific, even though they are commonly encountered with anaerobic infections. They can also occur in other types of infection and in the absence of infection, but they should make one suspect an anaerobic infection. Three types of malignancy have a special association with anaerobic infections—bronchogenic carcinoma, carcinoma of the colon, and uterine cancer.

CLINICAL SPECIMEN COLLECTION AND TRANSPORT

Specimen collection and transport are important considerations if the surgeon wishes to document the roles of anaerobes in an infection.[1-3] The best anaerobic bacteriology laboratory is necessarily limited by the nature of the specimen submitted and the care that was taken in transporting it. Table 6-7 lists the recommended methods of specimen collection for a variety of anaerobic infections (also see Chapter 12, Fig. 12-1).

Ideally, all types of specimens should be cultured for anaerobes for these simple reasons: (1) anaerobes are commonly involved in a variety of infections; (2) any type of infection may involve these organisms; and (3) many nonanaerobic organisms (especially streptococci) will grow better under anaerobic conditions than aerobically. There are practical limitations, however. Anaerobes are so prevalent as normal flora that no specimen likely to be contaminated with normal flora should be cultured for anaerobic organisms. This only imposes an unnecessary chore on the bacteriology laboratory and provides data that can be seriously misleading. The following types of specimens should *not* routinely be set up for anaerobic culture: gingival or oral swabs, gastric contents, small bowel contents, feces, expectorated sputum, voided urine, vaginal or endometrial swabs, and bronchoscopic brushings when specially protected brushes are not available. In certain instances, exceptions will have to be made. For example, in suspected "blind loop syndrome" quantitation of the aerobic or facultative and anaerobic flora of the small bowel of afferent

TABLE 6-7. RECOMMENDED SPECIMEN COLLECTION METHODS FOR ANAEROBIC CULTURE

Source	Procedure
Pulmonary	Percutaneous transtracheal aspiration or direct lung puncture. Medi Tech double catheter and bronchial brush for bronchoscopic specimens
Pleural	Thoracentesis
Urinary tract	Suprapubic percutaneous bladder aspiration
Abscesses	Needle and syringe aspiration of closed abscess. Use of swabs is much less desirable
Female genital tract	Use culdocentesis to obtain specimens, when possible, after decontaminating the vagina with povidone iodine. Medi Tech double catheter and bronchial brush or sterile swab for uterine cavity specimens (not suitable for postpartum endometritis)
Sinus tracts or draining wounds	Aspiration by syringe and small plastic catheter introduced as deeply as possible through decontaminated skin orifice. Specimen obtained at surgery from depths of wound or underlying bone lesion always preferable. Curettings and tissue biopsies provide excellent material

gastric loop contents may be important in diagnosis and in guiding therapy.

The most important consideration is to protect the organisms in the specimen from exposure to oxygen. Even brief exposure will kill some species. Whenever possible, obtain a specimen by needle and syringe—bubbles of air or gas should be expelled from both. After collection the needle can be plunged into a solid rubber stopper (as for a blood gas analysis), and the syringe itself will serve as the transport vehicle. Plastic syringes, however, will eventually permit air to diffuse through the plastic. Thus, unless specimens transported by plastic syringe can be received in the laboratory and set up in anaerobic culture within 20 to 30 minutes, this procedure is not satisfactory. Most often a gassed-out transport tube represents the optimum type of transport. Such tubes should incorporate an oxidation-reduction indicator, such as resazurin which turns pink on exposure to even trace amounts of oxygen, in a small amount of liquid or agar nonnutritive medium in the bottom of the tube. The specimen is inoculated through the rubber stopper into the tube. Although anaerobes will survive in this type of atmosphere for several days, cultures should be set up within 2 to 3 hours, or the tube refrigerated (15C) to avoid the overgrowth of coexistent facultative organisms.

When it is impossible to use a needle and syringe to obtain a specimen, a swab must be used, although it is always less satisfactory. The swab is put up in an anaerobic atmosphere, and the stick of the swab is imbedded in the rubber stopper. A companion tube contains a deep column of semisolid transport medium such as Cary and Blair medium in an anaerobic atmosphere. The swab is removed from its container at the last possible moment and then inserted in the specimen. Then the stopper is removed from the tube containing the transport medium and the swab and stopper inserted into that tube. Although both the swab and the transport medium are exposed to air briefly, the swab ends up at the bottom of the semisolid medium, where conditions remain quite anaerobic, despite the manipulations. A number of other types of transport setups, many of them commercially available, can be used (Chapter 12).

It is important that the specimen be examined directly by Gram stain to determine the suitability of the specimen (by noting the types of cells present, for example) and to gain immediate information about the types and number of bacteria present. Certain of the anaerobes, such as *C. perfringens* and many of the gram-negative anaerobic bacilli, have distinctive morphologic characteristics. Because anaerobes grow more slowly than facultative or aerobic bacteria, and because it may take quite a while to complete the bacteriologic examination of a specimen from a polymicrobial mixed infection (as is commonly true in anaerobic infections), it is helpful to be able to determine the infecting organisms in a matter of minutes.

Special Collection Problems

Aspiration Pneumonia

Obtaining a proper specimen when aspiration pneumonia is suspected is a major problem. If there is a complicating empyema, the empyema fluid will ordinarily reflect the bacterial flora of the parenchymal disease, and information obtained from blood cultures may be useful if bacteremia is present. However, most cases of aspiration pneumonia or other anaerobic pulmonary infection are not complicated by bacteremia. Even when bacteremia occurs, only one or two of the many organisms present are cultured. Thus, at least in patients who are seriously ill, it is often desirable to do percutaneous transtracheal aspiration to bypass normal upper respiratory tract flora and to obtain the true infecting flora. Patients with severe hypoxia, hemorrhagic diathesis, or severe intractable cough should not be subjected to this procedure. If bronchoscopy is indicated to remove aspirated particulate matter, a double-sheathed bronchial brush may permit the retrieval of a reliable specimen for anaerobic and aerobic culture. (The effectiveness of this procedure is not yet established.) Without meticulous care and the use of such a double protected brush, however, normal and transient oral flora, which may or may not actually be involved in the aspiration pneumonia, will be inadvertently cultured.

Female Genital Infection

In the case of female genital tract infections with cul de sac abscess, culdocentesis after decontamination of the vaginal wall with povidone iodine should yield the etiologic agents. Some claim that a few drops of material obtained by culdocentesis, without a cul-de-sac collection, will accurately reflect the bacteriology of the deeper infection. The double-protected bronchoscopy brushes may be used to obtain material from the endometrial cavity in the case of endometritis. This would not be reliable in postpartum endometritis, since there is significant contamination of the endometrial cavity with vaginal flora after delivery.

SPECIAL DIAGNOSTIC TESTS

Direct gas liquid chromatography of clinical specimens may, occasionally, provide important clues to the presence of certain gram-negative anaerobic bacilli.[3] Presence of large amounts of butyric acid in the absence of isobutyric or isovaleric acids is indicative of the presence of *Fusobacterium* species. The presence of succinic acid in a specimen that shows only gram-negative bacilli on Gram stain is indicative of *Bacteroides*. The presence of both succinic and isobutyric acid in a specimen indicates that *Bacteroides* is present. Fluorescent antibody procedures have been developed for identification of *Actinomyces* and of certain gram-negative anaerobic bacilli in clinical material. The reagents for *Actinomyces* are not generally available, and it is not yet clear how valuable and reliable fluorescent antibody procedures are for identification of gram-negative anaerobic rods.

Serologic tests are not yet practical diagnostic aids. Commercial polyvalent gas gangrene antitoxin, or its *C. sordellii* antitoxin component, will neutralize the toxin produced by *C. difficile*, the cause of pseudomembranous colitis related to antimicrobial therapy. Thus, the use of such antibody to block the cytopathic effect of *C. difficile* toxin in tissue culture constitutes a diagnostic test. Both the organism and its toxin may be present in the absence of pseudomembranous colitis; therefore, it is necessary to demonstrate the presence of the typical plaques or pseudomembrane in addition to the toxin.

PROTOTYPIC INFECTIONS

In general, anaerobic infections are characterized by abscess formation and tissue destruction. Some prototypic infections will be discussed here, and some are covered in greater detail in other chapters.

BRAIN ABSCESSES

Brain abscess begins as an acute suppurative encephalitis and eventually becomes localized and encapsulated; 90 percent of brain abscesses yield anaerobic bacteria. The most important underlying condition is chronic otitis media, with or without mastoiditis. Infection of the lung or pleural space is the second most common underlying condition for anaerobic brain abscess, and chronic sinusitis is third. Other underlying conditions include dental or oral infection, infection in the tonsillar or pharyngeal area, congenital heart disease, and trauma. Gram-negative anaerobic bacilli and anaerobic and microaerophilic streptococci are the most common etiologic agents; however, anaerobes of all other types occasionally may be found (Chapter 28).

ASPIRATION PNEUMONIA

Aspiration pneumonia, a common postoperative complication, involves oral anaerobic bacteria in almost all cases. The three major anaerobes found are the *B. melaninogenicus–B. asaccharolyticus* group, *Fusobacterium nucleatum*, and anaerobic cocci.

There is a distinct difference, however, between aspiration pneumonia occurring in the community and that occurring within the hospital. Community-acquired aspiration pneumonia (ie, an individual aspirating after a cerebrovascular accident at home) involves primarily anaerobic bacteria from the oral flora and thus is ordinarily best treated with penicillin G. *B. fragilis* or other beta lactamose-producing anaerobes may be recovered from 15 percent of the cases, but many patients with *B. fragilis* as part of a mixed flora will nonetheless respond to penicillin.

Aspiration within the hospital frequently involves, in addition to anaerobes of the oral flora, potential nosocomial pathogens which have colonized the upper respiratory tract. This includes such organisms as *S. aureus* and a variety of gram-negative bacilli such as *Klebsiella, Enterobacter, Serratia, Pseudomonas,* and *Proteus.* Colonization of the upper respiratory tract with these nosocomial pathogens is more common in the very ill, elderly patients who have received antimicrobial drugs, and those hospitalized for some time. Therapy for this type of aspiration pneumonia, of course, is much more difficult. In addition to penicillin G, one must use aminoglycosides and, when *S. aureus* is present, a penicillinase-resistant penicillin or other appropriate agent. The earliest manifestation of the disease is pneumonitis alone. Without effective therapy, necrotizing pneumonia or lung abscess, either of which may be complicated by empyema, can occur. Because aspiration is the background for this type of pneumonia, the disease involves dependent pulmonary segments. The major cause for aspiration is compromised consciousness but dysphagia accounts for some cases. Principal causes of compromised consciousness include alcoholism, cerebrovascular accident, general anesthesia, drug ingestion, and seizure disorder. The dysphagia may be related to neurologic disorder or esophageal stricture. Certain nonanaerobic bacteria, such as *S. aureus* and *Klebsiella pneumoniae,* are more likely to induce abscess formation than other organisms but among the anaerobes there seems to be no particular difference with regard to species of anaerobe involved as to whether or not there will be necrotizing pneumonia or abscess formation (Chapter 30).

INTRA-ABDOMINAL INFECTION

Intra-abdominal infection, particularly peritonitis and intra-abdominal abscess, is discussed in Chapter 34. Anaerobes can be recovered from the majority of such infections but are seldom recovered in pure culture.[12] Most infections are mixed with both anaerobes and facultative or aerobic bacteria. In most of these infections, the source of the organism is the bowel flora, particularly the flora of the colon. Accordingly, the *B. fragilis* group, and *B. fragilis* and *B. thetaiotaomicron* in particular, is recovered regularly. Other gram-negative anaerobic rods may be found on occasion. Anaerobic cocci are commonly found, as are clostridia, especially *C. perfringens* and *C. ramosum.* Among the aerobes, *E. coli, Klebsiella,* and enterococci are encountered most commonly in patients who have not had their bowel flora modified by prior antimicrobial therapy or disease.

POSTABORTAL SEPSIS

Anaerobes are important in postabortal sepsis. Although clostridia account for only a small percentage of these infections, they often cause the most severe and dramatic illnesses. Clostridial infection of the uterus starts as a localized chorioamnionitis with invasion in the placenta of a dead fetus. This process, known as fetal emphysema, is relatively benign, but the gaseous vaginal discharge, crepitus of the uterine wall, and striking radiographic findings may make it difficult to distinguish from more serious infections. The next stage is a low-grade endometritis with vaginal discharge and uterine tenderness, with or without gas formation. The most severe form of this process extends beyond the endometrium to the uterine muscle and results in necrosis, which may be accompanied by perforation, peritonitis, and bacteremia. The patient is toxic, exhibits tachycardia out of proportion to the fever, and has uterine and abdominal pain and foul gaseous vaginal discharge that reveals numerous clostridia on direct Gram stain. A unique and dramatic clinical picture accompanies severe clostridial sepsis—hemolytic anemia, hemoglobinemia, hemoglobinuria, disseminated intravascular coagulation, bleeding tendency, bronze-colored skin, hyperbilirubinemia, shock, and anuria. *C. perfringens* is the key pathogen in patients with sepsis and hemolytic anemia. It may also be important in less severe cases of postabortal sepsis, along with anaerobic streptococci, gram-negative anaerobic bacilli (including, at times, *B. fragilis*), other clostridia, aerobic streptococci (most often group A), and coliforms.

GAS GANGRENE

A classic, but fortunately uncommon, variety of anaerobic infection is clostridial myonecrosis, or gas gangrene.[16] The term gas gangrene should be limited to those infections that invade muscle and produce massive necrosis of tissue. It is a clinical syndrome, and clostridial species other than *C. perfringens* may be involved. Gas gangrene usually manifests itself with a sudden appearance of pain and heaviness in the region of an injury. The onset may be so sudden that it suggests a vascular accident. The pain steadily increases in severity but remains localized, spreading as the infection itself spreads. Soon local edema and a thin hemorrhagic exudate can be noted. The tachycardia is out of proportion to the slight elevation of temperature. The skin is tense, white, often marbled, colder than normal, and very tender. Bronze discoloration increases with time. Local swelling and toxemia increase gradually, and the serous discharge becomes more profuse. Bullae filled with dark red or purplish fluid appear, and gas becomes manifest, although usually in relatively small amounts. A peculiar sweet smell may be present. The patient may remain clear mentally with a profound terror of impending death; a toxic delirium is also characteristic. Later, there may be overwhelming prostration and toxemia. As time goes on, there may be a drop in blood pressure. The patient has a peculiar gray pallor, weakness, and profuse sweating.

The evidence of the disease at the skin surface and the clinically demonstrable gas are relatively minor compared to the extensive involvement of underlying muscle, which can be seen only at operation. At first the muscle is pale and edematous, but later the color changes, the blood supply is lost, contractility disappears, and gas may be seen. As the disease progresses, the muscle becomes red with mottled purple and the consistency becomes pasty or mucoid. Finally, the muscle is diffusely gangrenous, dark greenish purple or black, friable, and even liquefied.

C. perfringens is present in 80 percent of cases, *C. novyi* in 40 percent, *C. septicum* in 20 percent, and *C. bifermentans*, a few. *C. histolyticum*, and *C. fallax* are uncommon. The diagnosis of clostridial myonecrosis is made clinically. When material can be obtained for Gram stain, the characteristic large, relatively broad, gram-positive (or gram-variable) bacilli may be an important clue, as is disruption of white blood cells caused by the action of the toxin. Definitive identification of clostridia in the wound is not of great value, however, because many wounds, particularly traumatic wounds, may be colonized with these organisms without evidence of infection. It is crucial to keep in mind that the infection may spread rapidly and irreversible tissue changes may develop in a matter of hours. Accordingly, immediate operative exploration is indicated when suspicion exists. It is important to recognize also that gas gangrene may occur after elective surgery, especially operations on the lower limbs, bowel, and gallbladder. A common error is to leave casts, splints, or dressings undisturbed. At the slightest suspicion of infection, they must be removed and the wound thoroughly inspected.

PSEUDOMEMBRANOUS COLITIS

The primary cause of antimicrobial agent–induced pseudomembranous colitis is now known to be the toxins of *C. difficile*. Whether the postoperative pseudomembranous colitis sometimes seen prior to the antimicrobial era was also due to this organism is unknown. Similarly, it is not known whether ischemic colitis may be caused by this organism and its toxin. Essentially all antimicrobial agents with the exception of vancomycin are capable of inducing this complication, but it is seen most often after clindamycin, lincomycin, ampicillin, and less often the cephalosporins. The entire spectrum of clinical colitis can be seen ranging from a relatively mild diarrhea to severe intractable diarrhea, toxic megacolon, perforation of the colon, shock, and sometimes death. The sine qua non of antibiotic-associated pseudomembranous colitis is the presence of the distinctive elevated yellowish plaques on the colonic mucosa, or frank pseudomembrane. Recovery of *C. difficile*, even in high numbers, and demonstration of the cytotoxin of this organism, even in high titer, do not necessarily establish the diagnosis, because these may be seen on occasion in the course of antimicrobial therapy without any evidence of colon pathology. Proctoscopic examination is the best way to establish the diagnosis. It must be kept in mind, however, that some lesions, particularly early in the course of the illness, may be found only on the right side of the colon so that colonoscopy may be necessary.

The toxin of *C. difficile* is cytopathic for numerous tissue culture cell lines. The cytopathic effect can be abolished by prior incubation of the toxin with commercial polyvalent gas gangrene antitoxin or the antitoxin to *C. sordellii*, one of the components of the polyvalent mixture. Antitoxin to the toxin of *C. difficile* is difficult to prepare and is not generally available. An enterotoxin is also produced.

Various factors determine the likelihood of an individual developing pseudomembranous colitis on antimicrobial therapy. A toxin-producing strain of *C. difficile* must be present in the colon either as a component of the indigenous flora or as the result of nosocomial spread. *C. difficile* must either be resistant to the agent being used or would have to survive in small numbers until the agent was discontinued. In the latter case, *C. difficile* then would multiply and produce sufficient toxin to cause the disease before the normal flora could be reestablished. The offending antimicrobial agent would presumably have had to suppress the normal colonic flora sufficiently to permit overgrowth by the toxin-producing organism; this means not only an appropriate antibacterial spectrum but also sufficient levels of drug in the colonic lumen itself. Presumably, the host might have antitoxic immunity, which could prevent the disease regardless of the amount of toxin produced—this remains to be established.

INTESTINAL OVERGROWTH SYNDROMES

Bowel bacterial overgrowth syndromes (blind loop syndrome) may result from prior operations, such as production of an afferent loop or ileal bypass for obesity, and operation may be required to correct the cause of bacterial overgrowth in the bowel. The steatorrhea and macrocytic anemia, which are important findings in this process, are a result of deconjugation of bile acids and adsorption of vitamin B_{12}, usually high in the small bowel. Various anaerobes, notably members of the *B. fragilis* group, are important in this regard, along with other types of organisms (Chapter 38).

INFECTION IN MALIGNANCY

The strong association between *C. septicum* infection and malignancy should be mentioned. Carcinoma of the colon, in particular, should be suspected in patients who have infection with *C. septicum*.

ACTINOMYCOSIS

Actinomycosis is frequently grouped with fungal infections because of its clinical resemblance. *A. israelii* is actually an anaerobic bacterium which is part of the normal pharyngeal flora and is the usual cause of actinomycosis in people, although *A. naeslundi* or other members of the genus, as well as *Arachnia*, have been implicated in human disease. *A. bovis* is primarily a pathogen of swine and cattle. The bacterium is an anaerobic gram-positive rod which grows in thin filamentous strands at 37C. Tangled masses of organisms form macroscopic specks known as sulfur granules, which are the hallmark of the infection.

Actinomycosis is a chronic suppurative infection producing abscess cavities, separated by bands of fibrosis and interconnected by fistulous tracts. At the periphery of the lesion, granulomas consisting of large, lipid-laden macrophages can sometimes be found imparting a yellow color to the tissue. Spread may be hematogenous but is usually by direct extension.

Three main types of infection are recognized—cervicofacial, thoracic, and abdominal.[14] Cervicofacial disease usually begins in the mouth or oropharynx, commonly the result of a break in the normal protective barriers (eg, gingivitis). The infection extends into adjacent bone and burrows through soft tissues, producing multiple abscesses with interconnecting fistulas and sinus tracts that drain to the skin surface. Pus expressed from the sinus tracts frequently contains the sulfur granules, the matted masses of organisms which are characteristic of actinomycosis. There is little pain until the infection is far advanced.

Pulmonary actinomycosis is a chronic fibrosing and abscess-forming infection, which frequently resembles tuberculosis. As in any aspiration pneumonia, the abscesses may also contain multiple organisms from the mouth. Direct involvement of the pleura and adjacent ribs is common, but free pleural effusions are rare. The symptoms of pulmonary infection are mild fever, cough, and the production of purulent sputum. With more chronic disease, anemia and weight loss are common.

Abdominal actinomycosis frequently begins as a fistula on the abdominal wall. The organism gains access to the peritoneal cavity either by hematogenous spread from the oral pharynx or by direct penetration of the bowel mucosa (from within by a sharp object such as a fishbone or from without by a penetrating wound). Appendicitis may be a primary source of abdominal actinomycosis.

There have been recent reports of chronic endometrial actinomycosis, most frequently related to intrauterine devices used for contraception. The infection may spread to the adjacent fallopian tubes.

Osteomyelitis caused by actinomycosis is indistinguishable from hematogenous osteomyelitis caused by other bacteria, and can be found in any bone in the body.

Examination of fresh pus from draining sinuses frequently shows the characteristic sulfur granules (Fig. 6-2). They are easiest to find on gauze dressings used to

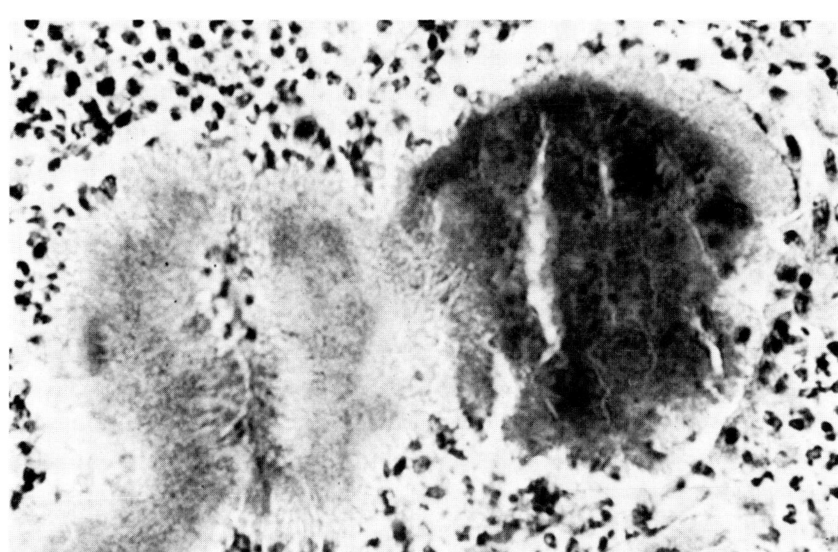

Fig. 6-2. Abdominal actinomycosis. "Sulfur granule" expressed from purulent material draining from fistula. Note the fine filaments of the organisms at the periphery (×472).

cover sinuses, and appear as small 1- to 2-mm yellow granules. Crushed granules stained with Gram stain show gram-positive branching filamentous organisms.

Direct anaerobic culture of pus of resected tissue will frequently yield the organism, although *Actinomyces* is quite fastidious. Small, white mycelial colonies appear in 2 to 5 days and can be subcultured under strict anaerobic conditions.

Skin tests and serology play no role in the diagnosis.

The best treatment is prolonged use of penicillin. High dose intravenous therapy is given for 2 to 3 weeks, followed by oral penicillin for 6 to 12 months. Incision and drainage of abscesses should be done only after institution of penicillin coverage. Clindamycin, and sometimes a tetracycline, or erythromycin can be used in penicillin-sensitive patients.

TREATMENT OF ANAEROBIC INFECTIONS

There are three principles of treatment of anaerobic infections: (1) make the tissue environment hostile for anaerobic proliferation; (2) check the spread of anaerobic bacteria to healthy tissues; and (3) neutralize the toxins.

To control the local environment, a variety of surgical measures includes: debridement of dead tissue, removal of foreign bodies, drainage of pus, elimination of obstructions, release of trapped gas, excision of malignancies, improvement of circulation to the part, and improved oxygenation of tissues. The surgeon must also obtain material by biopsy or aspiration for diagnosis.

Antimicrobial therapy is also important to prevent the spread of infection. In vitro susceptibility tests, properly performed, serve as a good guide to drug therapy for anaerobic infections. Table 6-8 lists the most common anaerobic bacteria and their susceptibility to various agents. In serious anaerobic infections, antimicrobial therapy must be intensive and prolonged, because these infections have a tendency to relapse if therapy is discontinued too soon. In the case of anaerobic pulmonary infections, therapy is usually required for several weeks. Liver abscess and other intra-abdominal infections may require even more prolonged therapy.

B. fragilis is a particular problem; it is both the most commonly encountered of all anaerobes and the most resistant to antimicrobial agents. The susceptibility of *B. fragilis* to a number of different antimicrobial agents is shown graphically in Figure 6-3. The beta-lactamase produced by the *B. fragilis* group is one of the major means by which this organism manifests resistance to certain antimicrobial agents. The beta-lactamases produced are primarily cephalosporinases, but also account for significant destruction of penicillins. Other anaerobic bacteria also produce beta-lactamases (Table 6-9). Anaerobes particularly resistant to one or more antimicrobial agents are listed in Table 6-10.

The nature of the various organisms in mixed infections will influence the choice of drugs. Drugs active against anaerobic bacteria in vitro may be quite inactive against accompanying aerobic or facultative organisms, and vice versa. Other factors that influence choice of drugs include the toxicity of the various agents, whether or not the patient is allergic to given agents, the lack of penetration of the central nervous system (ie, by clindamycin), the excellent bactericidal activity of metronidazole, and the renal and hepatic functional status of the patient. As noted earlier, penicillin G may work perfectly well in an anaerobic pulmonary infection in which *B. fragilis* is part of a mixed flora. This may relate to significant reduction of the bacterial load by the penicillin G so that the body can handle the *B. fragilis* that persists. On the other hand,

TABLE 6-8. SUSCEPTIBILITY OF ANAEROBIC BACTERIA TO ANTIMICROBIAL AGENTS *

	Antimicrobial Agent						
Bacteria	***Penicillin***	***Chloramphenicol***	***Clindamycin***	***Erythromycin***	***Tetracycline***	***Metronidazole***	***Vancomycin***
Bacteroides fragilis group	1	3 †	3	1–2	1–2	3	1
Other Bacteroides	2 †	3	3	3	2–3	3	1
Fusobacterium varium	2 †	3	1–2	1	2–3	3	1
Other *Fusobacterium* sp	4	3	3	1	3	3	1
Microaerophilic and anaerobic cocci	3–4	3	2–3	2–3	1–2	2	3
Actinomyces and *Eubacterium*	4	3	2–3	3	2–3	1–2	2–3
Clostridium perfringens	4 †	3	3 †	3	2	3	3
Other *Clostridium* sp	3	3	2	2–3	2	2–3	2–3

Symbols: 4 = Drug of choice; 3 = Good activity; 2 = Moderate activity; 1 = Poor or inconsistent activity

* Only drugs which might be used therapeutically are included; not all of these agents are routinely used clinically for anaerobic infections and not all are FDA approved.

† A few strains are resistant.

Aminoglycosides, such as gentamicin and kanamycin, are generally quite inactive against the majority of anaerobes. The activity of erythromycin varies significantly according to the testing procedure. Erythromycin and vancomycin are not currently approved by the Food and Drug Administration for anaerobic infections. Other penicillins and cephalosporins are frequently less active than penicillin G. Ampicillin, carbenicillin, and cephaloridine are roughly comparable to penicillin G on a weight basis, but the high blood levels safely achieved with carbenicillin make it effective against 95% of the strains of *Bacteroides fragilis.* Cefoxitin, a compound resistant to penicillinase and cephalosporinase appears promising; it is active vs 90% of *B. fragilis* group strains. One third of the strains of *Clostridium* sp. other than *C. perfringens* are resistant to cefoxitin. Cefamandole is active vs. most anaerobes other than those in the *B. fragilis* group. Doxycycline and minocycline are more active than other tetracyclines, but susceptibility testing is indicated to ensure activity.

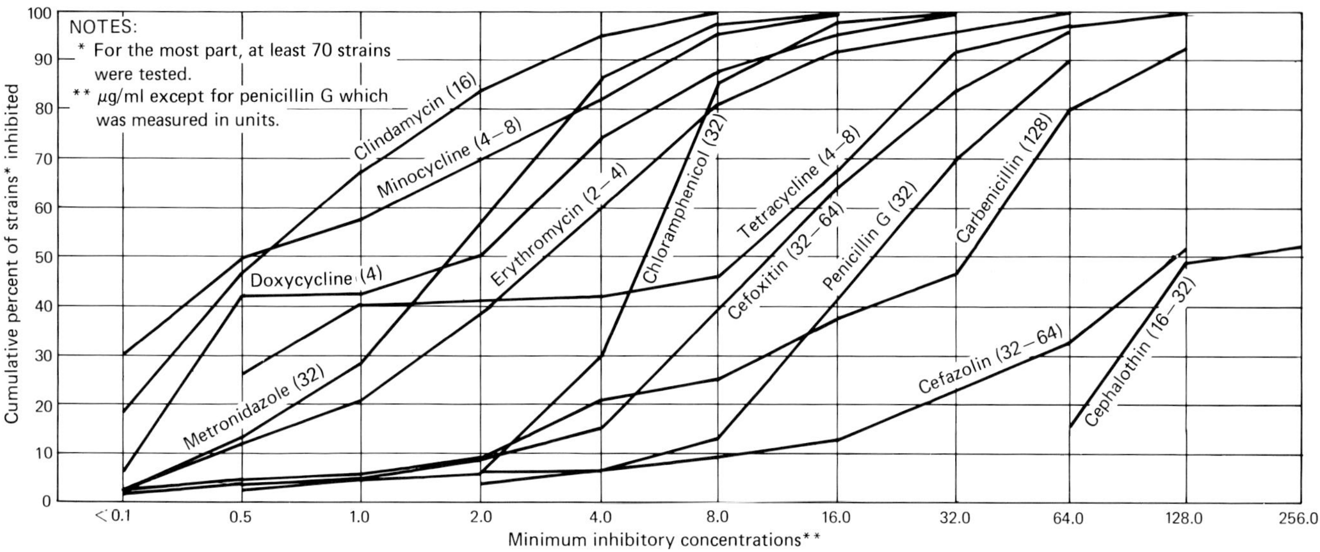

Fig. 6-3. **Susceptibility of *Bacteriodes fragilis* to antimicrobial agents. (Figures in parentheses are usual maximum serum levels.)**

TABLE 6-9. BETA-LACTAMASE-PRODUCING ANAEROBES

Bacteroides fragilis group
B. melaninogenicus–B. asaccharolyticus
B. oralis
B. bivius
B. disiens
B. ruminicola
B. splanchnicus
Clostridium ramosum
C. clostridiiforme

TABLE 6-10. OTHER RESISTANT ANAEROBES

Bacteroides ruminicola—β lactam drugs, tetracycline
B. splanchnicus—penicillin
B. urcolyticus—penicillin, clindamycin
Fusobacterium varium—clindamycin
F. naviforme—penicillin
F. mortiferum—penicillin
Peptococcus—clindamycin
Clostridium ramosum—tetracycline, clindamycin
Other non-*perfringens* clostridia—clindamycin, cefoxitin
Actinomyces, Arachnia—metronidazole

at times such infections involving *B. fragilis* will not respond to penicillin G, so that patients who are very ill with suspected anaerobic pulmonary infection, in whom the bacteriology is not yet worked out, should also received therapy adequate to cover *B. fragilis.* In the case of hospital-acquired aspiration pneumonia, additional therapy may be required for the nonanaerobic bacteria present. Penicillin G remains an excellent drug for anaerobic infections other than those involving *B. fragilis* and related organisms. In serious infections of these types, however, penicillin G should be given in high dosage (10 to 20 million units per day in average-sized adults) because certain of the anaerobes, such as the cocci and *B. melaninogenicus* strains, may have relatively high minimal inhibitory concentrations (5 to 15 units per ml).

In patients with antimicrobial agent–associated pseudomembranous colitis caused by *C. difficile,* discontinuation of the offending antimicrobial agent is the first step. About half of the patients will respond to cholestyramine, a bile acid-binding resin which also binds the toxin of *C. difficile.* In sicker patients, oral vancomycin (500 mg given at 6 hour intervals) should be given for 10 days to 2 weeks. Considerably smaller doses have been used in Great Britain with apparently good results. Patients should be observed carefully for at least 4 to 6 weeks after discontinuation of vancomycin therapy, because relapse can occur.

PREVENTION

The major principles of prophylaxis of anaerobic infections are to avoid conditions that reduce the redox potential of the tissues and prevent the introduction of anaerobes from mucosal surfaces into tissues. Adherence to important surgical principles such as achievement of good hemostasis, avoidance of dead space, gentle handling of tissues during operation, and avoidance of contamination of clean body cavities (for example, using an extraperitoneal approach for drainage of adnexal abscess when possible) is essential. In traumatic wounds, the most effective prophylaxis is thorough debridement and cleansing of the wound, elimination of foreign bodies and dead space, and reestablishment of good circulation. This type of wound management must be carried out as early as possible following the injury. The systemic use of prophylactic antimicrobial agents has not ordinarily been helpful except where there must be significant delay before definitive management of the wound can take place, as in battlefield wounds.

Bathing causes a significant reduction in transient skin organisms, such as *C. perfringens.* A shower seems to yield even greater reduction in skin bacterial count than a tub bath. Iodophors, such as povidone iodine, are sporicidal and are effective in removing *C. perfringens* from skin, provided there is sufficient contact time. Compresses applied for 15 minutes are highly effective. This type of procedure is extremely useful prior to elective surgery, such as hip surgery.

Precautions to minimize the possibility of aspiration will help prevent anaerobic pulmonary infection. Patients should be kept in the head-down position during and immediately following tonsillectomy. Care should be observed in feeding feeble or confused patients, and the head of the bed should be elevated for a time after feeding by gastric tube.

It is clear that prophylactic antimicrobial therapy may be useful in a variety of settings in which anaerobes can participate in infections, such as for patients undergoing bowel surgery. Both oral neomycin plus oral erythromycin, and oral neomycin plus oral tetracycline, have been used effectively in this setting. The principle is to use these drugs for a short period of time so that there is relatively little opportunity for overgrowth of resistant organisms. Parenteral administration of antibiotics for prophylaxis in this setting has also been recommended by some, either alone or together with an oral preoperative bowel preparation (Chapters 23 and 39).

In gallbladder surgery, the possibility of serious clostridial complications must be kept in mind. This problem may be minimized by avoiding trauma to the liver bed and by the prophylactic use of penicillin, which carries little risk of superinfection with resistant organisms.

Conditions predisposing to puerperal sepsis are premature rupture of the membranes, prolonged labor, and postpartum hemorrhage. If labor does not develop following premature rupture of the membranes and the patient is kept at rest in bed, infection is unlikely to occur. With rare exceptions, cesarean section should be performed electively or after not more than 8 to 12 hours of labor. During labor, particularly with ruptured membranes, pelvic and rectal examinations should be kept to a minimum. During delivery, trauma should be minimized and lacerations repaired with accepted surgical principles. Retained portions of the placenta should be removed immediately following the third stage of labor. Excessive blood loss should be corrected immediately postpartum.

BIBLIOGRAPHY

Finegold, SM: Anaerobic Bacteria in Human Disease. New York, Academic, 1977.

Mansheim BJ, Kasper DL: Infections produced by non-sporulating anaerobic bacteria: pathogenisis, microbiology, and clinical manifestations. In Weinstein L, Fields BN (eds): Seminars in Infectious Disease. Vol 2. New York, Stratton Intercontinental Medical Book Corp., 1979, p. 1.

REFERENCES

1. Dowell VR Jr, Hawkins TM: Laboratory Methods in Anaerobic Bacteriology. Bacteriological technics. DHEW Publication No (CDC) 74–8272. Washington, DC, GPO, 1974.
2. Holdeman LV, Cato EP, Moore WEC (eds): Anaerobe Laboratory Manual, 4th ed. Blacksburg, VA, Virginia Polytechnic Institute and State University, 1977.
3. Sutter VL, Citron DM, Finegold SM: Wadsworth Anaerobic Bacteriology Manual, 3rd ed. St Louis, Mosby, 1980.
4. Rosebury T: Microorganisms Indigenous to Man. New York, McGraw-Hill, 1962.
5. Anderson CB, Marr JJ, Ballinger WF: Anaerobic infections in surgery: clinical review. Surgery 79:313, 1976.
6. Balows A, DeHaan RM, Dowell VR Jr, Guze LB (eds): Anaerobic Bacteria: Role in Disease. Springfield, IL, Thomas, 1974.
7. Finegold SM: Anaerobic Bacteria in Human Disease. New York, Academic, 1977.
8. Gorbach SL, Bartlett JG: Anaerobic infections. N Engl J Med 290:1177, 1237, 1289, 1974.
9. Saksena DS, Block MA, McHenry MC, Truant JP: Bacteroidaceae: anaerobic organisms encountered in surgical infections. Surgery 63:261, 1968.
10. Sim FH: Anaerobic infections. Orthop Clin North Am 6:1049, 1975.
11. Smith L DS: The Pathogenic Anaerobic Bacteria, 2nd ed. Springfield, IL, Thomas, 1975.
12. Swenson RM, Lorber B, Michaelson TC, Spaulding EH: The bacteriology of intra-abdominal infections. Arch Surg 109:398, 1974.
13. Willis AT: Clostridia of Wound Infection. London, Butterworths, 1969.
14. Weese WC, Smith IM: A study of 57 cases of actinomycosis over a 36 year period. A diagnostic "failure" with good prognosis after treatment. Arch Intern Med 135:1562, 1975.
15. Kasper DL, Finegold SM: Virulence factors of anaerobic bacteria (Symposium). Rev Infect Dis 1:245, 1979.
16. MacLennan JD: The histotoxic clostridial infections of man. Bacteriol Rev 26:177, 1962.
17. Paavonen J, Valtonen VV, Kasper DL, Malkamaki M, Makela PH: Serological evidence for the role of *Bacteroides fragilis* and Enterobacteriaceae in the pathogenisis of acute pelvic inflammatory disease. Lancet 1:293, 1981.

CHAPTER 7
Microorganisms Infrequently Encountered in Surgery

DALE N. GERDING

THIS chapter is a potpourri of microorganisms rarely encountered by most surgeons and not comprehensively discussed elsewhere in this text. The organisms range from conventional gram-negative and gram-positive bacteria to *Mycobacteria, Nocardia,* spirochetes, rickettsiae, chlamydiae, and *Mycoplasma.* Some cause infections that are specifically related to surgical procedures, particularly in immunosuppressed patients, and many are likely to require surgical consultation for diagnosis or treatment. The discussion of each organism is designed to provide the essentials of identification, pathogenesis, clinical illness, diagnosis, and treatment. Special emphasis has been placed on the clinical features that are of surgical interest and importance.

The number of microorganisms known to cause disease in humans continues to expand, as does knowledge of the type of infection caused by previously known pathogens. These newer aspects of infectious disease have been emphasized, particularly as they apply to the immunocompromised patient. Because of the large number of pathogenic organisms, however, it is not possible to discuss them all. The selecton is somewhat arbitrary, but it is designed to include the organisms that surgeons in the Western world will encounter. Discussions of taxonomy have been minimized because of controversy in this area. Newer nomenclature has been used, but older names and synonyms are included to reduce confusion.

GRAM-POSITIVE BACTERIA

GENUS BACILLUS

Bacillus organisms are aerobic spore-forming bacilli, which are usually gram-positive but may be gram-variable. The majority are nonpathogenic for people, with the notable exception of *B. anthracis,* and are commonly found in soil, water, dust, feces of animals, and animal products. *Bacillus* species have been recognized recently as causative agents of infection, particularly in immunosuppressed patients.

Bacillus Anthracis

Morphology and Identification

Bacillus anthracis (Table 7-1) is the cause of human and animal anthrax. It is a rod-shaped, gram-positive bacillus 1 $\mu m \times 3\text{–}10\ \mu m$. Although it grows best under aerobic conditions it can also grow anaerobically, potentially causing confusion with clostridial organisms. The organism grows well on ordinary culture media at 37C. *B. anthracis* is nonmotile and forms capsules in sodium bicarbonate agar incubation with 5 percent CO_2. Both a gamma phage test and fluorescent-antibody stain are available from the Center for Disease Control for rapid identification. Good bacteriologic safety techniques are essential in handling suspected anthrax specimens; one must especially avoid aerosol production when working with material containing spores.

Epidemiology and Pathogenesis

Approximately 20,000 to 100,000 cases of anthrax occur annually in the world; less than ten occur in the United States each year. Most cases result from contact with animal products, especially goat and sheep hides, hair, wool, and meat. Most recent American cases have been acquired by handlers of imported wool and yarns. Anthrax is acquired by the deposition of *B. anthracis* spores directly into the skin, by inhalation of spores and, rarely, by consumption of contaminated meat. Infection may be confined to local skin lesions or extend to regional lymph nodes in the lung or gastrointestinal tract with production of toxin and necrosis, hemorrhage, and edema.

Clinical Manifestations

The majority of infections are acquired by the cutaneous route and usually remain localized. After a 1- to 7-day incubation, typical skin lesions evolve through an initial papule, which progresses to a vesicle or ring of vesicles, followed by development of a depressed ulcer covered by black eschar. Most lesions occur on the hands, arms, or head and they heal with the formation of a scar. The respiratory syndrome usually begins as a mild, nonspecific, flulike illness with a nonproductive cough. It pro-

TABLE 7-1. CHARACTERISTICS OF INFECTIONS DUE TO MICROORGANISMS ENCOUNTERED INFREQUENTLY BY SURGEONS

Organism	Infection Name	Spread via animal contact	Spread via arthropod vector	Spread via air, food, soil or water	Normal human flora or carrier	Patient to patient transmission
Gram-positive bacteria						
Bacillus anthracis	Anthrax	+++	0	+	0	0
Bacillus species		0	0	++	++	0
Corynebacterium diphtheriae	Diphtheria	0	0	0	+++	+++
Corynebacterium species		0	0	0	+++	0
Listeria monocytogenes	Listeriosis	++	0	+	++	+
Erysipelothrix rhusiopathiae	Erysipeloid	+++	0	+	0	0
Gram-negative bacteria						
Francisella tularensis	Tularemia	+++	+++	+	0	0
Pasteurella multocida		+++	0	+	+	0
Streptobacillus moniliformis	Rat bite fever	+++	0	+	0	0
Spirillum minor	Rat bite fever	+++	0	+	0	0
Eikenella corrodens		0	0	0	+++	0
Bordetella pertussis	Pertussis	0	0	0	+	+++
Hemophilus influenzae		0	0	0	+++	++
H. ducreyi	Chancroid	0	0	0	+	+++
Hemophilus species		0	0	0	+++	+
Calymmatobacterium granulomatis	Granuloma inguinale	0	0	0	+	+++
Brucella species	Brucellosis	+++	0	++	0	0
Vibrio cholerae	Cholera	0	0	+++	+	++
V. parahemolyticus		0	0	+++	0	0
L+ vibros		0	0	+++	0	0
Campylobacter fetus		+++	0	++	+	++
Acinetobacter calcoaceticus		0	0	++	+++	+
Legionella pneumophila	Legionnaires' disease	0	0	+++	0	+
Acid-fast bacteria						
Mycobacterium tuberculosis	Tuberculosis	+	0	0	0	+++
M. bovis	Bovine tuberculosis	++	0	++	0	+++
* *Mycobacteria* of groups I–IV	"Atypical" tuberculosis	+	0	+++	++	0
Mycobacterium leprae	Leprosy	0	0	0	0	+++
Nocardia asteroides	Nocardiosis	0	0	+++	+	0
Spirochetes						
Leptospiral species	Leptospirosis	+++	0	+++	0	0
Borrelia species	Relapsing fever	+	+++	0	0	0
Treponema pallidum	Syphilis	0	0	0	+++	+++
Rickettsia						
Rickettsia rickettsii	Rocky Mountain spotted fever	+	+++	+	0	0
R. typhi	Murine typhus	++	+++	+	0	0
Coxiella burnetii	Q fever	+++	+	+++	0	0
Chlamydiae						
Chlamydia psittaci	Psittacosis	+++	0	+++	0	++
C. trachomatis	LGV, trachoma, NGU	0	0	0	0	+++
Mycoplasma						
Mycoplasma pneumoniae		0	0	0	+++	+++

0 = Not recognized; + = rare; ++ = occasional; +++ = most frequent.
* See Table 7-2.
† For serious infections.

gresses to development of severe respiratory distress with fever, rales, and occasionally pleural effusion and subcutaneous edema of the upper torso. Meningitis can also develop. Gastrointestinal anthrax may be of importance to surgical consultants because its symptoms resemble an acute surgical abdomen with elevated leukocyte count, nausea, vomiting, fever, abdominal pain, and occasionally bloody diarrhea.

Diagnosis

A history of animal or animal product contact, particularly in a geographic area endemic for anthrax, should arouse

Disease in normal host	Disease in immunosuppessed host	Usual sites of infection	Secondary infection sites	Surgical importance	Antimicrobial treatment
+++	+	Skin	Lung, GI	Excision not indicated	Penicillin
+	+++	CNS, eye	Lung, GI	Immunosuppressed host	Tetracycline
+++	+	Pharynx	Skin	Respiratory distress	Antitoxin
+	+++	Endocarditis	CNS, bone	Prosthetic device infection	Variable
++	+++	CNS	Blood	Renal transplantation	Ampicillin
+++	+	Skin	Blood, CNS	Skin and wound infection	Penicillin
+++	+	Skin	Lung, eye	Skin ulcer	Streptomycin
+++	++	Skin	Blood, bone	Animal bite infection	Penicillin
+++	+	Skin, blood	—	Animal bite infection	Penicillin
+++	+	Skin, blood	—	Animal bite infection	Penicillin
+++	+	Skin	Oral cavity	Trauma, abdominal surgery	Ampicillin
+++	+	Pharynx, bronchi	Lung	Childhood infections	Erythromycin
+++	+	Pharynx, bronchi	Ear, CNS	Childhood infections	Chloramphenicol†
+++	+	Genitals	Mucosa, lymphatics	Genital lesions	Sulfonamides
+++	++	Blood, endocarditis	Vagina, skin	Vaginitis, immunosuppressed host	Variable
+++	+	Genitals	Lymphatics, bone	Genital lesions	Tetracycline
+++	+	Blood	Bone, spleen	Chronic abscesses and osteomyelitis	Tetracycline
+++	+	Intestinal	—	Diarrheal illness	Tetracycline
+++	+	Intestinal	—	Diarrheal illness	Usually none
+++	++	Wound, blood	—	Marine wound infection	Variable
+++	++	Intestinal	Blood	Diarrheal illness	Erythromycin
+	+++	Lung, urine	Wounds, blood	Immunosuppressed host, wounds	Variable
+++	++	Lung	—	Renal transplantation	Erythromycin
+++	+++	Lung	Bone, GU, GI	Extrapulmonary surgery	Isoniazid, rifampin
+++	+	Lung	Bone, GU, GI	Extrapulmonary surgery	Isoniazid, rifampin
+++	+	Lung	Skin, wounds	Surgical treatment	Variable
+++	+	Skin, nerve	Nose, eye	Reconstructive surgery	Dapsone
+++	+++	Lung	Skin, brain	Immunosuppressed host	Sulfonamides
+++	+	Blood	—	Confusion with other diagnosis	Penicillin
+++	+	Blood	—	Confusion with other diagnosis	Tetracycline
+++	+	Genitals	CNS, vascular	Confusion with other diagnosis	Penicillin
+++	+	Vascular	—	Confusion with other diagnosis	Tetracycline, chloramphenicol
+++	+	Vascular	—	Confusion with other diagnosis	Tetracycline, chloramphenicol
+++	+	Vascular	Lung, liver, heart	Confusion with other diagnosis	Tetracycline, chloramphenicol
+++	+	Lung	Spleen	Confusion with other diagnosis	Tetracycline
+++	+	Genital	Eye	Genital infection	Tetracycline
+++	+	Lung	Many	Confusion with other diagnosis	Erythromycin, tetracycline

CNS = Central nervous system; GI = Gastrointestinal; GU = Genitourinary; LGV = Lymphogranuloma venereum; NGU = Nongonococcal urethritis

suspicion. Diagnosis is dependent on isolation of *B. anthracis* from clinical material. Moistened swabs should be used to obtain material from vesicular skin lesions and from under the edge of eschars. The diagnosis of anthrax may also be established by a fourfold rise in indirect hemagglutination titer in paired sera.

Treatment and Prognosis

Penicillin, administered orally for mild cases but intravenously or intramuscularly in severe cases, is the best drug for the treatment of anthrax. Local excision of cutaneous lesions can lead to spread of infection. Topical antibiotics should also be avoided. The expected survival in treated cutaneous anthrax is over 99 percent. In contrast, pulmonary anthrax is almost always fatal, despite antibiotic therapy, while gastrointestinal anthrax is fatal 25 to 50 percent of the time.

Bacillus Species

Morphology and Identification

Bacillus species (Table 7-1) other than anthrax are responsible for a small but increasing number of human infections. These organisms are indistinguishable on Gram stain from the anthrax bacillus, and differentiation requires detailed biochemical testing. *B. subtilis* and *B. cereus* are most frequently associated with human disease.[1,2]

Epidemiology and Pathogenesis

Human infection caused by these organisms is extremely rare and, except for eye infections, occurs almost exclusively in immunosuppressed hosts.[3] The exception to this rule is food poisoning caused by *B. cereus,* which is due to an enterotoxin.[4]

Clinical Manifestations and Diagnosis

A variety of systemic infections with *Bacillus* species have been reported, including endocarditis, pneumonia, baçteremia, eye infections, wound infections and urinary tract infections.[1-3] There are two types of *B. cereus* food poisoning—an acute upper gastrointestinal syndrome that resembles staphylococcal food poisoning, and an acute diarrheal illness similar to *Clostridium perfringens* food poisoning. Fried rice is often implicated. Diagnosis is made by isolation of the organism from suspect foods or the stool; however, *B. cereus* organisms may be normal inhabitants of the stool.[4] Diagnosis of systemic illness is based on the isolation of *Bacillus* species from blood or body fluids.

Treatment and Prognosis

Antibiotic therapy is indicated only for systemic infection. Unlike anthrax bacillus, many bacillus species are resistant to penicillins and cephalosporins, and in vitro studies have demonstrated that tetracyclines, gentamicin, kanamycin, and chloramphenicol have been most effective against a variety of strains.[5] In general, *B. subtilis* tends to be penicillin- and cephalosporin-sensitive, while *B. cereus* is most resistant to these drugs. *B. cereus* food poisoning is self-limited and does not require antibiotic therapy.[4]

GENUS *CORYNEBACTERIUM*

Organisms of the genus *Corynebacterium* (Table 7-1), with the exception of the diphtheria bacillus, are seldom pathogenic for man. These organisms are gram-positive rods, non-spore-forming, non-acid-fast, nonmotile, and nonencapsulated. They are aerobic or microaerophilic and, when grown on nutritionally deficient media, exhibit terminal clubbing from which the group derives its name.

Corynebacterium diphtheriae

Morphology and Identification

C. diphtheriae (Table 7-1) are gram-positive, irregularly staining rods that are 0.3–0.8 μm × 1–8 μm. Confirmation of *C. diphtheriae* requires isolation in pure culture and biochemical and toxigenicity testing. In the laboratory, cultures are grown on both inhibitory media such as tellurite media or Löeffler's media as well as conventional blood agar. Three colonial forms—mitis, gravis, and intermedius—can be distinguished on tellurite media. On biochemical testing, diphtheria organisms are nonmotile, produce acid (but not gas) from glucose and maltose, usually reduce nitrate to nitrite, and are gelatin-, urea-, indole-, and trehalose-negative. Presumptive identification can be made when L- and V-shaped organisms (Chinese characters) and granules that appear as polar bodies are seen on Löeffler alkaline methylene blue stain.

The presence of diphtheria toxin can be tested for by an in vivo guinea pig inoculation test or by an in vitro gel-diffusion test. A positive toxigenicity test is essentially proof that the organism is *C. diphtheriae* because only *C. ulcerans* can also produce a toxin that is neutralized by diphtheria antitoxin.

Epidemiology and Pathogenesis

Diphtheria is a worldwide disease, but only about 200 cases per year are reported in the United States, usually in epidemic settings.[6] Inadequately immunized persons are most often affected, especially children who have failed to be immunized and older adults whose immunity has waned.[7] The disease occurs most often in the colder months of the year, and it is thought to be spread by droplets and close personal contact. Convalescent or healthy carriers are the presumed reservoir of disease between epidemics. The most frequent site of illness is the upper respiratory tract, although skin infections occur.[8]

The lethal nature of the disease is primarily related to the production of an exotoxin, an acidic globular protein (molecular weight about 62,000) which acts by interfering with polypeptide synthesis in the cell.[9] The production of toxin is mediated by parasitization of the diphtheria organism by specific bacteriophage. Local invasiveness of the organism is probably necessary for clinical illness.

Clinical Manifestations

The majority of patients exhibit upper respiratory symptoms of sore throat, nonproductive cough, low-grade fever, and malaise. In severe cases, cervical adenopathy may be prominent with additional soft tissue swelling. Most characteristic is a thick adherent membrane in the pharynx with severe local inflammation and edema. The membrane may appear gray, green, or black and consists primarily of fibrin, necrotic epithelium, lymphocytes, and polymorphonuclear leukocytes. Local concomitant infection with group A streptococci is frequent. Pharyngeal edema and membrane formation may be sufficiently severe to cause respiratory obstruction. Occasionally the ear, eye, and genitalia are infected. Also, infection of preexisting skin lesions such as stasis ulcers or burns can occur in temperate climates, although it is more common in the tropics.

Myocarditis and polyneuritis, manifestations of diphtheria toxemia, appear one or more weeks after the onset of clinical illness. Congestive heart failure, heart block, or other cardiac arrhythmias may be evident. Polyneuritis is most frequent in the cranial nerves, and patients exhibit difficulty in swallowing and have a nasal voice.

Diagnosis

The diagnosis is established by isolation of *C. diphtheriae* and proof of toxin production. Pharyngeal swabbings, or preferably portions of pharyngeal membranes, should be submitted to the laboratory for culture. The laboratory must be informed of the suspicion of diphtheria so that the specimens can be cultured on either Löeffler or tellurite media. Clinical diagnosis of the disease is particularly difficult in mild cases when a pharyngeal membrane is not present. In patients who have the late manifestations, such as congestive heart failure, heart block, or polyneuritis, it may be impossible to prove the etiology. A history of pharyngeal infection will help establish the diagnosis.

Treatment and Prognosis

Specific therapy is directed at neutralizing toxin by the use of a horse antitoxin; 30,000 to 40,000 units of antitoxin are injected intramuscularly in moderately severe cases. Severely ill patients can be treated with up to 80,000 units. Because approximately 10 percent of patients will develop allergic reactions to horse serum, a careful history of allergy should be taken, and tests for hypersensitivity to horse serum should be done before administration. Antibiotic treatment is an adjunct to antitoxin and is used to eliminate the organism from the pharynx and prevent spread to other persons. Penicillin or erythromycin are preferred and can be used to treat asymptomatic carriers.[11]

Although immunization has reduced the frequency of diphtheria, the mortality has only recently declined from 10 to 6 percent.[6,10] Most deaths are the result of either respiratory obstruction by the pharyngeal lesion or subsequent myocarditis.

Prevention

Diphtheria is usually prevented by immunization with diphtheria toxoid, a formalin detoxified preparation commonly administered in childhood. Immunity, however, is not lifelong and requires repeated booster shots in later life.

Corynebacterium Species

Morphology and Identification

Corynebacteria (Table 7-1) other than *C. diphtheriae* are usually saprophytic or weakly pathogenic for man. They are frequently reported from pharyngeal, conjunctival, or skin isolates as "diphtheroids." They can be distinguished from *C. diphtheriae* on the basis of morphology, biochemical reactions, failure to produce an exotoxin, and hemolysis.

Epidemiology and Pathogenesis

Members of the genus *Corynebacterium* are normal inhabitants of the pharynx, skin, and conjunctivae. With a few exceptions, they are pathogenic only in immunologically compromised patients. A localized skin eruption, characterized by mild inflammation, scaling, and weeping in body folds or intertriginous areas and termed erythrasma has been attributed to *C. minutissimum. C. haemolyticum* and *C. ulcerans* may be confused with *C. diphtheriae* in the laboratory, particularly because *C. ulcerans* strains occasionally produce diphtheria toxin. More recently, bacteremia with a previously unidentified *Corynebacterium* organism has been described in immunosuppressed patients or those with prosthetic devices.[12,13] *C. acnes* and *C. granulosum* are anaerobic species frequently found in acne, but their pathogenetic importance is not fully established.

Treatment and Prognosis

Erythrasma is usually treated with topical antibacterial soaps, but erythromycin may be required in severe cases.

Unlike *C. diphtheriae*, most *Corynebacterium* species have exhibited resistance to commonly used antibiotics such as penicillin G,[12–14] and susceptibility testing is essential. Most successful treatments of diphtheroid infections, however, have included penicillin G with the addition of an aminoglycoside.[14] The newer *Corynebacterium* species that have been found to cause bacteremia in cancer patients have been sensitive only to vancomycin.[13]

LISTERIA AND *ERYSIPELOTHRIX*

Although *Listeria* and *Erysipelothrix* differ in their pathogenicity and the type of disease they cause, they will be discussed together because of their similar morphologic and cultural appearances, and because both are associated with disease in animals as well as people.

Listeria monocytogenes

Morphology and Identification

The genus *Listeria* is of uncertain affiliation. These small, gram-positive coccobacillary organisms frequently appear in pairs and chains and may be confused with diplococci. They are not encapsulated, they lack spores and are motile when grown at 18 to 20C. They can be grown on ordinary laboratory media, usually aerobically, but they are also facultatively anaerobic. Growth may be enhanced by prior refrigeration of the specimens at 4C. On sheep blood agar there is a characteristic narrow zone of beta-hemolysis around the colonies. Organisms are usually catalase-positive, they hydrolyze esculin and produce acid, but not gas, from glucose, levulose, trehalose, and salicin. Purulent conjunctivitis results from instillation of the organism in the eye of guinea pigs or rabbits.

Epidemiology and Pathogenesis

L. monocytogenes is an ubiquitous organism that causes disease in both animals and people.[15,16] It has been isolated from animals, birds, water, sewage, and soil, and is carried in the stool in a small proportion of patients; the carriage rate is increased among close contacts of patients with listeriosis.[15] Although animal contact is associated with the disease, the majority of cases occur in urban dwellers during late summer; it is an early winter disease in animals. The organism does not produce toxins. Immunity to it is mediated by the T-lymphocyte and macrophage system, as it is for other intracellular infections such as tuberculosis. *Listeria* meningitis does not differ pathologically from acute meningitis caused by other pyogenic organisms. Normal people may be infected with *Listeria*, but most cases are associated with immunologic compromise or advanced age. *L. monocytogenes* can also cause abortion or perinatal infection in both mother and child. Infection in the mother is usually benign and nonspecific, whereas the newborn has signs of meningitis and frequently hepatosplenomegaly and a rash.[17,18] The importance of underlying malignant disease, particularly lymphoma and leukemia, as an associated factor in *Listeria* infection has been emphasized.[19,20] More recently listerial meningitis and bacteremia without meningitis have been reported in kidney transplant recipients.[21-23]

Clinical Manifestations and Diagnosis

Both normal and immunosuppressed patients will have typical symptoms of septicemia or meningitis. Diagnosis is based almost entirely on the isolation and identification of *L. monocytogenes* from infected tissues or body fluids. Occasionally, the organism may be isolated from skin lesions in the newborn. Serologic tests are not clinically useful. Physicians should always be alert to the possibility of *Listeria* when diphtheroids are reported from Gram smears or cultures of spinal fluid.

Treatment and Prognosis

Death from *Listeria* infection is most common in the neonatal period, particularly if the infection is contracted transplacentally. Listeriosis in immunosuppressed patients, particularly kidney transplant recipients, has been associated with a remarkably low mortality (5 to 10 percent).[21,22] This may be related to the higher frequency of *Listeria* bacteremia without meningitis in this group of patients. The organism is sensitive to a large number of antibiotics including ampicillin, penicillin, erythromycin, tetracycline, and gentamicin.[24] Although it is inhibited readily by these drugs, there may be a wide discrepancy between the minimal inhibitory concentration and the minimum bactericidal concentration for penicillin and ampicillin. The addition of an aminoglycoside to penicillin or ampicillin demonstrates synergistic killing in vitro,[25] but the clinical benefit is unclear. Penicillin G or ampicillin in high intravenous doses are still the best treatment for *Listeria* infections. If combination penicillin–aminoglycoside treatment is elected, the aminoglycoside should be administered intrathecally or intraventricularly to assure adequate concentrations in the cerebrospinal fluid in meningitis. Renal transplant recipients should be treated for at least 3 weeks; there is a relapse rate of 35 percent when shorter periods are used.[23]

Erysipelothrix rhusiopathiae

Morphology and Identification

E. rhusiopathiae (Table 7-1), also designated *E. insidiosa*, is the only member of the genus *Erysipelothrix*. The organism is a slender, gram-positive rod 0.2–0.4 μm × 0.5–2.5 μm. The organism can be grown on ordinary bacteriologic media. It develops circular transparent colonies, which may produce a green appearance around the margin when grown on blood agar. The organism is nonmotile, does not produce spores, does not produce catalase, is nonhemolytic, and is inhibited by potassium tellurite, thus enabling it to be distinguished from *L. monocytogenes* and *Corynebacterium* species, with which it is most often confused.

Epidemiology and Pathogenesis

E. rhusiopathiae is common in nature and is the cause of swine erysipelas. In humans, erysipeloid is the most common form of infection. This inflammatory eruption usually occurs on the hands as a purplish erythema, with sharply demarcated margins that are irregular and slightly raised. Histologic examination reveals inflammation of the dermis with gram-positive bacilli identifiable on Gram stain. Fish handlers, butchers, veterinarians, fishermen, abattoir workers, and cooks are most susceptible to infection because of their contact with potentially contaminated fish and animal products. Local infection is thought to occur by primary inoculation through skin injury. A more severe form of disease with fever, systemic illness and septicemia, and occasionally endocarditis, arthritis, and meningitis is also described. The systemic form may occur with or without the presence of skin lesions.[26,27]

Clinical Manifestations

The majority of patients have the previously described lesions of the hands; edema may be severe enough to restrict finger motion. Lymphangitis and lymphadenitis or other systemic signs of illness are ordinarily absent. Itching, burning, and tenderness are typical. Signs and symptoms of systemic illness and endocarditis cannot be distinguished from those caused by other organisms. Both normal and abnormal cardiac valves can be involved in endocarditis.[28]

The diagnosis of cutaneous infection can readily be made by the typical appearance of the skin lesions, and can be confirmed from biopsy specimens taken from the advancing margin of a lesion. The biopsy sample should be submitted for both histologic examination and culture in glucose infusion broth. Diagnosis can also be made by injection and aspiration of normal saline at the margin of the lesion. The organism is readily grown from ordinary blood culture media in cases of septicemia or endocarditis.

Treatment and Prognosis

E. rhusiopathiae is typically sensitive to pencillin, cephalosporins, erythromycin, and clindamycin, but not to vancomycin or to aminoglycoside.[28] Localized skin lesions can be treated with a single intramuscular injection of long-acting benzathine penicillin or with oral erythromycin. Penicillin G is the best treatment for endocarditis and should be administered in high doses because the reported mortality in endocarditis is approximately 50 percent.

GRAM-NEGATIVE BACTERIA

Francisella tularensis

Morphology and Identification

F. tularensis (Table 7-1) is a genus of uncertain affiliation. It is also known as *Brucella tularensis* or *Pasteurella tularensis*. The organisms are small, coccobacillary, gram-negative, nonmotile, unencapsulated, and non-spore-forming, 0.2 μm × 0.2–0.7 μm. The organism cannot be grown on ordinary media and requires isolation on blood-glucose-cysteine agar or similar supplemented media. If the specimens are expected to contain contaminating organisms, it may be necessary to add penicillin or polymyxin B to the media to suppress their growth. Because of the pathogenicity of this organism, its isolation in hospital laboratories should be accompanied by extreme caution. Although the organism may be recovered from animals after inoculation, this practice is also potentially dangerous. Smooth, gray colonies appear on selective media within 18 to 24 hours. Biochemical identification is not necessary or recommended, as the organism can be identified by a slide agglutination test.

Epidemiology and Pathogenesis

F. tularensis is the cause of tularemia in people. The organism is a parasite of numerous mammals (cottontail rabbit, beaver, muskrats, moles, squirrels, rats, mice).[29] The most frequent arthropod vectors are the tick and the deerfly.[30,31] Although the majority of the 200 American cases per year come from the lower Mississippi Valley region, there are regular reports of cases from both the East and West coasts. Most infections are thought to be caused by passage of the organism through the skin, either via scratches or breaks in the skin during the handling of contaminated animal products or by entry at the time of a vector bite. A pneumonic form of the disease may be acquired by inhalation of the organism. Necrosis is common in both the lymph nodes and lung. The organisms are not visible on ordinary dye-stained sections of clinical specimens and require direct or indirect fluorescent antibody techniques.

Clinical Manifestations

Four types of tularemia are traditionally described. The most common, the ulceroglandular form, appears 80 to 90 percent of the time, followed by the nonspecific "typhoidal" form of tularemia. Oculoglandular tularemia is the most rare, occurring in less than 1 percent of cases. The fourth type, pneumonic tularemia, may occur as an isolated event or in association with any of the other three forms.

Ulceroglandular disease is characterized by a cutaneous ulcer at the site of inoculation and local lymphadenopathy. Oculoglandular tularemia is associated with conjunctivitis with local lymphadenopathy; the typhoidal form of disease exhibits only nonspecific febrile symptoms that are occasionally accompanied by nonproductive cough. Patients have a high fever, 40 to 41C, and abrupt onset. Severe headache is not unusual, and hepatomegaly and splenomegaly are usually present. Tularemia pneumonia presents with a lobar consolidation, frequently with accompanying respiratory distress. Pleural effusion accompanies pneumonia in over 50 percent of patients, but cavity and abscess formation are rare.[32] Meningitis, osteomyelitis, and endocarditis seldom occur.

Diagnosis

Because of the difficulty of isolating the tularemia organism, the diagnosis frequently hinges on a high index of clinical suspicion. A history of animal contact, particularly with rabbits, or tick or insect bites, is particularly important, as is examination for the presence of tender lymphadenopathy and skin ulceration. Occasionally, the organism can be recovered from routine blood cultures. If tularemia is suspected, laboratory personnel should be alerted to prepare the special media for inoculation of material from draining lymph nodes or ulcers at the patient's bedside. Culture of sputum on special media will occasionally yield the organism. Gram stain is usually not helpful.

In the majority of patients, the diagnosis is reached retrospectively by use of a serum agglutination test. Titers become positive after 10 to 14 days with peak titers of 1:1280 at 4 to 8 weeks of illness. A serial rise in agglutinin titers at 1- to 2-week intervals is diagnostic. A skin test for tularemia is also available and becomes positive sooner than the agglutination test; unfortunately, there is no commercial supplier.[33] The differential diagnosis is difficult because it includes all the rare ulceroglandular diseases (eg, cat-scratch fever, *Yersinia pseudotuberculosis, Pasteurella multocida* bite infection, plague, chancroid, melioidosis, and sporotrichosis).

Treatment and Prognosis

The mortality rate with untreated tularemia pneumonia may be as high as 30 percent; the mortality with untreated ulceroglandular disease is only about 5 percent. Streptomycin, the most effective antibiotic, is usually administered for at least 1 week. Other aminoglycosides should also be effective but clinical experience is limited. Chloramphenicol and tetracycline will inhibit but not eradicate *F. tularensis,* and relapses may occur after treatment. Lifelong immunity seems to result after clinical tularemia, but the mechanism has not been elucidated.

Pasteurella multocida

Morphology and Identification

P. multocida (Table 7-1), also known as *Pasteurella septica,* is a gram-negative bacillus 1–1.8 $\mu m \times 0.3$–$0.5\ \mu m$, which is nonmotile, non-spore-forming, and bipolar staining. It is a facultative anaerobe which grows on ordinary media and is oxidase- and catalase-positive and citrate-negative, does not liquefy gelatin, and reduces methylene blue. Other *Pasteurella* species which are essentially avirulent for man, *P. ureae* and *P. haemolytica,* can be distinguished from *P. multocida* by biochemical testing. Caution must be exercised in the identification of *P. multocida* in the laboratory because of the wide variability of morphologic, cultural, and biochemical characteristics.[34,35]

Epidemiology and Pathogenesis

P. multocida is a normal inhabitant of the upper respiratory and digestive tracts of healthy animals and birds. It is the cause of cholera in fowl and hemorrhagic septicemia in cattle and other animals.[34] Human infection is associated with close contact with animals, particularly bites from cats and dogs (cat bite fever).[36-38] Rare cases of pneumonia, meningitis, peritonitis, and septicemia have been reported.[39] In patients with respiratory infection, the organism is usually associated with bronchiectasis, chronic bronchitis, and bronchogenic carcinoma.[39] On pathologic examination, specimens exhibit evidence of acute inflammation that is indistinguishable from that caused by other pyogenic organisms.

Clinical Manifestations and Diagnosis

The majority of patients have acute cellulitis with purulent drainage, lymphangitis, and regional adenopathy, associated with a recent animal bite or scratch, particularly when caused by a cat. Occasionally, acute and chronic cough develop with or without evidence of pulmonary infiltration and consolidation. Severe septicemia can also develop, particularly in patients who are immunosuppressed. In addition, alcoholics can develop spontaneous bacterial peritonitis. Physicians should be suspicious of *P. multocida* when Gram stain of an infected animal bite or scratch shows gram-negative coccobacillary organisms. Routine culture techniques will identify the organism.

Treatment and Prognosis

P. multocida is susceptible to penicillin G, related compounds, and the tetracyclines but is generally resistant to the macrolides (eg, erythromycin).[40] Local infections should be drained and penicillin administered. The use of penicillin for the empiric treatment of patients with animal bites is an unsettled issue, but selective use has been recommended for deep bites that involve tendon or bone. Others recommend the uniform use of systemic antibiotics for any animal wound that requires suturing.[37,38] The prognosis is excellent in localized infections, and death is rare except in immunocompromised patients.

Streptobacillus moniliformis and Spirillum minor

These two gram-negative organisms will be discussed together because of their similar propensity to cause rat bite fever. *S. moniliformis* and *Spirillum minor* (Table 7-1) belong to different bacterial genera, and each causes a somewhat different clinical illness.

Morphology and Identification

S. moniliformis is a gram-negative, 1 μm × 1–5 μm pleomorphic bacillus which often forms long filaments. It is aerobic or facultatively anaerobic. Growth medium must be supplemented with blood, serum, or ascitic fluid to support growth. In addition to conventional bacterial colonies, cell wall deficient L-forms can also be seen. The presence of sodium polyanetholsulfonate in blood culture medium may inhibit growth of the organism.[41] *Spirillum minor* is also a gram-negative bacillus, 2–5 μm in length with two to six spirals and bipolar tufts of flagella. The organism has not been cultivated in vitro. Identification is dependent upon its appearance on wet mounts examined with a dark-field microscope, or on blood films stained with Giemsa or Wright stains.

Epidemiology and Pathogenesis

Disease caused by *S. moniliformis* (streptobacillary fever) is rare but is still the most common type of rat bite fever in the United States. Most illness is associated with a rodent bite or the bite of an animal (weasel, cat) that has fed on infected rodents. This organism is also thought to have been the cause of a large milkborne epidemic of streptobacillary fever in Haverhill, Massachusetts. Many reported cases in the United States derive from bites of experimental rats in the laboratory.[42] *Spirillum minor,* the causative organism of spirillary fever (Sodoku), was first described in Japan but is also sporadically reported from the United States, Asia, and Europe. It too is contracted from rat bites.

Both organisms are thought to disseminate through the bloodstream, although *S. moniliformis* infection may be restricted to the site of the bite and local lymph nodes. Examination of infected tissue reveals only a nonspecific chronic inflammatory response, with microorganisms visible. In fatal cases, the organism has disseminated to various organs.

Clinical Manifestations

Clinical symptoms after a streptobacillary infection tend to occur earlier than in the spirillary form of the disease. Chills, fever, malaise, headache, and rash occur within 10 days of the rat bite. About one-fourth of the patients with streptobacillary fever have local lymphangitis and lymphadenitis. The original site of the bite is usually healed but may still be quite tender. Migratory polyarthritis is present in half the patients with streptobacillary fever, but is unusual in spirillary fever. Patients with spirillary fever usually have no symptoms until at least 7 days after being bitten. The rash in spirillary fever is usually purplish red in color and macular, and occurs with approximately the same frequency (75 percent) as in streptobacillary fever. False-positive serologic test results occur for syphilis in approximately 25 percent of streptobacillary fevers and 50 percent of spirillary fevers.

Diagnosis

Definitive diagnosis in streptobacillary fever depends on the isolation of *S. moniliformis* from blood, the site of the bite, skin pustules, or joint fluid. If there is no recent rodent bite, the differential diagnosis must include Rocky Mountain spotted fever, Rickettsialpox, meningococcemia, syphilis, and the viral exanthems. A serum agglutination test for *S. moniliformis* may be useful if cultures are negative; titers of 1:80 are diagnostic. The diagnosis of spirillary fever requires a demonstration of *S. minor* in a dark-field preparation of infected exudate or blood. Blood films stained with Giemsa or Wright stains may also reveal the organism. If these initial examinations fail to demonstrate the organism, the only diagnostic recourse is to inoculate mice and guinea pigs.

Treatment and Prognosis

Mortality in untreated streptobacillary fever may exceed 10 percent, while mortality in spirillary fever is approximately one-half of that. Penicillin is the best treatment for both infections. Streptomycin, tetracycline, and chlortetracycline have been effective alternatives; however, the choice should be based on susceptibility testing of *S. moniliformis.*[43] The use of penicillin prophylactically at the time of a rat bite has been recommended, but its ability to prevent rat bite fever is unproven.

Eikenella corrodens

Morphology and Identification

E. corrodens (Table 7-1) is a recently identified pathogen of man that is facultatively anaerobic and grows best under increased carbon dioxide tension. In the past, this organism has been termed HB-1 and *Bacteroides corrodens*. More recently, the strictly anaerobic *B. corrodens* has been separated from the microaerophilic *E. corrodens*. *E. corrodens* is a nonmotile, small, gram-negative bacillus that grows slowly on sheep blood agar plates. Colonies are small (0.5 mm) at 24 hours and typically do not reveal pitting or corroding of the surface until at least 48 hours of incubation. The organisms are oxidase-positive and urease-negative.

Epidemiology and Pathogenesis

E. corrodens is a member of the normal oral flora of man and may also be a normal resident of the fecal flora. Most clinical infections have implicated oral or gastrointestinal secretions as the source of the infective organism. Breaks in normal mucosal integrity, eg, lacerations of the oral mucosa, periodontal infection, bites, and abdominal operations, permit invasion of tissue. In addition, there seems to be a unique relationship among *E. corrodens*, cutaneous abscesses, and the practice of subcutaneous or intravenous injection of methylphenidate (cf: amphetamine).[44] The majority of infections are indolent abscesses, which frequently reveal multiple organisms, particularly anaerobic bacteria and streptococci, in addition to *Eikenella*.

Clinical Manifestations and Diagnosis

Most patients will have abscesses of the head and neck, particularly the mouth, and dental abscesses. Other sites of infection include abdominal abscesses, endocarditis, meningitis, and osteomyelitis.[44,45] Cutaneous abscesses are frequently associated with drug abuse or with trauma to the hands from teeth. Diagnosis is based on Gram stain and culture of abscesses. Patients typically have a rather quiescent, indolent history of abscess formation after trauma or injury, particularly to the head, neck, and hands. Abscess material may be particularly foul smelling, which suggests that the infection is anaerobic in origin. Because of this the patient may be empirically treated with clindamycin for a presumptive diagnosis of anaerobic abscess and fail to respond because of the resistance of *E. corrodens* to clindamycin and lincomycin.

Treatment and Prognosis

Surgical drainage combined with appropriate antimicrobial treatment, usually with ampicillin or penicillin, results in rapid cure of abscesses. Alternate antibiotics are tetracycline and possibly erythromycin or chloramphenicol; however, some strains can be resistant to the latter two drugs. Organisms typically exhibit high resistance to methicillin, clindamycin, lincomycin, and metronidazole.[44,46] In vitro susceptibility tests should be performed to determine optimal antibiotic therapy for endocarditis in the penicillin-allergic patient.[47]

Bordetella pertussis

Morphology and Identification

B. pertussis (Table 7-1) is a minute coccobacillus, 0.2 to 0.3 μm by 0.5–1.0 μm. It is nonmotile and produces smooth, pearly, glistening, small colonies on Bordet-Gengou medium. Along with *B. parapertussis* and *B. bronchiseptica*, *B. pertussis* is the cause of whooping cough. In addition to culture techniques, immunologic diagnosis can be made using a fluorescent-antibody staining technique either on direct nasopharyngeal smears or on specimens obtained from culture media.

Epidemiology and Pathogenesis

Whooping cough is largely a disease of unimmunized young children. The disease is acquired by droplet spread from clinical cases or even adult carriers.[48] The frequency of pertussis has decreased since the advent of widespread immunization in childhood. Immunity is not lifelong, however, and side effects of the vaccine prohibit its use in older children and adults, which leads to susceptibility with increasing age. Although several toxins and humoral factors are produced by the organism, including endotoxin and a lymphocytosis-promoting factor, the role of these products in the pathogenesis of clinical illness is not known. Infection appears to be limited primarily to the upper respiratory tract and bronchi, where large numbers of organisms are found enmeshed in a mucosal exudate. Bronchopneumonia is unusual.

Clinical Manifestations

Whooping cough has been divided into three phases, which follow an incubation period of approximately 1 to 3 weeks. The initial or catarrhal phase of the illness also lasts 1 to 3 weeks and is characterized by rhinorrhea, conjunctivitis, and generalized upper respiratory symptoms. Next the paroxysmal stage begins and lasts an additional 2 to 6 weeks with severe episodic coughing. The disease acquires its name from the characteristic crowing (whooping) sound made during inspiration after coughing spells. A child may appear remarkably well between the seiges of coughing, but vomiting or cyanosis during paroxysms suggests the diagnosis.[49] A third phase of convalescence lasts an additional 2 to 3 weeks.

In infants under the age of 6 months, the disease does not have typical symptoms and the child may present only with coughing, gurgling, and respiratory distress. Furthermore, in older children and in adults the manifestations are difficult to distinguish from viral upper respiratory infection. There is speculation that adenoviruses may cause a syndrome similar to whooping cough.[50]

Diagnosis

Culture for *B. pertussis* should be performed by using long, thin, nasopharyngeal swabs, which should be plated on Bordet-Gengou medium at the bedside or taken immediately to the laboratory. Growth is slow and usually does not occur for 48 to 96 hours. Fluorescent antibody studies may be performed immediately on direct swabs.

Treatment and Prognosis

Treatment of the infected patient is designed primarily to assure adequate oxygenation and nutrition. Antibiotics do not alter the clinical course of the illness, and certain antibiotics do not even eliminate the organism.[49-51] Ten to 14 days of erythromycin is recommended in an effort to reduce spread of infection to other susceptible persons. Tetracycline and chloramphenicol are effective but potentially more toxic, and ampicillin is ineffective.[51] The fatality rate is approximately 5 per 1,000. The ultimate treatment is prevention by means of adequate immunization of children. Chemoprophylaxis with erythromycin has been recommended, especially for those with inadequate immunization as children. The efficacy of this practice has not been unequivocally documented.

GENUS *HAEMOPHILUS*

Haemophilus influenzae

Morphology and Identification

H. influenzae (Table 7-1) are minute gram-negative rods 0.2–0.3 μm × 0.5–2.0 μm and coccobacillary in appearance. They are notoriously difficult to recognize on Gram stains of clinical material and may appear to be gram-positive. Both encapsulated and unencapsulated types have been described in clinical illness, but of the six capsular types, type b is by far the most frequent pathogen. Laboratory culture requires the presence of the so-called X and V factors in media. The X factor is supplied by the heme portion of hemoglobin and the pyridine nucleotide, nicotinamide adenine dinucleotide, is the V factor. The organism grows aerobically, does not produce spores, and produces acid from glucose and sucrose.

Epidemiology and Pathogenesis

H. influenzae is a normal inhabitant of the upper respiratory tract, particularly in young children. The organism usually causes upper respiratory infection from the age of 6 months to about 3 years. Typical infections include epiglottitis, otitis media, tracheobronchitis, laryngitis, and pneumonia, but cellulitis, arthritis, pericarditis, osteomyelitis, and meningitis also occur frequently.[52] Bacteremia may accompany any of these infections. Among adults, pneumonia due to *H. influenzae* is becoming increasingly frequent.[53] The virulence of the organism is thought to be associated with the capsule; however, the precise mechanism by which a normal respiratory inhabitant becomes pathogenic is not known. Immunity is related to the development of specific antibodies to the capsule, which are lacking in young children but are present in most adults and older children.

Clinical Manifestations

Most patients are young children whose symptoms begin with nonspecific upper respiratory symptoms, cough, hoarseness, fever, and occasionally stridor. Acute epiglottitis has a rapid onset. The pharynx becomes beefy red, and the epiglottis is swollen and may have complete obstruction necessitating tracheostomy. Signs and symptoms in meningitis cannot be distinguished from illness caused by other pyogenic organisms.

Diagnosis

Diagnosis is dependent upon the isolation and identification of the organism from infected exudates or body fluids such as sputum, throat swabs, and cerebrospinal fluid. Caution must be exercised in the interpretation of Gram smears because the organism may appear gram-positive and may resemble diplococci. For spinal fluid specimens, rapid detection of *H. influenzae* may be accomplished by the use of counterimmunoelectrophoresis.

Treatment and Prognosis

During the 1970s, *H. influenzae* resistant to ampicillin have become sufficiently prevalent to contraindicate the empiric use of ampicillin for serious infections.[54,55] Most physicians favor the use of either chloramphenicol or chloramphenicol together with ampicillin for serious infections. Alternative antibiotics to chloramphenicol for treatment of meningitis are the subject of active investigation. Although cefamandole has shown good in vitro activity against *H. influenzae,* its clinical efficacy has not been encouraging.[56] Rifampin and trimethoprim-sulfamethoxazole have been used successfully for the eradication of the pharyngeal carriage state.[57] Attempts to develop a vaccine that is effective against *H. influenzae* have been hampered by poor antibody response in children under 18 months of age, the group most likely to benefit from such a vaccine.

Other *Haemophilus* Species

Other species of the genus *Haemophilus* that are known or suspected to cause disease in people include *H. parainfluenzae, H. haemolyticus, H. parahaemolyticus, H. aphrophilus, H. aegyptius,* and *H. ducreyi.* In addition, *H. vaginalis (Corynebacterium vaginale)* is also included in the *Haemophilus* genus by Bergey's manual; however, this categorization is questioned. All the organisms are gram-negative coccobacilli and differ from *H. influenzae* in the extent of their dependence on X or V factors for growth and in their biochemical reactions.

Haemophilus ducreyi

Chancroid, a soft, painful, venereal ulcer, is caused by *H. ducreyi* (Table 7-1). Lesions are more frequent in the male and usually occur under the foreskin or around the corona of the glans penis, and occasionally on the penile shaft. Inguinal adenopathy may or may not be present. Special techniques using media containing blood or serum are required to culture *H. ducreyi.* Demonstration of small, gram-negative coccobacilli on direct Gram smear of the lesion may be used as presumptive diagnosis of chancroid if a dark-field examination for syphilis is negative.[58] Gram stains of aspirates of inguinal nodes may also be used to establish the diagnosis. Although chancroid appears to be declining in incidence in Western countries, it was frequent in servicemen in Vietnam. Treatment of early ulcers with soap and water may be effective. However, sulfonamides have become the standard drug treatment, with tetracycline as an alternative; in some instances, the simultaneous use of both drugs may be required.[58,59] In some particularly resistant infections in Vietnam, systemic kanamycin or cephalothin was used successfully, coupled with povidone-iodine topical cleansing.[60] Drainage of fluctuant inguinal abscesses may be useful.[58]

Haemophilus Aphrophilus

H. aphrophilus (Table 7-1) can be found among the normal oral and pharyngeal flora and is occasionally the cause of endocarditis, brain abscess, bacteremia, meningitis, pneumonia, or soft tissue abscesses. It may be difficult to distinguish from *Actinobacillus actinomycetemcomitans*, which can cause similar clinical illness.[61] Patients with *H. aphrophilus* infection have a high frequency of trauma, oropharyngeal infection, and underlying malignancies or chemotherapy for cancer.[62] Results of in vitro antimicrobial susceptibility testing of *H. aphrophilus* suggests that chloramphenicol, tetracycline, streptomycin, and gentamicin may be effective drugs. Susceptibility to penicillin G and ampicillin is variable and the preferred treatment, particularly for endocarditis, remains unsettled.[62] Susceptibility testing should be performed by the agar dilution or broth dilution method because disk susceptibility testing appears to be unreliable.

Haemophilus parainfluenzae

A prominent feature of recently recognized acute and subacute bacterial endocarditis caused by *H. parainfluenzae* is the high incidence of major arterial occlusion secondary to emboli. This organism can be regularly isolated from the upper respiratory tract of healthy persons and only rarely causes human disease. It requires V, but not X, factor for growth and may be particularly difficult to recognize in blood cultures because of its failure to produce a cloudy medium. Blind subculturing to chocolate agar with incubation under CO_2 may be the only method of identifying the organism from blood. Combination treatment with a penicillin (ampicillin) and an aminoglycoside appears to be most effective.[63,64]

Other *Haemophilus* Species

H. vaginalis is a member of the normal vaginal flora; it has been implicated as the cause of vaginitis,[65] and has been associated with transient bacteremias associated with childbirth, particularly when surgical intervention was required.[66] *H. aegyptius* has been the cause of acute conjunctivitis. *H. haemolyticus*, *H. parahaemolyticus*, and *H. paraphrophilus* are all found in the upper respiratory tract and have been implicated as causes of bacteremia and possibly pharyngitis.

Calymmatobacterium granulomatis

Morphology and Identification

This small, pleomorphic, gram-negative rod, formerly known as *Donovania granulomatis*, causes granuloma inguinale. It is extremely difficult to culture this organism, which requires either inoculation of egg yolks or egg yolk slants. On Wright stain, the organisms appear blue and exhibit bipolar staining (Donovan bodies) and are frequently found lying within the vacuoles of large phagocytic cells.

Epidemiology and Pathogenesis

Fewer than 100 cases of granuloma inguinale are reported in the United States per year, mostly in the southeastern states. Over 90 percent of the time the disease is localized to the genital and groin area and traditionally has been thought to be disseminated by sexual contact; however, the rate of transmission appears to be quite low. The organism has been isolated from stools, raising the possibility of acquisition from the patient's own flora. The ulcer base is infiltrated with mononuclear cells with large macrophages filled with organisms. Lesions begin as papules, which slowly ulcerate. Infection may extend from the genital area with development of large inguinal nodes. Occasionally, lesions have been noted in bones, joints, and liver.

Clinical Manifestations and Diagnosis

Patients are rarely seen during the acute stage of the illness, which is characterized by papules and small ulcers on the vulva, perineum, groin, glans penis, or penile shaft. Later lesions are hypertrophic and may resemble carcinoma. Lesions are typically long-standing, destructive, and painless, but not insensitive.[67] Diagnosis is accomplished by microscopic examination of Wright or Giemsa stained smears of scrapings or biopsies at the advancing margin of ulcerative lesions. Dark-field examination should be performed to rule out syphilis. Although complement-fixation serologic tests are available, they lack specificity and cross-react with other venereal diseases. Granuloma inguinale is considered a probable premalignant lesion, and carcinoma must always be suspected in hypertrophic lesions.[68]

Treatment and Prognosis

A number of antibiotic regimens have been successful, including tetracycline, chloramphenicol, erythromycin, streptomycin, and gentamicin. Oral treatment with tetracycline is usually continued for 10 to 20 days. The disease may reappear years later, despite adequate treatment. Treatment of late lesions may result in stricture of the urethra, vagina, or anus.

GENUS *BRUCELLAE*

Members of the genus *Brucellae* are the causative organisms of brucellosis (formerly undulant fever) in man. They primarily infect the genitourinary tract of a variety of animals and are associated with abortion. Species pathogenic for man and their usual animal hosts are *B. abortus* (cattle), *B. suis* (swine), and *B. melitensis* (sheep and goats); however, there is a wide overlap in the susceptibility of various animals to *Brucella* species. More recently, *B. canis* (dogs) has also been associated with disease in humans.

Brucella Species

Morphology and Identification

The organisms are short, coccobacillary, gram-negative rods that are nonmotile, strict aerobes, some of which require the addition of CO_2 for growth. Growth of *Brucellae* on ordinary media is slow. A special medium such as albimi brucella broth facilitates growth. Cultures of body fluids should be held for 21 days before being reported as negative. Organisms are catalase-positive, and strains pathogenic for humans are also oxidase-positive. Differentiation of the various *Brucellae* species is accomplished by biochemical and metabolic testing, as well as specific agglutinating sera.

Epidemiology and Pathogenesis

Human brucellosis is acquired by contact with infected animals or animal products. In the early 1970s in the United States, swine were the most frequent animal source of brucellosis; however, in 1976 and 1977 cattle were the most common source.[69] The majority of cases in the United States occur in adult males who work in meat packing plants.[69,70] Other sources of brucellosis include ingestion of unpasteurized dairy products and consumption of foreign cheese, particularly goat cheese from Mexico. From 1967 to 1977, 17 cases in the United States have been attributed to *B. canis* acquired through contact with dogs. The organism probably causes infection by entering the body through breaks in the skin or by ingestion or inhalation. Organisms spread rapidly, are phagocytosed by macrophages and polymorphonuclear leukocytes and multiply within phagocytic vacuoles.[71] Pathologic specimens reveal the presence of suppurative and nonsuppurative granulomas containing multinucleated giant cells as well as frank abscesses.

Clinical Manifestations

The diagnosis is particularly difficult to make if a history of animal contact has not been obtained because the symptoms are nonspecific—fever, chills, sweats, malaise, weakness, body aches, anorexia, and weight loss. Headache is reported in about half the patients. Lymphadenopathy, splenomegaly, and hepatomegaly can be evident in up to 25 percent of patients but the results of physical examination are usually normal. Occasionally, patients will exhibit symptoms of dysuria, testicular pain, arthralgias, respiratory symptoms, visual disturbances, tinnitus, loss of balance, and mental depression. Because of nonspecificity of acute symptoms, the differential diagnosis in acute brucellosis includes a variety of bacterial, parasitic, viral, and fungal diseases.

Diagnosis

The majority of brucellosis infections are diagnosed by demonstration of a serologic rise in agglutinating antibody to *B. abortus* antigen. Agglutinating titers almost always exceed 1:160 within 2 to 3 weeks of acute illness. Titers may remain elevated for years, and their significance in chronic brucellosis can be difficult to interpret. Blood is the most frequent source of the organism during the acute phase, while aspirates of bone, joint fluid, or soft tissue abscess may reveal the organism in chronic brucellosis.

Treatment and Prognosis

Mortality is low with antimicrobial therapy in brucellosis, and even without treatment most patients recover spontaneously. Most of the deaths are associated with infective endocarditis. If acute brucellosis is diagnosed or suspected, antimicrobial therapy should be instituted. In vitro susceptibility testing suggests that the tetracycline antibiotics, as well as erythromycin, gentamicin, kanamycin, streptomycin, and rifampin, are quite active against *Brucellae* organisms.[72] Patients are usually treated with a tetracycline for 3 to 4 weeks; however, relapses may be reduced when combination therapy with tetracycline and streptomycin is used.[70] More recently, trimethoprim-sulfamethoxazole has also proved effective. Herxheimer-like reactions may occur with the initiation of antimicrobial therapy and are best treated by administration of glucocorticoids.

GENUS *VIBRIO*

Organisms of the genus *Vibrio* are currently divided in at least three categories: (1) *Vibrio cholerae,* (2) the so-called "nonagglutinable" (NAG) or "noncholera" (NCV) vibrios, and (3) the halophilic vibrios, which include *V. parahaemolyticus, V. alginolyticus,* and an unnamed lactose fermenting (L+) vibrio. In addition, a fourth organism, *Campylobacter fetus* (formerly *Vibrio fetus*), is a related vibrio-like organism that is currently classified in the family Spirillaceae.

Vibrio cholerae and NCV (Noncholera Vibrios)

Morphology and Identification

The *V. cholerae* organism is a short, slightly curved, 0.5 μm × 1.5–3.0 μm gram-negative, motile rod, which is facultatively anaerobic and oxidase-positive. Both nonselective and selective media should be used for the initial isolation of the organism from stool. Nutrient or gelatin agars are suitable for nonselective media, and thiosulfate citrate bile salts (TCBS) agar or tellurite taurocholate gelatin agar (TTGA) are used for selective isolation. Most strains will grow on MacConkey agar. However, some selective media may fail to grow the organism, eg, *Salmonella–Shigella,* eosin methylene blue, and brilliant green agars. Identification is usually performed by inoculation to Kligler iron agar followed by slide agglutination tests with specific polyvalent antisera against *V. cholerae.* Direct fluorescence microscopy on stool specimens using fluorescein-labeled, type-specific antibody can also be used for rapid presumptive diagnosis. The two major *V. cholerae* serotypes, Inaba and Ogawa, may be distinguished by slide agglutination, and the El Tor and classical biotypes can be differentiated by phage susceptibility, polymyxin B susceptibility, and tube hemolysis. NCV vibrios are indistinguishable morphologically or biochemically from *V. cholerae,* but fail to agglutinate with *V. cholerae* antiserum.[73]

Epidemiology and Pathogenesis

Man is the only known host of *V. cholerae,* and the disease is endemic to portions of India and Bangladesh. Periodic pandemics have swept the world since 1800. Cases have been sporadic in Western Europe and the United States since 1960, with a small number of cases reported in Louisiana in 1978. The major mode of transmission appears to be infected water. Asymptomatic cases usually outnumber clinical cases, so that control is difficult. A gallbladder-carrier state may develop but its importance in promulgation of the disease is unknown. The pathogenesis of clinical cholera is one of the best known of all infectious diseases. Illness results from the action of a protein enterotoxin which binds to small bowel epithelial cells and stimulates production of adenylcylase leading to increased concentrations of intracellular cyclic AMP and secretion of electrolytes into the small bowel. The enterotoxin does not cause cell death.

Clinical Manifestations and Diagnosis

The patient with cholera typically has no fever or abdominal pain, but has abrupt, watery diarrhea without blood or mucous, with initial signs of fluid depletion, including poor skin turgor, thready pulse, low blood pressure, tachycardia, and tachypnea. Most adults remain alert, but children may exhibit stupor and convulsions in severe cases. Although many patients have mild illness with relatively small amounts of fluid loss, up to 1 liter per hour may be lost from the gastrointestinal tract. Diarrhea may continue for as long as 7 days. Where the disease is endemic, a presumptive diagnosis can be made on the basis of the clinical evidence. Ultimate diagnosis is established by culture of the organism from stool and identification with specific agglutinating antisera. Diarrhea which is caused by toxin-producing *E. coli* can mimic cholera but is usually not as severe.

Treatment and Prognosis

The mainstay of cholera treatment is fluid and electrolyte replacement. For severely ill patients and those unable to take oral fluids, intravenous replacement is necessary, but oral therapy has become an accepted treatment for those less seriously ill.[74] The failure rate of oral therapy (15 to 20 percent) is highest in those patients with the greatest amount of diarrhea (greater than 20 ml per kg per hour). For oral replacement, either glucose (20 gm per liter) or sucrose (40 gm/liter) is required to facilitate the uptake of sodium by the intestinal epithelium.[75] Concentrations of electrolytes in the oral solution should be approximately 90–100 mEq of sodium, 10–25 mEq of potassium, 65–70 mEq of chloride, and 24–45 mEq of bicarbonate per liter.[74,75] The duration and volume of diarrhea can be reduced by the use of antibiotics. Tetracycline is usually used, but organisms are also susceptible to ampicillin, chloramphenicol, and sulfonamides. The mortality rate in treated cholera should be under 1 percent.

Halophilic Vibrios

Morphology and Identification

The most important organism in this group is *V. parahaemolyticus*, which is one cause of acute diarrhea associated with seafood consumption.[76,77] In addition, *V. alginolyticus* has been found in bacteremias and wound infections associated with a marine environment. More recently, an unnamed lactose-fermenting (L+) vibrio has also been implicated as the cause of bacteremia and wound infections in people exposed to seawater.[78] The organisms are gram-negative, facultative anaerobes that require 1 to 3 percent sodium chloride in media for growth, hence the "halophilic" grouping. TCBS agar is usually used for isolation. Suspect colonies should be picked and transferred to Kligler iron agar or triple sugar iron agar. The three types of halophilic vibrios can be distinguished by their ability to ferment lactose and sucrose.

Epidemiology

Infection with all these organisms is associated either with exposure to seawater or ingestion of seafoods. Gastroenteritis caused by *V. parahaemolyticus* is the most common cause of food poisoning in Japan. In the United States, all cases have been reported from eastern or Gulf Coast states. Most Japanese infections are associated with eating raw seafood, while in the United States infections have been associated with cooked crab, shrimp, lobster, or oysters.[76] Most patients exhibit cramping diarrhea, which begins 6 to 36 hours after ingestion of the suspect food. About one-half of the patients have vomiting and one-fourth have fever.[77] Symptoms usually subside spontaneously after 24 to 48 hours. Both *V. alginolyticus* and L+ vibrios have been isolated from infected wounds of persons working in or near seawater and L+ vibrios have also been isolated from seawater, particularly in warm weather months when the frequency of gastroenteritis peaks.

Pathogenesis

The pathogenesis of *V. parahaemolyticus* infection does not appear to be due to a choleralike enterotoxin but rather to invasion of the gastrointestinal mucosa. In contrast, L+ vibrios resemble *Yersinia* and *Salmonella* organisms in their ability to cause bacteremia via a gastrointestinal portal.

Clinical Manifestations

Patients with *V. parahaemolyticus* infection present with cramping, watery diarrhea with occasional vomiting and nausea. Blood and mucus may be found in the stool. Patients do not have bacteremia and usually have a history of recent seafood ingestion. Patients with skin or wound infections exhibit an intense cellulitis at the site of entry of the organism. Patients with L+ vibrio wound infections may also exhibit signs of systemic infection, including fever and chills, and have positive blood culture results. Patients with L+ vibrio bacteremia, not associated with wound infection, may exhibit erythematous or ecchymotic areas on the extremities which form bullae or vesicles and then become necrotic ulcers. On biopsy, these lesions reveal a vasculitis in the skin and subcutaneous tissues.

Diagnosis

Diagnosis of *V. parahaemolyticus* gastroenteritis can be made by isolation of the organism from stool and from suspect seafoods. Patients with *V. parahaemolyticus* gastroenteritis may have red cells and leukocytes in stool on microscopic examination. Diagnosis of L+ vibrio infection is made from blood or wound cultures.

Treatment and Prognosis

V. parahaemolyticus food poisoning or gastroenteritis is a self-limited disease in the majority of patients and does not require treatment; the efficacy of antibiotics in severe cases is unknown. Antibiotic treatment is strongly recommended for treatment of L+ vibrio infections, but the optimal regimen is not known. Both organisms are susceptible to broad spectrum antibiotics including ampicillin, cephalosporins, gentamicin, tetracycline, and chloramphenicol. Prognosis in *V. parahaemolyticus* gastroenteritis is excellent. In contrast, the mortality rate with L+ vibrio infection approaches 50 percent in bacteremic patients.[78]

GENUS *CAMPYLOBACTER*

Campylobacter fetus

Morphology and Identification

C. fetus, formerly called *Vibrio fetus*, is a non-spore-forming, microaerophilic, spirally curved gram-negative rod that is motile by means of a single polar flagellum. Although multiple subspecies of *C. fetus* are recognized, only two, *intestinalis* and *jejuni*, are associated with the majority of human disease. The organism can be recovered from ordinary blood culture medium as well as thioglycolate, trypticase soy, and beef heart infusion broths, and grows well on sheep blood agar plates under 5 percent carbon dioxide. It tolerates anaerobic conditions but fails to grow under atmospheric conditions. Recovery of the organism from stool in outbreaks of diarrhea has been facilitated by selective media containing vancomycin, polymyxin B, and trimethoprim.[79]

Epidemiology and Pathogenesis

C. fetus is a well-known pathogen of animals, causing abortion in cattle and sheep and enteritis in calves and pigs. Although some cases in humans may be related to animal contact, there are large numbers of patients who give no history of this contact and for which the etiology remains unknown. At least one outbreak has been attributed to contaminated water and cases of bacteremia are presumed to be acquired by the gastrointestinal route. Occasionally, foods have been implicated as a source of gastroenteritis outbreaks, and household contacts have acquired the disease. The pathogenic mechanism of disease remains unexplained, as there is no evidence of either enterotoxin production or invasiveness of the organism, but the disease resembles infections by *Yersinia*, *Salmonella*, and L+ vibrios.[80]

Clinical Manifestations and Diagnosis

Gastrointestinal illness is characterized by abdominal cramping and pain, diarrhea, headache, and fever in approximately 50 percent of patients. Symptoms usually last 1 to 4 days. Infants, pregnant women, and elderly individuals may be at increased risk; among older patients, predisposing debilitating illness is common. Clinical features of the disease are nonspecific, and diagnosis is based on isolation of the organism from blood, stools, or body fluids.

Treatment and Prognosis

The majority of gastrointestinal infections are self-limited and resolve within 4 days without treatment. For persisting diarrhea, erythromycin has been used. In vitro susceptibility suggests that erythromycin, gentamicin, chloramphenicol, and tetracycline are active against the organism and that the organisms may be resistant to ampicillin, penicillin, cephalothin, and carbenicillin.[81] Patients treated for less than 4-week periods have had relapses.[82]

GENUS *ACINETOBACTER*

Acinetobacter Calcoaceticus

Morphology and Identification

Two varieties of this organism cause disease in people: *A. calcoaceticus* var. *anitratus* (formerly *Herellea vaginicola*) and *A. calcoaceticus* var. *lwoffi* (formerly *Mima polymorpha*). The organisms are short, plump, gram-negative rods or coccobacillary forms. They are strict aerobes, do not form spores, and grow readily on simple laboratory media without enrichment or supplementation. Organisms are nonmotile, oxidase-negative, and catalase-positive. The two varieties can be distinguished by their oxidative metabolism of various carbohydrates.

Epidemiology and Pathogenesis

A. calcoaceticus is a ubiquitous organism that is found in soil and water, in both wet and dry environments, and has been isolated from the normal skin, conjunctiva, genitourinary tract, and occasionally pharynx of people. Its pathogenic potential for debilitated and hospitalized patients has been realized only within the last 15 years.[83,84] Infections have been reported primarily from pulmonary sources, wounds, urinary tract, and occasionally cellulitis. Bacteremias have been reported from all these foci. Most patients have undergone instrumentation or manipulation of the respiratory tract or urinary tract, or have had prior surgical procedures. The organism probably causes infection from either the patient's own indigenous flora or is acquired from environmental sources or cross-contamination by hospital personnel or equipment.[84]

Clinical Manifestations and Diagnosis

Most patients have nosocomial respiratory, urinary, or wound infection and exhibit fever, chills, and occasionally hypotension that is indistinguishable from sepsis from other gram-negative organisms. Diagnosis is based on culture isolation of the organism from sputum, urine, blood, or body fluids.

Treatment and Prognosis

Acinetobacters are resistant to a large number of antimicrobials. Most are susceptible to the aminoglycosides, particularly tobramycin and kanamycin, and may also be susceptible to trimethoprim-sulfamethoxazole, carbenicillin, colistin, minocycline, and tetracycline. Susceptibility testing should determine the therapy. For cases resistant to aminoglycosides, the combination of an aminoglycoside and carbenicillin may be synergistic. Mortality in cases of pneumonia or septicemia ranges from 20 to 50 percent and is probably related to the underlying illnesses of the patients and the relative resistance of the organism to most antimicrobials.

GENUS UNKNOWN

Legionnaires' Bacillus *(Legionella pneumophila)*

Morphology and Identification

The name *Legionella pneumophila* has been proposed for the unclassified organism responsible for a large common-source outbreak of respiratory illness which occurred at the American Legion Convention in Philadelphia in July 1976.[85,86] Similar outbreaks and sporadic cases of this illness have been found elsewhere. The organism is a gram-negative bacillus, 0.3–0.4 μm × 2–3 μm, with fastidious growth requirements, which were responsible for the initial failure to isolate it. The first isolates were grown in embryonated chicken eggs, but more recently Mueller–Hinton agar containing 1 percent hemoglobin and 1 percent IsoVitaleX or F-G agar which contains L-cysteine hydrochloride and soluble ferric pyrophosphate have been successful.[87]

The organisms grow optimally at 35C under 2.5 percent CO_2. Although laboratory personnel have rarely been infected by the organism, it should be handled only in laboratories with adequate safety facilities until additional epidemiology data is available.

Epidemiology

The epidemiology of Legionnaires' disease is being actively researched. Evidence of both epidemic outbreaks and hyperendemic disease in certain geographic areas of the country have been established. Epidemic disease has occurred during the warm weather months from July through October, while sporadic cases in endemic areas have occurred throughout the year. Several outbreaks have implicated air conditioning cooling towers as the possible source of the organism. Elsewhere, recent construction has implicated the soil as a possible source. Nosocomial infections, particularly in renal transplant recipients, have been prominent in a newly constructed hospital in California.[88,89] Smokers seem to be more susceptible than nonsmokers to Legionnaires' disease. The incubation period ranges from 2 to 10 days.

Pathogenesis

It is presumed that the organism is acquired by inhalation. The characteristic pathologic findings are limited to the lung where either unilateral or bilateral lobar bronchopneumonia is most often found. The cellular exudate consists of polymorphonuclear neutrophils and macrophages with some areas of coagulative necrosis, but rarely formation of abscesses.[90] Bacteria can be seen by using Dieterle or Gram stain of unfixed tissue imprints.

Clinical Manifestation

In the early phases of illness, Legionnaires' disease cannot be distinguished from other respiratory infections. The patient complains of weakness, malaise, muscle aches, anorexia, mild headache, and occasional dry cough. This is usually followed within a day by the onset of rapidly rising fever, rigors, increasing nonproductive cough with pleuritic pain, and in some instances diarrhea.[91] Altered mentation and obtundation may be a prominent feature in some patients. Rales are usually audible on chest examination, and chest roentgenograms reveal either patchy interstitial infiltrates or discrete areas of consolidation. About half the patients have unilateral involvement; small pleural effusions may be present; cavitation is usually not found. Leukocytosis is common, and hyponatremia, hypophosphatemia, and abnormal liver function tests have been described. Extrathoracic spread to heart, kidney, liver, and spleen has been reported in immunosuppressed or debilitated patients.

Diagnosis

In hyperendemic areas, or during an epidemic, the clinical presentation may be sufficiently unique to make the diagnosis; however, in sporadic cases diagnosis is difficult. Serologic conversion remains the mainstay of diagnosis, and the indirect fluorescent antibody test has been used most frequently. A fourfold rise in titer of paired serum specimens is required for unequivocal diagnosis; however, plague, tularemia, and leptospirosis can also cause fourfold titer rises. During an outbreak, a single titer of $\geq$ 1:256 is required when paired specimens are not available. Other methods of diagnosis are being evaluated, and include the direct immunofluorescent staining of sputum, pleural fluid, transtracheal aspirates, and bronchial washings, all of which have been positive in small numbers of cases.[92] Diagnosis by means of direct culture of lung biopsy specimens remains difficult but should improve with the more widespread use of appropriate media. In the nonepidemic situation, diseases such as psittacosis, Q fever, mycoplasma infection, and influenza can mimic the symptoms of Legionnaires' disease.

Treatment and Prognosis

Mortality in the original Philadelphia outbreak was 16 percent. The number of deaths in subsequent epidemic outbreaks has been reduced because of more rapid recognition of the disease and institution of antimicrobial therapy. In vivo and in vitro susceptibility tests suggest that rifampin and erythromycin are the most effective antimicrobial drugs.[93,94] Among clinical cases, erythromycin has been the mainstay of therapy, usually at a dosage of 2 gm daily, for at least 3 weeks.[88] In addition to antimicrobial therapy, treatment has been directed at maintaining adequate oxygenation with the use of intubation and supportive ventilation.

GENUS *AEROMONAS*

The genus *Aeromonas* consists of motile gram-negative organisms that are commonly isolated from water, soil, food, and a variety of environmental sources. These organisms are often confused with pseudomonads or vibrios because of their origins. Another point of similarity is that one of the *Aeromonas* species, *A. hydrophila,* produces a clinical syndrome that closely resembles that of *P. aeruginosa* septicemia. In contrast to the pseudomonads and other nonfermentative organisms, however, members of the genus *Aeromonas* use carbohydrates fermentatively but are oxidase-positive. Two species of *Aeromonas* have been implicated in human infection—*A. hydrophila* and *A. shigelloides*. *A. hydrophila* has been the cause of an increasing number of human infections including infected traumatic wounds, septicemia, meningitis, osteomyelitis, and postoperative infections.[96] Because of the aquatic nature of these organisms, some infections have been related to trauma and concomitant history of exposure to soil or water (eg, fish handlers).

A. hydrophilia induces two extremely interesting clinical syndromes; (1) a relatively slowly progressing myonecrosis, characterized by liquefaction of muscle in patients with hematologic malignancies, and (2) a syndrome of rapidly progressing necrotizing vasculitis, possibly mediated by endotoxins or exotoxins liberated from the organism and accompanied by cutaneous lesions that are indistinguishable from those observed with *P. aeruginosa* septicemia.[97]

A. shigelloides has been found alone or in associatic with *Shigella* organisms isolated from patients with acute gastroenteritis. Bacteremic and meningitic infections have also been described. *A. hydrophilia* is susceptible to chloramphenicol, the aminoglycosides, tetracycline, and trimethoprim-sulfamethoxazole. Most strains are resistant to the penicillins.[97a]

Miscellaneous Gram-Negative Rods

No distinctive clinical patterns can be observed with a number of miscellaneous gram-negative rods that are occasionally isolated from surgical and systemic infections. *Alcaligenes faecalis* has been isolated from ear cultures, urine, and blood. The genus *Achromobacter* refers to organisms that are often misidentified unless specific biochemical criteria are used. *Achromobacter* strains have been isolated from blood, bronchial washings, and urine. Strains of *Flavobacterium*, particularly *F. meningosepticum*, are free-living organisms found in soil and water that will cause epidemics of meningitis in premature infants. A number of species of *Moraxella* have been designated, and the majority that have been studied have been from either the blood, urine, or upper respiratory secretion.

ACID-FAST BACTERIA

GENUS *MYCOBACTERIA*

The diseases caused by organisms in this genus are summarized in Table 7-2. Other saprophytic organisms exist but are rarely pathogenic.

Mycobacterium tuberculosis and *Mycobacterium bovis*

Morphology and Identification

M. tuberculosis and *M. bovis* are slightly curved or straight rods that are 0.2–0.6 μm × 1–10 μm. With the other mycobacteria, they exhibit the property of resistance to the decolorizing effect of acid-alcohol. The organisms do not stain readily by Gram method but are usually considered to be gram-positive. Because of the slow growth characteristics of tubercle bacilli, special handling procedures are required to control contaminants. Most laboratories use an egg medium such as Lowenstein-Jensen as well as the clear Middlebrook 7H-11 media. From 3 to 8 weeks may be required to detect growth of *M. tuberculosis* colonies, which are usually cream-colored, dry, and wrinkled in appearance. Preliminary screening of cultures to separate *M. tuberculosis* from other *Mycobacteria* is done by means of the niacin test. The identification of acid-fast bacilli in clinical specimens is an important diagnostic procedure, but can be misleading if acid-fast contaminants are present.

Epidemiology

Tuberculosis is contracted almost exclusively by airborne transmission of infected droplets from patients with active

TABLE 7-2. MYCOBACTERIA MOST PATHOGENIC FOR MAN

Group*	Species	Disease Name	Primary Infection Site	Human Saphrophyte	Need for Surgical Treatment
Tuberculosis	*M. tuberculosis*	Tuberculosis	Pulmonary	No	Rare
Complex	*M. bovis*	Bovine tuberculosis	Pulmonary	No	Rare
I Photochromogens	*M. kansasii*	None	Pulmonary	Yes	Occasional
	M. marinum	"Swimming pool granuloma"	Skin	No	Occasional
II Scotochromogens	*M. scrofulaceum*	Scrofula†	Cervical adenitis	Yes	Usual
III Nonphotochromogens	*M. avium complex (M. avium-intracellulare)*	None	Pulmonary	Yes	Frequent
IV Rapid growers	*M. fortuitum*	None	Skin, wound	Yes	Usual
	M. chelonei	None	Skin, wound	Yes	Usual
Unclassified	*M. leprae*	Leprosy	Skin	No	Occasional
	M. ulcerans	Buruli ulcer	Skin	No	Usual

* Groups I to IV as classified by E. H. Runyon

† Scrofula is also frequently caused by *M. kansasii, M. avium-intracellulare* and *M. tuberculosis.*

pulmonary disease. Although bovine tuberculosis may be acquired by the ingestion of contaminated milk, this risk has been all but eliminated by the practice of milk pasteurization. Although tuberculosis may be acquired from contact with infected animals, person-to-person infection is the most common mode of spread. There are currently 30,000 new cases of active tuberculosis reported in the United States each year, approximately 13.5 cases per 100,000 population. Tuberculosis occurs most frequently in major metropolitan areas, the southern United States, areas of high American Indian population, and among lower socioeconomic groups.[97b]

Pathogenesis

Primary tuberculosis infection begins with the inhalation of tubercle bacilli into the alveoli of the lung, where local intracellular and extracellular multiplication takes place. This initial site of infection can be sufficiently prominent to be seen on chest roentgenogram, but usually goes unrecognized. From the local pulmonary site of infection, organisms spread via the lymphatics to hilar lymph nodes and via the bloodstream to all parts of the body. The acute inflammatory cells are replaced by a lymphocytic and histiocytic response, which develops into the characteristic tubercle or granulomatous reaction, frequently with necrosis of central areas. The development of an active cellular immunity might be the rate-limiting factor in control of the initial infection. Factors responsible for active dissemination and spread of tuberculosis at the time of initial infection are not clear. Some patients develop frank pulmonary infiltration or tuberculous pneumonia, while others develop widespread metastatic lesions which, because of their millet-seed appearance, have been called miliary tuberculosis. Patients who have initial hematogenous spread to distant organs usually have no symptoms with the initial infection but may activate disease in these areas at a much later date. Common sites of extrapulmonary involvement include bones, joints, kidneys, adrenal glands, and meninges. Production of cavities in the lung at the site of active infection is common and develops as a result of the emptying of a caseous pulmonary lesion. Pulmonary cavities are the source of large numbers of mycobacterial organisms. Although active disease in adults is most common in the apical and posterior segments of the upper lobes, disease in children may occur anywhere in the lung. The higher oxygen tension in the upper lobes of adults probably favors the growth of the organism in this area. In patients who have effectively controlled their primary infection, calcification of initial parenchymal lung lesions and lymph nodes occurs (Ghon complex).

Clinical Manifestations and Diagnosis

Most patients with active tuberculosis initially have insidious nonspecific symptoms, which include general malaise and fatigue, anorexia, weight loss, low-grade fever, and night sweats. Patients seldom complain of cough during the early phase of the illness; however, as pulmonary lesions progress, cough becomes a more prominent symptom and hemoptysis is common. Cavitary pulmonary tuberculosis can usually be established by the finding of acid-fast organisms in sputum, but in noncavitary disease, the number of organisms expectorated may not be sufficient to be detected by smear.

Extrapulmonary tuberculosis may be even more insidious and difficult to diagnose than pulmonary disease. Patients with tuberculous meningitis usually have an indolent, semiacute course characterized by headache and stiff neck. Cerebrospinal fluid shows mononuclear cells, a low glucose, and an elevated protein, but acid-fast organisms are seen in only about 20 percent of cases. Diagnosis usually depends on evidence of tuberculous disease in other organ systems and the presence of a positive tuberculin skin test.

Patients with tuberculous genitourinary infection usually have asymptomatic pyuria for many years, or may present with the acute onset of dysuria and hematuria. Parenchymal calcification of the kidney may be present but is overemphasized as a sign of renal tuberculosis.[98] Cultures of urine are effective in confirming urinary tract infection, but slow growth of the organism often makes initial empiric treatment necessary.

Female genital tract infections appear as low-grade chronic pelvic inflammatory disease.[99] The presentation of gastrointestinal tuberculosis is often confused with carcinoma of the colon or Crohn disease. Patients have anorexia, weight loss, and signs of intermittent bowel obstruction. Radiographic gastrointestinal contrast studies may show either hypertrophy or ulceration, or both.[100,101] Tuberculous peritonitis is characterized by ascites and fever. Ascitic fluid shows mononuclear leukocytosis and elevated protein. Peritoneal biopsy is usually required for diagnosis, although a large volume of ascitic fluid may yield the organism on culture.[102] Skeletal tuberculosis usually involves chronic pain in the spinal area, although the disease can also involve the hips, pelvis, knees, or long bones. Diagnosis is best established by needle biopsy of bone or synovium.[103]

The diagnosis of all forms of tuberculosis is heavily dependent on the establishment of a positive delayed hypersensitivity skin test. The test is normally applied with intermediate strength (5 tuberculin units) of purified protein derivative (PPD), which is injected intradermally. The presence of 10 mm or more of induration at 48 to 72 hours constitutes a positive result. Induration of 5–10 mm is equivocal and may be indicative of disease caused by *Mycobacteria* other than *M. tuberculosis.* Negative skin test results have been found in up to 17 percent of patients with active tuberculosis.[104]

Treatment and Prognosis

The treatment of tuberculosis has been improved by effective chemotherapeutic drugs (Table 7-3 and Chapter 18). The organism has shown a propensity to develop resistance when single drugs are used for therapy. When a proper regimen of multiple chemotherapeutic drugs is prescribed and adhered to, however, an almost uniformly successful result is achieved. Isoniazid has become the mainstay of antituberculous treatment and is frequently coupled with rifampin, ethambutol, or streptomycin.[105] Most treatment regimens have continued for 18 months; however, recent studies suggest that the duration of therapy can be reduced without increase in the number of relapses. Treatment for up to 2 years may be required for extrapulmonary tuberculosis, and three drugs have been recommended for the initial treatment of tuberculous meningitis. The need for thoracic operations in the treatment of tuberculosis has decreased to almost negligible levels as the effectiveness of antimicrobial chemotherapy has increased.[106] Most operative intervention is performed for nonpulmonary tuberculosis, such as bowel obstruction or perforation in intestinal tuberculosis. For treatment of tuberculosis of the spine, operation may be required to decompress the spinal cord, for drainage of exceptionally large paravertebral abscesses, and occasionally to stabilize a badly destroyed weight-bearing joint. An operation to diagnose extrapulmonary tuberculosis is also frequently required, particularly for intestinal and skeletal disease.

Mycobacteria of Groups I–IV

Morphology and Identification

Nontuberculous mycobacteria, formerly called atypical mycobacteria, have been classified by Runyon into four distinct groups. The species most frequently pathogenic for man are shown in Table 7-2 along with their disease name, the most frequent site of infection, their potential to be saprophytic in man, and the need for surgical intervention. They can be differentiated in the laboratory by their pigmentation and growth characteristics. In addition to the species listed, there are a large number of mycobacterial species that are probably strictly saprophytic, such as *M. gordonae* and *M. smegmatis,* which can be found in clinical specimens but are not known to be pathogenic for people.[107] In addition, *M. simiae, M. szulgai,* and *M. xenopi* have also been found to be rare causes of pulmonary disease.

Epidemiology and Pathogenesis

In contrast to infection caused by members of the tuberculosis complex, people appear to acquire infection with these organisms either from their own saprophytic flora or from the widespread exposure to the organism in nature. Person-to-person spread has not been documented. *M. marinum,* for example, has been found in a variety of water sources including seawater, aquariums, fish tanks, and swimming pools. Infection is probably acquired by abrasion of the skin and subsequent exposure to the organism, which causes disease in fish. *M. intracellulare* has been found in soil as well as in cattle and swine; however, the exact mode of acquisition, particularly in the areas of high skin test reactivity in the southeastern coastal states, remains speculative. Similarly, *M. kansasii* has been isolated from water and raw milk, but specific vehicles of transmission in individual cases are usually obscure. *M. scrofulaceum* and *M. gordonae* are commonly found in water, foods, and soil, and are readily isolated from the respiratory secretions of normal people. *M. fortuitum* has a widespread distribution similar to that of *M. scrofulaceum. M. ulcerans,* the cause of Buruli ulcer, has been described only in Africa, Asia, Australia, and Mexico, where the organism is thought to be acquired from soil. *M. marinum* causes chronic granulomatous skin nodules and ulcers, which occur most frequently in the cooler extremities, and *M. scrofulaceum,* although occasionally a pulmonary pathogen, is usually the cause of cervical lymphadenitis in children. *M. fortuitum* has been associated most often with cutaneous abscesses and wound infections usually at the site of breaks in the skin, and *M. chelonei* has been associated with wound infections at the time of cardiovascular surgery, particularly sternal osteomyelitis, as well as contamination of porcine heart valves at the time of implantation.[108,109]

Clinical Manifestations and Diagnosis

The clinical presentation of *M. kansasii* and *M. intracellulare* mimics that of pulmonary tuberculosis. *M. marinum* causes chronic skin nodules and ulceration, which may be present for many years, and *M. ulcerans* produces extensive granulomatous ulceration of skin and underlying tissue. *M. fortuitum* infections usually present as chronic nodules or draining ulcers at the site of previous trauma. *M. scrofulaceum* shows remarkably little evidence of systemic infection and only a relatively asymptomatic cervical adenitis in children.[110]

Diagnosis of groups I to IV skin infection is best determined from biopsy samples from the margin of the lesion, and examination for acid-fast organisms and granulomas as well as culture for mycobacteria. The causative role of groups I to IV organisms in pulmonary infection may be particularly difficult to demonstrate, because even the most pathogenic of the nontuberculous mycobacteria, *M. kansasii,* may be a saprophyte in the sputum.[111] The presence of a nontuberculous mycobacteria in sputum must be correlated with the illness of the patient and roentgenographic evidence for active pulmonary disease before a diagnosis can be made. Reactivity to the intermediate-strength five TU tuberculin skin test (PPD-S) is usually between 5 and 10 mm in diameter in patients with nontuberculous mycobacterial infection. Greater specificity of the skin test reaction may be achieved by using antigens specific for the mycobacterial species in question.

Treatment and Prognosis

The response to drug therapy of the nontuberculous mycobacteria is extremely variable. *M. kansasii* is the most responsive; however, it is not as susceptible as *M. tuberculosis.* Multiple drug regimens which contain rifampin have been most successful in the treatment of *M. kansasii* pulmonary infections.[107] Triple drug therapy with isoniazid, ethambutol, and rifampin is well tolerated and should be successful in more than 90 percent of cases. Duration of therapy is usually 18 to 24 months. Surgical intervention is only occasionally required as an adjunct to medical treatment. In contrast, *M. avium–intracellulare* is usually resistant to most antituberculous drugs and the use of four to six drugs simultaneously has resulted in bacteriologic conversion in less than 50 percent of patients. Resection of residual diseased segments coupled with chemotherapy is usually recommended for progressive localized *M. avium–intracellulare* pulmonary infections.[107,112] Infection caused by *M. scrofulaceum* and *M. fortuitum* usually requires resection because the organisms are highly resistant to antituberculous drugs.[113] The management of *M. marinum* is difficult to assess because the disease is frequently self-limited. A variety of chemotherapeutic, operative, and irradiation treatments have been applied; however, the results are difficult to evaluate. Successful regimens include traditional antituberculous drugs (rifampin and ethambutol) (Table 7-3), trimethoprim–sulfamethoxazole, minocycline, and tetracycline (Chapter 18, Table 18-42).[107,114,115]

Mycobacterium Leprae

Morphology and Identification

M. leprae is the causative organisms of leprosy (Hansen disease). The organism is an obligate-intracellular, acid-fast bacillus, which is more readily decolored than tuberculosis organisms. Because of this the organism is not dependably stained by the Ziehl-Nelsen method. The Fite method or Fite-Faraco stain is recommended.[116] The organism has never been grown reliably on artificial media. Propagation of the organism in the footpads of mice has been achieved by the injection of infected human material and is a useful confirmatory diagnostic procedure.

Epidemiology and Pathogenesis

Leprosy is primarily a disease of tropical and subtropical areas. In the United States, the majority of endemic cases are reported from Texas, California, Hawaii, and occasionally Louisiana. The average annual incidence in the United States is 0.67 cases per million population.[117] Most of the cases reported in the United States are acquired elsewhere, primarily in Mexico and the Philippines. Leprosy is probably spread directly from person to person, via either respiratory droplets or direct skin contact. Three forms of the disease—tuberculoid, borderline (dimorphous), and lepromatous—have been described. Histologically, patients with tuberculoid leprosy demonstrate epithelioid cell proliferation and typical granuloma formation. Those with borderline leprosy have both an epithelioid and histiocyte cellular response, while those with lepromatous leprosy have only a histiocytic response without demonstrable granulomas. Lymphocytes are frequent in tuberculoid lesions but scanty or absent in lepromatous lesions. Cellular invasion and destruction of nerves is commonly demonstrated in tuberculoid leprosy, while lepromatous leprosy demonstrates only the presence of organisms within the nerves. In the early stages of leprosy, the disease may be indeterminate, ie, the type of reactivity is not yet apparent, and only a nonspecific perivascular mononuclear cell infiltrate may be present.[116]

Clinical Manifestations

The presence of skin lesions accompanied by sensory loss should arouse the suspicion of leprosy, particularly in patients from endemic areas. The organism has a propensity to involve the cooler areas of the body including the peripheral subcutaneous nerves, nasopharyngeal mucous membranes, testes, and the anterior third of the eye. The early sign of leprosy is a hypopigmented skin macule, which may or may not be associated with sensory loss. Patients with tuberculoid disease frequently have a large anesthetic single skin lesion which is raised, scaly, and has a sharp, erythematous margin. In dimorphous or borderline leprosy skin lesions are more widespread than in tuberculoid. In lepromatous leprosy, skin lesions are much smaller and more widely distributed, and diffuse nodular, macular, or plaquelike disease may be present. Loss of the eyebrows is common in lepromatous leprosy, as is a continuous bacteremia.[118] Corneal nerves may be involved, as well as other structures of the anterior eye with potential loss of visual acuity, glaucoma, and blindness.[119] In addition to the three basic types of leprosy, at least two types of reactive episodes have been described early in the course of treatment: the reversal reaction (fever, erythema, edema, neuritis) and erythema nodosum leprosum (red, hot, tender skin nodules).

Diagnosis

Material for diagnosis usually consists of skin scrapings or biopsies. Although nasal secretions are often positive for the organism, diagnosis of the disease depends on the demonstration of acid-fast organisms within the nerves on skin biopsies. The lepromin skin test is frequently used to differentiate the stage or type of leprosy; however, this test has not been useful in the diagnosis. Patients with tuberculoid disease are normally reactive to lepromin, while those with lepromatous disease lack cutaneous reactivity.

Treatment and Prognosis

Dapsone is the primary antimicrobic for the treatment of leprosy. Two other drugs, clofazimine and rifampin, are both effective, although neither has been evaluated as long as dapsone. Plastic and reconstructive surgery is invaluable in the rehabilitation of patients with severe nerve involvement. Prophylactic dapsone treatment of family members has been recommended, particularly if they are under the age of 25.[120]

GENUS *NOCARDIA*

Nocardia asteroides

Morphology and Identification

Members of the genus *Nocardia* are of the family Nocardiaceae, which shares the order Actinomycetales with both the Mycobacteriaceae and Actinomycetaceae. *Nocardia* have previously been considered fungi; however, they are clearly bacteria. Although this discussion will focus on disease caused by *N. asteroides,* occasional infections caused by *N. caviae* and *N. brasiliensis* also occur in the United States. *Nocardia* organisms are aerobic, nonmotile, nonspore-forming, unencapsulated bacteria that are 0.5–1 μm in diameter and have a variable length. Classically, the organisms exhibit thin, filamentous morphology, frequently with branching. They are gram-positive and are also acid-fast; however, exposure to acid alcohol solutions used in the traditional Ziehl-Neilsen staining procedure for mycobacteria should be brief or it will decolorize *Nocardia.* Organisms can be grown in 3 to 10 days on media that is used for mycobacterial culture, on fungal culture

TABLE 7-3. TREATMENT OF MYCOBACTERIAL DISEASE IN ADULTS AND CHILDREN

	Dosage*		Most common side effects*	Tests for side effects*	Remarks*
	Daily	*Twice weekly*			
FIRST-LINE DRUGS					
Isoniazid	5–10 mg/kg up to 300 mg PO or IM	15 mg/kg PO or IM	Peripheral neuritis, hepatitis, hypersensitivity	SGOT/SGPT (not as a routine)	Bactericidal. Pyridoxine 10 mg as prophylaxis for neuritis; 50–100 mg as treatment
Ethambutol	15–25 mg/kg PO	50 mg/kg PO	Optic neuritis (reversible with discontinuation of drug; very rare at 15 mg/kg), skin rash	Red-green color discrimination and visual acuity†	Use with caution with renal disease or when eye testing is not feasible
Rifampin	10–20 mg/kg up to 600 mg PO	Not recommended	Hepatitis, febrile reaction, purpura (rare)	SGOT/SGPT (not as a routine)	Bactericidal. Orange urine color. Negates effect of birth control pills
Streptomycin	15–20 mg/kg up to 1 g IM	25–30 mg/kg	8th nerve damage, nephrotoxicity	Vestibular function, audiograms;† BUN and creatinine	Use with caution in older patients or those with renal disease
SECOND-LINE DRUGS					
Viomycin	15–30 mg/kg up to 1 g IM		Audiotory toxicity, nephrotoxicity, vestibular toxicity (rare)	Vestibular function, audiograms;† BUN and creatinine	Use with caution in older patients. Rarely used with renal disease
Capreomycin	15–30 mg/kg up to 1 g IM		8th nerve damage, nephrotoxicity	Vestibular function, audiograms;† BUN and creatinine	Use with caution in older patients. Rarely used with renal disease
Kanamycin	15–30 mg/kg up to 1 g IM		Auditory toxicity, nephrotoxicity, vestibular toxicity (rare)	Vestibular function, audiograms;† BUN and creatinine	Use with caution in older patients. Rarely used with renal disease
Ethionamide	15–30 mg/kg up to 1 g PO		GI disturbance, hepatotoxicity, hypersensitivity	SGOT/SGPT	Divided dose may help GI side effects
Pyrazinamide	15–30 mg/kg up to 2 g PO		Hyperuricemia, hepatotoxicity	Uric acid, SGOT/SGPT	Combination with an aminoglycoside is bactericidal
Para-aminosalicylic acid	150 mg/kg up to 12 g PO		GI disturbance, hypersensitivity, hepatotoxicity, sodium load	SGOT/SGPT	GI side effects very frequent making cooperation difficult
Cycloserine	10–20 mg/kg up to 1 g PO		Psychosis, personality changes, convulsions, rash	Psychologic testing	Very difficult drug to use. Side effects may be blocked by pyridoxine, ataractic agents or anticonvulsant drugs

* Check product labelling for detailed information on dose, contraindications, drug interaction, adverse reactions, and monitoring.
† Initial levels should be determined on start of treatment.

From American Thoracic Society[114]

media such as Sabouraud's dextrose agar, or on blood agar plates.

Epidemiology and Pathogenesis

Nocardia organisms are found in soil around the world. The primary route of organism acquisition is inhalation and most patients develop pulmonary disease, but breaks in the skin may result in local inoculation of the organism. Widespread dissemination from the initial site of infection is common, particularly extension to the meninges and brain. Although healthy people can acquire nocardiosis, at least half the patients appear to have significant underlying predisposing disorders. The most frequent of these are corticosteroid therapy, chronic pulmonary disease or tuberculosis, leukemia, lymphoma, collagen-vascular disease, and organ transplantation.[121-123] Localized pneumonitis frequently results in tissue necrosis with abscess formation. Granulomas are rare, and the microscopic appearance of the lesion is nonspecific. Direct extension from lung to chest wall is common as is abscess formation at distant sites, particularly the brain.

Clinical Manifestations and Diagnosis

The classic presentation of pulmonary nocardiosis is a progressive necrotizing and cavity-forming infection. Patients usually have a subacute course that is characterized by fever and cough with purulent sputum. The appearance on chest roentgenogram is particularly variable, with manifestations that mimic tuberculosis, acute lobar consolidation, cavitary abscesses, pleural effusions, empyema, and hilar lymphadenopathy.[124] In addition, solitary nodules may be present. Because of the nonspecificity of the presentation, diagnosis may be particularly difficult. If acid-fast smears and cultures of sputum are not productive, more invasive techniques should be pursued, particularly in immunosuppressed patients. Fiberoptic bronchoscopy with brushing and biopsy has been particularly useful, but open lung biopsy may be required.[123] Where subcutaneous nodules and abscesses are present, direct needle aspiration with microscopic examination and cultures should be performed. A brain abscess should be suspected in anyone with a *Nocardia* infection, and axial tomography or technetium brain scanning should be performed if symptoms suggest the possibility. A biopsy specimen from the brain will be needed if the diagnosis cannot be made from another site. Serologic tests have not been useful.

Treatment and Prognosis

The traditional treatment of nocardial infections has been sulfonamides, which should be administered in a dosage sufficient to result in peak serum concentrations of 12–15 mg per 100 ml. Prolonged treatment is usually necessary, ranging from 6 to 12 months. More recently, the combination trimethoprim-sulfamethoxazole has been successfully used,[125] but experience is limited. Susceptibility testing suggests that minocycline, doxycycline, gentamicin, and amikacin may have activity, but they have not been used much.[126,127] Trimethoprim-sulfamethoxazole may be a particularly attractive choice for the treatment of brain abscess because both drugs penetrate well into cerebrospinal fluid. Although immunosuppressed patients can be successfully treated, even with adequate treatment, mortality remains 25 to 45 percent.[128] Mortality is higher in patients who have acute courses of infection, those treated with corticosteroids or other antineoplastic drugs, and those with widely disseminated disease.[128] Abscesses of the brain and other distant sites often must be drained.

SPIROCHETES

GENUS *TREPONEMA*

Treponema pallidum

Morphology and Identification

Although this discussion will focus on *T. pallidum*, the causative organism of syphilis, two other *Treponema* organisms also cause disease in humans. They are *T. pertenue*, which is the cause of yaws, a communicable disease of skin and bones found in tropical regions, and *T. carateum*, which causes pinta, a communicable disease of the tropical Americas characterized by hypopigmented skin lesions. *T. pallidum* is a slender, tightly coiled helical organism 6–20 μm × 0.09–0.18 μm. The organism has not been successfully cultured in vitro, and identification is dependent upon observation of typical motility on dark-field microscopy. The organism can be maintained in the laboratory by intratesticular injection in mature rabbits, and can be stained by specific fluorescein-conjugated antisera as well as by silver impregnation methods on tissue specimens.

Epidemiology and Pathogenesis

Humans are believed to be the only natural host of *T. pallidum*, and infection is thought to occur only by direct contact with infected lesions, usually during sexual intercourse. Congenital syphilis is acquired by the fetus in utero. Most new syphilis cases occur in young persons in the sexually active age groups from 15 to 39. Reported cases of syphilis reached a low point in the United States in the late 1950s but since that time have been gradually increasing. Approximately 5 percent more new cases were reported in 1978 than in 1977. Organisms are thought to enter the body by direct inoculation through the skin or mucous membrane, from which lymphatic and hematogenous spread occurs. Infection is characterized by an endarteritis with vascular inflammatory cell-cuffing of a mononuclear cell type and, in some cases, development of frank granuloma formation, which may demonstrate necrosis.

Clinical Manifestations and Diagnosis

Clinical disease is classically divided into three stages: primary, secondary, and tertiary syphilis. The chancre is the typical lesion of primary syphilis, which begins an average of 21 days after inoculation as a papule that eventually erodes and develops a smooth base with raised firm borders. Lesions are usually single, located on the skin or mucous membranes of the genital area, and painless. Primary lesions can occur at extragenital sites, usually the oral cavity, anus, breasts, and hands. Regional lymphadenopathy in the area of the chancre is common. The chancre usually heals within 3 to 6 weeks without treatment. A pelvic examination must be performed in females to locate the primary chancre, which is often asymptomatic.

Secondary syphilis occurs 6 weeks to 6 months following the primary chancre. Secondary syphilis is characterized by a variety of dermatologic manifestations, including macular, papular, and papulosquamous eruptions which are usually symmetric, mucous membrane lesions, and lymphadenopathy. The skin lesions on the plantar and volar aspects of the hands and feet are most characteristic. Condylomata lata are wartlike lesions of the anogenital area, which are highly infectious. Alopeica may occur, as well as localized infection of the eye, liver, or meninges.[129] The patient with secondary syphilis frequently exhibits nonspecific systemic symptoms such as malaise, headache, sore throat, arthralgias, and low-grade fever. Skin lesions heal without treatment in 4 to 12 weeks.

The patient then enters the latent phase of syphilis during which he or she remains infectious, probably for at least the first year. During the first 4 years of latency (early latency), the patient may develop relapses with mucocutaneous lesions typical of secondary syphilis. In late latency, the patient is considered noninfectious, except for the possibility of maternal fetal transmission or blood transfusion.

Tertiary or late syphilis is the final stage of the disease and is considered noninfectious. Manifestations of tertiary syphilis are of three major types: (1) the gumma or granulomatous syphilitic lesion, which usually occurs in skin or bone, (2) cardiovascular syphilis, in which the basic lesion is aortitis, and (3) neurosyphilis, in which the manifestations may be either primarily meningovascular or general paresis. Patients with neurosyphilis can also have tabes dorsalis, in which degeneration of the posterior columns of the spinal cord occurs.

In addition, newborns with early congenital syphilis can have mucocutaneous lesions much like those of secondary syphilis, as well as nasal purulent discharge and bone lesions. Hepatosplenomegaly is common. Later manifestations of congenital syphilis include dental abnormalities (Hutchinson incisors) and skeletal abnormalities (saddle nose, saber shins, and perforated nasal septum).

Diagnosis

The diagnosis of syphilis can be established by positive dark-field microscopy of lesions of primary, secondary, or congenital syphilis. Although dark-field examination is the most certain way of diagnosis, it requires experience and skill in interpretation and is not generally available. Serologic tests therefore have become the most widespread method of syphilis diagnosis. The serologic tests are of two major types, the nontreponemal or reagin tests such as the Venereal Disease Research Laboratory (VDRL) or Rapid Plasma Reagin (RPR), and the treponemal tests, of which the fluorescent treponema antibody-absorption (FTA-ABS) is the most frequently used. Although the nontreponemal tests are less specific than the treponemal tests, they continue to be used more frequently because of their low cost. They are also useful in following the course of the disease because the results become negative with treatment, whereas the FTA-ABS does not.[130] Because false-positive VDRL tests are common (leprosy, aging, collagen-vascular disease, and intravenous drug abuse), positive results should always be confirmed with the FTA-ABS. In general, false-positive reactions with the FTA-ABS are rare, but the test is positive in nonsyphilitic treponemal diseases such as yaws and pinta.

Treatment and Prognosis

Recommended treatment regimens for the various stages of syphilis are available.[131] In general, early syphilis is treated with a long-acting penicillin, such as benzathine penicillin G, which is administered intramuscularly in a dosage of 2.4 million units. Alternate regimens include aqueous or procaine penicillin G, tetracycline, and erythromycin. For syphilis of more than one year's duration, benzathine penicillin G, 2.4 million units, is administered weekly for 3 weeks. Following treatment the patient should be followed every three months with quantitative VDRL to assure that treatment has been effective. Patients with early syphilis should be evaluated for 1 year, and those with late syphilis for 2 years. Follow-up of case contacts is the major mode of epidemiologic control of syphilis.

GENUS *BORRELIA*

Borrelia **Species**

Morphology and Identification

Borrelia organisms cause relapsing fever. The causative organisms are gram-negative helical, 0.2–0.5 μm × 3–20 μm. They are considered microaerophilic or anaerobic and require complex special media for growth. *B. recurrentis* which is cosmopolitan in distribution is spread by the human body louse. Three species in the United States are spread by ticks and are named after their respective tick vectors, *B. parkeri, B. turicatae,* and *B. hermsii.*

Epidemiology and Pathogenesis

Man is infected by *Borrelia* through the bite of a tick or a louse. Lice acquire the organism by ingesting blood from an infected human and are carriers for life. Humans become infected when bitten by a louse, which is subsequently crushed to release the organism into the abraded skin. A variety of mammalian animals, most often rodents, are probably the source of tick contamination with *Borrelia* organisms in the United States. Tickborne relapsing fever is endemic to western and southwestern states.[132]

Ticks are infectious without being crushed, and the infected person is frequently unaware of a tick bite. Most cases in the United States occur in the summer among campers and hikers in the western part of the country. The incubation period following the bite is approximately 7 days. The spleen is the most frequently involved organ during infection, with splenomegaly and large numbers of spirochetes demonstrable histologically. Immunity is probably humoral.

Clinical Manifestations and Diagnosis

Tickborne and louseborne relapsing fever have similar symptoms characterized by the sudden onset of spiking fever up to 41C, accompanied by headache, myalgias, and arthralgias. Gastrointestinal and upper respiratory symptoms may also be present. Splenomegaly and hepatomegaly are common. A macular truncal rash occurs in about one-fourth of the patients. Symptoms usually subside in 3 to 6 days but last as long as 17 days, followed by an afebrile interval which lasts an average of 6 to 10 days, at which time the patient once again experiences a febrile episode.[133] The afebrile intervals become longer, and relapses milder, as the disease evolves. The mechanism of the relapse is not well explained but is thought to be related to the serial emergence of different serotypes of *Borrelia* organisms during the illness. Wright or Giemsa stained blood smears are often positive on direct examination, but mouse inoculation may be necessary for diagnosis when numbers of organisms are low, as in relapses or afebrile intervals.

Treatment and Prognosis

Drugs currently recommended for the treatment of relapsing fever include tetracycline, erythromycin, and chloramphenicol. Single oral dose treatment regimens with tetracycline and erythromycin have been successful in the treatment of the *B. recurrentis* infection. Patients generally respond more slowly to penicillin G than to tetracycline or erythromycin. The Jarisch-Herxheimer reaction is frequent after the initial administration of an antibiotic, especially if the antibiotic is given during a febrile episode. This reaction is probably mediated by the release of endotoxin. The reaction should be expected and can be fatal in louseborne relapsing fever.[134] Ninety-five percent or more of patients will recover with treatment.

GENUS *LEPTOSPIRA*

Leptospira interrogans

Morphology and Identification

Only a single species, *L. interrogans*, is currently included in the genus *Leptospira* in *Bergey's Manual of Determinative Bacteriology*. Approximately 150 different serotypes of this organism, which causes clinical leptospirosis in man, have been described. The organisms are helical in shape and tightly coiled, 6–20 μm × 0.1 μm, and have a characteristic hook at one or both ends. The organisms are faintly stained with most aniline dyes but can be seen by darkfield microscopy. Culture of the organisms requires special media containing 10 percent serum, such as Fletcher semisolid or Stuart liquid media.

Epidemiology and Pathogenesis

Leptospirosis is a disease of animals, and people acquire it by contact with animals or water contaminated by animal urine. Wild rodents, especially rats, and domestic animals (dog, cat, swine, cattle, horses) are usually responsible for infection in man. Traditionally, the disease has occurred most often in occupations with high animal exposures (farmers, packing plant workers, and veterinarians). More recently, an increasing number of cases are reported among campers, hikers, and swimmers, particularly those who swim in ponds and creeks potentially contaminated by animal urine.[135] The organisms probably enter the body through breaks in the skin and possibly through the respiratory tract. Since the diagnosis is difficult, the disease is probably underreported. Approximately 100 cases per year are reported in the United States, mostly from the south and southeastern states. The mechanism of leptospiral disease production in man is unknown. In fatal cases, organisms are found in the kidney with destruction of tubular epithelium, and hepatocellular degeneration can also be found.

Clinical Manifestations and Diagnosis

Following an incubation period of 7 to 10 days, patients develop an acute febrile illness characterized by headache, severe myalgia, chills, and in some cases nausea, vomiting, and abdominal pain. Nuchal rigidity and meningismus occur frequently, and lumbar puncture reveals cerebrospinal fluid pleocytosis, as well as elevated protein.[136,137] Severe cases with hepatic and renal dysfunction have been referred to as Weil disease. The diagnosis of leptospirosis can be extremely difficult because of the nonspecificity of symptoms, particularly in mild cases. A history of exposure to animals should make the physician suspect the diagnosis. The presentation mimics influenza, viral meningitis, infectious hepatitis, mononucleosis, glomerulonephritis, and viral or mycoplasma pneumonia.[138] Because of the difficulties in isolating the organism, all diagnostic tests are retrospective. The most frequently used serologic test is macroscopic agglutination, but indirect hemagglutination is also in use. Macroscopic agglutination titers should show either a fourfold rise or on single specimens a titer of $\geq$ 1:200. Of the serotypes currently reported in the United States, the most frequent are icterohaemorrhagiae, canicola, and pomona.

Treatment and Prognosis

The benefits of antibiotic treatment for leptospirosis are debatable. The disease is often not diagnosed until late in its course, when there appears to be little benefit from antimicrobial therapy. For early cases, there may be some benefit from penicillin G or tetracycline, which are effective in vitro. Other methods of treatment remain supportive, including renal dialysis when necessary. In severe cases, with combined renal and hepatic failure, mortality may be as high as 10 to 40 percent.

RICKETTSIEAE

Organisms of the tribe Rickettsieae, pathogenic for humans, are included in two genera, *Rickettsia* and *Coxiella*. A variety of worldwide illness is caused by these organisms which are minute, 0.3–0.6 μm × 0.8–2 μm, gram-negative coccobacillary obligate intracellular parasites. Some characteristics of disease caused by these organisms are summarized in Table 7-4. All are transmitted by an arthropod vector, with the possible exception of Q fever, and all are associated with a nonhuman mammalian host for that vector. The three organisms that are the most frequent cause of disease in the United States will be discussed. They are *R. rickettsii*, the cause of Rocky Mountain spotted fever; *R. (mooseri) typhi*, the cause of murine typhus; and *C. burnetii*, the cause of Q fever.

GENUS *RICKETTSIA*

Rickettsia rickettsii

Morphology and Identification

R. rickettsii is the cause of Rocky Mountain spotted fever, probably the most important rickettsial illness in the United States. Because of the dangers and difficulties in identification of rickettsial organisms, isolation is not routinely performed in laboratories. Growth of the organism requires embryonated eggs or cell culture lines and is reserved for well-equipped, experienced research laboratories. Tissue diagnosis of rickettsial illness is usually made by demonstration of the organism in sections using immunofluorescent techniques or Giemsa or Gimenez stains.

Epidemiology and Pathogenesis

Rocky Mountain spotted fever is somewhat a misnomer in the United States, because the majority of cases occur in the Middle Atlantic states. North Carolina, Virginia, Tennessee, and Oklahoma reported the most cases in the years 1975 to 1977.[139] Since the early 1960s, the incidence has risen steadily. In 1977, there were 1,115 reported cases for an incidence of 0.5 cases per 100,000 population. The usual mode of acquisition of the disease is by the bite of a tick. The common tick, *Dermacentor andersoni*, the dog tick, *D. variabilis* and the Lone Star tick, *Amblyoma americanum* are all capable of transmitting Rocky Mountain spotted fever and are distributed in virtually all parts of the United States.[140] The organism is passed transovarially within the ticks, and mammals serve only as supportive hosts for the tick population. The majority of disease occurs in children and young adults during the summer months when ticks are most active; however, in warm southern states the disease may also occur during the winter. Disease may also be acquired by skin abrasions, inhalation, and blood transfusion. The pathogenesis and pathology of all rickettsial diseases is similar because the organism proliferates in the endothelial cells which line the small blood vessels. This leads to perivascular infiltration and bleeding accompanied by thrombosis. Virtually any organ system can be affected, but the skin typically demonstrates a rash as a result of the vasculitic process.

Clinical Manifestations and Diagnosis

The initial presentation is nonspecific, consisting of fever, headache, myalgias, and often mental confusion, usually accompanied by a rash by the second or third day of the illness. The rash is typically maculopapular and petechial and begins on the extremities at the wrists and ankles and spreads proximally, typically involving both palms and soles. The symptoms are frequently confused with those of measles and meningococcal meningitis. Diagnosis is usually made by one of two serologic methods available. Complement fixation tests using specific rickettsial antigens are the most specific means of making the diagnosis; however, the Weil-Felix test is generally more available and depends upon the agglutination of OX-19, OX-2, and OX-K strains of *Proteus vulgaris* by antibodies produced by patients with rickettsial disease. In Rocky Mountain spotted fever, titers greater than 1:160 to either OX-19 or OX-2 are diagnostic. Titers do not normally become positive for a week to 10 days, so diagnosis is frequently made on the basis of the clinical picture. Biopsies of skin lesions with staining by immunofluorescence technique may be positive as early as 4 to 5 days after the onset of the illness.[141]

Treatment and Prognosis

Although specific antimicrobial therapy is available for Rocky Mountain spotted fever, the difficulties and delays in making the diagnosis and initiating therapy are probably responsible for the relatively constant fatality rate, which remains at approximately 5 percent. Both tetracycline and chloramphenicol have been effective and should be instituted promptly and at high dosages. Intravenous therapy is recommended in severe cases, but mild illness may be treated orally. The practice of taking prophylactic tetracycline before potential exposure does not seem to prevent Rocky Mountain spotted fever.

Rickettsia (mooseri) typhi

Morphology and Identification

R. typhi is the causative organism of murine or endemic typhus. The organism is similar to *R. prowazekii*, the causative organism of epidemic typhus (Table 7-4).

Epidemiology and Pathogenesis

Murine typhus is an endemic disease of rodents, affecting about 10 percent of rats,[142] and is transmitted to people by a rat flea bite. Only about 25 cases are reported yearly in the United States, mostly in the South and Southwest. As with the other rickettsial diseases, the pathologic finding is a vasculitis; however, the extent and severity of the disease is generally milder than that of epidemic typhus.

Clinical Manifestations and Diagnosis

Patients typically develop a sudden onset of fever and headache. A pink macular rash appears in the truncal area between the fourth and eighth days of illness which, in contrast to Rocky Mountain spotted fever, spreads peripherally from the trunk. The rash usually remains maculopapular but in severe cases may become petechial. Muscular aches are common, and profound stupor and coma can ensue.[143] Clinically, the disease cannot be distinguished from epidemic typhus or Brill-Zinsser disease. The disease is usually diagnosed by Weil-Felix titer to Proteus OX-19 of 1:160 or greater. Complement-fixing antibodies are also available and appear at 8 to 12 days after the onset of illness.

TABLE 7-4. CHARACTERISTICS OF SOME HUMAN RICKETTSIAL DISEASES

Organism	Disease	Geographic location	Arthropod vector	Mammal host	Weil-Felix Agglutination			Rash
					OX-19	*OX-2*	*OX-K*	
Spotted fever group								
R. rickettsii	Rocky Mountain spotted fever	Western hemisphere	Tick	Rodents, dogs, foxes	+++*	+++*	0	+
R. sibirica	Tick typhus	Siberia, Mongolia	Tick	Rodents	+++*	+++*	0	+
R. australis	Tick typhus	Asia, Australia	Tick	Rodents, Marsupials	+++*	+++*	0	+
R. akari	Rickettsialpox	N. America, Russia, Africa, Korea	Mite	Mouse	0	0	0	+
Typhus fever group								
R. prowazekii	Epidemic typhus	Worldwide	Human body louse	Human	+++	+	0	+
R. prowazekii	Brill-Zinsser disease	N. America, Europe	Reactivation of epidemic typhus years after first attack	Human	0 or +++	0	0		
R. typhi (mooseri)	Murine typhus	Worldwide	Flea	Rodents	+++	0	0	+
Other Rickettsia								
Coxiella burnetti	Q fever	Worldwide	Tick	Rodents, cattle, sheep, goats	0	0	0	0
R. tsutsugamushi	Scrub typhus	Asia, Australia, Pacific	Mite	Rodents	0	0	+++	+

+++ = Strong reaction (≥1:160 dilution).
* Either OX-19 or OX-2 agglutination can occur with Rocky Mountain spotted fever and tick typhus.

Treatment and Prognosis

The best treatment is with either tetracycline or chloramphenicol, and in general the prognosis is excellent. Relapses, which can occur in patients treated early in the disease, respond to reinstitution of therapy.

GENUS *COXIELLA*

Coxiella burnetii

Morphology and Identification

C. burnetii is the causative organism of Q fever. The organism differs somewhat from other Rickettsiae in that it is resistant to physical and chemical agents, and can survive in dust and excreta as well as water and milk. In addition, the Weil-Felix agglutinations fail to respond to infection with *C. burnetii.*

Epidemiology and Pathogenesis

Q fever is worldwide in distribution and is associated with cattle and sheep farms. Ticks are responsible for maintaining the disease in animals, but human infection is acquired primarily by inhalation of dust contaminated by infected animals, by drinking raw milk,[144] or by skin contact with infected animal products (eg, placenta). The disease probably spreads via the bloodstream, and pathologic findings are most frequent in the lung and liver. Peribronchial mononuclear infiltrates are seen in the lung with interstitial pneumonitis, and in the liver most of the infiltration is histiocytic with hepatic cell necrosis.[145] In addition, frank granulomatous formation may be evident.

Clinical Manifestations

Q fever is an acute illness characterized by headache, chills, fever, myalgia, and malaise. Pneumonitis, hepatomegaly, and splenomegaly are present. In patients with atypical pneumonia or infectious hepatitis, the diagnosis of Q fever should always be considered. In contrast to those with the other rickettsial illnesses, patients with Q fever do not have a rash. Severe cases may be complicated by endocarditis.

Diagnosis

Diagnosis is aided greatly by a history of contact with animals, particularly sheep, goats, or cattle; however, the disease may be difficult to differentiate from brucellosis or leptospirosis, which are also acquired from animals. Attempts to isolate the organism from blood or other tissues are usually not made because of the danger of laboratory infection. The most frequent mode of diagnosis is by complement-fixation serologic titers or agglutination tests. In patients with chronic infection such as endocarditis, complement-fixation titer to phase 1 antigen has been the most helpful diagnostic test.[146] Fourfold rises in serologic titers during convalescence are diagnostic.

Treatment and Prognosis

Most patients with acute Q fever have a self-limited illness, lasting 1 to 3 weeks, with a mortality under 1 percent. Both chloramphenicol and tetracycline are effective in vitro, but response to treatment is not as dramatic as with the other rickettsial diseases. Q fever endocarditis remains the most serious complication and requires long-term chronic treatment with either tetracycline or possibly trimethoprim-sulfamethoxazole. Even so, the prognosis is poor and there is some question whether the disease can ever be cured. Prosthetic valve replacement may be required in cases of hemodynamic instability.

CHLAMYDIACEAE

GENUS *CHLAMYDIA*

Chlamydia psittaci

Morphology and Identification

Organisms of the genus *Chlamydia* are coccoid (0.2–1.5 μm diameter) gram-negative obligate intracellular parasites. The chlamydial organisms have both DNA and RNA but are restricted to an intracellular existence because they are incapable of synthesizing ATP and must derive this energy source from their host cells. *C. psittaci* is the causative organism of human psittacosis and similar infections in nonpsittacine birds, in which it is called ornithosis. Isolation of the organism can be accomplished by use of embryonated eggs or cell culture lines; however, extreme caution should be exercised in performing these techniques because of danger of infection of laboratory personnel. Most laboratories rely on serologic diagnosis using a complement-fixation test for psittacosis.

Epidemiology and Pathogenesis

Psittacosis is a disease acquired almost solely by contact with birds and bird products. The majority of cases in the United States occur in people with pet birds (parrots, parakeets, and cockatoos), pet shop workers and poultry plant workers. Domestic and wild pigeons, as well as turkeys, however, are a significant source of the disease.[147] Birds may transmit illness and still appear well. Human infection is acquired by inhalation of droplets or direct contact with infected bird tissues. The disease can also be spread from patient to patient during the acute illness. The organism spreads from the lung via the bloodstream to reticuloendothelial organs. Pathologic examination shows a lobar pneumonia, which is polymorphonuclear early in the disease but is later mononuclear. Cellular inclusions may be visible in large mononuclear cells and stain purple with Giemsa and red with Gimenez stain. Next to the lung, evidence of infection is seen most frequently in the liver and spleen.

Clinical Manifestations and Diagnosis

Patients develop chills, fever, malaise, and headache usually 1 to 2 weeks after exposure. Cough is a prominent feature, but purulent sputum is not. Nausea, vomiting, mental confusion, and delirium may occur in severe cases. An interstitial pneumonitis is seen on roentgenograms of the chest. Because of difficulties of isolating the psittacosis organism, diagnosis is normally made by complement-fixation serologic titers. A fourfold or greater rise in titer during the period from acute illness to convalescence is diagnostic; however, a single titer of $\geq$ 1:16 is frequently considered significant. Differential diagnosis is often difficult without evidence of exposure to birds, and includes such diverse causes of pneumonia as Q fever, mycoplasma pneumonia, influenza, blastomycosis, and histoplasmosis.

Treatment and Prognosis

Tetracycline is the preferred drug for the treatment of psittacosis. Chloramphenicol and penicillin G have also been used, but they are not as effective as tetracycline. Treatment should be continued for 14 days. Mortality is 1 percent in treated patients.

Chlamydia trachomatis

Morphology and Identification

Isolation of *C. trachomatis* is usually accomplished in nonreplicating cell culture lines such as HeLa or McCoy cells, using antibiotics to inhibit other organisms. Centrifugation of the inoculum is required to increase the tissue culture infection rate. *C. trachomatis* cellular inclusions can be identified with the use of iodine stains, and this staining property distinguishes the organisms from *C. psittaci.*[148] Use of cell culture techniques has enhanced the ability of laboratories to isolate *C. trachomatis,* which is the causative organism of a number of clinical illnesses including trachoma inclusion conjunctivitis, lymphogranuloma venereum, nongonococcal urethritis and other genital infections, and neonatal pneumonia.

Epidemiology and Pathogenesis

The epidemiology of *C. trachomatis* infection varies with the type of infection. Specific serotypes have been implicated as the cause of lymphogranuloma venereum, while another group of serotypes are the cause of trachoma. Still a third group consisting of eight serotypes is associated with nongonococcal urethritis, cervicitis, salpingitis, conjunctivitis, and neonatal pneumonia.[148]

Trachoma. Trachoma is thought to spread from person to person by direct contact with secretions from the eyes. It is a disease that is endemic in families in certain underdeveloped areas of Africa, Asia, and Latin America. In the United States, the disease is most common in the Southwest. Trachoma begins as a hyperemic infiltrative lesion of the conjunctiva under the lids, usually in children under 10 years of age. Part of the pathologic development in trachoma may be related to secondary bacterial infections which occur frequently. The classic cobblestone appearance of the palpebral conjunctiva is evident in well-established disease.

Lymphogranuloma Venereum. Lymphogranuloma venereum is transmitted by sexual contact and is most frequent in tropical areas of Africa and Asia. There are usually less than 1,000 cases reported annually in the United States, most of which are acquired outside the country; however, the disease is endemic in the southeastern United States. Lymphogranuloma venereum usually begins with a nonspecific granulomatous genital vesicle or ulcer, from which the organisms spread to regional groin lymph nodes. Central radiating areas of necrosis are common in lymph nodes, which are usually filled with epithelioid cells and giant cells. Frank purulent drainage may occur in severe cases. Lymphatic obstruction may result in genital edema. Involvement of the rectum and perirectal tissues can lead to the formation of hemorrhagic mucosal lesions and eventually fibrotic stricture, mucosal ulceration, and fistula formation.

Nongonococcal Urethritis. Nongonococcal urethritis is also contracted by sexual contact, as are cervicitis, salpingitis, and epididymitis.[149-151] Neonatal conjunctivitis and pneumonia probably occur by direct contact at the time of birth.[152]

Clinical Manifestations and Diagnosis

Diagnosis of trachoma is usually established by typical clinical signs but should be confirmed with Giemsa, iodine, or immunofluorescent stains of conjunctival scrapings, or by culture of the responsible agent.

Lymphogranuloma venereum is also diagnosed by the clinical appearance of inguinal adenopathy and isolation of *C. trachomatis* from lymph node aspirates. Direct Giemsa or iodine stain smears may be helpful where cultures are not available. The complement-fixation serologic test is the most widely used diagnostic test; however, it does cross-react with other *Chlamydia*. Single titers $\geq$ 1:16 are usually considered significant.

Complement fixation titers are also elevated in *C. trachomatis* genital infections, conjunctivitis, and neonatal pneumonia. The only completely reliable diagnostic method is isolation of the organism in cell culture or embryonated eggs. Organisms that grow on cell culture are presumptively identified to be *C. trachomatis* by demonstrating iodine-stained cytoplasmic inclusions. In urethritis, a serous discharge that contains few polymorphonuclear leukocytes favors nongonococcal rather than gonococcal etiology.

Treatment and Prognosis

The treatment for trachoma has been difficult, largely because of the problem of regular administration of antibiotics to patients in underdeveloped countries. Tetracycline, erythromycin, rifampin, and sulfonamides are all effective against *C. trachomatis*, which differs from *C. psittaci* in its susceptibility to sulfonamides. Improvement in hygienic conditions is probably as important as the antimicrobial therapy in the control of trachoma. For lymphogranuloma venereum, treatment with either tetracycline or sulfonamides for 2 to 4 weeks has been recommended; however, the long-term complications of rectal stricture may not be prevented by these measures. Fluctuant lymph nodes should be drained by needle aspiration. For the treatment of chlamydial urethritis, tetracycline is recommended with a minimum course of 7 days. Some authors have recommended prolonged treatment for as long as 21 days. Erythromycin is also effective. The sexual partners of males with urethritis should also receive treatment. Nongonococcal urethritis can be prevented by a single dose of minocycline.

MYCOPLASMATACEAE

GENUS *MYCOPLASMA*

Mycoplasma pneumoniae

Morphology and Identification

Although other *Mycoplasma* species have been implicated as potential causes of disease in the genitourinary tract,[153] *M. pneumoniae* is primarily a respiratory tract pathogen. The mycoplasmas are the smallest organisms capable of independent existence and are about 125–250 nm in largest, and is pleomorphic. *M. pneumoniae* is filamentous. All *Mycoplasma* species lack a true cell wall and are enclosed only by a single triple-layered membrane. Special culture media are required for the isolation of *Mycoplasma* because cholesterol or other sterols are required. Serum and yeast extract is usually included in the medium. *M. pneumoniae* grows aerobically, but requires 2 to 3 weeks for isolation.

Epidemiology and Pathogenesis

M. pneumoniae infections occur throughout the world's temperate zones. Most cases occur in people between the age of 5 and 25 years and are unusual in preschool children and the elderly. High rates of mycoplasma infection have typically been described in college students and military recruits, and case clustering occurs in families.[154] Inhalation of droplets from infected patients is the method of spread. An interstitial pneumonia with acute bronchiolitis accompanied by mononuclear cell infiltrates results.

Clinical Manifestations and Diagnosis

Patients usually have an insidious onset of upper respiratory symptoms accompanied by fever and cough. Occasionally, there are chills. Fever persists for 8 to 10 days, and typically the cough remains dry and nonproductive. Headache is a frequent accompaniment, but myalgias and arthralgias occur in only about 20 percent of patients. On physical examination, rales are heard in about three-fourths of the patients. About 20 percent have a rash. Bullous or hemorrhagic myringitis occurs in about 10 percent. Other manifestations of mycoplasma infection include cold-agglutinin hemolytic anemia, gastroenteritis, hepatitis, pericarditis, myocarditis, and erythema multiforme.[154,155] Meningitis and meningoencephalitis are rarely described. The major differential diagnosis of *M. pneumoniae* is pneumonia caused by psittacosis, Q fever, various viruses, and Legionnaires' bacillus. Because of the difficulty and time required to culture the organism, presumptive diagnoses are frequently made on the basis of a positive cold-agglutinin titer of 1:32 or greater. Specific complement-fixation serologic tests are also available and are much more specific than the cold-agglutinin. More unusual manifestations of pulmonary mycoplasma infection include lung abscess and pleural effusion.

Treatment and Prognosis

Mycoplasma organisms are sensitive to erythromycin and the tetracyclines, but are resistant to penicillin, cephalosporins, and chloramphenicol.[156] Clinical studies have shown that pneumonia resolves more rapidly in patients treated with either erythromycin or tetracyclines. Persistence of mycoplasma organisms in the sputum of patients during antibiotic therapy has been described; in spite of this, the patients appear to respond to treatment. The spectrum of mycoplasma infection varies from asymptomatic infection to fatal pneumonia; however, most patients gradually recover after 7 to 10 days of illness whether antibiotic treatment is used or not.

BIBLIOGRAPHY

Buchanan RE, Ribbons NE (eds): Bergey's Manual of Determinative Bacteriology. Baltimore, Williams and Wilkins, 1974.

Hoeprich PD (ed): Infectious Diseases. Hagerstown, Harper and Row, 1977.

Lennette EH, Spaulding EH, Truant JP (eds): Manual of Clinical Microbiology. Washington, American Society for Microbiology, 1974.

Mandell GL, Douglas RG Jr, Bennett JE: Principles and Practice of Infectious Diseases, Vol I and II New York: John Wiley, 1979.

Wilson GS, Miles AA: Topley and Wilson's Principles of Bacteriology, Virology and Immunity. Baltimore, Williams and Wilkins, 1968.

REFERENCES

GRAM-POSITIVE BACTERIA

Genus *Bacillus*

1. Farrar EW: Serious infections due to "non-pathogenic" organisms of the genus bacillus. Am J Med 34:134, 1963.
2. Turnbull PCB, French TA, Dowsett EG: Severe systemic and pyogenic infections with *Bacillus cereus*. Br Med J 1:1628, 1977.
3. Pennington JE, Gibbons ND, Strobeck JE, Simpson GL, Myerowitz RL: Bacillus species infection in patients with hematologic neoplasia. JAMA 235:1473, 1976.
4. Terranova W, Blake PA: *Bacillus cereus* food poisoning. N Engl J Med 298:143, 1978.
5. Coonrod JD, Leadley PJ, Eickhoff TC: Antibiotic susceptibility of bacillus species. J Infect Dis 123:102, 1971.

Genus *Corynebacterium*

6. Center for Disease Control: Diphtheria Surveillance. Summary Report No. 12 issued July 1978.
7. McCloskey RV, Eller JJ, Green M, Mauney CU, Richards SEM: The 1970 epidemic of diphtheria in San Antonio. Ann Intern Med 75:495, 1971.
8. Pedersen AHB, Spearman J, Tronca E, Bader M, Harnisch J: Diphtheria on Skid Road, Seattle, Washington, 1972–1975. Public Health Rep 92:336, 1977.
9. Collier RJ: Diphtheria toxin: mode of action and structure. Bacteriol Rev 39:54, 1975.
10. Munford RS, Ory HW, Brooks GF, Feldman RA: Diphtheria deaths in the United States, 1959–1970. JAMA 229:1890, 1974.
11. McCloskey RV, Green MJ, Eller J, Smilack J: Treatment of diphtheria carriers: Benzathine penicillin, erythromycin and clindamycin. Ann Intern Med 81:788, 1974.
12. Hande KR, Witebsky FG, Brown MS, Schulman CB, Anderson SE Jr, Levine AS, MacLowry JD, Chabner BA: Sepsis with a new species of *Corynebacterium*. Ann Intern Med 85:423, 1976.
13. Pearson TA, Braine HG, Rathbun HK: *Corynebacterium* sepsis in oncology patients. Predisposing factors, diagnosis, and treatment. JAMA 238:1737, 1977.
14. Johnson WD, Kaye D: Serious infections caused by diphtheroids. Ann NY Acad Sci 174:568, 1970.

LISTERIA

15. Bojsen-Moller J: Human listeriosis. Diagnostic, epidemiological and clinical studies. Acta Pathol Microbiol Scand (B) 229:1, 1972.
16. Nieman RE, Lorber B: Listeriosis in adults: a changing pattern. Report of eight cases and a review of the literature, 1968–1978. Rev Infect Dis 2:207, 1980.
17. Bottone EJ, Sierra MF: *Listeria monocytogenes:* Another look at the "Cinderella among pathogenic bacteria." Mt Sinai J Med NY 44:42, 1977.
18. Visintine AM, Oleske JM, Nahmias AJ: *Listeria monocytogenes* infection in infants and children. Am J Dis Child 131:393, 1977.
19. Louria DB, Hensle T, Armstrong D, Collins HS, Blevens A, Krugman D, Buse M: Listeriosis complicating malignant disease. A new association. Ann Intern Med 67:261, 1967.
20. Buchner LH, Schneierson SS: Clinical and laboratory aspects of *Listeria monocytogenes* infections. With a report of ten cases. Am J Med 45:904, 1968.
21. Ascher NL, Simmons RL, Marker S, Najarian JS: *Listeria* infection in transplant patients. Five cases and a review of the literature. Arch Surg 113:90, 1978.
22. Schröter GPJ, Weil R III: *Listeria monocytogenes* infection after renal transplantation. Arch Intern Med 137:1395, 1977.
23. Watson GW, Fuller TJ, Elms J, Kluge RM: *Listeria* cerebritis: relapse of infection in renal transplant patients. Arch Intern Med 138:83, 1978.
24. Wiggins GL, Albritton WL, Feeley JC: Antibiotic susceptibility of clinical isolates of *Listeria monocytogenes*. Antimicrob Agents Chemother 13:854, 1978.
25. Moellering RC Jr, Medoff G, Leech I, Wennersten C, Kunz LJ: Antibiotic synergism against *Listeria monocytogenes*. Antimicrob Agents Chemother 1:30, 1972.

ERYSIPELOTHRIX

26. Scully RE, Galdabini JJ, McNeely BU: Case records of the Massachusetts General Hospital. Weekly clinicopathological exercises. Case 16—1978. N Engl J Med 298:957, 1978.
27. Grieco MH, Sheldon C: *Erysipelothrix rhusiopathiae*. Ann NY Acad Sci 174:523, 1970.
28. Simberkoff MS, Rahal JJ Jr: Acute and subacute endocarditis due to *Erysipelothrix rhusiopathiae*. Am J Med Sci 266:53, 1973.

GRAM-NEGATIVE BACTERIA

Francisella tularensis

29. Young LS, Bickness DS, Archer BG, Clinton JM, Leavens LJ, Feeley JC, Brachman PS: Tularemia epidemic: Vermont, 1968. Forty-seven cases linked to contact with muskrats. N Engl J Med 280:1253, 1969.
30. Guerrant RL, Humphries MK Jr, Butler JE, Jackson RS: Tickborne oculoglandular tularemia. Case report and review of seasonal and vectoral associations in 106 cases. Arch Intern Med 136:811, 1976.

31. Klock LE, Olsen PF, Fukushima T: Tularemia epidemic associated with the deerfly. JAMA 226:149, 1973.
32. Miller RP, Bates JH: Pleuropulmonary tularemia. A review of 29 patients. Am Rev Resp Dis 99:31, 1969.
33. Buchanan TM, Brooks GF, Brachman PS: The tularemia skin test. 325 skin tests in 210 persons: serologic correlation and review of the literature. Ann Intern Med 74:336, 1971.

Pasteurella multocida

34. Carter GR: Pasteurillosis. *Pasteurella multocida* and *Pasteurella hemolytica.* Adv Vet Sci 11:321, 1969.
35. Heddleston KL, Wessman G: Characteristics of *Pasteurella multocida* of human origin. J Clin Microbiol 1:377, 1975.
36. Hubbert WT, Rosen MN: I. *Pasteurella multocida* infection due to animal bite. Am J Pub Health 60:1103, 1970.
37. Francis DP, Holmes MA, Brandon G: *Pasteurella multocida.* Infections after domestic animal bites and scratches. JAMA 233:42, 1975.
38. Tindall JP, Harrison CM: *Pasteurella multocida* infection following animal injuries, especially cat bites. Arch Dermatol 105:412, 1972.
39. Hubbert WT, Rosen MN: II.*Pasteurella multocida* infection in man unrelated to animal bite. Am J Pub Health 60:1109, 1970.
40. Rosenthal SL, Freudlich LF: In vitro antibiotic sensitivity of *Pasteurella multocida.* Health Lab Sci 13:246, 1976.

Streptobacillus moniliformis and *Spirillum minor*

41. Lambe DW, McPhedran AM, Mertz JA, Stewart P: *Streptobacillus moniliformis* isolated from a case of Haverhill fever: biochemical characterization and inhibitory effect of sodium polyanethol sulfonate. Am J Clin Pathol 60:854, 1973.
42. Cole JS, Stoll RW, Bulger RJ: Rat-bite fever. Report of three cases. Ann Intern Med 71:979, 1969.
43. Roughgarden JW: Antimicrobial therapy of rat-bite fever. A review. Arch Intern Med 116:39, 1965.

Eikenella corrodens

44. Brooks GF, O'Donoghue JM, Rissing JP, Soapes K, Smith JW: *Eikenella corrodens,* a recently recognized pathogen: infections in medical-surgical patients and in association with methylphenidate abuse. Medicine 53:325, 1974.
45. Dorff GJ, Jackson LJ, Rytel MW: Infections with *Eikenella corrodens.* A newly recognized human pathogen. Ann Intern Med 80:305, 1974.
46. Robinson JVA, James AL: In vitro susceptibility of *Bacteroides corrodens* and *Eikenella corrodens* to ten chemotherapeutic agents. Antimicrob Agents Chemother 6:543, 1974.
47. Geraci JE, Hermans PE, Washington JA II: *Eikenella corrodens* endocarditis: report of cure in two cases. Mayo Clin Proc 49:950, 1974.

Bordetella pertussis

48. Nelson JD: The changing epidemiology of pertussis in young infants. The role of adults as reservoirs of infection. Am J Dis Child 132:371, 1978.
49. Olson LC: Pertussis. Medicine 54:427, 1975.
50. Baraff LJ, Wilkins J, Wehrle PF: The role of antibiotics, immunizations, and adenoviruses in pertussis. Pediatrics 61:224, 1978.
51. Bass JW, Klenk EL, Kotheimer JB, Linnemann CC, Smith MHD: Antimicrobial treatment of pertussis. J Pediatr 75:768, 1969.

GENUS *HAEMOPHILUS*

Haemophilus influenzae

52. Todd JK, Bruhn FW: Severe *Haemophilus influenzae* infections. Am J Dis Child 129:607, 1975.
53. Wallace RJ Jr, Musher DM, Martin RR: *Haemophilus influenzae* pneumonia in adults. Am J Med 64:87, 1978.
54. Syriopoulou V, Scheifele D, Smith AL, Perry PM, Howie V: Increasing incidence of ampicillin resistance in *Haemophilus influenzae.* J Pediatr 92:889, 1978.
55. Ward JI, Tsai TJ, Filice GA, Fraser DW: Prevalence of ampicillin- and chloramphenicol-resistant strains of *Haemophilus influenzae* causing meningitis and bacteremia: national survey of hospital laboratories (NY). J Infect Dis 138:421, 1978.
56. Steinberg EA, Overturf GD, Wilkins J, Baraff LJ, Streng JM, Leedom JM: Failure of cefamandole in treatment of meningitis due to *Haemophilus influenzae* type b. J Infect Dis 137 (Suppl):S180, 1978.
57. Kirven LA, Thornsberry C: Minimum bactericidal concentration of sulfamethoxazole-trimethoprim for *Haemophilus influenzae:* correlation with prophylaxis. Antimicrob Agents Chemother 14:731, 1978.

Haemophilus Ducreyi

58. Hammond GW, Slutchuk M, Scatliff J, Sherman E, Wilt JC, Ronald AR: Epidemiologic, clinical, laboratory, and therapeutic features of an urban outbreak of chancroid in North America. Rev Infect Dis 2:867, 1980.
59. Kerber RE, Rowe CE, Gilbert KR: Treatment of chancroid. A comparison of tetracycline and sulfisoxazole. Arch Dermatol 100:604, 1969.
60. Marmar JL: The management of resistant chancroid in Vietnam. J Urol 107:807, 1972.

Haemophilus Species

61. Page MI, King EO: Infection due to *Actinobacillus actinomycetemcomitans* and *Haemophilus aphrophilus.* N Engl J Med 275:181, 1966.
62. Bieger RC, Brewer NS, Washington JA II: *Haemophilus aphrophilus:* a microbiologic and clinical review and report of 24 cases. Medicine 57:345, 1978.
63. Lynn DJ, Kane JG, Parker RH: *Haemophilus parainfluenzae* and *influenzae* endocarditis: a review of forty cases. Medicine 56:115, 1977.
64. Chunn CJ, Jones SR, McCutchan JA, Young EJ, Gilbert DN: *Haemophilus parainfluenzae* infective endocarditis. Medicine 56:99, 1977.
65. Pheifer TA, Forsyth PS, Durfee MA, Pollock HM, Holmes KK: Nonspecific vaginitis: role of *Haemophilus vaginalis* and treatment with metronidazole. N Engl J Med 298:1429, 1978.
66. Venkataramani TK, Rathbun KH: *Corynebacterium vaginale (Haemophilus vaginalis)* bacteremia: Clinical study of 29 cases. Johns Hopkins Med J 139:93, 1976.

CALYMMATOBACTERIUM GRANULOMATIS

67. Lal S, Nicholas C: Epidemiological and clinical features in 165 cases of granuloma inguinale. Br J Vener Dis 46:461, 1970.
68. Stewart DB: The gynecological lesions of lymphogranuloma venereum and granuloma inguinale. Med Clin N Amer 48:773, 1964.

Genus *Brucella*

BRUCELLAE SPECIES

69. Center for Disease Control: Brucellosis Surveillance, Annual Summary 1977, issued December 1978.
70. Buchanan TM, Faber LC, Feldman RA: Brucellosis in the United States, 1960–1972. An abattoir-associated disease. I. Clinical features and therapy. Medicine 53:403, 1974.
71. Elberg SS: Immunity to brucella infection. Medicine 52:339, 1973.
72. Hall WH, Manion RE: In vitro susceptibility of Brucella to various antibiotics. Appl Microbiol 20:600, 1970.

Genus *Vibrio*

VIBRIO CHOLERAE AND NONCHOLERAE VIBRIOS

73. Highes JM, Hollis DG, Gangarosa EJ, Weaver RE: Noncholera vibrio infections in the United States. Clinical epidemiologic, and laboratory features. Ann Intern Med 88:602, 1978.
74. Pierce NF, Sack RB, Mitra RC, Banwell JG, Brigham KL, Fedson DS, Mondal I: Replacement of water and electrolyte losses in cholera by an oral glucose-electrolyte solution. Ann Intern Med 70:1173, 1969.
75. Palmer DL, Koster FT, Islam AFMR, Rahman ASMN, Sack RB: Comparison of sucrose and glucose in the oral electrolyte therapy of cholera and other severe diarrheas. N Engl J Med 297:1107, 1977.

VIBRIO SPECIES

76. Barker WH Jr: *Vibrio parahaemolyticus* outbreaks in the United States. Lancet 1:551, 1974.
77. Bolen JL, Zamiska SA, Greenough WB III: Clinical features in enteritis due to *Vibrio parahaemolyticus.* Am J Med 57:638, 1974.
78. Blake PA, Merson MH, Weaver RE, Hollis DG, Heublein PC: Disease caused by a marine Vibrio. Clinical characteristics and epidemiology. N Engl J Med 300:1, 1979.

Genus *Campylobacter*

CAMPYLOBACTER FETUS

79. Skirrow MB: *Campylobacter* enteritis: a "new" disease. Br Med J 2:9, 1977.
80. Guerrant RL, Lahita RG, Winn WC Jr, Roberts RB: Campylobacteriosis in man: Pathogenic mechanisms and review of 91 bloodstream infections. Am J Med 65:584, 1978.
81. Butzler JP, Dekeyser P, Lafontaine T: Susceptibility of related vibrios and Vibrio fetus to twelve antibiotics. Antimicrob Agents Chemother 5:86, 1974.
82. Bokkenheuser V: Vibrio fetus infection in man. I. Ten new cases and some epidemiologic observations. Am J Epidemiol 91:400, 1970.

Genus *Acinetobacter*

ACINETOBACTER CALCOACETICUS

83. Glew RH, Moellering RC Jr, Kunz LJ: Infections with *Acinetobacter calcoaceticus (Herellea vaginicola):* clinical and laboratory studies. Medicine 56:79, 1977.
84. Buxton AE, Anderson RL, Werdegar D, Atlas E: Nosocomial respiratory tract infection and colonization with *Acinetobacter calcoaceticus.* Epidemiologic characteristics. Am J Med 65:507, 1978.

LEGIONNAIRES' BACILLUS

85. Fraser DW, Tsai TR, Orenstein W, Parkin WE, Beecham HJ, Sharrar RG, Harris J, Mallison GF, Martin SM, McDade JE, Shepard CC, Brachman PS: Legionnaires' disease: description of an epidemic of pneumonia. N Engl J Med 297: 1189, 1977.
86. McDade JE, Shepard CC, Fraser DW, Tsai TR, Redus MA, Dowdle WR: Legionnaires' disease: isolation of a bacterium and demonstration of its role in other respiratory disease. N Engl J Med 297:1197, 1977.
87. Feeley, JC, Gorman GW, Weaver RE, Mackel DC, Smith HW: Primary isolation media for Legionnaires' disease bacterium. J. Clin Microbiol 8:320, 1978.
88. Kirby BD, Snyder KM, Meyer RD, Finegold SM: Legionnaires' disease: clinical features of 24 cases. Ann Intern Med 89:297, 1978.
89. Bock BV, Kirby BD, Edelstein PH, George WL, Snyder KM, Owens ML, Hatayama CM, Haley CE, Lewis RP, Meyer RD, Finegold SM: Legionnaires' disease in renal-transplant recipients. Lancet 1:410, 1978.
90. Winn WC Jr, Glavin FL, Perl DP, Keller JL, Andres TL, Brown TM, Coffin CM, Sensecqua JE, Roman LN, Craighead JE: The pathology of Legionnaires' disease. Fourteen fatal cases from the 1977 outbreak in Vermont. Arch Pathol Lab Med 102:344, 1978.
91. Center for Disease Control: Legionnaires' disease: diagnosis and management. Ann Intern Med 88:363, 1978.
92. Broome CV, Cherry WB, Winn WC Jr, MacPherson BR: Rapid diagnosis of Legionnaires' disease by direct immunofluorescent staining. Ann Intern Med 90:1, 1979.
93. Thornsberry C, Baker CN, Kirven LA: In vitro activity of antimicrobial agents on Legionnaires' disease bacterium. Antimicrob Agents Chemother 13:78, 1978.
94. Edelstein PH, Meyer RD: Susceptibility of *Legionella pneumophila* to twenty antimicrobial agents. Antimicrob Agents Chemother 18:403, 1980.
95. Haley CE, Cohen ML, Halter J, Meyer RD: Nosocomial Legionnaires' disease: A continuing common-source epidemic at Wadsworth Medical Center. Ann Intern Med 90:583, 1979.

GENUS *AEROMONAS*

96. Washington JA II: *Aeromonas hydrophila* in clinical bacteriological specimens. Ann Intern Med 76:611, 1972.
97. Ketover BP, Young LS, Armstrong D: Septicemia due to *Aeromonas hydrophila:* clinical and immunologic aspects. J Infect Dis 127:284, 1973.

97a. Overman TL: Antimicrobial susceptibility of *Aeromonas hydrophila.* Antimicrob Agents Chemother 17:612, 1980.

ACID-FAST BACTERIA

Genus *Mycobacteria*

MYCOBACTERIUM TUBERCULOSIS AND BOVIS

97b. Glassroth J, Robins AG, Snider DE Jr: Tuberculosis in the 1980s. N Engl J Med 302:1441, 1980.

98. Christensen WI: Genitourinary tuberculosis: review of 102 cases. Medicine 53:377, 1974.
99. Klein TA, Richmond JA, Mishell DR Jr: Pelvic tuberculosis. Obstet Gynecol 48:99, 1976.
100. Tabrisky J, Lindstrom RR, Peters R, Lachman RS: Tuberculous enteritis. Review of a protean disease. Am J Gastroenterol 63:49, 1975.
101. Schulze K, Warner HA, Murray D: Intestinal tuberculosis: experience at a Canadian teaching institution. Am J Med 63:735, 1977.
102. Dineen P, Homan WP, Grafe WR: Tuberculous peritonitis:

43 years' experience in diagnosis and treatment. Ann Surg 184:717, 1976.
103. Davidson PT, Horowitz I: Skeletal tuberculosis. A review with patient presentations and discussion. Am J Med 48:77, 1970.
104. Holden M, Dubin MR, Diamond PH: Frequency of negative intermediate-strength tuberculin sensitivity in patients with active tuberculosis. N. Engl J Med 285:1506, 1971.
105. Johnston RF, Wildrick KH: "State of the art" review. The impact of chemotherapy on the care of patients with tuberculosis. Am Rev Respir Dis 109:636, 1974.
106. Strieder JW, Laforet EG, Lynch JP: The surgery of pulmonary tuberculosis. N Engl J Med 276:960, 1967.

MYCOBACTERIA OF GROUPS I–IV

107. Wolinsky E: Nontuberculous mycobacteria and associated diseases. Am Rev Respir Dis 119:107, 1979.
108. Robicsek F, Daugherty HK, Cook JW, Selle JG, Masters TN, O'Bar PR, Fernandez CR, Mauney CU, Calhoun DM: *Mycobacterium fortuitum* epidemics after open-heart surgery. J. Thorac Cardiovasc Surg 75:91, 1978.
109. Tyras DH, Kaiser GC, Barner HB, Laskowski LF, Marr JJ: Atypical mycobacteria and the xenograft valve. J Thorac Cardiovasc Surg 75:331, 1978.
110. Lincoln EM, Gilbert LA: Disease in children due to mycobacteria other than *Mycobacterium tuberculosis.* Am Rev Respir Dis 105:683, 1972.
111. Rauscher CR, Kerby G, Ruth WE: *Mycobacterium kansasii* in Kansas: saprophyte or infection? Chest 66:162, 1974.
112. Yeager H Jr, Raleigh JW: Pulmonary disease due to *Mycobacterium intracellulare.* Am Rev Respir Dis 108:547, 1973.
113. Hand WL, Sanford JP: *Mycobacterium fortuitum*—a human pathogen. Ann Intern Med 73:971, 1970.
114. American Thoracic Society. Treatment of mycobacterial disease. Am Rev Respir Dis 115:185, 1977.
115. Zeligman I: *Mycobacterium marinum* granuloma. A disease acquired in the tributaries of Chesapeake Bay. Arch Dermatol 106:26, 1972.

MYCOBACTERIUM LEPRAE

116. Mansfield RE, Binford CH: The histopathologic diagnosis of leprosy. Southern Med J 69:986, 1976.
117. Golden GS, McCormick JB, Fraser DW: Leprosy in the United States, 1971–1973. J Infect Dis 135:120, 1977.
118. Drutz DJ, Chen TSN, Lu WH: The continuous bacteremia of lepromatous leprosy. N Engl J Med 287:159, 1972.
119. Jacobson RR, Trautman JR: The diagnosis and treatment of leprosy. Southern Med J 69:979, 1976.
120. Filice GA, Fraser DW: Management of household contacts of leprosy patients. Ann Intern Med 88:538, 1978.

Genus *Nocardia*

NOCARDIA ASTEROIDES

121. Frazier AR, Rosenow EC III, Roberts GD: Nocardiosis. A review of 25 cases occurring during 24 months. Mayo Clin Proc 50:657, 1975.
122. Krick JA, Stinson EB, Remington JS: Nocardia infection in heart transplant patients. Ann Intern Med 82:18, 1975.
123. Palmer DL, Harvey RL, Wheeler JK: Diagnostic and therapeutic considerations in *Nocardia asteroides* infection. Medicine 53:391, 1974.
124. Balikian JP, Herman PG, Kopit S: Pulmonary nocardiosis. Radiology 126:569, 1978.
125. Cook FV, Farrar WE Jr: Treatment of *Nocardia asteroides* infection with trimethoprim-sulfamethoxazole. Southern Med J 71:512, 1978.
126. Bach MC, Sabath LD, Finland M: Susceptibility of *Nocardia asteroides* to 45 antimicrobial agents in vitro. Antimicrob Agents Chemother 3:1, 1973.
127. Wallace RJ Jr, Septimus EJ, Musher DM, Martin RR: Disk diffusion susceptibility testing of *Nocardia* species. J Infect Dis 135:568, 1977.
128. Presant CA, Wiernik PH, Serpick AA: Factors affecting survival in nocardiosis. Am Rev Resp Dis 108:1444, 1973.

SPIROCHETES

Genus *Treponema*

TREPONEMA PALLIDUM

129. Drusin LM: The diagnosis and treatment of infectious and latent syphilis. Med Clin North Am 56:1161, 1972.
130. Sparling PF: Diagnosis and treatment of syphilis. N Engl J Med 284:642, 1971.
131. Center for Disease Control: Recommended treatment schedules for syphilis. 1976.

Genus *Borrelia*

BORRELIA SPECIES

132. Boyer KM, Munford RS, Maupin GO, Pattison CP, Fox MD, Barnes AM, Jones WL, Maynard JE: Tick-borne relapsing fever: an interstate outbreak originating at Grand Canyon National Park. Am J Epidemiol 105:469, 1977.
133. Southern PM Jr, Sanford JP: Relapsing fever. A clinical and microbiological review. Medicine 48:129, 1969.
134. Butler T, Jones PK, Wallace CK: *Borrelia recurrentis* infection: single-dose antibiotic regimens and management of the Jarisch-Herxheimer reaction. J Infect Dis 137:573, 1978.

Genus *Leptospira*

LEPTOSPIRA INTERROGANS

135. Center for Disease Control: Leptospirosis surveillance. Annual Summary 1976, issued April 1978.
136. Edwards GA, Domm BM: Human leptospirosis. Medicine 39:117, 1960.
137. Heath CW Jr, Alexander AD, Galton MM: Leptospirosis in the United States. N Engl J Med 273:857, 915, 1965.
138. Thorsteinsson SB, Sharp P, Musher DM, Martin RR: Leptospirosis: an underdiagnosed cause of acute febrile illness. Southern Med J 68:217, 1975.

RICKETTSIEAE

Genus *Rickettsia*

RICKETTSIA RICKETTSII

139. D'Angelo LJ, Winkler WG, Bregman DJ: Rocky Mountain spotted fever in the United States, 1975–1977. J Infect Dis 138:273, 1978.
140. Hattwick MAW, O'Brien RJ, Hanson BF: Rocky Mountain spotted fever: epidemiology of an increasing problem. Ann Intern Med 84:732, 1976.
141. Woodward TE, Pedersen CE Jr, Oster CN, Bagley LR, Romberger J, Snyder MJ: Prompt confirmation of Rocky Mountain spotted fever: identification of rickettsiae in skin tissues. J Infect Dis 134:297, 1976.

RICKETTSIA TYPHI (MOOSERI)

142. Woodward TE: A historical account of the rickettsial diseases with a discussion of unsolved problems. J Infect Dis 127:583, 1973.

143. Gastel B (ed): Clinical conference at the Johns Hopkins Hospital. Murine typhus. Johns Hopkins Med J 141:303, 1977.

Genus *Coxiella*

COXIELLA BURNETTII

144. Hart RJC: The epidemiology of Q fever. Postgrad Med J 49:535, 1973.
145. Dupont HL, Hornick RB, Levin HS, Rapoport MI, Woodward TE: Q fever hepatitis. Ann Intern Med 74:198, 1971.
146. Wilson HG, Nielson GH, Galea EG, Stafford G, O'Brien MF: Q fever endocarditis in Queensland. Circulation 53:680, 1976.

CHLAMYDIACEAE

Genus *Chlamydia*

CHLAMYDIA PSITTAII

147. Center for Disease Control: Psittacosis surveillance. Annual Summary 1975–1977, issued December, 1978.

CHLAMYDIA TRACHOMATIS

148. Schacter J: Chlamydial infections. N Engl J Med 298:428, 490, 540, 1978.
149. Holmes KK, Handsfield HH, Wang SP, Wentworth BB, Turck M, Anderson JB, Alexander ER: Etiology of nongonococcal urethritis. N Engl J Med 292:1199, 1975.
150. Mårdh PA, Ripa T, Svensson L, Westrom L: *Chlamydia trachomatis* infection in patients with acute salpingitis. N Engl J Med 296:1377, 1977.
151. Berger RE, Alexander ER, Monda GD, Ansell J, McCormick G, Holmes KK: *Chlamydia trachomatis* as a cause of acute "idiopathic" epididymitis. N Engl J Med 298:301, 1978.
152. Beem MO, Saxon EM: Respiratory-tract colonization and a distinctive pneumonia syndrome in infants infected with *Chlamydia trachomatis*. N Engl J Med 296:306, 1977.

MYCOPLASMATACEAE

Genus *Mycoplasma*

153. Taylor-Robinson D, McCormack WM: The genital mycoplasmas. N Engl J Med 302:1003, 1063, 1980.

MYCOPLASMA PNEUMONIAE

154. Denny FW, Clyde WA Jr, Glezen WP: *Mycoplasma pneumoniae* disease: clinical spectrum, pathophysiology, epidemiology and control. J. Infect Dis 123:74, 1971.
155. Murray HW, Masur H, Senterfit LB, Roberts RB: The protean manifestations of *Mycoplasma pneumoniae* infection in adults. Am J Med 58:229, 1975.
156. Shames JM, George RB, Holliday WB, Rasch Jr, Mogabgab WI: Comparison of antibiotics in the treatment of mycoplasmal pneumonia. Arch Intern Med 125:680, 1970.

CHAPTER 8
Mixed and Synergistic Infections

DAVID H. AHRENHOLZ and RICHARD L. SIMMONS

IN the past, emphasis in the discipline of infectious diseases was on the study of diseases caused by individual pathogenic organisms. Koch's postulates are easily fulfilled only if a single species can be grown in pure culture and reinoculated to produce a specific disease. For this reason, most traditional textbooks of infectious disease are organized according to the individual etiologic agents and their microbiologic characteristics. Similarly, surgeons frequently refer to the infections they treat as being caused by individual species of staphylococci, streptococci, *Escherichia coli,* and so on.

It is increasingly apparent, however, that many of the infections treated by surgeons are associated with mixtures of organisms rather than single pathogens. Three trends have directed attention to this fact: (1) the discovery of antibiotic therapy effective against pyogenic cocci, so that life-threatening diseases caused by other pathogens now predominate, (2) the increased frequency of opportunistic infections, and (3) the increased recognition of the role of anaerobic bacteria as copathogens.

The majority of surgical infections result from breaks in the normal cutaneous or mucosal barriers that permit the endogenous mixed flora on these surfaces to penetrate and infect the surrounding tissue. In this sense, most surgical infections are opportunistic infections, ie., caused in part by bacteria not generally considered to be pathogens. There is little understanding of how the individual microbial components of such complex mixtures interact with each other or with the tissue defenses, but a profound simplification of the normal cutaneous and mucosal flora occurs after inoculation into tissues, and certain bacteria frequently emerge as principal copathogens.

Mixed and synergistic surgical infections usually contain anaerobic bacteria for two reasons: (1) the inocula contain mixed anaerobes, and (2) surgical infections take place in anaerobic environments, where blood supply is deficient and necrotic debris is plentiful. Even if aerobes are present in the initial inoculum, they soon consume all the available local oxygen. At that point, facultative organisms can switch to anaerobic metabolism, while the strict aerobes cannot survive. Finally, anaerobic fermentative metabolic pathways release a variety of complex organic compounds that can serve as substrates for other anaerobic bacteria.

MIXED BACTERIAL COLONIZATION OF BODY SURFACES

Most body tissues are isolated from contact with bacteria, and the presence of bacteria in these areas is pathognomonic of infection. Exceptions are the skin and mucous membrane surfaces of the respiratory, alimentary, and external genital tracts. These surfaces represent two different types of physical barriers to bacterial invasion, the cornified skin and the mucosa-lined surface. The skin is specifically modified to resist water loss and withstand abrasion. It loses most of its resistance to bacterial invasion if subjected to prolonged contact with moisture. The mucosa-lined tracts retain their effectiveness as microbial barriers under wet conditions, but this ability is rapidly lost if they are allowed to dry completely.

The microbial ecology of the skin and the mucosa-lined tracts is only partially understood. Many resident and transient microbial species coexist on the skin, and mechanisms exist for reestablishing a fairly stable population of mixed microbes whenever the balance has been temporarily disturbed (Chapter 3). Only *Staphylococcus epidermidis* and diphtheroids survive as residents on the rather dry, lipid-rich, mildly acidic, nutritionally deprived surfaces of normal glabrous skin (Chapters 3 and 25). Fecal gram-negative bacilli and oral streptococci, which frequently contaminate normal skin, survive only transiently unless moisture is constantly provided. Even then, colonization is impossible unless the normal flora is displaced or eradicated. For example, the vaginal organisms deposited on the skin of the neonate during delivery are rapidly replaced by the normal cutaneous flora from the environment.[1]

The mucosa-lined surfaces possess a more complex ecosystem. The oral cavity becomes inoculated with bacteria within hours of birth by nursing or contact with environmental surfaces.[1] The ability of bacteria to adhere to surfaces is a prerequisite to survival within the mouth, since the oral cavity is constantly washed by saliva and intermittently exposed to the abrasive effects of eating, toothbrushing, and dental flossing. Different types of bacteria are better able to adhere to each type of surface. *Streptococcus sanguis* organisms have such a high affinity for dental enamel that chewing only temporarily displaces them. *Streptococcus salivarius* has a similar affinity for the tongue and oral mucosa. *Streptococcus mutans*, the organism most frequently associated with dental caries, has surprisingly little intrinsic affinity for dental enamel, and its survival as a pathogen depends on a complex set of interactions with other flora. Dental plaque begins as a storage form of glucose for *S. sanguis*, within the confines of which huge numbers of aerobic and anaerobic bacteria can grow. *S. mutans* releases acids during growth that remain in contact with dental enamel under a blanket of plaque and etch it away, exposing dentin. Numerous aerobic and anaerobic bacteria now can invade and destroy the exposed dentin, resulting in dental caries.[2]

Anaerobic organisms flourish in the oral cavity, not only on exposed plaque-covered surfaces but especially within the gingival cleft, where the oxygen tension is very low. The fermentative metabolic pathways utilized release a variety of complex organic compounds which then become substrates for other bacteria. The majority of oral organisms have never been isolated or characterized because they require extremely low oxygen environments and complex organic substrates for growth. For the same reason, mixed bacterial infections most commonly flourish in anaerobic environments, where blood supply is poor and organic debris is abundant.

The remainder of the gastrointestinal tract is also sterile at birth but becomes contaminated almost synchronously with the oral cavity. The empty stomach represents an effective acidic deterrent to the development of a resident gastric population of bacteria. With each food bolus, the pH temporarily rises, and oral bacteria traverse the stomach to the small bowel.

Bacteria resident in the small bowel must adhere to bowel mucosa or be washed away by the fecal stream. Because of the rapid transit time of intestinal contents, bacterial populations remain low and are supplemented by the intermittent influx of oral microorganisms. A few specifically adherent bacteria have been identified—eg, travelers' diarrhea is caused by an adherent, enterotoxigenic strain of *E. coli*. The ability to adhere to small bowel mucosa is associated with cell surface antigens, and diarrhea is produced by an enterotoxin, each property being coded separately by the bacterial genome. If the organism has only the surface antigen or only the ability to produce the toxin, disease does not result.[3] Travelers' diarrhea can be prevented if purified cell surface antigen is ingested before the pathogenic *E. coli*.

In the colon, bacterial adherence to the mucosa is not a critical factor in disease production because the flow of the fecal stream is intermittent. Here, aerobic bacteria rapidly remove available oxygen, and multiple species of anaerobes flourish, outnumbering aerobes 1,000 to 1 (Chapter 3). Bacteria in stool number $10^{11.5}$ per gram of feces, representing 500 or more species.[4] Bacteria comprise half the total weight of feces.

The significance of the normal colonic microbial interactions in man is poorly understood. Clearly, the normal gastrointestinal flora inhibits the colonization by pathogenic bacteria (eg, *Salmonella, Shigella, Pseudomonas*).[5] No detectable nutritional effects other than excessive water and electrolyte loss are noted in patients who have undergone colectomy. In ruminant animals, such as cattle, however, anaerobic bacteria in the foregut break down cellulose into fatty acids and alcohols, which are directly absorbed into the bloodstream. The bacteria are then digested in the hindgut and serve as a significant source of nutrients. There is little evidence for such beneficial interactions between man and his colonic flora. Bacterial growth is probably a secondary phenomenon as the colon absorbs water and stores feces before evacuation.

The male genital tract, except for the distal urethra, remains sterile throughout life in the absence of infection. The female tract, however, becomes colonized by fecal organisms early in life. During the childbearing years, lactobacilli come to predominate. Their presence usually inhibits the growth of other organisms, but during pregnancy, the vaginal secretions change, and overgrowth by *Candida albicans* or other organisms frequently results. Vaginal secretions represent too little flow to physically remove bacteria, and bacterial adherence to the vaginal mucosa is not essential to colonization. Virulent strains of the gonococcus, however, have surface pili and a high affinity for urethral mesothelium. Nonpiliated strains of gonococcus have a much lower affinity for genitourinary epithelium and are much less virulent.[6]

BACTERIAL COMPETITION

The microbial world is generally characterized by a fierce competition for available nutrients, especially under aerobic conditions. Any aerobic organism that gains a temporary advantage will multiply and displace other organisms by sheer weight of numbers. Not every species, however, can metabolize every available energy source. If oxygen and sufficient glucose are available in a given microenvironment, inoculation of aerobic organisms will result in a bacterial population explosion, as glucose is actively transported across the bacterial cell wall and used as a rich energy source. Use of all other energy sources is repressed by specific genetic control mechanisms. As the glucose is depleted, enzymes for transport and utilization of other substrates are derepressed or induced by specific organic compounds. The first bacterial species to produce the enzymatic machinery to utilize a secondary energy source will proliferate. This sequence may be repeated endlessly. One of the reasons *Pseudomonas* species are so ubiquitous in nature is that they carry the genetic information to use over 100 organic substrates for energy.

Aerobic organisms in the presence of oxygen preferentially oxidize organic substrates to carbon dioxide and water. This results in the highest energy yield and permits exponential growth. Under anaerobic conditions, fermentative processes must be utilized, typically producing less than 5 percent of the energy available by oxidative metabolism. Thus, obligate anaerobes rarely show the explosive growth potential of aerobes even under ideal conditions and may require days or weeks for culture in vitro.

Anaerobic metabolism, in addition, produces many complex organic end products. Usually these products can be utilized as energy sources by another microorganism.

Complex bacterial interactions are thus characteristic of anaerobic environments. Surgical infections, which occur under conditions of injury and tissue death, frequently provide a relatively anaerobic environment. Since polymicrobial contamination is inevitable whenever the mechanical barriers of skin or mucosa are breached, many surgical infections are initially mixed infections. The mixture tends to persist when anaerobic metabolism fosters complex substrate production.

Although all bacterial interactions seem to be characterized by competition for available nutrients, this competition is more illusory than real. Most bacteria have but one response to the presence of nutrients—rapid growth and reproduction. Those that reproduce most rapidly are most successful. Some bacteria do, however, have other competitive mechanisms for survival in mixed colonies. Some secrete antibiotics: the bacteriocins of *Bacillus* species, for example, are locally bacteriostatic or bactericidal. In fact, all naturally occurring antibiotics are microbial products and facilitate survival of the organism.

Other bacteria rely on their ability to rapidly alter the available nutrients into forms that impair the growth of their competitors. For example, lactobacilli, which are very acid tolerant, rapidly convert glucose to lactic acid. This process has a low energy yield but has two advantages: it removes glucose available for the growth of other bacteria and produces an acidic environment that is inhibitory to most other bacterial species. Similarly, *S. mutans* in the mouth rapidly converts ingested sucrose to dextran polymer, which is unsuitable as an energy source to most other bacteria. The dextran in this case acts as a surface to which a variety of bacteria can adhere secondarily, but only those that produce dextranase can use the material for growth.[7]

If a bacterial species can occupy all the available binding sites on a surface, it can successfully dominate the microenvironment. *S. sanguis* has a high affinity for tooth enamel and can prevent colonization of the teeth by introduced *S. mutans*. If *S. sanguis* is removed by toothbrushing, *S. mutans* will adhere readily to the teeth. However once *S. mutans* becomes established, the dextran it elaborates creates a new area for bacterial adherence.[8]

The preceding examples of bacterial competition illustrate the general principle of *amensalism*, in which interacting bacteria derive no benefit from the interaction. Examples of true *parasitism*, in which the parasite derives benefit at the expense of the host, are rare in bacterial interactions. A few intracellular parasites of bacteria are known, such as *Bdellovibrio* which attacks *E. coli*. However, bacterial interactions become remarkably altered when one organism produces an end product that another organism can use as a substrate for growth. This is an example of *commensalism*—mutual association with benefit to one partner without adverse effects on either. Often the bacteria are found in association only because the substrate that the dependent partner consumes is rare or nonexistent elsewhere. The association can become *symbiotic* when both partners benefit from the association, a common occurrence. Many bacteria are rapidly inhibited by the accumulation of their metabolic end products. A second organism that removes these end products allows the continued growth of the first organism.[9]

MICROBIAL SYNERGISM

A useful term in describing microbial interactions is "synergism," an effect on the host found in the presence of two or more organisms not seen with either organism alone. Many bacteria involved in synergistic infections are not considered typical pathogens, ie, organisms capable in pure culture of invading a normal host. Opportunistic organisms are those that can establish an infection only in a host with impaired defense mechanisms. Trauma, especially extensive burns, neoplastic disease, collagen-vascular disease, and chemotherapy, can all alter the host defense mechanisms and allow the establishment of opportunists. The term "opportunistic synergism" probably best describes the sequence of events in which a pathogenic organism invades a host, establishes a disease, and suppresses local or systemic host defenses to the extent that an opportunistic organism can become established. These synergistic effects have been recently reviewed by Mackowiak.[10] Virtually any opportunistic organism can produce disease if host defenses are sufficiently impaired. By extension of this concept, the organisms need not even be synchronously present. For example, rheumatic fever after group A streptococcal infection resulting in valvular heart damage can predispose to bacterial endocarditis years later. In this chapter, we will emphasize synergistic infections, where two bacteria synchronously produce an effect not seen with either alone. As noted above, not all bacterial synergistic actions produce disease.

Mechanisms of Microbial Synergism

Mackowiak[10] identifies four principal mechanisms of microbial interactions that are synergistic:

1. One organism may facilitate transmission to or colonization of the host by a second organism.
2. The organism may lower local or systemic host resistance, allowing invasion by a second organism.
3. One organism may provide growth factors for another organism.
4. One organism may increase the virulence of another.

Increased Transmission

Synergistic mechanisms may have only an indirect effect on the host. In the broadest sense, some microbial interactions merely increase the transmission of a virulent organism. For example, *Treponema pallidum* is a virulent organism capable of penetrating intact skin, but it is extremely sensitive to oxygen and dies rapidly on exposed surfaces. Nevertheless, the open chancre of primary syphilis has a redox potential of −180 to −250 mv and is teeming with the spirochetes, which are readily transmitted by direct contact. Apparently *Fusobacteria, Bacteroides,* and anaerobic streptococci, which are regularly isolated from these lesions, serve to maintain the low redox potential necessary for survival and transmission of the spirochete.

In man, influenza virus produces changes that increase the susceptibility of patients to secondary pyogenic pneumonia. Initially, this was thought to be due to edema and cellular debris producing suitable culture material for the secondary bacterial pathogens. There is now increasing evidence that primary viral infections produce anatomic alterations in the tracheal epithelium, allowing adherence of bacterial pathogens. Fainstein et al[11] found an increased adherence of *Staphylococcus aureus, Haemophilus influenzae,* and *Streptococcus pneumoniae* to tracheal epithelium both in naturally acquired acute respiratory illness and in volunteers inoculated with influenza virus vaccine. To produce clinical influenza in swine, a virus and *H. influenzae* must be inoculated intranasally.[12]

Eichenwald et al[13] found that simultaneous infection with a respiratory virus and a bacterial pathogen in the nasopharynx of infants results in a much greater spread to the surrounding environment of both organisms. These organisms may then infect other children nearby. Children with a marked rhinorrhea exhibit a stuffy-nose syndrome, with frequent sneezing, snorting, and coughing. Asymptomatic children may also disseminate bacteria and have been called "cloud babies." In both groups, the ability to spread organisms is correlated with the presence of both a respiratory virus and a bacterial pathogen. In the first group, it is possible that the severe rhinorrhea found when both organisms are present results in increased coughing, which spreads the organisms. In asymptomatic infants, the presence of a virus allows persistence of pathogenic bacteria that would otherwise be readily eliminated. These increased numbers of pathogens are spread to the local environment, and the incidence of infection increases.

Lowered Host Resistance

Breakdown in Local Defense. There is a time-dependent factor in many synergistic interactions. Commonly, the presence of one organism alters the local conditions so that a second organism can become established. The first organism is then no longer required to maintain the disease. If the order of introduction of these organisms is reversed, the disease does not result.

Certainly the most common form of bacterial interaction occurs when a pathogenic organism causes a break in anatomic defenses, which subsequently allows one of a variety of opportunistic organisms to invade the host. This anatomic deformity can be either chronic scarring or an acute open lesion. Acute rheumatic fever that follows a streptococcal infection can produce chronic changes in the heart valves that predispose to late bacterial endocarditis. Because the events in this chain of action are widely separated in time, they probably no longer fit the definition of true synergistic infection. A similar example is the damage to fallopian tubes caused by gonorrhea that predisposes women to recurrent salpingitis. The scarring is a permanent anatomic change. The salpingitis in the scarred tubes is usually a mixed bacterial infection with organisms less virulent than the gonococcus.

Any pathogen that produces an open lesion of a cutaneous or mucosal surface can permit secondary invasion by other organisms. A classic example is foot rot in sheep, a synergistic infection in which *Fusobacterium nodosus* causes a chronic epidermal irritation that allows subsequent invasion of the tissues by both *Fusobacterium necrophorum* and *Corynebacterium pyogenes.* Both of the latter bacteria are required to maintain the infection. *F. nodosus* is not required if the sheep are kept in muddy pastures so that maceration of the skin can occur.[14]

Liver granulomas of turkeys and liver abscesses of cattle cause large economic losses. In turkeys, the causative organism is a gram-positive anaerobe, probably *Catenabacterium* species.[14] Gastrointestinal inoculation of the bacterium into germ-free animals does not cause disease unless a desquamating streptococcus has already been introduced orally. Similarly, liver abscesses of cattle are caused by *F. necrophorum,* which commonly colonizes the rumen. When cattle are given feed lot diets, the normal commensal balance is disrupted, and the acid-producing bacteria can overgrow to produce ruminal ulcers. Liver granulomas only occur in the presence of such ulcers.[14]

In humans, there is evidence that nematodes break down local mucosal barriers to allow bacterial infections to develop. The nematode *Strongyloides* can carry enteric bacteria from the intestine to various internal organs during its migration from the bowel. Polymicrobial septicemia is said to be suggestive of *Strongyloides* enteric infection.[15] *Trichinella spiralis* and *Nematospiroides dubius* possibly transmit *Salmonella typhimurium,* and the *Fasciola* liver fluke may carry *Salmonella dubein* in cattle.

LoVerde et al[16] have reviewed the evidence of an association between *Schistosoma* species and *Salmonella.* They present evidence that *Salmonella* have pili that allow specific adherence to the tegument of the male schistosomes. This interaction may allow the establishment and persistence of *Salmonella* infections in man. The mucosal lesions produced by the worms may contribute to the disease as well. Many more prosaic examples can be cited. Typhoid perforations of the distal ileum, perforated amebic ulcers, and actinomycotic abscesses all lead to polymicrobial intraabdominal infections.

Shope found that the swine lungworm acts as an intermediate host for swine influenza virus. Overt influenza may be triggered by migration of *Ascaris* larvae through the lungs. The lungworms serve a similar function for hog cholera virus. Swine influenza virus can survive similarly in a murine population within *Strongyloides ratti.*[12]

All these examples represent a breach of the local physical barriers to microbial invasion. Many infections seen in clinical surgical practice result when prior tissue damage so impairs local host defenses or so alters the tissue microenvironment that superinfection takes place. The classic example is the indolent diabetic foot ulcer produced by trauma to a relatively ischemic and neuropathic area. Colonization of the lesion with mixed flora may be stable for prolonged periods until a predominant set of pathogens emerges, usually for reasons unknown. A similar set of circumstances surrounds the sudden emergence of necrotizing fasciitis, or other gangrenous infections, in decubitus ulcers that may have been present for years. Secondary *Candida* or *Pseudomonas* infections of sinus tracts, fistulas, and open wounds have a similar pathogenesis.

Secondary infections of chronic visceral abscesses and necrotic granulomas are more exotic examples of breakdown in local defense. Secondary bacterial infection of an amebic liver abscess, an aspergilloma in an old tuberculous cavity, or invasive pulmonary aspergillosis emerging from a resolving pyogenic lung abscess in a transplant recipient are sometimes seen.

Breakdown of Systemic Defenses. A variety of pathogens (eg, measles virus, Epstein-Barr virus, cytomegalovirus, *M. tuberculosis,* and *H. capsulatum*) are capable of suppressing cell-mediated immunity (Table 8-1).[10] Cytomegalovirus infections increase the lethality of *Pseudomonas, Staphylococcus,* and *Candida* infections in mice, and bacterial superinfection of cytomegalovirus-infected patients in a common lethal syndrome in recipients of organ transplants.[17] Other infections (eg, influenza, measles, mumps, and herpesvirus) can produce a nonspecific suppression of fixed and circulating phagocytic cells. Malaria and influenza have been implicated in the suppression of humoral immunity, but exact mechanisms are unclear.

Temporary depression of cell-mediated immunity occurs in a variety of infections.[10] The mechanisms causing this depression are unknown, and there is little direct evidence that this increases the risk of secondary infections. An exception is the increased incidence of tuberculosis during epidemics of measles. Measles in malnourished infants in some tropical countries is associated with herpetic ulcerations of the mouth, which in turn become infected by mixed oral flora, leading to the gangrenous infection known as "noma" (chancrum orum).[18] Adenoviral infections are more frequent after smallpox and typhoid vaccination. The commonly observed activation of herpes labialis during pyogenic infections suggests that this is a result of a temporary depression of cell-mediated immunity. Conversely, resistance to experimental herpes infections is increased by BCG or *Corynebacterium parvum* inoculation, both documented stimulators of cell-mediated immunity.[10]

Many microorganisms, especially viruses, nonspecifically impair the reticuloendothelial system, which may allow secondary invasion by opportunistic organisms (Table 8-2).[10] Suppression of phagocytosis is transient and species specific and may be directly related to the quantity of virus present. Viruses apparently can produce a metabolic block in the glycolytic pathway in the phagocytic cell to prevent phagocytosis.[10]

There are experimental studies to show that infection by a phagocytosis-suppressing virus followed by bacterial infection produces a higher mortality rate than is found with the individual organisms alone. This occurs only when the viral infection precedes the bacterial infection. Organisms that produce a chronic hemolytic state, such as *Plasmodium* and *Bartonella,* may also impair phagocytosis by iron overload of the reticuloendothelial system.[10]

In addition, the capsule from many types of bacteria is capable of blocking phagocytosis. The presence of encapsulated organisms, such as *Bacteroides fragilis* or *Bacteroides melaningogenicus,* may therefore prevent phagocy-

TABLE 8-1. STUDIES DEMONSTRATING SUPPRESSION OF CELL-MEDIATED IMMUNITY DURING INFECTIONS

Infection	Animal Studied	In Vitro Studies *	In Vivo Studies *	Immunogen †
Influenza	Man		+	T, H, C, Cx, Tr
Parainfluenza	Mouse		+	*Listeria monocytogenes*
Measles	Man		+	T
Infectious mononucleosis	Man	+	+	C, SK, SD
Herpes simplex	Man	+		HSV-1
Cytomegalovirus	Man	+	+	M, P, PM
Tuberculosis	Man		+	T, H, C, M
Histoplasmosis	Man	+		H
Leprosy	Man	+	+	L, T, C, Tr, P
Syphilis	Man	+		P
Pertussis	Man		+	T
Streptococcus	Man		+	T
Trypanosomiasis	Rabbit	+	+	T
Toxoplasmosis	Mouse		+	*Schistosoma mansoni*
Live virus vaccines ‡	Man	+	+	H, C, P, PM

From MacKowiak PA: N Engl J Med 298:21, 1978.

* + denotes type of study.

† C, *Candida;* Cx, coccidioidin; H, histoplasmin; HSV-1, herpes simplex virus Type 1; L, lepromin; M, mumps; P, phytohemagglutinin; PM, pokeweed mitogen; SD, streptodornase; SK, streptokinase; T, tuberculin; Tr, trichophyton.

‡ Rubeola, rubella, mumps, and attenuated influenza virus vaccines.

TABLE 8-2. STUDIES DEMONSTRATING SUPPRESSION OF THE RETICULOENDOTHELIAL SYSTEM DURING VIRAL INFECTIONS

Infection	Animals Studied	In Vitro Studies *	In Vivo Studies *	Phagocyte Challenge
Influenza	Mouse, guinea pig	+	+	*Haemophilus influenzae Bacillus anthracis,* Baker's yeast, *S. aureus, S. pneumoniae, Staphylococcus epidermidis*
Parainfluenza	Mouse	+		*H influenzae, S. aureus*
Adenovirus	Man	+		*Neisseria meningitidis*
Sandfly fever	Man	+		*S. aureus,* aggregated albumin
Mumps	Guinea pig	+		*Bacillus anthracis*
Reovirus	Mouse		+	*S. aureus*
Herpes simplex	Man	+		Endotoxin
Measles	Man	+		Endotoxin

From MacKowiak PA: N Engl J Med 298:21, 1978. * + denotes type of study.

tosis of other organisms present within a mixed inoculum.[19] A few bacteria secrete substances (leukocidins) that are directly cytocidal to phagocytic cells—*S. aureus, F. necrophorum,* and group A *Streptococcus pyogenes.*[20]

Microorganisms can alter the humoral immune system as well. Antibody production may be inhibited or enhanced, or the complex interactions of immunoregulation may be disturbed. The agents known to be associated with inhibition of antibody production are listed in Table 8-3. The mechanisms of suppression are unknown, but hypotheses include: (1) an infection of the B lymphocytes themselves, (2) competitive inhibition of noncommitted antibody-producing cells, and (3) neoplastic transformation by viruses.[10] In addition, interferon induced by viral infection may suppress antibody synthesis.

Malaria in the experimental animal impairs humoral immunity by an unknown mechanism, resulting in protection from spontaneous autoimmune disease. Malaria also enhances the oncogenic potential of certain viruses, eg, induction of lymphomas in mice is enhanced by *Plasmodium berghei* infection. Dengue is normally a mild febrile illness but becomes hemorrhagic fever if the patient has circulating heterologous dengue antibodies.[21] This may occur by passive transfer of antibodies from mother to child or by prior infection with a heterologous strain. Similarly, unusually severe respiratory syncytial viral infections can occur in those persons previously inoculated with an attenuated vaccine.[22]

Certain microorganisms may stimulate IgA blocking antibodies that protect secondary pathogens from circulating IgM. The secondary invaders are coated with IgA, thereby blocking IgM attachment, which normally would result in death of the cells by phagocytosis or complement activation.

Nutritional Synergism

The third mechanism by which microbes interact occurs when one organism provides a growth factor for another organism. For example, tetanus spores inoculated into normal viable tissue will not germinate unless other facultative bacteria are present to provide the proper oxidation-reduction potential. This is probably the major mechanism by which aerobic and anaerobic bacteria interact in mixed surgical infections. Most species of anaerobic bacteria are so sensitive to oxygen that even a few minutes exposure to room air is lethal. Even *B. fragilis,* the most common anaerobic pathogen in man, is unable to grow in such conditions, although it can survive for extended periods of time in contact with oxygen. Similarly, *Clostridium botulinum* normally cannot germinate in such acid foods as tomato juice. In the presence of *Cladosporium* or *Penicillium* species, the clostridial spores will germinate, grow, and produce toxin.[23]

Infections involving *Toxoplasma gondii* and cytomegalovirus are common in patients with disseminated cancer. In these infections, both organisms occupy the same cells, and the *Toxoplasma* rosettes tend to form around the cytomegalovirus inclusion bodies. There is speculation that *Toxoplasma* derives nutrients in this way.[24]

Several other well-documented examples are known. In the synergistic gangrene of Meleney, the microaerophilic, nonhemolytic *Streptococcus* thrives only if hyaluronidase and a heat-labile growth factor usually provided by *S. aureus* are present.[14] *Bacteroides melaninogenicus* has a requirement for vitamin K which facultative diphtheroids apparently provide in many mixed infections.[25]

In fusospirochetal gingivitis, four types of organism are typically isolated. These include *Treponema microdentium,* a small *Fusobacterium,* an anaerobic hemolytic *Streptococcus,* and an anaerobic *Vibrio.* Combinations of three or fewer of these organisms usually fail to produce characteristic necrotic lesions. Socransky et al [26,27] showed that *T. microdentium* requires isobutyrate, polyamines, and a low redox potential for growth. The organism could be grown in the presence of a facultative diphtheroid accompanied by either a *Fusobacterium* or a motile, gram-negative, anaerobic rod *(Bacteroides).*

Conferred Virulence

The fourth mechanism of microbial synergism occurs when one organism confers increased virulence onto another microorganism. *Entamoeba histolytica* usually exists as a commensal organism in the large intestine, feeding on bacteria and superficial mucosal cells. It can become highly invasive in laboratory animals only if allowed to associate for 6 to 12 hours with certain bacteria before inoculation. This suggests that some virulence factors are derived from the intestinal bacteria.[9]

The best example, however, is the transmission of antibiotic resistance factors between organisms. This is especially common among the Enterobacteriaceae but has also been demonstrated from *E. coli* to *B. fragilis*. Transmissible drug resistance was discovered in Japan in 1959, when a strain of *Shigella* resistant to chloramphenicol, tetracycline, streptomycin, and sulfonamides was isolated from a patient with dysentery.[28] Since that time, resistant strains have been found throughout the world to most of the commercially available antibiotics. Strains resistant to ampicillin, kanamycin, neomycin, chloramphenicol, streptomycin, tetracycline, sulfonamides, and penicillin are especially common. Multiple antibiotic resistance is usually transmitted to an extrachromosomal plasmid consisting of two parts. The first part is an r-determinant, which codes for resistance to one or more antibiotics. The resistance transfer factor (RTF) is an independent sex factor responsible for the formation of sex pili. Pili-bearing bacteria attach to nonpili-bearing cells and transfer the resistance plasmid by conjugation. The recipient cell now becomes fertile and, after forming its own sex pili, can further transmit the resistance factor.

Transmission of drug resistance is different from selection of drug-resistant organisms, in that multiple drug resistance is usually transmitted. This is especially important in diseases being treated with multiple antibiotics because emergence of resistant strains requires multiple sequential mutations, whereas antibiotic resistance can be transmitted in one step during conjugation.[28]

Gram-positive organisms are also capable of transmitting a plasmid for the enzyme beta-lactamase. This splits the lactam ring of penicillin, conferring penicillin resistance. Gram-positive cells do not undergo conjugal transfer but rely upon transduction by a viral vector. As viral phage particles are formed in a bacterial cell, they sometimes incorporate parts of the bacterial genome, including plasmids keying for beta-lactamase. These phage particles can then specifically attach to phage-susceptible strains of bacteria. After attachment, the genetic contents are injected into the cell, which can now elaborate beta-lactamase. The cell is not always killed after injection of the viral genome if the viral genome is incomplete or if the cell undergoes lysogeny in which a specific repressor for expression of the viral genome is elaborated, preventing cell lysis. The virally injected DNA can then undergo recombination with the bacterial genome to allow replication and expression of the antibiotic resistance plasmid. These resistance mechanisms are described in greater detail by Joklik and Willett.[28]

Even in the absence of direct transmission from one

TABLE 8-3. STUDIES DEMONSTRATING SUPPRESSION OF THE HUMORAL IMMUNE SYSTEM BY AGENTS OR MEDIATORS INVOLVED IN HUMAN INFECTIONS

Agent or Mediator	Animal Studied	In Vitro Studies *	In Vivo Studies *	Immunogen
Influenza virus	Mouse		+	*S. pneumoniae*
Lymphocytic choriomengitis virus	Mouse		+	Ovalbumin, human serum albumin, sheep erythrocytes
Junin virus	Guinea pig		+	Human erythrocytes
Newcastle disease virus	Rabbit	+		Egg albumin, bovine serum, albumin
Malaria	Man, mouse		+	Tetanus toxoid, sheep erythrocytes, *Salmonella typhi* (O antigen)
Trypanosoma brucei	Mouse		+	Sheep erythrocytes
Toxoplasma gondii	Mouse		+	Sheep erythrocytes
Trichinella spiralis	Mouse		+	Sheep erythrocytes
Endotoxin	Rabbit, mouse		+	*Neisseria meningitidis*, actinophage, sheep erythrocytes
Interferon	Mouse	+	+	Sheep erythrocytes, concanavalin A, phytohemagglutinin, lipopolysaccharide

From MacKowiak PA: N Engl J Med 298:21, 1978.

* + denotes type of study.

organism to another, bacteria producing penicillinase, cephalosporinase, or other extracellular enzymes that inactivate antibiotics can protect otherwise sensitive copathogens from these antibiotics. The best examples are penicillin-resistant mixed infections with *S. aureus*, where the extracellular penicillinase protects the penicillin-sensitive copathogens.[29] This also probably occurs with *Bacteroides* infections, since virulent *B. fragilis* strains elaborate many enzymes, including a penicillinase and cephalosporinase.

DIAGNOSTIC CLUES TO MIXED BACTERIAL INFECTIONS

The mixed infections of greatest importance to surgeons contain bacteria or fungi, and anaerobes are usually present. The findings suggestive of anaerobic infection are also associated with many mixed infections. The clinical clues to anaerobic infections provided by Finegold are equally applicable to mixed infections (Table 8-4).[31] Especially suggestive are a foul odor, gangrene or obvious tissue necrosis, or gas in the tissue, or discharge.[31]

Infections of tissue in proximity to a mucosal surface characteristically contain mixed flora. These include dental infections, aspiration pneumonia, lung abscess, bronchiectasis, peritonitis, intraabdominal abscess, wound infection following bowel surgery or trauma, perirectal or ischial rectal abscess, gas-forming and/or necrotizing soft tissue infections, infections following human bites, and many nongonococcal gynecologic infections. Although in the past, most cutaneous infections were caused by *S. aureus*, mixed infections are becoming more common (Chapter 25).

When the Gram stain shows a mixture of morphologic types of bacteria, the definitive diagnosis of mixed bacterial or fungal infections still depends on the cultural isolation of multiple organisms. Failure to isolate more than one organism is usually because of inadequate anaerobic technique. Since abscesses are often polymicrobial, it is important that all abscesses be cultured for both aerobes and anaerobes, but it is useless to culture for mixed organisms when specimens are contaminated with normal flora, such as throat cultures, gingival or vaginal swabs, expectorated sputum, gastric contents, small bowel contents, or feces. Specimens contaminated with normal flora will be reported as mixed infections in error. Culture results of tissue biopsy specimens are more reliable. The collection and transport of specimens for anaerobic cultures have been described (Chapter 12). The pathogenic aerobes are relatively easy to culture and identify, and the clinician is aware of their presence early. The surgeon depends on the Gram stain to indicate a mixed infection until the anaerobic cultures are examined and reported (usually 48 hours).

In many mixed infections, the limitations of the laboratory will prevent the identification of many of the organisms present, especially if a wound is freshly contaminated with feculent flora. Not every organism is virulent, however, and, with time, only a few species persist. For this reason, sequential culturing of most mixed infections is important to identify the microflora that emerge in the face of surgical or antimicrobial therapy.

TABLE 8-4. CLINICAL CLUES TO POSSIBLE MIXED BACTERIAL INFECTION

I. Clinical setting suggestive of infection due to colonization by bacteria normally resident on mucosal or skin surfaces
   A. Soft tissue infection due to acute or chronic skin breaks, especially of perineal region and feet
   B. Intraabdominal infection due to a perforated viscus
   C. Gynecologic infections after instrumentation or operation
   D. Soft tissue infections of head and neck due to mucosal trauma or disease
   E. Infection after human or animal bite
II. Infection associated with malignancy or other process resulting in tissue destruction
III. Necrotic tissue, gangrene, pseudomembrane formation
IV. Gas in tissues or discharges
V. Foul-smelling discharge

Adapted from Finegold SM: Anaerobic Bacteria in Human Disease, 1977, p 41. Courtesy of Academic Press.

PRINCIPLES OF TREATMENT OF MIXED BACTERIAL INFECTIONS

Little is known about optimal antimicrobial therapy of mixed bacterial infections. Historical evidence suggests that many infections caused by or contaminated by mixed bacterial organisms will resolve if adequately drained and debrided and if antimicrobial therapy is directed against the principal aerobic pathogens. For example, a recent report utilizing cefamandole for the treatment of a large number of mixed bacterial infections shows that many *Bacteroides*-associated infections respond to this drug, which has limited in vitro effectiveness against the majority of *Bacteroides* strains.[32] The treatment of the major aerobic pathogens in mixed infections is thought by some to break the synergistic interaction between aerobe and anaerobe, with resolution of the infection—particularly if the predisposing local environment is altered by surgical means.

A similar experience has been gained by treating only the anaerobic component of a mixed infection. Thadepalli et al[33] reported 12 patients with intraabdominal or pelvic abscesses containing mixtures of aerobes and anaerobes who were treated successfully with clindamycin alone. Similarly, Leigh[34] indicated that it was only necessary to treat *Bacteroides* in certain mixed infections. Gorbach and Bartlett[35] found 31 cases in the literature of mixed aerobic and anaerobic infection that responded to therapy with clindamycin alone, despite the presence of various resistant aerobes in the mixed infection. However, there are many instances of failure to cure anaerobic mixed infections with limited spectrum antibiotics, and breakthrough bacteremia frequently occurs if important pathogenic components of the mixture are not eliminated. An example is the high incidence of *Bacteroides* bacteremia reported when antimicrobial therapy for peritonitis does not include an agent effective against *Bacteroides* organisms.[36] Similarly, Solomkin et al[37] report a number of patients dying of metastatic disseminated candidiasis whose regional infection involved a mixed bacterial and *Candida* peritonitis. When the bacteria were eliminated, the *Candida* remained, resulting in disseminated infection.

Thadepalli et al[38] have clearly shown that patients who received clindamycin and kanamycin for the treatment of mixed intraperitoneal infections did better than those who received cephalothin and kanamycin—a regimen not very effective against bowel anaerobes. Stone and Fabian[39] recently reported improved clinical results in patients treated with metronidazole and gentamicin, indicating better results from treatment of both anaerobes and aerobes in mixed infections. Several recent randomized studies have noted a failure of response to penicillin or cephalosporin-aminoglycoside regimens in women with mixed pelvic infections, whereas combinations of clindamycin and an aminoglycoside were effective.[40] Finegold states, "At present, it is my feeling that therapy should be directed against all significant components of a mixed flora in seriously ill patients."[31]

PATHOGENS IN MIXED BACTERIAL INFECTIONS

It is sometimes difficult to decide which organisms are major pathogens in mixed infections. There is little question about the pathogenicity of the pyogenic cocci, the enteric gram-negative facultative organisms, pseudomonads, or mycobacteria. The pathogenic role of other bacteria, discussed in Chapter 7, is variable.

Most debate centers around the role of the anaerobic bacteria in mixed infections. Finegold[31] defines a bacterial species as a significant pathogen requiring treatment if: (1) there is repeated isolation of the same organism from a patient over a period of time, (2) the organism is grown in pure culture, or (3) if the Gram stain or quantitative culture shows that one organism predominates. With these criteria in mind, Finegold[31] lists certain anaerobic organisms that are pathogens. Despite traditional doubts concerning virulence, infections with such organisms should be treated (Tables 6-1 and 8-5).

B. fragilis is the most commonly isolated anaerobe in clinical infections and is most resistant to antimicrobial agents.[31] It is isolated in pure culture more often than any other anaerobic organism, and few surgeons doubt its virulence. Other *Bacteroides* species, such as *B. thetaiotaomicron* appear virulent, whereas *B. ovatus* and *B. ruminocoli* are less often associated with infection. *B. melaninogenicus,* which is commonly found in mixed bacterial infections, is so dependent on other organisms to supply growth factors that, alone, it is rarely capable of causing disease.[31]

Of the anaerobic gram-positive cocci, *Fusobacterium nucleatum, F. necrophorum,* and *F. varium* are commonly found as part of the mixed flora and are capable of causing infections in pure culture. The microaerophilic streptococcus can also cause infection if not eliminated, although the viridans group of streptococci is less pathogeneic.[31]

TABLE 8-5. MAJOR ANAEROBIC COPATHOGENS FOUND TO BE PART OF MIXED BACTERIAL INFECTIONS

Gram-negative bacilli
Bacteroides fragilis *
B. melaninogenicus *
Fusobacterium nucleatum *
F. necrophorum
F. varium
F. mortiferum
Gram-positive cocci *
Peptococcus (especially *P. magnus, P. asaccharolyticus, P. prevotii*)
Peptostreptococcus (especially *P. anaerobius, P. intermedius,*† *P. micros*)
Microaerophilic cocci and *streptococci*
Gram-positive spore-forming bacilli
Clostridium perfringens *
C. ramosum
C. septicum
C. novyi
C. histolyticum
C. sporogenes
C. sordellii
Gram-positive non-spore-forming bacilli
Actinomyces
Arachnia
Eubacterium (especially *E. lentum, E. limosum, E. alactolyticum*)
Bifidobacterium eriksonii

From Finegold SM: Anaerobic Bacteria in Human Disease, 1977, p 68. Courtesy of Academic Press.
* These five organisms or groups of organisms account for two thirds of all clinically significant anaerobic isolates.
† *P. intermedium* is actually microaerophilic and belongs in the genus *Streptococcus.*

Most clostridial species, including *Clostridium perfringens* and *C. ramosum,* clearly can cause serious infections,[41] as can *Actinomyces* species, *Arachnia,* and *Bifidobacterium eriksonii.*[42]

In general, most gram-positive anaerobic cocci are significant pathogens and should be eradicated as part of the mixed bacterial flora. In contrast, the gram-negative anaerobic cocci seem to lack virulence. Many bacteria are benign and not capable of causing infection by themselves, including most species of *Bifidobacterium* and *Eubacterium,* most anaerobic lactobacilli (with the exception of *Lactobacillus catenaforme*), *Propionibacterium,* and most spirochetes, except *T. pallidum.* None need be treated in immunocompetent hosts.[31]

ANTIBIOTIC CHOICE IN THE TREATMENT OF MIXED INFECTIONS

The appropriate antibiotic choice depends on the in vitro susceptibility of the organisms (see Chapter 18). Multiple agents have proven their value in the treatment of life-threatening polymicrobial infections, particularly in the hospitalized and immunocompromised patient. Many authors advocate single drug therapy to exclude drug interaction or antagonism and decrease the incidence of drug reactions. Minor infections within an outpatient setting are typically treated with a single agent.

In general surgical infections, common bacterial mixtures include the Enterobacteriaceae, enterococci, and *B. fragilis,* which are typically responsive to an aminoglycoside, ampicillin, and clindamycin, respectively. Many clinicians use the combination of an aminoglycoside and clindamycin, because they feel that the enterococcus is so seldom a primary pathogen that its chemotherapeutic eradication is unnecessary. Enterococci are important synergistic partners in experimental models[43] and occasionally emerge as a single pathogen after other organisms are eliminated from clinical infections.[44] For this reason, we include ampicillin in the treatment of mixed infections that contain enterococci.

Whether to treat *Candida* found as part of a mixed bacterial infection is currently unclear, since *Candida* frequently colonizes superficial wounds and sinus tracts. We prefer short-term therapy with modest doses (0.5 mg per kg per day) of amphotericin combined with surgical and antibacterial therapy when *Candida* is part of a mixed infection deep within tissue or is isolated from multiple sites during the treatment of bacterial infections.[45]

Whether antibiotic treatment of anaerobes, isolated from a mixed infection, is always indicated in conjunction with the treatment of the major aerobes encountered is a controversial point. Clindamycin is effective against the two major anaerobic components of mixed bacterial infections, the gram-positive anaerobic cocci and *B. fragilis.* It is available in oral and parenteral forms and is effective against most aerobic gram-positive cocci. Its major disadvantage is a moderate incidence of pseudomembranous enterocolitis—a disadvantage it seems to share with many other agents.[46] Most of the penicillins and the cephalosporins are effective against most gram-positive anaerobes from mixed bacterial infections. Some of the new cephalosporins, including cefoxitin and moxalactam, and cefamandole, in high doses, are effective against many strains of *B. fragilis* as well.

Chloramphenicol is the most effective agent against anaerobes in vitro and is a very effective clinical agent in mixed infections. There are reports, however, of chloramphenicol therapeutic failures in the treatment of *B. fragilis* infections and of inactivation of the drug by the bacteria, which are sensitive to it in vitro.[35]

Metronidazole and rifampin have wide anaerobic spectra but have not been widely utilized in the United States for the treatment of anaerobic infections. Neither should be used alone, but when used in combination with a drug directed against the principal aerobic copathogens, they have proved to be effective. Metronidazole has excellent activity against most anaerobes, except *Actinomyces, Propionibacterium, Eubacterium,* and certain other microaerophilic organisms.

Rifampin is very active against most gram-positive and gram-negative anaerobic bacteria. Only *F. varium, Fusobacterium mortiferum,* certain strains of *Eubacterium,* and certain *Clostridia,* including *C. ramosum,* are resistant.[31] However, there is little experience utilizing rifampin to treat mixed anaerobic infections.

Neither metronidazole nor rifampin should be used alone to treat mixed infections because of the risk of emergence of resistant organisms. The aminoglycosides have no activity against anaerobic and experimental *B. fragilis* infections.

HUMAN MIXED INFECTIONS

In human mixed infections, the sources of bacteria are principally the oral, enteric, or soil flora. These bacterial populations contain significantly different groups of organisms and will be discussed separately.

MIXED INFECTIONS WITH ORAL FLORA

The oral flora contain large numbers of the viridans group of streptococci, including *S. sanguis, S. salivarius,* and *S. mutans,* which have little ability to invade tissues. In a gingival crevice, anaerobes such as *Bacteroides* (especially *B. melaninogenicus*), *Viellonella, Actinomyces,* and the spirochetes, including *Spirillum* and *Treponema* species, proliferate. Most of these organisms are of low virulence alone but, as a mixture, are responsible for such destructive lesions as necrotizing gingivitis, noma, and tropical ulcer. They also have been isolated from a variety of peritonsillar and pharyngeal space and otogenic cerebral abscesses.[47-49]

Much of the evidence for the synergistic interactions of oral microorganisms has been published in the dental literature and is summarized in Table 8-6.[26,27,49-57] These disease processes were originally described as fusospirochetal diseases because of the prominent findings of fusiform bacteria and spirochetes in the lesions. In necrotizing gingivitis, for example, four zones of tissue destruction are noted. The deepest zone consists of healthy tissue being invaded by spirilliform organisms. Superficial to this is a necrotic zone, followed by a leukocyte-rich zone and, at the surface, a bacterial zone. This suggests active invasion of the tissues by the fusospirochetal flora.

Fusobacterium necrophorum appears to be one of the most pathogenic organisms present. It produces an exotoxin capable of killing leukocytes (leukocidin). It can also produce a hemolysin and a cytoplasmic toxin and has a number of cell wall proteolytic enzymes.

Corynebacterium pyogenes is a diphtheroid that appears to serve as a facultative organism in the anaerobic fusospirochetal infection, and it lowers the redox potential, allowing the growth and proliferation of anaerobes. Roberts[51,52] found that it is capable of secreting a growth factor for *F. necrophorum,* and MacDonald et al[53] found that it produced vitamin K, a growth requirement of *B. melaninogenicus.*

Most of the oral spirochetes have been exceptionally difficult to study because they have not been cultured in vitro. This probably is a result of their strict metabolic requirements for survival and growth. For example, *Treponema microdentium* was found to require isobutyrate, polyamines, and a lowered redox potential for growth.[55] These requirements may be supplied all or in part by diphtheroids and fusobacteria or *Bacteroides*. *B. melaninogenicus* is a questionably virulent organism which has rather strict growth requirements, including vitamin K and hemin. In addition, *B. melaninogenicus* (like *B. fragilis*) produces an antiphagocytic capsule capable of protecting surrounding organisms from neutrophil phagocytosis. Socransky and Gibbons[27] noted that, in guinea pigs, mixtures of fusiform bacteria and spirochetes were insufficient to produce typical necrotizing infections in the absence of *B. melaninogenicus*, illustrating the complex interactions that take place in some mixed bacterial infections. Experimentally, the typical necrotizing lesions are best produced by spirochetes, diphtheroids, fusiform rods, and the gram-negative anaerobic rods, as listed in Table 8-6. On occasion, one or more of these organisms may be omitted if the local environment provides suitable conditions for growth of the other organisms.

Necrotizing Gingivostomatitis (Trench Mouth)

With better oral hygiene, these diseases are becoming less frequent. Necrotizing gingivostomatitis characteristically occurs in young adults under conditions of stress, poor nutrition, and poor oral hygiene. It is extremely painful, with rapid invasion of the gingiva around the teeth producing pockets of necrosis. Ultimately, there is a breakdown of the dental ligament and surrounding bone, with loss of the teeth. The disease is prevented by daily plaque removal and good periodontal care. For acute treatment, warm water lavage with gum debridement and scaling of the teeth results in dramatic symptomatic relief and rapid healing. In patients with fever, lymphadenopathy,

TABLE 8-6. MECHANISMS OF BACTERIAL SYNERGISM IN FUSOSPIROCHETAL INFECTIONS

Interacting Organisms	Mechanisms	References
Organisms usually present: a spirochete (*Treponema* or *Spirillum* species), a diphtheroid (*Corynebacterium* species), a fusiform rod *(Fusobacterium)*, a gram-negative anaerobic rod *(Bacteroides)*.		
Fusobacterium necrophorum	Destroys leukocytes (leukocidin)	51, 52
	Also produces a hemolysin and cytoplasmic toxin	50
	Produces cell wall-bound proteolytic enzymes	50
	Produces viable L-form after penicillin therapy	50
Corynebacterium pyogenes	Lowers pH for anaerobes	51, 52
	Growth factor for *F. necrophorum*	51, 52
	Provides vitamin K for *B. melaninogenicus*	53
Diphtheroids with either *Fusobacterium* or gram-negative anaerobic rod *(Bacteroides)*	*T. microdentium* requires isobutyrate, polyamines, and lowered Eh for growth	26
Treponema microdentium	Invades surrounding tissue, allowing other bacteria to proliferate	53
Bacteroides melaninogenicus or *B. fragilis*	Encapsulated forms produce an antiphagocytic capsule	27
B. melaningogenicus required for experimental fusospirochetal infection in guinea pigs	Unknown	27
F. necrophorum liver abscesses are potentiated by *B. melaninogenicus, B. fragilis,* or *F. nucleatum*	Unknown	

or septicemia, penicillin or erythromycin is given orally. These agents are of little benefit without effective local care, however. Any abscessed tooth pockets are drained as an adjuvant to this therapy.

Vincent's Angina

A similar disease, Vincent's angina or Vincent's stomatitis, can involve the tonsils, pharynx, tongue, or oral mucosa. The onset is usually sudden with mild fever. A pseudomembranous ulcerative process is found, accompanied by pain, lymphadenopathy, difficulty in eating, and foul breath. These pharyngeal infections may be severe enough to be confused with diphtheria. However, a direct wet smear examination under darkfield microscopy reveals the spirochetal flora.

Peritonsillar Abscess

Peritonsillar and deep pharyngeal space abscesses caused by mixed oral flora produce intense local pain, swelling, and systemic toxicity. These lesions tend to dissect through adjacent tissue planes and may cause septicemia or even airway obstruction. The agents may be streptococci or mixed aerobic and anaerobic or only anaerobic species. Therapy is high-dose penicillin and surgical drainage with daily debridement (Chapter 27).

Tropical Ulcer

Tropical ulcer is a fusospirochetal infection with oral flora but typically occurs on the ankle following injury or abrasion. Malnutrition and skin maceration are common predisposing factors. Pain, fever, toxemia, and marked disability are characteristic. The ulcer rapidly enlarges and may extend deeply, with destruction of underlying muscle, tendon, or bone. Treatment requires large doses of parenteral penicillin and local debridement. Oral tetracycline or, more recently, metronidazole has also proved effective. Even after control of the infection, however, a large granulating tissue defect remains which often requires skin grafting (Chapter 25).

Human Bite Infections

Human bite infections result from the inoculation of mixed oral flora into tissue planes. These most frequently occur on the hand, especially after fist fights, or in the relatively avascular cartilage of the ear. These infections usually represent spreading abscesses which require adequate surgical drainage, especially in the hand, where extensive tissue loss may result in permanent disability (Chapter 43).

MIXED INFECTIONS WITH ENTERIC FLORA

Of the hundreds of species of bacteria that inhabit the gastrointestinal tract (Chapter 3), some are especially virulent. Meleney et al,[56] in 1932, was the first to observe that combinations of enteric flora produced an increased mortality when injected intraperitoneally into dogs. Altemeier [57] supported these findings.

Firm experimental evidence has been gathered for the synergistic nature of intraperitoneal infections.[58-60] Feces from grain-fed rats inoculated intraperitoneally consistently failed to produce intraperitoneal infection. The colonic flora of animals fed meat, however, became very similar to that of the human, and 27 species could be isolated from rat feces. Intraperitoneal implantation of feces [58,59] in a double-gelatin capsule containing barium sulfate and anaerobic growth media resulted in a two-stage intraperitoneal infection. The first stage consisted of free peritonitis characterized by *E. coli* septicemia and large numbers of *E. coli* in the peritoneal fluid. Lesser numbers of *B. fragilis*, *F. necrophorum*, and enterococci were isolated. Other isolates of the original 27 species were rare. Later the animals formed intraperitoneal abscesses consisting of larger numbers of *B. fragilis* and lesser numbers of *E. coli*, *F. necrophorum*, and enterococci.[58-60]

In a subsequent study, the facultative aerobes *E. coli* and enterococcus and the obligate anaerobes *B. fragilis* and *F. necrophorum* were mixed in various combinations before intraperitoneal implantation.[60] The highest mortality was associated with a free peritonitis stage usually due to *E. coli* septicemia. However, abscesses were only consistently produced if a mixture of an anaerobe and a facultative aerobe was inoculated intraperitoneally.

These initial studies were further supported by experiments in which animals were treated with either an aminoglycoside (effective against *E. coli* but not *B. fragilis*) or clindamycin (effective against anaerobes but not aerobes) and various other antibiotics, alone or in combination. Antibiotics effective against *E. coli* prevented lethal septicemia but had no effect on the incidence of abscesses. Antibiotics effective against anaerobes had no effect on *E. coli* septicemia but virtually eliminated subsequent abscesses. Combinations of antibiotics effective against both classes of organisms resulted in the lowest mortality and the lowest residual infection rate. Clearly, the pattern of infection of the mixture depended on both aerobic and anaerobic organisms.[43]

The mechanisms of interaction in mixed enteric infections are listed in Table 8-7. Facultative organisms, such as *E. coli* and *Enterococcus*, can consume local oxygen and lower the redox potential. In addition, there is evidence to suggest that the facultative organisms can secrete specific growth factors, such as vitamin K, for *Bacteroides* species; *B. melaninogenicus* requires vitamin K for growth. In addition, the truly pathogenic anaerobes, such as *B. fragilis*, have an inducible superoxide dismutase system, which may be protective in nonreduced environments.

Bacteroides species apparently have a number of virulence factors that make them good synergistic partners. They secrete a variety of extracellular enzymes, including pronases, penicillinases, lipases, and heparinases. Extracellular beta-lactamases protect both the *Bacteroides* organisms and any other bacteria from the effects of penicillin or cephalosporin antibiotics. The variety of digestive enzymes elaborated by *Bacteroides* species breaks down tis-

TABLE 8-7. MECHANISMS OF BACTERIAL SYNERGISM AMONG MIXED ENTERIC ORGANISMS

Organisms	Mechanisms
Organisms usually present: facultative gram-negative rod *(E. coli, Klebsiella),* anaerobic gram-negative rod *(B. fragilis),* facultative gram-positive cocci *(Enterococcus),* anaerobic gram-positive rods or cocci (*Peptostreptococcus* or *Peptococcus*).	
Facultative organisms, such as *E. coli* or *Enterococcus*	Lowers redox potential Secretes growth factors, possibly vitamin K, especially for *Bacteroides* species May release catalase to protect *Bacteroides* species
B. fragilis, B. melaninogenicus	Produces an antiphagocytic capsule Elaborates penicillinases or cephalosporinases Elaborates other digestive enzymes Produces heparinase to stabilize fibrin deposits and decrease influx of antibiotics, antibodies, and complement

sue, which becomes a good culture medium for all other organisms in a mixed infection. In addition, *Bacteroides* heparinase may stabilize local fibrin deposits, preventing influx of antibiotics, antibodies, and complement and allowing abscess formation.[61] Ingham et al [49] presented data that encapsulated *Bacteroides* species (especially *B. fragilis* and *B. melaninogenicus*) protect aerobic bacteria from phagocytosis and believed that the capsule blocked phagocytosis. Finally, Tofte et al [62] have reported that *Bacteroides,* when incubated in normal serum with *E. coli,* can compete for opsonins and thereby reduce phagocytosis of *E. coli.*

Intra-abdominal Infections

Mixed enteric infections usually originate from a break in the bowel mucosa, releasing the organisms into the surrounding tissue and producing peritonitis or soft tissue abscesses. The symptoms manifested are determined largely by the duration and intensity of inflammation before the release of bacteria, the quantity of inoculum released, and the source of the inoculum, since the distal gastrointestinal tract contains far more virulent mixtures of bacteria than do gastric or duodenal contents (Chapter 34).

Gangrenous Soft Tissue Infections

Necrotizing fasciitis can be produced by mixed enteric organisms. This form of gangrenous soft tissue infection spreads along the fascial cleft between superficial and deep fascia, leaving the overlying skin intact. During the Civil War, this disease was called "hospital gangrene," and Meleney and others attributed it to group A beta-hemolytic streptococci either alone or in combination with *S. aureus.*[63] However, in the antibiotic era, this disease is caused by mixtures of facultative and anaerobic enteric flora, which colonize traumatized or ischemic sites on the lower trunk.[64,65]

In general, soft tissue infections occurring below the waist are caused by mixed enteric organisms, and those above the waist are caused by mixed gram-positive or oral organisms (Chapter 25).

Especially in diabetics and others with compromised immune defenses, this can be a very virulent infection. The immunodepressed patient presents with minimal constitutional symptoms, and the physician notes only a draining wound with intact surrounding skin that may or may not be anesthetic. Suddenly, however, the patient develops vascular collapse, and death may rapidly ensue. Opening the wound reveals extensive subcutaneous necrosis hidden by the deceptively intact skin (Chapter 25).

Progressive Synergistic Gangrene (Meleney's Cutaneous Synergistic Gangrene)

Brewer and Meleney,[66] in 1926, first described an unusual chronic progressive cutaneous infection following drainage of an appendiceal abscess and reviewed 18 cases in the literature. The infection is characterized by a painful, tender area of erythema and swelling, with a central purplish zone that expands slowly with central gangrene. It was inexorably progressive until wide total excision was performed. Progressive synergistic gangrene has become, for surgeons, the prototype of synergistic soft tissue infections—even though it is now so rare that few surgeons have seen a case, and its character may have changed in the antibiotic era.

The original studies of Meleney demonstrated that this lesion was a result of a synergistic infection with a microaerophilic streptococcus (originally *Streptococcus evolutus* and now probably *Streptococcus intermedius*) and

S. aureus.[66] In the original study, coliforms were isolated but were not felt to be pathogenic organisms. Both the streptococcus and staphylococcus could be recovered from the central necrotic area, but the reddened edge contained only the streptococcus. Meleney found subsequently that the infection could be reproduced in dogs only by the synchronous injection of both organisms. Unique synergistic partners are seldom found in the current antibiotic era. Enteric gram-negative organisms, especially *Proteus* species, are commonly found as part of the flora, and *Enterobacter aerogines* is also a frequent isolate.

Meleney, in 1945, reported successful treatment of this infection with penicillin, and many antibiotics have led to successful resolution. There are even multiple cases reported of spontaneous cure without specific therapy, but debridement and antimicrobial therapy probably should be combined for the most prompt results.

BIBLIOGRAPHY

Finegold SM: Anaerobic Bacteria in Human Disease. New York; Academic, 1977.

REFERENCES

1. Drasar BS, Hill MJ: Human Intestinal Flora. London, Academic Press, 1974.
2. MacDonald J, Socransky S, Gibbons R: Aspects of the pathogenesis of mixed anaerobic infections of mucous membranes. J Dent Res 42:529, 1963.
3. Evans DG, Satterwhite TK, Evans DJ Jr, Dupont HL: Differences in serological responses and excretion patterns of volunteers challenged with enterotoxigenic *Escherichia coli* with and without the colonization factor antigen. Infect Immun 19:883, 1978.
4. Skinner FA, Carr JG (eds): The Normal Microbial Flora of Man. New York, Academic Press, 1974.
5. Donaldson RM Jr: Normal bacterial populations of the intestine and their relation to intestinal function. N Engl J Med 270:938, 994, 1050, 1964.
6. Tramont EC, Hodge WC, Gilbreath MJ, Ciak J: Differences in attachment antigens of gonococci in reinfection. J Lab Clin Med 93:730, 1979.
7. Gibbons RJ: Ecology and cariogenic potential of oral streptococci. In Wannamaker LW, and Matsen JM (eds): Streptococci and Streptococcal Diseases, Recognition, Understanding and Management. New York, Academic Press, 1972, p 355.
8. Shulman JA: Streptococci of the viridans group. In Mandell GL, Douglas RG, Bennett JE (eds): Principles and Practices of Infectious Diseases. New York, Wiley, 1979, Vol 2, p 1612.
9. Williams REO: Benefit and mischief from commensal bacteria. J Clin Pathol 26:811, 1973.
10. MacKowiak PA: Microbial synergism in human infections [2nd of 2 parts]. N Engl J Med 298:83, 1978.
11. Fainstein V, Musher DM, Cate TR: Bacterial adherence to pharyngeal cells during viral infection. J Infect Dis 141:172, 1980.
12. Easterday BC: Animal influenza. In Kilbourne ED (ed): The Influenza Viruses and Influenza. New York, Academic Press, 1975, p 449.
13. Eichenwald HF, Kotsevalov O, Fasso LA: Some effects of viral infection on aerial dissemination of staphylococci and on susceptibility to bacterial colonization. Bacteriol Rev 25:274, 1961.
14. Roberts DS: Synergic mechanisms in certain mixed infections. J Infect Dis 120:720, 1969.
15. Walker-Smith JA, McMillan B, Middleton AW, Robertson S, Hopcroft A: Strongyloidiasis causing small bowel obstruction in an aboriginal infant. Med J Aust 2:1263, 1969.
16. LoVerde PT, Amento C, Higashi GI: Parasite-parasite interaction of *Salmonella typhimurium* and *Schistosoma.* J Infect Dis 141:177, 1980.
17. Simmons RL, Matas AJ, Rattazzi LC, Balfour HH Jr, Howard RJ, Najarian JS: Clinical characteristics of lethal cytomegalovirus infection following renal transplantation. Surgery 82:537, 1977.
18. Whittle HC, Smith JS, Kogbe GI, Dossetor J, Duggan M: Severe ulcerative herpes of mouth and eye following measles. Trans R Soc Trop Med Hyg 73:66, 1979.
19. Ingham HR, Freeman R, Wilson RG: Anaerobic breast abscesses. Lancet 1:164, 1979.
20. Fales WH, Warner JF, Teresa GW: Effects of *Fusobacterium necrophorum* leukotoxin on rabbit peritoneal macrophages in vitro. Am J Vet Res 38:491, 1977.
21. Monath TP: Flavovirus (St. Louis encephalitis and dengue). In Mandell GL, Douglas RG, and Bennett JE (eds): Principles and Practices of Infectious Diseases. New York, Wiley, 1979, Vol 2, p 1248.
22. Kim HW, Canchola JG, Brandt CD, Pyles G, Chanock RM, Jensen K, Parrott RH: Respiratory syncytial virus disease in infants despite prior administration of antigenic inactivated vaccine. Am J Epidemiol 89:422, 1969.
23. Huhtanen CN, Naghski J, Custer CS, Russell RW: Growth and toxin production by *Clostridium botulinum* in moldy tomato juice. Appl Environ Microbiol 32:711, 1976.
24. Gelderman AH, Grimley PM, Lunde MN, Rabson AS: *Toxoplasma gondii* and cytomegalovirus: mixed infection by a parasite and a virus. Science 160:1130, 1968.
25. Gibbons RJ, MacDonald JB: Hemin and vitamin K compounds as required factors for the cultivation of certain strains of *Bacteroides melaninogenicus.* J Bacteriol 80:164, 1960.
26. Socransky SS, Loesche WJ, Hubersak C, MacDonald JB: Dependency of *Treponema microdentium* on other oral organisms for isobutyrate, polyamines, and a controlled oxidation-reaction potential. J Bacteriol 88:200, 1964.
27. Socransky SS, Gibbons RJ: Required role of *Bacteroides melaninogenicus* in mixed anaerobic infection. J Infect Dis 115:247, 1965.
28. Joklik WK, Willett HP (eds): Zinsser Microbiology, 17th ed. New York, Appleton-Century Crofts, 1980.
29. Fong IW, Engelking ER, Kirby WMM: Relative inactivation by *Staphylococcus aureus* of eight cephalosporin antibiotics. Antimicrob Agents Chemother 9:939, 1976.
30. Rudek W, Haque R: Extracellular enzymes of the genus *Bacteroides.* J Clin Microbiol 4:458, 1976.
31. Finegold SM: Anaerobic Bacteria in Human Disease. New York, Academic Press, 1977.
32. Glanges E, Crenshaw CA, Webber CE: A clinical and bacteriologic evaluation of cefamandole therapy in serious skin and skin structure infections. Surg Gynecol Obstet 150:502, 1980.
33. Thadepalli H, Gorbach SL, Broido PW, Norsen J, Nyhus L: Abdominal trauma, anaerobes, and antibiotics. Surg Gynecol Obstet 137:270, 1973.
34. Leigh DA: *Bacteroides* infections. Lancet 2:1081, 1973.
35. Gorbach SL, Bartlett JG: Anaerobic infections. N Engl J Med 290:1177, 1237, 1289, 1974.
36. Fry DE, Garrison RN, Polk HC Jr: Clinical implications in bacteroides bacteremia. Surg Gynecol Obstet 149:189, 1979.

37. Solomkin JS, Flohr AB, Quie PG, Simmons RL: The role of *Candida* in intraperitoneal infections. Surgery 88:524, 1980.
38. Thadepalli H, Gorbach SL, Broido P, Norsen J: A prospective study of infections in penetrating abdominal trauma. Am J Clin Nutr 25:1405, 1972.
39. Stone HH, Fabian TC: Clinical comparison of antibiotic combinations in the treatment of peritonitis and related mixed aerobic-anaerobic surgical sepsis. World J Surg 4:415, 1980.
40. Sen P, Apuzzio J, Reyelt C, Kaminski T, Levy F, Kapila R, Middleton J, Louria D: Prospective evaluation of combinations of antimicrobial agents for endometritis after cesarean section. Surg Gynecol Obstet 151:89, 1980.
41. Armfield AY, Felner JM, Thompson FS, McCroskey LM, Balows A: Comparison of clinical and bacteriologic data from *Eubacterium filamentosum* and *Clostridium innocuum*. Bacteriol Proc [abst M266] p 109, 1971.
42. Georg LK, Robertstad GW, Brinkman SA, Hicklin MD: A new pathogenic anaerobic *Actinomyces* species. J Infect Dis 115:88, 1965.
43. Weinstein W, Onderdonk A, Bartlett J, Louie TJ, Gorbach SL: Antimicrobial therapy of intraabdominal sepsis. J Infect Dis 132:282, 1975.
44. Gibbs RS, Listwa HM, Dreskin RB: A pure enterococcal abscess after cesarean section. J Reprod Med 19:17, 1977.
45. Solomkin JS, Simmons RL: *Candida* infections in surgical patients. World J Surg 4:381, 1980.
46. Bartlett JG, Chang TW, Gurwith M, Gorbach SL, Onderdonk AB: Antibiotic-associated pseudomembranous colitis due to toxin-producing clostridia. N Engl J Med 298:531, 1978.
47. Ferreira MC, Araujo WC, Otto SS, Uzeda M: Anaerobic and facultative microbial organisms in chronic tonsillitis. Ear Nose Throat J 58:35, 1979.
48. Flodstrom A, Hallander HO: Microbiological aspects on peritonsillar abscesses. Scand J Infect Dis 8:156, 1976.
49. Ingham HR, Selkon JB, Roxby CM: Bacteriological study of otogenic cerebral abscesses: Chemotherapeutic role of metronidazole. Br Med J 2:991, 1977.
50. Langworth BF: *Fusobacterium necrophorum:* Its characteristics and role as an animal pathogen. Bacteriol Rev 41:373, 1977.
51. Roberts DS: The pathogenic synergy of *Fusiformis necrophorus* and *Corynebacterium pyogenes.* I. Influence of the leucocidal exotoxin of *F. necrophorus.* Br J Exp Pathol 48:665, 1967.
52. Roberts DS: The pathogenic synergy of *Fusiformis necrophorus* and *Corynebacterium pyogenes.* II. The response of *F. necrophorus* to a filterable product of *C. pyogenes.* Br J Exp Pathol 48:674, 1967.
53. MacDonald JB, Socransky SS, Gibbons RJ: Aspects of the pathogenesis of mixed anaerobic infections of mucous membranes. J Dent Res 42:529, 1963.
54. Hill G, Osterhout S, Pratt P: Liver abscess production by non-spore-forming anaerobic bacteria in a mouse model. Infect Immun 9:599, 1974.
55. Smith DT: Fusospirochetal disease of the lungs produced with cultures from Vincent's angina. J Infect Dis 46:303, 1930.
56. Meleney F, Olpp J, Harvey H, Zaytseff-Jern H: Peritonitis: II. Synergism of bacteria commonly found in peritoneal exudates. Arch Surg 25:709, 1932.
57. Altemeier W: The pathogenicity of the bacteria of appendicitis peritonitis. An experimental study. Surgery 11:374, 1942.
58. Weinstein WM, Onderdonk AB, Bartlett JG, Gorbach SL: Experimental intra-abdominal abscesses in rats: Development of an experimental model. Infect Immun 10:1250, 1974.
59. Onderdonk AB, Weinstein WM, Sullivan NM, Bartlett JG, Gorbach SL: Experimental intra-abdominal abscesses in rats: Quantitative bacteriology of infected animals. Infect Immun 10:1256, 1974.
60. Onderdonk AB, Bartlett JG, Louie T, Sullivan-Seigler N, Gorbach SL: Microbial synergy in experimental intra-abdominal abscess. Infect Immun 13:22, 1976.
61. Gesner BM, Jenkin CR: Production of heparinase by *Bacteroides.* J Bacteriol 81:595, 1961.
62. Tofte RW, Peterson PK, Schmeling D, Bracke J, Kim Y, Quie P: Opsonization of four *Bacteroides* species: Role of the classical complement pathway and immunoglobulin. Infect Immun 27:784, 1980.
63. Meleney F: Bacterial synergism in disease processes with confirmation of synergistic bacterial etiology of certain type of progressive gangrene of abdominal wall. Ann Surg 94:961, 1931.
64. Giuliano A, Lewis F Jr, Hadley K, Blaisdell FW: Bacteriology of necrotizing fasciitis. Am J Surg 134:52, 1977.
65. Stone HH, Martin JD Jr: Synergistic necrotizing cellulitis. Ann Surg 175:702, 1972.
66. Brewer GE, Meleney FL: Progressive gangrenous infection of the skin and subcutaneous tissues, following operation for acute perforative appendicitis. A study in symbiosis. Ann Surg 84:438, 1926.

CHAPTER 9
Fungi of Surgical Significance

SCOTT F. DAVIES AND GEORGE A. SAROSI

BIOLOGY OF THE FUNGI

Fungi are among the most primitive eukaryotic organisms.[1-3] They are classified as protists, as are algae and protozoa. These simple life forms do not show differentiation of cells into organs or specialized tissues; rather, a single cell is capable of regenerating the entire organism. Even large fungi are best thought of as collections of individual cells rather than as complex organisms.

Fungi require organic nutrients, so they must either live in organic debris or invade other living species. The majority live on decaying matter in soil or are pathogenic only to plants. Of the thousands of fungal species, only a few can cause disease in mammals. Even then, infection is an incidental part of the fungi's life cycle and the illness is usually mild.

The majority of fungi of medical importance grow as molds in nature. A mold is a fungus that is growing in long filaments called hyphae, often divided into cells by septae. The hyphae grow out from the surface of solid media as a tangled mass with many side branches and form an aerial growth called a mycelium; this is the visible fungus colony on a culture plate. Specialized branches of hyphae, called conidiophores, develop on the hyphae of most fungi; they are primarily reproductive structures and produce conidia, which are often referred to as spores. In general, spores are called microconidia if they are unicellular and macroconidia if they are multicellular, but there are a wide variety of names used for specific structures. The spores are small, easily aerosolized, and are usually the infectious particles (Fig. 2-12 to 2-14).

Some fungi grow only as yeasts, which are unicellular organisms that reproduce by budding. Buds may break off from the parent cell or remain attached, forming so-called pseudohyphae.

Many of the fungi of major medical importance are dimorphic. They can grow either as mycelia or as yeasts, depending on their environment. Thermal dimorphic fungi, including *Histoplasma capsulatum, Blastomyces dermatitidis, Paracoccidiodes brasiliensis,* and *Sporothrix schenckii,* grow in soil at ambient temperatures as mycelia but in infected mammalian tissue at 37C as yeast. *Coccidioides immitis* is often referred to as a tissue dimorphic fungus. The mycelial phase is found in nature, but the tissue form consists of large spherules which rupture and release multiple endospores, each of which can mature into a new spherule. The morphologic conversion from soil phase to tissue phase of growth is more complicated than that of the thermal dimorphic fungi. It is the result of a combination of environmental conditions and not solely of changes in temperature.

Many of the major fungal diseases occur only in highly specialized geographic areas. Soil in these endemic areas has been enriched by an organic nitrogen source, frequently by bird or bat droppings, and serves as a reservoir for fungal growth. Within an endemic area, it is common for many cases of a given fungal disease to occur in close temporal proximity. Such instances are sometimes incorrectly called epidemics. As there are no secondary cases, and no evidence of person-to-person spread, however, they are perhaps better thought of as outbreaks in various locales rather than as epidemics of illness.

GENERAL CLASSIFICATION OF FUNGAL DISEASE

The number of fungi that cause invasive disease in humans is small. These fungi are not easily classified but will be considered here in three major groups, according to the usual mechanism by which they cause infection.[1] Fungal diseases acquired by inhalation of organisms include diseases caused by the dimorphic pathogenic fungi—histoplasmosis, blastomycosis, coccidioidomycosis, and paracoccidioidomycosis, and also cryptococcosis.[2] Diseases caused by ubiquitous fungi that can colonize mucosal surfaces but can invade only under special circumstances include aspergillosis and mucormycosis, caused by opportunistic molds, and candidiasis, caused by opportunistic yeast.[3] Fungal diseases that are ordinarily initiated by the inoculation of organisms into subcutaneous tissues include sporotrichosis and mycetoma.

There are also many other essentially avirulent fungi, which have been associated with invasive infection in severely immunocompromised patients. These include members of the genera *Torulopsis, Rhodotorula, Hansenula, Geotrichum, Penicillium,* and others. Infection in these instances has little to do with the biology of the fungal organisms, but reflects a total lack of any resistance in an immunoincompetent patient who serves essentially as an organic nutrient for the organism. These infections will not be discussed further.

Actinomycosis and nocardiosis are not fungal diseases. They are caused by higher bacteria. *Actinomyces* species resemble diphtheroids, and *Nocardia* species resemble mycobacteria. The organisms grow in long filaments resembling fungal hyphae, but they can be distinguished by the narrow diameter of the strands (1 μm or less), which compares with a diameter of at least 4 μm for hyphae of fungal organisms. These bacteria are discussed in Chapters 6 and 7, respectively.

INTRODUCTION TO THE DIAGNOSIS OF FUNGAL DISEASES

Only in rare instances can the diagnosis of an invasive fungal infection be made on clinical evidence alone. Rhinocerebral mucormycosis and lymphocutaneous sporotrichosis are two examples. In all other cases, a variety of diagnostic tests must be used to make a definitive diagnosis. A summary of the available diagnostic tests and their usefulness in specific fungal diseases is presented in Table 9-1.

Serology

Serologic tests measure the level of specific antibody to a fungal organism by complement-fixation assay, immunodiffusion, and other methods. Positive test results support a clinical impression but are rarely diagnostic. In general, the titer is proportional to the likelihood of infection by the particular organism. Negative results, however, seldom rule out the diagnosis. Cross-reactions between related fungi can also be confusing.

Skin Tests

Intradermal skin tests were the first diagnostic tests used for fungal diseases. Skin tests are easy to perform, and the antigens for histoplasmosis and coccidioidomycosis are standardized. A positive skin test merely means that the patient has had an infection at some time. The frequency of positive results in an area endemic for a specific fungus is so high that these tests are more valuable in epidemiologic work than they are in making a specific diagnosis.

Pathologic Examination

Definitive diagnosis of a specific invasive fungal infection generally requires direct demonstration of the organism histopathologically or cultural isolation of the organisms from infected tissue. Examination of potassium hydroxide digested sputum or pus from patients with possible fungal infections can be extremely helpful. The strong alkali dissolves the inflammatory cells and the mucus but leaves the fungal elements intact. This technique is especially useful in demonstrating the characteristic organisms of *B. dermatitidis* and *C. immitis* in freshly digested sputum or pus. Examination of KOH-treated cerebrospinal fluid after addition of a drop of India ink is useful in the diagnosis of cryptococcosis.

Although such direct examination of specimens may sometimes be helpful, biopsy and histopathologic examination after fixation and staining adds greatly to the diagnostic yield. The routine hematoxylin and eosin stain fails to stain many of the fungi, but the demonstration of a granulomatous process may suggest a fungal infection and stimulate further diagnostic work-up. Special stains greatly facilitate the histopathologic identification of specific organisms. The best available special stain for screening for fungi in tissue sections is the Gomori methenamine silver (GMS) stain, which colors all fungi and the filaments of *Actinomyces* and *Nocardia* a dark brown or black. It also stains old or dead (nonviable) fungal particles. In spite of the dark color of the stain, which can obscure the details of the various fungal elements, many of the fungi have specific morphologic features that allow recognition. Unfortunately, not everything that stains with GMS is a fungus. The parasite *Pneumocystis carinii* stains readily and, because of its size and avidity for the silver stain, has frequently been confused with *Histoplasma capsulatum* or with other yeast.

TABLE 9-1. VALUE OF DIAGNOSTIC TESTS IN CERTAIN MYCOTIC DISEASES

Disease	Culture	Smear (sputum, pus, etc.)	Skin test	Serology (C.F. precipitin, etc.)	Histopathology
Histoplasmosis	4+	0	2+	2+	3–4+
Blastomycosis	4+	4+	1+	0	4+
Coccidioidomycosis	4+	4+	4+	4+	4+
Paracoccidioidomycosis	4+	4+	2+	2+	4+
Cryptococcosis	4+	4+ India ink	0	4+ Antigen	3+
Aspergillus					
Invasive	1+	0	0	0	4+
Fungus ball	4+	2+	0	3+	4+
Mucormycosis	1+	0	0	0	2–3+
Candidiasis	1+	0	0	1–2+	2+
Sporotrichosis	4+	0	0	1–2+	1+

Legend: 0, not useful; 1, rarely useful; 2, occasionally of some use; 3, useful; 4, very useful.

Of other special stains available, Mayer's mucicarmine stain renders the mucopolysaccharide capsule of *Cryptococcus neoformans* a bright carmine. Because *C. neoformans* is the only encapsulated pathogenic fungus, the use of this stain is a specific diagnostic tool. Occasionally, the much larger yeasts of *B. dermatitidis* are also stained by this method, but the color is always a pale red and never the brilliant bright carmine seen with the cryptococcal capsule. One other frequently used stain is the Gridley stain, which stains mucin and elastin as well as fungi. Morphologic detail is good, but nonviable organisms are not stained.

Culture

While the direct identification of some fungi can be made by the preceding tests, identification by culture should be attempted whenever possible and may be the only means of making a specific diagnosis. Specimens are inoculated onto Sabouraud agar or other special fungal media, and observed for at least 1 month because most fungi grow slowly. Most cultures are kept at room temperature for primary isolation of pathogenic fungi. Although it is usually more difficult, incubation and isolation may be attempted at 37C when the yeast form of a thermal dimorphic fungus is the suspected pathogen.

When growth begins, a tentative identification is made by examining teased and mounted specimens for the size, shape, and septation of the hyphae, and the morphology of any spores or other specialized structures that are seen. Potassium hydroxide is used for mounting in most cases. When *Aspergillus* species are examined, however, tap water is the best mounting media, because strong alkali could damage the delicate structure of the conidiospores needed for identification.

Because most pathogenic fungi are acquired by inhalation of spores, laboratory work with these organisms in the mycelial phase is hazardous and must be done only in biohazard hoods.

FUNGAL DISEASES ACQUIRED BY INHALATION OF FUNGAL ORGANISMS

HISTOPLASMOSIS

Histoplasma capsulatum induces a primary infection in the lung where the fungus replicates within the macrophages.[5] Fungemia is common and self-limited, but results in seeding of reticuloendothelial organs throughout the body.[6] The ability of the organism to cause progressive disease in one or several sites results in a variety of clinical manifestations.

Etiology

H. capsulatum is a thermal dimorphic fungus. At 25C on Sabouraud agar it grows as a fluffy white to brown septate mycelium, which bears microconidia and characteristic tuberculate macroconidia. The organism is free-living in nature in this mycelial phase. Since it replicates as a small (2–4 μm) yeast at 37C, this is the form in which organisms are seen intracellularly within macrophages in histopathologic preparations of infected tissue.

Epidemiology

H. capsulatum has been isolated from the soil in more than 50 countries. It is most common in temperate climates along river valleys and has been found in North, Central, and South America, India, and Southeast Asia. It is rare in Europe and probably not present in Australia.

The most heavily endemic area is the east central United States bordering the Mississippi and Ohio rivers. The center of disease activity is in Ohio, Kentucky, Indiana, Illinois, Tennessee, Missouri, and Arkansas. Many bordering states have a substantial amount of histoplasmosis, and the endemic area also extends eastward into Virginia and Maryland. Although the organism is widely distributed in these areas, the concentration of the fungus is variable from site to site. Heavy concentrations are found in excrement of chickens and of pigeons, starlings, and other wild birds. Fungus-laden soil is most common in rural areas but may also be found in urban areas where starlings roost. Exposure of small groups of people to heavy inocula of organisms results in small outbreaks of symptomatic disease. Sources of such exposure include chicken coops, other farm buildings, and frequently starling roosts. "Cave fever" caused by inhalation of infected bat guano is a well known variation on this theme. Large outbreaks of histoplasmosis have been associated with excavation of infected soil for construction of roads or buildings. Progressive dissemination after a primary respiratory infection is rare. Only one case of disseminated disease was seen among more than 6,000 cases in an urban epidemic in Mason City, Iowa.

Infection is almost universal in highly endemic areas because any disturbance of the soil may scatter the infectious spores (microconidia) into the air. Over 90 percent of people living in some areas have had a primary pulmonary histoplasma infection before age 20.

Pathogenesis and Pathology

Inhalation of microconidia results in patchy areas of interstitial pneumonitis. The spores are engulfed by macrophages and multiply intracellularly in the yeast phase.[5] The draining lymph nodes are quickly involved, and hematogenous spread of the organism occurs with clearance by reticuloendothelial cells throughout the body. Specific lymphocyte-mediated cellular immunity develops within 7 to 14 days and results in rapid limitation of spread with necrosis and granuloma formation in involved areas.[7] Humoral antibody also develops but is of little protective value.

The histology of individual lesions depends on the adequacy of the host cellular immune response. In disseminated infection, macrophages may be crowded with organisms and show no tendency to form aggregates. In contrast, the granulomas in the lung and in the reticuloendothelial organs after a normally limited primary spread are well developed with epitheloid histiocytes, giant cells, and central necrosis. Older lesions may show dense, surrounding fibrosis, and eventually may calcify.

Clinical Manifestations

Primary Pulmonary Histoplasmosis. Primary pulmonary histoplasmosis usually has few symptoms.[8] Chest roentgenograms, even in asymptomatic cases, can show patchy nonsegmental areas of basal pneumonitis and prominent hilar adenopathy; pleural effusions are uncommon. Some patients, however, are symptomatic within 1 to 2 weeks after exposure. They have an influenza-like illness with fever, chills, myalgias, and a nonproductive cough. Regardless of the presence or absence of symptoms, a primary fungemia generally occurs; organisms can be recovered from blood and bone marrow without implying progressive dissemination. The calcified granulomas commonly found in spleens and livers of patients from endemic areas, result from this primary self-limited fungemia and not from true dissemination.

Following exposure to a large infecting inoculum, a more diffuse pulmonary involvement may occur, with an extensive nodular infiltrate on chest roentgenogram. Most of these patients are symptomatic, but they usually recover uneventfully. Rarely, the illness will continue for weeks to months, with a remitting and relapsing course.

The chest roentgenogram often reveals a return to normal after a primary pulmonary infection, but a variety of residual abnormalities can be seen. Initial soft infiltrates may "harden" and leave one or several nodules. Central necrosis may lead to a dense core of calcium (a target lesion), but this is not universal, especially in adults. Infrequently, alternate periods of activity followed by healing may result in characteristic concentric rings of calcium as the lesion slowly enlarges. Lymph node calcification, either in association with a parenchymal nodule or as a solitary finding, is common. Finally, small punctate "buckshot" calcifications may be scattered over both lung fields, a pattern characteristic of a heavy primary exposure with uneventful recovery (Chapter 30).

Primary histoplasmosis has several uncommon local complications within the chest. An extensive fibrosing process in the mediastinum can cause vascular compression and result in a superior venacaval syndrome. Involvement of the pericardium may result in pericarditis with eventual constriction. Involvement of the esophagus can cause a traction diverticulum. If a calcified node erodes through a bronchus, hemoptysis and a broncholith may result.

Chronic Cavitary Histoplasmosis. Upper lobe cavitary histoplasmosis closely resembles reinfection tuberculosis in its roentgenographic appearance. The mechanism of infection, however, is not endogenous reactivation; instead, it is the direct result of a primary infection in abnormal lungs, typically the lungs of middle aged, male smokers who have central lobular emphysema.[9] Acute pulmonary histoplasmosis in this setting usually resolves without sequelae, but infected air spaces persist in a few cases. A progressive fibrosing cavitary process then develops, which may gradually destroy adjacent areas of the lung. Specific antifungal chemotherapy is required. Although bilateral upper lobe involvement is characteristic, cavitary disease may occur in other parts of the lung. Chronic cough is a common clinical symptom, although some patients are asymptomatic. Constitutional symptoms, including weight loss, increase as the illness progresses, although fever need not be present. The coexistence of cavitary histoplasmosis with either tuberculosis or with bronchogenic carcinoma is common.

Disseminated Histoplasmosis. Disseminated histoplasmosis refers to any progressive extrapulmonary infection.[10] In children, it can occur as an overwhelming postprimary spread with no tendency to granuloma formation despite the presence of massive numbers of organisms in all reticuloendothelial tissues. High fever, lymphadenopathy, hepatosplenomegaly, disturbance of bone marrow function, and a fulminant course can cause death within weeks. Among adults, dissemination is most common in elderly men who have a smoldering, subacute, clinical illness many months long, with moderate fever, hepatosplenomegaly, skin and mucous membrane lesions, and weight loss. Disseminated histoplasmosis also occurs as an opportunistic infection in the immunosuppressed patient; high dose glucocorticoid therapy is an important predisposing factor.[11] The degree of granulomatous response in the immunosuppressed patient can vary from almost nothing (the infantile form) to a considerable amount.

It is important to note that fewer than one-half of patients with disseminated histoplasmosis have a cough, dyspnea, or other pulmonary symptoms.[10,12] The chest roentgenogram may be normal or it may show a diffuse interstitial infiltrate which suggests a hematogenous process. Although at least one-third of nonimmunosuppressed patients will have a localized interstitial infiltrate on chest x-ray, such a finding is unusual in the immunosuppressed patient in whom there is usually no history of a preceding respiratory illness. The mechanism of infection may be endogenous reactivation. The clinical picture of disseminated histoplasmosis is extremely variable and nonspecific. Persistent fever is the only finding common to nearly all patients.

Progressive extrapulmonary histoplasmosis may begin with a more localized infection. These cases include central nervous system histoplasmoma, meningeal histoplasmosis, and isolated gastrointestinal histoplasmosis, which usually involves the terminal ileum.

Diagnosis

Morphology and Laboratory Identification. Histopathologic specimens that reveal macrophages crowded with small yeast are diagnostic of histoplasmosis. These organisms are easily seen in routine hemotoxylin and eosin sections. With well-developed granulomas, the yeast forms may be rare, larger, and seen only in GMS stained sections. Differentiation in these cases must be made from *C. neoformans* (has a capsule seen on mucicarmine staining), *B. dermatitidis* (has characteristic wide-necked budding), and occasionally from endospores of *C. immitis* or yeast forms of *S. shenckii.*

The organism can frequently be cultured from the sputum in primary or in chronic cavitary histoplasmosis, although it is almost never identified in KOH preparations. Bone marrow aspirate and fragments of liver biopsied by needle are frequently culture-positive in disseminated histoplasmosis. If there are skin lesions, culture of a skin biopsy is easy and the results are reliable. Blood culture results may also be positive in disseminated histoplasmosis but should be requested specifically for fungal cultures, because they may have to be held for a longer time than routine bacterial cultures.

Although the organism is easy to grow from infected tissue specimens, identification may take several weeks. In suspected disseminated disease, this is too long and treatment must be instituted quickly.

Skin Test and Serology. Skin testing is performed with histoplasmin, a mycelial antigen. The skin test is generally positive 2 to 3 weeks after a primary pulmonary infection and remains positive for many years. Most inhabitants of an endemic area will have a positive skin test, and therefore the test is not of diagnostic use in those areas.

Complement-fixing serologic reactions become positive to mycelial and then to yeast antigens 3 to 4 weeks after primary infection. The titers usually decrease over 3 to 12 months but occasionally remain positive at a high dilution for years. Nonetheless, titers against the yeast antigen of 1:16 or greater in the appropriate clinical setting suggest a recent infection. A rising titer is diagnostic. Unfortunately, complement-fixation tests may be negative in 50 percent or more of the patients with disseminated histoplasmosis, although a high titer in an individual patient with an obscure febrile illness may suggest the diagnosis.

Immunodiffusion testing for precipitating antibodies to H or M antigens is specific for histoplasmosis, and positive reactions suggest recent infection. A negative test does not exclude histoplasmosis.

Surgical Importance

Histoplasmosis is a common cause of a solitary pulmonary nodule. If it is noncalcified, thoracotomy is often required to exclude bronchogenic carcinoma. Amphotericin B is not required after the excision of such a nodule.

Specific antifungal chemotherapy is probably also unnecessary if a mediastinal mass has been biopsied to exclude lymphoma and histoplasmosis is documented. Large caseous masses should be removed.[13,14] No surgical therapy is generally effective in cases where fibrosing mediastinitis has caused a superior venacaval syndrome. Thoracotomy is often necessary for diagnosis, however, and vascular bypass procedures have been performed in some patients with severe symptoms. Treatment with amphotericin B is generally recommended only if operative specimens are culture-positive. Operation should rarely be necessary in chronic cavitary histoplasmosis. An exception might be hemoptysis localized to a specific large cavity.

The diagnosis of disseminated histoplasmosis often depends on a biopsy of a skin lesion, a mucosal ulcer, or a vocal cord ulceration. The specimen should be cultured, as well as submitted, for histopathology. Open liver biopsy may be indicated in some patients; however, bone marrow aspirate and trephine biopsy should precede laparotomy if a disseminated infection is suspected.

Disseminated histoplasmosis may also be of importance as an opportunistic infection among renal transplant recipients and other immunosuppressed patients.

Therapy

The usual primary pulmonary infection requires no therapy, but amphotericin B may be used for severe or prolonged infections.[15] A total course of 500 mg may be adequate in this situation.[16] Rarely, a massive primary exposure may result in acute respiratory failure with marked hypoxia. Oxygenation and ventilatory support may be required, and use of amphotericin B is mandatory.

Progressive chronic cavitary histoplasmosis requires full therapy with amphotericin B, as does disseminated histoplasmosis.

BLASTOMYCOSIS

Blastomycosis, also known as North American blastomycosis, to distinguish it from paracoccidioidomycosis or South American blastomycosis, refers to infection by *Blastomyces dermatitidis.* Primary infection is in the lung, where large central inflammatory masses can mimic carcinoma. Involvement of skin, bone, and prostate gland are prominent features of disseminated blastomycosis; reticuloendothelial organs are seldom involved.

Etiology

B. dermatitidis is a thermal dimorphic fungus. At 25C it grows on Sabouraud agar as a septate mycelium, with a variable colony form, which ranges from white and fluffy to tan and smooth. Microconidia are present on the hyphae, but they have no characteristic identifying features. At 37C on blood agar the organism grows as a large 8–20 μm yeast, which can be identified by its doubly refractile wall and its characteristic wide-necked single budding. These are the organisms seen extracellularly in histopathologic preparations of infected mammalian tissue.

Epidemiology

B. dermatitidis is endemic in the southeastern and south central regions of the United States. Disease activity extends northward along the western shores of Lake Michigan and is also present in Minnesota, North Dakota, and bordering Canadian provinces. Its exact ecologic niche is uncertain because isolations of the mycelial phase from nature have been infrequent. The organism is a soil saprophyte which infects only after direct, intimate exposure. The disease occurs most frequently in rural areas among those with outdoor jobs or interests, predominantly males aged 20 to 50.

Pathogenesis and Pathology

The infectious microconidia are inhaled into the lung, where a vigorous acute suppurative response occurs. Cell-mediated immunity develops later, and the tissue reaction at the time of diagnosis of pulmonary blastomycosis has a mixed pyogenic and granulomatous nature. Acute pulmonary blastomycosis is self-limited in a majority of cases, although the tendency to heal is probably not as pronounced as it is with histoplasmosis.

Hematogenous spread does not always occur during pulmonary infection as it does in histoplasmosis; favored sites of spread are skin, bone, and prostate rather than liver and spleen.[17]

Clinical Manifestations

Primary Pulmonary Blastomycosis. Acute pulmonary blastomycosis is a variably symptomatic illness.[18] Patchy areas of alveolar consolidation usually affect one or both lower lobes. Hilar adenopathy may occur, but pleural involvement and cavitation are rare. If present, the symptoms are like acute pneumonia and include high fever, productive cough, pleuritic chest pain, and myalgias. Symptoms may vary in intensity and duration but usually last less than 2 weeks. Radiographic evidence often persists for up to 3 months (Chapter 30).[19]

Progressive primary infections with continued suppuration and eventual necrosis and cavitation are rare. Involvement of the pleural space may occur with unmistakable empyema formation. Acute miliary spread may occur throughout the body; massive pulmonary involvement can lead to respiratory failure.

Chronic Pulmonary Blastomycosis With or Without Involvement of Distant Sites. Most clinical cases of blastomycosis present as chronic pulmonary blastomycosis.[20] Many of these patients give no history of an antecedent acute pneumonia, but have chronic respiratory symptoms of weeks to months duration. Chronic cough, low-grade fever, night sweats, weight loss, and a variable amount of dyspnea are the common complaints. The chest roentgenogram may reveal a single large mass, often perihilar in location. This pattern is responsible for the fact that blastomycosis is misdiagnosed as carcinoma of the lung more often than any other fungal disease.[21] The most common finding on chest roentgenogram is fibronodular infiltrates, often with small cavities and stringy fibrosis extending toward the hila, which may mimic tuberculosis. A rare roentgenographic finding is a single large cavity, which may resemble a primary lung abscess (Chapter 30).[19]

Involvement of distant sites is common in chronic pulmonary blastomycosis; two-thirds of the patients have skin involvement, one-third have bone involvement, and one-fifth have genitourinary tract involvement.[20] The occurrence of infection in these sites, in association with a chronic pulmonary infection, can be helpful in suggesting the presence of blastomycosis and in providing an easily accessible source of diagnostic material.

Isolated Involvement of Distant Sites. Isolated involvement of skin, bone, or genitourinary tract can occur without any history or evidence of respiratory tract infection. This probably represents reactivation of sites seeded during primary asymptomatic infection.

Skin Infection. The characteristic lesions of skin infection are raised, warty, crusted lesions with irregular borders on the face and upper extremities. The lesions can mimic basal cell carcinoma, but the small microabscesses at the periphery of the lesions are a distinguishing feature (Fig. 25-29).

Skeletal System. Bone is the second most common distant site of infection in blastomycosis.[20] The spine is most frequently involved, followed by the ribs, skull, and long bones. Involvement of the spine mimics tuberculosis, with involvement of adjacent vertebrae and destruction of the intervening disc space. Osteolytic and osteoblastic processes may be seen on roentgenogram, but periosteal proliferation is unusual. Long bones are involved near the epiphysis, and the infection can extend directly to an adjacent joint space (Chapter 43).

Genitourinary System. Unlike tuberculosis, blastomycosis rarely involves the kidney or ureter or any part of the female genitourinary tract. The prostate, epididymis, and less frequently testes, however, become involved and can result in a scrotal or prostatic mass, hematuria, pyuria, or bladder outlet obstruction.[22] Venereal transmission may result in a self-limited ulceration in a sexual partner.[23]

Diagnosis

Morphology and Laboratory Identification. The yeast can frequently be seen in the sputum, in aspirates of skin lesions, or in prostatic secretions. The organisms can be positively identified in KOH preparations, although cytology specimens treated with Papanicolaou stain are superior.

Histopathologic examination of biopsy specimens of infected tissue also reveals the characteristic 8–20 μm yeast of blastomycosis with doubly refractile walls and wide-necked single budding. The organism is seldom seen in hematoxylin and eosin stained sections; silver and PAS stains are best for diagnosis.

In the laboratory, *B. dermatitidis* grows slowly, often requiring a month or more. The plates must be sealed to prevent drying during the long incubation period. The organism is sensitive to cyclohexamide, so this antibiotic should not be used in the culture media.

Diagnosis of blastomycosis ultimately depends on observing the typical morphology of the yeast form, either directly in clinical specimens or in the converted 37C yeast phase of an organism isolated as a mycelium by culture at 25C.

Skin Test and Serology. Neither skin nor serologic tests are useful in blastomycosis. The complement-fixing titers are neither specific (a rise in titer against *H. capsulatum* is more common than a rise in titer against *B. dermatitidis* in blastomycoses) nor sensitive (50 to 75 percent of cases are negative). Immunodiffusion may be specific but is so insensitive that negative results are expected. Serologic tests are useful only when a high antibody titer might initiate the gathering of specimens for direct examination and culture (Table 9-1).

Surgical Importance

Blastomycosis can present as a mass (up to 10 cm) in the chest. Fever and night sweats suggest a chronic inflammation. If the diagnosis is confirmed from cytologic specimens, thoracotomy is not necessary. Amphotericin B will be required if a resected mass is proved to be chronic pulmonary blastomycosis.

Surgery is rarely necessary to drain a large abscess or an empyema.

Skin lesions can mimic basal cell carcinoma, but microabscesses at the periphery of the lesion should suggest the correct diagnosis. Aspiration of the lesion will ordinarily establish the diagnosis, and the lesions will respond to amphotericin B.

Blastomycosis in the spine usually resembles tuberculosis, but an osteolytic lesion can suggest myeloma or other malignant disease. Aspiration of the bone lesions may be necessary.

If a needle biopsy of a prostate nodule reveals characteristic yeast forms, treatment with amphotericin B is mandatory.[22] Prostatic involvement can also look like bladder outlet obstruction. Testicular involvement can mimic a tumor, but more often the presence of tender swelling will indicate an infection.

Treatment

Acute pulmonary blastomycosis probably does not require treatment in all cases. Treatment with a total course of 2 gm amphotercin B should be given if the patient is severely ill, if the illness progresses under observation, or if there is no improvement after 2 to 3 weeks. Long-term evaluation is always necessary, however, because systemic disease can develop much later despite a self-limited primary infection. Patients with chronic pulmonary disease, or disease at distant sites should also receive a total dose of 2 gm of amphotericin B (Chapter 18).[24] A second course of amphotericin B should be used in the 10 percent of patients who have a relapse.

COCCIDIOIDOMYCOSIS

Coccidioidomycosis is caused by the fungus *Coccidioides immitis*. Symptomatic pulmonary illnesses occur in almost half of all exposed people. Although the majority of primary infections resolve, many patients develop disseminated disease with central nervous system, skeletal, and cutaneous involvement. Disseminated coccidioidomycosis is a chronic illness with many relapses.

Etiology

C. immitis is a tissue dimorphic fungus. In the soil and on laboratory culture media, the fungus grows as a septate mycelium with numerous side branches. Spore formation occurs along the hyphae; thick-walled arthrospores develop, which alternate with empty cells. When the infecting arthrospores are inhaled into the mammalian lung, they develop into spherules characteristic of the tissue phase of growth. Spherules are round, thick-walled structures, which grow to 30–80 μm in diameter and reproduce by progressive cleavage of the cytoplasm with formation of multiple endospores (as many as 10^5 per mature spherule). Each spherule eventually ruptures; the endospores are released into the tissue where each, again, has the potential to mature into another spherule and repeat the cycle.

Epidemiology

C. immitis is endemic in the southwestern United States, particularly in the San Joaquin Valley of California and in southern Arizona and New Mexico. Nevada, Utah, and southwest Texas have some disease activity. The disease is also endemic in areas of Mexico adjoining these southwestern states and in several areas of Central and South America. The specific habitat favoring fungal growth is the desert soil in a semiarid climate with hot dry summers and mild winters with moderate rainfall.

The arthrospores are scattered long distances by the wind. Exposure to the fungus is an almost universal occurrence in highly endemic areas; 80 percent of nonimmune persons who move to such areas develop a primary pulmonary infection within 5 years.

Pathogenesis and Pathology

The infecting particle is the arthrospore, and infection occurs only by inhalation. The arthrospore is so infective that a casual exposure such as driving through an endemic area can cause a primary pulmonary infection. In exceptional cases, infection has occurred after exposure to arthrospore-contaminated articles shipped to nonendemic areas.

The arthrospore elicits an exudative response with polymorphonuclear cells predominating in the lung alveoli. Rupture of developing spherules liberates great numbers of endospores, most of which are phagocytosed and rapidly destroyed. Some of the endospores always survive and mature into new spherules.

Within 1 to 2 weeks, a specific cell-mediated immunity develops, which is directed against the maturing spherules. Such specific cell-mediated immunity is essential in arresting the infection. A mixed granulomatous and pyogenic tissue response is seen in histopathologic specimens obtained at this stage of the infection.

If the cell-mediated response is inadequate, a fulminant miliary illness can result. In less extreme cases, a few endospores may be deposited at distant sites and reactivation can occur weeks or even years later. Meningitis is the most frequent and the most ominous presentation; bone and skin are other sites of late activation.

Clinical Manifestations

Primary Pulmonary Coccidioidomycoses. Sixty percent of patients with a primary pulmonary infection have minimal or no symptoms.[25,26] The other 40 percent have a febrile pulmonary illness that resembles influenza and lasts 1 to 3 weeks. Chest pain, often pleuritic, is a common complaint but is often short-lived. Cough is usually quite mild. Weight loss and anorexia are common, as are myalgias, arthralgias, headache, and fatigue. Dyspnea is unusual in an uncomplicated pulmonary infection. The chest roentgenogram can show an alveolar infiltrate (usually at one of the lung bases) or a single nodular density.

Primary pulmonary infection resolves without any sequelae 95 percent of the time; the other 5 percent will have abnormal findings on chest x-rays, most commonly with solitary thin-walled cavities. Only one or two patients in 1,000 will develop disseminated disease. Dissemination occurs most commonly in black and Filipino men, diabetics, and pregnant women.

Manifestations of cell-mediated immunity, such as erythema nodosum, erythema multiforme, and frank arthritis, occur in up to 20 percent of all patients with pulmonary coccidioidomycosis, a much higher incidence than other fungal infections. Such clinical features are of favorable prognostic significance, being most common in white women. In endemic areas, "desert rheumatism," "valley fever," and "the bumps" are recognized clinical syndromes.

Sterile but painful pleural effusions occur in 5 to 10 percent of the patients with primary pulmonary disease.[27] Fifty percent of the time, the effusions are accompanied by erythema nodosum or erythema multiforme, suggesting that they are manifestations of hypersensitivity.

The persistent single asymptomatic thin-walled cavity is the most common residium.[28] Residual solitary pulmonary nodules must be differentiated from bronchogenic carcinoma.[29] Occasionally, a patient with coccidioidomycosis may have a chronic fibronodular cavitary infiltrate that mimics tuberculosis (Chapter 30).

Disseminated Coccidioidomycoses. Persistent or recurrent fever can signal the onset of disseminated disease. Rapid progression with development of meningitis, multiple bony lesions, and verrucous cutaneous lesions like those of blastomycoses can occur (Fig. 25-29).[30] Although it is rare, patients have an even more fulminant postprimary miliary spread with respiratory failure. Clinically recognizable defects in cell-mediated immunity are frequent in these patients; past high doses of prednisone are an important predisposing factor.[31,32]

For most patients, however, the onset of disseminated infection with *C. immitis* is more insidious. While it usually follows the primary pulmonary infection by either weeks or months, it may occur much later. In many instances, the primary pulmonary infection has been asymptomatic and cannot be adequately dated. Coccidioidal meningitis is the most frequent manifestation of extrapulmonary disease.[33] A granulomatous process at the base of the brain entraps cranial nerves and obstructs the flow of cerebrospinal fluid. Headache may be the only symptom, but the level of consciousness is usually disturbed, especially with obstructive hydrocephalus. Fever and stiff neck are not common. The cerebrospinal fluid reveals a moderate leukocytosis (often less than 500 cells) with a predominance of mononuclear cells. Organisms are rarely seen, and cultures are frequently sterile. Diagnosis may depend on the demonstration of complement-fixing antibodies in the spinal fluid. Skeletal disease occurs in 10 to 20 percent of the patients with extrapulmonary disease. Single or multiple nonreactive lytic lesions appear in long bones, spine, or skull. Bony involvement may spread to involve adjacent meninges, joints, or skin with the development of a draining fistula. Skin lesions appear in those with widespread dissemination. Individual lesions, like those of blastomycoses, often mimic basal cell carcinoma. Renal involvement is similar to tuberculosis except for less ureteral involvement. Prostate and epididymis are seldom involved.

Diagnosis

Morphology and Laboratory Identification. Histopathologic specimens are diagnostic if the large spherules or spherule fragments can be identified in hematoxylin and eosin or silver-stained sections. Spherules are diagnostic if identified in KOH-treated specimens such as sputum or pus. The organisms can be cultured on Sabouraud agar or on blood agar without difficulty, but the arthrospores are highly infectious. Because similar arthrospores exist in other saphrophytic fungi, routine cultures themselves are not diagnostic. After injection of the mycelial elements into mice, the characteristic tissue phase spherule will develop. Because of these difficulties and because cultures are seldom positive in coccidioidal meningitis (where they would be most helpful), cultural identification is not of great clinical importance. Reliance on direct demonstration of organism and on skin tests and serology is adequate for management of most patients.

Skin Test and Serology. Skin testing is performed with coccidioidin, prepared from the mycelial phase of growth. A positive test (5 mm induration) is present in most patients with primary disease from 2 to 20 days after infection. Failure to develop a positive test is predictive of progressive disseminated infection. Loss of established skin test reactivity often precedes late dissemination. Successful chemotherapy returns skin test positivity, and relapse is likely if the skin test remains negative. Antigenic material from the tissue phase of growth, named spherulin, has recently become available for skin testing. Spherulin has been useful in epidemiologic studies because it is a more specific and more sensitive skin test. It is not certain, however, whether it will have the full prognostic importance of coccidioidin.

Complement-fixing antibodies are also of great clinical importance because mild infections do not develop these antibodies.[34] Severe but self-limited primary infections in the lung may have a mild elevation in titer, which disappears in 6 months or persists at levels 1:8 or less. Persistent titers of 1:16 or greater, and especially gradually rising titers, usually mean present or impending dissemination. Successful drug therapy results in a fall in complement-fixing antibody titers, which often accompanies the development of a positive skin test.

Complement-fixing serologic titers in the cerebrospinal fluid are of particular diagnostic importance in coccidioidal meningitis. These titers are positive in 95 percent of patients, many of whom have isolated meningeal disease and negative cerebrospinal fluid cultures and could not be diagnosed by other noninvasive means.

Immunodiffusion may identify antibodies that appear earlier and are quite specific. This type of antibody usually disappears within a month but is of no prognostic importance even if it persists for a long time (Table 9-1).

Surgical Importance

Coccidioidomycosis is a common cause of a solitary pulmonary nodule in endemic areas. Residual nodules rarely calcify, and thoracotomy may be required to exclude bronchogenic carcinoma.

Thin-walled cavities caused by coccidioidomycosis are common in endemic areas and ordinarily require no therapy. Resection of such cavities may be necessary, however, to control recurrent hemoptysis or symptomatic superinfection. Resection may be indicated for a growing cavity or one that is subpleural in location or crosses fissure lines. Rupture into the pleural space may produce an empyema with bronchopleural fistula. This is a serious complication that requires pleural drainage and later operative closure of the bronchopleural fistula, under amphotericin B coverage.

A surgical procedure may be required for diagnosis. Biopsies of skin or bony lesions may be undertaken with a presumptive diagnosis of basal cell carcinoma or metastatic carcinoma, respectively.

Neurosurgical placement of an Ommaya reservoir may be needed to treat some patients with coccidioidal meningitis.[35,36]

Finally, immunosuppressed patients, including transplant recipients and other patients on high-dose prednisone, may develop disseminated coccidioidomycosis as a result of endogenous reactivation or progressive primary infection.

Therapy

Amphotericin B is less effective against *C. immitis* than against any other pathogenic fungi, but it is still the best available treatment.[24] Treatment is indicated in primary pulmonary coccidioidomycosis only in patients whose immune status or racial backgrounds place them at high risk of dissemination, ie, immunosuppressed patients, diabetics, pregnant women, and black and Filipino men. Treatment is especially advisable when pulmonary infection is severe, persistent, or progressive. The usual total dose of amphotericin B is 500 mg to 2 gm.

All patients undergoing resection of coccidioidal pulmonary lesions for any indication should also receive amphotericin B coverage, with 500 mg administered prior to operation and an additional 500 mg afterward.

Disseminated disease always demands prompt and aggressive therapy. An initial course of 2.5 gm is employed. If remission is not obtained, prolonged courses of 4–5 gm are indicated.

Coccidioidal meningitis should be treated intrathecally with amphotericin B until complement-fixing antibody levels in the cerebrospinal fluid are negative. The skin test may revert to positive as well, although this is not always the case. Sclerosing complications may limit intrathecal administration of the drug at the lumbar site and an alternate route of administration (intracisternal or intraventricular via Ommaya reservoir) may have to be used.[35,36] Patients with isolated coccidioidal meningitis should also receive a total dose of 1 gm of systemic amphotericin B.

The use of amphotericin B is not always successful.[24] Miconazole or ketoconazole may be of use in patients who have failed to improve with amphotericin B.[4,37] Their exact roles in treatment are not defined.[4,24,37]

PARACOCCIDIOIDOMYCOSIS

Paracoccidioidomycosis (South American blastomycosis) is caused by *Paracoccidioides brasiliensis.* Asymptomatic pulmonary infection is produced when the organism is inhaled, and disseminated disease is characterized by involvement of the oral and pharyngeal mucosa and cervical adenopathy.

Etiology

P. brasiliensis is a thermal dimorphic fungus. The mycelium, which grows at 25C on laboratory media (and soil), has no specific identifying features. In mammalian tissue and on blood agar at 37C, the fungus converts to a yeast phase which buds in a characteristic fashion with multiple buds around the periphery of the parent cell, each with a thin neck.

Epidemiology

An endemic region exists in Brazil, Colombia, and Venezuela with scattered cases from other areas of South and Central America. Most cases are asymptomatic.

Pathogenesis and Pathology

When inhaled, the infectious spores provoke an acute inflammatory response similar to that seen in blastomycosis. If progressive pulmonary disease occurs, the pathologic picture includes mixed granulomatous and suppurative processes. Mucocutaneous lesions demonstrate pseudoepitheliomatous hyperplasia with areas of granuloma formation, but also with microabscesses. Both the lung and the skin pathology resemble that seen in blastomycosis.

The fungus can spread throughout the body during a primary infection. The distinctive tendency for oral and pharyngeal lesions in disseminated disease, long thought to imply ingestion as a mechanism of infection, is now thought to represent distant spread. The fungus favors this site for growth because of a slight temperature differential.

Clinical Manifestations

A primary asymptomatic self-limited illness is inferred by the frequency in endemic areas of positive skin tests and incidental findings at autopsy.[38,39] Progressive pulmonary disease presents with fever, weight loss, productive cough, and increasing shortness of breath over a period of weeks to months. The chest roentgenogram reveals nodular areas that may be confluent and most often involve the lower lobes. Fibrosis can occur as areas of the lung are destroyed. Cavitation occurs in one-third of the cases.

Disseminated paracoccidioidomycosis classically presents with multiple oral and pharyngeal ulcerations and cervical adenopathy. The lesions are initially painless, but the granulomatous process eventually invades lip, palate, epiglottis, and gingiva with loss of teeth. Pulmonary involvement may be minimal or absent.

Widely disseminated disease also occurs with the lymph nodes, spleen, intestine, and skin as preferred sites. Bone and central nervous system involvement occurs only occasionally.

Diagnosis

Morphology and Laboratory Identification. The diagnosis depends on the forms in sputum, purulent secretions, or tissue biopsy. The pathognomonic feature is multiple peripheral budding with thin-necked attachment on a 15–40 μm parent cell.

The mycelium grows slowly on yeast extract agar at 25C. It has no characteristic spores, and conversion to the typical yeast form by culture on blood agar at 37C is necessary before positive identification can be made.

Skin Test and Serology. Skin testing has no important clinical role in paracoccidioidomycosis. The skin test results are generally positive in mild disease but may be negative with far advanced terminal illness.[40]

The complement fixation test is positive in 80 percent of patients with active infection and generally negative after successful therapy. An immunodiffusion test developed by Restrepo is even more sensitive and specific.[39,40]

Surgical Importance

Biopsy of specimens from mucocutaneous lesions or of lymph nodes may be needed to make a specific diagnosis. Progressive pulmonary disease can generally be diagnosed from the sputum. Surgery has no major role in therapy.

Therapy

Effective chemotherapeutic agents include sulfonamides, amphotericin B, and possibly miconazole.[41] Many of these patients have a relapse after therapy is stopped. Some patients must be maintained on sulfanomides for up to 5 years.

CRYPTOCOCCOSIS

Cryptococcosis is caused by the encapsulated yeast *Cryptococcus neoformans.* The primary pulmonary infection rarely produces a clinical illness, and most patients have subacute or chronic meningitis, which is associated with an underlying disease so often that in Europe it is referred to as "signal malade."

Etiology

C. neoformans exists both in nature and in infected mammalian tissue as a 4–20 μm budding yeast. Its distinctive feature is its thick carbohydrate capsule; it is the only pathogenic yeast that is encapsulated (Fig. 2-10).

Epidemiology

Cryptococcal organisms are distributed worldwide, in both urban and rural areas. They are most frequently associated with pigeon droppings.

Pathogenesis and Pathology

In the lung, the organism produces its carbohydrate capsule, which inhibits phagocytosis and the recruitment of inflammatory cells. Nonetheless, the innate infectivity of the organism is not great and the cellular immune response, although minimal, generally limits the local infection. In immunocompromised patients, hematogenous spread of organisms may occur so that cryptococcal infection later becomes active at a distant site, most commonly the meninges. Postulated explanations for meningeal predilection include a decreased phagocytic response in the cerebrospinal fluid, where cerebrospinal fluid and amino acid concentrations may also be more optimal for yeast growth. Skin, bone, and occasionally visceral organs can become involved. A miliary form of cryptococcosis can occur in immunosuppressed patients.

The lesions are either myxomatous or granulomatous. Myxomatous lesions have masses of encapsulated organisms lying free in the tissues, without inflammatory response. The lesions appear gelatinous or mucoid, often resembling myxomatous neoplasms. Other lesions are typically granulomatous, with fewer organisms. The mixed pyogenic and granulomatous response seen in blastomycosis and coccidioidomycosis does not occur, however, nor does the lymphocytic and fibrotic response around the periphery of the lesion which is seen in histoplasmosis.

Clinical Manifestations

Primary Pulmonary Cryptococcosis. Patients usually have no symptoms, although if an active focus erodes into an airway there may be a transient heavy discharge of mucoid sputum laden with organisms. If present, fever is modest.

Chest roentgenograms usually show a localized discrete infiltrate in one of the lower lobes without hilar adenopathy. As a rule, the infiltrates completely resolve without cavitation or residual nodules (Chapter 30).

Central Nervous System Cryptococcosis. Eighty percent of diagnosed cases of cryptococcosis involve the central nervous system without a history or clinical evidence of respiratory involvement.[42–44] Headaches that gradually increase in frequency and severity, and mild fever and meningeal signs, are usually present. Abnormal laboratory findings are usually confined to the cerebrospinal fluid with increased pressure, high protein, low glucose, and a variable lymphocytic pleocytosis, usually less than 200 cells. India ink preparation of spinal fluid is positive in half of the culture-proven cases (Fig. 2-10).

Without specific treatment, rapid deterioration and death will result. About half of patients have an underlying disease, such as lymphoma, leukemia, and diabetes, or any disorder treated with high-dose steroids.[45,46] These patients have a poor prognosis. Other negative prognostic factors include less than 20 white blood cells per mm^3 in the cerebrospinal fluid, the presence of organisms on India ink preparation, positive cultures of blood or other extraneural specimens in association with meningitis, and high titers of cryptococcal antigen in cerebrospinal fluid or serum.

Less commonly,[2] patients have a single focus in the brain, a mass lesion, with signs of increased intracerebral pressure (nausea, vomiting, changes in level of consciousness) and focal neurologic signs.

Bone Involvement. Although cryptococcosis can involve the skull, vertebrae, and long bones, it occurs much less frequently than in blastomycosis or coccidioidomycosis. Roentgenograms show a destructive focus, without much periosteal reaction, which is often indistinguishable from neoplasm.

Cutaneous Involvement. A variety of skin lesions are produced by hematogenous spread rather than by inoculation, and occur in conjunction with disseminated disease. Specific diagnosis is impossible without biopsy.

Disseminated Cryptococcosis. Rapid hematogenous spread to many organs occurs primarily in immunosuppressed patients. High fever is common. Diffuse lung involvement can lead to respiratory insufficiency. Liver and bone marrow involvement can also be documented. The cerebrospinal fluid is usually involved. Diagnosis in these cases is usually made from a blood culture or on examination of the bone marrow.

Diagnosis

Morphology and Laboratory Identification. Histopathologic material is diagnostic if a yeast form (4–20 μm), with a thick unstained capsular halo, can be demonstrated with hematoxylin and eosin, or silver stain. The mucicarmine stain brightly outlines the carbohydrate capsule. India ink preparation permits rapid identification of an encapsulated yeast in the cerebrospinal fluid or other body fluids.

Cultures of cerebrospinal fluid, blood, urine, or aspirates of bony or skin lesions are diagnostic of cryptococcosis if an encapsulated yeast is recovered. *C. neoformans* grows readily at 25C and at 37C on Sabouraud agar and other media.

Interpretation of sputum cultures is more difficult because other cryptococcus species occasionally colonize the respiratory tract. Even *C. neoformans* can be recovered from the sputum of a debilitated patient without an invasive infection.

The final differentiation of *C. neoformans* from other cryptococcal species depends on its virulence for mice, or on biochemical and physiologic characteristics similar to those used when identifying bacteria.

Skin Testing and Serology. No reliable skin test antigen is available for clinical use. The tube precipitin method is the best serologic procedure, but it is unreliable.

Cryptococcosis is the only fungal infection where measurement of a fungal antigen is important. Capsular material in serum and cerebrospinal fluid can be detected by a sensitive latex-fixation method, which is specific if controls for rheumatoid factor are included. Cryptococcal antigen is of diagnostic and also prognostic importance. Initial high levels of antigen, or failure of the antigen level to decrease during therapy, indicate the likelihood of treatment failure or early relapse.

Surgical Importance

A nodule resected to exclude the possibility of bronchogenic carcinoma can be a cryptococcal lesion. A spinal tap should be done in such patients to determine if the spinal fluid is involved, but treatment is not necessary if the findings are negative.

Bone lesions can mimic neoplasm; diagnosis depends on aspiration or an open biopsy. Diagnosis of cutaneous cryptococcosis may also depend on biopsy.

Cryptococcal meningitis is an important opportunistic infection in renal transplant recipients and other immunosuppressed patients, so the onset of chronic headaches should prompt the performance of a spinal tap.[45,47] Disseminated cryptococcosis is also in the differential diagnosis of generalized systemic infections in such patients and can mimic cytomegalovirus infection.

Therapy

All patients who have *C. neoformans* isolated from any site should have a spinal tap done to exclude meningeal involvement. Some patients will be asymptomatic even when *Cryptococcus* has been identified in sputum or in a pulmonary nodule. These people do not require treatment if their cerebrospinal fluid is free of the organism. All patients, however, who have extrapulmonary involvement require full treatment. The best treatment is combined therapy with amphotericin B, 0.3 to 0.5 mg per kg per day, and 150 mg per kg per day of 5-Fluorocytosine.[48] Twelve of 16 patients with culture-proven cryptococcal meningitis responded to the lower dose, despite the presence of poor prognostic features in many cases.

Relapses must be treated with combination therapy. Intrathecal administration of amphotericin B is usually not required, but it can be tried in patients who are responding poorly to conventional therapy.

OPPORTUNISTIC FUNGAL DISEASES

Opportunistic fungal diseases are caused by ubiquitous fungi, which are ordinarily nonpathogenic and invade tissue only under conditions of local or systemic host immunoincompetence.

ASPERGILLOSIS

Aspergillosis refers to infection by any of the numerous members of the genus *Aspergillus.* These fungi have a low pathogenicity for healthy individuals. Although they can readily colonize mucosal surfaces, these organisms do not invade people unless the normal defense mechanisms are altered. Common sites for local infection are the external ear, the orbit and paranasal sinuses, and the lung, especially if there are abnormal airways or preexisting cavities.[49] In addition, an allergic response to *Aspergillus* organisms growing in the thick bronchial secretions of asthmatics may contribute to their symptomatology. Dissemination of the disease occurs only in severely immunosuppressed patients.

Etiology

There are more than 300 species of *Aspergillus*. The majority of human infections are caused by *A. fumigatus*. Occasionally, infections are caused by *A. niger, A. clavatus, A. flavus,* or *A. nidulans.* At 25C to 37C the fungus is a fast-growing mycelium on Sabouraud agar and on other laboratory media. A white fluffy mycelium appears first and quickly turns green to dark green, or brown, as spores form. The hyphae are thick, septate, and have branches that spread out at acute angles, in a fingerlike manner. Expanded knoblike sporeheads are located at the end of specialized hyphae or conidiophores. Identification of a particular species is difficult and usually depends on the structure of the sporeheads.

The *Aspergillus* species are among the most common fungi. Spores are present in all environments, and any small source of organic debris serves as a nidus for growth.

Pathogenesis and Pathology

The organisms are inhaled and may be recovered from the sputum of uninfected patients after heavy exposure. In external otitis, the organism colonizes the superficial keratinized layer of the skin and evokes little or no inflammatory response. True invasive infections occur in the middle ear, the paranasal sinus, and the contents of the orbit. Histopathology reveals a mixed inflammatory exudate with acute and chronic inflammatory cells. As a rule, the density of the organism is low, and special stains must be used to find hyphae.

Perhaps the most characteristic lesion produced by *Aspergillus* species is the intracavitary fungus ball, or aspergilloma. Matted masses of aspergilli grow in preexisting cavities which communicate with airways. The cavity colonized by the fungus is usually an inactive residual lesion secondary to tuberculosis, fungal disease, sarcoidosis, carcinoma, or bronchiectasis. Although there may be some inflammatory infiltration (with many eosinophils) around the cavity, the fungus does not invade adjacent lung parenchyma.

In allergic bronchial aspergillosis, the bronchi are dilated and full of mucus plugs. Hyphae and eosinophils are seen within the inspissated mucus, but fungi never invade the dilated bronchial walls, which are heavily infiltrated with eosinophils and other inflammatory cells.

In disseminated aspergillosis, widespread necrosis of tissue occurs, especially in the lung where there may be multiple wedge-shaped areas of bronchial pneumonia. Growth within blood vessels may cause thrombosis, with necrosis of further tissue and subsequent cavitation as the necrotic material is expectorated. Multiple metastatic abscesses are in the brain, liver, and heart.

Aspergillus endocarditis most commonly follows cardiac surgery. The vegetations are large, bulky, and friable, and frequently embolize to major arteries.

Clinical Manifestations

Ear, Paranasal Sinuses, and Orbit. Colonization of the oral pharynx causes no symptoms. Limited disease in the external ear causes pain and redness. When a paranasal sinus is invaded, local swelling and erythema result. Focal osteomyelitis should be considered when tenderness is severe. In the sinuses as well as in the nose and on the palate, the organism may grow as a large, bulky, soft tissue mass (which can bleed profusely). Once *Aspergillus* infection has become established in the paranasal sinuses, extension to the orbit and to the central nervous system is possible. Proptosis and ophthalmoplegia may be the dominant signs of orbital invasion. Sudden onset of a stroke indicates the involvement of an intracranial vessel, with distal hemorrhagic infarction. Patients who survive this complication usually develop abscesses with signs of increased intracranial pressure.

Aspergilloma. The major clinical feature of intracavitary fungus balls is hemoptysis, which can be profuse and sometimes even life-threatening, especially if blood is aspirated.[50] In the absence of hemoptysis, the patient's symptoms are generally related to the underlying chronic cavitary pulmonary disease, and are determined by the extent of pulmonary destruction present before the appearance of the fungus ball. The fungus ball will not invade deeply into the lung, nor will it lead to disseminated disease.

Allergic Bronchopulmonary Aspergillosis. Most patients with allergic bronchopulmonary aspergillosis have episodic dyspnea that is related to their underlying asthma. The clinical course of their asthma, however, is punctuated by intermittent bouts of increased anatomic obstruction of bronchi because the organisms proliferate in the thick mucus characteristic of asthma. When this happens, fever and cough are common and active infiltrates are usually seen on the chest roentgenogram. Mucous plugs are frequently expectorated, and pleuritic chest pain and peripheral blood eosinophilia are common. In the early stages of bronchopulmonary aspergillosis, the patients are relatively asymptomatic between acute exacerbations of bronchial plugging, except for the symptoms of their underlying asthma. Later on, however, the repeated attacks of bronchial plugging can result in gradual destruction of bronchial mucosa with eventual development of saccular bronchiectasis. When this occurs, the symptoms of infective bronchiectasis can dominate the clinical picture with continuous production of purulent sputum, even during the interval between episodes of bronchial plugging. Scanty hemoptysis comes from bronchiectatic lesions.

Invasive Aspergillosis. The invasive form of aspergillosis has become common in patients on cancer chemotherapy or steroids. The first symptoms of the invasive form of aspergillosis are usually like acute pulmonary infection, with fever, cough, dyspnea, mild hemoptysis, and pleuritic pain. The chest roentgenogram may show rapidly cavitating infiltrates in any of the lung fields; because the fungus frequently grows intravascularly, the picture may resemble pulmonary embolus with a wedge-shaped area of infarction. Dissemination to the central nervous system, heart, liver, and skin can occur.

Diagnosis

Morphology and Laboratory Identification. The diagnosis of invasive infection often depends on the histopathologic demonstration of the organism in infected tissue. *Aspergillus* organisms grow in tissue as thick (5–8 μm) septate hyphae, which have an acute angle of branching. They may be evident in hematoxylin and eosin-stained sections but are easier to see in silver-stained sections if the density of organisms is low.

The organisms are not fastidious, but a positive sputum culture does not indicate invasive infection and a negative culture does not preclude it. A positive culture of a bronchial plug from an asthmatic patient strongly suggests bronchopulmonary aspergillosis. A positive culture from a metastatic site is diagnostic. The results of blood cultures are almost uniformly negative, even in cases of endocarditis.

Skin Test and Serology. Skin tests are of minimal use only in allergic bronchopulmonary aspergillosis—a wheal and flare reaction is elicited in asthmatics with or without the syndrome.

Serum precipitins are found in 70 to 90 percent of the patients with allergic bronchopulmonary aspergillosis, and are also found in 15 to 20 percent of asthmatics without it.[51] Precipitating antibodies, to one or more *Aspergillus* antigens, are always found in patients with aspergilloma but rarely in patients with invasive aspergillosis.

An increase in total IgE level (>1500 ng per ml) is often present in bronchopulmonary aspergillosis and other types of allergic asthma, but a high level of IgE (>15,000 ng per ml) strongly suggests infection. High levels of specific IgE and IgG antibodies directed against aspergillosis, as measured by radioimmunoassay, are diagnostic.[51]

Surgical Importance

Invasive sino-orbital disease often requires aggressive debridement in combination with amphotericin B therapy.

Significant hemoptysis is an indication for resection of a cavity with a fungus ball, if the underlying pulmonary disease is not too severe. Resection is curative, and amphotericin B is not required.[52,53] An operation is not indicated in an asymptomatic patient.

Although the diagnosis of invasive pulmonary aspergillosis can sometimes be made by transbronchial biopsy, an open biopsy of the lung may be needed for diagnosis. Aspiration or open biopsy of distant metastatic sites of infection may be required to establish the diagnosis in other instances.

Aspergillus endocarditis may present with occlusion of a major artery by a bulky embolus (eg, with a cold pulseless extremity) and thus may mimic other surgical conditions. Endocarditis can occur on prosthetic valves as an early postoperative infection.

Ordinarily, operation is not used for either diagnosis or management of allergic bronchopulmonary aspergillosis.

Treatment

Invasive sino-orbital disease is treated with excision of the infected tissue. Concomitant amphotericin B may be of some value, but the drug probably does not have to be continued after the wound is healed.

Aspergillomas seldom require resection; most require no treatment.[52,53]

Amphotericin B is the only effective treatment of invasive pulmonary or widely disseminated aspergillosis.[54,55] When aggressive diagnostic methods have been used so that amphotericin B is started early, cure is possible. Glucocorticoid therapy, preferably on an alternate-day schedule, can be used successfully to treat allergic bronchopulmonary aspergillosis.[56]

MUCORMYCOSIS

Mucormycosis, a term used synonymously with phycomycosis and zygomycosis, refers to infection by any of several genera of fungi, including *Mucor, Rhizopus,* and *Absidia.* These organisms are ubiquitous in nature and lack any ability to invade a healthy person. Under special circumstances, these organisms invade the nose, sinuses, and other facial structures of ketoacidotic diabetics, the lungs of leukemics or transplant patients, or the necrotic body surface of burned patients.[57-59]

Etiology

Mucor, Rhizopus, and *Absidia* are the three genera of the family Mucoraceae which tend to cause human disease. All grow rapidly at 37C as fluffy white mycelia and will grow on all routine culture media without cyclohexamide. The hyphae are thick (average diameter 10–15 μm) and nonseptate. Side branches are rare and often arise at right angles to their parent hyphae. Determination of the genus is done morphologically; speciation is extremely difficult. These fungi are found throughout the world and are associated with almost all decaying organic material.

Progressive facial infection in diabetics is caused by members of the genus *Rhizopus,* most commonly *R. arrhizus* or *R. oryzae.*

Pathogenesis and Pathology

Everyone is regularly exposed to airborne spores of these fungi, which settle on the skin or are inhaled. However, there is no tendency for invasion, except in the specialized settings of diabetic ketoacidosis, severe immunosuppression (especially hematologic malignancy), or severe burns. The histopathology of infected tissue reveals many polymorphonuclear cells and much necrosis. The organism tends to directly invade arteries, which causes infarction of tissue, adding to the area of necrosis. There is little granuloma formation.

Clinical Manifestations

Rhinocerebral Mucormycosis. The most fulminant fungal infection of man is rhinocerebral mucormycosis. Diabetic ketoacidosis provides a unique opportunity for *Rhiozpus* species, which grow best at acid pH in a high-glucose environment.[57] Hyperglycemia also inhibits the function of phagocytic cells. Rarely, patients with metabolic acidosis of other etiologies, or severely immunosuppressed patients, are infected.

Infection begins in the nose with a dark, blood-tinged discharge from both nostrils. Necrosis of the nasal septum and the turbinates occurs, with rapid spread to the paranasal sinuses. Ulceration and necrosis of the palate, periorbital cellulitis, direct invasion of the orbit, eye, and brain can follow. Major arterial thrombosis adds to the extent of tissue destruction. Early focal neurologic findings include cranial nerve palsies. These are soon followed by generalized seizures and a deteriorating level of consciousness. The entire process usually culminates in death within 1 week.

Leukocytosis is often observed, but fever may not be prominent. Roentgenograms of the sinuses reveal opacification and air fluid levels. Biopsy of the tissue usually shows only suppuration and necrosis; the organisms may be difficult to find in the biopsy sections. Organisms can often be cultured from infected tissue, but the clinical picture should be diagnostic.

Pulmonary Mucormycosis. Pulmonary mucormycosis begins as acute pneumonia, with superimposed signs of pulmonary infarction. Fever, cough, and dyspnea are often accompanied by hemoptysis and pleuritic pain. The most characteristic roentgenographic finding is a wedge-shaped area of infiltration, which may cavitate. Most patients have had lymphoma or acute leukemia, but many cases also have been reported in transplant patients.[58,59] The disseminated disease most often presents as pulmonary disease with metastatic brain abscesses; liver, spleen, pancreas, kidney, and skin (ecthyma gangrenosum) may be involved.

Cutaneous Mucormycosis. Isolation of organisms from skin or wounds does not imply infection, although both local and invasive soft tissue infection has occurred.[60] Contaminated elastoplast has been implicated as a source of infection.[61] Patients with extensive burns can develop a rapidly fatal invasive infection.

Gastrointestinal Mucormycosis. Gastrointestinal mucormycosis is a rare condition that is associated with severe protein malnutrition, especially in children. The organisms invade the bowel wall and eventually cause hemorrhage, bowel infarction, peritonitis, and death. Most cases have been discovered only at autopsy.

Diagnosis

Morphology and Laboratory Identification. The diagnosis depends on the histologic demonstration of the broad nonseptate hyphae found in diseased tissue. Unlike other fungi, they are stained better in routine hematoxylin and eosin sections than in sections stained with silver methenamine or other special stains.

Positive cultures must be interpreted cautiously because the organisms are ubiquitous and can occasionally be recovered from the skin, sputum, and throat of healthy people.

Skin Test and Serology. Skin or serologic tests are of no value in diagnosis.

Surgical Importance

Aggressive debridement of all necrotic tissue is an integral part of the management of rhinocerebral mucormycosis. It is often necessary to examine lung tissue to establish the diagnosis of pulmonary mucormycosis. The choice between transbronchial biopsy via a fiberoptic bronchoscope and open lung biopsy depends on the clinical situation.

Cutaneous mucormycosis is of particular importance in severely burned patients. Initial control of bacterial infection may be followed by invasive fungal disease.

Mucormycosis can also occur in any necrotic tissue. Because the fungus readily grows on elastoplast, it should not be applied directly to any wound, especially where tissue damage has occurred.

Treatment

Rhinocerebral mucormycosis has an 80 percent mortality. Successful therapy must include control of ketoacidosis, debridement of necrotic tissue, and use of amphotericin B.

Pulmonary mucormycosis is also usually fatal, although therapy, including amphotericin B and resection of necrotic lung tissue during a diagnostic thoracotomy, has been reported.

CANDIDIASIS

Candidiasis refers to infection by any species of the genus *Candida*. *Candida* organisms are part of the normal bowel flora of man and are also constant inhabitants of the mouth, pharynx, and upper airways. A wide variety of clinical illnesses can be caused by these organisms, including mucocutaneous, peritoneal, and other invasive infections with septicemia and seeding of kidney, meninges, heart, joints, and other distant sites.[62,63] Invasive infections occur only in patients with altered local or systemic immunity.

Etiology

Clinical candidiasis is most frequently caused by *C. albicans*. Other *Candida* species including *C. parapsilosis*, *C. tropicalis*, *C. stellatoidea*, *C. guilliermondii*, and *C. krusei* can also be involved in human infections.

C. albicans is a normal inhabitant of the gastrointestinal tract of humans, living in balance with the bacterial flora. It is also found in the mouth and upper airway, and in moist intertriginous skin. It is not found in soil. Other *Candida* species are normal inhabitants of the skin and mucous membranes. *Candida* organisms grow rapidly at room temperature on Sabouraud and other routine media, appearing within 24 to 48 hours as white, pasty, smooth colonies. The organisms grow in tissue with a characteristic mixture of yeast forms, pseudohyphae formed by elongated buds, and true hyphae.

Pathogenesis and Pathology

Although *Candida* organisms ordinarily live in equilibrium with their host and do not cause disease, a variety of local or systemic factors can alter that harmony. The absence of competing bacterial flora permits local overgrowth of *Candida* in the oral cavity of infants, resulting in thrush. Alteration of vaginal flora by pregnancy, diabetes, or broad-spectrum antibiotics may lead to vaginal candidiasis. Moist macerated skin in intertriginous areas is especially subject to *Candida* overgrowth, resulting in candidal dermatitis.

Invasive candidiasis is the most important clinical form of the disease. Recognized predisposing factors include malnutrition, broad-spectrum antibiotics, systemic steroids, hyperalimentation, indwelling catheters, and immunosuppression. Invasion of the bloodstream can be transient and self-limited or can result in seeding of distant organs, establishment of multiple microabscesses, and death from progressive infection.

The organism normally grows on body surfaces as a yeast. When an overgrowth of yeast occurs in a given area, there is an associated acute inflammatory reaction. When tissue invasion occurs, mycelial growth begins and both yeast and hyphae can be seen. In recently established microabscesses, yeast forms predominate and there is a polymorphonuclear response similar to that of bacterial organisms spread hematogenously. In chronic intestinal ulcerations or more established metastatic foci of infection, mycelial forms predominate and there may be some granulomatous response.

Clinical Manifestations

Cutaneous Candidiasis. Cutaneous candidiasis involves the moist intertriginous areas of the groin, intramammary and gluteal folds, axillae, interdigital spaces, and adjacent areas of skin. Paronychial infection and chronic infection of the nails afflicts those whose hands require frequent immersion. The lesions are generally moist, erythematous, and pruritic, with satellite vesicles surrounding the sharp margins.

Mucocutaneous Candidiasis. Thrush consists of oral mucosal patches of a white exudate composed entirely of *Candida* yeast and hyphae. The mucosa underneath is red and oozing, and may become ulcerated. Oral candidiasis occurs in people with diabetes, in asthmatics who are treated with inhalational steroids, and in patients being treated with systemic steroids, broad-spectrum antibiotics, and antineoplastic drugs (who are at risk of developing invasive disease).

Candida esophagitis may occur as a direct extension of oral candidiasis; patients usually complain of dysphagia. The diagnosis can be confirmed by esophagoscopy or sometimes by barium swallow, which shows a ragged mucosa but no loss of esophageal distensibility.

Diabetes and antibiotic therapy also predispose to vaginal candidiasis, as do pregnancy and the postmenopausal state. The mucosa is red and covered with patches of whitish exudate. Pustular lesions and ulcerations occur in severe cases. Pruritis may be severe, and there is a white to yellow vaginal discharge.

Candida organisms are part of the bronchial flora in all chronic lung conditions including chronic bronchitis and bronchiectasis and are thought to contribute to chronic productive cough in some instances. *Candida* yeast rarely causes severe pneumonia.[64]

Chronic mucocutaneous candidiasis is a distinct clinical syndrome with widespread superficial infection of nails, skin, and mucous membranes.[65] It occurs primarily in children with immunodeficiency diseases or polyendocrine deficiences.

Invasive Candidiasis. Overgrowth of candida organisms in the mouth, esophagus, bowel, bladder, or on the skin can result in deep penetration into the tissue and intermittent seeding of organisms into the bloodstream.[66] Indwelling plastic intravenous catheters, especially when used for hyperalimentation, may permit direct seeding.

Transient fungemia with *Candida* is probably of little significance in a normal host. However, the same patients who have overgrowth on mucosal surfaces or who require long-term intravenous therapy often have serious underlying diseases and are being treated with antibiotics, steroids, and immunosuppressive agents. In these patients, hematogenous spread of *Candida* organisms may result in the establishment of multiple microabscesses in multiple organs. About half of these patients have an underlying lymphoma or leukemia.[67] The clinical picture includes fever, chills, and renal failure. Macronodular skin lesions and endopthalmitis may be clues to the diagnosis. Seventy-five percent of these patients die despite therapy.

Patients with the septicemic form of candidiasis often have multiple cerebral microabscesses. Other patients may develop meningitis after an episode of candidemia. Any neurologic signs in patients at risk for systemic invasive candidiasis should be investigated to rule out infection of their central nervous system with *Candida.*

Candida endocarditis occurs among drug addicts, on the damaged valves of patients with previous bacterial endocarditis, or on long-term antibiotic therapy, and as an early postoperative infection on prosthetic valves. Vegetations are large and bulky, and embolic events often involve major arteries. Patients with *Candida* septicemia generally develop numerous cardiac microabscesses rather than endocarditis.

Intra-abdominal *Candida* infections may be a complication of peritoneal dialysis or of secondary bacterial peritonitis treated with broad-spectrum antibiotics.[68,68a] The prognosis is good with relatively low doses of amphotericin B, but only if the perforation is recognized, surgically sealed, and chemotherapy promptly instituted. If the culture report of *Candida* is overlooked in the polymicrobial infection, lethal candidiasis can result.[68a]

Diagnosis

Morphology and Laboratory Identification. The definitive diagnosis probably requires histopathologic confirmation of tissue invasion. The distinctive feature is the combination of yeast, pseudohyphae, and hyphae in the tissues. Organisms are readily visualized in hematoxylin and eosin and Gomori methenamine silver-stained sections.

This organism is relatively easy to culture. *C. albicans* can be distinguished from other yeast by its ability to sprout mycelium after incubation in serum for 2 hours. Further speciation is based on mycelial morphology and biochemical tests.

While cultural identification is easy, assessing the significance of a positive culture is extraordinarily difficult. *Candida* organisms are regularly found in stool, sputum, mouth, throat, bronchial washings, the urine of patients with indwelling catheters—all without implying disease. Positive blood cultures most often indicate invasive disease, except when fungemia associated with an intravenous catheter disappears after removal of the device. *Candida* cultures from wounds and drain sites sometimes forecast deep tissue infections, and should not be ignored.

Skin Test and Serology. *Candida* organisms are part of our normal flora; therefore, a positive skin test, or serologic evidence of an antibody response to the organism, has little meaning.

Surgical Importance

Invasive candidiasis is an important opportunistic infection and occurs in debilitated patients who are receiving hyperalimentation. It is especially common among patients who have had multiple abdominal operations and long courses of broad-spectrum antibiotics.[68,68a]

Candida peritonitis is of obvious surgical importance. In the absence of peritoneal dialysis, it implies a breach in the integrity of the gastrointestinal tract.

Candida endocarditis occurs on prosthetic valves in the early postoperative period or on previously damaged valves.

Therapy

Oral candidiasis can be treated with oral nystatin. *Candida* esophagitis can also be treated with oral nystatin, but if there is no response after 48 hours, the infection should be treated with intravenous amphotericin B in doses of 0.25–0.5 kg per day for 2 weeks. Vaginal or skin infections can be controlled with local nystatin. *Candida* in the bladder can be treated by discontinuance of catheter drainage; when this cannot be done, irrigation with a solution of 50 mg of amphotericin B in one-liter solution of 5 percent glucose may be helpful.

Meningitis requires the use of amphotericin B. Endocarditis usually requires a combination of amphotericin B and operative removal of the valve. If there is clear-cut evidence of invasive candidiasis including hematogenous skin lesions, endophthalmitis, or multiple positive blood cultures, full treatment with amphotericin B is necessary. In systemic candidiasis, a combination of flucytosine and amphotericin B may be helpful, although this has not been well documented.[24]

Prevention

Candida seems to be an infection of endogenous origin which benefits from changes in ecologic balance between host defenses and competitive bacteria. Traditionally, one is advised to prevent candidiasis by avoidance of radiation, immunosuppression, antibiotics, indwelling catheters, and radical surgery. Sometimes these agents are necessary. Oral nystatin in high doses appears to be useful in reducing the numbers of *Candida* in the intestine and can reduce the incidence of fungemia in various populations of immunodepressed patients. Oral ketoconazole may prove to be useful in preventing *Candida* colonization.[68b]

FUNGAL DISEASES ACQUIRED BY SUBCUTANEOUS INOCULATION

SPOROTRICHOSIS

Sporotrichosis refers to any infection by the thermal dimorphic fungus *S. schenckii.* Suppuration, ulceration, and a slow proximal lymphatic spread follow subcutaneous inoculation of spores. A rare pulmonary form is caused by inhalation of the spores.

Etiology

Sporothrix schenckii is a thermal dimorphic fungus. At 25C it grows as a mycelium of delicate hyphae whose side branches are capped by clusters of small oval spores arranged like the petals of a flower. At 37C the organism grows as a yeast, in which form it infects mammalian tissue.

Epidemiology

S. schenckii is distributed worldwide in association with decaying vegetation, most notably rotting wood, sphagnum moss, and rich humus soil.

Pathogenesis and Pathology

The organism grows at the site of inoculation and spreads proximally along the lymphatic system. The skin overlying the nodules may reveal pseudoepitheliod proliferation. The nodules themselves have a mixed granulomatous and suppurative reaction similar to that seen in blastomycosis. Unlike the situation in blastomycosis, however, the causative organisms are extremely sparse and are usually not seen in histopathologic sections, even with special stains.

The asteroid body, although not common, is considered characteristic of sporotrichosis when it is seen. It consists of an oval basophilic material. Asteroid bodies are felt to represent specific immune proteins associated with the yeast in the tissues.

Clinical Manifestations

Cutaneous and Lymphatic Sporotrichosis. Cutaneous and lymphatic sporotrichosis is an occupational disease of gardeners and others who are commonly traumatized by contaminated thorns, branches, and wood splinters. Epidemics among underground miners and forestry workers were caused by contaminated support timbers and sphagnum moss, respectively.[69,70]

A minor puncture wound, usually on the hand or foot, directly introduces the spores into the subcutaneous tissues. A small nodule develops, grows slowly, and attaches to the overlying skin as it becomes partially necrotic. Superficial ulceration (the sporotrichotic chancre) usually follows the initial inoculation by 2 to 3 weeks. Additional subcutaneous nodules develop along the draining lymphatics in the succeeding weeks. Each nodule becomes thick and indurated and attaches to the overlying skin as it grows—each may eventually ulcerate (Chapter 25).

The course of the infection varies, often with periods of activity followed by regression. Eventually, spontaneous resolution may occur, especially in patients with fixed cutaneous sporotrichosis, with only a primary lesion. There is no tendency for spread along lymphatics, possibly because of some degree of previously acquired immunity to the fungus. Patients with lymphocutaneous sporotrichosis do not have fever or other constitutional symptoms and generally have little disability.

Pulmonary Sporotrichosis. Inhalation of these spores occasionally results in a chronic pulmonary infection similar to other inhalational fungal infections.[71,72] Nodular infiltrates, often with cavitation, most commonly involve the apices but also occur in other parts of the lung. Symptoms may include productive cough and dyspnea. Weight loss is common as the disease progresses.

Disseminated Sporotrichosis. Dissemination is rare in sporotrichosis. Immunosuppression and protein malnutrition are possible predisposing factors to dissemination. Eighty percent of the cases involve bone or joints, although any organ can be affected.[73]

Diagnosis

Morphology and Laboratory Identification. Histopathologic specimens only rarely demonstrate the yeast, which are 3–5 μm in size and oval in shape. Although the clinical diagnosis of the lymphocutaneous form is easy, definitive diagnosis of all forms depends on culture of the organism. Material aspirated from nodules along lymphatics, joints, or bony lesions should be cultured on Sabouraud agar and blood agar at 25C. Colonies appear as brown to black mycelia within several days.

Skin Test and Serology. Sporotrichin is a skin test antigen that is not usually used in the diagnosis of individual cases, although it is useful in epidemiologic studies.

Available serologic tests include agglutination, immunodiffusion, and complement fixation tests. High titers of agglutinating or complement-fixing antibody suggest an infection (the complement-fixation test is the least sensitive).[74]

Surgical Importance

If the lymphocutaneous form of sporotrichosis is suspected, a biopsy of one of the nodules should not be taken. The yeast is seldom found histopathologically, and the increased tendency for spread after a biopsy is too great. The lesion should be aspirated for a culture.

Resection of chronically infected lung tissue has been part of the management of many successfully treated cases of pulmonary sporotrichosis.

Therapy

The lymphocutaneous form of the disease should be treated with a saturated solution of potassium iodide in doses of up to 10 drops three times a day for at least 4 weeks after the visible lesions have healed.

Treatment of pulmonary sporotrichosis or disseminated sporotrichosis is more controversial. Most authorities recommend a total dose of amphotericin B of 2.5–3 gm; however, some cases of pulmonary sporotrichosis have responded to potassium iodide. There are no controlled studies of the various forms of therapy. Many of the successfully treated cases have combined amphotericin B, potassium iodide, and resection of the chronically infected lung.

MYCETOMA

Mycetoma (maduromycosis) is the result of subcutaneous inoculation of some fungal spores. The resulting reaction produces swelling, multiple abscesses, and sinus tracts with purulent drainage that contains granules or grains.

Etiology

Mycetoma is caused by a wide variety of soil organisms including many true fungi (eumycotic mycetoma) and also several species of *Actinomyces* (actinomycotic mycetoma) (Chapter 25).

Epidemiology

Mycetoma is primarily a tropical disease of India, Central Africa, and Mexico. *Allescheria boydii* is the most commonly reported agent in the southern United States. Mycetoma is initiated by the direct inoculation of spores into subcutaneous tissues. It is most common in rural areas among malnourished persons who go shoeless. Although mycetoma occurs most commonly on the foot (madura foot), it may also occur on the hand, the buttocks, and other areas.

Pathogenesis and Pathology

Purulent abscesses develop which burrow deeply into the involved tissue, invading soft tissue, fascia, and bone. Extensive fibrosis develops, and sinus tracts communicate between individual abscesses and also drain to the surface. Histopathologic examination shows multiple abscesses, which contain many neutrophils and occasional granules made up of the organisms themselves, the morphologic characteristics of which permit etiologic diagnosis. The tissue surrounding the abscesses contains granulomatous elements and much fibrosis.

Clinical Manifestations

The primary lesion is a small, painless, subcutaneous swelling, which slowly enlarges in a tumorlike fashion. Progression is slow, but eventually the swelling will suppurate and drain to the surface. When the lesion is on the foot, the entire foot eventually becomes swollen and studded with multiple sinus tracts. The pus expressed from the orifices of the sinus tracts reveals the small granules which may be up to 5 mm in size. Eventually, the arch of the foot is lost and the sole becomes convex (Fig. 25-27).

Mycetoma usually remains localized to an extremity. There are no constitutional symptoms nor even regional adenopathy. Extensive involvement, while it does not impair general health, can be disfiguring and disabling.

Diagnosis

Demonstration of granules permits a general diagnosis of mycetoma in a patient with a localized area of multiple abscesses and draining sinuses. Experienced laboratories can identify the organism from the morphology of the granule; however, culture may be necessary to identify the exact agent. Of particular importance is the differentiation of actinomycotic from eumycotic mycetoma, because the former may respond to antibiotics.

A deep biopsy sample is best for culture because superficial material is often contaminated by multiple bacteria and fungi. Granules obtained from such a biopsy are washed, crushed, and plated at 25C aerobically, and at 37C both aerobically and anaerobically.

Skin test and serology are not useful in the diagnosis of mycetoma.

Surgical Importance

Early cases of actinomycotic mycetoma can sometimes be cured with limited drainage and antibiotics. Because mycetoma can remain a localized process for a long time, a conservative approach is generally taken. Amputation is necessary for some advanced cases.

Therapy

Actinomycotic mycetoma may respond to penicillin or tetracycline. Eumycotic mycetoma is resistant to chemotherapy because the infection invades deep into the soft tissues and bone. Local excision is rarely helpful, even in early cases. Ketoconazole may prove to be a useful adjunct.[68b]

Actinomycosis and nocardiosis are diseases of higher bacteria which resemble fungal infections, and can cause infections that are identical to mycetoma (Chapters 6 and 7).

BIBLIOGRAPHY

Emmons CW, Binford CH, Utz JP: Medical Mycology, 3rd ed. Philadelphia, Lea & Febiger, 1977.

Mandell GL, Douglas RG Jr, Bennett JE (eds): Mycoses, Section F (Part III). In Principles and Practice of Infectious Diseases. New York, John Wiley & Sons, 1979, pp. 1979–2084.

Medoff G, Kobayashi GS: Strategies in the treatment of systemic fungal infections. N Engl J Med 302:145, 1980.

Odds FC: Candida and Candidosis. Baltimore, University Park Press, 1979.

Rippon JW: Medical Mycology: The Pathogenic Fungi and the Pathogenic Actinomycetes. Philadelphia, Saunders, 1974.

REFERENCES

1. Conant NF, Smith DT, Baker RD, Callaway JD: Manual of Clinical Mycology. Philadelphia, Saunders, 1971.
2. Emmons CW, Binford CH, Utz JP: Medical Mycology, 3rd ed. Philadelphia, Lea & Febiger, 1977.
3. Rippon JW: Medical Mycology: The Pathogenic Fungi and the Pathogenic Actinomycetes. Philadelphia, Saunders, 1974.
4. Codish SD, Tobias JS, Monaco AP: Recent advances in the treatment of systemic mycotic infections. Surg Gynecol Obstet 148:435, 1979.

HISTOPLASMOSIS

5. Howard DH: Intracellular growth of *Histoplasma capsulatum.* J Bacteriol 89:518, 1965.
6. Goodwin RA Jr, Des Prez RM: State of the art: histoplasmosis. Am Rev Respir Dis 117:929, 1978.
7. Howard DH, Otto V, Guptka RK: Lymphocyte-mediated cellular immunity in histoplasmosis. Infect Imm 4:605, 1971.
8. Goodwin RA Jr, Des Prez RM: Pathogenesis and clinical spectrum of histoplasmosis. S Med J 66:13, 1973.
9. Goodwin RA Jr, Owens FT, Snell JD, Hubbard WW, Buchanan RD, Terry RT, Des Prez RM: Chronic pulmonary histoplasmosis. Medicine 55:413, 1976.
10. Sarosi GA, Voth DW, Dahl BA, Doto IL, Tosh FE: Disseminated histoplasmosis: results of long-term follow-up. A Center for Disease Control cooperative mycoses study. Ann Intern Med 75:511, 1971.
11. Davies SF, Khan M, Sarosi GA: Disseminated histoplasmosis in immunologically suppressed patients. Occurrence in a nonendemic area. Am J Med 64:94, 1978.
12. Smith JW, Utz JP: Progressive disseminated histoplasmosis: a prospective study of 26 patients. Ann Intern Med 76:557, 1972.
13. Dukes RJ, Grimlan CV, Dines DE, Payne S, MacCarty RL: Esophageal involvement with mediastinal granuloma. JAMA 236:2313, 1976.
14. Strimlan CV, Dines DE, Payne WS: Mediastinal granuloma. Mayo Clin Proc 50:702, 1975.
15. Parker JD, Sarosi GA, Doto IL, Bailey RE, Tosh FE: Treatment of chronic pulmonary histoplasmosis. N Engl J Med 283:225, 1970.
16. Naylor BA: Low-dose amphotericin B therapy for acute pulmonary histoplasmosis. Chest 71:404, 1977.

BLASTOMYCOSIS

17. Laskey W, Sarosi GA: Endogenous activation in blastomycosis. Ann Intern Med 88:50, 1978.
18. Sarosi GA, Hammerman KJ, Tosh FE, Kronenberg RC: Clinical features of acute pulmonary blastomycosis. N Engl J Med 290:540, 1974.
19. Laskey W, Sarosi GA: The radiological appearance of pulmonary blastomycosis. Radiol 126:351, 1978.
20. Witorsch P, Utz JP: North American blastomycosis: a study of 40 patients. Medicine 47:169, 1968.
21. Poe RH, Vassallo CL, Plessinger VA, Witt RL: Pulmonary blastomycosis versus carcinoma—a challenging differential. Am J Med Sci 263:145, 1972.
22. Bissada NK, Finkbeiner AE, Redman JF: Prostatic mycosis: nonsurgical diagnosis and management. Urology 9:327, 1977.
23. Craig MW, Davey WN, Green RA: Conjungal blastomycosis. Am Rev Respir Dis 102:86, 1970.
24. Medoff G, Kobayashi GS: Strategies in the treatment of systemic fungal infections. N Engl J Med 302:145, 1980.

COCCIDIOIDOMYCOSIS

25. Drutz DJ, Catanzaro A: Coccidioidomycosis. Part I. Am Rev Respir Dis 117:559, 1978.
26. Drutz DJ, Catanzaro A: Coccidioidomycosis. Part II. Am Rev Respir Dis 117:727, 1978.
27. Lonky SA, Cantazaro A, Moser KM, Einstein H: Acute coccidioidal pleural effusion. Am Rev Respir Dis 114:681, 1976.
28. Winn WA: A long-term study of 300 patients with cavitary-abscess lesions of the lung of coccidioidal origin. An analytical study with special reference to treatment. Dis Chest 54:Suppl 1:268, 1968.
29. Sarosi GA, Parker JD, Doto IL, Tosh FE: Chronic pulmonary coccidioidomycosis. N Engl J Med 283:325, 1970.
30. Bayer AS, Yoshikawa TT, Galpin JE, Guze LB: Unusual syndromes of coccidioidomycosis: diagnostic and therapeutic considerations; a report of 10 cases and review of the English literature. Medicine 55:131, 1976.
31. Deresinski SC, Stevens DA: Coccidioidomycosis in compromised hosts. Medicine 54:377, 1974.
32. Rutala PJ, Smith JW: Coccidioidomycosis in potentially compromised hosts: the effect of immunosuppressive therapy in dissemination. Am J Med Sci 275:283, 1978.
33. Ellner JJ, Bennett JE: Chronic meningitis. Med 55:341, 1976.
34. Smith CE, Saito MT, Beard RR, Hepp RM, Clark RW, Eddie BU: Serological tests in the diagnosis and prognosis of coccidioidomycosis. Am J Hyg 52:1, 1950.
35. Diamond RD, Bennett JE: A subcutaneous reservoir for intrathecal therapy of fungal meningitis. N Engl J Med 288:186, 1973.
36. Graybill JR, Ellenbog C: Complications with the Ommaya reservoir in patients with granulomatous meningitis. J Neurosurg 38:477, 1973.
37. Stevens D: Miconazole in the treatment of systemic fungal infections. Am Rev Respir Dis 116:801, 1977.

PARACOCCIDIOIDOMYCOSIS

38. Pan-American Health Organization 1972: First Pan-American Symposium on paracoccidioidomycosis. Medellin, Colombia 25–27 October 1971. Scientific Publication No 2540. Washington, DC, World Health Organization.
39. Restrepo A, Robledo M, Giraldo R, Hernandez H, Sierra F, Gutierrea F, Londono F, Lopez R, Calle G: The gamut of paracoccidioidomycosis. Am J Med 61:33, 1976.
40. Restrepo AM, Robledo MV, Ospina SC, Restrepo MA, Correa AL: Distribution of paracoccidioides sensitivity in Colombia. Am J Trop Med Hyg 17:25, 1968.
41. Stevens DA, Restrespo AM, Cortes A, Betancourt J, Galgiani JN, Gomez I: Paracoccidioidomycosis (South American blastomycosis): treatment with miconazole. Am J Trop Med Hyg 27:801, 1978.

CRYPTOCOCCOSIS

42. Berger MP, Paz J: Diagnosis of cryptococcal meningitis. JAMA 236:2517, 1976.
43. Diamond RD, Bennett JE: Prognostic factors in cryptococcal meningitis. A study in 111 cases. Ann Intern Med 80:176, 1974.
44. Goodman JS, Kaufman L, Koenig MG: Diagnosis of cryptococcal meningitis. Value of immunologic detection of cryptococcal antigen. N Engl J Med 285:434, 1971.
45. Kaplan MH, Rosen PP, Armstrong D: Cryptococcosis in a cancer hospital: clinical and pathological correlates in 46 patients. Cancer 39:2265, 1977.
46. Khan MA, Sbar S: Cryptococcal meningitis in steroid treated systemic lupus erythematosis. Postgrad Med J 51:660, 1975.
47. Schroter GPJ, Temple DR, Husberg BS, Weil R III, Starzl TE: Cryptococcosis after renal transplantation: report of ten cases. Surgery 79:268, 1976.
48. Utz JP, Garriques IL, Sande MA, Warner JF, Mandell GL, McGehee RF, Duma RJ, Thadomy S: Therapy of cryptococcosis with a combination of flucytosine and amphotericin B. J Infect Dis 132:368, 1975.

ASPERGILLOSIS

49. Young RC, Bennett JE, Vogel CL, Carbone PP, De Vita VT: Aspergillosis: the spectrum of the disease in 98 patients. Medicine 49:147, 1970.
50. British Tuberculosis Association: Aspergillus in persistent lung cavities after tuberculosis. Tubercle (London) 49:1, 1968.
51. Wang JL, Patterson R, Rosenberg M, Roberts M, Cooper BJ: Serum IgE and IgG antibody activity against *Aspergillus fumigatus* as a diagnostic aid in allergic bronchopulmonary aspergillosis. Am Rev Respir Dis 117:917, 1978.
52. British Tuberculosis Association: Aspergilloma and residual tuberculosis cavities—the results of a resurvey. Tubercle (London) 51:227, 1970.
53. Varkey B, Rose HD: Pulmonary aspergilloma: a rational approach to treatment. Am J Med 61:626, 1976.
54. Aisner J, Wiernik PH, Schimpff SC: Treatment of invasive aspergillosis: relation of early diagnosis and treatment to response. Ann Intern Med 86:539, 1977.
55. Hammerman KJ, Sarosi GA, Tosh FE: Amphotericin B in the treatment of saprophytic forms of pulmonary aspergillosis. Am Rev Respir Dis 109:57, 1974.
56. Rosenberg M, Patterson R, Roberts M, Wang J: The assessment of immunologic and clinical changes occurring during corticosteroid therapy for allergic bronchopulmonary aspergillosis. Am J Med 64:599, 1978.

PHYCOMYCOSIS

57. Abramson E, Wilson D, Arby RA: Rhinocerebral phycomycosis in association with diabetic ketoacidosis. Report of two cases and a review of clinical and experimental experience with amphotericin B therapy. Ann Intern Med 66:735, 1967.
58. Hammer GS, Bottone EJ, Hirschman SZ: Mucormycosis in a transplant recipient. Am J Clin Pathol 64:389, 1975.
59. Meyer RD, Rosen P, Armstrong D: Phycomycosis complicating leukemia and lymphoma. Ann Intern Med 77:871, 1972.
60. Jain JK, Maokowitz A, Kjilanani PV, Lauter CB: Localized mucormycosis following intramuscular corticosteroid. Case report and review of the literature. Am J Med Sci 275:209, 1978.
61. Gartenberg G, Bottone EJ, Keusch GT, Weitzman I: Hospital-acquired mucormycosis *(Rhizopus rhiaopodiformis)* of skin and subcutaneous tissue: epidemiology, mycology, and treatment. N Engl J Med 299:1115, 1978.

CANDIDIAL INFECTIONS

62. Edwards JE Jr, Lehrer RI, Stiehm ER, Fischer TJ, Young LS: Severe candidal infections: clinical perspective, immune defense mechanisms, and current concepts of therapy. Ann Intern Med 89:91, 1978.
63. Murray HW, Fialk MA, Roberts RB: Candida arthritis: a manifestation of disseminated candidiasis. Am J Med 60:587, 1976.
64. Masur H, Rosen PP, Armstrong D: Pulmonary disease caused by *Candida* species. Am J Med 63:914, 1977.

65. Kirkpatrick CH, Smith TK: Chronic mucocutaneous candidiasis: immunologic and antibiotic therapy. Ann Intern Med 80:310, 1974.
66. Gaines JD, Remington JS: Disseminated candidiasis in the surgical patient. Surgery 72:730, 1972.
67. Bodey GP: Fungal infections complicating acute leukemia. J Chronic Dis 19:667, 1966.
68. Bayer AS, Blumenkrantz MJ, Montgomerie JZ, Galpin JE, Coburn JW, Guze LB: Candida peritonitis. Report of 22 cases and review of the English literature. Am J Med 61:832, 1976.
68a. Solomkin JS, Flohr AB, Quie PG, Simmons RL: The role of *Candida* in intraperitoneal infections. Surgery 88:524, 1980.
68b. Restrepo A, Stevens DA, Utz JP (eds): First International Symposium on Ketoconazole. Rev Infect Dis 2:519, 1980.

SPOROTRICHOSIS

69. DuToit, CJ: Sporotrichosis on the Witwaterstrand. Proc Mine Med Off Assoc 22:111, 1942.
70. Powell KE, Taylor A, Phillips BJ, Blakey DL, Campbell GD, Kaufman L, Kaplan W: Cutaneous sporotrichosis in forestry workers. Epidemic due to contaminated *Sphagnum* moss. JAMA 240:232, 1978.
71. Jay SJ, Platt MR, Reynolds RC: Primary pulmonary sporotrichosis. Am Rev Respir Dis 115:1051, 1977.
72. Mohr JA, Patterson CD, Eaton BG, Rhoades ER, Nichols NB: Primary pulmonary sporotrichosis. Am Rev Respir Dis 106:260, 1972.
73. Wilson DE, Mann JJ, Bennett JE, Utz JP: Clinical features of extracutaneous sporotrichosis. Medicine 46:265, 1967.
74. Karlin JV, Nielson HS Jr: Serological aspects of sporotrichosis. J Infect Dis 121:316, 1970.

CHAPTER 10
Viruses

STEPHEN C. MARKER and RICHARD J. HOWARD

GENERAL PROPERTIES OF VIRUSES

ANATOMY

Viruses are a unique class of infectious agents, ubiquitous in nature, which infect all types of plants and animals. They were originally distinguished by their extremely small size and because they are obligate intracellular parasites, although some small bacteria share these features. Animal viruses range in diameter from 18 nm to 230 x 300 nm. Their essential size and structure are discussed in Chapter 2. The distinctive nature of viruses lies in their rather simple composition and organization and their mode of replication. A complete virus particle or virion may be simply regarded as genetic material surrounded by a coat that protects the internal genetic information from the environment and functions as a vehicle for transmission from one host to another.

The genetic material of viruses is either DNA or RNA, never both. Viruses differ from bacteria, plants, and animals in that they lack the machinery for independent metabolism; they must use the metabolic machinery of the host cells and hence are obligate intracellular parasites.

REPLICATION

Replication of viruses involves a series of ordered sequential steps: (1) Adsorption of the virus onto the cell membrane. For enveloped viruses, such as the herpesviruses, the outer membrane of the virus appears to fuse with the cell membrane. (2) Penetration of the virus into the cell. Penetration can occur by pinocytosis or by fusion of the viral and cell membranes, leaving the nucleocapsid inside the cell. (3) Uncoating—removal of the viral protein coat by host enzymes, leaving the bare nucleic acid. (4) Reproduction of viral RNA usually occurs in the cytoplasm, whereas reproduction of viral DNA occurs in the nucleus. (5) Synthesis of the proteins of the viral coat or capsid occurs in the cytoplasm. The viral DNA or RNA has the necessary information for the protein coat, and messenger RNA (mRNA) is synthesized (transcribed) from the viral DNA or RNA. Alternatively, viral RNA may actually be mRNA. (6) The proteins of the viral coat (capsid) are assembled in the nucleus of DNA viruses and in the cytoplasm for RNA viruses, and the nucleic acid is inserted into the empty capsid, forming the mature nucleocapsid. The mature virus then leaves the cell when the cell lyses, or it may acquire a host membrane coat as it buds from the surface of the cell (Fig. 10-1). When a cell lyses, it literally bursts apart, releasing thousands of virus particles at once. Lysis always results in the death of the cell; budding viruses may be released over a prolonged period, and the cell does not necessarily die. For DNA viruses, the viral DNA must be transcribed into mRNA, which is then translated on host ribosomes in the cytoplasm.

CLASSIFICATION OF VIRUSES

Unlike bacteria, which are classified according to their chemical and physical properties, viruses are divided into two groups according to the type of nucleic acid—RNA or DNA (Fig. 10-2). They are further divided according to the symmetry of their capsid and subdivided by whether the nucleocapsid is naked or surrounded by a membrane envelope. Enveloped viruses are sensitive to ether and other organic solvents because lipids in the membrane are dissolved by the solvent and the virus can no longer adsorb onto the host cell. Viruses are further divided according to size. Viruses grouped according to these criteria generally have similar antigenic determinants, growth characteristics, and host range.

PRINCIPLES OF DIAGNOSIS OF VIRAL INFECTIONS

The techniques available for the direct and indirect identification of viruses include: (1) viral isolation, (2) measurement of antiviral antibodies during the course of an infection, (3) histologic examination of infected tissues, (4) detection of viral antigens in lesions, and (5) electron microscopic examination of fluids and tissue extracts for virus. Evidence of a virus, found by any of these techniques, does not prove that it is the etiologic agent for a given disease. Some viruses, such as the herpesvirus, may persist in human hosts for long periods, and some, such as the enteroviruses, may be isolated from asymptomatic people. In patients with clinical illness, these viruses may be innocent bystanders.

Specimens must be handled properly to ensure the greatest likelihood of viral identification (Chapter 12). The normal procedures of most operating rooms are geared for bacterial isolation only, and special arrangements must be made by the surgeon. Specimens for isolation should

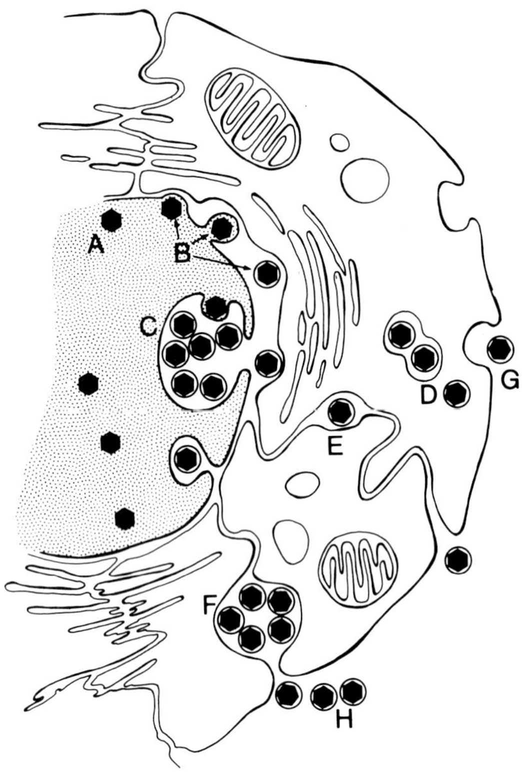

Fig. 10-1. **Envelopment and release of herpesvirus. Replication of viral DNA occurs in the nucleus. Viral proteins are synthesized in the cytoplasm and transported to the nucleus, where assembly takes place. Virus approaches the nuclear membrane (A), which thickens and progressively envelops the nucleocapsid (B). The viral envelope pinches off, leaving the nuclear membrane intact and the enveloped virus free in the perinuclear cisterna. The nucleocapsid can also acquire an envelope by budding into nuclear vacuoles (B). These vacuoles appear to be indentations of the nuclear membrane and are continuous with the perinuclear cisterna (C). The enveloped virus then is transported through the cytoplasm in vacuoles (D), which fuse with the surface membrane to release the virus to the extracellular space (G). Alternatively, the virus reaches the cell surface by traversing the cisternae of the endoplasmic reticulum (E,F) to the cell surface (H). (Reproduced, with permission, from Jawetz E, Melnick JL, Adelberg EA:** ***A Review of Medical Microbiology,*** **13th ed. Los Altos, Calif., Lange Medical Publications, 1978.)**

be promptly inoculated into the appropriate cell line. Alternatively, they may be stored at refrigerator temperature (4C). The virologist should be told that viruses are suspected, so that appropriate cell lines may be inoculated.

For detection of viral antigens in tissues by immunofluorescence, small pieces of tissue must be immediately snap-frozen in liquid nitrogen. This technique requires having liquid nitrogen in the operating room or nearby so that no time is lost in freezing the tissue. For electron microscopy, the tissue specimen must be placed into a proper fixative such as glutaraldehyde, which is not commonly available in the operating room unless special arrangements have been made.

VIRUS ISOLATION AND IDENTIFICATION

The isolation of virus requires proper collection of specimens, transportation to the laboratory, and inoculation into animals or appropriate cell lines. Bacteria must be removed from potentially contaminated material by addition of antibiotics, filtration, or centrifugation.

Tissue culture methods are most widely used for virus identification. Many cell lines (ie, human, monkey, hamster) are used, since some viruses replicate on some cell lines and may not grow at all on others. Virus identification depends on the effects produced in tissue culture. Viruses may cause histologic alterations of the host cells called cytopathic effects, ie, lysis of cells, rounding of cells, multinucleated cells (Fig. 10-3). Some viruses (eg, rubella) produce no direct cytopathic effect but can be detected by their interference with the cytopathic effect of a second challenge virus (viral interference). Other viruses (myxoviruses) cause changes in the cell membrane so red cells will stick to the cell surface (hemadsorption). The identity of an isolated virus can be confirmed by using specific antisera, which inhibit viral growth.

Animal inoculation is frequently used to isolate neurotropic viruses causing encephalitis. Infant mice are inoculated intracerebrally. If the mouse dies and if bacteria are not cultured from the brain, the death is presumably due to a virus. Virus isolated from the mouse brain can be identified by specific antisera, which neutralize the virus and prevent death of a subsequently inoculated infant mouse.

HISTOLOGIC EXAMINATION OF TISSUE

Histologic examination of biopsy and autopsy tissues may reveal cellular inclusion bodies typical of viral infection (Fig. 10-4). DNA viruses usually produce intranuclear inclusions surrounded by a clear halo. With RNA viruses, inclusion bodies are seen in the cytoplasm where RNA viruses replicate. Some viruses (eg, measles) produce both intranuclear and intracytoplasmic inclusions. Inclusion bodies are believed to be either masses of closely packed virus particles that can be seen by electron microscopy to mature within the inclusion body or a remnant of earlier virus replication. Inclusion bodies may be of considerable diagnostic aid. For instance, the Negri body is an intracytoplasmic inclusion in nerve cells that is pathognomonic for rabies (Fig. 10-4).

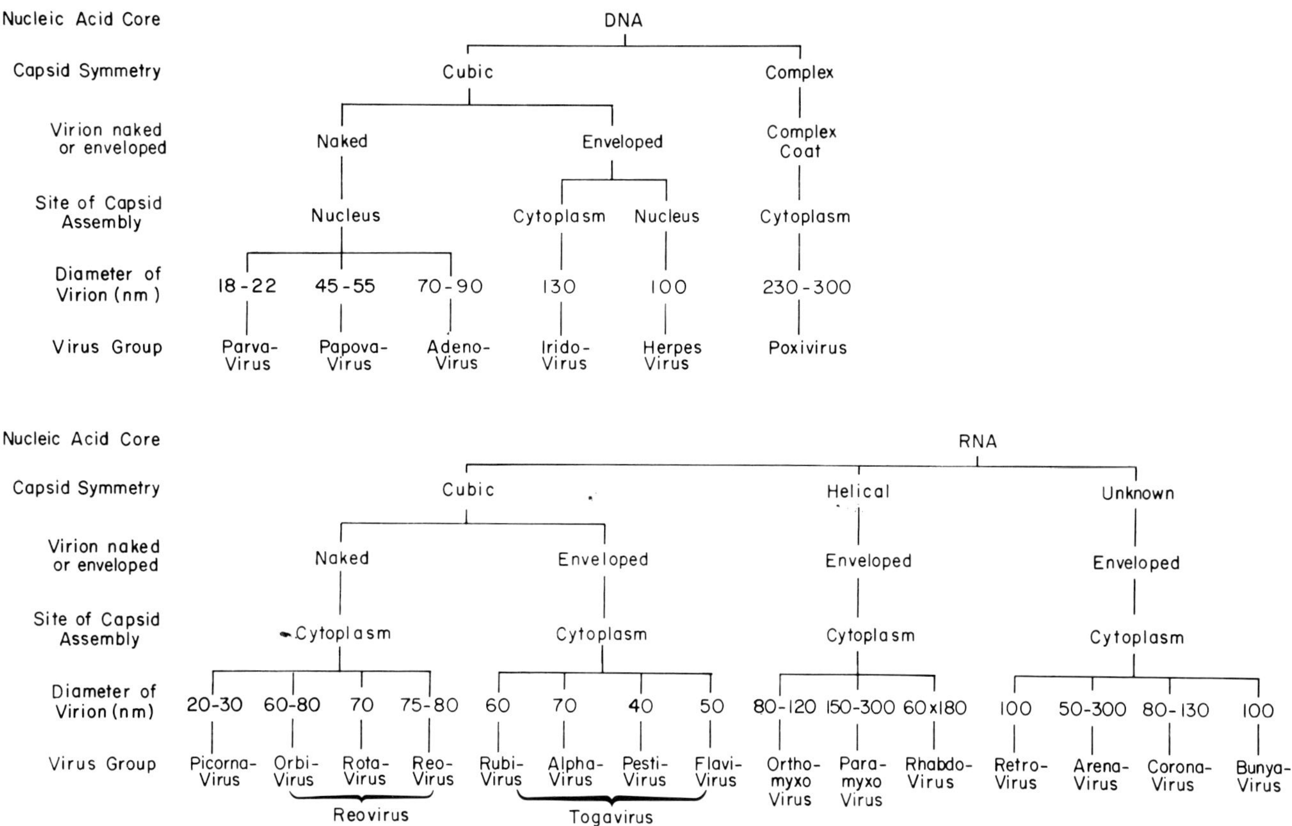

Fig. 10-2. **Classification of viruses. Viruses are divided into two groups according to their nucleic acid, DNA or RNA. They are subdivided according to the symmetry of their nucleocapsid and whether or not the nucleocapsid is surrounded by an outer membrane (envelope).**

ELECTRON MICROSCOPIC EXAMINATION

Typical virus particles can be seen by electron microscopy in body fluids, tissues, and tissue extracts. They are observed more easily in body fluids and tissue extracts after concentration of virus by ultracentrifugation, evaporation, or ultrafiltration. Only after concentration by ultracentrifugation was hepatitis B virus observed in urine specimens of patients with serum hepatitis. Electron microscopic examination permits diagnosis within a matter of hours in patients with vesicular lesions such as those produced by the poxviruses or herpesviruses. Myxoviruses (influenza) can be identified just as rapidly in respiratory secretions.

DETECTION OF VIRAL ANTIGENS IN TISSUES

Viral antigens can be detected in biopsy and autopsy specimens by reacting frozen sections with flourescein-labeled antiviral antibody (direct immunofluorescence) and examining the specimen for fluorescence under ultraviolet light. Because formalin fixation can destroy viral antigens, fresh frozen (preferably in liquid nitrogen) specimens must be used. Alternatively, antiviral antibody can be applied to the frozen tissue section followed by a fluorescein-labeled antigammaglobulin (indirect immunofluorescence). The specimen is then examined for fluorescence under ultraviolet light.

SEROLOGIC DIAGNOSIS

Several procedures are available for detection of serum antibody against virus (Table 10-1). The neutralization test is generally not used for routine laboratory testing, because other tests (complement fixing, hemagglutination inhibition) are much easier to perform and require less time.

Two or more serum samples taken several days or weeks apart are required to establish proof of an active viral infection, since a rising titer to the virus must be demonstrated. Antibody to a virus detected in a single serum sample only means that the individual has been infected with that virus at some time, past or present.

HOW VIRUSES CAUSE DISEASE

Viruses cause disease through a variety of mechanisms. A given virus can cause more than one illness. For instance, varicella-zoster virus can cause zoster, chicken pox, and encephalitis. Measles virus can cause measles or the slow virus infection, subacute sclerosing panencephalitis. The disease depends on the status of the host (age, immune competence) as well as the virus (inoculum, route of infection).

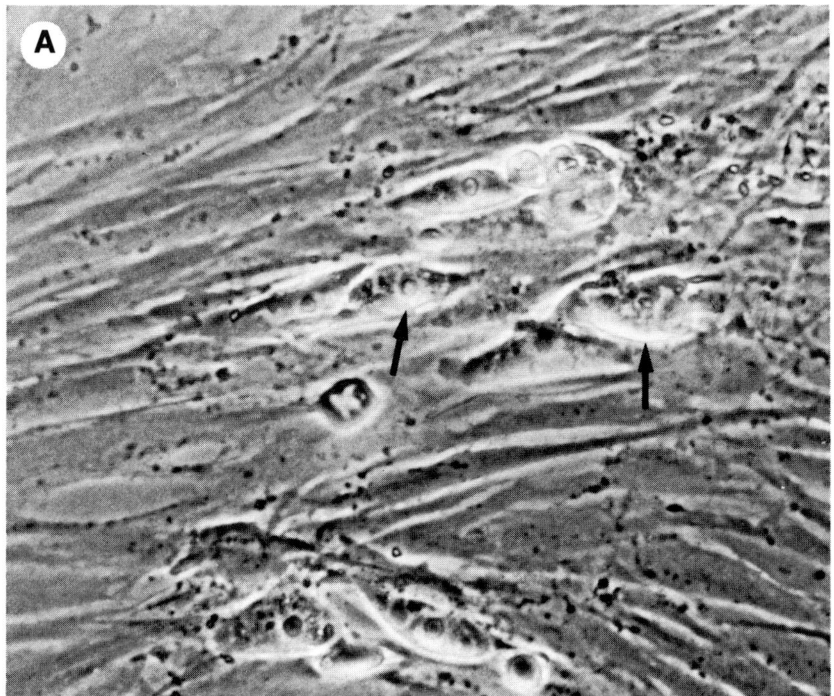

Fig. 10-3. Cytopathic effects produced by herpesviruses. A. Cytomegalovirus-infected fibroblasts. Infected cells are enlarged and rounded (arrows), (×80). B. Rhesus monkey kidney cells infected with *Herpesvirus hominis.* The infected cells are rounded. Several cells have died and have lifted off the flask, leaving clear spaces where a confluent monolayer had been (×80). C. Plaques produced by poliovirus *(left)* and by an echovirus *(right).* (After Hsuing and Melnick) (Reproduced, with permission, from Jawetz E, Melnick JL, Adelberg EA: *Review of Medical Microbiology,* 13th ed. Los Altos, Calif., Lange Medical Publications, 1978.)

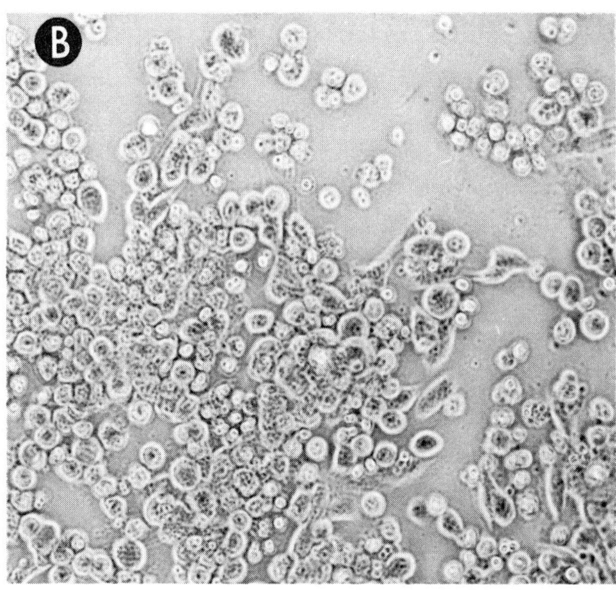

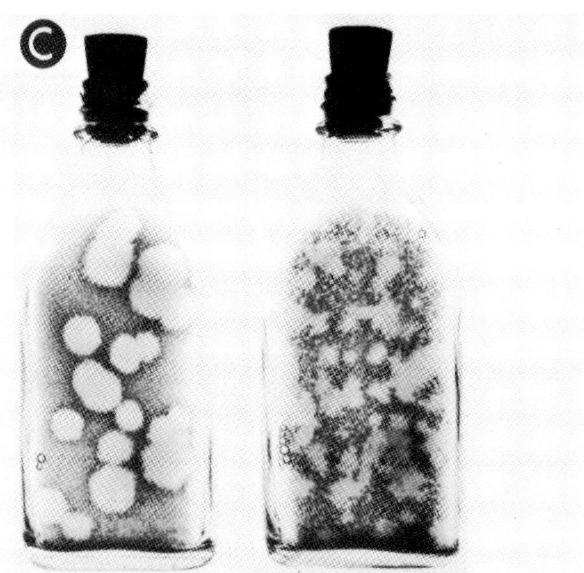

Cell Lysis

When the replication of nonbudding viruses is completed, cells may lyse to release new virions. This lysis results in cell death. Death of a sufficient number of cells in an organ can cause such severe organ dysfunction that the host dies.

Altered Cell Function

During cellular infection, various metabolic processes may be altered to replicate virus. Thus, cell DNA and RNA synthesis may cease or be altered, with cessation of production of cellular proteins. This interference by virus with normal cell machinery can alter cell function and even cause death. For example, influenza and cytomegalovirus infect polymorphonuclear leukocytes and macrophages and inhibit their phagocytic ability. This decreased phagocytic ability renders the infected host more susceptible to bacterial invasion, with the result that death of the host may actually be due to bacterial superinfection.

Congenital Malformations

Several viruses are known or are suspected to cause congenital malformations in humans and experimental animals. The embryo or fetus may be infected by transplacental transfer from the mother. Congenital defects

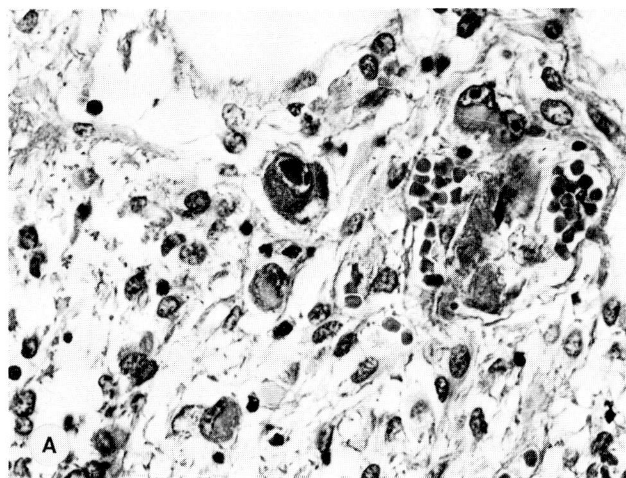

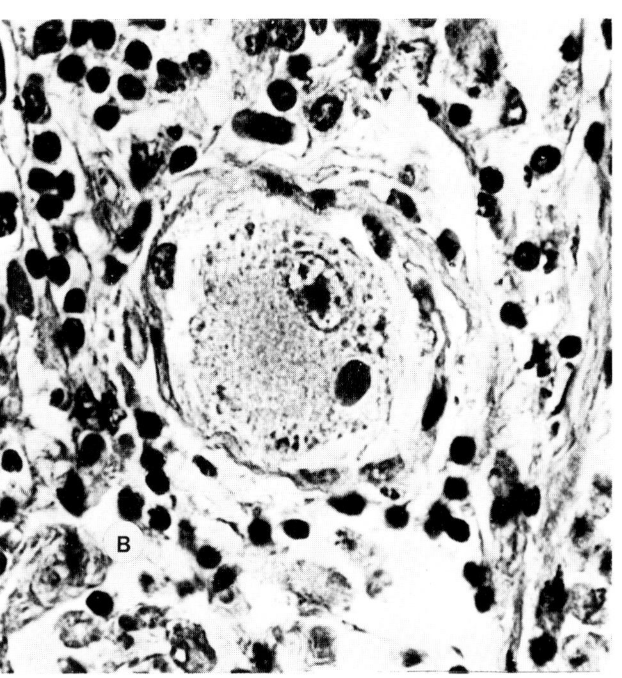

Fig. 10-4. A. Intranuclear inclusions in glial cells infected with cytomegalovirus. The eosinophilic intranuclear inclusion is surrounded by a clear halo (×435). B. Cytoplasmic inclusion (Negri body) in ganglion cell infected with rabies virus (×696). (Courtesy of Dr JH Sung, Dept. of Neuropathology, University of Minnesota.)

TABLE 10-1. SEROLOGIC TESTS FOR DIAGNOSIS OF VIRAL INFECTIONS

Test	Basis of Test
Complement-fixation	Virus–antibody complexes bind complement, making it unavailable for lysis of sheep red blood cells, which have been sensitized by addition of anti-sheep red blood cell antibody
Neutralization	Addition of specific antibody to virus neutralizes its infectivity for animals or for cells in tissue culture
Hemagglutination-inhibition	Some viruses can agglutinate red blood cells. Addition of antiviral antibody to the virus prevents them from agglutinating erythrocytes
Precipitation	Antiviral antibody and virus results in a solid precipitate. In the immunodiffusion or counterelectrophoresis system, the precipitation takes place in agar, forming a visible line
Immunofluorescence	Antiviral antibody will react with viral antigen in tissue culture cells in which the virus is growing. If rabbit antihuman gammaglobulin labeled with fluorescein isothiocyanate is added to the cells, they will fluoresce under ultraviolet light. They will not fluoresce if antiviral antibody was not present in the test serum
Radioimmunoassay	A radioactive antigen forms antigen–antibody complexes, which can be separated from the uncomplexed antigen. The quantity of uncomplexed antigen then is detected by the amount of radioactivity it emits. The presence of antibody reduces the amount of radioactivity in the unbound fraction.

Used with permission from: Howard RJ, Balfour HH Jr, Simmons RL: The Surgical Significance of Viruses. *Curr Probl Surg* 14:1, 1977.

usually occur with exposure to the teratogen during the early period of fetal development. Most viruses causing congenital malformations affect the nervous system, but some (eg, rubella) cause defects that require operative correction (eg, cardiac defects).

Chromosome Damage

Chromosome damage such as breakage, fragmentation, and rearrangement can be caused by viral infection. Abnormal chromosomes and changes in chromosome number have also been reported. Several viruses (measles, rubella, herpesvirus, influenza, mumps, adenoviruses) have been demonstrated to cause chromosomal injury. For most viruses, such injury is observed only in infection of primary cell cultures. Chromosome breaks during natural infection have been observed in peripheral blood leukocytes of patients with measles and chickenpox. Chromosome damage may be important in the cause of congenital malformations by viruses.

Altered Immune Function

Some viruses cause an alteration of immune function of the host, including changes in serum gammaglobulin concentrations, increased and decreased humoral and cell-mediated immunity, and increased and decreased phagocytic capacity of polymorphonuclear leukocytes and macrophages. Many human viruses, such as cytomegalovirus, rubella, and measles, produce these variations in immune capacity. Decreased immune function can lead to increased susceptibility to bacterial and fungal superinfection.

Immune Response to the Virus as a Cause of Disease

Although the immune response to infectious agents such as viruses usually serves to rid the host of the infection, such immune responses paradoxically can lead to disease. Circulating virus can persist until the host mounts an immune response against it. The resultant antibody binds the virus, and these virus–antibody complexes are filtered out by the reticuloendothelial system. Some circulating virus–antibody complexes are not removed from the blood but remain in the circulation for the life of the host. These complexes can attach to basement membranes, notably in the renal glomeruli and small arterioles. Here, they activate the complement system, leading to an inflammatory response. Virus–antibody complexes can cause glomerulonephritis (lymphocytic choriomeningitis virus and lactic dehydrogenase virus in mice) and arteritis (Aleutian mink disease). Proof of the participation of virus–antibody complex in the pathogenesis of disease exists most convincingly in experimental animals, but hepatitis has been reported to cause immune complex glomerulonephritis in people. The dengue shock syndrome is also probably caused by virus-antibody complexes; it occurs only in people with antibody to dengue virus.

Increased Cell Proliferation and Oncogenesis

Another mechanism whereby viruses can cause disease is cellular proliferation—controlled or uncontrolled. Controlled cellular proliferation occurs in lymphatic tissue during infection with Epstein-Barr virus (the etiologic agent of infectious mononucleosis) and other viruses. This enlarged lymphoid tissue may cause surgical illness by blocking the lumen of hollow viscera (causing appendicitis) or may serve as the lead point in intussusception. Benign proliferation of virus-infected duct epithelial cells may be a cause of congenital biliary atresia.

Viruses may also cause tumors through the induction of uncontrolled cellular proliferation. Viruses cause a variety of tumors in animals and have been strongly implicated in a number of human tumors as well. The best evidence for the viral etiology of human cancer exists in the cases of nasopharyngeal carcinoma and Burkitt lymphoma, both of which are believed to be due to Epstein-Barr virus. Virally produced tumors may not all be malignant; for example, human warts are caused by a virus.

Difficulties arise in studying oncogenic viruses, since some animal and human viruses may cause in vitro malignant cell transformation only in cells from species other than the one naturally infected by the virus. Cell transformation is a term referring to in vitro cell cultures in which the cells take on properties akin to tumors, ie, uncontrolled growth, lack of contact inhibition, increased rate of multiplication, chromosomal abnormalities, lack of uniform cell size and shape. Yet viruses that cause in vitro cell transformation may not cause any tumors in intact animals. Conversely, some viruses that cause tumors in vivo do not cause in vitro cell transformation.

The process whereby viruses cause cell transformation and tumors involves changes found in the early stages of other viral infections, such as adsorption, penetration, and uncoating. However, the DNA or RNA is not replicated. Instead, viral DNA is physically integrated into cellular DNA. The integrated viral DNA (provirus) is replicated along with cellular DNA during cell division. The viral nucleic acid of oncogenic RNA viruses cannot be incorporated into host DNA. Instead, an RNA-directed DNA polymerase (reverse transcriptase) intrinsic to the virion allows DNA to be synthesized using the viral RNA as a template. This DNA is then integrated into the cellular DNA and replicated during cell division.

PATTERNS OF VIRAL INFECTIONS

Viruses can cause at least three different patterns of infection—acute, persistent, and slow. Some viruses can cause more than one type of infection under appropriate conditions (Fig. 10-5).

Acute Infections

Viruses can cause three basic patterns of acute infection—localized, disseminated, and inapparent.

Localized Infection

In a localized infection, virus remains localized near the site of entry—skin, respiratory tract, or gastrointestinal tract. Virus may spread to neighboring cells by diffusion and cell-to-cell contact, forming a single lesion or group of lesions, such as warts. At no time does it enter the bloodstream. The common cold and viral gastroenteritis can be regarded as localized infections.

Disseminated Infection

For many viral illnesses, the virus usually undergoes multiplication at its site of entry. Progeny viruses then enter the blood and lymphatics and are disseminated throughout the body. The virus then may reach the target organ (eg, the skin in exanthematous diseases) or it may undergo a

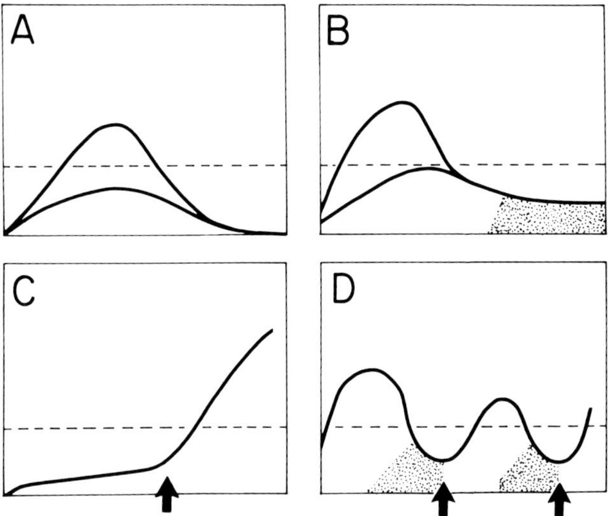

Fig. 10-5. **Patterns of viral infections. Dashed line—threshold of apparent infection (clinical disease). Solid line—course of disease. Stippled area—presence of occult virus. Arrows—activation of virus in original host. A. Acute viral infection with acute clinical course followed by long-lasting immunity (measles, poliovirus). Some acute viral infections may not become clinically evident but may still lead to long-lasting immunity (polio). B. Viral infections can also be clinical or subclinical. Virus may persist after the illness, or there may be a long latent infection during which virus is present in small quantity (adenoviruses, influenza). C. Viral infection can be latent for long periods before it is activated. These "slow" viral infections are characterized by kuru and cancer viruses. D. Viruses can be reactivated periodically, giving rise to clinical disease. In between clinical manifestations, the virus is latent as in fever blisters *(Herpesvirus hominis)* and zoster or "shingles" (varicella-zoster). (Drawn with permission from Jawetz E, Melnick JL, Adelberg EA: *A Review of Medical Microbiology,* 13th ed. Los Altos, Calif., Lange Medical Publications, 1978.**

further multiplication. A secondary viremia then takes place, and the virus goes to a target organ and produces clinical disease. Usually, clinical signs and symptoms of illness begin only after the virus is disseminated and has attained maximal titers in the blood. Measles and rubella are examples of this type of acute infection.

Inapparent Infection

Transient viral infection can occur without causing clinical illness. People with inapparent infections represent an unrecognized source of viral spread throughout a population. Inapparent infections also confer immunity on the host and represent an important source of "natural" immunity. Examples of inapparent infection include anicteric viral hepatitis and poliomyelitis. Before the use of the polio vaccine, there were an estimated 100 inapparent infections for every paralytic case of poliomyelitis.

Persistent Infections (Latent Infections)

In persistent viral infections, clinical disease does not occur, or occurs infrequently. An equilibrium is achieved between virus and host in different ways, depending on the virus and host. Since virus replication occurs within cells, it is unavailable to the host's protective immune response until it leaves the cell. Thus, persistence can continue as long as the virus does not destroy the cell or interfere with its essential cellular functions. Under these circumstances, cells can continue to replicate virus. Persistence may also occur if the viral genome is incorporated into and replicates along with the cellular genome, or if replication of separate viral genomes occurs without viral maturation. The viral genome persists in the host cell, but it is not entirely transcribed and no virus is produced. Oncogenic (tumor-producing) viruses exist in the cell in this manner.

The herpesviruses are the best known persistent human viruses that can be reactivated by different stimuli. Herpes simplex virus is reactivated by stimuli such as heat (fever blisters), actinic radiation, and stress. Cytomegalovirus, a member of the herpesvirus family, is reactivated by immune reactions, immunosuppressive drugs such as those used to prevent transplant rejection, and cancer chemotherapeutic agents. Varicella-zoster, which causes zoster, is latent in the dorsal root ganglia. When appropriately stimulated, it migrates along the dorsal nerve to the skin epithelial cells, where it proliferates and causes the vesicular lesions typical of zoster.

Slow Infections

Slow viral infections involve those viruses that require prolonged periods—up to several years—before disease becomes clinically apparent. Virus multiplication is not necessarily slow, but the disease develops over a prolonged period. In people, these are all neurologic illnesses.

VIRAL INFECTIONS AS THE CAUSE OF SURGICAL ILLNESS

ACUTE CONDITIONS

Viruses are alleged to either cause or participate in the pathogenesis of several illnesses that may require operative treatment. Some of these diseases are listed in Table 10-2, but evidence is scanty. This problem has been reviewed in detail by Howard, Balfour, and Simmons.[1]

Proving that a surgical illness is caused by a virus can be difficult. The most obvious method is to culture the virus from the patient—especially from the affected tissues. However, live virus may no longer be available for culture by the time operation or autopsy is performed. It may already have been eliminated or subsequent overgrowth by bacteria may make detection impossible. Neither culture nor histologic evidence of tissue infection is proof that the virus caused the actual illness, since it may have found the diseased tissue a fertile soil in which to replicate. Similarly, viruses cultured from other tissues (secretions, urine, or feces) may not be related to the disease being studied but may be innocent passengers. Some viruses may even be present in the individual in a latent form and be reactivated by the surgical illness rather than cause it.

Epidemiologic studies can provide evidence of a correlation between virus infection and a disease process, but they do not prove causation. Carefully performed epidemi-

TABLE 10-2. SURGICAL DISEASES IN WHICH A VIRAL PATHOGENESIS HAS BEEN PROPOSED

Disease	Virus
Appendicitis	Enterovirus Adenovirus Coxsackie B Hepatitis Other or unspecified
Mesenteric adenitis	Adenovirus Unspecified Measles
Ileocecal intussusception	Adenovirus Other
Pancreatitis	Mumps Hepatitis Cytomegalovirus Other
Gastrointestinal ulcers	Cytomegalovirus
Regional enteritis	Unidentified RNA virus
Ulcerative colitis	Cytomegalovirus
Constrictive pericarditis	Coxsackie B

ologic studies are undoubtedly one of the best methods of establishing viruses as the cause of surgical illness. Few carefully performed epidemiologic studies of viral disease have been carried out. In fact, many of the reports cited in Table 10-2 present only one or a few cases showing some evidence of viral infection, but these isolated reports can indicate where epidemiologic studies should focus.

One reason that epidemiologic investigations must be relied on is that Koch's postulates are not easy to fulfill for viral infections. Some viruses (hepatitis virus A and B) have not been successfully grown in tissue culture. Many viruses causing disease in humans do not produce illness in common laboratory animals. Finally, attempting to produce the original illness in humans by inoculating the original virus is obviously unacceptable.

CONGENITAL MALFORMATIONS

A variety of agents may be important in the etiology of congenital malformations, including drugs, chemicals, infections, radiation, and genetic factors. Maternal age and maternal disease are important also. From studies on viral teratogenesis in experimental animals, it has been determined that: (1) Defects occur only in the presence of a fully infective virus. (2) Defects result from the death of cells in primordial tissues or from the inhibition of growth of specific tissues. For example, it is known that rubella and cytomegalovirus inhibit the division of cells in tissue culture and cause chromosome breaks. (3) If embryos are inoculated after a critical stage of development, the defect no longer occurs. For a defect to arise in a certain organ system, the viral infection must be present at the time the organ system is actively undergoing differentiation and development. (4) Each virus produces a different range of host defects. This may be due to different viral receptor sites on developing cells. (5) The likelihood of a defect developing during embryonic viral infections is proportional to the size of the virus inoculum.[2]

Whether a viral infection of a pregnant female or the developing fetus results in a congenital defect depends on a number of factors: (1) the maternal immune status, (2) the particular virus, (3) the strain of the virus, (4) the maternal-fetal host susceptibility, and (5) the developmental stage of the fetus. Virus may gain access to the developing embryo transplacentally following maternal infection or via an ascending infection through the vagina. The lack of fetal immune response may allow proliferation of the virus in the developing fetus for a prolonged period without challenge from the host.

Proving that a virus is a teratogen in humans can be difficult. Retrospective studies depending on a maternal history of illness or postpartum serologic correlation are unreliable.[3] Prospective studies are more reliable but more difficult. For valid studies, accurate recordings of illness, culture data from the mother, and determination of serial antibody levels to detect subclinical infections during the early months of pregnancy must be obtained. Since major embryonic development is essentially complete during the first trimester, these prospective studies must focus their primary attention on this early period. By the time of the first visit to a physician, the viral infection may already have occurred. These studies require the inoculation of specimens into a wide variety of cell lines and a search for antibodies against a battery of viruses. Otherwise, the viruses causing anomalies may not be found. Prolonged follow-up examination of the infant is required, since anomalies may not be recognized at birth. Many viral infections that could possibly produce congenital defects fail to give rise to easily identifiable syndromes or a complex of malformations.

Virus-caused congenital malformations that may require surgical correction later probably represent a minority of anomalies due to viral infections. Most congenital defects due to viral infections affect the central nervous system, producing microcephaly, mental retardation, deafness, and other uncorrectable lesions. Congenital viral infection can also result in infection of the fetus without producing congenital anomalies. Rubella, cytomegalovirus, influenza, coxsackievirus B, and mumps are the main viral causes of congenital malformations.[1]

INFECTIONS FOLLOWING OPEN HEART OPERATION AND BLOOD TRANSFUSION (NOT DUE TO HEPATITIS)

A syndrome that resembles infectious mononucleosis can develop after open heart procedures with extracorporeal perfusion. Variously called the postperfusion syndrome, posttransfusion syndrome, or the postpump syndrome, it is most often characterized by fever, erythematous rash, hepatomegaly, splenomegaly, eosinophilia, and atypical lymphocytes in the peripheral blood. However, the heterophil test is negative.[4,5] Usually the postperfusion syndrome appears within 3 to 5 weeks of operation and is almost always self-limited and not fatal. It may lead to unnecessary hospitalization, however, and to an expensive search for a source of fever. The syndrome is unusual in adults, but as many as 10 percent of children and young adults can be affected. In some centers, this syndrome has been traced to the use of fresh blood for perfusion, and a similar syndrome can be observed in patients who receive transfusions of fresh whole blood even though they do not undergo cardiac operation. Both Epstein-Barr virus and cytomegalovirus have been implicated in the etiology of the posttransfusion and postperfusion syndromes. These syndromes have also been attributed to reexacerbation of rheumatic fever, an autoimmune response to traumatized cardiac tissue, an inflammatory response to blood in the pericardial sac, and a cellular immunologic response to the transfused white blood cells.

The most likely cause of this syndrome is infection with cytomegalovirus. Significant increases in cytomegalovirus antibody titers occur in as many as 3 to 60 percent of patients undergoing open heart operations even though the incidence of clinical postperfusion syndrome is significantly lower. It is estimated that only one in every 10 patients who have postoperative cytomegalovirus develops the postperfusion syndrome.

Still unknown is whether the transfused blood is the source of virus or whether the blood transfusion and trauma of the operative procedures lead to reactivation of endogenous latent virus in the patient. Several studies have implicated the transfused blood as the source of viral infection. Armstrong et al [6] were able to isolate cytomegalovirus for 28 days from whole blood stored at 4C and from fresh frozen plasma for up to 97 days. Thus, fresh whole blood does not necessarily have to be used for live virus to be transfused.

The anticytomegalovirus antibody levels of 187 blood donors for 24 patients undergoing open heart surgery were studied prospectively by Klemola et al.[7] None of the 24 blood recipients had prior detectable antibody to cytomegalovirus, but 14 developed antibody after the operation. There was no significant difference in anticytomegalovirus antibody titers between the donors who gave blood to the 14 patients who had anticytomegalovirus antibody titers after operation and those who donated blood to the 10 patients who did not have postoperative antibody titers. However, all 14 patients who developed evidence of cytomegalovirus infection had received fresh blood from at least three seropositive donors.

A number of similar epidemiologic studies of the postperfusion syndrome have been published.[8,9] Most are consistent with the idea that cytomegalovirus and to a lesser extent Epstein-Barr virus and herpes simplex virus cause disease within the first 2 to 3 postoperative months. The virus itself can sometimes be cultured from the blood or urine, but proof of the infecting agent is most consistently found in change in antibody titer. Seroconversion to one or more viruses most often occurs without illness, but the clinical syndrome is almost always followed by seroconversion after recovery. In contrast, viral infections have only rarely been reported following other operative procedures, such as cancer operations, hysterectomy, and operations for trauma.

The majority of postoperative viral infections appear to be asymptomatic, but the illnesses reported are so nonspecific that the symptoms and signs might well be attributed to a variety of insignificant problems. Most have been detected by seroconversion, and no extensive culture studies have been done. Furthermore, there has been no attempt at an extensive prospective epidemiologic study examining the incidence of viral infections in a variety of surgical procedures, and no careful attempt to correlate minor clinical illness with viral screening has been undertaken. Such a study would give a truer picture of the incidence and significance of viral infections in the postoperative period. In addition, the relative role of exogenous sources of virus and its reactivation from latent endogenous sites might be obtained. One cannot assume that such infections are not of clinical significance, because it is known that certain viruses so impair host defenses that serious and even lethal bacterial infections can supervene. Viral cultures and serologic studies are seldom obtained in patients who develop febrile illness in the postoperative course; however, extensive bacteriologic and fungal studies usually are obtained.

INFECTIONS IN COMPROMISED HOSTS AFTER OPERATION

The clinical problems of opportunistic infections of all types are discussed in Chapter 47. Only a few epidemiologic points need be made here. Members of the herpesvirus family have commonly been isolated from patients with neoplastic disease. Patients with malignancies of hematologic origin are particularly susceptible to infections with the herpesviruses. Cytomegalovirus occurs more commonly in patients with leukemias, whereas varicella-zoster is found more frequently in patients with Hodgkin disease and non-Hodgkin lymphomas. Zoster (manifested clinically as shingles) occurs in 8 to 25 percent of patients with Hodgkin disease and in 97 percent of patients with non-Hodgkin lymphomas.[10,11] The incidence of zoster increases dramatically in patients who have had a splenectomy or receive radiotherapy or chemotherapy.[10-13] Zoster is an important prognostic sign, since it is sometimes a harbinger of recurrent disease.[12] Zoster and cytomegalovirus infections also occur in patients with solid tumors, but less often, and most victims have received radio or chemotherapy.[14]

The occurrence of viral infections in cancer patients is not known to be associated with a poor prognosis except for those patients who have disseminated zoster. It is interesting that viral infections are discovered to be important contributors to complex illnesses only when they are associated with characteristic clinical pictures such as rashes (eg, zoster). Viruses that cause malaise, hepatic malfunction, or fever will easily be missed because the illness will be attributed to the neoplasm, bacterial infection, chemotherapeutic drugs, or other causes. Thorough postmortem examinations are sometimes not performed in patients who die of cancer, and little note may be taken of the nonspecific inflammatory changes induced by viral illnesses. Only when careful systemic epidemiologic studies are carried out will the true importance of viral infections be determined.

Viral Infections Following Transplantation

Immunosuppressive agents are known to increase the susceptibility to viruses. Members of the herpesvirus family have been found most frequently following renal transplantation (Chapter 47). Of the herpesviruses, cytomegalovirus has been reported most frequently. Hill et al [15] and Hedley-Whyte and Craighead [16] were the first to report cytomegalovirus infection in renal allograft recipients, and a series of careful epidemiologic studies has shown an incidence of 70 to 90 percent. Many patients are asymptomatic, but a number of important clinical illnesses are caused by cytomegalovirus (Chapter 47). The source of infection in transplant patients may be different from that of patients having cytomegalovirus after open heart operations. In the latter instance, transfusion of fresh blood is the most likely source of the viral infection, whereas transplant recipients appear to reactivate latent viral infection. The distinction is not entirely clear, however, since transplant recipients also receive many blood transfusions that can harbor the virus. In addition, Ho et al [17] and Betts et al [18] have indicated that the donor kidney may be the source of virus. They showed a higher incidence of infections in the recipients whose living related donors had antibody to cytomegalovirus before transplantation than in those whose donors did not have antibody.

Although most emphasis has been placed on cytomegalovirus by transplant groups, other herpesviruses are clinically important in transplant recipients as well. Cutaneous zoster is common, but it is usually a self-limited illness with mild transient fever (or none at all) and without leukopenia or signs of rejection. Disseminated chickenpox, however, has occurred in several patients never previously exposed to the virus, with an occasional death. A few children have developed mild chickenpox despite a previous episode of the disease. Previously uninfected children should receive zoster immune plasma if they are exposed to chickenpox.

Herpes simplex is common in transplant recipients. It usually appears in the early posttransplant months and is characterized by cold sores or vesicular eruption of the buccal mucosa, pharynx, or genitalia. Herpes esophagitis is associated with dysphagia, and the virus has been cultured from ulcers of the esophagus and ileum.[19] The cold sores can become necrotic and can be slow to heal. Only rare cases of disseminated herpes, herpes encephalitis, and herpes hepatitis have occurred in transplant recipients. Like most viral infections in transplant recipients, antibodies can develop in the absence of clinical illness.

Several groups have recovered Epstein-Barr virus from renal allograft recipients. Virus was not closely associated with clinical illness. However, recent evidence suggests that the Epstein-Barr virus is the etiologic agent in posttransplant lymphoproliferative disorders, including malignant lymphoma.[20,20a]

Viruses have also been implicated in the pathogenesis of complications previously thought to be due to technical error. Coleman et al [21] observed a new papovavirus, designated as the BK virus, by electron microscopy from the urine of five renal transplant recipients and cultured the virus from two of these. Four patients remained healthy, but one had ureteral obstruction. This last patient, and one of five other patients, had ureteral obstruction more than 100 days after transplantation and had viral inclusions in the ureteral endothelium. The virus was not identified, however. Coleman and colleagues also described three recipients of liver homografts who required revision of the cholecystojejunostomy because of cystic duct obstruction. Cytomegalovirus was isolated from the cystic duct in all three instances. Whether it had any role in the etiology of the cystic duct obstruction is not known.

In addition to causing morbidity during the period after transplantation, viral infection may be responsible for chronic active hepatitis, retinitis, and intestinal ulceration many years after apparent successful transplantation.

PREVENTION AND TREATMENT OF VIRAL INFECTIONS

VIRAL VACCINES

Vaccines are preparations of live attentuated, or killed, virus that elicit a protective immune response. Generally, attentuation of virus is accomplished by multiple passages in tissue culture, which permits selection of mutant virus strains whose pathogenicity is lowered. Live viral vaccines have the advantage of eliciting a more vigorous immune response because of some limited multiplication of virus within the host. In addition, live vaccines may be administered orally or intranasally, facilitating an immune response at the natural site of infection. Killed viral vaccines must be administered parenterally but cannot transmit disease. The viral vaccines that have been developed thus far are against acute infections (ie, rubella, smallpox, measles, poliovirus, hepatitis B). Viral vaccines against members of the herpesvirus family, the infections seen most commonly by the surgeon, are in the early stages of development.[21a,21b]

PASSIVE IMMUNIZATION

Passive immunization uses infusions of plasma containing protective antibody or purified immunoglobulin prepared from this plasma. Although passive immunization is effective in the prevention of hepatitis and varicella-zoster, the protection is short-lived because of the normal degradation of gammaglobulin.

CHEMOTHERAPY OF VIRAL INFECTIONS

The chemotherapy of bacterial infection takes advantage of the differences in biochemical make-up and metabolic requirements of bacterial and mammalian cells—the former can be killed or inhibited, and the latter remain unharmed. Until recently, many scientists believed that a safe and effective antiviral agent could not be produced, because viruses use the host cells' own synthetic and metabolic machinery for replication. It has been difficult to find agents that are effective against viral infections and are not highly toxic to the mammalian cells. Recently, however, investigators have identified many differences between the replicative cycle of viruses and of mammalian cells. Some viruses rely on unique enzymes not present in the uninfected cell, and some have nucleotides in their nucleic acid that are not normal components of mammalian nucleic acids. Still, there are few effective and safe antiviral agents available. These are discussed in Chapter 18.

INTERFERON

Interferons are cellular proteins produced in response to viral infections or chemical agents that confer resistance to viral infection. To be effective, cells must be exposed to interferon before infection. This exposure establishes an antiviral state that is mediated by a second protein induced by interferon. This second protein inhibits viral replication by interfering with transcription of the viral genome or the translation of messenger RNA into viral proteins. Although not virus-specific, interferon is species-specific, so that any attempt at using interferon in the prevention or treatment of viral infections requires large-scale production from human cell lines, with a resultant great production cost. Also, the half-life of interferon after injection is short (10 minutes). Experimental studies, however, have shown interferons to be effective in prevention of viral infections in animals, and they may prove useful in the prevention of viral infections in people at high risk. A second possible approach is the use of synthetic agents that can elicit endogenous interferon production. Few clinical trials with interferon have been attempted and the results are equivocal (Chapter 18).

From what is understood of its mechanism of action, interferon should be effective only when given before viral infection. How can it be efficacious in chronic viral infections? With some chronic viral infections, such as chronic hepatitis B virus, new cells must be constantly infected to maintain the production of hepatitis B virus. Protecting these new, previously uninfected cells from viral replication would diminish the amount of virus detected in the serum.

TRANSFER FACTOR

Transfer factor is one of the many humoral agents (lymphokines) derived from lymphocytes of human beings. It can be extracted from lymphocytes in vitro and can transfer immunity from an immune cell to a nonimmune one. It is dialyzable, stable on prolonged storage, and has a molecular weight of less than 10,000. It is inactivated by heat (56C for 30 minutes) but not by trypsin or DNase. Its effects appear to be antigen-specific, ie, it will confer specific immunity to a given antigen to a population of nonimmune cells. Transfer factor transfers cell-mediated but not humoral immunity. The understanding of the chemical nature and mode of action of transfer factor has been hampered because there is no reliable animal model or in vitro assay, so that all testing of purified transfer factor preparations must be done in human volunteers.

Transfer factor is being used clinically to treat patients with infections, malignancies, and immunodeficiency diseases. It has been used to treat patients with chronic hepatitis B and one patient with cytomegalovirus retinitis, but the results are inconsistent.[22-24]

LOWER RESPIRATORY TRACT SYNDROMES

A dozen viruses, representing hundreds of antigenically different strains, provide enough variation for a lifetime of recurrent respiratory illness. Fortunately for diagnostic purposes, a half-dozen viruses account for most of the lower respiratory tract diseases. Frequently, a tentative etiologic diagnosis can be established by knowing the patient's age, the community epidemiology, and the location and severity of respiratory symptoms in the patient.

Influenza, respiratory syncytial virus, parainfluenza, and adenovirus account for the most serious viral lower respiratory tract infections in normal people, whereas cytomegalovirus is the main viral respiratory pathogen in the immunosuppressed patient. Winter epidemics of influenza in adults with febrile illness and myalgia are readily recognized. Winter epidemics of severe respiratory illness, sometimes requiring hospitalization of infants (bronchiolitis), are caused by respiratory syncytial virus. Sporadic pneumonia in adults, associated with conjunctivitis or pharyngitis, may be due to adenovirus. Laryngotracheobronchitis, or croup, which occurs sporadically or as epidemics at any time of the year, may be caused by parainfluenza virus.

INFLUENZA

Etiology and Epidemiology

The structure and replication of the influenza virion provide a basis for understanding the virus epidemiology, serologic tests, and the preparation of vaccines (Fig. 10-6). The hemagglutinin polypeptide is the major specific antigen of the virus envelope and is responsible for the attachment of the virus to cells, and antibody against the hemagglutinin provides protection against infection. Unfortunately, it can undergo dramatic antigenic variations from year to year, accounting for the lack of protective immunity between major epidemic strains of influenza.[25] The four major antigenic types of human influenza hemagglutinin are designated H0, H1, H2, H3, in order of their temporal appearances in 1933, 1947, 1957, and 1968. In 1977, Hsw appeared briefly in a few people in the United States. This hemagglutinin was more closely related to the hemagglutinin of swine influenza than human. Between epidemics there may be minor antigenic changes in the hemagglutinin, but protection against these intrapandemic strains remains substantial.

The neuraminidase polypeptide has undergone antigenic change once since 1933. The two human influenza neuraminidases are designated N1 and N2. The only major change occurred in 1957 with the appearance of the Asian (H2/N2) epidemic. The N1 antigen reappeared in 1976 as the neuraminidase of U.S.S.R. influenza (H1/N1). The

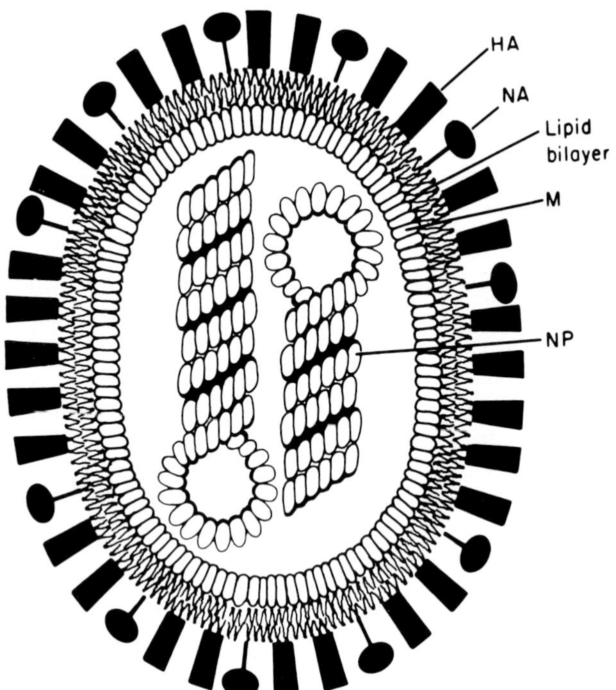

Fig. 10-6. **Structure of influenza virus. Schematic of the influenza virion. This enveloped RNA virus is approximately 100 nm in diameter and contains eight species of polypeptide. The major structural proteins are hemagglutinin (HA), neuraminidase (NA), matrix protein (M), and nucleoprotein (NP).**

protective role of antibody against this protein is still speculative, but antibody may decrease shedding of the virus.[26]

A third virus polypeptide, the nucleoprotein, is antigenically stable and provides a serologic basis for separating the influenza viruses into types A, B, and C. This antigenic classification also corresponds to the distinctive epidemiologic and clinical characteristics of these three viruses.

The segmented RNA genome of the influenza virion permits it to readily exchange genetic material with other influenza virions. This recombination potential and the existence of many influenza strains in birds and animals have led to the speculation that highly selected, recombinant, animal-human strains of influenza virus are the source of new human pandemic strains. In fact, the Hong Kong influenza virion is related to the equine and duck hemagglutinin.

The reemergence in 1976 of an H1/N1 influenza virion, A/U.S.S.R./76, has shown the possible cyclical nature of influenza antigenic variation. H1/N1 influenza had not been isolated in the interval from 1957 to 1976. The relatively short time that influenza strains have been available for study (since 1933) prevents any exact knowledge of the limitations in antigenic variation to be expected in the future for influenza A.

Incidence and Clinical Manifestations

The clinical features of influenza A are often sufficiently distinct to permit a tentative diagnosis based on community epidemiology, age of the patient, and symptoms (Table 10-3) [27-29] The disease is not sporadic and appears only during discrete 1- to 2-month epidemics that usually receive wide news coverage. The abrupt onset of chills, fatigue, myalgia, and headache are typical. The acute febrile phase of the disease is over in 3 to 5 days, and convalescence is usually complete in 7 to 10 days. Coryza is not prominent, and pharyngitis may occur, but seldom with a purulent exudate. Laryngitis with hoarseness is common, and croup in children may be severe.

Pneumonia is the real threat of influenza.[30] Fatal influenza penumonia may occur in previously normal young adults and is particularly common in pregnant women, in the elderly, and in patients with preexisting cardiac or respiratory disease. Deaths may occur in the absence of bacterial superinfection. The respiratory distress of viral pneumonia appears within 24 hours of the initial symptoms and progresses rapidly. Combined influenza and bacterial pneumonia account for 80 percent of severe or fatal pneumonias during influenza epidemics. Often, these patients have had a period of improvement followed by return of fever and increased cough and sputum production. *Staphylococcus aureus* and *Streptococcus pneumoniae* are the primary bacterial pathogens.

Diagnosis

Confirmation of the diagnosis is readily obtained by virus culture. Pharyngeal secretions or sputum show influenza cytopathic effect within 2 to 4 days when inoculated onto susceptible cells in culture, such as primary monkey kidney cells. Direct examination of desquamated cells in pharyngeal secretions with fluorescein-conjugated anti-influenza antibody can provide an immediate diagnosis. A rise in influenza hemagglutinin-inhibition or complement-fixation serum antibodies can also confirm the diagnosis but entails a 2-week delay to obtain a convalescent serum.

Treatment

Amantadine (Chapter 18) may have a role in treatment of acute illness or prophylaxis. Severe influenza pneumonia may require mechanical ventilatory support with tracheostomy. In pure influenza pneumonia, one would expect the pulmonary pathology to resolve if the patients could be maintained perhaps only for another day or two. For this reason prolonged support (eg, membrane oxygenation and other heroic measures) needs evaluation.

Prevention

Three preventive measures may be instituted during influenza epidemics.

1. Specific immunization with influenza vaccine may be 80 percent effective in preventing infection, but the main protective effects of influenza vaccination probably only last 1 year; people with functionally significant cardiac or pulmonary disease, and health professionals, should probably receive yearly influenza immunization. Influenza vaccine composition is updated each year to contain the most current antigens.

2. In-hospital isolation of acute respiratory illness during influenza epidemics is needed, because influenza will spread rapidly on hospital wards among patients and staff.[31]

TABLE 10-3. FEATURES OF COMMON VIRAL ILLNESSES

Organism	Incubation Period	Period of Communicability	High-Risk Patients	Control
		LOWER RESPIRATORY INFECTIONS		
Influenza A	1–3 days	Before onset >1 week	Cardiac or pulmonary diseases	Annual vaccine; Amantadine hydrochloride for high-risk patients
Parainfluenza	2–6 days	Unknown; virus recoverable >1 week	Children with congenital stridor from abnormalities of larynx	None
Respiratory syncytial virus	3–7 days	Unknown; virus recovered >1 week	Infants	None
Adenoviruses	5–6 days, adults	For long periods, but greatest during first days	None	Military recruits receive vaccine for types 4 & 7
		GASTROENTERITIS		
Rotavirus	1–3 days	Unknown; virus found in stool for 8 days	Children <6 years	None
Norwalk virus	2 days	Unknown	None	None
		HEPATITIS		
Hepatitis B	6 weeks–6 months	Virus in blood for years, even without hepatitis	Medical personnel	Human hepatitis B immune globulin; vaccine in development
Hepatitis A	15–40 days	Uncertain; most communicable 1 week before or after onset of jaundice	Adults	Immune serum globulin
Hepatitis non A-non B	2 weeks	Virus persists in blood even after acute infection	Multiply transfused patients	None
		ENCEPHALITIS		
Rabies	3–8 weeks to 1 year	Cats and dogs—3–5 days before onset		Human rabies immune globulin and vaccine
Herpes simplex	4 days (range 2–12 days)	During active cutaneous lesions	Newborns, burn patients, other skin disease	Vidarabine for hepatitis and encephalitis; 5-iodo-2′-deoxyuridine for hepatitis
		CONGENITAL INFECTIONS		
Congenital cytomegalovirus		Not highly contagious. Infants may have high virus titers in urine	Pregnant women; immunosuppressed patients	Live attenuated vaccine in development
Rubella	5–21 days		Fetuses; gestational infection causes congenital anomalies	Live attenuated vaccine at 15 months, or all immune, nonpregnant women
		CUTANEOUS INFECTIONS		
Varicella	10–21 days	1 day before rash until crusts form 6–7 days	Nonimmune patients who received immunosuppressive drugs; newborns whose mothers develop chicken pox 4 days before birth	Live attenuated vaccine in development

3. Amantadine hydrochloride provides specific chemoprophylaxis for influenza A.[32] The dose is 200 mg/day, and it is remarkably safe. Amantadine hydrochloride should be considered for high-risk patients and close household or hospital ward contacts of influenza A index cases (Chapter 18).

PARAINFLUENZA

Etiology

Parainfluenza viruses are members of the paramyxovirus group that includes human measles and mumps viruses and some animal pathogens such as canine distemper virus and Newcastle disease virus. Among the many common properties of this virus group are a lipid-containing envelope surrounding a helical nucleocapsid that in turn contains a single-stranded RNA genome.

Epidemiology

The salient epidemiologic features are listed in Table 10-3. Parainfluenza virus may spread in hospitals and other institutions such as nursing homes.[33,34] Among the three common antigenic types of parainfluenza virus, there is more seasonal variation than with either respiratory syncytial virus or influenza. Parainfluenza type 3 is the most prevalent and can be isolated at all times of the year. Type 3 is associated with pneumonia or bronchiolitis in infants, croup in children age 1 to 2 years, and tracheobronchitis in older children. Epidemics of type 3 may occur most often in the spring and early summer. Infections with types 1 and 2 occur in the fall.[35,36]

Clinical Manifestations and Treatment

Parainfluenza viruses are the responsible pathogen in up to half of all cases of severe croup. Influenza A also causes croup. Croup, or laryngotracheobronchitis, may require surgical attention for several reasons. This entity may be confused with the surgical emergency of acute *Haemophilus influenza* epiglottitis. The two diseases may be differentiated by the higher fever, greater apprehension, and protective positioning in patients with epiglottitis. Lateral neck roentgenograms and direct observation at the time of tracheostomy will also confirm the diagnosis of epiglottitis (Fig. 10-7). When convinced that the disease is croup and *not* epiglottitis, the epiglottis can be directly inspected with gentle (to avoid laryngospasm) use of a tongue blade.

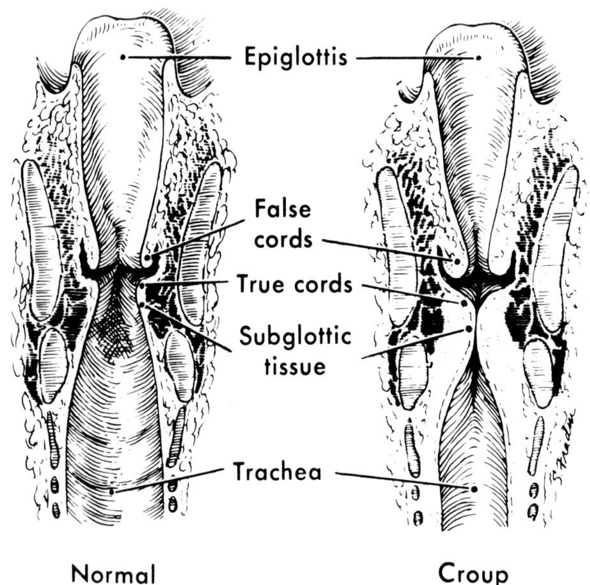

Fig. 10-7. **Site of laryngeal inflammation and swelling during viral croup. (Reproduced with permission, from Krugman S, Ward R, Katz SL (eds): *Infectious Diseases of Children,* 6th ed. St Louis, Mosby, 1977.)**

This maneuver, however, is extremely dangerous in the child with epiglottitis, who requires emergency tracheostomy, and should not be done when that disease is suspected. The child should be taken directly to the operating room, with physicians in constant attendance for an emergency tracheostomy.

Children with congenital stridor, caused by tracheal webs and other anatomical forms of laryngeal obstruction, may rapidly develop life-threatening airway obstruction from an otherwise mild episode of viral croup. When a child develops croup, a history of congenital stridor should be sought. Patients known to have anatomical airway obstruction should be warned about the need for immediate medical attention and intensive observation for even mild episodes of croup. Finally, the upper airway obstruction that occurs during croup may require mechanical ventilation, usually by endotracheal tube, but occasionally by tracheostomy.

Parainfluenza virus infections are extremely common in children. Fifty percent have been infected with parainfluenza 3 by age 1 and 90 percent by age 2. Second infections with the same antigenic type occur in both children and adults. The degree of protection against clinical illness conferred by the first infection is not clear, although there seems to be some benefit.

Diagnosis

The laboratory diagnosis of these infections may be done by virus isolation or serology. Typical parainfluenza cytopathic effect appears 2 to 5 days after inoculation of sensitive cells, such as primary monkey kidney cells. Infected cells adsorb sheep red blood cells and release hemagglutinating virus into the supernatant. A rise in hemagglutination inhibition, or complement fixation, may occur after infection but may not distinguish the type of parainfluenza virus.

Prevention

Progress in the development of an effective parainfluenza vaccine has been difficult. Inactivated vaccines have not been effective, and live, attenuated strains have been too virulent at times.

RESPIRATORY SYNCYTIAL VIRUS

Etiology

Respiratory syncytial virus is antigenically distinct from the paramyxoviruses, and only one major serotype is recognized.

Epidemiology

Respiratory syncytial virus is the most common pathogen implicated in lower respiratory tract disease in children (Table 10-3). It causes yearly epidemics of lower respiratory disease manifested by bronchiolitis and pneumonia in infants, more commonly in boys.[37] The virus has a high propensity for intrahospital spread and may cause serious nosocomial infection of infants and children.[38] The death rate from respiratory syncytial virus bronchiolitis among otherwise normal infants is less than 1 percent, but it is 4 to 5 percent when associated with congenital heart diseases.

Patients are susceptible to repeated respiratory syncytial virus infections. In a 10-year prospective study of children in a research day care program the attack rate for first infections was 98 percent, for second infections 75 percent, and for third infections 65 percent. Immunity induced by a single infection had no effect on illness with reinfection 1 year later; however, a considerable reduction in severity occurred with the third infection. Age did not have an independent effect on severity.

Clinical Manifestations

Bronchiolitis can occur as a distinct clinical entity, but more frequently signs of bronchopneumonia and upper respiratory illness are also present. It is more frequent and severe in infants less than 1 year old. The most distinctive clinical findings are the result of air trapping from bronchiolar obstruction. Wheezing and hyperinflation of the lungs are evident on clinical and radiographic examination. Respiratory rates of over 50 per minute and hypoxia are both common. Hypoxia may not be clinically evident but is always present and must be treated in severe cases. The symptoms are frequently confused with those caused by a vascular ring.

Diagnosis

Diagnosis is established by culture of pharyngeal secretions in sensitive cells such as HEp-2 cells. The virus is labile, and thus specimens should be inoculated into cultures immediately after collection.

Prevention

Early attempts at vaccination with a purified formalin-inactivated vaccine did not decrease the severity of infection, but resulted in increased disease severity during natural infection. This paradoxical response to inactivated vaccine has shifted vaccine emphasis to live, attenuated viruses. Early trials with live vaccines showed insufficient attenuation with reversion to wild type virus. At the present time, there is no approved respiratory syncytial virus vaccine.

ADENOVIRUSES

Adenovirus infection is a rather uncommon cause of severe sporadic lower respiratory tract disease, which is only rarely fatal. However, these viruses are common causes of upper respiratory illness in children. Associations with keratoconjunctivitis, the combination of conjunctivitis, fever, and pharyngitis, or acute respiratory disease among military recruits, add to the clinical picture of adenovirus infections. Less commonly, they may be associated with intussusception and rarely with hemorrhagic cystitis. Hospital and clinic epidemics of adenovirus keratoconjunctivitis can occur from contaminated ophthalmologic instruments and solutions.

There are 44 serologically distinct types of adenovirus, and infection with one type provides no protection against the other types. Children commonly become infected with several endemic types early in life and they may intermittently shed the virus from the intestinal tract for several years. Adenoviruses can be cultured from almost half of resected tonsils. Thus, adenoviruses apparently have the ability to produce a latent infection, but the mechanisms of latency are not yet worked out.

Type-specific immunity to adenoviruses is long lasting and more protective than the immunity provided by prior infection with other lower respiratory tract pathogens (Table 10-3). Live virus vaccines to types 4 and 7 can reduce acute respiratory disease in military recruits.

Specific diagnosis may be made by culturing the virus from respiratory secretions or stool. Because latent virus can be reactivated during other illnesses, however, isolation of the virus may not be diagnostic of acute infection caused by adenovirus. A group reaction complement-fixation assay can also be useful to detect a rise in antibody, following recovery. A rise in serum antibody or demonstration of basophilic intracytoplasmic inclusions in lung tissue are more specifically diagnostic than virus isolation from stool.

GASTROINTESTINAL SYNDROMES

After respiratory infections, gastroenteritis is the next most common viral disease in people. Two recently described viruses, rotavirus and the Norwalk agent, account for the majority of these illnesses. Rotaviruses cause disease in children, and the Norwalk agent causes disease in both children and adults. Their recent isolation has opened the door for accurate diagnostic tests, prevention, and more accurate assessment or treatment. A viral or infectious etiology for Crohn disease is still tenuous.[39]

ROTAVIRUS

Rotavirus (formerly called orbivirus, duovirus, reovirus-like agent, and infantile gastroenteritis virus) is the major pathogen responsible for acute gastroenteritis in children. It occasionally causes gastroenteritis in adults. The virus is readily demonstrated by electron microscopy of feces during the acute illness 4 to 8 days after the onset of symptoms. Although serologic procedures, including complement-fixation and immunofluorescence assays, show an antibody rise with acute infection, the tests are not yet readily available. At least two serotypes of rotavirus are recognized, and recurrent infections may occur.

Rotaviruses are highly transmissible and can cause epidemic gastroenteritis in hospitals, especially in the winter months. Their surgical significance arises mainly from their extreme prevalence—eventually everyone sustains these infections, including surgical patients. The differential diagnosis of abdominal diseases requiring operation may include diseases caused by these common pathogens. Specific knowledge of their presentation and natural course can be a diagnostic aid. Surgical patients with short bowel syndrome or ileostomy may rapidly develop fluid and electrolyte imbalance during these infections.

Development of a vaccine for human rotaviruses has been impeded by lack of an in vitro cell culture method. The great success of animal rotavirus vaccines promises success with the human strains when technical problems are overcome.

NORWALK VIRUS

The Norwalk virus may cause adult gastroenteritis and has been identified by electron microscopy as a 27 nm diameter virus.[40] Rotavirus is larger and is primarily a disease in children. Epidemic adult gastroenteritis has been called winter (September to March) vomiting disease. In the Norwalk, Ohio epidemic in 1969, the disease affected 50 percent of the elementary school students with nausea and vomiting, and to a lesser extent low-grade fever and diarrhea. There was short-term malabsorption of D-xylose, lactose, and fat following infection. Leukocytes were not found in the stool during acute infection. Immunity to reinfection lasts for at least 14 weeks. More than one antigenic type of virus has been demonstrated by cross-challenge experiments between viruses isolated from various epidemics. An unusual discrepancy between long- and short-term immunity to the Norwalk virus has been demonstrated. This is compatible with the hypothesis that some persons may have a genetically determined susceptibility to infection with these viruses.

HEPATITIS

Hepatitis is of major surgical significance because surgeons are at high risk of developing infection with hepatitis B. These are common, serious postoperative infections because both hepatitis B and non A-non B hepatitis (hepatitis C) can be transmitted by blood products. The other causes of hepatitis are of lesser significance but are often part of the differential diagnosis (hepatitis A, Epstein-Barr virus, cytomegalovirus, and rarely, a fulminant herpes simplex infection and neonatal coxsackievirus B).

HEPATITIS B

Etiology

The agent responsible for hepatitis B has been identified by electron microscopy (Fig. 10-8). Hepatitis B is caused by a DNA virus. Three particles have been demonstrated in infected serum. In 1970, a particle (the Dane particle) 42 nm in diameter was identified (Fig. 10-8).[41] In addition, smaller spherical particles 22 nm in diameter and filaments with a diameter of 22 nm and 200–400 nm long were also seen. The 42-nm Dane particle represents the complete virus, and the smaller spheres and filaments represent excess coat or surface protein. The surface protein is HBsAg (hepatitis B surface antigen), whereas the core material is HBcAg (hepatitis B core antigen) (Table 10-4). The core of the virus contains DNA and a DNA polymerase. HBeAg, the e antigen, is closely linked to the polymerase or is the polymerase itself. The concentration of particles in serum is approximately 3.4×10^{13}/ml.

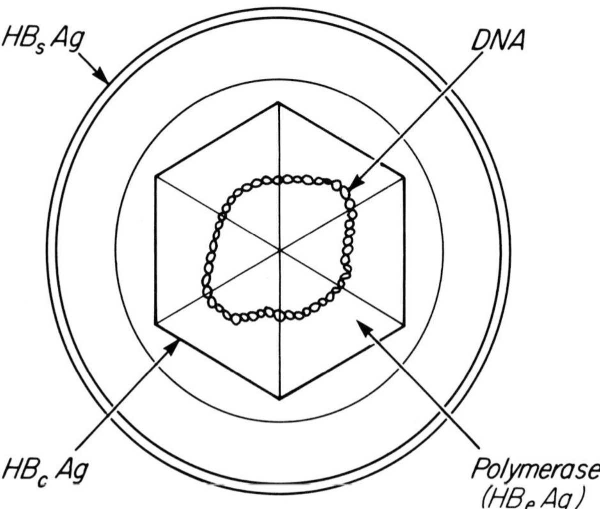

Fig. 10-8. **A schematic drawing of hepatitis B virus (diameter 42 nm). Outer rings constitute the surface antigen (HBsAg). The inner 28-nm hexagonal core (HBcAg) contains the DNA polymerase, which is closely associated with the e antigen (HBeAg) and the circular DNA. (Drawn after Krugman S: *Hepatitis, current status of etiology and prevention.* Hosp Prac, November 1975.)**

Epidemiology

Hepatitis B is a serious hazard to the health of surgeons, other medical personnel, and patients. It is a common nosocomial infection because of its ability to persist in the blood for indefinite periods. It is readily transmitted by blood or blood products, but it is also found in other body fluids—saliva, urine, semen, and stool. Human bites and sexual contact have been implicated in the transmission of hepatitis B. It was recently estimated that 6.5 million units of blood were transfused annually in the United States.[42] From these transfusions, there were an estimated 120,000 instances of jaundice and 14,000 deaths. The number of cases of transfusion hepatitis may be substantially greater, since an estimated 90 to 99 percent of cases are anicteric. Most cases of transfusion hepatitis B can be prevented by routinely screening donor blood for HBsAg. Approximately 60 to 90 percent of post-transfusion hepatitis is now due to non A-non B hepatitis. Roughly 5 to 10 percent of those who contract hepatitis become chronic carriers.

In 1975 in Minnesota, the incidence of hepatitis B was 132 cases per 100,000 population for hospital personnel compared to 24.5 cases per 100,000 for Minnesota citizens as a whole. The incidence was greater for dialysis technicians (9,615 cases per 100,000 per year) and clinical laboratory personnel (553 cases per 100,000 per year). For physicians, the incidence was 228 cases per 100,000 per year. The presence of dialysis facilities was an important factor. Hospitals with dialysis units had an incidence of 558 cases per 100,000 per year compared to 15 cases per 100,000 per year for hospitals without dialysis facilities.

Clinical Manifestations

Following an incubation period of 40 to 60 days, longer if immune globulin has been given, anorexia, fever, urti-

TABLE 10-4. SIGNIFICANCE OF SELECTED DIAGNOSTIC TESTS IN HEPATITIS B

HBsAg	Hepatitis B surface antigen. Tests for this antigen are readily available for clinical use. HBsAg is usually present in the serum at the onset of clinical illness and may persist for 3 to 4 months. Antibody to this antigen appears in serum after the antigen is gone. Persistence of HBsAg beyond 4 months usually indicates the onset of a prolonged carrier state. Rarely, the antigen will disappear after being present for 1 to 6 years. This lipoprotein aggregates into 20-nm particles that are visible in serum by electron microscopy.
HBsAg/adw ayw adr ayr	The hepatitis B surface antigen shows some antigenic heterogeneity that has been useful for epidemiologic studies. As yet, there is no firm association between these antigenic subtypes and specific hepatitis syndromes or complications. The prevalence of each antigenic type varies from place to place. The "a" determination is shared by all hepatitis B viruses, whereas the d, y, w, and r are subtype specific.
Anti-HBs	Hepatitis B surface antibody. This antibody appears late—1 to 2 months after HBsAg is no longer detectable. The presence of this antibody indicates recovery and immunity to hepatitis B.
HBcAg	Hepatitis B core antigen is found within the core of the nuclei of hepatocytes, but it has not been found free in the serum of patients with hepatitis. However, antibody is readily detected early in acute infection.
Anti-HBc	Hepatitis B core antibody. This antibody appears about 1 week after the onset of hepatitis, rises to high titers for several months, then eventually becomes nondetectable. Thus, this antibody appears early during infection, while viremia is still present.
HBeAg	Hepatitis B e antigen appears in serum during the acute stage of hepatitis B, is gone by early convalescence. It is only found in serum that contains HBsAg, DNA polymerase, and Dane particles. It may represent whole virus. This antigen when present in serum may indicate greater infectivity. Most patients with chronic active hepatitis are HBeAg positive.
Anti-HBe	Hepatitis B e antibody appears after the viremia abates and persists for 1 to 2 years. This may be a good indicator of lack of infectivity.

caria, arthralgia, arthritis, myalgia, coryza, nausea, and malaise occur as prodromal symptoms of the icteric phase. Fever may precede jaundice for a week. Dark urine, jaundice, vomiting, abdominal pain, mental depression, bradycardia, and pruritis can all occur in the acute phase and can last weeks to several months. Complete recovery is the rule. Rarely, fulminant hepatitis and death ensue. Ninety percent of hepatitis patients recover completely, about 10 percent develop chronic persistent hepatitis, and less than 1 percent develop chronic active hepatitis.

In chronic persistent hepatitis, the patient is asymptomatic with mild hepatomegaly and persistently or recurrently elevated liver enzymes. There is no progression to cirrhosis. HBsAg persists in the serum in chronic persistent hepatitis, although it may clear after several years. Chronic active hepatitis often progresses to cirrhosis after chronic and recurrent episodes of jaundice and abnormally elevated hepatic enzymes.

Diagnosis

Table 10-4 lists the diagnostic serologic procedures that can be done for hepatitis B and their significance.[43] The various antigens associated with the hepatitis virus may be present in serum obtained prior to the onset of jaundice. Sensitive assays for HBsAg detect this antigen as early as 6 days after exposure to infectious virus.

Prevention

Prevention of hepatitis B depends on early and rapid detection of individuals who have hepatitis B infections. All potential blood donors must be screened for the presence of HBsAg and most likely in the future for e antigen as well. Those who are positive must be excluded from donation of blood or plasma products. Patients who are in high-risk groups, such as those on hemodialysis or those who have received frequent transfusions, as well as all who have clinical manifestations of hepatitis, should be screened for HBsAg. Positive patients should be isolated for the duration of their hospitalization or until the acute illness subsides. Hepatitis isolation consists of placing the patient in a room that is private or occupied by other patients whose sera contain HBsAg. The patient's personal articles are used only by the patient, and all linen and other materials that come into contact with secretions from the patient are double-bagged before autoclaving.

Personnel wear gowns and gloves for direct care or when drawing blood or handling other body fluids. In addition to gowns and gloves, masks are worn when manipulating arteriovenous shunts or during other procedures that may result in aerosolization of blood. In the operating room, double-gowning is recommended; in addition, the use of two pairs of gloves is recommended, whenever possible, to minimize parenteral exposure. Tissue penetration by contaminated surgical instruments is the route of acquisition of hepatitis B for most surgeons. Any means of preventing inadvertent needle or scalpel cuts (such as the use of retractors instead of hands) is of value.

The staff members are not permitted to eat, drink, or smoke in any areas of patient care or in the clinical laboratory, where serum specimens from hepatitis patients are received. Specimens sent to the clinical laboratory are identified as coming from a high-risk source and are sent in ziplock bags. If spills of blood or body fluids from HBsAg-positive patients occur, they are cleaned up with 1 percent sodium hypochlorite solution.

In a cooperative Veterans Administration study, 419 persons with needle-stick exposure to HBsAg-positive serum were randomly selected to receive either hepatitis B immune globulin (HBsAb titer 1:100,000 by passive hemagglutination) or immune serum globulin (HBsAg titer <1:8).[44] Both globulin preparations were given as a 5-ml dose as soon as possible after exposure and again 28 days later. Clinical hepatitis developed in 1.4 percent of the hepatitis B immune globulin recipients and in 5.9 percent of the immune serum globulin recipients ($p = 0.016$). The hyperimmune globulin was obviously effective.

In another collaborative study with 757 subjects,[45,46] three globulin preparations were compared: normal titer (HBsAb titer 1:50 by passive hemagglutination), intermediate titer (HbsAb titer 1:5000), and high titer (HbsAb titer 1:500,000). During the two and a half years of this study, the titers in this globulin preparation decreased to 1:100,000. Three ml of the globulin solution was administered as soon as possible after exposure and again 25 to 35 days later. In this study, the high-titer globulin delayed the onset of hepatitis B, but did not significantly decrease its occurrence or severity. It was thought that this difference from earlier studies may have resulted from the proteolytic digestion of the particular high-titer globulin preparation during the study period. An effective hepatitis B vaccine should soon be available for high risk persons, such as male homosexuals, hospital personnel, patients who require frequent transfusions, patients with renal failure, and children of HBsAg-positive mothers.[21b,46a]

Because some health personnel following acute hepatitis B may have long-term HBsAg antigenemia, there has been some concern that they may be infectious to others. The risk is exceedingly small, and no restrictions of activity are recommended. Any decision to limit the activities of a health care worker must be based on evidence that the individual is associated with the transmission of hepatitis B to others. Such transmission from health care professionals who were HBsAg-positive has not been regularly found.[47] However, sporadic outbreaks of hepatitis B have been linked to medical personnel.

Despite advances in immune prophylaxis,[21b] the major deterrent to this infection is scrupulous technique in handling potential infectious blood or tissue. The question is frequently asked whether a patient is a potential transmitter of this disease. When one is exposed to HBeAg-positive blood, hepatitis commonly results. Hepatitis less often results from exposure to HBsAg-positive, HBeAg-negative blood. When antibodies to HBs appear, the patient has recovered and is immune.

HEPATITIS A

Infection with hepatitis A virus, infectious hepatitis, is often in the differential diagnosis of acute liver disease. The responsible virus has been identified as an enterovirus. Although there are clinical differences between hepatitis A and hepatitis B virus infections, the precise identification of these infections is best done by specific laboratory tests. Distinction between these two infections is clinically important for prognostic and public health reasons.

Hepatitis A has a shorter incubation period (15–40 days) than hepatitis B (50–180 days) (Table 10-3). Hepatitis A is present in feces and is spread predominantly by the intestinal-oral route. The sources of epidemics are frequently food handlers. The disease is most communicable for 1 week before the onset of jaundice to 1 week after. The signs, symptoms, and laboratory features of hepatitis A are similar to those of hepatitis B. The symptoms of hepatitis A are prevented by the administration of standard human immune serum globulin.

Viremia persists for only a few days before and after the onset of jaundice, and this accounts for the occasional parenteral transmission of this virus. Chronic hepatitis A antigenemia has not been observed and would not be expected from an enterovirus. Almost all patients with hepatitis A recover completely. The disease is especially mild in children. In young adults, the fatality rate is about 1 to 2 per 1,000 cases.

The diagnosis can be specifically confirmed by measuring hepatitis A-specific IgM antibody or a rise in immune adherence antibody.

NON A-NON B HEPATITIS (HEPATITIS C)

Non A-non B hepatitis may be the cause of 60 to 90 percent of all posttransfusion hepatitis in the United States. In a prospective study of 108 multiply transfused, open heart surgery patients, eight cases of non A-non B hepatitis developed.[48] The clinical illness associated with non A-non B virus is less severe than hepatitis B, although epidemiologically they are similar because parenteral exposure is required for transmission. As with hepatitis B, a chronic viremia and chronic liver disease may be sequelae of non A-non B hepatitis, and chronic viremia and chronic active hepatitis may develop after inapparent or mild illness.

The responsible virus was transmitted to volunteers in the 1950s, and more recently to chimpanzees.[49] At the moment, there is no specific serologic assay available for this virus, and the diagnosis rests on the exclusion of better characterized viruses (hepatitis A and B, Epstein-Barr virus, and cytomegalovirus). However, a presumptive virus causing non A-non B hepatitis has been identified by electron microscopy.

ENCEPHALITIS

The pathogen responsible for viral encephalitis can be accurately determined in only 20 to 40 percent of patients, but a precise etiologic diagnosis is important for public health and therapeutic reasons. Surgical consultation may be sought for five reasons: (1) brain biopsy may be required for diagnosis, (2) the viral encephalitis may mimic other surgically amenable diseases that can cause sudden onset of diffuse cerebral dysfunction, (3) transducers to monitor intracranial pressure may be required, (4) decompression may be needed, and (5) organ transplantation from these patients has raised the possibility of transmitting the encephalitis with the transplanted organ.[50] Although rabies is an extremely rare cause of viral encephalitis, over 30,000 courses of postexposure prophylaxis are administered in this country each year following animal bites that frequently require surgical attention.

RABIES

One case of human rabies occurs each year in the United States, although animal rabies is fairly widespread (Fig. 10-9). After a prodrome including fever, malaise, and headache, hyperactivity and diffuse cerebral dysfunction occur, followed by coma and death. Five to 20 percent may show progressive paralysis. Occasionally, there is no history of animal bite. Diagnosis may be confirmed by virus culture from secretions, cerebrospinal fluid, or brain, demonstration of rabies antigen in cornea or skin, or rise in rabies antibody. It is incurable. At postmortem examination typical intracytoplasmic inclusions called Negri bodies can be seen in the brain (Fig. 10-4B).

When and how to prevent it is the problem. Three products are available for prophylaxis: antirabies hyperimmune human globulin, a killed vaccine prepared in duck embryo cells, and a purified killed vaccine prepared in human diploid cells.[50a] The latter product has recently been licensed and should replace the vaccine prepared in duck embryo cells. It is currently recommended by the United States Public Health Service. This vaccine requires fewer doses than the duck embryo vaccine.

A unique report from Iran, where 17 villagers were attacked by a rabid wolf and sustained severe head and neck wounds, clearly showed the superiority of immune serum plus vaccine as opposed to vaccine alone.[51] The combined use of rabies vaccine and hyperimmune serum is widely accepted. In that 1955 study from Iran, only one of 12 persons who received rabies immune serum (rabbit origin) and vaccine developed rabies, whereas three of five persons who received vaccine alone died.

Who should receive rabies prophylaxis? Tables 10-5 and 10-6 summarize the principles involved. Every exposure to rabies must be individually evaluated, and this evaluation should include the country and specific locality of the exposure. In the United States, bites from wild animals, excluding rodents or lagomorphs (squirrels, rats, mice, rabbits) should be considered as rabies exposure and treatment with vaccine plus serum begun. Bites from domestic dogs and cats that are suspected to be rabid, proved rabid, or escaped should be considered as rabies exposures. If the dog or cat is healthy at the time of biting, it may be observed for 10 days for signs of rabies before starting prophylaxis. In other domestic animals such as cows, horses, or goats, the decisions are more difficult. The duration of rabies virus excretion prior to the onset of clinical illness in domestic animals varies with species. At times, this period of infectious virus excretion may not be reliably known.

Other factors to consider include: (1) the circumstances of the biting—an unprovoked attack is more likely to mean the animal is rabid; (2) the vaccination status of the biting animal—a properly immunized animal has only a minimal chance of transmitting the virus; and (3) the presence of rabies in the region—adequate laboratory documentation of a lack of rabies in the domestic species may be considered by local health officials.

Finally, but perhaps most important, local treatment of the wound is a critical part of prophylaxis after exposure. The wound should be thoroughly scrubbed with soap and water. Rinsing the wound with quaternary ammo-

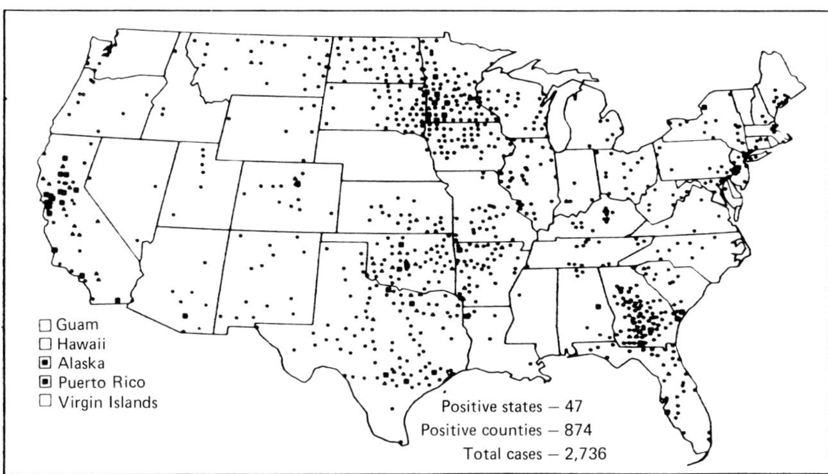

Fig. 10-9. **Counties reporting wild animal rabies, 1977.**

TABLE 10-5. GENERAL CONSIDERATIONS IN RABIES EXPOSURE

Rabies occurs in many wild animals, bats, and domestic animals, such as dogs, cats, and cattle, but rarely, if ever, in rodents.

A dog or cat that remains healthy for 10 days after a bite does not have rabies, and prophylaxis for a person bitten by that animal is not indicated.

A negative fluorescent antibody (FA) examination of an animal brain in an experienced laboratory is reliable evidence that the animal did not have rabies.

Saliva of a rabid animal on an open wound (usually a bite) or mucous membrane constitutes exposure to rabies.

A decision to inititate postexposure prophylaxis is based upon balancing two probabilities: (1) that rabies virus was introduced into an exposed person, and (2) that a serious reaction to prophylaxis material might occur.

From the Committee on Trauma, American College of Surgeons.

nium compounds (1 percent zephiran) after the soap has been removed has also been recommended. The principles of rabies postexposure prophylaxis are shown in Table 10-6.

After significant rabies exposure, the wound should be washed thoroughly with soap and water. Human rabies immune globulin should then be administered in a dose of 20 IU/kg, with half the dose infiltrated at the site of the wound and the rest given intramuscularly. A 1 ml dose of human diploid cell rabies vaccine should be given at the same time and repeated on days 3, 7, 14, and 28 after the first dose. A sixth dose on day 90 is optional.[51b]

HERPES SIMPLEX ENCEPHALITIS

Herpes simplex encephalitis is a rare but devastating disease, which can begin with focal neurologic symptoms that suggest surgical disease. There is also evidence to suggest vidarabine may improve survival, so a specific diagnosis is essential. At present, surgical biopsy of the affected area in the brain is the only reliable diagnostic test, although a radioimmunoassay for herpesvirus-specific glycoprotein in cerebrospinal fluid may be available soon.

Fever, headache, behavioral disturbances, and lethargy usually precede coma and seizures. A febrile encephalitis with focal neurologic findings, which may be confirmed by electroencephalogram, radioisotopic brain scan, or by computerized axial tomography (occasionally the latter may fail to demonstrate focal encephalitis) suggest this pathogen. Angiograms may be required to rule out vascular or mass lesions. The cerebrospinal fluid often reveals an elevated pressure, some leukocytosis, and red blood cells. Brain biopsy histology may show nonspecific necrosis, perivascular inflammation, and focal microglial proliferation or may show intranuclear inclusions specific for herpesvirus infection. Herpes simplex may be readily cultured from brain biopsy tissue or demonstrated by immunofluorescense. Rising serum antibody levels may be demonstrated, but are not diagnostic. Also, cerebrospinal fluid antibody measurements have not been diagnostically useful.

Adenine arabinoside (Ara-A) has shown some efficacy in a placebo-controlled study, reducing the mortality from 70 to 28 percent.[52] The drug is now licensed for use in this disease. Because diagnosis is so difficult, therapeutic trials are unreliable and much more work is needed to develop reliable diagnostic procedures and effective therapy (Chapter 18).

ARBOVIRAL ENCEPHALITIS

Summer epidemics of La Crosse, St. Louis, and Western equine encephalitis may occur in the United States. Other arboviral encephalitides are uniquely distributed about the world, and specific location, epidemiologic, and clinical data are essential to narrow the suspected diagnosis. Their surgical significance rests in the differential diagnosis of acute cerebral dysfunction, at times with focal findings, and the occasional need for surgical biopsy and pressure monitoring.

La Crosse encephalitis is almost exclusively a disease of children, most commonly boys between the ages of 5 and 9 years. The mosquito vector, *Aedes triseriatus*, feeds only during the daytime, breeds in the basal tree holes of hardwood trees, and travels only a few hundred yards from the breeding site. Thus, disease usually occurs in localized areas, and physicians in those areas become highly adept at diagnosis on clinical grounds. Acute febrile encephalitis with peripheral leukocytosis and difficult-to-control focal seizures highlight the illness. Most patients recover completely. Diagnosis is confirmed by a rise in serum antibody to the La Crosse virus.

St. Louis encephalitis occurs in epidemics. In 1975, a total of 1,815 cases were reported to the Center for Disease Control. Those cases were predominantly from Illinois, Ohio, and Mississippi. The vectors are *Culex* mosquitos, principally *C. pipiens* in the central and southern states. These species thrive in urban areas and are thus amenable to vector control. The disease begins abruptly with fever and headache, progressing to confusion, tremors, and coma. The disease is more common in adults and has a 20 percent mortality among documented cases. The illness lasts approximately 2 weeks and may be biphasic with a few days of improvement interspersed between the prodromal symptoms and actual encephalitis. Leukocytosis of the cerebrospinal fluid is common.

CONGENITAL AND NEONATAL VIRAL INFECTION

Cytomegalovirus is now the major intrauterine viral infection responsible for serious fetal damage. One symptom of fetal cytomegalovirus infection, neonatal hepatitis, may be included in the differential diagnosis of biliary atresia. Cytomegalovirus chorioretinitis and sensorineural hearing loss may come to the attention of ophthalmologists and otolaryngologists respectively. Congenital rubella has become rare since the advent of an effective vaccine, and

TABLE 10.6. PRINCIPLES OF RABIES POSTEXPOSURE PROPHYLAXIS

Animal Species	Condition of Animal at Time of Attack	Treatment
Household pets: dogs and cats	Healthy and available for 10 days of observation	None unless animal develops rabies. At first sign of rabies in animal, treat patient with RIG and HDCV. Symptomatic animal should be killed and tested as soon as possible.
	Rabid or suspect	RIG and HDCV
	Unknown (escaped)	Consult public health officials, if treatment indicated, give RIG and HDCV
Wild animals: skunks, bats, foxes, coyotes, racoons, bobcats, other carnivores	Regard as rabid unless proved negative by laboratory tests. If available, animal should be killed and tested as soon as possible.	RIG and HDCV
Other animals: livestock, rodents, lagomorphs (e.g., rabbits, hares)	Consider individually. Local and state public health officials should be consulted on the need for prophylaxis. Bites by the following almost never call for antirabies prophylaxis: squirrels, hamsters, guinea pigs, gerbils, chipmunks, rats, mice, other rodents, rabbits, and hares.	

GENERAL MEASURES: All bites and wounds should be thoroughly cleansed immediately with soap and water. If vaccine treatment is indicated, both rabies immune globulin (RIG) and human diploid cell rabies vaccine (HDCV) should be given as soon as possible, regardless of interval after exposure. (The administration of RIG is the more urgent procedure. If HDCV is not immediately available, start RIG and give HDCV as soon as it is obtained.) If either RIG or HDCV is unavailable, substitute antirabies serum equine (ARS) and/or duck embryo vaccine (DEV), respectively. Do not exceed recommended RIG or ARS dose. Common local reactions to DEV do not contraindicate continued treatment. Vaccine use should be discontinued if test results of animal tissues for rabies antigen, using fluorescent reagents, are negative.

From MMWR, June 13, 1980.

cataracts and patent ductus arteriosis from congenital rubella are rare. However, the question of therapeutic abortion for intrapartum rubella and intrapartum vaccination still occurs. Genital herpes simplex at the time of parturition can cause fatal neonatal infection so that the timing of cesarean section to avoid such catastrophic infections is important. Fetal disease from intrapartum chickenpox is rare, although maternal chickenpox near the time of parturition can lead to a fatal infection of the newborn.

CONGENITAL CYTOMEGALOVIRUS

One percent of all newborns will have acquired cytomegalovirus infection before or at the time of birth.[53] The extent of illness caused by this infection is variable and may depend on the gestational age when infection occurs (Table 10-3). Severe congenital infection with resultant microcephaly, hepatosplenomegaly, jaundice, thrombocytopenia, and psychomotor retardation may result from infection early in pregnancy, perhaps in the first and second trimesters. Severe congenital cytomegalovirus infections occur in 1 of every 1,000 live births. Silent congenital infection is so named because the affected infants appear normal at birth and are identified only through screening programs to detect cytomegalovirus IgM or cytomegalovirus viruria at birth. These infants have a 20 percent chance of severe sensorineural hearing loss. Silent congenital infections occur in 6 of every 1,000 births. At the time of parturition, about 5 to 10 percent of women shed cytomegalovirus from the urine or cervix. These infected secretions may be the source for the neonatal acquisition of cytomegalovirus infection by 1 percent of newborns. These perinatal infections are frequently asymptomatic and have no known long-term consequences, but some are manifested by respiratory infection, including pneumonia and, less commonly, hemolytic anemia.

All three groups of infected infants shed virus for several years after birth. Cytomegalovirus infection is fairly common, and most adults have antibody. As with the other herpesviruses, however, cytomegalovirus remains latent following a primary infection and can be reactivated and shed during pregnancy. This reactivated virus is the most likely source for the perinatal acquisition of virus. It seems unlikely that reactivated virus is responsible either for severe congenital infection or silent congenital infection. Rather, in these diseases, the damage is more likely from a primary cytomegalovirus infection of the nonimmune pregnant woman.

Since the virus is known to be shed in high concentrations from the urine of infected infants, the potential for infections of hospital staff exists. Fortunately, cytomegalovirus is not highly contagious, and most hospital staff are immune. The greatest risk is to nonimmune pregnant women who have intimate contact with infected infants, such as changing diapers.

Although many congenital anomalies have been associated with congenital cytomegalovirus infection, such as inguinal hernia, cleft palate, and diaphragmatic hernia, there is no firm evidence for such associations.

The diagnosis of the severe or silent congenital infection is best established by culture of the urine for cytomegalovirus or determination of cytomegalovirus-specific IgM in the first week of life. Perinatally infected infants begin to shed virus and develop cytomegalovirus antibodies several weeks later.

Cytomegalovirus is a herpesvirus and, with a DNA of 100 million daltons, contains enough genetic information to provide for considerable antigenic variation, although distinct subclasses with antigenic similarity are not clearly defined. The role of this antigenic variation in the protective immunity developed after infection is not yet defined.

HERPES SIMPLEX

Maternal genital herpes simplex infection at the time of parturition can result in severe neonatal herpes simplex infection. If active genital herpes infection is recognized before birth, a cesarean section may prevent infection of the infant (Table 10-7). Prolonged rupture of membranes in the face of active genital herpes has a poor prognosis. The typical appearance of genital herpes is a vesiculopapular rash with crusting. The diagnosis in atypical cases can be confirmed by culture or by finding multinucleated giant cells in scrapings from the base of the lesions—Tzanck preparation. Active genital herpes early in pregnancy and even well into the third trimester usually resolves uneventfully before term.

Neonatal infection has a broad clinical spectrum and can affect skin, brain, eye, or oral cavity or may be disseminated. The herpetic skin vesicles are lacking in at least one-third of the infants, making the diagnosis difficult at times. The prognosis depends on the system of major clinical involvement and the gestational age of the infant (Table 10-7). Onset is usually from 6 to 20 days after birth. Neither adenine arabinoside nor acyclovir therapy has proved effective (Chapter 18). Topical 2 percent adenine arabinoside eye ointment is highly effective for the keratitis that may be a part of the neonatal infection. Newborns can acquire herpes simplex as a nosocomial infection and should be protected from active labial herpes among hospital staff, visitors, and of course from active neonatal herpes in other infants.

RUBELLA

Fortunately, the widespread use of a live attenuated vaccine has made congenital rubella a rare disease. Surgical

TABLE 10-7. CLINICAL SPECTRUM AND OUTCOME OF 298 CASES OF NEONATAL HERPETIC INFECTION *

		Outcome in Infants		
Clinical Group	**No. Cases**	***Died***	***Survived with Sequelae***	***Survived without Apparent Sequelae***
I. Disseminated				
Without CNS involvement	98 (5) †	90 (2)	1 (1)	7 (2)
With CNS involvement	96 (17)	68 (6)	15 (6)	13 (5)
II. Localized ‡				
CNS	51 (10)	19 (3)	24 (6)	8 (1)
Eye	15 (3)	0	6 (2)	9 (1)
Skin	33 (3)	1	8	24 (3)
Oral cavity	3 (1)	0	0	3 (1)
III. Asymptomatic	2	0	0	2
Total	298 (39)	178 (11)	54 (15)	66 (13)

* An additional 13 cases could not be classified due to insufficient data.

† Numbers in parenthesis refer to patients treated with systemic antiviral agents.

‡ Classified according to major site of involvement if more than one site was infected.

Taken with permission from Nahmias AJ, Visintine AM, Reimer CB, Del Buono I, Shore SL, Starr SE: Herpes simplex virus infection of the fetus and newborn. *Prog Clin Biol Res* 3:63–77, 1975.

correction of congenital rubella cataracts and cardiac anomalies is now uncommon. Therapeutic abortion is sometimes indicated after accidental vaccination or primary disease during pregnancy. The infection begins with a mild prodromal period of upper respiratory symptoms and occipital lymphadenopathy. The maculopapular rash begins on the face and spreads rapidly, lasting about 3 days, with a mild fever. Rubella is usually more severe in adults and can be accompanied by joint and muscle pain.

The teratogenic effects of rubella infection are greatest in the first trimester of pregnancy (Table 10-3). Congenital rubella can be diagnosed by finding rubella-specific IgM in the sera of infected infants or by culturing the virus. Rubella is readily discovered from cerebrospinal fluid and pharyngeal secretions in the first year and can often be recovered for several years. Cataracts are common at birth and are usually bilateral. The corneal opacities are central and involve all but the outermost layers of the lens. The most common cardiac defect is patent ductus arteriosis (58 percent), ventricular septal defect (17 percent), tetralogy of Fallot (7 percent), atrial septal defect (6 percent), and pulmonary valvular stenosis (6 percent).

The last epidemic in the United States occurred in 1965 and resulted in more than 30,000 congenitally affected infants. Since the live attenuated rubella vaccine was first used, the incidence of congenital infection has dramatically decreased. The vaccine is theoretically teratogenic if inadvertently administered to pregnant women, and it has been recovered from fetuses aborted after vaccination. If a woman is inadvertently vaccinated during pregnancy, the risk of damage to the fetus is quite small (<5 percent). Nevertheless, every precaution should be taken to ensure that women are not pregnant when vaccinated, and do not become pregnant for 8 weeks after vaccination.

Isolated incidences of rubella are difficult to diagnose, and should be confirmed by testing paired acute and convalescent sera for rubella antibody. One week after the rash, significant antibody can be found.

VIRUS INFECTIONS WITH CUTANEOUS SIGNS

Among the classic exanthems of childhood, chickenpox remains a substantial hazard to immunosuppressed surgical patients. Warts and laryngeal papillomatosis may require surgical therapy. Herpes simplex and vaccinia may produce fatal infections in burn patients. Rubeola, rubella, erythema infectiosum, Epstein-Barr virus, and enteroviruses produce rashes that may be confused with drug eruptions.

VARICELLA ZOSTER

Chickenpox, although a common, usually innocuous epidemic childhood infection, can cause life-threatening infection in immunosuppressed patients. Varicella-zoster human immune plasma or globulin can protect high-risk patients who have been exposed to chickenpox. Most people have naturally acquired immunity by the time they are adults. It is young patients, particularly children who have had surgery plus chemotherapy for malignancies and renal transplant recipients, who are at greatest risk. Of course, immunosuppressed adults are at risk too if they are among the 2 to 5 percent of people who have not had childhood chickenpox. The newborn child, whose mother developed chickenpox 4 days before or 2 days after the child's birth, may develop severe varicella with a 20 percent mortality.

In the normal host, varicella begins with a vesicular-pustular rash on the trunk, which spreads and increases in intensity for 5 days. Fever is common in the last 3 days of rash. Occasionally, a child will have fresh vesicles for longer than 7 days.

In the immunocompromised host, the disease may be fulminant, resulting in death within 1 to 2 days of onset. More commonly, the infection begins like an ordinary case of chickenpox, but the rash and fever progress more rapidly, more intensely, and longer than normal. An ominous sign is the onset of varicella pneumonia, which can be fatal for immunosuppressed patients. Encephalitis and hepatitis can occur but do not usually cause death. Bacterial superinfection can also occur and is usually caused by streptococci.

Intense supportive therapy is needed after chickenpox occurs, because no specific therapy is available. Immunosuppressive drugs should be withheld after exposure and certainly after the onset of the eruption. Steroid administration should not be abruptly decreased or stopped. The likelihood of infection varies with the duration and intensity of exposure.

Zoster, or shingles, is a common manifestation of latent varicella-zoster virus. Though it may occur in people with normal immune systems, it is more common in immunosuppressed patients. The rash may be preceded or accompanied by pain at the site of the eruption, fever, and headache. The distribution of the vesiculopustular eruption is along spinal sensory nerve paths. An inflammatory neuritis occurs, and functional impairment is possible. Most commonly, the rash begins to heal 5 to 7 days after onset, but severe postherpetic neuralgia occurs in 20 percent and may last from a few months to a year.

In the immunosuppressed, fever and prolonged eruption are more common. Cutaneous dissemination, vesicular eruption outside the primary and immediately adjacent dermatomes, is not by itself an ominous sign. Most immunosuppressed patients handle shingles fairly well and eventually recover. The severely suppressed, such as those with stage IV Hodgkin disease, occasionally cannot contain the infection and after several weeks of continuous eruption develop fatal varicella pneumonia or encephalitis.

A placebo-controlled study of adenine arabinoside for the treatment of shingles has been reported. There was some reduction in pain and virus yield from the vesicular lesion, although the drug has not been approved for this purpose. Acyclovir has not yet had an adequate trial (Chapter 18).

An attenuated varicella vaccine has been developed

by Takahashi in Japan and by Merck Sharp and Dohme in the United States.[21a]

HERPES SIMPLEX

We discussed herpes simplex virus as a cause of severe neonatal disease and encephalitis. Herpes simplex virus may also severely affect burned patients in a manner similar to that described as Kaposi varicelliform eruption—herpes simplex infection of patients with eczema. Skin that has been damaged, as in burns or eczema, facilitates the local invasion by the herpes simplex virus. These severe local infections may disseminate to cause multiple organ involvement, most classically herpes hepatitis with acute liver failure. The only protection against this illness is isolation from persons with active herpetic lesions. Acyclovir may prove to be effective therapy (Chapter 18).

WARTS AND LARYNGEAL PAPILLOMAS

Epithelial growths caused by human papova viruses are extremely common and occasionally require surgical attention. For example, laryngeal papillomas require early surgical diagnosis and treatment, and a squamous cell carcinoma can arise from long-standing warts. The common wart (verruca vulgaris) is especially troublesome in the nailbed or on the sole of the foot (plantar warts), and small flat warts on the face and hands of children (verruca plana juvenilia) and filiform warts are common variants. Genital warts (condyloma acuminata) are especially troublesome and recurrent.

It has become apparent recently that there are several biochemically and serologically distinct papovaviruses responsible for these various clinical warts.

VIRUSES AND THE ETIOLOGY OF CANCER

The discovery that several—perhaps most—malignant tumors of animals, as well as leukemias and lymphomas, are caused by transmissable oncogenic viruses has led to a wide search for similar agents in human neoplasms.[1,54] In animals, proving that a virus is indeed oncogenic is confounded by: (1) the frequent requirement for a second or helper virus, because many oncogenic viruses are incomplete or defective, or (2) the fact that the oncogenic virus must first be triggered by a variety of metabolic, hormonal, or chemical factors or radiation before it can cause malignant tumors. Gross [54,55] speculated that oncogenic viruses are latent infections vertically transmitted from one generation to another until they are triggered by some stimulus. Epidemiologically, they are akin to slow virus infections of man, in that they can be vertically transmitted and must reside a long time in the host before causing clinical disease.

Despite an extensive search for viruses that cause human tumors, none has yet been found. By indirect means, viruses have been implicated as a cause of Burkitt lymphoma, nasopharyngeal carcinoma, breast cancer, carcinoma of the cervix, leukemia, Hodgkin disease, and lymphoma.[1,20a] In studying presumed human cancer viruses, indirect kinds of evidence must be used, since Koch's postulates cannot be fulfilled with human subjects. Even if one could perform such an experiment, inoculating a putative oncogenic virus into humans (or primates), one might have to wait years for the tumor to develop or the kind of circumstances that would trigger the virus might not exist.

Thus, indirect means of looking for human oncogenic viruses must be used. Indirect methods of study include epidemiologic, electron microscopy, serologic, and biochemical.[1] Despite these sophisticated experimental techniques, evidence for a viral etiology of human cancer has only rarely been found.

BIBLIOGRAPHY

Debré R, Celers J (eds): Clinical Virology: The Evaluation and Management of Human Viral Infections. Philadelphia, Saunders, 1970.

Howard RJ, Balfour HH Jr, Simmons RL: The surgical significance of viruses. Curr Probl Surg 14:1, 1977.

Mandell GL, Douglas RG Jr, Bennett JE (eds): Viral Diseases, Section A (Part III). In Principles and Practice of Infectious Diseases. New York, Wiley, 1979, pp 1079–1460.

REFERENCES

VIRAL INFECTIONS AS CAUSE OF SURGICAL ILLNESS

1. Howard RJ, Balfour HH Jr, Simmons RL: The surgical significance of viruses. Curr Probl Surg 14:1, 1977.
2. Blattner RJ: The role of viruses in congenital defects. Am J Dis Child 128:781, 1974.
3. Brown GC: Recent advances in the viral aetiology of congenital anomalies. Adv Teratol 1:55, 1966.

INFECTIONS FOLLOWING TRANSFUSION (NOT INCLUDING HEPATITIS)

4. Foster KM: Post-transfusion mononucleosis. Aust Ann Med 15:305, 1966.
5. Reyman TA: Postperfusion syndrome; a review and report of 21 cases. Am Heart J 72:116, 1966.
6. Armstrong D, Ely M, Steger L: Post-transfusion cytomegaloviremia and persistence of cytomegalovirus in blood. Infect Immun 3:159, 1971.
7. Klemola E, Von Essen R, Paloheimo J, Furuhjelm V: Cytomegalovirus antibodies in donors of fresh blood to patients submitted to open heart surgery. Scand J Infect Dis 1:137, 1969.
8. Perham TGM, Caul EO, Conway PJ, Mott MG: Cytomegalovirus infection in blood donors—a prospective study. Br J Haematol 20:307, 1971.
9. Henley W, Henley G, Scruba M, Joyner CR, Harrison FS Jr, Von Essen R, Paloheimo J, Klemola E: Antibody responses to the Epstein-Barr virus and cytomegaloviruses after open heart surgery. N Engl J Med 282:1068, 1970.

INFECTIONS IN COMPROMISED HOST AFTER OPERATION

10. Sokal JE, Firat D: Varicella-zoster infection in Hodgkin's disease. Am J Med 39:452, 1965.

11. Schimpff S, Serpick A, Stoler B, Rumak B, Mellin H, Joseph JM, Boock J: Varicella-zoster infection in patients with cancer. Ann Intern Med 76:241, 1972.
12. Wilson JF, Marsa GW, Johnson RE: Herpes zoster in Hodgkin's disease. Cancer 29:461, 1972.
13. Goffinet DR, Glatstein EH, Merigan TC: Herpes zoster-varicella infections and lymphomas. Ann Intern Med 76:235, 1972.
14. Duval CP, Casazza AR, Grimley PM, Carbond PP, Rowe WP: Recovery of cytomegalovirus from adults with neoplastic disease. Ann Intern Med 64:531, 1966.
15. Hill RB Jr, Rowlands DT Jr, Rifkind D: Infectious pulmonary disease in patients receiving immunosuppressive therapy for organ transplantation. N Engl J Med 271:1021, 1964.
16. Hedley-Whyte ET, Craighead JE: Generalized cytomegalic inclusion disease after renal homotransplantation. N Engl J Med 272:473, 1965.
17. Ho M, Suwansirikul S, Dowling JN, Youngblood LA, Armstrong JA: The transplanted kidney as a source of cytomegalovirus infection. N Engl J Med 293:1109, 1975.
18. Betts RF, Freeman RB, Douglas RG Jr, Talley TE, Rundell B: Transmission of cytomegalovirus infection with renal allograft. Kidney Int 8:387, 1975.
19. Montgomerie JZ, Becroft DMO, Croxson MD, Doak PB, North JDK: Herpes simplex virus infection after renal transplantation. Lancet 2:876, 1969.
20. Marker SC, Ascher NL, Kalis JM, Simmons RL, Najarian JS, Balfour HH Jr: Epstein-Barr virus antibody responses and clinical illness in renal transplant recipients. Surg 85:433, 1979.
20a. Hanto DW, Sakamoto K, Purtilo DT, Simmons RL, Najarian JS: The Epstein-Barr virus in the pathogenesis of post-transplant lymphoproliferative disorders: clinical, pathologic and virologic correlation. Surgery 1981, in press.
21. Coleman DV, Mackenzie EF, Gardner SD, Pounding JM, Amer B, Russell WJ: Human polyomavirus (BK) infection and ureteric stenosis in renal allograft recipients. J Clin Pathol 31:338, 1978.
21a. Ha K, Baba K, Ikeda T, Nishida M, Yabuuchi H, Takahashi M: Application of live varicella vaccine to children with acute leukemia or other malignancies without suspension of anticancer therapy. Pediatrics 65:346, 1980.
21b. Szmuness W, Stevens CE, Harley EJ, Zang EA, Oleszko, WR, William DC, Sadovsky R, Morrison JM, Kellner A: Hepatitis B vaccine: Demonstration of efficacy in a controlled clinical trial in a high-risk population in the United States. N Engl J Med 303:833, 1980.
21c. Pazin GJ, Armstrong JA, Lam MT, Tarr GC, Jannetta PJ, Ho M: Prevention of reactivated herpes simplex infection by human leukocyte interferon after operation on the trigeminal root. N Engl J Med 301:225, 1979.
22. Tong MJ, Nystrom AS, Redeker AG, Marshall GJ: Failure of transfer-factor therapy in chronic active type B hepatitis. N Engl J Med 295:209, 1976.
23. Shulman ST, Schulkind ML, Ayoub EM: Transfer-factor therapy of chronic active hepatitis. Lancet 2:650, 1974.
24. Rytel MW, Aaberg TM, Dee TH, Heim LH: Therapy of cytomegalovirus retinitis with transfer factor. Cell Immunol 19:8, 1975.

LOWER RESPIRATORY TRACT SYNDROMES

25. Kilbourne ED: The molecular epidemiology of influenza. J Infect Dis 127:478, 1973.
26. Stuart-Harris CH: Immunity to influenza. J Infect Dis 126:466, 1972.
27. Stuart-Harris CH, Schild GC: Influenza: The Viruses and the Disease. Littleton, MA, Publishing Sciences Group, 1976.
28. Knight V, Kasel JA: Influenza Viruses. In Knight V (ed): Viral and Mycoplasmal Infections of the Respiratory Tract. Philadelphia, Lea & Febiger, 1973, p 87.
29. Kilbourne ED (ed): The Influenza Viruses and Influenza. New York, Academic, 1975.
30. Center for Disease Control: Influenza—United States. MMWR 26:50, 1977.
31. Report of the Committee on Infectious Diseases, 18th ed. Evanston, Ill., American Academy of Pediatrics, 1977.
32. Galbraith AW: Therapeutic Trials of Amantadine (Symmetrel) in General Practice. In Oxford JS, Williams JD (eds): Chemotherapy and Control of Influenza. London, Academic, 1976, p 81.
33. Center for Disease Control: Parainfluenza outbreaks in extended care facilities—United States. MMWR 27:475, 1978.
34. Mufson MA, Mocega HE, Krause HE: Acquisition of parainfluenza 3 virus infection by hospitalized children. I. Frequencies, rates and temporal data. J Infect Dis 128:141, 1973.
35. Glezen WP, Denny FW: Epidemiology of acute lower respiratory disease in children. N Engl J Med 288:498, 1973.
36. Chanock RM, Parrott RH: Parainfluenza Viruses. In Horsfall FL Jr, Tamm I (eds): Viral and Rickettsial Infections of Man. Philadelphia, Lippincott, 1965, p 741.
37. Brandt CD, Kim HW, Arrobio JO, Jeffries BC, Wood SC, Chanock RM, Parrot RH: Epidemiology of respiratory syncytial virus infection in Washington, DC. III. Composite analysis of eleven consecutive yearly epidemics. Am J Epidemiol 98:355, 1973.
38. Hall CB, Douglas RG Jr, Geiman JM, Messner MK: Nosocomial respiratory syncytial virus infections. N Engl J Med 293:1343, 1975.

GASTROINTESTINAL SYNDROMES

39. Gitnick GL, Rosen VJ: Electron microscopic studies of viral agents in Crohn's disease. Lancet 2:217, 1976.
40. Kapikian AZ, Wyatt RG, Dolin R, Thornhill TS, Kalica AR, Chanock RM: Visualization by immune electron microscopy of a 27-nm particle associated with acute infectious nonbacterial gastroenteritis. J Virol 10:1075, 1972.

HEPATITIS

41. Robinson WS, Lutwick LI: The virus of hepatitis B. N Engl J Med 295:1168, 1976.
42. Holzbach RT, Leon MA: Posttransfusion viral hepatitis and the hepatitis associated antigen (HAA). Ohio State Med J 67:329, 1971.
43. Deinhardt F: Predictive value of markers of hepatitis virus infection. J Infect Dis 141:299, 1980.
44. Seeff LB, Wright EC, Zimmerman HJ, Alter HJ, Dietz AA, Felsher BF, Finkelstein JD, Garcia-Pont P, Gerin JL, Greenlee HB, Hamilton J, Holland PV, Kaplan PM, Kiernan T, Koff RS, Leevy CM, McAuliffe VJ, Nath N, Purcell RH, Schiff ER, Schwartz CC, Tamburro CH, Vlahcevic Z, Zemel R, Zimmon DS: Type B hepatitis after needle-stick exposure: prevention with hepatitis B immune globulin: final report of the Veterans Administrative Cooperative Study. Ann Intern Med 88:285, 1978.
45. Prince AM, Szmuness W, Mann MK, Vyas GN, Grady GF, Shapiro FL, Suki WN, Friedman EA, Avram MM, and Stenzel KH: Hepatitis B immune globulin: final report of a controlled, multicenter trail of efficacy in prevention of dialysis-associated hepatitis. J Infect Dis 137:131, 1978.
46. Grady GF, Lee VA: Hepatitis B immune globulin—preven-

tion of hepatitis from accidental exposure among medical personnel. N Engl J Med 293:1067, 1976.

46a. Maupas P, Barin F, Chiron JP, Coursaget P, Goudeau A, Perrin J, Denis F, Diop Mar I: Efficacy of hepatitis B vaccine in prevention of earlier HBsAg carrier state in children. Controlled trial in an endemic area (Senegal). Lancet 1:289, 1981.

47. Alter HJ, Chalmers TC, Freeman BM, Lunceford JL, Lewis TL, Holland PV, Pizzo PA, Plotz PH, Meyer WJ: Health-Care workers positive for hepatitis B surface antigen: are their contacts at risk? N Engl J Med 292:454, 1975.

48. Alter HJ, Purcell RH, Holland PV, Feinstone SM, Morrow AG, Moritsugu Y: Clinical and serological analysis of transfusion-associated hepatitis. Lancet 2:838, 1975.

49. Alter HJ, Purcell RH, Holland PV, Popper H: Transmissable agents in non-A non-B Hepatitis. Lancet 1:459–463, 1978.

RABIES AND OTHER CAUSES OF ENCEPHALITIS

50. Houff SA, Burton RC, Wilson RW, Henson TE, London WT, Baer GM, Anderson LJ, Winkler WG, Madden DL, Sever JL: Human-to-human transmission of rabies virus by corneal transplant. N Engl J Med 300:603, 1979.

50a. Plotkin SA: Rabies vaccination in the 1980s. Hosp Prac, November, 1980, p 65.

51. Habel K, Koprowski H: Laboratory data supporting the clinical trial of antirabies serum in persons bitten by a rabid wolf. Bull WHO 13:773, 1955.

51a. Meyer HM Jr: Rabies vaccine. J Infect Dis 142:287, 1980.

52. Whitley RJ, Soong SR, Dolin R, Galasso GJ, Ch'ien LT, Alford CA: Adenine arabinoside therapy of biopsy-proved herpes simplex encephalitis. National Institute of Allergy and Infectious Disease Collaboration Antiviral Study. N Engl J Med 297:289, 1977.

CONGENITAL INFECTIONS

53. Reynolds DW, Stagno S, Stubbs KG, Dahle AJ, Livingston MM, Saxon SS, Alford CA: Inapparent congenital cytomegalovirus infection with elevated cord IgM levels. Causal relation with auditory and mental deficiency. N Engl J Med 290:291, 1974.

VIRUSES AND CANCER

54. Gross L: Viral etiology of cancer and leukemia: a look into the past, present, and future. Cancer Res 38:485, 1978.

55. ———: Cancer and slow virus diseases—some common features. N Engl J Med 301:432, 1979.

CHAPTER 11
Surgical Parasitology

LEE S. MONROE

IT IS not the purpose of this chapter to present in encyclopedic fashion the multitude of parasitoses that could conceivably be encountered by the surgeon. For example, opportunistic infections, such as pneumocystosis, toxoplasmosis, or strongyloidiasis, which may become rampant in the immunosuppressed or deficient patient, are discussed in Chapter 47. On the other hand, the chapter will focus on infections that may present as (or develop) a surgical problem during the parasitism. As modern travel has the potential of introducing exotic infection to the United States, it is important that the clinician be acquainted with certain problems that are not indigenous to this country. A summary of the life cycle and the methods of diagnostic study will be included with each organism.

PROTOZOA

Entamoeba histolytica

Amebiasis has a worldwide distribution and is without a doubt the most important of the parasitic problems regularly encountered by the surgeon in the United States.

Life Cycle, Pathogenesis, and Pathology

Infection with *E. histolytica* is acquired by the ingestion of food or water contaminated with mature cysts. The vegetative form, the trophozoite, is destroyed by hydrochloric acid, whereas the cyst survives gastric transit. Upon exposure to the alkaline milieu of the small bowel, excystation and division occur to form eight metacystic trophozoites (amebic form), which become lodged within the crypts of the cecum. In this locale, the trophozoites usually feed, grow, and multiply as commensals. As fecal material solidifies, encystation of the ameba takes place. The cyst nucleus undergoes two successive mitotic divisions, giving rise to four nuclei in the mature stage. The cyst acquires two types of food inclusions (glycogen masses and chromatoidals), which gradually dissipate. Cysts of *E. histolytica* in cool moist surroundings may remain viable for a month and are resistant to the common germicides as well as chlorinated water. Fortunately, they are destroyed by heat over 50C.[1] Potentially contaminated water should be boiled.

Most trophozoites inhabit the colonic mucosa as commensals, but active tissue invasion will occur under certain conditions. Factors such as the strain or virulence of the organism and host resistance are commonly cited [2] as influencing the ability of the trophozoite to invade. Malnutrition, avitaminosis, dietary factors (a fish or wheat diet), or steroid administration may predispose to infection.[3-5] Bacteria of the gut play a permissive role in the development of invasive amebiasis. Phillips et al [6,7] found that infection did not occur in the germ-free guinea pig until the intestinal tract was contaminated with bacteria (eg *C. perfringens* or *B. subtilis*).

The trophozoites of *E. histolytica* apparently vary considerably in their invasive capability. Trophozoites with invasive properties have a "fuzzy" surface comprised of complex membranous dendritic extensions, which contain lytic enzymes.[8] On contact such surface-active lysosomes are probably released, destroying tissue cells and defensive macrophages and lymphocytes.

Probably as a combination of these factors, *E. histolytica* penetrates the depths of the colonic crypts at separate localities. The initial invasion is usually unaccompanied by inflammatory reaction, and with progressive involvement the muscularis mucosa is penetrated and lateral spread begins. Overlying surface epithelium is then breached, and typical circumscribed flask-shaped ulcers are formed (Fig. 11-1). Ulcers eventually involve the muscularis and become confluent. At this time, bacterial invasion with inflammatory cell reaction is the rule. Although amebic ulcers may be disseminated, they are usually limited to the cecum. Less commonly, there is involvement of the rectosigmoid and other parts of the colon; rarely, the ulcerations may appear in the ileum near the ileocecal junction.[9] On occasion, tissue reaction includes an exuberant fibroblastic, eosinophilic, and lymphocytic response. Such lesions (amebomas) occur in 1 to 5 percent of cases of amebic colitis and may mimic adenocarcinoma or inflammatory bowel disease (Fig. 11-2).[9,10]

With the invasion of trophozoites, mesenteric venules may be entered and the amebae swept into the portal circulation. Most trophozoites are eradicated, but when circumstances are favorable tiny colonies coalesce to form an abscess. Portal hemodynamics favor the right lobe. Within the abscess, trophozoites accumulate at the periphery while the central portion contains variable amounts of blood, necrotic hepatic cellular debris, and leukocytes. The physical appearance of the fluid from an amebic hepatic abscess depends on the age of the lesion. With lesions

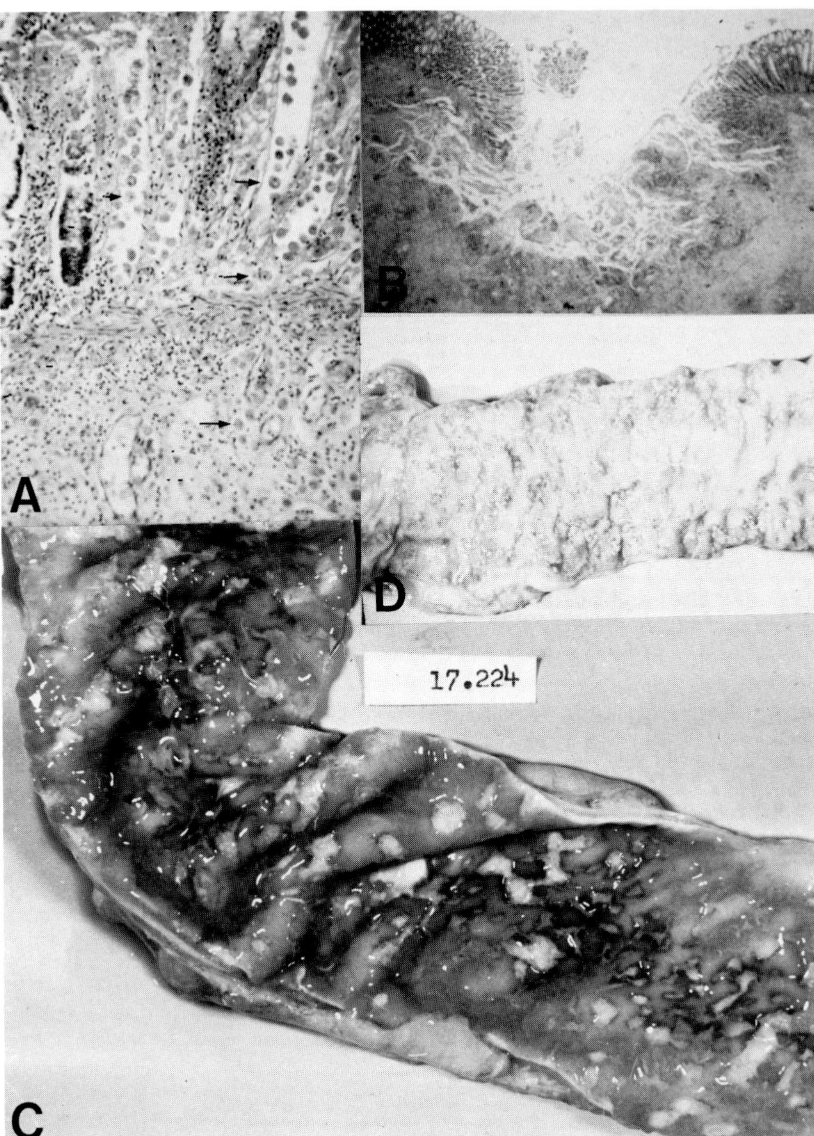

Fig. 11-1. Amebic colitis. A. Histologic section of a colon showing trophozoites of *E. histolytica* within the crypts, lamina propria, and submucosa; little inflammatory response is present. B. Typical flask-shaped ulcer. C. Gross appearance of ulcers in amebic colitis (chronic phase), with normal mucosa between areas of ulceration. D. Secondarily infected amebic colitis grossly resembling chronic ulcerative colitis. (Courtesy of Rudolfo Céspedes.) (Figs. 11-1–11-7 from Monroe LS: Amebiases. In Bockus HL (ed): *Gastroenterology.* Philadelphia, Saunders, 1976, p 165.)

of short duration, 3 weeks or less, the aspirate is thick, usually of a dark red appearance, and usually bacteriologically sterile. When abscesses are older, the contents are often of thinner consistency and may have a marbled appearance (caused by blood streaking) or be pale yellow (Fig. 11-3). The aspirate of such amebic hepatic abscesses, unless secondarily infected, is odorless (in contrast to abscesses produced by anaerobes), a finding that is important to the surgeon who is attempting to determine the etiology of a lesion at the operating table. Amebic abscesses are multiple in 30 percent of the cases, and the majority of single lesions usually arise from a coalition of smaller lesions. Trophozoites of *E. histolytica* collect on the periphery of an abscess and therefore are best demonstrated in the last material to be aspirated.

An enlarging amebic hepatic abscess may rupture into surrounding structures, to produce such complications as bronchohepatic fistula, empyema, pericarditis, or peritonitis (Chapter 36). As a secondary, rare complication to such abscess, metastatic involvement (via the bloodstream) can occur in nearly any part of the body, particularly the lungs, brain, spleen, and kidneys.

Clinical Manifestations

The identification of amebic forms in stool (cysts or trophozoites) does not necessarily indicate infection. In fact, the majority of *E. histolytica* exist as commensals within the gut and are not responsible for any pathologic change. On the other hand, when invasion of the intestine occurs, the resulting symptoms are widely variable. Indeed, some patients without intestinal complaints can harbor invasive trophozoites, which produce symptoms only after invading the liver. Mild diarrhea is the most common manifestation of intestinal involvement. The onset after exposure averages 7 days, and stools are usually watery or poorly formed. As a rule, the initial accompanying systemic manifestations are not prominent, as with the bacillary dysenteries. Acute cecal involvement can produce right lower quadrant pain and localized tenderness, which simulates acute appendicitis. In certain parts of the world, particularly in tropical

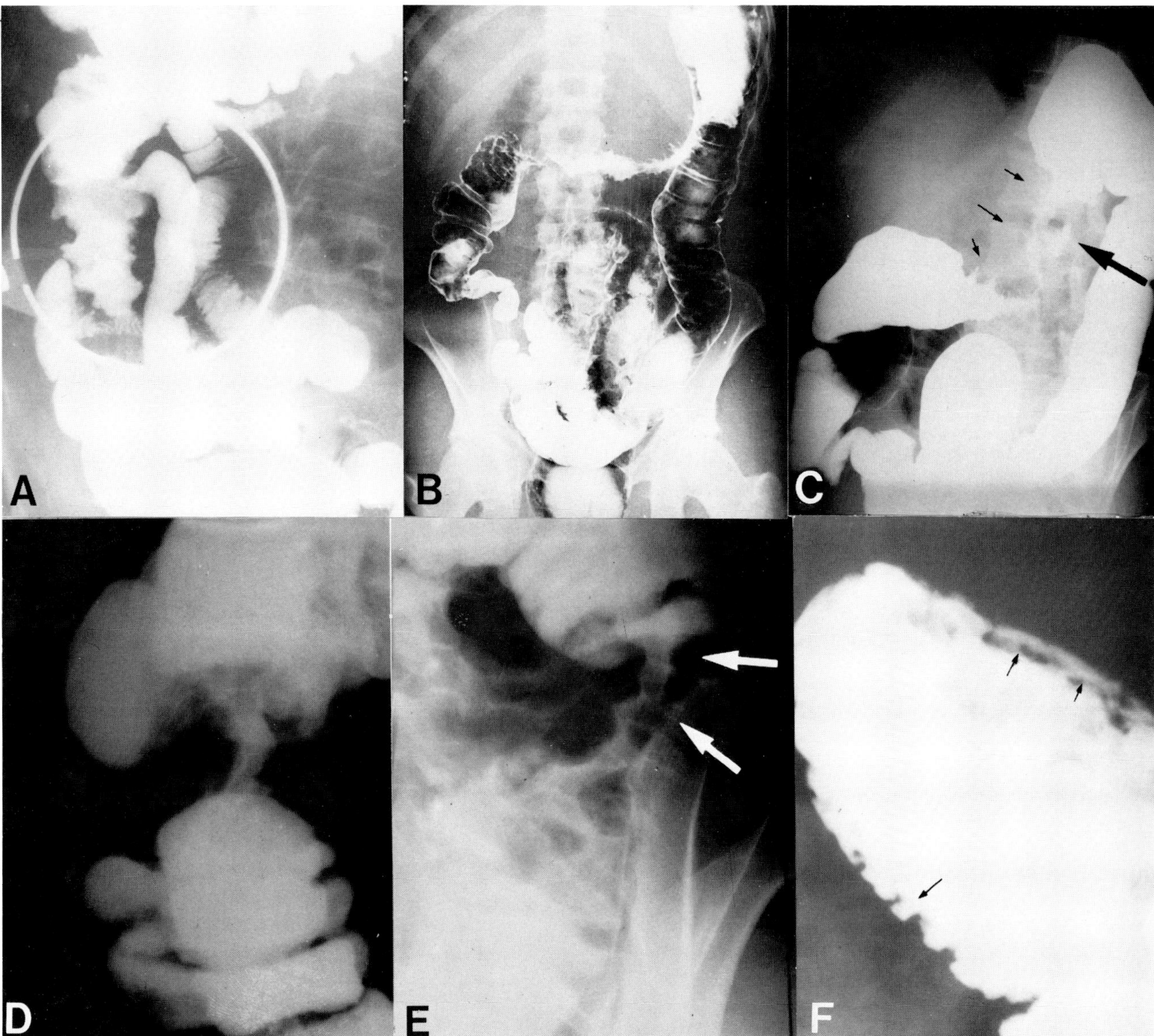

Fig. 11-2. **Radiographic appearance of amebic colitis and amebic granuloma. A. Conical cecum of amebic cecitis. B,C. Segmental involvement of the transverse colon. Note similarity to granulomatous colitis. D. Amebic granuloma (ameboma) of ascending colon, which simulates carcinoma. E. Amebic granuloma, descending colon. F. Collar-button and undermined amebic abscesses. (A–D courtesy Jorge Lega-Siccar, E,F courtesy Robert Berk.)**

zones, acute dysentery with bloody diarrhea, dehydration, and electrolyte losses may occur. Such a fulminant process is more common in the malnourished, elderly, or immunosuppressed patient.[11]

Complications of intestinal amebiasis include perforation, hemorrhage (rare), stenosis, granuloma, and hepatic abscess formation. Chapter 36 contains a detailed description of the clinical manifestation and treatment of amebic liver abscesses (Fig. 11-4). Only a few additional points are discussed here. Secondary infection is reported in 10 to 30 percent of cases.[12] It is probable that modern bacteriologic methods will find coliforms and anaerobes to be the most common offenders; however, staphylococci and streptococci are the most frequently reported organisms. Such secondary infection should be suspected when the patient is unusually toxic, does not respond to antiamebal drugs, and when the liver aspirate is malodorous. Any region of the body can be involved by metastatic amebiasis, and this event is rather uniformly antedated by an amebic hepatic abscess. Brain, lung, and kidney are among the rare sites of such secondary involvement.

Diagnosis

It is paramount for the clinician to be aware of the possibility of amebiasis among the jungle of etiologies that produce such symptoms as diarrhea, hepatomegaly, right upper quadrant pain, right basilar pulmonary lesions. The requisite diagnostic maneuvers are relatively simple. The most precise diagnosis requires the demonstration of some form of *E. histolytica,* and fortunately coprology or examination

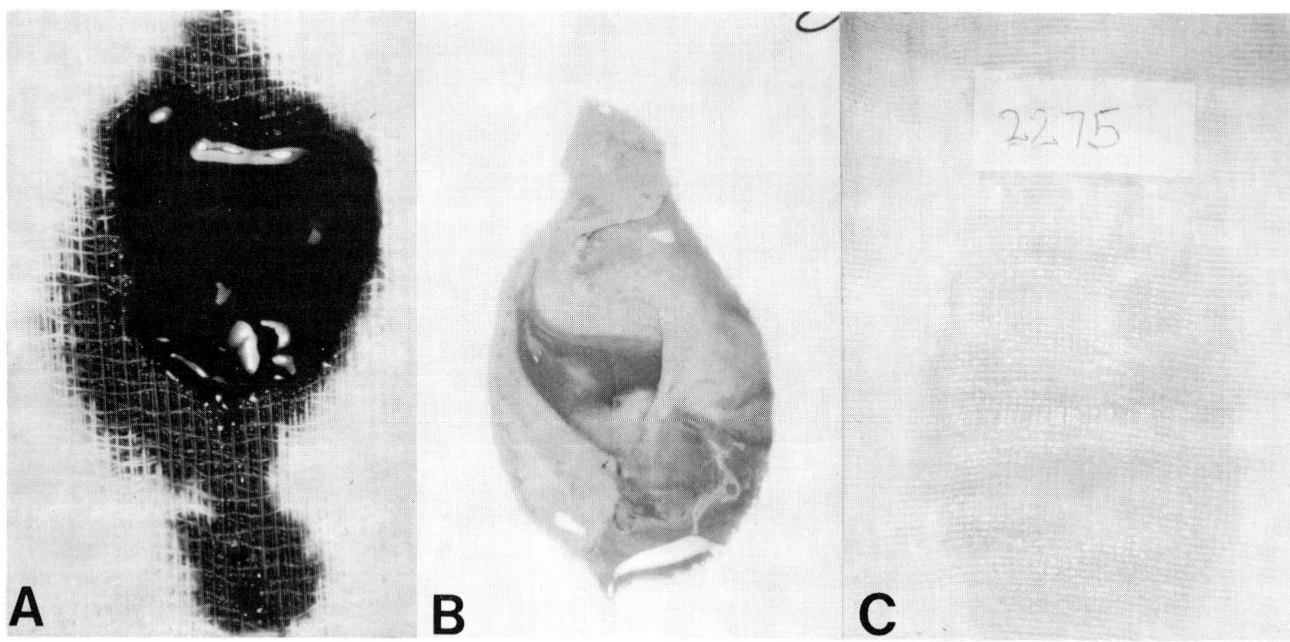

Fig. 11-3. Gross appearance of aspirate from amebic liver abscess. A. Acute (symptoms less than 2 weeks), B. subacute (symptoms less than 3 months), and C. chronic liver abscess (symptoms for longer than 3 months). The aspirate of the chronic abscess has a watery appearance. (Courtesy SJ Powell, Durban, South Africa.)

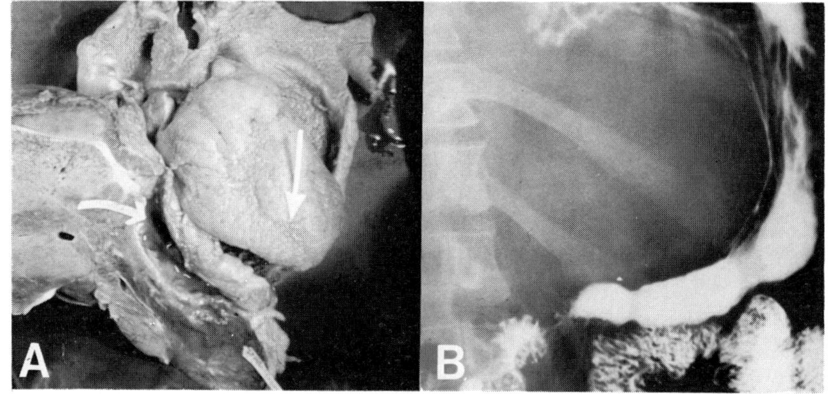

Fig. 11-4. A. Section through the liver showing abscess of the left lobe with perforation into the pericardium and secondary pericarditis. B. Radiograph showing lateral displacement of the stomach by a large left lobe abscess.

of an aspirate is a rapid method. It is important, however, to remember that the majority of persons who harbor *E. histolytica* in the gut have no significant pathology that can be attributable to the organism; also, the demonstration of an amebic form does not necessarily indicate that the symptoms are related. In the stool, amebae may appear intermittently, influenced adversely by medications (mineral oil, kaolin, bismuth, antibiotics) or hypertonic enemas. At the time of sigmoidoscopy, the examining physician should obtain multiple specimens by scraping or aspiration from a suspicious lesion, and such material should be prepared in a saline mount for prompt examination. Pending such microscopy, a heating pad, turned to low setting, makes an ideal slide storage area; the warmth helps preserve the motility of trophozoites. To obtain specimens from an ulcerating lesion of the bowel or skin, the clinician should scrape or aspirate the overhanging margins where the greatest concentration of amebae lie.

In the study of the dysenteric state, laboratory attention should be focused on the demonstration of trophozoites. The ideal material for this purpose is obtained either at sigmoidoscopy or from warm liquid stools after a saline cathartic (sodium sulfate or buffered phosphosoda). Alicna and Fadell [13] have demonstrated that the examination of three specimens on successive days will greatly increase the accuracy of coprology. Trophozoites will be scarce in solid stools, but cyst recovery can be enhanced by using a concentration technique (formalin ether or zinc sulfate). Whenever possible, a positive specimen should be preserved by a permanent staining technique (trichrome or iron hematoxylin). Remember that coprology is a poor method for confirming the presence of an amebic hepatic abscess (less than 50 percent of stools are positive); for this purpose scanning techniques and serology are required (Chapter 36).

Spurred by the development of axenic antigen, which has greatly improved specificity, serologic study has become increasingly important for diagnosis. The tests available from the parasitology division of the Center for Disease Control include precipitin, indirect hemagglutination, complement fixation, latex agglutination, and fluorescent antibody (Table 11-1). Usually, however, the results must be obtained within a short period, so it is important to have serologic testing available to every hospital laboratory. The precipitin test (agar gel diffusion) and the latex agglutination are optimal and avoid the technical difficulties of the other procedures.[14] The agar gel diffusion (done by the Ouchterlony technique) can be done with commercially available axenic antigens, although it requires 48 hours to read. The latex agglutination test, also commercially available, employs antigen-coated particles, and the results are available in less than 1 hour. As both the agar gel diffusion and latex agglutination tests are positive in over 98 percent of the cases with amebic liver abscess, a negative result is also important. Rarely, a case is found that does not develop circulating antibodies to tissue invasion and a false-negative result ensues. Another rare source of false-negative serology is the presence of fulminant infection with antigen excess and binding of circulating antibody. In symptomatic intestinal amebiasis, 70 to 90 percent of serologic tests are positive. In the commensal state, a lower percentage of serologic tests are positive.

Circulating antibodies may persist for years; therefore, in endemic areas, a positive result is not necessarily an indication of a currently active infection. In the United States, however, where the background of infection is extremely low, a positive test is most often accompanied by invasive amebiasis.

Scanning (ultrasound, isotopic, and computerized axial tomography) techniques have been improved to vastly simplify the diagnosis of amebic hepatic abscess (Fig. 11-5) (Chapter 36). Roentgen study of the colon gives important clues (Fig. 11-2). Classical amebic typhlitis is characterized by a conical, stiff-appearing cecum, which is unassociated with involvement of the ileum. It is also important to recognize that an ameboma can manifest a con-

TABLE 11-1. SEROLOGIC TESTS FOR HELMINTHIC AND PROTOZOAL INFECTION

Parasitic infection	Tests available
Protozoa	
Amebiasis	CF, P, H, FA
American trypanosomiasis (Chagas)	CF, H
Nematodes	
Ascariasis/toxocariasis	BF, H
Trichinosis	BF
Cestodes	
Cysticercosis	H
Echinococcosis	CF, BF, H
Trematodes	
Clonorchiasis	CF
Fascioliasis	CF
Schistosomiasis	CF, BF, H, FA

P = precipitin; CF = complement fixation; BF = Bentonite flocculation; H = indirect hemagglutination; and FA = indirect fluorescent antibody. Available at the Center for Disease Control, Atlanta, Georgia.

Fig. 11-5. A. Anterior scintiscan of patient with a huge right lobe abscess. B. Lateral scan. C. High gain ultrasound scan allowing cross-sectional visualization of the liver in the same patient. The fluid-containing abscess appears as a sonulecent (dark, clear) area.

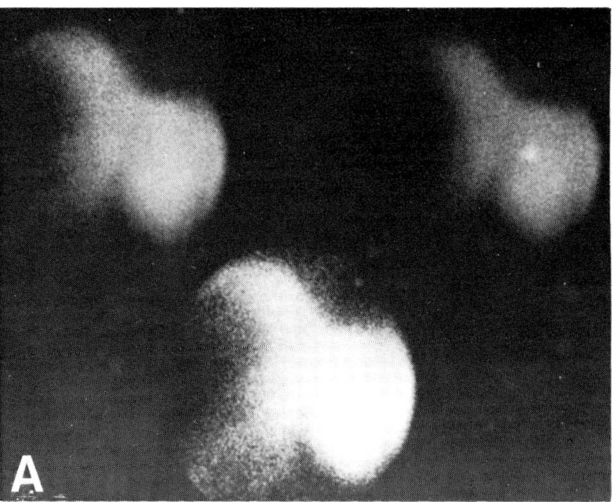

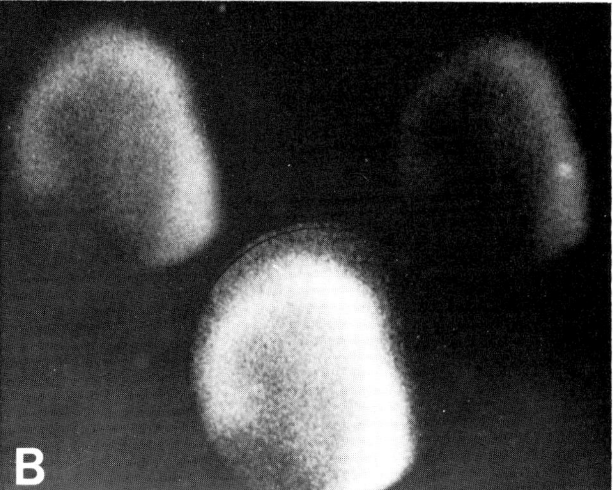

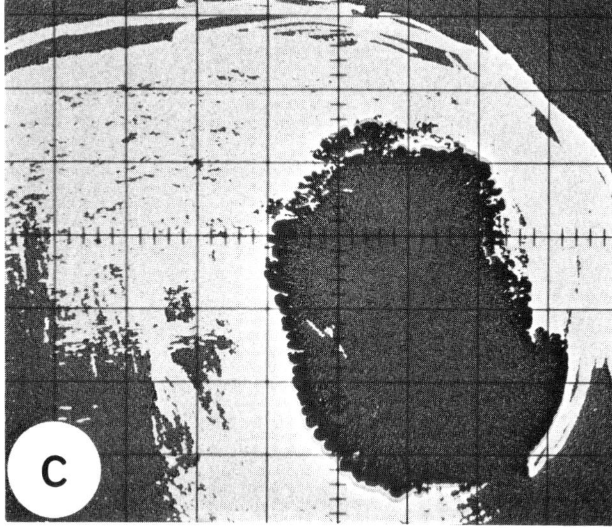

figuration identical to carcinoma or the segmental involvement of Crohn disease.

On rare occasions, colonscopy is useful to differentiate ameboma, carcinoma, or inflammatory bowel disease. The ulcers of amebic colitis can be biopsied through the endoscope.

A therapeutic trial was formerly an important step in the diagnosis of liver abscess. With current scanning and serologic techniques, it is seldom necessary. Further, if metronidazole were to be used in such a regimen, the clinician should be alert to the fact that this drug is effective in certain anaerobic infections [15] so that a clinical response would not necessarily indicate *E. histolytica* as the culprit.

Treatment

The drugs used in the medical treatment of amebiasis are outlined in Table 11-2.[16-18] Most drugs that eliminate cysts

TABLE 11-2. DRUG THERAPY OF ENTAMOEBA HISTOLYTICA

Drugs	Average adult dose (grams)	Duration (days)	Clinical indications	Adverse effects
Direct-acting luminal amebicide				
Quinidine derivatives				
Diiodohydroxyquin, USP	0.65 (3 times daily)	20	Commensal state	Diarrhea, mild iodism, interference with thyroid function tests, subacute myeloptic neuropathy rare
Iodochlorhydroxyquin, USP	0.25 (3 times daily)	10	Commensal state	
Arsenical derivatives				
Carbarsone, USP	0.25 (2 times daily)	10	Commensal state	Potentially toxic to liver and kidneys
Glycobiarsol, USP	0.50 (3 times daily)	7	Commensal state	
*†*Diloxanide furoate*	0.50 (3 times daily)	10	Commensal state	Occasional mild gastrointestinal upset
Indirect-acting luminal amebicides				
Antibiotics				
*Tetracycline, USP	0.50 (4 times daily)	10	Symptomatic intestinal	Diarrhea, staining of teeth in children to 8 years old and in newborn when given to mother after fourth month gestation
Oxytetracycline, NF	0.50 (4 times daily)	10	Symptomatic intestinal	Diarrhea, alteration of bacterial flora
Erythromycin, USP	0.50 (4 times daily)	5–7	Symptomatic intestinal	Diarrhea, alteration of bacterial flora
Tissue amebicide mainly active in the liver				
4-Aminoquinilone				
Chloroquine phosphate, USP	0.50 (2 times daily) then	2	Extraintestinal	Nausea, vomiting, diarrhea, skin eruptions, blood dyscrasias rare
	0.25 (2 times daily)	21		Corneal opacity uncommon, retinal injury when dosage greater than 100 gm
Tissue amebicides effective at all sites				
Nitroimidazole derivatives				
*Metronidazole	0.75 (3 times daily)	10	Symptomatic intestinal and extraintestinal	Diarrhea, vomiting, dizziness, dark urine, depression. Fall in blood pressure with alcohol. Leukopenia
Emetine	0.065 (IM) daily (1 mg/kg)	10	Symptomatic intestinal and extraintestinal	Diarrhea, painful injection site, neuropathy. Potentially toxic to heart, liver, and kidneys
†Dehydroemetine	0.065 to 0.1 (IM) daily (1 to 1.5 mg/kg)	10	Symptomatic intestinal and extraintestinal	

* Drug of choice

† Obtainable from the Parasitology Diseases Division, Center for Disease Control, Atlanta, Georgia.

or trophozoites from the gut do not destroy tissue-invading trophozoites. For example, using diiodohydroxyquin because cysts were found in the stool does not guarantee that amebic liver involvement will not develop. Thus, it is my practice to always include a direct-acting luminal amebicide (ie, diiodohydroxyquin), an indirect-acting amebicide (ie, tetracycline), and a drug active against trophozoites within tissue (metronidazole, emetine, chloroquine).

The surgeon is most often called upon to see a patient suffering from a complication of primary intestinal involvement. Drug therapy should be instituted if emergency tests indicate amebiasis in a perforation of the colon (particularly the cecum), resulting from an "idiopathic" inflammatory process. If such diagnostic testing (serology and stool study) is not immediately available, treatment with a tissue-active drug should be started in the interim.

The treatment of amebic hepatic abscess should be varied depending on the particular situation. Although aspiration of an abscess is a routine procedure in certain parts of the world, local experience with the morbidity and mortality of secondarily infected abscesses has led to a selective approach. Aspiration is undertaken when: (1) there are manifestations of impending perforation, (2) the response to appropriate antiamebics is unsatisfactory in 72 hours, and (3) in left lobe abscess to prevent pericarditis unless response is prompt and dramatic. Open drainage is safer for left lobe abscesses. The techniques of aspiration and open drainage are described in Chapter 37. The abscess should be evacuated as completely as possible, and the last bit of aspirate, which contains the highest concentration of trophozoites, should be submitted for microscopy immediately. Systemic tissue-active amebicides are always indicated in liver abscess and usually have been given before aspiration is undertaken. Bacterial cultures should always be carried out to detect superinfections.

Abscesses that metastasize to distant organs (ie, brain, lung, kidney) carry a high mortality. The treatment, in addition to tissue-active antiamebicides, usually requires surgical drainage of the lesion.

Balantidium coli

Balantidiasis is caused by a ciliated protozoan, *B. coli,* which commonly infects primates, rats, and swine, and has a worldwide distribution. Man, on occasion, can acquire the infection and sometimes develops perforation of the colon or appendix.

Morphology, Life Cycle, and Pathology

The trophozoites of *B. coli* are large, measuring 50–200 μm in their long axis, and as a result can be seen with the naked eye in fresh saline mounts. Configuration of the motile form is slightly lemon-shaped with a prominent cytostome visible at the narrow end. The prominent macro- and micronucleus are distinctive features in stained specimens (Fig. 11-6).[1] Furthermore, in fresh preparations activity of the cilia produces prominent eddy currents about the living organism. The cysts are somewhat smaller than the motile forms and have a prominent macronucleus and refractile cyst wall (Fig. 11-6).

The life cycle of *B. coli* is probably similar to *E. histolytica,* except that many parts of the colon are commonly involved. Protein starvation, vitamin deficiency, and alcoholism may play a permissive role in the establishment of infection. More than 50 percent of infected humans have lived near swine.[19]

Within the colon, *B. coli* most often exists as a harmless commensal; however, when invasion of the epithelium occurs, sloughing ulcers are formed (Fig. 11-6). These do not acquire the overhanging edge often produced by amebic ulceration and are accompanied by an unusual amount of vascular thrombosis and bleeding. In histologic sections, trophozoites may be seen teeming in the exudate and penetrating below the submucosa of an ulcer. Some investigators have reported a hyaluronidase-like substance secreted from the trophozoite and have suggested that this may facilitate tissue invasion. On rare occasions, ulcers of the cecum or appendix may deepen with perforation and the development of peritonitis. Distant metastasis of the parasite is reported, but it is extremely rare.[20]

Clinical Manifestations

Balantidiasis must be considered in any acute diarrheal condition, but especially when the following clinical features are found: (1) close contact with pigs, (2) residence in a tropical area (although the condition has been reported in the United States and Canada), (3) malnutrition, and (4) acute diarrhea with a prominent amount of blood and mucus in the stool. Perforation of a balantidial abscess is often heralded by abdominal pain, rigidity, and diminished bowel sounds. Before the use of tetracyclines in such an acute abdomen, mortality was in the neighborhood of 30 percent.

Diagnosis

Unless the patient has received prior antibiotic treatment, the diagnosis is easily made by examination of material aspirated from ulcerating lesions at the time of proctosigmoidoscopy. Balantidiasis should be considered whenever discrete ulcers with intervening normal mucosa are observed. It should enter into the differential diagnosis of granulomatous colitis and amebiasis. Fortunately, in the usual dysenteric case, the wet preparation teems with organisms, and trophozoites can be identified with the naked eye. The diarrheal stool produced by *B. coli* often has a diffusely bloody or blood-streaked appearance. When stools are solid or semiformed, cysts are found on examination of the stool. As with amebiasis, eosinophilia is not a feature of the infection.[21]

Treatment

For the carrier state or invasive balantidial colitis, the primary treatment is oxytetracycline (average adult dose of 0.5 gm four times a day for 10 days), and an alternate drug is diiodohydroxyquin (0.650 gm three times a day for 20 days). It is needless to observe that in any acute diarrheal condition, fluid and electrolyte replacement is equal in importance to drug therapy. If the clinical signs of perforation appear during the course of an acute balantidial colitis, prompt laparotomy is indicated. Rapid preliminary restoration of fluid and electrolyte balance may be

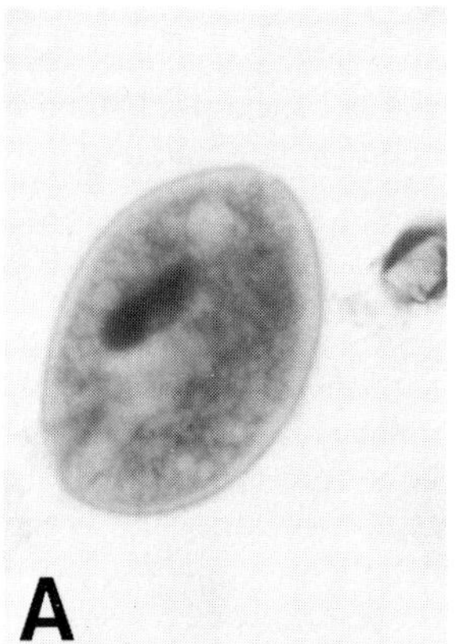

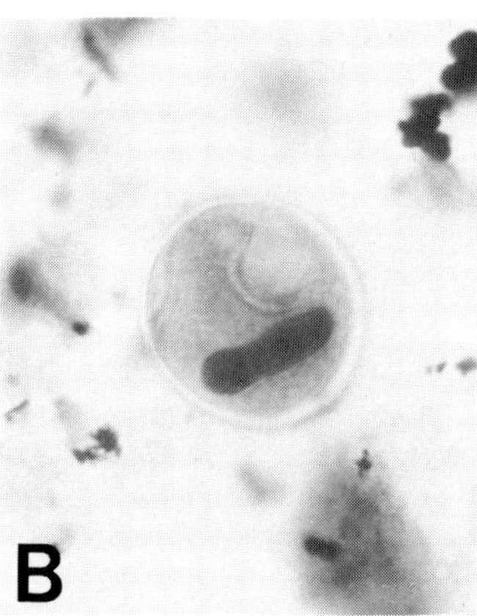

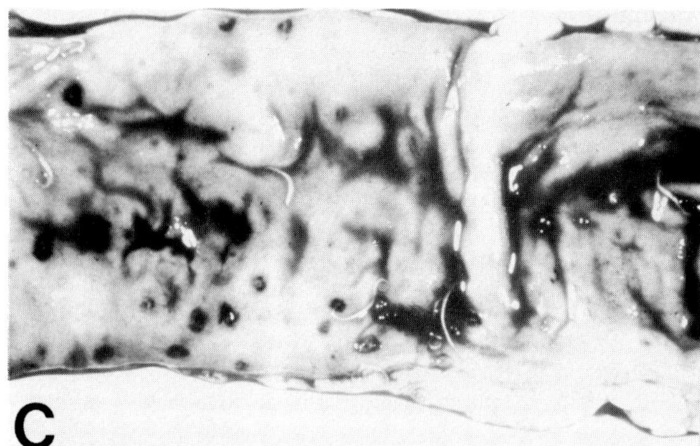

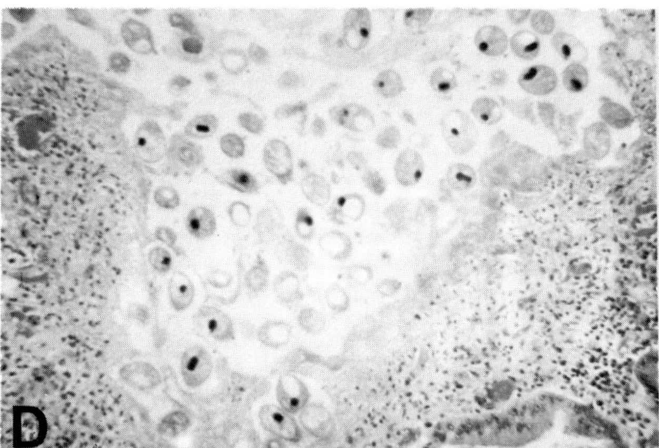

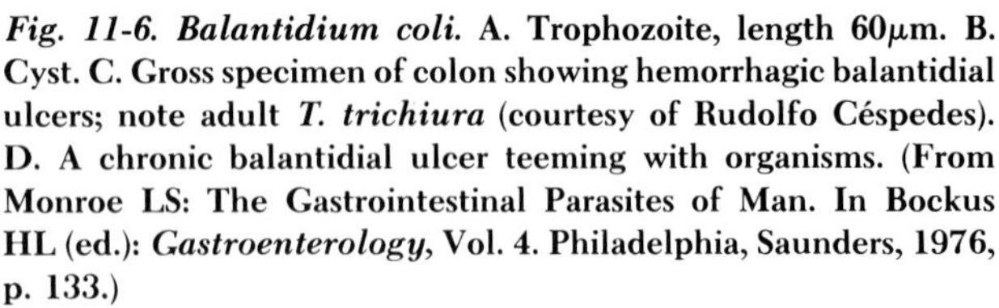

Fig. 11-6. Balantidium coli. **A. Trophozoite, length 60μm. B. Cyst. C. Gross specimen of colon showing hemorrhagic balantidial ulcers; note adult *T. trichiura* (courtesy of Rudolfo Céspedes). D. A chronic balantidial ulcer teeming with organisms. (From Monroe LS: The Gastrointestinal Parasites of Man. In Bockus HL (ed.): *Gastroenterology*, Vol. 4. Philadelphia, Saunders, 1976, p. 133.)**

life saving, because many of these patients are nearly moribund at the time of intestinal perforation.

Trypanosoma cruzi

Infection with *T. cruzi* may result in such gastrointestinal or urinary tract hypomotility that operative intervention is required. American trypanosomiasis (Chagas disease) afflicts approximately 7 million people in the Western Hemisphere, with South America and particularly Brazil harboring the majority of cases. Chagas disease extends northward through Central America to Mexico and is occasionally documented in the southern and southwestern United States.[22,23]

Morphology and Life Cycle

T. cruzi is the only trypanosome to exhibit both leishmanial and trypanosomal stages in man. In the Wright-stained blood smear, the trypanosome assumes a U or C shape and the organism approximates 15–20 μm in length. A posterior kinetoplast and a large centrally placed nucleus characterize the trypanosomal form, while the leishmania contains a large eccentrically placed nucleus with a rod-shaped kinetoplast.[1]

The vertebrate hosts of *T. cruzi* include man and various wild and domestic animals—at least 40 species of triatomids (reduviid bugs) transmit the infection (Fig. 11-7).[24] Infection with Chagas disease is favored by unsanitary rural living conditions and, in particular, primitive habitations containing chinks and cracks that provide hiding for the triatomids. These biting insects emerge at night to seek a blood meal. While feeding, the triatomid defecates, and if the feces contains infective metacyclic forms, the protozoa enter the subcutaneous tissues through the punctured skin. Infection can also be introduced through abraded skin, the conjunctiva, by blood transfusion or, rarely, congenitally via the placenta. Once within the host, the trypanosomes enter macrophages and transform to leishmanias. In turn, the leishmanias spread to local nodes where the parasites multiply by binary fission. From these sites, intermediate forms (crithidial and leptomonas) are carried by the blood and lymph to distant sites throughout the body.

Pathology and Clinical Manifestations

At the original site of infection, an inflammatory reaction characterized by lymphocytes, plasma cells, reticulum cells, and fibroblasts arises. This locus appears as an erythematous nodular (or ulcerated) lesion called a chagoma and is associated with enlargement of regional lymph nodes. An even more common initial lesion is a unilateral facial and orbital edema associated with conjunctivitis (Romaña's sign) (Fig. 11-7). Although the associated fever may continue, the local lesions usually subside within 30 days. In approximately 25 percent of cases, local signs are lacking and the signs of invasion are easily confused with a variety of febrile disease states.[25] During the acute invasive phase, the patient may remain febrile from 4 to 5 weeks, and hepatosplenomegaly may persist for months. In the acute phase, myocarditis may develop with cardiac enlargement, congestive heart failure, and the appearance of first-degree heart block and T wave inversion.

Patients recovering from acute Chagas disease (some are asymptomatic) have a positive complement-fixation test (Machado-Guerreiro reaction). Months to years later, the subacute or chronic manifestations may appear with the development of electrocardiographic conduction defects and arrythmias. Congestive heart failure may result.

The inflammatory reaction that attends leishmanial invasion produces degeneration of ganglion cells—a late

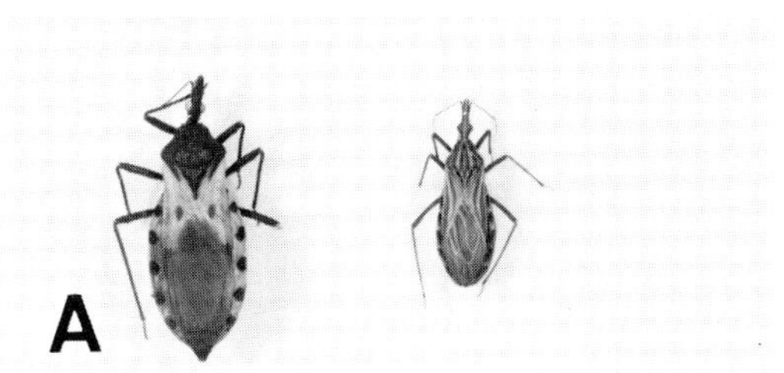

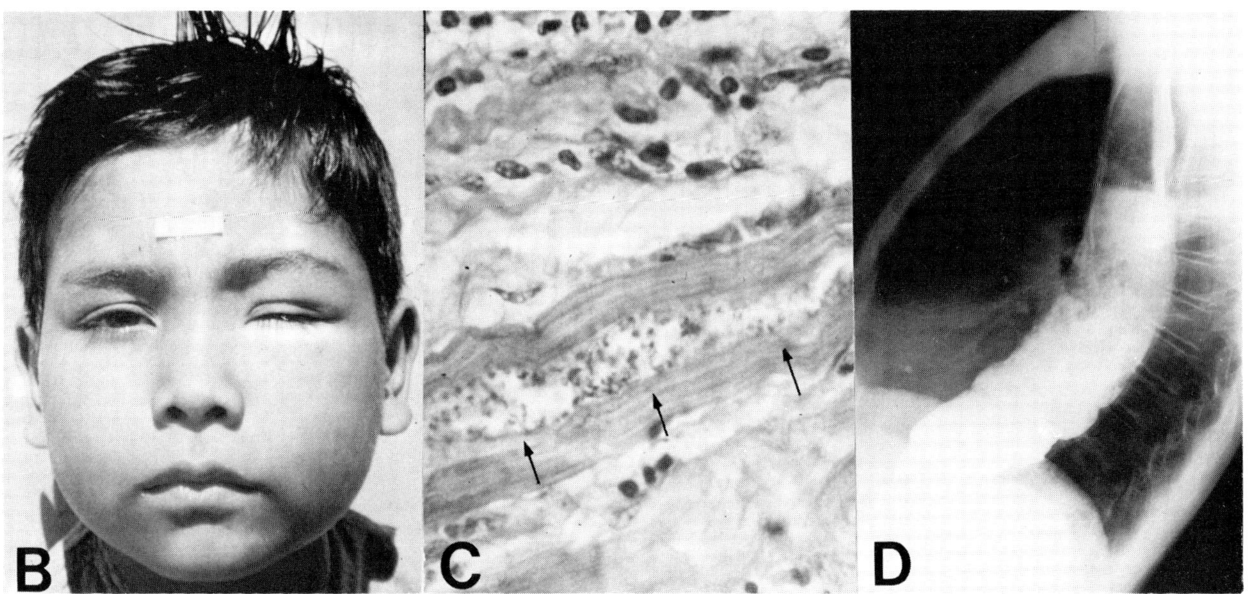

Fig. 11-7. A. Adult (upper) and nymph of triatoma, ***Rhodnius prolixus;*** B. Unilateral facial cellulitis, Romaña's sign. C. Pseudocyst (Leishmanial forms) in the myocardium. D. Megaesophagus caused by Chagas disease (Courtesy Rudolfo Cépedes.) (From Monroe LS: The Gastrointestinal Parasites of Man. In Bockus HL (ed.): *Gastroenterology*, Vol. 4. Philadelphia, Saunders, 1976, p. 133.)

feature of visceral Chagas disease. The symptoms resulting from such loss of ganglion cells are variable. In mild cases, patients may be asymptomatic. Gastrointestinal symptoms develop late and may not appear until 2 to 20 years after the acute infection has subsided. "Megas" of various organs develop, especially the colon and esophagus. Stomach, small bowel, ureters, and bladder are afflicted less often.

With the development of megacolon, the patient develops a slowly progressing constipation. Esophageal stasis may not produce symptoms but often gives rise to dysphagia and regurgitation similar to achalasia. As in the latter condition, secondary complications of aspiration pneumonitis, abscess, and carcinoma may arise.

Diagnosis

The appearance of a lesion suggesting a chagoma or Romaña's sign should, in an endemic area, immediately raise suspicion. Within the first 6 weeks (during the febrile period), the demonstration of trypanosomes in the blood smear or lymph node aspirate is confirmatory. Also during this acute period, xenodiagnosis * is positive in upward of 80 percent of cases.

In the subacute and chronic stages of the disease, the indirect hemagglutination and complement-fixation tests are the most frequently used. Within the first 2 months, the indirect hemagglutination test is most often positive; later, the complement-fixation is positive in over 90 percent of those originally infected (Table 11-1).

In the late stages, the roentgen appearance of the megaesophagus is indistinguishable from that of achalasia (Fig. 11-7), and the manometric profile is similar. The roentgen configuration of Chagas megacolon is one of uniform dilatation and atony, resembling secondary megacolon rather than Hirschsprung disease with the narrow bowel segments demonstrable in this latter condition.

Treatment

Although patients with acute Chagas disease are often treated with such antitrypanosomal drugs as nitrofurans, 8-aminoquinolones, and metronidazole, there is no currently satisfactory medical treatment.[24] An investigational drug, Bayer 2052, is available from the Parasitology Division, Center for Disease Control.[16] With the development of megaesophagus, the patient should be treated as for achalasia. This includes elevation of the head of the bed to prevent nocturnal regurgitation and the institution of bag or balloon dilation (bouginage is not satisfactory, as the lower sphincter will not be sufficiently weakened by this procedure). It is doubtful that surgery is often warranted in view of the generally satisfactory results reported from dilation—45 percent cured, 51 percent improved.

* An uninfected triatomid is allowed to bite and consume blood from a suspected case. The feces of the insect is then examined for metacyclic trypanosomes at biweekly intervals for a period of 2 months before the test is declared negative.

When surgery is undertaken, a Heller procedure or subtotal esophagectomy has been advocated.[26] Ferriera-Santos [26] reports carcinoma in 10 percent of 75 cases of esophageal surgery for Chagas disease.

Softeners (such as dioctyl succinate) and enemas have value to prevent impaction. Particularly in children, such enemas should be of physiologic saline to avoid water intoxication. Rarely, hemorrhage from a stercoraceous ulcer, obstruction, or perforation will mandate surgery. Patients who are completely obstipated are usually poor risks and may require proximal colostomy for decompression and the removal of impacted stool. Resection of the rectosigmoid is a more definitive procedure when the patient's condition permits.

HELMINTHS

NEMATODES

Anisakis marina

Fully developed (third stage) ascaris-type larvae of the genus *Anisakis* are capable of producing an ulcerative and granulomatous lesion of both the upper and lower gastrointestinal tracts (anisakiasis). Originally described as "Herringworm disease," it is contracted by the ingestion of raw or partially cooked marine fish.[27] Although the majority of cases have been reported from The Netherlands or Japan, the infection may be considered in any maritime area where raw fish is consumed, ie, Mexico and California.

Morphology and Life Cycle

The adult *A. marina* is a nematode inhabiting the intestinal tracts of whales, porpoises, seals, and sea lions. Although the details of the life cycle are largely unknown, the immature eggs are probably discharged with the feces into the sea, where larvae develop within plankton, which are eaten by fish. The marine mammal acquires the infection through this fish diet (Fig. 11-8). The third stage larvae that inhabit fish or accidentally infect people are slender and measure 1–2 cm in length. A larval tooth and three labia characterize the anterior portion. In histologic cross-section the lateral cords, forming a Y-shaped structure, are a distinctive feature.[28] The apparent recent increase in reported cases may have been due to the changes in the methods of fish preparation, eg, no longer filleting fish immediately after a catch. The refrigeration of whole fish allows larvae to migrate from the gut mesenteries into the musculature.

Pathology and Clinical Features

Following consumption of infected raw fish, the larvae burrow into the gut mucosa, where an ulcerative and granulomatous lesion is formed. The stomach is more often involved than the small bowel and colon. Perforation is rare but may occur at any site from the stomach to the colon. Repeated invasion with subsequent sensitization may help enhance tissue reactivity. Histologically, the lesion appears as an eosinophilic granuloma, and occasionally the etiology is recognized when the larva is identified within the reactive tissue.

Crampy abdominal pain and fever are primary manifestations and may persist for months. Perforation is accompanied by signs of peritonitis.

Diagnosis

Although it is rare for the diagnosis to be made before laparotomy, anisakiasis should be considered whenever a patient who eats raw fish develops acute and chronic abdominal symptoms.[29] In chronic infection, roentgen study may reveal stenotic lesions of the bowel simulating Crohn disease. Ishimura et al,[30] in a review of presumed regional enteritis in Japan, found 13 of 50 to have been caused by *A. marina*. Other than the identification of the larva within the lesion, there is no reliable way to diagnose the infection.[31] Eosinophilia is inconstant, varying from 3 to 34 percent.

Treatment

In that rare circumstance in which the clinician is highly suspicious of anisakiasis, a medical trial with thiabendazole might prove worthwhile. Most patients undergo resection of the afflicted portion of the intestinal tract without a preoperative diagnosis. Operation carries a high mortality, and staphylococcal enteritis is a common complication.

Phocanema decipiens

The "codworm" or "seal worm" known as *Phocanema decipiens* (*Ascaris decipiens*, *Porrocaecum decipiens*, and *Terranova decipiens*) is a close relative of *A. marina*. The morphology of the infective third- and fourth-stage larvae is similar to *A. marina* and is characterized by an anterior portion with three prominent lips having dentigerous ridges (Fig. 11-9). The cuticle is thick, with fine transverse striations.[32] The life cycle is identical to that of *A. marina*, and most infections occur following the ingestion of Pacific halibut or cod.[33] These nematodes do not invade, and most infections involve the stomach transiently, are seen on gastroscopy, or the worms are coughed up. Removal of the helminths with the biopsy forceps has produced symptomatic relief.

Angiostrongylus costaricensis

In Central America, an occasional eosinophilic granuloma in the terminal ileum, appendix, or cecum is caused by this nematode. In 1971, Morera and Cespedes described *A. costaricensis* (a metastrongylid), defined its life cycle, and located the adults in the mesentery of the small bowel.[34,35]

Morphology and Life Cycle

The adult male and female *A. costaricensis* range from 20–33 mm in length and possess a cephalic extremity that lacks a buccal capsule. The morphologic details of the adults and larvae forms are best described by Morera.[36]

The adult worms inhabit the mesenteric arterioles of various species of rats. Embryonated eggs enter the bowel and exit with the feces. The intermediate larval stages

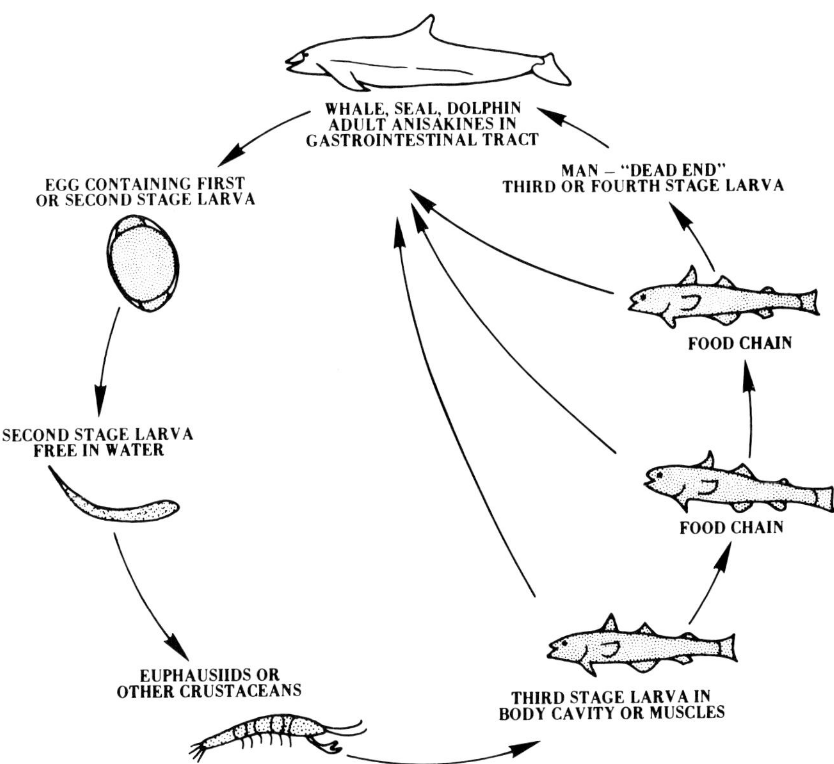

Fig. 11-8. Suspected life cycle of anisakine larvae (Courtesy of Armed Forces Institute of Pathology 76-6006.)

develop within the common garden slug, and the infective third-stage larvae are extruded with the slime as the mollusk travels. Rats and people acquire the infection through the ingestion of contaminated vegetables. From the gut, the larvae pass through the local lymphatics and penetrate the lumen of the mesenteric arteries, where maturation occurs (Fig. 11-10).

Pathology and Clinical Features

A granulomatous tissue response with abundant eosinophils and plasma cells develops in the mesentery, bowel wall, and lymphatics. Although the condition has been recognized from the terminal ileum to the ascending colon, the appendix and cecum are most commonly invaded. The adults reside in the vessels at a distance from the bowel wall and will not be included in the usual surgical specimen.

Abdominal pain and fever are the earliest symptoms. A mass in the right lower quadrant suggests an appendiceal abscess or tumor. Leukocytosis is variable, sometimes reaching 50,000 white blood cells per mm ^{3}. Roentgen examination may reveal a stenotic lesion of the bowel. Eosinophilia is usually a prominent feature and may give a clue to diagnosis.

Diagnosis and Treatment

Because the eggs and larvae of *A. costaricensis* are not recognized in the stool, most cases are diagnosed as a bowel lesion before operation. A precipitin reaction has been developed for the diagnosis; however, clinical correlation is lacking.[37] When a partial obstruction of the ileum or a mass that resembles an appendiceal abscess is associated with an eosinophilia and occurs within an endemic area (Central America), this diagnosis should be considered. Most of these patients do well after resection of the inflammatory mass and the involved mesentery.

Ascaris lumbricoides

The large nematode *A. lumbricoides* is the most prevalent helminthic infection. In certain parts of the world, more

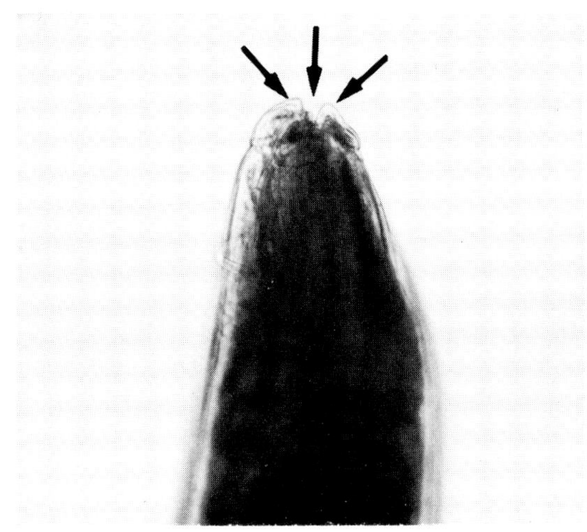

Fig. 11-9. Phocanema species, showing three prominent lips. This specimen was coughed up by a Mexican woman 48 hours after the ingestion of raw fish.

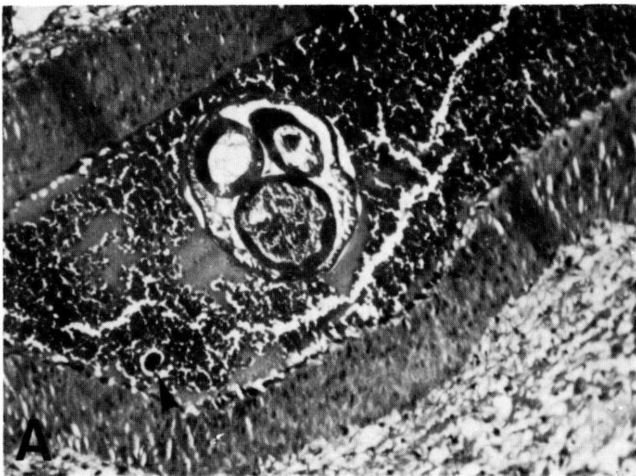

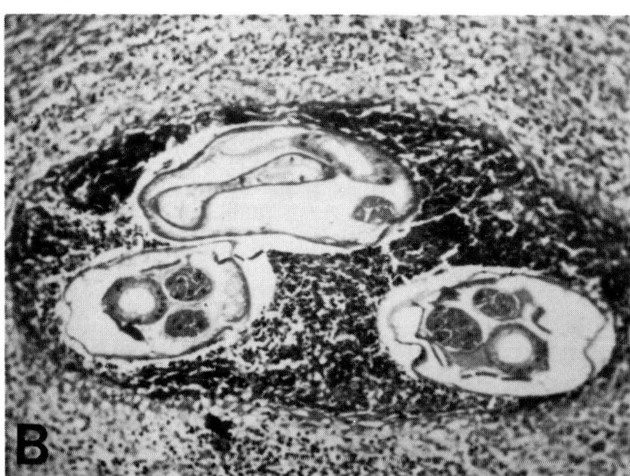

Fig. 11-10. An adult *Angiostrongylus costaricensis* is shown in A. the lumen of a colonic mesenteric artery, and in B. vascular space with surrounding inflammatory reaction. The arrow points to a thin-walled ovoidal egg. (Courtesy Rudolfo Céspedes.) (From Monroe LS: The Gastrointestinal Parasites of Man. In Bockus HL (ed.): *Gastroenterology*, Vol. 4. Philadelphia, Saunders, 1976, p. 133.)

than 90 percent of the population harbor the parasite. The condition is ubiquitous but is more common in humid tropical areas, particularly when night soil is used as a fertilizer. Accumulations of these worms produce intestinal obstructions. The helminth has a propensity for entering small orifices—a habit that frequently produces a biliary tract or a pancreatic manifestation.

Morphology and Life Cycle

The adult male *A. lumbricoides* resembles a large pale earthworm, measuring 15–31 cm in length and 2–4 mm in diameter, and is easily identified by a sharp central curve to the tail, and the presence of a pair of copulatory spicules.[1] The female is somewhat larger, and a single fertile female can extrude an average of 200,000 eggs per day, so the concentration of eggs in the feces is enormous.

Fertilized eggs pass via the feces; they are extremely resistant to the usual methods of water purification and may retain their infectious potential for up to 6 years.[38] When ingested, the larvae erupt and penetrate the small intestine wall to reach the mesenteric lymphatics or portal venules. They proceed to the lungs and, after a few days, rupture into the alveolar spaces. The larvae then migrate up the bronchial tree, are swallowed, and reach the small intestine, where maturation occurs in about 70 days.

The morphology of the eggs of ascaris species is variable (Fig. 11-11). The unfertilized ova are slightly longer than the fertilized eggs and lack a distinctive internal structure. Fertilized eggs have two outer envelopes, and as maturation proceeds internal cellular division takes place.

Clinical Manifestations and Diagnosis

Maximal larval migration occurs 5 to 6 days after infection, through pulmonary arteries, and is often accompanied by pulmonary symptoms. Patients develop chills, fever, cough, dyspnea, and asthmatic attacks. Examination reveals corresponding bronchial rales, and roentgen examination may demonstrate the changes of a bronchopneumonia or an infiltrate that suggests miliary tuberculosis. After about 10 days, the symptoms begin to subside, over a period to 3 weeks. The degree of symptomatology is related to previous exposure, which produces sensitization, and the size of the original larval inoculum.

By far the most troublesome complication of ascariasis is the development of intestinal obstruction (Fig. 11-12). Ascarids have a tendency to intertwine themselves. In infants, as few as 10 worms can occlude the ileum, the most vulnerable site in all age groups. When obstruction occurs, abdominal distention, nausea and vomiting, and variable degrees of obstipation develop. Abdominal scout films can be helpful, and stool studies (if stool can be obtained from the rectal ampulla by digital exam) should reveal *Ascaris* eggs. A soft periumbilical mass has been described. Intestinal obstruction is sometimes associated with intussusception or volvulus.

Perforation of the bowel, secondary to ascarid obstruction, may occur at any level. For example, an ascarid intruding into the lumen of the appendix may produce an abscess with perforation. *A. lumbricoides* also has a propensity to invade the site of a recent intestinal anastomosis, with subsequent perforation. When the helminth enters into the peritoneal cavity, localized or generalized peritonitis may occur. On occasion, ascarids may enter the peritoneum without inducing pain, but will produce a syndrome characterized by an abdominal mass, leukocytosis, and fever. Such entry occasionally occurs without a demonstrable site of gut perforation.

Ascarids may migrate into the biliary and pancreatic tree, causing cholangitis and pancreatitis. In localities such as the Far East where worm burdens are highest, such hepatic infections are called "Hong Kong liver." In addition, the irritant effects of eggs produce granulomatous lesions and an exuberant cholangitis with pylephlebitis. Such involvement of the biliary system is usually accompanied by hepatomegaly and liver tenderness. Leukocystosis

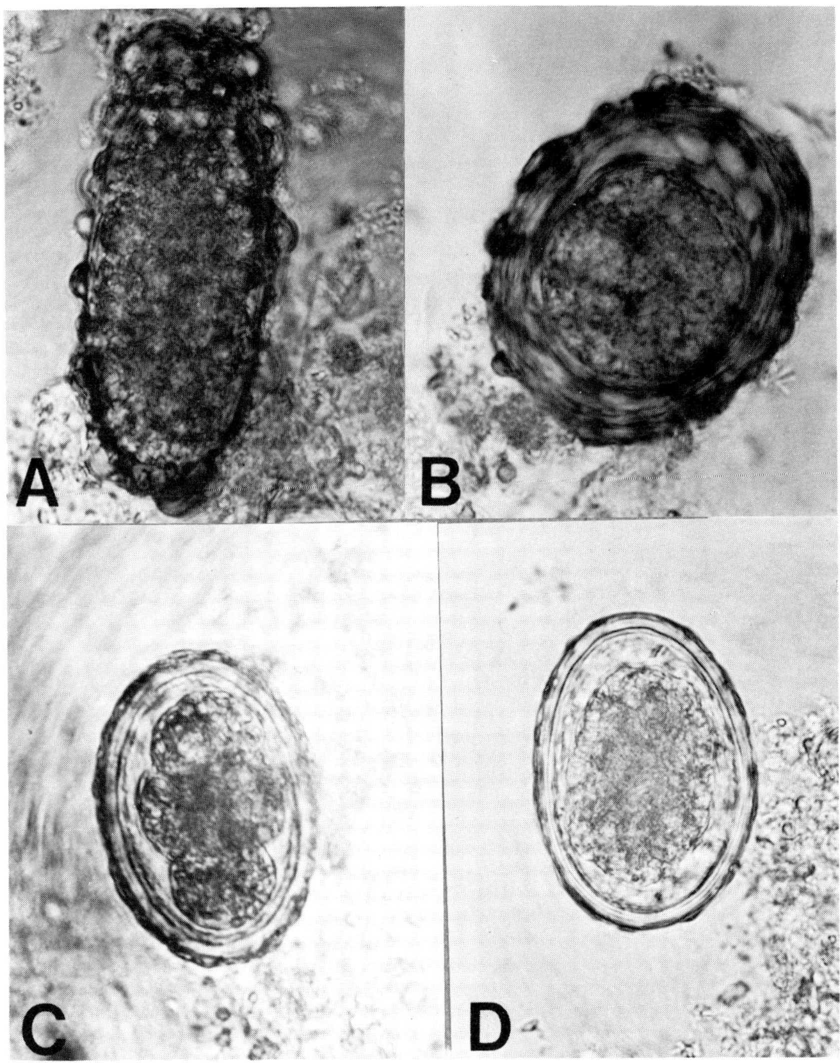

Fig. 11-11. Morphologic variations in the eggs of *Ascaris lumbricoides:* A. unfertilized, B. fertilized, C. 4-cell state, and D. decorticate egg (actual length 50–90 μm). (From Monroe LS: The Gastrointestinal Parasites of Man. In Bockus HL (ed): *Gastroenterology,* Vol. 4. Philadelphia, Saunders, 1976, p. 133.)

varies from 12,000 to 20,000 white blood cells per mm^3, and eosinophilia is usually mild. Rarely, ascarids reach an arterial lumen, pulmonary parenchyma, eustachian tube, or larynx.

Treatment

Uncomplicated intestinal ascariasis requires only the administration of an appropriate drug (levamisole,[39] mebendazole, and pyrantel pamoate are currently preferred, with piperazine derivatives being an effective alternative) (Table 11-3). Such drug therapy is 77 to 100 percent effective, and the side effects are minimal. If complications that require operations occur, medical therapy should be instituted after recovery.

Intestinal obstruction produced by ascariasis is an emergency. If it is recognized, nonoperative therapy is sometimes effective. This consists of: (1) fluid and electrolyte replacement, (2) nasogastric suction for the relief of distention and vomiting, and (3) enemas with physiologic saline to remove ascarids that clog the colon. If vomiting subsides within 4 to 6 hours, suction is discontinued and drugs (Table 11-3) are instilled via the nasogastric tube. On the other hand, if obstruction is not relieved within 24 hours, an operation should be undertaken. The simplest procedure is to milk the worm bolus from the ileum into the large bowel. Enemas can complete the evacuation most easily if the bolus of worms is small. When the obstruction in the ileum cannot be dislodged, resection with end-to-end anastomosis is recommended. A simple enterotomy to extract the ascarids frequently leads to infection and disruption of suture lines.

If biliary or pancreatic ascariasis is suspected and eggs are in the stool, primary drug treatment should be initiated. When symptoms do not abate after 3 weeks, an exploration is in order. Removal of helminths from the biliary or pancreatic systems may be instrumental in relieving the manifestations of acute cholangitis or pancreatitis. Surgical cholangiography and pancreatography are important to rule out the presence of residual helminths. Little can be done with the development of ascaris liver abscess, other than using drugs and operative cleansing of the ductal system.

Helminths in ectopic locations will seldom be diagnosed preoperatively. When they are encountered, simple

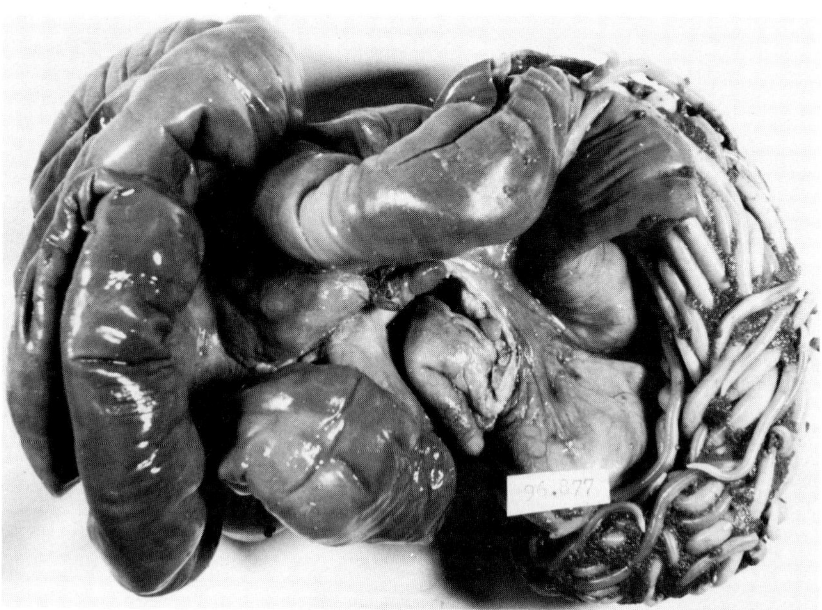

Fig. 11-12. Autopsy specimen of ascarids producing intestinal obstruction and bowel necrosis (Courtesy of Rodolfo Céspedes.)

removal usually suffices with a search subsequently for residual infecting worms.

Dirofilaria Species

Infection with *Dirofilaria* sp. (heartworm) is cosmopolitan in certain carnivores, including dogs and cats. In people, this parasitosis may appear as a subcutaneous swelling, a coin lesion of the lung, or rarely as an adult parasite within the cardiovascular system. More than 70 cases of human dirofilariasis have been recognized.[40]

Life Cycle and Pathology

The adult worm is most often found within the right heart and pulmonary artery of a dog, where microfilariae are released into the bloodstream. Mosquitoes are intermediate hosts to the microfilariae and transmit the infection to definitive hosts, including man. As man is a poor host, it is unusual to have adult parasites develop within the pulmonary artery or right heart, and as a rule, involvement is not associated with symptoms. Microfilaremia does not occur within humans, and the parasite typically produces a pulmonary infarct [40,41] or subcutaneous mass.[42,43]

D. tenuis produces a subcutaneous inflammatory swelling in the raccoon and is believed by some to be the chief cause of cutaneous masses caused by dirofilariasis in people (Fig. 11-13). *D. conjunctivae,* a related species, relies on the raccoon as a host and can produce an inflammatory mass of the eye in humans. The intermediate host of *D. conjunctivae* is the flea.[44] In humans, *D. immitis* microfilariae produce an infarct within the small branches of the pulmonary artery. The resultant roentgen picture may appear as a coin lesion, which simulates early cancer. Inflammation is characterized by fibrosis with masses of eosinophils and plasma cells. When recognized, the adult helminth has a finely cross-striated cuticle with inner thick tall muscular cords (Fig. 11-13) Although absence of longitudinal ridges on the cuticle would indicate *D. immitis,* exact species identification depends on the morphology of the caudal portion of the adult male.

Clinical Features and Diagnosis

Heartworms in the dog can produce cor pulmonale or pulmonary disease. In humans, less than six cases of right heart involvement have been reported. The infection is usually asymptomatic but may cause subcutaneous masses or pulmonary coin lesions. Other than the identification of a helminth within infected tissue, there is no reliable diagnostic tool. Serologic tests using antigen from *D. immitis* have satisfactory sensitivity, but the specificity is not satisfactory.

Treatment

Although drugs are used to treat canine heartworm, the disease in humans does not require treatment except to exclude cancer or explain subcutaneous masses.

Dracunculus medinensis

Infection with the nematode *D. medinensis* occasionally produces an erythematous, serpiginous tract in the subcutaneous tissue. Blisters usually develop in the skin of the lower extremities, where the gravid female discharges larvae (Fig. 11-14). Dracunculiasis occurs predominantly in Africa and Asia, although cases have been reported from the West Indies to South America.[45]

The adult females are extremely long, 70–120 cm, in contrast to the tiny male, which averages 12–29 mm.[45] The larvae, discharged from the gravid female, enter a freshwater cyclops. People are infected by drinking water containing such parasitized copepods. Within the gut, the larvae penetrate the intestinal wall to enter the retroperitoneal tissues, where maturation and fertilization occur. After about 12 months, the females migrate to the subcutaneous tissues and subsequently penetrate the skin to discharge their larvae. Infection is usually recognized by the appearance of either a long subcutaneous tract or cutaneous blister (Fig. 11-15A). At times, a portion of the nematode may protrude from the skin.

Treatment consists of dissection and removal of the worm. The classic maneuver of winding the protruding

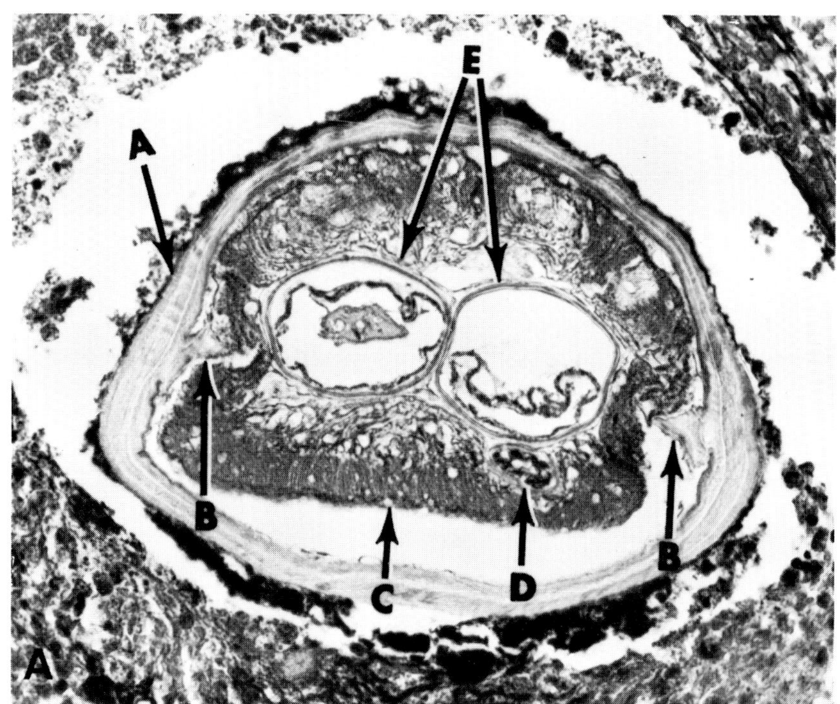

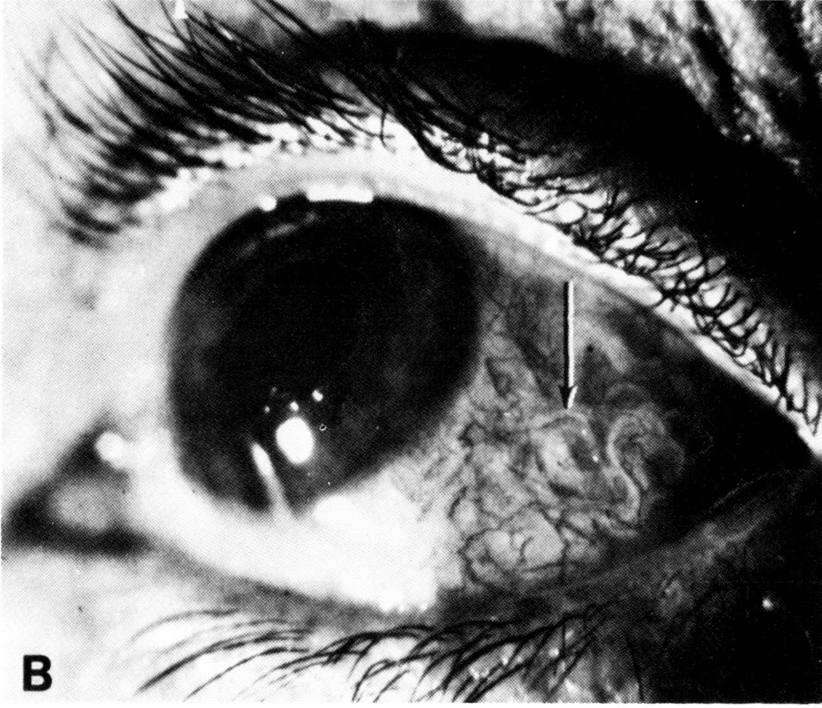

Fig. 11-13. **A. Lung, *D. immitis*, immature female. A. cuticle, B. cuticular ridge, C. muscle, D. intestine, and E. uterus. B. *D. tenuis* in conjunctiva of eye. (Courtesy of Armed Forces Institute of Pathology 71–11563 and 74–6351–2.)**

nematode on a stick is not recommended, because the worm can rupture, with a resultant violent tissue reaction (Fig. 11-15B). Thiabendazole and metronidazole are effective in killing the worm but should not be substituted for removal.

Enterobius vermicularis

A plague to nervous parents, the ubiquitous pinworm is rarely the cause of any concern to the surgeon. The importance of *E. vermicularis* lies in the fact that the helminth can be incidentally found in surgical specimens, particularly the appendix or fallopian tubes. In addition, it should be considered as a rare cause of inflammatory reactions in these areas.

The adults (Fig. 11-16, A and B) inhabit the right colon (cecum and appendix) and the adjacent small bowel. The gravid females migrate to the rectum and during the night pass through the sphincter to deposit their eggs on the perineal surfaces. Eggs are relatively resistant to drying and disinfectants, and when ingested complete the simple oral-anal cycle. The symptoms of infection are usually ex-

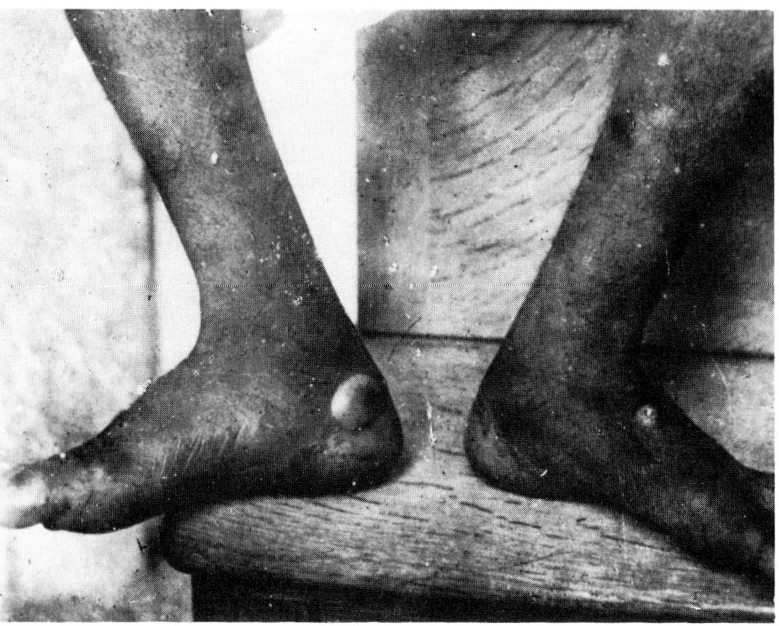

Fig. 11-14. Typical blister produced by a gravid female of *D. medinensis* after approaching the skin surface to discharge larvae. (Courtesy Armed Forces Institute of Pathology N-81418.)

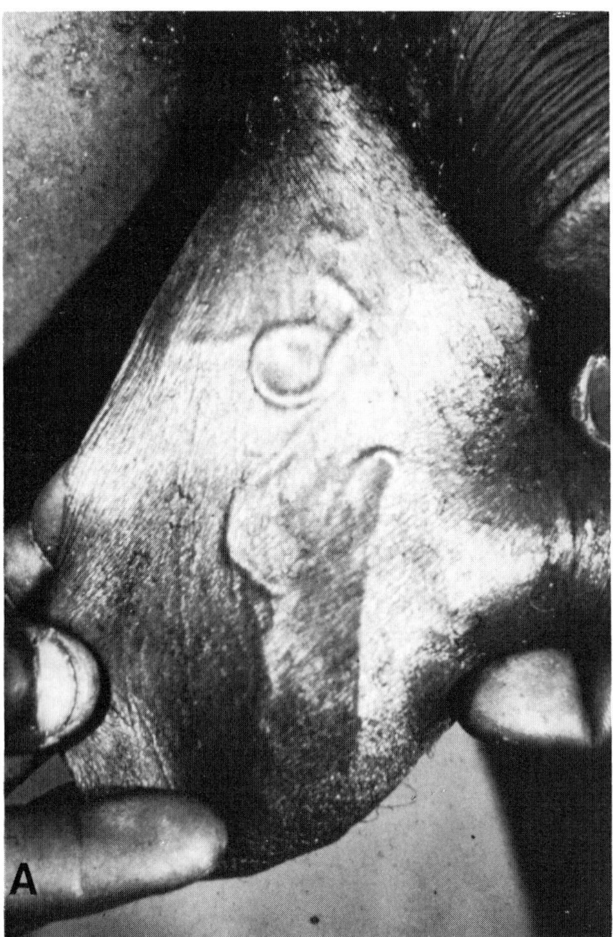

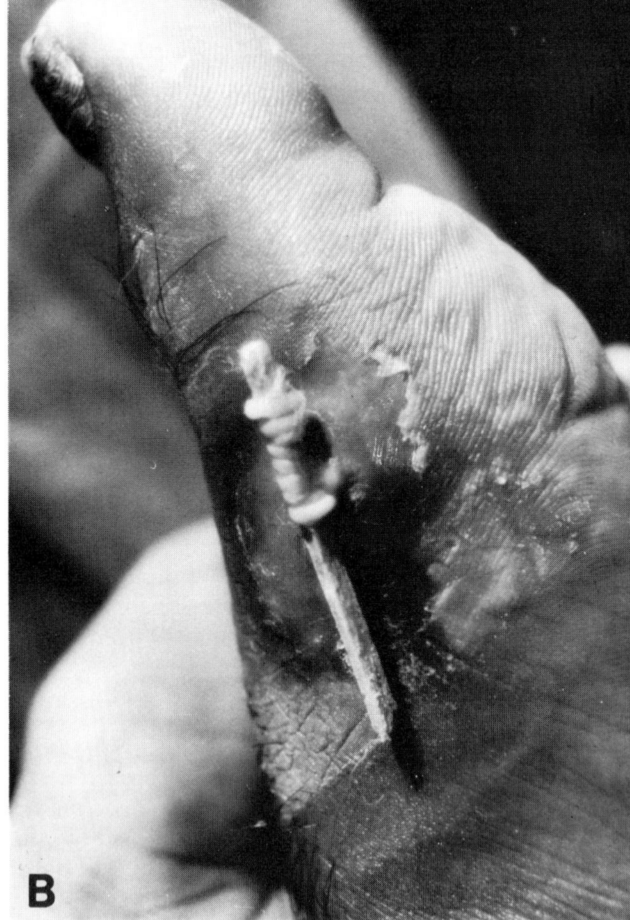

Fig. 11-15. D. medinensis. A. The tortuous tract of the female is evident in the subcutaneous tissue of the scrotum. (Courtesy Armed Forces Institute of Pathology, 67–1563–6; contributed by Dr. Everett L. Schiller.) B. The folk remedy of winding the protruding *D. medinensis* on a stick—not recommended.

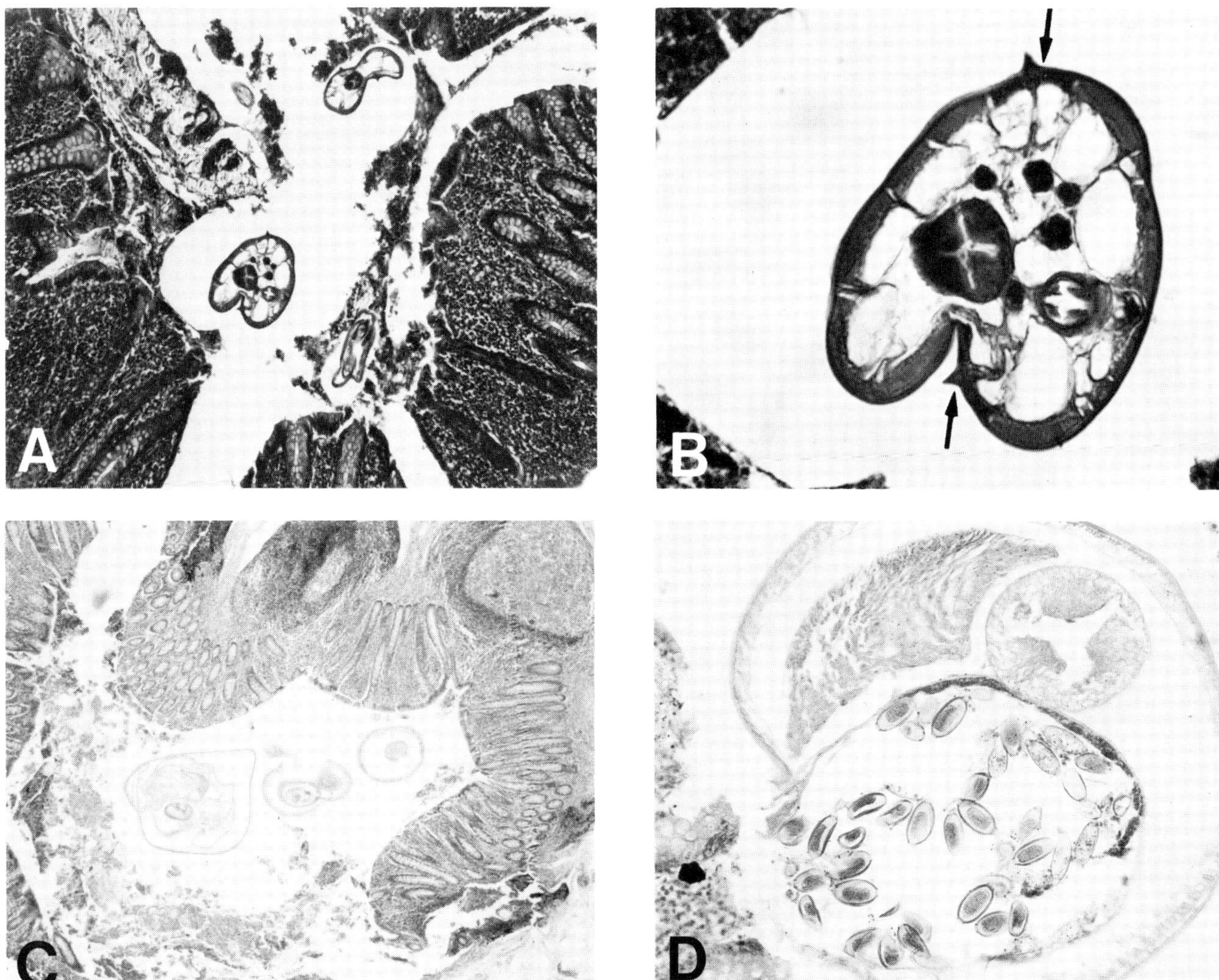

Fig. 11-16. A. An appendix containing transverse sections of *E. vermicularis* (×47). B. Enlarged (×190), the lateral alae is apparent. C. An appendix containing transverse sections of female *T. trichiura* (×47). D. Enlarged to show eggs with bipolar plugs (×190).

ceedingly mild and are limited to a pruritus produced by the ovipositing female. The role of enterobiasis in the production of acute appendicitis is probably minimal, but convincing cases are reported.[46] Migrating gravid females may pass through the vagina and produce an endometritis, salpingitis, or granulomatous nodules within the peritoneal cavity.[47] The diagnosis of enterobiasis is based on the recovery of typical eggs in stool specimens, from fingernail dirt, or by the cellophane tape technique (clear adhesive tape is placed sticky side down on the uncleansed perineum and then transferred to a slide for microscopic examination). Drug treatment is outlined in Table 11-3 and one of those listed should be given to all members of a family.

Gongylonema pulchrum

The plasmid nematode *G. pulchrum,* the scutate threadworm, is a cosmopolitan parasite of ruminants and other mammals. In humans the adult helminths occasionally burrow beneath the submucosa of the stomach, esophagus, and oral cavity to be seen as serpiginous submucosal elevations.[48] Occasionally, the patient may become aware of the infection and remove the worm manually. Parasitism is rare because infection requires the ingestion of viable larvae contained within a dung beetle, or water contaminated by infected disintegrating insects. Larvae penetrate the walls of the mammalian stomach or duodenum and apparently migrate upward to the esophagus and buccal cavity. The adult female is easily identified by the characteristic bosses on the anterior end. The egg is thick-walled and embryonated. Removal of the adult from the submucosal tunnels is followed by rapid healing.

Onchocerca volvulus

Infection with the filarial nematode, *O. volvulus,* is an important parasitic infection in Africa and in Central

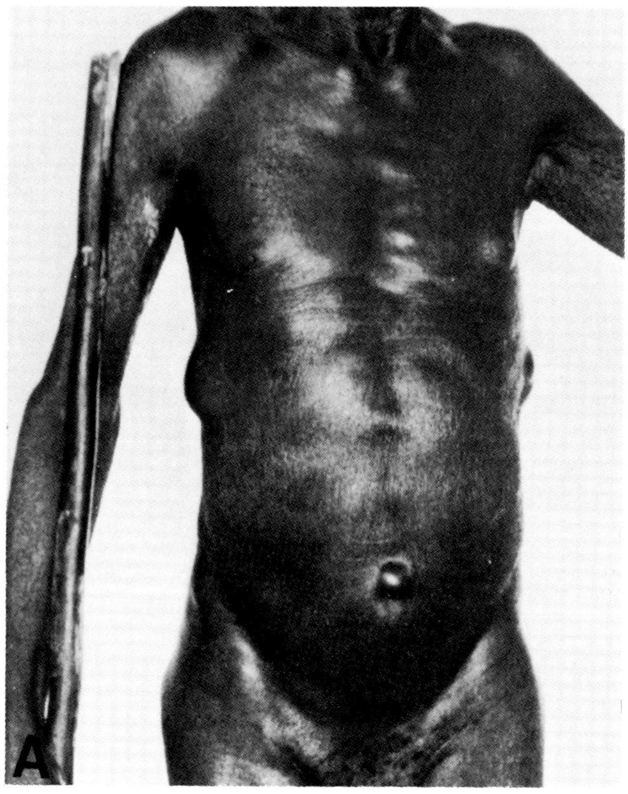

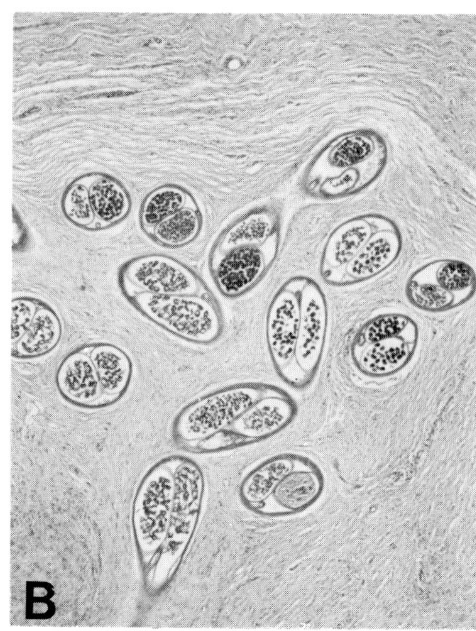

Fig. 11-17. **A. These subcutaneous nodules are caused by *O. volvulus*. (Courtesy Armed Forces Institute of Pathology 68–10071–3). B. Coiled worm within dense scar tissue (×17).**

America. It produces subcutaneous nodules and microfilaria, which give rise to important cutaneous and ocular lesions. It has been estimated that 50 million persons are infected in Equatorial Africa and 200,000 in Central and South America.[49]

Morphology, Life Cycle, and Pathology

The adults of *O. volvulus* are long (to 50 cm) slender nematodes that form masses to form nodules within the subcutaneous tissue (Fig. 11-17). These onchocercomas release microfilariae, which can either infect the flies of the Simuliidae family or cause ocular and cutaneous reactions within the host. Although these lesions are usually located in the subcutaneous tissue above the waist, they may also be found adherent to periosteum and in bone. Microfilariae produce ocular lesions, which are characterized pathologically as limbitis, uveitis, and optic atrophy. Furthermore, microfilariae produce edema and lichenification of the skin.

Diagnosis

The demonstration of microfilariae from bloodless skin snips, involved skin, or aspiration of subcutaneous nodules confirms the diagnosis. An eosinophilia in the range of 35 percent is usually present. When a patient resides in an endemic zone, the appearance of subcutaneous nodules should raise clinical suspicion. Frequent cross-reactions limit serologic diagnostic methods.

Treatment

Chemotherapy with drugs such as diethylcarbamazine, which are active against microfilariae, has limited value because of the rather violent allergic reactions attending the death of microfilariae.[49] The chief method is surgical removal of the subcutaneous onchocercomas. This measure reduces the number of microfilariae and diminishes the danger of ocular damage. The removal of onchocercomas can be easily accomplished using local anesthesia—the lesions are enclosed in a fibrous layer that usually offers a definite cleavage plane.

Thelazia californiensis

The eyeworm is a nematode which, in the western United States, parasitizes the conjunctiva of animals and occasionally man. The adult worm is slender, white, measures 5–17 mm in length, and has a characteristic oral zone with two rings of sessile papillae.[50] It is suspected that the larva is arthropod-borne, probably by members of the housefly family, but details of the life cycle are unknown. The worm can be seen in the conjunctival sac; the helminth often exits and can be removed using an eye forceps. The closely related *T. callipaeda*, the Oriental eyeworm, has a similar clinical picture.

Toxocara canis and *T. cati*

The ascarids, *T. canis* and *T. cati* commonly infect domestic dogs and cats, as well as related wild species. Children playing in contaminated areas may become infected by the ingestion of eggs. The life cycle is abortive in humans and larvae do not mature into adult helminths. The larvae penetrate the intestinal wall and produce eosinophilic granulomas and abscesses of the liver (Fig. 11-18). Less

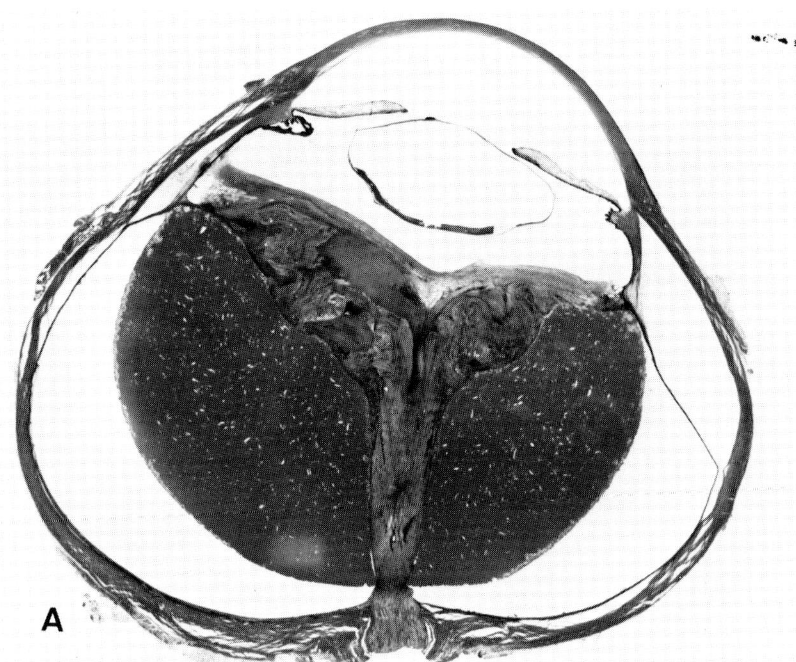

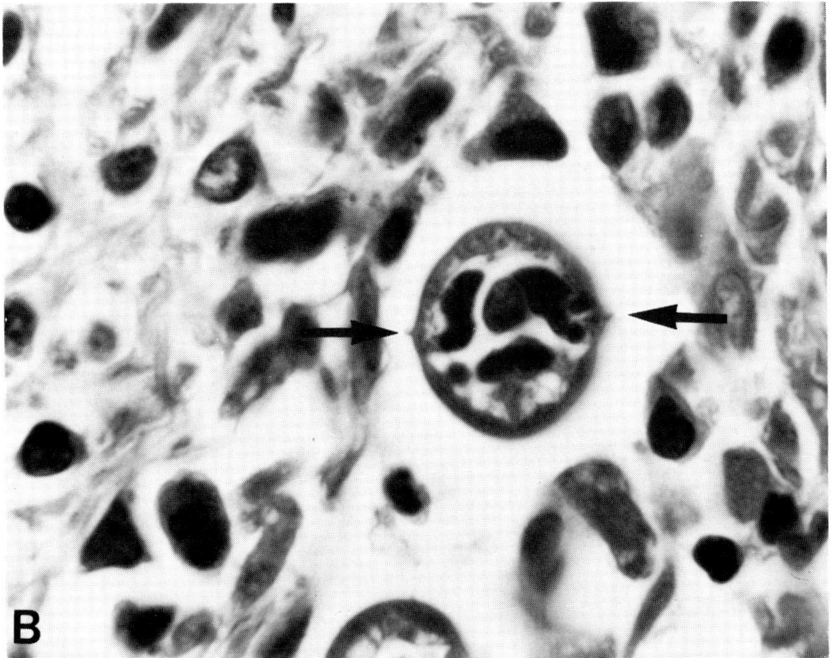

Fig. 11-18. A. An enucleated eye showing a preretinal inflammatory mass produced by visceral larvae migrans of *T. canis*. The retina is totally detached (×2.24). B. A transverse section of *T. canis* in the liver, showing tiny lateral alae. (Courtesy Armed Forces Institute of Pathology 55–22087 and 69–4372.)

commonly, larvae may reach the central nervous system, lung, or rarely the eye (Fig. 11-18A). At this latter site, the larvae may produce a severe chorioretinitis or endophthalmitis, which ends in blindness. Such lesions are usually unilateral, and enucleation is sometimes carried out with the presumptive diagnosis of retinoblastoma or other malignancy.[51]

The diagnosis of toxocariasis should be suspected when a child develops cough, hepatomegaly, lymphadenopathy, and lung infiltrates, and on laboratory examination a hypergammaglobulinemia and persistent eosinophilia is documented. Suspicion is further heightened if household pets can be shown to harbor *Toxocara* species and if the child is known to eat dirt. Stool examination is, of course, worthless, as the larvae do not develop into adults. Liver biopsy may be diagnostic, and such material should be serially sectioned. Because the lesions are unevenly distributed, failure to find the larvae or granuloma does not rule out the diagnosis. With ocular involvement, the larvae can occasionally be seen by slit-lamp examination. Eye lesions are unilateral, and the absence of calcifications favors a parasitic rather than a neoplastic etiology. A number of serologic procedures are available at the Center for Disease Control for the diagnosis of visceral larvae migrans.[52] Because of cross-reactivity, positive results are only suggestive.

TABLE 11-3. DRUG THERAPY OF COMMON HELMINTH INFECTIONS OF SURGICAL INTEREST

Organism	Drug	Average Adult Dose	Days	Adverse reactions and Comments
NEMATODES				
Ascaris lumbricoides	Pyrantel pamoate (Antiminth)	11 mg/kg (max. 1 g)	1	Occasional: nausea, vomiting, rash, fever, headache
	Mebendazole (Vermox)	0.1 gm 2 times daily	3	Occasional: diarrhea and abdominal discomfort
	Piperazine citrate (Antepar)	0.175 gm/kg (max. 3.5 gm)	2	Occasional: dizziness, nausea, vomiting, urticaria. Rare visual disturbances, ataxia, exacerbation of epilepsy
	Levamisole	150 mg	1	Occasional: headache, nausea and vomiting—may be the drug of choice, but confirmatory reports lacking
Enterobius vermicularis	Mebendazole * (Vermox)	0.100 gm	1—repeat in 2 wks	See above
	Pyrantel pamoate (Antiminth)	11 mg/kg (max. 1 gm)	1—repeat in 2 wks	See above
Trichuris trichuria	Mebendazole (Vermox)	0.100 gm	3–4	See above
	Thiabendazole (Mintezol)	0.025 gm/kg 2 times daily	2	Common: dizziness, nausea, and vomiting. Occasional: rash, leukopenia, hallucinations. Rare: Stevens-Johnson syndrome, shock
Taenia solium	Niclosamide (Yomesan)	2.0 gm in a single dose	1	Occasional: nausea, abdominal discomfort
	Paromomycin (Humatin)	1 gm every 15 min. for four doses	1	Common: abdominal discomfort, nausea
TREMATODES				
Clonorchis sinensis	Chloroquine (Aralen)	0.250 gm (3 times daily)	42	Occasional: nausea, vomiting, confusion, corneal opacities, ocular palsies, retinitis. Rare: blood dyscrasias, 8th nerve damage, discoloration of mucous membranes and nails
Fasciola hepatica	Bithionol	0.030 to 0.050 gm/kg on alternate days—10–15 doses		Common: skin eruption, urticaria, photosensitivity, nausea, vomiting, diarrhea
Paragonimus westermani	Bithionol	as for *F. hepatica*		See above
Schistosoma mansoni, hematobium, japonicum	See under *Schistosomes* (Table 11-4)			

* Probable drug of choice

Primary treatment of toxocariasis consists of preventing reinfections, ie, separation of the patient from infected pets and the prevention of dirt eating. If additional infection can be prevented, most patients begin to improve within weeks. Therapy should continue for the lifespan of the larvae (months to years). Treatment with thiabendazole (Table 11-3) might shorten the period of invasion. Additional rapid clinical improvement following the use of corticosteroids has been suggested.[53] If a larvae can be identified by slit-lamp examination, thiabendazole has been used, on rare occasions, with probable benefit.

Trichuris trichiura

Infection with whipworm, *T. trichiura*, a cosmopolitan nematode, is commonly asymptomatic. Occasionally, however, particularly in children, the infection may be fulminant and lead to colonic ulceration and rectal prolapse.

Morphology and Life Cycle

Averaging 30–50 mm in length, the adult worms (Fig. 11-19) are narrowed in their anterior portion. The male is characterized by its coiled posterior end and by a spicule projecting from the caudal portion.[54] The eggs are a deep brown color, and are distinguished by bipolar plugs and an ovoidal shape (Fig. 11-16, C and D). The life cycle is simple and parallels that of *Enterobius vermicularis.* Excreted in the feces, the eggs maturate, and when they are ingested, larvae erupt and begin their development within the villi of the small intestine. Within 30 days the parasites migrate to the proximal colon, where they reside with their slender esophagi burrowed beneath the mucosa. These helminths may survive as long as 3 years.[55]

Clinical Manifestations

Trichuriasis is seldom accompanied by symptoms. Severe infection can initiate diarrhea, debility, and blood loss. When more than 800 helminths are present, iron deficiency can be expected. Furthermore, in children infection of the rectosigmoid may precipitate diarrhea, tenesmus, and rectal prolapse. Rarely, ulcerations produced by infection will lead to perforation with the signs of peritonitis.

Diagnosis

The eggs of *T. trichiura* are easily recognized. Adults rarely may be identified in the mucosa of a rectal prolapse or during colonoscopic examination (Fig. 11-19).

Treatment

Mebendazole is a well-tolerated anthelminthic drug; 100 mg twice a day for 4 days will cure 90 percent of adults (Table 11-3).

The surgeon may be called for advice regarding a patient (usually a child) with rectal prolapse. The etiology can often be established with identification of adult whipworms residing within the prolapsed mucosa. The first maneuver is gentle digital replacement of the prolapsed segment. Next, oral drugs are used to prevent tenesmus and treat the infection. If a patient with severe trichuriasis and diarrhea develops signs of intestinal perforation, laparotomy should be undertaken. Unfortunately, trichuriasis is seldom a pure infection, and the clinician should always be alert to the necessity of treatment for an additional pathogen such as hookworm or *Ascaris.* Drug therapy should follow any operation to eradicate residual helminths.

CESTODES

Echinococcus granulosa

Hydatid disease or echinococcosis is an important parasitic infection of man and other animals (dogs, wolves, and cats). Humans usually become infected by the ingestion of viable eggs that originate in dog feces. The larvae produce cystic lesions, 75 percent of which arise in the liver (Chapter 36).

The condition is cosmopolitan but is particularly prevalent where sheep are raised in South America, South Africa, and Central Europe. Sixty-nine cases have recently been reported in the United States.[56]

Morphology and Life Cycle

The adult *E. granulosus* is a small tapeworm, measuring 3–6 mm in length with three proglottids (Fig. 11-20). The rostellum has a double crown of hooks, and the scolex

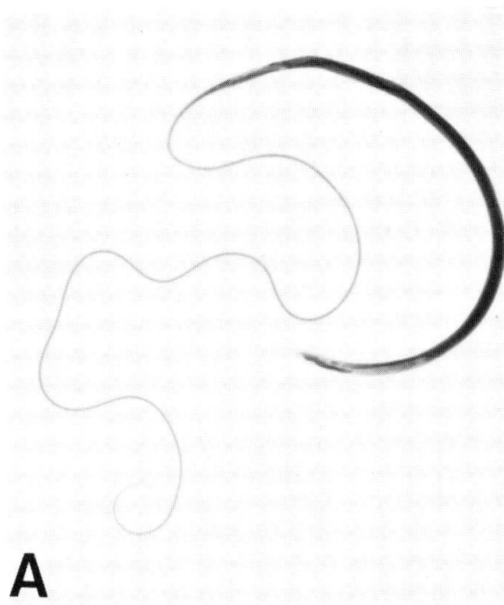

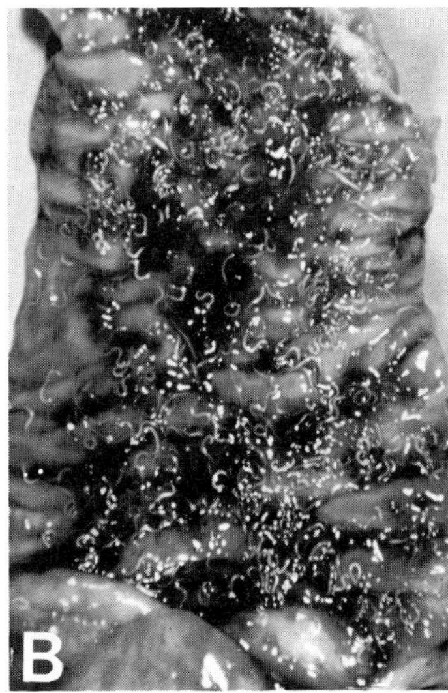

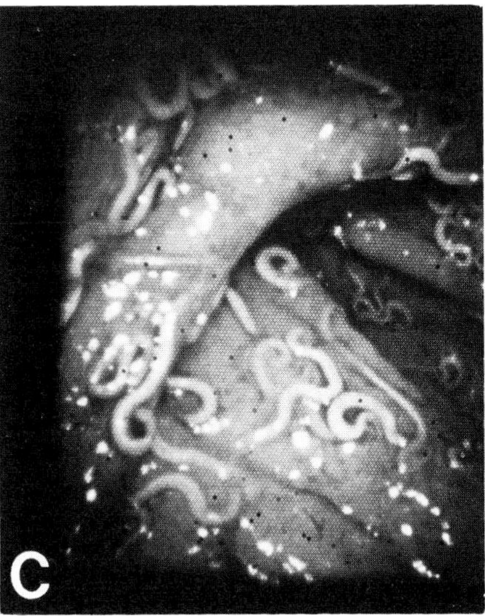

Fig. 11-19. **A. Adult *Trichuris trichiura* (length 50 mm). B. An autopsy specimen of colon heavily infected with *T. trichiura* (courtesy Rudolfo Céspedes). C. Colonoscopic view of *T. trichiura* in situ in cecum (courtesy McCaffery TD: *Gastrointest Endosc* 21:172, 1975.) (From Monroe LS: The Gastrointestinal Parasites of Man. In Bockus HL (ed): *Gastroenterology,* Vol. 4. Philadelphia, Saunders, 1976, p. 133.)**

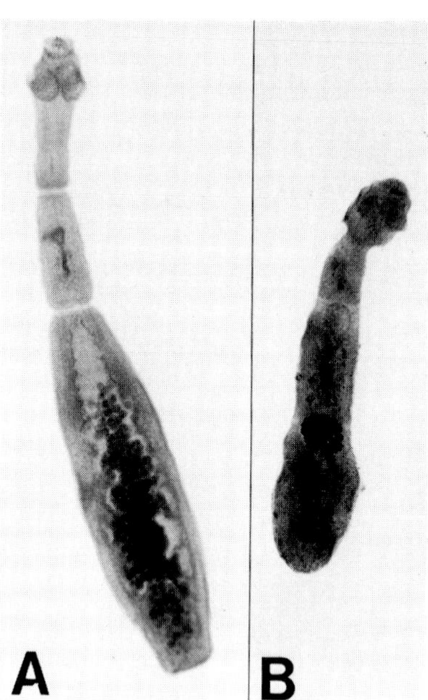

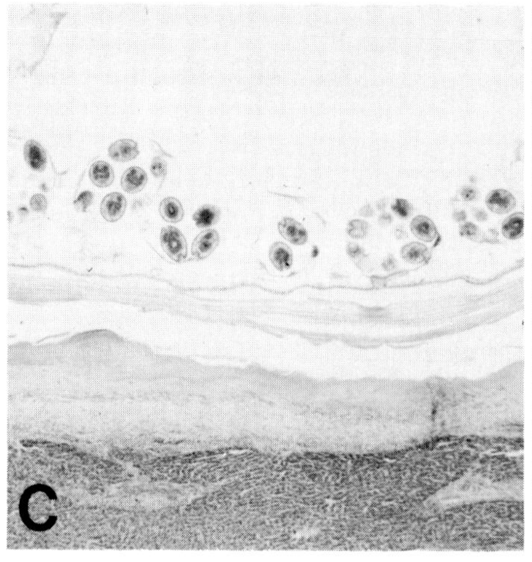

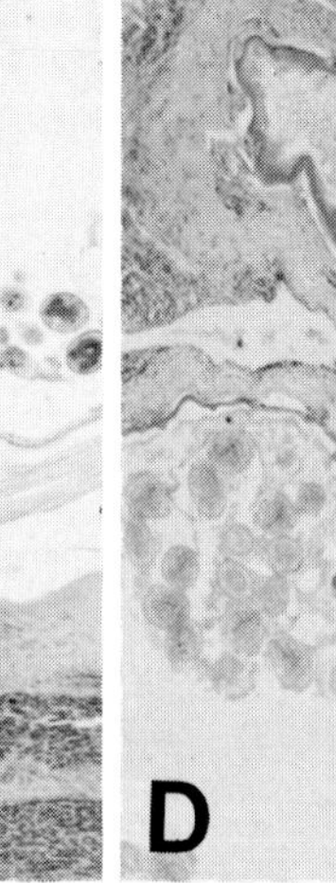

Fig. 11-20. A. Adult *Echinococcus granulosus*, length 6 mm. B. Adult *E. multiocularis*, length 4 mm. C. Wall of echinococcus cyst showing germinative membrane and scolices. D. Alveolar hydatid showing budding of the cyst. (From Monroe LS: The Gastrointestinal Parasites of Man. In Bockus HL (ed): *Gastroenterology*, Vol. 4. Philadelphia, Saunders, 1976, p. 133.)

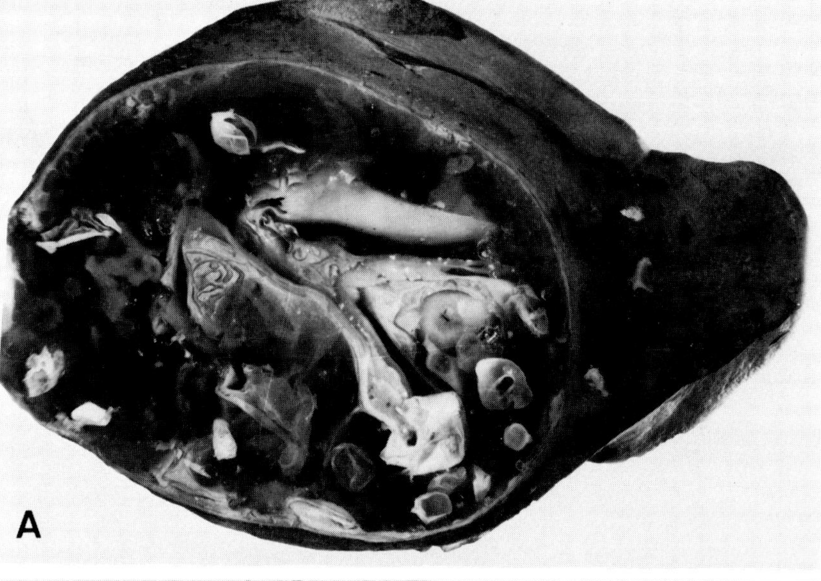

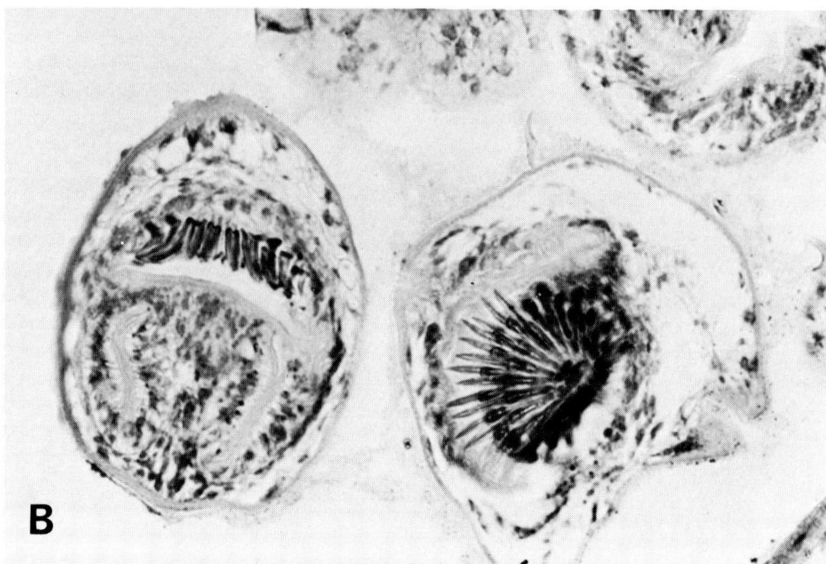

Fig. 11-21. A. A large unilocular hydatid cyst of the liver, with free daughter cysts in fluid. B. Scolices and *E. granulosis* in the brood capsule. (Courtesy Armed Forces Institute of Pathology N-31977 and 70–8831.)

has four suckers. The eggs cannot be distinguished from other *Taenia* species.[57]

Eggs or sloughed proglottids are passed in the feces of the definitive host and when ingested by an intermediate host (usually sheep), including man, the larvae usually pass to the liver but also to the lung, spleen, central nervous system, and bone. In the liver the cysts grow slowly, averaging 2–3 cm a year, until they reach a huge size and contain several liters of fluid. The fully developed cyst (Fig. 11-21) contains a peripheral zone of fibrous tissue that may calcify, an intermediate chitinous layer, and an inner germinal layer which produces brood capsules and proscolices. When such scolices break loose into the hydatid fluid they, along with free daughter cysts, are termed "hydatid sand" (Fig. 11-21).

Clinical Aspects and Diagnosis

In approximately 80 percent of the cases, the cysts involve the right lobe of the liver and are multiple 25 percent of the time. The pressure of hydatid cyst fluid is high (averaging 40–80 cm of water), and the pressure on the biliary tree produces jaundice in approximately one-third of the patients. After many years without symptoms, the cysts are finally found as an abnormal mass during a routine physical examination. Vilardel[58] described pain, resembling that of biliary colic, in one-half of 98 patients with hydatid liver cysts. Other manifestations included eosinophilia in 55 percent, palpable mass in 53 percent, fever in 27 percent, and pruritus in 24 percent. The hydatid cysts appear as a smooth rounded mass, which may be tender but is not characteristically hard. Uncommonly, vascular compression may produce a Budd-Chiari syndrome or splenomegaly. A hydatid liver cyst will perforate the biliary tree approximately 25 percent of the time. Uncommonly, rupture can occur into the gastrointestinal tract, pleural or peritoneal space (Chapter 36).

Serologic testing is of definitive value in confirming the diagnosis of echinococcosis. The intradermal (Casoni test) and indirect hemagglutination together give a positive reaction in 92 percent of known cases.[59] The Casoni test is false-positive, however, in about 18 percent of cases.[58] The complement-fixation test is positive in a smaller percentage.

Immunoelectrophoresis with cyst fluid antigen is positive in approximately 85 percent of cases. Unfortunately, serologic procedures, while important diagnostically, do not indicate whether or not a cyst is enlarging. This distinction must be made using clinical evidence (observed enlargement, tenderness). Radiographically, the presence of a densely calcified cyst is an important clue to a dormant cyst.

Treatment

A densely calcified hydatid cyst that is not producing symptoms can be observed, and operation deferred. In the majority of cases, however, an operation is recommended because of the danger of rupture of the cyst and progressive destruction of liver mass. Details of treatment are given in Chapter 36.

Echinococcus multilocularis

An unusual but serious variant of echinococcus disease is produced by *E. multilocularis* in southern Germany, Switzerland, and the U.S.S.R. near the Bering Sea. The adult *E. multilocularis* is smaller than *E. granulosis* (Fig. 11-20). The larvae of *E. multilocularis* cannot produce a confined colony of organisms as does *E. granulosis*. The alveolar hydatid proliferates by exuberant budding—a feature that makes this infection behave as if it were a malignancy (Fig. 11-20).

The intermediate hosts of *E. multilocularis* are small rodents, while the definitive hosts are usually foxes and other members of the dog family. Man usually becomes the accidental intermediate host by eating vegetable material contaminated by egg-containing feces.

In over 90 percent of patients, the liver is involved and is gradually destroyed by invasive cystic masses. Diagnostic measures as for *E. granulosis* are of value. Needle biopsy should not be done because of the danger of spread of infection. Surgical resection of the infected portion of the liver is the only hope for cure (Chapter 37).

Multiceps multiceps

The larval stages of this cestode have a predilection for the eye and brain of the intermediate host, and when people are accidentally infected, chorioretinitis and brain cysts result.

Morphology and Life Cycle

The dog and wolf are definitive hosts. The adult *M. multiceps* is long, 40–60 cm, and has a pyriform scolex armed with a double row of hooklets.[60] The eggs are identical to those of other *Taenia* species. The life cycle is similar to that of *E. granulosis*. The usual intermediate hosts are various domestic herbivores in which the larvae prefer to infect the brain, meninges, and ocular structures. In this locale, the larvae develop into a bladder worm (coenurus), which is characterized by multiple scolices projecting from the inner cyst wall (Fig. 11-22) in contrast to the single scolex seen in the cysticercus produced by *C. cellulosae*.

Clinical Features and Diagnosis

In man, coenurosis most frequently produces a basal leptomeningitis often associated with a hydrocephalus. As a result, the symptoms frequently include suboccipital headache associated with vomiting. Lumbar puncture is nondiagnostic and reveals, as a rule, an increase in pressure (greater than 150 mm water), an elevated protein concentration, and a pleocytosis. Clinically, it is impossible to distinguish coenurosis from cysticercosis or hydatid involvement of the central nervous system. The differential diagnosis may include tuberculosis or a space-occupying tumor. Eosinophilia is seldom seen, and serologic tests have little value. To further complicate diagnosis, cysts may be "sterile" and not contain scolices; these are often confused with those of *E. granulosa* or *C. cellulosae*. In contrast to cysticercosis, coenurus cysts seldom calcify.

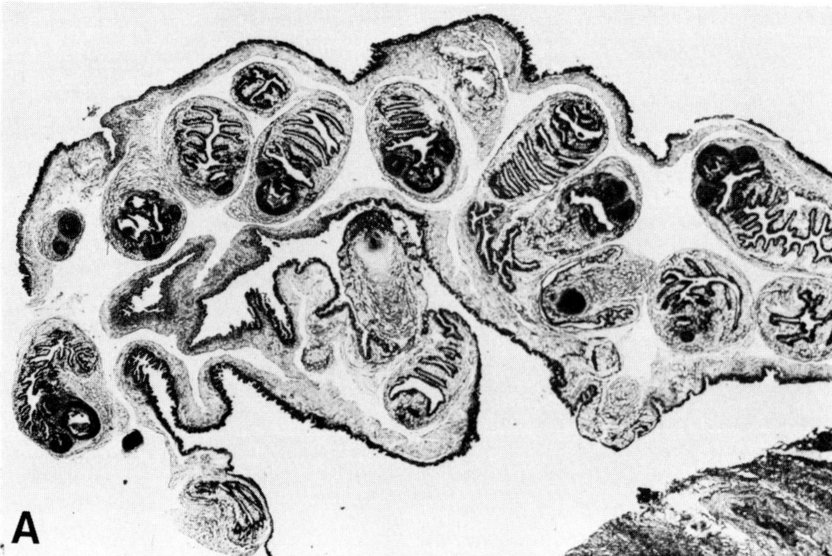

Fig. 11-22. A. Section of a coenurus from a rabbit demonstrating the thin cyst wall and the numerous scolices (×12.75). B. Coenurus of the eye displacing the vitreous humor (×2.25). (Courtesy Armed Forces Institute of Pathology 69–4736 and 72–5162.)

Computerized axial tomography should be of great diagnostic help as in cysticercosis. A chronic coenurosis leptomeningitis may involve the lumbosciatic nerve roots and produce a chronic pain syndrome. Diagnosis can be made by the recognition of cysts, which may be extremely difficult.

The eye is less often involved. The coenurus attaches to the surrounding structures (Fig. 11-22). The visual defect produced correlates with the degree of chorioretinal damage.

Treatment

There is no known medical treatment for coenurosis. The majority of cases are diagnosed after operative intervention and histologic study. The usual preoperative diagnoses include internal hydrocephalus (cause unknown), glioma, meningioma, or tumor of the orbit.

Sparganosis

Human infection with the second larval stage of the subgenus *Spirometra,* a cestode group closely related to *Diphyllobothrium,* is a rare cause of an inflammatory mass developing in the muscular or subcutaneous tissues. The anterior portion of the sparganum is grooved vertically to produce two lips; moreover, the larva has neither scolex nor internal organs, while the body is covered with a tegument 5–15 μm in thickness (Fig. 11-23).[61] The adult cestodes (17 species are capable of human infection) inhabit the intestinal tracts of dogs and cats. The larvae pass through a cyclops to enter their intermediate vertebrate hosts, particularly frogs and snakes. Infection of humans may occur following ingestion of the infected cyclops or flesh-containing sparganum. Liberated plerocercoid larvae transit the gut wall and pass through the circulation to enter the muscles or subcutaneous tissues, where an inflammatory reaction gradually ensues. Direct migration from infected flesh into bruised human ocular tissue is an important source of infection in Vietnam and Thailand, where the natives often use raw frog meat as a poultice.[62]

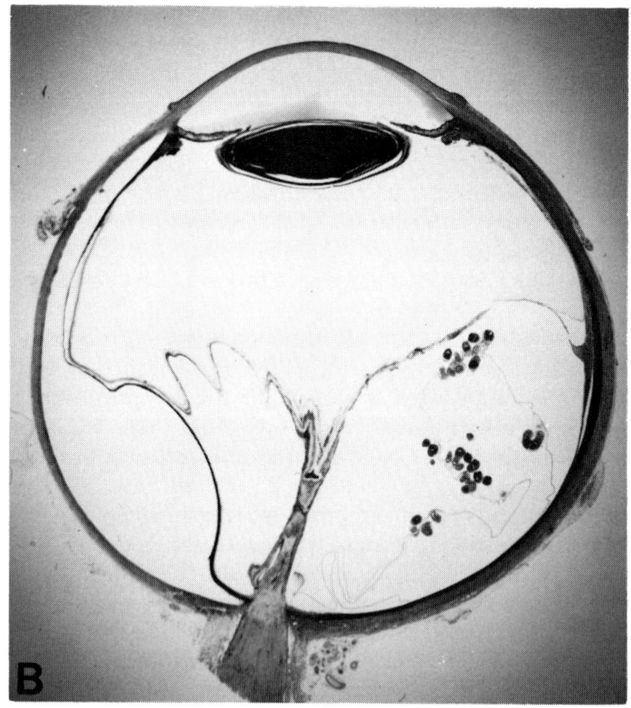

An inflammatory mass should be excised with removal of the spargana.

Taenia solium and *Cysticercus cellulosae*

Wherever undercooked pork is consumed, infection with *T. solium* will be encountered. When humans become the intermediate host, the larval form of the parasite, *C. cellulosae* becomes an important cause of space-occupying intracranial lesions.[63]

Morphology and Life Cycle

The adult *T. solium* is characterized by a scolex having four suckers and a rostellum encircled by a double row

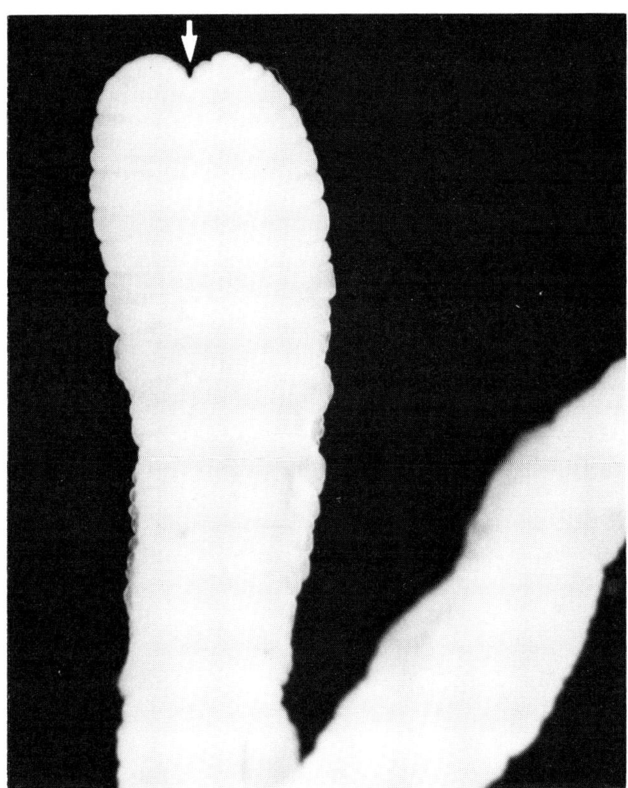

Fig. 11-23. **The anterior end of a sparganum demonstrating the bothrium ×18. (Courtesy Armed Forces Institute of Pathology 70–7390.)**

of hooklets.[64] The gravid proglottid is distinguished by having fewer lateral uterine branches (7 to 13) than does the corresponding proglottid of *T. saginata.* The adult *T. solium* resides in the upper gut of man, the only known definitive host. When living proglottids are passed in the feces, they may be ingested by a variety of mammalian intermediate hosts. Within the gut of the intermediate host the eggs hatch, penetrate the wall, and migrate throughout the body to develop in 60 to 90 days as infective bladder worms.

When eggs are accidentally ingested, man becomes the accidental intermediate host, with the development of cysticerci within tissues. As a rule, however, man acquires the adult *T. solium* through the ingestion of *C. cellulosae* present in raw or undercooked meat, especially in countries where meat inspection is uncertain, for example, Mexico.

Clinical Features

People are seldom aware that they are harboring an adult *T. solium.* Mild aberrations of appetite, abdominal discomfort, and diarrhea are reported. Cysticercosis produces symptoms referable to the site: brain, heart, lungs, muscles, liver, and eye (Fig. 11-24). No tissue is immune to invasion. When nonvital structures, such as the subcutaneous tissue, are involved, the patient may be unaware of infection or note pain, tenderness, and generalized malaise. The most serious complication of cysticercosis is the development of a cerebral lesion with the resultant edema and gliosis. Such diverse conditions as brain tumor, pseudotumor, luetic meningitis, or the cerebral atrophies may be mimicked. On the other hand, silent cerebral cysticercosis can develop, the diagnosis being made by the roentgen visualization of end-stage intracranial calcifications.

Diagnosis

As the eggs of various *Taenia* species are indistinguishable, the recognition of *T. solium* infection rests with the identification of the typical scolex or gravid proglottid. The definitive histologic diagnosis of cysticercosis depends on the demonstration of an invaginated scolex with four suckers and two rows of hooklets.

The sudden appearance of subcutaneous nodules associated with acute central nervous system complaints (particularly Jacksonian convulsions) should suggest cysticercosis. Computerized axial tomography is often a diagnostic aid (Fig. 11-25). In the eye, examination may reveal a mobile cysticercus within the vitreous. With end-stage lesions, calcifications may be seen scattered throughout skeletal muscles or within the brain (Fig. 11-26). It should be remembered that such calcified lesions are rarely, if ever, symptom-producing, and that active *C. cellulosae* are not radiopaque. Eosinophilia is variable and is rarely helpful. The Center for Disease Control provides a hemag-

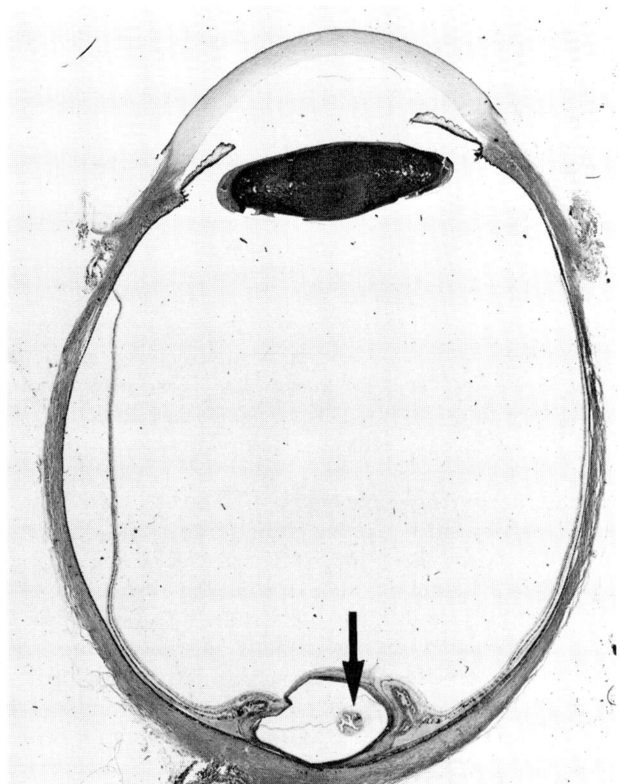

Fig. 11-24. **Cysticercus between the retina and the vitreous (×16.2). (Courtesy Armed Forces Institute of Pathology 74–12712.)**

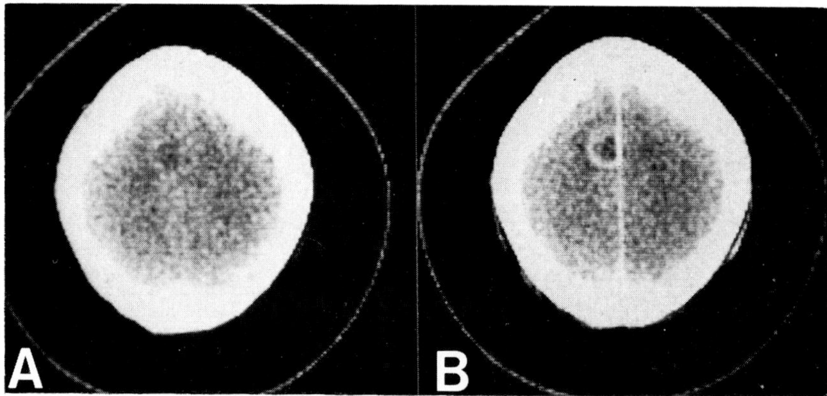

Fig. 11-25. Computerized axial tomography (CAT) scan showing lesion of cysticercosis in left superior cerebral hemisphere adjacent to the falx. Tomogram A. without contrast infusion; B. with Renografin infusion (courtesy Marcus Drupp). (From Monroe LS: The Gastrointestinal Parasites of Man. In Bockus HL (ed): *Gastroenterology,* Vol. 4. Philadelphia, Saunders, 1976.)

glutination test for cysticercosis. Cross-reaction occurs with other tapeworms.

Treatment

The medical therapy of intestinal *T. solium* is listed in Table 11-3. The surgeon is most frequently consulted for the problem of cysticercosis. As a rule, simple excision of subcutaneous masses suffices for diagnostic purposes. Unresected *C. cellulosae* will die and calcify without producing symptoms and will not require treatment. On the other hand, when the brain is involved, the signs of a focal expanding intracranial lesion will often demand operative intervention. The cystic character may suggest a benign lesion, but an operation should not be withheld unless it is apparent that the lesion is mild and not life-threatening. Calcified cysticerci in the central nervous system is not by itself a surgical indication because the *C. cellulosae* are dead. In such a case with a neurologic disorder, a different etiology should be sought.

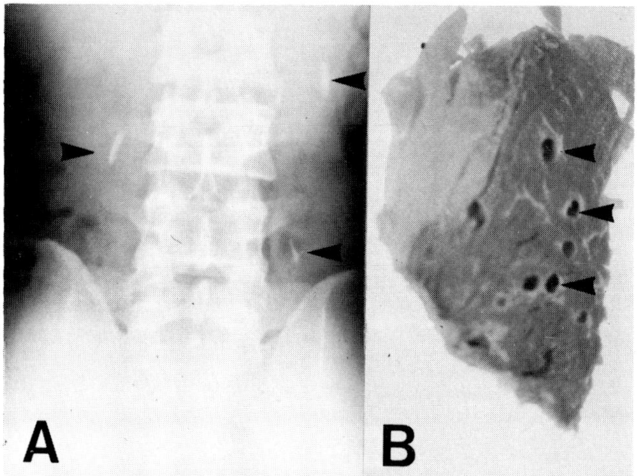

Fig. 11-26. A. Radiograph showing "rice grain" calcifications in skeletal muscles, produced by larvae of *Taenia solium.* B. Skeletal muscle of a hog infected with cysticerci of *T. solium* (measly pork). (From Monroe LS: The Gastrointestinal Parasites of Man. In Bockus HL (ed): *Gastroenterology,* Vol. 4. Philadelphia, Saunders, 1976.)

TREMATODES

Clonorchis sinensis

Infection with the Chinese liver fluke, *C. (Opisthorchis) sinensis* is common in the areas of Asia bounded by the China Sea. An autopsy series from Hong Kong found evidence of clonorchiasis in 65 percent of deaths. Inasmuch as the adult flukes may survive in biliary passages for more than 20 years, the condition is frequently detected in Asiatics who have moved long ago from other areas.

Morphology and Life Cycle

The average adult *C. sinensis* ranges from 10 to 25 mm in length and has an anterior and ventral sucker. The eggs are small, averaging 27–35 μm, and have a prominent "shoulder" adjacent to the operculum.[65] The boss, which is often illustrated in texts at the anopercular end of the egg, is not a reliable morphologic feature and should not be depended upon for diagnosis.

Cats, pigs, camels, rats, and dogs are important reservoir hosts of *C. sinensis.* On reaching water with the feces, the eggs are ingested by snails and undergo metamorphosis. After 4 to 5 weeks, cercariae emerge and penetrate freshwater fish where metacercariae encyst in the flesh. People (and other flesheaters) acquire the infection from undercooked fish. The metacercariae are released, penetrate the duodenal mucosa to migrate to the biliary tree, seeking as a rule the smaller branches of the left lobe of the liver where maturation occurs (Fig. 11-27).

Pathology and Clinical Manifestations

Although mild asymptomatic infections are common, the presence of *C. sinensis* in the biliary passages provokes a marked inflammatory reaction, edema, and later progressive fibrosis with proliferation of ductal epithelium. A portal-type cirrhosis with its complications, ascites and varices, may follow. More frequently, complications of clonorchiasis include the development of biliary calculi centering about eggs or adults and the occurrence of acute suppurative cholangitis. The latter condition, cholangiohepatitis, can be acute or chronic and is associated with intrahepatic stones, abscesses, and ductal strictures. The incidence of cholangioma is reported by Hou[66] to be increased in clonorchiasis—in fact, 15 percent of primary carcinoma of the liver in Hong Kong may be induced

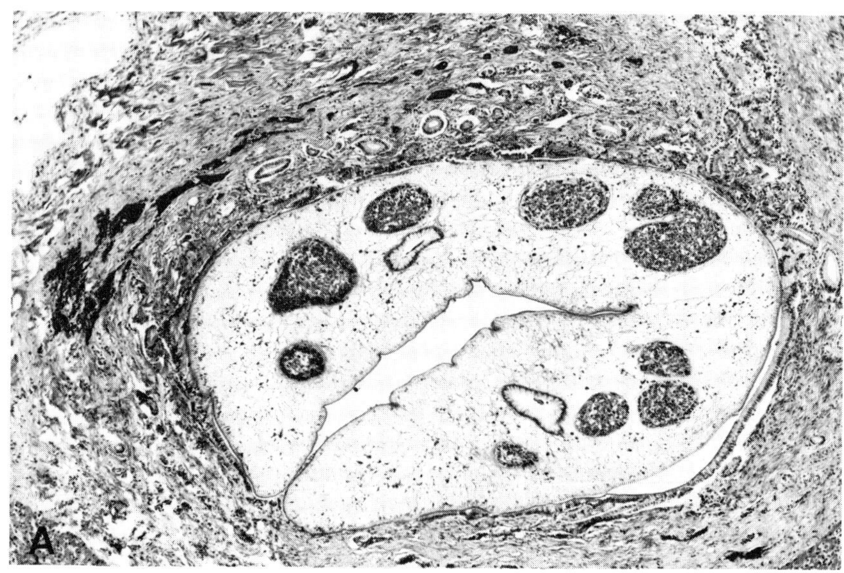

Fig. 11-27. A. Section through posterior portion of *C. sinensis* in a bile duct, showing testis and cecae (×31.5). B. T-tube cholangiogram showing ductular dilatation and numerous parasites. (Courtesy Armed Forces Institute of Pathology 74–11157 and 69–5522–3.)

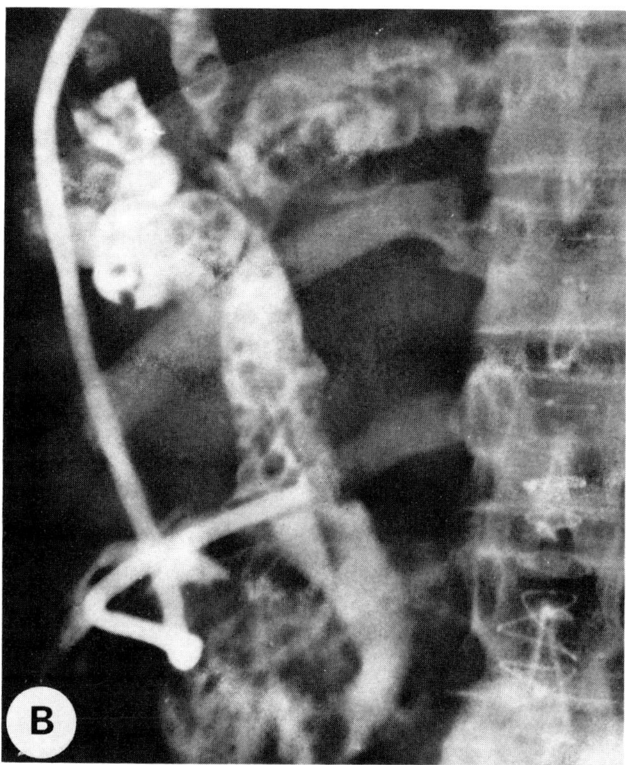

by this infection. The presence of *C. sinensis* within the pancreatic ductal system has been found in as many as 37 percent of autopsy reports of clonorchiasis, but the pancreatitis produced is usually mild.

There is no characteristic pattern to the infection produced by *C. sinensis,* and symptoms may occur before eggs are detectable in the stool. Many light infections are asymptomatic. A tender, enlarged liver accompanied by chills, fever, and malaise are frequent early signs in heavy infections. Fluctuating jaundice is usually obstructive in character, and eosinophilia to 40 percent may accompany the illness. Right upper quadrant and epigastric pain, of a colicky nature, may simulate or be caused by associated cholelithiasis and choledocholithiasis. Late rare manifestations of advanced disease are like decompensated cirrhosis.

Diagnosis

Clonorchiasis should be suspected when a patient develops signs of hepatic, biliary, or pancreatic disease and has eaten raw Cyprinoid freshwater fish from an endemic area. Eosinophilia indicates a possible parasitic etiology. The final diagnosis depends on finding the tiny operculated egg in the stool. A concentration technique (such as the formalin-ether method) will facilitate recovery of the eggs. Serologic tests have been described but are not available clinically. Retrograde endoscopic cholangiography should prove to be a useful tool in delineating the strictures and stones associated with cholangiohepatitis.

Treatment

There is no satisfactory drug treatment for clonorchiasis, although chloroquine diphosphate (Aralen) is usually given for 6 weeks (Table 11-3). Emetine can be given as for amebiasis but has a low therapeutic index.

Exploration of the common bile duct with removal of flukes, detritus, and associated stones has been of value in advanced cases of cholangiohepatitis. Symptomatic cholelithiasis, developing in a parasitic locus, would require cholecystectomy. Operative cholangiography, common duct exploration, and lavage should probably be carried out whenever cholecystectomy is performed.

Fasciola hepatica

Human infection with *F. hepatica* (fascioliasis) occurs wherever sheep are raised. Forty-nine cases were reported from England in 1968, which demonstrates the problem wherever parasitized water plants (particularly watercress) are ingested.[1,67-69] Because humans are poor hosts for the parasite, the flukes frequently localize ectopically in subcutaneous tissue, lung parenchyma, peritoneum, brain, and stomach rather than the usual site—the biliary tree.

Morphology, Life Cycle, and Diagnosis

The adult *F. hepatica* has a broadly ovoidal shape with a distinctive ephalic cone (Fig. 11-28). The average length (30 mm) and the branching intestinal cecae are distinguishing features. The eggs of *F. hepatica* are operculated, large, and easily confused with those of other trematodes (Fig. 11-28). The animal hosts of *F. hepatica* include sheep, goats, cattle, and a variety of wild herbivores. Eggs are passed with the feces. When they reach water, the eggs maturate to develop miracidiae, which penetrate snails and eventually acquire the cercarial form. Such cercariae leave the snail and encyst on aquatic plants, which are food for grazing animals. When consumed by the definitive host, including man, the larvae hatch, transit the intestinal tract to traverse the peritoneal surfaces, and enter the liver to finally arrive in the biliary tree. Ectopic migration can occur to any organ but is particularly frequent in subcutaneous tissue. In herbivores, the flukes within the biliary tree evoke an intense inflammatory reaction with a predominant eosinophilic component. Local abscesses are common, and the term "sheep liver rot" describes the infected organ.

In man, the larval migration is accompanied by eosinophilia, which subsides as the fluke matures. The ingestion of contaminated water plants (particularly watercress) is followed within 7 to 14 days by a febrile illness and an eosinophilia. The appearance of a coin lesion in the lung or a mass in the subcutaneous tissues should further increase suspicion. Mature eggs are rarely seen in the stool, and coprology is of little value. The ultimate diagnosis is usually made by recovery of the adult trematode at the time of biliary exploration. The larvae can occasionally be identified when removed from their aberrant site. Serology is available from the Parasitology Division of the Center for Disease Control (Table 11-1); however, there are cross-reactions with other trematodes.

Treatment

Whenever fascioliasis is diagnosed, medical treatment should be instituted with bithionol and emetine (Table 11-3), but clinical proof of their efficacy is scarce. The surgeon may encounter flukes at the time of cholecystectomy. In such a case, operative cholangiography and common duct exploration should be undertaken for the removal of residual helminths. When an eosinophilic granuloma is removed from the lung, serologic testing should be performed, and if it is positive, medical treatment should be given.

Paragonimus westermani

Infection with the lung fluke *P. westermani* and closely related species, is widely distributed in areas of the Far East. Man acquires the disease after eating freshwater crustaceans or their juice. Lesions may develop in the lungs, subcutaneous tissue, spinal canal, brain, liver, pancreas, and peritoneal surfaces. Some of its manifestations may require surgical intervention.

Morphology, Life Cycle, and Pathology

The adult *P. westermani* resides in man and a variety of domesticated and wild animals. The adult flukes average 7.5–20 mm in length and have an elongate oval shape (Fig. 11-29).[70] There are anterior and ventral suckers. The adults, which reside in pulmonary cysts, exit the body via sputum or feces, and upon reaching water the miracidia hatch to enter snails, the usual pattern for trematodes. After further development, cercariae emerge from the

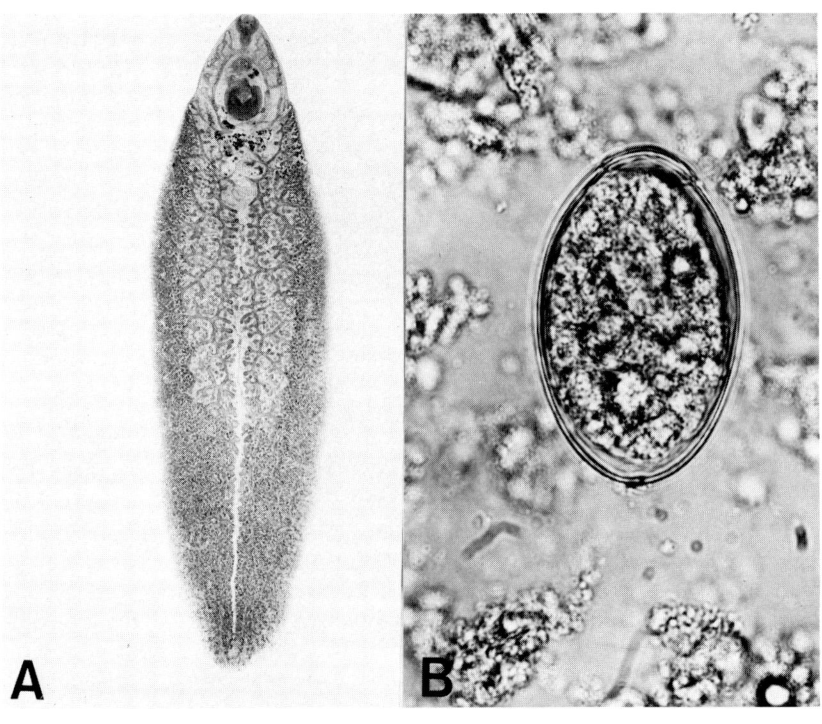

Fig. 11-28. **A. Adult *Fasciola hepatica* (actual length 25 mm). B. Egg of *F. hepatica* (actual length 130 μm). (From Monroe LS: The Gastrointestinal Parasites of Man. In Bockus HL (ed): *Gastroenterology*, Vol. 3. Philadelphia, Saunders, 1965.)**

snails and encyst as metacercariae in the gills and muscles of crustaceans. When ingested by an appropriate definitive host, the metacercariae penetrate the upper small intestine and enter the abdominal cavity, from which they may penetrate the diaphragm, enter the pleural cavity, and invade the lungs. It requires about 70 days for the flukes to mature and produce eggs. After such an odyssey, it is not surprising that larval forms may reach widespread ectopic areas in the body, ie, liver (Fig. 11-30), bone, pancreas, subcutaneous tissue.

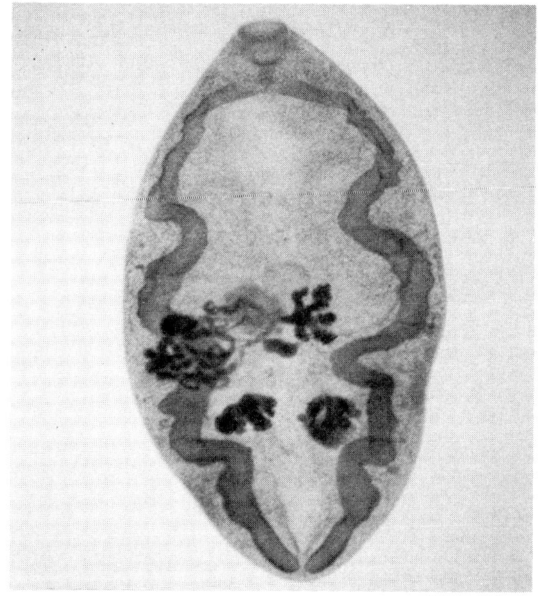

Fig. 11-29. An adult *P. westermani* (×10).

The oval pulmonary parasitic cysts, averaging 0.6–3.3 cm in greatest dimension, are thin-walled and usually discernible as firm masses at or near the pleural surface.[71] On section, one and occasionally more flukes may be seen. The lung parenchyma surrounding the cysts is hemorrhagic. The inflammatory reaction shows varying numbers of neutrophils and mononuclear cells with eosinophils predominating. Charcot-Leyden crystals may be seen in the necrotic center of such a cyst. Inflammatory changes peripheral to the cyst may lead to bronchitis, peribronchitis, and bronchopneumonia. The contents of a ruptured cyst enter the bronchi and produce a cough and many times bronchopneumonia. The foreign protein may stimulate a granulomatous reaction with giant cells of the Langhans type and, as a late event, ossification of the granuloma and cysts can occur.

When the brain is involved, the parasites usually die and form a pseudocavity in the cerebral substance, which may contain only liquified residue, foreign body granuloma, and possibly a few eggs.[72] The circumscribed lesions usually involve the brain bilaterally but also have a predisposition to localize in the right temperoparietal and occipital areas. Lesions involving the spinal canal commonly occur in the epidural area of the thoracic vertebrae and involve the arachnoid.

Although no region escapes infection, cutaneous paragonomiasis has a predilection for the subcutaneous tissue of the trunk. A typical cyst would appear in the abdominal wall and measure 2–3 cm in diameter. Histologically, the parasite and eggs can be identified in about 50 percent

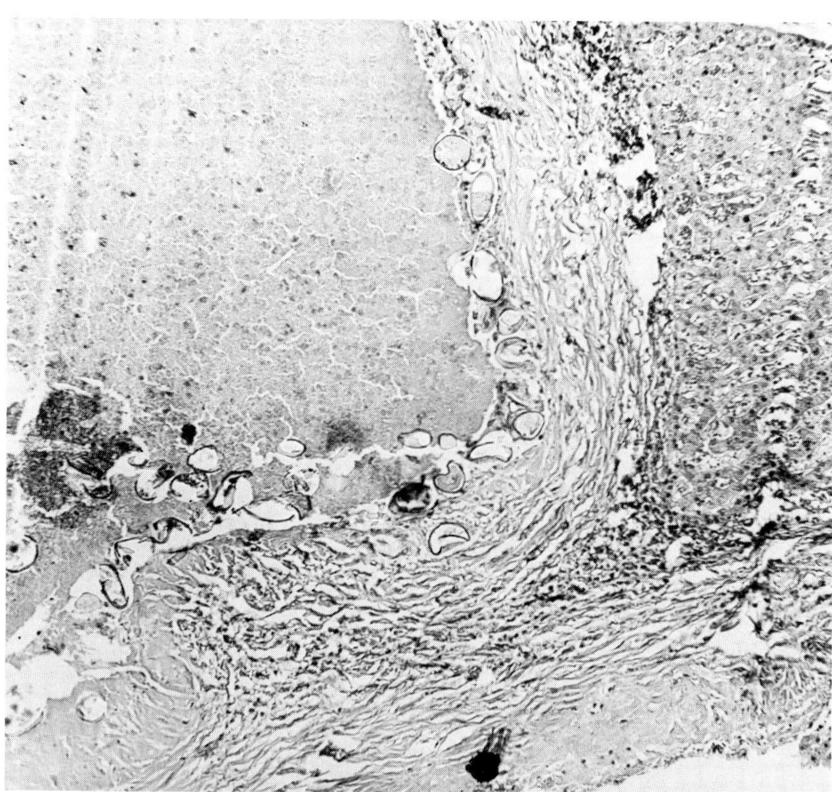

Fig. 11-30. A cyst of *P. westermani* in the liver. The inner surface of the fibrotic wall is lined by eggs (×88). (Courtesy Armed Forces Institute of Pathology 64–1846.)

of cases. Granulomata with foreign body giant cells and eosinophilia dominate the tissue response.

Clinical Manifestations

With pulmonary involvement, cough with the production of blood-tinged sputum is a cardinal complaint. The condition is often chronic, extending over years; aside from periodic bouts of pleuritic pain, patients as a rule show relative well-being. Examination of the sputum should be done repeatedly by concentration techniques and direct smear when the patient is from an endemic area.

On roentgen examination the peripheral circumscribed pulmonary lesions of paragonimiasis are often typical coin lesions, and the differential diagnosis includes the infectious granulomas, tumor, and other parasites. In at least 40 percent of the cases, the roentgenographic picture is indistinguishable from tuberculosis. Examination of sputum and stool for typical eggs is an important diagnostic measure when evaluating an Asiatic with such an x-ray picture.

Cerebral paragonimiasis may initiate with progressive neurologic symptoms and signs of a space-occupying intracranial lesion. The most common first sign is a Jacksonian or grand mal seizure. Headache, hemiplegia, and nuchal rigidity occur to a lesser degree. The clinical picture, of course, depends on the anatomy of the compromised structures. In the past, ventriculography and pneumoencephalography were tools that gave diagnostic aid. The coaxial computerized scan should be the most effective diagnostic tool. Simple roentgen examination of the skull may show calcification, and again the diagnostic possibilities would include cysticercosis; additional clues hinge on historical and laboratory findings. The development of a spastic paraplegia with the attendant motor and neurologic phenomena may herald spinal paragonimiasis. Occasionally, eggs can be demonstrated in the spinal fluid.

Diagnosis

The large operculated egg in sputum confirms the diagnosis. In stool, however, the large trematode eggs of other species may be similar. A complement-fixation test is available from the Center for Disease Control; however, there is cross-reactivity with other trematodes.

Positive skin tests persist for years.[71] Skin testing should always be performed after serologic testing because the skin test antigen may produce antibodies.

Treatment

Bithionol should be used as soon as the diagnosis is made—the cure rate is 90 percent (Table 11-3). An operation is still indicated for a localized, space-occupying, intracranial or spinal lesion.

Schistosoma mansoni

Schistosomiasis is the most important parasitic infection of people.[72,72a] In 1947, Stoll estimated that there were 29 million cases of *S. mansoni,* 39 million of *S. haematobium,* and 46 million of *S. japonicum* infections in the world. *S. mansoni,* along with *S. haematobium,* is found in the Nile Basin and other parts of Africa. Foci also exist in Central and South America (particularly Puerto Rico). Although the vectors are present, the condition is not acquired within the continental United States.

Morphology and Life Cycle

S. mansoni is a trematode and the adults reside within the venous radicles of the hemorrhoidal plexus.[73] The paired worms are usually located in the vasculature near the rectum and sigmoid. Eggs with a subterminal spine (Fig. 11-31) are deposited in the immediate submucosal area. On transiting the mucosa, the eggs mix with the stool, reach water, and the miracidium develops to enter a snail.[74] Within the snail, division and metamorphosis occur, with the release of a forked-tailed cercariae. These motile cercariae penetrate the exposed skin or when swallowed transit the gut to enter local lymphatics, from whence they migrate to the lungs. From this latter site, the schistosomules reach the liver, probably via the bloodstream. Maturation continues, and the developing adults migrate against the blood current to their final habitat. From cutaneous penetration to final maturation and egg deposition requires approximately 40 to 50 days.

Pathology and Clinical Features

Within minutes to hours after entry of cercariae into the skin, an urticarial rash may develop; the eruption can last for several days. Symptoms are usually absent during the stage of larval migration to early oviposition.[73] Beginning with the onset of sustained oviposition, however, symptoms of the acute stage commence with fever, abdominal pain, and diarrhea. Fever is usually remittent, with afternoon elevations, and continues for approximately 2 weeks. During this period, physical findings may include a generalized lymphadenopathy and a mild hepatomegaly. Periorbital edema and transitory urticarial rashes may also be present during this stage. A leukocytosis in the range of 20,000 white blood cells per mm^3 is accompanied by a eosinophilia with values averaging 30 to 75 percent.[73] In the chronic stage, tissue alterations caused by *S. mansoni* can be attributed to the adult worms, their eggs, toxic products, and the host's reaction to the parasitism. Probably the most significant pathology is produced by the eggs which stimulate fibroblasts and induce granulomas or pseudotubercules with phlebitis in the liver, intestine, lungs, bladder, heart, and other organs.[75] Within the colon, this leads to a progressive fibrosis with mucosal ulceration and occasionally inflammatory polyps and papillomata. Eggs that circulate into the liver induce phlebitis and allergic hyperreactive proliferation within the portal tracts. A concentric fibrosis occurs about the portal tracts and, in association, reticulin fibers proliferate in an "onion skin" configuration (Fig. 11-32). A Symmers fibrosis can be produced, with the liver appearing "as if a number of clay pipe stems had been thrust at various angles through the organ" (Fig. 11-33). Portal hypertension with congestive splenomegaly, hypersplenism with anemia, leukopenia, and thrombocytopenia may ensue. This cirrhosis is presinusoidal, so that the measurement of wedged hepatic vein pressure does not reflect the elevated portal vein pressure.

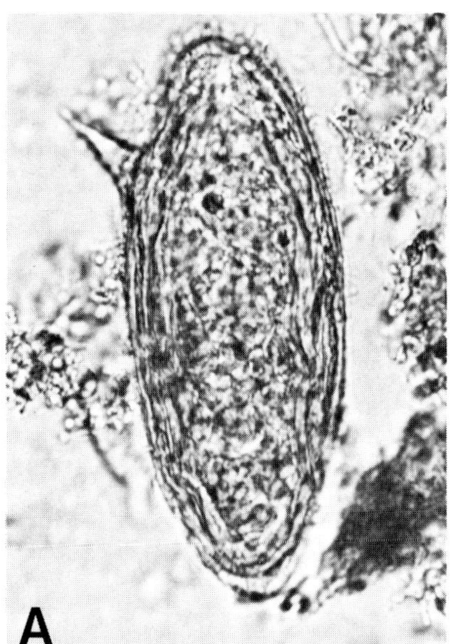

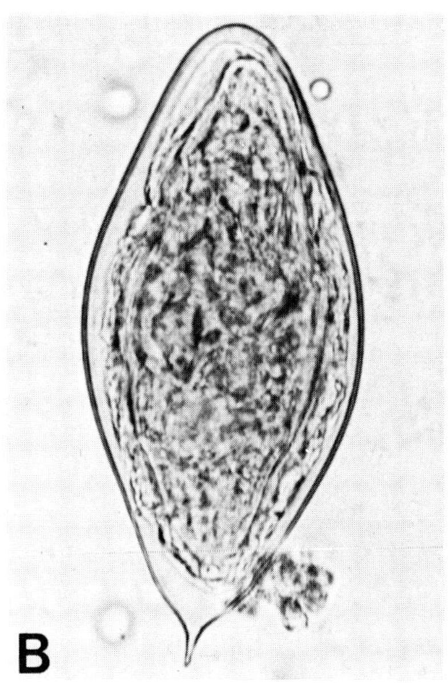

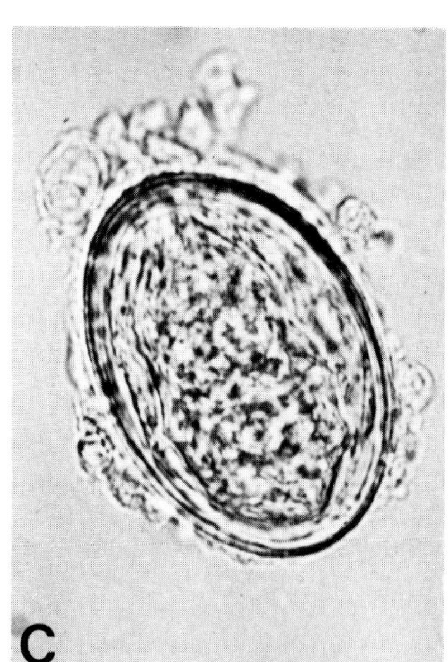

Fig. 11-31. Eggs of A. *S. mansoni,* B. *S. haematobium,* and C. *S. japonicum* (×342).

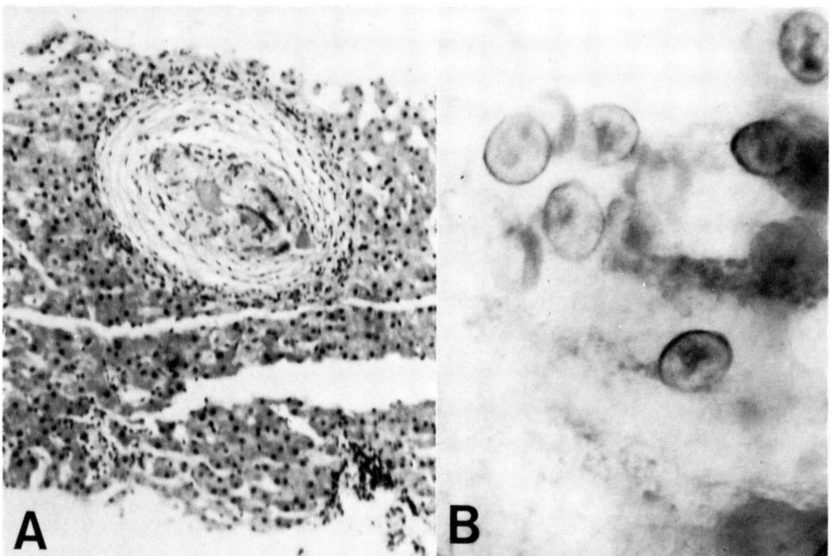

Fig. 11-32. A. Percutaneous liver biopsy of patient with *S. japonicum* infection. Concentric fibrosis is evident about the portal area, with remnants of an egg positioned centrally. B. Rectal biopsy (unstained) on the same patient containing numerous eggs of *S. japonicum.* C. Rectal biopsy of a patient with *S. mansoni* showing submucosal eggs, edema, and fibrosis (×153).

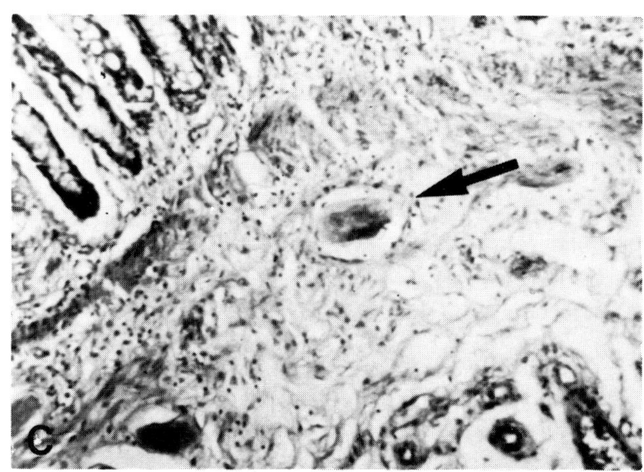

In the severe case, garden variety portal or postnecrotic cirrhosis develops. The adult worms inhabit chiefly the hemorrhoidal plexus, so they contribute little to the hepatic pathology.

In advanced cases, bleeding from esophageal varices occurs. Inasmuch as parenchymal function remains good because of adequate perfusion of the lobule, these bleeding episodes are usually well tolerated by the patient. In fact, liver function study results are only mildly disturbed in most cases.[73]

Cardiopulmonary schistosomiasis produces a spectrum of pathologic changes including the development of diffuse minute arteriovenous fistulas with deficient oxygenation.[73]

The appearance of the rectosigmoid mucosa is variable, and many mild cases may appear normal even though

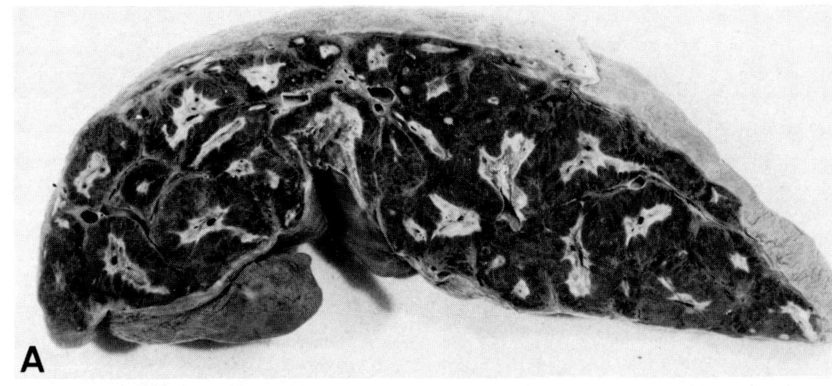

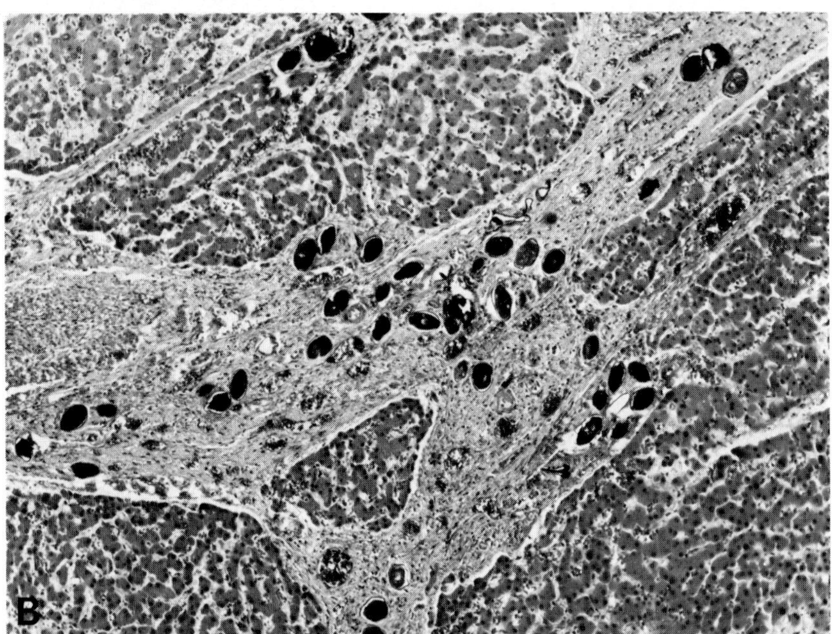

Fig. 11-33. **A. A liver showing classic Symmers pipestem fibrosis. The lobular architecture is preserved, while the parenchyma may be distorted by bands of fibrous tissue in the smaller portal areas. B. Eggs in a bland area of mature fibrosis (×58.75). (Courtesy Armed Forces Institute of Pathology 83437 and 749593.)**

superficial ulcerations and progressive thickening of the mucosa may mimic granulomatous colitis, inflammatory stricture, or carcinoma.[74] Hyperplastic (inflammatory) polyps of the colon can develop under the stimulus of eggs within the mucosa and simulate the pseudopolyps of chronic ulcerative colitis. Such polyps can disappear with medical treatment (niridazole).[76]

Diagnosis

The diagnosis of *S. mansoni* is most easily made by biopsy of the rectal mucosa. Multiple specimens are best taken from an upper rectal valve. Observation of the flickering flame cell or motility of the miracidium gives a clue to its viability. After treatment, the exterior shell may remain intact for months to years, although the egg is nonviable. This differentiation is important because the mere presence of eggs does not indicate the need for treatment. Coprology is much less successful, so it should not be used in lieu of biopsy to help identify eggs.

Serologic studies (complement-fixation, precipitin, and Bentonite flocculation, available through the Center for Disease Control) have been used chiefly in public health surveys, but may be useful in sporadic cases.[77]

Treatment

Drugs used in the treatment of *S. mansoni* are outlined in Table 11-4. Niridazole (Ambilhar) is administered orally in a single daily dose, and toxicity is evidenced by vomiting, cramps, dizziness, and headaches. Glucose 6-phosphate dehydrogenase–deficient patients may exhibit a hemolytic anemia. Central nervous system manifestations (convulsions and psychosis) are rarely seen.

Stibocaptate, antimony sodium dimercaptosuccinate, is an alternative drug but is contraindicated in renal, cardiac, and liver disease not caused by schistosomiasis. Toxic manifestations include vomiting, albuminuria, and purpura, and are indications for stopping the drug.[16]

The toxicity of available drugs must be weighed against the prognosis in each case. In the debilitated poor-risk patient, it is often wise to withhold specific treatment and to rely instead on supportive measures. Even in highly endemic areas, it is estimated that less than 10 percent of cases develop portal hypertension or the tumoral form of the disease.

Bleeding esophageal and gastric varices, secondary to portal hypertension, is a common complication of hepatosplenic schistosomiasis. As a rule, these patients tolerate hemorrhage better than patients with portal hypertension from portal cirrhosis, and encephalopathy and functional renal failure rarely ensue. Such hemorrhages usually respond to blood replacement, pitressin, and esophageal tamponade. When bleeding episodes become frequent, a variety of surgical procedures have been proposed. Portal caval shunt has been widely used. Some authors,[75] however, believe that there is an unacceptably high incidence of hepatic encephalopathy and liver failure associated with this procedure. Splenorenal shunts avoid these complications but have a higher incidence of shunt thrombosis. In endemic areas, splenectomy is favored. Prata [75] lists the following advantages of splenectomy: (1) elimination of the discomfort of a large abdominal swelling, (2) immediate correction of hypersplenism, (3) cure of infantilism, (4) improvement in the general state of the patient, and (5) reduction in portal pressure by about 40 percent. Ligation of esophageal varices has been proposed but is seldom indicated because the bleeding usually arrests with conservative measures.

Inflammatory and granulomatous lesions may produce obstructive or compressive lesions of the bowel or peritoneum. These masses, which resemble tumors, may become large and require resection for relief.

Schistosoma haematobium

Infection with *S. haematobium* is common in the valley of the Nile and in many areas of Africa, the Middle East, and southwestern India. The life cycle is similar to that of *S. mansoni* and *S. japonicum.* The adult worms lodge in the vascular plexus of the pelvis and bladder. *S. haematobium* is the chief cause of urogenital schistosomiasis with its exudative and granulomatous involvement of the bladder and ureters. Obstructive uropathy with hydroureter and hydronephrosis may ensue, but in the young it is reversible with medical treatment (Fig. 11-34). Masses of eggs with surrounding connective tissue frequently produce a bilharzioma, which may simulate an exophytic tumor.[73,78]

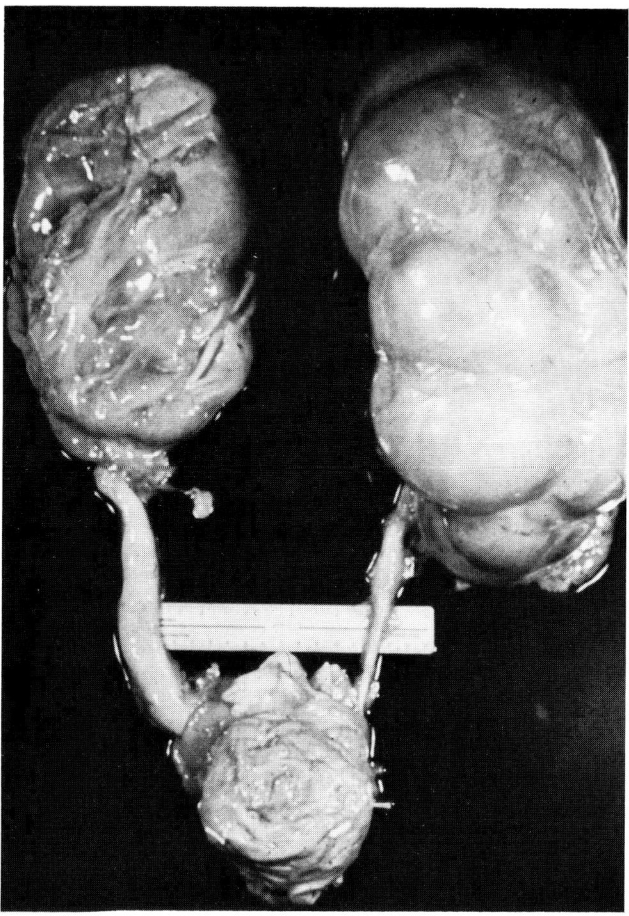

Fig. 11-34. **Schistosomal obstructive uropathy with bilateral hydronephrosis in an Egyptian. The bladder is calcified. (Courtesy Armed Forces Institute of Pathology 76–2330.)**

TABLE 11-4. DRUGS USED IN THE TREATMENT OF SCHISTOSOMIASIS

Drug	Adult Dose
	Schistosoma mansoni
Niridazole (Ambilhar)*	25 mg/kg (maximum 1.5 gm) Given daily in a single oral dose for 5–7 days
Antimony sodium dimercaptosuccinate (Stibocaptate)*	8 mg/kg IM, once or twice a week for 5 doses
	Schistosoma japonicum
Antimony potassium tartrate 0.5% solution	8, 12, 16, 20, and 24 ml given IV on alternate days. Followed by 28 ml IV on alternate days for 10 doses
Niridazole*	As for *S. mansoni,* give for 10 days
	Schistosoma haematobium
Niridazole*	As for *S. mansoni*
Antimony sodium dimercaptosuccinate (Stibocaptate)*	As for *S. mansoni*

* Available from the Parasitology Division, Center for Disease Control, Atlanta.

Radiography can demonstrate calcified eggs in the bladder wall. Ulceration of the bladder often produces hematuria, and inflammatory polyps may simulate carcinoma. In addition, there is a high incidence of malignancy associated with schistosomal bladder disease; of these 50 percent are squamous cell, 40 percent transitional cell, and 10 percent adenocarcinoma.[78] *S. haematobium* rarely causes cirrhosis but along with the other species can involve the central nervous system to produce Jacksonian epilepsy or the manifestations of tranverse myelitis. The diagnosis of *S. haematobium* is made by identifying typical eggs (Fig. 11-31) in rectal biopsy, in a centrifuged urine specimen or in histologic sections. In addition to medical treatment (Table 11-4), an operation to relieve chronic obstructive uropathy or associated neoplasm is often lifesaving.

Schistosoma japonicum

The Oriental blood fluke, *S. japonicum*, is encountered in the Far East. The basic life cycle is common to all the schistosomes. The adults reside in the tributaries of the inferior mesenteric veins. As with *S. mansoni*, the liver and intestinal tract are chiefly involved, although infection of the central nervous system can be severe. Diagnosis is best made via rectal biopsy with recovery of eggs having a tiny lateral spine which is often not seen (Fig. 11-31). These infections are highly resistant to treatment, and tartar emetic, despite its toxicity, is the best drug (Table 11-4).

PENTASTOMIDAS

Controversy exists as to whether pentastomids are arthropods or constitute a phylum that is intermediate between the annelids and the arthropods.[79] The members of this group (Fig. 11-35) superficially resemble helminths, live in the respiratory tree of reptiles and birds and the nasopharynx of carnivores, while the larvae parasitize many orders of vertebrates. The families Porocephalidae and Linguatulidae of the order Porocephalida are of medical importance to humans. In certain areas in Africa and Malaysia, nearly 50 percent of natives have evidence of larval infection.[80] Eggs passed from the respiratory passages in the saliva and in the feces of snakes may be accidentally ingested by man. Within the human intestinal tract, the larvae (Fig. 11-35) penetrate the gut wall and encyst within the peritoneal cavity, liver, mesentery or, rarely, the lung and eye. In most of these localities, the immature forms seldom produce symptoms but may be demonstrated as small curled "C-shaped" radiodensities. Significant symptoms are produced, however, when the third-stage larvae of Linguatula are acquired by people directly through the ingestion of raw or partially cooked liver or lymph nodes from sheep or goats (a dietary item of the Lebanese). These ingested larvae migrate directly from the stomach, where they attach themselves to the nasopharynx. Within a few hours, coughing, pain, nasal discharge, and wheezing may develop (Halzoun syndrome). Most people recover within 7 to 10 days, but edema of the upper respiratory passages can produce total obstruction. In this event, emergency tracheotomy may be necessary. Halzoun should be consid-

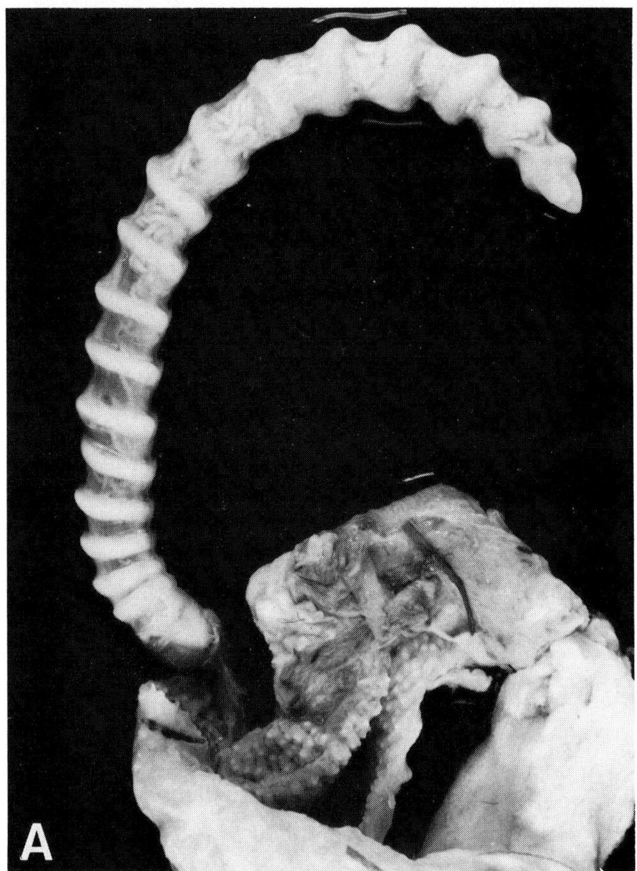

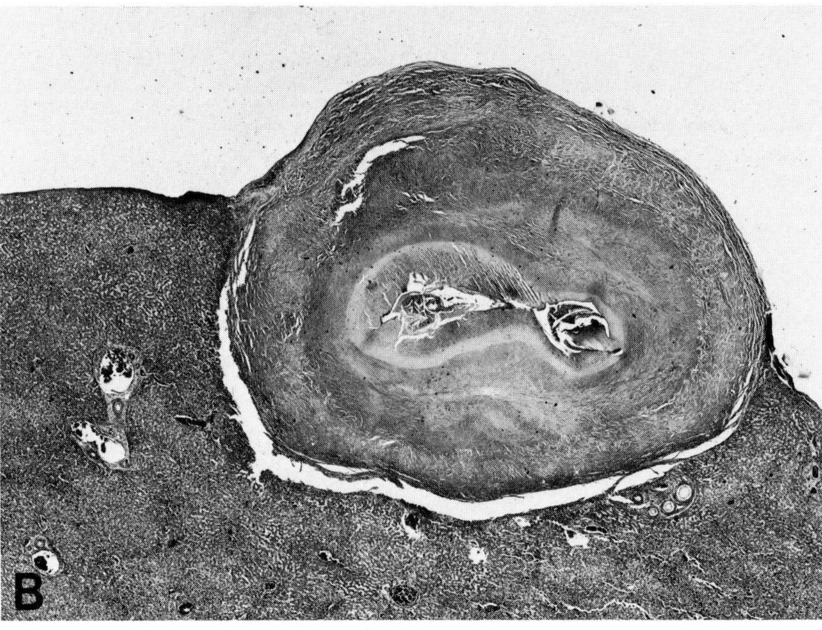

Fig. 11-35. **A. Adult female *A. armillatus* attached to the respiratory epithelium of a rock python from Zaire (×0.975). B. Encysted degenerating pentastomid larva in the liver (×9). (Courtesy Armed Forces Institute of Pathology 72–8881 and 75–7732.)**

ered when respiratory symptoms or distress occurs within minutes to hours after the ingestion of raw liver or lymph nodes. Rarely, third-stage larvae can be recovered.

SUBCUTANEOUS HELMINTHS

The surgeon is often called upon to excise a subcutaneous nodule or to biopsy an inflammatory serpiginous cutaneous lesion. As these may be parasitic in origin, it is important to understand the diverse etiologies. Table 11-5 outlines the most important of the helminths that produce skin lesions. Some of these are discussed in Chapter 25. For lesions produced by arthropods, a parasitology text should be consulted.[1]

In making a diagnosis of a cutaneous or subcutaneous parasitic infection, it is important to take a careful medical history, ie, the ingestion of undercooked chicken or fish for gnathostomiasis; the exposure to stagnant water in association with avian schistosomiasis, and the geographical location of the patient. Furthermore, the physical characteristics of the lesion—subcutaneous nodule, creeping eruption, or patchy edema—may indicate its cause. For example, the most common etiology of creeping eruption is exposure of the skin to the infective larvae of hookworms that infect animals, ie, *Ancylostoma braziliense* and *A. caninum.* In the biopsy of all migrating lesions (including the deep subcutaneous lesions produced by gnathostomosis), it should be remembered that the larvae are usually ahead of the advancing inflammatory tract they produce and that tissue excised for biopsy must include this region. Unfortunately, it is seldom possible to make species identification from biopsy material, and the pathologist must usually be content with recognition of the family or genus. Several subcutaneous parasitic diseases have already been discussed. (See sections on *Dirofilaria immitis* and *tenuis; Dracunculus medinesis; Onchocerca volvulus;* spiruroids [*Gongylonema* and *Thelazia*]; as well as sparganosis and cysticercosis, caused by cestodes; and *F. hepatica, P. westermani, S. mansoni, S. japonicum,* and *S. haematobium*).

Ancylostoma duodenale and *Necator americanus* (Human Hookworm)

The skin of the lower extremity is usually involved when the filariform larvae of hookworm species gain entrance to the body. The lesion is a tiny purplish macule that is intensely pruritic and persists for several days. Histologically, edema with a neutrophilic and inflammatory infiltrate is present. Secondary infection produces a condition known as ground itch (Fig. 11-36).[81,82]

Ancylostoma braziliensis and *A. caninum* (Nonhuman Hookworm)

Infection with the larvae of the dog and cat hookworm produces a cutaneous lesion, which is indistinguishable from infection with the human species.[83] Involvement is often on the trunk, as many persons acquire the infection while sun bathing on a beach contaminated with animal feces. The lesion is more chronic than those produced by human hookworms, and a pruritic inflammatory migrating tunnel is often observed. The histology is entirely similar to those of human hookworm. In biopsy material, the larvae can be identified by small double lateral alae (Fig. 11-36). Thiabendazole (see under *Trichiura,* Table 11-3) is usually effective in treatment, as is local freezing.

Strongyloides stercoralis

Penetration of the skin by infective filariform larvae can produce lesions identical to those of hookworm species. Such lesions usually occur on the lower extremities but may occur in the perianal area when hemorrhoidal tags or redundant mucosa promotes the collection of stool.

Gnathostoma spinigerum

Infection with this nematode is an unusual cause of "larva migrans" in humans and is endemic in Southeast Asia,

TABLE 11-5. HELMINTHIC INFECTIONS PRODUCING CUTANEOUS LARVAE MIGRANS AND SUBCUTANEOUS LESIONS IN MAN

Organism	Characteristic Skin Lesion
Nematodes	
Dirofilaria immitis, D. tenuis (nonhuman)	Subcutaneous mass
Dracunculus medinensis	Subcutaneous, migrating tunnel
Human Hookworm	
Ancylostoma duodenale	Ground itch
Necator americanus	(purplish macules, pruritic, urticaria)
Nonhuman Hookworm	
A. braziliense	Creeping eruption (pruritic,
A. caninum	migrating, inflammatory tunnel)
Gnathostoma spinigerum (nonhuman)	Migrating subcutaneous masses, intermittent urticaria, creeping eruption (rare)
Onchocerca volvulus	Subcutaneous masses (nonmigrant)
Spiruroids (nonhuman)	
Gongylonemia	Subcutaneous masses (rare)
Physaloptera	
Thelazia	Ground itch
Cestodes	
Taenia solium (cysticercosis)	Subcutaneous masses
Sparganosis (nonhuman)	Subcutaneous masses
Trematodes	
Fasciola hepatica	Subcutaneous masses
Paragonimus westermani	Subcutaneous masses
Schistosoma (human)	
mansoni, haematobium, and *japonicum*	Urticarial, patchy
Avian schistosomes (nonhuman)	Swimmers itch (urticarial)
Fresh and salt water	

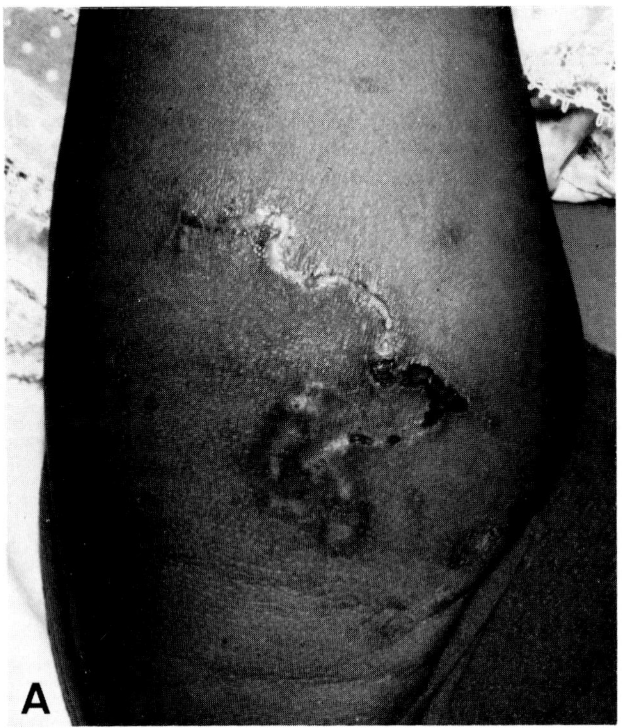

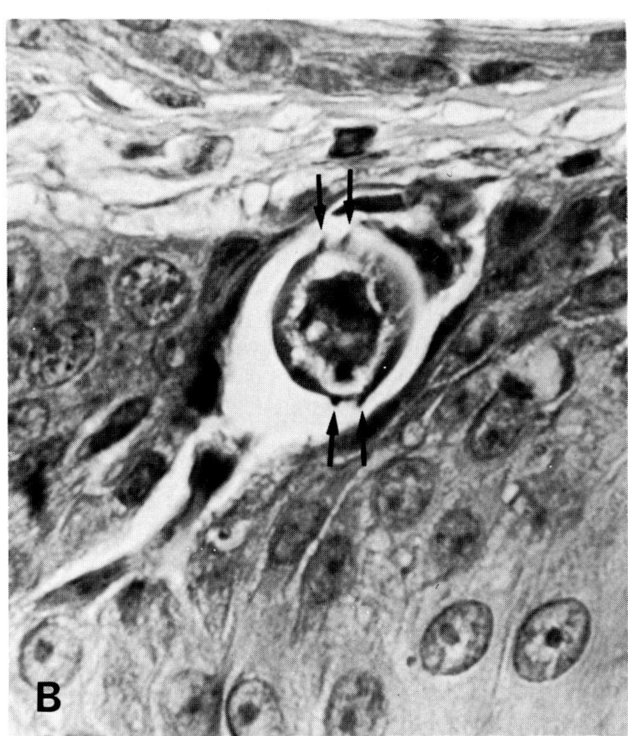

Fig. 11-36. A. Creeping eruption on the thigh of a Brazilian child. B. Creeping eruption with histologic section demonstrating small double alae of *Ancylostoma* sp (×697) (Courtesy Armed Forces Institute of Pathology 74–8291–2 and 75–9908.)

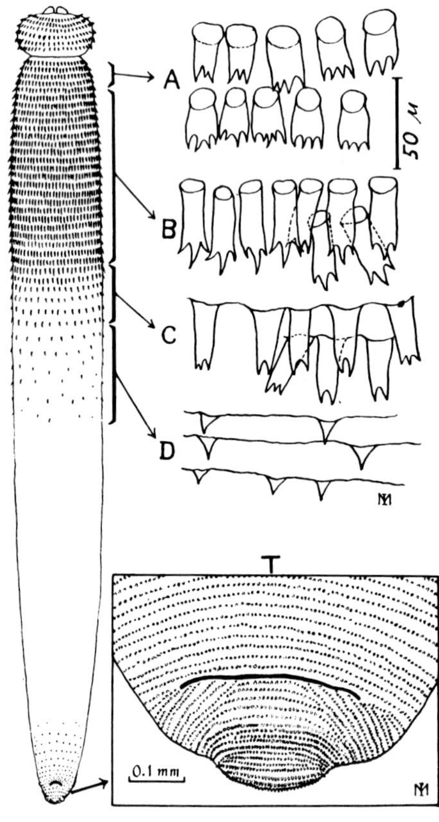

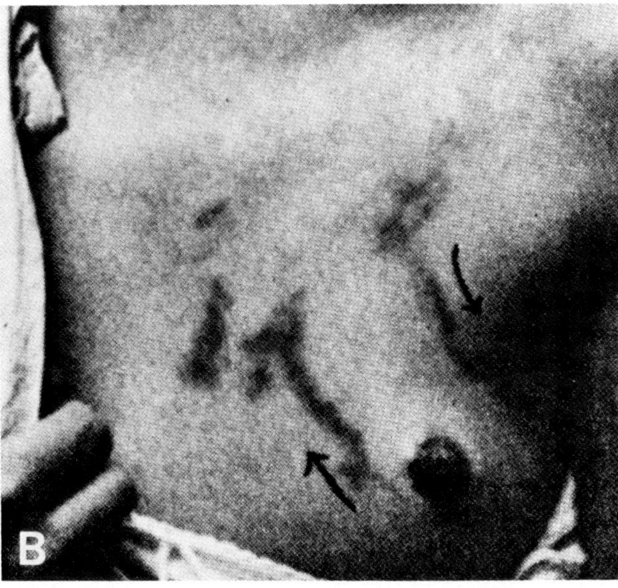

Fig. 11-37. A. Depiction of an adult female *G. spinigerum*, showing distribution of cuticular spines. Inset: magnified ventral vein of terminal end (T) covered by minute spines. B. Creeping eruption caused by larva between the epithelial layers. Movement can be as swift as 1 cm per hour. (Courtesy Armed Forces Institute of Pathology 75–10895–1 and 75–10895–9.)

India, and China.[84] The adult nematodes inhabit the gastric wall of wild and domestic members of the dog and cat family. The life cycle requires the passage of larvae through a cyclops and a wide variety of secondary intermediate hosts (freshwater fish and other animals, particularly chickens, which consume fish). Within 48 hours of the ingestion of infected foods (undercooked fish or chicken), allergic and abdominal symptoms ensue, and cutaneous manifestations begin in approximately 1 month. The typical lesion is subcutaneous rather than cutaneous, as with hookworm species and appears as a rounded, erythematous bulging, which is intensely pruritic. The appearance of lesions is periodic, and usually the larvae will migrate, occasionally as rapidly as 1 cm per hour, for 1 week and then become dormant for 2 to 6 weeks (Fig. 11-37). The central nervous system is rarely involved by this parasite.[85]

Avian schistosomes (Nonhuman)

Dermatitis produced by invasion with the cercariae of nonhuman schistosomes is characterized by intense pruritis and the appearance of patchy uriticarial macules and papules. The lesions disappear after 7 to 10 days, leaving pigmented residual spots. The condition should be suspected when a rash appears after the patient has been swimming in fresh, salt or brackish water. Treatment consists of systemic antihistamines and local antipruritic medications (calamine lotion) and local corticosteroids.[86]

ACKNOWLEDGMENT

In the preparation of this chapter the aid of G. E. Cosgrove, A. C. Olson, Jr., and M. H. Hauser of the Parasitology Study Group of the San Diego Zoo Hospital is gratefully acknowledged.

BIBLIOGRAPHY

Binford CH, Connor DH (eds.): Pathology of Tropical and Extraordinary Diseases, Vol. 1 & 2. Washington, AFIP, 1976, p. 308.

Hunter GW, Swartzwelder JC, and Clyde DF: Tropical Medicine. Philadelphia, Saunders, 1976.

Mandell GL, Douglas RG Jr, Bennett JE (eds.): Protozoal Diseases, Section G (Part III). In Principles and Practice of Infectious Diseases, vol II. New York, Wiley, 1979, pp. 2085–2153.

Mandell GL, Douglas RG Jr, Bennett JE (eds.): Diseases Due to Helminths, Section H (Part III). In Principles and Practice of Infectious Diseases, vol II. New York, Wiley, 1979, pp. 2155–2198.

REFERENCES

PROTOZOA

1. Faust EC, Russel PF, Jung RC: Craig and Faust's Clinical Parasitology, 8th ed. Philadelphia, Lea and Febiger, 1970.
2. Neal RA: Pathogenesis of amebiasis. In Cahill KM (ed): Clinical Tropical Medicine, Vol II. Baltimore, Baltimore Univ. Park Press, 1972, p 134.
3. Elsdon-Dew R: Factors influencing the pathogenecity of *Entamoeba histolytica*. Proceedings of the World Congress of Gastroenterology. Baltimore, Williams and Wilkins, 1959, p 770.
4. Villarejos VM: Studies on the pathogenecity of *Entamoeba histolytica* and other ameba species. Dissertation for PhD, Tulane University, New Orleans, 1961.
5. Teodorovic S, Ingals JW, Greenbergh L: Effects of corticosteroids on experimental amoebiasis. Nature (London) 197:86, 1963.
6. Phillips BP, Gorstein F: Effects of different species of bacteria on the pathology of enteric amebiasis in monocontaminated guinea pigs. Am J Trop Med 15:863, 1966.
7. Phillips BP, Wolfe PA, Bartgis IL: Studies on the ameba-bacteria relationship in amebiasis. Am J Trop Med 7:392, 1958.
8. El-Hashimi W, Pittman F: Ultrastructure of *Entamoeba histolytica* trophozoites obtained from the colon and from in vitro cultures. Am J Trop Med 19:215, 1970.
9. Connor DH, Neafie RC, Meyers WM: Amebiasis. In Binford CH, Connor DH (eds): Pathology of Tropical and Extraordinary Diseases, Vol 1. Washington, DC, AFIP, 1976, p 308.
10. Tucker PC, Webster PD, Kilpatrick ZM: Amebic colitis mistaken for inflammatory bowel disease. Arch Intern Med 135:681, 1975.
11. Juniper K: Amoebiasis. Clinics of Gastroenterology 7:3, 1978.
12. Lamont NH, Pooler NR: Hepatic amoebiasis: a study of 250 cases Q J Med 27:389, 1958.
13. Alicna AD, Fadell BJ: Advantage of purgation in recovery of intestinal parasites and their eggs. Am J Clin Pathol 31:139, 1959.
14. Monroe LS, Korn ER, Fitzwilliam SJ: A comparative study of the latex agglutination and the gel diffusion precipitin tests in the diagnosis of amebic liver abscess. Am J Gastroenterol 58:52, 1972.
15. Galgiani JN: Metronidazole for anaerobic bacterial infections. Drug Ther Nov:155, 1978.
16. The Medical Letter: Drugs for parasitic infections. 20:17, 1978.
17. Monroe LS: Amebiasis. In Bockus HL (ed): Gastroenterology, Vol 4. Philadelphia, Saunders, 1976, p 195.
18. Krogstad DJ, Spencer HC, Healy GR: Current concepts in parasitology: amebiasis. N Engl J Med 298:262, 1978.
19. Baskerville L, Yusufuddin A, Ramchand S: *Balantidium* colitis. Report of a case. Am J Dig Dis 15:727, 1970.
20. Cespedes R, Rodriguez O, Valverde O, Fernandez J, Gonzales FU, Jara JWP: Estudio de un caso anatomoclinico masivo con lesiones y presencia del parasito en el intestino delgado y pleura. Acta Medica Cost 10:135, 1967.
21. Neafie RC: Balantidiasis. In Binford CH, Conner DH (eds): Pathology of Tropical and Extraordinary Diseases, Vol I. Washington, DC, AFIP, 1976, p 325.
22. Woody NC, Woody HB: American trypanosomiasis. In clinical and epidemiologic background of Chagas' disease in the United States. J Pediadtr 58:568, 1961.
23. WHO: Chagas' disease: report of a study group. WHO Tech Rep Ser No 202. Geneva, 1960.
24. Edgcomb JH, Johnson CM: American trypanosomiasis (Chagas' disease). In Binford CH, Connor DH (eds): Pathology of Tropical and Extraordinary Diseases. Vol I. Washington, DC, AFIP, 1976, p 244.
25. Andrade ZA, Andrade SG: Chagas' disease (American trypanosomiasis). In Marcial-Rojas RA (ed): Pathology of Protozoal and Helminthic Diseases. Baltimore, Williams and Wilkins, 1971, p 69.
26. Ferreira-Santos R: Tratamento cirurgico do megaesofago. In

Cancado JR (ed): Doenca del Chagas. Belo Horizonte, Minas Gerais, 1968, Chap 29, p 592.

ANISAKIASIS

27. Van Thiel PH, Kuipers FC, Roskam RT: A nematode parasitic to herring, causing acute abdominal syndromes in man. Trop Geogr Med 12:97, 1960.
28. Yokogawa M, Yoshimura H: Clinicopathologic studies on larval antisakiasis in Japan. Am J Trop Med 16:723, 1967.
29. Yoshimura H: Parasitic granuloma with special reference to clinical pathology of anasakis-like larva infection in the digestive apparatus of man. Jpn J Parasitol 15:32, 1966.
30. Ishimura H, Hawasaka H, Kikuchi Y: Acute regional ileitis in Hokkaido with special reference to intestinal anisakiasis. Sapporo Med J 32:183, 1967.
31. Arean VM: Anisakiasis. In Marcial-Rojas RA (ed): Pathology of Protozoal and Helminthic Disease. Baltimore, Williams and Wilkins, 1971, p 846.

PHOCANEMA

32. Little MD, Most H: Anisakid larva from the throat of a woman in New York. Am J Trop Med Hyg 22:609, 1973.
33. Margolis L: Public health aspects of "codworm" infection: A review. J Fish Res Bd Can 1977, p 887.

ANGIOSTRONGYLUS COSTARICENSIS

34. Morera P, Cespedes R: *Angiostrongylus costaricensis* n. sp. (Nematoda: Metastrongyloidea) a new lungworm occurring in man in Costa Rica. Rev Biol Trop 18:173, 1971.
35. Morera P, Cespedes R: *Angiostrongilosis abdominal.* Acta Med Cost 14:159, 1971.
36. Morera P: Life history and redescription of *Angiostrongylus costaricensis.* Morera and Cespedes, 1971. Am J Trop Med and Hyg 22:613, 1973.
37. Sauerbrey M: A precipitin test for the diagnosis of human abdominal angiostrongyliasis. Am J Trop Med Hyg 26:1156.

ASCARIS

38. Pawlowski ZS: Ascariasis. Clin Gastroenterol 7:157, 1978.
39. Moens M, Dom J, Burke WE, Schlossberg S, Schuermans V: Levamisole in ascariasis. A multicenter controlled evaluation. Am J Trop Med Hyg 27:897, 1978.

DIROFILARIA SPECIES

40. Tuazon RA, Firestone F, Blanstein AU: Human pulmonary dirofilariasis manifesting as a "coin" lesion. A case report. JAMA 199:45, 1967.
41. Gershwin LJ, Gershwin ME, Kritzman J: Human pulmonary dirofilariasis. Chest 66:92, 1974.
42. Blecka LJ, Miller A, Graf EC: Human subcutaneous dirofilariasis in Illinois. JAMA 240:245, 1978.
43. Beaver PC, Samuel WN: Dirofilariasis in Canada. Am J Trop Med Hyg 26:329, 1977.
44. Harrison EG, Thompson JH: Dirofilariasis. In Marcial-Rojas RA (ed): Pathology of Protozoal and Helminthic Diseases. Baltimore, Williams and Wilkins, 1971, p 903.

DRACUNCULUS MEDINENSIS

45. Neafie RC, Connor DH, Meyers WM: Dracunculiasis. In Binford CH, Connor DH (eds): Pathology of Tropical and Extraordinary Diseases, Vol 2. Washington, DC, AFIP, 1976, p 397.

ENTEROBIUS VERMICULARIS

46. Duran-Jorda F: Appendicitis and enterobiasis in children: a histological study of 691 appendices. Arch Dis Child 32:208, 1957.
47. Moreno E: Enterobiasis (Oxyuriasis, Pinworm Infection). In Marcial-Rojas RA (ed): Pathology of Helminthic and Protozoal Diseases. Baltimore, Williams and Wilkins, 1971, p 760.

GONGYLONEMA PULCHRUM

48. Marcial-Rojas RA: Other rare spirurids which infect man. In Marcial-Rojas RA (ed): Pathology of Protozoal and Helminthic Diseases. Baltimore, Williams and Wilkins, 1971, p 864.

ONCHOCEREA VOLVULUS

49. Connor DH, Neafie RC: Onchocerciasis. In Binford CH, Connor DH (eds): Pathology of Tropical and Extraordinary Diseases, Vol II. Washington, DC, AFIP, 1976, p 360.

THELAZIA

50. Marcial-Rojas RA: Other rare spirurids which infect man. In Marcial-Rojas RA (ed): Pathology of Protozoal and Helminthic Diseases. Baltimore, Williams and Wilkins, 1971, p 866.

TOXOCARA CANIS AND CATI

51. Arean VM, Crandall CA: Toxocariasis. In Marcial-Rojas RA (ed): Pathology of Protozoal and Helminthic Diseases. Baltimore, Williams and Wilkins, 1971, p 808.
52. Glickman L, Schantz P, Dombroske R, Cypess R: Evaluation of serodiagnostic tests for visceral larva migrans. Am J Trop Med Hyg 27:492, 1978.
53. Krupp IM: A pet disease: visceral larva migrans. Drug Therap May:143, 1978.

TRICHURIS TRICHIURA

54. Ramirez-Weiser RR: Trichuriasis. In Marcial-Rojas RA (ed): Pathology of Protozoal and Helminthic Diseases. Baltimore, Williams and Wilkins, 1971, p 658.
55. Neafie RC, Connor DH: Trichuriasis. In Binford CH, Connor DH (eds): Pathology of Tropical and Extraordinary Diseases, Vol II. Washington, DC, AFIP, 1976, p. 415.

ECHINOCOCCUS GRANULOSIS AND MULTILOCULARIS

56. Miller CW, Ruppanner R, Schwabe CW: Hydatid diseases in California: study of hospital records, 1960 through 1969. Am J Trop Med Hyg 20:904, 1971.
57. Sparks AK, Connor DH, Neafie RC: Echinococcosis. In Binford CH, Connor DH (eds): Pathology of Tropical and Extraordinary Diseases, Vol II. Washington, DC, AFIP, 1976, p 530.
58. Vilardel F: Echinococcus (hydatid) cysts of the liver. In Bockus HL (ed): Gastroenterology, Vol III. Philadelphia, Saunders, 1976, p 570.
59. Poole JB, Marcial-Rojas RA: Echinococcosis. In Marcial-Rojas (ed): Pathology of Protozoal and Helminthic Diseases. Baltimore, Williams and Wilkins, 1971, p 635.

MULTICEPS MULTICEPS

60. Sparks AK, Neafie RC, Connor DH: Coenurosis. In Binford CH, Connor DH (eds): Pathology of Tropical and Extraordinary Diseases, Vol II. Washington, DC, AFIP, 1976, p 543.

SPARGANOSIS

61. Sparks AK, Neafie RC, Connor DH: Sparganosis. In Binford CH, Connor DH (eds): Pathology of Tropical and Extraordinary Diseases, Vol II. Washington, DC, AFIP, 1976, p 534.
62. Transurat P: Sparganosis. In Marcial-Rojas RA (ed): Pathology of Protozoal and Helminthic Diseases. Baltimore, Williams and Wilkins, 1971, p 585.

TAENIA SOLIUM

63. Marquez-Monter H: Cysticercosis. In Marcial-Rojas RA (ed): Pathology of Protozoal and Helminthic Diseases. Baltimore, Williams and Wilkins, 1971, p 592.
64. Sparks AK, Neafie RC and Connor DH: Cysticercosis. In Binford CH, Connor DH (eds): Pathology of Tropical and Extraordinary Diseases, Vol II. Washington, DC, AFIP, 1976, p 539.

CLONORCHIS SINENSIS

65. Dooley JR, Neafie RC: Clonorchiasis and opisthorchiasis. In Binford CH, Connor DH (eds): Pathology of Tropical and Extraordinary Diseases, Vol II. Washington, DC, AFIP, 1976, p 509.
66. Hou PC: The relationship between primary carcinoma of the liver and infestation with *Clonorchis sinensis.* J Pathol Bacterial 72:239, 1956.

FASCIOLA HEPATICA

67. Norton RA, Monroe L: Infection by *Fasciola hepatica* acquired in California. Gastroenterology 41:46, 1961.
68. Ashton WLG, Boardman PL, Everall PH, Houghton AWJ: Human fascioliasis in Shropshire. Br Med J 3:500, 1970.
69. Hardman EW, Jones RLH, Davies AH: Fascioliasis—a large outbreak. Br Med J 3:502, 1970.

PARAGONIMUS WESTERMANI

70. Meyers WM, Neafie RN: Paragonimiasis. In Binford CH, Connor DH (eds): Pathology of Tropical and Extraordinary Diseases, Vol II. Washington, DC, AFIP, 1976, p 517.
71. Chung CH: Human paragonimiasis (pulmonary distomiasis, endemic hemoptysis). In Marcial-Rojas RA (ed): Pathology of Protozoal and Helminthic Diseases. Baltimore, Williams and Wilkins, 1971, p 504.

SCHISTOSOMIASIS

72. Stoll NR: This wormy world. J Parasit 33:1, 1947.
72a. Warren KS: The relevance of schistosomiasis. N Engl J Med 303:203, 1980.
73. Marcial-Rojas RA: *Schistosomiasis mansoni.* In Marcial-Rojas RA (ed): Pathology of Protozoal and Helminthic Diseases. Baltimore, Williams and Wilkins, 1971, p 373.
74. Mendes TF: The schistosomiases. In Bockus HL (ed): Gastroenterology, Vol. 4. Philadelphia, Saunders, 1976, p. 220.
75. Prata A: *Schistosomiasis mansoni.* Clin Gastroenterol 7:49, 1978.
76. Nebel OT, el Masry NA, Castell DO, Farid Z, Fornes MJ, Sparks HA: Schistosomal disease of the colon: a reversible form of polyposis. Gastroenterology 67:939, 1974.
77. Kagan IG, Norman L: Serodiagnosis of parasitic diseases. In Blair JE, Lennette EH, Truant JP (eds): Manual of Clinical Microbiology. Bethesda, American Society for Microbiology, 1970, p 453.
78. McCully RM, Barron CN, Cheever AW: Schistosomiasis (bilharziasis). In Binford CH, Connor DH (eds): Pathology of Tropical and Extraordinary Diseases, Vol II. Washington, DC, AFIP, 1976, p 482.

PENTASTOMIDAS

79. Hopps HC, Keegan HL, Price DL, Self JT: Pentastomiasis. In Marcial-Rojas RA (ed): Pathology of Protozoal and Helminthic Diseases. Baltimore, Williams and Wilkins, 1971, p 970.
80. Meyers WM, Neafie RC, Connor DH: Pentastomids. In Binford CH, Connor DH (eds): Pathology of Tropical and Extraordinary Diseases, Vol II. Washington, DC, AFIP, 1976, p 546.

SKIN LESIONS

81. Meyers WM, Neafie RC, Connor DH: Ancylostomiasis. In Binford CH, Connor DH (eds): Pathology of Tropical and Extraordinary Diseases, Vol II. Washington, DC, AFIP, 1976, p 421.
82. DeLeon E, Maldonado JF: Uncinariasis (ancylostomiasis). In Marcial-Rojas (ed): Pathology of Protozoal and Helminthic Diseases. Baltimore, Williams and Wilkins, 1971, p 734.
83. Meyers WM, Neafie RC: Creeping eruption. In Binford CH, Connor DH (eds): Pathology of Protozoal and Extraordinary Diseases, Vol II. Washington, DC, AFIP, 1976, p 437.

GNATHOSTOMIASIS

84. Swanson VL: Gnathostomiasis. In Marcial-Rojas RA (ed): Pathology of Protozoal and Helminthic Diseases. Baltimore, Williams and Wilkins, 1971, p 871.
85. Swanson VL: Gnathostomiasis. In Binford CH, Connor DH (eds): Pathology of Tropical and Extraordinary Diseases, Vol II. Washington, DC, AFIP, 1976, p 471.
86. Hunter GW: Schistosome cercarial dermatitis and other rare schistosomes that may infect man. In Marcial-Rojas (ed): Pathology of Protozoal and Helminthic Diseases. Baltimore, Williams and Wilkins, 1971, p 450.

CHAPTER 12
Laboratory Diagnosis of Infections

HENRY H. BALFOUR, JR. AND DONNA J. BLAZEVIC

A MICROBIOLOGY laboratory is essential for establishing the etiology of infectious diseases. The clinical picture is often sufficient to narrow the differential diagnostic possibilities to several microorganisms, but it is unwise to rely solely on clinical data to diagnose and treat surgical infections. Knowledge of how to use the diagnostic microbiology laboratory is vital for the surgeon. This chapter will not make the reader a microbiologist, but details for various procedures will be given so that the surgeon can correctly interpret the results received from the diagnostic microbiology laboratory. In addition, a working knowledge of the techniques for each type of culture will provide insight into the limitations of the diagnostic procedures.

COLLECTION OF SPECIMENS

Specimen collection and transport are the foundation for reliable microbiologic diagnosis. A culture report is only as good as the specimen cultured. If specimens are inappropriately collected and transported, the etiologic agent can be lost and other organisms that are actually contaminants may be erroneously considered as pathogens.

GENERAL PRINCIPLES

Knowledge of normal flora is important for developing a rational approach to the collection of specimens and interpretation of the results. The skin, upper respiratory tract, intestinal tract, female genital area, and open wounds all have or develop normal microbial flora. The presence of normal flora is a problem but may be circumvented or minimized in one of the following ways.

1. Look only for organisms whose presence may be pathogenic, such as group A beta hemolytic streptococci or *Corynebacterium diphtheriae* in the throat. Indicate this to the microbiology laboratory when sending the specimen for culture.

2. Cleanse the area with an appropriate disinfectant to eliminate surface flora or contaminants. This is especially important when obtaining material from wounds.

3. Completely bypass areas of normal flora to reach tissue or body cavities not normally colonized with microbial agents. An example would be aspirating the bladder to obtain a urine sample for culture.

4. Use quantitation as a means of determining probable disease association, such as quantitative clean-catch urine specimens or bacterial counts from Gram stains of tissues.

Adequate equipment and materials are important in the collection and transport process, and new equipment and transport systems are being devised constantly (Fig. 12-1). Some prove to be valuable, but the laboratory must continuously evaluate them. Their adoption by a hospital should depend not on the laudatory literature supplied by the manufacturer but on actual clinical trial within the immediate environment.

Another important part of the collection process is the use of an appropriate requisition form. A completed requisition slip should accompany each specimen. Be sure to let the laboratory personnel know the diagnostic considerations, and fill in all requested information. The laboratory personnel can do a much better job with a specimen if they know the suspected organism (if possible), the clinical diagnosis, and recent antibiotic therapy.

COLLECTION OF SPECIMENS FOR BACTERIAL, FUNGAL, AND PARASITIC EXAMINATION

Abscesses

If possible, prepare the abscess surface with povidone-iodine solution and let dry. Aspirate 1–5 ml of purulent material with a sterile syringe and needle. Expel air from the syringe and inject the sample into an anaerobic vial, which can also be used for aerobic and fungal cultures. If a vial is not available, put a rubber cork on the end of the needle and send the specimen in the syringe to the laboratory immediately. Swabs should not be used because (1) the amount of material collected is too small, (2) swabs provide an inadequate sample of the total specimen, (3) contamination with surface flora is common, and (4) exposure to air, which is unsatisfactory for anaerobic cultures, is unavoidable.

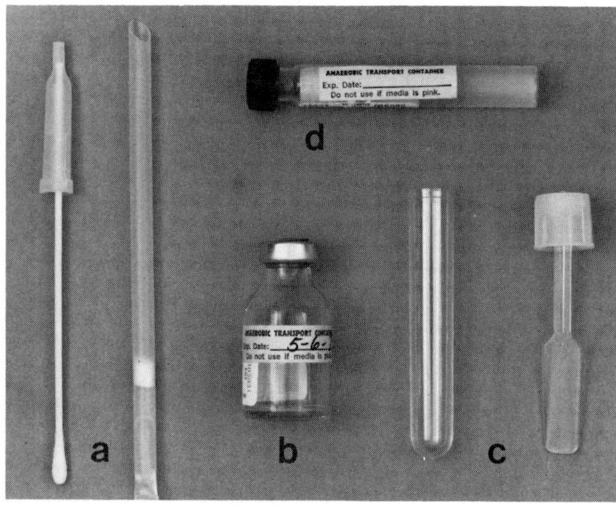

Fig. 12-1. **Devices useful for collection and transport of specimens. A. Culturette swab and tube (Marion Scientific, Kansas City, Missouri). B. Anaerobic transport vial (Gibco Diagnostics, Madison, Wisconsin). C. Swube paddle and tube (BBL, Cockeysville, Maryland). D. Anaerobic transport tube (Gibco Diagnostics).**

Actinomyces

See next section on anaerobic cultures.

Anaerobic Cultures

Collect specimens in special anaerobic containers as supplied by the laboratory. Routinely culture all abscesses and body fluids, except cerebrospinal and joint fluids, which rarely are infected with anaerobes. If anaerobes are specifically suspected, also culture wounds, drainage, endometrium, tissue, cerebrospinal fluid, and joint fluid. If urine is to be cultured for anaerobes, it must be obtained by suprapubic aspiration.

Whenever possible, aspirate material for culture. Expel air from the syringe and inject the specimen into an anaerobic vial. Put tissue samples into an anaerobic tube specifically designed for this purpose and follow the instructions for use of the particular tube. Specimens obtained for anaerobic culture may also be used for routine and fungal cultures.

The following specimens *should not be* cultured for anaerobes because they come from areas of the body that contain anaerobes as normal flora: mouth, throat, sputum, bronchial washings (unless collected by a covered brush system), skin, cervix, urethra, vagina, and stool.

Blood Cultures

Proper preparation of the skin is critical before performing a venipuncture. The following procedure is recommended: Scrub the venipuncture site for 2 minutes with povidone-iodine surgical scrub, dry it with sterile gauze, and then cover the site with povidone-iodine solution and allow it to dry. Do not touch the venipuncture site after cleansing, unless your finger has been similarly cleaned or you are wearing sterile gloves. Follow the directions established for the blood culture collecting device in use; this should include both an aerobic and an anaerobic bottle.

A frequent question is how many blood cultures should be drawn. In cases of suspected acute sepsis, acute untreated bacterial pneumonia, meningitis, or acute bacterial endocarditis, obtain two sets of blood cultures from separate sites (left and right arms) before starting empirical therapy. For cases of fever of unknown origin or suspected subacute bacterial endocarditis, obtain three sets of blood cultures on the first day. Draw the samples at least 60 minutes apart. If the culture results are negative after 24 hours, draw two to three more. If five or six blood cultures are negative, special culture techniques may be needed. Data indicate that patients with suspected acute infections rarely have positive blood culture results after five to six negative sets. Although previous antimicrobial therapy may delay the growth of organisms, more than five or six cultures do not increase the yield of positives. There is almost no information on the proper guidelines to follow in cases of suspected infection after various types of operations. One must assume in these cases that cultures of blood will be valuable any time conditions change.

Body Fluid Culture, Except Urine and Cerebrospinal Fluid

For percutaneous collection, prepare the skin as for blood cultures. In any case, the fluid should be aspirated with a sterile syringe and needle. Expel air from the syringe, and inject the sample into an anaerobic vial. If a vial is not available, put a rubber cork on the end of a needle, and send the specimen to the laboratory immediately. Do not collect the specimen on swabs, and do not use blood culture systems for these samples.

Bronchoscopic Washing

Collect the washings using a covered brush system and place in an anaerobic tube or other anaerobic collection vial. If no anaerobic vial is available, a sterile syringe technique, as described in the previous section, can be used.

Bullous Lesions, Cellulitis, Petechiae, or Vesicles

Again, the skin is cleansed as for blood cultures. The lesion must not be ruptured during preparation. Aspirate sample material with a sterile syringe and needle; do not use swabs. Inject the material into a sterile tube, or place a cork on the needle and transport the syringe to the laboratory. If no aspirate is available, sterile normal saline for injection (without preservative) may be injected and aspirated at the lesion edges.

Petechiae present special collection problems. After cleansing the skin, excoriate the lesion with a needle. This material can be used to inoculate a chocolate agar plate or to prepare a smear for Gram stain directly at the bedside. Swabs are not acceptable because of possible contamination with surface flora.

Catheters

To culture venous or arterial catheters, disinfect the entry site, remove the catheter, clip off the tip, and drop it aseptically into a sterile container. Do not culture Foley catheters, because a positive result does not correlate with urinary tract infection. If infection is suspected, culture the urine.

Cerebrospinal Fluid

Gloves, gown, and mask must be worn to avoid contamination of the cerebrospinal fluid with respiratory or other flora because inadvertent introduction of respiratory streptococci into the cerebrospinal fluid sample will alter the results and confuse the diagnosis. Wearing the mask prevents unnecessary exposure to *Mycobacterium tuberculosis* or meningococcus.

Prepare the skin as for a blood culture, drape the surrounding skin with sterile linen, and collect 2–5 ml of cerebrospinal fluid in a sterile, screw-capped (leakproof) tube. Ideally, separate tubes should be collected for culture, cell counts, and chemical determinations.

Cervix

Use a speculum lubricated with water, not petroleum products, to examine the cervical os, and collect a culture sample. Insert a swab into the distal portion of the cervical os, rotate gently, and allow it to remain for 10 to 30 seconds so that it is saturated. For gonococcal cultures, immediately inoculate a warm (room temperature) Thayer-Martin agar plate at one edge. Send the plate to the laboratory immediately. For nongonococcal cultures, place the specimen in a Culturette tube (Marion Scientific Corporation, Kansas City, Missouri) or other satisfactory transport system.

Endometrium

Insert a speculum, visualize the cervical os. Remove the mucous plug, wipe the cervical os with povidone-iodine solution, and aspirate material by needle and syringe or by a double lumen catheter. The catheter technique involves first making a slight cut in the end of a No. 16 straight rubber catheter. Insert the catheter through the cervical os, pass a No. 8 infant feeding tube or intravenous catheter through the lumen of the rubber catheter to avoid contamination by normal flora, and aspirate the material. If an anaerobic culture is desired, expel air from the syringe and inject the material into an anaerobic vial. If the specimen is to be cultured only for aerobic and facultative organisms, place the aspirate in a sterile tube.

Do not collect the specimen on swabs because it will be contaminated with normal cervical and vaginal flora.

Eye

Collect culture samples from the eye by retracting the lower lid and blotting the conjunctiva or pus with a swab. Avoid the lid margins and eyelashes, or the sample may be contaminated. Place the swab into a Culturette tube or other suitable transport system.

Fungal Cultures

For culture of blood see the previous section, blood cultures.

Systemic Fungi

When systemic fungi such as *Histoplasma, Blastomyces,* or yeast are suspected, collect the specimen as described for bacterial culture from appropriate sites.

For the culture of dermatophytes from skin, cleanse the area with 70 percent alcohol, scrape off some skin at the active border of the lesion (including some healthy skin), and place the scrapings in a dry sterile container. The same procedure should be used for nails, except that the initial portions of the nails should be discarded and deeper scrapings sent for culture.

Gonococcal Cultures

In females, collect cervical specimens using the method previously described. In addition, if there is purulent material in the urethra, swab it and inoculate it directly onto a warm Thayer-Martin agar plate. If no purulent material is seen in the urethra, collect an anal sample by inserting a swab approximately 3 cm into the anal canal. Move the swab from side to side to sample the crypts and leave it for 10 to 30 seconds to allow for absorption of organisms. Inoculate it directly onto a warm Thayer-Martin plate. Do not make a smear, because gonococcal infection cannot be confirmed or ruled out by Gram staining material from this source. Send the culture to the laboratory immediately.

In males, collect a sample of the urethral exudate with a swab. If no exudate is present, use a sterile bacteriologic loop and gently scrape the mucosa of the anterior urethra. Alternately, a flexible wire swab may be inserted into the urethra. Inoculate the specimen directly onto a warm Thayer-Martin plate and also prepare a smear. An anal culture should also be collected.

Malarial and Other Blood Parasites

Blood collected from the finger or earlobe should be used to prepare both thick and thin films when malaria or other parasites are suspected. The thick films need to dry at room temperature for 8 to 12 hours before stains may be performed. Collect two sets of films approximately 8 hours apart each day for 3 days.

Mycobacteria Cultures

Sputum. Do not submit a 24-hour specimen of sputum for mycobacteria cultures. Collect the first morning sputum on three separate days, and send each separately (see section on sputum collection that follows). Refrigerate specimens until they are sent to the laboratory. If the patient is not producing sputum, induce its production by having the patient inhale a warm aerosol of sterile 1 percent aqueous sodium chloride. The best time for this procedure is in the morning before breakfast. Induced sputum is superior to a gastric specimen, but a combination of both will give more positive culture results than either will alone.

Gastric washings. The specimen should be collected through a nasogastric tube 30 minutes after induction of sputum. If the specimen is not sent to the laboratory within 1 day, the acid should be neutralized by adding about 100 mg of powdered sodium carbonate.

Urine. A 24-hour specimen of urine should not be used for culture. Collect the first morning midstream urine on three separate days, and send each as a separate specimen (see section on urine collection). The specimens should be refrigerated if there is a delay in sending them to the laboratory.

Nasopharynx

Cultures of the nasopharynx are only indicated for diagnosis of streptococcal disease in infants, for *Bordetella pertussis* (whooping cough), and to detect carriers of *Neisseria meningitidis.* The patient should be comfortably seated, with the head tilted back. A flexible wire swab is inserted through a nasal speculum into the posterior nasopharyngeal area. The swab is gently rotated and allowed to remain in place for 20 to 30 seconds. The swab is placed in a Culturette tube or other satisfactory transport system. If *B. pertussis* is suspected, immediately inoculate fresh Bordet-Gengou plates previously ordered from the microbiology laboratory. If the culture is being used to detect *N. meningitidis* carriers, be sure to indicate this on the request slip.

Nocardia

See section on fungi.

Nose

Samples from the nose are taken by swabbing the anterior nares with a sterile swab and placing it in a Culturette tube or other satisfactory transport system.

Peritoneal Fluid

See body fluid section.

Pinworm Ova

A Swube paddle (Falcon, Division of Becton, Dickinson & Co., Oxnard, CA) can be used to collect the pinworm ova specimen in the morning before the patient has bathed or defecated. Hold the paddle by its cap and remove it from the tube. Separate the buttocks and press the tacky surface against several areas of the perianal region. Replace the paddle in the tube and send it to the laboratory. Three consecutive morning specimens should be collected to ensure detection of pinworm infection.

Pleural Fluid

See body fluid section.

Skin

See bullous lesions, cellulitis, petechiae, or vesicles

Sputum

Expectorated sputum is not recommended for routine bacterial culture because of unavoidable contamination with upper respiratory flora. The high incidence of staphylococci and gram-negative rods in the oral cavity of hospitalized individuals and the presence of potential pathogens as normal upper respiratory flora make interpretation of sputum cultures difficult. The presence of 10 epithelial cells per low-power field on Gram stain of sputum indicates extensive oropharyngeal contamination. These specimens should not be cultured.

A sputum culture is distinctly valuable if a pathogen that rarely contaminates the mouth or pharynx is isolated. For example, the pathogenic dimorphic fungi, *M. tuberculosis, Pneumocystis carinii, Strongyloides stercoralis,* and cytomegalovirus can be diagnosed from sputum cultures alone.

Have the patient gargle with water and then cough deeply to expectorate the material into a sterile container. A transtracheal aspirate may be necessary in seriously ill or debilitated patients.

Stool

Stool Bacterial Culture

Stool cultures are useful for isolation of *Salmonella, Shigella,* and *Campylobacter* species routinely. In special cases culture for *Yersinia, Vibrio,* or *Clostridium difficile* may be indicated. A test for *C. difficile* toxin may also be indicated for diagnosis of antibiotic-associated colitis. Acute typhoid fever is best diagnosed from blood cultures because the bacteria are rarely found in the stool during the acute phase of the illness. Diarrhea caused by enterotoxigenic *E. coli* cannot be diagnosed by stool culture. *S. aureus* and *C. albicans* must be present in large numbers in Gram stain of the feces to justify a diagnosis of staphylococcal or candidal enteritis; isolation of either organism alone is not sufficient—they are part of the normal fecal flora.

The specimen should be collected in a sterile bedpan or on newspaper over the toilet seat. Place a portion in a sterile nonpaper container, with a lid. Send the specimen to the laboratory immediately. If a rectal swab must be used instead of a stool, insert the swab 3 cm into the anal canal and leave it in for 20 to 30 seconds. Place the swab in a Culturette tube or other transport system. One specimen should be tested during the acute illness.

Request a smear for fecal leukocytes; their presence will differentiate bacterial gastroenteritis from nonspecific, toxic, or viral diarrhea. In the absence of fecal leukocytes, more than one stool culture cannot be justified.

Stool for Ova and Parasites

Stool samples to test for ova and parasites should be collected in the same manner as for bacterial culture. Specimens should not be mixed with urine or toilet bowl water because this destroys the protozoan trophozoites. A maximum of three normally passed specimens should be collected on three alternate days; the parasites are not passed consistently. If no parasites are found after three tests, one saline-purged stool may be obtained, or rectal biopsy material can be submitted. If all four specimens reveal no ova and parasites, the patient probably does not have an intestinal parasitic infection. Stools from patients receiving antidiarrheal compounds, antibiotics, antacids, oils, bismuth, or barium are unsuitable for examination. Wait at least 7 days after barium or bismuth administration before collecting a specimen suspected of containing parasites. Never transport stools in an incubator, because it enhances the disintegration of trophozoites. Liquid or soft stools should be brought to the laboratory immediately, whereas formed stools can be refrigerated.

It is important to tell the laboratory which organism you suspect (eg, *Shistosoma, Giardia*). The patient's travel history will assist the laboratory personnel to perform optimal examinations of each specimen.

Throat

Culture samples from the throat can be taken with the help of a tongue blade and bright light. Swab both tonsillar areas, posterior pharynx, and areas of inflammation, ulceration, or exudation. Place the swab in a Culturette tube or other transport device. If *C. diphtheriae* is suspected, the swab should be rubbed firmly over the lesion, or if possible, inserted beneath the tonsillar membrane. Consult the microbiology laboratory for the appropriate medium to be inoculated at the bedside. Send the culture to the laboratory immediately.

Transtracheal Aspirate

Transtracheal aspirate is valuable only when anaerobic pneumonia or lung abscess is suspected. It is not a routine culture technique, and is best done by an experienced individual. Aspirate the material from the transtracheal catheter with a sterile syringe. Expel air, and inject the sample into an anaerobic vial.

Urethra

See gonococcal cultures.

Urine

Because overnight incubation in the bladder yields the highest bacterial counts, the first morning urine sample is the best specimen to culture.

For clean-catch or midstream specimens, either assist the patient or give both verbal and written instructions, which include the following for females: Have the patient remove her undergarments and wash her hands with soap and water—dry them with a disposable paper towel. With one hand, the patient or nurse should spread the labia and keep them apart for the rest of the procedure. Using a fresh povidone-iodine swab for each movement, wipe the inner labial tissues down one side from front to back; then wipe the other side from front to back. With another fresh swab, wipe center from front to back. Repeat until thoroughly clean, and finally dry the area with sterile gauze. Have the patient void a small amount of urine into the toilet or a bedpan. Stop the flow briefly, and then continue the flow into a sterile specimen container. A few drops are adequate for culture, but 5–10 ml are ideal. Be careful not to touch the inner part of the container or lid while the container is being capped.

In males: Have the patient wash his hands with soap and water and dry them with a disposable paper towel. Retract the foreskin, if necessary. Using a povidone-iodine swab, clean the glans and meatus thoroughly and wipe with sterile gauze. Void a small amount into the toilet or a bedpan. Stop the flow briefly, and then have the patient void 5–10 ml into a sterile specimen container.

In infants or small children: After cleaning the periurethral tissues, place a sterile urine bag over the labia or penis to collect urine. If no urine is present after 30 minutes, reclean the patient and attach a new bag. If it is impossible to obtain urine or if the culture yields a mixture of organisms, a suprapubic aspiration is recommended.

The suprapubic tap is the most desirable technique for infants and small children. The suprapubic area should be scrubed with povidone-iodine surgical scrub. Paint the area with povidone-iodine solution and allow it to dry. Using a sterile syringe and needle, aspirate a few milliliters of urine from the bladder. Inject the urine into a sterile container. If an anaerobic culture is desired, expel the air and inject the sample into an anaerobic vial.

All specimens should be refrigerated if there is to be a delay in transport to the laboratory. Urine for culture should never be taken from a bedpan or urinal, nor should a specimen be brought from home because any contaminants will have multiplied and false-positive results are common.

Venereal Disease

If *Chlamydia* or *Gonococcus* is suspected, the appropriate sections in this chapter should be consulted.

TABLE 12-1. WHICH PATIENTS TO STUDY FOR VIRAL INFECTIONS AND WHAT TO COLLECT

General Disease Category	Specimens Recommended for Viral Cultures
Neonatal	Throat swab, fresh morning urine; vesicular fluid or swabs if rash is present
Respiratory (index or lower respiratory tract involvement)	Throat swab
Central nervous system	Throat swab; stool or rectal swab (stool is preferable); urine, CSF, biopsy material; vesicular fluid if available
Gastrointestinal	Throat swab, stool or rectal swab
Exanthems	Throat swab; stool or rectal swab; vesicular fluid if present
Fever of unknown origin	Throat swab; urine; stool; heparinized blood
Infections in immunocompromised patients	Throat swab, urine, heparinized blood, bronchial washings

Haemophilus ducreyi. Special chocolate agar (with and without vancomycin) should be ordered from the laboratory before collection and should be present at the patient's bedside for immediate incubation. The ulcer base should be cleansed thoroughly with a sterile gauze pad moistened in sterile saline. A sterile swab moistened in sterile saline should then be applied to the cleansed ulcer base and immediately rolled at the edge of the chocolate plate. Only then should it be rolled at the edge of the plate with vancomycin. The plates should be taken to the laboratory immediately. A direct smear is not indicated because other gram-negative bacteria, eg, *Bacteroides fragilis,* have morphology similar to *H. ducreyi.*

Syphilis. Serologic tests are best for the diagnosis of syphilis. Many laboratories do not even perform dark-field examinations for syphilis because substantial expertise is required to differentiate *Treponema pallidum* from saprophytic treponemes.

When obtaining specimens from open lesions, always wear rubber gloves. First remove surface crusts or scabs, cleanse several times with a saline-soaked gauze sponge. Dry the surface and abrade it until it bleeds. Remove the blood by gentle sponging, and when a serum exudate appears touch it with a No. 1 coverslip. Invert the coverslip on a slide, and seal the edges with Vaseline or other suitable sealing material. Immediately send the specimen for dark-field examination. Delay will result in loss of motility of the spirochetes.

Wounds

To collect culture samples from closed wounds, use the technique described in the section on bullous lesions.

For open wounds, clean the sinus tract opening or wound surface with a sterile water-soaked sponge. Be careful not to use bacteriostatic saline. Curettings of the wound are best because the contribution of the surface flora is minimized. Alternatively, aspirate the material with a sterile syringe and needle or catheter. Do not use swabs. If little fluid is present, inject a small amount of sterile water, and aspirate. Place any material into a sterile container. If an anaerobic culture is desired, expel air bubble from the syringe and inject the sample into an anaerobic vial or place curettings into an anaerobic tube. Send the specimen to the laboratory immediately, and indicate the site of the wound on the request slip.

Viruses

We recommend collecting viral specimens from all patients who have the general types of infection listed in Table 12-1. Collect the specimens as outlined in Table 12-2. When submitting specimens for viral culture, always send an additional serum sample for acute viral antibody titers. If no virus is isolated, submit a second serum 2 to 6 weeks later. The diagnosis can then be made by finding an antibody titer rise, as described later in this chapter.

TRANSPORTATION OF SPECIMENS

Although some specific directions for specimen transport were already included, they are worth repeating because even when the sample is obtained by the best technique available, the organisms might be altered or lost during inappropriate storage and transportation. Some organisms, including enteric gram-negative rods, anaerobes, and myxo- and herpes group viruses, do not survive outside of the body for long and are particularly susceptible to drying. Culturette tubes contain a small amount of Stuart's medium in a capsule, which is broken after a swab has been inserted in the tube, to provide enough liquid medium to keep the specimen moist.

When the specimen collected is a body fluid, many organisms will proliferate in the fluid at room temperature. For example, the number of *E. coli* in contaminated urine will double every 20 minutes at room temperature. If the urine specimen cannot be delivered to the laboratory within 20 minutes after collection for bacterial culture or within 4 hours for viral isolation, the sample should be held in a refrigerator (4C). Refrigerator temperatures are deleterious to the types of fastidious bacteria that may be found in body fluids, and specimens containing these must be delivered to the laboratory immediately. Specimens should not be frozen for storage.

Serum samples for antibody titers may be shipped, if necessary, at room temperature if the sera have been separated from the clot. Most serologic tests measure IgG antibody, which is extremely stable unless the specimen is grossly contaminated with bacteria. Even IgM can usually survive shipment at room temperature. Sera may also be stored or shipped frozen, but whole blood should never be frozen because hemolysis renders complement-fixation tests impossible.

For anaerobic cultures, particularly those placed in

TABLE 12-2. COLLECTION OF SPECIMENS FOR VIRAL DIAGNOSIS

Specimen	Method
Throat swab	Swab posterior pharynx briskly with two sterile, dry, cotton-tipped applicators. (If respiratory syncytial virus is suspected, it may be preferable to insert one swab into the nasopharynx and use the other to swab the posterior pharynx. They can be sent to the laboratory as one specimen.) Insert the tips of the applicators into a sterile tube containing medium suitable for bacteriologic cultures such as trypticase soy or Hank's balanced salt solution. Culturette tubes are acceptable.
Rectal swab	Insert two cotton-tipped applicators at least 3 cm into the rectum. The swab should be stained with stool. Transport as a throat swab.
Vesicular lesions	If vesicles are intact, aspirate at least six lesions with a 25-gauge needle attached to a tuberculin syringe. Replace the hub on the needle. Label the syringe appropriately and send to the laboratory.
Urine, stool, cerebrospinal fluid, biopsy, or autopsy	Collect in sterile containers. At least 1 gm of tissue or stool, 2 ml of spinal fluid, and 20 ml of urine are adequate.
Heparinized blood (for viral isolation)	Draw at least 10 ml of blood and place in a heparinized tube at once; shake gently to insure anticoagulation.
Serum (for antibody tests)	Two specimens are preferred; the first should be collected as soon after onset of acute illness as possible, and the second two to six weeks later. Collect 7 ml of blood, if possible, in a plain (not anticoagulated) tube. Avoid hemolysis and do not freeze.

tubes, rapid transportation is essential because the anaerobic atmosphere can become aerobic and the fastidious anaerobes will be lost.

A good clinical microbiology laboratory will have arranged for messenger services and timed specimen pickup; these are critically important. It is an excellent idea to monitor the time from collection of specimens to the time the laboratory has logged them in. In the case of urine cultures, more than 20 minutes from collection to receipt in the laboratory is unsatisfactory. This could be solved by arranging to have the urine specimens put on ice after collection and during transportation to the laboratory.

BEST METHODS OF LABORATORY DIAGNOSIS

In addition to appropriate collection and transportation of microbiology specimens, one should also have a working knowledge of the best laboratory procedures for making an accurate diagnosis of each microbial agent. A summary of the optimal methods is given in Table 12-3.

DIRECT MICROSCOPIC EXAMINATION

Direct Gram stains of certain clinical specimens are extremely valuable (Fig. 12-2). One of the most useful is Gram-staining the spinal fluid sediment, which can give the diagnosis of *H. influenzae, N. meningitidis,* or *S. pneumoniae* meningitis. If organisms are seen on the Gram stain, a Quellung test with specific polyvalent antiserum will establish the diagnosis almost immediately. It is also very useful to perform Gram stains on purulent exudates to determine immediately the types of organisms involved and their relative numbers. Because you may want or need to perform a Gram stain yourself, a satisfactory method is given in Table 12-4. The Gram stain is especially useful where anaerobes are suspected. Finding pleomorphic gram-negative rods suggests the presence of *B. fragilis,* and appropriate therapy with chloramphenicol or clindamycin can be instituted (Fig. 12-3).

A Gram stain can give not only rapid information as to the class and general morphology of the organism, but also important quantitative information. For example, in mixed infections, the most prevalent organism cannot always be gleaned from a culture because after bacteria are inoculated onto medium, the rates of growth differ. If a large number of a slow-growing organism were present in the wound, only a few organisms may become apparent on the culture plate. A smaller number of a fast-growing organism may proliferate and appear to be more impor-

TABLE 12-3. CLINICAL MICROBIOLOGY LABORATORY DIAGNOSIS

Agent	Best Method for Diagnosis
Bacteria	Isolation of organisms on agar or in broth media; direct Gram stains of certain specimens valuable
Chlamydiae	Inoculation into cell culture and identification of inclusion bodies in infected cells
Fungi	Isolation of organisms on selective media, such as Saboraud's; detection of antigen by latex agglutination useful for *Cryptococcus;* India ink preparation of cerebrospinal fluid; KOH preparation of direct specimens
Mycobacteria	Culture definitive but slow; acid-fast stains of sputum or lymph nodes valuable
Mycoplasma pneumoniae	Serology; four-fold or greater rise in complement-fixing titers or elevated cold agglutinins
Parasites	
Helminths	Identification of ova or larvae in stool preparations
Protozoa	Direct microscopic identification of organisms in stool, tissue, or blood specimens; specific stains sometimes useful
Rickettsia	Serology: fourfold rise in complement-fixing tests or elevated *Proteus* agglutinins
Viruses	Isolation in cell cultures or fourfold rise in serum antibody titers

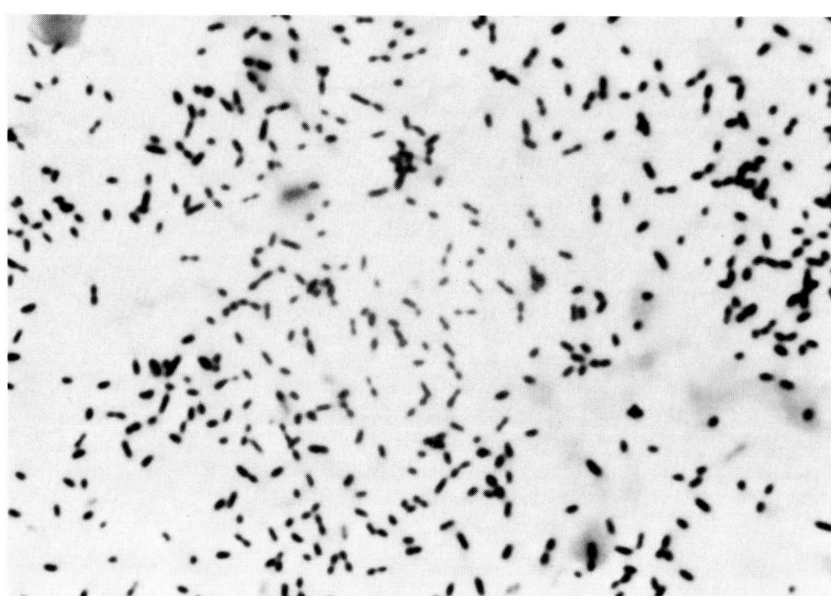

Fig. 12-2. Gram stain of cerebrospinal fluid showing typical gram-positive diplococci, indicating the presence of *Streptococcus pneumoniae.* (Courtesy of Louise Hofherr, University of Minnesota, Minneapolis.)

tant on culture. The truly predominant organism may be identifiable on initial smear and Gram stain.

Direct examination of the specimen in actinomycosis may demonstrate the presence of the diagnostic sulphur granules. If these are seen, an acid-fast stain should also be performed. *Actinomyces* are not acid-fast, and this distinguishes them from *Nocardia,* which are acid-fast and may produce a similar granule.

Direct examination of all specimens sent for fungal cultures should be performed. This is best done by suspending a portion of the specimen in a potassium hydroxide solution. The potassium hydroxide dissolves the tissue elements and reveals the fungal hyphae or mycelium. Although a specific identification of the fungus cannot always be made, its presence in the tissue indicates a fungal infection and thus helps to determine that any fungus subsequently isolated is not a contaminant.

TABLE 12-4. METHOD OF GRAM STAINING

Procedure: Prepare smear and fix with heat.

1. Flood slide with crystal violet (solution A). Add about 3 drops solution B. Wash with tap water.
2. Flood slide with iodine. Wash with tap water.
3. Decolorize with acetone-alcohol until no more purple is seen in the washings (about 10 seconds, depending on thickness of smear). Wash with tap water.
4. Flood slide with safranin. Wash with tap water. Blot dry with clean blotter, bibulous paper, or paper towel.

Reagents	
Solution A—crystal violet	
Crystal violet, CI 42555	20 gm
Distilled water	2,000 ml
Solution B—sodium bicarbonate	
$NaHCO_3$	100 gm
Distilled water	2000 ml
Iodine (dilute 1 : 10 for working solution)	
Iodine crystals	100 gm
Potassium iodide (KI)	5 gm
Sodium hydroxide pellets	20 gm
Distilled water	500 ml
Add sodium hydroxide pellets slowly to 50 ml water. After pellets have dissolved, add iodine and potassium iodide. Add 300–400 ml water and mix until iodine goes into solution. Dilute to total of 500 ml. Dilute 1 : 10 before using.	
Acetone Alcohol	
Acetone	1,000 ml
Alcohol (95% ethyl)	1,000 ml
Safranin	
Safranin O, CI 50240	40 g
Distilled water	2,000 ml

BACTERIAL IDENTIFICATION

For bacteria, microbiology laboratories use various media and atmospheres for isolation of organisms. The media most commonly employed include 5 percent sheep blood agar for growth of most organisms, MacConkey agar, or eosin methylene blue for gram-negative rods, and trypticase soy or thioglycollate broth for more fastidious organisms or those present in smaller numbers. Many laboratories also include media such as colistin-nalidixic acid agar or phenylethyl alcohol agar for isolation of gram-positive organisms. The majority of bacterial species will grow in the media mentioned. Some, such as *H. influenzae,* require special growth factors that are present in chocolate agar. *N. gonorrhoeae* and meningitidis are particularly fastidious and require either chocolate or Thayer-Martin agar and incubation in CO_2. This emphasizes again the need to specify, on the requisition slip, the clinical diagnosis and what organisms are suspected. Culture techniques for anaerobic bacteria are discussed in Chapter 6.

After isolation, organisms are identified on the basis of colonial morphology, Gram stain, biochemical and serologic tests. Isolation and identification of commonly isolated bacteria is relatively rapid, within 24 to 48 hours. Some particularly fastidious anaerobes may require several

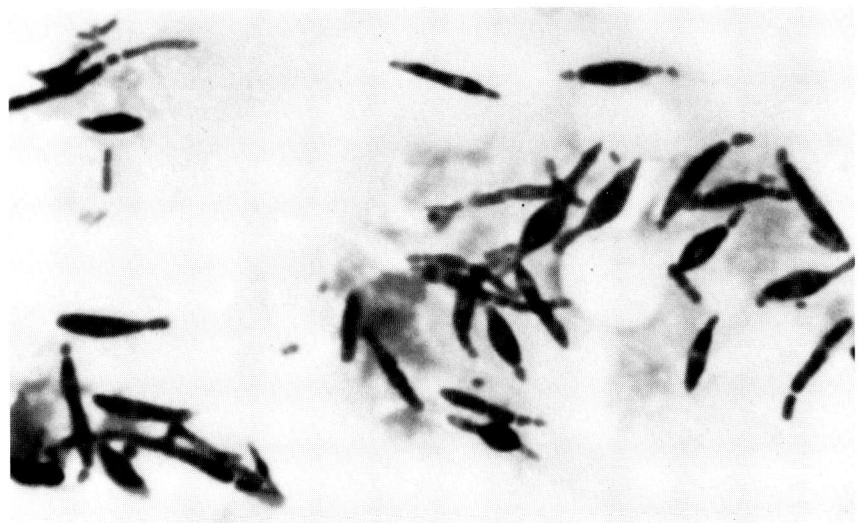

Fig. 12-3. **Gram stain showing extreme pleomorphism often seen with *Bacteroides fragilis.* (Courtesy of Karen Viskochil, University of Minnesota, Minneapolis.)**

weeks before a definitive identification can be made.

If one suspects the presence of a certain organism and the laboratory does not report it, consultation with the laboratory personnel is recommended. If a fastidious organism was suspected and not indicated on the requisition slip, the proper medium may not have been inoculated, or the specimen collection and transport may have been imperfect. It is tremendously useful to the laboratory to obtain feedback on patients who appear to have classic diseases but in whom the causative organism was not found. An example would be a patient with scarlet fever from whom group A beta-hemolytic streptococci were not isolated. Only through a continual feedback between the clinician and the laboratory can optimal service for the patient be provided.

Quantitative cultures are occasionally of great value. The best example is urine, where a properly collected specimen containing 100,000 colonies or more of a single gram-negative rod is statistically linked to urinary tract infection, whereas a culture with colony counts lower than that or a culture containing mixed organisms is usually not indicative of a bona fide infection. Here again, not only the quantity of organisms present but the method of specimen collection is critical. For example, culturing any quantity of bacteria in a suprapubic tap would be significant, whereas greater than 100,000 colonies of mixed skin flora such as alpha streptococci or *Corynebacterium* species in a clean-catch sample from a woman would probably be insignificant.

Recently, quantitative cultures of tissue in burns and other wounds have been used to determine when to graft or otherwise secondarily close open wounds. Wounds containing more than 100,000 organisms per gram of tissue are probably associated with sepsis, whereas a bacterial level less than 100,000 indicates that sepsis is unlikely. For accuracy, the tissue submitted to the laboratory should weigh at least 0.5 gm, which would be a piece measuring about $2 \times 1 \times 0.5$ cm. The tissue is weighed on an analytic balance and the bacterial count determined by direct culture after homogenization. More recently, a semiquantitative technique has been devised, which involves the examination of Gram-stained material under an oil immersion lens.

Legionella pneumophila (Legionnaires' disease bacillus) may be isolated using special media (Fig. 12-4). However, only lung biopsy or pleural fluid are satisfactory specimens for culture at the present time. Sputum and bronchial washings are contaminated with normal respiratory flora that will overgrow the slower-growing *L. pneumophila.* For detection of the organism in these latter specimens, the direct fluorescent antibody technique can be used. Antiserum for this test is available from the Center for Disease Control. In addition to culture and immunofluorescence tests, serologic detection of antibody production may be used to diagnose Legionnaires' disease. These tests are available through local state departments of health.

Counterimmunoelectrophoresis has been developed to provide rapid diagnosis of meningitis caused by *H. influenzae, S. pneumoniae,* and *N. meningitidis.* The test is usually performed on cerebrospinal fluid. The direct Gram stain of cerebrospinal fluid and the quellung test is simpler and more accurate than counterimmunoelectrophoresis, except in cases where the patient has already been treated with antibiotics. In these patients, when organisms can no longer be seen on Gram stain or isolated on culture, the counterimmunoelectrophoresis may be positive and give a definitive diagnosis.

The detection of antibody-coated bacteria in urine has been deemed useful in diagnosing upper tract infection. If no antibody-coated bacteria are found in the urine of a patient with a urinary tract infection, this may be considered a bladder infection. However, the distinction between upper and lower urinary tract infection is not absolute. This test is not useful with yeast infections, because these organisms fluoresce almost all the time, and thus false-positive results occur. The test has not been shown to be of value in children. For performance of the test, the urine should be sent to the laboratory before antibiotic therapy has been initiated; bacteria must be

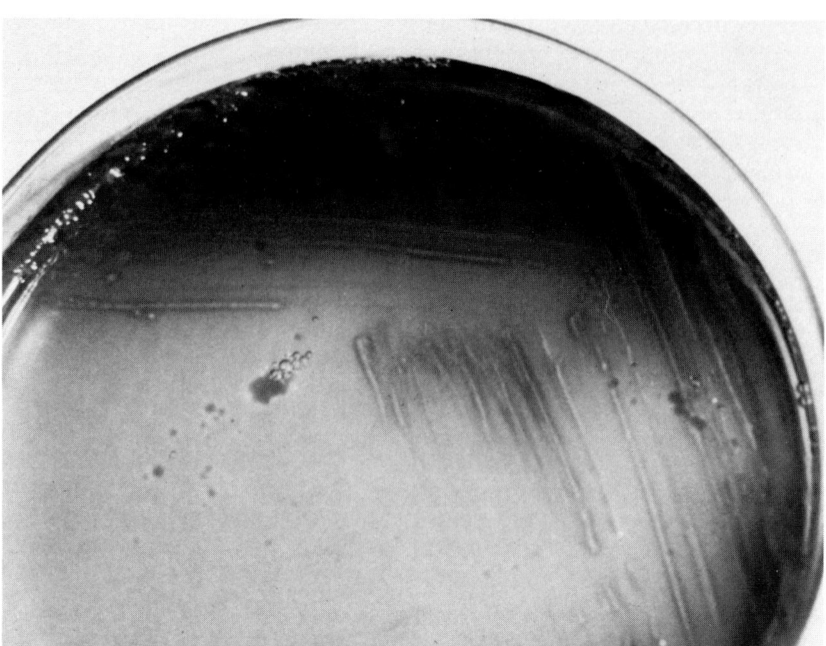

Fig. 12-4. **Colonies of *Legionella pneumophila* (Legionnaires' bacillus) growing on special F-G medium, 48 hours. The organism produces a characteristic brown pigment in the medium.**

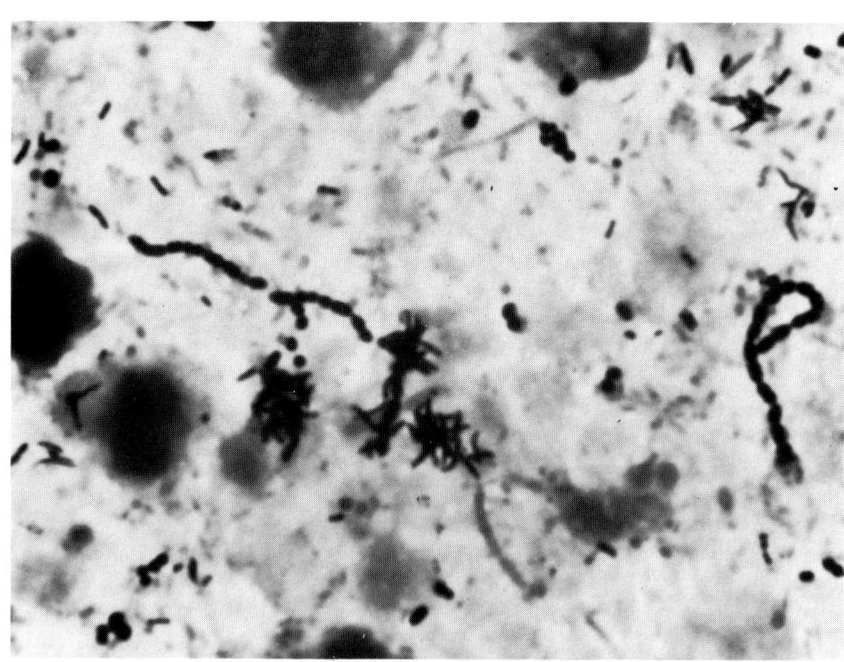

Fig. 12-5. **Gram stain of peritoneal fluid showing various rods, pleomorphic rods, and cocci typical of fecal flora. (Courtesy of Louise Hofherr, University of Minnesota, Minneapolis.)**

present in the urine. If the bacteria are coated with antibody (human immunoglobulin), a fluorescein-labeled antihuman immunoglobulin will attach to the cells and fluoresce under the fluorescence microscope.

Interpretation of culture results when several organisms have been isolated is difficult. An example of this is a culture of peritoneal fluid. Often, the specimen will contain many fecal organisms, especially when the infection has just begun. In these cases, it should suffice for the laboratory to report the culture as "mixed fecal flora" (Fig. 12-5). Isolation and identification of all the anaerobic organisms is tedious, time-consuming, and expensive. It is impossible to be certain which organisms are the initial pathogens in mixed infections because relatively avirulent organisms can act synergistically in mixture. Selection of appropriate antimicrobial therapy is therefore complex. If fecal-like flora are present, the clinician can assume the presence of *B. fragilis*, the most antibiotic-resistant of the anaerobes, and treatment should include an appropriate antibiotic such as clindamycin or chloramphenicol. Recently, a fluorescent antibody test for direct detection of *B. fragilis* in clinical specimens has been developed. This may prove to be useful and obviate the necessity of making assumptions about the content of the culture.

Isolation and identification of facultative organisms, such as *E. coli*, from peritoneal fluid is simpler than with anaerobes, but the interpretation of the importance of each in a mixed infection is still difficult. Predominance does not necessarily equate with clinical significance.

Wound cultures also present problems of interpretation when several organisms are isolated. However, if the specimen has been collected so as to eliminate any contaminating surface flora, the isolated organisms will take on more significance. We again emphasize the importance of proper collection of specimens to obtain worthwhile results.

Chlamydiae

Chlamydiae Culture

To diagnose nongonococcal urethritis in males, insert a swab of 2–5 cm into the urethra. In females, swab the cervix. If synovitis is present, aspirate the joint. Place the specimen *immediately* into the transport medium appropriate for *Chlamydiae* supplied by the laboratory and send it directly to the laboratory. Lung tissue obtained by biopsy or autopsy should be treated in the same way.

These intracellular bacteria grow only in living cells and are transmitted by direct contact. Nongonococcal urethritis and cervicitis, trachoma and lymphogranuloma venereum, inclusion conjunctivitis in adults and children, and inclusion blennorrhea and pneumonia in infants are caused by *Chlamydiae*. There are two species of *Chlamydiae*—*C. trachomatis*, which consists of 15 serotypes, and *C. psittaci*, which produces the zoonosis psittacosis. These organisms can be isolated in embryonated eggs, but certain cell cultures, such as McCoy, have been shown to be ideal. The presence of *Chlamydiae* is detected approximately 2 days after inoculation by finding typical cytoplasmic inclusion bodies after the cell cultures have been stained with iodine. In the case of conjunctivitis, typical cytoplasmic inclusion bodies may be seen in Giemsa-stained conjunctival scrapings.

Mycobacterial Identification

The most important agent is *M. tuberculosis*, but the so-called atypical organisms also cause scrofula and pneumonia. The definitive method of diagnosis is culture, which unfortunately is extremely slow. Six weeks or more may be required for isolation and identification of some of the mycobacteria. For this reason, selective stains, including modifications of the Ziehl-Nielson acid-fast procedure and fluorescent staining of the organisms, have achieved importance. Neither of these stains differentiates between *M. tuberculosis* and the atypical mycobacteria.

Mycoplasma Identification

Mycoplasma pneumoniae can be grown on cell-free medium (eg, Hayflick), but growth of these organisms is relatively slow and definitive identification takes approximately 3 weeks. For this reason, routine cultures for *Mycoplasma* are rarely done, and serologic techniques are used to make the diagnosis. A fourfold or greater rise in *M. pneumoniae* complement-fixing titers is diagnostic. A nonspecific test, the cold-agglutinin titer, is readily available in most laboratories, and if titers are elevated or rising a presumptive diagnosis of *M. pneumoniae* infection can be made. Some children will not develop elevated cold agglutinins in the presence of mycoplasmal infection. Conversely, adults may have positive cold agglutinins associated with *Chlamydia* or nonmycoplasmal infections.

PARASITIC IDENTIFICATION

Helminth infections are best identified by a parasitologist skilled in microscopic morphologic identification of characteristic ova or larvae. These are found in stool preparations that have been collected as outlined in the preceding section.

Protozoa are identified directly by microscopic examination of the specimen and are rarely cultured. Either PAS or Gridley modified hematoxylin and eosin stain that employs naphthol green B should be used to aid the histologic diagnosis when amebic liver abscess is suspected.

In an immunocompromised patient in whom *Pneumocystis carinii* infection is suspected, a methenamine silver stain on material obtained from bronchoscopy, bronchial brushings, or lung biopsy may be extremely useful. Giemsa stain may also disclose the presence of organisms, but in our experience methenamine silver has been better.

Malarial and other blood parasites are identified by microscopic examination of the blood by an experienced parasitology technologist. Periodic specimens are needed to ensure detection of all the stages needed to identify each species.

RICKETTSIAL IDENTIFICATION

Rickettsiae can be grown in embryonated eggs and some tissue cultures, but for practical purposes, serologic techniques are used for diagnosis. Nonspecific tests such as *Proteus* agglutinins are sometimes helpful, but the definitive method is to document a fourfold or greater rise in complement-fixing antibody to the specific organism in question. These latter tests are usually only available at the Center for Disease Control. The most important organism in the United States is *Rickettsia rickettsiae*, the cause of Rocky Mountain spotted fever. The rash of this infection is characteristic, being maculopapular, purpuric, sometimes bullous, and frequently involving both palms and soles. Because the illness progresses fairly rapidly, antimicrobial therapy with tetracycline or chloramphenicol is usually begun before serologic confirmation of the diagnosis is made.

FUNGAL IDENTIFICATION

The diagnosis of fungal diseases frequently requires histopathologic, serologic, morphologic, and culture techniques. Fungi are usually isolated on selective media designed to suppress more rapidly growing bacteria so that the fungi can have an opportunity to multiply and be identified. Fungi grow more slowly than bacteria, and cultural isolation may require 4 to 6 weeks.

For *C. neoformans* it may be possible to demonstrate

the presence of encapsulated yeast in spinal fluid sediment by the use of India ink. Although other yeasts may produce capsules, these are not found in spinal fluid, so a positive India ink test is virtually diagnostic of *C. neoformans* meningitis. However, organisms are not always demonstrable in spinal fluid, and serologic techniques have been developed. The one in vogue is the latex agglutination test for identification of cryptococcal antigen. The antigen test can be positive in the absence of culturable cryptococci and thus may prove to be more sensitive.

VIRUSES

Viral Isolation Techniques

Most clinical virology laboratories rely on cell cultures to isolate viruses. Confluent monolayers of cells are prepared in tubes or plates (Fig. 12-6). As soon as the specimen is received in the laboratory, antibiotics are added (usually a combination of penicillin, gentamicin, and amphotericin B) to prevent bacterial and yeast overgrowth. A small portion of each specimen, approximately 0.2 ml, is inoculated into at least two tubes or two wells of the appropriate cell lines. Because no single line will support the growth of all human viruses, a combination of cell lines (typically three) is used: (1) cynomolgus monkey kidney, which best supports the growth of myxoviruses and enteroviruses, (2) a continuous line of human epithelial cells (HEp-2), which are ideal for isolation of respiratory syncytial and adenoviruses, and (3) a diploid fibroblast cell line (human foreskin cells or MRC-5), which best supports the growth of human cytomegalovirus. The inoculated cells are examined microscopically at least every other day for the presence of cytopathic effect produced by virus. If cytopathic effect is observed, the technologist can frequently recognize it as typical of a particular virus. For example, the cytopathic effect produced by cytomegalovirus (Fig. 12-7) is distinctive. The type of cytopathic effect and ability to grow in certain cell lines often suggest the presumptive virologic diagnosis. As soon as cytopathic effect is detected, the phy-

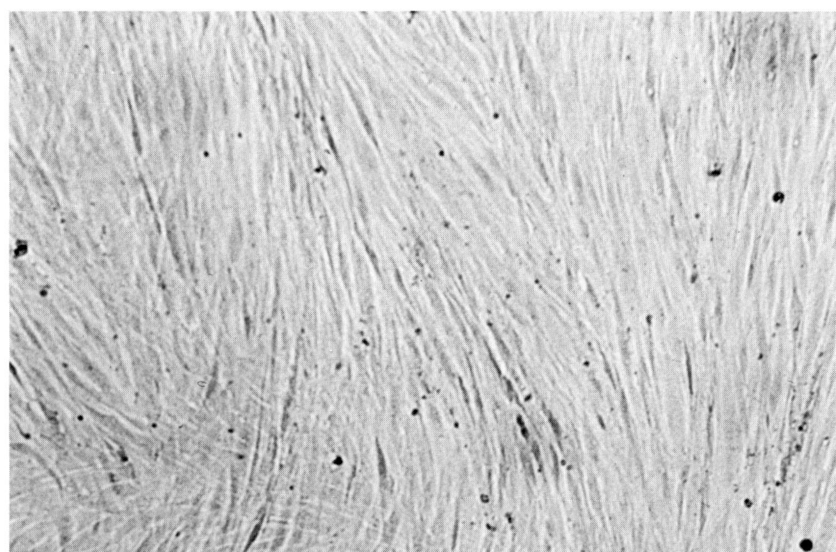

Fig. 12-6. **Uninfected monolayer of human skin-muscle fibroblast cells (106×, unstained).**

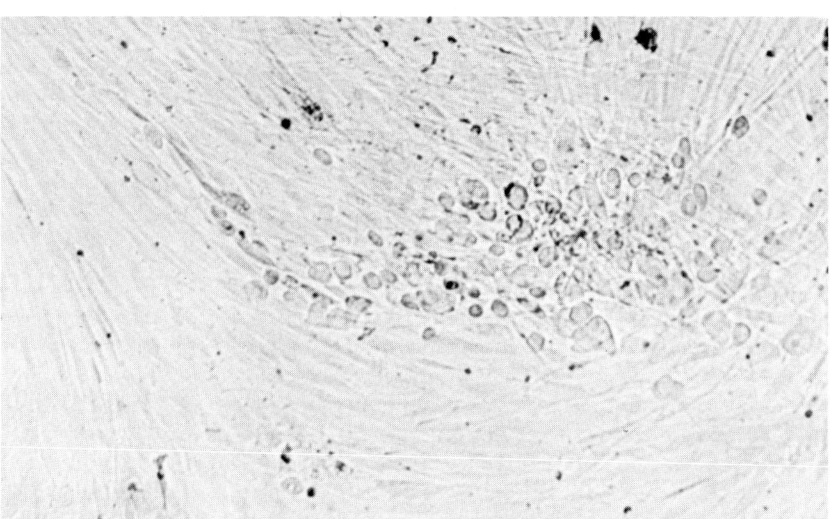

Fig. 12-7. **Same cells as Fig. 12-6, inoculated 2 weeks previously with a throat swab from an infant with pneumonitis. A large focus of enlarged refractile cells in the center is typical of human cytomegalovirus (106×, unstained).**

sician can be phoned and informed that an isolation has been made. This can usually be accomplished within a week except for cytomegalovirus, which is relatively slow-growing and may require 4 weeks of observation before cytopathic effect is seen.

In addition to examining the cells for cytopathic effect, monkey kidney cells are tested periodically for the presence of hemagglutinating agents. A small amount of the nutrient medium covering the cell monolayer is aspirated and mixed with guinea pig red blood cells at several temperatures. If a hemagglutinating virus is present, a smooth sheet forms as the red cells settle to the bottom of the well. The sheet develops because the virus causes the cells to stick together like a lattice instead of descending individually and forming a button at the bottom of the well. A positive hemagglutination test is presumptive evidence for the presence of certain orthoviruses or paramyxoviruses, such as influenza A and B, parainfluenza types 1, 2, and 3, or mumps. The reason for performing hemagglutination is that some hemagglutinating viruses do not produce recognizable cytopathic effects during the observation period and would not be detected by direct microscopic examination of the cell cultures.

Viral Serologic Tests

The measurement of serum antibodies has two major clinical applications: (1) diagnosis of acute viral illness when virus cannot be recovered from clinical specimens or is present only in the stool, and (2) determination of immune status. Because rubella may be teratogenic, assessment of rubella immunity is necessary for unvaccinated women of childbearing age. In the future, it may be necessary to check immune status in rubella vaccinees and possibly in recipients of measles and mumps vaccine as well. In these instances, the diagnostic virology laboratory can assist in deciding which patients need reimmunizations.

Six serologic procedures are commonly used to measure viral antibodies.

1. Complement fixation (CF) is the method most frequently used by viral diagnostic laboratories. Although not as sensitive as most of the other methods, it has the advantage of measuring antibodies to some groups rather than single types of virus. For example, CF tests can be done for adenovirus and in most instances will detect infection with any of the more than 30 adenovirus serotypes.

2. Hemagglutination-inhibition (HI) testing is sensitive and relatively specific. Rubella and measles antibodies are most commonly measured by the HI method. Since HI antibodies persist for life, the HI test is useful for determination of immune status. CF antibodies often decline to undetectable levels several years after infection, and hence the CF test is not as useful as the HI procedure for the determination of immune status.

3. Immunofluorescence is quite sensitive in the hands of experienced technologists. For antibody determinations, indirect immunofluorescence is the technique most often employed.

4. Neutralizing antibodies are usually measured by incubating serial dilutions of the patient's serum with virus and then inoculating the virus-serum mixtures into cell cultures. If antibody is not present, the virus produces cytopathic changes in the cells. The antibody titer is usually expressed as the highest dilution of serum that prevents the development of cytopathic effect in 50 percent of the inoculated cell cultures. This method is sensitive and very specific.

5. Precipitin testing can be done by simple diffusion or counterimmunoelectrophoresis. It is specific but relatively insensitive.

6. Radioimmunoassay can be used to identify viral antigens or antibodies. This technique is probably the most sensitive method available for detection of viral antibodies and antigens, but does require expensive equipment and carries a small risk of exposure to radioactivity.

Enzyme-linked immunospecific assay (ELISA) is an exciting new method, which may prove to be sensitive and specific for identifying both viral antibodies and antigens. Commercial kits are now available for rubella antibody tests by the enzyme-linked immunospecific assay method.

Interpretation of Virology Results

The significance of viral isolation varies according to the source of the specimen (Table 12-5). Isolation of virus from any of the sites in the first group listed is diagnostic of a viral infection in that area. For example, isolation of herpes simplex from corneal scrapings is diagnostic of herpes keratitis. Because viruses can be found in stool specimens of asymptomatic persons, especially children, isolation of virus from stool alone is not diagnostic.

Viral Antibody Titers

A fourfold rise or decline in serum antibody titer is considered diagnostic of a recent infection (Table 12-6). Although paired specimens are preferred, a single titer can sometimes be useful. A high titer suggests a recent infection, whereas a negative titer during convalescence excludes

TABLE 12-5. SIGNIFICANCE OF VIRAL ISOLATION

Source of Positive Culture	Interpretation
Autopsy Blood Biopsy tissue Cerebrospinal fluid Exudates and transudates Eye Cervix Skin lesions	Virtually diagnostic of infection in the site cultured
Throat* Urine*	Virus isolated is probably associated with clinical illness
Stool*	Virus isolated is possibly associated with clinical illness

* Isolation of virus from these specimens would be diagnostic if accompanied by serologic evidence of homologous virus infection.

TABLE 12-6. SIGNIFICANCE OF VIRAL ANTIBODY TITERS

	Interpretation
SEROLOGIC RESPONSES IN PAIRED SERA	
Fourfold rise in titer	Diagnostic of recent infection
Fourfold decline in titer	Diagnostic of relatively recent infection
High but unchanging titers, eg, mumps CF titers of 64*	Suggestive of recent infection
SEROLOGIC FINDINGS IN A SINGLE SERUM	
High titer, eg, adenovirus CF titer of 128*	Suggestive of recent infection
Rubella HI† titer of ≥8*	Patient immune to rubella
Varicella-zoster IF‡ titer of ≥8*	Patient immune to varicella

* Reciprocal of serum dilution
† HI = Hemagglutination-inhibition
‡ IF = Indirect immunofluorescence

that particular virus. The presence of serum antibody usually connotes immunity. For example, it is extremely rare for individuals with detectable rubella hemagglutination-inhibition antibodies to subsequently develop clinical rubella.

BIBLIOGRAPHY

Finegold SM, Martin WJ, Scott EG: Bailey and Scott's Diagnostic Microbiology, 5th ed. St Louis, Mosby, 1978.

Krugman S, Ward R, Katz SL: Infectious Diseases of Children, 6th ed, St Louis, Mosby, 1977.

Lennette EG, Spaulding EH, Truant JP: Manual of Clinical Microbiology, 2nd ed. Washington, DC, American Society for Microbiology, 1974.

Matsen JM, Ederer GM: Specimen collection and transport. Human Pathol 7:297, 1976.

Moffet HL: Clinical Microbiology. Philadelphia, Lippincott, 1975.

Koneman EW, Allen SD, Dowell VR Jr, Sommers HM: Color Atlas and Textbook of Diagnostic Microbiology. Philadelphia, Lippincott, 1979.

PART III: HOST DEFENSES

CHAPTER 13 Host Defenses

JONATHAN L. MEAKINS, DAVID C. HOHN, THOMAS K. HUNT, AND RICHARD L. SIMMONS

THE natural history of each infection can be conceptualized on an anatomic basis, ie, on the basis of the body's attempt to localize infection to the original site or, if that is not possible, to regionally confine the process. When regionalization fails, invasion of the bloodstream takes place, and septicemia must be controlled using all homeostatic mechanisms.

At the site of injury, the body mounts the classical inflammatory response to contain invasion of bacteria. The usual result is control and resolution of the potential infection. When infection becomes established, the inflammatory response attempts to contain and localize the process. Suppuration and spontaneous drainage is an obviously successful resolution of this response, although suppuration is frequently not required for local control.

Failure to localize leads to cellulitis or some degree of lymphangitis. The infecting organism passes through the lymphatic channels, resulting in regional lymphadenopathy secondary to local inflammation and reactive edema which effectively blocks lymph flow. Suppuration can occur in the attempt to regionalize the infection. Cutaneous and pulmonary infections are commonly controlled by these processes. Streptococcal lymphangitis and lymphadenitis, mesenteric lymphadenopathy with acute nonperforated appendicitis, and the Ghon complex in tuberculosis are common examples of the body's attempt to regionalize and contain an infection. Although in some situations this process cannot take place (eg, pleural cavity, brain), the concept is useful.

Some infections are not contained by these attempts to localize or regionalize, and systemic invasion results. When bacteremia does take place, there are a variety of responses, including fever, chills, and cardiovascular collapse. The reticuloendothelial system (RES) attempts to clear the bloodstream of opsonized bacteria by active phagocytosis and is the last line of defense against invasive sepsis. These echelons of defense are an integral part of homeostasis, just as the maintenance of cardiovascular stability is a homeostatic mechanism that prolongs life until sepsis can be controlled.

To be effective, host defense requires the integrated and efficient function of the component parts. The failure of any segment of the system can result in a septic process, as is apparent in the congenital immunologic deficiencies that affect single-cell or cell enzyme systems and frequently result in persistent, recurrent, or lethal sepsis.

The inflammatory response is the basic delivery system. The classic signs of inflammation—rubor, dolor, tumor, and calor—can be explained by examining the vascular, cellular, and molecular components of the response. Inflammation is also the effector system of almost all aspects of immunologic injury.

The vascular changes are largely mediated through vasoactive amines, notably the kinin system, histamine, and serotonin. The release of these subtances is coordinated to produce the vascular and endothelial changes, which then allow delivery of the humoral and cellular components to the inflammatory response. The precise sequence of action is not completely understood, but a synthesis follows.

The vascular response, initially vasoconstriction, takes place within minutes of the insult and is then followed in 10 to 30 minutes by a persistent vasodilation. The overt cutaneous signs are the triple response of Lewis. The vasodilation is accompanied by changes in the vessel wall and, subsequently, blood flow. There is stasis of blood with increased margination and adherence to the endothelial lining by polymorphonuclear leukocytes. Endothelial changes allow diapedesis of the polymorphonuclear leukocytes into the inflammatory focus. The vessel wall changes, and increased capillary pressure produces increased vascular permeability allowing delivery of plasma proteins, notably immunoglobulins, complement, and fibrinogen. In addition, there is breakdown of some large protein molecules and increased fluidity of the tissue ground substance, all of which contribute to the "tumor" associated with inflammation.

The cellular exudate parallels the fluid exudate and initially is almost exclusively polymorphonuclear leukocytes. After the first 24 hours, monocytes tend to replace neutrophils as the predominant phagocytic cell. When activated, the monocyte becomes an activated macrophage and, as such, is a more effective phagocyte. However, the macrophage also processes bacterial and other antigens before delivery to the lymphocyte for production of specific antibody. As the inflammatory process develops, the lymphatics, in part secondary to local swelling, enlarge, and lymphatic flow increases, aiding delivery of antigen to the regional lymph nodes.

For purposes of this discussion, the inflammatory exudate is directed against microbial invasion. The humoral opsonic component is made up of complement and immunoglobulins. The role of complement is a multifaceted one; it aids immune adherence, bacterial cytolysis, polymorphonuclear leukocyte chemotaxis, and phagocytosis. Immunoglobulins, notably IgG and IgM, together with complement are involved in polymorphonuclear leukocyte bacterial phagocytosis. Bacterial cytolysis can be effected by complement and immunoglobulin, but these play a modest role in the control of invasive bacteria. The crucial role of complement is to attract polymorphonuclear leukocytes to the area of the bacteria and then together with IgG provide opsonization of the bacteria for effective polymorphonuclear leukocyte phagocytosis and subsequent bacterial killing (Figs. 13-7, 13-8). In the absence of complement or immunoglobulins, phagocytosis is substantially decreased. Fibrin polymerization facilitates localization of the infection in abscesses and also supplies a matrix against which neutrophils can phagocytize bacteria that are not opsonized. Thus, the humoral and cellular components work together to control bacterial growth.

Polymorphonuclear leukocytes are the initial cellular response to an insult. They are actively phagocytic when delivered to the inflammatory focus. With ingestion, the bacterium is encased in a membrane-lined sac, the phagosome, which becomes a phagolysosome when fused with the enzyme-rich contents of polymorphonuclear leukocyte lysosomes. These lysosomes contain the multiple enzymatic and metabolic processes that result in bactericidal action. The polymorphonuclear leukocyte is the initial killer cell and is essential to maintenance of intact host defense. The inability to contain the microbial invasion, whether because of decreased numbers or decreased delivery, is a critical factor, which allows active microbial invasion to take place.

The second line of phagocytic response is the monocyte, which is activated at an area of inflammation to an aggressive phagocytic and bactericidal long-lived cell, the macrophage. As with polymorphonuclear leukocytes, macrophage chemotaxis and phagocytosis require antibody and complement. Following ingestion and digestion, the microbial antigen is processed by the macrophage and transported locally or regionally to lymphocytes for production of specific antibody. The involved cells can be derived from bone marrow (B) or thymus (T) lymphocytes. The B cells are responsible for production of specific antibodies and T cells for production of specifically sensitized lymphocytes. These lymphocytes play a major role in protection against intracellular parasites through the macrophage, which becomes the effective microbicidal cell when activated.

The role of cell-mediated immunity in the traditional

TABLE 13-1. EFFICACY OF THREE COMPARTMENTS OF HOST DEFENSE IN COUNTERING INFECTIOUS ORGANISMS

Humoral	Cell-mediated	Phagocytic
Bacteria:	Bacteria:	Bacteria:
Pneumococcus	*Mycobacteria*	*Staphylococcus* *
Streptococcus	*Listeria*	*Klebsiella*
Hemophilus	*Brucella*	*Aerobacter*
Meningococcus	*Salmonella*	*Serratia*
Pseudomonas	*Staphylococcus* *	*Proteus*
		Probably most other enteric and anaerobic bacteria
Toxins:	Fungi:	Fungi:
Diphtheria	*Candida* *	*Candida* *
Tetanus	*Aspergillus*	
	Histoplasma	
	Mucor	
Viruses:	Viruses:	
Polio	*Vaccinia*	
Hepatitis	Cytomegalic inclusion disease	
Rubella	Most others	
Others		
	Parasites:	
	Pneumocystis carinii	

* Many infectious agents are attached by two compartments of host defense; selecting the predominant compartment may not be possible.

sense has not been addressed. In surgical practice, its most significant role is transplantation biology and tumor resistance. The anti-infective role is limited to intracellular parasites. The antimicrobial action of cell-mediated immunity takes place through a complex system of recognition and cell activation involving different cells and numerous humoral mediators. Simplified, the cell-mediated antimicrobial system is based on recognition of antigen by T lymphocytes and subsequent macrophage attraction and stimulation. If the body has not had previous experience with the specific organism, time is required before sensitized lymphocytes are produced. In this situation, the arc will work somewhat in reverse; that is, the bacterial antigen will be processed by macrophages and delivered to lymphocytes for production of specifically sensitized T cells, which will then deliver effector cells to the site of infection.

When the host has had experience with a specific microbe, specific T cells are attracted to the focus of infection where they are more specifically activated to produce lymphokines, a family of soluble humoral mediators, some of which can affect macrophages. The lymphokines of specific interest are migration inhibition factor and macrophage activation factor. Migration inhibition factor attracts macrophages to the infection and keeps them in the area, and macrophage activation factor turns them into activated cells capable of effective antibacterial function. The process and mechanism of intracellular killing is similar to polymorphonuclear leukocytes. Failure of T cell function or congenital absence of T cells results in failure to mount an effective antimicrobial response against intracellular parasites.

Cell-mediated immunity is a specific reaction to an antigen or to antigen on cell or microbe surfaces. Delayed hypersensitivity is a cell-mediated immune phenomenon. The failure to respond appropriately can be a reflection of an alteration of the specific cell-mediated immune reaction or to a nonspecific failure of the sequence required to produce the positive skin test reaction.

Humoral systems, phagocyte function, and cell-mediated immunity have specific organisms, or classes of organisms, against which they are most effective (Table 13-1). It should be clear that usually two of the three listed compartments of host defense are involved against invading microbes and that the predominant system is listed. For example, in the absence of specific antibody, the pneumococcus is not phagocytized by polymorphonuclear leukocytes; however, once present, phagocytosis and intracellular killing proceed rapidly. The key to this defense is the specific antibody, although control of the actual infection is a two-compartment effort.

BIBLIOGRAPHY

Alexander WJ, Good RA (eds.): Fundamentals of Clinical Immunology. Philadelphia: Saunders, 1977.

Gallin JI, Quie PG (eds.): Leukocyte Chemotaxis: Methods, Physiology, and Clinical Implications. New York, Raven Press, 1978.

Howard RJ: Host defense against infection, Part 1. Curr Probl Surg 17 (5):267, 1980.

Howard RJ: Host defense against infection, Part 2. Curr Probl Surg 17 (6):319, 1980.

Root RK: Humoral immunity and complement. In Mandell GL, Douglas RG Jr, Bennett JE (eds.): Principles and Practice of Infectious Diseases. New York: John Wiley & Sons, 1979, pp 21–62.

A. Local Host Defenses

JONATHAN L. MEAKINS

The primary goal of the local host defense system is the *prevention of lodgement* of pathogenic microorganisms. The modified homunculus in Figure 13-1 indicates the routes of access of microbes to the body. All surfaces have highly specialized systems for regulation of their permanent and transient flora or for maintenance of their sterile environment. Although the components of this defense system vary for different organs, certain common factors are present: (1) a biologic wall, eg, skin and mucous membranes, (2) specialized surface cell functions, eg, macrophages, cilia, (3) local secretions, including those that provide specific local immunity, and (4) the normal microbial flora which, by being more adapted to the environ-

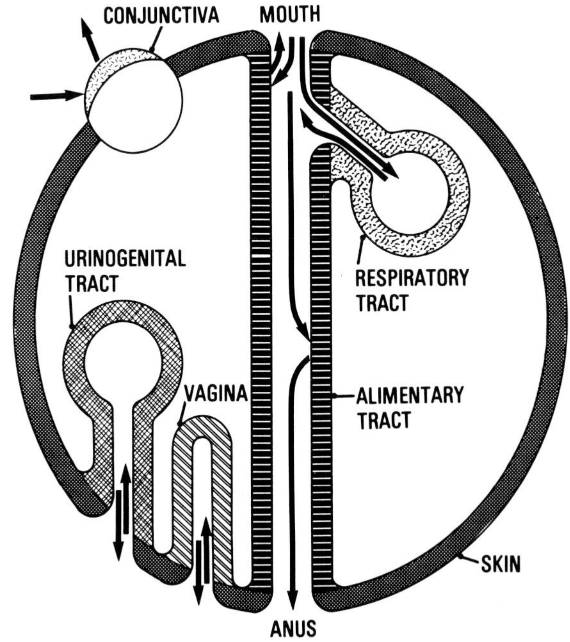

Fig. 13-1. **A modified homunculus, demonstrating the different epithelial surfaces and their relationship to the outside world.**

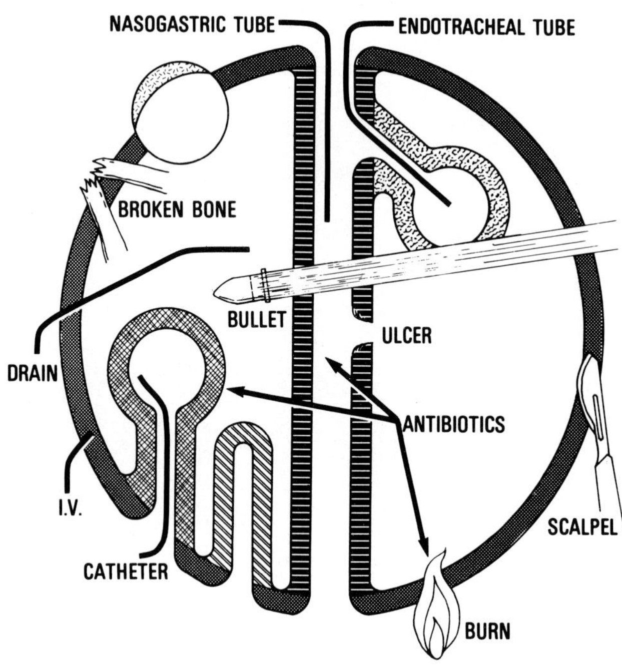

Fig. 13-2. **The epithelial disruptions induced by trauma, disease, and therapy, which permit microbial invasion.**

ment, successfully compete with and thereby control colonization by pathogens.

The alteration of these protective interrelated systems in clinical practice is schematically represented in Figure 13-2. It is apparent that many routine therapeutic devices bypass or alter natural environmental defenses, increasing the probability of infection.

THE SKIN

The skin presents a barrier to the external environment and has specific antibacterial mechanisms. Absorption of microorganisms through normal skin does not occur. At each juncture where the skin becomes internalized, a structural and functional alteration in the epithelium leads to a modification of the protective mechanisms.

The skin is in general a hostile environment for microbial growth (Chapters 3, 25). Although there are sufficient nutrients for growth and survival, there is inadequate water. The pH of skin is normally between 5 and 6, and where bacteria flourish an alkaline environment is found. It is not clear if the alkalinity is a cause of bacterial growth or a result of it, but it is probably a combination of factors. The constant regeneration of skin and its desquamation contribute to elimination of transient or potentially pathogenic organisms.

The skin has specific antibacterial substances, although their precise nature is unclear.[1] Acetone extracts of normal skin lipids have some antimicrobial factors.[2] The free fatty acids on the skin, themselves products of bacterial degradation, also have antibacterial properties.[2] *S. pyogenes* is sensitive to some of these lipids and is rarely found on uninfected skin.

The resident flora lives in the stratum corneum and in a limited way in and around orifices of the glands of the skin. The sebum of sebaceous glands does not appear to have intrinsic major antibacterial properties.

The population density of the resident flora varies depending on environmental features. On skin of forearm and abdomen, there are 10^2 organisms per cm^2; on the forehead, 10^4, and in most intertriginous areas such as the axilla, groin, and foot, 10^6. Wherever skin becomes moist, bacterial populations increase so that skin adjacent to wet wounds, the perineum, and the backs of bedridden patients frequently develop an infective dermatitis. The addition of other factors that may damage skin, such as uncontrolled pancreatic, duodenal, gastric, or small bowel fistulae, produces environments conducive to infections. The skin is difficult to infect; both destruction of integrity and moisture are required and, of course, one leads to the other (Chapter 25).

Interestingly, *S. aureus* persists more effectively on fingertips and hands than in other areas.[3] Surgeons must maintain their own benign resident skin flora free from pathogenic transient flora, because hands are the most significant carriers of infection in hospitals. The sources of transient flora are the perineum and anterior nares of the personnel and the wounds of patients. Constant reminders regarding handwashing are required to develop this lost but valuable habit.

EYE

There is a modest indigenous bacterial flora in the conjunctival surface of the eye, largely *S. epidermidis* and lactobacillus, with fewer *H. influenza* and *S. aureus.*[4] Infections are unusual because of a combination of the mechanical, chemical, and immunologic properties of tears.[5,6]

Tears are isotonic, pH 7.35, and reflect blood urea and glucose levels. They are produced at about 12 μl per minute, with about 6 μl in each eye. A flow rate greater than 100 μl per minute will exceed the capacity of the eye. Blinking maintains an even wetness and promotes distribution of a tear film, which is structured into three layers; superficial lipid, middle aqueous, and deep mucous. The protein content is between 0.67 and 2 gm per 100 ml divided relatively equally between albumin, globulin, and lysozyme. Lysozyme, which has both bacteriolytic and bacteriostatic properties, is found in highest concentration in tears.

The immunoglobulins IgA, IgG, and IgE are all found in tears, but IgA predominates. IgA is made by conjunctival and lacrimal plasma cells and acts to inhibit bacterial adherence to conjunctival epithelium. Tears can then wash away bacteria, reducing colonization.[6] IgG has an important but incompletely defined role in control of colonization and infection. Specific IgG picornavirus neutralizing antibody can be produced rapidly (1 to 3 days) by eye-associated lymphoid tissue in response to a specific local viral challenge. Its presence and concentration accurately parallel the course of the infection.[4]

RESPIRATORY TRACT

The respiratory tract, which extends from the anterior nares through the alveolus (Fig. 13-3), counteracts colonization by a variety of methods. Common to most parts are a moist surface, a mucous blanket, a mucociliary mechanism, and immunoglobulin A.

In addition to protecting itself from infection, the respiratory tract must cope with a considerable organic and nonorganic particulate matter. The respiratory tract provides innumerable convolutions and directional changes, providing opportunity for airborne particles to impact or settle onto the surface mucous layer overlying the respiratory epithelium. Once in contact with mucosa, they are moved toward the pharynx via mucociliary action (Fig. 13-3) and coughing (Chapter 30).

NASOPHARYNX

The nose is better designed to filter particulate matter including microbes from the air than is the mouth. The hairs, turbinates, and physical convolutions of the nose function to generate turbulence such that particulate matter of all sizes, but particularly those in the 10-μm range, strike the nasal and pharyngeal mucosa. They are then swept posteriorly by mucociliary action in the mucous blanket of the nasal mucosa to the pharynx. The mucociliary blanket clears the nose every 14 minutes.[7]

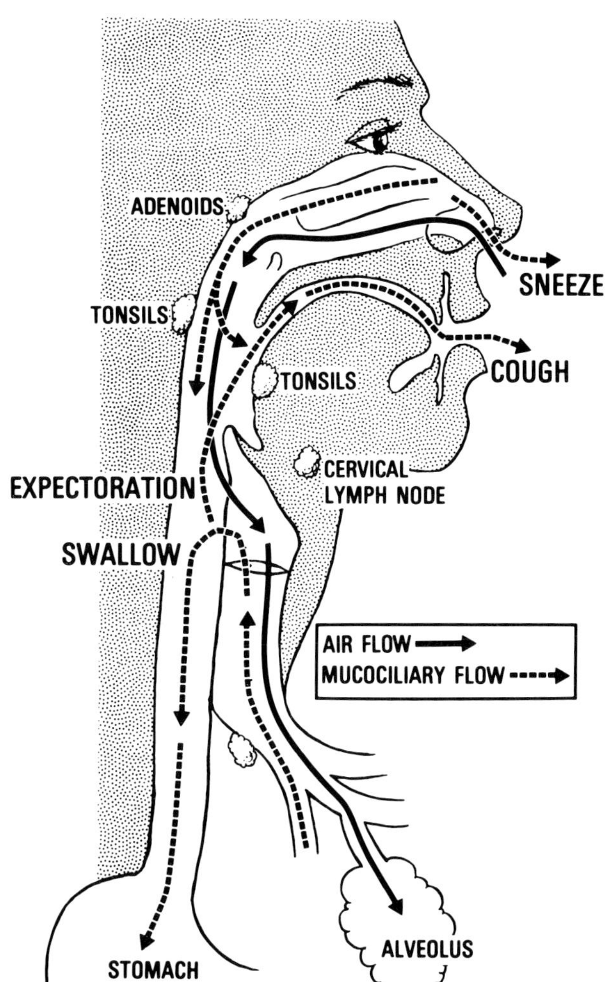

Fig. 13-3. **The natural environmental clearance mechanisms in the normal respiratory tract.**

The anatomical arrangements to produce air turbulence around a richly vascularized mucosa provide for humidification and warming as well as filtration of inspired air. Dry air impairs ciliary action. In northern climates, artificial humidification of air in homes during the winter will reduce the incidence of colds. Bacterial infection of the nose is rare without a previous viral infection that damaged the mucosa. Viruses, the major infecting agents in the nose and pharynx, attach to receptors on the mucosal cells. As in the lower bronchopulmonary tree, bacterial invasion can follow viral infection after the mucociliary barrier is broken.

LARYNX

The larynx, apart from its control over voice, acts essentially as an air conduit. All the defenses of the nasopharynx are present—the mucous blanket for entrapment, ciliary action, immune mechanisms, and normal flora to prevent colonization. In addition, irritants in the larynx are removed principally by an induced cough reflex.

A defective cough mechanism seriously impairs respiratory tract defenses, especially if an altered gag reflex is also present. Cough will be muted by the presence of an indwelling nasogastric tube and obliterated by an endotracheal tube or tracheostomy. Not only are the upper airway defenses bypassed, but aspiration and pooling of bronchial secretions will result (Fig. 13-4).

TRACHEOBRONCHIAL TREE

Particulates contaminating inhaled air are captured by the superficial mucous blanket, which glides over the ciliated respiratory epithelium. These cilia (200 per cell) beat regularly in coordinated sequence within a fluid medium.[8] The tips of the cilia push the gel-like mucous layer, guiding it toward the pharynx. In humans, the superficial mucous blanket moves at almost 15 μm per minute, with the proximal rates greater than more distal rates because of the greater volume of mucous within the larger bronchi.[9]

Matsuyama [10] used rabbit tracheal explants to show how ciliary action removes bacteria to the laryngeal end of the explant. Ultraviolet irradiation eliminates the ciliary action, allowing inoculated surface bacteria to invade. The logical extension of these studies suggests that any drug, process (viral infection), or mechanical device that interferes with mucociliary clearance places the patient severely at risk of infection.

The ciliated epithelium only extends into the terminal bronchiolar region. Material deposited in the terminal respiratory units are removed by alveolar macrophages, which function primarily to prevent lodgement of contaminants rather than to fight active infection. Alveolar macrophages behave as though they are in a perennially

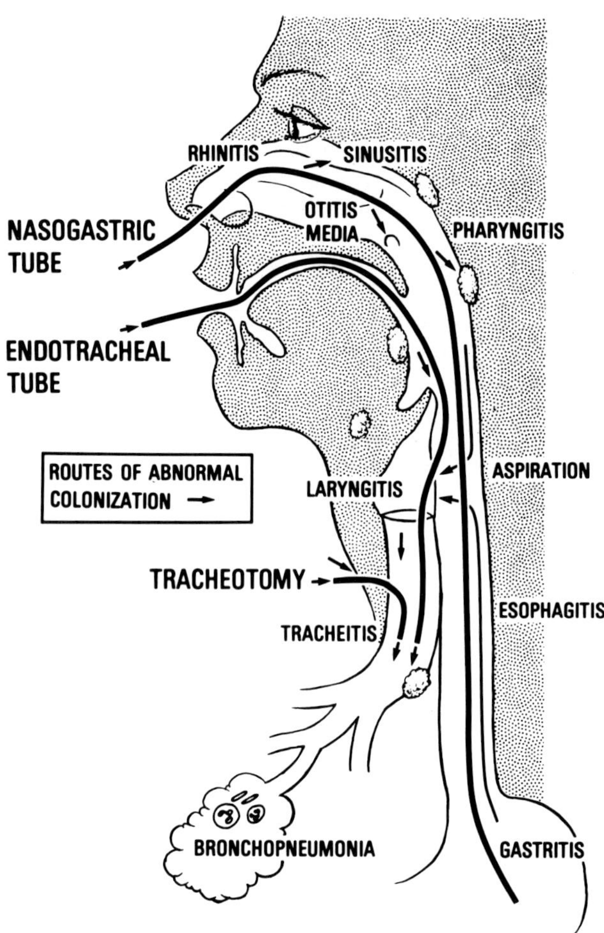

Fig. 13-4. **The alteration of anatomy and interference with natural bacterial clearance mechanisms in respiratory tract and their infectious complications.**

activated state.[11] Underlying cell-mediated immunity to a variety of airborne antigens may induce a high local concentration of macrophage-activating lymphokines.[12] After phagocytosis, macrophages migrate to the mucociliary area, after which they are swept upward.[13] The macrophage can also migrate through the interstitium to terminal respiratory bronchioles or to lymphatic channels, thence to lymph nodes. The lymphatic route is used least, generally when the other systems are overburdened. Some particulate matter, eg, silica particles, rest permanently in the alveoli because they injure macrophages. This is apparent when comparing the lungs of a city dweller to a country resident or a smoker to a nonsmoker.

LOCAL IMMUNITY

There are, in addition, immunologic antibacterial mechanisms that prevent microbial lodgement and clear the organisms that get through the mechanical and biologic barriers (see subsequent section on IgA). In the upper respiratory tract, these include the immunoglobulins IgA and IgE and small molecular weight mediators; in the lower tract, IgG, IgM, and large molecular weight mediators are present.[14] IgA is the most important defense against new or transient bacteria in the nasopharynx and tracheobronchial tree, interfering with the ability of bacteria to adhere to mucosal cells. Protective local immunity can be present in excess of systemic immunity to previously encountered respiratory antigens.[12]

The defense mechanisms of the respiratory tract are not solely the physical, cellular, and immunologic characteristics of the mucociliary lining of the tracheobronchial tree. Some secretions have antibacterial or antiviral properties—lysozyme and interferon are probably the most important.

THE ALIMENTARY TRACT

OROPHARYNX

The squamous epithelium of the oropharynx generally provides a strong mechanical barrier against bacterial ingress. Two areas, however, have particularly thin epithelium, the gingival margin and the tonsillar crypts; invasive infection is most likely to originate in these areas. Considering the wealth of bacterial flora in the mouth, it is surprising that there are not more infections. It is also striking how well the mucous membranes within a mouth heal after ordinary trauma. This may be due to an epithelial growth factor in saliva.

Saliva constantly bathes the mouth to maintain a specific environment and contains mucin, lysozyme, and IgA. Lysozyme has antibacterial properties; bacteria become entrapped in the mucin and are thereby easily swallowed; and IgA has the ability to prevent adherence of bacteria to mucous membranes.[12] Postoperative parotitis was once a common postoperative problem. It has been eliminated by careful attention to systemic hydration, which facilitates salivary flow, and by adequate oral hygiene, which removes inspisated secretions behind which infection could develop.

The normal mixed flora of the mouth is itself an important defense mechanism. These flora do not, in general, cause disease except in lung abscesses, peridontal disease, and human bites. With adequate oral hygiene, the normal flora prevents colonization with more pathogenic bacteria. A clear example of the value of the normal oral flora was seen when penicillin lozenges became available for the treatment of (bacterial) pharyngitis. Rather than control the infection, the lozenges merely eliminated the normal flora and allowed *Candida* to flourish. One mechanism by which the normal flora inhibit fungal overgrowth is to reduce the salivary glucose to a level insufficient to support *Candida*.[15]

ESOPHAGUS

The esophagus is essentially a conduit, which becomes infected only when obstructed or when systemic defenses are compromised. The swallowed bacteria are propelled more rapidly than they can reproduce.

STOMACH

The pH of the stomach provides an inhospitable environment for the growth of bacteria. There is electron microscopic evidence that some bacteria reside normally within the stomach, but their role and growth characteristics are as yet undefined. Because of the acid environment, even ulceration of the stomach in the face of systemic sepsis does not contribute to bacterial invasion.

The stomach is not always sterile, however. Food or blood neutralize the acid and permit microbial survival. The patient with achlorhydria no longer has an acid barrier. Obstruction of the stomach, or the small bowel, leads to a higher pH and can produce a feculant or foul secretion, a result of bacterial overgrowth. As a rule, however, systemic infection does not result if the mucosal lining is intact.

SMALL AND LARGE BOWEL

An increasing gradient in the numbers of bacteria exists within the gastrointestinal tract from the ligament of Treitz to the anus. To a limited extent the mechanical barrier of the mucous membranes is effective in preventing bacterial invasion; however, some bacteria can penetrate the gastrointestinal epithelium (eg, tubercule bacilli, *Salmonella*). The propulsive motion of the gastrointestinal epithelium keeps the bacterial population of the small bowel in check, but in more stagnant areas of the distal ileum, proximal to the ileocecal valve or within the colon, bacterial numbers increase markedly. Bacteria make up a large part of the total weight of the intestinal contents (Chapter 3).

The normal flora of the gastrointestinal tract is the single most important factor inhibiting colonization by potential pathogens.[16] The anaerobic environment, the competition for nutrients, and a variety of antimicrobial substances produced by the normal flora all act to restrain the proliferation of pathogens. The ecologic balance is delicate, however; even hospitalization leads to colonization of the lower gastrointestinal tract with hospital organisms, and antimicrobial agents can facilitate the overgrowth of organisms which cause serious disease (eg, *Clostridium difficile* pseudomembranous colitis).[17]

In germ-free animals the anatomical structure of the gastrointestinal tract is markedly different from that seen in animals more normally colonized. The cecum only attains 50 percent of normal weight in these animals. It returns to its normal size and configuration after colonization. Without normal flora, there is no evidence of normal lymphoid maturation, and it is likely that the normal flora act as an immunologic stimulant for the submucosal lymphoid tissues. These lymphoid tissues secrete IgA (and to a lesser extent IgM). Although IgA cannot opsonize bacteria for lysis, bacteria coated with IgA cannot adhere to intestinal mucosa, a step necessary for invasion.

THE URINARY TRACT

The urinary tract is normally sterile except at the urethral orifice. The periodic mechanical flushing effect of urine flow usually keeps the proximal urethra clear. Urine itself has a mild bacteriostatic effect because of its high urea content, high osmolality, high ammonia concentration, urinary IgA, and the acid pH.[18] Elevated urinary glucose levels support bacterial growth. Sodium, potassium, and organic acids have no inhibitory effect on bacterial growth.

Although urine contains IgG and IgA, the IgG probably has no antibacterial role. Secretory IgA acts primarily to prevent bacterial adherence to urothelium in the urethra, where colonization with fecal flora is common.[19] Both prostatic fluid and semen contain poorly characterized antimicrobial substances.[20]

One of the most important defenses against urinary infection is anatomical. The male urethra is long, and the meatus is distant from the anus; urinary tract infections are unusual in normal men. In the female, the urethra is short and its orifice is close to the fecal stream, and normal women can have urinary tract infections. Trauma to the urethra from whatever cause, changes in urine and urinary dynamics during pregnancy, and heavy colonization easily overwhelm the other defenses [21] (Chapter 45).

FEMALE GENITAL TRACT

Like other mucosal lined spaces, the female genital tract offers a mechanical barrier to bacterial infection in the form of a thick squamous epithelium and a mucous plug within the cervix. IgA and lysozyme are among its secretions. In the adult (and newborn), an acid pH and a glycogen-rich desquamation foster the growth of lactobacilli (Döderlein's bacillus), which in turn competes successfully with pathogenic bacteria. The prepubertal vagina is alkaline, and its flora is made up of staphylococci, streptococci, coliforms, and diphtheroids.

BIBLIOGRAPHY

Ganguly R, Waldman RH: Local immunity and local immune responses. Prog Allergy 27:1, 1980.

REFERENCES

1. Aly R, Maibach HI, Shinefield HR, Strauss W: Survival of pathogenic microorganisms on human skin. J Invest Dermatol 58:205, 1972.
2. Aly R, Maibach HI, Rahman R, Shinefield HR, Mandel AD: Correlation of human in vivo and in vitro cutaneous antimicrobial factors. J Infect Dis 131:579, 1975.
3. William REO: Healthy carriage of *Staphylococcus aureus:* its prevalence and importance. Bacteriol Rev 27:56, 1963.
4. Langford MP, Stanton GJ, Barber JC, Baron S: Early-appearing antiviral activity in human tears during a case of picornavirus epidemic conjunctivitis. J Infect Dis 139:653, 1979.
5. Walter JB, Israel MS: General Pathology, 3rd ed. London, Churchill, 1970, p 414.
6. Newell FW: Physiology and biochemistry of the eye. In Newell FW: Ophthalmology Principles and Concepts, 4th ed. St Louis, Mosby, 1978.
7. Proctor DF, Andersen I, Lundgvist G: Clearance of inhaled particles from the human nose. Arch Intern Med 131:132, 1973.
8. Rhodin JAG: Ultrastructure and function of the human tracheal mucosa. Am Rev Respir Dis 93 (suppl):1, 1966.
9. Santa Crus R, Landa J, Hirsch J, Sackner M: Tracheal mucous velocity in normal man and patients with obstructive lung

disease; effects of terbutaline. Am Rev Respir Dis 109:458, 1974.
10. Matsuyama T: Point inoculation of cultivated tracheal mucous membrane with bacteria. J Infect Dis 130:508, 1974.
11. LaForce FM: Effect of aerosol immunization with RE 595 *Salmonella minnesota* on lung bactericidal activity against *Serratin marcescens, Enterobacter cloacae* and *Pseudomonas aeruginosa*. Am Rev Respir Dis 116:241, 1977.
12. Ganguly C, Waldman RH: Local immunity and local immune defenses. Prog Allergy 27:1, 1980.
13. Hocking WG, Golde DW: The pulmonary-alveolar macrophage (Part I). N Engl J Med 301:580, 1979.
14. Cohan AB, Gold WM: Defense mechanisms of the lungs. Ann Rev Physiol 37:325, 1975.
15. Knight L, Fletcher J: Growth of *Candida albicans* in saliva: stimulation by glucose associated with antibiotics, corticosteroids and diabetes mellitus. J Infect Dis 123:371, 1971.
16. Donaldson RM Jr: Normal bacterial populations of the intestine and their relation to intestinal functions. N Engl J Med 270:938, 994, 1050, 1964.
17. Bartlett JG, Gorbach SL: Pseudomembranous enterocolitis (antibiotic-related colitis). Adv Intern Med 22:455, 1977.
18. Kaye D: Host defense mechanisms in the urinary tract. Urol Clin NA 2:407, 1975.
19. Burden DE: Immunologic reaction to urinary infection: the nature and function of secretory immunoglobulins. In Williams DT, Chisholm GD (eds): Scientific Foundations of Urology. Chicago, Yearbook Medical Publishers, 1976.
20. Stamey TA, Fair WR, Timothy MM, Chung HK: Antibacterial nature of prostatic fluid. Nature 218:444, 1968.
21. Stamey TA: Pathogenisis and Treatment of Urinary Tract Infections. Baltimore, Williams and Wilkins, 1980.

B. The Phagocytes

DAVID C. HOHN

The system of phagocytic leukocytes, along with the humoral and cellular immune systems, comprise the major constituents in systemic host resistance to infection. The circulating blood phagocytes are the granulocytes (neutrophils, eosinophils, and basophils) and the monocytes. The noncirculating phagocytic system, previously referred to as the reticuloendothelial system (RES), is comprised of tissue macrophages, which are present in all tissues and are especially numerous in the spleen, liver (lining the sinusoids), and lung (alveolar macrophages lining the distal air sac). These cells not only phagocytose and kill microbes, they also participate in all microbial and nonmicrobial inflammatory reactions, where they are essential for wound healing and the disposal of immune complexes, injured cells, and foreign material. Unfortunately, under certain circumstances, the cells can themselves contribute to tissue injury (eg, gouty arthritis).

Disposal of most bacteria and fungi is accomplished by phagocytosis, which is the single most important process in the control of infection. Each step in the phagocytosis and killing is also a potential crack in the armor of host defense. Many of these cracks have been detected by recognition of a variety of inherited disorders of phagocytic function. Furthermore, acquired disorders of phagocytic function may occur in response to the stress of injury, sepsis, and malnutrition.

GRANULOCYTES

Morphology and Metabolism

Polymorphonuclear cells have segmented nuclei and are called granulocytes because of the granules found within the cytosol. Basophils possess granules that stain deep blue-black with Wright stain, because they contain heparin. They also contain histamine and other substances that cause contraction of smooth muscle and increase the permeability of small blood vessels. Eosinophils have granules that stain red or orange with Wright stain. Their functions are not known, but they are dramatically increased in numbers during parasitic infections, and they may have some role in protection against parasitic infections like schistosomiasis.[1]

Neutrophils are the most common granulocyte. There are at least two types of cytoplasmic granules. The azurophil (purple-staining) granules constitute 10 to 20 percent of the total population and are electron dense (Fig. 13-7). The specific granules are smaller (less than 0.2 μm), stain pink, and are electron lucent.

The azurophil granules are typical lysosomes containing various hydrolytic enzymes with optimal activity at about pH 5 (amylase, alpha and beta glucosidase, β glucuronidase, elastase, neutral proteases, collaginase, and cathepsin D). These enzymes collectively can break down organic material into building blocks of amino acids, sugars, and nucleotides. Azurophil granules also contain lysozyme and myeloperoxidase, which may actually kill bacteria. Lysozyme hydrolyzes the muramic-N-acetyl glucosamine bond found in the mucopeptide coat of all bacteria. Myeloperoxidase is an enzyme that is capable of complexing with hydrogen peroxide and using it to effect oxidations of various types. Azurophil granules also contain some nonenzymatic materials including the cationic proteins, a group of antibacterial proteins with highly positive charges, a protein that causes inflammation when injected into the skin, and sulfated mucopolysaccharides with highly negative charges.

Specific granules contain some lysozyme and lactoferrin, a protein that contains a heme group with strong affinity for ferric iron. All bacteria need iron to grow, and lactoferrin is thought to reduce free iron concentration to far below the required levels. Lactoferrin may also play a part in killing bacteria.[2]

The nucleus of the granulocyte is subdivided into a number of lobes. When the demand for neutrophils is high during bacterial infection, many young cells are mobilized from the bone marrow and have a nucleus that is elongated and twisted upon itself (band or stab cells). The functional significance of the multisegmented nucleus is unknown. Within the nucleus the chromatin is clumped, suggesting that much of the genome is inactive. There is virtually no incorporation of tritiated thymidine into cellular DNA, and these cells are end cells that do not divide. It is unlikely that neutrophils can synthesize ribosomes, since the nucleolus in which ribosomal synthesis normally occurs is missing. Protein synthesis is thought to occur, however, and RNA is present.

Within the neutrophil cytoplasm, there are large numbers of small electron-dense particles thought to be composed of glycogen, which serves as the major energy source for the cell as a substrate in glycolysis. The rate of glycogen breakdown is not greatly affected by oxygen, and during phagocytosis there are great increases in the rates of glycogen breakdown, glucose uptake, and lactate output. Total cell glycogen decreases. Phagocytosis cannot occur unless energy from glycolysis is available; only a few mitochondria are present in mature neutrophils. Neutrophils can move and take up bacteria in the total absence of oxygen. The rate of bacterial killing under these circumstances may be abnormally low, because hydrogen peroxide cannot be generated under anaerobic conditions. Neutrophils can metabolize glucose by the hexose monophosphate shunt, and reliance on this route of metabolism may rise to as much as 30 percent of total glucose utilization after the cell has phagocytosed bacteria.[2]

Granulopoiesis and Its Disorders

Normal Granulopoiesis

Maturation of neutrophils in the marrow requires approximately 14 days. During the early phases of maturation, proteins are synthesized and assembled into the azurophil granules. During the myelocyte stage, the smaller specific granules are assembled.[3] With further maturation, there is a reduction in mitochondrial content, an increase in glycogen stores, and glycolytic metabolism becomes the predominant energy source for movement and phagocytosis.

Normal bone marrow maintains an extraordinary capacity for granulopoiesis. Daily cell turnover of neutrophils in a 70-kg man is in the order of 126 billion cells, with a circulating half-life of approximately 6 hours and with maintenance of function in tissues for 1 to 2 days.[4]

Release from the bone marrow requires that the neutrophil has acquired sufficient plasticity and motility to negotiate the marrow sinuses and enter the circulation. During periods of stress and infection, a less mature neutrophil reserve, which includes band forms and occasionally metamyelocytes, is released into the circulation. These immature neutrophils are less deformable and less motile than mature cells and may also ingest particles and kill bacteria less efficiently.

Disorders of Neutrophil Production

Neutropenia arises as a result of decreased marrow production or increased destruction of cells. Although the etiology of many of the neutropenias is unclear, a number of autoimmune mechanisms have been described. Neutropenias may be sustained or cyclic, and the clinical significance of the defect depends on the degree of neutropenia, the periodicity of the cycle, and whether monocytes are also deficient. The number of neutrophils migrating into tissues decreases strikingly when the absolute neutrophil count falls below 1500 per mm.[3] If adequate monocyte counts are maintained, the clinical consequences of neutropenia are relatively mild in otherwise normal subjects.[5] Such patients, however, may be profoundly susceptible to infection when undergoing operation if microbial contamination is present, and they should be covered with broad-spectrum antibiotics. In neutropenic patients with documented hypersplenism, splenectomy should be considered. In contrast to the selective neutropenias, patients deficient in both neutrophils and monocytes are highly susceptible to infections, and even with optimal antibiotic management and granulocyte transfusion therapy, mortality from sepsis remains high.

Neutrophil Migration

Normal Migration

Following release from the marrow, only about half of the intravascular granulocytes circulate. The remainder are sequestered in small vessels or become adherent to the endothelium of larger vessels constituting the "marginated" pool of leukocytes. The marginated cells are released after administration of catecholamines or corticosteroids, and this probably accounts for the transient neutrophilia that follows stress or hypovolemic shock.

In acute inflammatory conditions, neutrophils migrate into tissues within a few hours. This unidirectional migration of leukocytes in response to a diffusion gradient of chemical attractant is referred to as chemotaxis. The simplest method for studying chemotaxis in vivo is the skin window technique of Rebuck and Crowley.[6] A sterile glass coverslip is placed over a standard skin abrasion and is periodically removed, stained, and replaced. Microscopic examination and counting of adherent leukocytes provides an estimate of the number and type of cells arriving in the wound. Neutrophils move rapidly and are present in large numbers by 4 hours; monocytes migrate more slowly and become the predominant cell type within 12 to 24 hours. A similar pattern of leukocyte response is seen in surgical wounds where neutrophils arrive early and are replaced by monocytes in several days.

Most studies of chemotaxis have employed the in vitro Boyden chamber technique, wherein two chambers are separated by a filter membrane with pore size small enough to allow leukocyte passage by migration but not by sedimentation. Leukocytes are placed in the upper chamber, and a source of chemotactic factor in the lower chamber. The number of leukocytes migrating through the filter is determined microscopically, and a chemotactic index can be calculated. With a standard chemoattractant, this system allows assessment of the cellular motility; when normal cells are used, it can be used to study chemotactic factor activities.[7] Recently, chemotaxis has been studied by allowing leukocytes to migrate on plastic dishes beneath a layer of nutrient gel. Cells are loaded in a small well cut in the agarose, and chemotactic factor is loaded in an opposing well a short distance away.[8] This system allows study of cellular and humoral response and is relatively simple to perform.

Normal chemotactic function requires that adequate quantities of soluble chemotactic factors be generated and that leukocytes be capable of directional migration toward these factors. Chemotactic disorders involving both cellular and humoral mechanisms have been recognized. Leukocyte motion (and the associated phagocytic behavior) appears to be generated by a contractile cytoplasmic protein system comprised of actin and myosin, which is activated by cell surface contact and by interaction of chemotactic substances with receptors on the cell membrane.

Chemotactic factors can be generated by clotting of blood, injured tissues, interaction of injured tissues and bacteria with complement, direct release of bacterial peptides, and antigen stimulation of lymphocytes (Fig. 13-5). While many of these chemotactic factors may be produced locally in response to injury and infection, the complement-derived constituents appear to be most important. The C3a and C5a peptides are cleaved from C3 and C5 through the action of nonspecific proteases liberated from injured tissues and by the interaction of bacteria with the antibody-dependent hemolytic complement pathway or the alternative properdin pathway (see subsequent section on complement). It now appears that C5a is the more active and important of these complement-derived components. In addition to activating complement components, bacteria may also liberate substances with direct chemotactic activity toward leukocytes. Lymphokines derived from antigen-stimulated lymphocytes are probably more important in chronic inflammatory conditions than in acute injury and infection.

Leukocyte migration is dependent on glycolysis for energy metabolism and proceeds normally under anoxic conditions. Motility is maintained for several hours in glucose-free media and is unaffected by mild acidosis to pH values of 6.5. Phagocytosis of particles, however, does impair capacity for subsequent migration. It is evident that leukocytes are well equipped to migrate into the hypoxic, acidotic, and relatively hypoglycemic tissues surrounding a surgical wound or an area of localized infection. Furthermore, tissue injury and infection produce a variety of substances capable of attracting leukocytes even in complement-depleted hosts.[9]

A number of substances present in serum and in leukocyte granules also serve to inhibit the chemotactic response. These chemotactic inhibitors may prevent excessive activation of chemotactic mechanisms and may also serve to retain the leukocytes in an area of inflammation after they have been attracted. An additional mechanism to retain leukocytes is the refractoriness of a leukocyte to further respond to chemotactic agents in the presence of a high concentration of the same, or a different chemotactic factor—a process called chemotactic deactivation.[10] Furthermore, many bacterial and viral toxins can inhibit leukocyte locomotion.[11]

Disorders of Leukocyte Migration

A variety of intrinsic and acquired disorders of leukocyte motility have been recognized. In these conditions, the infections tend to be recurrent and prolonged, and there is poor response to appropriate antibiotics. The infections most commonly involve soft tissues including the skin, while pulmonary, hepatic, and renal infections may also occur. Systemic septicemia and meningitis are uncommon in these patients. The pathogens seen in patients with chemotactic and granulocyte function defects are characteristically *S. aureus* (by far the most common organism), *S. epidermidis*, gram-negative enteric bacilli, and fungi. In contrast, patients with immunoglobulin abnormalities are subject to septicemia and meningitis with organisms such as *S. pneumoniae* (pneumococcus), *H. influenzae*, and group A streptococci.[5]

Chemotactic disorders may be secondary to an intrinsic or acquired cellular disorder, deficiency in production of chemotactic factors, or the presence of inhibitors of cells or chemotactic factors as outlined in Table 13-2. Association of a cellular chemotactic defect with severe pyo-

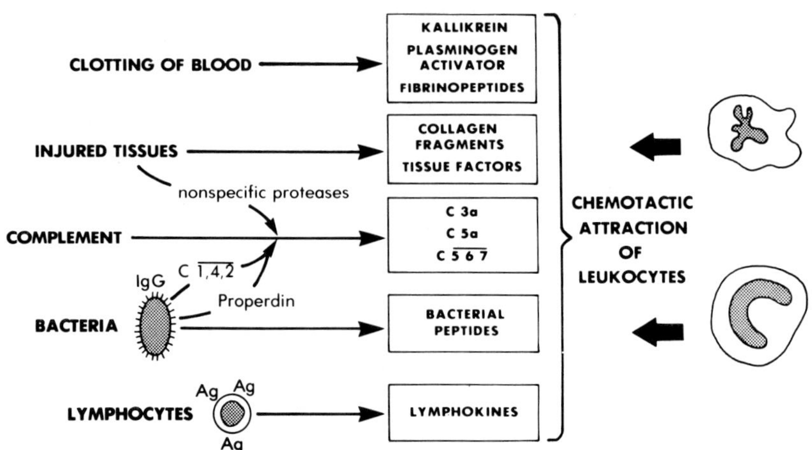

Fig. 13-5. Major mechanisms for generation of chemotactic factors.

TABLE 13-2. LEUKOCYTE MOTILITY DISORDERS

CELLULAR DEFECTS
- Congenital
  - Hyper-IgE syndrome
  - Lazy leukocyte syndrome
  - Chediak-Higashi syndrome
- Acquired
  - Trauma and burns
  - Malnutrition
  - Tumors
  - Infections
  - Diabetes mellitus

HUMORAL DEFECTS
- Chemotactic factor deficiency
  - C3 deficiency
  - C5 deficiency or dysfunction
- Inhibitors of chemotactic factors
  - Cirrhosis
  - Hodgkin disease
  - IgA
- Inhibitors of cell migration
  - Steroids
  - Serum inhibitors

derma and elevated levels of IgE has been an increasingly recognized clinical syndrome (Job syndrome or Hill-Quie syndrome),[12] and disordered leukocyte motility may partially explain the unusual susceptibility to infection seen in diabetics.[13] Transient impairment of chemotaxis has also been described in trauma, burns, and malnutrition and is seen as well with malignant tumors.[14,15] Overwhelming infection may also cause impairment of the chemotactic response.

Deficiency of chemotactic factor generation or cellular inhibitors of chemotaxis are relatively uncommon. Inhibitors of chemotactic factor activity have been described in the sera of patients with cirrhosis, Hodgkin disease, and in anergic patients when levels of immune globulin A are elevated. IgA may itself be an inhibitor.[16-18]

Patients with recurrent or persistent infections, particularly where there is a lifelong or family history, should be screened for genetically transmitted chemotactic disorders. Vigorous nutritional therapy, aggressive management of serious infections, early skin grafting in burn patients, and avoidance wherever possible of the use of corticosteroids contributes to the preservation or restoration of leukocyte migration.

Opsonization for Phagocytosis

Normal Opsonization

After leukocytes are attracted to the area of inflammation through the process of chemotaxis, recognition and ingestion of offending organisms normally occurs. The ingestion process is facilitated by humoral factors called opsonins, which bind to the microbial surface and interact with receptors on the surface of the phagocyte to accelerate ingestion. Opsonization permits the leukocyte to recognize which particles need to be ingested, and in the absence of opsonins, most organisms are neither ingested nor effectively eliminated by phagocytes.

The major opsonic mechanisms are shown in Figure 13-6. Antibodies of the IgG subclass are opsonic when bound in sufficient concentration to the surface of a microbial cell. Normal serum has relatively little IgG-dependent opsonic activity, whereas serum from hyperimmunized subjects contains considerable amounts.[19] In the presence of an intact complement system, the opsonic activity of small amounts of bound IgG is greatly amplified.[20] This is accomplished by antibody activation of the classical C142 hemolytic complement sequence, which results in proteolytic cleavage of C3 to yield a highly opsonic fragment called C3b. Fixation of C3b to the microbial surface greatly enhances the rate of uptake by phagocytic cells. Opsonization also occurs in the absence of IgG and appears to be largely due to direct interaction of bacteria with properdin, which also cleaves C3 and promotes C3b fixation (see subsequent section on complement). It is important to distinguish these microbial opsonins from the nonspecific tissue opsonin described by Saba and DiLuzio [21] and in Chapter 17. These investigations have

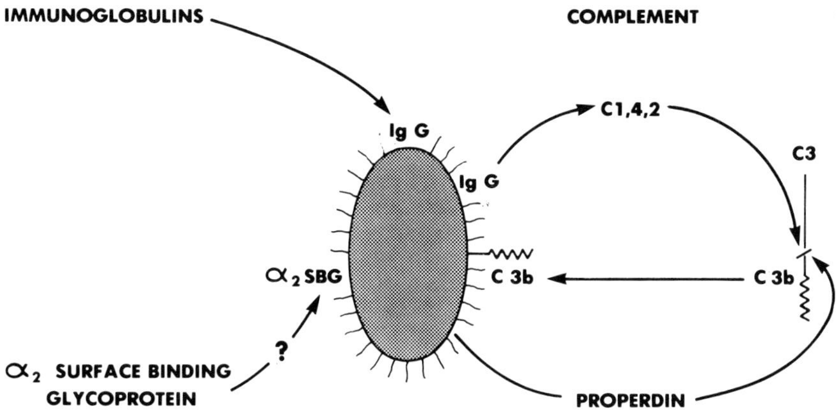

Fig. 13-6. Mechanisms of bacterial opsonization. The major opsonin for bacteria is the complement fragment C3b, which results from the activation of the complement cascade by either the classical (C_1,4,2) or the alternative (properdin) pathways. Opsonization by specific antimicrobial immunoglobulin is less commonly utilized. Whether α_2 surface-binding glycoprotein (fibrinectin) can function as a microbial opsonin is controversial.

shown that effective phagocytosis of circulating nonmicrobial particulate matter by the reticuloendothelial system requires opsonization by an α_2 surface-binding glycoprotein which does not function as a bacterial opsonin. In patients with posttraumatic depletion of α_2 surface-binding glycoprotein, however, repletion by administering cryoprecipitated plasma fraction may lead to clinical improvement in septicemic patients.[22]

Disorders of Opsonization

The kinds of infection typically encountered in patients with opsonin deficiency tend to involve virulent encapsulated bacteria including pneumococci, *P. aeruginosa*, streptococci, or *H. influenzae*. Unlike patients with chemotactic disorders, these patients are typically susceptible to bacteremias, meningitis, and respiratory tract sepsis.[5]

A number of patients with genetic complement deficiency states have been identified and found to have defective opsonization and recurrent pyogenic infections (Table 13-3). The presence of adequate levels of C3 is particularly important in this regard, and patients with genetic C3 deficiency, hypercatabolism of C3, or defective C3 activation mechanisms may have opsonin deficiencies with associated infections. Patients with immune globulin deficiency or specific antibody deficiency may also opsonize bacteria ineffectively and be subject to infections.[23] Deficiencies of gamma globulin and certain of the complement constituents may be treated with globulin or infusions of fresh frozen plasma.

Alexander et al [24] have extensively studied the opsonic system following major burn injury, trauma, and infection. Depressed opsonic capacity has been found early in the burn injury period, but there has been poor correlation between opsonic index and incidence of infection in burn patients. Patients with overwhelming infection have also been shown to be deficient in opsonic components, and it has been postulated that this is due to consumption of available opsonins. Others, however, have been unable to convincingly demonstrate that consumptive opsoninopathy occurs clinically.

TABLE 13-3. OPSONIN DISORDERS

CONGENITAL DEFECTS
- Complement disorders
  - C3 deficiency or hypercatabolism
  - Properdin system disorders
- Immunoglobulin deficiency

ACQUIRED OR TRANSIENT DISORDERS
- Low birth weight infants
- Systemic lupus erythematosis
- Cirrhosis
- Glomerulonephritis
- Burn injury
- Overwhelming sepsis (opsonic consumption?)
- α_2 surface glycoprotein deficiency (?)

INAPPROPRIATE OPSONIZATION
- Autoimmune anemias
- Autoimmune thrombocytopenia
- Autoimmune leukopenias

Although opsonins may not be totally depleted during infection, there is good evidence that complement is activated in the serum. C5a serum levels are increased in surgical sepsis, and C5a receptors on circulating leukocytes are lost in direct proportion to the loss of neutrophil function.[24a] Similar events probably occur during cardiopulmonary bypass.[24b]

Ingestion and Degranulation

Normal Leukocyte Ingestion and Degranulation

After the phagocytes have been attracted to the area of inflammation and after the bacteria have been coated with opsonic proteins, the opsonized bacteria attach to surface receptors on the leukocytes, triggering ingestion. The phagocytes have receptors for C3b and for the Fc portion of IgG. Once attachment has taken place, pseudopodia are extended around the organism, encasing it in a phagocytic vacuole which is lined by the invaginated cell membrane (Fig. 13-7). An integrated series of morphologic and metabolic changes then occur, which convert the phagocytic vacuole into a microbicidal trap.

Mature granulocytes and monocytes contain at least two distinct populations of cytoplasmic granules, which contain a variety of hydrolytic, digestive, and antimicrobial proteins and enzymes described previously. These granules now approach and then fuse with the membrane of the phagocytic vacuole, discharging their contents in contained proximity to the sequestered organism (Fig. 13-8).

Coincident with the morphologic changes occurring during phagocytosis, there is also a profound increase in oxidative metabolism, the so-called respiratory burst of phagocytosis. In addition to augmentation of oxygen consumption, increased production of hydrogen peroxide and superoxide and increased glucose oxidation via the hexose monophosphate shunt also occur.[25] The critical enzyme in the oxidative burst is an NADPH-linked, cyanide-resistant oxidase (primary oxidase), which reduces oxygen to superoxide (Fig. 13-9). Superoxide then combines with two hydrogen ions (the dismutation reaction) to form hydrogen peroxide. The $NADP^+$ produced during the production of oxygen is reduced back to NADPH by the enzyme system of the hexose shunt. Phagocytosis therefore activates a self-regenerating enzyme system which consumes oxygen and produces hydrogen peroxide and superoxide (H_2O_2 and O_2^-). Both of these substances are highly reactive agents and either directly or indirectly produce potent antimicrobial activity.[25]

Disorders of Ingestion and Degranulation (Table 13-4)

Leukocytes from patients with a rare genetic leukocyte disorder known as chronic granulomatous disease (CGD) are devoid of oxidase activity, so that killing of a variety of common bacteria and fungi by CGD leukocytes is impaired.[26] CGD patients are profoundly susceptible to infection, especially by *S. aureus*, *E. coli*, *Pseudomonas*, *Salmonella*, *Serratia*, and fungi.

Impaired uptake of opsonized particles and microorganisms has been recognized in several clinical settings. Leukocytes from patients with high levels of circulating

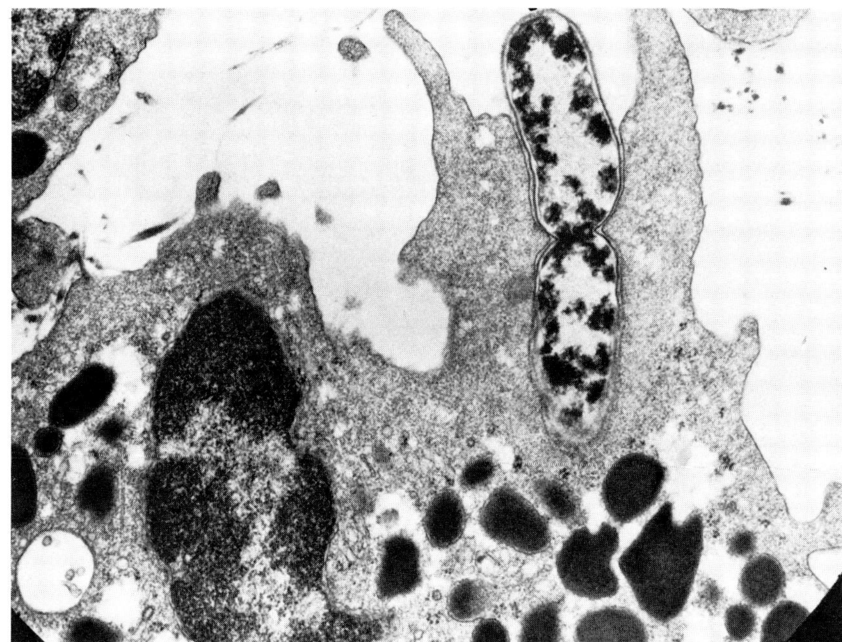

Fig. 13-7. Bacteria (arrow) in the process of being ingested by a neutrophil. The electron-dense azurophil granules can be seen in the cytoplasm. (Courtesy DF Bainton, MD, University of California, San Francisco.)

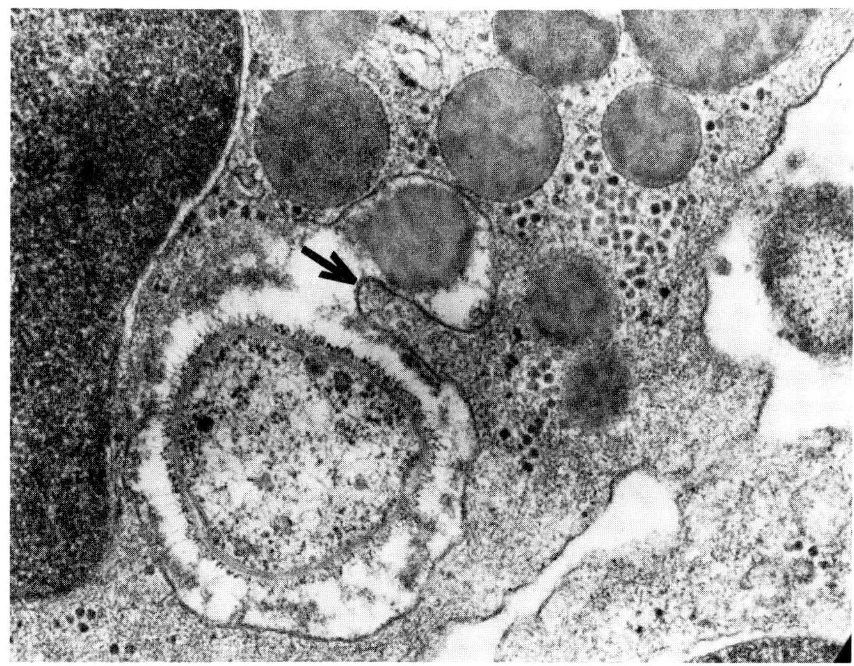

Fig. 13-8. Neutrophil degranulation. Arrow indicates point of fusion between the granule membrane and that of the phagocytic vacuole. (Courtesy DF Bainton, MD, University of California, San Francisco.)

immune complexes may exhibit impaired ingestion,[27] as may cells from patients with diabetic acidosis or nonketotic hyperosmolar conditions.[28] Overwhelming infection may lead to a high percentage of immature neutrophils and band forms, and these cells may ingest organisms less avidly than their mature counterparts.[4] Acquired defects in fusion of granules with the phagocytic vacuole have not been found in surgical patients, however. Impaired degranulation does occur in a rare genetic leukocyte disorder known as the Chediak-Higashi syndrome. Hereditary deficiency of myeloperoxidase, a leukocyte granule enzyme, has been reported and may predispose to fungal septicemias.[29] Hyperactive degranulation may be a part of inflammatory conditions such as gout, rheumatoid arthritis, silicosis, and immune complex nephritis, and the hydrolytic enzymes may attack host tissue contributing to the inflammatory cycle.

Microbicidal Mechanisms of Leukocytes

The oxygen-NADPH oxidase microbicidal system is the most important microbicidal mechanism within the neutrophil, but there are others (Table 13-5). The microbicidal systems can be divided into two large categories: those

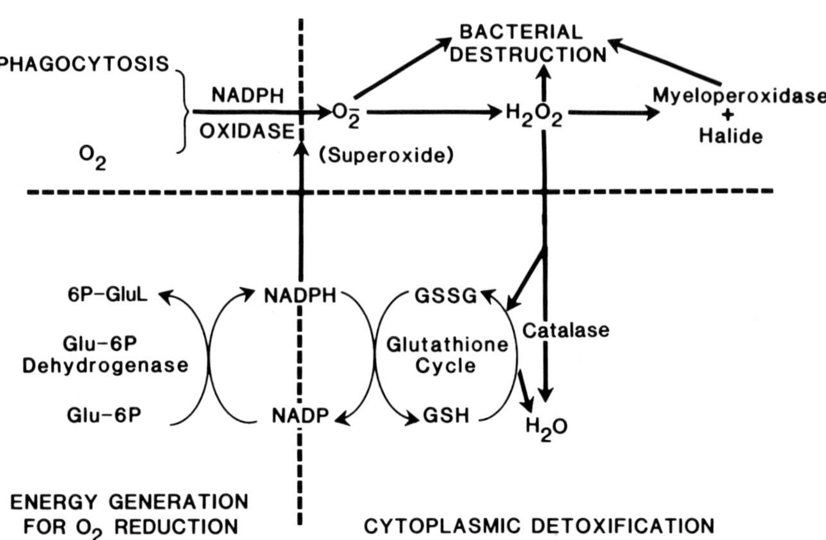

Fig. 13-9. Metabolic pathway of the leukocyte primary oxidase system. The interaction between phagocytosis and bacterial destruction is schematically outlined. Phagocytosis stimulates the production of superoxide and hydrogen peroxide which, in conjunction with the myeloperoxidase-halide system, leads to bacterial destruction within the phagosome. Excess hydrogen peroxide, which could damage the cell, is detoxified by catalase and the glutathione cycle. The energy for both H_2O_2 production and detoxification is provided by the hexose monophosphate shunt. Other bactericidal mechanisms are listed in Table 13-5.

that depend on molecular oxygen for generation of microbicidal moieties and those that function equally well in the absence of oxygen and are oxygen-independent.

Oxygen-Dependent Microbicidal Mechanisms

Hydrogen Peroxide. Although hydrogen peroxide itself has some bactericidal activity, it becomes manifest only at concentrations greater than 0.5 mM.[30] Whether such high concentrations of peroxide are regularly achieved in the phagocytic vacuole is doubtful. Klebanoff et al,[31] however, have demonstrated that the toxicity of hydrogen peroxide is profoundly augmented in the presence of halide ions and myeloperoxidase, a hemoprotein present in the granules of neutrophils and monocytes. During phagocytosis, myeloperoxidase is delivered to the phagocytic vacuole through the process of degranulation, and hydrogen peroxide is generated by the leukocyte-oxidase system. Chloride is normally present in the leukocyte vacuole and probably functions as the halide in this system. The myeloperoxidase-hydrogen peroxide-halide system has broad antimicrobial activity (Fig. 13-9).

TABLE 13-4. SOME DISORDERS OF LEUKOCYTE INGESTION, DEGRANULATION, AND MICROBICIDAL FUNCTION

CONGENITAL DEFECTS
Chronic granulomatous disease (CGD)
G6PD deficiency (severe)
Myeloperoxidase deficiency
Chediak-Higashi syndrome (defective degranulation)
ACQUIRED DEFECTS
Septicemia
Burn and traumatic injury
Malnutrition
LOCAL DEFECTS
Impaired killing due to tissue hypoxemia
Phagocytic engorgement

The precise mode of microbial death still remains somewhat vague. The myeloperoxidase–H_2O_2 system does result in halogenation of microbial surfaces; amino acids in the cell wall are converted to aldehydes; and finally, the myeloperoxidase system may generate other toxic oxygen radicals such as singlet oxygen.

Superoxide. The discovery that superoxide (O_2^-) is generated in high concentrations by phagocytes has led to speculation that superoxide anion itself may be a microbicidal agent.[32] Thus far, the evidence for direct superoxide-mediated bacterial killing is relatively weak.

Hydroxyl Radical. A number of recent studies have suggested that hydroxyl radical (OH·) may be an important intracellular microbicide. This highly unstable radical reacts almost instanteously with most organic molecules. Enzyme systems that produce hydroxyl radicals have been demonstrated to kill bacteria, and hydroxyl radicals can be formed during the interaction of superoxide and hydrogen peroxide, both of which are present in the leukocyte vacuole.

Singlet Oxygen (O_2*). Singlet oxygen is another highly reactive oxidizing agent which has been implicated in killing of bacteria by phagocytes,[25] although rigorous proof is still absent. This species differs from molecular oxygen only in the distribution of electrons around the two oxygen nuclei.

Oxygen-Independent Microbicidal Systems

Among the identified oxygen-independent microbicidal agents is acid, which is formed in the phagocytic vacuole and can directly kill certain acid-sensitive organisms. Lactoferrin, present in the leukocyte granule, exerts a microbistatic effect by chelation of iron required for microbial growth. Lysozyme is an abundant leukocyte granule enzyme which digests cell wall constituents, contributing to killing and particularly to digestion of the ingested organisms.[32a] Leukocyte granules also contain a group of

TABLE 13-5. LEUKOCYTE MICROBICIDAL MECHANISMS

OXYGEN-DEPENDENT KILLING MECHANISMS
Hydrogen peroxide (H_2O_2)
H_2O_2 + halide + myeloperoxidase
Superoxide anion (O_2^-)
Hydroxyl radicals ($OH\cdot$)
Singlet oxygen (O_2^*)
OXYGEN-INDEPENDENT KILLING MECHANISMS
Acid
Lactoferrin
Lysozyme
Granule cationic proteins

highly cationic proteins, which bind to the surface of ingested organisms and mediate microbial killing. The cationic proteins possess striking microbial specificity.[33] Emerging evidence suggests that this latter system may be of major importance in the antimicrobial armamentarium of the leukocyte.

THE MONOCYTE-MACROPHAGE SYSTEM

Maturation of Monocytes and Differentiation to Macrophages

Mononuclear phagocytes arise from an undifferentiated stem cell, which also gives rise to cells of the granulocytic series. As monoblasts mature and form a complex Golgi apparatus and definite granule populations, they are identified as promonocytes. With maturation of promonocytes to monocytes, there is a reduced nuclear-cytoplasmic ratio, increased phagocytic capacity, and increased activity of acid hydrolases.[34] The intravascular half-life of blood monocytes is approximately 8.4 hours. Approximately two-thirds of the total blood monocyte pool circulates, while the remainder is marginated on vascular endothelium. Monocytes undergo a continual one-way exodus from the vascular compartment into tissues and organs, where they differentiate into mature tissue macrophages. Tissue macrophages are also produced in situ through mitosis. The major types of tissue macrophages are listed in Table 13-6. Collectively, the monocyte-macrophage system is the functional equivalent of what was originally called the reticuloendothelial system (RES).

TABLE 13-6. TYPES OF TISSUE MACROPHAGES

Macrophages of lymphoid tissue
Pleural and peritoneal macrophages
Alveolar macrophages
Connective tissue macrophages (histiocytes)
Microglial cells of nervous system
Hepatic macrophages (Küpffer cells)
Macrophages of splenic sinusoids

During maturation, macrophages increase in size with the development of one or more large nuclei, numerous cytoplasmic lysosomes, and mitochondria, and lose mitotic activity. In addition, macrophages become capable of synthesizing proteins, including complement factors C2 and C3, and they also generate a plasminogen activator, prostaglandin E2, and endogenous pyrogen. Functional and metabolic differentiation of maturing tissue macrophages is partially determined by the organ in which the cells reside. For example, circulating monocytes and most tissue macrophages depend largely on glycolytic energy metabolism. The alveolar macrophage, however, loses phagocytic activity, develops numerous mitochondria, and depends predominantly on oxidative energy sources. Küpffer cells of the liver and splenic macrophages have high phagocytic capacities, and macrophages in wounds appear to release factors that stimulate repair. Tissue macrophages are capable of survival for several months.[35]

Functions of Monocytes and Macrophages

Scavenger Function

The major identified functions of the monocyte-macrophage system are outlined in Table 13-7. While it has been long recognized that mononuclear phagocytes serve as scavengers of damaged cells and debris and of inorganic and organic foreign material, there has been relatively little recent study of this important subject. Macrophages are involved in the debridement of injured cells from wounds as well as in the remodeling of tissue during embryogenesis. Particulate foreign substances are ingested by phagocytic mechanisms, while soluble materials and macromolecules undergo pinocytic uptake. Monocytes contain lysosomal hydrolytic enzymes, lipase, and large quantities of lysozyme. Hydrolytic enzyme content is markedly increased during the process of macrophage "activation." These enzymes are capable of digestion of most ingested substrates. It is not known whether the process of ingestion of foreign material alters other functional characteristics of the macrophage such as microbicidal activity or immune processing function.[36]

Microbicidal Function

Monocytes and macrophages also possess a broad spectrum of microbicidal activity toward bacteria, fungi, viruses, and various facultative intracellular parasites. Rates of ingestion and killing of common bacterial pathogens by monocytes are substantially lower than for granulocytes. Monocytes, however, play the principal role in ingestion and killing of intracellular pathogens such as *Pneumocystis carinii, Mycobacterium, Salmonella, Listeria, Cryptococcus, Toxoplasma, Plasmodium,* and *Brucella.* The antibacterial mechanisms of the human blood monocyte probably resemble those of granulocytes with both oxidative and peroxidative mechanisms as well as oxygen-independent microbicidal mechanisms (Table 13-5, Fig. 13-9). The clinical importance of the monocyte-macrophage system in resistance to infection is illustrated by the substantial mi-

TABLE 13-7. BIOLOGIC FUNCTIONS OF THE MONOCYTE-MACROPHAGE SYSTEM

Scavenger function
Microbicidal activity
Cooperative immune processing
Cytotoxic activity
Regulation of granulopoeisis
Generation of pyrogen
Synthesis of complement (C2,C3), prostaglandin E2, and plasminogen activator
Generation of mediators of wound repair—collagen synthesis, angiogenesis

crobial resistance shown by patients suffering from various neutropenic disorders.[37]

Immune Function

Macrophages are essential in the modulation of both humoral and cell-mediated immunity.[38] With regard to humoral immunity, most complex antigenic materials are first processed by macrophages, which eliminate certain immunogenic materials and retain other antigens in a native or partially degraded state. The antigen-sensitized macrophage then interacts in a complex fashion with immunocompetent lymphocytes. For certain types of antigens, interaction of macrophages with T-lymphocytes is essential for a maximal antibody production by B-lymphocytes.[38] Macrophages are essential for optimal mitogenic responses by T-lymphocytes and for the generation of T-helper cells.[38] Conversely, stimulated lymphocytes release products called lymphokines, which strongly influence macrophage function and metabolism. Stimulation of a lymphocyte by exposure to antigen may cause release of factors which result in activation of macrophages with enhancement of metabolic, protein-synthetic, and antimicrobial activities.[37]

Macrophages are also involved in expression of cell-mediated immune responses, including delayed hypersensitivity response and allograft rejection. In these responses, macrophages are attracted to the site of inflammation by antigen-induced lymphokines released from lymphocytes and are maintained there by migration inhibitory factors (MIF). Macrophages are then locally activated by macrophage activation factors (MAF), which stimulate phagocytosis, digestion of debris and foreign antigens, and release of hydrolytic enzymes (Section 13 C).

Other Functions of Macrophages

Monocytes and macrophages also participate in a variety of cytotoxic reactions, which can be directed against allograft cells, host cells in autoimmune disorders, and tumor cells. Some of these mechanisms require prior attachment of specific antibodies, while others depend on non-specific macrophage activation. The actual cytotoxic mechanisms are poorly understood. Although intimate cell contact is necessary,[39] phagocytosis is not required for cytotoxicity.

Monocytes and macrophages also participate in regulating granulopoiesis by elaboration of humoral colony stimulating activity (CSA). Evidence suggests that CSA is a heterogeneous group of glycoproteins, which probably stimulate both granulocyte and monocyte proliferation. Monocyte CSA elaboration may be induced by endotoxin or certain nucleotides. As shown by Leibovich and Ross,[40] macrophages induce fibroblast proliferation and collagen synthesis in healing wounds, and macrophage-dependent factors may be involved in stimulation of angiogenesis in wounds as well. Monocytes are instrumental in regulation of febrile responses through the release of endogenous pyrogens, and macrophages synthesize a variety of important compounds including complement factors C2 and C3, plasminogen activator, and prostaglandin E2 (Table 13-7).

While the predominant biologic function of the monocyte-macrophage system is phagocytosis of debris and microorganisms, an increasing number of macrophage-dependent biologic activities is being recognized.[38] It is also likely that disorders of immunity caused by monocyte dysfunction may be identified. The mononuclear phagocyte system is of crucial importance in defense against opportunistic infections, particularly in patients who are compromised by virtue of trauma, malnutrition, chronic infection, or immunosuppression.

Metabolic and Physiologic Characteristics of Monocytes and Macrophages

Energy Metabolism

The circulating blood monocyte is largely dependent on glycolytic energy metabolism, as are granulocytes. During the process of differentiation into tissue macrophages, however, mitochondria are produced and mitochondrial oxidative respiration becomes a more prominent feature of the cell. This is particularly true of pulmonary alveolar macrophages.

Like neutrophils, mononuclear cells also contain cyanide-insensitive oxidase activity, increase their respiration with phagocytosis, and generate hydrogen peroxide and superoxide anion in their oxidative burst. Variable quantities of peroxidase are present in monocytes as well, depending on the degree of differentiation and the location of the cell. In this regard, alveolar macrophages are nearly devoid of peroxidase activity. Macrophages from patients with chronic granulomatous disease are incapable of post-phagocytic augmentations in respiratory function and also have defective microbicidal activity.

Efforts to demonstrate oxygen-independent microbicidal systems in the monocyte have been less convincing than in the granulocyte. Low concentrations of cationic proteins with antimicrobial activity have been demonstrated by some investigators. In summary, the oxidative metabolic killing mechanisms of monocytes appear to resemble those found in the granulocytes, and monocytes may also possess oxygen-independent killing pathways.[35]

Migration of Monocytes and Macrophages

Both granulocytes and monocytes possess the capacity to migrate toward various chemical attractants (Fig. 13-5).

Monocytes migrate more slowly, but their movement can be sustained for rather prolonged periods. Fixed macrophages in tissues retain migratory capacity. For these reasons, granulocytes infiltrate inflammatory foci early and are followed over a period of hours to days by a gradual influx of mononuclear phagocytes.[41]

"Activation" of Macrophages

Activated macrophages are those which display increased pinocytic activity, contain increased amounts of various hydrolytic enzymes, and adhere and spread readily on glass surfaces. Respiratory function and glucose metabolism may be increased. Activated cells are capable of accelerated phagocytic activity, increased microbial killing, and enhanced cytotoxic activity against tumor cells. Under most circumstances, the activation process requires intimate participation of immune lymphoid cells,[42] and infection with facultative intracellular parasites *(Toxoplasma, Mycobacterium)* can lead to their proliferation.

The biologic significance of macrophage activation remains to be determined, and as yet no clinical disorders of macrophage activation have been recognized.

Monocyte and Macrophage Dysfunction

Relatively few monocyte function disorders have been recognized. Defects in monocyte migration have been reported in patients with mucocutaneous candidiasis, in viral infections, in major burn injury, and in some patients with malignant tumors. In patients with cancer, serum inhibitors of chemotaxis have been demonstrated. Administration of corticosteroids causes impaired migration of monocytes into areas of skin abrasion.

Impaired microbicidal capacity has been recognized in monocytes from patients with chronic granulomatous disease in whom normal postphagocytic activation of oxidative metabolism does not occur. This defect in monocytes parallels that seen in neutrophils from these patients. Mononuclear phagocytes from patients with hereditary deficiency of granule myeloperoxidase also have a microbicidal defect toward fungi. Certain patients with viral infection, lymphoma, and myelomonocytic leukemia have been shown to have impaired microbicidal activity.[35]

Finally, patients with severe malnutrition display impaired cell-mediated immunity and are often incapable of mounting delayed cutaneous hypersensitivity responses. Whether this is due to defective function of mononuclear phagocytes or of lymphoid cells remains to be determined.

Means for quantitative assessment of mononuclear phagocytic function are becoming available, and it can be anticipated that further disorders of monocyte and macrophage function will be recognized in the future.

BIBLIOGRAPHY

Moller G (ed): Role of macrophages in the immune response. Immunol Rev 40:3–255, 1978.

Weissmann G, Samuelsson B, Paoletti R (eds): Advances in Inflammation Research (vol 1). New York, Raven Press, 1979.

Weller PF, Goetzl EJ: The regulatory and effector roles of eosinophils. Adv Immunol 27:339, 1979.

REFERENCES

GRANULOCYTES

1. Mahmoud AAF, Warren KS, Grahm RC Jr: Antieosinophil serum and the kinetics of eosinophilia in *Schistosomiasis mansoni*. J Exp Med 142:560, 1975.
2. Murphy P: The Neutrophil. New York, Plenum, 1976.
3. Cline MJ: The White Cell. Cambridge, Harvard Univ. Press, 1975.
4. Walker RI, Willemze R: Neutrophil kinetics and the regulation of granulopoiesis. Rev Infect Dis 2:282, 1980.
5. Stossel TP: Phagocytosis. N Engl J Med 290:717, 774, 833, 1974.
6. Rebuck JW, Crowley JH: A method of studying leukocytic functions in vivo. Ann NY Acad Sci 59:757, 1955.
7. Gallin JI, Quie PG (eds): Leukocyte Chemotaxis: Methods, Physiology, and Clinical Implications. New York, Raven, 1978.
8. Nelson RD, Fiegel VD, Simmons RL: Chemotaxis of human polymorphonuclear neutrophils under agarose: morphological changes associated with the chemotactic response. J Immunol 117:1676, 1976.
9. Wilson DM, Ormrod DJ, Miller, TE: Role of complement in chemotaxis: study of a localized infection. Infect Immunity 29:8, 1980.
10. Nelson RD, McCormack RT, Fiegel VD, Herron M, Simmons RL, Qu'e PG: Chemotactic deactivation of human neutrophils: relation to stimulation of oxidative metabolism. Infect Immunity 23:282, 1979.
11. Wilkinson PC: Leukocyte locomotion and chemotaxis: effects of bacteria and viruses. Rev Infect Dis 3:293, 1980.
12. Hill HR, Estensen RD, Hogan NA, Quie PG: Severe staphylococcal disease associated with allergic manifestations, hyperimmunoglobulinemia E and defective neutrophil chemotaxis. J Lab Clin Med 88:796, 1976.
13. Hill HR, Warwick WJ, Dettloff J, Quie PG: Neutrophil granulocyte function in patients with pulmonary infection. J Pediatr 84:55, 1974.
14. Clark RA: Disorders of granulocyte chemotaxis. In Gallin JI, Quie PG (eds): Leukocyte Chemotaxis: Methods, Physiology, and Clinical Implications. New York, Raven, 1978, p 329.
15. Meakins JL, McLean APS, Kelly R, Bubenik O, Pietsch JB, MacLean LD: Delayed hypersensitivity and neutrophil chemotaxis: effect of trauma. J Trauma 18:240, 1978.
16. DeMeo AN, Anderson BR: Defective chemotaxis associated with a serum inhibitor in cirrhotic patients. N Engl J Med 286:735, 1972.
17. Ward PA, Berenberg JL: Defective regulation of inflammatory mediators in Hodgkin's disease: Super normal levels of chemotactic-factor inactivator. N Engl J Med 290:76, 1974.
18. Van Epps DE, Palmer DL, Williams RC: Characterization of serum inhibitors of neutrophil chemotaxis associated with anergy. J Immunol 113:189, 1974.
19. Young LS, Armstrong D: Human immunity to *Psuedomonas aeruginosa* in in vitro interaction of bacteria, polymorphonuclear leukocytes, and serum factors. J Infect Dis 126:257, 1972.
20. Johnston RB Jr, Klemperer MR, Alper CA, Rosen FS: The enhancement of bacterial phagocytosis by serum: the role of complement components and two cofactors. J Exp Med 129:1275, 1969.
21. Saba TM, DiLuzio NR: Reticuloendothelial blockade and recovery as a function of opsonic activity. Am J Physiol 216:197, 1969.

22. Saba TM: Prevention of liver reticuloendothelial systemic host-defense failure after surgery by intravenous opsonic glycoprotein therapy. Ann Surg 188:142, 1978.
23. Rosen FS, Alper CA, Janeway CA: The primary immunodeficiencies and the serum complement defects. In Nathan DG, Oski FA (eds): Hematology of Infancy and Childhood. Philadelphia, Saunders, 1974, p 529.
24. Alexander JW, Ogle CK, Stinnett JD, MacMillan BG: A sequential prospective analysis of immunological abnormalities and infection following severe thermal injury. Ann Surg 188:809, 1978.
24a. Solomkin JS, Jenkins MD, Nelson RD, Chenoweth D, Simmons RL: Neutrophil dysfunction in sepsis: II. Evidence for the role of complement activation products in cellular deactivation. Surgery 90:319, 1981.
24b. Chenoweth D, Cooper SW, Hugli TE, Stewart RW, Blackstone EH, Kirklin JW: Complement activation during cardiopulmonary bypass: evidence of generation of C3a and C5a anaphylatoxins. N Engl J Med 304:497, 1981.
25. Babior BM: Oxygen-dependent microbial killing by phagocytes. N Engl J Med 298:659, 1978.
26. Quie PG, White JG, Holmes B, Good RA: In vitro bactericidal capacity of human polymorphonuclear leukocytes: diminished activity in chronic granulomatous disease of childhood. J Clin Invest 46:668, 1967.
27. Turner RA, Schumacher HR, Meyers AR: Phagocytic function of polymorphonuclear leukocytes in rheumatic diseases. J Clin Invest 52:1632, 1973.
28. Drachman RH, Root RK, Wood WB Jr: Studies on the effect of experimental nonketotic diabetes mellitus on antibacterial defenses. I. Demonstration of a defect in phagocytosis. J Exp Med 124:227, 1966.
29. Lehrer RI, Cline MJ: Leukocyte myeloperoxidase deficiency and disseminated *Candidiasis:* the role of myeloperoxidase in resistance to *Candida* infection. J Clin Invest 48:1478, 1969.
30. McRipley RJ, Sbarra AJ: Role of the phagocyte in host-parasite interactions. XII. Hydrogen peroxide-myeloperoxidase bactericidal system in the phagocyte. J Bacteriol 94:1425, 1967.
31. Klebanoff SJ: Myeloperoxidase-halide-hydrogen peroxidase antibacterial system. J Bacteriol 95:2131, 1968.
32. Babior BM, Curnett JT, Kipnes RS: Biological defense mechanisms: evidence for the participation of superoxide in bacterial killing by xanthine oxidase. J Lab Clin Med 85:235, 1975.
32a. Elsbach P: Degradation of microorganisms by phagocytic cells. Rev Infect Dis 2:106, 1980.
33. Odeberg H, Olsson I: Antibacterial activity of cationic proteins from granulocytes. J Clin Invest 56:1118, 1975.

MONOCYTE-MACROPHAGE SYSTEM

34. Nichols BA, Bainton DF: Differentiation of human monocytes in bone marrow and blood. Sequential formation of two granule populations. Lab Invest 29:27, 1973.
35. Cline MJ, Lehrer RI, Territo MJ, Golde DW: Monocytes and macrophages: functions and diseases. Ann Intern Med 88:78, 1978.
36. van Furth R, van Waarde D, Thompson J, Gassmann AE: The regulation of the participation of mononuclear phagocytes in inflammatory responses. In Glynn LE, Schlumberger HD (eds): Bayer-Symposium VI, Experimental Models of Chronic Inflammatory Diseases. Berlin, Springer-Verlag, 1977, p 302.
37. Unanue ER, Cerottini JC: The function of macrophages in the immune response. Semin Hematol 7:225, 1970.
38. Pierce CW: Macrophages: modulators of immunity. Am J Pathol 98:10, 1980
39. Keller R: Cytostatic and cytocidal effects of activated macrophages. In Nelson DS (ed): Immunobiology of the Macrophage. New York, Academic, 1976, p 487.
40. Leibovich SJ, Ross R: The role of the macrophage in wound repair. Am J Pathol 78:71, 1975.
41. Snyderman R, Mergenhagen SE: Chemotaxis of monocytes. In Nelson DS (ed): Immunobiology of the Macrophage. New York, Academic, 1976, p 323.
42. Mackaness GB: The influence of immunologically committed lymphoid cells on macrophage activity in vivo. J Exp Med 129:973, 1969.

C. The Lymphocytes and Cell-Mediated Immunity

RICHARD L. SIMMONS

Many microbes, especially those that live within the host cell, cannot be effectively eliminated by opsonization and phagocytosis. The principal means of acquired resistance to these microbes resides in the action of specifically sensitized thymus-derived (T) lymphocytes (Table 13-1).[1] Cell-mediated immunity refers to this system even though immune cells (eg, antibody-manufacturing B cells) and nonimmune cells (eg, phagocytes of all types) participate in all aspects of host defense. Specifically sensitized T lymphocytes act in concert with many other specific and nonspecific cellular and humoral systems in performing their function.

THE IMMUNE APPARATUS

At birth, human beings are already immunologically competent and have undergone a complex developmental process. All lymphocytes are derived from a single hemopoietic stem cell, found in the extra-embryonic yoke sac, which begins to proliferate early in embryonic life. The resulting stem cells migrate to various centers of differentiation, within which progenitor cells form erythrocytes, eosinophils, basophils, neutrophils, and lymphoid cells depending on the local microchemical environment. Further proliferation of these progenitor stem cells apparently depends on the action of poietins, which tend to expand the populations of specialized cells in the way that erythropoietin acts on the erythrocyte line (Fig. 13-10).[2]

The lymphoid cell line develops as a dual system within two primary (or central) lymphoid tissues. The thymus governs the development of cellular immunity. In birds, the bursa of Fabricius governs the development of humoral immunity, but the bursa exists as a clearly defined

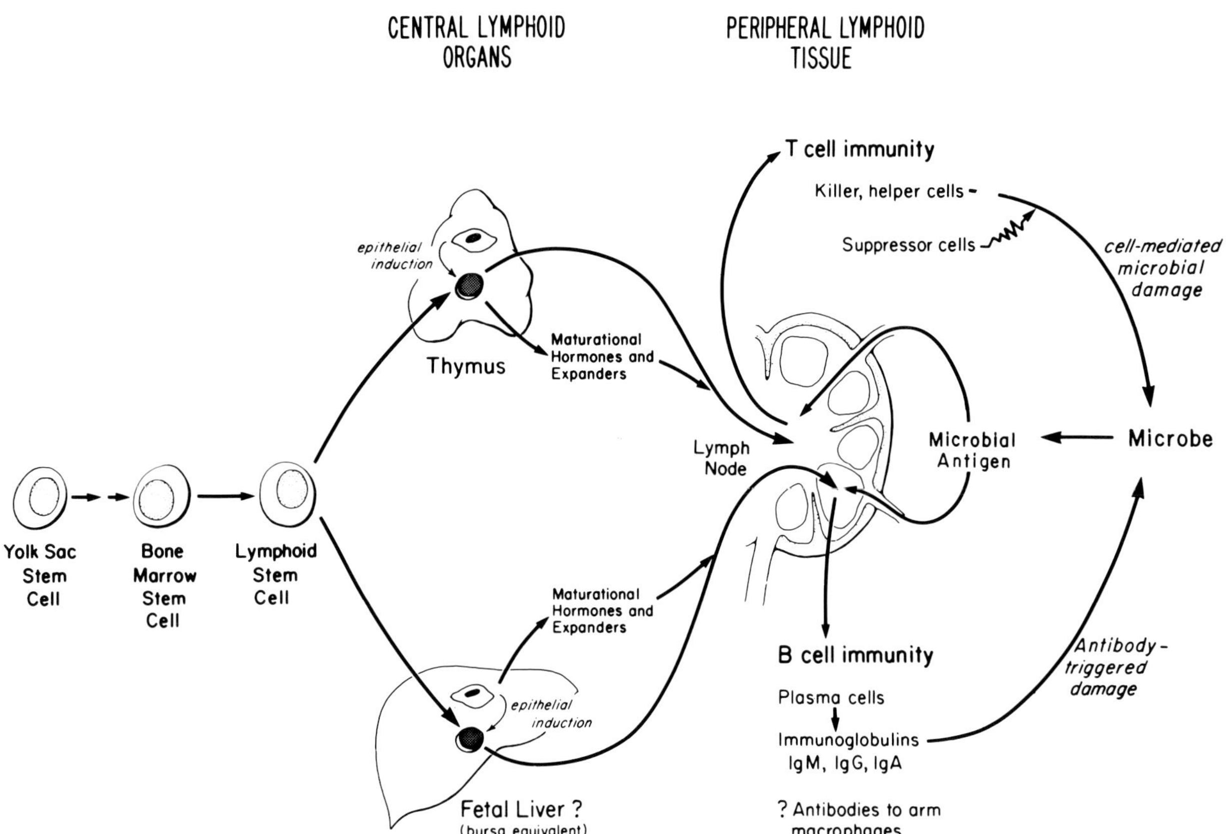

Fig. 13-10. **Summary of the extraordinarily complex developmental sequences of the immune system. Certain of the known reducers, expanders, growth factors, and sites of maturation needed to establish the T and B cell lines are presented. Much of this takes place before birth; consequently, human beings are fully competent with established peripheral lymphoid populations in the lymph nodes, Peyer patches, and spleen. (Modified from Foker JE, Simmons RL, Najarian JS: Principles of immunosuppression. In Sabiston DC Jr (ed): *Davis-Christopher Textbook of Surgery.* Philadelphia, Saunders, 1977, p 506.)**

central lymphoid structure only in birds. The equivalent of the bursa of Fabricius has not been defined in mammals, but there is evidence that it exists, perhaps within the fetal liver or within the bone marrow itself.

Both the thymus and the bursa (or its equivalent) are responsible for the further development of the peripheral lymphoid tissues, ie, spleen, lymph nodes, and Peyer patches. Certain areas of the lymph node depend on the functional presence of the thymus or bursa. The paracortical regions between the cortical germinal centers and the medulla are dependent on the thymus, while the germinal centers themselves and the medullary cord lymphoid tissue are under the developmental control of the bursal equivalent. Therefore, thymectomy early in the neonatal period results in failure of development of the paracortical regions of the lymph nodes. In chickens, bursectomy leads to failure of development of germinal centers and medullary cord lymphoid tissues.

During ontogeny, the thymus is the site of a vigorous lymphocyte proliferation, and many of these cells migrate to the paracortical areas of lymph nodes. All lymphocytes that were once dependent on the thymus for their development are called T cells. Similarly, lymphocytes developing a commitment for immunoglobulin synthesis under the influence of the bursa or its mammalian equivalent are known as B cells.

The combined function of the dual lymphoid system is the source of the body's specific immunologic response. Once the lymphocytes (T or B cells) have migrated to the peripheral lymphoid tissue, they are fully immunocompetent. It is likely that Burnet's clonal selection theory holds true, ie, a state of preparedness for a certain antigen or group of related antigens exists within the genome of each lymphoid cell so that it is only capable of responding to a narrow range of antigenic specificities.[3] Conversely, only a small percentage of the lymphocytes in the body can respond to a specific antigen. The B cells appear to be relatively sessile, but their end products, antibodies, can interact with foreign antigens at distant sites. The T cells responsible for cell-mediated immunity are more peripatetic and must migrate to the periphery in order to neutralize foreign antigens. Table 13-8 lists some distinguishing characteristics of human T and B lymphocytes.[4] In addition to the characteristics listed, there is mounting evidence that certain subpopulations of these cells carry specific marker proteins on their surfaces, which correlate with the function of the cell itself. These differentiation antigens have permitted investigators to delete certain cells from mixed populations in order to identify cells that perform certain well-defined functions (ie, cell-mediated cytotoxicity or proliferation in response to antigens).[5]

Besides the T and B cells, other populations of lympho-

TABLE 13-8. DISTINGUISHING CHARACTERISTICS OF HUMAN T AND B LYMPHOCYTES

	T lymphocytes	B lymphocytes
Maturation of precursor cells	Thymus	Fetal liver Gut-associated lymphoid tissue (?) Bone marrow (?)
Location in lymph nodes	Deep cortical region	Germinal centers and medullary cords
Electrophoretic mobility	High	Low
Forms rosettes with sheep erythrocytes	Yes	No
Surface receptor for Fc of IgG	No in most; yes for small sub-population	Yes
Surface receptor for C3b	No	Yes
Presence of surface immuno-globulin	No	Yes
Responsiveness to:		
PHA and Con-A	High	Low
Pokeweed mitogen	High	High, in presence of T lymphocytes
E. coli lipopolysaccharide	Low	High
Basis of surface specificity and capacity to combine with antigen	V region Ig on cell surface constituents	IgM or IgM and IgD, other immunoglob-ulins

Modified from Alexander WJ, Good RA (eds): Lymphocytes and their function. In *Fundamentals of Clinical Immunology.* Philadelphia, Saunders, 1977, p 20.

cytes exist. Some are called K (killer) cells, because they can participate in the lysis of target cells to which specific antibody has been bound. K cells themselves do not appear to bear receptors for the specific cellular antigens but instead carry receptors for C3b, and the Fc portion of the IgG molecule. A fourth type of cell is now called the NK (natural killer) cell. This cell may be a type of T cell, which appears to have the capacity to lyse certain foreign cells such as tumor cells or virally infected cells. Some evidence supports the idea that they may be activated by interferon and secrete interferon after activation.

EVENTS DURING THE INDUCTION OF IMMUNITY

Mature lymphocytes appear to sit in a state of immunologic readiness. The first step is the recognition of the foreign molecule to which the lymphocyte is genetically programmed to respond. This first phase of the immunologic response has been called the afferent arc. It involves the processing and recognition of the immunogens and the early phases of response.

Macrophages are absolutely necessary in order for T lymphocytes to respond to an antigen.[6] Figure 13-11 illustrates three of the possible mechanisms by which macrophages present the antigen for recognition by the lymphocyte. Most evidence supports the idea that macrophages actually bind the antigens to their cell surfaces. Only when the lymphocyte recognizes the complex produced by macrophage surface and bound antigen does it make an optimal response. Furthermore, the macrophage can release soluble mediators which influence lymphocyte responses, and recent information suggests that the macrophage can, under certain circumstances, help to regulate or modulate the extent of lymphocyte response.

RECOGNITION OF THE IMMUNOGEN BY LYMPHOCYTES

The center of the immune response lies in the reaction of the lymphocyte to the immunogen. This most certainly requires direct interaction of the lymphocyte with the antigen or its products, since the most striking aspect of the immune response is its specificity. For each unique stimulus, a distinctive population of immune cells is activated. The specificity of the immune response provides an important clue to the nature of the antigen receptors on the antigen recognition cells. The receptor sites must be at least as discriminatory as the antibody-combining sites or the cellular recognition sites on hypersensitive cells. Probably, the receptors on B lymphocytes are antibodies because immunoglobulins have been demonstrated on the cell surface. The antigen-recognizing molecule on T cells has been more difficult to demonstrate, but most evidence now supports the idea that T cells possess specific antigen

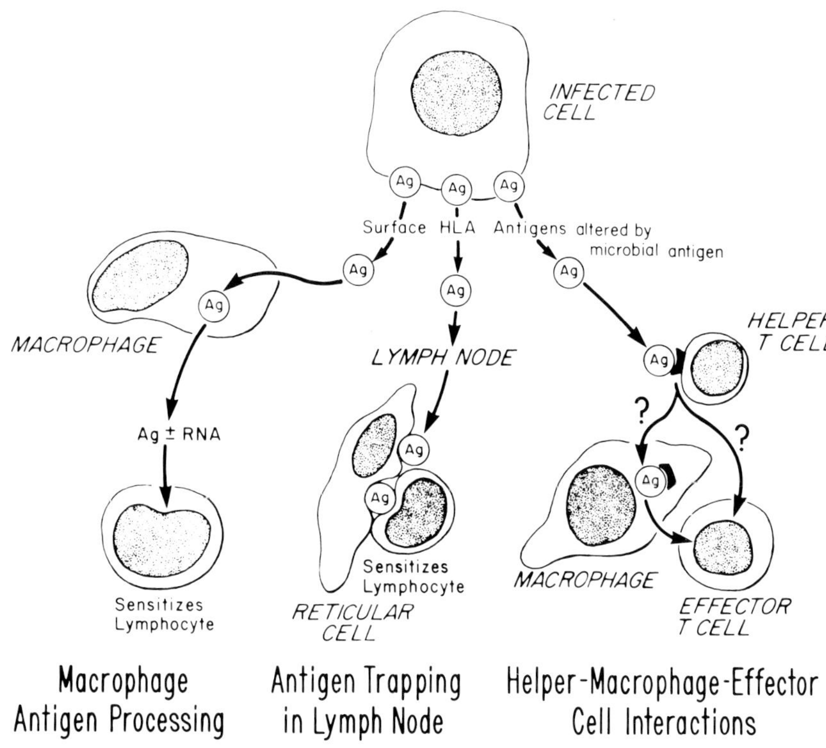

Fig. 13-11. **Three possible mechanisms of antigen processing and presentation. Macrophages may first need to process the microbial antigens and pass them in more immunogenic form to lymphocytes. The processing may or may not require the attachment of an RNA molecule. The antigen may not need to be internalized, however, and may need to be presented only on the surface of the lymph node reticular cells. This may facilitate sensitization of the lymphocytes. More recently, it has been found that maximum sensitization may require an even more complex interaction. In this scheme, the antigen is first recognized by a helper T cell, which in turn may pass it to a macrophage for processing or directly to an effector T cell to produce sensitization. Some of these helper-macrophage-effector cell studies have utilized transplantation antigens, and these conclusions may be applicable only to allograft immunity. It is clear, however, from the extensive experimental data that the cell–cell interactions involved are complex and not yet understood. (Modified from Simmons RL, Foker JE, Lower RR, Najarian JS: Transplantation. In Schwartz SI, Shires GT, Spencer FC, Storer EH (eds): *Principles of Surgery* (3rd ed). New York, McGraw-Hill, 1979, pp 383–473.)**

receptors similar to the variable portion of the heavy chain of the immunoglobulin molecule (see Section D). Antibodies to these sites (anti-idiotypes) interfere with immune responses.

How recognition molecules on either T or B cells are induced during lymphocyte development is unknown. Burnet's clonal selection theory proposes that clones of lymphocytes specifically reactive to an antigen arise, probably by somatic mutation, before any actual experience with the antigen itself.[3] Thus, the lymphocytes are precommitted and equipped with recognition molecules to the antigen before the initial encounter with it. An alternative, and currently less favored, theory would have an instructional role for the antigen in the first exposure with the individual's lymphocytes, with the recognition sites and sensitivity resulting from the exposure.

CELLULAR INTERACTIONS IN THE AFFERENT ARC

When lymphocytes encounter appropriate foreign antigens, the clones of cells precoded to these antigens respond in two essential ways—proliferation and differentiation. Thus, there is an increase in the numbers of specifically sensitized cells, either actively manufacturing antibody (B cells or the end cell of the B cell line-plasma cells) or being capable of interacting directly with the foreign antigen (T cells). The lymphocytes, however, do not act individually in any immunologic response. A great deal of cellular cooperation is required, and such cooperation is not confined to the enlistment of immunologically nonspecific cells such as macrophages, neutrophils, and platelets into the inflammatory response. Extensive lymphocyte-lymphocyte interaction is needed for the development of maximum lymphocyte proliferative activity and the differentiation of the cells into mature effector T cells or antibody-producing B cells. The cooperation occurs both between subpopulations of T cells and between T and B cells.

The requirement for cooperation between T and B cells was established by showing that neither cell population alone could mount an immune response to certain antigens, whereas mixtures of the two cell types resulted in the production of high levels of antibody.[7] Because B cells are the precursors of antibody-forming cells, and T cells do not synthesize readily detectable amounts of immunoglobulin, the T cells must serve as "helper cells," which assist B cells to differentiate into producers of antibody. Response to most antigens requires this cooperation, and a suspension of B cells alone or lymphocytes from athymic mice in tissue culture will not effectively produce antibodies to these antigens unless T cells are added. Therefore, T-cell recognition of at least a portion of the antigen is necessary for the production of specific antibody by the B cell. Not all T cells can function in this role, only the subgroup of helper T cells (T_H). Production of IgG, IgE, and probably IgA also seems to require aid from T_H cells for full efficiency.

Although T_H cells are also needed for the development of cell-mediated immunity, a second subpopulation of lymphocytes (T_E cells) act as effectors in these responses. The T_H cell is required for the T_E cell to fully develop the capacity to inflict cell damage. Obligate intracellular pathogens such as viruses are prominent among the antigens that require T_H-T_E cell cooperation for induction of effective immunity.

LYMPHOCYTE DIFFERENTIATION AND PROLIFERATION

Both lymphocyte proliferation and differentiation result from the activation of lymphocyte clones by appropriate immunogens. Although it is not clear whether or not a cell must proliferate in order to differentiate further, lymphoid differentiation to antibody-producing cells is usually accompanied by cellular proliferation. When the B cell proliferates, morphologic differentiation accompanies the proliferation, and the end result is a plasma cell busily engaged in making specific antibody.

Activation of T cells by appropriate antigens most often stimulates the transformation of these cells into lymphoblasts with accompanying DNA synthesis and subsequent mitosis. The T cell that proliferates most is the helper T cell (T_H), which recognizes the antigen but develops little capacity to eliminate it. The cell that differentiates and acquires the capability to inflict cytotoxic damage, the effector T cell (T_E), undergoes relatively little proliferation. This has been best shown in mice, where the proliferating but noncytotoxic T_H cells bear one differentiation antigen (Lyt 1) on their surface, and the destructive but nondividing T_E cells have different (Lyt 2) membrane markers.[8]

An analogous system almost certainly exists for human lymphocytes.[8a] Not only do the two cell types respond differently, but different antigenic configurations can sometimes be shown to stimulate the T_H and T_E cells to different degrees. For example, the antigens governed by the A and B subloci of the HLA major histocompatibility complex induce cytotoxicity, while the D antigens promote proliferation. The proliferation of the T_H cells appears to be an important mechanism by which the immune response is amplified. The susceptibility to intracellular pathogens of persons treated with drugs that interfere with cell proliferation may reside in this mechanism.

CELLULAR REGULATION OF THE IMMUNE RESPONSE

There is evidence that yet another T cell subpopulation can inhibit either the development of antibody-producing B cells or the generation of T_E cells by interacting directly or indirectly with T_H cells. These regulatory lymphocytes have been called suppressor T (T_S) cells.[7]

Much current information suggests that the interaction of certain precursor T cells with antigen induces a dual response in other lymphocyte subpopulations.[9] On the one hand, T_H cells cooperate with T_E cells and B cells to eliminate the antigen. On the other, feedback circuits are set up among cooperating T_S cells, which limit the immune response. Thus, immune reactions are regulated by messages passed among different types of immunologic cells.[9,9a]

EXPRESSION OF IMMUNITY: MICROBIAL DESTRUCTION

The stimulation by antigens of sensitized cells or antibodies marks the beginning of the active disposal of the foreign microbe. The role of antibodies after their production by B cells will be discussed in Section D of this chapter. They are of primary importance in the elimination of encapsulated bacteria, bacterial toxins, and many viruses. Cell-mediated immunity is most important in the response to the pathogens listed in Table 13-1.

TABLE 13-9. PRIMARY T-CELL IMMUNODEFICIENCIES

Hematopoietic hypoplasia (reticular dysgenesis)
Thymic hypoplasia (DiGeorge syndrome)
Severe combined immunodeficiency
Immunodeficiency with enzyme deficiency
Combined immunodeficiency presenting as the Letterer-Siwe syndrome
Short-limbed dwarfism with immunodeficiency and cartilage-hair hypoplasia
Immunodeficiency with thrombocytopenia and eczema
Immunodeficiency with ataxia-telangiectasia
Chronic mucocutaneous candidiasis
Immunodeficiency with thymoma
Episodic lymphopenia with lymphocytotoxin

Adapted from Stiehm ER: Immunodeficiency disorders: general considerations. In Stiehm ER, Fulginiti VA (eds): *Immunologic Disorders in Infants and Children.* Philadelphia, Saunders, 1973, p 145.

ROLE OF SPECIFICALLY IMMUNIZED LYMPHOCYTES IN MICROBIAL HOST DEFENSE

The efferent limb in lymphocyte-mediated immunity has both an immunologically specific (recognition) phase and an immunologically nonspecific (effector or amplification) phase. The recognition phase occurs when the sensitized T_E cell engages the antigen; the second phase of antigen elimination is more complex.

One method of antigen elimination is direct cell mediated cytotoxicity. Specifically sensitized T_E cells are capable of killing virally infected cells, and the mechanism has been much studied.[10] Direct contact between the sensitized lymphocyte and the target cell appears to be important. The ameboid lymphocyte contacts the target cells with its uropod and remains attached for 10 minutes. The lymphocyte then moves off, and 10 to 20 minutes later the target cells lyse. The mechanism of cell membrane damage has not been identified, although most evidence favors the idea that interaction of cell surfaces is important in directly damaging the target cell. Soluble cytotoxic factors that have been found during lysis appear to play little role.

The antigens recognized by T cells on the surfaces of virus-infected target cells are specific, not only for the virus but also for the major histocompatibility antigen systems of the host itself.[10] In fact, immune T cells from certain animals recognize and kill virus infected target cells only if donors of the killer cells and target cells share the major histocompatibility antigen system. The viral antigen is thought to alter or interact with self-antigen on the cell surface, and only then provide a target which immune T_E cells can recognize.

Although specifically sensitized cytotoxic T cells can kill cells infected with intracellular pathogens (viruses, bacteria), it is unlikely that this is the major method of control.

In order to halt virus replication and spread, lysis of target cells would be necessary before assembly of virus within them. Thus, recognizable viral-induced changes in the infected cell membranes would have to occur early after infection. With some viruses this does happen. Ectromelia (mousepox) infected L cells, for example, become susceptible to immune T cell destruction about 3 hours after infection. Similarly, vaccinia virus may not reproduce in the early hours after infection.[1] Most viruses, however, do not conform to this scenario. In addition, the mechanism is inefficient and requires more specifically sensitized cells at the site of inflammation than can be shown to be present. Furthermore, lysis of host cells will release more virus. Finally, cells infected with bacteria do not display bacterial antigens on their cell surface.

A more popular postulate is that a small number of specifically sensitized T_H or T_E cells recognize the antigen, interact with it, and thereby trigger the influx and activation of nonsensitized mononuclear cells, which truly eliminate the antigen.

EFFECTOR MOLECULES (LYMPHOKINES) RELEASED BY SENSITIZED LYMPHOCYTES ENCOUNTERING ANTIGEN

The release of cytotoxic factors by lymphocytes infiltrating a site of infection would be the most direct way to damage infected cells, but probably not the most efficient since nonspecific cell killing would result. Several other kinds of molecules are released by specifically sensitized T cells which encounter an immunogen, and these products (lymphokines) serve to activate and enlist macrophages, polymorphonuclear leukocytes (PMNs), lymphocytes, etc., and thus amplify the initial cellular response.[11] Several lymphokines have been identified, but it is not yet clear whether there is a small number of molecules with multiple functions or whether a different molecule is specific for each function. Some of the best-studied lymphokines are depicted in Figure 13-12.

A host of activities has been ascribed to the lymphokines.[11] Neutrophils, basophils, and eosinophils are attracted by them. Growth inhibitory and cytotoxic activities against target cells have been described in vitro. Several lymphokines affect lymphocytes themselves and can be shown under suitable experimental conditions to stimulate mitosis and increase antibody production. Transformed lymphocytes also release a vascular permeability factor in addition to the cytotoxic lymphokines. Little is known about the permeability factor(s) and its possible effect on an inflammatory reaction. Tissue edema is, however, a prominent feature of delayed hypersensitivity reactions, and it may act in concert with the vascular permeability factors released by complement activation and neutrophil and platelet participation in the efferent arc of microbial elimination.

THE SENSITIZED LYMPHOCYTE AND THE ACTIVATED MACROPHAGE

Macrophages seem to be very active participants in cell-mediated reactions to certain microbes; their role does not end with antigen processing. Two of the most investigated lymphokines, migration inhibitory factor (MIF) and chemotactic factor (CF), have similar properties and may be the same molecule. By attracting macrophages and then inhibiting their escape, the CF and MIF activities released by lymphocytes recruit increased numbers of macrophages to the area.

Another lymphokine, macrophage activating factor (MAF), has also been described. Macrophages resemble lymphocytes in that they have resting and activated states. In the activated phase, macrophage cytoplasm has the appearance of great activity both morphologically and enzymatically. Phagocytosis, pinocytosis, as well as bacteriostatic and tumoricidal activities are increased. Many enzymes, including the digestive enzymes found in lysosomes, are elevated. Macrophages found at the site of delayed hypersensitivity reactions appear to be in the

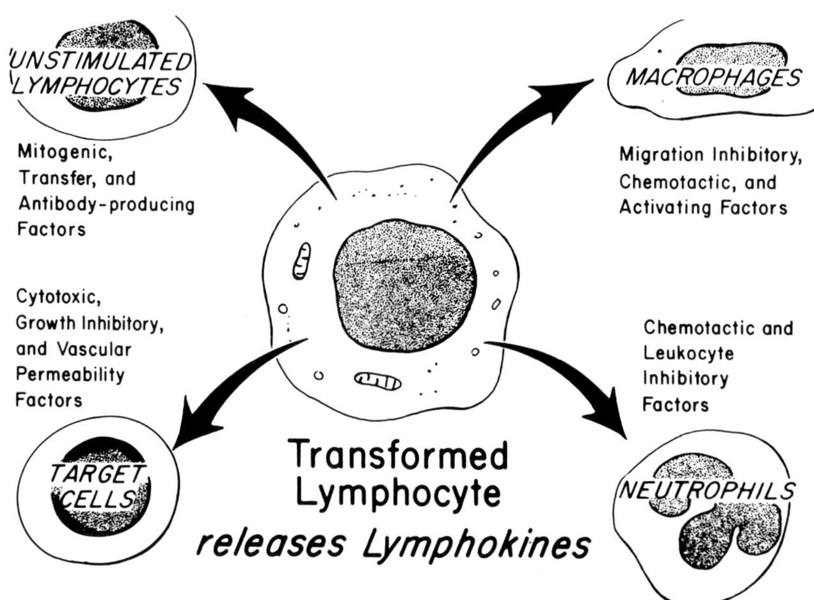

Fig. 13-12. Activated (transformed) lymphocytes give off a variety of biologically active molecules (lymphokines). A number of properties have been ascribed to these lymphokines from cell culture experiments. These activities have obvious importance to host defenses. Chemotactic and migration inhibitory activity for macrophages and neutrophils, activating factors for lymphocytes, cytotoxicity for target cells, and vascular permeability factors all contribute to the inflammatory process. (From Simmons RL, Foker JE, Lower RR, Najarian JS: Transplantation. In Schwartz SI, Shires GT, Spencer FC, Storer EH (eds): *Principles of Surgery* (3rd ed). New York, McGraw-Hill, 1979, pp 383–473.)

activated state. The most important difference between a resting and an activated macrophage in terms of resistance to infection is the greatly increased capacity of the activated cell to inhibit or kill intracellular pathogens. This capacity is nonspecific: thus, macrophages activated in the course of infection due to one pathogen can inhibit or kill unrelated intracellular pathogens.[12] Macrophages activated by different means, however, may have different functional capacities. For example, certain populations of activated macrophages are capable of inhibiting tumor cells but lack the capacity to kill intracellular pathogens. Furthermore, the biochemical mechanism by which macrophages acquire increased microbicidal activity under the influence of the T_E cells is not yet clear; the halide-myeloperoxidase-H_2O_2 system probably plays a role.

The presence of activated macrophages appears to be the most important factor in resistance to many infectious agents. But the heterogeneity of the immune response against microbial infections is almost axiomatic, and it is impossible to attribute a single mechanism of resistance to any one immunologic response. For example, with certain worms both antibody-mediated damage and cell-mediated expulsion of the damaged worms are necessary.

CELL-MEDIATED IMMUNITY AND GRANULOMATOUS INFLAMMATIONS

Granulomatous inflammations are chronic, predominantly mononuclear host reactions to persisting, poorly degradable tissue irritants. The type, intensity, duration, and resolution of the granulomatous inflammations depends on the physical characteristics, chemical reactivity, and biologic activity of the irritant as well as the ensuing host response.[12] The hypersensitivity granulomas, ie, those seen most commonly in granulomatous infections, are evoked by slowly released antigens, which induce cellular immunity. Early in the lesion, microbial products or tissue and plasma-derived chemical mediators may participate in cell recruitment and mobilization; however, in the subsequent phase, locally secreted lymphokines mobilize, attract, and activate the various cellular components (neutrophils, macrophages, fibroblasts, T and B lymphocytes, plasma cells, eosinophils, and basophils). The ultimate result of the cell activation is the removal, containment, and eventual elimination of antigens, antigen-antibody complexes, and replicating invaders from the tissues. Such granulomatous inflammations, therefore, are not an exaggerated host reaction but a defensive mechanism for aggregating lymphokine-activated macrophages at the site of invasion by organisms not normally destroyed by opsonization and phagocytosis. Such organisms, if unchecked, tend to cause an insidiously developing chronic disease, with parasitism of the mononuclear phagocytic system and miliary spread.[12]

Though the granulomatous reaction is essentially a beneficial tissue response against noxious irritants, the exaggerated prolonged inflammations and the inadvertent release of lysosomal enzymes can cause considerable tissue destruction, liquefaction, and severe organ derangement. Fibrotic tissue repair may often aggravate the disease to the point of becoming the major cause of pathology, as seen in schistosomiasis and the pneumonitides. Thus, whereas the granulomatous response is highly protective against replicating invaders, when it is formed in response to inanimate or noninvasive agents such as schistosome eggs, it may be more detrimental than helpful. In any case, the key element in any granulomatous response seems to be the extent and degree of macrophage activation. Minimal or moderate activation will result in a quiescent lesion with minor or negligible tissue destruction and reparative fibrosis. Conversely, high levels of macrophage activation, whether induced by inanimate silica or live tubercle bacilli, will result in lysosomal enzyme-mediated tissue damage and detrimental reparative fibrosis.[13]

CELL-MEDIATED IMMUNITY ON MUCOSAL SURFACES

Until recently cell-mediated immunity on secretory surfaces has not been recognized.[14] Although it seems to function at least partially independently of systemic cell-mediated immunity, research has been hampered by difficulty in obtaining cells in sufficient quantity from secretions. The first convincing evidence that local cell-mediated immunity could be correlated with protection in vivo came with the work of Yamamoto et al,[15] who demonstrated that protection against tuberculosis in immunized mice correlated best with lung cell immunity rather than peritoneal cellular immunity. Later, Henney and Waldman [16] demonstrated cell-mediated immunity in the respiratory tract lymphocytes to dinitrophenylated human IgG. This cell-mediated immunity appears to be mediated by T cells, and immunization to enhance the effects of local cellular immunity can be induced with various aerosol immunizing agents. Local cellular immunity may be relatively short-lived compared with antibody responses and may wane after several weeks. All known subpopulations of T lymphocytes are present in Peyer patches, and lymphocytes removed from such gut-associated lymphoid tissue (GALT) respond appropriately in vitro.[14]

Cell-mediated immunity associated with mucosal surfaces can exert a protective action in a variety of ways, ie, the production of lymphokines, the activation of local (eg, alveolar) macrophages, as well as direct cytotoxic function against intracellular organisms. This research is in its embryonic phases.

OTHER MECHANISMS OF CELLULAR IMMUNITY AGAINST INTRACELLULAR MICROBES

Recruitment of Specifically Sensitized Cells

It is possible that the specifically immune T_E cell, upon encountering the antigen that elicited its maturation, can recruit specifically sensitized cells from unsensitized lymphocytes in their environment. Recruitment of lymphocytes producing cellular hypersensitivity may be accomplished in several ways. A recognition molecule manufactured and released by the specifically sensitized cell could be attached to the cell surfaces of adjacent cells. Such factors would quickly convert lymphoid cells into specific cells, which on encountering the antigen could transform and become metabolically active. The impressment of the cells in this manner would allow quick amplification of the number of sensitized cells.

One recognition molecule that could be transferred from lymphocyte to lymphocyte could be specific antibody, but it has not yet been established that cytophilic antibody can enlarge the lymphocyte population specifically sensitized to a microbial antigen.

A second recognition molecule that may expand the sensitized cell population is the transfer factor described by Lawrence.[17] Transfer factor is dialyzable material of less than 10,000 molecular weight, which can be extracted from specifically sensitized lymphocytes and will convert previously unsensitized lymphocytes to a specific antigen-responsive state both in vitro and in vivo. When the converted lymphocytes are subsequently exposed to the specific antigen, they will transform and proliferate. Transfer factor itself appears not to be an immunoglobulin but has a polypeptide-polynucleotide composition, although it is resistant to pancreatic ribonuclease (RNase). Transfer factor may act as a transmitter of immunologic information. Much controversy revolves around its presence and nature, however, and some writers regard it as transferred antigen or question its importance in the control of infection.

Another potential mechanism for recruitment of specifically sensitized cells would be by transfer of the information needed to produce a recognition molecule. In addition to the possible role of RNA in the transfer of processed antigenic information from macrophage to lymphocyte, RNA from sensitized cells may enlist other lymphocytes into specific immunity. Mannick and Egdahl [18] found that RNA from the nodes of rabbits immunized to skin allografts conferred the capacity to produce transfer reactions on normal lymphoid cells when they were injected into the skin of the graft donor. In later experiments, they demonstrated that rabbit spleen cells exposed in vitro to RNA extracted from the lymph nodes of immune rabbits would sensitize isogenic rabbits to subsequent grafts from the skin donor. These RNA extracts would confer sensitivity to the immunizing antigen on lymph node cells as measured by the ability to inhibit the migration of macrophages or the production of delayed skin hypersensitivity. The obvious conclusion has been that the transfer and incorporation of a messenger RNA (mRNA) will establish immunity in lymphoid cells. Although these experiments suggest such a conclusion, more understanding of the development of immunity at the molecular level will be needed before it can be established. In addition, it has not been shown that the RNA comes from lymphocytes. The RNA could be from macrophages.

The recruitment, or horizontal expansion, of sensitized cells is an appealing concept, and certain evidence suggests it may be true; however, it has not been established for immunity in general, and its role in microbial elimination is unknown.

Antibody-Dependent Cellular Cytotoxicity and NK Cells

A previous discussion made mention of subpopulations of lymphocytes capable of cellular lysis. K cells can lyse cells to which antibody is bound. NK cells can lyse certain tumor cells and virally infected cells. Their role in effective cell-mediated immunity to pathogenic microbes is unknown.[4]

EVALUATION OF DEFICIENCIES IN CELL-MEDIATED IMMUNITY

Deficient cell-mediated immunity has been identified in a number of clinical conditions. The primary T cell deficiencies—some congenital, some idiopathic—are noted in Table 13-9. Table 13-10 lists some of the diseases that have been characterized as secondary T cell deficiency states, using one or more of the clinical tests described below.[19]

Individuals susceptible to viral, protozoal or intracellular bacterial infections should be studied for defects in cell-mediated immunity.[19] Screening tests should include total peripheral blood lymphocyte counts and evaluation of lymphocyte morphology. A roentgenogram of the chest (PA and lateral) should show a thymic shadow; its absence suggests thymic hypoplasia. A right-sided aortic arch is often seen in congenital thymic hypoplasia.

Recall Skin Tests. Delayed skin tests can evaluate cellular immunity to microbial agents or vaccine antigens. Antigens specific for mumps, trichophyton, purified protein derivative (PPD), *C. albicans* (dermatophytin), tetanus toxoid, and streptokinase-streptodornase (SK:SD) are injected intradermally and the induration measured at 24 and 48 hours (Table 13-11). Traditionally, erythema alone is not a good indication of reactivity. All adults and children over age 10 should be positive to one or more antigens, but even normal infants will not respond.

DNCB Sensitization. Active sensitization with 2,4-dinitrochlorobenzene (DNCB) can also be used to assess cellular immunity. Since unpleasant burns and scars may occur during sensitization, this procedure is recommended only in unusual circumstances in infants or children. Stiehm [20] recommends a vesicant dose of DNCB, 0.05 ml of a 10 percent solution in acetone (30 percent in adults), applied to the volar surface of the forearm on filter paper 1 cm in diameter. A test dose (0.05 ml of 0.1 percent solution of DNCB in acetone) is applied at the same time as a presensitization control. The filter papers are removed after 24 hours; the control is read at 48 hours after application for erythema, induration, and vesiculation. Patients are challenged 14 to 21 days later with the test dose. The filter paper (1 cm in diameter) is applied to a different area and kept in place for 24 hours; the reaction is read 48 hours after application. Skin reactions are graded: (0) no reaction, (+) erythema only, (++) erythema and induration, (+++) vesiculation, (++++) bullae and ulceration. Only (++) or greater reactions are accepted as evidence of sensitization. Repeat testing is indicated if the initial test is negative. A positive test is seen in 95 percent of normal subjects.

T Cell Enumeration. The first advanced test, requiring a special laboratory, is estimation of the number of T lymphocytes in the peripheral blood.[21] For reasons not yet understood, T cells have a surface receptor for sheep erythrocytes. Mononuclear cell preparations from periph-

TABLE 13-10. SECONDARY T CELL IMMUNODEFICIENCY STATES

Disorder	T cell defects
Infection	
Rubella (congenital)	May have decreased T cells, PHA, MLC
Measles	Transient suppression of delayed hypersensitivity; decreased PHA
Leprosy	Decreased delayed hypersensitivity; decreased response to *M. leprae;* decreased PHA, T cells
Tuberculosis	Decreased delayed hypersensitivity; decreased T cells; decreased MIF
Coccidioidomycosis	Decreased delayed hypersensitivity; lymphocyte blastogenesis, MIF to coccal antigen
Acute viral infection	Lymphopenia; decreased T cells, decreased PHA in some
Congenital cytomegalovirus	Specific unresponsiveness to cytomegalovirus
Malignancy	
Hodgkin disease	Suppression of delayed hypersensitivity; decreased PHA; serum factors suppress T cells
Acute leukemia	Decreased delayed hypersensitivity; decreased PHA
Chronic leukemia	Serum factors inhibit PHA
Nonlymphoid	Variable decrease in delayed hypersensitivity; suppression of PHA, MLC, T cells; immunosuppressive factors present
Myeloma	Increased suppressor T cells (macrophages ?)
Autoimmune disease	
Systemic lupus erythematosus	Decreased delayed hypersensitivity; decreased T cells, PHA, MLC; decreased suppressor cells in animal models and in humans
Rheumatoid arthritis	Decreased delayed hypersensitivity; decreased PHA, MLC
Chronic active hepatitis	Decreased delayed hypersensitivity; decreased lymphocyte cytotoxicity, decreased T cells; mitogen response normal to decreased
Protein-losing states	
Protein-losing enteropathy	Decreased delayed hypersensitivity; decreased T cells, PHA, MLC
Other disorders	
Diabetes	Decreased PHA, MLC normal
Alcoholic cirrhosis	Decreased PHA
Malnutrition	Lymphopenia; decreased T cells; decreased delayed hypersensitivity
Burns	Decreased delayed hypersensitivity; lymphopenia
Sarcoidosis	Decreased delayed hypersensitivity; decreased PHA; inhibitory plasma factor
Uremia	Decreased delayed hypersensitivity; serum blocking factors suppress PHA, MLC
Aging	Decreased delayed hypersensitivity; decreased mitogen response, decreased T cells
Subacute sclerosing panencephalitis	Specific unresponsiveness to measles antigen; blocking factor present in some

PHA = phytohemagglutinin stimulation of lymphocytes
MLC = allogeneic cell stimulation of lymphocyte

Adapted from Ammann AJ, Fundenberg HH: Immunodeficiency diseases. In Fundenberg HH, Stites DP, Caldwell JL, Wells JV: *Basic and Clinical Immunology, (3rd ed).* Los Altos, Lange Publications, 1980, pp 409–441.

eral blood are incubated with sheep cells first at 37C and then at 0C, spread on a slide and examined by light microscopy. About 55 to 75 percent of peripheral lymphocytes will form rosettes (E rosettes). Alternate methods give a lower percentage of T cells and are sometimes termed "active" rosettes. This may measure a subpopulation of T cells, possibly effector T lymphocytes. Antisera specific for T lymphocytes can be used in immunofluorescence or in cytotoxicity assays to identify T cells.[20]

Patients with T cell defects (eg, severe combined immunodeficiency) have few (<15 percent) T cells, a peripheral lymphopenia, and a very low absolute number of T cells. Patients with partial T cell defects (eg, Wiskott–Aldrich syndrome, DiGeorge syndrome) have moderately depressed T cell numbers (15 to 40 percent). Patients with secondary cellular immunodeficiency (eg, malnutrition, viral disease) have depression of T cells in proportion to the severity of the cellular immune defect.

A depression of E-rosetting T cells is said to be the most sensitive index of a subtle T cell defect, but some patients with profound T cell defects have normal numbers of E-rosetting cells.

Lymphocyte Proliferation. Cellular immunity can be evaluated by determining the ability of the patient's lymphocytes to proliferate in vitro under the influence of antigens, allogeneic cells, or mitotic agents such as phytohemagglutinin or pokeweed. Mitogens activate lymphocytes nonspecifically via receptors on the cell membrane. Lymphocyte reactivity can best be assayed by measuring the incorporation of radioactive thymidine into dividing cells. The absolute count and the ratio of counts to the unstimulated control, the stimulation index, is recorded.

The ability to respond to specific antigens can be determined by substituting allogeneic lymphocytes (from another person) for the mitogen. Allogeneic lymphocytes are treated with mitomycin or x-irradiation so they cannot react to the cells being tested in the mixed leukocyte culture (MLC). Every normal individual will react to histocompatibility antigens that he or she lacks, even without prior sensitization (a positive MLC).

Serum factors may influence the proliferative lymphocyte response to mitogens or antigens. Specific or nonspecific inhibitors have been reported. Specific inhibitors are usually antibody to the antigen. Nonspecific inhibitors may be antibodies directed against lymphocytes or poorly characterized nonimmunoglobulin substances. These are seen in uremia, certain malignancies, leprosy, hepatitis, and ataxia-telangiectasia (Tables 13-9, 13-10).

Lymphocyte Mediator Assays (Lymphokines). Assays for lymphokines can be used to assess lymphocyte effector function. Macrophage migration inhibition factor (MIF) is assayed by incubating sensitized lymphocytes with antigen for 3 to 5 days and assessing the concentrated supernatant for its ability to inhibit the migration of guinea pig peritoneal cells from a capillary tube.

Lymph Node Biopsy. The morphologic appearance of a biopsied lymph node also provides information about the cellular immune system. Deficiencies of lymphocytes in the thymic-dependent deep cortical region, histiocytic infiltration, and cellular disorganization are noted in cellular immunodeficiencies. A lymph node biopsy is unnecessary if there is unequivocal laboratory evidence of cellular immunodeficiency. There is some risk of infection from the procedure in severe immunodeficiency states.

Enzyme Assays for Adenosine Deaminase and Nucleoside Phosphorylase. Patients with combined immunodeficiency should have assays for adenosine deaminase (ADA) and nucleoside phosphorylase in lysed erythrocytes, since absence of either of these enzymes identifies genetic variants of autosomal recessive combined immunodeficiency.[22,23]

Thymic Hormone Assays. Circulating thymic hormone is absent or very depressed in combined immunodeficiency and DiGeorge syndrome, and for atypical patients in which these diagnoses are being considered, assay of thymic activity may be of diagnostic value. Serial assays may also be of use in following response to reconstitution

TABLE 13-11. COMMON SKIN TESTS *

	Initial Strength	Second Strength	Third Strength
PPD	1:10,000	1:1,000	1:100
Trichophyton	1:1,000	—	1:10
Candida	1:1,000	1:100	1:10
SK:SD	50 μ:12.5 μ/ml	400 μ:100 μ/ml	1,000 μ:200 μ/ml
Normal Response:	5 mm or more of induration at 24 or 48 hours Anergy (A): no response (0/5) Relative anergy (RA): single response (1/5) Normal (N): two or more responses (2^+/5)		

* 0.1 ml intradermally. Mumps antigen is also sometimes used.

From Stiehm ER: Immunodeficiency disorders: general considerations. In Stiehm ER, Fulginiti VA (eds): *Immunologic Disorders in Infants and Children,* Philadelphia, Saunders, 1973, p 145.

or other therapies. Two assays for thymic hormone have been described, both utilizing spleen cells of thymectomized or nude mice.[24,25]

BIBLIOGRAPHY

Cohen S, Pick E, Oppenheim JJ (eds): Biology of the Lymphokines. New York, Academic Press, 1979.

Fudenberg HH, Stites DP, Caldwell JL, Wells JV (eds): Basic and Clinical Immunology (3rd ed). Los Altos, Lange Medical Publications, 1980.

REFERENCES

1. Wing EJ, Remington JS: Lymphocytes and macrophages in cell-mediated immunology. In Mandell GL, Douglas RG Jr, Bennett JE (eds): Principles and Practice of Infectious Diseases, Vol 1. New York, Wiley, 1979, p 83.
2. Simmons RL, Foker JE, Lower RR, Najarian JS: Transplantation. In Schwartz SI, Shires GT, Spencer FC, Storer EH (eds): Principles of Surgery. New York, McGraw-Hill, 1979, p 383.
3. Burnet FM, Fenner F: Genetics and immunology. Heredity (Lond) 2:289, 1948.
4. Alexander WJ, Good RA (eds): Lymphocytes and their function. In Fundamentals of Clinical Immunology. Philadelphia, Saunders, 1977, p 20.
5. Douglas, SD: Cells involved in immune responses. In Fudenberg HH, Stites DP, Caldwell JL, Wells JV (eds): Basic and Clinical Immunology (3rd ed). Los Altos, Lange Medical Publications, 1980, p. 96.
6. Pierce CW: Macrophages: modulators of immunity. Am J Pathol 98:10, 1980.
7. Tada T, Okumura K: The role of antigen-specific T cell factors in the immune response. Adv Immunol 28:1, 1979.
8. Cantor H, Boyse EA: Functional subclasses of T lymphocytes bearing different Ly antigens. I. The generation of functionally distinct T cell subclasses is a differentiative process independent of antigen. J Exp Med 141:1376, 1975.

8a. Chess L, Schlossman SF: Human lymphocyte subpopulations. Adv Immunol 25:213, 1977.

9. Cantor H, Gershon RF: Immunological circuits: cellular composition. Fed Proc 39:2058, 1979.

9a. Katz DH: Adaptive differentiation of lymphocytes: theoretical implications for mechanisms of cell–cell recognition and regulation of immune responses. Adv Immunol 29:137, 1980.

10. Zinkernagel RM, Doherty PC: MHC-restricted cytotoxic T cells: studies on the biological role of polymorphic major transplantation antigens determining T-cells restriction-specificity, function and responsiveness. Adv Immunol 27:52, 1979.
11. Rocklin RE, Bendtzen K, Greineder D: Mediators of immunity: lymphokines and monokines. Adv Immunol 29:55, 1980.
12. Boros DL: Granulomatous inflammations. Prog Allergy 24:183, 1978.
13. Blanden RV, Hapel AJ, Doherty PC, Zinkernagel RM: Lymphocyte-macrophage interactions and macrophage activation in the expression of antimicrobial immunity in vivo. In Nelson DS (ed): Immunobiology of the Macrophage. New York, Academic, 1976, p 367.
14. Ganguly R, Waldman RH: Local immunity and local immune responses. Prog Allergy 27:1, 1980.
15. Yamamoto K, Anacker RL, Ribi E: Macrophage migration inhibition studies with cells from mice vaccinated with cell walls of *Mycobacterium bovis* BCG: relationship between inhibitory activity of lung cells and resistance to airborne challenge with *Mycobacterium tuberculosis,* H37Rv. Infect Immun 1:595, 1970.
16. Henney CS, Waldman RH: Cell-mediated immunity shown by lymphocytes from the respiratory tract. Science 169:696, 1970.
17. Lawrence HS: Transfer factor. In Dixon FJ Jr, Kunkel HG (eds): Advances in Immunology, Vol II. New York, Academic, 1969, p 195.
18. Mannick JA, Egdahl RH: Transformation of nonimmune lymph node cells to state of transplantation immunity by RNA. A preliminary report. Ann Surg 156:356, 1962.
19. Fudenberg H: Basic and Clinical Immunology (3rd ed). Los Altos, Lange Medical Publications, 1980.
20. Stiehm ER: Immunodeficiency disorders: general considerations. In Stiehm ER, Fulginiti VA (eds): Immunologic Disorders in Infants and Children, 2nd ed. Philadephia, Saunders, 1980, in press.
21. Strober S, Bobrove AM: Assays for T and B cells. In Vyas GN, Stites DP, Brecher G (eds): Laboratory Diagnosis of Immunologic Disorders. New York, Grune and Stratton, 1975, p 71.
22. Meuwissen HJ, Pollara B, Pickering RJ: Combined immunodeficiency disease associated with adenosine deaminase deficiency. J Pediatr 86:169, 1975.
23. Giblett ER, Ammann AJ, Wara DW, Sandman R, Diamond LK: Nucleoside-phosphorylase deficiency in a child with severely defective T-cell immunity and normal B-cell immunity. Lancet 1:1010, 1975.
24. Dardenne M, Bach JF: The sheep cell rosette assay for the evaluation of thymic hormones in biologic activity of thymic hormones. Rotterdam, Kooyker, 1975, p 235.
25. Lewis V, Twomey JJ, Goldstein G, O'Reilly R, Smithwick E, Pahwa R, Pahwa S, Good RA, Schulte-Wisserman H, Horowitz S, Hong R, Jones J, Sieber O, Kirkpatrick C, Polmar S, Bealmear P: Circulating thymic hormone activity in congenital immune-deficiency. Lancet 2:471, 1977.

D. Humoral Immunity to Infection and the Complement System

JONATHAN L. MEAKINS
RICHARD L. SIMMONS

The preceding section discussed the cellular components of the immune response not only to infection but to other foreign materials. This section will address the humoral components of the immune response, made up principally of immunoglobulins and complement. Historically, immunologists were divided into two camps. One, led by Metchninkoff, championed the cellular components as most important in control of infection. The other, led by Ehrlich, proposed that humoral factors were more significant. Almoth Wright in 1903 initiated resolution of the controversy by demonstrating that neutrophil phagocytosis (cellular) was dependent on particle opsonization (humoral). The resolution of the early arguments as to which component of immune response was most important was that they act in conjunction in support of one another. Although immune response is presented as a series of separate components, they interact closely with one another.

IMMUNOGLOBULINS

All immunoglobulins (antibodies) are manufactured by cells of the B cell line, which terminates with the plasma cell. Interaction with a T_H cell is required for active primary immunization of a B cell to most antigens, but there are exceptions. After sensitization, the clone of B cells which bear genetically programmed receptors for the antigens undergoes proliferative expansion with the concurrent manufacture and release of large quantities of immunoglobulin. The initial concept was that an immunoglobulin was specifically produced for each specific antigenic molecule. It is, however, probable that large families of immunoglobulin molecules are produced in response to the various antigenic configurations of a single complex molecule each derived from a separate B cell clone. So-called natural antibodies probably represent antibodies to cross-reacting antigenic specificities elicited by previously encountered antigens.[1,2]

IMMUNOGLOBULIN STRUCTURE

The basic immunoglobulin (Ig) molecule is a heterogeneous family of glycoproteins which despite their diversity share many structural properties, biologic functions, and origins. There are five classes of immunoglobulins (Table 13-12), each defined by their heavy chain (α, γ, μ, δ, ϵ). The basic structure of Ig molecules is made up of pairs of polypeptide chains of unequal size (Fig. 13-13). There are two light (L) and two heavy (H) chains, which are held together by strong noncovalent forces and interchain disulphide bonds. The basic unit of the Ig molecule is L_2H_2, which may be considered as a monomer of two light and two heavy chains. This basic four-chain unit can, with utilization of further bonding or other molecular pieces, form even larger units (IgA, sIgA, IgM) (Fig 13-14). The light and heavy chains are composed of regions or domains, formed of somewhat more than 100 amino acid residues.

The amino acid residues in the amino-terminal domains of the light and heavy chains fold to form the antigen-binding sites (Fig. 13-13). The balance of the molecule, ie, the Fc fragment, binds to Ig (Fc) receptors on cells or proteins. This reaction produces the effector function mediating the body's response to the presence of the antigen-antibody complexes. The antigen-binding region, the amino-terminal domains, is heterogeneous in primary structure and is termed the variable (V) region. The remaining domains, progressing to the carboxyl end of the molecule, are less variable and are called the constant (C) region. The constant domains in the heavy chain, Fc end of Ig molecule, perform specific functions vis-à-vis Fc receptors. The B cell clones which synthesize the immunoglobulins are genetically programmed to the synthesis of a single light chain variable region and a single heavy chain variable region. These domains determine the specificity of the antigen and in each Ig molecule are identical.

Within this basic structure, there are five major classes of Ig molecules, and each has distinct physiochemical,

TABLE 13-12. SELECTED PROPERTIES OF HUMAN IMMUNOGLOBULINS

	IgG	IgA	IgM	IgD	IgE
Molecular weight	150,000	160,000 and polymers	900,000	200,000	185,000
Normal serum concentration (μg/ml)	8–16	1.5–4	0.5–2	0.00004	0–0.4
Percent total immunoglobulin	80	13	6	0.002	1
Sedimentation coefficient	7S	7S, 9S, 11S	19S	8S	7S
Serum T½ (days)	23	5.8	10	2.8	2.3
Valency for antigen binding	2	2 (polymers ?)	5(10)	2	?

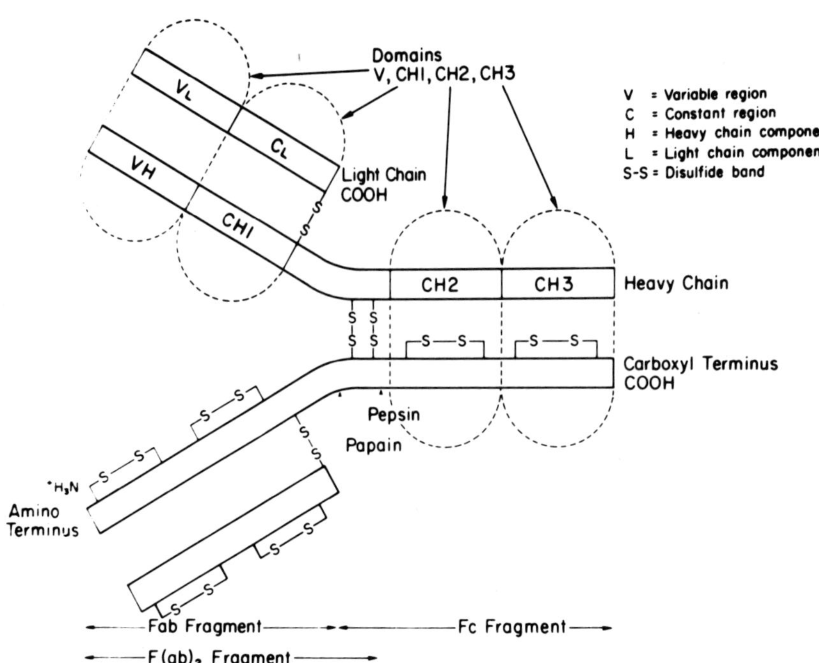

Fig. 13-13. **Four-chain structure of an IgG molecule. (From Alexander JW, Good RA: The immunoglobulins. In *Fundamentals of Clinical Immunology.* Philadelphia, Saunders, 1977, p 69.)**

physiologic, and antigenic properties (Tables 13-12, 13-13). It is the constant regions of the heavy chains that differ between classes and determine all class-specific properties. Different types of heavy chains are designated by Greek letters and correspond to the Ig class of immunoglobulin. The variable regions and light chains are not class specific. There are two types of light chains, kappa and lambda.

The Ig molecule is susceptible to enzymatic attack (Fig. 13-13) and gives rise to specific molecular fragments made up of intact domains. The Fab, $F(ab)_2$, and Fc fragments result from enzymatic reactions in the hinge region. Papain digestion produces the Fab and Fc fragments. The Fab has an intact light-chain and amino acid terminal as well as one constant heavy-chain domain. It contains a single intact antigen-combining site. The Fc fragment is the region that fixes to skin and cell receptors and initiates complement activation. Pepsin digestion gives the $F(ab)_2$ fragment, similar to Fab molecule except the cleavage includes disulphide bonds and protein of Fc fragment. It also has an antigen-combining site.

Immunoglobulin Classes (Table 13-12)

Immunoglobulin G (IgG)

IgG is the most abundant immunoglobulin, comprising about 85 percent of the total Ig. IgG has a molecular weight of 150,000 and is widely distributed throughout the intravascular and extravascular spaces. Antibodies of the IgG class provide antiviral and antibacterial protection. They are used therapeutically against bacterial infections, viral infections, and for their antivenom and antitoxin activities.

IgG has four different subclasses, numbered 1 through 4 in order of abundance. The significance of these four

TABLE 13-13. BIOLOGIC PROPERTIES OF ANTIBODIES BY IMMUNOGLOBULIN CLASS

	IgG	IgA	IgM	IgD	IgE
Complement activation					
Classical pathway	++	0	++++	0	0
Alternate pathway	+	+	+	+	+
Opsonic activity	++++	0	+	0	0
Lytic activity *	++	0	++++	0	0
Inhibition of bacterial adherence	+	+++	+	?	?
Viral neutralization	+++	+++	++	?	?
Reaginic activity	0	0	0	0	++++
Placental transfer	++++	0	0	0	0

* Through activation of complement after combining with cellular antigens.

Adapted from Alexander JW, Meakins JL: A physiologic basis for opportunistic infection. *Ann Surg* 176:273, 1972.

classes is not clear. Antibodies of the IgG class bind to and are actively transported across the placenta to the fetus, accounting for neonatal immunoglobulin levels equivalent to those of the mother. They subsequently decrease and, with exposure to the outside world, the child is producing IgG by the fourth month in adequate quantities. The serum levels are in dynamic equilibrium throughout life responding appropriately to stimuli. Generally levels decrease with advanced age.

The biologic effectiveness of IgG resides in large part with its opsonic capacity. The Fab component binds to antigen, and the Fc component interacts with the Fc receptors on phagocytic cells, either neutrophils, monocytes, or macrophages, with subsequent ingestion of the antigenic cell, particle, or antigen-antibody complex. Two molecules of IgG bound to a particulate antigen are, in addition, able to fix and activate the classic complement pathway (see subsequent section).

Immunoglobulin M (IgM) (Fig. 13-14)

IgM, originally referred to as macroglobulin, is the largest of the immunoglobulins, with a molecular weight in the region of 900,000 daltons. The large size is a result of polymerization of five Ig molecules into a pentameter $(L_2H_2)_5$ with a single J chain (Fig. 13-14).[3] Because of its size, it is found only in the intravascular space. The 18 to 19S molecule is formed by polymerization of 5.7S subunits joined by disulphide bonds. It has a half life of 5 to 6 days. IgM is the major component of the primary response to an antigen and is the first peak of immunoglobulin produced. IgM production declines on the basis of feedback mechanism secondary to increasing IgG production. Some IgM antibody production appears T cell–independent, and antibodies to T cell–independent antigens are usually of this class.

IgM is a potent activator of complement; a single molecule is able to initiate the classical complement sequence. Monomer subunits of IgM occur on the surface of many B lymphocytes and may have an important role as antigen receptors for these cells.

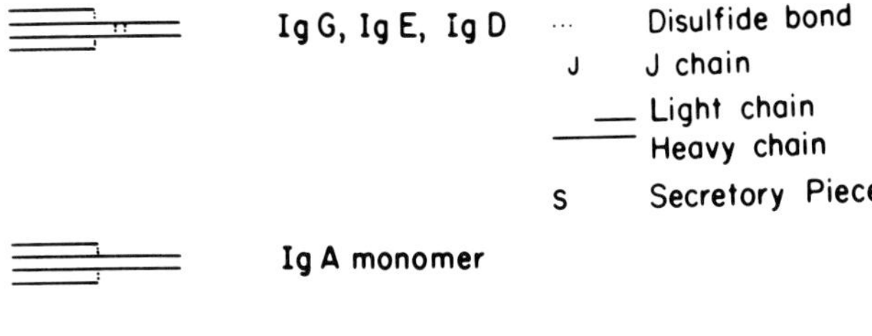

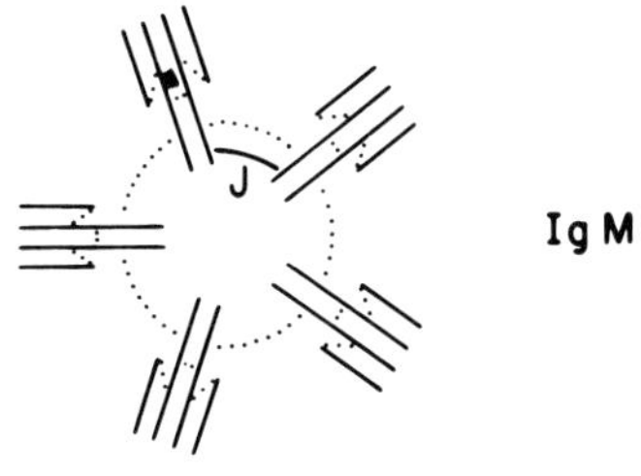

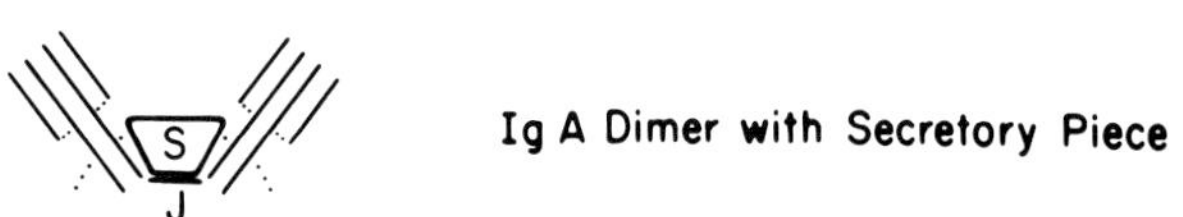

Fig. 13-14. **Schematic structures of the immunoglobulin classes. Disulfide bonds may differ from those shown for individual subclasses. (From Alexander JW, Good RA: The immunoglobulins. In *Fundamentals of Clinical Immunology.* Philadelphia, Saunders, 1977, p 69.)**

Immunoglobulin E (IgE) (Table 13-12)

Reagin, present in minute amounts in the serum (0.003 mg/ml), is an important mediator of acute allergic response as exemplified by the Prausnitz-Kustner test. It has the lowest synthetic rate of known Ig classes. Antibodies of this class are the chief antigen-specific mediators of immediate type hypersensitivity reactions (reaginic) and are, therefore, extremely potent biologic effectors. The Fc portion of the molecule fixes specific receptors on mast cells and basophils, which are thus sensitized to release histamine and other mediators when exposed to antigen. IgE is an important mediator of respiratory allergic disease. These globulins may be important in the protection of the respiratory tract against microbial infection.

Immunoglobulin D (IgD)

IgD is present in relatively low concentrations in normal human plasma, less than 1 percent that of IgG. No distinct biologic function has been ascribed to IgD.

Immunoglobulin A (IgA) and Local Mucosal Immunity

Antibodies can be produced by lymphoid tissues associated with mucosal surfaces, and IgA is secreted onto those surfaces. IgA in external secretions has a structure different from IgA and serum where it is a minor component.[4] The contents of IgA in various mucosal fluids differ from site to site. An inflammation of the mucosal surface markedly changes those concentrations, especially during the transudation of serum proteins.

IgA and Secretory IgA Structure. IgA exists as a monomer in serum. Secretory IgA (S-IgA), however, exists in multiple polymeric forms with increasing sedimentation coefficients up to 185. Most S-IgA exists in the dimeric form, molecular weight of 380,000, which possesses a unique secretory piece or component (SC), also called T component or transport piece (Table 13-12; Fig. 13-14). Secretory component is a nonimmunoglobulin glycoprotein (molecular weight 58,000) bound to the light immunoglobulin chains by disulfide bonds. Dimeric IgA also has a J chain (molecular weight 23,000–26,000) consisting of a single amino acid chain. These J chains are also found in dimeric serum IgA and IgM.[4]

SC probably mediates transport of IgA (and probably IgM) across epithelial surfaces and may also be important in the absorption of antigens from mucosal surfaces. SC is also thought to be responsible for the greater resistance of S-IgA to digestion by proteolytic enzymes. IgG does not react with SC and is thus not protected from proteolysis.

Most S-IgA is synthesized locally in plasma cells underlying the epithelium of secretory surfaces. The dimeric IgA then reaches the mucosal surface by passing through intracellular channels or between the epithelial cells. SC is synthesized by the epithelial cells and combines with the dimeric IgA molecule. The S-IgA molecule is thus produced.[4]

Antimicrobial Activity of IgA. Secretory IgA can bind to viral and bacterial antigens to which the animal is immune, but it can neither fix complement in the normal way nor can it serve as an opsonin for phagocytosis.[4] Recently, however, Burritt et al [5] have shown that the Fc fragment of IgA can bind complement and might, under proper conditions, have the capacity to activate complement and lyse bacteria. Adinolfi et al [6] have shown that secretory IgA antibody is capable of bacterial lysis in the presence of complement and lysozyme. Burdon has found a heat-stable component of complement necessary for IgA-mediated bacterial lysis. This new complement component appears to be different from any other previously described.[7] What is not known is whether complement is active and activatable within the complex milieu of intestinal and respiratory fluids.

Equally controversial as the role of IgA in the complement-mediated immunolysis of bacteria is the suggestion that IgA antibodies can function as opsonins. Since IgM is present in biologic fluids, much of the opsonization shown may be due to contamination by IgM.

However these controversies are resolved, most evidence currently supports the idea that IgA acts primarily to prevent the adherence of pathogenic bacteria to epithelium. Similar properties are possessed by other immunoglobulin classes. This mechanism probably operates as a first line of defense against many, if not all, mucosal pathogens, which normally invade by adhering to and colonizing the epithelium prior to deeper invasion.[8]

Klein et al [9] have suggested another mechanism of S-IgA protection, namely, the inhibition of some bacterial enzyme activity involved in the pathogenesis of disease. These observations, however, were restricted to the pathogenesis of dental lesions.

S-IgA and Local Immunity. Parenterally administrated vaccines can elicit an S-IgA response, but levels of local antibody are usually low and result in only partial protection. The direct application of vaccines to the mucosal surface elicits a greater degree of local immunity as well as a moderate degree of systemic immunity.[10] The level of S-IgA correlates with antimicrobial protection, but preexisting secretory antibody activity interferes with secondary immunization response. In addition, the response of the mucosal immune system to bacterial antigens is so short-lived that local immunity to gonorrhea, for example, disappears promptly, and there is often no booster effect following reinfection.

The local immunity achieved by the use of topical vaccines has been studied extensively and the results reviewed by Regamey et al: [11] (1) A higher dose of antigen is required compared to parenteral immunization; (2) repeated immunization is required; (3) dose of vaccine, size of particles and aerosol vaccines, living conditions before exposure to antigen, and age of recipients influence the outcome of immunization; (4) attenuated nonparenteral vaccines are usually not transmissable to contacts, produce few side effects, and are suitable for mass application; and (5) serum antibodies do not always reflect the state of immunity generated by nonparenteral vaccine.

Secretory Humoral Immunity in IgA Deficiency States. IgA is not the only mucosal immunoglobulin. IgG-containing cells lie immediately below the surface epithelium of the nasal mucosa and the gingival tissues. Local synthesis of IgG is present in bladder, kidney, and urinary tract. In addition, IgM-producing cells predominate over IgG-producing cells within salivary glands and the gastrointestinal tract. In IgA deficiency, IgM usually predominates in mucosal secretions. IgE is also synthesized in secretory organs. The tonsils, adenoids, bronchial and mesenteric lymph nodes, and lamina propria of the gastrointestinal and respiratory tract mucosa contain a large number of IgE-producing cells.

IgA is the most common isolated immunoglobulin deficiency.[12] Most patients are normal without increased incidence of mucosal infections, with protection probably mediated by IgM. Patients with selective IgA deficiencies have IgA-bearing peripheral blood lymphocytes but lack IgA-producing plasma cells. As a group, patients with selective IgA deficiency have some abnormalities (hereditary ataxia-telangectasia and recurrent viral and bacterial infections of the respiratory tract, resulting in chronic bronchitis and bronchiectasis). There is also more frequent association with allergic disorders, ear infections in children, autoimmune phenomena, malabsorption, and cancer. *Giardia lamblia* infections are particularly common in this group of patients. Patients deficient in secretory component also have chronic intestinal candidiasis.[13]

FUNCTIONS OF THE CIRCULATING IMMUNOGLOBULINS

Antibodies play almost no role in the prevention or eradication of infection of intracellular pathogens once cells have become successfully invaded. The primary role, therefore, is directed against pathogens in an extracellular location. Specific antibodies promote the following events: (1) opsonization for destruction by phagocytic cells, (2) activation of cell-free lysis by the complement system, (3) neutralization of toxins, (4) inhibition of attachments of microbes to susceptible host cells, and (5) virus neutralization (Table 13-13). IgG is the most abundant immunoglobin in the extravascular fluids, and is the most important immunoglobin in tissue infection. IgM is a pentameric intravascular molecule and cannot leave normal vessels. It is an effective bacterial agglutinator and stimulant of the classic complement-dependent cytolytic system. Its role is as a first line of specific immune defense against bacteremia.

IMMUNIZATION

Active Immunization

Immunoglobulins were the first form of host support via manipulation of the immune system against infections. Jenner's cowpox experiments predicted a valuable approach to control of infectious diseases. The apparent eradication of smallpox worldwide is testimony to the power of this approach. The concept of active immunization has been extended to include tetanus, diphtheria, pertussis, polio, measles, and rubella in the general population, as well as anthrax, cholera, plague, rabies, Rocky Mountain spotted fever, typhoid, typhus, yellow fever, and influenza in selected persons. There is evidence to suggest that *Pseudomonas* heptavalent vaccines can protect burn patients from *Pseudomonas* infections. At present, because of the high incidence of pneumococcal infection following splenectomy, it is appropriate that all splenectomized patients should receive the polyvalent pneumococcal vaccine. The goal in both of these instances is to raise available opsonizing antibodies to the level that will allow enough opsonization of the infecting bacteria to take place to resolve or abort the infectious process.

Passive Immunization

Serotherapy was once utilized in pneumococcal infection. The opsonizing antibody allowed the pneumococcus to be ingested and killed by neutrophils. Recollection of the polio epidemics of 30 years ago brings to mind the value of gammaglobulin (IgG) as a protective measure in these disastrous situations. Currently, passive immunoprophylaxis is useful for botulism, diphtheria, viral hepatitis, measles, rabies, tetanus, pseudomonas sepsis, and varicella zoster. In most cases, hyperimmune IgG of human origin is available.

B CELL IMMUNODEFICIENCIES

Agammaglobulinemia was first diagnosed by Bruton in 1952, and this was the first description of any type of true immunodeficiency. This autosomal recessive condition responds well to the administration of immunoglobulins every 2 weeks. Similarly, patients with hypogammaglobulinemia of either an acquired or a congenital nature can be treated in this manner. Surgery in these patients can safely be conducted with preoperative administration of immunoglobulin and correct use of antibiotics. Some primary and secondary B cell immunodeficiency diseases are listed in Tables 13-14 and 13-15.

COMPLEMENT

Antibodies are highly efficient and highly specific methods for recognizing antigenic microorganisms. By themselves, they can sometimes inhibit clinical interactions between microbe and host necessary for bacterial virulence. They cannot, however, by themselves eliminate invaders from the body. For this, antibodies require phagocytes to ingest and digest the opsonized organisms, and the complement system to amplify opsonization or lysis. Antibodies have a second disadvantage: response to a new antigen requires a complicated cellular response, so that antibodies may not be detected for many days. A far more primitive and nonspecific humoral defense mechanism is the complement system. This is comprised of a number of components always present within the circulation, which can be activated by a variety of microbial and other stimuli. It can act independently of, as well as in concert with, the humoral and cellular immune systems.

COMPLEMENT COMPONENTS

Complement is not a single substance; it is a group of proteins in blood and interstitial fluid with smaller quantities on mucosal surfaces. The components themselves are listed in Table 13-16. All are inactive and without known biologic activity.

Interaction of these normally inactive substances with microbial cell surfaces or antigen-antibody complexes

TABLE 13-14. PRIMARY B CELL IMMUNODEFICIENCIES

Isolated B Cell Immunodeficiency Diseases	Combined T Cell and B Cell Immunodeficiency Diseases
Sex-linked infantile hypogammaglobulinemia	Severe combined immunodeficiency
Transient hypogammaglobulinemia of infancy	Cellular immunodeficiency with abnormal immunoglobulin synthesis (Nezeloff syndrome)
Sex-linked immunodeficiency with hyper-IgM	Immunodeficiency disease with enzyme deficiency
Selective IgA deficiency	Immunodeficiency with eczema and thrombocytopenia (Wiskott-Aldrich syndrome)
Selective IgM deficiency	Immunodeficiency with thymoma
Selective deficiencies of IgG subclasses	Immunodeficiency with ataxia-telangiectasia
	Immunodeficiency with short-limbed dwarfism
	Episodic lymphocytopenia with lymphotoxin (immunologic amnesia)

From Stiehm ER: Immunodeficiency disorders: general considerations. In Stiehm ER, Fulginiti VA (eds): *Immunologic Disorders in Infants and Children,* Philadelphia, Saunders, 1973, p 145.

TABLE 13-15. SECONDARY B CELL DISORDERS

Disorder	B cell
INFECTION	
Rubella (congenital)	May have hypogammaglobulinemia or selective immunoglobulin deficiencies; no response to rubella immunization; decreased response to multiple antigens
Leprosy	Decreased B cells in some, increased in others; increased antibody
Chronic infection	Increased immunoglobulins
Congenital cytomegalovirus	Elevated IgM, IgA
MALIGNANCY	
Hodgkin disease	Immunoglobulins normal to increased; decreased antibody response to certain antigens
Acute leukemia	Variable immunoglobulin levels
Chronic leukemia	Variable immunoglobulin levels
Nonlymphoid	Variable immunoglobulin levels
Myeloma	Impaired antibody response; decreased immunoglobulins
AUTOIMMUNE DISEASE	
Systemic lupus erythematosus	Immunoglobulins usually elevated; increased antibody titers to multiple antigens
Rheumatoid arthritis	Immunoglobulin levels usually increased, normal antibody response to antigens
Chronic active hepatitis	Immunoglobulins increased
PROTEIN-LOSING STATES	
Nephrotic syndrome	Decreased IgG; IgM and IgA may be decreased; antibody response decreased
Protein-losing enteropathy	Hypogammaglobulinemia frequent
OTHER DISORDERS	
Burns	Decrease in all immunoglobulins; normal antibody response
Sarcoidosis	Increased immunoglobulins; normal antibody response
Splenectomy	Immunoglobulins normal; decreased antibody response to whole organisms; normal antibody response to purified antigens
Sickle cell disease	IgM may be decreased; decreased antibody response to whole organisms with normal response to purified antigens
Aging	Increased IgG (IgA in some); increased B cells; decreased IgG response to certain antigens

PHA = phytohemagglutinin stimulation of lymphocyte; MLC = allogeneic cell stimulation of lymphocytes

Adapted from Ammann AJ, Fundenberg HH: Immunodeficiency diseases. In Fundenberg HH, Stites DP, Caldwell JL, Wells JV: *Basic and Clinical Immunology, (3rd ed).* Los Altos, Lange Publishing, 1980, pp 409–441.

leads to the formation of several proteolytic enzymes, which cleave other components, forming new enzymes until a cascade of reactive substances is produced. Two pathways of activation have been described—the classical pathway and the alternative pathway. The early events in the two pathways are not the same but both converge at the third complement component (C3), after which the pathways are identical (Fig. 13-15). In the classical pathway, the initiators (Table 13-16) interact with antigen-antibody complexes leading to C3 activation; in the alternative pathway, the initiators (Table 13-16) interact with other plasma factors, which then activate C3. Figure 13-16 schematically outlines the classical pathways and the final common pathway leading to cell lysis; however, most antimicrobial activity of complement activation does not derive from direct bacteriolysis through either pathway. The

TABLE 13-16. MOLECULAR WEIGHTS AND SERUM CONCENTRATIONS OF COMPLEMENT COMPONENTS

Component	Molecular Weight (Daltons)	Serum Concentration * (μg/ml)
Initiators		
Classical pathway		
C1q	400,000	180
C1r	180,000	?
C1s	86,000	110
C2	117,000	25
C4	206,000	640
Alternate pathway		
Initiating factor (IF)	150,000	?
Properdin	184,000	25
Properdin factor B	93,000	200
Properdin factor D	24,000	?
Effectors		
C3	180,000	1,600
C5	180,000	80
C6	95,000	75
C7	110,000	55
C8	163,000	80
C9	79,000	230
Inhibitors		
C1	90,000	180
C3b inactivator	100,000	25
C6	?	?
C3a, C5a inactivator	300,000	?

* Serum concentrations given are the means in adults.

From Root RK: Humoral immunity and complement. In Mandell GL, Douglas RG Jr, Bennett JE (eds): *Principles and Practice of Infectious Diseases.* New York, Wiley, 1979, p 23.

ultimate effect of activation of the C3–9 terminal cascade is multifold: vasodilation, chemotaxis of phagocytic leukocytes into the contaminated region, and the opsonization of the microbes so that phagocytosis can take place (Fig. 13-16).[14]

THE CLASSICAL PATHWAY

The Initiating Events

Activation of complement components proceeds by a highly ordered sequence of events. The usual initial event for activation of the classical pathway is the interaction of the components of C1 with the Fc fragment of one molecule of IgM combined with antigen on a cell surface, or two molecules of IgG side by side (a so-called antibody doublet) (Figs. 13-16, 13-17.) Binding of antibody to antigen effects a conformational change in the antibody molecule, exposing the Fc fragment for interaction with either Clq or Fc receptors on phagocytic cells. IgA, IgE, IgD and some IgG subclasses do not bind C1 and therefore do not activate the classical complement pathway.[15] Although most microorganisms that activate complement do so directly through the alternative pathway (Fig. 13-16), under some circumstances some microorganisms (lipid A or endotoxin, staphylococcal protein A) or plasmin may activate C1 directly without participation of antibody.[16]

C1 is itself a complicated molecular complex, composed of three subunits termed C1q, C1r, C1s. The complex interactions of C1 with C4 have been diagrammed by Frank [17] (Fig. 13-17).

The activation of $\overline{C1}$ leads to the activation of C2 in a manner similar to that by which C4 is activated (Fig. 13-18). C2 is cleaved by enzymatic action of $\overline{C1}$ into two components, C2 and C2b. C2b is released into the environment, and C2a binds to C4b on the cell surface (Fig. 13-18). The $\overline{C4a2a}$ complex in turn activates C3, leading to the release of C3a with its multiple biologic activities (chemotaxis, vasodilation) and to $\overline{C3b}$, which binds to the cell surface and is the opsonin for phagocytes (Table 13-17).

One essential to the understanding of the complement cascade is the fact that the cascade itself acts as an amplification system, so that the binding of only a few molecules of antibody permits the activation through enzymatic mechanisms of large amounts of complement. Amplification occurs at two important points along the cycle: (1) activated $\overline{C1}$ enzymatically cleaves many molecules of C4 so that many molecules of $\overline{C4b}$ are deposited on the cell membrane for each molecule of antibody. (2) Many C3b molecules are produced. C3b is the critical molecule in the whole cascade (see next section).

THE ALTERNATIVE PATHWAY

Activators of the Alternative Complement Pathway

Endotoxin, polysaccharides, aggregates of Ig, zymosan (fungal cell surface), and teichoic acids C on pyogenic cocci have all been shown capable of activating this pathway.

TABLE 13-17. BIOLOGIC EFFECTS OF COMPLEMENT FRAGMENTS RELEASED DURING SEQUENTIAL ACTIVATION OF THE SYSTEM

Mediator	Effect
C4a	Release of serotonin
C2b	Kininlike activity
C4b	Immune adherence
C3a	Anaphylatoxin, vascular effect; chemotaxis; leukocyte mobilization
C3b	Opsonization; immune adherence; release of platelet factor 3
C5a	Most potent chemotactic factor; Opsonin for *Candida* (?); C5b may attach to platelets, active distal components, and cause platelet lysis as an innocent bystander
$\overline{C567}$	Chemotaxis
$\overline{C8}$	Initiates lytic process; inserted into membrane
$\overline{C9}$	Completes lytic process

Adapted from Alexander JW, Good RA: *Fundamentals of Clinical Immunology.* Philadelphia, Saunders, 1977, Chap 7, p 80.

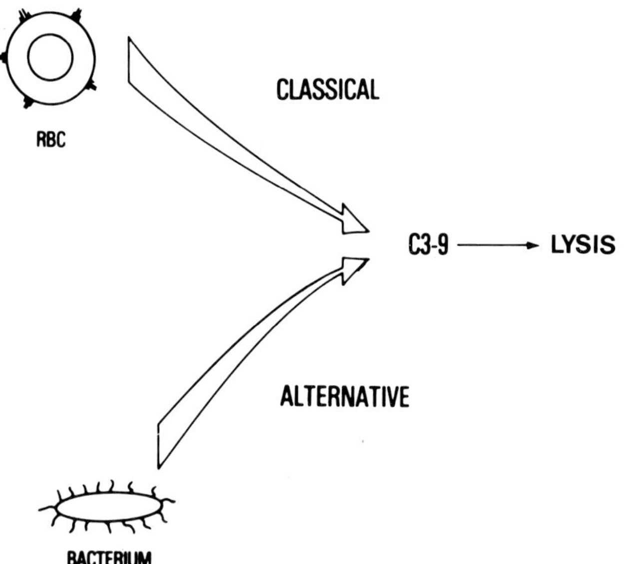

Fig. 13-15. Two pathways of complement activation converge at the level of the complement component C3. These pathways then engage C5–C9 and lead to lysis of bacteria or sensitized erythrocytes (RBC). (Adapted from Frank MM: The complement system in host defense and inflammation. *Rev Infect Dis* 1:483, 1979.)

The alternative pathway is probably the major pathway of activation of the terminal complement components when antibody is absent.[18]

The Initiators

Table 13-16 includes a list of the four initiators of the alternate pathway. Each is analogous to one of the classical pathway initiators.

Properdin factor D is analogous to C1; properdin factor B is analogous to C2. To activate D, one requires initiating factor, properdin, and one of the activators described in the previous section. In addition, $C3\overline{b}$ is required. Figure 13-19 demonstrates the interaction of B, $\overline{D}$, and cell-bound $C3\overline{b}$. $C\overline{462a}$ enzymatically degrades C3, leading to the production of many $C3\overline{b}$ molecules for opsonization and many C3a molecules to enhance the inflammatory response. $C\overline{3bBb}$ is capable of cleaving C3 into C3a and $C3\overline{b}$ as in the classical pathway. $\overline{D}$ acts to stabilize the $C\overline{3bBb}$ complex.[17]

It is obvious that some C3b must be formed before the alternative pathway can be initiated. This may be a function of other proteolytic enzymes, including plasmin and neutrophil lysozomal proteases.[19]

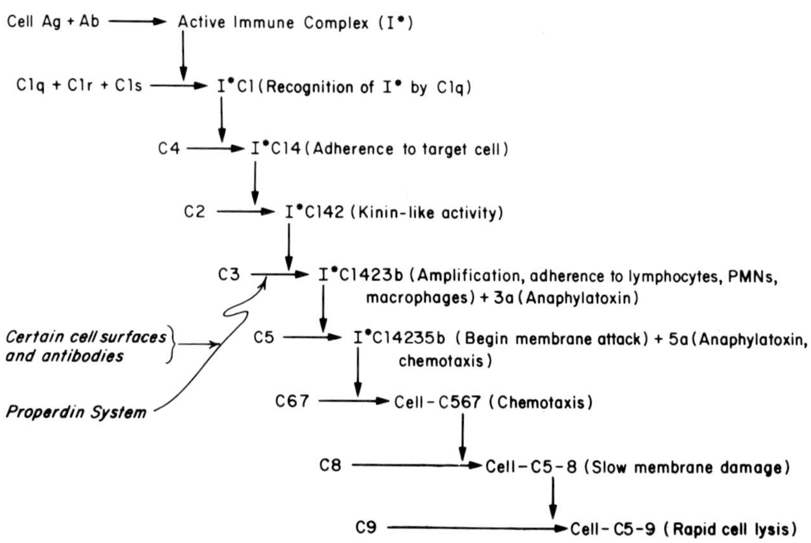

Fig. 13-16. The complement pathways and the biologic activity released at each step. The classical pathway begins with a specific antigen-antibody reaction. The properdin pathway is triggered by a more nonspecific interaction between cell surfaces and the molecules that comprise the properdin systems. Both pathways, however, converge at the C3 step, where most of the biologic activity associated with complement activation begins. Amplification also occurs at several steps, but it is greatest at C3. The subsequent steps lead to the molecular condensation of the target cell surface, which ultimately results in membrane damage and lysis. There are several other important consequences of complement activation. The presence of these molecules on the target cell surface makes them adherent to other cells. Macrophages, platelets, polymorphonuclear leukocytes, and lymphocytes adhere and increase the damage to the target cells. The steps through C5 are largely enzymatic in nature; the C3 and C5 components, for example, are split during activation, releasing chemotactic and vasoactive molecules (anaphylatoxins). Attachment of the C5b molecule to the cell begins the condensation ending in membrane damage; this seems to occur away from the immune complex. Interaction of the C6, C7 components results additionally in the release of another chemotactic factor. The activation of the complement pathway, therefore, contributes to many of the features seen in infection; cellular infiltrates, adherent PMNs and platelets, thrombosed vessels, interstitial edema, and cellular damage. (From Simmons RL, Foker JE, Lower RR, Najarian JS: Transplantation. In Schwartz SI, Shires GT, Spencer FC, Storer EH: *Principles of Surgery (3rd ed).* New York, McGraw-Hill, 1979, pp 383–473.)

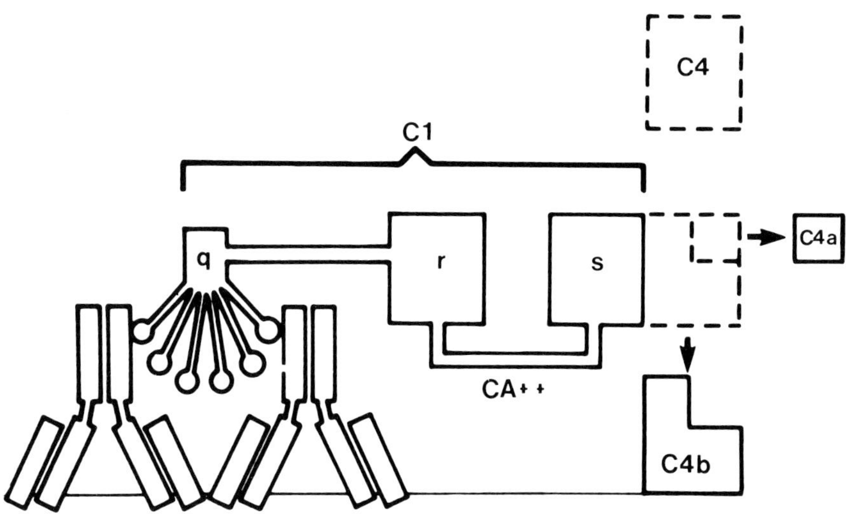

Fig. 13-17. Detail of the earliest steps in the classical complement pathway. Shown is an IgG antibody doublet bound by its variable region combining sites to the membrane of a sensitized erythrocyte. The Fc fragments of the two IgG molecules are free to interact with a binding site on subunit q of C1. In the presence of calcium, subunits q, r, and s of C1 are held together in a macromolecular complex. Also shown is the fact that fluid-phase C4 can interact with C1s. This interaction leads to cleavage of C4 into a small fragment (C4a) and a larger fragment (C4b), which is bound by covalent bonds to the cell membrane. (Adapted from Frank MM: The complement system in host defense and inflammation. *Rev Infect Dis* 1:483, 1979.)

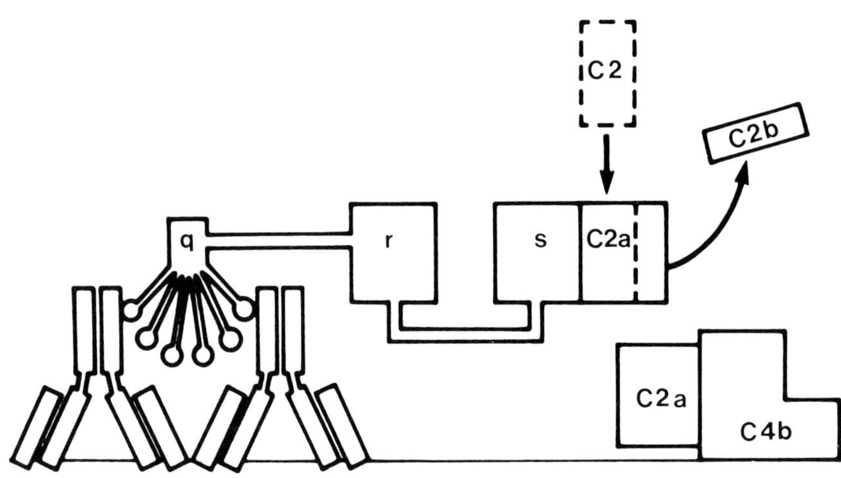

Fig. 13-18. Further details of the activation of the classical complement pathway. In the presence of cell-bound C4b, the complex of immunoglobulin and activated C1 interacts with and cleaves C2 into two fragments. The smaller fragment, C2b, is released into the fluid phase. The larger fragment, C2a, associates with the cell-bound C4b to form a new enzyme complex composed of these two protein fragments and termed C3 convertase. (From Frank MM: The complement system in host defense and inflammation. *Rev Infect Dis* 1:483, 1979.)

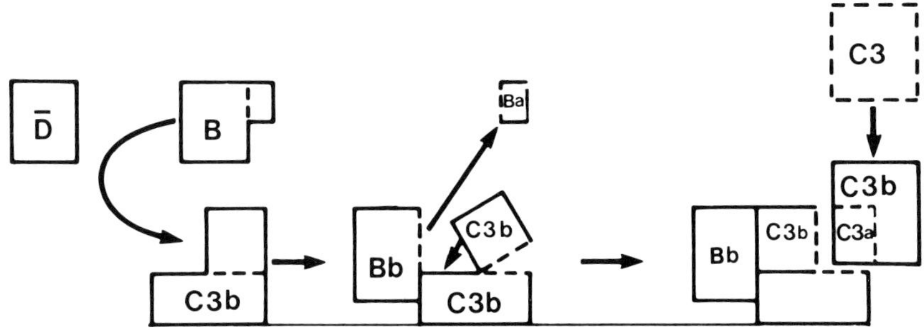

Fig. 13-19. Schematic analysis of alternative pathway activation. Cell-bound C3b can interact with properdin factor B in the presence of activated properdin factor D. Activation is shown by a superscript bar. The factor B is cleaved into two fragments, Bb and Ba. The Ba is released into the fluid phase. Bb binds to C3b. Here, it is shown as causing an allosteric change in C3b such that the combination of Bb and C3b forms a protein configuration analogous to the complex of C4b and C2a. This complex, like the classical pathway convertase, is capable of coordinating with C3 and cleaving it into two fragments, C3a and C3b. (From Frank MM: The complement system in host defense and inflammation. *Rev Infect Dis* 1:483, 1979.)

EFFECTORS OF THE COMPLEMENT CASCADE (C3–9) (Table 13-17)

C3b

Although C1q and C4b may neutralize some viruses, the distal complement components are responsible for most of the biologic effects of the cascade. The C3b molecule is the critical one:

1. The C3b molecule acts to amplify the system by being produced in large quantity, and serves as an enzyme cleaving further C3 molecules into C3a and C3b.

2. It serves as a key subcomponent with properdin factor $\overline{B}$, leading to even further formation of C3b through C3 cleavage (Fig. 13-19).

3. It mounts a proteolytic attack on the C5 molecule, perpetuating the cascade.

4. Interaction of C3b with B lymphocytes may also mediate the release of lymphokines from the lymphocytes, thereby recruiting other cells into the inflammatory response.

5. Most importantly, $C3\overline{b}$ is the most potent biologic opsonin. Phagocytic neutrophils and both fixed and wandering macrophages possess cell surface receptors for C3b, enabling bacteria to be phagocytosed and killed.

Despite the essential role of C3b in the opsonization of microbes for phagocytosis by both fixed and wandering phagocytes, the mere binding of C3b on the microbe to the C3b receptor on a fixed macrophage does not guarantee phagocytosis. Even this process can be amplifed by either activation of the macrophages or a few molecules of specific IgG or IgM bound to the cell surface. Otherwise, the presence of C3B inactivator (see subsequent section) can interfere with normal phagocytosis.

Lysis of Bacteria

When C3b is deposited on the surface of a microbe in proximity to $\overline{C4bC2a}$ (or the analogous $\overline{C3bBb}$) (Fig. 13-19), C5 is cleaved into two fragments. C5a is released into the fluid phase, and C5b binds to the cell surface where it interacts with C6 and C7 to produce a $C\overline{567}$ complex on the cell membrane. This complex is not an enzyme but is actually inserted into the lipid bilayer of the cell membrane. This complex in turn binds C8 and then C9. The interaction leads to the formation of a damaged site or lesion in the surface of the cell, through which osmotically active materials are able to pass with ultimate osmotic lysis.

Inflammatory Mediators

C3a and C5a are soluble cleavage products of C3 and C5 respectively. They share similar properties: both are chemotactic for neutrophils and macrophages (C5a > C3a), and both are anaphylotoxins, acting as vasodilators and releasing histamine from basophils and most cells (C3a > C5a). C5a can, in addition, trigger a respiratory burst from phagocytic cells. The $C\overline{567}$ complex seems to possess some chemotactic properties as well (Table 13-17).

INHIBITORS AND REGULATORS OF COMPLEMENT ACTIVATION

At first glance, it would seem that complement would be a self-perpetuating system in which ultimate depletion of complement components would be an inevitable consequence of its activation. This does not normally occur. There are several mechanisms by which the complement cascade is regulated. For example, C4b is loosely bound to target cells, and when unbound, it loses biologic activity. Its activity can be perpetuated only if it is continually produced by C1 esterase. In addition, there are inhibitors of the complement system within serum (Table 13-16):

1. C1 esterase inhibitor can enzymatically disrupt $C1\overline{qrs}$ by binding to C1s. If C1s esterase inhibitor is absent, hereditary angioneurotic edema results.[20]

2. C3b inactivator cleaves $C3\overline{b}$ into two inactive components, C3c and C3d. $C3\overline{b}$ can be attacked even when bound to cells. Since $C3\overline{b}$ is the critical component in the perpetuation of the cascade, C3b inactivator is the most potent inhibitor of the system. When C3b inactivator is missing, C3 becomes depleted and such patients are severely susceptible to bacterial infections.

3. There are also serum inhibitors to C6, C3a, and C5a in serum (Table 13-16).

ADVERSE EFFECTS OF COMPLEMENT ACTIVATION

Like other host defense mechanisms, activation of the complement cascade plays an important role in the pathogenesis of some of the secondary manifestations of systemic infection. For example, the activation of complement within the blood can lead to a number of damaging effects: disseminated intravascular coagulation, vasodilation, and shock. Platelets and leukocytes becomes aggregated and embolize to critical areas of blood flow. This not only depletes essential complement components and leukocytes necessary for localization, opsonization, and lysis of the microbes; it also leads to development of hypotension, altered pulmonary capillary permeability (shock lung), and intravascular disseminated coagulation (Chapters 16, 17). Furthermore, in diseases in which antigen-antibody complexes circulate, tissue damage occurs because of complement activation at sites of antigen-antibody deposition (eg, the renal glomerulae and joints). In short, many of the secondary effects of infections are mediated by the complement cascade activated to an excessive degree.

DEFECTS OF THE COMPLEMENT SYSTEM AND THE CONSEQUENCES TO HOST DEFENSE

Table 13-18 lists the known defects in the complement system as summarized by Root.[2] Patients with recurrent infections should be screened for complement deficiencies, the most serious of which is C3 deficiency.[21] Absence of this pivotal component results in recurrent infections with encapsulated and gram-negative bacteria—a picture similar to that seen in agammaglobulinemia. C3 deficiency is a rare congenital disorder, but acquired deficiencies due

TABLE 13-18. DEFECTS OF THE COMPLEMENT SYSTEM AND CONSEQUENCES TO HOST DEFENSE

Component	Associated Diseases	Effects on Host Defenses *
C1		
C1q	Combined immunodeficiency	Major †
C1r	SLE, glomerulonephritis	Minor †
C1s	SLE	Minor †
C1 inhibitor	HAE (hereditary angioedema)	None
C4	SLE (systemic lupus erythematosus)	Minor †
C2	None, discoid LE, SLE, anaphylactoid purpura, Hodgkin, dermatomyositis, congenital with bacterial infections	Minor † to none
C3	Hereditary deficiencies cirrhosis, SLE, nephritis, immune complex disorders	Major †,‡
C3b inactivator	Bacterial infections	Major ‡
C5	SLE, bacterial infections	Major ‡
C5 "dysfunction"	Bacterial infections, diarrhea, eczema (Leiner syndrome)	Major ‡
C6	None, neisserial infections	Minor †
C7	None, Raynaud, neisserial infections	Minor ‡
C8	None, SLE, neisserial infections	Minor ‡
Alternate pathway	Sickle cell disease, splenectomy (?)	Major †,‡

* Major effects on host defenses are manifest by severe, recurrent bacterial infections, whereas minor effects are marked by infrequent infections.
† Effects on host defense appear to be mediated as much or more by the associated disease rather than by the complement deficiency per se.
‡ Effects on host defense are mediated primarily by the complement deficiency.

From Root RK: Humoral immunity and complement. In Mandell GL, Douglas RG Jr, Bennett JE (eds): *Principles and Practice of Infectious Diseases.* New York, Wiley, 1979, p 27.

to decreased production (eg, liver disease) or excessive utilization (eg, C3b inactivation deficiency, lupus erythematosus) have been described. Alexander et al [22] have described a state of consumptive opsonopathy, an acquired syndrome in which the opsonin is depleted by repeated or continuous gram-negative bacteremia.

C5 deficiency has been discovered in several patients who behave like patients with hypogammaglobulinemia with recurrent infections of the upper and lower respiratory tract.

BIBLIOGRAPHY

Fundenberg HH, Stites DP, Caldwell JL, Wells JV (eds): Basic and Clinical Immunology (3rd ed). Los Altos, Lange Medical Publications, 1980.

Müller-Eberhard HJ, Schreiber RD: Molecular biology and chemistry of the alternative pathway of complement. Adv Immunol 29:1, 1980.

REFERENCES

1. Fitch FW: Selective suppression of immune responses: regulation of antibody formation and cell-mediated immunity by antibody. Prog Allergy 19:195, 1975.
2. Root RK: Humoral immunity and complement. In Mandell GL, Douglas RG, Bennett JF (eds): Principles and Practice of Infectious Diseases. New York, Wiley, 1979, p 21.
3. Alexander JW, Good RA (eds): The immunoglobulins. In Fundamentals of Clinical Immunology. Philadelphia, Saunders, 1977, p 69.
4. Ganguly R, Waldman RH: Local immunity and local immune responses. Prog Allergy 27:1, 1980.
5. Burritt MF, Calvanico NJ, Mehta S, Tomasi TB Jr: Activation of the classical complement pathway by Fc fragment of human IgA. J Immunol 118:723, 1977.
6. Adinolfi M, Glynn AA, Lindsay M, Milne CM: Serological properties of yA antibodies to *Escherichia coli* present in human colostrum. Immunology 10:517, 1966.
7. Burdon DW: The bactericidal action of immunoglobulin. Am J Med Microbiol 6:131, 1973.
8. Freter R: Mechanism of action of intestinal antibody in experimental cholera. II. Antibody-mediated antibacterial reaction at the mucosal surface. Infect Immun 2:556, 1970.
9. Klein JP, Schöller M, Frank RM: Inhibition of glucosyltransferase by human salivary immunoglobulin A. Infect Immun 15:329, 1977.
10. Perkins JC, Tucker DN, Knopf HLS, Wenzel RP, Kapikian AZ, Chanock RM: Comparison of protective effect of neutralizing antibody in serum and nasal secretions in experimental rhinovirus type 13 illness. Am J Epidemiol 90:519, 1969.
11. Regamey RH, Hennessen W, Hulse EC, Perkins FT: International symposium on vaccination of man and animals by the

nonparenteral route. Proc 14th Int Congr Int Assoc of Biol Standardizations, Douglas, Isle of Man, 1975. Dev Biol Standard, Vol 33. Basel, Karger, 1976.
12. Ammann AJ, Hong R: Selective IgA deficiency and autoimmunity. Clin Exp Immunol 7:833, 1970.
13. Strober W, Krakauer R, Klaeveman HL, Reynolds HY, Nelson DL: Secretory component deficiency. A disorder of the IgA immune system. N Engl J Med 294:351, 1976.
14. Simmons RL, Foker JE, Lower RR, Najarian JS: Transplantation. In Schwartz SI, Shires GT, Spencer FC, Storer EH: Principles of Surgery. New York, McGraw-Hill, 1979, p 383.
15. Rapp HJ, Borsos T: Molecular Basis of Complement Action. New York, Appleton, 1970.
16. Cooper NR, Morrison DC: Binding and activation of the first component of human complement by the lipid A region of lipopolysaccharides. J Immunol 120:1862, 1978.
17. Frank MM: The complement system in host defense and inflammation. Rev Infect Dis 1:483, 1979.
18. Götze O, Müller-Eberhard HJ: The alternative pathway of complement activation. Adv Immunol 24:1, 1976.
19. Ward PA, Zvaifler NJ: Complement-derived leukotactic factors in inflammatory synovial fluids of humans. J Clin Invest 50:606, 1971.
20. Donaldson VH, Evans RR: A biochemical abnormality in hereditary angioneurotic edema: absence of serum inhibitor of C1-esterase. Am J Med 35:37, 1963.
21. Alper CA, Abramson N, Johnston RB Jr, Jandl JH, Rosen FS: Increased susceptibility to infection associated with abnormalities of complement-mediated functions and of the third component of complement (C3). N Engl J Med 282:349, 1970.
22. Alexander JW, McClellan MA, Ogle CK, Ogle JD: Consumptive opsoninopathy: possible pathogenesis in lethal and opportunistic infections. Ann Surg 184:672, 1976.

E. The Defenses of the Wound

THOMAS K. HUNT

A surgical or traumatic wound is obviously a physical breach of the armor of host defense, and about 5 to 10 percent of surgical wounds will become infected.[1] Table 13-19 shows that there has been a general improvement in wound infection rates over the past 20 years. The reasons for the decrease are not totally clear. A more rational use of prophylactic antibiotics must take some credit, but so must improved anesthesia management, improved physiologic support of patients, improved means of measuring oxygenation and cardiac function, improved nutrition, better surgical techniques, and probably many other factors. Diminution of external contamination has probably had a fairly minor role, since few improvements of operating room design and cutaneous antiseptics have been generally adopted during that 20 years. Adoption of antibiotic bowel and urinary tract preparation has undoubtedly contributed to the diminution of infection. One of the more important questions in surgical care today is, "How far can this trend be exploited? Can wound infections be eliminated totally?"

VULNERABILITY OF THE WOUND

A large portion of human bacterial infections originate in some kind of wound. Yet we do not fully understand why wounds are so susceptible. At one time, it seemed enough to say that the protective epithelial barrier had been broken and that the infection resulted from bacteria introduced into the break. Now, this view is obviously inadequate. For instance, the immunosuppressed and malnourished patient clearly is more susceptible than the normal patient.[2-4] Furthermore, the way the wound is made greatly influences its susceptibility. Wounds made with the electrocautery are roughly twice as susceptible to infection as those made with a cold knife.[5] Avulsed wounds are more susceptible then cleanly cut ones.[6] Wounds of the face are less susceptible than those of the normal foot. Wounds made in the ischemic foot are vastly more susceptible yet. Traumatized patients are clearly more infectable than normals.[7] In addition, wounds are susceptible to only a few of the many bacteria that contaminate them. Obviously, local conditions within the wound can foil the host defenses.

Some explanations for the vulnerability of wounds lie in the physiology of injury itself. When the wound is made, ruptured vessels bleed and then thrombose back to the nearest through-flowing vessel. In normal connective tissue and dermis, this creates a space of 50 to 100 μm of unperfused tissue. Because of the normal differences in capillary density, the space is larger in the extremities than in the face, and larger in connective tissue than in parenchymatous organs. Infectability is closely and *inversely* related to the blood flow through the injured and contaminated tissue.

The end result is local hypoxia, hypercarbia, acidosis, low glucose (except in diabetics), and usually increased lactic acid concentration. These environmental conditions are also characteristic of many natural spaces (the appendix, gallbladder, middle ear), especially those that have become obstructed. They are also characteristic of infarcts.

To reach the inaccessible portions of a wound, a phagocyte must be able to travel long distances under its own power. The most mobile of all the defensive cells is the polymorphonuclear leukocyte, and these cells are the first line of defense against infection in injured tissue.

The adequacy of the defense, then, must rest on such factors as how many granulocytes can be delivered, how rapidly they can arrive, how competent they are when they arrive, how well they can function in the abnormal environment of injured tissue, and how much of a task there is for them to do. Each leukocyte has a finite capacity for seeking out, ingesting, and killing bacteria. In examining experimental studies on infected wounds, one finds that there is a critical inoculum of about 10^6 bacteria above which infection is likely to result.[8] By the end of the first few hours after injury, fluid from normal wounds contains

TABLE 13-19. INCIDENCE OF INFECTION (PERCENT) IN RELATION TO WOUND CLASSIFICATION *

	Five Hospitals (1964)	Foothills Hospital (1973)	University of California Hospitals (1975)
Distribution of operations (total)	(15,613)	(23,649)	(7,570)
Clean	74.8	76.4	64.6
Clean-contaminated	16.5	17.5	22.3
Contaminated	4.3	3.2	7.9
Dirty	3.7	2.9	5.2
Incidence of wound infection (total)	7.4	4.8	2.1
Clean	5.0	1.8	1.4
Clean-contaminated	10.8	8.9	3.6
Contaminated	16.3	21.5	4.3
Dirty	28.5	38.3	—

* These are examples of infection rates in the four-category classification system. The rates in the five hospitals are based on 1964 data. General rates are thought to be only slightly lower today. However, the Foothills Hospital and University of California hospitals data support our belief that infection rates can and should be considerably lower today. The infection rates for "dirty" cases in the University of California study are not given because liberal use of secondary and delayed primary closure make the figure meaningless. This is also part of the reason why the heavily contaminated category rate is so low. But delayed primary closure does not affect the statistic for clean-contaminated cases.

From Cruse JPE, Foord R: *Arch Surg* 107:206, 1973; and Howard JM et al: *Ann Surg* 160(Suppl):1, 1964; University of California data given courtesy of A Giulliano, MD, and TK Hunt, MD.

approximately 10^6 granulocytes per ml. Obviously, the probability that an infection will result from any given inoculum will rise if fewer or less competent granulocytes can be delivered within the first few hours after injury and contamination.

Granulocytes are initially attracted into the wound by complement factors, especially C5a, which are released as a result of the injury, even in the absence of contamination or infection. The natural defense mechanism, therefore, contains a brigade of leukocytes, which arrive in the wound on suspicion. The cells that arrive first and encounter bacteria are activated to amplify the chemotactic response. They also secrete neutrophil-immobilizing factors, which prevent the egress of inflammatory cells.[9] Since almost all wounds are contaminated while far fewer become infected, this nonspecific inflammatory reaction is usually sufficient to ward off infection. An infection results when the initial response to injury, plus the augmented response to contamination, is unable to contain the initial contamination.

THE WOUND LEUKOCYTE

In order to reach the wound space, leukocytes must marginate on the damaged vascular endothelium. They must then migrate through the endothelial wall (diapadesis) and through tissue to reach the site of injury. Studies of leukocytes taken from the extracellular fluid of small, relatively atraumatic wounds reveal that despite this difficult journey, the cells arrive as well prepared to deal with bacteria as their fellow circulating cells that have not made the trip.[10] However, even normal bloodborne leukocytes, when placed in an in vitro environment that is as hypoxic as a wound space, are clearly less capable of killing bacteria than normal leukocytes kept in an arterial, or even venous, pO_2.[11] Figure 13-20 shows the effect of lowering environmental pO_2 on bactericidal capacity of normal leukocytes, and Figure 13-21 shows the effect of oxygen supply on wound infections in vivo.

Leukocytes appear to be able to migrate into hypoxic wounds. In fact, more granulocytes enter infected hypoxic wounds than hyperoxic ones. Although microbicidal capacity is less, hypoxic leukocytes ingest organisms normally.[12] The white cell seems to migrate normally at a pH of 7.1 or 7.2, which is characteristic of wounds. Other leukocyte functions have not been well tested at varying pH. Their ability to work in the hypercarbic atmosphere of perhaps 60 to 100 torr, which characterizes wounds, is also not well measured.

The microbicidal defect of hypoxic leukocytes results from failure of the oxidative bactericidal pathway (see section B). The well-known oxidative killing mechanism of leukocytes is impaired by chronic granulomatous disease (CGD), in which the cells lack the primary oxidase which converts dissolved oxygen to superoxide, from which it is changed to other high-energy oxygen derivatives. In the absence of oxygen, which is the critical substrate for the primary oxidase, microbicidal activity of normal PMNs is identical to that of CGD cells incubated in the air.[11] One might speculate from the preceding data that organisms killed primarily by the oxidative killing mechanisms and not by intrinsic systems, such as granular cationic protein, lysozyme, and others, might be pathogenic, not so much by their own "strength" but because, within the hypoxic human wound, they have found a crack in the

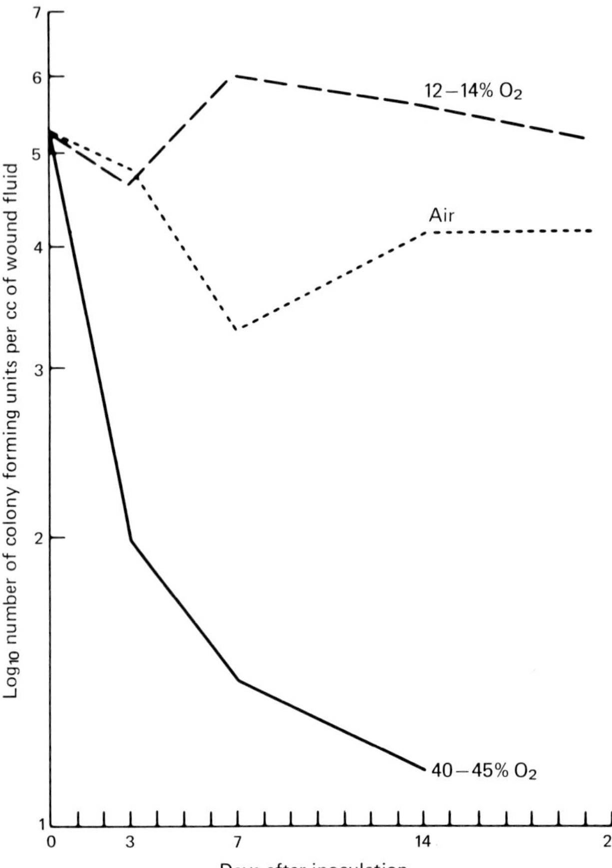

Fig. 13-20. **Staphylococci (502-A) were inoculated into wire mesh cylinder wounds in the backs of rabbits. One group of animals breathed 12 to 14 percent oxygen constantly. Others breathed air and 40 to 45 percent oxygen at 3, 7, and 14 days after inoculation. Wound fluid was aspirated and culture counts performed.**

body's armor. In fact, most of the organisms found in human wound infections are those killed largely by the oxidative killing pathway. This is particularly true of *S. aureus*, *E. coli*, and *Klebsiella*.[13] These bacteria, together with the anaerobes, are most pathogenic in a hypoxic environment and constitute the vast majority of organisms isolated from human wound infections. Organisms that are not killed primarily by the oxidative mechanism more often cause infection in patients who have suppressed cellular immunity and chronic exposure to infection, eg, patients with severe burns.

The journey from the blood vessel to the edge of the wound is also a critical event, and disorders of chemotaxis are important pathologic conditions which impair resistance to wound infection. A variety of conditions may contribute (see section B), ranging from defects in complement activation to the inability of immature cells to deform and squeeze through tissue interstices.

Leukocytes have a finite capacity to ingest and digest foreign material, devitalized tissue, and bacteria. Their capacity to ingest bacteria can be overwhelmed by devitalized tissue. There are, thus, two reasons for irrigating certain wounds—to remove bacteria and to remove foreign body and dead tissue that would sap the phagocytic capacity of leukocytes if allowed to remain.

CLINICAL DETERMINANTS OF WOUND INFECTION (Table 13-20)

Wounds made with the electrocautery or with a laser are more susceptible to wound infection than wounds made with the cold knife.[5] This fact presumably relates to the lateral diffusion of energy and the devitalization of tissue to the sides of the wound. Those closed with tapes are less likely to become infected than those closed with sutures.[14] This undoubtedly relates to the foreign body of the suture, which joins the outside of the wound to the wound space, as opposed to the tape, which rests solely on the outside of the wound. In at least one study, stapled wounds seem to be more prone to infection than wounds closed with tape (Chapter 22).[15] Table 13-20 lists some factors that are related to the cause of wound infections.

The presence of hypovolemia, vasoconstrictors, or anticomplement substances enhance wound infection when given in the first few hours after wounding.[2] This corresponds to the period in which oxygenation is most important and probably to the period in which bloodborne components such as complement, nonspecific antibody, and white cells are most urgently needed. Ischemia, in the determinative period, is therefore particularly detrimental.

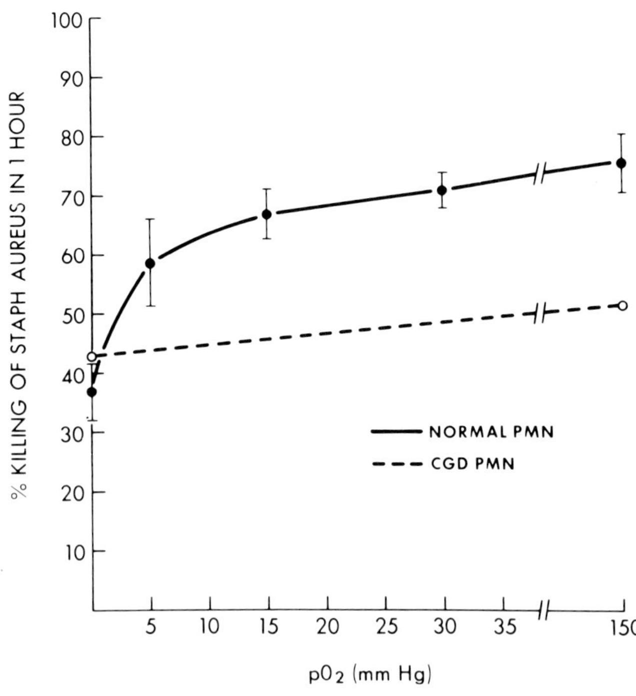

Fig. 13-21. **Percent killing of staphylococci (502-A) mixed with leukocytes and wound fluid. The rate of kill is obviously diminished at low pO_2. Anoxic leukocytes are equivalent to leukocytes taken from children with symptomatic chronic granulomatous disease. This is a large and significant decrement.**

TABLE 13-20. FACTORS RELATED TO WOUND INFECTION

Contamination
Cautery
Technique of dividing tissue
Dead tissue
Foreign body
Suture size
Suture material
Type of closure (suture, tapes, staples, clips)
Corticosteroid therapy
Ischemia
Hypoxia
Blood viscosity
Catecholamines
Prophylactic antibiotics
Preoperative shave
Diabetes
Delayed closure
Dead spaces
Drains
Dressings

There is disagreement about whether diabetes increases susceptibility to infection. Certainly, well-controlled diabetics have no higher infection rates than normal patients. However, diabetics operated upon under emergency conditions with high blood sugars are particularly susceptible to infection, and the reasons for this susceptibility are not fully known. Some of it certainly has to do with neuropathy and ischemia. Whether or not leukocyte phagocytic function is defective in hyperglycemia is being studied and debated.[16]

Obese patients are more likely to become infected than nonobese patients.[5] Whether this relates to diabetes or the mass of subcutaneous tissue that must be cut, the extra sutures that are often required, the lower arterial pO_2 that such patients characteristically have, hypertension, vasoconstriction, or other factors is unknown. Heavily contaminated subcutaneous tissue should be treated by delayed wound closure techniques to reduce the incidence of infection.[17]

Aged patients become infected more frequently than young ones.[18] Numerous immune mechanisms have been found to fade with age, but which ones relate to wound infection is unclear.

The degree of injury, both local and remote, from the wound is particularly important. If shock is induced by bleeding in an experimental animal and the blood immediately reinfused, healing and resistance to infection are not likely to be impaired. If blood volume remains significantly depressed, however, infection and poor healing are more likely. While this is largely a blood volume effect, blood viscosity changes are thought to play a part as well.[7]

Even the traditional preoperative shave has its effect. Those patients who are shaved the night before the operation are twice as likely to get wound infections as those who are shaved immediately before it. Those who are not shaved at all seem to be the most protected.[14] Long hair can be clipped with a barber shear.

Much is made of sutures and wound infection. In general, inert materials enhance infection less than absorbable or highly reactive suture. Large sutures enhance infection more than small.[14] In practice, however, the way the suture is used is more important. Too many, too large, too tight, or carelessly placed sutures strangulating large bits of tissue are all probably more important in enhancing infection than is the material of which the suture is made. Nevertheless, the best combination is good suture material and good surgery. Chapters 20 and 23 discuss the principles of the prevention of wound infection in greater detail.

BIBLIOGRAPHY

Hunt TK (ed): Wound Healing and Wound Infection: Theory and Surgical Practice. New York, Appleton-Century-Crofts, 1980.

Hunt TK, Dunphy JE (eds): Fundamentals of Wound Management. New York, Appleton-Century-Crofts, 1979.

REFERENCES

1. Altemeier WA, Burke JF, Pruitt BA, Sandusky WR: Manual on Control of Infection in Surgical Patients. American College of Surgeons. Philadelphia, Lippincott, 1976.
2. Burke JF: Infection. In Hunt TK, Dunphy JE (eds): Fundamentals of Wound Management. New York, Appleton-Century-Crofts, 1979, p 170.
3. Burke JF (ed): Surgical Physiology. Philadelphia, Saunders, in press.
4. Meakins JL: Host defense mechanisms, wound healing, and infection. In Hunt TK, Dunphy JE (eds): Fundamentals of Wound Management. New York, Appleton-Century-Crofts, 1979, p 242.
5. Cruse PJE, Foord R: A five-year prospective study of 23,649 surgical wounds. Arch Surg 107:206, 1973.
6. Cardany CR, Rodeheaver GT, Thacker J, Edgerton MT, Edlich RF: The crush injury: a high risk wound. J Am Coll Emerg Phys 5:965, 1976.
7. Hunt TK, Zederfeldt BH, Goldstick TK, Conolly MB: Tissue oxygen tensions during controlled hemorrhage. Surg Forum 18:3, 1967.
8. Elek SD: Experimental staphylococcal infections in the skin of man. Ann NY Acad Sci 65:85, 1956.
9. Weisbart RH, Golde DW, Spolter L, Eggena P, Rinderkneckt H: Neutrophil migration inhibition factor from T lymphocytes (NIF-t): a new lymphokine. Clin Immunol Immunopathol 14:441, 1979.
10. Hohn DC, Ponce B, Burton RW, Hunt TK: Antimicrobial systems of the surgical wound. I. A comparison of oxidative metabolism and microbicidal capacity of phagocytes from wounds and from peripheral blood. Am J Surg 133:597, 1977.
11. Hohn DC, MacKay RD, Halliday B, Hunt TK: The effect of O_2 tensions on the microbicidal function of leukocytes in wounds and in vitro. Surg Forum 27:18, 1976.
12. Hunt TK, Linsey M, Grislis G, Sonne M, Jawetz E: The effect of differing ambient oxygen tensions on wound infection. Ann Surg 181:35, 1975.
13. Babior BM: Oxygen-dependent microbial killing by phagocytes (first of two parts). N Engl J Med 298:659, 1978.
14. Conolly WB, Hunt TK, Zederfeldt B, Cafferata HT, Dunphy JE: Clinical comparison of surgical wounds closed by suture and adhesive tapes. Am J Surg 117:318, 1969.

15. Edlich RF, Rodeheaver GT, Thacker JG, Edgerton M: Technical factors in wound management. In Hunt TK, Dunphy JE (eds): Fundamentals of Wound Management. New York, Appleton, 1979, p 364.
16. Mowat AG, Baum J: Chemotaxis of polymorphonuclear leukocytes from patients with diabetes mellitus. N Engl J Med 284:622, 1971.
17. Verrier ED, Bossart J, Heer FW: Reduction of infection rates in abdominal incisions by delayed wound closure techniques. Am J Surg 138:22, 1979.
18. Gardner ID: The effect of aging on susceptibility to infection. Rev Infect Dis 2:801, 1980.

F. Alterations of Host Defenses in the Surgical Patient

JONATHAN L. MEAKINS

The primary immunodeficiencies have been discussed in the preceding sections in their appropriate categories: (1) antibody or B-cell deficiency, (2) cellular or T-cell deficiency, (3) phagocytic cell dysfunction, (4) disorders of complement, and (5) combined immunodeficiency disorders. A system of nomenclature has been proposed by a committee of the World Health Organization.[1]

ACQUIRED IMMUNODEFICIENCY IN SURGICAL PATIENTS

Much more common and of greater general clinical significance but less well defined are acquired defects of host defense. As in patients with congenital defects, the characteristic feature of acquired defects is also recurrent infection, but it has been difficult to identify the cause of the susceptibility except that it is the result of injury or stress in its broadest sense. Unlike congenital defects, in which a single defect usually accounts for the clinical manifestations, acquired defects involve more than one component of host defense.

BURNS

Recurrent infections, frequently life-threatening, are characteristic sequellae of thermal injury, and many of the components of the immune response are abnormal.[2] Thermal injury has, in fact, become the prototype of acquired derangement of host defenses because of the magnitude and breadth of the abnormalities. All defects return to normal following resolution and healing of the burn wound.

Humoral Responses

Immunoglobulins of all classes are reduced following thermal injury.[3,4] The early reductions are likely to be secondary to generalized catabolism, leakage into the burn wound and its underlying interstitial spaces, as well as some dilution by the enormous volumes of fluids required for resuscitation. Alexander and Moncrief[5] have shown that the primary humoral response to an antigen was reduced, although the anamnestic response to tetanus was earlier and greater than normal.

Complement levels are only slightly reduced after burns but become increasingly depressed if sepsis supervenes. Alexander et al[6] have shown that a consumptive opsonopathy occurs during infection.

Cellular Responses

Macrophage and reticuloendothelial system function is difficult to study in humans. Most animal studies indicate that reticuloendothelial function is somewhat depressed and that there is a reduced ability to deliver monocytes to an inflammatory focus after thermal injury.

Cell-mediated immunity is markedly altered following thermal injury. Both man and the experimental animal can accept skin allografts and even xenografts.[7,8] Pigskin xenografts have survived for prolonged periods in patients with burns over 30 percent of the body surface.[8] Burned patients are anergic to recall skin test antigens. Recovery of all these responses follows coverage of the burn wound.

Neutrophil function is similarly depressed following a major burn injury. Bactericidal function is abnormal, and such dysfunction sometimes coincides with the development of septic episodes.[2] Chemotaxis is defective in direct proportion to burn size and depth.[9] Neutrophil bactericidal function improves with nutritional support and the incidence of septicemia falls.[10] Once the burn wound is covered, neutrophil function returns to normal.

THE TRANSPLANT PATIENT

Transplantation became common clinical practice with the development of immunosuppressive regimens effective in preventing or treating rejection. The resultant pharmacologic immunosuppression induced a sizable risk of serious sepsis. Although more dexterous use of immunosuppression has reduced their incidences, infection remains the major cause of death.[11]

The principal immunosuppressive agents utilized in transplantation are corticosteroids and azathioprine. Steroid effects include reduced lymphoid proliferation, lympholysis of B and T cells in high concentrations, reductions in antibody formation, inhibition of neutrophil and monocyte chemotaxis, suppression of the inflammatory response, and prolongation of tissue allografts with concomitant effects on the efferent and afferent arcs of cell-mediated immunity. Azathioprine can reduce or abolish the delayed hypersensitivity response, the nonspecific inflammatory response, antigen processing, and the primary antibody and anamnestic response. Bone marrow suppression with significant leukopenia is the major potential complication leading to infection. The increased incidence of sepsis in this population is clearly a function of alteration of host defense mechanisms. Infections include all bacterial species as well as viral, fungal, and protozoal infestations (Chapter 47).

PATIENTS WITH INFECTIONS

Chapter 8 has reemphasized the interaction between various microbial agents and the effects produced by infection itself on the defenses against subsequent or superinfection (Tables 8-1 to 8-3).[11a]

All infected patients do not have reduced host defenses; in fact many bear neutrophils wirh enhanced chemotactic and bacteriocidal activity.[11b] Patients with more serious infections, however, show a depression in neutrophil function that is associated with increased susceptibility to subsequent infections.[11c]

IDENTIFICATION OF THE SURGICAL PATIENT WITH ACQUIRED DEFECTS OF HOST DEFENSE

In clinical practice, there are a number of situations in which one could predict an increased probability of sepsis—advanced age, major operation, trauma, diabetes, uremia, cancer, poor nutrition, severe pancreatitis, hemorrhagic shock, and sepsis, among many. Every patient in these categories does not, however, have detectable abnormalities of host defense, nor do they all develop infection. Identification of those likely to develop infection is an important task, in order to institute appropriate preventive measures and therapeutic adjustments. In addition, the development of a simple screening test to define a high-risk population would permit the selection of a population appropriate for further study of the critical defects. Selection of this population is difficult.

Investigations of primary immunodeficiencies involved a defined population of patients: those persons with recurrent infections. In surgical practice, investigations are usually instituted after the infection has already started. The discovered abnormalities may or may not have been present before the infectious episode and may be the result rather than the cause of the problem. Patients with potential for abnormalities of host defenses are a large and heterogeneous group. The approach of testing everyone is unrewarding and expensive.

Using the recall skin test antigens, defining the skin test results as in Table 13-11, and sepsis as a positive blood culture or an abscess identified at surgery or autopsy, we have shown that patients who are anergic (A) and relatively anergic (RA) had a significantly increased incidence of sepsis and death compared to those whose skin tests were normal (N).[12–14] (Table 13-21 A, B). The results have been confirmed.[15–18] These data show that skin testing preoperatively identified a group of patients at risk for increased sepsis and mortality following surgery. Sequential skin testing indicates that patients who become anergic and recover normal responses have a higher ratio of sepsis *while* anergic, but have much improved mortality rate compared to those who *remain* anergic.[13]

Regardless of the patient population studied (preoperative, postoperative, intensive care,[12,13] trauma,[19,20] all general surgical, nonoperative surgical, cancer,[21] gastrointestinal bleeding [22]), the presence of altered responses to skin tests with recall antigens has predictive value for patient sepsis and mortality and identifies a patient population unusually sensitive to major infection.

Cutaneous responses to recall antigens—delayed hypersensitivity reactions (DHR)—are classically considered to be a reflection of cell-mediated immunity. The infections for which cell-mediated immunity is effective are rare in surgical patients, and the organisms that produce sepsis in anergic patients are common bacteria. Host response against these organisms is mediated via the humoral and phagocytic components of host defense. This suggests that even though the delayed hypersensitivity reaction is altered and correlates with increased rate and

TABLE 13-21.A. CLINICAL OUTCOME ACCORDING TO SKIN TEST RESPONSES IN TWO PROSPECTIVE STUDIES: SEPSIS AND MORTALITY FOLLOWING INITIAL SKIN TEST

Patients Studied	Response	Number	Sepsis (%)	Mortality (%)
Preoperative (322)	Anergy	21	4 (19.0)	7 (33.3)
	Relative anergy	21	5 (23.8)	7 (33.3)
	Normal	280	13 (4.6)	12 (4.3)
Postoperative after trauma (115)	Anergy	71	44 (62.0)	24 (33.8)
	Relative anergy	25	15 (60.0)	6 (24.0)
	Normal	19	5 (26.3)	1 (5.3)
No operation (83)	Anergy	23	5 (21.7)	11 (47.8)
	Relative anergy	4	1 (25.0)	1 (25.0)
	Normal	56	0 (0.0)	1 (1.8)

TABLE 13-21.B. CLINICAL OUTCOME ACCORDING TO SKIN TEST RESPONSES IN TWO PROSPECTIVE STUDIES: SEPSIS AND MORTALITY IN 1,776 PATIENTS BASED UPON LEAST REACTIVE SKIN TEST

Skin Test	Patients	Sepsis (%)	Mortality (%)
Normal	1172	88 (7.5)	25 (2.1)
Relative anergy	178	57 (32)	27 (15)
Anergy	426	200 (47)	149 (35)

severity of infectious complications, the defect may be a general one and other anti-infective aspects of host defense are likely to be abnormal.

IMMUNOLOGIC STUDIES IN ANERGIC SURGICAL PATIENTS

In conjunction with skin testing, numerous measures of host defense have been assessed in normal and anergic patients. Mixed lymphocyte culture, lymphocyte response to the phytohemagglutinin [23] and pokeweed mitogens, cell-mediated lympholysis, and lymphocyte generation of blastogenic factor were all normal.[12] In four anergic patients, a serum inhibitor of their mixed lymphocyte culture was present.[12] Anergic patients had a reduction in the total lymphocyte count and number of rosetting T lymphocytes.[24]

Neutrophil chemotaxis is reduced in patients with altered skin test responses and returns toward normal with recovery of normal responses.[24-26] This evolution of chemotaxis to normal is more clearly seen in trauma patients. Following major injury, neutrophil chemotaxis is reduced to anergic levels within hours of the injury (Fig. 13-22). Recovery of normal neutrophil chemotaxis can take weeks.[19,20] The prompt appearance of defective neutrophil chemotaxis suggests that it is mediated by a serum factor. Neutrophil adherence is significantly increased and is directly correlated with chemotaxis.[25]

Anergic serum was found to consistently inhibit the chemotaxic responses of normal cells.[27] One inhibitor was found in all sera and has pI = 6.2, $S_{20,w}$ = 5.3, and MW = 110,000. The other was found only in anergic sera and has pI = 4.6, $S_{20,w}$ = 9.4, MW = 310,000. The data suggest that the decreased PMN chemotaxis observed in anergy is the result of the de novo appearance of the larger PMN chemotaxis inhibitor and that decreased neutrophil chemotaxis and skin test anergy correlated highly with increased sepsis and mortality in the surgical patient.

Solomkin et al [27a] have shown that defects in neutrophil chemotaxis in infected surgery patients are associated with both elevated C5a levels in plasma and loss of C5a receptors on neutrophils. Exposure of normal neutrophils to patient plasma reduces the number of C5a receptors on normal neutrophils and also impairs normal neutrophil function.

Chenoweth et al [27b] have shown similar results in patients undergoing open heart operations.

Lymphocyte chemotaxis [23] was studied to assess whether or not anergy might be caused by a failure of recruitment of lymphocytes to the area of antigen deposition. Lymphocytes from anergic patients migrated less well than did control lymphocytes. Simultaneous determinations of lymphocyte and neutrophil chemotaxis demonstrated that the two are highly correlated. Anergic sera, which decreased control neutrophil chemotaxis, also decreased normal lymphocyte chemotaxis. The failure of delayed hypersensitivity in surgical patients probably does not reflect classical defects in cell-mediated immunity. The defect resides in the chemotactic response, in the ability of the cell either to read the chemotactic gradient or to respond by cell migration.

Not every anergic patient has every defect. In general, however, 90 percent of anergic patients had increased neutrophil adherence, decreased neutrophil and lymphocyte chemotaxis, and a circulating inhibitor of chemotaxis of both cells. There may also be some defects in phagocytosis and bactericidal capacity. All these defects disappear as skin test responses return to normal.

ETIOLOGIC FACTORS IN ANERGY

Studies of preoperative patients support the association of skin test anergy with the subsequent development of sepsis. In other patients, however, it becomes difficult to say that sepsis is a result rather than a cause of abnormal host defenses. In some patients, sepsis is obviously a major factor in the development of anergy and associated defects

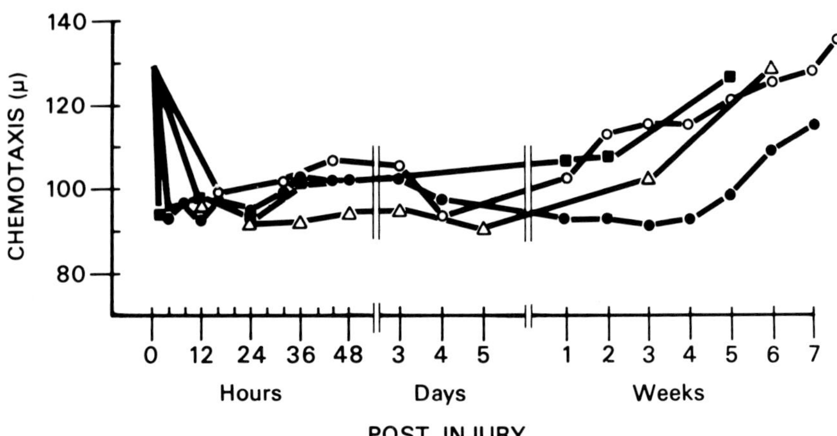

Fig. 13-22. **Neutrophil chemotaxis in four patients with blunt trauma from time of admission to recovery. Chemotaxis abnormal at *first* examination 2 to 12 hours after injury. Recovery of normal chemotaxis takes weeks.**

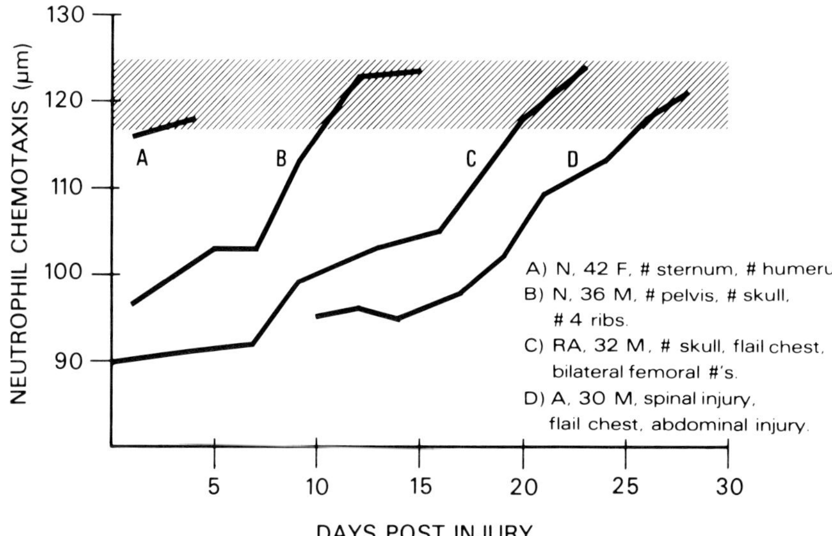

Fig. 13-23. **Recovery of neutrophil chemotaxis following injury of varying severity in patients of similar age. (From Meakins JL, McLean APH, Kelly R, et al: Delayed hypersensitivity and neutrophyl chemotaxis: effect of trauma. *J Trauma* 18:240, 1978.)**

in host defense. In these patients, eradication of the septic process is immediately followed by recovery of normal skin test reactions.[28]

The pathogenesis of anergy in surgical patients is difficult to completely sort out because multiple factors can contribute. Several clinical correlations can be made, however. Anergy following blunt trauma develops as a function of the age of the patient and the severity of injury. Neutrophil chemotaxis is reduced after major trauma, as a result of the action of a serum factor. The duration of abnormality is a function of the severity of the injury (Fig. 13-23). Following gastrointestinal hemorrhage, development of anergy is related to clinical measures of blood volume such as pulse and the total volume of blood and colloid solutions administered and is unrelated to nutrition or etiology of bleeding.[22] In cancer patients, on the other hand, nutritional measures seem more important in the anergic state than blood volume or site of origin.[21] In each of these patient populations, the anergic state precedes infection.

Malnutrition independently contributes to immune defects. In many of the patients with multifactorial problems, and frequently in those with sepsis, malnutrition is a component of the surgical illness. Abnormal body composition compatible with malnutrition is clearly associated with anergy. The restoration of body composition to normal with total parenteral nutrition is associated with restoration of skin test responses.[29] While not the only cause of anergy, malnutrition may be a significant contributing factor, and in some instances the only etiologic factor.

OTHER FACTORS PRODUCING ACQUIRED IMMUNODEFICIENCY

Operation and Anesthesia

It becomes very difficult to separate the effects on the immune response of operation from that due to anesthesia. Operation suppresses leukocyte counts and antibody production for 72 hours. Phagocytosis, allergic responses and skin reactivity may be depressed. Neutrophil chemotaxis is not affected by anesthetics or superficial operation but is reduced by abdominal or cardiac operation.[30-32] At present, these cannot be related directly to the development of bacterial infection, although they may be important in the spread of tumor cells. Anesthetic gases do appear to adversely affect B cell, T cell, and phagocyte function. What this transient insult means for the patient is not clear.

Immunosuppressive Effect of Pharmacologic Agents

Many drugs, by design or inadvertence, have immunosuppressive properties. The adrenocortical steroids have been the cornerstone of immunosuppressive therapy since their development. Their effects are global—reduced lymphoid proliferation, lympholysis of B and T cells in high concentrations, reduction in antibody formation, inhibition of neutrophil and monocyte chemotaxis, suppression of inflammation, prolongation of tissue allografts with concomitant effects on afferent and efferent arcs of cell-mediated immunity. Clearly, one of the side effects of steroid usage is the development of infectious complications.

The purine antagonists, azathioprine and 6-mercaptopurine, have significant immunosuppressive properties and have been, together with the corticosteroids, the agents that have allowed clinical transplantation to become a reality. The development of viral infection is common in these patients. If dosage is not carefully controlled, bone marrow suppression and neutropenia frequently lead to bacterial or fungal infection.[11] The infectious complications of cancer chemotherapy drugs are also largely related to bone marrow suppression and resultant neutropenia. Neutrophil function does not otherwise seem grossly affected.

Antibiotics may have immunosuppressive properties and may theoretically be working at odds with therapy. The high incidence of superinfection in patients on antibiotic therapy, particularly the development of *Candida* infections, has been ascribed in part to antibiotic-mediated immunosuppression. The major practical difficulty relates to bone marrow suppression, which results occasionally from many antibiotics. The idiosyncratic irreversible bone marrow aplasia caused by chloramphenicol is the best known of these effects.

Other classes of drugs, of which the salicylates are the best known and most important, may have some immunosuppressive activity.

Malnutrition and Acquired Immunodeficiency

A broad range of immunodeficiencies involving most components of the immune response are induced by malnutrition.[33,34] Their relationship to infection seems intuitively clear but has been difficult to prove. The question has been raised as to whether malnutrition decreases the immune response or infection precipitates malnutrition. The interaction of infection, malnutrition, and immunodeficiency is probably a vicious circle, each making the next stage worse.

Malnutrition can be shown to decrease phagocytic and bactericidal function, decrease complement levels and antibody responses, reduce lymphocyte response to mitogens, and obviate delayed hypersensitivity responses (Chapter 19). The use of total parenteral nutrition [35-38] and oral hyperalimentation [10] will restore host defenses to normal and reduce the associated rates of sepsis. The malnourished patients are usually anergic, and restoration of body cell mass restores cutaneous responses to normal in about a third.

Disease States Associated with Immunosuppression

Many disease states have a high incidence of infectious sequelae. Infections are even more common as treatment prolongs the lifespan of patients with metabolic derangements (diabetes, uremia), neoplastic disease (leukemias, lymphomas, advanced solid tumors), or altered physiologic states. An additional concern is that therapy may itself further reduce resistance, ie, cancer chemotherapy, immunosuppression. In advanced cancer or diabetes, there are secondary anatomical, physiologic, and nutritional alterations, all of which directly affect the local or systemic response to infection.

Today's surgeons are presented with a vastly different patient population from their predecessors. The natural histories of many illnesses are being altered, and new surgical situations constantly appear. The patient in end-stage renal failure is just one example. Transplantation, hemodialysis, and chronic ambulatory peritoneal dialysis have completely altered the inevitable outcome of kidney failure but have substituted a new set of potential problems. Alteration of host resistance is almost universal in these patient groups.

TABLE 13-22. ANERGIC PREOPERATIVE PATIENTS: COMPARISON OF OUTCOME WITH LEVAMISOLE OR PLACEBO

	Levamisole (19)	Placebo (20)
Sepsis	3 (16)	9 (45)
Mortality	2 (10)	5 (25)
Improved skin test	14 (74)	12 (60)
Improved chemotaxis	11/16 (69)	9/18 (50)

TREATMENT OF ACQUIRED IMMUNODEFICIENCIES IN SURGICAL PATIENTS

GENERAL PHYSIOLOGIC MAINTENANCE

Physiologic derangements are important in the development of infection, since such disturbances lead to acquired defects in host defense. Restoration of Bernard's "Milieu Interieure" has broader implications than simply the maintenance of vital signs. The restoration and maintenance of blood volume, good tissue perfusion, adequate pO_2, and a physiologic acid base balance are essential for the delivery and adequate function of the humoral and cellular responses to infection. Similarly, clean technically perfect operations have immunobiologic implications in the delivery and function of the mediators of host defense to the operative field.[39] Following recovery from the acute phase of injury and early respiratory insufficiency, sepsis is the major cause of death in the trauma patient. It is therefore of considerable significance that all aspects of a patient's physiology be supported with equal enthusiasm, starting from the moment he or she enters the emergency room.

THE OPERATION

Operative correction of the underlying disease frequently corrects the defects in host defense. Drainage of infection, control of hemorrhage, relief of bowel obstruction, and resection of cancer, with no other treatment, lead to conversions of skin test from anergy to relatively anergic or normal.[12,28,40] Although the skin test responses are accompanied by improvement in a patient's general physiologic state, the effects are obviously due to changes at the cellular and molecular level. The persistence of anergy frequently indicates that there are complications that require attention.[28] In our experience,[28] anergy that continues after drainage of an abscess suggests inadequate drainage, another focus of sepsis, *or* both.

For this reason, major operations, when directed at the cause of the anergic state, must not be deferred "to build the patient up." Total parenteral nutrition is a valuable support for the catabolic septic patient. Cure of the primary disease may be the better solution.

NUTRITION

For many reasons, one of them immunologic, total parenteral nutrition was probably the single most significant development in surgical care in the 1970s. However, it is as yet not possible to state the role of nutrition in maintenance and support of the immune system. Infection and malnutrition have been linked for centuries.

Each thrives upon the other. Infection contributes or aggravates malnutrition, and malnutrition aids in providing the susceptible host for an infection. In our studies, sepsis is both a cause and a result of malnutrition. The causative component relates primarily to the extraordinary metabolic demands of infected patients and their subsequent catabolism (Chapters 15 and 16). In anergic patients, about a third respond to total parenteral nutrition by converting skin tests to normal.[29] The balance of patients do not change skin tests and, significantly, their body composition remains the same. Total parenteral nutrition is therefore required to maintain body cell mass and presumably also helps maintain, although not augment, host defense.

Studies in man and animal have shown that malnutrition induces a variety of abnormalities of host defense, all of which can be corrected by nutritional replenishment.[10,35-38,40] The route of nutritional support is said to be important in burn patients, whose neutrophil function is improved, and infection and mortality rates reduced, by enteric nutrition rather than total parenteral nutrition.[10]

IMMUNOMODULATING AGENTS

We still do not have effective direct means of stimulating the immune system during an acute situation. Vaccines have not proved efficacious in most common bacterial diseases. The most active research in modulation of the immune response is in cancer therapy, where *C. parvum*, Bacille Calmette-Guerin (BCG), glucan, levamisole, and a host of other pharmacologic or microbial products are being tested (Table 13-22). The effort is directed toward stimulating immune responses, or restoration of abnormal immune response to normal and as a means of controlling or curing cancer. These immunomodulating agents are discussed in Chapter 19.

BIBLIOGRAPHY

Howard RJ: Effect of burn injury, mechanical trauma, and operation on immune defenses. Surg Clin North Am 59:199, 1979.

Simmons RL (ed): Surgical Aspects of Immunology (symposia). Surg Clin North Am 59(2):183, 1979.

REFERENCES

1. Fudenberg HH, Good RA, Goodman HC, Hitzig W, Kunken HG, Roitt IM, Rosen FS, Rowe DS, Seligmann M, Soothill JR: Primary immunodeficiencies: Report of a World Health Organization Committee. Pediatrics 47:927, 1971.
2. Alexander JW, Meakins JL: A physiologic basis for opportunistic infection. Ann Surg 176:273, 1972.
3. Arteison G, Hogman CF, Johnson SGO, Killander J: Changes in immunoglobulin levels in severely burned patients. Lancet 1:546, 1969.
4. Ritzmann SE, McLung C, Falls D: Immunoglobulin levels in burned patients. Lancet 1:1152, 1969.
5. Alexander JW, Moncrief JA: Alterations of the immune response following severe thermal injury. Arch Surg 93:75, 1966.
6. Alexander JW, McClelland MA, Ogle CK, Ogle JD: Consumptive opsonopathy. Possible pathogenesis in lethal and opportunistic infections. Ann Surg 184:672, 1976.
7. Kay GD: Prolonged survival of a skin homograft in a patient with very extensive burns. Ann NY Acad Sci 64:64, 1957.
8. Polk HC: Prolongation of xenograft survival in patients with pseudomonas sepsis: a clarification. Surg Forum 19:514, 1968.
9. Warden GD, Mason AD, Pruitt BA: Suppression of leukocyte chemotaxis in vitro by chemotherapeutic agents used in management of thermal injuries. Ann Surg 181:363, 1975.
10. Alexander JW: Emerging concepts in control of clinical infection. Surgery 75:934, 1974.
11. Matas A, Simmons RL, Najarian JS: Sepsis in renal transplant recipients. In Hardy JD (ed): Critical Surgical Illness. Philadelphia, Saunders, 1980, p 552.
11a. MacKowiak PA: Microbial synergism in human infections (part 2). N Engl J Med 298:83, 1978.
11b. Barbour AG, Crain DA, Solberg CO, Hill HR: Chemiluminescence by polymorphonuclear leukocytes from patients with active bacterial infection. J Inf Dis 141:14, 1980.
11c. Solomkin JS, Bauman MP, Nelson RD, Simmons RL: Neutrophils dysfunction during the course of intraabdominal infection. Ann Surg 194:9, 1981.
12. MacLean LD, Meakins JL, Taguchi K, Duignan JP, Dhillon KS, Gordon J: Host resistance in sepsis and trauma. Ann Surg 182:207, 1975.
13. Pietsch JB, Meakins JL, MacLean LD: Delayed hypersensitivity response: application in clinical surgery. Surgery 82:349, 1977.
14. Christou NV: Alterations in host defense mechanisms of surgical and trauma patients with particular reference to polymorphonuclear function and predisposition to sepsis and mortality. PhD Thesis, McGill University, 1980.
15. Johnson WC, Ulrich F, Meguid MM, Lepak N, Bowe P, Harris P, Alberts LH, Nabseth DC: Role of delayed hypersensitivity in predicting postoperative morbidity and mortality. Am J Surg 137:536, 1979.
16. George C, Robin M, Carlet J, Rapin M, Landais C, Sabatier C: Tests cutanés explorant l'immunité cellulaire chez les malades en reanimation. Nouv Press Méd 7:2541, 1978.
17. McLoughlin GA, Wu AV, Saporoschetz I, Nimberg R, Mannick JA: Correlation between anergy and a circulating immunosuppressive factor following major surgical trauma. Ann Surg 190:297, 1979.
18. Buzby GP, Mullen JL, Matthews DC, Hobbs CL, Rosato EF: Prognostic nutritional index in gastrointestinal surgery. Am J Surg 139:160, 1980.
19. Meakins JL, McLean APH, Kelly R, Bubenik O, Pietsch JB, MacLean LD: Delayed hypersensitivity and neutrophil chemotaxis: effect of trauma. J Trauma 18:240, 1978.
20. Christou NV, McLean APH, Meakins JL: Host defense in blunt trauma: interrelationships between kinetics of anergy and depressed neutrophil function, nutritional status and sepsis. J Trauma 20:833, 1980.
21. Meakins JL, Christou NV, Hallé C, MacLean LD: Influence of cancer on host defense and susceptibility to infection. Surg Forum 30:115, 1979.
22. Christou NV, Meakins JL, Gotto D, MacLean LD: Influence of gastrointestinal bleeding on host defense and susceptibility to infection. Surg Forum 30:46, 1979.
23. Christou NV, Meakins JL: Delayed hypersensitivity: a mecha-

nism for anergy in surgical patients. Surgery 86:78, 1979.
24. Meakins JL, Pietsch JB, Bubenick O, Kelly R, Rode H, Gordon J, MacLean LD: Delayed hypersensitivity: indicator of acquired failure of host defenses in sepsis and trauma. Ann Surg 186:241, 1977.
25. Christou NV, Meakins JL: Neutrophil function in surgical patients: neutrophil adherence and chemotaxis and cutaneous anergy. Ann Surg 190:557, 1979.
26. Zigmond SH, Hirsch JG: Leukocyte locomotion and chemotaxis. J Exp Med 137:387, 1973.
27. Christou NV, Meakins JL: Neutrophil function in surgical patients: two inhibitors of granulocyte chemotaxis associated with sepsis. J Surg Res 26:335, 1979.
27a. Solomkin JS, Jenkins MD, Nelson RD, Chenoweth D, Simmons RL: Neutrophil dysfunction in sepsis: II. Evidence for the role of complement activation products in cellular deactivation. Surgery 90:319, 1981.
27b. Chenoweth DE, Cooper SW, Hugli TE, Stewart RW, Blackstone EH, Kirklin JW: Complement activation during cardiopulmonary bypass: evidence of generation of C3a and C5a anaphylotoxins. N Engl J Med 304:497, 1981.
28. Meakins JL, Christou NV, Shizgal HM, MacLean LD: Therapeutic approaches to anergy in surgical patients: surgery and levamisole. Ann Surg 190:286, 1979.
29. Spanier AH, Pietsch JB, Meakins JL, MacLean LD, Shizgal HM: The relationship between immune competence and nutrition. Surg Forum 27:332, 1976.
30. Bubenik O, Meakins JL: Neutrophil chemotaxis in surgical patients. Effect of cardiopulmonary bypass. Surg Forum 27:267, 1976.
31. Slade MS, Simmons RL, Yunis EJ, Greenberg LJ: Immunodepression after major surgery in normal patients. Surgery 78:363, 1975.
32. Howard RJ, Simmons RL: Acquired immunodeficiencies after trauma and surgical procedures. Surg Gynecol Obstet 139:771, 1974.
33. Alexander JW: Nutrition and surgical infection. In ACS Manual of Surgical Nutrition, chap 19. Philadelphia, Saunders, 1975.
34. Susskind RM: Immune status of the malnourished host. In Dick G (ed): Immunological Aspects of Infectious Disease. Lancaster, England, MTP Press, 1979.
35. Dionigi R, Zonta A, Dominioni L, Gnes F, Ballabio A: The effects of total parenteral nutrition on immunodepression due to malnutrition. Ann Surg 185:467, 1977.
36. Law DK, Dudrick SJ, Abdou NI: Immunocompetence of patients with protein-calorie malnutrition. The effects of nutritional repletion. Ann Intern Med 79:545, 1973.
37. Law DK, Dudrick SJ, Abdou NI: The effects of dietary protein depletion on immunocompetence. The importance of nutritional repletion prior to immunologic induction. Ann Surg 179:168, 1974.
38. Copeland EM, MacFadyen BV, Dudrick SJ: Effect of intravenous hyperalimentation on established delayed hypersensitivity in the cancer patient. Ann Surg 184:60, 1976.
39. Edlich RF, Rodeheaver GT, Thacker JG, et al: Technical factors in wound management. In Hunt TK, Dunphy JE (eds): Fundamentals of Wound Management. New York, Appleton, 1979.
40. Daly JM, Dudrick SJ, Copeland EM: Intravenous hyperalimentation: effect on immunocompetence in cancer patients. JAMA, 1981, in press.

CHAPTER 14
Events in Early Inflammation

JOHN F. BURKE

THE early period of inflammation must be described rather than defined in terms of exact time, because the various reactions depend on the animal studied, the injury, and the interval between injury and observation. Early inflammation is comprised of various events occurring in the blood vascular system, the lymphatic system, and the interstitial tissues.

Changes in vascular permeability have been the most extensively investigated aspect of early inflammation, but the causes of the vascular response remain incompletely understood.[1-3]

Regardless of the cause of the inflammatory response (bacterial invasion, introduction of antigens,[4,5] or trauma such as heat or a severe blow,[6,7]), the sequence of vascular events during early inflammation and these phases of vascular permeability after injury provide a useful framework on which to construct an overall view of the sequential development of early inflammation. Figure 14-1 illustrates the relation of early inflammatory events in the lymphatics and in the interstitial area both to the vascular response and to each other. The interrelationships between the causes and effects of physical and chemical changes in this period have yet to be completely elucidated. No causal connection has been established, for example, between alterations in the chemical structure of the ground substance and changes in capillary permeability.

VASCULAR RESPONSE

The blood vascular system plays a predominant role in early inflammation. It makes the initial response to the injury, informs other defenses of the injury, and subsequently reacts to the effects of host resistance. Whereas the vascular bed continuously adjusts to various physiologic stimuli by vasodilation and vasoconstriction, injury induces a degree of vasodilation that exceeds the normal physiologic limits. As a result, vascular permeability increases and large amounts of plasma proteins pass into the interstitial fluid.

During the past 20 years, we have witnessed an intensive attempt to understand the fluctuations in vascular permeability that occur in the area of a developing inflammatory lesion. In 1961, Majno et al [8] demonstrated that both capillaries and venules took part in this periodic increase. Whereas the vascular change is usually biphasic, involving an *immediate* and a *delayed* response, three other patterns may occur (Fig. 14-1). For example, depending on the severity of injury the fluctuation may consist of only a single phase,[9] or there may be periods of normal or nearly normal permeability between repeated periods of increased permeability.[10,11] It is believed that two independent chains of events elicit the immediate and delayed responses.

THE IMMEDIATE RESPONSE

The immediate response is a single, defined process that occurs within minutes of tissue injury and lasts no more than one-half hour. It is most reliably explained as the result of the chemical action of a specific mediator. The mediator appears to be serotonin in the rat and histamine in the guinea pig. The uniformity in onset and duration of the immediate response and the fact that this response can be blocked with appropriate histamine or serotonin blocking agents add weight to the belief that there is a specific mediator involved.[12] Venules 20–30 μm in diameter [13] are most extensively involved, but other small venules (<100 μm in diameter) also play an important role.[8,14] Ultrastructural studies have demonstrated that adjacent endothelial cells contract, thereby widening the intercellular junctions.[15] Protein-containing plasma then leaks through the gaps between endothelial cells and filters through the basement membrane.[8,14,16]

THE DELAYED RESPONSE

The delayed phase of increased vascular permeability varies considerably in time of onset, magnitude, and duration, and is therefore more difficult to characterize (Fig. 14-1). It may occur without a preceding immediate phase, and is not affected by complete blocking of the immediate response. The delayed response may consist of either a single episode or a number of episodes, over a few hours to more than a day, depending on the strength and nature of the injury.[16] For example, if inflammation is the result of bacterial infection [3] or mild thermal injury,[12] the delayed response begins several hours after injury and continues for 2 to 3 hours. In such injuries, an immediate response usually precedes the delayed response, with an interval of low or normal permeability that lasts 1 hour or more between the two phases. In the case of a hypersensitivity reaction elicited by injection of tuberculin into a

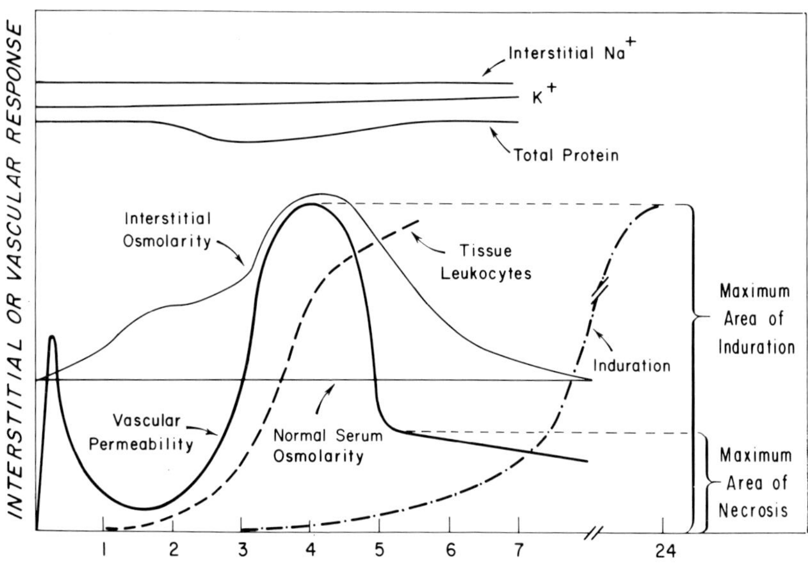

Fig. 14-1. A comparison of the time of occurrence of events in early inflammation. Changes in interstitial composition (osmolarity, electrolyte, and protein concentration) are compared with changes in vascular permeability and development of induration and tissue leukocytosis.

sensitized guinea pig, however, the delayed phase does not begin until 6 hours after the immediate response and lasts more than 40 hours.[17] In studies of the inflammatory response to graded doses of ultraviolet light, Logan and Wilhelm[10] have shown that the intensity of stimulus needed for a maximum immediate response or a maximum delayed response differs considerably.

Capillaries or venules are both involved in the delayed response.[18-20] Widening of the intercellular junctions between endothelial cells occurs, but the integrity of the endothelial cells remains unaltered. The mechanism by which intercellular junctions widen is unknown. There is no evidence that the delayed phase is triggered by a specific chemical substance in the same way that the immediate response is triggered by serotonin or by histamine. The delayed response cannot be inhibited by any known blocking agent. Evidence is accumulating that an evolving series of chemical and physical alterations in the interstitial area probably mediate the delayed response.

The efficiency with which various types of injury generate alterations in connective tissues, ground substance, and interstitial fluid might explain the variation in both time of onset (1 to 8 hours) and duration (2 to more than 40 hours) of the delayed response. Similarly, the fact that the delayed phase sometimes consists of more than one episode of increased permeability could be explained by the presence of more than one mode of injury—eg, bacterial and immunologic—each with a different period of action. There is a direct relation between the variability of the delayed response and the type of stimulus. The pattern of delayed response to ultraviolet radiation, for example, is generally consistent; its intensity is proportional to the stimulus. In contrast, the response pattern after immunologic injury with tuberculin differs considerably.

RESPONSE TO VASCULAR DAMAGE

The differences between the immediate response and the delayed response strongly suggest that the early evolution of an inflammatory lesion involves two separate processes. In fact, however, the biphasic pattern of increased vascular permeability occurs only when the stimulus cannot cause immediate destruction of the vascular endothelial cells. When these cells are destroyed, a third process takes place—vascular permeability immediately increases as a result of destruction of the vessel wall. The duration of increased permeability in this case depends on how long it takes before thrombosis prevents further flow in the destroyed vessel. This type of vascular alteration occurs after strong chemical injury, severe thermal injury, surgical incision, and crushing injury. When vessel destruction is incomplete, it is possible to have both an immediate increase in permeability due to vascular destruction and an immediate histamine or serotonin response plus a typical delayed response in the residual, viable tissues. Severe bacterial injuries may produce this type of response. In addition, several agents, such as bacterial toxins, ultraviolet radiation, and less severe chemical injuries, cause vessel destruction over a long period, further complicating attempts to understand early vascular responses in tissue injury.

INTERSTITIAL RESPONSE

Four aspects of interstitial response during early inflammation have been isolated and studied: (1) alterations in the interstitial fluid, (2) leukocyte accumulation, (3) development of induration, and (4) the overall ability of the tissue to protect itself against the injury in the "decisive period." Figures 14-1 and 14-2 illustrate temporal relationships between these responses and changes in vascular permeability.

ALTERATIONS IN INTERSTITIAL FLUID

Early changes in the interstitial fluid in the area of injury are substantial. They probably result from several influ-

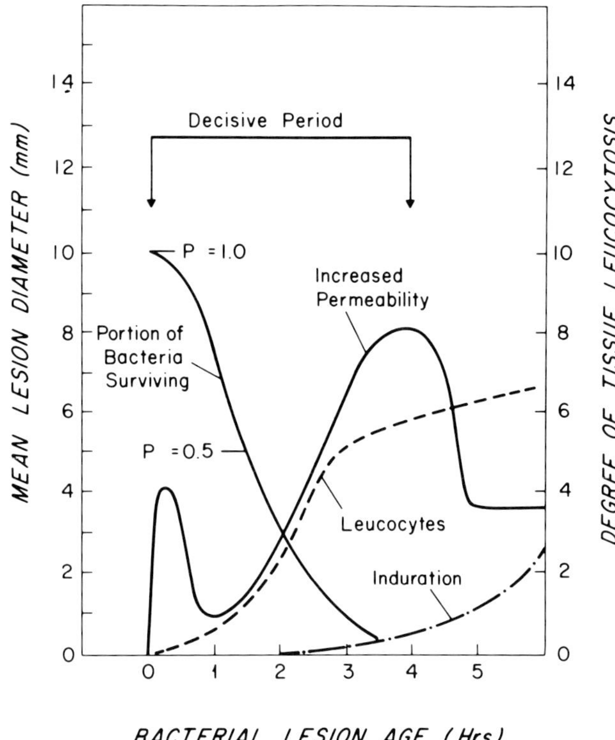

Fig. 14-2. **The period of active tissue antibacterial activity (decisive period) compared with the arrival of leukocytes in the tissue, the beginning of induration, and the phases of vascular permeability. P is a curve representing the estimated proportion of infecting bacteria surviving. Tissue defensive activity and bacterial control are seen to be far advanced before tissue leukocytosis, induration, or delayed permeability are changed.**

ences, including both alterations in collagen and the glycosaminoglycan ground substance, alterations of cells such as fibroblasts and muscle cells that are typically present in the area of inflammation, as well as from the increase in vascular permeability discussed earlier. Furthermore, since interstitial fluid is obtained by means of an implanted reservoir, artifacts can be introduced. It is now clear, however, that the normal composition of interstitial fluid is similar to that of plasma, except that the total protein concentration is much lower in interstitial fluid.[21,22] The protein concentrations in interstitial fluid are similar to those in regional lymph.[23]

We studied changes in interstitial fluid composition in the first several hours of bacterial inflammation in guinea pigs [22] and found a slow, steady increase in the potassium concentration, which leveled off at about 7 hours. This increase did not coincide with the time of increased vascular permeability or the period of increased osmolarity. At the same time, other interstitial electrolyte concentrations and the serum electrolyte concentration remained stable (Fig. 14-1). The reservoir was implanted adjacent to the panniculus carnosus, and although the additional potassium ions appeared to be released from damaged cells, especially muscle cells, it was not apparent whether the cellular damage was the result of the bacterial invasion or the presence of the reservoir. No consistent change was seen in the total protein concentration of the interstitial fluid when compared with control samples. Within 3 hours after inflammation began, however, it decreased by about 10 percent in several animals, returning to normal within the next 2 hours (Fig. 14-1). The increased protein known to extravasate from the inflamed vessels, therefore, does not appear to stay in the fluid phase but may be rapidly fixed in the affected interstitial area.

These studies substantiate earlier experiments in which we used microdensitometry to estimate the total protein concentration of interstitial fluid in situ during early inflammation, following infection with staphylococci.[22,23] A decrease in dry mass of the inflammatory exudate occurred at about 3 hours, and we interpreted this as indicating either an increase in water concentration or a decrease in protein concentration. This interpretation was strengthened by the fact that there was no evidence of containment of the area of developing inflammation by fibrin blockade within the first 6 hours.

Investigators have widely held that the increase in vascular permeability in early inflammation causes a high protein concentration in the vascular exudate. Our finding of a stable or slightly decreased protein concentration in interstitial fluid is inconsistent with this belief, and two explanations can be offered. First, extravasated protein would not be detectable in the lymphatics or in the implanted reservoir if it were "fixed" near its point of extravasation. Second, if there were an overall increase in volume but not an increase in the protein-water ratio from the permeable vessel, the protein concentration would stay the same, even though the total amount of protein extravasated would increase.

Of considerable interest is the fact that the osmotic pressure of the interstitial fluid begins to rise soon after bacterial injury.[21,22] It levels off somewhat after about 1 hour, rises steeply at 2 hours, peaks between 4 and 5 hours, and approaches the normal level between 6 and 7 hours (Fig. 14-1). In bacterial lesions, it coincides almost exactly with the delayed response of increased vascular permeability. Increased osmolarity has also been observed in experimental burns,[24] and it is thought to be caused by the formation of small molecules from larger molecules, triggered partly by uncontrolled enzymatic activity. Changes in the affinity for water and electrolytes, on the part of collagen and of glycosaminoglycans in the ground substance, could also explain local changes in osmolarity in the inflamed area.

ACCUMULATION OF LEUKOCYTES

Initially, the cellular response in the inflamed area is slight. Late in the first hour, however, neutrophils begin to marginate (aggregate) along the walls of the vessels in the inflammatory area; these leukocytes migrate into the interstitial area [25,26] within the second to the sixth hour (Figs. 14-1, 14-2). Heavy infiltration occurs in the tissue that will become necrotic, and the density decreases toward the periphery of the inflammation. Leukocytes have not been proved to cause either increased vascular permeability or alterations in interstitial fluid, although they accumulate throughout the period when these changes develop.[27,28]

INDURATION

The precise nature of induration is not understood, nor is there much known about the forces by which water and solute are kept in the inflamed area during healing. In experimental staphylococcal lesions, induration, as evidenced by tissue thickening with increased water concentration, becomes apparent 4 to 5 hours after bacterial injury, increases rapidly from 10 to 20 hours, and peaks at 24 hours (Fig. 14-1). In the guinea pig, infection with pyogenic bacteria produces a mature lesion from 24 to 36 hours after inflammation begins.[29] The extent of the delayed permeability response at approximately 3.5 hours, however, predicts how large the indurated area will be long before any of the traditional signs of inflammation have become apparent. In addition, the extent of permeability that persists at 5 hours predicts the extent of the necrotic area in the center of the mature lesion, and this is long before thrombosis and necrosis actually develop.[26,27]

LYMPHATIC RESPONSE

Even though the inflammatory response appears to be dominated by the blood vascular system, the lymphatic vascular system and the involved interstitial area also play important roles. Although the importance of the lymphatic system in the maintenance of fluid homeostasis is recognized [30-32] and a substantial amount is known about the flow rates of lymph,[33-35] its protein composition, and the fluid exchange between the blood and the interstitium,[33-37] there is still a great deal to learn about the unidirectional flow of interstitial fluids and the mechanisms controlling the permeability of the lymphatic capillaries. Much more emphasis has been placed on understanding the mechanisms by which the blood vascular system responds to provide increased flow of fluids, proteins, and cells into the interstitial area than on understanding how these substances are removed.

Because of the structural arrangement and the thinness of adjacent endothelial cells, water and crystalloids continuously pass across blood capillary walls to provide oxygen and nutrients to all tissue.[38-40] In addition, the plasma proteins that permeate the interstitial area leak through the blood capillary walls; the amount of protein lost from the plasma is about 4 percent of the total circulating protein. Whereas most resorption of water and crystalloid occurs at the venous limb of the blood capillaries, this is not true in the case of plasma proteins. Plasma proteins are cleared from the extravascular compartment and returned to the circulation through lymphatic vessels.[41,42] Without drainage by the lymphatic system, a gradient of colloid osmotic pressure across the blood capillary wall would not exist, because the relative concentration of interstitial colloid would become similar to that of plasma. As a result, water and electrolytes would no longer be resorbed into the venous limb, and intravascular volume would be lowered by a widespread fluid shift. The end result would be increased tissue edema. Proper function of the lymphatic system avoids this and also results in constant movement of lymphocytes throughout the body.[43]

Of the several components of the lymphatic system, the most important for the purposes of this chapter are the lymph nodes and the lymphatic capillaries. Although in some cases lymph is channeled directly into a vein from collecting vessels,[44] it must usually pass through at least one lymph node before it reaches the bloodstream.[45,46] Lymph is channeled into each node by afferent lymph vessels on the node surface; reflux is prevented by a valve at the junction of the afferent vessel with the node. A subcapsular sinus receives the lymph from the afferent lymphatics, and the fluid is then directed through radial sinuses that pass between nodules of lymphocytes in the cortex of the node. The radial sinuses branch into many anastomosing vessels in the medulla of the node, pursuing a radial course toward the hilus. Intermediate sinuses communicate with the subcapsular sinus at the hilus, where lymph is channeled into the efferent lymphatic.

Lymph nodes consist principally of supporting connective tissue, a reticular cell stroma, and lymphoid cells. In the stroma, a fibrous reticular meshwork serves both as a support for nerves and blood vessels and as a framework for the phagocytic and nonphagocytic reticular cells, including macrophages, lymphocytes, plasma cells, and other free and fixed cells. It may be that the crisscross arrangement of the reticular meshwork aids filtration of the lymph by slowing its flow. The cortical area contains nodular and diffuse lymphoid tissue. The nodules are composed of densely packed lymphocytes and have prominent pale germinal centers that frequently contain many large lymphoblasts. In addition, interconnected strands of densely packed lymphocytes extend from the cortex into the hilus. "Retothelial cells" [47] line the sinuses, which extend tortuously through the node.

Each lymph node contains a dense network of blood vessels; arteries enter at the hilus and then branch to the cortex and medulla. The medulla is also richly supplied with fenestrated capillaries, which allow larger molecules to pass rapidly across the endothelium. In this manner, antigens in the bloodstream can be transferred directly to the site of antibody formation. In the cortex, venules function importantly in lymphocyte recirculation.[48]

In the early 1930s, Drinker et al [45] demonstrated the efficiency of the lymph node as a filter for microorganisms. They channeled a perfusate heavily loaded with streptococci through the popliteal and iliac lymph nodes in sequence. They found that although the popliteal lymph node was ineffective, the iliac node blocked the streptococci successfully. More than 30 years later, Hall [48] demonstrated that the lymph nodes also produce cells that are involved in the propagation and dissemination of the immune response. The immunologic functions of the lymph node are discussed in Chapter 13.

The function of the lymphatic system depends on an easy access of fluid and large molecules, as well as white cells from the interstitial area to the lymphatic system. This transfer appears to take place almost exclusively at the level of the lymphatic capillary, where protein molecules and cells enter the system via specialized intercellular junctions between the lymphatic capillary cells. This flow of large particles and cells is facilitated by an absent, or irregular, basement membrane at the lymphatic capillary level and a system of one-way valves allowing flow in but not out of the capillary[41] (Figs. 14-3, 14-4). The lymphatic capillary endothelial cell is held in place by anchoring fibrils, which extend from the external cell membrane into the connective tissue (Figs. 14-3, 14-4, 14-5). These fibrils maintain the lumen of the lymphatic capillary even when the pressure in the interstitial space exceeds that in the capillary lumen. The anchoring fibrils extend along all abluminal surfaces except at the intercellular junctions where the cells are overlapped (Figs. 14-4, 14-6). At the overlap, the outer cell is supported but the inner cell is not. This means that if the pressure is greater outside the vessel, the inner overlapped cell portion acts as the movable portion of a simple flap valve and swings into the lumen, allowing fluid, large particles, and cells to enter (Fig. 14-6). If, however, the pressure is greater inside the vessel, the unsupported overlapped portion is pushed against the external supported portion, making a tight seal. In this way, the specialized overlapped cell junction of the lymphatic capillary endothelial cells, in coordination with the special distribution of the anchoring fibrils, creates a simple system maintaining the flow of fluid, particles, and cells[48,49] into the lymphatic system but not in reverse (Fig. 14-6).

Although the role of the lymphatic capillaries in acute inflammation is obviously important, the mechanisms by which the capillaries function to control local infection and to prevent its dissemination still require investigation. To study the structural alterations in lymphatic capillaries during the early phase of inflammation, we injected 0.002 ml bacterial suspensions into the ears of guinea pigs and albino mice; each injection contained approximately 10^6 viable *S. aureus.* We then examined the resultant lesions at intervals from 1 to 24 hours with electron microscopy and cinephotography.[50] In the first 4 hours after introduction of the bacteria, the patency of the lymphatic capillaries remained intact. Within the lesions and in their immediate vicinity, we observed an increased number of gaps between endothelial cells in the small blood vessels, as well as both red blood cells and leukocytes passing across the vessel wall. Other investigators have reported these

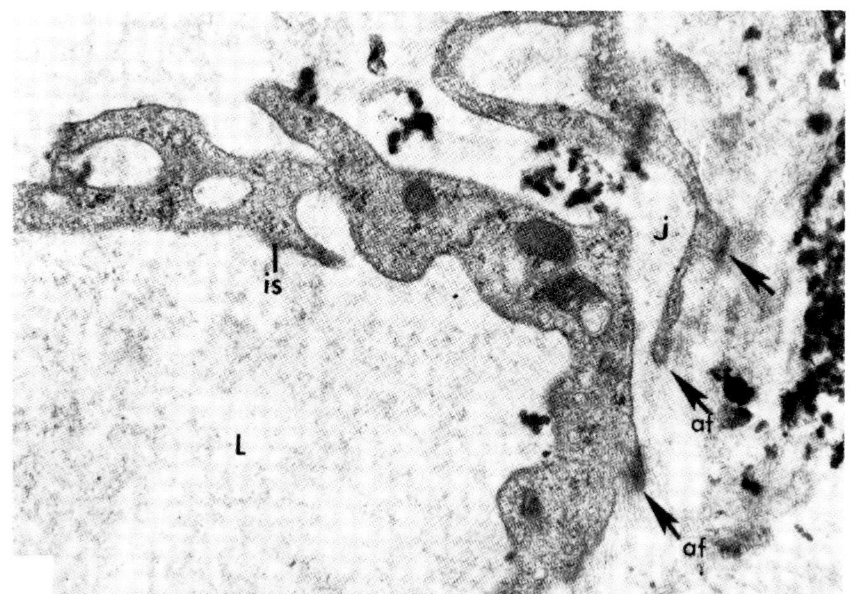

Fig. 14-3. **A patent intercellular junction (j) of a lymphatic capillary; anchoring filaments (af) are attached along the abluminal endothelial surface *(arrows).* The inner segment (is) acts as a "one-way flap valve" by swinging into the lumen (L) to allow free passage of fluids and particulate components (×21,024). (From Leak LV, Burke JF: Fine structure of the lymphatic capillary and the adjoining connective tissue area. *Am J Anat* 118:785, 1966.)**

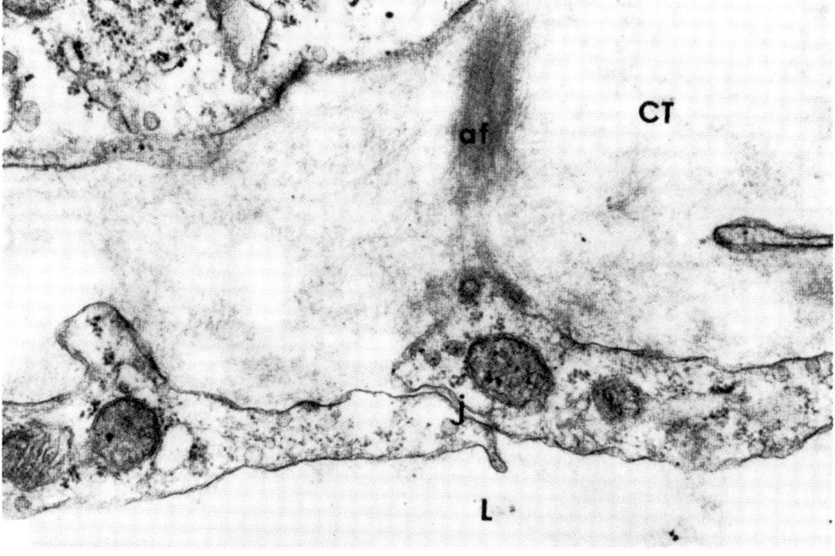

Fig. 14-4. **Part of the terminal cell process that comprises the cell junction (j) of the lymphatic capillary wall, containing anchoring filaments (af) that extend into the connecting tissue (CT) area (×18,000). (From Leak LV, Burke JF: Ultrastructural studies on the lymphatic anchoring filaments. *J Cell Biol* 36:129, 1968.)**

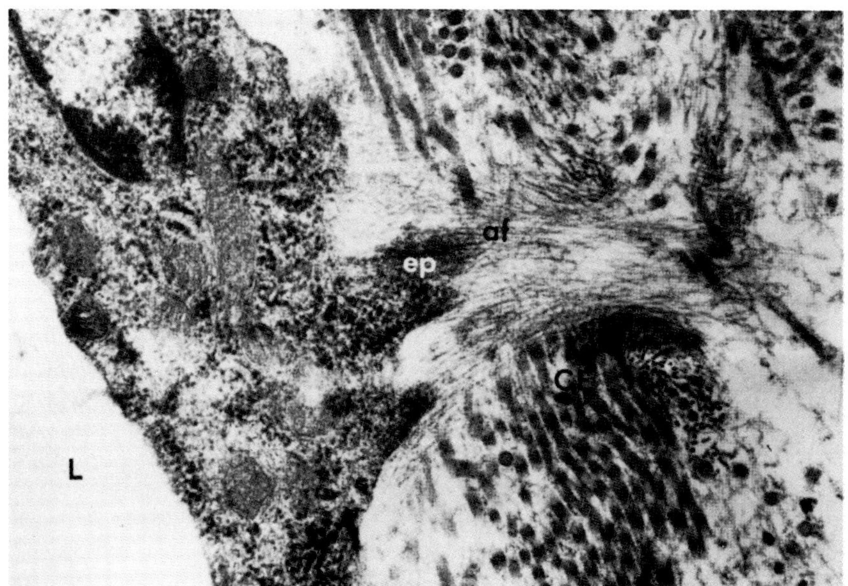

Fig. 14-5. The anchoring filaments (af) emanate from the lymphatic endothelial processes (ep) and extend into the adjoining interstitium for varying distances among collagen bundles (CF). L = lymphatic lumen (×20,016). (From Leak LV, Burke JF: Ultrastructural studies on the lymphatic anchoring filaments. *J Cell Biol* 36:129, 1968.)

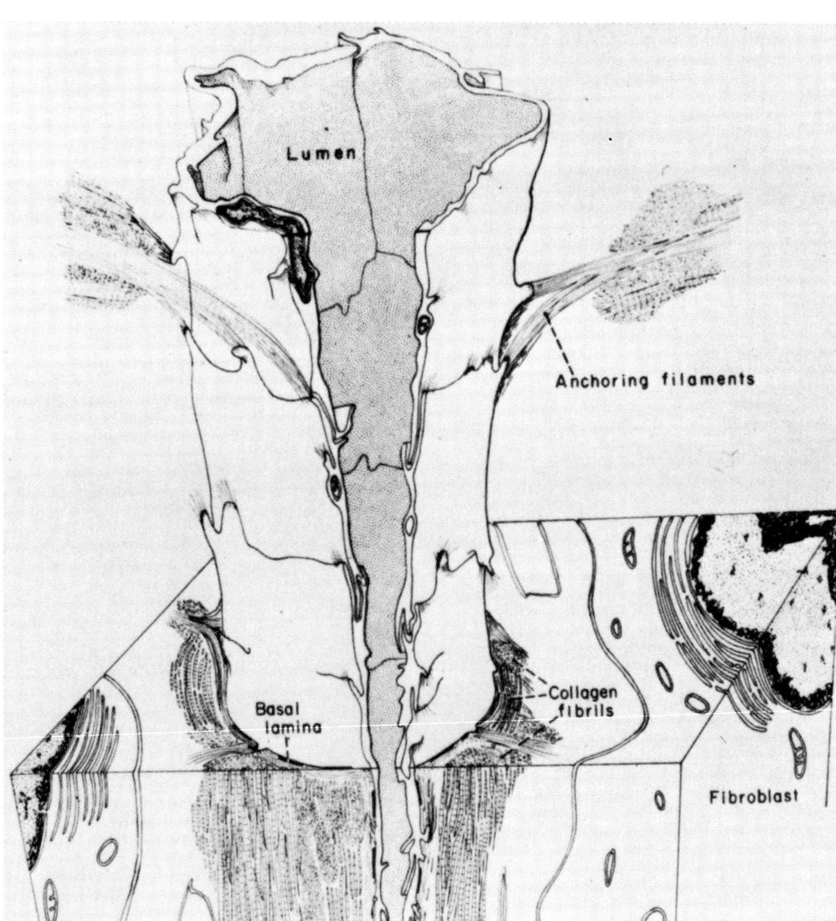

Fig. 14-6. A three-dimensional interpretive diagram of a lymphatic capillary showing its relationship to the surrounding interstitium (reconstructed from collated electron micrographs). The lymphatic anchoring filaments appear to originate from the endothelial cell surface and extend among collagen bundles, elastic fibers, and cells of the adjoining tissue area, thus providing a firm connection between the lymphatic capillary wall and the surrounding connective tissue. An irregular basement lamina and collagen fibers are indicated. (From Leak LV, Burke JF: Ultrastructural studies on the lymphatic anchoring filaments. *J Cell Biol* 36:129, 1968.)

same alterations after other types of injury.[6,21,50–54]

At the same time, there is a rapid increase in the number of patent junctions in the lymphatic capillaries, followed by dilatation to several times their normal size. Excess interstitial fluid, proteins, cells, and invading toxic bacterial or viral agents are constantly removed by this mechanism.

In similar experiments, we studied the flow of electron-dense material from the interstitial space, where it was injected into the lymphatic capillary lumen. Figure 14-7 shows an electron-dense flocculent material in the interstitial area similar to dense substance in the lymphatic lumen. Lymphatic anchoring filaments maintain the close association between the lymphatic wall and the connective tissue despite the gaps between adjacent endothelial cells. In the development of bacterial infection, the lymphatic endothelium initially suffers no obvious cellular damage up to 4 hours; the organelles and the longitudinal orientation of the cytoplasmic filaments are not altered. In contrast, after thermal injury the lymphatic endothelium, the blood vessels, and the interstitial area all suffer immediate cellular damage.

Flow of an increased amount of fluid and plasma proteins in the interstitial area during bacterial infection is manifested by an electron-dense, flocculent reticular meshwork (Fig. 14-7). In addition, electron-dense filaments presumed to be fibrin form dense aggregates throughout the interstitium. Within 24 hours of bacterial infection, the interstitium contains large amounts of fibrin near the lymphatic wall and frequently extends into the lumen of the lymphatic vessel through the widened intercellular junctions. At 24 hours, the lymphatic endothelial cells are still essentially intact, with few structural alterations. At the same time, leukocytosis and destruction of cells can be seen in the connective tissue.

The integrity of the lymphatic system is maintained by several factors. The anchoring filaments, which provide stability between the lymphatic capillary wall and the interstitial area, are particularly important. Also important are the overlapping endothelial cells, which can slide past each other for distances of several microns when fluid transport needs to be increased during inflammation (Fig. 14-6). Decompensation of the lymphatic capillary and therefore disruption of its tubular integrity would develop only if extreme interstitial edema were to take place. This usually occurs only if a collecting trunk or lymph node develops mechanical obstruction.

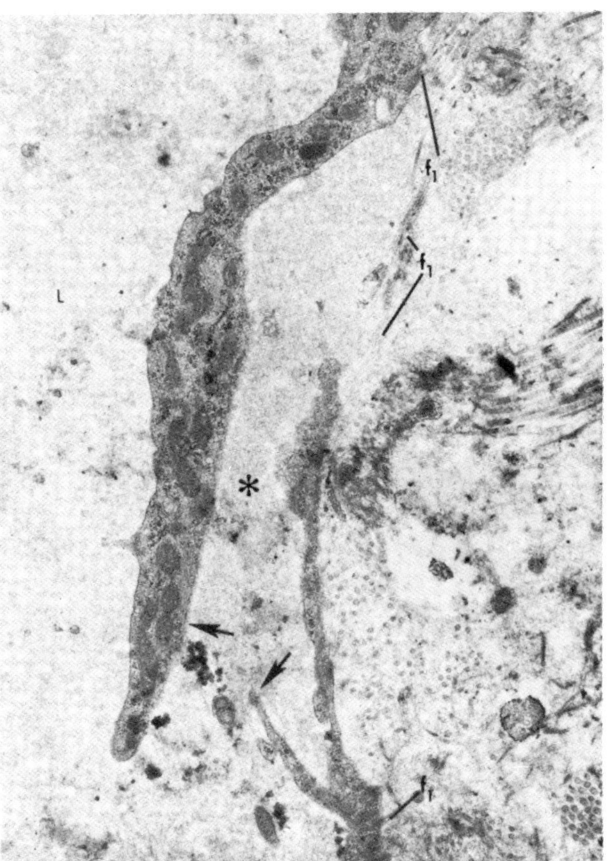

Fig. 14-7. **A patent intercellular junction *(arrow)* in a lymphatic capillary 1 hour after bacterial infection. The electron-dense flocculent material within the intercellular cleft (*) is continuous with the lymphatic lumen (L). The anchoring filaments (f) are observed along the connective tissue front of the vessel (×14,400).**

EARLY INFLAMMATION AND WOUND INFECTION

The two primary factors in infection are the involved host resistance and the infecting bacteria; resistance of the host to bacteria is intimately involved with the early inflammatory process. If, as is believed, bacterial infection results from overwhelming of the host's ability to prevent multiplication of pathogens, two principal means of preventing infection must be followed: (1) the number of bacteria in the environment must be reduced as much as possible, as in aseptic surgery, and (2) the host's defenses must be maintained, or if necessary improved, so that the remaining bacteria can be resisted successfully. Coordination of the two approaches is a prerequisite for an optimal result.

Extensive precautions are now taken to protect the surgical patient from bacterial contact (Chapter 21 and 24). In addition, to maintain or to improve the host's defenses, other steps must be followed, including use of meticulous surgical technique and repair of any physiologic abnormalities.

Meticulous surgical technique is important because it has been shown that the condition of the tissue is crucial in the prevention or development of a bacterial lesion.[55,56] The surgeon must avoid unnecessary damage to the tissue through mechanical trauma or ischemia. While the number of bacteria required to create a suppurative wound is usually in the millions, such a wound can be created by small numbers of pathogens in the presence of necrotic or traumatized tissues, inaccurate hemostasis, or retained blood clots. Tissue should be gently manipulated with noncrushing instruments, and strong retraction should not be used. Hemostasis must be accurate and complete to reduce tissue damage and the possibility of hematoma. Foreign bodies should be avoided unless absolutely necessary. The amount of suture material used must be kept to a minimum. Tissues must be accurately approximated to prevent both strangulation and dead space. If these principles are followed, the incision should be most resistant to bacterial invasion, and healing should proceed at an optimal rate. Any factor that delays wound healing also increases the likelihood of infection.

In infection prevention, maintenance of normal physiology and repair of systemic abnormalities are as important as avoidance of tissue trauma. Normal perfusion in the area of the wound is essential for the mobilization of local host defenses. During low cardiac output and systemic hypoperfusion, not only is the resistance of the wound reduced but also compromised function of the brain, heart, and kidneys will lessen the patient's overall bacterial defenses. This can be especially dangerous if the wound is contaminated. Circulatory failure must be prevented or promptly corrected to avoid wound sepsis.

The devastating effects of hypotension on host resistance are widely recognized. It is incorrect to rely on urinary flow and the return of normal central arterial pressure as indications that an adequate level of circulation has been achieved, because in such cases the skin and peripheral muscle mass may still be underperfused. As a result, inadequate oxygenation, decreased local leukocytosis, and failure of circulating antibodies to reach the site of infection, as well as other factors, can allow proliferation of bacteria. Further, if the wound area is vasoconstricted as a result of hypovolemia, preventive antibiotics will not be able to penetrate the tissues where they are needed.

In addition to normal circulatory function, it is necessary to have normal respiratory function and adequate gas exchange, to provide sufficient tissue oxygen as well as acid-base balance, electrolyte balance, and normal overall hydration, to support normal leukocyte function. As an example, leukocyte mobility is reduced if intracellular potassium concentrations are low.

The energy-supplying systems are significant contributors to the level of host resistance, and must remain intact if infection is to be avoided. Malnutrition (especially protein depletion) is a particular threat. In acute starvation, lymphocyte deficiencies, lymphopenia, and immunoprotein deficiencies may develop, but immune competence can rapidly be restored with return of adequate nutrition. However, during sepsis, the nutritional needs of the patient increase and bacterial resistance decreases; this results in a vicious cycle, which can most effectively be stopped by treatment of both the infection and the defect in resistance. A similar situation may develop in a vitamin deficiency. Vitamins A and C, for example, both contribute to natural immunity. Vitamin A is required for a complete inflammatory response, and it also contributes to the development of specific antibody; vitamin C is believed to be a significant factor in the superoxide formation required for the oxidative killing mechanism of leukocytes (Chapter 13). The B vitamins are needed for energy production and are thought to have an important role in the immune system. In the surgical patient, the probability of infection is heightened more by preoperative protein depletion than by postoperative depletion, and part of the complete preoperative workup should include clinical and laboratory assessment for malnutrition and vitamin deficiencies.

Several other physiologic abnormalities and disease states also seriously compromise host resistance. For example, Cushing disease, Addison disease, hepatic disease, diabetes mellitus, leukemia, obesity, and agammaglobulinemia all make it more difficult for the patient to combat infection. Agammaglobulinemia, complement defects, and hormonal imbalances can create serious deficits in the patient's defenses. Retardation of the inflammatory response by excess adrenal corticosteroids is recognized; large doses of these hormones weaken antibacterial defenses.

Antibacterial resistance may also be diminished by severe trauma. Inhibition in this case results from catecholamine release, inadequate oxygenation of leukocytes, hypovolemia, and suppression of humoral and specific cell-mediated immune responses. Patients with severe burns are particularly affected; for example, in these patients, even allograft rejection may be suppressed at times of severe infection or malnutrition. Patients who have experienced physical trauma must be supported to reduce the stimuli for catecholamine release, restoration and maintenance of blood volume, and adequate nutrition.

Patients often have heavily contaminated wounds, and subsequent infection is almost guaranteed if primary wound closure is completed. Surgical experience has demonstrated that the incidence of wound infection may be substantially reduced by ensuring the free drainage of contaminated material and foreign bodies. Two techniques, delayed primary and secondary closure, have been used. In delayed primary closure, the wound surface should first be thoroughly debrided and left open to drain into the dressings. The wound is closed on the fourth or fifth day if no infection has developed. Secondary closure is used for wounds that are infected when first examined and for wounds that become infected before delayed primary closure can be accomplished. This approach usually involves a waiting period of at least 10 days, during which time granulation tissue is forming. After granulation, one of two types of secondary closure may be accomplished. In simple closure, the two granulating surfaces are brought together without excision of any tissue. However, a better functional result is usually achieved if the granulations and indurated scar tissue are excised first, followed by apposition of the two surfaces. This would be the best procedure, for example, in patients with a surgical incision that is heavily contaminated by drainage from an underlying abscess.

ENHANCEMENT OF HOST RESISTANCE BY ANTIBIOTICS

Aseptic techniques, gentle accurate tissue handling, and maintenance of normal physiology are of critical importance in preventing the development of bacterial infection in the surgical wound. Unfortunately, these goals are seldom achieved, so a small but significant number of wound infections continue to be seen. It is therefore reasonable to explore the possibilities of increasing host resistance, but aside from the principles elaborated previously, no specific means are available (Chapter 19).

There is, however, an adjunctive method which, although it does not directly increase host resistance, supplements this resistance by reducing bacterial viability in the wound. This method is the use of an antibiotic to prevent the establishment of an infection rather than to treat an infection that is already established. This type of antibiotic use has been called preventive antibiotics (prophylaxis) and is based on the biologic principles of early inflammation outlined previously. Since there is a period of intense, highly effective host antibacterial activity, which begins immediately on arrival of bacteria in the tissue and contains the bacteria—if they are to be contained—in less than 4 hours (Fig. 14-2), there is reason to believe that any supplement to this host resistance should be delivered during the period of active host antibacterial activity. In this way, the two antibacterial activities, antibiotics and host resistance, will have an additive, or synergistic, effect in preventing the development of a bacterial lesion. The effectiveness of this method has been proved in the experimental laboratory [57] and extensively in the clinic (Chapter

23).[58] It represents a special case in surgery of the decisive period and has been called "the effective period of preventive antibiotics." The exact opposite is seen if an agent such as local ischemia produced by adrenalin is used to decrease host resistance rather than to supplement it. Figure 14-8 demonstrates the time relationships of increased host resistance caused by antibiotics and decreased host resistance caused by adrenalin ischemia. Figure 14-9 shows the histology of a control wound and a wound contaminated with staphylococcal organisms, contrasted with those in an animal given an antibiotic 3 hours after staphylococcal contamination of a surgical incision. Although the wound in the animal given penicillin before wound contamination is slightly different from the saline control, it is markedly different from the histologic appearance of the contaminated wound without antibiotic and a contaminated wound given antibiotics 3 hours following contamination. Prevention of the development of a bacterial lesion is maximum if the antibiotic is in the tissue before the bacteria arrive, and its effect disappears if it is not given until 3 or 4 hours following bacterial contamination. These biologic relations are important in surgery, for the time of contamination during an operation is during the proce-

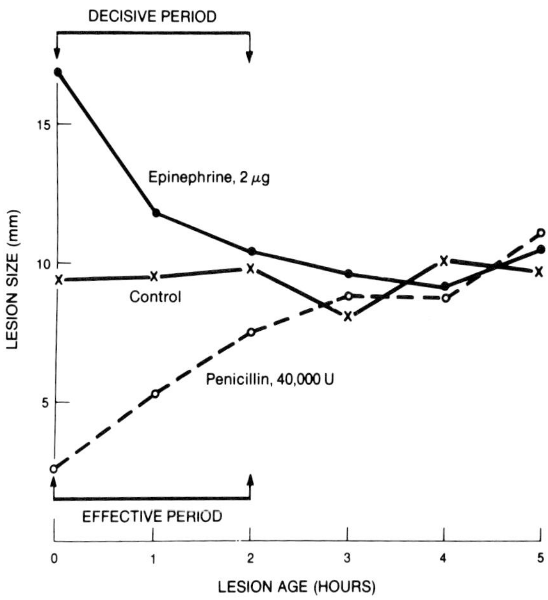

Fig. 14-8. Lesion size after inoculation of bacteria as a function of systemic antibiotic administration, or epinephrine-induced ischemia.

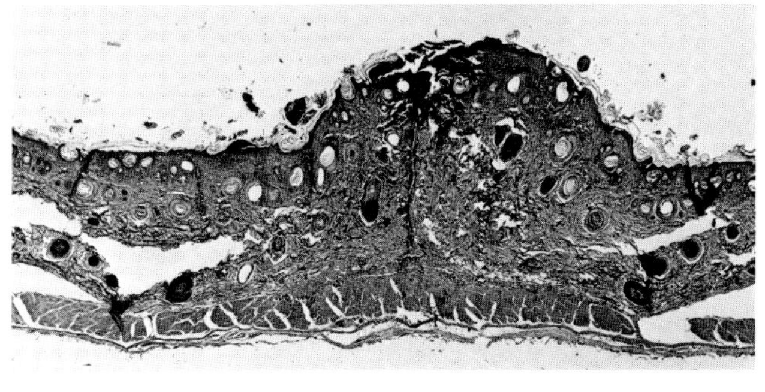

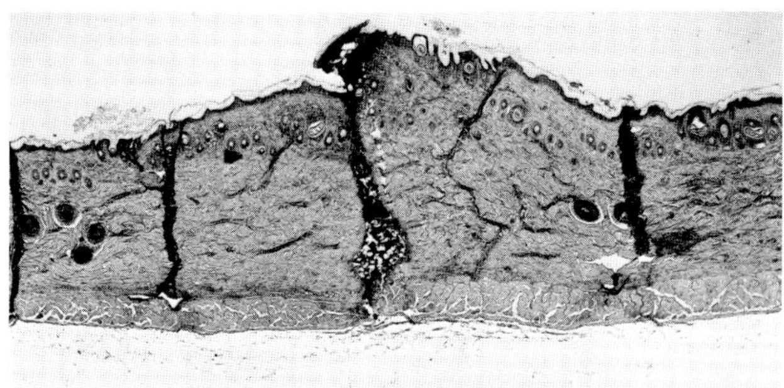

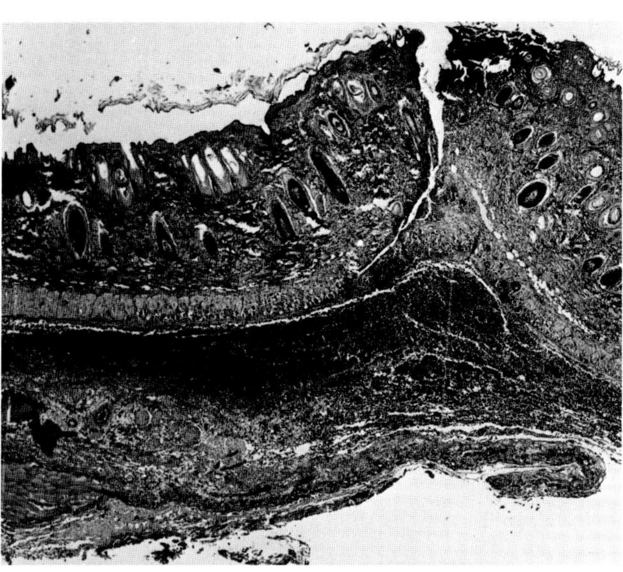

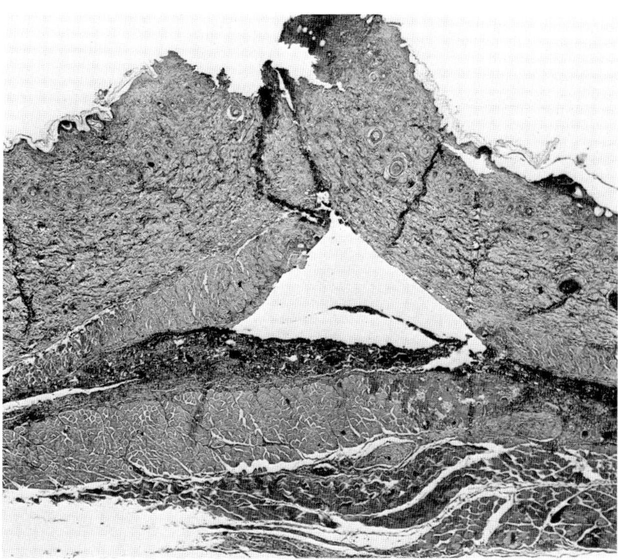

Fig. 14-9. **A. Control incision, contaminated with sterile normal saline. B. Incision contaminated with 0.1 ml of live staphylococcal suspension; no penicillin given. C. Penicillin, 20,000 units, followed by contamination of the incision with 0.1 ml of staphylococcal suspension. D. Incision contaminated with 0.1 ml of staphylococcal suspension, followed in 3 hours by 20,000 units penicillin (×29.25). (From Burke JF: The effective period of preventive antibiotic action in experimental incisions and dermal lesions. *Surgery* 50:161, 1961; and Hunt TK, Dunphy JE: Fundamentals of Wound Management. New York, Appleton-Century-Crofts, 1979, pp 204–205.)**

dure itself. An antibiotic may therefore be given preoperatively so that bactericidal concentrations will be present in the tissue when the bacteria arrive. It also indicates that for prevention alone there is no need to give antibiotics after bacterial contamination.

BIBLIOGRAPHY

Burke JF, Miles AA: The sequences of vascular events in early infective inflammation. J Pathol Bacteriol 76:1, 1958.

Weissman G, Samuelsson B, Paoletti R: Advances in Inflammation Research. New York, Raven, 1979.

REFERENCES

1. Ramsdell SG: Use of trypan blue to demonstrate immediate skin reaction in rabbits and guinea pigs. J Immunol 15:305, 1928.
2. Rawson RA: The binding of T-1824 and structurally related diazo dyes by the plasma proteins. Am J Physiol 138:708, 1943.
3. Burke JF, Miles AA: The sequence of vascular events in early infective inflammation. J Pathol Bacteriol 76:1, 1958.
4. Flax MH: Experimental allergic thyroiditis in the guinea pig. II. Morphologic studies of development of disease. Lab Invest 12:199, 1963.
5. Smith JB, Pedersen NC, Morris B: The role of the lymphatic system in inflammatory responses. Ser Hematol 3(2):17, 1970.
6. Cotran RS: The delayed and prolonged vascular leakage in inflammation. II. An electron microscopic study of the vascular response after thermal injury. Am J Pathol 45:589, 1965.
7. Leak LV, Kato F: Electron microscopic studies of lymphatic capillaries during early inflammation. I. Mild and severe thermal injuries. Lab Invest 26:572, 1972.
8. Majno G, Palade GE, Schoefl GI: Studies on inflammation. II. The site of action of histamine and serotonin along the vascular tree: a topographic study. J Biophys Biochem Cytol 11:607, 1961.
9. Wilhelm DL, Mason B: Vascular permeability changes in inflammation: the role of endogenous permeability factors in mild thermal injury. Br J Exp Pathol 41:487, 1960.
10. Logan G, Wilhelm DL: The inflammatory reaction in ultraviolet injury. Br J Exp Pathol 47:286, 1966.
11. Elder JM, Miles AA: The action of the lethal toxins of gas-gangrene clostridia on capillary permeability. J Pathol Bacteriol LXXIV:133, 1957.
12. Majno G, Palade GE: Studies on inflammation. I. The effect of histamine and serotonin on vascular permeability: an electron microscopic study. J Biophys Biochem Cytol 11:571, 1961.
13. Cotran RS, Remensnyder JP: The structural basis of increased vascular permeability after graded thermal injury—light and electron microscopic studies. Ann NY Acad Sci 150:495, 1968.
14. Majno G, Shea SM, Leventhal M: Endothelial contraction induced by histamine-type mediators: an electron microscopic study. J Cell Biol 42:647, 1969.
15. Cotran RS, LaGattuta M, Majno G: Studies on inflammation: fate of intramural vascular deposits induced by histamine. Am J Pathol 47:1045, 1965.
16. Baumgarten A, Wilhelm DL: Vascular permeability responses in hypersensitivity. I. The tuberculin reaction. Pathology 1:301, 1969.
17. Wells FR, Miles AA: Site of the vascular response to thermal injury. Nature 200:1015, 1963.
18. Wells FR: The site of vascular response to thermal injury in skeletal muscle. Br J Exp Pathol 52:292, 1971.
19. Cotran RS: Studies on inflammation: ultrastructure of the prolonged vascular response induced by *Clostridium oedematiens* toxin. Lab Invest 17:39, 1967.
20. Burke JF: An implanted reservoir for continuous sampling of interstitial fluid. J Surg Res 4:195, 1964.
21. Vakili C, Ruiz-Ortiz F, Burke JF: Chemical and osmolar changes of interstitial fluid in acute inflammatory states. Surg Forum 21:227, 1970.
22. Burke JF, Leak LV: Lymphatic capillary function in normal and inflamed states. In Viamonte M, Koehler PR, Witte M, Witte C (eds): Progress in Lymphology, 2nd ed. Stuttgart, Thieme, 1970, p 81.
23. Burke JF, Friberg U: A microradiographic study of developing staphylococcal inflammation using ultra-soft roentgen rays. Surg Forum 12:38, 1961.
24. Arturson G, Mellander S: Acute changes in capillary filtration and diffusion in experimental burn injury. Acta Physiol Scand 62:457, 1964.
25. Steele RH, Wilhelm DL: The inflammatory reaction in chemical injury. II. Leucocytosis and other histological changes induced by superficial injury. Br J Exp Pathol 51:265, 1970.
26. Miles AA: Nonspecific defense reactions in bacterial infections. Ann NY Acad Sci 66:356, 1956.
27. Logan G, Wilhelm DL: Vascular permeability changes in inflammation. I. The role of endogenous permeability factors in ultraviolet injury. Br J Exp Pathol 47:300, 1966.
28. Willoughby DA, Giroud JP: The role of polymorphonuclear leukocytes in acute inflammation in agranulocytic rats. J Pathol 98:53, 1969.
29. Evans DG, Miles AA, Niven JSF: The enhancement of bacterial infections by adrenaline. Br J Exp Pathol 29:20, 1948.
30. Mayerson HS, Patterson RM, McKee A, LeBrie SJ, Mayerson P: Permeability of lymphatic vessels. Am J Physiol 203:98, 1962.
31. Grotte G: Passage of dextran molecules across the blood-lymph barrier. Acta Chir Scand, Suppl 211:1, 1956.
32. Allen L: Lymphatics and lymphoid tissue. Ann Rev Physiol 29:197, 1967.
33. Bollman JL, Cain JC, Grindlay JH: Techniques for the collection of lymph from the liver, small intestine, or thoracic duct of the rat. J Lab Clin Med 33:1349, 1948.
34. Lascelles AK, Morris B: Surgical techniques for the collection of lymph from unanaesthetized sheep. Q J Exp Physiol 46:199, 1961.
35. Hall JG, Morris B, Woolley G: Intrinsic rhythmic propulsion of lymph in the unanaesthetized sheep. J Physiol 180:336, 1965.
36. Kinmonth JB, Harper RAK, Taylor GW: Lymphangiography by radiological methods. J Faculty Radiol 6:217, 1955.
37. Bellman S, Odén B: Experimental micro-lymphangiography. Acta Radiol 47:289, 1957.
38. Flexner LB, Gellhorn A, Merrell M: Studies on rates of exchange of substances between the blood and extravascular fluid. I. The exchange of water in the guinea pig. J Biol Chem 144:35, 1942.
39. Merrell M, Gellhorn A, Flexner LB: Studies on rates of exchange of substances between the blood and extravascular fluid. II. The exchange of sodium in the guinea pig. J Biol Chem 153:83, 1944.
40. Chinard FP, Vosburgh GJ, Enns T: Transcapillary exchange of water and of other substances in certain organs of the dog. Am J Physiol 183:221, 1955.
41. Leak LV, Burke JF: Fine structure of the lymphatic capillary and the adjoining connective tissue area. Am J Anat 118:785, 1966.

42. Leak LV: Electron microscopic observations on lymphatic capillaries and the structural components of the connective tissue-lymph interface. Microvasc Res 2:361, 1970.
43. Hall JG, Morris B, Moreno GD, Bessis MC: The ultrastructure and function of the cells in lymph following antigenic stimulation. J Exp Med 125:91, 1967.
44. Askar OM: "Communicating lymphatics" and lympho-venous communications in relation to deep venous occlusion of the leg. Lymphology 2:56, 1969.
45. Drinker CK, Field ME, Ward HK: The filtering capacity of lymph nodes. J Exp Med 59:393, 1934.
46. Yoffey JM, Courtice FC: Lymphatics, Lymph and the Lymphomyeloid Complex. New York, Academic, 1970.
47. Mori Y, Lennert K: Electron Microscopic Atlas of Lymph Node Cytology and Pathology. Berlin, Springer-Verlag, 1969, p 4.
48. Hall JG: Studies of the cells in the afferent and efferent lymph of lymph nodes draining the site of skin homografts. J Exp Med 125:737, 1967.
49. Hurley JV, Ham KN, Ryan GB: Acute inflammation: a topographical and electron-microscope study of increased vascular permeability in bacterial and chemical pleurisy in the rat. J Pathol Bacteriol 93:621, 1967.
50. Leak LV, Burke JF: Ultrastructure of lymphatic capillaries (Abstract). J Appl Physics 36:2620 1965.
51. Hurley JV, Ham KN, Ryan GB: The mechanism of the delayed prolonged phase of increased vascular permeability in mild thermal injury in the rat. J Pathol Bacteriol 94:1, 1967.
52. Marchesi VT: The passage of colloidal carbon through inflamed endothelium. Proc R Soc (Biol) 156:550, 1962.
53. Movat HZ, Fernando NVP: Acute inflammation: the earliest fine structural changes at the blood-tissue barrier. Lab Invest 12:895, 1963.
54. Moval HZ, Fernando NVP: Allergic inflammation. I. The earliest fine structural changes at the blood-tissue barrier during antigen-antibody interaction. Am J Pathol 42:41, 1963.
55. Miles AA, Miles EM, Burke JF: The value and duration of defence reactions of the skin to the primary lodgement of bacteria. Br J Exp Pathol 38:79, 1957.
56. Elek SD: Experimental staphylococcal infections in the skin of man. Ann NY Acad Sci 65:85, 1956.
57. Burke JF: The effective period of preventive antibiotic action in experimental incisions and dermal lesions. Surgery 50:161, 1961.
58. Burke JF: Preventive antibiotic management in surgery. Ann Rev Med (WP Kreeger, ed), 24:289, 1973.

PART IV: SYSTEMIC RESPONSES TO INFECTION

CHAPTER 15

Thermoregulatory Responses and Metabolism

DOUGLAS W. WILMORE AND LOUIS H. AULICK

THE invasion of the body by microorganisms initiates a wide variety of host responses. First, local penetration of tissue stimulates mobilization of phagocytes, initiates an inflammatory response at the local site, and may activate additional local host immunologic mechanisms. If the infection progresses, fever, tachycardia, and other systemic responses occur; these more generalized reactions may reflect *direct* effects of the infective process on cellular function or *indirect* effects resulting from homeostatic adjustments to these alterations in function. These systemic events represent the interaction of all these processes and may be categorized into two general areas—thermoregulatory and metabolic adjustments. The predominant alteration in thermoregulation is fever, and the principal changes in metabolism relate to the regulation of glucose, nitrogen, and trace elements.

Several general characteristics describe the systemic events that occur after infection.

1. The systemic responses to infection appear rather stereotyped and can be produced after the administration of a wide variety of microorganisms or their toxins. The systemic responses to infection are similar in many respects to the events that follow injury.

2. The magnitude of the responses vary with the extent and duration of infection.

3. The complex sequence of systemic events that follow infection appears to be interrelated in time, and hence sequential studies must be performed to locate the response precisely within this time.

4. Although the systemic responses to infection are stereotyped, these processes are significantly modulated by the physiologic reserve of the individual. The magnitude of the responses to infection depends on age and sex of the individual, previous nutritional status, function of vital organs, immunologic memory, and associated disease processes. The classic responses to infection have been observed in young, previously healthy, well-nourished, active adults with no other associated medical problems. However, these patients are rarely admitted to surgical services. Surgeons usually see patients at extremes of life who are hospitalized because of associated disease processes (such as degenerative diseases, cancer, gastrointestinal and cardiovascular disease) and have additional stress (usually an operation or injury) which limits physiologic, biochemical, or immunologic responses to infection. Thus, infection complicating the recuperative course of surgical patients may not evoke the standard textbook systemic response. Limitations of a patient's capacity to respond to infection may greatly affect host recovery or survival.

5. As infection progresses, additional functional limitations may be imposed on one or more specific organs, which further impair the host systemic responses. This can be observed in patients with severe pneumonia and marked pulmonary dysfunction which causes hypoxemia, and it can be associated with circulatory failure and hypotension related to severe gram-negative sepsis.

In spite of the complexities involved in unraveling and understanding the systemic responses to infection in critically ill surgical patients, a large body of investigative and clinical data is available to aid our understanding of these host defense mechanisms. This chapter will review the common systemic alterations associated with pyrogenic bacterial infections. Chapter 16 discusses these metabolic changes in terms of the hemodynamic responses they invoke.

FEVER

BODY TEMPERATURE AND TEMPERATURE MONITORING

The mechanisms for control of body temperature are extremely efficient, but alteration in the setpoint or derangements in sensitivity of the central thermostat are almost universally associated with infection or inflammation. Elevation of body temperature is such a sensitive and reliable indicator of the presence of disease that thermometry is one of the most common and frequent procedures used in hospitalized patients.

Core or central body temperature (the temperature of internal tissues) reflects the balance between metabolic heat production and surface heat loss. In general, physicians refer to a "normal body temperature" (37C, 98.6F), but this is not considered the true average or mean body temperature because of the wide variations in the temperature of various body tissues (eg, skin and subcutaneous tissue may be 2 to 6C cooler than visceral organs). Because there is no practical way to determine mean body temperature, clinicians rely for convenience on a single measurement of internal temperature and equate this value with body temperature.

Oral or rectal temperature taken in a group of healthy individuals demonstrates the usual bell-shaped distribution curve. The normal temperature for any one individual will vary as much as 1C throughout the day, and this temperature is affected by food intake and level of physical activity. The highest temperatures are usually observed in the afternoon; temperature falls with sleep and reaches its lowest value in the early morning. Oral (or axillary) temperatures average about 0.65C (1.2F) lower than rectal temperature, which is the accepted standard for clinical thermometry, but there are wide variations in this relationship. Although a normal active individual may demonstrate a central temperature ranging between 36 and 40C under ordinary conditions, a quiet person with a rectal temperature above 37.5C (99.5F) or an oral temperature above 37.0C (98.6F) should be suspected of harboring an inflammatory or infectious process until proven otherwise.[1]

But what does rectal temperature really measure? The temperature of the rectum is determined by: (1) local metabolism, (2) the temperature of the arterial blood delivered to this area and the rate of blood flow, and (3) conductive heat exchange between rectum and surrounding tissue. Eichna et al[2] compared rectal temperatures of resting subjects with intracardiac and various intravascular temperatures. They found that rectal temperature was 0.2 to 0.3C higher than right heart temperature in afebrile individuals, but that it could exceed intracardiac temperature by as much as 0.8C in febrile patients. Femoral artery blood temperature was equivalent to intracardiac temperatures, and Eichna argued that these two intravascular temperatures offered the best index of average body temperature.

Cooper and Kenyon[3] placed thermocouples on the aorta during thoracic operations and compared para-aortic blood temperatures (an indirect measurement of central intravascular temperature) with rectal and esophageal temperatures. Esophageal temperature at the level of the heart was a more reliable index of aortic blood temperature than the rectal temperature. Moreover, rectal temperature was always higher than aortic temperature and responded slowly to rapid fluctuations in central blood temperatures. Molnar and Read[4] also confirmed that rectal temperature was slower than esophageal and stomach temperatures to respond to fluctuations in arterial temperature.

In spite of these limitations, rectal temperature (taken 5 to 10 cm above the anal sphincter) is the most practical method of monitoring core temperature in the critically ill patient. However, the rectal temperature response to alterations in body heat content is slow, and its relationship to that of the arterial blood that perfuses the temperature control center in the brain is altered in an unpredictable manner with the onset of a fever. While the esophagus is a better location for more accurate central temperature monitoring, it is practical only in the operating room. Tympanic temperature has also been utilized as an index of central body temperature. While it will follow body temperature changes more rapidly than rectal measurements, it is more sensitive to variations in ambient temperatures, and the probe is difficult to position comfortably. With the use of thermal dilution cardiac output catheters, a central intravascular thermistor is available for continuous monitoring of mixed venous blood temperature. Rectal temperatures may range from 0.2 to 0.8C above these central intravascular values in both healthy individuals and febrile patients.[5] The temperature of venous blood from brain and liver will usually be higher than that observed in the right heart or aorta, reflecting the contribution of these particular organs to the heat input of the body.

BODY HEAT BALANCE

Body temperature reflects a balance between the heat produced and the heat lost, and under usual conditions body heat balance is a finely regulated physiologic process. Approximately two-thirds of the heat produced in the basal state occurs in the brain and visceral organs. Metabolic heat production will increase above basal levels for a variety of reasons. First, body metabolism increases slightly (10 to 15 percent) following food ingestion. This is known as the specific dynamic action of food, lasts for several hours, and uses approximately 10 percent of the ingested calories. Second, environmental cold stress or the rise in hypothalamic setpoint temperature with a fever will cause an increase in skeletal muscle activity (unconscious tensing to uncontrollable shivering and involuntary movements) and thereby increase metabolic heat production. When stimulated by a cold environment, calorigenic hormones (primarily the catecholamines) are liberated to aid heat production and mobilize body fuels. Third, the greatest increase in metabolism occurs during physical exercise, when levels of heat production may reach four to five times basal rates.

To maintain thermal equilibrium, heat loss must equal metabolic and environmental heat gains. Body heat loss is regulated by physiologic adjustments in sweating and cutaneous blood flow as well as by behavioral means (covering up with a blanket in a cool room or moving into the shade on a hot day). Based on the low thermal conductivity of deep body tissue, the body must rely heavily on the circulation to carry metabolic heat from the deeper tissues where it is produced to the skin and respiratory surfaces where it can be dissipated. The wide range of vasomotor adjustments, plus the high heat conductivity and specific heat of blood, make this system ideally adapted for its thermoregulatory role. Cutaneous vasodilation will increase the rate of heat delivery to the body surface where, if skin temperatures exceed ambient temperatures, heat is dissipated primarily by radiation and convection. In warmer environments most, if not all, body heat is lost by the evaporation of sweat.

The primary means of heat conservation is vasoconstriction of the skin. The magnitude of cutaneous vasomotion is best appreciated in the fingers, where blood flow is primarily superficial. In response to a cold challenge, finger blood flow will drop to approximately one one-hundredth that found in a hot environment. Reduced surface circulation greatly increases the insulative layer of the body, causing a rise in body heat storage and central temperatures.

Many adaptations to alterations in internal temperature or to the external thermal environment are determined by behavioral changes. To retain heat, an individual will curl up to minimize exposed surface area and add clothing or bed covers to provide additional insulation. Conversely, if heat is to be lost, an individual will move into a cooler environment, remove clothing, drink cold liquids, and extend the extremities to maximize effective body surface area and promote heat exchange. Behavioral thermoregulation is available to most awake, alert hospitalized patients, but many individuals who are receiving critical care cannot make these important behavioral adjustments. Because these patients frequently have additional derangements in physiologic means of thermoregulation, they are extremely vulnerable to changes in the thermal environment.

CENTRAL NERVOUS SYSTEM CONTROL AND TEMPERATURE "SETPOINT"

Central control of body temperature resides predominately within the hypothalamus. Cells within both the preoptic region of the anterior hypothalamus and the posterior hypothalamus receive a variety of extrinsic and intrinsic temperature information, integrate this sensory input, and initiate a coordinated effector response. Thermoreceptors in the skin and body core provide neurogenic afferents which ultimately reach and effect hypothalamic thermoregulatory activity. Thermosensitive cells have also been identified in the preoptic region of the hypothalamus; these alter their intrinsic firing rates with changes in local temperature. These cells are of two distinct populations: warm-sensitive cells will increase firing rates during a rise in local temperature, and cold-sensitive neurons will increase their firing frequency upon cooling. Like the rest of the body, hypothalamic temperature varies as a function of changes in local heat production and loss. Vascular heat transfer appears to be a primary means of reducing hypothalamic temperature. As a consequence, any variation in body heat content that changes arterial blood temperature can ultimately affect hypothalamic thermoregulatory activity. Therefore, circulatory as well as neurogenic factors contribute to the afferent limb of hypothalamic temperature control.

Numerous mathematical and engineering models have been devised to explain the hypothalamic temperature controller. The most commonly used system, however, involves a comparison between an intrinsic reference or "setpoint" signal and one from the sensor(s) of actual body temperature (eg, hypothalamic, core, mean body). The thermoregulatory output from such a controller would be qualitatively and quantitatively related to both the direction and the magnitude of the differences in these two signals.[6] Physiologic control of body temperature is therefore analogous to a thermostat, which compares room temperature to a set value and then activates either the heater or air conditioner until the thermal environment returns to the reference value of the thermostat. Likewise, the body's central reference temperature is not a fixed value but can be adjusted up or down by seasonal or daily circadian rhythms, environmental stress, body injury, and infection. Regardless of the cause for the shift in setpoint temperature, the body will continue to thermoregulate in a normal manner around this new central reference value.

Fever is explained by a rise in hypothalamic setpoint temperature, which initiates both physiologic and behavioral thermoregulatory mechanisms to elevate and hold central body temperature at a higher level. When the reference temperature is normal, the individual is considered *normothermic* when body temperature matches setpoint, *hypothermic* when it drops below setpoint, and *hyperthermic* when body temperature exceeds the normal central reference level.

PYROGENS—THE AFFERENT MEDIATORS OF FEVER

Fever is one of the earliest recognized signs of inflammation and infection. During the late eighteenth and early nineteenth centuries, it was realized that injection of a variety of solutions or putrified material into an animal caused fever. Clinical studies at this time also supported the relationship between fever and infection. Semmelweiss introduced endometrial secretions of patients with puerperal fever into female rabbits immediately after delivery and observed fever and lethal sepsis.[7] Billroth and his students demonstrated that the injection of filtrates of pus caused elevations in body temperature when administered to animals.

With the contributions of Lister and Pasteur to the germ theory of disease, scientists moved into a new bacteriologic era by describing many features of the newly discovered microorganisms. A constant feature of the bacterial studies was that the organisms secreted a substance into the culture media which was regularly pyrogenic in animals and would often invoke a leukocyte response. At the turn of the century, it was realized that bacteria produced pyrogenic factors in addition to the exotoxins which were excreted by the microorganisms into the culture media. A new toxin was described, which was tightly anchored to, if not a part of, the cell wall. This substance was called endotoxin and was later biochemically characterized as a lipopolysaccharide.

In addition to the pyrogenic substances associated with microorganisms, products of the hosts's own cells can serve as signals to stimulate fever. For example, a patient with a simple long bone fracture regularly developed "posttraumatic fever," yet without an open wound or other source of obvious contamination, a bacterial etiology of this febrile response was highly unlikely. In 1948, Bennett and Beeson[8] developed techniques to exclude endotoxin from their test system and reported that a fever-inducing pyrogen could be extracted from rabbit granulocytes. Further studies revealed that the leukocyte substance was regularly pyrogenic, while similar extracts from a wide variety of tissues carried no fever-inducing effect. In addition, the host pyrogen (called endogenous pyrogen) differed in many respects from the pyrogen of microbial origin.[9]

A number of investigators have contributed to knowledge of endogenous pyrogen. Tissue pyrogen does not exist in storage form in host cells but is synthesized shortly before being liberated into the bloodstream. Activation occurs following a variety of stimuli, which include exogenous pyrogens (endotoxin), viruses, bacteria, antigen–antibody complexes, and specific steroids. These stimulators cause cells to synthesize and then liberate the pyrogen. Granulocytes were once thought to be the only cell type with the capacity to elaborate endogenous pyrogen, but monocytes and macrophages—all cells capable of phagocytosis—also serve as a pyrogenic source. When stimulated, these cells produce and release a heat-labile protein of 100,000 to 200,000 molecular weight, which produces a prompt monophasic fever spike.

Partial species cross-reactivity to this substance has been observed, but tolerance in the animal does not develop after repeated injection. In contrast, an animal becomes unresponsive or tolerant after repeated injections of endotoxin. The fever response to injection of endogenous pyrogen into the central nervous system is much greater than the response to a comparable intravenous dose. Although the presence and activity of tissue pyrogen have been demonstrated in man,[10] repeated attempts to assay circulating pyrogen during high fevers have been unsuccessful, hampering definition of the specific role of tissue pyrogen in human infection and injury.

More recently, other properties have been attributed to endogenous pyrogens. For example, leukocyte endogenous mediator is closely related to (or may be the same as) endogenous pyrogen, but has effects other than the induction of fever.[11] When injected into normal rats, leukocyte endogenous mediator has specific and direct effects in the liver to promote hepatic uptake of plasma zinc and iron, increase plasma copper (elevate ceruloplasm), and stimulate hepatic uptake of plasma amino acids, which are used in the synthesis of acute-phase proteins. Thus, the inflammatory cells involved in phagocytosis appear to regulate (either directly through organ effects or indirectly through the central nervous system) body redistribution of trace elements and nitrogen, and stimulate acute-phase protein synthesis to participate in the host defense mechanisms.

HOW PYROGENS AFFECT THE CENTRAL THERMOSTAT

As previously noted, body temperature is maintained by a delicate balance between heat production and heat loss. The central thermostat located in the hypothalamus controls the physiologic, biochemical, and behavioral adjustments of the body to alterations in external and internal temperatures. Fever is the result of an upward adjustment of this central regulatory apparatus, and heat loss from the body is diminished or heat gain increased. When body temperature has risen to a new setpoint, thermoregulation occurs around this higher temperature (Fig. 15-1).

The central nervous system is essential for the febrile response.[12] The response is not observed in experimental animals after hypothalamic ablation or in animals with

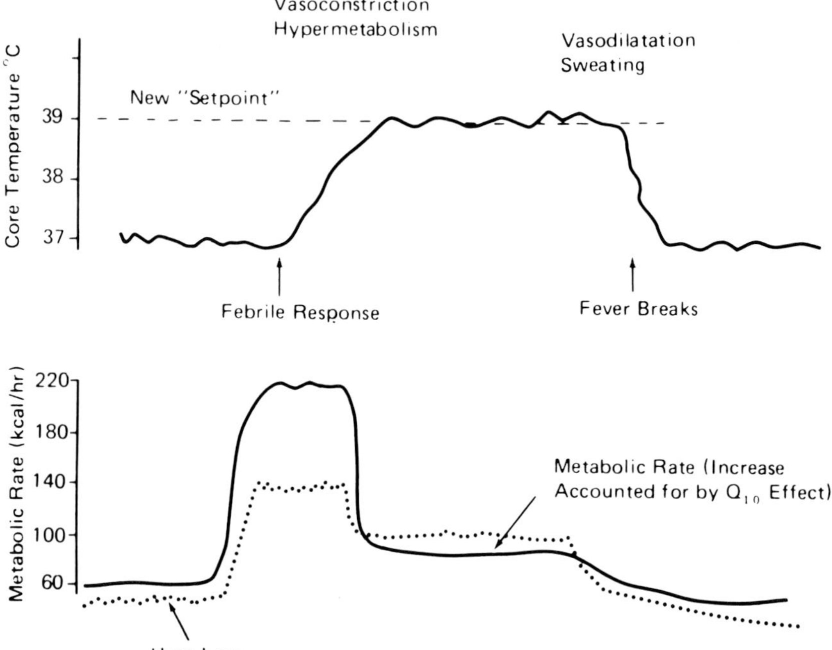

***Fig. 15-1.* The response of body temperature, heat production (metabolic rate), and cutaneous heat loss to a pyrogenic fever.**

electrically created lesions placed in the preoptic area. The febrile response in man does not occur after intravenous pyrogen administration if a proximal tourniquet cuff precludes delivery of the substance to the brain. In rabbits, the response to pyrogen is much more pronounced when the substance is infused into the carotid artery than when the same dose is given intravenously. When the substance is injected directly into the thermoregulatory area, only one one-hundredth of the intravenous dose of pyrogen is required to produce the same fever. Finally, if the hypothalamus of the animal is heated by a thermode placed in the preoptic area during the latent period before the onset of fever, the fever response is abated. This suggests that the increased setpoint temperature called for, following administration of pyrogen, is provided by the local warming of the neuronal pool, and systemic thermoregulatory adjustments are unnecessary.

The exact biochemical mechanisms by which pyrogens interact with the thermoregulatory apparatus to effect alterations in thermoregulation are not known, and is an area of vigorous investigation.[13] The cells of the preoptic area change their rate of firing when fever develops in response to injection of pyrogens, and these neurophysiologic alterations appear to parallel the apparent setpoint shift. Alterations in ionic balance, changes in local concentrations of monoamines (norepinephrine and 5-hydroxytryptamine) and increased synthesis of prostaglandins have all been suggested as local hypothalamic effectors or mediators of the setpoint shift response. An association between prostaglandin activity, hypothalamic temperature reset, and fever rests on the following: (1) injection of minute amounts of protaglandin E into the hypothalamus causes fever; (2) after administration of endotoxin or endogenous pyrogen, prostaglandin levels increase in the cerebral spinal fluid, suggesting increased central nervous system synthesis or release; and (3) commonly used antipyretics (aspirin and indomethacin) inhibit prostaglandin synthesis. In spite of this apparent evidence, there are also strong arguments against the role of prostaglandin involvement in normal hypothalamic temperature regulation.[10]

With the upward shift in the hypothalamic setpoint, two mechanisms are used by the body to achieve an increase in core temperature.[14] Vasoconstriction by the cutaneous vessels limits heat loss. This may be the first adjustment by individuals who are in a warm or thermally neutral environment. Increased heat production, manifested by shivering and associated with an increased oxygen consumption, can also occur, especially if the individual is exposed to a cool ambient temperature. Frequently, both of these mechanisms operate together to increase body heat content and achieve the new setpoint temperature. Once this new reference temperature is achieved, temperature regulation will function in a normal manner around this elevated new level. The metabolic rate at this new equilibrium (following the initial responses and associated shivering) should be accounted for by the effect of the increased body temperature on metabolism (Q_{10} effect). When the infection clears, the setpoint returns to normal, and central nervous system mechanisms are activated to aid heat loss. Cutaneous vasodilatation and sweating cause body temperature to fall, and metabolic activity returns to normal. Thus, a new thermal equilibrium is achieved, and lower body temperatures are maintained around a normal hypothalamic setpoint.

THE BACTERIOSTATIC EFFECTS OF FEVER

Although fever is a common sign of infection, it is not clear that an elevated body temperature itself provides any benefit to the host. Induced hyperthermia was once used in the treatment of poliomyelitis, neurosyphilis, and gonorrheal infection, because of the in vitro sensitivity of the infecting organisms to elevated temperatures. More recently, the beneficial effects of fever have been demonstrated in fish and desert iguanas, ectotherms that adjust body temperatures by behavior. These species move into warm or cold environments to achieve higher or lower body temperatures. Iguanas were infected with live bacteria and then placed in incubators at 38C (their normal body temperature), 40 to 42C temperatures which would mimic a fever response, and 34 and 36C which would simulate hypothermia.[15] A positive correlation existed between the lizard's temperature and survival rate following bacteremia; more than 80 percent of the warmest animals lived after infection, compared to survival rates of less than 40 percent in the 38C animal group and less than 20 percent in the 34C animals. When the fever was reduced by sodium salicylate, seven out of seven animals died following bacteremia.[16] In eight additional infected animals, salicylates were administered but the lizards were housed in a warm incubator, thereby preventing a fall in body temperature. Only one of eight warm animals died, demonstrating that the increased mortality after administration of salicylate was not the direct effect of drugs on the microorganisms but rather of the reduction of body temperature.

In similar studies in bacteremic rabbits, survival from infection increased as the magnitude of the fever increased up to 2.25C.[17] When the fever response was greater than 2.25C, the mortality rate increased. This evidence from mammals does not demonstrate a causal relationship between fever and survival, but the association between fever and survival is similar to that observed in patients: The lack of a febrile (and leukocyte) response after infection is, in general, associated with a poor prognosis.

The specific mechanisms augmented by fever to aid host defenses are unknown, but several nonspecific factors that may aid host immunity have been suggested. Van't Hoff described the physical law that the rate of biochemical reactions increases with heating. For ordinary temperatures, the velocity of chemical reactions increases approximately two to threefold for every 10C rise in temperature (Q_{10} effect). Thus, the reaction rate of a variety of host defense mechanisms may be accelerated by the febrile state. The half-life of endotoxin is reduced during fever. Fever in ectotherms increases the mobility of leukocytes into the site of infection, and fever appears to increase the iron requirements of pathogenic bacteria for growth.[15] Because serum iron levels fall during infection, this biochemical alteration caused by the febrile response decreases, in relative quantities, the iron available for metabolism by microorganisms.[18]

OTHER EFFECTS OF FEVER AND REQUIREMENTS FOR FEVER TREATMENT

Marked increases in body catabolism and cardiac output have served, in the past, as clinical indications for the need for antipyretics in infected febrile patients. Metabolism and body temperature are interdependent. As body temperature rises, there is an increase in the rate constant for chemical reactions. This Q_{10} effect accounts for a 10 to 13 percent increase in heat production for each degree centigrade rise in body temperature, although there is wide variation in this relationship in actual practice.[1] The patient with a fever of 40C may demonstrate, therefore, an increase in oxygen consumption of 30 to 35 percent because of the elevation in body temperature alone.

To distinguish the difference between the direct effects of infectious disease and the effect of increased tissue temperature on body catabolism, Beisel and associates [19] studied healthy men placed in a hot chamber, adjusted to increase the subject's rectal temperature over 18 hours to 39.4C and maintain that temperature for 6 hours. The adrenal responses and alterations in nitrogen metabolism during artificial hyperthermia resembled changes during infectious disease. Negative balance of nitrogen, potassium, and magnesium was produced by a combination of reduced dietary intake, increased urinary excretion, and increased sweat losses. With induced hyperthermia, there was greater surface electrolyte loss (through profuse sweating) than cutaneous losses which accompany the hyperthermia of infectious disease. In spite of this increase in body catabolism induced by fever, current methods of nutritional support are more than adequate to offset the wasting of body tissue during infectious illness.

There is a well-known effect of fever on heart rate. In general, with each 1C rise in body temperature, the pulse rate increases approximately 10 beats per minute. The accompanying increase in cardiac output reflects an increased burden on the circulation to support both rising metabolic demands and a thermoregulatory increase in surface blood flow.

The febrile course during an infectious disease is a valuable indicator of the effect of treatment, and it is argued that antipyretics interfere with this clinical indicator and thus hamper use of core temperatures as an accurate reflection of the course of the infection. If the febrile response does not impose great discomfort, or strain the cardiovascular reserve of the patient, treatment is rarely necessary. In trauma patients (with or without infection), we support the fever response by maintaining patients in a warm environment. We consider a normal (37.0C) or subnormal rectal temperature as one of the earliest indications of gram-negative bacteremia.

There are situations, however, when lowering the body temperature is of vital importance, specifically during heat stroke, postoperative or interoperative malignant hyperthermia, delirium or seizure activities associated with fever, and cardiocirculatory failure associated with hyperpyrexia. The body temperature can be lowered by sponging the body with alcohol, by increasing airflow over the body, or by using cooling blankets. *Without pharmacologically altering the central setpoint (using chlorpromazine or related medications or morphine), cooling the surface will only stimulate additional vasoconstriction and increase heat production (through shivering).* In cases of severe hyperthermia (> 41C), rubbing the skin to promote vasodilatation, or immersion of the patient into an ice bath should be considered life-saving.

CLINICAL MANIFESTATIONS OF FEVER

At one time, many of the infectious diseases could be diagnosed by their characteristic fever patterns. In this era of sophisticated medical practice, diagnosis of specific infection is best made by microbiologic techniques. The fever pattern is unreliable. Several factors may affect the temperature of critically ill patients. First, the temperature of the room may affect the core temperature of the patient. Responsive, oriented individuals will inform the hospital staff if they are too hot or too cold. In critically ill patients, often unresponsive or sedated while receiving ventilatory support, behavioral adaptation to ambient temperature may not be possible. Air conditioning (< 28C) is an additional stress for critically ill patients who have alterations in temperature regulation (such as sepsis, head injury, thermal trauma, or multiple injury).[20] The best rule of thumb during treatment is that patient comfort should be achieved. Those patients who cannot communicate with the nursing staff should be cared for in thermally neutral (28 to 30C) environments. Shivering should never be allowed, because of the added physiologic stress it places on the critically ill patient. If reduction of body temperature is a desired goal, drugs that lower central setpoint should be administered before ambient cooling is instituted.

Salicylates are the most common antipyretic administered to febrile patients, but their method of action is still unknown. Salicylates are effective in attenuating or eliminating the fever resulting from a systemic injection of bacterial or leukocyte pyrogen. Myers and Tytell [21] have suggested that the salicylate effect in the central nervous system may be caused by alterations of the ionic balance across the cell membrane in the hypothalamic area. Other salicylate-like antipyretics are acetaminophen, phenacetin, antipyrine, and aminopyrine.

Some general anesthetics have a pronounced effect in diminishing sympathetic outflow from the central nervous system. This is usually ascribed to the nonspecific depression of the central nervous system by the agent rather than to selective action on thermal regulatory centers. The hypothermia that frequently accompanies major operations is the combined result of decreased heat production that occurs secondary to general anesthesia and the increased heat loss that occurs in patients with depressed thermoregulatory capacities undergoing operations in the cool operating room.

Morphine has a pronounced effect on decreasing heat production; narcotic administration may be associated with a prompt fall in body temperature. Although small doses of morphine exert minimal effects on heat production and heat loss, morphine can have a pronounced effect on sympathetic outflow from the brain and greatly diminish heat production when given in an anesthetic dose in the operating room or administered repeatedly to patients who are on a ventilator. Chlorpromazine and similar tranquilizers can also cause a fall in heat production, while amphetamines increase oxygen consumption, mainly by an increase in central nervous system activity rather than direct stimulation of the thermal regulatory areas. Other commonly used drugs can affect central setpoint: 1-methyl-dopa causes a slight reduction in core temperature of normal men studied in a cool room; atropine diminishes the rate of sweating and in large doses causes hyperthermia and can also affect central thermal regulatory areas, resulting in a decrease in heat production.[22]

Dehydration in infants is usually associated with fever once referred to as inanition fever. The febrile response is greater if the dehydrated patient is hypertonic (ie, hypernatremic). Moyer [23] reproduced this finding in rats and found a decrease in oxygen consumption with hypo-osmolar dehydration, a rise in oxygen consumption during hyperosmolar dehydration, and no change in metabolic rate during isotonic dehydration.[23] This effect may be mediated by the central nervous system, because injection of sodium into the thermoregulatory center causes a prompt rise in body temperature. A similar association between oxygen consumption and extracellular sodium concentration has been observed in vitro, presumably through the stimulation of the Na^+K^+ membrane pumps that are accelerated by the increased sodium concentration in the medium.[24]

Alcohol is the most frequent cause of accidental hypothermia in the elderly patient. Alcohol causes cutaneous vasodilation and suppresses shivering, thereby increasing heat loss and decreasing heat production during cold exposure.[25] Alcohol also blocks hepatic gluconeogenesis, resulting in hypoglycemia and diminished glucose flow from the liver to peripheral tissues. The hypoglycemia is potentiated if the subject has been exercising or has partially or totally fasted. Thus, an unconscious hypothermic patient may be somnolent not because of excess alcohol ingestion but because of hypoglycemia.

Hypothermia is frequently associated with gram-negative bacteremia. Cutaneous vasodilation may occur in patients with sepsis to promote increased heat loss. However, gram-negative infection also blunts hepatic gluconeogenesis and other hepatic metabolic functions, which may account for a major reduction in the heat produced in support of the core temperature in traumatized patients. The hypoglycemia associated with severe infection [26] may also limit heat production, as the lack of available glucose substrate may create a significant fuel deficit.

METABOLIC ALTERATIONS—ANABOLIC PATTERNS DURING SYSTEMIC CATABOLIC WASTING

GENERALIZED RESPONSES

Body wasting is one of the most recognized consequences of infection. Prolonged fever, hypermetabolism, alterations in protein economy, anorexia, and the extended nature of many infections contribute to the loss of body tissue. These effects are compounded in the critically ill patient with multiple system organ failure, whose gastrointestinal tract will not accept enteral feeding. In spite of this generalized catabolic setting, increased synthesis occurs with increased production of inflammatory cells, acute-phase reactant proteins, albumin, new glucose, and immunoglobulins. These synthetic functions occur primarily within the liver and in the area of inflammation.

Hypermetabolism is a common consequence of infection—metabolic rates may rise 10 to 20 percent with mild infections, and 40 to 60 percent in patients with severe sepsis.[27] The hypermetabolism returns to normal with resolution of the disease. While fever may account for some of the extra heat produced (approximately a 13 percent increase in basal metabolic rate per 1C), additional energy is required for mechanical and synthetic work of the body. Studies of respiratory gas exchange and nitrogen balance have been performed in hypermetabolic infected patients to determine the mixture of oxidized metabolic fuels during the fed and fasting state.[28] Because glycogen stores are limited and no other available storage form of carbohydrate exists in the body, stored glycogen is readily utilized in the early phase of infection; thereafter, body fat and protein become the primary oxidized energy sources. At this time, approximately 85 percent of the body fuel arises from body fat, and 15 to 20 percent of the oxidized energy arises from nitrogen. That fat is the major oxidized body fuel is revealed in the respiratory exchange ratio (RQ) in infected patients, which approaches 0.7, like the ratio observed during long-term starvation.

Marked body loss of protoplasmic elements occurs during infection, resulting in negative balances of nitrogen, potassium, phosphorus, magnesium, sulfur, and zinc.[29] Losses of these substances occur primarily through increased urinary excretion, and the magnitude is proportional to the severity of the illness (Table 15-1). Intracellular mineral loss is also roughly proportional to the negative nitrogen balance. These deficits in metabolic balance may be related to diminished food intake with infection. Unlike the compensatory events that result in reduced nitrogen excretion in starved men, however, elevated nitrogen loss continues at a high level in infected patients until the disease is resolved, demonstrating that

TABLE 15-1. URINARY NITROGEN EXCRETION IN NORMAL AND FASTED SUBJECTS DURING FEBRILE INFECTION AND HYPERTHERMIA

Treatment	Urinary N gm/day
Normal *	13
Normal + cortisol (25–30 mg/day)	13
Fasted: 72 hr	7–11
28 days	4
Typhoid fever	18–25
Pneumonia	20–25
Meningitis	20–30
Tularemia	16–17
Sepsis	16–22
Hyperthermia: 1 day	15
following day	20

* Intake 14–15 gm, N and 2,500–2,800 cal/day

Adapted from references 19, 29, 51, 57, 58, 62, and 67.

the regulation of body protein economy is severely altered by infection. With resolution of the infection, nitrogen and mineral losses return toward normal. Additional evidence that these deficits are not solely the consequence of diminished food intake is found in controlled feeding studies; energy source, protein, and other nutrients that maintain balance before the onset of infection fail to offset the increased losses during the catabolic phase of infective illness. With resolution of the infection, anabolism once again predominates and body nitrogen and mineral stores are replenished.

Hypermetabolism, negative balance of essential elements, alterations in protein and water economy, and diminished or absent food intake contribute to loss of body weight. If the weight loss is minimal, it may be of no significance to the patient, but if it is severe and protracted, the loss of protoplasmic mass may greatly limit the host responses to infection. Because of the known relationships between malnutrition and infection and the availability of current modalities to maintain or replete body mass, every effort should be made to limit weight loss to no more than 10 percent of the preillness weight.

ALTERATIONS IN GLUCOSE DYNAMICS

Blood glucose is generally elevated in infected patients, and glucose tolerance curves may demonstrate prolonged disappearance after a glucose load. These observations have resulted in descriptive terms, such as "diabetes of infection," which suggest an insulin-deficient state. Moreover, the concept of insulin deficiency was appealing, for it helped explain the increased protein catabolism in critically ill patients. Over the past 10 years, however, a large quantity of data has been gathered in humans, which has improved understanding of carbohydrate metabolism following infection and does not support this thesis.

The first important piece of information comes from respiratory gas exchange data indicating that fat, not carbohydrate, is the major oxidized body fuel.[28] At first glance, this information may appear somewhat contradictory to the implications that have been drawn from well-known nitrogen loss data. Urinary nitrogen excretion increases during a critical illness, and the quantity of nitrogen lost can be generally related to the extent of infection (Table 15-1). The major component of urinary nitrogen is urea, and ureagenesis has been closely linked to gluconeogenesis in starved man. Thus, it was generally assumed that the large quantity of urea excreted after infection and injury reflected increasing rates of gluconeogenesis. Taken together with the results from respiratory gas exchange studies, these data suggest glucose is produced at an accelerated rate but is not totally oxidized.

More direct measurements of the rate of glucose production in infected patients are now available. Long and associates [30] administered C^{14}-glucose and calculated glucose turnover from a multicompartment model. They concluded that glucose flow through the extracellular fluid compartment was increased during infection and that the accelerated rate of gluconeogenesis could not be easily blunted by glucose administration. Further results demonstrated that injury and infection did not impair the ability of the body to oxidize glucose, a finding consistent with respiratory gas data which yielded respiratory exchange ratio values greater than one with progressive carbohydrate loading in severely injured and infected patients. Gump and coworkers [31] catheterized the hepatic vein and estimated splanchnic blood flow by a dye extraction technique. Net hepatic (splanchnic) glucose production (determined from arterial-hepatic vein concentration differences multipled by an estimated flow) was elevated in patients with intra-abdominal infection, and hepatic gluconeogenesis could not be depressed in some of the patients following glucose administration. Moreover, no correlation occurred between net hepatic glucose uptake or production and blood glucose levels in the seriously ill patients. Finally, Long and associates [32] studied the conversion rate of l-alanine to glucose in infected surgical patients. Using C^{14}-l-alanine as a marker to determine the conversion rate of alanine to glucose, the authors found that glucose synthesis from alanine was increased in the patients with intra-abdominal infection. Moreover, the increased alanine conversion rate was not suppressed to normal levels when the patients received exogenous glucose. These data taken together demonstrate that gluconeogenesis is increased in infected patients, and confirm the animal studies demonstrating the increased production of hepatic glucose that follows infection (Figs. 16-10, 16-11).[33]

Although hyperglycemia is the usual response after an infection, a fall in blood glucose can occur, reflecting an imbalance between glucose production and cellular use.

TABLE 15-2. PLASMA GLUCOSE IN BACTEREMIC BURN PATIENTS (Mean ±SE)

Group	N	Age (years)	% Total Body Surface Burn	Postburn Day Studied	Plasma Glucose (mg/100 ml)
Normals (no burns)	12	26	—	—	70±2
Burn patients (no bacteremia)	17	29	42	9	113±5
Burn patients (gram-positive bacteremia)	4	30	62	10	112±7
Burn patients (gram-negative bacteremia)*	16	28	72.5	10	129±9
Burn patients (gram-negative bacteremia)*	5	22	70	12	68±2

* Data from Wilmore, DW, Mason AD Jr, Pruitt BA Jr: Impaired glucose flow in burned patients with gram negative sepsis. *Surg Gynecol Obstet* 143:720, 1976.

The association between gram-negative infection and hypoglycemia was first studied in infected burned rats.[34] Progressive hypoglycemia occurred after the burn wound was seeded with *P. aeruginosa*. This was attributed to impaired hepatic gluconeogenesis, apparently from a direct effect of endotoxin on key gluconeogenic enzymes. These studies were subsequently confirmed and extended in other animal models with other types of microorganisms.[35]

But does this imbalance in glucose metabolism occur in man? The answer is clearly yes, although alterations in glucose production or disposal secondary to severe infection may not consistently cause hypoglycemia because of apparent compensatory mechanisms which maintain blood glucose. Hypoglycemia occurs in infected adults [36-38] and children,[39] but only five of 21 burn patients with gram-negative bacteremia developed hypoglycemia after a 6-hour fast (Table 15-2). All these patients had a stable hyperdynamic circulation and exhibited normal blood pressure and urinary output at the time of study. Occasionally, hypoglycemia (30 to 40 mg per 100 ml) has been observed in other patients (particularly injured children) with gram-negative bacteremia while they are receiving intravenous glucose solutions.

The etiology of this imbalance in glucose production and disposal is multifaceted and a major area of research in many laboratories. Alterations in hepatic blood flow during "septic shock," the toxic effect of endotoxins on the liver, and accelerated peripheral disposal of glucose are factors that may participate in this glucose imbalance syndrome. It should be realized that the hypoglycemia of infection is frequently masked by glucose infusion, and when present is usually seen only in the most critically ill patients. Hyperglycemia in association with accelerated hepatic glucose production is the usual response.

PROTEIN AND AMINO ACID METABOLISM

The increased excretion of urea nitrogen during infection reflects accelerated catabolism of amino acids derived from body protein, primarily skeletal muscle. The increased degradation of skeletal muscle protein is associated with increased urinary excretion of 3-methylhistadine, creatine, and creatinine, all nonmetabolized substances that are liberated from skeletal muscle during catabolism.[29] In addition, prelabeling muscle protein of experimental animals with a tagged amino acid demonstrates accelerated metabolism and utilization of these substances following infection.[40] Amino acids move, via the bloodstream, from peripheral protein stores to the liver where they are used for two fundamental synthetic processes: (1) gluconeogenesis and (2) synthesis of new protein (Figs. 16-10 and 16-13).

Gluconeogenic amino acids (primarily alanine and glutamine) are deaminated in the liver, their carbon skeleton utilized to synthesize glucose and the nitrogen residue converted to urea. Amino acids may provide 10 to 30 percent of the 3-carbon precursors for glucose synthesis,[32] with the remaining gluconeogenic substrate accounted for by the use of glycerol and the recycling of glucose through the Cori pathway, which provides lactate and pyruvate. Alanine accounts for a major quantity of amino acids released from the periphery, yet alanine represents no more than 10 percent of the skeletal muscle protein.[41] It has been proposed that de novo synthesis of alanine must occur, and two metabolic pathways have been suggested for intracellular muscle cell alanine synthesis: (1) a proposed glucose-to-alanine cycle [41] and (2) protein degradation and transamination.[42] Although the specific mechanisms for alanine synthesis in skeletal muscle after infection have not been studied, the progressive muscle wasting that occurs in the infected patient supports the thesis that peripheral protein degradation predominates, a finding similar to that observed during the post-traumatic metabolic response (Figs. 16-8, 16-10, 16-13).

The second requirement for hepatic utilization of the amino acids mobilized from peripheral stores is the synthesis of acute-phase plasma proteins.[43] Infection liberates mediators, which directly (or indirectly, through the sympathetic nervous system) stimulate hepatic production of acute phase proteins including alpha$_1$-antitrypsin, alpha$_2$-acid glycoproteins, haptoglobin, fibrinogen, C-reactive proteins, ceruloplasmin, and the third component of complement (C3). The specific functions of many of these acute-phase reactants is poorly understood, but evidence is accumulating that they participate in host defenses, minimize local tissue damage, and possibly amplify hormonal and cell-mediated host responses. The production rate and accumulation of these substances is generally related to the severity of infection, and accelerated synthesis occurs when infection is superimposed during starvation or after protein-calorie malnutrition, suggesting that these hepatic synthetic processes are preferred pathways for substrate use during various forms of stress.

As previously mentioned, the transport of amino acid substrate from the periphery to the liver occurs by the bloodstream, and characteristic alterations in blood amino acid concentrations occur following infection.[44] In those infections that do not primarily affect the liver, there is a prompt reduction in the total concentration of amino acids in the blood.[29] While the amino acid pattern may vary depending on the infecting organism involved, the plasma aminogram usually shows decreased levels of most free amino acids and increased concentrations of phenylalanine (and frequently tyrosine). The phenylalanine-tyrosine ratio is increased in a variety of infections and febrile conditions and may serve as an index of the catabolic response to infection.[44] This unique response cannot be explained by reduced conversion of phenylalanine to tyrosine or diminished clearance of phenylalanine from the plasma.[45] However, the biologic necessity for this elevation may occur, because this amino acid serves as the essential precursor for catecholamines, which are used at increasing rates during acute illness. Plasma amino acid concentrations characterized by high phenylalanine concentrations and low branched chain amino acid levels are associated with hepatic coma. It has been hypothesized that alterations in mentation and progressive obtundation that occur during infection may be related to similar plasma amino acid imbalances.[46] Other amino acid pathways have not been investigated in such precise detail as phenylalanine, although increased amino acid turnover of almost all amino acids probably exists and may be accompanied by increased oxidation (such as has been described with alanine) or increased diversion into a specialized metabolic pathway (such as increased tryptophan metabolism via the kynurenine pathway). (Figs. 16-8, 16-9)

LIPID METABOLISM

Fat is the major fuel utilized by infected patients and is mobilized from peripheral stores, particularly during periods of inadequate nutritional support. Lipolysis is thought to be mediated by the heightened sympathetic activity, which is a potent stimulus for fat mobilization. Free fatty acids, which serve as the principal fuel for liver and skeletal muscle, disappear at an increased rate early in the clinical course of most infection, and the rates of triglyceride and cholesterol synthesis within the liver are accelerated.[29] Despite increased hepatic production, peripheral utilization may also rise, and serum levels of all lipid moieties may remain normal or even decline in the infected host. Gallin et al [47] observed normal concentrations of total serum lipids in patients with gram-positive infection but found striking elevations of total lipids, triglycerides, and fatty acids in patients with infection caused by gram-negative bacilli. Similar observations were reported by Griffiths et al [48] in their investigations of gram-negative sepsis in the dog (Fig. 16-11).

More recently, Carpentier et al [49] have measured the rate of lipolysis in septic surgical patients and attempted to explain the regulatory mechanisms of the increased fat mobilization. Glycerol turnover was increased 195 percent in the group of infected patients, and fat breakdown was not diminished by administration of glucose, a substrate which significantly limited lipolysis in normal controls. More important, while the absolute serum concentrations of glycerol correlated well with fat turnover in normal individuals, no such relationship could be established between plasma glycerol concentrations and the rate of lipolysis in infected individuals. Thus, during infection, plasma concentrations of fat moieties are not indicative of turnover rates of the lipid components.

Another alteration in fat metabolism after infection has been described. In normal people, starvation results in progressive "ketosis," with the liver forming acetoacetate and beta-hydroxybuturate from the mobilized free fatty acids. These water-soluble lipid fuels will reduce amino acid mobilization from skeletal muscle and serve, in part, as a fuel for the central nervous system, thus sparing glucose. In contrast, ketosis appears to be limited during starvation in the infected organism. Thus, Neufeld et al [50] observed diminished hepatic ketone production in infected starved rats, and Border et al [51] found minimal hepatic ketone release in septic patients during transhepatic substrate flux studies. The exact mechanism for this response is not known, but this phenomenon demonstrates the increased reliance of the body on beta-oxidation of fatty acids which provide a 2-carbon fuel source for oxidative metabolism during infection (Fig. 16-10).

MINERAL METABOLISM

The changes in balance of magnesium, inorganic phosphate, zinc, and potassium generally follow alterations in nitrogen balance. Although iron-binding capacity of transferrin is usually unchanged in early infection, iron virtually disappears from the plasma, especially during severe pyrogenic infections; similar alterations are also observed with serum zinc.[29] These decreases cannot be accounted for by losses of these minerals from the body. Rather, both iron and zinc accumulate in the liver, and this appears as another host defense mechanism. Administration of these minerals to the infected host, especially in the early phase, is contraindicated, for increased serum concentrations may impair host resistance. Unlike the alterations of iron and zinc, copper levels generally rise, and the increased plasma concentration can be ascribed almost entirely to the increased ceruloplasmin produced by the liver.

HORMONAL RESPONSES DURING INFECTION

In healthy people, metabolism is finely balanced between anabolic and catabolic processes. These events are primarily under hormonal control; insulin acts as the principal anabolic agent, while glucocorticoids, glucagon, and catecholamines serve to integrate catabolic responses. When infection occurs, humoral signals arise from the invaded tissue and reach the hypothalamus.[52] Subsequent alterations in hypothalamic afferent activity cause a variety of thermal, circulatory, respiratory, and metabolic adjustments. Many of the investigations describing systemic response to infection have relied on the intravenous administration of pyrogenic substances, which may not provide stimuli totally analogous to those that occur during invasive infection.[53] This is because the infective tissue also releases products of intracellular metabolism, which can serve as additional circulatory mediators. In addition, hypovolemia, hypotension, and alterations in normal acid-base balance can occur, and these derangements will initiate additional homeostatic adjustments. Bed rest, restraint, and pain serve as other factors that modify the hypothalamic responses to infection, primarily through neurogenic afferent input.

GLUCOCORTICOID RESPONSE

With hypothalamic stimulation, increased adrenal corticotropic hormone secretion from the pituitary occurs, causing glucocorticoid liberation from the adrenal cortex.[54] With severe infection, initial blood concentrations of corticoids are elevated and return slowly to normal after the acute phase. Measurements of cortisol turnover indicate that the adrenal cortisol secretion may increase from two to five times normal and return to baseline levels during convalescence.[29] Elevated cortisol concentrations are also associated with periods of cardiovascular instability and hypotension, and can occur during hepatic dysfunction when deconjugation processes are impaired. During stable, prolonged, infectious illness the serum cortisol remains in the high–normal range, and this stable state replaces the usual normal circadian rhythm.

Although the specific effects of corticoids are well known, their role in the metabolic response to infection appears to be the promotion of events in concert with other hormones. Glucocorticoids stimulate gluconeogenesis, and when blood concentrations are elevated they also increase skeletal muscle proteolysis,[55] providing amino acid precursors to be utilized for new glucose. This hormone, however, merely facilitates in this catabolic function (some say permissive), and adrenal ablation studies demonstrate that catabolic responses still occur in adrenalectomized, stressed animals that receive a maintenance dose of cortisol.[56] Moreover, administering large doses of glucocorticoids to fed [57] or fasting [58] control subjects failed to increase urinary urea excretion or accelerate total body nitrogen loss. Thus, cortisol participates with other hormones to facilitate gluconeogenesis and mobilize 3-carbon glucose precursors. It is not *the* catabolic *hormone,* but acts with other hormonal stimuli to promote the transfer of substrate from carcass to liver.

THE PANCREATIC HORMONES

Glucagon, a primary gluconeogenic hormone released from the pancreatic alpha cell, is also elevated promptly during infection and returns to normal during convalescence.[59] The stimuli for this response may be increased sympathetic nervous system activity, increased concentrations of 3-carbon amino acid glucose precursors, or a direct effect of the microorganism or its by-products on the endocrine pancreas. Simultaneous insulin levels remain normal or fall during the acute phase of infection.[26,59,60] Suppression of insulin secretion results from the influence of the adrenergic nervous system or circulating catecholamines on pancreatic beta cells. This frequently occurs in the early phase of infection but is also associated with episodes of hypotension or cardiovascular instability accompanying severe sepsis. In chronic stable infections, insulin rises to normal or elevated levels, despite a low insulin-to-glucagon ratio, a hormonal relationship considered to indicate a call for gluconeogenesis. The elevation of serum insulin levels has been described as insulin resistance, although the experimental support of the concept is incomplete. The interaction between the pancreatic hormones (high glucagon, low insulin) and the participation of other glucoregulatory hormones (cortisol and catecholamines) during infection favor increased hepatic glucose production. With time and convalescence, blood levels of pancreatic hormones return to normal. During late convalescence after severe infection, the insulin response to glucose may be quite low, similar to the response observed during prolonged starvation.

CATECHOLAMINES

While the clinical course of the septic patients is characterized by increased sympathetic nervous system activity (such as hyperpnea, tachycardia, fever) few studies are available to quantitate this response following a variety of infections. Groves and his colleagues [61] measured plasma epinephrine and norepinephrine in patients after uneventful major operations, and in similar patients with severe postoperative infection. These serial measurements revealed that the patients with complications had mean arterial plasma levels of catecholamines near the upper limits of normal, while the catecholamine values were significantly elevated in the septic individuals. Norepinephrine was consistently greater than epinephrine. The increase in plasma catecholamines did not appear in response to circulatory reflexes, because it occurred when blood pressure was normal and there were no other clinical indices to suggest hypovolemia. In our studies, of 10 bacteremic, normotensive, trauma patients, the normal relationship between urinary catecholamine excretion and oxygen consumption that occurs in the noninfected trauma patients appeared disturbed. High levels of catecholamines were present during sepsis but oxidative processes were attenuated.[62] This suggests that sepsis results in an inability of the body to respond appropriately to this calorigenic hormone. Because catecholamines are central to the metabolic and cardiovascular adjustments to infection, the inappropriate nature of this response in infected trauma patients may limit appropriate homeostatic adjustments to severe infection and injury.

OTHER HORMONAL RESPONSES

Thyroid Function

Thyroid function is altered by the stress of acute infection. Protein-bound iodine levels and hormone concentrations of thyroxine (T_4) and triiodothyronine (T_3) fall, while the serum levels of reverse T_3 rise.[63] Kinetic studies of these hormones demonstrate accelerated disappearance of T_3 and T_4 during acute illness.[64] In spite of the low serum concentrations of active thyroid hormones, the pituitary elaboration of thyrotropin-releasing hormone does not increase as it does during hypothyroidism.[65] This suggests that associated adjustments have also occurred in the hypothalamus, which limits thyrotropin-releasing hormone release from the pituitary and, ultimately, the output of thyroid hormone. Thyrotropin-releasing hormone is also markedly inhibited during the administration of dopamine, a commonly used vasoactive agent administered to septic patients during cardiovascular instability. These alterations in thyroid hormone concentration appear at a time when concentrations of thyroid-binding proteins are also altered; the interrelationships between free and bound hormone and the effects of these low serum concentrations on tissue metabolism in criticially ill patients are not known. Thus, apparent biochemical hypothyroidism occurs following acute infection. It has been suggested that the iodine derived from thyroid hormone may play an important role in the bactericidal function of the phagocytic cell, but this hypothesis remains to be proved.

Growth Hormone

Growth hormone has both anabolic and catabolic effects, and one major action of this hormone is to augment fat mobilization and oxidation. During infection or administration of pyrogen, growth hormone increases,[66] but unlike other hormones, this elevation continues into convalescence.[29] Although the precise actions of growth hormone during acute infection are not known, it appears that the prolonged elevation serves to promote anabolism during convalescence.

Aldosterone and Antidiuretic Hormone

Alterations in fluid volume and extracellular electrolyte concentrations occur during infection concurrent with changes in the hormones that regulate salt and water metabolism. Increases in aldosterone, which may not parallel the early rise in cortisol, become evident after fever has begun, persist into convalescence, and then gradually abate. The effect of aldosterone to retain sodium and water can be augmented by increased secretion of antidiuretic hormone, which also aids water retention. Extracellular fluid and total body sodium can thus increase during illness, but these volume and compositional changes are returned to normal during convalescence; these adjustments are heralded by a large and often prolonged diuresis.[67]

TABLE 15-3. THE EFFECT OF HIGH-CALORIC FEEDINGS ON NITROGEN BALANCE IN PATIENTS WITH TYPHOID FEVER

Number of patients	4
Number of periods of study	8
Duration of each study (days)	6
Range of maximum temperature (°F)	101.7 – 103.8
Heat production (kcal/day)	2059
Food calories (kcal/day)	2756
Nitrogen intake (gm/day)	14.3
Nitrogen balance (gm/day)	−3.29

Adapted from Coleman W, DuBois EF: Clinical colorimetry. VII. Calorimetric observations on the metabolism of typhoid patients with and without food. *Arch Intern Med* 15:887, 1915.

REVERSING OR MINIMIZING THE CATABOLIC RESPONSES

NUTRITION FOR THE INFECTED PATIENT

For centuries, starvation was the accepted treatment for patients with fever, and frequently included water deprivation. In 1884, Graves [68] suggested that the deleterious effects of starvation compounded the consequences of disease. He recommended a diet for patients with hypermetabolism secondary to infection and thyrotoxicosis that was considered revolutionary for the times. Although the nutritional intake consisted of only sugar water, meat broths, toast crumbs, and jellies, and probably provided no more than 300 calories per day, this meager oral diet therapy became the accepted means of nutritional support. Graves was convinced of the value of nutrition for critically ill patients, and late in life suggested that his own epitaph read "He feeds fever." In the later 1800s a milk diet for typhoid fever was proposed,[69] and later Peabody advocated the more liberal use of standard oral feedings. However, it was not until the classic studies of Coleman and DuBois,[70] in the early 1900s, that nutritional management of the infected patient was based on scientific fact. Using both direct and indirect calorimetry and additional techniques of energy and nitrogen balance, a variety of patients with typhoid fever were studied during their acute and convalescent phases. The balance calculations and heat transfer data were correlated with alterations in body weight and core and surface temperatures. The impact of food intake on heat production during the febrile period was also assessed.

The conclusions of Coleman and DuBois still describe the interactions between nutritional intake and fever: (1) Body fuels are oxidized to the same end-products as in health, and the laws of the conservation of energy apply to fever patients; (2) the specific dynamic action of protein and carbohydrate is much smaller in the febrile patient with typhoid fever than in the healthy individual; and (3) increased breakdown of protein occurs in infected patients, and the negative nitrogen balance cannot be offset by positive energy balance at the levels of protein intake utilized for normals (Table 15-3).

The specific dietary requirement suggested by Coleman was food equivalent to 4,000 calories per day in a 70-kg man.[69] The diet was high in carbohydrate and protein, based on the studies that demonstrated "carbohydrate protects body protein better than any other foodstuff," and nutrients were provided by meals and interval feedings. Thus, it became accepted that partial starvation was detrimental to the patient's welfare. It was "not only desirable but necessary" that the typhoid patient be given sufficient exogenous nutrients to equal energy expenditure. Physicians of this period repeatedly noted the difficulties in patients' acceptance of hypercaloric oral feedings, and care was taken to provide a variety of palatable food preparations. It was difficult to maintain palatability and taste by reducing dietary fat intake below 20 to 30 percent of the total caloric intake, although carbohydrate provided the greatest reduction of nitrogen losses in the early studies and in subsequent investigations by Lusk.[71]

The development of nutritional support for critically ill patients who cannot eat parallels, but lags by some 50 years, the evolution of dietary therapy for infected patients, who could be maintained by oral intake. While the body's catabolic response could be offset by high-caloric, high-nitrogen feedings, techniques of nutrient delivery and product availability remained the single deterrent for providing adequate nutritional support for the critically ill hospitalized patient. These final hurdles were overcome by the development of a technique for central venous cannulation and infusion of hypertonic nutrient solutions,[72] the formulation and evolution of techniques for administration of defined bulk-free formula enteral diets,[73] and the development of a safe fat emulsion for intravenous administration.[74] Product development has since flourished.

For those critically ill patients who can eat, nutritional support requires a major commitment of the physician and nursing staff and an obligatory full-time commitment of a dietitian or nurse specialist. The unpredictable and variable clinical course of the critically ill patient and the frequent interruption of intake necessitated by repeated operations, treatment procedures, and prolonged diagnostic testing require the strictest of nutritional bookkeeping to insure appropriate intake. Even when "on paper" balance is achieved, inadequate nutrition may result from diarrhea, drug-nutrient interaction, or micronutrient deficiencies or toxicities.

Anorexia and food boredom remain as they were 75 years ago—a significant problem for the seriously ill patient who can eat. The hospital diet, adjusted for the patient's previous dietary preferences and taste, must be supplemented by interval liquid nutrient feedings. When patients cannot eat enough, tube feedings may be used. Most diets can be administered through soft feeding tubes using low-volume continuous administration of hypotonic dietary solutions. Both volume and concentration can be increased with time to achieve caloric intakes that exceed energy demands. If small nasogastric feeding tubes are utilized, bulk-free elemental diets may be necessary.

One unique application of the use of elemental diets is the placement of a 16-gauge polyethylene catheter into the jejunum during an operation on the upper or lower gastrointestinal tract.[75] Immediately following operation, dilute nutrient solutions are infused at low rates, and the volume is slowly increased over the next several days to provide the fluid, electrolyte, and nutrient requirements by enterostomy feeding, thus obviating the need for intravenous support of postoperative patients beyond the first few postoperative days. There are no reported comparisons of this technique with intravenous support.

In some patients, enteral feedings may be inadequate or impossible, and intravenous nutritional support is indicated. This is particularly true in individuals with more than 10 percent body weight loss in whom nutritional intake remains inadequate and resolution of the catabolic process is not immediately forthcoming.[27] Parenteral nutrition is also indicated in the debilitated, malnourished, or thin patient, who has limited body fuel stores and inadequate food intake by the enteral route. Even in the face of tremendous energy requirements in the critically ill patient, parenteral feeding techniques can provide more than enough calories and nitrogen to prevent significant negative energy and nitrogen balance.

THE EFFECT OF GLUCOSE AND GLUCOSE INSULIN THERAPY

Over the past 75 years, many testimonials have appeared supporting the use of glucose or glucose and insulin therapy during critical illness. As previously noted, Coleman[69] and Lusk[71] preferred carbohydrate for its superior nitrogen-sparing capacity. Benn and associates in England, Darrow in this country, and many others administered dextrose and antitoxin in the treatment of diphtheria.[76] Some groups favored the simultaneous administration of insulin with the glucose, but not all agreed, and this contention was extensively studied and actively debated.[76]

What are the physiologic advantages provided by glucose therapy? Cardiac function and circulatory status may improve in patients with refractory congestive heart failure, hypovolemic shock, or gram-negative septicemia.[77] Liver function may stabilize or improve, but it is not known if this effect is the result of a provision of additional cellular energy or the increased exposure of the hepatocyte to high insulin levels, a hormone thought by some to induce hepatic cell regeneration and replication.[78] In recent years, Allison's group[79] in England have stimulated renewed interest in glucose-insulin administration, reporting the protein-sparing and potassium-retaining effects of this therapy in a wide variety of disease processes. In burn patients with infection, dextrose-insulin infusions resulted in a prompt natriuresis and nonosmotic diuresis.[79] The movement of glucose into the cells is thought to restore the adenosine triphosphate-dependent sodium-potassium pump, which may become energy-deficient during critical illness. Failure of the cell pump results in an increased accumulation of intracellular sodium and water, often referred to as the "sick cell syndrome."

Curreri and associates[80] confirmed the intracellular cation dysequilibrium in critically ill patients, and noted that supracaloric feedings administered to extensively injured patients returned the abnormally elevated erythrocyte cation concentration to normal. Further studies in burn patients confirmed a decrease in active erythrocyte membrane cation transport; restoration of sodium-potassium cell pump activity was achieved by the provision of carbohydrate in the diet.[78] McDougal and associates[81] extended these studies, demonstrating that hepatic transport of indocyanine green dye (a marker incorporated by active hepatic membrane transport) is improved with the addition of carbohydrate to the parenteral feedings that follow infection.

In all recent studies that involve glucose or glucose and insulin therapy, generous quantities of protein and other essential nutrients have been simultaneously administered with the carbohydrate. Omission of the protein of high biologic value from the diet would eventually lead to hospital-induced kwashiorkor, further impairing hepatic function.

Early investigators favored high carbohydrate diets in patients with infection, noting that carbohydrate provided greater protein sparing than fat. More recent studies evaluating the interaction of fat and carbohydrate calories were reported by Long and associates,[82] using intravenous diets. Hypermetabolic patients were infused with a constant dose of amino acids (11.7 gm per m^2 per day) and received a varying proportion of calories delivered as a soybean emulsion or glucose. The use of carbohydrate resulted in a rapid decrease in nitrogen excretion, while comparable doses of fat calories failed to have a similar effect. As carbohydrate calories increased, nitrogen excretion decreased. Addition of insulin further blunted nitrogen loss. Within the period of these studies, there was no evidence of adaptation to the infused fat, which exceeded 2,000 calories per day in some patients. European investigators have reported increased nitrogen excretion from infected or traumatized patients when fat is substituted isocalorically for carbohydrate.[83]

These studies in critically ill patients, however, are contrasted to the investigations in either normal or chronically depleted patients where no alteration in nitrogen excretion was found after a period of adaptation when intravenous fat was substituted for carbohydrate.[84] The differences in these studies may be reconciled by the fact that hypermetabolic patients have neurohormonal signals, which accelerate gluconeogenesis and override the ability of the body to adapt metabolically to starvation or variations in energy sources. In the critically ill patients, intravenous fat is a satisfactory source of essential fatty acid and

TABLE 15-4. SYSTEMIC RESPONSES TO INFECTION

Response	Clinical Manifestation	Liabilities	Clinical Implications
Upward shift in central reference temperature or body's "thermostat"	Controlled elevation of body temperature (fever) Increased Q_{10} Increased metabolic rate (Q_{10} effect of fever)	Increased energy costs Increased circulatory demands CNS derangement (malaise, seizures, etc.) Normal room temperature perceived as cold and causes shivering Increased insensible water loss	Support a *reasonable* (< 40C) febrile state by providing exogenous fuel and a warm thermal environment When heat unloading patients with excessive body temperature, modify central setpoint Maintain hydration
Body catabolism	Weight loss Loss of lean body mass Weakness Increased urinary excretion of nitrogen, K^+, PO_4^{-3}	Loss of functional body proteins and other intracellular components limiting physiologic reserve	Adequate nutritional support to achieve nitrogen equilibrium Exercise
Increased gluconeogenesis	Hyperglycemia Glucosuria Osmotic diuresis	Increased energy cost Hyperosmolality Excessive fluid loss Inability to conserve protein by formation of ketone bodies	Minimize gluconeogenesis by administration of exogenous dietary carbohydrate Control hyperglycemia with insulinization
Increased acute-phase protein synthesis	Alterations in serum protein concentrations	Skeletal muscle proteolysis Alteration in osmotic pressure with fall in serum albumin	Provide adequate nutritional support with protein of high biologic value Vitamin supplementation
Trace mineral distribution	Decreases in serum concentrations of Zn^{+2} and Fe^{+3} and increase of Cu^{+2}		Administration of Zn^{+2} and Fe^{+3} (not indicated during the acute phase)

provides additional calories to meet energy expenses, thus stabilizing body fat or increasing body weight. It should not be administered to the exclusion of carbohydrate in the hypermetabolic critically ill patient.

ADJUNCTIVE MEASURES

Deposition and incorporation of amino acids into skeletal protein is facilitated by active muscular activity. Critically ill patients have marked limitations of their activity and require a planned exercise program to maintain an active and functional skeletal mass. With the help of physical therapists, simple isometric exercise can be accomplished while the patient remains in bed. These exercises may aid the vitality of the muscles and help restore nitrogen balance across the skeletal muscle bed after caloric and nitrogen equilibrium have been achieved. Technologic advances, such as air-fluidized and water beds, provide improved methods for patient care yet discourage active use of muscle groups. These devices provide unique suspension systems for patients, which simulate the antigravity state, and can increase the breakdown of lean body mass if regular and special exercises are not instituted.

Every effort should be made to resolve the infective process, diminish wound contamination, and aid wound healing. Judicious use of antibiotics, operative drainage of abscesses, and well-planned operative procedures remain the mainstay in limiting postinfective or posttraumatic catabolism. Cold ambient temperature, pain, anxiety, and hypovolemia are potent afferent stimuli, which accentuate the metabolic response to injury and infection; these factors can be minimized by careful management. Following resolution of the initiator of the hypermetabolic response, the patient's appetite seems to improve, spirits rise, and increased exercise is possible. Convalescence heralds a rebuilding of body mass, a gain in weight, and the patient's return to an active and productive life.

Invasive infection directly alters cellular function and elaborates circulating mediators, both of which modify hormonal regulation. The integrated sum of all these responses is expressed in the body's systemic adjustments to infection. The major systemic events following infection fall into two broad categories: thermoregulatory and metabolic alterations. There is a growing body of evidence to suggest that these systemic responses facilitate host defense. If they are not a set of responses with a purpose they are certainly associated with a positive result—resolution of the infective process. The systemic responses, however, are not without their liabilities (Table 15-4). Comprehensive understanding of the neuroendocrine basis for thermoregulatory and metabolic alterations that occur after infection is necessary for appropriate clinical management and restoration of normal function.

BIBLIOGRAPHY

Dinarello CA, Wolff SM: Pathogenesis of fever in man. N Engl J Med 298:607, 1978.

Moore FD: Metabolic Care of the Surgical Patient. Philadelphia, Saunders, 1959.

Wilmore DW: The Metabolic Management of the Critically Ill—Support Plan. New York, Plenum, 1977.

Wilmore DW, Aulick LH, Pruitt BH Jr: Metabolism during the hypermetabolic phase of thermal injury. In Advances in Surgery, Vol 12. Yearbook Medical Publishers, 1978, pp 193–225.

Wilmore DW, Goodwin C, Aulick LH, Powanda MC, Mason AD Jr, Pruitt BA Jr: Effect of injury and infection on visceral metabolism and circulation. Ann Surg 192:4, 1980.

REFERENCES

1. DuBoise EF: Fever and the Regulation of Body Temperature. Springfield, Ill, Thomas, 1948.
2. Eichna LW, Berger AR, Rader B, Becker WH: Comparison of intracardiac and intravascular temperatures with rectal temperatures in man. J Clin Invest 30:353, 1951.
3. Cooper KE, Kenyon JR: A comparison of temperatures measured in the rectum, oesophagus and on the surface of the aorta during hypothermia in man. Br J Surg 44:616, 1957.
4. Molnar GW, Read RC: Studies during open-heart surgery on the special characteristics of rectal temperature. J Appl Physiol 36:333, 1974.
5. Wilmore DW, Aulick LH, Pruitt BA Jr: Metabolism during the hypermetabolic phase of thermal injury. Advances in Surgery, Vol 12. Yearbook Medical Publishers, 1978, pp 193–225.
6. Hammell HT: Regulation of internal body temperature. Ann Rev Physiol 30:641, 1968.
7. Westphal O, Westphal U, Sommer T: The history of pyrogen research. In Schlessinger D (ed): Microbiology. Washington, DC, American Society of Microbiology, 1977, pp 221–238.
8. Bennett IL Jr, Beeson PB: Studies on the pathogenesis of fever. I. The effect of injection of extracts and suspensions of uninfected rabbit tissues upon the body temperature of normal rabbits. J Exp Med 98:477, 1953.
9. Atkins E, Bodel P: Fever. N Engl J Med 286:27, 1972.
10. Dinarello CA, Wolff SM: Pathogenesis of fever in man. N Engl J Med 298:607, 1978.
11. Wannemacher RW Jr, DuPont HL, Pekarek PS, Powanda MC, Schwartz A, Hornick RB, Beisel WR: An endogenous mediator of depression of amino acids and trace metals in serum during typhoid fever. J Infect Dis 126:77, 1972.
12. Snell ES, Atkins E: The Mechanism of Fever in the Biological Basis of Medicine. New York, Academic, 1968, pp 397–419.
13. Bligh J: Temperature Regulation in Mammals and Other Vertebrates. Amsterdam, North-Holland, 1973.
14. Buskirk ER, Thompson RH, Rubenstein M, Wolff SM: Heat exchange in men and women following intravenous injection of endotoxin. J Appl Physiol 19:907, 1964.
15. Kluger MJ: The evolution and adaptive value of fever. Am Sci 66:38, 1978.
16. Bernheim HA, Kluger MJ: Fever: effect of drug-induced antipyresis on survival. Science 192:237, 1976.
17. Kluger MJ, Vaughn LK: Fever and survival in rabbits infected with *Pasteurella multocida*. J Physiol 282:243, 1978.
18. Grieger TA, Kluger MJ: Fever and survival: the role of serum iron. J Physiol 279:187, 1978.
19. Beisel WR, Goldman RF, Joy RJT: Metabolic balance studies during induced hyperthermia in man. J Appl Physiol 24:1, 1968.
20. Liljedahl SO, Birke G: The nutrition of patients with extensive burns. Nutr Metab 14(suppl):110, 1972.
21. Myers RD, Tytell M: Fever: reciprocal shift in brain sodium to calcium ratio as the set-point temperature rises. Science 178:765, 1972.
22. Lomax P: Drugs and body temperature. Int Rev Neurobiol 12:1, 1970.
23. Moyer CA, Nissan S: Alterations in the basal oxygen consumptions of rats attendant upon three types of dehydration. Ann Surg 154:51, 1961.
24. Nissan S, Aviram A, Czaczkes JW, Ullmann L, Ullmann TD: Increased O_2 consumption of the rat diaphragm by elevated NaCl concentrations. Am J Physiol 210:1222, 1966.
25. Freinkel N, Arky RA, Singer DL, Cohen AK, Bleicher SJ, Anderson JB, Silbert CK, Foster AE: Alcohol hypoglycemia. IV. Current concepts of its pathogenesis. Diabetes 14:350, 1965.
26. Wilmore DW, Mason AD Jr, Pruitt BA Jr: Impaired glucose flow in burned patients with gram negative sepsis. Surg Gynecol Obstet 143:720, 1976.
27. Wilmore DW: The Metabolic Management of the Critically Ill—Support Plan. New York, Plenum, 1977.
28. Duke JH Jr, Jorgensen SB, Broell JR, Long CL, Kinney JM: Contribution of protein to caloric expenditure following injury. Surgery 68:168, 1970.
29. Beisel WR: Metabolic response to infection. Annu Rev Med 26:9, 1975.
30. Long CL, Spencer JL, Kinney JM, Geiger JW: Carbohydrate metabolism in men: effect of elective operations and major injury. J Appl Physiol 31:110, 1971.
31. Gump FE, Long CL, Killian P, Kinney JM: Studies of glucose intolerance in septic injured patients. J Trauma 14:378, 1974.
32. Long CL, Kinney JM, Geiger JW: Nonsuppressability of gluconeogenesis by glucose in septic patients. Metabolism 25:193, 1976.
33. Wannemacher RW Jr, Neufeld HA, Canonico PG: Hepatic gluconeogenic capacity and rate during pneumococcal infection in rats. Fed Proc 35:343, 1976.
34. LaNoue KF, Mason AD Jr, Daniels JP: The impairment of glucogenesis by gram negative infection. Metabolism 17:606, 1968.
35. McCallum RE, Berry LJ: Effects of endotoxin on gluconeogenesis, glycogen synthesis and liver glycogen synthase in mice. Infect Immun 7:642, 1973.
36. McFadzean AJS, Yeung RTT: Hypoglycaemia in suppurative pancholangiitis due to *Clonorchis sinesis.* Trans R Soc Trop Med Hyg 59:179, 1965.
37. Berk JL, Hagen JF, Beyer WH, Gerber MJ: Hypoglycemia of shock. Ann Surg 171:400, 1970.
38. Rackwitz R, Jahrmärker H, Prechtel H: Hypoglykämie Wahrend Kreislaufschock. Klin Wochenschr 52:605, 1974.
39. Yeung CY: Hypoglycemia in neonatal sepsis. J Pediatr 77:812, 1970.
40. Wannemacher RW Jr, Powanda MC, Dinterman RD: Amino acid flux and protein synthesis after exposure of rats to either *Diplococcus pneumoniae* or *Salmonella typhimurium.* Infec Immun 10:60, 1974.
41. Felig P: Amino acid metabolism in man. Annu Rev Biochem 44:933, 1975.
42. Garber AJ, Karl IE, Kipnis DM: Metabolic interrelationships and factors controlling skeletal muscle protein degradation and the selective synthesis and release of alanine and glut-

amine. In Greene H, Holliday M, Munro H (eds): Clinical Nutrition Update: Amino Acids. Chicago, American Medical Association, 1977, pp 10–20.
43. Powanda MC: Changes in body balances of nitrogen and other key nutrients: description of underlying mechanisms. Am J Clin Nutr 30:1254, 1977.
44. Wannemacher RW Jr: Key role of various individual amino acids in host response to infection. Am J Clin Nutr 30:1269, 1977.
45. Herndon DN, Wilmore DW, Mason AD Jr, Pruitt BA Jr: Abnormalities of phenylalanine and tyrosine kinetics: significance in septic and nonseptic burned patients. Arch Surg 113:133, 1978.
46. Freund HR, Ryan JA Jr, Fischer JE: Amino acid derangements in patients with sepsis: treatment with branched chain amino acid rich infusions. Ann Surg 188:423, 1978.
47. Gallin JI, Kaye D, O'Leary WM: Serum lipids in infection. N Engl J Med 281:1031, 1969.
48. Griffiths J, Groves AC, Leung FY: Hypertriglyceridemia and hypoglycemia in gram-negative sepsis in the dog. Surg Gynecol Obstet 136:897, 1973.
49. Carpentier YA, Askanazi J, Elwyn DH, Jeevanandam M, Gump FE, Hyman AI, Burr R, Kinney JM: Effects of hypercaloric glucose infusion on lipid metabolism in injury and sepsis. J Trauma, 1981 (in press).
50. Neufeld HA, Pace JA, White FE: The effect of bacterial infections on ketone concentrations in rat liver and blood and on free fatty acid concentrations in rat blood. Metabolism 25:877–884, 1976.
51. Border JR, Chenier R, McManamy RH, LaDuca J, Seibel R, Birkhahn R, Yu L: Multiple systems organ failure: muscle fuel deficit with visceral protein malnutrition. Surg Clin North Am 56:1147, 1976.
52. Chambers WW, Koenig H, Koenig R, Windle WF: Site of action in the central nervous system of a bacterial pyrogen. Am J Physiol 159:209, 1949.
53. Berry LJ: Bacterial Toxins, Critical Reviews in Toxicology, vol 5. Cleveland, Chemical Rubber Company Press, 1977, pp 239–318.
54. Egdahl RH: The differential response of the adrenal cortex and medulla to bacterial endotoxin. J Clin Invest 38:1120, 1959.
55. Thomas FM, Munro HN, Young VR: Effect of glucocorticoid administration on the rate of muscle protein breakdown in vivo in rats, as measured by urinary excretion of N^{r}-methylhistidine. Biochem J 178:139, 1979.
56. Ingle DJ, Meeks RC, Thomas KE: The effect of fractures upon urinary electrolytes in non-adrenalectomized rats and in adrenalectomized rats treated with adrenal cortex extract. Endocrinology 49:703, 1951.
57. Beisel WR, Sawyer WD, Ryll ED, Crozier D: Metabolic effects of intracellular infections in man. Ann Intern Med 47:744, 1967.
58. Owen OE, Cahill GF Jr: Metabolic effects of exogenous glucocorticoids in fasted man. J Clin Invest 52:2596, 1973.
59. Rocha DM, Santeusanio F, Faloona GR, Unger RH: Abnormal pancreatic alpha-cell function in bacterial infections. N Engl J Med 288:700, 1973.
60. Rayfield EJ, Curnow RT, George DT, Bisel WR: Impaired carbohydrate metabolism during a mild viral illness. N Engl J Med 289:618, 1973.
61. Groves AC, Griffiths J, Leung F, Meek RN: Plasma catecholamines in patients with serious postoperative infection. Ann Surg 178:102, 1973.
62. Wilmore DW, Long JM, Mason AD Jr, Skreen RW, Pruitt BA Jr: Catecholamines mediator of the hypermetabolic response to thermal injury. Ann Surg 180:653, 1974.
63. Burger A, Suter P, Nicod P, Vallotton MB, Vagenakis A, Braverman L: Reduced active thyroid hormone levels in acute illness. Lancet 1:653, 1976.
64. Wartofsky L, Martin D, Earll JM: Alterations in thyroid iodine release and the peripheral metabolism of thyroxine during acute falciparum malaria in man. J Clin Invest 51:2215, 1972.
65. Talwar KK, Sawhney RC, Rastogi GK: Serum levels of thyrotropin, thyroid hormones and their responses to thyrotropin releasing hormone in infective febrile illnesses. J Clin Endocrinol Metab 44:398, 1977.
66. Davidson MB, Mager M, Killian P, Braun A: Metabolic and thermal responses to piromen in man. J Clin Endocrinol Metab 32:179, 1971.
67. Moore FD: Metabolic Care of the Surgical Patient. Philadelphia, Saunders, 1959.
68. Graves RJ: Clinical Lectures on the Practice of Medicine. London, New Sydenham Society, 1884 (reprinted from the second edition).
69. Coleman W: Diet in typhoid fever. JAMA 53:1145, 1909.
70. Coleman W, DuBois EF: Clinical calorimetry. VII. Calorimetric observations on the metabolism of typhoid patients with and without food. Arch Intern Med 15:887, 1915.
71. Lusk G: The Elements of the Science of Nutrition. Philadelphia, Saunders, 1906.
72. Dudrick SJ, Wilmore DW, Vars HM, Rhoads JE: Long-term total parenteral nutrition with growth, development, and positive nitrogen balance. Surgery 64:134, 1968.
73. Stephens RV, Randall HT: Use of a concentrated, balanced liquid elemental diet for nutritional management of catabolic states. Ann Surg 170:642, 1969.
74. Wretlind A: Complete intravenous nutrition. Theoretical and experimental background. Nutr Metab 14(Trippe):1, 1972.
75. Page CP, Ryan JA Jr, Haff RC: Continual catheter administration of an elemental diet. Surg Gynecol Obstet 142:184, 1976.
76. Martin E: Dextrose Therapy in Everyday Practice. New York, Hoeber, 1937.
77. Clowes GHA Jr, O'Donnell TF Jr, Ryan NT, Blackburn GL: Energy metabolism in sepsis: treatment based on different patterns in shock and high output state. Ann Surg 179:684, 1974.
78. McDougal WS, Heimburger S, Wilmore DW, Pruitt BA Jr: The effect of exogenous substrate on hepatic metabolism and membrane transport during endotoxemia. Surgery 84:55, 1978.
79. Hinton P, Allison SP, Littlejohn S, Lloyd J: Electrolyte changes after burn injury and effect of treatment. Lancet 2:218, 1973.
80. Curreri PW, Wilmore DW, Mason AD Jr, Newsome TW, Asch MJ, Pruitt BA Jr: Intracellular cation alterations following major trauma: effect of supranormal caloric intake. J Trauma 11:390, 1971.
81. McDougal WS, Wilmore DW, Pruitt BA Jr: Glucose dependent hepatic membrane transport in nonbacteremic and bacteremic thermally injured patients. J Surg Res 22:697, 1977.
82. Long JM III, Wilmore DW, Mason AD Jr, Pruitt BA Jr: Comparison of carbohydrate and fat as caloric sources. Surg Forum 26:108, 1975.
83. Woolfson AMJ, Heatley RV, Allison SP: Insulin to inhibit protein catabolism after injury. N Engl J Med 300:14, 1979.
84. Jeejeebhoy KN, Anderson GH, Nakhooda AF, Greenberg GR, Sanderson I, Marliss EB: Metabolic studies in total parenteral nutrition with lipid in man. Comparison with glucose. J Clin Invest 57:125, 1976.

CHAPTER 16
Hemodynamic and Metabolic Responses

MARC S. VISNER, FRANK B. CERRA, AND ROBERT W. ANDERSON

THE normal systemic responses to infection include hyperpyrexia and tachycardia, which are self-limited and frequently do not require treatment. During severe and inadequately controlled infection, however, the physiologic responses to even localized infections can become life-threatening, because they result in inadequate perfusion and fueling of vital organs and tissues. Although organ system dysfunction can in some cases result from hemodynamic derangements (such as renal failure associated with hypovolemia), most organ failure in patients with uncontrolled sepsis is due to metabolic abnormalities. In these circumstances, the circulatory abnormalities reflect the general metabolic disorder.

This chapter emphasizes the circulatory and metabolic responses to gram-negative bacillary infections. The physiologic responses to these infections have been thoroughly studied and are of obvious clinical importance. Although endotoxin itself has no direct effect on myocardium or vascular smooth muscle, endotoxin can activate endogenous mediators, which are capable of inducing both circulatory and metabolic abnormalities.

Whether or not a given infection leads to a life-threatening systemic circulatory response depends largely on the patient's underlying health. The elderly or debilitated patient with chronic disease, trauma, or burn is most susceptible to this type of insult. Degenerative diseases, immunologic disorders (either primary or iatrogenic), malignancies, aplastic anemia, hepatic disease, and the collagen disorders can all contribute to decreased host resistance and worsen the prognosis of serious infections. In children, prematurity and congenital defects are important risk factors; in elderly patients, cardiac disease, reduced pulmonary function, and poor renal function predispose to the development of severe infection and worsen the prognosis when infection occurs. Freid and Vosti [1] found that the mortality in 270 patients with gram-negative bacteremia was 86 percent in patients with rapidly fatal underlying diseases, 46 percent in patients with ultimately fatal diseases, and 16 percent in patients in otherwise good health. Additional studies by Meakins et al [2] have emphasized the importance of immunologic competence in determining the clinical outcome of severe infection.

PATTERNS OF CIRCULATORY RESPONSES TO SEPSIS

SEPSIS AND ENDOTOXEMIA IN ANIMAL MODELS

The circulatory abnormalities complicating serious human infection are difficult to reproduce in animal models. The hemodynamic response to endotoxin alone is species-specific. An extensively utilized model has been the hemodynamic response of the dog to a lethal intravenous bolus of endotoxin. The dog manifests hypotension within the first minute, the apparent result of hepatic venous constriction and decrease in systemic venous return (Fig. 16-1). The blood pressure returns to near normal levels within the first hour. Subsequently, a progressive decline in cardiac output accompanied by intense peripheral vasoconstriction leads to profound hypotension and death.[3] Bloody diarrhea frequently occurs within the first several hours, and severe hemorrhagic necrosis of the intestinal mucosa is a characteristic postmortem finding. This vascular intestinal injury was at one time attributed to the hepatic venoconstriction. However, dogs that have previously undergone hepatectomy, hepatic devascularization, or portosystemic decompression manifest the same mortality and intestinal pathology even though they are spared the precipitous initial episode of hypotension.[3] Pulmonary vascular resistance and pulmonary artery pressure are both increased during the initial episode of hypotension in dogs. Pretreatment with goat antiplatelet serum, inducing thrombocytopenia, obliterates the initial pulmonary hypertension but does not prevent early systemic hypotension and fall in cardiac output.[4]

The hemodynamic response of the subhuman primate to the infusion of endotoxin or live bacteria is quite different from the response of the dog. Circulatory failure evolves over a period of 3 to 6 hours and is characterized by a gradually decreasing cardiac output without a precipitous early decline in blood pressure. Total peripheral resistance falls progressively during a 3-hour infusion of gram-negative organisms and continues to decline thereafter.[5,6] Hypotension often does not occur except as a preterminal event. Oxygen consumption and arteriovenous oxygen

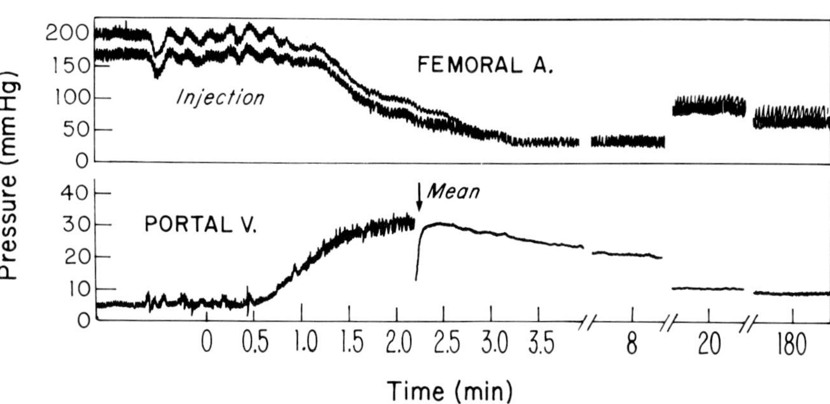

Fig. 16-1. The hemodynamic response of the dog to a lethal intravenous bolus of *E. coli* endotoxin is illustrated. The fall in femoral artery pressure occurs at 1 minute and is associated with an increase in portal venous pressure. At 20 minutes, the portal pressure has returned nearly to baseline levels, and the blood pressure has partially recovered. A subsequent decline in blood pressure is apparent at 3 hours. This second phase of hypotension is unrelenting and eventually fatal. (From McLean LD, Weil MH: Hypotension (shock) in dogs produced by *Escherichia coli* endotoxin. *Circul Res* IV:546, 1956)

(A-VO_2) differences are normal or increased. The fall in cardiac output and the failure of the A-VO_2 difference to narrow limit the usefulness of this model, because both these findings are opposite to the abnormalities often observed in human sepsis.

RELEVANCE OF ANIMAL MODELS FOR HUMAN RESPONSES

A broad spectrum of circulatory responses to infections in humans has been described, but few data are available describing the circulatory response to a bolus injection of endotoxin. No immediate hypotension has been observed in those few experiments performed in healthy volunteers.[7] In addition, the early phases of the circulatory response to infection have seldom been studied because such patients are not often monitored hemodynamically until they have already demonstrated instability of their arterial pressure. Thus, an early and precipitous hypotensive response to clinical infection has never been documented.

The individual patient's response seems to depend on the seriousness of his infection, his preexisting fluid and metabolic status, and the functional reserve of his cardiovascular system. One of the most common patterns of hemodynamic response in humans is characterized by elevated cardiac output, decreased peripheral resistance, and decreased oxygen extraction and utilization by the tissues. This pattern of response has not been successfully reproduced in animals. The failure to simulate this response in animal models is not only a problem of species difference but is probably also related to the rate of toxin infusion. In the clinical setting, a number of interactive factors determine the extent and the rate at which bacteria and their toxins are disseminated systemically. Clearly, this is different from a bolus injection of endotoxin used in the laboratory. The animal models that have come the closest to reproducing the hyperdynamic human response have been those in which a more indolent form of infection has been created (intraperitoneal abscess[8] and hindlimb cellulitis[9]).

The inability of animal models to simulate the spectrum of the human circulatory response to infection underlies the need to study this response at the bedside. Here both ethical and practical difficulties are encountered, because various invasive procedures are necessary to quantitate hemodynamic responses. Blood vessels must be catheterized to measure cardiac output, arterial pressure, pulmonary and systemic resistances, and right- and left-sided ventricular filling pressures. The clinician, however, cannot justify the risk and expense of making these measurements unless there is already some evidence that hemodynamic abnormalities are present. By the time the most overt signs of these abnormalities (usually arterial hypotension) appear, however, the systemic circulatory response may already be life-threatening. Furthermore, if a more complete description of the cardiovascular reserves of the patient is desired, interventions that have not been proved justifiable in even the critically ill patient may be required. For example, the mechanics of cardiac muscle can be analyzed from the dimension and pressure data provided by cardiac catheterization and ventriculography—procedures rarely feasible in the critically ill patient. Newly developed radionuclide imaging techniques may provide the necessary noninvasive means of obtaining comparable data.

PATTERNS OF HUMAN RESPONSE TO INFECTION

Since 1940, a wealth of hemodynamic and metabolic data has become available from patients with serious infections, particularly septicemia. The analysis of these data has led clinical investigators to the following conclusions: (1) circulatory insufficiency in sepsis differs hemodynamically from shock states that accompany trauma and hemorrhage; (2) hemodynamic abnormalities in sepsis are usually accompanied by metabolic derangements in the peripheral tissues; (3) the inability of the circulatory system and the peripheral metabolic machinery to meet the energy demands of the tissues can result from either a decrease in cardiac output or a decrease in oxygen utilization by the tissues; and (4) the pattern of circulatory insufficiency in which cardiac output is decreased is usually associated with a rapid death if cardiac output cannot be augmented.

The patient with a serious surgical infection, such as peritonitis, who becomes hypotensive will usually manifest one of two hemodynamic patterns.

1. In one pattern, the cardiac output is high and the peripheral vascular resistance is low (the hyperdynamic or high-flow state). The patient is warm and pink; cardiac output is increased by as much as 400 percent, oxygen consumption is normal or decreased, and A-VO_2 differences are diminished resulting in abnormally high venous oxygen contents.

2. In the low-flow state, hypotension occurs in the presence of decreased cardiac output and often greatly increased peripheral vascular resistance. The extremities are cool, mottled, and cyanotic. This pattern of circulatory insufficiency is similar to that seen in hemorrhagic shock, in which hypovolemia and decreased venous return are the cause of low cardiac output and hypotension. Sympathetic tone is dramatically increased, and peripheral vasoconstriction sustains perfusion of the brain and heart. The pattern of endotoxic shock in canine models is in many respects similar to this hypodynamic response in man.

This simple classification scheme has taken a long time to evolve. In 1941, Ebert and Stead [10] reported eight cases of circulatory failure accompanying serious gram-positive infection. Neither Trendelenberg position nor transfusion reversed the hypotension. The authors concluded that depletion of blood volume was not the primary cause of the hemodynamic derangements.

Ten years later, Waisbren [11] defined two distinct clinical patterns in a group of 29 patients with gram-negative bacteremia. One group appeared toxic, hot, dry, and flushed; blood pressure was normal and peripheral pulses were bounding. Waisbren designated a second group of patients as being in a shocklike state. They appeared critically ill and were cold, clammy, and lethargic. They remained hypotensive until their infections were controlled.

In 1966, Clowes et al [12] reported quantitative hemodynamic and metabolic data from 25 surgical patients with fulminating peritonitis. Nine of these patients eventually died of their sepsis; twelve recovered promptly from their infections. All 12 had elevated cardiac indices, averaging 3.5 liters per minute per M^2, and in only two was hypotension present at any time. Often in this group, intravenous fluid administration was necessary to replace third-space losses before cardiac output increased. In contrast, deaths occurred in nine patients who either never responded to their infections with increased cardiac output or failed to sustain high output because of intercurrent complications.

MacLean et al [13] confirmed these observations in a study of 56 patients with apparent septic shock. Two distinct groups of patients were identified (Figs. 16-2, 16-3). Twenty-eight patients were classified as being in early septic shock; 24 survived. The clinical presentation among the survivors was characterized by: (1) hyperventilation with arterial pH exceeding 7.40, (2) elevated cardiac output, (3) high central venous pressure, (4) low peripheral vascular resistance, (5) elevated blood volume, (6) hypotension, (7) oliguria, (8) warm, dry extremities, and (9) arterial blood lactate accumulation (Fig. 16-2). A second group of patients initially had: (1) low central venous pressure, (2) low cardiac output, (3) high peripheral resistance, and (4) cold, cyanotic extremities. If the patients in this second group were identified early, they were usually alkalotic and survived after replacement of volume deficits and treatment of their infections. If they were acidotic when initially studied, neither fluids nor vasopressors augmented their cardiac outputs, and most died (Fig. 16-3).

Siegel et al [14] also recognized that the hemodynamic response of patients with severe infections could be categorized on the basis of high or low cardiac outputs. In addition, these investigators made the important observation that those patients with the highest cardiac outputs manifested abnormally high venous oxygen contents and diminished A-VO_2 differences. When oxygen consumption was correlated with cardiac output, a higher cardiac output was observed at each level of oxygen consumption in the hyperdynamic group compared to seriously ill, nonseptic patients. Siegel's group also analyzed myocardial function by evaluating left ventricular stroke work as a function of central venous pressure. They concluded that even those patients with elevated cardiac outputs had compromised myocardial function with depressed Starling curves. The patients with high flows, however, had better myocardial function than the hypodynamic patients who had cardiac indices of less than 2.4 liters per minute per M^2. Treatment with isoproterenol or digitalis improved the myocardial performance of some patients in both groups. In contrast to the preceding reports, this study did not conclude that the hypodynamic state was necessarily attended by a poor prognosis. Instead, the patients who demonstrated the most severe abnormalities in oxygen utilization and extraction were the least likely to survive.

No one knows how to predict which of the two hemodynamic patterns will be found in a given patient with uncontrolled infection. In the few animal models in which the hyperdynamic state has been successfully reproduced, almost equal numbers of animals have manifested the hyperdynamic or hypodynamic response. This would suggest that one pattern does not necessarily evolve into the other, but that instead a variety of host factors may determine which circulatory response will become manifest. Clinical studies do not generally control for the type or severity of the septic insult, but these studies also suggest that patients can initially present with either pattern of response. There is some data from MacLean et al [13] that those patients who were hypovolemic at the time their circulatory abnormalities were discovered were more likely to have low cardiac outputs and elevated peripheral vascular resistances. Certainly, in the clinical setting of intra-abdominal sepsis, there are often large third-space fluid losses. Delay in replacing these losses and correcting electrolyte and acid-base abnormalities can lead to a low-flow pattern that is refractory to pharmacologic intervention. Among dogs with septic hindlimb cellulitis, those developing elevated cardiac outputs within the first 24 to 48 hours had less volume loss into their septic extremity than dogs with low cardiac outputs.[9] The cardiovascular performance of the hyperdynamic animals also seemed to be extremely sensitive to depletion of intravascular volume. They demonstrated a 50 percent greater decrease in cardiac output during a period of controlled hemorrhage when compared to dogs without sepsis. Besides fluid status, there are pre-

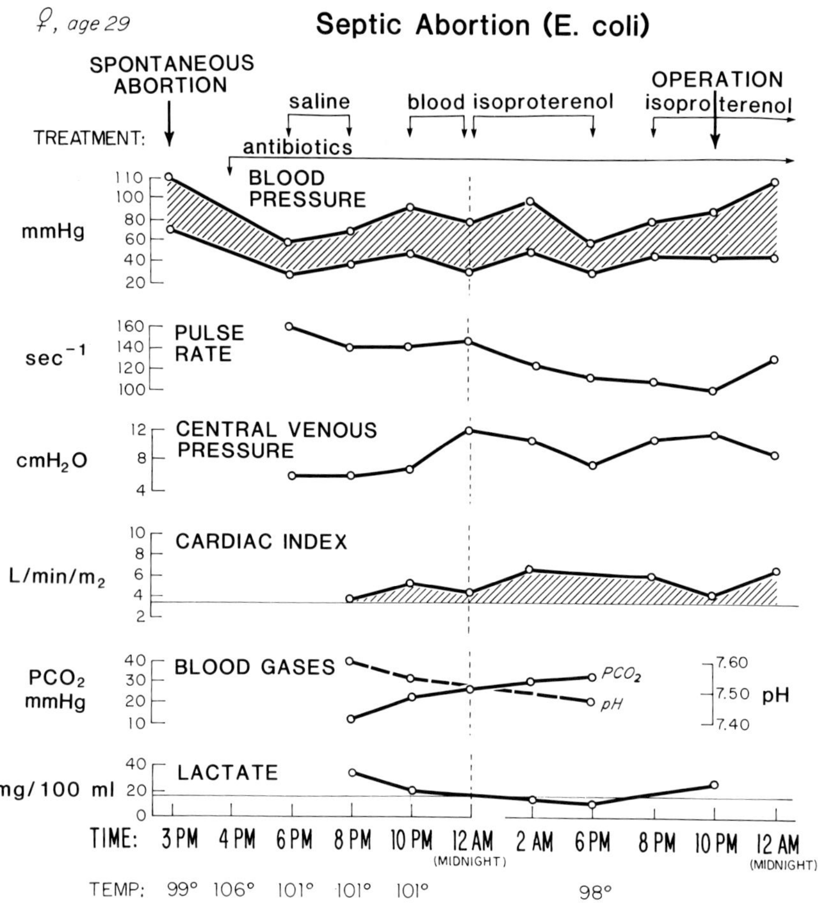

Fig. 16-2. **This 29-year-old woman was 12 weeks pregnant and was admitted to the hospital after 24 hours of shaking chills with a blood pressure of 110/70 mm Hg. She passed the products of what was thought to be a complete abortion. Antibiotics were administered after blood cultures were obtained. Two hours later, she spiked a temperature of 106F, and her blood pressure fell to 85/45 mm Hg with only scant urine output. Her blood pressure continued to decline. At 8:00 P.M. her blood pressure was 70/40 mm Hg, blood lactate level was 34 mg/dl, pO_2 was 78 mm Hg, pH 7.58, pCO_2 16 mm Hg. The cardiac index was 3.75 L/min/M^2 with a central venous pressure of 6 cm H_2O. With the infusion of saline and blood, the central venous pressure rose to 12 cm H_2O and the cardiac index to 3.9 L/min/M^2. However, the patient remained hypotensive with a blood pressure of 80/40 mm Hg. Inotropic support was instituted with isoproterenol. This resulted in a prompt response in both blood pressure (100/50 mm Hg) and cardiac index (6.5 L/min/M^2). Urine volume increased to 120 ml/min and blood lactate fell to 15.2 mg/dl.**

The following day, the patient was weaned from isoproterenol, but during the evening her blood pressure fell to 60/35 mm Hg. The extremities were cool and cyanotic, and urine output fell to 20 ml/min. Lactate rose to 27.5 mg/dl. Blood cultures from the previous day grew out *E. coli.* Isoproterenol was restarted, restoring the blood pressure to 110/50 and the cardiac output to 6.9 L/min/M^2. Immediate operation was performed to evacuate the uterus. The patient subsequently recovered. (Modified from MacLean LD, Mulligan WG, McLean APH, Duff JH: Patterns of septic shock in man—a detailed study of 56 patients. *Ann Surg* 166:543, 1967.)

sumably other host factors (such as preexisting cardiovascular disease, nutritional status, and hormonal environment) that determine which of the two responses will be observed.

Siegel et al [15-19] have been instrumental in classifying the circulatory response in septic patients into more meaningful physiologic categories than simply hyperdynamic or hypodynamic. Arterial and central venous catheterization are necessary to obtain the data for proper physiologic staging. The variables determined are cardiac index (CI), pulmonary dispersive volume (Td) (a reflection of pulmonary blood volume), cardiac mixing time (Tm) (a reflection of ventricular ejection fraction and contractility), ventricular ejection time (ET), right atrial pressure (RAP), total peripheral resistance (TPR), arterial and central venous blood gases, A-VO_2 difference, and oxygen consumption index (O_2CI). The oxygen consumption index is calculated as a product of cardiac index and A-VO_2 difference (Table 16-1).

The primary variables are then analyzed according to the method of Siegel et al [18,19] and a physiologic response state determined. In this classification system, the data are compared to those of a group of nonstressed, preoperative general surgery patients who fasted overnight. They comprise a reference (R) or control state. Each variable is then normalized in terms of standard deviations from

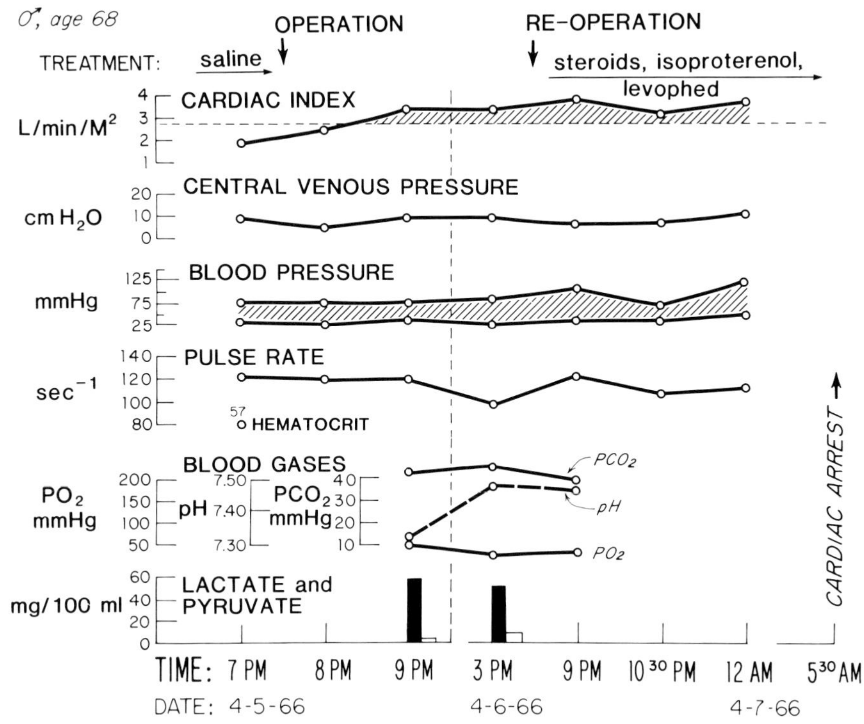

Fig. 16-3. This 68-year-old man was admitted to the hospital with a 12-hour history of abdominal pain and vomiting. Physical examination revealed abdominal signs of peritonitis, and an abdominal roentgenogram was suggestive of small bowel obstruction. Initially, the blood pressure was not obtainable, and the CVP was 0 cm H_2O. There was no urine present in the bladder. Following the infusion of 1,500 ml of saline, the blood pressure was 70/40. At operation, an internal herniation of small bowel was reduced, and 2,000 ml of blood-tinged fluid was removed from the peritoneal cavity. During the subsequent 12 hours, the patient remained hypotensive with only minimal improvement in cardiac output. At reoperation, a necrotic segment of small bowel was resected. Following this procedure, the patient's cardiac index remained low, and the lactate-pyruvate ratio remained abnormally high despite pressors and steroids. He died following a cardiac arrest early the next morning. (Modified from MacLean LD, Mulligan WG, McLean APH, Duff JH: Patterns of septic shock in man—a detailed study of 56 patients. *Ann Surg* 166:543, 1967.)

its corresponding value in the reference control state. In this way, the deviation from the reference control state can be measured in standard deviational units.

By clustering techniques, the data from critically ill patients with a variety of illnesses have resulted in a description of four prototypic stress response states (A, B, C, D) (Fig. 16-4, Table 16-2). The *A state* represents the normal balanced stress response state seen in compensated sepsis or after a significant insult such as major elective general surgery or trauma. The *A state* is characterized by a balanced physiologic response consisting of increased cardiac output and heart rate, an increase in contractility, and decreases in mean pulmonary transit time and cardiac ejection time. There is a normal relationship between cardiac output and peripheral vascular resistance (vascular tone), and the A-VO_2 difference is normal or slightly increased. Oxygen consumption is therefore generally increased. The *D state* is at the opposite extreme of the physiologic spectrum and is characterized by low cardiac output, high peripheral resistance, wide A-VO_2 difference, and reduced oxygen consumption on the basis of poor peripheral perfusion.

The *B state* represents a state of unbalanced vascular tone characterized by a large increase in cardiac output and a reduction in total peripheral resistance that is disproportionate to this increase in flow. The A-VO_2 difference is narrowed, primarily from a failure of venous desaturation, resulting in an absolute reduction in oxygen consumption, which cannot be explained on the basis of poor tissue perfusion. Some degree of metabolic acidosis is commonly present. This state is also characteristic of patients with early multiple organ failure and is associated with increased mortality if the metabolic derangement cannot be corrected. The *C state* is characterized by respiratory

TABLE 16-1. DESCRIPTION OF THE ELEVEN PARAMETERS USED TO DETERMINE SIEGEL'S "PHYSIOLOGIC RESPONSE STATE" *

Parameters	Derivation
CARDIOVASCULAR DESCRIPTORS	
HR	Arterial cannula
MAP	Arterial cannula
ET	Arterial cannula
RAP	CVP catheter
CI	Dye dilution curve analysis
Td	Dye dilution curve analysis
Tm	Dye dilution curve analysis
METABOLIC DESCRIPTORS	
AV DIF	Arterial and mixed venous blood samples
VpH	Mixed venous blood sample
$VpCO_2$	Mixed venous blood sample
VpO_2	Mixed venous blood sample

HR = Heart rate; MAP = Mean arterial pressure; ET = Cardiac ejection time; RAP = Right atrial pressure; CI = Cardiac Index; Td = Pulmonary dispersive time; Tm = Cardiac mixing time; AV DIF = A-VO_2 difference; VpH = Venous pH; $VpCO_2$ = Venous carbon dioxide tension; VpO_2 = Venous oxygen tension.

* The physiologic descriptors necessary for clinical classification in the R, A, B, C, D system of Siegel can be obtained after placement of arterial and central venous catheters. Td and Tm are time constants derived from the analysis of the dye dilution curve used to compute CI. Td is the pulmonary dispersive time—the mean transit time of dye-containing blood across the pulmonary vascular bed: Td × CI, therefore, approximates the pulmonary blood volume. Tm is the time constant for washout of dye-containing blood from the left ventricle. During each interval Tm, the amount of dye in the left ventricle decays by a factor l/e. Tm is therefore a descriptor of ventricular ejection; low values of Tm correlate with high left ventricular ejection fractions.

failure noncompensable by ventilator support that is superimposed on the B state with hypotension and profound metabolic and respiratory acidosis. Death almost inevitably ensues.

If the appropriate physiologic and metabolic parameters are measured in an individual patient, the data can be statistically compared to the five prototypic states (R, A, B, C, D) and the patient's similarity and dissimilarity to each prototypic state measured in terms of a Euclidian distance from each of these states. Consequently, the existing physiologic state of the patient can be precisely defined and categorized in terms of the state to which the patient has the most resemblance (the shortest distance) at that

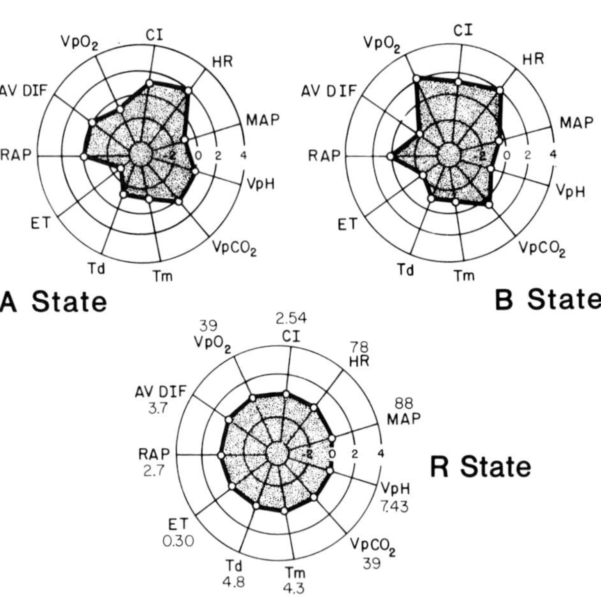

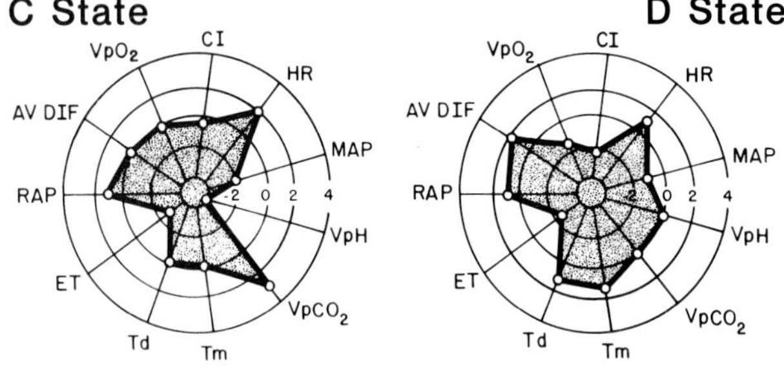

Fig. 16-4. **Siegel's physiologic response states: The heavy circle in the central polar plot represents the R physiologic state. The mean values for each of the physiologic parameters among the patients classified in the R state are shown. In the four corners of the figure are the polar plots of the means of the physiologic parameters in states A, B, C, and D. Each of the parameters has been normalized in terms of standard deviations from its mean value in the R state. Abbreviations and units: CI—cardiac index (liters/min/M²); HR—heart rate (beats per min); MAP—mean arterial pressure (mm Hg); VpH—venous pH; $VpCO_2$—venous carbon dioxide tension (mm Hg); VpO_2—venous oxygen tension (mm Hg); T_m—cardiac mixing time (see footnote, Table 16-1) (sec); Td—pulmonary dispersive time (see footnote, Table 16-1) (sec); ET—cardiac ejection time (sec); AV diff—A-VO_2 difference (volumes percent); RAP—right atrial pressure (cmH_2O).**

TABLE 16-2. DESCRIPTION OF SIEGEL'S FOUR PHYSIOLOGIC RESPONSE STATES[15-19]

State	Description	Parameters
A	Compensated stress response to trauma, surgery, or well-controlled sepsis	↑ HR ↑ CI ↓ Td ↓ Tm ↓ ET
B	Incipient metabolic dysfunction occurring in the face of high flow	↑ HR ↓ ET ↓ Td ↓ Tm ↑ CI ↑ VpO_2 ↓ AV-DIF ↓ VpH
C	Respiratory decompensation superimposed on already existing metabolic deficits	↑ HR ↓ VpH ↑ $VpCO_2$ ↓ MAP ↓ ET
D	Pattern of primary myocardial dysfunction	↑ HR ↑ Tm ↑ Td ↑ AV-DIF ↓ ET ↓ BP ↑ RAP ↓ CI ↓ MAP ↓ VpO_2

See also Figures 16-4, 16-5.

moment. By taking the ratio of the distance of the patient to the D state relative to the A state, the D/A ratio, a measure of cardiovascular adequacy, is determined. Likewise, the relationship between the B state of metabolic insufficiency and the C state of respiratory insufficiency can be represented in the C/B ratio and provides an indication of the patient's balance of metabolic and respiratory function. Thus, the data can be reduced to state distances and their ratios. By plotting these parameters over time, it is possible to plot the patient's physiologic trajectory during his clinical course. The course of the patient's physiologic response can be precisely and statistically quantified and compared to known response trajectories from other states of disease and stress. This pathophysiologic classification of an acutely ill patient provides a useful means of monitoring the clinical course and efficacy of therapeutic maneuvers. Multivariate mapping of the patient's physiologic state increases the discriminatory power of the analysis. Specific combinations of abnormalities often signal early changes that cannot be characterized by the monitoring of any single parameter.

Figure 16-5 depicts the clinical course of a 62-year-old man with peritonitis. The three studies represented show his progression from a compensated A state stress response to a B state of metabolic decompensation (with

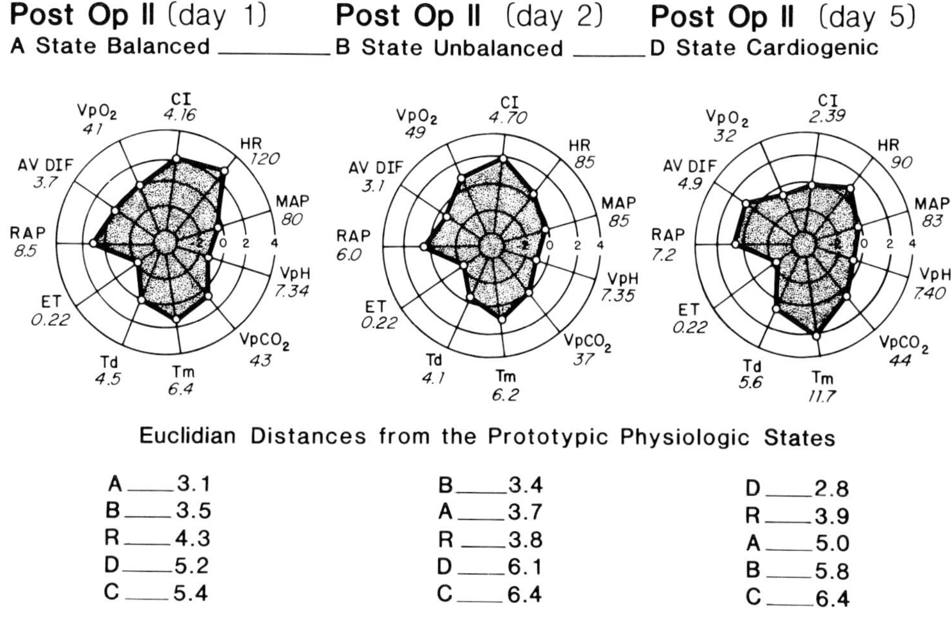

Fig. 16-5. **The clinical progress of a 62-year-old man with small bowel infarction is mapped by physiologic coordinates. The patient developed peritonitis, sepsis, and abdominal wound dehiscence. He underwent ileostomy, colostomy, tracheostomy, and repair of his dehiscence as a second operative procedure (Op II). The changing physiologic patterns, together with their distances from each prototypic state, are illustrated. The patient's course was marked by transition from a compensated A response to a B state of metabolic imbalance and finally to a D state of cardiac decompensation. (Abbreviations: see Fig. 16-4 and Table 16-1.)**

narrowing of the A-VO_2 difference and increased cardiac index) and thence into the D state, with myocardial dysfunction (low cardiac index and prolonged Tm). This pattern of deterioration demonstrates the cardiovascular vulnerability of the hyperdynamic septic patient who manifests a state B metabolic imbalance. The early recognition of metabolic derangements should alert the clinician to the possibility of impending cardiovascular decompensation. The use of inotropic agents to support this hyperdynamic response can be considered if the metabolic abnormalities are intractable. In Figure 16-5, the Euclidian vector distance (the square root of the sum of squares of individual parameter distances) in each of the three illustrated physiologic states from each of the five prototypic states is noted. The clinician can use these distances as well as the D/A and C/B ratios to follow the patient's progress in much the same way that a pilot charts the course of an aircraft in terms of known beacons and potentially dangerous landmarks.

THE PATHOPHYSIOLOGY OF SEPTIC SHOCK

Until recently, there has been a conceptual obstacle to the description and comprehension of the circulatory response to sepsis in the clinical setting. Difficulty arises when one attempts to define circulatory abnormality and insufficiency without regard for the interrelationship between the circulatory system and the metabolic processes it serves. In 1899, Crile [20] first created a model of hemorrhagic shock in the dog and demonstrated the effect of hypovolemia on arterial pressure. Blalock [21] emphasized the importance of hypovolemia in traumatic shock in his experimental studies of 1930. From these beginnings, our conception of shock has evolved to include those states of cardiovascular insufficiency in which there is adequate blood volume and blood pressure but in which cardiac output is so diminished that the viscera and peripheral tissues suffer ischemic injury on the basis of low flow. Metabolic abnormalities then develop with accumulation of toxic products as the function of the ischemic organs deteriorates. In this conception, the critical abnormality in shock is the failure of the circulatory system to meet the metabolic demands of the tissues with appropriate regional blood flow.

In septic shock there is growing evidence that the metabolic abnormalities induced by infection lead to circulatory deficits, rather than vice versa. During serious infections, human tissues often demonstrate what appears to be a diminished ability to utilize the oxygen delivered to their capillary beds. This is manifested by a decreased A-VO_2 difference in the face of increased metabolic needs. The mediators of this deficit, whether exogenous or endogenous, have not been completely defined, but their net effect is to increase the demands on the cardiovascular system. When these demands are not met, septic shock occurs.

The following discussion will consider the evidence for and against this point of view and will describe the abnormalities of the circulatory response to sepsis in terms of the responses of three principal target areas of pathophysiology—the heart, the peripheral vasculature, and the metabolic function of the peripheral tissues. The goal of this description is the synthesis of the known dysfunction in these three areas into a model capable of describing those patterns of response that are observed clinically.

CARDIAC FUNCTION IN THE INFECTED HOST

The role of the heart in the evolution of the circulatory response toward shock is controversial, whether the initiating insult is sepsis, trauma, or hemorrhage. The problem in determining whether circulatory failure is the result of cardiac dysfunction or abnormalities in the peripheral vasculature is compounded by the dependence of cardiac loading on the status of the peripheral vascular beds. The performance of the heart is in part determined by the venous return that fills the ventricles and the peripheral resistance against which the ventricles eject. Abnormalities in venous capacity that decrease venous return will in turn decrease cardiac output. Similarly, increased peripheral arteriolar resistance impedes systolic shortening of the myocardial fibers.

Our ability to determine whether the contractility of cardiac muscle is abnormal during serious infection is limited by our inability to define quantitatively the inotropic reserves of the heart independent of loading conditions. Those indices of cardiac contractility that have been examined during infection are each, to some extent, dependent on preload and afterload, and therefore not true measures of inotropic state.

Evidence for Myocardial Dysfunction in Septic Shock

Clinical studies describing circulatory abnormalities associated with infection have documented some degree of primary myocardial dysfunction.[15-17] The hemodynamic measurements have been derived from relatively noninvasive techniques and provide only a coarse description of inotropic reserves. In addition, most data suggest that cardiac dysfunction occurs relatively late in the course of the developing circulatory and metabolic abnormalities.

Similarly, dogs infused with endotoxin manifest delayed deterioration of ventricular function. Hinshaw et al [22-25] have reported the most extensive data, using a model in which the heart of the endotoxin-treated animal is isolated in cross-circulation with a normal animal. The purpose of such a model is to control the peripheral capacity and resistance that determine loading of the ventricular myocardium. The obvious disadvantage of isolating the heart is abrogation of humoral and neurogenic pathways that might influence cardiac performance in the intact septic animal.

The data from these experiments are similar to data from many clinical studies purporting to demonstrate ventricular dysfunction during the intermediate and late phases of serious infection. In each instance, an abnormal relationship between preload, afterload, and cardiac output or work is demonstrated. Usually, the filling pressure of either ventricle is normal or increased during decreased afterload (low systemic blood pressure). That cardiac output and work are decreased is taken as evidence that myocardial inotropic state is decreased. There are pitfalls in drawing conclusions from this type of data, and the clinical management of the septic patient can be misguided by an uncritical interpretation. One important problem is that of reliably assessing preload. This parameter is most commonly estimated by measuring ventricular filling pressures. Central venous catheterization can be used to measure right atrial pressure, while pulmonary artery catheterization is used to measure pulmonary capillary wedge pressure as an estimate of left atrial pressure. The measurement of atrial pressures, however, is not itself a measurement of preload or diastolic fiber length. Filling pressures estimate diastolic lengths and volumes only if it is assumed that there is a constant and predictable relationship between pressure and volume. If, however, there is an abnormality in myocardial compliance, pressure is not a reliable measure of preload. Alyono et al [26] have demonstrated in a model of hemorrhagic shock that acute loss of diastolic compliance can occur in response to a severe hypotensive insult. Furthermore, the measurement of pulmonary capillary wedge pressure may underestimate end diastolic left ventricular pressure in congestive heart failure and chronic pulmonary disease.[27] Therefore, data demonstrating an abnormal relationship between cardiac output, atrial pressures, and arterial pressures are indirect evidence, at best, that myocardial dysfunction is present and should be regarded cautiously.

Mechanisms for Myocardial Dysfunction in Septic Shock

Investigators who report abnormal inotropic cardiac performance have suggested numerous mechanisms, all of which are consistent with the concept that if the performance of the heart is impaired at all, the abnormality develops late (in both a temporal and physiologic sense) and is not a primary cause of circulatory failure. The proposed mechanisms also predict that those patients with preexisting cardiovascular disease are at substantially greater risk of developing cardiac failure in the course of a septic illness.

The mechanisms most frequently invoked fall into three general categories: (1) peripheral hemodynamic abnormalities, (2) abnormalities induced by circulating toxins, and (3) abnormal myocardial metabolism.

Cardiac Failure Caused by Peripheral Hemodynamic Changes

Hinshaw et al [24] demonstrated inotropic failure 4 to 6 hours after the induction of endotoxin shock in dogs. If the heart is isolated and coronary perfusion pressure and flow are maintained at baseline levels, there is less measurable cardiac dysfunction.[28] These results suggest that myocardial ischemia is exacerbated by prolonged hypotension. In fact, coronary perfusion is dependent on systemic blood pressure and diastolic interval, both of which are reduced in the usual endotoxemia preparation. In the clinical situation, these problems will be exacerbated by preexisting coronary artery disease. The hyperdynamic response characterized by elevated cardiac output and decreased peripheral resistance may be as poorly tolerated as strenuous exercise by the patient with ischemic heart disease. This may be one host variable that influences which patient will be able to sustain a hyperdynamic response and which patient has insufficient reserve to do so.

Cardiac Failure Due to Circulating Toxins

At present, there is no evidence that endotoxin itself is capable of altering the mechanical performance of cardiac muscle. There is evidence, however, that one or more endogenous mediators may influence the inotropic state of the heart in response to infection. The catecholamines are an important class of circulating mediators that can alter cardiac inotropism. In fact, Goodyer [29] and Urschel et al [30] have demonstrated that in dogs subjected to endotoxemia, cardiac contractility may be augmented during the first few hours and that this augmentation can be abolished with pharmacologic sympathetic blockade. The role of catecholamines and sympathetic tone in determining the course of the hemodynamic response to sepsis or any other type of stress cannot be overemphasized. The sympathetic and adrenal responses of the host also help determine whether the peripheral vasculature will be constricted or dilated and thus to some degree determine the basic pattern of circulatory response. Metabolic data, however, indicate that receptor sites become less responsive to the hormonal milieu as the severity of the septic process increases.

Blalock [31] was the first to show that circulating toxins can influence the systemic hemodynamic response to a peripheral insult. He demonstrated a toxic factor in the thoracic lymph of dogs subjected to crushing limb trauma. The injection of lymph from traumatized dogs into healthy animals caused progressive hypotension and death. Lefer [32] demonstrated that a similar toxic factor, myocardial depressant factor, may be responsible for depression of myocardial function in hemorrhagic, endotoxic, and splanchnic artery-occlusion shock in dogs. Myocardial depressant factor is a relatively small polypeptide (10,000 daltons), which can be detected by its negative inotropic effect on isolated cat papillary muscle. It appears to be released by the action of lysosomal acid hydrolases within the splanchnic circulation after 3 to 4 hours of ischemia.[33] The existence of myocardial depressant factor has been disputed by some investigators, who could not demonstrate its existence in similar experiments.[34] Other investigators have also identified humoral factors with the same or different chemical characteristics, which they believe are released in response to endotoxin shock and have a negative cardiac inotropic effect.[35] The majority of these substances have been found to originate within the splanchnic circulation of the dog. They can therefore be most easily demonstrated during the hypersensitive response of the splanchnic viscera of the dog to ischemic insult. Lovett et al [36] have, however, demonstrated the presence of myocardial depressant factor in the sera of patients with severe infections. No matter how this controversy is settled, the effects of myocardial depressant factors have only been demonstrated to occur late in the course of sepsis, and only when the subject has already sustained significant visceral injury. Treatment aimed at mitigating the effects of such factors would therefore be largely supportive and ineffective in preventing the precipitating pathologic processes in septic shock.

Inotropic Failure Caused by Defective Cardiac Metabolism

The role of defective myocardial fueling on cardiac dysfunction during infection has only recently been investigated. While the peripheral tissues appear relatively incapable of extracting and using oxygen during severe infections, the heart is less likely to manifest this defect. The ever-changing metabolic demands of the heart are normally met by changes in coronary flow. The coronary bed dilates in response to the metabolic demands of increased cardiac work. The A-VO_2 difference across the coronary bed remains relatively wide and fixed. Cerra et al (unpublished data) have, however, demonstrated some degree of narrowing of the A-VO_2 difference across the coronary circulation in (B state) septic patients.

Glucose and insulin derangements also may have some effect on cardiac performance in sepsis. Clowes et al [8] have demonstrated that animals with pericecal abscesses can have either elevated or depressed cardiac outputs. Animals that do not respond with increased cardiac output rarely survive. Although serum glucose levels are elevated, serum insulin levels in the hypodynamic responders are lower than the levels in the hyperdynamic responders. Clowes et al [8,37] have demonstrated a similar correlation in surgical patients with septic complications. Although this difference in insulin levels may be an epiphenomenon, the intravenous administration of glucose, insulin, and potassium can substantially improve the cardiovascular status of subjects with hypodynamic septic shock.[8] Clowes et al [8] therefore postulated that a permissive level of insulin must be present for normal cardiac performance. Whether this phenomenon is mediated by direct or secondary effects of insulin on the myocardium remains unclear.

THE PERIPHERAL AND VISCERAL VASCULAR BEDS IN THE INFECTED HOST

The Vascular Beds in the Hyperdynamic State

Total peripheral vascular resistance can either be increased or decreased in response to systemic infection. Decreased peripheral vascular resistance can occur as a response to localized infection such as an abscess or as a response to severe septicemia. In either case, cardiac output is usually normal or elevated. This hyperdynamic state has only rarely been observed in animal preparations and then only when sepsis has been induced by a localized infection (ie, septic hindlimb cellulitis,[9] pericecal abscess,[8] or the ischemic, infected gallbladder[38]).

Studies in animal models support the thesis that vasodilation does not simply serve the metabolic demands of infected tissues. In fact, systemic vasodilation may be mediated by circulating factors and serve little or no local adaptive purpose. Hermreck and Thal [9] examined the effects of a septic hindlimb preparation on regional blood flow in dogs. Although systemic oxygen consumption increased only 12 percent, the average increase in cardiac output was 50 percent. Blood flow in the septic limb increased 81 percent, but this increase could not account for the overall rise in cardiac output. Renal blood flow increased 50 percent, while flow through the splanchnic organs was estimated to increase 38 percent on the basis of narrowed A-VO_2 difference across the splanchnic bed (splanchnic oxygen consumption was assumed to be constant or increased). Blood flow to the nonseptic limb decreased 39 percent, and the authors inferred that this reflected a generalized decrease in flow to nonseptic skin and skeletal muscle.[9]

Hermreck and Thal[9] suggested that a vasodilating substance is released from the septic limb and that an interaction between the response to this substance, the response to other endogenous vasoactive substances, and local metabolic demands determines flow in each peripheral vascular bed. To confirm the existence of such a substance, they perfused either the contralateral (nonseptic) hindlimb or an isolated limb from another animal with venous blood from the septic limb. The nonseptic limbs assumed the hemodynamic characteristics of the septic leg when perfused with septic venous blood.

Gump et al[39] used portal vein catheterization to demonstrate increased splanchnic blood flow in patients with intra-abdominal infections. In those patients whose cardiac output was increased during infection, mean splanchnic blood flow was nearly double that of patients with normal cardiac output values. Forty-two percent of the increased cardiac output could be accounted for by flow through the splanchnic bed.

Pigs with pericecal abscesses demonstrated two types of hemodynamic responses. The hyperdynamic responders showed only slight increases in total hepatic blood flow, but there was a 96 percent increase in hepatic arterial flow, and a concomitant increase in hepatic oxygen consumption of 26 percent.[40] In the hypodynamic responders, total hepatic flow decreased only slightly, but hepatic arterial flow dropped significantly, and hepatic oxygen consumption decreased by 29 percent. The authors suggested that the increased mortality in the low flow group might be partly determined by decreased hepatic oxygen utilization and oxidative metabolism.

These data reveal a trend in sepsis; regional blood flow is not directly related to the metabolic demands for oxygen and substrate. The region of sepsis, however, seems to command a greater share of the augmented cardiac output. In addition, the splanchnic viscera and liver can receive increased blood flow even if no intra-abdominal infection exists.

To what extent this redistribution of blood flow is adaptive is unclear. One could postulate that vasodilation is simply a physiologic response to the increased metabolic demands of the tissues being perfused. For this to be the case, three criteria must be fulfilled: (1) the metabolic demands must be increased, (2) increased flow must reach those areas where demand is increased, and (3) the tissues must be capable of extracting and utilizing the energy substrates delivered during this response.

Oxygen extraction, however, eventually falls in severely ill septic patients who have decreased peripheral resistance. Thus, the critical pathophysiologic problem in these patients appears to be the inability of the tissues to burn fuels that are being circulated at high flows. There are three alternative schemes that could explain this finding: (1) the peripheral vasodilation and increased blood flow is unnecessary and is therefore an inappropriate response to the metabolic demands, (2) increased flow is necessary but is not being distributed to areas of high metabolic demands (ie, arteriovenous communications are open that bypass vascular beds where the rate of metabolism demands increased blood flow), or (3) the increased flow is demanded by the energy requirements of the tissues, but the tissues are unable to extract or utilize the oxygen provided by the increased flow.

That severely ill septic patients who are hyperdynamic and vasodilated develop progressive and eventually irreversible metabolic derangements indicates that the metabolic demands of their tissues are not being met, despite increased cardiac output. Thus, the metabolic and circulatory responses are not properly balanced.

It has been attractive for investigators to propose arteriovenous shunting as a mechanism by which blood flow (cardiac output) can be increased and the tissues remain relatively underperfused. This proposition has been examined using two experimental techniques. Finley et al[41] used the washout of labeled xenon to measure capillary flow in hyperdynamic septic patients and found that capillary flow increases in parallel with cardiac output. This finding does not support the existence of arteriovenous shunting. In animal models, Wright et al[42] have made similar observations using a xenon washout technique. Archie,[43] using radiolabeled microspheres, did not demonstrate increased arteriovenous shunting in dogs administered endotoxin.

Cerra et al[44] have collected metabolic data from severely ill septic patients that also indicate that the progressive metabolic derangements are not the result of inadequate perfusion. Lactate levels rise in these patients, but pyruvate levels rise concomitantly. The pyruvate-lactate ratio, which falls dramatically in patients with lactic acidosis due to low flow, is near normal levels in septic patients. Thus, the hyperdynamic response to sepsis seems to be a response to altered intermediary metabolism rather than inadequate perfusion. Why the tissues do not utilize the increased flows of substrates and oxygen will be discussed in a subsequent section.

The Vascular Beds in the Hypodynamic State

A vasoconstrictive response is usually present in patients who do not respond to their infections with increased cardiac output. These patients may be temporarily benefited by this response if coronary and cerebral perfusion can be maintained only in this fashion. The perfusion of the coronary circulation in patients with preexisting ischemic heart disease, even at the expense of intense vasoconstriction and low flow elsewhere, can sometimes be a desirable therapeutic objective. At some point, however, this response becomes pathologic. The kidneys and splanchnic viscera are adversely affected by decreases in flow, and the circulating products of anaerobic metabolism can become toxic.

The vasoconstrictive response to infection seems to develop in the patient with preexisting cardiovascular disease and reduced cardiac reserves, and in the patient whose cardiovascular reserves are exhausted by the prolongation or severity of the hyperdynamic response. The status of the peripheral vascular beds in the low-output response to sepsis resembles that observed following a hypovolemic insult such as hemorrhage. This intense vasoconstriction is also present in canine models of sepsis created by the intravenous injection of endotoxin. Presumably, this response is a feature of the final common pathway in almost all forms of irreversible circulatory insufficiency. It may represent the sympathetic and adrenal response to prolonged imbalance between circulatory performance and metabolic demands. When present for short periods of time, this response is potentially life-saving in that it sustains cerebral and coronary perfusion. When the response is necessary for more than several hours, the damage done to the peripheral vascular beds and their end organs may eventually cause death. The canine splanchnic viscera are extremely sensitive to this type of vasoconstrictive insult. Dogs develop sloughing of the intestinal mucosa during shock induced by hemorrhage or endotoxemia. Human intestinal mucosa is not so vulnerable, but irreversible ischemic damage to the kidneys, intestines, liver, and other organs can occur during prolonged intense vasoconstriction.

The irreversibility of vasoconstrictive injury to the viscera is possibly mediated by an imbalance between the sensitivity of the precapillary and postcapillary small vessels to catecholamines.[45] The arterioles may lose their responsiveness to adrenergic stimulation, perhaps in response to ambient acidosis or an energy deficit. If the postcapillary sphincters remain sensitive and continue to constrict, a so-called stagnant ischemia will result where blood flows into capillary beds without a route for egress. The capillary beds will dilate, and fluid will leak into the interstitial space. If the integrity of the capillaries themselves is destroyed, interstitial hemorrhage will result. This scenario is consistent with both the hemorrhagic infarction of intestinal mucosa observed in shocked dogs and many of the pathologic changes that are found in patients who die with septic shock.

Data from small animal experiments suggest that endotoxin modifies the sensitivity of peripheral vascular beds to the constrictive effects of catecholamines. Zweifach et al [46] have demonstrated in the rat mesoappendix that the terminal arterioles and venules exhibit a greatly augmented and prolonged vasoconstrictive response to epinephrine and norepinephrine when the animal is first injected with a sublethal dose of endotoxin. After larger doses of endotoxin, the vascular hyperactivity is of briefer duration and is followed by a phase of hyporeactivity. With lethal doses of endotoxin, the terminal arterioles and venules can become completely refractory to epinephrine, while heightened reactivity persists in larger arteries and veins. The end result is pooling of stagnant blood in distended capillaries and venules, accompanied by the appearance of petechiae. Whether this modulation of the peripheral vascular response to catecholamines contributes to the ischemic insult perpetuated by vasoconstriction in humans with refractory shock and gram-negative septicemia is speculative.

THE METABOLIC COMPONENT OF THE SYSTEMIC SEPTIC RESPONSE

Chapter 15 has outlined the metabolic response to infection. It now appears that metabolic defects underlie the hemodynamic manifestations of infections. Septic patients do not utilize oxygen appropriately, in spite of more than adequate delivery. This abnormal relationship between oxygen delivery and extraction is to be contrasted to the relationship in nonseptic patients whose cardiovascular system is stressed. In nonseptic individuals, when the limits of the cardiovascular response are reached, tissue oxygen extraction is next augmented by widening of A-VO_2 differences (reduced venous oxygen content). In maximal states of exercise, therefore, both cardiac output and A-VO_2 differences are increased. Oxygen delivery and extraction are balanced. Similarly, primary cardiac decompensation in a nonseptic patient is accompanied by immediate widening of the A-VO_2 difference manifested by decreased venous hemoglobin saturations. Septic patients, however, fail to augment their desaturation of hemoglobin when the demand for delivery is increased. The A-VO_2 difference becomes inappropriately narrow for the level of cardiac output (Fig. 16-6).[47]

These paradoxical observations in the high-flow state of human sepsis are best understood if one conceptualizes the hemodynamic derangements as secondary phenomena initiated by a primary defect in intermediary metabolism. The tissues cannot use the oxygen and substrate supplied to their capillary beds. Thus, the hyperdynamic state may be a response to unmet metabolic demands of tissues that are intrinsically unable to use fuel supplies appropriately.

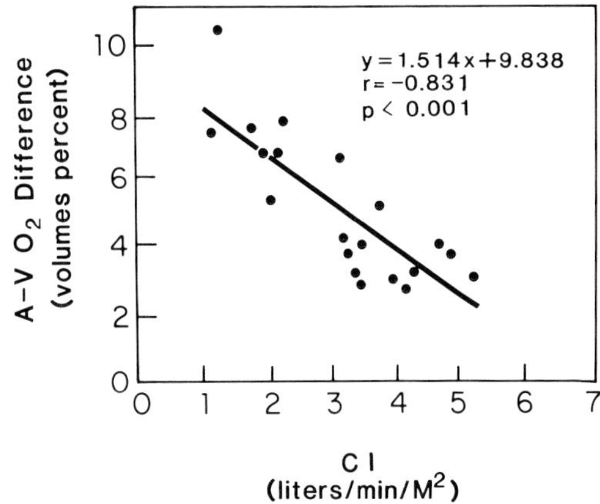

Fig. 16-6. **The data demonstrate the negative correlation between cardiac index (CI) and A-VO_2 difference during severe clinical infection. (From Duff JH, Groves AC, McLean APH, LaPointe R, MacLean LD: Defective oxygen consumption in septic shock. *Surg Gynecol Obstet* 128:1051, 1969.)**

The narrow A-VO_2 difference is simply a manifestation of this peripheral metabolic defect.

That this defect in metabolism has the net effect of limiting the septic patient's total oxygen utilization is clearly demonstrated by clinical data. Septic patients with increased cardiac output and increased venous oxygen content *(B state)* have depressed total oxygen utilization (measured as the product of cardiac output and A-VO_2 difference).[17] This reduced oxygen utilization is not flow related and not accompanied by an oxygen debt. There is no excess lactate production relative to pyruvate. The decrease in the ability of the tissues to utilize oxygen may eventually result in the hyperdynamic physiologic response. The cause of this hemodynamic derangement may be the body's incorrect interpretation of developing energy deficits as a manifestation of inadequate flow.

The defect in oxygen extraction cannot be accounted for by a reduced capacity of the hemoglobin molecule to deliver oxygen to the tissues, ie, a shift to the left of the oxygen-hemoglobin dissociation curve. There is no evidence that bacterial infection directly affects the dissociation of oxygen from hemoglobin. Johnson et al [48] demonstrated a 26 percent decrease in 2, 3 dephosphoglycerate (2, 3 DPG) in baboons subjected to endotoxemia. They calculated that this deficit in itself would shift the oxygen-hemoglobin dissociation curve 2.9 mm Hg to the left at the P_{50} point and thereby decrease oxygen delivery by 11 percent. This abnormality alone, however, could not account for the severe circulatory and metabolic derangements that resulted in the death of their animals.

Watkins et al [49] studied nine septic patients and detected decreased 2, 3 DPG levels and left-shifted oxygen-hemoglobin dissociation curves in seven of the nine. They found, however, that this abnormality was entirely preventable if hypophosphatemia, alkalosis, and transfusion of 2, 3 DPG–poor blood were avoided. They stressed that this abnormality could be detrimental to septic patients, in that a small decrease in oxygen extraction would have to be compensated by a large increase in cardiac output.

The Metabolic Time Course

The overall peripheral problem in hyperdynamic septic states is not one of maldistribution of flow, but one of defective oxidative cellular metabolism. These relationships between metabolism and physiology became apparent when the metabolic data were correlated with the physiologic state classification system.[17]

The most informative data come from septic patients who are categorized by physiologic criteria as group A or group B (Fig. 16-7, Table 16-2). Group A patients demonstrate a hyperdynamic response. Heart rate, cardiac index, and cardiac contractility (as measured by ejection and mixing times) are all increased. Group B patients are also hyperdynamic, but oxygen extraction is diminished, venous pH is low, and thus some degree of metabolic decompensation has occurred.

When the metabolic profiles of the septic and nonseptic trauma–general surgery patients, categorized by the state classification, were compared, several patterns emerged (Fig. 16-7), from which deviant pathways of intermediate metabolism could be inferred (Figs. 16-8, 16-9). The metabolic profiles were obtained from patients who were nutritionally supported on a commercial amino acid mix (Aminosyn), administered with glucose in a ratio of 100 glucose calories per gram of administered protein nitrogen. The protein was administered at a rate of 1 gm per kg body weight every 24 hours by constant infusion.

One of the first observable features of metabolic derangement in sepsis is the appearance of hyperglycemia (250 to 300 mg per dl). It is refractory to the administration of exogenous insulin and aggravated by exogenous glucose

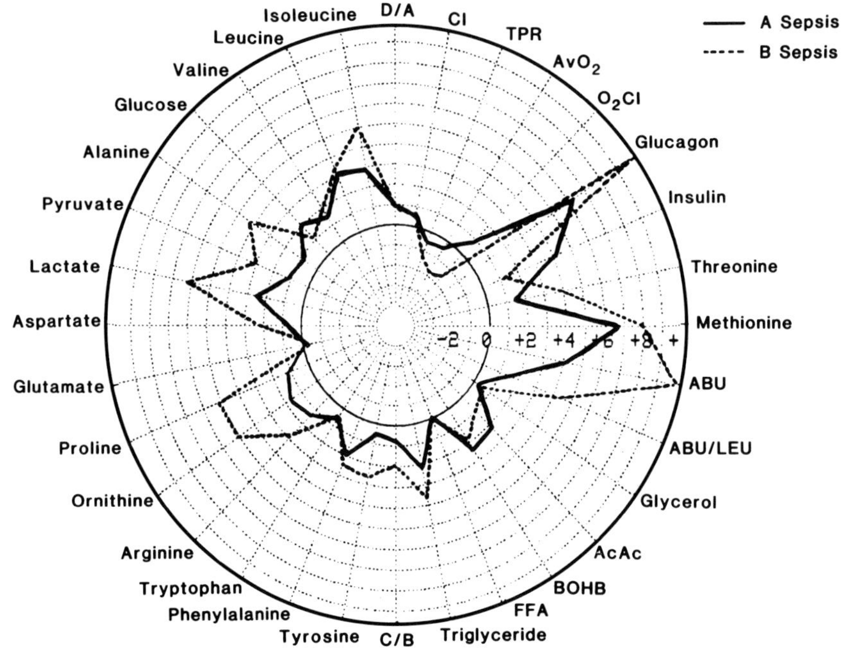

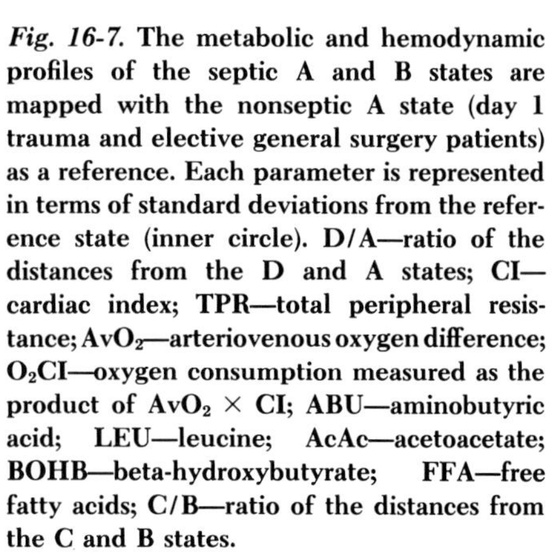

Fig. 16-7. **The metabolic and hemodynamic profiles of the septic A and B states are mapped with the nonseptic A state (day 1 trauma and elective general surgery patients) as a reference. Each parameter is represented in terms of standard deviations from the reference state (inner circle). D/A—ratio of the distances from the D and A states; CI—cardiac index; TPR—total peripheral resistance; AvO_2—arteriovenous oxygen difference; O_2CI—oxygen consumption measured as the product of $AvO_2 \times CI$; ABU—aminobutyric acid; LEU—leucine; AcAc—acetoacetate; BOHB—beta-hydroxybutyrate; FFA—free fatty acids; C/B—ratio of the distances from the C and B states.**

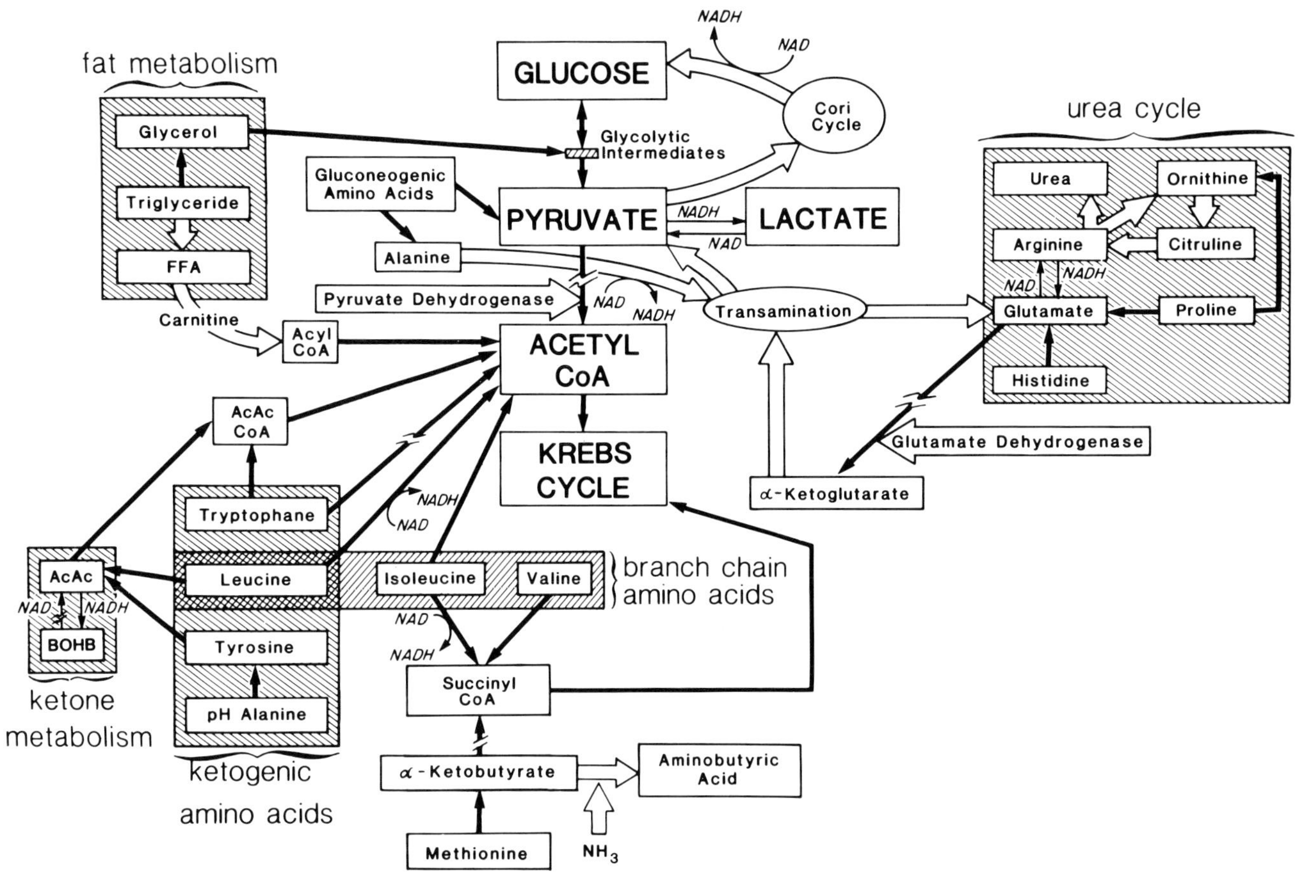

Fig. 16-8. The major catabolic pathways for fats, glucose, and selected amino acids through acetyl coenzyme A (acetyl Co-A) are illustrated. Those pathways that seem to be blocked in sepsis are represented by interrupted arrows. Pathways with enhanced substrate flow are represented by broad open arrows. The oxidative conversion of pyruvate to acetyl Co-A is blocked, and substrates that must enter the Krebs cycle via pyruvate cannot be utilized normally. The branch chain amino acids can enter the Krebs cycle distal to pyruvate and can, therefore, be coupled with oxidative phosphorylation when other substrates cannot. The availability of alpha-ketoglutarate as an intermediate in the Krebs cycle may be limited by a block in the oxidative conversion of glutamate and by increased utilization in transamination reactions. NAD—nicotinamide-adenine dinucleotide; NADH—reduced form of NAD; AcAc—acetoacetate; BOHB—beta-hydroxybutyrate.

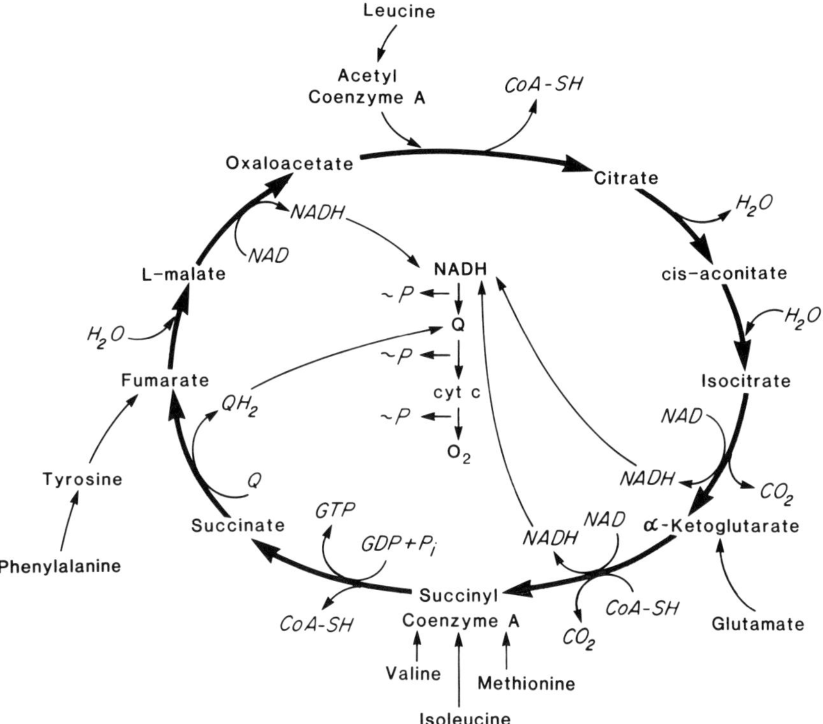

Fig. 16-9. The reactions of the Krebs (citric acid) cycle are illustrated. If the regeneration of nicotinamide-adenine dinucleotide within the mitochondrion is blocked, those reactions dependent on the conversion of NAD to its reduced form NADH will be impeded. The regeneration of NAD from NADH is coupled to oxidative phosphorylation and requires the normal functioning of the chemical processes that transport hydrogen ions across the inner mitochondrial membrane. The stoichiometry of the citric acid cycle is such that for every acetyl coenzyme A molecule that is consumed, two molecules of carbon dioxide are produced, one molecule of guanosine triphosphate (GTP) is generated from guanosine diphosphate (GDP), three pairs of electrons are removed from NADH, and one pair of electrons is removed from ubiquinol (Q). Each pair of electrons removed from NADH will account for the production of three molecules of adenosine triphosphate (ATP) from adenosine diphosphate (ADP) by oxidative phosphorylation. Each pair of electrons removed from Q will yield two molecules of ATP. ~P—high energy phosphate bond; NADH—reduced form of NAD; cyt C—cytochrome C.

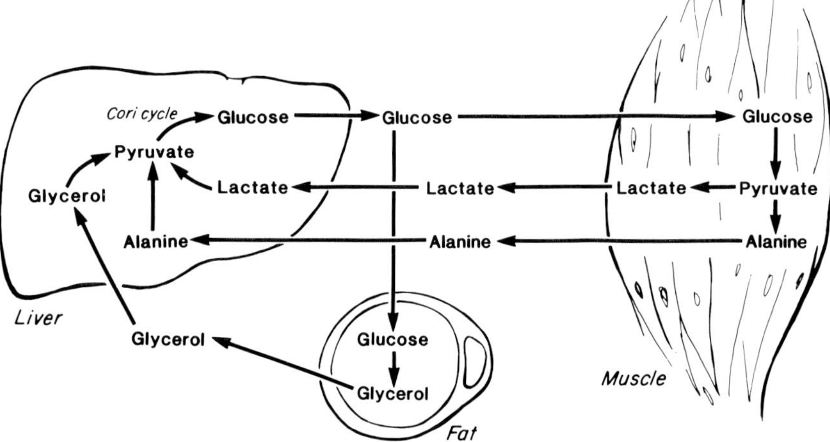

Fig. 16-10. Glucose recycling during sepsis: In the septic patient, glucose is oxidized to pyruvate and lactate in muscle. Lactate can be cycled through the liver and converted back to glucose via the Cori cycle. Pyruvate can also be converted to alanine in the periphery, and alanine can be circulated back to the liver for gluconeogenesis. Glucose is converted to glycerol in fat cells; the glycerol is circulated back to the liver where it is used to synthesize glucose again.

administration so that a hyperosmolar state can be produced. Attempting to control the hyperglycemia with exogenous insulin results in the use of high quantities of regular insulin, sometimes up to 40 units per hour by continuous infusion. Even with these doses, it is difficult to maintain the blood sugar below 200 mg per dl. This increase in glucose pool size is associated with an increase in mass flow of glucose to the periphery [50,51] and an increased turnover of glucose through the Cori, alanine, and glycerol cycles (Fig. 16-10). Experiments using C14 labeled glucose and alanine infusions further indicate that there is an increase in the gluconeogenic response, which cannot be suppressed by the administration of exogenous glucose.[52]

This hyperglycemia coincides in time with elevations of lactate, pyruvate, and alanine, which rise proportionately in a constant relationship with one another. For a given level of lactate, there are predictable levels of pyruvate and alanine. The initial lactate-pyruvate ratio is normal. As the septic state evolves, lactate and pyruvate rise proportionately, but the lactate-pyruvate ratio remains constant.[44,53] Liaw et al [54] have recently shown that the lactate-pyruvate ratio remains constant within muscle cells as well, ie, there is no excess of lactate production relative to pyruvate. This observation provides strong supporting evidence that the metabolic defect is not the result of a perfusion-related deficit.

The serum triglyceride level also rises progressively, and the serum can become hyperlipemic (Fig. 16-11). A prolonged clearance time of administered triglyceride can be demonstrated, and there is evidence for increased hepatic lipogenesis.[55,56] The free fatty acid levels become inappropriately high for the level of glucose, and there is increased glycerol turnover. Initially, there are large amounts of circulating ketone bodies. The beta-hydroxybutyrate level is initially increased. Relative to trauma-hypermetabolic man, the acetoacetate levels are also increased in sepsis (Fig. 16-7). As the patient proceeds toward death, the acetoacetate level progressively falls while the beta-hydroxybutyrate level remains the same or rises. The beta-hydroxybutyrate-acetoacetate ratio, therefore, progressively increases toward death. If measurements are made on the day of death, however, the acetoacetate level is barely detectable, and the beta-hydroxybutyrate level has fallen precipitously.

The serum branch chain amino acid levels are of considerable interest: leucine, isoleucine, and valine levels are reduced relative to overnight fasting man [44] but increased relative to trauma-hypermetabolic man [57] (A state, Fig. 16-7). In fact, a common feature of the early systemic septic response seems to be an increase in muscle catabolism with an apparent utilization of branch chain amino acids as an energy source.[58-60] As the infection evolves, however, the peripheral tissues become less capable of catabolizing the branch chain amino acids, and their levels in the blood eventually begin to rise and are extemely high on the day of death (B state, Fig. 16-7). The hepatic clearance of the branch chain amino acids is reduced in sepsis.[61] The levels of aromatic amino acids (phenylalanine, tyrosine, and tryptophane) are elevated and continue to rise as the patient deteriorates, despite increased hepatic clearance.

The levels of the sulfur-containing amino acids threonine and methionine, as well as their breakdown product,

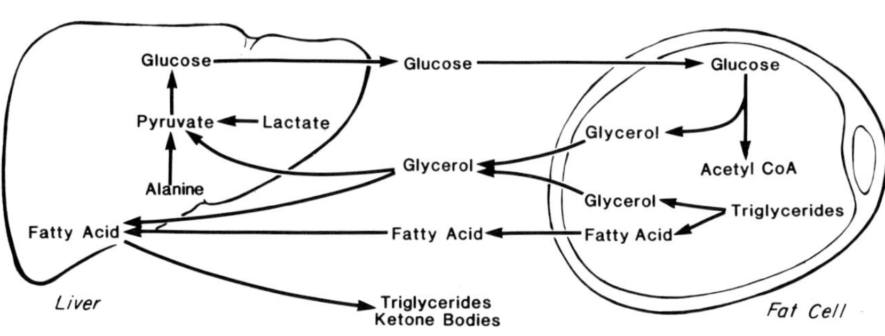

Fig. 16-11. Fat metabolism in sepsis: Because the peripheral tissues are unable to oxidatively metabolize long chain fatty acids in sepsis, and because hepatic triglyceride production is increased, serum triglyceride and fatty acid levels are elevated. Fatty acids cleared by the liver are synthesized into triglycerides and ketone bodies. The glycerol that is split off triglyceride or manufactured from glucose in the fat is cycled back to the liver for triglyceride synthesis or conversion back to glucose.

aminobutyric acid, rise progressively during uncontrolled serious infections, as do the levels of aspartate, glutamate, proline, ornithine, arginine, and ammonia. Correlated with a rise in these amino acids is a progressive increase in urea excretion in the urine.

The onset of serious sepsis, therefore, is associated with abnormalities in the plasma substrate levels of glucose, fat, and amino acids. In the patients who survive, the plasma substrate levels eventually go back toward that for overnight fasting man. If sepsis is uncontrolled, the levels continue to rise up to the moment of death. The exceptions are the ketone bodies and glucose, which tend to fall until they reach low plasma levels on the day of death.

The exogenous nutritional support that a patient is receiving can influence the plasma substrate levels. If albumin is the sole source of intravenous protein, isoleucine levels and isoleucine-leucine ratios fall drastically because albumin and plasma protein fractions are deficient in isoleucine.[62] When exogenous amino acids are used, the effect in survivors and nonsurvivors is much different. In both cases, there is some increase in plasma substrate levels as a function of the amino acid load. The levels most affected are glycine, alanine, lactate, pyruvate, and the aromatic amino acids. The effect is more prominent in survivors, with little effect in nonsurvivors.[62,63] In addition, exogenous amino acid support seems to profoundly influence the levels of prealbumin, transferrin, and retinol-binding protein in survivors, whereas there is little effect in patients who eventually die.[64]

As has been pointed out, during sepsis there is a tight correlation in time between inappropriately low peripheral vascular resistance for the existing cardiac output, decreased O_2 consumption, and unbalanced metabolism. This relationship can be further emphasized by analyzing one amino acid in detail. Proline cannot be catabolized by muscle and is mainly catabolized by liver. Proline levels in sepsis rise in an exponential fashion as death approaches.[53] As the proline level rises, the total peripheral resistance falls in a tight linear relationship (Fig. 16-12). This rise in proline level is also associated with a fall in the oxygen consumption index and progressive rises in both lactate and pyruvate levels with constancy of the lactate-pyruvate ratio.[53] In the hepatic degradation pathways of proline, it is converted to an intermediate, which then comes into equilibrium with ornithine and glutamate. The action of glutamate dehydrogenase can convert glutamate into α-ketogluterate, which enters the Krebs cycle (Fig. 16-8). Plasma glutamate concentration, likewise, rises exponentially as death approaches. This is associated with linear rises in proline, ornithine, and ammonia, and simultaneous falls in total peripheral resistance and oxygen consumption.[53]

Endocrine Responses in Sepsis*

The glucagon and insulin response in sepsis and multiple systems organ failure may underlie some of the substrate abnormalities. Early in the course, there is a rapid elevation in circulating glucagon levels (A state, Fig. 16-7). Although insulin levels are increased, there is an increase in the glucagon-insulin ratio.[57] This phenomenon coincides with the onset of hyperglycemia and elevated free fatty acid levels. The insulin levels are inappropriately low for the glucose level. As sepsis progresses, the high glucagon-insulin ratio persists (B state, Fig. 16-7).[57]

The metabolic and circulatory deficits in sepsis cannot as easily be correlated with adrenal function. The cortisol levels in stressed patients are elevated relative to overnight fasting man, but the levels do not discriminate between the presence or absence of sepsis. Similarly, the excretion of epinephrine, norepinephrine, and their derivatives are increased with all kinds of stress, and no specific septic pattern has been found. In patients who die, the norepinephrine levels remain increased, while the epinephrine levels drop toward zero,[65] a finding compatible with sustained sympathetic activity in all kinds of critically ill patients. Sympathetic tone is one of the most potent stimuli to glucagon production, and there is a close correlation between catecholamine excretion rate and glucagon levels.[66,67]

Causes of Metabolic Dysfunction

Sepsis appears to induce progressive abnormalities in metabolism coincident with the development of the physiologic abnormalities.[44,53] The characteristic changes of

* See also Chapter 15.

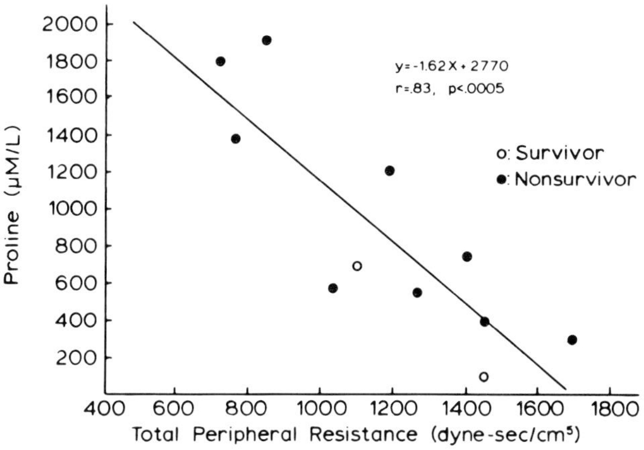

Fig. 16-12. **The data demonstrate the correlation in time of rising plasma proline levels and decreased total peripheral resistance. Inasmuch as decreased peripheral resistance is an important hallmark of the hemodynamic abnormalities attending the B state of sepsis, rising serum proline levels are a reliable predictor of metabolic and hemodynamic deterioration. (From Cerra FB, Caprioli J, Siegel JH, McMenamy RR, Border JR: Proline metabolism in sepsis, cirrhosis and general surgery: the peripheral energy deficit. *Ann Surg* 190:577, 1979.)**

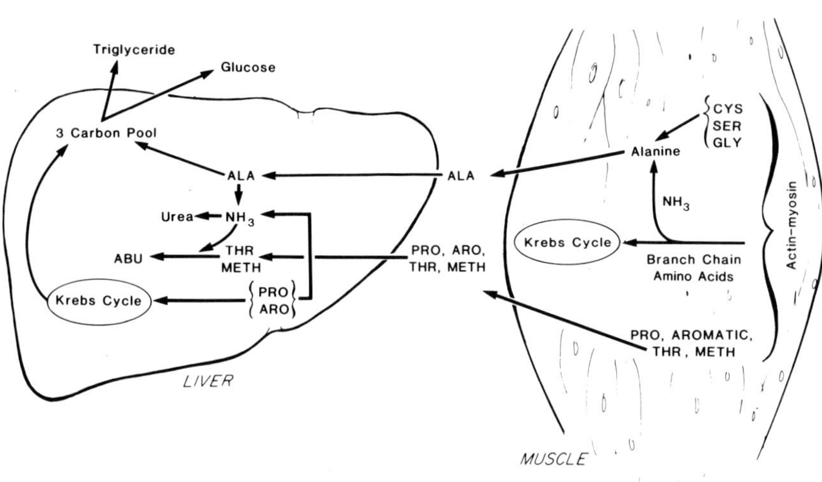

Fig. 16-13. **The flow of amino acid substrates between the periphery and liver during sepsis is illustrated. The branch chain amino acids can enter the Krebs cycle and be catabolized in the periphery. Proline (PRO), threonine (THR), methionine (METH), and the aromatic amino acids (ARO) cannot be interconverted or catabolized by muscle. They are released into the bloodsteam for processing by the liver. In the liver, METH and THR are preferentially converted to aminobutyric acid (ABU) rather than entering the Krebs cycle. Nitrogen from PRO and ARO is channeled into urea synthesis. The carbon skeletons of PRO and ARO are eventually cycled back into glucose and triglycerides by the liver. Similarly, the carbon skeletons of those amino acids (CYS—cystine, SER—serine, GLY—glycine) that can be converted to alanine (ALA) in the periphery are eventually recycled into the 3-carbon pool for gluconeogenesis.**

hyperglycemia, elevation of lactate and pyruvate with a constant lactate-pyruvate ratio, progressive elevation of triglycerides, the progressive increase in the beta-hydroxybutyrate-acetoacetate ratio, and the amino acid profile characteristics described become progressively more apparent as the unbalanced physiology (B state) emerges. The data indicate a progressive inability to burn glucose, fat, ketone bodies, and finally protein as the septic process unfolds. Early in the clinical course, there seems to be an increase in the utilization of branch chain amino acids by the periphery. As death approaches, the ability to utilize branch chain amino acids for energy production also declines. The clinical correlation of this protein-based energy production economy is seen in the rapidly declining muscle mass in these patients at a time when fat mass does not seem to be as rapidly declining. Other clinical indicators of reduced protein synthesis are also apparent—the onset of hypoalbuminemia, anergy, intestinal mucosal ulceration, and the failure of wound healing.

The regulation of metabolism normally proceeds through a combination of local factors with modulation, when necessary, by the neurohumoral systems. The result is a coordinated interorgan flow of substrate in accordance with demand. Thus, the liver produces glucose, which is essential for red cell and brain function and can be burned by other organs, such as muscle. Ketone bodies are produced by the liver and become a preferred source of fuel for other organs (eg, muscle). The liver, however, has no capacity to metabolize ketone bodies. Free fatty acids and glycerol are mobilized from adipose tissue and become sources for ketone body formation by the liver and are a primary fuel for the heart and skeletal muscle. The liver has a large capacity for the catabolism of aromatic and sulfur-containing amino acids but only takes up branch chain amino acids in accordance with its needs for protein synthesis and not for energy production. Muscle, on the other hand, can not only use branch chain amino acids for protein synthesis but can also use them for energy production.

Neuroendocrine modulation normally increases this interorgan, balanced substrate flow in accordance with existing demand. The substrate flow remains balanced in healthy people who are under stress. In patients with sepsis, however, there appears to be a progressive ineffectiveness of the normal hormonal modulating mechanisms and eventually a failure of the primordial metabolic machinery itself. Increased hepatocellular gluconeogenesis increases the mass flow of glucose to the periphery, where glucose oxidation is impaired. There is subsequent recycling of lactate, pyruvate, alanine, and glycerol back to the liver, thereby increasing the substrate the liver uses for gluconeogenesis (Fig. 16-10). Simultaneous increased hepatic production of triglycerides coincides with reduced use of triglyceride and fatty acid in the periphery (Fig. 16-11). The primary energy substrate thus becomes muscle protein. The branch chain amino acids seem to be preferentially burned in the mitochondria for energy production, but since the branch chain amino acids released from muscle cannot be preferentially removed from the actin-myosin, all the amino acids must be released (Fig. 16-13). Some unburned amino acids are converted to alanine and sent back to the liver which then makes more glucose. The amino acids that muscle cannot catabolize or interconvert (such as proline, methionine, threonine, and the aromatic amino acids) are released into the bloodstream. The liver, in its own tendency to use nonoxidative catabolic pathways, cannot properly metabolize them. The nitrogen-containing components of proline and the aromatic amino acids are used for urea synthesis, while their carbon skeletons eventually enter the 3 carbon pool and are recycled into glucose. Methionine and threonine are metabolized to alpha-ketobutyrate which, rather than entering the Krebs cycle, combines with ammonia to form aminobutyric acid. The result is a protein-based energy economy with muscle wasting and a progressively unbalanced amino acid pattern which the liver can no longer normalize. In such a setting, hepatic protein synthesis seems to become progressively inefficient.

All data point to a primary defect in mitochondrial function underlying these changes in substrate metabolism. The mitochondrial defect appears to be an energy deficit associated with a progressive fall in redox potential and a progressive preference for nonoxidative pathways of catabolism. Muscle from septic patients demonstrates a reduction in high-energy phosphate-containing compounds, a finding consistent with this hypothesis.[68] The fall in redox potential may be related to an inability to regenerate adenine nucleotide (NAD) from NADH, with a subsequent progressive failure of the NAD/NADH dependent systems (Figs. 16-8, 16-9). One of the most sensitive systems is the pyruvate dehydrogenase system for the conversion of pyruvate to acetyl Co-A. The entrance of acetyl Co-A into the Krebs cycle is, of course, the cornerstone for the entrance of glucose, fat, and ketone bodies into the process of oxidative phosphorylation. This inhibition of pyruvate dehydrogenase on a progressive basis would account for the observed alterations in lactate, pyruvate, and glucose. In addition, the high NADH concentrations would, with the reduced redox potential of the mitochondria, account for the decreased utilization of fatty acids by an inhibition of the fatty acid decarboxylase enzymes and subsequent reduced entry through acetyl Co-A. The reduced redox state would also favor the ketone bodies being present in the form of beta-hydroxybutyrate rather than in the utilization form of acetoacetate, because their interconversion is NAD/NADH–dependent. There is some indication, however, that acetoacetate may not be utilized until late in the course of progressive sepsis.

The branch chain amino acids, likewise, enter oxidative metabolic pathways through NAD/DADH-dependent systems, and during the course of uncontrolled sepsis their usefulness as fuels progressively declines. (Figs. 16-8, 16-13). Glutamate dehydrogenase also seems to be inhibited during infection. This inhibition is consistent with the proline data analysis described previously and seems to be primarily a hepatic phenomenon. The increased formation of aminobutyric acid from ammonia and alpha-ketobutyrate is consistent with failure to regenerate NAD and maintain redox potential.

The net result is the progressive inability of substrate to enter the mitochondria for high-energy phosphate production. This energy deficit would also account for the seemingly progressive inability of hormones to modulate the metabolic machinery. Such an energy deficit with a reduction in cytosol ATP would severely inhibit the cyclic AMP system through which most of the hormones act in their process of modulating metabolism.[69]

Several hypotheses have been proposed to explain the derangement in mitochondrial function, but all involve the hydrogen ion shuttle systems across the mitochondrial membrane. There has been an increased interest in calcium metabolism and its action as a messenger in cellular function of both a metabolic and contractile nature. Hydrogen ion transport has been shown to be intimately involved with the sodium-calcium pump across the mitochondrial membrane. This energy-dependent mechanism seems to be involved in all tissues except liver, kidney, lung, and smooth muscle.[70] Certainly a lack of high-energy phosphate would inhibit this sodium-calcium pump, with a progressively reduced ability for removal of hydrogen ion from the mitochondria. Whether or not this phenomenon would be a primary or secondary abnormality is as yet uncertain.

A second hypothesis for the reduced ability for hydrogen ion transport across the mitochondria is concerned with the malate-asparate shuttle.[71] An elevation of long chain fatty acid acyl-Co-A esters serves to inhibit the malate-asparate shuttle and the subsequent transport of hydrogen ions across the mitochondrial membrane. This would produce the resultant fall in mitochondrial redox potential and all its consequences. Recent studies have also shown that the plasma carnitine is not deficient in patients with sepsis. There is some experimental evidence to indicate, however, that intracellular carnitine is deficient in the systemic septic response.[72] An intracelluar deficiency of carnitine could result in an excess of fatty acid acyl-Co-A esters and the inhibition of the malate-asparate shuttle.

MEDIATORS OF THE CIRCULATORY RESPONSE TO ENDOTOXIN

The foregoing sections have emphasized the complexity of the pathophysiologic circulatory and metabolic response to infection. The mediators of this response are less well understood. Investigators have focused their attention on the ways in which the body responds to endotoxin, since gram-negative bacillary infection remains the most frequent cause of septic shock. But all data support the idea that endotoxin is not the prime inducer of the metabolic defects that accompany the septic state. These abnormalities appear to be a host response to many different types of invasive organisms.

Endotoxin has not been demonstrated to have a direct effect on either the heart or vascular smooth muscle, but the host's defenses against gram-negative bacterial infection can have secondary effects that are deleterious to the organism as a whole (Fig. 16-14). As Thomas [73] has stated, "our arsenals for fighting off bacteria are so powerful and involve so many defense mechanisms, that we are in more danger from them than from the invaders. . . . These macromolecules (endotoxin) are read by our tissues as the very worst of bad news. When we sense endotoxin, we are likely to turn on every defense at our disposal."

Although endotoxin is commonly characterized as a lipopolysaccharide, it also contains both protein and noncovalently bound lipid (Chapter 5), both of which may modulate interactions with host mediator systems.[73a] Endotoxin is the outermost of the three layers of cell wall of gram-negative bacteria. It exists as a high molecular weight aggregate (10^6 daltons) and is often particulate. The lipopolysaccharide component of the molecule is responsible for most of its toxicity. The polysaccharide complex consists of a core region and an O antigen region. The O antigen is an oligosaccharide and is specific for the bacterial species. The lipid moiety of LPS (lipid A) has a diglucosamine backbone with both ester and amide linked fatty acids as well as pyrophosphate groups. A variety of chemical preparations of endotoxin are available, and each has a unique chemical composition and invokes a unique set of host responses. The species of bacteria from which endotoxin is prepared will also determine its effects on the host. Lipid A can be chemically modified (eg, by binding to polymyxin B or by hydrolysis), often leading to loss of biologic activity.

The humoral responses that have been studied in most detail and that have the most bearing on the circulatory response to sepsis involve the serum complement and coagulation systems. The complement system can be activated by one of two pathways. The classic pathway is activated by the interaction of antigen with IgG or IgM antibody. This complex activates C1, the first complement component, which via the catalysis of C4 and C2 (C4 + C2 → C42) activates C3 and the physiologically active terminal components through C9. Endotoxin is capable of initiating this classic pathway without the presence of antibody. The lipid A region of the molecule is probably essential for this response. The alternative pathway of activation requires the interaction of properdin with serum factors B and D as well as C3b (Chapter 13, Figs. 13-13 through 13-19).

Activation of the complement cascade releases a number of pharmacologically active mediators (eg, anaphylatoxins C3a, C5a, which trigger the release of histamine from mast cells; Table 13-17, Fig. 13-16), and some of the hemodynamic consequences of endotoxin administration in animals can be abrogated by prior depletion of complement. Cobra venom from Naja Naja (CoF) complexes with serum factor B and the terminal components of complement and effectively decomplements test animals. From et al [74] compared the hemodynamic response to endotoxin in normal dogs to dogs previously decomplemented with CoF. They found that although the immediate hypotensive phase of response could be abrogated, the progressive hypotension that ensues after the first hour is unaffected. In contrast, Garner et al [75] demonstrated that decomplemented dogs remained normotensive for as long as 3 hours after the administration of endotoxin. The usual depletion of platelets, clotting factors, and leukocytes within the first hour was partially abrogated by decomplementation. Ulevitch et al [76] did similar experiments in Rhesus monkeys and found that decreases in cardiac output and total peripheral resistance could not be prevented by prior decomplementation.

The significance of endotoxin activation of complement during human gram-negative infection is not known. McCabe,[77] however, has demonstrated that humans with gram-negative bacteremia and hypotension have decreased serum levels of complement. Reduced levels of complement were not demonstrated in patients with bacteremia who did not become hypotensive. Fearson et al [78] have demonstrated that patients with gram-negative bacteremia and hypotension have normal levels of C1, C4, and C2, but decreased levels of C3 and the terminal complement components, as well as decreased levels of factor B and properdin. On the basis of these data, it appears that complement activation by the alternative pathway may participate in the human circulatory response to gram-negative bacteremia.

The response of the coagulation system to endotoxin has also been implicated in the development of circulatory abnormalities (Fig. 16-14). In 1928, Shwartzman [79] demonstrated that two doses of endotoxin administered 24 hours apart could cause local hemorrhagic tissue injury (the local

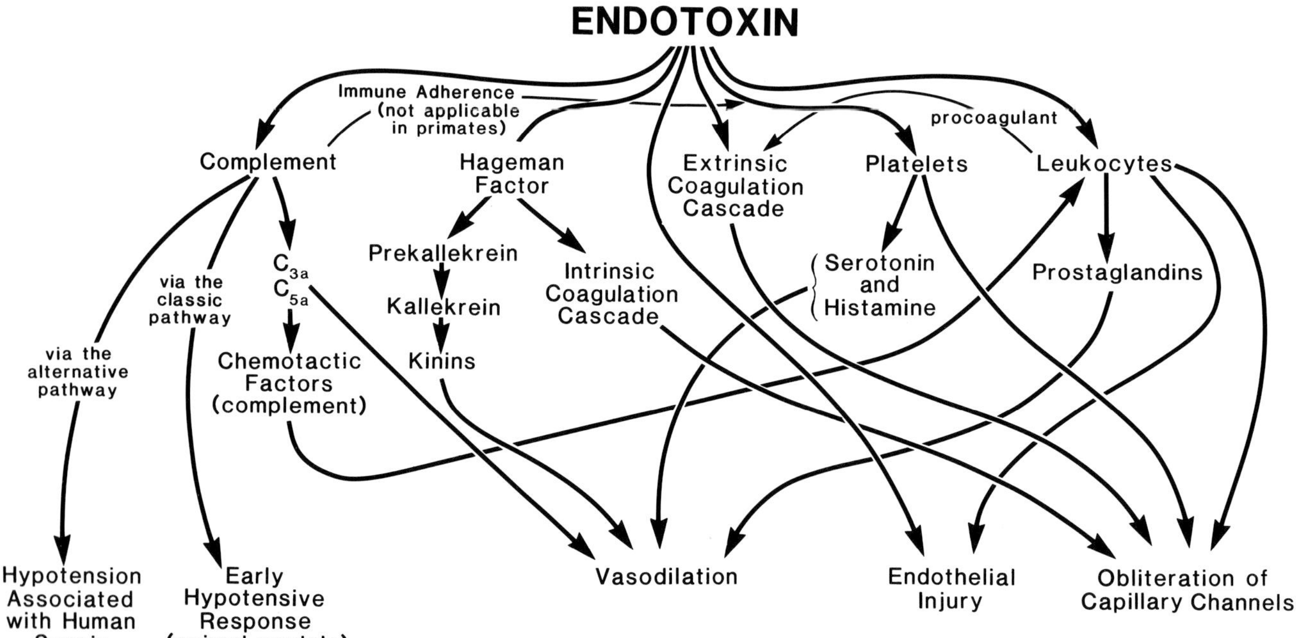

Fig. 16-14. **The mediators of endotoxin-induced tissue damage.**

Shwartzman reaction). A single intravenous dose of endotoxin is capable of causing a generalized Shwartzman reaction, in which occlusive fibrin thrombi are lodged in the capillary beds of the lungs, liver, and spleen. These patterns of injury are consistent with the pathologic changes associated with the consumption coagulopathy referred to as disseminated intravascular coagulation (DIC).

Many patients who die of sepsis will demonstrate coagulopathy in the terminal stage of their disease, with decreased levels of clotting factors and platelets. Autopsy findings frequently demonstrate occlusive thrombi in the vascular beds. McKay et al [80] electromicroscopically demonstrated free-floating fibrin strands in canine plasma 15 minutes after the administration of endotoxin. After 2 hours, occlusive masses of fibrin, leukocytes, and platelets were found in hepatic sinusoids. Horwitz et al [81] have demonstrated depletion of plasma levels of fibrinogen and accumulation of fibrinolytic products within 1 hour of giving endotoxin to baboons.

Whether these responses compromise regional perfusion by obliterating capillary beds, and whether they occur via extrinsic or intrinsic activation of the coagulation system or a combination of the two, has yet to be determined. Endotoxin can, however, accumulate within, and injure, vascular endothelial cells. The exposure of the basement membrane by this mechanism probably releases procoagulant material that initiates the extrinsic cascade. Similarly, the monocyte is susceptible to the lipid A component of endotoxin and may also release procoagulant material and contribute to disseminated coagulation via the extrinsic pathway.

The intrinsic activation of the coagulation system commences with the activation of Hageman factor. This protein may be pivotal in the development of circulatory abnormalities because it is also capable of converting prekallikrein to kallikrein, thereby initiating the pathway that leads to the production of kinins, which have potent vasodilatory effects (Fig. 16-17). Kimball et al [7] administered endotoxin to human volunteers and demonstrated tachycardia, hyperpyrexia, and increased bradykinin levels within 30 to 60 minutes. Robinson et al [82] studied patients undergoing either cystoscopy or transurethral prostate resection and found that those with assayable endotoxin in their blood after operation demonstrated decreased peripheral vascular resistance and decreased levels of prekallikrein. In Rhesus monkeys, the response to lipid A is characterized by decreases in cardiac output and total peripheral resistance with increased plasma levels of bradykinin.[83] When a lipid-poor fraction of endotoxin is tested, bradykinin levels are not significantly increased and vasoconstriction, rather than vasodilation, occur during the first hour.

Endotoxin also interacts with cellular elements of the host (Fig. 16-14), and several of these interactions may contribute to the pathophysiologic circulatory response. Thrombocytopenia and leukopenia are common results of endotoxin administration. In rabbits, platelets accumulate within the pulmonary and hepatic capillaries.[84] The early hypotensive response in this species can be abrogated by sulfapyrazone, which blocks platelet aggregation and the release of platelet substances.[85] As already mentioned, thrombocytopenic dogs given endotoxin do not manifest the early pulmonary hypertension that otherwise accompanies the initial episode of systemic hypotension. Because platelets are capable of releasing the vasoactive substances histamine and serotonin, platelet deposition and lysis in the capillary beds may contribute to the hemodynamic response to endotoxemia. In vitro experiments indicate that complement must be present for platelets to aggregate when exposed to endotoxin. The platelets of primates lack immune adherence sites and are not activated by complement fixation. This may explain why large doses of endotoxin are required to induce thrombocytopenia in primates. There are no hard data demonstrating that platelets are capable of mediating a circulatory response in primates.

Leukopenia is a prominent early response to endotoxemia, as leukocytes are sequestered in capillaries, particularly in the pulmonary beds. In Rhesus monkeys, the neutrophils are sequestered in the pulmonary capillary bed and are degranulated within 15 minutes of endotoxin administration. The capillary endothelium is injured at sites of adherence suggesting a possible etiology for pulmonary lesions associated with endotoxemia.[86] Pingleton et al,[87] however, demonstrated the same endotoxin-induced pulmonary vascular lesions in neutropenic animals.

Besides contributing to the injury of vascular endothelium, white cells may also release products capable of mediating hemodynamic abnormalities. The mononuclear cells (macrophages and monocytes) are capable of releasing both procoagulant (the activator of the extrinsic coagulation system) and prostaglandins. Fletcher et al [88] found increased plasma levels of prostaglandins E and F (PGE, PGF) after administration of endotoxin in the baboon and correlated these levels with hemodynamic abnormalities. PGE levels fell as the cardiac output and blood pressure decreased. PGF levels were inversely related to cardiac output and arterial blood pressure and were positively correlated with pulmonary artery pressures. The intravenous administration of prostaglandin synthetase inhibitors (aspirin and indomethacin) decreased the circulating prostaglandin levels and dampened the hemodynamic response to endotoxin.[88]

Injuries to the vascular endothelium during endotoxemia may be mediated by the sequestration of leukocytes or by the direct effects of endotoxin itself (Fig. 16-14). Endotoxin accumulates in the vascular endothelium of dogs within 10 minutes, primarily in the small or medium-sized veins of the liver, spleen, and jejunum.[89] Mesenteric arteries in rabbits suffer endothelial damage within the first hour after endotoxin administration,[90] and endothelial cells can be found circulating in the bloodstream of rabbits within 5 minutes.[91] McKay et al,[80] however, could not demonstrate endothelial damage in response to endotoxin in Rhesus monkeys. It is not known to what extent this type of injury can account for hemodynamic abnormalities.

In summary, the host-mediated response to endotoxin is multifaceted. To what extent these responses contribute to the hemodynamic changes during clinical infection remains a speculative issue. The effects of endotoxin and endogenous mediators on metabolic mechanisms may be more important in determining the outcome of the systemic response to sepsis. Endotoxemia is only one component of the gram-negative insult, and it is unlikely that all the observed abnormalities can be attributed to this one molecule.

THE TREATMENT OF THE SYSTEMIC CIRCULATORY AND METABOLIC RESPONSE TO SEPSIS

Since a wide spectrum of physiologic patterns comprise the human circulatory response to sepsis, both hemodynamic and metabolic monitoring are the foundation upon which treatment must be based. The measurement of physiologic parameters defines the patient's pattern of response to sepsis and provides a means of determining the effects of therapy.

The awareness that patients with serious surgical infection are capable of pathologic circulatory and metabolic responses to this stress is paramount to the recognition of the earliest phases of the response. Careful and systematic physical examination is an important means of monitoring these patients before the obvious signs of cardiopulmonary and metabolic failure are apparent.

It must be understood, however, that the metabolic and cardiopulmonary effects of sepsis are present for a considerable period of time before their manifestation as symptoms and physical signs. In the appropriate clinical setting, therefore, a high index of suspicion must be present and an appropriate monitoring regimen instituted. The status of the patient's peripheral vascular beds is an important index of circulatory response to infection. A patient with an elevated core temperature, who is cold and clammy in the extremities and has thready pulses, is vasoconstricted. These signs should alert the clinician to a deterioration in the patient's circulatory response and prompt quantitative hemodynamic monitoring.

The patient whose response to infection is vasodilation and increased cardiac output has more subtle manifestations on physical examination. The symptoms and signs pertinent to organ systems other than the cardiovascular system often provide clues that an abnormal circulatory response is present. Thus, mental confusion, oliguria, tachypnea, and jaundice are signs that may parallel the manifestations of cardiovascular dysfunction when infection is uncontrolled. Such signs are indications for more quantitative hemodynamic monitoring.

The most informative and most readily accessible directly monitored hemodynamic parameters are arterial blood pressure, right and left ventricular filling pressures, and cardiac output. Blood pressure analysis by plethysmography is often adequate, but when peripheral arterial pressure is not a valid measure of aortic pressure (as in the profoundly vasoconstricted patient) or when arterial pressure is sufficiently labile so that intermittent checks with an arm cuff are necessary at an impractical frequency, monitoring via arterial catheterization is indicated. For this purpose, a cannula can be introduced into the radial artery and advanced centrally. An arterial port can, in addition, provide ready access for blood sampling (rather than repeated venipunctures) and for the determination of cardiac output by dilution techniques. Arterial thrombosis, distal embolization, and intravascular infection are, however, potential complications (Chapter 24).

Central venous catheterization, usually via an antecubital, subclavian, or internal jugular vein, provides access for the measurement of right ventricular filling pressures (catheter tip in the superior vena cava or right atrium) or left ventricular filling pressures (tip wedged in a pulmonary capillary). The pulmonary capillary wedge pressure is a useful estimator of left atrial pressure, particularly in settings of passive pulmonary edema. However, during severe pulmonary disease or the adult respiratory distress syndrome, the wedge pressure may under- or overestimate left atrial and left ventricular filling pressures. The central venous or pulmonary artery catheter can also be used as an injection port for determination of cardiac output. The measurement of cardiac output, central venous pressure, and arterial pressure is sufficient for the calculation of total peripheral resistance (TPR):

$$\text{TPR} = \frac{(\text{arterial pressure}) - \text{right atrial pressure}}{\text{Cardiac output}}$$

The patient's fluid status can be assessed initially based on physical examination, laboratory values (hematocrit, serum osmolality, and serum sodium), and ventricular filling pressures. These data, along with the measurement of A-VO_2 difference, provide the essentials for physiologic classification in the framework devised by Siegel and his colleagues (Figs. 16-4, 16-5).

Several decisions must then be made to govern the overall strategy of patient management. First, it must be determined to what extent the patient's overall deterioration is a reversible process. The underlying disease, the etiology of the infection, and the likelihood of controlling the infection will most often determine what the optimal outcome can be if the cardiovascular abnormalities are reversed.

The patient's greatest vulnerabilities must next be considered. Circulatory insufficiency threatens each organ system to a different degree, depending on what interventions are made by the physician. The patient will tolerate an insult to a given organ system less well if there is preexisting disease within that system. Thus, the patient with preexisting renal insufficiency will be at greater risk of developing acute renal failure after a period of low renal blood flow. Similarly, patients with arteriosclerotic ischemic heart disease are at greater risk of suffering myocardial ischemia or infarction as the result of decreased arterial pressure and coronary perfusion pressure.

GENERAL PRINCIPLES OF HEMODYNAMIC MANIPULATION

The overriding principle of hemodynamic manipulation is to allow oxygen delivery to be equal to tissue demand (Fig. 16-15). Unfortunately, there is no good clinical

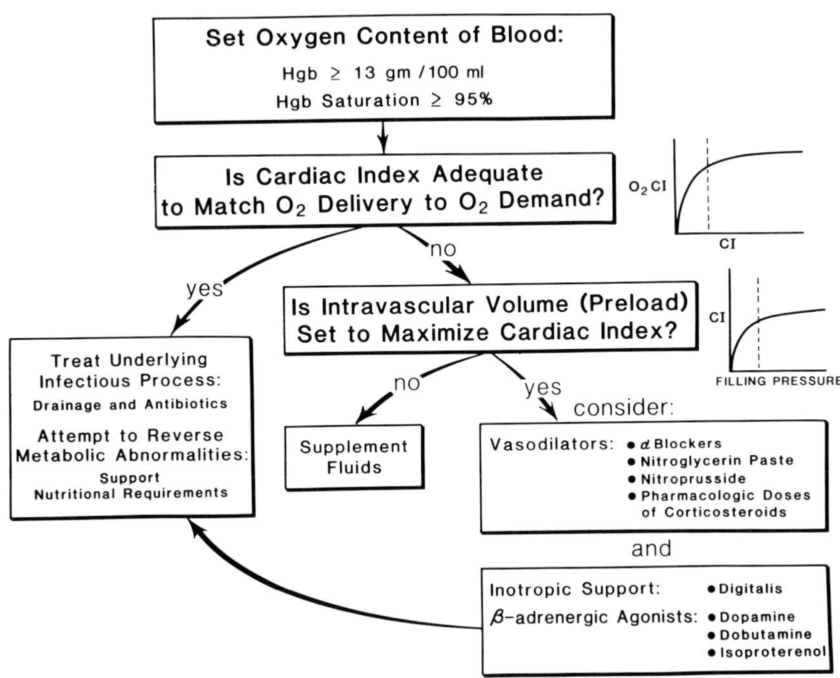

Fig. 16-15. An outline approach to physiologic monitoring and treatment of systemic sepsis: the adequacy of cardiac index must first be considered. If cardiac index needs to be augmented (oxygen utilization is not maximized), an increase in preload should first be attempted. Secondary measures to increase cardiac index include afterload reduction and inotropic support. In the patient with adequate cardiac index, efforts should be directed toward supporting nutritional requirements and stabilizing metabolic derangements. Untreated septic foci will thwart all these maneuvers; drainage and antibiotics are, therefore, the most important aspect of treatment in all patients.

method to indicate exactly what the tissues want to consume. There are two clinically useful methods, however, for being reasonably certain that delivery is optimal. The first is to increase cardiac index and observe the change in oxygen consumption ($CI \times AV\ DIF = O_2CI$). When the O_2CI is no longer increasing with increasing increments of cardiac index, optimization of demand and delivery is probably present. The second method is to combine O_2CI determinations with the lactate-pyruvate ratio. Then O_2CI is increased by raising the cardiac output so that there is no excess lactate relative to pyruvate (usually at an O_2CI 130 ml per M^2). Oxygen delivery and demand will then have been optimized.

The former concepts are predicated on the assumptions that blood oxygen content is adequate and that the distribution of blood flow at the tissue-blood interface is normal. Blood oxygen content can be normalized by maintaining a hemoglobin of 13 gm per dl and a reasonable PAO_2, ie, a PAO_2 that maintains ≥ 95 percent hemoglobin saturation. In that setting, oxygen delivery becomes a function of cardiac output and peripheral distribution. In sepsis, as has been shown, the problem does not seem to be one of flow distribution. Oxygen delivery manipulation, therefore, ultimately becomes that of manipulation of cardiac output.

The manipulation of cardiac output must always occur in combination with optimal preload to minimize the adverse effects of the other two methods of increasing cardiac output—afterload reduction and inotropic augmentation. Optimized preload, at a given setting of contractility and afterload, occurs when there is no longer an increase in cardiac output for a given increase in ventricular preload. Once this has been achieved and oxygen delivery is still inadequate, contractility or afterload therapy can be instituted. Once instituted, the preload again needs to be optimized and the adequacy of oxygen delivery assessed.

TREATMENT OF THE PATIENT WITH INADEQUATE CARDIAC OUTPUT

The first diagnostic consideration in treating a patient with inadequate cardiac output is whether intravascular volume is adequate (Fig. 16-15). If the available data suggest the patient can tolerate intravenous fluids, they should be administered. Caution must be exercised since even transient volume overload in combination with the pulmonary abnormalities that often accompany sepsis can result in pulmonary edema (increased interstitial pulmonary fluid). One available strategy is to supplement the adult patient's calculated basal crystalloid requirement with plasma or additional crystalloid while monitoring the myocardial response to that fluid load with pulmonary capillary wedge pressure measurements. A patient who is deficient in coagulation factors should receive fresh frozen plasma so as not to further dilute his stores.

If the patient with inadequate flow fails to improve his cardiac index despite optimization of left ventricular filling pressures, afterload-reducing and inotropic interventions should be considered. If the patient has not already been digitalized to improve contractility and ejection fraction, this can be a valuable maneuver. Since vasoconstriction at some point is deleterious to both the end organs receiving low flow and to the heart ejecting against increased afterload, vasodilator drugs are a logical choice as the next mode of therapy, either alone or in combination with inotropes. The drugs that have most commonly been used in this setting are phenoxybenzamine (a long-acting alpha adrenergic blocker), phentolamine (a short-duration alpha adrenergic blocker administered as a constant infusion), and nitroglycerine. Cerra et al[92] have recently demonstrated the efficacy of treating septic patients with nitroglycerin paste to augment their cardiac output and decrease their peripheral resistance. Nitroprusside, a short-acting agent with direct effects on vascular smooth muscle, is now commonly used to treat myocardial failure. This agent often dramatically reduces both preload and afterload while augmenting cardiac output. It must be administered as a constant infusion, and the patient's arterial pressure must be closely monitored by means of an arterial catheter. Investigators have also advocated pharmacologic doses of corticosteroids for vasodilation in this setting, but their efficacy in this area remains largely unproven in humans. A vasoconstricted patient administered one of these agents may respond with a decrease in arterial pressure although cardiac output is improved. This fall in blood pressure may not be detrimental. However, if the patient is vulnerable to myocardial ischemia, his coronary bed may be maximally dilated when he is vasoconstricted in order to support coronary metabolic needs. A fall in peripheral vascular resistance and thus coronary perfusion pressure may be poorly tolerated by such a patient, although cardiac work and cardiac metabolic demands may be decreased. Similarly, a patient with preexisting cerebrovascular disease may not tolerate the fall in central perfusion pressure that may accompany vasodilator therapy. Furthermore, the use of vasodilator therapy requires that an adequate contractility reserve be present in the ventricle. If not, profound hypotension in the absence of increased forward flow can occur. Almost always, afterload reduction in sepsis requires the administration of additional fluid to readjust preload as the afterload reduction agent is applied to maximum effect. Close monitoring of filling pressures and arterial pressures is required. An inotropic agent must often be administered at the same time the afterload agent is applied.

In patients in whom afterload reduction fails to improve flow, an additional inotropic pharmacologic agent should be considered. The sympathomimetic drugs, dopamine, isoproterenol, and dobutamine can provide inotropic support with variable dose-dependent effects on the peripheral vasculature. Dopamine has a unique advantage in that there appears to be a specific renal receptor for this agent through which renal blood flow is augmented. This agent also causes little or no vasoconstriction in the splanchnic circulation. At doses greater than 10 μg per kg per minute, however, dopamine mimics the vasoconstrictive action of levarterenol on the peripheral vascular bed. It is ill advised to use any vasoconstrictive drug in hypodynamic patients, especially if they are already vasoconstricted.

Berger et al [93] have reported successful results after circulatory augmentation with an intra-aortic balloon pump in two patients with sepsis and low-flow refractory to medical treatment. The advantages of this intervention are that: (1) it improves cardiac performance without increasing myocardial oxygen demands, (2) coronary perfusion is augmented without further constriction of the peripheral vascular bed, and (3) cardiac afterload is reduced during ejection. On the other hand, the procedure introduces another foreign body into the arterial tree in the presence of sepsis. It is a costly procedure in terms of both human and financial resources and should be approached judiciously in a patient whose sepsis is associated with irreversible disease in other organ systems.

TREATMENT OF THE PATIENT WITH ELEVATED CARDIAC OUTPUT

The state B patient with elevated cardiac index (usually > 5 L per minute per M^2), decreased total peripheral resistance (< 800 dyne cm^5), and narrowed A-VO_2 difference (< 3 volume percent) represents an interesting dilemma in management. Although not usually in immediate jeopardy, the patient in this category is often refractory to treatment and may eventually exhaust his cardiac reserves and progress to the low-flow state or develop hypotension despite an elevated cardiac output. Inotropic support for this type of patient may therefore be a useful prophylactic measure. However, it should again be emphasized that cardiac output is adequate if, and only if, oxygen consumption has been maximized. This may require flows in excess of 5 L per minute per M^2. The cardiac output should be augmented by the means described above until maximal oxygen utilization is attained. This task becomes impossible, however, in septic patients who eventually die. The previous discussion of the physiologic and metabolic derangements associated with sepsis also indicates that there is seldom a role for the use of vasoconstrictor agents to support blood pressure. The problem is one of maintaining an adequate cardiac output. If this cannot be done by the manipulation of preload, contractility, and afterload, death ensues and is unaffected by the addition of vasoconstrictor agents.

TREATMENT OF THE METABOLIC ABNORMALITIES

If the thesis is accepted that the high flow and low resistance response to sepsis is the result of metabolic derangement, then in theory treatment should be instituted to correct or prevent the responsible metabolic abnormalities. Because these derangements have yet to be completely defined biochemically, and the prime movers are unknown, rational definitive therapy is not presently available. There are, however, several basic guidelines for the metabolic management of seriously ill patients. The majority of patients demonstrating a pathologic circulatory response to infection are catabolic with large deficits in nitrogen balance that cannot be reversed by exogenous nutritional support until the infection begins to resolve itself. During this hypermetabolic phase when the energy production economy seems to be primarily protein-based, the most that can be achieved is a degree of protein sparing. Because of abnormalities in fuel utilization, this seems to be best achieved by providing high amino acid loads (2.0 to 3.0 gm per kg every 24 hours), with approximately 100 glucose calories per gram of administered protein nitrogen (eg, 3.7 percent amino acids in 15 percent glucose), together with multivitamins and adequate trace elements. The use of standard total parenteral nutrition during this hypermetabolic phase of sepsis is usually detrimental and produces fatty infiltration of the liver. Exogenous insulin administration (except in patients with diabetes mellitus), in an effort to regulate the serum glucose, only seems to potentiate the hepatic steatosis. The maximum tolerable protein load can be clinically assessed by the blood urea nitrogen-creatinine ratio. In the absence of hypovolemia, a prerenal azotemia in which the blood urea nitrogen exceeds that which is proportionate to the existing creatinine by 20 mg per dl (eg, creatinine of 3.0 mg per dl and a blood urea nitrogen of 90 mg per dl) probably indicates that maximum use of the exogenous amino acids has occurred.

During the hypermetabolic phase, hypertriglyceridemia is present along with a reduced triglyceride clearance. The use of currently available intravenous fats during this time serves no purpose, does not seem to improve nitrogen balance, and can potentiate pulmonary failure and cause reticuloendothelial blockade.

Once the glucose intolerance subsides, standard total parenteral nutrition can be safely and effectively employed. Likewise, intravenous fat can be safely used to replenish long chain fatty acids and to provide an additional source of calories. In the patient who is recovering from a severe septic episode, it is usually advisable to continue the intravenous nutritional support for a considerable period of time after oral nutrition has been reestablished. A program of physical therapy and exercise also seems to be advisable during this convalescence.

Intravenous protein nutrition cannot be given in the form of standard albumin-containing colloid solutions, which are deficient in the branch chain amino acids. Even the commercially available protein hydrolysates and mixtures of crystalline amino acids do not provide the septic patient the substrates that can be used most efficiently. Experimental trials with solutions rich in branch chain amino acids are needed to verify the evidence that these substrates are often the only fuel that the septic patient can burn in the peripheral tissues.

Clowes et al [8] have demonstrated both in an animal model (cecal ligation in the pig) and in patients that when the low-flow response is present and serum insulin levels are low, the intravenous administration of glucose, insulin, and potassium may improve hemodynamic status. This is manifested by as much as a threefold rise in cardiac output, with concomitant decreases in ventricular filling pressures. These investigators administer 1.5 units of insulin per kg body weight over 10 minutes with 10 meq of potassium and 1 gm per kg of glucose. The hemodynamic effects cannot be explained on the basis of the correction of hypoglycemia, since blood glucose levels were high prior to infusion in their studies.

The use of corticosteroids in the treatment of sepsis remains controversial. Schumer [94] in a double-blind prospective study showed that mortality in patients with positive blood cultures and hypotension (patients in so-called septic shock) was reduced in groups receiving either methylprednisolone or dexamethasone. In 86 saline-treated patients, the mortality was 28.4 percent while in 86 patients treated with steroids, mortality was 10.4 percent. This study, however, did not demonstrate a physiologic basis for this difference. Patients dying with hypotension did not necessarily die of circulatory abnormalities. Complications of steroid therapy including gastrointestinal hemorrhage, hyperosmolar diabetes, and psychosis occurred in 5 percent of the treated patients. Because of the expense and potential complications of high dose corticosteroids, investigative efforts should be directed toward identifying those groups of patients who are most likely to benefit from their use and those who are at greatest risk of complications. Although there is evidence in animal models, particularly in dogs, that administration of corticosteroids prior to endotoxin can protect the animals somewhat from severe vasoconstriction, no such hemodynamic improvements have been consistently documented in clinical trials. In patients with a high-flow response to sepsis, evidence has already been cited suggesting that the enzyme systems of intermediary metabolism are modulated to favor gluconeogenesis over oxidative glucose utilization. Corticosteroids may exacerbate this metabolic derangement.

If the hypermetabolic state recurs, if the pulmonary failure begins to worsen, or if the physiology again begins to deteriorate (particularly with recurrence of the B state), another septic focus may be present. A thorough search must be immediately instituted. The patient should be recultured, and intravascular catheters should be replaced. If no new source of sepsis is identified, a reexploration in the vicinity of the previously drained source is usually in order.

If the treatment regimens outlined are followed, renal failure requiring hemodialysis is unusual. If it does occur, the best policy seems to be to continue the support regimens as outlined. The frequency and technique of dialysis should be adjusted to control the fluid load and prevent uremia. This sometimes requires daily or twice daily dialysis.

It should once more be emphasized that many patients who demonstrate profound hemodynamic abnormalities in response to infection will die of their infection whether or not their circulatory status is improved by proper management. If the septic process remains uncontrolled, the function of the circulatory system as well as of other organ systems is likely to deteriorate. Adherence to the principles of adequate surgical eradication of septic foci, and effective antibiotic treatment based on careful and systematic culture of infected tissues and fluids, remain fundamental in treating the patient with serious infection. The early recognition of poorly controlled infection by careful monitoring of the patient will no doubt contribute to the prevention of the serious organ system derangements that may result from sepsis.

BIBLIOGRAPHY

Cerra FB, Siegel JH, Coleman B, Border JR, McMenamy RR: Septic autocannibalism: A failure of exogenous nutritional support. Ann Surg 192:4, 1980.

Crowley RA, Trump BF (eds.): Shock, Anoxia and Ischemia: Pathophysiology, Prevention and Treatment. Baltimore, Williams and Wilkins, 1981.

Moore FD: Metabolic Care of the Surgical Patient. Philadelphia, Saunders, 1959.

Siegel JH, Chodoff P (eds.): The Aged and High Risk Surgical

Patient. Medical, Surgical and Anesthetic Management. New York, Grune and Stratton, 1976.

REFERENCES

1. Freid MA, Vosti KL: The importance of underlying disease in patients with gram-negative bacteremia. Arch Intern Med 121:418, 1968.
2. Meakins JL, Pietsch JB, Bubenick O, Kelley R, Rode H, Gordon J, MacLean LD: Delayed hypersensitivity: indicator of acquired failure of host defenses in sepsis and trauma. Ann Surg 186:241, 1977.

CIRCULATORY RESPONSES TO INFECTION

3. MacLean LD, Weil MH: Hypotension (shock) in dogs produced by *Escherichia coli* endotoxin. Circul Res IV:546, 1956.
4. Bredenberg CE, Taylor GA, Webb WR: The effect of thrombocytopenia on the pulmonary and systemic hemodynamics of canine endotoxin shock. Surgery 87:59, 1980.
5. Guenter CA, Fiorica V, Hinshaw LB: Cardiorespiratory and metabolic responses to live *E. coli* and endotoxin in the monkey. J Appl Physiol 26:780, 1969.
6. Buckberg G, Cohn J, Darling C: *Escherichia coli* bacteremia shock in conscious baboons. Ann Surg 173:122, 1971.
7. Kimball HR, Melmon KL, Solfe SM: Endotoxin-induced kinin production in man (36302). Proc Soc Exp Biol Med 139:1078, 1972.
8. Clowes GHA Jr, O'Donnell TF Jr, Ryan NT, Blackburn GL: Energy metabolism in sepsis: treatment based on different patterns in shock and high output stage. Ann Surg 179:684, 1974.
9. Hermreck AS, Thal AP: Mechanisms for the high circulatory requirements in sepsis and septic shock. Ann Surg 170:677, 1969.
10. Ebert RV, Stead EA Jr: Circulatory failure in acute infections. J Clin Invest 20:671, 1941.
11. Waisbren BA: Bacteremia due to gram-negative bacilli other than the *Salmonella.* A clinical and therapeutic study. Arch Intern Med 88:467, 1951.
12. Clowes GHA Jr, Vucinic M, Weidner MG: Circulatory and metabolic alterations associated with survival or death in peritonitis: clinical analysis of 25 cases. Ann Surg 163:866, 1966.
13. MacLean LD, Mulligan WG, McLean APH, Duff JH: Patterns of septic shock in man—a detailed study of 56 patients. Ann Surg 166:543, 1967.
14. Siegel JH, Greenspan M, del Guercio LRM: Abnormal vascular tone, defective oxygen transport and myocardial failure in human septic shock. Ann Surg 165:504, 1967.
15. Siegel JH, Goldwyn RM, Friedman HP: Pattern and process in the evolution of human septic shock. Surgery 70:232, 1971.
16. Siegel JH, Farrell EJ, Goldwyn RM, Friedman HP: Myocardial function in human septic shock states. In Forscher BK, Lillehei RC, Stubbs SS (eds): Shock in Low- and High-Flow States. Amsterdam, Excerpta Medica, 1972, p 250.
17. Siegel JH, Cerra FB, Coleman B, Giovannini I, Shetye M, Border JR, McMenamy RH: Physiological and metabolic correlations in human sepsis. Surgery 86:163, 1979.
18. Siegel JH: Pattern and process in the evaluation of and recovery from shock. In Siegel JH, Chodoff P (eds): The Aged and High Risk Surgical Patient. Medical, Surgical and Anesthetic Management. New York, Grune and Stratton, 1976, p 381.
19. Siegel JH, Cerra FB, Peters D, Moody E, Brown D, McMenamy RH, Border JH: The physiologic recovery trajectory as the organizing principle for the quantification of hormonometabolic adaption to surgical stress and severe sepsis. Advan Shock Res 2:177, 1979.

PATHOPHYSIOLOGY OF SEPTIC SHOCK

20. Crile GW: An experimental research into surgical shock. Philadelphia, Lippincott, 1899.
21. Blalock A: Experimental shock: the cause of the low blood pressure produced by muscle injury. Arch Surg 20:959, 1930.
22. Hinshaw LB: Role of the heart in the pathogenesis of endotoxin shock. A review of the clinical findings and observations on animal species. Surg Res 17:134, 1974.
23. Hinshaw LB, Archer LT, Greenfield LJ, Guenter CA: Effects of endotoxin on myocardial hemodynamics, performance, and metabolism. Am J Physiol 221:504, 1971.
24. Hinshaw LB, Greenfield LJ, Owen SE, Black MR, Guenter CA: Precipitation of cardiac failure in endotoxin shock. Surg Gynecol Obstet 135:39, 1972.
25. Hinshaw LB, Archer LT, Black MR, Greenfield LJ, Guenter CA: Prevention and reversal of myocardial failure in endotoxin shock. Surg Gynecol Obstet 136:1, 1973.
26. Alyono D, Ring WS, Anderson RW: The effects of hemorrhagic shock on the diastolic properties of the left ventricle in the conscious dog. Surgery 83:691, 1978.
27. Rouchard RJ, Gault JH, Ross J Jr: Evaluation of pulmonary arterial end-diastolic pressure as an estimate of left ventricular end-diastolic pressure in patients with normal and abnormal left ventricular performance. Circulation 44:1072, 1971.
28. Elkins RC, McCurdy JR, Brown PP, Greenfield LJ: Effects of coronary perfusion pressure on myocardial performance during endotoxin shock. Surg Gynecol Obstet 137:991, 1973.
29. Goodyer AVN: Left ventricular function and tissue hypoxia in irreversible hemorrhagic and endotoxin shock. Am J Physiol 212:444, 1967.
30. Urschel CW, Serur JR, Forrester JA, Amsterdam EA, Parmley WW, Dembitsky W, and Sonnenblick EH: Myocardial contractility during hemorrhagic shock, endotoxemia, and ischemia. In Forscher BK, Lillehei RC, Stubbs SS (eds): Shock in low and high flow states. Amsterdam, Excerpta Medica 2, 1972, p 77.
31. Blalock A: A study of thoracic duct lymph in experimental crush injury and injury produced by gross trauma. Johns Hopkins Hosp Bull 72:54, 1942.
32. Lefer AM: Blood borne humoral factors in the pathophysiology of circulatory shock. Circ Res 32:129, 1973.
33. Wangensteen SL, Geissinger WT, Lovett WL, Glenn TM, Lefer AM: Relationship between splanchnic blood flow and a myocardial depressant factor in endotoxin shock. Surgery 69:410, 1971.
34. Greenfield LF, McCurdy JR, Hinshaw LB, Elkins RE: Preservation of myocardial function during cross-circulation in terminal endotoxin shock. Surgery 72:111, 1972.
35. Okada K, Kosugi I, Kitagaki T, Yamaguchi Y, Yoshikawa H, Kawashiwa Y, Kawakami S, and Senoy Y: Pathophysiology of shock. JPN Circ J 41:346, 1977.
36. Lovett WL, Wangensteen SL, Glenn TM, Lefer AM: Presence of a myocardial depressant factor in patients in circulatory shock. Surgery 70:223, 1971.
37. Clowes GHA Jr, Martin H, Walji S, Hirsch E, Gazitua R, Goodfellow R: Blood insulin responses to blood glucose levels in high output sepsis and septic shock. Am J Surg 135:577, 1978.
38. Perbellini A, Shatney CH, MacCarter DJ, Lillehei RC: A new

model for the study of septic shock. Surg Gynecol Obstet 147:68, 1978.
39. Gump FE, Price JB Jr, Kinney JM: Whole body and splanchnic blood flow and oxygen consumption measurements in patients with intraperitoneal infection. Ann Surg 171:321, 1970.
40. Imamura M, Clowes GHA Jr: Hepatic blood flow and oxygen consumption in starvation, sepsis and septic shock. Surg Gynecol Obstet 141:27, 1975.
41. Finley RJ, Duff JH, Holliday RL, Jones D, Marchuk JB: Capillary muscle blood flow in human sepsis. Surgery 78:87, 1975.
42. Wright CJ, Duff JH, McLean APH, McLean LD: Regional capillary blood flow and oxygen uptake in severe sepsis. Surg Gynecol Obstet 132:637, 1971.
43. Archie JP: Anatomic arterial-venous shunting in endotoxic and septic shock in dogs. Ann Surg 186:171, 1977.
44. Cerra FB, Siegel JH, Border JR, Peters DM, McMenamy RR: Correlations between metabolic and cardiopulmonary measurements in patients after trauma, general surgery and sepsis. J Trauma 19:621, 1979.
45. Lillehei RC, Longerbeam JK, Bloch JH, Manax WG: The nature of irreversible shock: Experimental and clinical observations. Ann Surg 160:682, 1964.
46. Zweifach BW, Nagler AL, Thomas L: The role of epinephrine in the reactions produced by the endotoxins of gram-negative bacteria. J Exp Med 104:2, 1956.
47. Duff JH, Groves AC, McLean APH, LaPointe R, and MacLean LD: Defective oxygen consumption in septic shock. Surg Gyn Obstet 128:1051, 1969.
48. Johnson G Jr, McDevitt NB, Proctor HJ: Erythrocyte 2, 3-Diphosphoglycerate in endotoxic shock in the subhuman primate: response to fluid and/or methylprednisolone succinate. Ann Surg 180:783, 1974.
49. Watkins GM, Rabelo A, Plzak LF, Sheldon GF: The left shifted oxyhemoglobin curve in sepsis: a preventable defect. Ann Surg 180:213, 1974.
50. Long CL: Energy balance and carbohydrate metabolism in infection and sepsis. Am J Clin Nutr 30:1301, 1977.
51. Long CL, Spencer JL, Kinney JM, Geiger JW: Carbohydrate metabolism in man: effect of elective operations and major injury. J Appl Physiol 31:110, 1971.
52. Long CL, Kinney JM, Geiger JW: Nonsuppressibility of gluconeogenesis by glucose in septic patients. Metabolism 25:193, 1976.
53. Cerra FB, Caprioli J, Siegel JH, McMenamy RR, Border JR: Proline metabolism in sepsis, cirrhosis and general surgery: the peripheral energy deficit. Ann Surg 190:577, 1979.
54. Liaw KY, Askanazi J, Michelsen CB, Kantrowitz LR, Furst P, Kinney JM: Effect of operative injury and sepsis on high energy phosphate activity and glycolytic activity in muscle and red cells. J Trauma, 20:755, 1980.
55. Beisel WR, Wannemacher RW: Metabolic response of the host to infectious disease. In Richards JR, Kinney JM (eds): Nutritional Aspects of Care in the Critically Ill. New York, Churchill-Livingstone-Longman, 1977, pp 135–161.
56. Wannemacher RW Jr, Dinterman RE, Hadick CL: Metabolic fuel utilization by skeletal muscle (SM) of Rhesus monkeys (RM) during pneumococcal sepsis. (Abstract) Fed Proc 37 (1):849, 1978.
57. Cerra FB, Siegel JH, Border JR, Wiles J, McMenamy RR: The hepatic failure of sepsis: Cellular versus substrate. Surgery 86:409, 1979.
58. Border JR, Chenier R, McMenamy RR, LaDuca J, Seibel R, Birkhahn R, Yu L: Multiple systems organ failure: muscle fuel deficit with visceral protein malnutrition. Surg Clin North Am 56:1147, 1976.
59. Border JR: Metabolic response to short term starvation, sepsis, and trauma. In Cooper L (ed): Surgery Annual. New York, Appleton, 1970.
60. Clowes GHA Jr, O'Donnell TF, Blackburn GL, Maki TN: Energy metabolism and proteolysis in traumatized and septic man. Surg Clin North Am 56:1169, 1976.
61. McMenamy RR, Border JR, Cerra FB, Moyer E, Reed R, Yu L: Splanchnic substrate balances and biochemical changes during sepsis. J Trauma 1981, in press.
62. Moyer ED, Border JR, Cerra FB: Unpublished data.
63. Cerra FB, Siegel JH, Coleman B, Border JR, McMenamy RR: Septic autocannabolism: a failure of exogenous nutritional support. Ann Surg 92:570, 1980.
64. Skillman JJ, Rosenoer VM, Smith PC, Fang MS: Improved albumin synthesis in postoperative patients by amino acid infusion. N Engl J Med 295:1037, 1976.
65. Benedict CR, Graham-Smith DC: Plasma noradrenaline and adrenaline concentrations and dopamine-beta-hydroxylase activity in patients with shock due to septicaemia, trauma and haemorrhage. Q J Med 47:1, 1978.
66. Wilmore DW: Carbohydrate metabolism in trauma. Clin Endocrinol Metab 5:731, 1976.
67. Wilmore DW, Long JM, Mason AD Jr, Skreen RW, Pruitt BA Jr: Catecholamines: mediator of the hypermetabolic response to thermal injury. Ann Surg 180:653, 1974.
68. Bergstrom J, Bostrous H, Furst P: Preliminary studies of energy rich phosphagens in critically ill patients. Crit Car Med 4:197, 1976.
69. Murad F: Cyclic nucleotides in cell injury. In Crowley RA, Trump BF (eds): Shock, Anoxia and Ischemia. Pathophysiology, Prevention and Treatment. Baltimore, Williams and Wilkins, 1981.
70. Carafoli E, Crompton M, Malsronm K, Sigel E, Salzmann M, Chiesi M, Affolter H: Mitochondrial calcium transport and the intracellular calcium homeostasis. In Semenya G, Carafoli E (eds); Biochemistry of Membrane Transport. Berlin, Springer Verlag, 1977, pp 535–551.
71. Shrago E, Shrey A, Ellison C: Regulation of cell metabolism by mitochondria transport system. In Hanse RW, Mehlman MA (eds): Gluconeogenesis. New York, Wiley, 1976, p 221.
72. Cerra FB, Aswald G, Border JR: Does the plasma carnitine matter in sepsis? J Surg Res 1981, in press.

MEDIATORS OF THE CIRCULATORY RESPONSES IN INFECTION

73. Thomas L: The Lives of a Cell: Notes of a Biology Watcher. New York, Viking, 1974, p 78.
73a. McCabe WR: Endotoxin: Microbiological, chemical, pathophysiologic and clinical correlations. In Weinstein L, Fields BN (eds): Seminars in Infectious Disease, (vol III). New York, Thieme-Stratton Inc., 1980, p 38.
74. From AHL, Gewurz H, Gruninger RP, Pickering RJ, Spink WW: Complement in endotoxin shock: effect of complement depletion on the early hypotensive phase. Infect Immun 2:38, 1970.
75. Garner R, Chater BV, Brown DL: The role of complement in endotoxin shock and disseminated intravascular coagulation: experimental observations in the dog. Br J Hematol 28:393, 1974.
76. Ulevitch RJ, Cochrane CG, Bans K, Herman CM, Fletcher R, and Rice CL: The effect of complement depletion on bacterial lipopolysaccharide. (LPS)-induced hemodynamic and hematologic changes in the rhesus monkey. Am J Pathol 92:227, 1978.

77. McCabe WR: Serum complement levels in bacteremia due to gram-negative organisms. N Engl J Med 288:21, 1973.
78. Fearson DT, Ruddy S, Schur PH, McCabe WR: Activation of the properdin pathway of complement in patients with gram-negative bacteremia. N Engl J Med 292:937, 1975.
79. Shwartzman G: Studies on *Bacillus typhosus*, toxic substances. I. Phenomenon of local skin reactivity to *B. typhosus* culture filtrate. J Exp Med 48:247, 1928.
80. McKay DG, Margaretten W, Csavossy I: An electron microscope study of endotoxin shock in rhesus monkeys. Surg Gyn Obstet 125:825, 1967.
81. Horwitz DL, Moquin RB, Herman CM: Coagulation changes of septic shock in the sub-human primate and their relationship to hemodynamic changes. Ann Surg 175:417, 1972.
82. Robinson JA, Klodnycky ML, Loeb HS, Racic MR, Gunnar RM: Endotoxin, prekallikrein, complement and systemic vascular resistance: sequential measurements in man. Am J Med 59:61, 1975.
83. Reichgott MJ, Melmon KL, Forsyth RP, Greineder D: Cardiovascular and metabolic effects of whole or fractionated gram-negative bacterial endotoxin in the unanesthetized Rhesus monkey. Circ Res 33:346, 1973.
84. Stetson CA, Jr: Studies on the mechanism of the Schwartzman phenomenon: certain factors involved in the production of local hemorrhagic necrosis. J Exp Med 93:489, 1951.
85. Evans G, Lewis AF, Mustard JF: The role of platelet aggregation in the development of endotoxin shock. Br J Surg 56:624 (Abstract), 1969.
86. Coalson JJ, Hinshaw LB, Guenter CA: The pulmonary ultrastructure in septic shock. Exp Mol Path 12:84, 1970.
87. Pingleton WW, Coalson JJ, Guenter CA: Significance of leukocytes in endotoxic shock. Exp Mol Path 22:183, 1975.
88. Fletcher JR, Ramwell PW, Herman CM: Prostaglandins and the hemodynamic course of endotoxin shock. J Surg Res 20:589, 1976.
89. Rubenstein HS, Fine J, Coons AH: Localization of endotoxin in the walls of the peripheral vascular system during lethal endotoxemia. Proc Soc Exp Biol Med 111:458, 1962.
90. McGrath JM, Stewart GJ: The effects of endotoxin on vascular endothelium. J Exp Med 129:833, 1969.
91. Gaynor E, Bouvier C, Spaet TH: Vascular lesions: possible pathogenic basis of the generalized Schwartzman reaction. Science 170:986–988, 1970.

THERAPY OF SEPTIC SHOCK

92. Cerra FB, Hasset J, Siegel JH: Vasodilator therapy in clinical sepsis with low output syndrome. J Surg Res 25:180, 1978.
93. Berger RL, Saini VK, Long W, Hechtman H, Hood W Jr: The use of diastolic augmentation with the intra-aortic balloon in human septic shock with associated coronary artery disease. Surgery 74:601, 1973.
94. Schumer W: Steroids in the treatment of clinical septic shock. Ann Surg 184:333, 1976.

CHAPTER 17
Organ Failure in Sepsis

SAMUEL R. POWERS JR. AND THOMAS M. SABA

DEDICATION

Co-author Dr. Thomas M. Saba would like to dedicate this chapter to his colleague, Dr. Samuel R. Powers Jr, who died several days after completing it. His tremendous personal effort to complete this work was remarkable. Dr. Powers was a leading academic surgeon and scientist in the field of trauma for more than 20 years.

SEQUENTIAL organ failure has recently been recognized as a frequently fatal complication of systemic sepsis.[1] Chapters 15 and 16 have extensively discussed the hemodynamic and metabolic responses to infection that can become manifest in the form of multiple organ failure. This chapter focuses on the complex response patterns of defense that operate to preserve organ function and their derangement.[2] Such responses include cardiovascular, pulmonary, renal, neural, hematologic, and metabolic adjustments, which are designed to selectively deliver blood to vital organs and maintain cellular function. Although the body's response to severe shock and trauma is initially protective, these adaptations may later contribute to persistent and progressive sequential organ failure,[3] refractory to conventional therapy, even with adequate hemodynamic and ventilatory support.

Clinical observation has long documented that shock and trauma can cause specific abnormalities of organ function. Clinicians, however, have only recently become aware of the sequential nature of multiple organ failure associated with sepsis.[4] The increased frequency of organ failure during sepsis appears to be related primarily to the fact that patients now survive the initial injury for extended periods because of sophisticated cardiovascular, pulmonary, and renal support systems.[1] Infection frequently supervenes, and as each new physiologic support system is brought into use, another organ system has the potential to fail.

An important factor in evaluating the mechanism of multiple organ failure is that failure of a particular organ is not necessarily at the site of infection.[5] Thus, a focus of wound sepsis may result in a failing organ distant to the site, a reflection of the systemic interaction of the products of bacterial infection with the tissue elements of the host. This interaction includes by-products of the immunologic response, triggering of the coagulation process, activation of the complement system, and a variety of cellular and humoral mediators. Indeed, the host response to infection may initiate a cascade phenomenon, which results in multiple organ failure.

With the exception of central nervous system injury, the predominant cause of late mortality in the injured patient, after initial successful resuscitation, is progressive organ failure, usually associated with local sepsis or bacteremia.[6] Sequential organ failure can develop even after a prolonged period of cardiovascular stability, normal pulmonary function, and adequate renal function.[7] The pattern of organ failure that insidiously develops is diffuse and can include respiratory distress, peripheral vascular instability, alterations in oxygen utilization, renal dysfunction, disruption of carbohydrate metabolism, and disturbances in reticuloendothelial function. With increasing duration of patient survival, there is also evidence of hepatic failure as well as cellular metabolic disturbances,[8] which are discussed in Chapters 15 and 16.

GENERAL PATHOLOGY OF SEQUENTIAL ORGAN FAILURE

Edema is a predominant pathologic finding, particularly in the lungs and peripheral tissue beds of the septic injured patient with organ failure. Such observations have suggested that altered microvascular-interstitial fluid balance may be a unifying mechanism in the etiology of this disorder.[9,10] Pulmonary interstitial edema in association with sepsis is related to altered pulmonary vascular permeability, with the bacteremic episode serving as a precipitating event that increases transvascular fluid flux and alters lung fluid balance.[11,12] Our ability to quantitatively investigate the mechanism of such events in the clinical setting is limited. Moreover, other vascular beds within the liver, intestine, brain, and kidneys may also be subjected to the same disturbances of altered vascular permeability, abnormal fluid balance, interstitial fluid accumulation, and organ dysfunction. A permeability defect may be compounded by alterations in hydrostatic and oncotic pressure gradients, although it is not totally dependent on their coexistence. For example, pulmonary edema following trauma in association with sepsis will occur without left heart failure. Similarly, changes in oncotic pressure will not necessarily lead to altered lung fluid balance. Thus, while hydrostatic and oncotic pressure alterations are factors in the pathogenesis of altered microvascular fluid balance and edema, other humoral and tissue factors may be mediating altered capillary function. These include the release of bacterial endotoxin, complement activation, immune complex deposition, leukostasis in the microcirculation, platelet disruption, fibrin embolization, fibrin split product generation, and altered endothelial cell adherence to the basement membrane. For example, sepsis is a powerful stimulant of intravascular coagulation, perhaps through the release of endotoxin. The presence of intravascular coagulation as a precipitating event in the development of pulmonary abnormalities has experimental support. Similarly, leukostasis in the pulmonary vascular bed in association with bacteremia, coupled with the deposition of immune complexes, may serve as a mechanism for activation of complement and release of other humoral factors which can alter the integrity of the microcirculation.

One aspect of the relationship of bacteria, endotoxin, fibrin microaggregates, altered platelets, and immune complexes in the pathogenesis of organ dysfunction with sepsis relates to the coexistence of reticuloendothelial systemic host defense failure (see subsequent section). Phagocytic cells of the liver and spleen are active in the clearance of the above factors from the vascular compartment and reticuloendothelial dysfunction occurs in both animals and man [13,14] after shock and trauma, especially in association with sepsis. The association of reticuloendothelial host defense failure in conjunction with cardiovascular and pulmonary failure may reflect an imbalance between bloodborne particulate matter observed during the bacteremic period and the reticuloendothelial phagocytic clearance capacity. In addition, disturbance of the RES function, combined with abnormalities of leukocyte function and immune responsiveness, can effectively undermine antibacterial defense as well as the afferent arc of the immune response. These will contribute to the development and persistence of sepsis.

The theme of this chapter is that the various organs which undergo sequential failure suffer from a common pathologic process whose focus of disturbance is the microcirculation. Indeed, failure of the microcirculation may truly represent the cardinal manifestation of the organ failure syndrome whether it is associated with hypovolemic or normovolemic episodes. As such, this syndrome results from an inability to utilize the existing vascular volume for adequate tissue perfusion and oxygenation. The lesion of the microcirculation is a combined vascular, cellular, and subcellular disruption.[15]

THE CLINICAL SETTING

The clinical setting for the development of sequential organ failure is remarkably constant. At least three factors are always present: (1) a focus of tissue destruction, (2) a low perfusion or ischemic episode, and (3) bacteremia or a site of local infection, usually with a gram-negative organism.

Although specific organ failures occur during systemic sepsis without primary damage to one specific organ, the presence of specific organ damage exaggerates the destructive consequences of the infection. For example, circulating myoglobin can contribute to the development of acute renal failure, and the presence of a pulmonary contusion or fat emboli will contribute to respiratory failure. Likewise, hepatic ischemia will potentiate the deranged metabolic functions of the liver in sepsis, and will accelerate all septic manifestations.

The common clinical course of a patient who develops sequential organ failure with sepsis is shown in Figure 17-1. First, there is an abrupt elevation of the temperature, which may be associated with a spiking leukocytosis or transient leukopenia. After a transient hypertensive episode, there is a fall in blood pressure which initially responds to intravenous fluid administration, but eventually this fluid appears to escape the vascular compartment, producing an increasingly positive fluid balance. Fluid requirements for maintenance of hemodynamic function are vastly in excess of what might be anticipated in relation to the size of the injury, the extent of fluid loss, or the size of the vascular compartment. This suggests a defect in microvascular integrity, which is manifested by changes in vascular permeability and endothelial cell function. Thereafter, a frequent early clinical sign of specific organ failure is a falling arterial Po_2 associated with a ventilation perfusion mismatch within the lung. This respiratory insufficiency is associated with fluid accumulation within the lung, which may be a result of altered permeability, secondary to lung injury from microembolization. A progressive deterioration of blood oxygenation is rapidly accompanied by a decrease in urine output, a falling creatinine clearance, and the production of an iso-osmotic urine. As the syndrome progresses, clinical jaundice becomes evident, and there is a rapid fall in the serum albumin level. Hepatic dysfunction, altered Krebs cycle activity, lactic acid accumulation, and an endocrine imbalance can all be part of the severe septic episode. In essence, it appears that there is an exaggerated metabolic demand placed on the body in the face of a limited capability to meet this demand. This includes inadequate substrate provision as well as decreased tissue oxygenation. Cognitive cerebral function deteriorates, and the patient lapses into a coma, with depressed tendon reflexes.

The cardiovascular consequences of this organ and metabolic disruption are a falling blood pressure, unresponsive to fluid administration, and progressive peripheral edema. Positive inotropic agents—initially successful in improving cardiac function—become ineffective, and the pulse pressure narrows, the systemic arterial pressure falls, and cardiovascular collapse develops. At postmortum examination, the patient is grossly edematous. Microscopic examination of visceral organs show signs characteristic of an alteration in that particular failing organ—the kidney shows acute tubular necrosis; the lung shows interstitial edema and alveolar flooding; the liver shows central lobular edema with cellular infiltration, and muscle tissue shows signs of diffuse edema.

The following material will attempt to summarize our current understanding, including new concepts that appear relevant to the pathogenesis of this disorder and several suggestions as to potential new modalities of therapy.

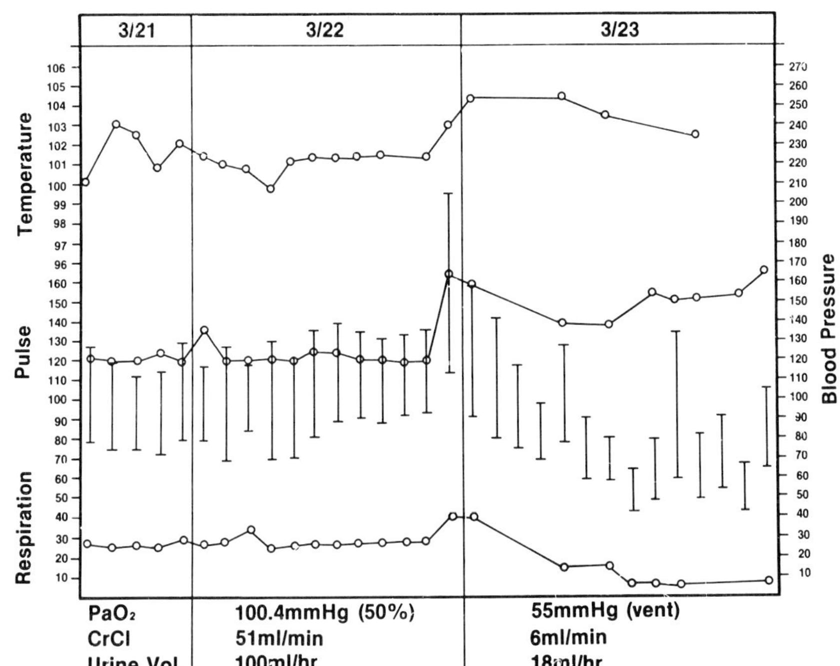

Fig. 17-1. Cardiovascular, renal, pulmonary, and temperature changes during onset of gram-negative septic shock. Data were obtained from a 20-year-old man after blunt abdominal trauma. (PaO_2 = arterial pO_2; CrCl = creatinine clearance.)

CARDIOVASCULAR (CARDIAC, PERIPHERAL VASCULAR) FAILURE IN SEPSIS

The hemodynamic response to systemic sepsis is discussed in Chapter 16.

Septic shock is characterized by hypotension during apparent adequate tissue perfusion—warm shock, since the skin and mucous membranes are generally warm, pink, and dry. These manifestations are at variance with those of hypovolemic and traumatic shock, where the hypotension is associated with cutaneous vasoconstriction leading to a pale, cold, clammy skin frequently characterized as cold shock. It is only in relatively recent times that bedside techniques for the measurement of cardiac output have demonstrated that patients in septic shock in distinction to those in hypovolemic shock have generally elevated cardiac outputs well above the normal range. It is because of the elevated cardiac output, decreased total peripheral resistance, and the associated increased total body oxygen consumption that septic shock has also been called hyperdynamic shock. Nevertheless, although the hypotensive state is relatively well tolerated because of the associated increased cardiac output, there comes a time when the perfusion pressure appears inadequate to maintain organ function. At this time, the hypotension fails to respond to positive inotropic drugs since the cardiac output is already at a hyperkinetic state. Increases in intravascular volume accomplished with intravenous crystalloid or colloid solutions are likewise ineffective, since the myocardium is already being driven to its maximum capability. Vasopressor agents may temporarily restore mean aortic pressure, but only at the expense of decreased perfusion to the kidneys, the peripheral tissue, and ultimately the splanchnic area. Increasing concentrations of vasopressor drugs result in peripheral cutaneous ischemia, acute renal failure, and gastrointestinal ulceration with hemorrhage. Since the maintenance of tissue perfusion depends on both an adequate perfusion pressure modulated by the cardiac output and a structurally intact peripheral microcirculation, these two factors will be considered separately.

CARDIAC FAILURE IN SEPSIS

As noted in Chapter 16, there is little convincing evidence of a failure of myocardial contractility as a result of systemic sepsis, and animal models seldom reproduce the clinical situation.

Sepsis may, however, have several indirect effects on myocardial function. The most important is on coronary blood flow. Any major decrease in coronary blood flow will result in a decreased oxygen delivery to the myocardium and could compromise myocardial function. The hemodynamic effects of systemic sepsis may have profound consequences on coronary blood flow. This is because diastolic hypotension is associated with a marked increase in heart rate. An increase in heart rate will, by encroaching on the diastolic interval, result in a decreased coronary blood flow. Myocardial perfusion takes place primarily during the diastolic interval—the period that begins with myocardial relaxation and ends with the onset of the next myocardial contraction. Since a substantial increase in heart rate decreases the diastolic interval, coronary blood flow must necessarily suffer. When this effect is combined with a decrease in perfusion pressure during diastole, the effects are compounded. An important distinction between septic shock and hypovolemic shock is the difference in diastolic pressure. Hypovolemia tends to maintain diastolic pressure by peripheral vasoconstriction even though systolic pressure will decline. Sepsis is associated with a decrease in peripheral vascular resistance and a fall in diastolic pressure. Thus, for any level of mean arterial pressure, coronary perfusion will be less in sepsis because of the lower diastolic pressure and shorter diastolic interval.

An additional secondary effect of sepsis on myocardial function relates to the development of a metabolic acidosis. This form of acidosis originates from excess lactic acid production due to hypoperfusion of the peripheral tissues and resultant anaerobic glycolysis. With a fall in arterial pH, the effects of endogenous catecholamines are inhibited, so that any possible positive inotropic effect originating from catecholamine release will be ineffective. Thus, hypotension, particularly the fall in diastolic pressure, tachycardia, and metabolic acidosis all act to impair myocardial contractility. These secondary effects suggest possible therapeutic modalities for improving myocardial function in the septic patient.

Therapy of Myocardial Depression in Sepsis

Understanding of the disturbed physiology of myocardial function in the septic state points the way to possible therapeutic approaches. All efforts are directed at improving oxygen delivery to the myocardium. Oxygen delivery is the product of the oxygen content of arterial blood and coronary blood flow. Oxygen content is improved when the hemoglobin concentration is raised to approximately 11 gm per dl by means of appropriate transfusion of packed red blood cells and when the oxygen saturation of the hemoglobin is maintained by means of adequate ventilatory support. Controlled ventilation with increased end-expiratory pressure will generally accomplish this end. The other determinant of oxygen delivery, ie, coronary blood flow, would be improved if it were possible to increase diastolic pressure and increase the diastolic interval by slowing the heart rate. Unfortunately, neither of these aims can be readily accomplished. Some improvement in coronary blood flow will result when agents such as isoproterenol are administered. These positive inotropic agents produce a shortening of the systolic interval and thereby, for any given heart rate, will result in an increase in the diastolic period. This increase probably accounts for the beneficial effects frequently seen with these drugs. Some of these agents, however, will also increase myocardial O_2 consumption. Furthermore, improvement in the myocardial response to both exogenous- and endogenous-positive inotropic substances will take place if the arterial pH is brought within normal limits. For this reason, sodium bicarbonate should be administered in sufficient quantities to restore a normal pH.

The cardiac output in patients with systemic sepsis who have been adequately resuscitated is generally far above normal. Since sepsis will be compounded by hypovolemia, it is essential to maintain the filling pressure of the left ventricle within a normal range. Traditional means for assessing this pressure have included the measurement of central venous pressure, usually an adequate guide in patients suffering from simple hypovolemia. This technique may be misleading in the septic patient. Systemic sepsis frequently results in an increase in pulmonary artery pressure (see section on pulmonary failure in sepsis). If the increase in pulmonary vascular resistance is due either to multiple microemboli or the presence of endothelial cell swelling, the filling pressure of the right heart will not be an accurate reflection of filling pressure of the left ventricle. Under these circumstances, an elevation of central venous pressure may be misinterpreted as fluid overload when, in fact, the elevated central venous pressure may be due to the increase in afterload on the right ventricle secondarily to the pulmonary artery occlusion. This distinction can best be ascertained with the use of a balloon-tipped flow-directed catheter (Swan-Ganz), which provides a direct estimate of pulmonary capillary wedge pressure and thereby left ventricular filling pressure. Ideally, any patient in refractory shock should have a Swan-Ganz catheter in place and should receive sufficient fluid resuscitation to maintain the pulmonary capillary wedge pressure within the range of 8 to 15 mm Hg. This is best accomplished with the use of crystalloid solution. The administration of albumin or plasma may be deleterious to the septic patient, since increases in capillary permeability, particularly in the pulmonary capillaries, are known to occur.[16] This increase in permeability allows the infused colloid to pass rapidly into the interstitium of the lungs, where it will attract and hold water, increasing the degree of interstitial pulmonary edema. Furthermore, as a result of the increased peripheral capillary permeability, any excess of infused saline solution will be sequestered in peripheral tissues producing gross, but relatively harmless, peripheral edema. This edema should not be confused with congestive heart failure. The presence of left heart failure is diagnosed by an elevation of the pulmonary capillary wedge pressure, not by an increased central venous pressure or the appearance of peripheral edema. This is an important distinction, because if heart failure is thought to be present, the proper treatment is fluid restriction and a diuretic. If the problem is volume sequestration due to increased capillary permeability, a diuretic will produce further volume depletion and a further decrease in left ventricular function. Diuretic therapy should be reserved for patients who demonstrate pulmonary edema in association with elevation of pulmonary capillary wedge pressure above 15 mm Hg. Heart failure in the septic patient rarely occurs in the absence of preexisting myocardial disease. The septic process per se does not usually produce left ventricular myocardial failure.

PERIPHERAL VASCULAR FAILURE IN SEPSIS

The peripheral circulation consists of major arteries, the arterioles that are normally responsible for much of the peripheral resistance and the microcirculation. Normally, the total vascular resistance is principally due to two components, the arteriolar resistance and the resistance of the microcirculation. Both of these components participate in the decreased vascular resistance associated with sepsis, although whether this is a primary failure of a peripheral regulatory mechanism or whether it is an attempt at compensation for impaired oxygen uptake by the peripheral tissues has yet to be determined (Chapter 16). In either case, the early phase of septic shock is characterized by a failure of the peripheral circulation to maintain sufficient vascular resistance to produce a normal blood pressure, even during elevated cardiac output. Clinical experience suggests that the difficulty is not associated with an inability of the arteriolar musculature to constrict in the presence of appropriate stimulation. Evidence for this statement is the immediate although transient response of the blood pressure to the use of vasopressor agents such as L-norepinephrine. Furthermore, the increased arterial blood pressure that results from the use of such pressor agents produces further manifestations of impaired peripheral circulation, such as cutaneous gangrene and acute renal failure. It is therefore equally possible that the low peripheral resistance in the septic patient is a normal compensatory mechanism designed to improve tissue perfusion in the face of a disordered microcirculation. This section will deal with the problems of the microcirculation associated with sepsis.

As noted in Chapter 16, patients in septic shock have elevated cardiac output and low total peripheral resistance. Despite these characteristics, there is evidence of impaired tissue oxygenation characterized by a metabolic acidosis in association with increased levels of plasma lactate. Oxygen extraction by the tissues is, however, diminished. One possible explanation for the failure to utilize oxygen may be a metabolic block at the mitochondrial level. This explanation is unlikely since increases in total blood flow in the septic trauma patient are associated with increases in oxygen uptake, whereas decreases in total oxygen delivery are generally associated with an overall decrease.[17] These findings suggest that the metabolic machinery is capable of utilizing some fraction of the increased quantity of oxygen provided by the peripheral circulation. The only consistent explanation for inadequate tissue oxygenation in the presence of adequate tissue perfusion is a disturbance in the fluid balance in the microcirculation, which interferes with the transport of oxygen from the red cell to the mitochondria. The occurrence of tissue edema may explain the tissue diffusion block.

Further evidence for incriminating the microcirculation as the site of physiologic disturbance is the loss of microvascular reactivity often associated with the septic shock state. The normal microcirculation can alter capillary blood flow over a wide range of values in response to the stimulus of increased oxygen demand. A standard method for assessing this responsiveness is to measure local blood flow following a short period of ischemia, such as would occur following the application of an arterial occlusion for a period of 2 minutes. This phenomenon, known as reactive hyperemia, results in one of the greatest blood flows that can be obtained through the peripheral circulation. An increase in total flow amounting to five times the resting value is common. Many patients in septic shock demonstrate a complete loss of the ability to increase blood flow following a period of ischemia. This loss of reactive hyperemia suggests a fundamental derangement in the reactivity of the microcirculation. Whether the failure of reactive hyperemia represents a paralysis of a normal control mechanism, or whether it is merely an indication that vasodilatation is already present, is not known. In any case, the association of a high perfusion rate, inadequate tissue oxygenation, a normal or elevated venous oxygen content coupled with a failure of microvascular reactivity all point to a fundamental disturbance of the microcirculation.

Several possible mechanisms could account for the observed disorganization of oxygen metabolism. The first would be the presence of precapillary arteriovenous shunts, which will divert blood away from nutritional capillaries directly into the venous bed. Although this explanation is attractive, since it will account for much of the observed data, there is little evidence that such precapillary shunts exist in skeletal muscle. Nevertheless, "absence of evidence is not evidence for absence." Therefore, this hypothesis [18] must still be considered.

A second possible explanation for the disruption of the microcirculation would be the presence of microemboli, which obliterate a significant fraction of the possible pathways for tissue perfusion. If such emboli were present, many of the available vascular channels would be occluded, and blood would pass through the remaining open channels at high velocity, leaving the oxygen content at the distal end of these capillaries significantly elevated. There is considerable evidence to support this hypothesis: (1) the demonstrated presence of microaggregates of fibrin, platelets, and macromolecules in the tissues of the septic patient; (2) demonstrated impairment of phagocytic clearance of particulate matter by the reticuloendothelial system in the septic state; large quantities of particulate matter can then embolize the peripheral circulation. In support of this hypothesis is the observation that the administration of an opsonic α_2 surface-binding glycoprotein (CIg; fibronectin) results in both a simultaneous improvement in microcirculatory blood flow and restoration or enhancement of the reactive hyperemic response.[19,20]

A third explanation for the disordered microcirculation relates to alterations in fluid distribution between the vascular space, interstitial space, and intracellular space. The most convincing evidence that such an abnormality regularly occurs in the septic patient is the frequent presence of massive peripheral edema. Peripheral edema is indicative of an accumulation of extravascular water within both the interstitial and intercellular compartments.

In order to understand the derangements in fluid dynamics across the capillary membrane, it is necessary to consider the Starling equation for transcapillary water equilibrium. This equation states that the movement of water across the capillary endothelium is a result of two opposing forces. The hydrostatic pressure gradient across the capillary tends to drive fluid from the vascular to the interstitial space. Conversely, the osmotic pressure gradient across the capillary due to the presence of plasma proteins tends to draw water from the interstitium into the vascular compartment. At an equilibrium state, these two forces will theoretically be balanced. The final equilibrium value for distribution of water also depends on the permeability of the capillary endothelium to water and on the reflection coefficient of the capillary to plasma proteins, principally albumin. If there was no movement of albumin across the capillary, ie, if the reflection coefficient were equal to 1, then the distribution of water would simply be determined by the difference between the hydrostatic pressure within the capillary and the oncotic pressure of the plasma proteins. In practice, the reflection coefficient is never precisely equal to 1, but is some value between 0 and 1. This implies that there is a continual loss of protein from the vascular space into the interstitial space, and if this were allowed to continue unchecked, the concentration of albumin in the interstitium would eventually reach the same value as that in the vascular bed. In this setting, the oncotic pressure difference between the vascular and interstitial space would disappear, and the vascular fluid would leak out into the interstitium as long as the pressure gradient would exist. Therefore, in order to maintain an osmotic pressure gradient across the capillary, it is necessary to remove the albumin that leaks into the interstitial fluid, and this is accomplished by means of the lymphatic system. The removal of protein by way of the lymph channels, therefore, is a necessary prerequisite to the maintenance of a capillary osmotic pressure gradient and the integrity of microvascular fluid balance. These factors are described by the Starling equation, which indicates that net transfer of water across the capillary endothelium (Q_f) is equal to the permeability of the capillary membrane to water (K_f) multiplied by the difference in hydrostatic pressure between the interstitium and the capillary ($P_c - P_i$) and the colloid osmotic pressure gradient ($\pi_c - \pi_i$). Thus:

$$Q_f = K_f[(P_c - P_i) - \sigma(\pi_c - \pi_i)]$$

where σ equals the reflection coefficient for albumin. The equation indicates that increases in net fluid flux will take place when there is an imbalance of the hydrostatic and oncotic forces as might result from either an increase in microvascular pressure or a decrease in plasma proteins, which would reduce plasma oncotic pressure.

Of particular interest in the septic state is the fact that interstitial edema will also take place when the reflection coefficient for albumin approaches 0 or when the lymphatic system is incapable of removing the albumin-containing fluid that leaks into the interstitium. This protein-rich interstitial fluid will further attract water from the vascular compartment. A further and generally unappreciated mechanism that will result in increased interstitial fluid relates to the number of capillaries being perfused at any given time. The Starling equation describes the transfer of fluid for a single capillary. Likewise, the reflection coefficient for albumin describes the rate of leakage of albumin through a single capillary. If the number of capillaries being perfused were to be suddenly increased, the net transport of albumin into the interstitium would be increased by the same proportion as the increase in the number of capillaries. If the capacity of the lymphatic system to remove protein from the interstitium did not increase at the same rate, albumin and hence interstitial fluid would accumulate in the interstitium. Evidence that such a mechanism is operative in the septic state is the rapid fall in serum albumin, which is uniformly noted in these patients. Furthermore, recovery from the septic state is generally accompanied by a rapid rise in serum albumin, indicating that protein is being recovered from the interstitial space and being transported back into the vascular compartment. It is not clear at present whether the increased interstitial edema and hypoalbuminemia is secondary to an increased permeability of the capillaries to albumin, a marked increase in the vascular exchange surface, or a limitation of the ability of the lymphatic system to remove excess protein.

In addition to increased interstitial edema during sepsis, intracellular edema also appears. One possible mechanism is a paralysis of the cell membrane sodium pump. Under normal circumstances, sodium leaks from the extra- to the intracellular compartments. Normal cells rapidly remove this sodium by means of the sodium-potassium ATPase system. Interference with this pump system may be due to either the products of bacterial sepsis or the direct action of endotoxins on the cell membrane.

Therapy for Disturbances of the Peripheral Circulation

Therapeutic efforts designed to increase arteriolar tone, such as the use of vasopressor agents, have been generally ineffective and are contraindicated in the septic state. This is not surprising, since these patients show evidence of inadequate tissue perfusion, such as a metabolic acidosis and lactic acidemia. Arteriolar vasoconstriction acts by further reducing perfusion, thereby compounding the problem. Likewise, using diuretics as the primary means to reduce interstitial edema is ineffective and is not based on an understanding of the physiologic disturbance. Since the Starling equation describes the distribution of fluid between the vascular and interstitial space rather than merely the quantity of fluid in the interstitial space, it is apparent that diuretics will reduce both the volume of the interstitial space and the vascular volume. Reductions in vascular volume will result in a fall in filling pressure of the left side of the heart and a subsequent fall in the cardiac output, further impairing the diminished tissue perfusion. Likewise, the administration of serum albumin or plasma proteins in the septic patient with permeability defects will produce an increase in protein concentration in both the interstitium and the vascular space. Since the concentration in the two compartments will remain in the equilibrium specified by the Starling equation, there will be a net increase in interstitial fluid as well as in vascular volume. Thus, the use of colloid solutions in the septic patient may be detrimental.

There are two promising advances in the treatment of the disordered microcirculation.[19-22] Both are based on the hypothesis that a large number of peripheral capillaries are obstructed by microemboli or endothelial swelling. Removal of particulate matter from the circulation may be enhanced by correction of the disordered reticuloendothelial system through the administration of cryoprecipitate,[19] as described elsewhere in this chapter. Preliminary evidence has indicated an improvement in limb blood flow, limb oxygen consumption,[14,20,23] and glomerular filtration rate following this therapy.[24]

To reduce the swelling of the capillary endothelial cells, hypertonic mannitol has been tried.[21,22] This substance distributes itself rapidly into the interstitial fluid so that it will exert its osmotic effect across the cell membrane. Removal of intracellular water should decrease tissue resistance and by reducing endothelial cell swelling will decrease resistance to blood flow in the microcirculation. Hypertonic mannitol [21] increases not only peripheral oxygen delivery but also peripheral oxygen consumption. Of perhaps more significance, hypertonic mannitol can restore normal microvascular reactivity, as indicated by the restoration of the reactive hyperemic response (Fig. 17-2).

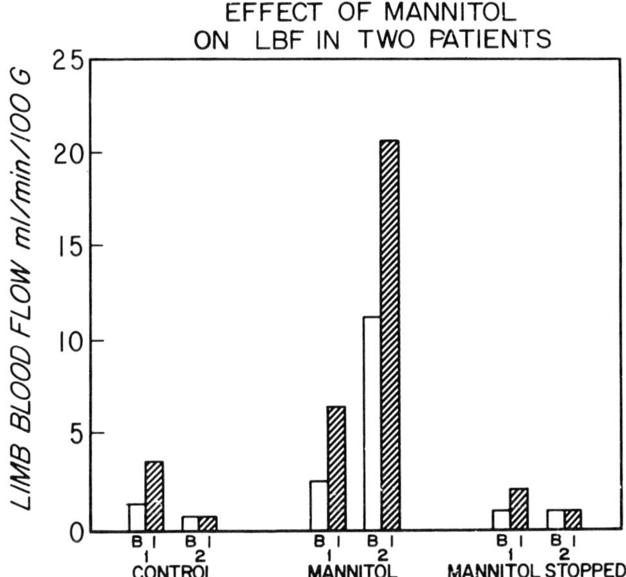

Fig. 17-2. **Limb blood flow prior to and during reactive hyperemia in septic surgical and trauma patients as influenced by hypertonic mannitol therapy. Limb blood flow was studied by venous occlusion plethysmography. Reactive hyperemia was studied after 2 minutes of ischemia. Flow during baseline (B) and after ischemia (I) in both subjects (No. 1, No. 2) is presented prior to (control) mannitol, 5 minutes after mannitol, and 60 minutes after mannitol was stopped.**

PULMONARY FAILURE IN SEPSIS

The respiratory distress syndrome is the leading immediate cause of death in most surgical intensive care units,[1] and systemic sepsis is most often the cause. About two-thirds of the septic patients who require endotracheal intubation for more than 48 hours with an inspired oxygen fraction of greater than 0.5 will die. Most of these patients who will not survive have severe systemic sepsis. Appropriate therapeutic maneuvers to correct this disorder will require definition of the basic pathologic disorder. Existing therapy has generally relied on mechanical ventilation, which supports gas exchange in much the same way that an artificial kidney supports renal function. In both cases, the physician waits for spontaneous remission of the disease. Recent studies have indicated that the primary pathologic disorder is not only centered around an abnormality of ventilation but is also a consequence of abnormalities in pulmonary perfusion. This insight has suggested new therapeutic modalities, which offer some promise of reversing the pathologic process during the time when ventilatory support is being maintained by artificial means.

Pathology

Acute respiratory failure was first described as a distinct clinical entity during World War II and was called traumatic wet lung. Subsequently, numerous investigators noted the occurrence of this disorder, called congestive atelectasis because of its pathologic picture.[25] At autopsy, the lungs were heavy, red, and boggy. Microscopically, they manifested collapse of alveolar spaces or flooding of open alveoli with protein-rich fluid material. The interstitial spaces were congested with fluid and red cells. This pathologic picture appears to be somewhat unique to human shock and sepsis, and it has yet to be effectively duplicated in an animal model, although recent reports are promising.

Clinically, the disorder presents as a subtle deterioration of oxygen transport. There is a fall in arterial Po_2 which initially responds to increased concentrations of inspired oxygen, but with the passage of time, higher and higher concentrations are required to maintain a marginal oxygenation. Ultimately, pure oxygen supplied by means of controlled ventilation is no longer adequate to maintain the arterial Po_2. During most of this period, the arterial Pco_2 is below normal, indicating that the problem is not simply one of inadequate ventilation but is rather the result of a ventilation-perfusion mismatch. Roentgenograms of the chest frequently show little or no abnormality in the early phases of this disorder. The chest roentgenogram is therefore an unreliable diagnostic technique. With advance of the disease, the lungs become diffusely opacified, with a fluffy alveolar pattern gradually spreading to confluent areas of increased radiodensity. In extreme cases, both lung fields appear uniformly white on the x-ray film (Fig. 17-3).

The clinical setting in which this disorder originates is characteristic. Frequently, the arterial Po_2 begins to deteriorate before there is evidence of systemic sepsis as judged by fever and leukocytosis. Indeed, a sudden fall in arterial Po_2 in a patient following severe trauma or intra-abdominal surgery is presumptive evidence that a focus of sepsis has developed. Thus, lung function appears to be one of a series of exquisitely sensitive indicators of the presence of a septic process in the seriously injured patient. If the septic focus can be promptly recognized and surgically evacuated, pulmonary function surprisingly returns to normal quite rapidly. Removal of an infected uterus or amputation of a gangrenous extremity may result in a return of the blood gas values to normal by the time the patient has reached the recovery room. This rapid recovery may not be surprising if one considers the efficiency of an intact liver and spleen reticuloendothelial system to clear bacteria as well as bacterial products such as endotoxin.[26,27] If a single bolus injection of a small dose of bacteria is given to a normal animal, the half-time of disappearance of the injected material is a few minutes. Thus, once the source of infection and sepsis has been removed, a normal reticuloendothelial phagocytic system will rapidly cleanse the blood of products of bacterial sepsis and injury.

Since it is not always possible to easily eradicate the source of sepsis, one must support pulmonary function and the reticuloendothelial system until the infection can be brought under control.

Physiopathology of Adult Respiratory Distress Syndrome

The exact etiology of the adult respiratory distress syndrome during sepsis has yet to be delineated. It is clear, however, that both pulmonary ventilation and perfusion are disturbed.

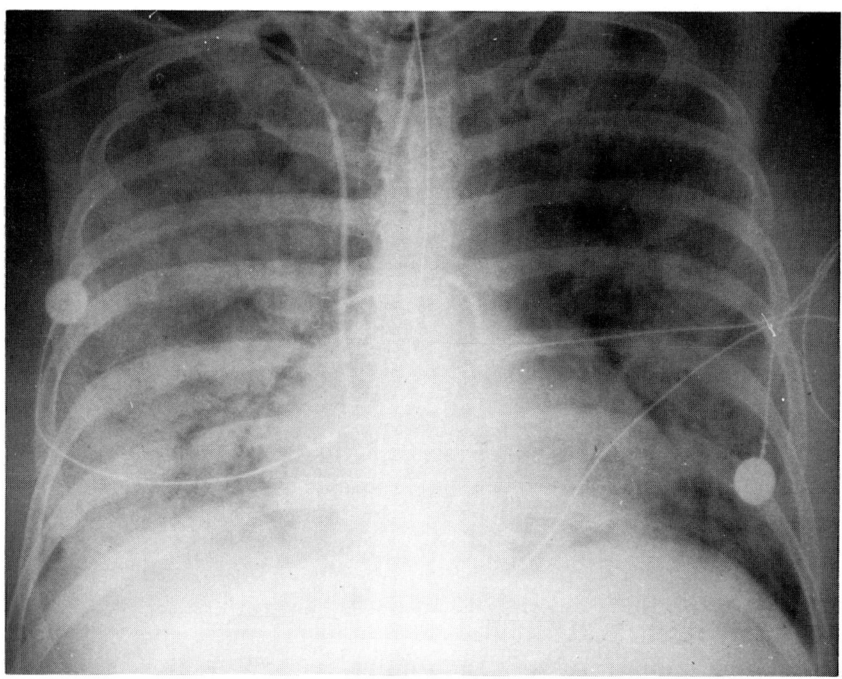

Fig. 17-3. **Film reflective of patient with adult respiratory distress syndrome. Typical uniformly white lung fields are shown. Note the position of the Swan-Ganz catheter in the pulmonary artery.**

Abnormalities of Ventilation

Disorders of ventilation were the first to be intensively studied in clinical settings, and disorders of ventilation were the first to be aggressively treated by means of mechanical ventilatory support. Evidence for disordered ventilation is a decrease in the resting lung volume (FRC), a decrease in pulmonary compliance, and an increase in intrapulmonary shunt or venous admixture.[28] Each of these factors is due, at least in part, to the occurrence of alveolar collapse. The most persuasive evidence that such collapse takes place is the observation that the functional residual capacity (FRC) is significantly reduced in these patients, frequently to levels 40 to 50 percent of normal. The determination of functional residual capacity is made by the technique of nitrogen washout. This is accomplished by suddenly changing the inspired gas from the therapeutic inspired oxygen concentration to pure oxygen. If the patient is inspiring a mixture of 50 percent oxygen, the other 50 percent of the inspired gas is nitrogen. To put this another way, half of the volume of gas in the lung at any moment consists of nitrogen. When the patient is suddenly switched to breathing pure oxygen, no further nitrogen enters the lungs and all nitrogen present will be washed out. If the expired gas is collected during the washout period, the amount of nitrogen in the expired gas can be measured, and since this was the amount of nitrogen present in the lungs, the lung volume can be calculated. The value obtained from the nitrogen washout can then be compared to the predicted FRC based on the patient's height and body weight.

Measurement of the lung volume does not distinguish between a uniform decrease of all alveoli and the total collapse of some of the alveoli with the others remaining at normal volume. Evidence that total collapse of some alveoli has taken place is provided by measurement of the intrapulmonary shunt. If no oxygen enters an alveolus, the pulmonary capillary blood flowing past the alveolus will not gain oxygen and the blood will enter and leave the alveolar unit with the same oxygen concentration. This concentration is identical with venous blood, and thus blood entering the pulmonary veins will be the same as if that portion of blood had not passed through the lungs at all. Thus, it is referred to as an intrapulmonary shunt. To make absolutely certain that blood flow is being measured past only non-ventilated alveoli, the patient is placed on pure oxygen. Under these circumstances, if there is any ventilation to these alveoli even at an extremely reduced level, the pure oxygen will eventually saturate any blood passing through the alveolus. Therefore, persistence of arterial oxygen desaturation during the breathing of pure oxygen is direct evidence of lack of alveolar ventilation of those units, and by inference, of either alveolar collapse or filling of the alveolus with fluid.[29] In practice, it is neither necessary nor desirable to place the patient on pure oxygen for very long, because 50 percent oxygen will increase the oxygen concentration of poorly ventilated alveoli to the point where peripheral arterial oxygen saturation will rise. Furthermore, it has been found that the breathing of pure oxygen for even a brief period may be deleterious to pulmonary function, especially in patients with the adult respiratory distress syndrome.

A decrease in pulmonary compliance is regularly noted in patients suffering from this disorder. In simple terms, the compliance is determined by measuring the patient's tidal volume and dividing it by the difference in airway pressure between inspiration and expiration. In practice, this is generally carried out when the patient is on a ventilator, so that the tidal volume is directly recorded and the change in airway pressure can be read from a pressure gauge. Compliance is defined as the tidal volume measured in liters divided by the change in airway pressure expressed as centimeters of water. A normal compliance for the average adult has the value of 0.1 L per cm H_2O. When alveolar collapse takes place, the remaining alveoli must be stretched to a greater extent to accommodate the same tidal volume. For example, if 50 percent of the alveoli are collapsed, a normal tidal volume will distend the remaining 50 percent of alveoli to twice the volume previously required. The pressure required to distend those alveoli to twice their previous size will be roughly twice as great. In other words, a doubling of the pressure will be required to attain the same tidal volume. When this is placed in the quantitative expression of compliance, it will appear that the compliance of the lung has fallen by half. It is important to realize that, in this idealized example, there is no abnormality of the remaining functioning alveoli. The apparent decrease in compliance is a reflection of the fact that the lung has become smaller, not stiffer. In reality, there is probably some decrease in compliance even of alveoli that are not collapsed. Nevertheless, clinical studies have demonstrated that, when the FRC is restored to normal, the measured compliance also approaches a normal value. Further evidence for the importance of alveolar collapse is gained from the observation that correction of this abnormality by increases in end-expiratory pressure (PEEP) is accompanied by a marked decrease in the measured intrapulmonary shunt. It thus appears that one significant component of the adult respiratory distress syndrome is collapse of alveolar units and that this can frequently be corrected by increasing end-expiratory airway pressure.[29]

Abnormalities of Perfusion

Abnormalities of the distribution of pulmonary perfusion have been emphasized only recently.[30] Even after mechanical ventilation with increased end-expiratory pressure has corrected the disordered ventilation and returned the resting lung volume to normal, many patients continue to show serious disorders of pulmonary gas exchange. Such abnormalities in the distribution of perfusion were not previously recognized because the routine measurements of arterial blood gases as carried out in most intensive care units will not detect this disorder.[30] Although occlusion of the pulmonary capillaries to ventilated alveoli has serious consequences in gas exchange, this does not result in a fall in arterial P_{O_2}. If no blood reaches an alveolus, no blood can leave it, and its contribution to the oxygen content of mixed pulmonary venous blood will be nil. The deleterious effect of occlusion of a pulmonary capillary to a well-ventilated alveolus is that the blood that might have been well oxygenated is now directed to other alveoli, which may themselves be underventilated.

To distinguish the increase in pulmonary venous admixture due to diversion of blood away from well-ventilated alveoli from that due simply to intrapulmonary shunt, an independent measurement of disordered perfusion is necessary, as can be done with inert gas studies.

Dead space is that portion of the ventilated respiratory tract where no gas exchange takes place. The trachea and bronchi are examples of normal dead space, and indeed the volume of the conducting airways is sufficient to account for approximately one-third of the normal tidal volume (ie, the normal dead space to tidal volume ratio is 1:3). If the blood flow to a ventilated alveolus is obstructed, no gas exchange will take place within that alveolus and it will become a part of the dead space. Occlusion of pulmonary capillaries to ventilated alveoli will therefore result in an increase in the dead space to tidal volume ratio. This number is easily and conveniently measured by collecting a sample of mixed, expired gas and arterial blood simultaneously. The partial pressure of carbon dioxide in both samples is then determined. If all of the respiratory tract were involved in gas exchange, the concentration of carbon dioxide in expired gas would be identical with that of arterial blood. On the other hand, if one-half of the respiratory tract did not participate in gas exchange, then expired gas from that region would consist of air that had not been altered by gas exchange, ie, with a carbon dioxide concentration of zero. The expired gas, which had come into equilibrium with alveolar capillary blood, would have a partial pressure of carbon dioxide identical to arterial blood. Since mixed expired gas would consist of 50 percent of each type, the expired gas would have a carbon dioxide partial pressure halfway between that of room air and arterial blood. Thus, the gradient of carbon dioxide concentration between expired air and arterial blood is a quantitative measure of the fraction of the tidal volume occupied by dead space. Repeated clinical studies have demonstrated that the dead space-tidal volume ratio is significantly elevated in the adult respiratory distress syndrome.

Further evidence for occlusion of pulmonary vasculature is obtained from the hemodynamic measurements of the pulmonary circulation. Recent studies have emphasized that the earliest physiologic change in patients who will subsequently develop the adult respiratory distress syndrome is an increase in pulmonary artery pressure and in the calculated pulmonary vascular resistance.[22] This measurement is therefore of great importance in following patients suffering from systemic sepsis. Calculation of pulmonary vascular resistance demands that measurements of pulmonary artery pressure, pulmonary venous pressure, and total cardiac output be obtained. These are conveniently obtained from a balloon-tipped flow-directed catheter with a thermistor. With this device, cardiac output is determined by means of the technique of thermal dilution, and the pressure drop across the pulmonary vascular bed is determined from the mean pulmonary artery pressure minus the pulmonary capillary wedge pressure. A sudden increase in pulmonary vascular resistance is frequently the earliest sign of impending pulmonary dysfunction. The exact mechanism for this disorder of the pulmonary microcirculation is unknown. Indirect evidence suggests that it is of two types. The first occurs from circulating particulate matter that becomes lodged in the terminal branches of the pulmonary microcirculation. The particulate matter may consist of fibrin aggregates, altered platelets, collagenous debris, fat, and possibly macromolecular immune complexes. A second mechanism is the occurrence of endothelial cell swelling. Such swelling may result from the direct action of products of the complement cascade—the coagulation cascade—including particularly the fibrinopeptides and substances released locally from platelets and marginated polymorphonuclear leukocytes. The significance of these two mechanisms of occlusion of the microcirculation have important therapeutic consequences, since on the one hand, the removal of particulate matter by enhancement of reticuloendothelial clearance would appear a rational choice, whereas in the case of cellular swelling, the removal of such cellular edema by means of hypertonic solutions would seem to offer promise.

Ventilation-Perfusion Mismatch

The preceding two sections have described disorders of ventilation, as evidenced by intrapulmonary shunt, and disorders of perfusion, as evidenced by increase in dead space. The measurements of shunt and dead space represent two ends of a spectrum of ventilation-perfusion abnormalities (Fig. 17-4). A true shunt represents a ventilation-perfusion ratio of zero, since there is no ventilation and perfusion remains intact. Likewise, true dead space represents a ventilation-perfusion ratio of infinity because ventilation is intact and perfusion is zero. In practice, most of the alveolo-capillary units fall somewhere between these two, and the distribution of ventilation-perfusion abnormalities reflects the disordered pulmonary function.

The interrelation of ventilation-perfusion abnormalities is best illustrated by considering a hypothetical experiment. If the main bronchus to one lung is suddenly occluded, no ventilation will take place in that lung and a true intrapulmonary shunt will have occurred. If this were to take place under normal circumstances, the occluded lung would rapidly become hypoxic and the vessels perfusing that lung would undergo hypoxic vasoconstriction. With an increased resistance to blood flow through the occluded lung, most of the blood would then pass to the normal lung, where it would be adequately oxygenated. Thus, the consequences of even a large unventilated region in otherwise normal lungs is well tolerated. Alternatively, if the main pulmonary artery to a lung is suddenly occluded, no gas exchange will take place through that lung and there will be a sudden increase in respiratory dead space. When this occurs, the blood originally intended for the occluded lung will pass to the other lung. As long as the ventilation of the other lung increases proportionately to the increase in blood flow, there will be no major discernible effect on peripheral oxygenation.

The interrelation between disordered ventilation and disordered perfusion is demonstrated when the two experiments are combined and one main bronchus is occluded at the same time that the opposite pulmonary artery is clamped. One lung will now receive no ventilation, the other will receive no perfusion, and overall gas exchange will fall to zero. Thus, the addition of areas of intrapulmonary shunting to areas of increased alveolar dead space are not only additive, but they also act to eliminate the compensatory mechanisms that would ordinarily correct for each individual abnormality. An example of this situation is seen in certain patients with head injury.[31]

THERAPY OF RESPIRATORY DISTRESS IN THE SEPTIC PATIENT

The single most important maneuver in correcting the disorders of gas exchange associated with the respiratory distress syndrome is to locate and remove the focus of sepsis. Indeed, other methods of therapy are merely techniques to sustain a reduced degree of pulmonary function while the septic focus is being eradicated. Therapy directed at the pulmonary lesion will only gain an additional short respite until the continuing effects of sepsis work their inexorable course. Nevertheless, appropriate therapeutic maneuvers properly applied may be life-saving in the acute situation and will therefore, allow ultimate survival of the patient.

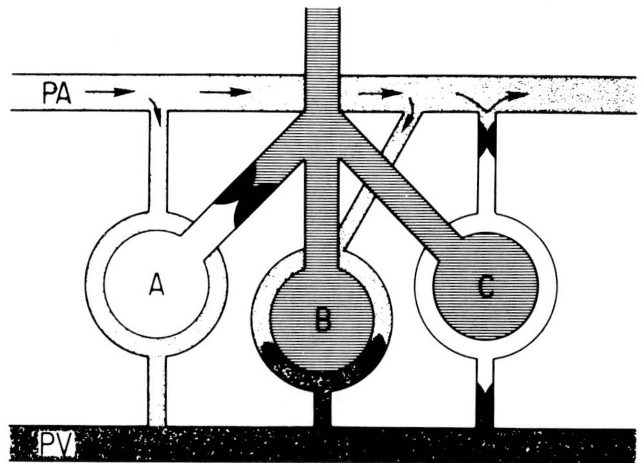

Fig. 17-4. **Diagrammatic presentation of three alveolar units presenting shunt (A), idealized normal (B), and dead space (C). The normal unit reflects adequate ventilation as well as vascular perfusion. Shunt is depicted as a perfused but nonventilated alveolus. Dead space is depicted as a ventilated but nonperfused alveolus. Consequently, the left and right units do not participate in gas exchange.**

Ventilatory Support

Satisfactory gas exchange across the alveolar capillary membrane first requires gas to fill all perfused regions of the lung. Since the respiratory distress syndrome is characterized by alveolar collapse and therefore an absence of alveolar ventilation to certain regions of the lung, restoration of alveolar volume is the first order of business. This can generally [29] be accomplished using a mechanical ventilator with increased levels of increased end-expiratory pressure. The aim of ventilatory support is to restore a normal lung volume (FRC). Unfortunately, the measurement of FRC is easily accomplished only in specially equipped research facilities. Therefore, indirect estimates of the efficacy of the increased end-expiratory pressure must be employed. The most direct evidence of an adequate end-expiratory pressure is a decrease of the intrapulmonary shunt to a level below 10 percent. One should select the lowest level of end-expiratory pressure that will provide this desired therapeutic result. Increases in end-expiratory pressure above the minimum needed to provide adequate arterial oxygenation may result in depression of cardiac output, rupture of damaged alveoli, and the production of a pneumothorax. Since the upper limit of acceptable end-expiratory pressure is determined by a fall in cardiac output, the cardiac output should be determined repeatedly by means of thermal dilution utilizing a Swan-Ganz catheter. Optimal levels of PEEP can therefore be defined as the lowest intrapulmonary shunt associated with the highest cardiac output.

Two additional parameters of mechanical ventilatory support are of great therapeutic importance. The first is the tidal volume, which is developed by the mechanical ventilator. If the patient is on controlled ventilation, the tidal volume necessary to maintain adequate gas exchange is greater than that required for spontaneous ventilation. The usual value required for mechanical ventilatory support is 12 ml per kg of body weight. The other important setting is related to the inspired oxygen concentration. Recent evidence suggests that increasing the inspired oxygen concentration above 50 percent offers little to the improvement of gas exchange and may cause further deterioration of pulmonary function. Oxygen concentrations above 60 percent impair mucosal ciliary activity, thereby inhibiting the clearance of mucous and particulate matter from the tracheobronchial tree. In general, then, one should limit the inspired oxygen concentration to 50 percent.

Therapy of Disordered Pulmonary Perfusion

Only recently have therapeutic efforts been directed at improving the distribution of perfusion within the lung. These efforts generally fall into two categories: (1) increasing the pulmonary capillary lumen by reducing endothelial cell swelling, and (2) enhancing removal of particulate matter from the circulation by supporting the reticuloendothelial system. Objective evidence for successful improvement of pulmonary perfusion is a decrease in the alveolar dead space and a reduction in the pulmonary vascular resistance. It is by these yardsticks that all therapeutic efforts must be judged. Decrease in dead space does not result in a corresponding decrease in intrapulmonary shunt. Nevertheless, the arterial Po_2 will generally improve, since the number of capillaries exposed for gas exchange has increased with a corresponding increase in surface area available for gaseous diffusion. This improvement will be reflected by an increase in arterial Po_2, even though the measured shunt remains unchanged.

Techniques for improving the distribution of perfusion are still experimental, and their promise remains to be verified. The administration of hypertonic mannitol is designed to reduce cellular swelling. Preliminary evidence indicates that mannitol will reduce alveolar dead space as well as the pulmonary vascular resistance in septic patients. The effect of a single intravenous injection of mannitol is, unfortunately, short-lived, and the respiratory and hemodynamic abnormalities return to their pretreatment value unless infection has been controlled. The mannitol is administered in a dose of 0.5 grams per kg of body weight as a 20 percent solution. If renal function is normal, approximately one-half of the injected dose will be excreted within 1 hour. It is therefore reasonable to repeat the dose at the end of a 2-hour period without significant risk of overexpansion of the vascular volume. Perhaps the most interesting conclusion to be drawn from the studies on hypertonic mannitol is that they lend indirect support to the concept of cellular swelling as a significant feature of the respiratory distress syndrome.

An additional experimental therapeutic approach has been the support of the reticuloendothelial system by the administration of opsonic α_2-surface binding (SB) glycoprotein (plasma fibronectin, cold insoluble globulin) [15] (see subsequent section). Many patients with respiratory insufficiency associated with sepsis have low circulating plasma fibronectin levels; correction of this deficiency by the administration of cryoprecipitate, which is rich in fibronectin, will partially correct the disorders of distribution of pulmonary blood flow in many patients. Whether the use of cryoprecipitate [19] will ultimately prove to be optimal therapy for disorders of pulmonary blood flow distribution remains to be determined. However, the initial success reported with this mode of treatment adds further support to the concept that a principal physiologic abnormality in patients with respiratory distress is a disorder of the microcirculation.

RENAL FAILURE IN SEPSIS

Acute renal failure (acute tubular necrosis; ATN) was the first organ system failure described in the seriously injured [5] and septic patient. Acute renal failure was the leading cause of death in adequately resuscitated combat casualties in the Korean conflict. Such deaths are now uncommon, but ATN is an important component in the cascade of sequential organ failure following systemic sepsis.

This disorder is associated with a fall in urine volume, which does not respond to increased fluid administration. Repeated attempts to restore urine volume by intravenous fluid loading expands the extracellular fluid volume and leads to severe peripheral edema. The fall in urine volume actually represents a final end-stage in the unsuspected, progressive deterioration of renal function. Recognition of the early evidences for acute renal failure is essential if progression is to be stopped.

PATHOLOGY OF ACUTE RENAL FAILURE

The gross pathologic findings of acute renal failure were well described at the end of World War II when this disorder was the main cause of death.[5,7] These findings consisted of severe swelling with increased interstitial pressure leading to a tense, swollen kidney. Microscopically, the picture is a combination of interstitial edema associated with necrosis of the renal tubular cells, most pronounced in the distal convoluted tubule. The latter finding was responsible for the early terminology of acute renal failure as distal tubular necrosis. More recent detailed pathologic studies, including electron microscopy, have indicated that the entire nephron is involved in the process, with the glomerulus being the center of pathologic abnormality. The pathologic process is characterized by the presence of proteinaceous casts in the renal tubule of involved nephrons, whereas adjacent tubule lumena are relatively empty. This pathologic picture is associated with the end-stage of acute renal failure and unfortunately does not provide insight into the early and potentially reversible phase.

PATHOPHYSIOLOGY OF ACUTE RENAL FAILURE

The precise details surrounding the development of acute renal failure are only poorly understood, but certain facts are known. The urine volume is not only a poor indication of impending renal dysfunction but may be completely misleading.[7] Consider the normal glomerular filtration rate of the average-size adult—120 ml per minute. This will provide 7,200 ml/hour. If the glomerular filtration were reduced to 10 percent of normal, the kidney would produce 720 ml of filtrate per hour. If only one-tenth of this filtrate (72 ml per hour) appeared as a final urine volume, it would still be normal. Since the kidney normally excretes less than 1 percent of the total glomerular filtrate, it is apparent that measurements of the final excretory product are a poor reflection of renal function.

A more important measurement of impaired renal function is the glomerular filtration, which can be estimated by the endogenous creatinine clearance (Fig. 17-5). This measurement requires only a measurement of serum and urine creatinine concentrations and the urine volume (Table 17-1). When the urine-plasma creatinine ratio is multiplied by the urine volume in milliliters per minute, creatinine clearance is quantitatively determined. A decrease in this value is the earliest sign of acute renal failure. Other estimates of renal function, such as the urine-plasma sodium ratio and the urine-plasma osmolar ratio are useful screening tests but may on occasion provide misleading information.

Acute renal failure in sepsis may be primarily the result of a redistribution of blood flow within the kidney. Total renal blood flow in the septic patient is probably normal, but the intrarenal distribution of blood flow is severely deranged. Under normal circumstances, the majority of renal blood flow passes to the superficial portion of the renal cortex. In impending acute renal failure, blood flow is diverted away from this superficial cortical region into the deep cortex or juxtamedullary region. Since the distal convoluted tubule of the majority of nephrons are found in the superficial cortical area, a preferential ischemia of the distal convoluted tubules is then produced. The distal tubule has important physiologic function, since it is the site of the macula densa and the juxtaglomerular apparatus. This region of the nephron is intimately involved in the control of glomerular filtration by means of a tubuloglomerular feedback mechanism. Decreased perfusion of this region is associated with the local release of renin, which activates the angiotensin system leading to intense vasoconstriction. Thus, the reduced blood flow to the outer cortex, coupled with intense vasoconstriction induced by the renin angiotensin system, may lead to ischemic damage of these two vital portions of the nephron. Furthermore, renin release results in secretion of aldosterone from the adrenal cortex, which enhances sodium reabsorption by the distal tubule. If the peritubular capillaries have insufficient flow to carry away the resorbed sodium, this ion will remain within the renal interstitium, leading to interstitial edema, increased intrarenal pressure, and further reduction of renal capillary blood flow. Whatever the exact mechanism leading to these changes may be, there is recent clinical evidence to suggest that maintenance of the glomerular filtration rate and reduction of interstitial edema protect the kidney in the septic patient.

PREVENTION OF ACUTE RENAL FAILURE IN THE SEPTIC PATIENT

Effective prophylaxis of acute renal failure depends on early recognition of disturbed renal function. The depressed glomerular filtration rate, observed before evidence of acute tubular necrosis has developed, can be reversed by the use of hypertonic mannitol.[32] Unfortunately, the period of time available for such reversals is only a few hours. If the glomerular filtration is allowed to remain at a low level for as little as 3 to 4 hours, therapeutic intervention will be unsuccessful. The exact mode of action of hypertonic mannitol is controversial, but it has been established that this agent will reduce renin release by the kidney under conditions of decreased renal perfusion. Furthermore, the hypertonic solution may both decrease cellular edema, permitting increased peritubular capillary perfusion, and reduce tubular swelling, improving tubular transport function. The effect of mannitol on the kidney is somewhat different from its effect on the lung or other organ systems. In the latter situation, the mannitol effect is usually completely over by 1 hour, and the organ function returns to its pretreatment state. On the other hand, the use of mannitol [32] for prevention of disordered renal function will frequently result in a significant increase in glomerular filtration rate, which is maintained for many hours. This finding suggests that hypertonic mannitol may interrupt a specific feedback mechanism, such as renin release, so that renal function will remain at a more normal level unless some additional insult takes place.

The beneficial effect of hypertonic mannitol is only secondarily related to its diuretic effect. The use of other diuretics, such as furosimide or ethacrynic acid, do not mimic the effects of mannitol and indeed may be deleterious to renal function. There is no evidence that these agents have any beneficial effect on glomerular filtration rate; in fact, if the diuresis results in vascular volume depletion, the glomerular filtration rate may actually fall. At present, there appears to be no indication for the use of loop diuretics to prevent renal failure in the septic patient. Adequate volume resuscitation, coupled with use of hypertonic mannitol, has virtually eliminated acute renal failure as a primary cause of death in the septic patient. Acute renal failure, when it occurs, is generally a terminal event associated with total disorganization of cellular metabolism.

RETICULOENDOTHELIAL SYSTEMIC FAILURE IN SEPSIS

Numerous studies have demonstrated the role of phagocytic cells in nonspecific host defense mechanisms and cellular immunity.[15,26] Central to the function of phagocytic cells is their ability to recognize foreign macromolecules, denatured proteins, and damaged tissue. Approximately 60 years ago, Aschoff introduced the term

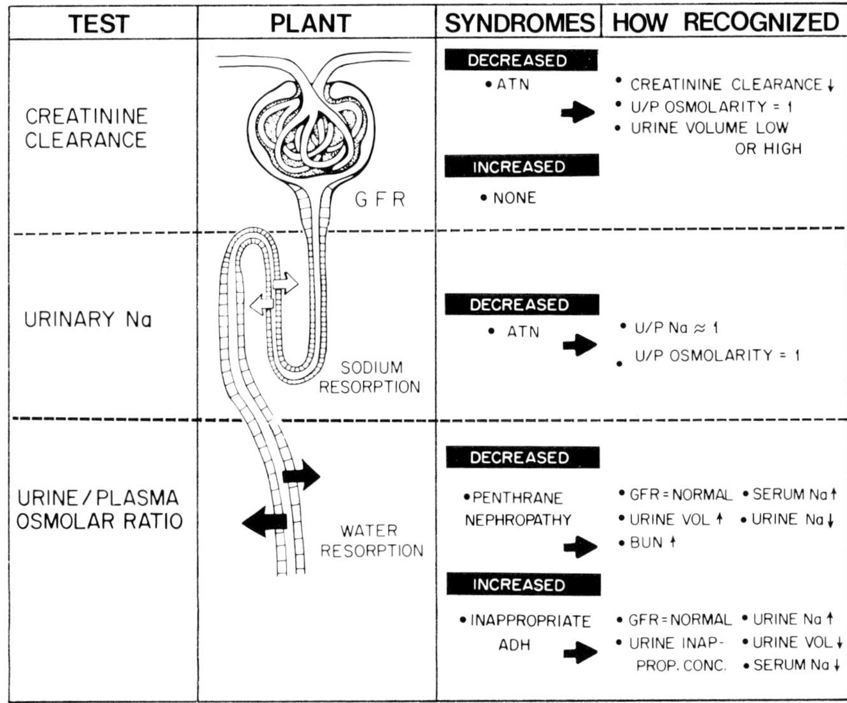

Fig. 17-5. **Presentation of three principal functions of the nephron with associated clinical tests corresponding to each of these functions. Control mechanisms identified participate in the maintenance of the internal environment following disturbances of the volume and composition of the extracellular space. The complete control system is obviously more complex than indicated, and additional factors such as prostaglandins and other vasoactive substances have been deleted.**

reticuloendothelial system (RES) to describe this diffuse system of sessile and wandering mononuclear macrophages, which comprise the phagocytic system.[33] Other descriptions of the RES have also included polymorphonuclear leukocytes which, although not anatomically part of the reticuloendothelial system, do effectively function as phagocytic cells in the host defense apparatus (Chapter 13).

The host phagocytic system can be generally visualized as occurring in three areas.[34] The first is local defense at the site of wound injury or infection. Here, both polymorphonuclear leukocytes and mononuclear phagocytic cells function to eliminate microbial invaders and remove dead and injured tissue. Such phagocytic cells play a major role in antibacterial defense and wound healing. Macrophages also participate in antigen uptake and processing and are thus participants in the afferent arc of the immune response.

If bacterial invasion is not contained to the local area of injury, the bacteria will pass into the lymphatic network. At this second stage, the process of lymphatic defense begins.[34] Lymph node macrophages provide an effective lymphatic barrier to the dissemination of bacteria into the blood. They also participate in antigen uptake, processing, and antibody production. Such antibodies can opsonize the microbes and, coupled with complement, form an ef-

TABLE 17-1. TYPICAL RESULTS FROM THE "ONE-HOUR RENAL FUNCTION TEST"

	Urine	Plasma	U/P	GFR (ml/min)
Common values obtained from oliguric patients with normal kidneys				
Creatinine (mg/100 ml)	100	1	100	
if urine volume = 30 ml/hr (0.5 ml/min)				50
Osmols (mOsm/L)	400	300	>1.3	
Sodium (mEq/L)	20	140	0.14	
Common values obtained from patients with acute renal failure				
Creatinine (mg/100 ml)	20	2	10	
if urine volume = 10 ml/hr (0.16 ml/min)				1.6 *
Osmols (mOsm/L)	300	290	1.03	
Sodium (mEq/L)	110	130	0.9	

* If urine volume = 100 ml/hr (1.6 ml/min), GFR = 16.

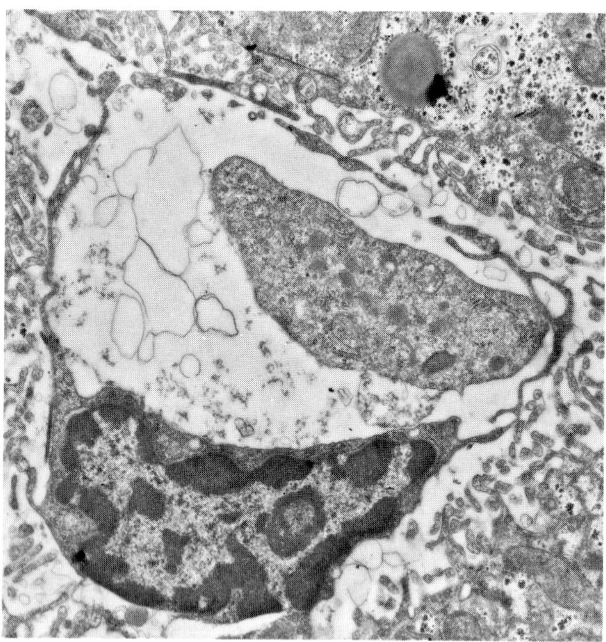

Fig. 17-6. **Electromicrograph of liver Küpffer cell before particle challenge. Readily apparent are collagen fibers, irregular nucleus of the Küpffer cell, minimal apparent cytoplasmic mass of the Küpffer cell, and a well-defined interstitial fluid space (space of Disse) between the endothelial barrier and hepatic parenchymal cells. Endothelial barrier is porous and freely permeable to the movement of fluid and proteins from the sinusoidal space (×19,019).**

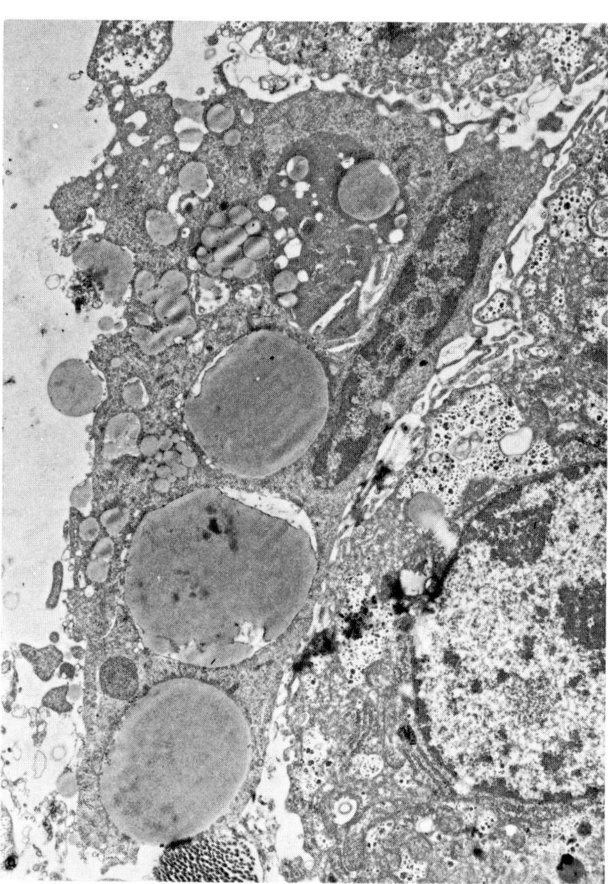

Fig. 17-7. **Electronmicrograph of liver Küpffer cell 15 minutes after intravenous injection of gelatin-coated reticuloendothelial test lipid particles. Rapid phagocytic uptake of the particulates, and vacuolization of the internalized particles, is present (×10,556).**

fective and specific antibacterial defense (Chapter 13). Lymphatic defense, however, can often be bypassed or overwhelmed by the bacterial load. When the bloodstream is invaded, the reticuloendothelial cells that line the vascular compartment provide the third echelon of phagocytic defense. Although tissue macrophages (eg, alveolar, peritoneal) have a diffuse distribution, the major population of reticuloendothelial cells consist of sessile macrophages localized in the liver, spleen and bone marrow, which are in direct contact with the vascular fluid.[26] There, they can rapidly remove bloodborne particulate and denatured material, including bacteria, viruses, tumor cells, endotoxin, fibrin, injured platelets, collagenous debris, and various other toxic and antigenic bloodborne particulate matter.[26,34] The splanchnic clearance (liver and spleen) accounts for about 90 percent of the total capacity of the reticuloendothelial system, and the Küpffer cells of the liver are especially efficient in this clearance role (Fig. 17-6), because 25 to 30 percent of the cardiac output passes by these cells every minute and they represent a large cellular population (Fig. 17-7).

This vital systemic defense clearance mechanism is influenced by numerous factors, including particulate size, particulate load, surface charge of the particle, metabolic status, splanchnic blood flow, and various bloodborne humoral factors called opsonic proteins. The major opsonic proteins for bacterial clearance are immunoglobulins and the C3b and C5b components of activated complement. In contrast, the major opsonic protein for nonbacterial entities is opsonic α_2-surface-binding (SB) glycoprotein,[19,35-37] which is identical to cold-insoluble globulin or plasma fibronectin.[15] Whether there are some naturally occurring particulates that can be efficiently cleared in the absence of serum opsonic activity remains to be documented, but their removal may also depend on the participation of cell-bound opsonic proteins on the surface of RES cells. Additionally, specific bacterial types, such as *Staphylococcus*, may be opsonized by plasma fibronectin for RES clearance.

In the present chapter, emphasis will be placed on opsonic α_2-surface-binding glycoprotein or plasma fibronectin as it relates to organ failure in patients with sepsis or bacteremia, because its modulation of reticuloendothelial clearance appears critical to the preservation of cardiovascular and pulmonary function. For example, depression of hepatic Küpffer cell and splenic reticuloendothelial cell phagocytic clearance of bloodborne particulates usually result in increased extrahepatic localization, especially in the lung and kidneys and probably in other peripheral beds. Organ microembolization undermines microvascular reactivity and organ integrity and this may be a contributing factor in the organ failure observed with overwhelming sepsis. An example would be the ventilation-perfusion mismatch, pulmonary edema, and altered gas exchange mechanisms observed in the septic injured patient with opsonic plasma fibronectin deficiency.[15,19,20,23]

RETICULOENDOTHELIAL PHAGOCYTIC DEPRESSION AFTER TRAUMA

The relationship between reticuloendothelial phagocytic activity and the physiopathology of shock and trauma is well established.[13,38,39] There are several lines of evidence: (1) colloid-induced reticuloendothelial blockade will decrease resistance to trauma and shock; (2) reticuloendothelial stimulation will increase resistance to experimental trauma and shock; (3) reticuloendothelial stimulation is observed in experimental states of adaptive tolerance to injury; and (4) deterioration of hepatic or splenic reticuloendothelial phagocytic clearance capacity occurs following trauma and shock and is usually proportional to the degree of injury. Following sublethal injury, the reticuloendothelial system usually undergoes phasic changes characterized by an early and severe phagocytic depression with a subsequent period of RES recovery and transient stimulation. In contrast, more severe trauma results in a progressive deterioration of reticuloendothelial function without recovery. Experimentally, survival following injury can be statistically correlated with organ deterioration and increased mortality.

Altered resistance to trauma, shock, and sepsis have been clearly documented following reticuloendothelial blockade. While colloid-induced reticuloendothelial blockade may be in part mediated by saturation of phagocytic cells, more recent evidence points to a humoral deficiency as the etiology of reticuloendothelial blockade.[15,26,35] Passage of denatured protein aggregates and collagenous debris into the bloodstream results in their rapid interaction with opsonic fibronectin.[26,35,40-42] This opsonized particulate complex is recognized by the reticuloendothelial cells, especially in the liver, and actively bound to receptors on the reticuloendothelial cell with subsequent ingestion. Depending on the nature of the particulate ingested, it can be destroyed, metabolized, degraded, or stored for an indefinite period. In the case of bacterial antigen whose opsonizing substance is mainly immunoglobulin, it can then be processed to implement immune responsiveness. Gelatin-coated colloids [35,42,43] appear to have a high affinity for opsonic protein, reflecting the fact that gelatin is denatured collagen.

Acute opsonic fibronectin depletion can be detected by bioassay or immunoassay after injection of denatured collagen-coated particulate matter into the blood.[35,42] If opsonins are depleted, liver reticuloendothelial clearance capacity falls. During this phase, animals demonstrate increased sensitivity to shock and trauma as well as to bacterial sepsis. This points to a key role for opsonic fibronectin in resistance to injury and organ dysfunction during bacteremia.[14,15] After major elective operations, patients demonstrate acute humoral opsonic fibronectin deficiency, followed by a rapid restoration to normal levels. Multiple trauma or severe burn patients demonstrate a more profound opsonic deficiency, the degree and persistence of which correlates with their clinical course in terms of organ failure, especially when combined with wound sepsis

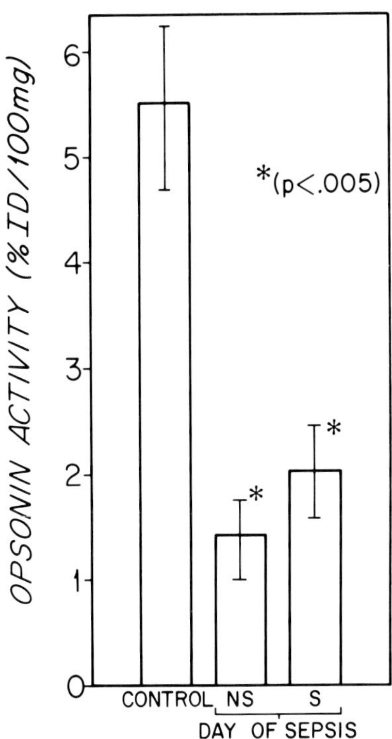

Fig. 17-8. **Bioassayable opsonic activity in surviving (S) and nonsurviving (NS) injured patients on the day of documented sepsis (blood cultures). The normal opsonin activity by in vitro liver slice bioassay with respect to Küpffer cell binding and uptake of isotopically labeled gelatin-coated test particles is 5.51 ± 0.79 percent injected dose per 100 mg of liver. Significant deficiency is observed on the day of sepsis. Data was obtained from four nonsurviving and seven surviving trauma patients with septicemia. (From Scovill WA, Saba TM, Kaplan JE, Bernard H, Powers SR Jr: Deficits in reticuloendothelial humoral control mechanisms in patients after trauma. *J Trauma* 16:898, 1976.)**

and bacteremia.[44-46] Survival after trauma is directly correlated with early restoration of opsonic activity.[15,19,20,44] All trauma patients, whether survivors or non-survivors, demonstrate profound depletion in opsonin activity with septicemia (Fig. 17-8). This deficiency actually develops prior to documented sepsis,[46] but a cause and effect relationship remains to be defined.

OPSONIC PROTEIN AND PLASMA FIBRONECTIN

Opsonic α_2SB glycoprotein is identical to cold-insoluble globulin (CIg) or plasma fibronectin.[40,41] The protein has a molecular weight of approximately 450,000 daltons and is comprised of two subunits, each about 220,000 to 230,000 daltons, held together by disulfide bonds. Opsonic protein (CIg; plasma fibronectin) is intimately associated with fibrinogen and fibrin and covalently binds to fibrin through coagulation factor XIII.[52] Plasma level in adults is usually 300 to 400 μg per ml, with a consistently lower level in serum due to its binding to fibrin, which can be accelerated in the cold. It will stimulate inert gelatin-coated particulate phagocytosis by monocytes and macrophages. Intravenous administration of monospecific antiserum to opsonic protein will decrease resistance to trauma,[15,45] and the purified protein will prevent reticuloendothelial dysfunction following surgical trauma in animals.[47]

CIg is antigenically related to a fibroblast cell surface glycoprotein called large external transformation sensitive protein (LETS), or cell surface fibronectin.[48,49] Cell surface fibronectin appears to play a role in cell-cell interaction and cell adherence to a substratum. While the plasma fibronectin is antigenically related to the cell surface fibronectin, there may be functional differences between these molecules.[15,49] One speculation is that the more soluble plasma form of the molecule may subserve an important role in host defense by the reticuloendothelial system, while the cell surface protein may mediate microvascular and tissue integrity.[15] This may include both fibroblast attachment to collagen and involvement in wound healing, as well as endothelial cell adherence to the basement membrane. Vascular endothelial cells, as well as fibroblasts, synthesize this molecule,[48-50] and vascular endothelial cells [15] may contribute to the plasma opsonic fibronectin pool. The fibroblast may elaborate this protein into lymph for modulating lymph node macrophage activity.[15] Reticuloendothelial cells or macrophages also produce fibronectin, and this may be a prime source for the opsonically active molecule in various sites.[15]

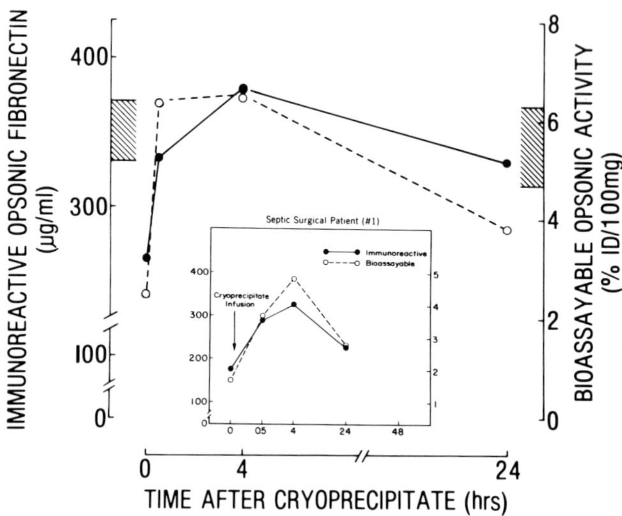

Fig. 17-9. **Reversal of opsonic fibronectin deficiency in septic surgical, trauma and burn patients (No. = 6) after intravenous infusion of plasma cryoprecipitate. Immunoreactive opsonic fibronectin was determined by electroimmunoassay and bioassayable opsonic activity was determined by standard liver slice phagocytic assay. Each patient was infused with 10 units of plasma cryoprecipitate in a total volume of 250 ml over a 60-minute infusion interval. Immunoreactive opsonic fibronectin levels in normal adults is typically 300 to 400 µg per ml. The first patient treated experimentally with cryoprecipitate to reverse the opsonic fibronectin deficiency (July, 1977) is shown in inset.**

REVERSAL OF HOST DEFENSE FAILURE BY CRYOPRECIPITATE

Plasma fibronectin is concentrated in cryoprecipitate, which also contains a high concentration of fibrinogen and factor VIII. Its level is decreased in patients with organ failure and disseminated intravascular coagulation[50] as well as in septic trauma and burn patients.[15,46] Opsonic deficiency in the injured septic patient can be reversed by this blood fraction.[19,23] Cryoprecipitate infusion into septic patients with organ failure and opsonic deficiency results in a rapid reversal of opsonic deficiency (Fig. 17-9) and improvement in organ function.[23,24] This includes pulmonary, renal, and peripheral vascular function. Such patients manifest a decrease in fever, normalization of leukocyte levels, and an improvement in pulmonary function as judged by requirements for positive end-expiratory pressure. There is a better matching of ventilation and perfusion with a significant decline in dead space and pulmonary shunt.[15,20] Peripheral vascular hemodynamic and oxygen consumption studies point to an increase in limb blood flow and improved reactive hyperemic response of the peripheral circulation.[14,20,23] The peripheral vascular hemodynamic alterations after cryoprecipitate are not dependent on an associated elevation in cardiac output. Even the glomerular filtration rate (GFR) improves.[24] The exact clinical utility of intravenous cryoprecipitate will, of course, require well-designed additional controlled studies with cryoprecipitate as well as opsonically active plasma fibronectin. Recent confirmatory clinical studies[53,54] that show reversal of opsonic fibronectin deficiency by cryoprecipitate infusion[19] are encouraging.

ORGAN FAILURE WITH SEPSIS AS RELATED TO OPSONIC FIBRONECTIN DEFICIENCY

Two interdependent physiologic mechanisms may explain improved organ function following replacement of opsonic fibronectin.[15] Opsonic fibronectin is important in the clearance of bloodborne particulates, which interfere with the microcirculation if they are not phagocytized. These particulates include collagenous debris associated with tissue damage,[15,42] fibrin associated with endotoxin-induced intravascular coagulation, and platelet debris, all of which appear as the by-products of infection.[19,44,51] Whether the opsonic protein is a regulator of bacterial phagocytosis in a manner analogous to immunoglobulin remains to be rigidly investigated, but its acceleration of *Staphylococcus* uptake by neutrophils, as observed in preliminary studies, suggests a potential role in augmenting granulocyte and macrophage antibacterial defense, in addition to augmenting removal of products of bacterial sepsis.[52]

The deleterious effects of circulating and embolizing microaggregates on the microcirculation are documented.[55,56] The normal reticuloendothelial system collaborates with other homeostatic mechanisms to preserve vascular patency following microaggregate formation during sepsis. Hepatic Küpffer cells can be demonstrated by immunofluorescent, as well as electronmicroscopic, techniques to contain microaggregates of fibrin following low-grade intravascular coagulation or challenge with intravenously infused fibrin. Furthermore, the reticuloendothelial system clears fibrin degradation products and fibrinogen-fibrin complexes, as well as blood thromboplastin and active thrombin. Modulation of reticuloendothelial function by stimulation or depression can alter such clearance mechanisms. Thus, the reticuloendothelial system interacts with the coagulation process before as well as after fibrin formation. When viewed from this perspective, the reticuloendothelial system subserves an important role in hemostatic homeostasis, since it is involved in the clearance of procoagulants from the vascular compartment, as well as the products of intravascular coagulation. The generalized Shwartzman response associated with fibrin deposition in the renal vascular bed after endotoxin or sepsis can be exaggerated by reticuloendothelial depression. Additionally, intravascular coagulation and platelet aggregation may be precipitating factors in the pathogenesis of posttraumatic pulmonary insufficiency.[55,56] One effect of microembolization may be endothelial injury, which is coupled with release of humoral mediators that may initiate microvascular lung fluid balance alterations. Indeed, it has been recently shown with the sheep lung lymph fistula model that the documented increase in lung vascular permeability with *Pseudomonas* bacteremia [11,12] can be exaggerated by experimental depletion of plasma opsonic fibronectin.[57] Moreover, the plasma opsonic fibronectin levels and RES function can be inversely correlated with lung localization of bloodborne particulates (Fig. 17-10).[13,45,58,59]

A second physiologic mechanism may also exist.[15] The soluble plasma fibronectin is probably in equilibrium with the insoluble cell surface fibronectin known to be a major adhesive glycoprotein holding cells to one another and to the basement membrane. Severe plasma fibronectin deficiency in septic patients with organ failure may lead to loss of tissue, or cell-surface fibronectin, which in turn would alter endothelial cell adherence to both the subendothelium and to adjacent cells. Such adherence alterations may increase capillary permeability, leading to organ interstitial edema. Cell surface fibronectin is sensitive to neutral proteases [60] released from human polymorphonuclear leukocyte granules. Leukocyte activation at a site of acute inflammation or leukostasis in the pulmonary or peripheral vascular bed may alter tissue integrity by proteolytic degradation of the tissue fibronectin and destruction of its adhesive capability. The leukopenia frequently observed in bacteremic patients may result from margination and leukostasis in the vascular bed. Additionally, immune complex deposition and associated complement activation may be involved in the microcirculation disruption. From this perspective, opsonic fibronectin deficiency may undermine microvascular integrity as well as limit particulate clearance by the reticuloendothelial system, resulting in further organ injury due to microvascular embolization. This process would be precariously imbalanced, especially in the trauma patient with wound sepsis and tissue injury, since the trauma-induced opsonic fibronectin deficiency and reticuloendothelial phagocytic depression would sensitize the host to the consequences of bacterial sepsis. Fibronectin has a high affinity for collagen,[61] fibrin-fibrinogen complexes,[62] and other particulates. Its depletion after trauma may be related in part to utilization during RES clearance of localized and bloodborne particulates in RES clearance and to sequestration at sites of injury.

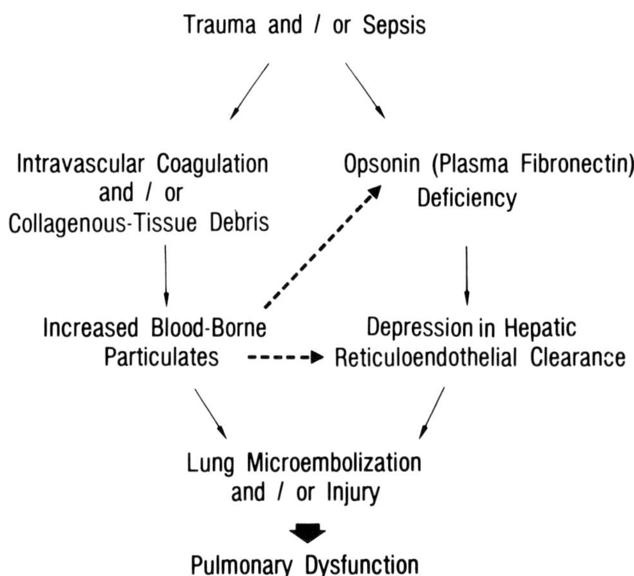

Fig. 17-10. **Relationship between trauma and sepsis and the development of lung injury. The central role for opsonic protein (plasma fibronectin) and reticuloendothelial system phagocytic clearance of products of bacterial sepsis, as well as collagenous debris, after trauma is emphasized. The influence of opsonic fibronectin deficiency resulting in systemic defense failure on lung embolization and injury is schematically presented. (From Niehaus G, Schumacker PT, Saba TM: Reticuloendothelial clearance of blood-borne particulates in sheep: relevance of lung microembolization and vascular injury. *Ann Surg*,** 191:479, 1980.)

Sophisticated techniques have been developed for monitoring and providing support to many vital organs. In contrast to the spectrum of diagnostic and prognostic parameters of cardiovascular, pulmonary, and renal function available, our ability to quantify the status of the host defense mechanism, as operationally executed by the reticuloendothelial system and its component macrophages, is limited, primitive, and not generally available clinically. Detailed studies of blood monocytes or circulating leukocytes derived from routine blood samples provide only a limited insight into the host defense apparatus. Additionally, complement and immunoglobulin levels as parameters of antibacterial resistance and immune status is not only limited to selected research or tertiary care facilities but also does not address the function of sessile reticuloendothelial cells in the liver and spleen. Colloid clearance techniques with isotopically labeled test particulates have limited clinical value. The dose of colloid necessary to effectively challenge the reticuloendothelial system may impair its function and deplete opsonic protein. The development of an immunoassay as well as the rapid (10 minute) immunoturbidimetric assay (Biodynamics/BMC, Indianapolis, Ind.) for opsonic fibronectin appears to provide an indirect, but sensitive and noninvasive, measure of reticuloendothelial function.[37,42,63] This is especially important since opsonic therapy as a modality of treatment for organ failure with sepsis using cryoprecipitate is acquiring rapid experimental support and specific component therapy using purified[15,19,20,23,24,53,54] opsonic fibronectin may have utility in the future. The importance has been repeatedly emphasized of basing such experimental therapy on the prevailing opsonic fibronectin levels in septic patients, and not providing excessive elevation of opsonic fibronectin, which may be counter productive.[14,15,23]

The availability of other drugs to manipulate the reticuloendothelial system also needs further study. Nonspecific RES stimulants such as zymosan, glucan, BCG, and *C. parvum*, have only limited clinical value (Chapter 19). Indeed, in many cases the associated hypertrophy and hyperplasia of the reticuloendothelial system, as elicited by such compounds, create other problems. Furthermore, the response time to such stimulants is quite delayed and of limited use in the septic patient with rapidly deteriorating organ function. Their use is obviously more important in the patient with malignant disease who also has disturbances of opsonic activity as well as macrophage function. In this setting, they appear to have value as judged by experimental and clinical studies in antitumor immunity as expressed by macrophage recognition and killing mechanisms. Since opsonic fibronectin levels are also disturbed in the cancer patient with macrophage dysfunction, it is possible that replacement therapy may have some short-term utility for such patients, especially during major operations, but this dimension remains to be fully investigated in controlled clinical studies.

It appears that the reticuloendothelial system and its component macrophages may be of central importance in the preservation of organ function during severe sepsis.[15,19] Patients with wound sepsis and bacteremia following severe burns or multiple trauma would be especially prone to the syndrome of multiple organ failure because of the trauma-induced opsonic fibronectin deficiency and related depression of the reticuloendothelial system, whose pattern of recovery may not have been complete after injury by the time the infection develops. Although continued emphasis needs to be directed toward elements of the host resistance apparatus that prevent infection from developing and spreading, it is obvious that the sequential organ failure with overwhelming infection and bacteremia may be a consequence of the products of wound inflammation and bacterial sepsis. As such, diagnostic and therapeutic approaches that can be used by the physician in evaluating circulating opsonic fibronectin and reticuloendothelial phagocytic function, as well as modulating its clearance capacity, need to be developed. We also need to further investigate the relationship between plasma fibronectin and a cell-surface fibronectin as it may influence vascular permeability in septic injured patients.[15] Indeed, an understanding of the physiology and physiopathology of the reticuloendothelial system,[26] coupled with quantitative approaches to monitor its status, should add a new dimension in the capacity to circumvent and treat organ failure in the septic surgical, trauma, or burn patient.

NONSPECIFIC MULTIPLE ORGAN FAILURE

In addition to the already mentioned specific organ failures associated with sepsis, there is a general deterioration of hepatic function, neural function, and gastrointestinal activity. Deterioration of these systems is generally terminal, and their pathogenesis has been discussed in other chapters. This discussion focused on disorders of the peripheral vascular, pulmonary, renal, and reticuloendothelial function. Moreover, it is suggested that failure of the reticuloendothelial systemic host defense clearance mechanism may be a pivotal event in the etiology of sequential organ failure, especially in the surgical, trauma, or burn patient with coexistent severe sepsis and intravascular coagulation. If cardiopulmonary and renal function can be supported in association with reversal of reticuloendothelial failure, while identification and correction of the septic focus is accomplished, patient mortality and morbidity will decline.

BIBLIOGRAPHY

Powers SR: Acute post-operative renal failure: Prophylaxis and management. In Sabiston DC (ed.): Textbook of Surgery. Philadelphia, Saunders, 1977, p 443.

Saba TM, Jaffe E: Plasma fibronectin (opsonic glycoprotein): Its synthesis by vascular endothelial cells and role in cardiopulmonary integrity after trauma as related to reticuloendothelial function. Am J Med 68:577, 1980.

REFERENCES

1. Moore FD, Lyons JH, Pierce EC, Morgan AP, Drinker PA, MacArthur JD, Dammin GJ: Post-traumatic pulmonary insufficiency. In Pathophysiology of Respiratory Failure and Principles of Respiratory Care After Surgical Operations, Trauma, Hemorrhage, Burns and Shock. Philadelphia, Saunders, 1969.
2. Moore FD: Convalescence: the metabolic sequence after injury. In Kinney JM, Egdahl RH, Zuidema CD (eds): Manual of Pre-operative and Post-operative Care, 2nd ed. Philadelphia, Saunders, 1971, p 19.
3. MacLean LD, Mulligan WG, McLean APH, Duff JH: Patterns of septic shock in man: a detailed study of 56 patients. Ann Surg 166:543, 1967.
4. Fulton RL, Jones CE Jr: The etiology of post-traumatic pulmonary insufficiency in man. Rev Surg 32:84, 1975.
5. Bywaters EGL, Beall D: Crush injuries with impairment of renal function. Br J Med 1:427, 1941.
6. Ladd M: Battle Casualties in Korea: Studies of the Surgical Research Team, Vol 4. U.S. Army Medical Service Graduate School. Walter Reed Medical Hospital, 1956, p 193.
7. Powers SR: Acute post-operative renal failure: prophylaxis and management. In Sabistan DCJ (ed): Textbook of Surgery. Philadelphia, Saunders, 1977, p 443.
8. Schumer W, Erve PR: Cellular metabolism in shock. Circ Shock 2:109, 1975.
9. Schlag G, Voight WH, Schnells G, Glatzl A: Die Ultrastruktur der menschlichen lunge in schock. I. Anaesthesist 25:512, 1976.
10. Gump FE, Mashima Y, Kinney JM: Water balance and extravascular lung water measurements in surgical patients. Am J Surg 119:515, 1970.
11. Brigham KL: Lung edema due to increased vascular permeability. In Staub NC (ed): Lungs and Water Solute. New York, Dekker, 1978, p 235.
12. Brigham K, Woolverton W, Blake L, Staub N: Increased sheep lung vascular permeability caused by *Pseudomonas* bacteremia. J Clin Invest 54:792, 1974.

13. Saba TM: Reticuloendothelial systemic host defense after surgery and traumatic shock. Circ Shock 2:91, 1975.
14. Saba TM, Scovill WA, Powers SR: Human host defense mechanisms as they relate to surgery and trauma. Surg Ann 12:1, 1980.
15. Saba TM, Jaffe E: Plasma fibronectin (opsonic glycoprotein): its synthesis by vascular endothelial cells and role in cardiopulmonary integrity after trauma as related to reticuloendothelial function. Am J Med 68:577, 1980.
16. Lucas CE, Weaver A, Higgins RF, Ledgerwood AM, Johnson SD, Bouwman DL: Effects of albumin versus non-albumin resuscitation on plasma volume and renal excretory function. J Trauma 18:564, 1978.
17. Powers SR Jr, Mannal R, Neclerio M, English M, Marr C, Leather R, Ueda H, Williams G, Custead W, Dutton R: Physiologic consequences of positive end-expiratory pressure (PEEP) ventilation. Ann Surg 178:265, 1973.
18. Gaehtgens P, Benner KU, Schickendantz S: Nutritive and non-nutritive blood flow in canine skeletal muscle after partial microembolization. Pflugers Archiv 361:183, 1976.
19. Saba TM, Blumenstock FA, Scovill WA, Bernard H: Cryoprecipitate reversal of opsonic alpha 2-surface binding glycoprotein deficiency in septic surgical and trauma patients. Science 201:622, 1978.
20. Scovill WA, Annest SJ, Saba TM, Blumenstock FA, Newell JC, Stratton HH, Powers SR: Cardiovascular hemodynamics after opsonic alpha-2-surface binding glycoprotein therapy in injured patients. Surgery 86:284, 1979.
21. Rhodes GR, Newell JC, Shah D, Scovill W, Tauber J, Dutton RE, Powers SR: Increased oxygen consumption accompanying increased oxygen delivery with hypertonic mannitol in adult respiratory distress syndrome. Surgery 84:490, 1978.
22. Powers SR Jr, Shah D, Ryon D, Newell J, Ralph C, Scovill W, Dutton R: Hypertonic mannitol in the therapy of the acute respiratory distress syndrome. Ann Surg 185:619, 1977.
23. Scovill WA, Saba TM, Blumenstock FA, Bernard H, Powers SR Jr: Opsonic α_2-surface binding glycoprotein therapy during sepsis. Ann Surg 188:521, 1978.
24. Annest SJ, Scovill WA, Blumenstock FA, Stratton HH, Newell JC, Paloski WH, Saba TM, Powers SR: Increased creatinine clearance following cryoprecipitate infusion in trauma and surgical patients with decreased renal function. J Trauma, 20:726, 1980.
25. Jenkins MT, Jones RF, Wilson B, Meyer CA: Congestive atelectasis—a complication of the intravenous infusion of fluids. Ann Surg 132:327, 1950.
26. Saba TM: Physiology and physiopathology of the reticuloendothelial system. Arch Intern Med 126:1031, 1970.
27. Rogers DE: Host mechanisms which act to remove bacteria from the blood stream. Bacteriol Rev 24:50, 1960.
28. Powers SR Jr, Burdge R, Leather R, Monaco V, Newell J, Sardar S, Smith EJ: Studies of pulmonary insufficiency in nonthoracic trauma. J Trauma 12:1, 1972.
29. Ashbaugh DC, Petty TL, Bigelow DB, Harris TM: Continuous positive pressure breathing (CPPB) in adult respiratory distress syndrome. J Thorac Cardiovasc Surg 57:31, 1969.
30. Stürm JA, Lewis FR Jr, Trentz O, Oestern H, Hempelman G, Tscherne H: Cardiopulmonary parameters and prognosis after severe multiple trauma. J Trauma 19:305, 1979.
31. Schumacker PT, Rhodes GR, Newell JC, Dutton RE, Shah DM, Scovill WA, Powers SR: Ventilation-perfusion imbalance after head trauma. Am Rev Respir Dis 119:33, 1979.
32. Valdes ME, Landau SE, Shah DM, Newell JC, Scovill WA, Stratton H, Rhodes GR, Powers SR Jr: Increased glomerular filtration rate following mannitol administration in man. J Surg Res 26:473, 1979.
33. Aschoff L: Reticuloendoethelial system. In Lectures on Pathology. New York, PB Hoeber, 1924.
34. Miles AA: Local defenses against infection and their relation to the general reticuloendothelial defenses. In Halpern BN (ed): Physiopathology of the Reticuloendothelial System. Springfield, Thomas, 1957, p 108.
35. Saba TM, Di Luzio NR: Reticuloendothelial blockade and recovery as a function of opsonic activity. Am J Physiol 216:197, 1969.
36. Blumenstock FA, Weber PB, Saba TM: Isolation and biochemical characterization of alpha-2-opsonic glycoprotein from rat serum. J Biol Chem 252:7156, 1977.
37. Blumenstock FA, Saba TM, Weber PB: Purification of α_2 opsonic glycoprotein from human serum and its measurement by immunoassay. J Reticuloendothel Soc 23:119, 1978.
38. Altura BM, Hershey SG: Reticuloendothelial function in experimental injury and tolerance to shock. Adv Exp Med Biol 33:545, 1972.
39. Zweifach BW, Benacerraf B, Thomas L: The relationship between the vascular manifestations of shock produced by endotoxin, trauma and hemorrhage. II. The possible role of the reticulo-endothelial system in resistance to each type of shock. J Exp Med 106:403, 1957.
40. Blumenstock FA, Saba TM, Weber P, Laffin R: Biochemical and immunological characterization of human opsonic α_2SB glycoprotein: Its identity with cold-insoluble globulin. J Biol Chem 253:4287, 1978.
41. Saba TM, Blumenstock FA, Weber P, Kaplan JE: Physiologic role for cold-insoluble globulin in systemic host defense: implications of its characterization as the opsonic α_2-surface-binding glycoprotein. Ann NY Acad Sci 312:43, 1978.
42. Blumenstock FA, Weber P, Saba TM, Laffin R: Electroimmunoassay of alpha-2-opsonic protein during reticuloendothelial blockade. Am J Physiol 232:R80, 1977.
43. Blumenstock FA, Saba TM, Weber P: Affinity method for rapid purification of opsonic α_2SB glycoprotein. In Schumer W, Spitzer JJ, Marshall BE (eds): Advances in Shock Research, Vol 2. New York, Liss, 1979, p 55.
44. Scovill WA, Saba TM, Kaplan JE, Bernard H, Powers SR Jr: Deficits in reticuloendothelial humoral control mechanisms in patients after trauma. J Trauma 16:898, 1976.
45. Kaplan JE, Saba TM: Humoral deficiency and reticuloendothelial depression after traumatic shock. Am J Physiol 230:7, 1976.
46. Lanser ME, Saber TM, Scovill WA: Opsonic glycoprotein (plasma fibronectin) levels after burn injury: Relationship to extent of burn and development of sepsis. Ann Surg 192:776, 1980.
47. Saba TM, Cho E: Reticuloendothelial systemic response to operative trauma as influenced by cryoprecipitate or cold-insoluble globulin therapy. J Reticuloendothel Soc 26:171, 1978.
48. Ruoslahti E, Vaheri A: Interaction of soluble fibroblast surface antigen with fibrinogen and fibrin. Identity with cold-insoluble globulin of human plasma. J Exp Med 141:497, 1975.
49. Yamada KM, Olden K: Fibronectin: adhesive glycoproteins of cell surface and blood. Nature 275:179, 1978.
50. Jaffe EA, Mosher DF: Synthesis of fibronectin by cultured human endothelial cells. J Exp Med 147:1779, 1978.
51. Mosher DF, Williams EM: Fibronectin concentration is decreased in plasma of severely ill patients with disseminated intravascular coagulation. J Lab Clin Med 91:729, 1978.
52. Mosher DF: Fibronectin. Progress in Hemostatis and Thrombosis 5:111, 1980.
53. Brodin B, Berghem L, Frigerg-Neilson S, Nordstrom H, Schildt B: Fibronectin in the treatment of septicemia—a preliminary report. Excerpta Medica, 7th World Congress of Anesthesiology, Hamburg, 1980, p 504.
54. Robbins AB, Doran JE, Reese AC, Mansberger AR: Cold-insoluble globulin levels in operative trauma: Serum depletion,

wound sequestration, and biological activity. Am Surg 46:663, 1980.

55. Malik AB, van der Zee H: Lung vascular permeability following progressive pulmonary embolism. J Appl Physiol 45:590, 1978.
56. Blaisdell FW, Lewis FR: Respiratory distress syndrome of shock and trauma: posttraumatic respiratory failure. Major Probl Clin Surg 21:1, 1977.
57. Niehaus G, Schumacker P, Saba TM: Influence of opsonic fibronectin deficiency on lung fluid balance during bacterial sepsis. J Appl Physiol, 49:693, 1980.
58. Niehaus G, Schumacker PT, Saba TM: Reticuloendothelial clearance of bloodborne particulates in sheep: Relevance to lung microembolization and vascular injury. Ann Surg, 191:479, 1980.
59. Saba TM: Effect of surgical trauma on the clearance and localization of blood-borne particulate matter. Surgery 71:675, 1972.
60. McDonald JA, Baum BJ, Rosenberg DM, Kelman JA, Brin SC, Crystal RG: Destruction of a major extracellular adhesive glycoprotein (fibronectin) of human fibroblasts by neutral proteases from polymorphonuclear leukocyte granules. Lab Invest 40:350, 1979.
61. Engvall E, Ruoslahti E: Binding of solute form of fibroblast surface protein, fibronectin, to collagen. Int J Cancer 20:1, 1977.
62. Mosesson MW: Cold-insoluble globulin (Clg): A circulating cell surface protein. Thromb Haemostas 38:742, 1972.
63. Saba TM, Albert WH, Blumenstock FA, Evanega G, Staehler F: Evaluation of a rapid immunoturbidimetric assay for opsonic fibronectin in surgical and trauma patients administered cryoprecipitate. J Lab Clin Med, in press, 1981.

PART V: ANTIMICROBIAL THERAPY

CHAPTER 18
Antimicrobial Agents

LEE D. SABATH, RICHARD L. SIMMONS, RICHARD J. HOWARD, AND DANIEL M. CANAFAX

THE appropriate use of antimicrobial agents in surgical practice is constantly changing as the agents and indications for the systemic use of antibiotics continue to evolve. The local and prophylactic uses of antimicrobial agents are more controversial and the resolution of conflicting concepts through well-designed trials may take time.

PRINCIPLES OF THERAPY

SELECTION OF ANTIBIOTICS

In most respects, the use of antibiotics in surgery does not differ from the use of antibiotics in general medicine. Knowledge of the infections most common in one's own practice, of the possible—and most likely—causative agents, and of the prevailing drug-sensitivity patterns of these agents in the community or hospital is required for the judicious selection of appropriate chemotherapeutic agents. Table 18-1[1] lists the pathogens most likely to cause infections in the various organs and tissues. Table 18-2 (p 362) lists the antimicrobial drugs of choice for each of the more common infecting organisms. In many surgical infections caused by mixtures of organisms, therapy should be directed at all potential pathogens that are capable of causing infections in pure culture (Chapter 8) and not assume that one strain is more important than another. A combination of several antibiotics may be required.

The data in Table 18-2 [1] are based on proved effectiveness and also on expected antibiotic resistance patterns. These patterns differ from one institution to another, so that it is important to know current local patterns of resistance. Tables 18-3 to 18-5 show the incidence of antibiotic resistance encountered at the University of Minnesota.

Precise Identification of the Infecting Organism

Knowledge of the most common infecting organism (Table 18-1) and its sensitivity pattern (Tables 18-3 to 18-5) will usually permit selection of the proper antibiotic for a given infection. Nevertheless, it is important to precisely identify the infecting organism or mixture of organisms. Rapid information on the morphology and staining characteristics of the bacteria can be gained by smear and stain of all aspirates, inflammatory exudates, and tissue biopsies. There is even occasional advantage in Gram stains of buffy coat smears in suspected cases of septicemia, and valuable information can be gained from smears of stool in patients with infectious diarrhea. There are, however, several pitfalls in the interpretation of the Gram stain.

1. If the preparation is carelessly obtained from superficial exudate or from contaminated mucosal surfaces, the findings may not truly reflect the infecting flora.
2. If fewer than 10^5 organisms per ml of exudate are present, Gram stains may not even reveal the organisms. During a clinically obvious or highly suspicious infection (eg, peritonitis), negative Gram stain results should be ignored until both the aerobic and anaerobic cultures are reported to be sterile. Concentration of the organisms by centrifugation may be necessary to detect low numbers of organisms, and special stains (acid-fast, fungal) may be necessary.
3. The need, in cases of deep infection, to start antibiotics prior to drainage can sometimes render the inflammatory exudate sterile. The Gram stain smear is therefore sometimes a better guide to therapy than the result of culture.

The exact nature of the infecting organism can usually be determined only by cultural isolation. The original choice of antibiotic therapy should always be compared with the results of culture and sensitivity testing. When interpreting laboratory reports of cultures, however, it is important to remember that different organisms pose different problems in bacterial identification for laboratory personnel. For example, some organisms *(Chlamydia, Treponema)* cannot be cultured in vitro. Some *Histoplasma, Nocardia, Mycobacterium,* and anaerobes grow slowly. Routine media will not support the growth of others (diphtheria). For these reasons, a clinically successful

TABLE 18-1. TABLE OF BACTERIA, FUNGI, AND SOME VIRUSES MOST LIKELY TO CAUSE ACUTE INFECTIONS

BLOOD (SEPTICEMIA)

Newborn Infants
1. *E. coli* (or other gram-negative bacilli)
2. *Streptococcus,* group B
3. *S. aureus*
4. *S. pyogenes* (group A)
5. Enterococcus
6. *L. monocytogenes*
7. *S. pneumoniae*

Children
1. S. pneumoniae
2. *N. meningitidis*
3. *H. influenzae*
4. *S. aureus*
5. *S. pyogenes* (group A)
6. *E. coli* (or other gram-negative bacilli)

Adults
1. *E. coli* (or other gram-negative bacilli)
2. *S. aureus*
3. *S. pneumoniae*
4. *Bacteroides*
5. *S. pyogenes* (group A)
6. *N. meningitidis*
7. *Candida albicans*
8. *N. gonorrhoeae*
9. Other *Candida* species

JOINTS
1. *S. aureus*
2. *S. pyogenes* (group A)
3. *N. gonorrhoeae*
4. Gram-negative bacilli
5. *S. pneumoniae*
6. *N. meningitidis*
7. *H. influenzae* (in children)
8. *M. tuberculosis* and other *Mycobacterium*
9. Fungi

MENINGES
1. Viral agents (enterovirus, mumps, and others)
2. *N. meningitidis*
3. *H. influenzae* (in children)
4. *S. pneumoniae*
5. *Streptococcus* group B (infants less than 2 months old)
6. *E. coli* (or other gram-negative bacilli)
7. *S. pyogenes* (group A)
8. *S. aureus* (after neurosurgery, brain abscess)
9. *M. tuberculosis*
10. *C. neoformans* and other fungi
11. *L. monocytogenes*
12. Enterococcus (neonatal period)
13. *Treponema pallidum*
14. *Leptospira*

ENDOCARDIUM
1. *Viridans* group of *Streptococcus*
2. Enterococcus
3. *Streptococcus bovis*
4. *S. aureus*
5. *S. epidermidis*
6. *C. albicans* and other fungi
7. Gram-negative bacilli
8. *S. pneumoniae*
9. *S. pyogenes* (group A)
10. Anaerobic streptococci

BONES (OSTEOMYELITIS)
1. *S. aureus*
2. *Salmonella* (or other gram-negative bacilli)
3. *S. pyogenes* (group A)
4. *M. tuberculosis*
5. Anaerobic streptococci (chronic)
6. *Bacteroides* (chronic)

SKIN AND SUBCUTANEOUS TISSUES

Burns
1. *S. aureus*
2. *S. pyogenes* (group A)
3. *P. aeruginosa* or other gram-negative bacilli)

Skin infections
1. *S. aureus*
2. *S. pyogenes* (group A)
3. Dermatophytes
4. *C. albicans*
5. Herpes simplex or zoster
6. Gram-negative bacilli
7. *T. pallidum*

Decubitus wound infections
1. *S. aureus*
2. *E. coli* (or other gram-negative bacilli)
3. *S. pyogenes* (group A)
4. Anaerobic streptococci
5. *Clostridium*
6. Enterococcus
7. *Bacteroides*

Traumatic and surgical wounds
1. *S. aureus*
2. Anaerobic streptococci
3. Gram-negative bacilli
4. *Clostridium*
5. *S. pyogenes* (group A)
6. Enterococcus

Eyes (cornea and conjunctiva)
1. Herpes and other viruses
2. *N. gonorrhoeae* (in newborn)
3. *H. aegyptius* (Koch-Weeks bacillus)
4. *S. pneumoniae*
5. *H. influenzae* (in children)
6. *Moraxella lacunata*
7. *S. aureus*
8. *P. aeruginosa*
9. Other gram-negative bacilli
10. *C. trachomatis*
11. *Chlamydiae* of inclusion conjunctivitis
12. Fungi

EARS

Auditory canal
1. *S. aureus*
2. *S. pyogenes* (group A)
3. *S. pneumoniae*
4. *P. aeruginosa* (or other gram-negative bacilli)
5. *H. influenzae* (in children)
6. Fungi

Middle ear
1. *S. pneumoniae*
2. *H. influenzae* (in children)
3. *S. pyogenes* (group A)
4. *S. aureus*
5. Anaerobic streptococci
6. *Bacteroides*
7. Other gram-negative bacilli (chronic)

(continued)

TABLE 18.1 ***(cont.)***

PARANASAL SINUSES
1. *S. pneumoniae*
2. *S. pyogenes* (group A)
3. *H. influenzae*
4. *Klebsiella* (or other gram-negative bacilli)
5. Anaerobic streptococci (chronic sinusitis)
6. *S. aureus* (chronic sinusitis)
7. *Mucor, Aspergillus* (especially in diabetics)

MOUTH
1. Herpes viruses
2. *C. albicans*
3. *Leptotrichia buccalis* (Vincent's infection)
4. *Bacteroides*
5. Mixed anaerobes
6. *T. pallidum*
7. *Actinomyces*

THROAT
1. Respiratory viruses
2. *S. pyogenes* (group A)
3. *N. meningitidis* or *N. gonorrhoeae*
4. *L. bucalis* (Vincent's infection)
5. *C. albicans*
6. *C. diphtheriae*
7. *B. pertussis*

LARYNX, TRACHEA, AND BRONCHI
1. Respiratory viruses
2. *S. pneumoniae*
3. *H. influenzae*
4. *S. pyogenes* (group A)
5. *C. diphtheriae*
6. *S. aureus*
7. Gram-negative bacilli

PLEURA
1. *S. aureus*
2. *S. pneumoniae*
3. *H. infuenzae*
4. Gram-negative bacilli
5. Anaerobic streptococcus
6. *Bacteroides*
7. *S. pyogenes* (group A)
8. *M. tuberculosis*
9. *Actinomyces, Nocardia*
10. Fungi

LUNGS

Pneumonia
1. Respiratory viruses
2. *M. pneumoniae*
3. *S. pneumoniae*
4. *H. influenzae*
5. *S. aureus*
6. *Klebsiella* (or other gram-negative bacilli)
7. *S. pyogenes* (group A)
8. *Rickettsia*
9. *C. psittaci*
10. *M. tuberculosis*
11. Anaerobic streptococci
12. *Bacteroides*
13. *P. carinii**
14. Fungi
15. *Legionella pneumophila*
16. Pittsburgh pneumonia agent

ABSCESS
1. Anaerobic streptococci
2. *Bacteroides*
3. *S. aureus*
4. *Klebsiella* (or other gram-negative bacilli)
5. *S. pneumoniae*
6. Fungi
7. *Actinomyces, Nocardia*

GASTROINTESTINAL TRACT
1. Gastrointestinal viruses
2. *Salmonella*
3. *E. coli*
4. *Shigella*
5. *Campylobacter fetus*
6. *Yersinia enterocolitica*
7. *S. aureus*
8. *V. cholerae*
9. *V. parahaemolyticus*
10. *T. pallidum* (anus)
11. *N. gonorrhoeae* (anus)
12. *C. albicans*

URINARY TRACT
1. *N. gonorrhoeae* (urethra)
2. *E. coli* (or other gram-negative bacilli)
3. *S. aureus* and *S. epidermidis*
4. *Enterococcus*
5. *C. albicans*
6. *Chlamydia* (urethra)
7. *T. pallidum* (urethra)
8. *T. vaginalis* (urethra)

FEMALE GENITAL TRACT

Vagina
1. *T. vaginalis**
2. *C. albicans*
3. *N. gonorrhoeae*
4. *S. pyogenes* (group A)
5. *H. vaginalis*
6. *T. pallidum*

Uterus
1. Anaerobic streptococci
2. *Bacteroides*
3. *N. gonorrhoeae*
4. *Clostridium*
5. *E. coli* (or other gram-negative bacilli)
6. Herpes virus, type II (cervix)
7. *S. pyogenes* (group A)
8. *Streptococcus,* groups B and C
9. *T. pallidum*
10. *S. aureus*
11. Enterococcus

Fallopian tubes
1. *N. gonorrhoeae*
2. *E. coli* (or other gram-negative bacilli)
3. Anaerobic streptococci
4. *Bacteroides*

MALE GENITAL TRACT

Seminal vesicles
1. Gram-negative bacilli
2. *N. gonorrhoeae*

Epididymis
1. Gram-negative bacilli
2. *N. gonorrhoeae*
3. *M. tuberculosis*

(continued)

TABLE 18.1 ***(cont.)***

Prostate gland
1. Gram-negative bacilli
2. *N. gonorrhoeae*

PERITONEUM
1. *E. coli* (or other gram-negative bacilli)
2. Enterococcus
3. *Bacteroides*
4. Anaerobic streptococci
5. *Clostridium*
6. *S. pneumoniae*
7. *Streptococcus* (group B)

* A protozoan.

From Abramowicz M (ed): *Handbook of Antimicrobial Therapy.* New Rochelle, Medical Letter, 1980, p 9.

TABLE 18-2. ANTIMICROBIAL DRUGS OF CHOICE

Infecting Organism	Drug of First Choice	Alternative Drugs
(NOTE: Because resistance may be a problem, susceptibility tests should be performed for those organisms preceded by an asterisk.)		
GRAM-POSITIVE COCCI		
* *S. aureus*		
Non-penicillinase producing	Penicillin G or V [1]	A cephalosporin [2]; clindamycin; vancomycin
Penicillinase producing	A penicillinase-resistant penicilin [3]	A cephalosporin [2]; vancomycin; clindamycin
S. pyogenes (group A and groups C and G)	Penicillin G or V [1]	An erythromycin [4]; a cephalosporin [2]
Streptococcus, group B	Penicillin G [1] or ampicillin	Chloramphenicol [5]; an erythromycin; a cephalosporin [2]
* *Streptococcus,* viridans group [6]	Penicillin G [1] with or without streptomycin	A cephalosporin [2]; vancomycin
S. bovis [6]	Penicillin G [1]	A cephalosporin [2]; vancomycin
Streptococcus, Enterococcus group		
Endocarditis [6] or other severe infection,	Ampicillin or penicillin G with gentamicin or streptomycin	Vancomycin with gentamicin or streptomycin
uncomplicated urinary tract infection [7]	Ampicillin or amoxicillin	Nitrofurantoin
Streptococcus, anaerobic	Penicillin G [1]	Clindamycin; a tetracycline [8]; an erythromycin; chloramphenicol [5]; a cephalosporin [2,9]
* *S. pneumoniae* (pneumococcus)	Penicillin G or V [1,10]	An erythromycin [4,10]; a cephalosporin [2]; chloramphenicol [5,10]; vancomycin
GRAM-NEGATIVE COCCI		
* *N. gonorrhoeae* [11]	A tetracycline [8] or penicillin G or amoxicillin	Ampicillin; spectinomycin; cefoxitin
N. meningitidis [12]	Penicillin G	Chloramphenicol [5]; a sulfonamide [13]
GRAM-POSITIVE BACILLI		
B. anthracis (anthrax)	Penicillin G	An erythromycin; a tetracycline [8]
C. perfringens (welchii) [14]	Penicillin G	Chloramphenicol [5]; clindamycin; a cephalosporin [2]; a tetracycline [8]
C. tetani [15]	Penicillin G	A tetracycline [8]; a cephalosporin [2]
C. diphtheriae [16]	An erythromycin	Pencillin G
L. monocytogenes	Ampicillin or penicillin G with or without gentamicin	Chloramphenicol [5]; a tetracycline [8]
ENTERIC GRAM-NEGATIVE BACILLI		
* *Bacteroides*		
Oropharyngeal strains	Penicillin G	Clindamycin; an erythromycin; a tetracycline [8]
Gastrointestinal strains	Clindamycin	Chloramphenicol [5,17]; cefoxitin [2]; metronidazole; a tetracycline [8]

(continued)

TABLE 18-2. *(cont.)*

Infecting Organism	Drug of First Choice	Alternative Drugs
Enterobacter	Gentamicin [18] or tobramycin [18]	Carbenicillin or ticarcillin; amikacin; cefamandole [2]; chloramphenicol [5]; a tetracycline [8]; trimethoprim-sulfamethoxazole
* *E. coli* [19]	Gentamicin [21] or tobramycin [21]	Ampicillin; carbenicillin or ticarcillin; a cephalosporin [2]; kanamycin; amikacin; a tetracycline [8]; trimethoprim-sulfamethoxazole; chloramphenicol [5]
* *K. pneumoniae* [19]	Gentamicin [21] or tobramycin [21]	A cephalosporin [2]; kanamycin; amikacin; a tetracycline [8]; trimethoprim-sulfamethoxazole; chloramphenicol [5]
* *P. mirabilis* [19]	Ampicillin [22]	A cephalosporin [2]; gentamicin or tobramycin; carbenicillin or ticarcillin; amikacin; trimethoprim-sulfamethoxazole; chloramphenicol [5]
* Other *Proteus* [19]	Gentamicin [18] or tobramycin [18]	Carbenicillin or ticarcillin; amikacin; a tetracycline [8]; trimethoprim-sulfamethoxazole [9]; chloramphenicol [5]; cefoxitin [2]
* *Providencia (Proteus inconstans)*	Amikacin	Gentamicin or tobramycin; carbenicillin or ticarcillin [9]; trimethoprim-sulfamethoxazole [9]; chloramphenicol [5]; cefoxitin [2] or cefamandole [2]
* *S. typhi* [23]	Chloramphenicol [5]	Ampicillin; amoxicilin [9]; trimethoprim-sulfamethoxazole [9]
* Other *Salmonella* [24]	Ampicillin or amoxicillin [9]	Chloramphenicol [5]; trimethoprim-sulfamethoxazole [9]
* *Serratia*	Gentamicin [18]	Amikacin; trimethoprim-sulfamethoxazole [9]; cefoxitin [2]; carbenicillin or ticarcillin
* *Shigella*	Trimethoprim-sulfamethoxazole	Chloramphenicol [5]; a tetracycline [8]; ampicillin
OTHER GRAM-NEGATIVE BACILLI		
* *Acinetobacter* (Mima, Herellea)	Gentamicin or tobramycin [9]	Kanamycin; amikacin; minocycline; doxycycline; trimethoprim-sulfamethoxazole [9]
Bordetella pertussis (whooping cough)	An erythromycin	
* *Brucella* (brucellosis)	A tetracycline [8] with or without streptomycin	Chloramphenicol [5] with or without streptomycin; trimethoprim-sulfamethoxazole [9]
Calymmatobacterium granulomatis (granuloma inguinale)	A tetracycline [8]	Streptomycin
Campylobacter (vibrio) fetus	An erythromycin [9]	A tetracycline [8]; gentamicin [9]; chloramphenicol [5]
* *F. tularensis* (tularemia)	Streptomycin [9]	A tetracycline [8]; chloramphenicol [5]
* *H. ducreyi* (chancroid)	Trisulfapyrimidines	A tetracycline [8]
* *H. influenzae*		
Meningitis, epiglottitis and other life-threatening infections	Chloramphenicol [5,25]	Ampicillin [25]; a tetracycline [8]
Other infections	Ampicillin or amoxicillin	A tetracycline [8]; trimethoprim-sulfamethoxazole; a sulfonamide; streptomycin; cefaclor [2]; cefamandole [2]
H. vaginalis	Metronidazole [9]	
L. pneumophila	An erythromycin [9] with or without rifampin [9,26]	A tetracycline [8,9]
Leptotrichia buccalis (Vincent's infection)	Penicillin G	A tetracycline [8]; an erythromycin
P. multocida	Penicillin G	A tetracycline [8]; a cephalosporin [2,9]

(continued)

TABLE 18-2. *(cont.)*

Infecting Organism	Drug of First Choice	Alternative Drugs
Pittsburgh pneumonia agent	An erythromycin [9] with or without rifampin [9,26]	Trimethoprim-sulfamethoxazole [9]; a tetracycline [8,9]
* *P. aeruginosa*		
Urinary tract infection	Carbenicillin or ticarcillin	Tobramycin; gentamicin; amikacin; a polymyxin
Other infections	Tobramycin or gentamicin with carbenicillin or ticarcillin [27]	Amikacin with carbenicillin or ticarcillin [27]
Pseudomonas (Actinobacillus) mallei (glanders)	Streptomycin with a tetracycline [8]	Streptomycin with chloramphenicol [5]
* *Pseudomonas pseudomallei* (melioidosis)	A tetracycline [8] with or without chloramphenicol [5,28]	Trimethoprim-sulfamethoxazole [9]; a sulfonamide
Spirillum minor (rat bite fever)	Penicillin G	A tetracycline [8]; streptomycin
Streptobacillus moniformis (rat bite fever; Haverhill fever)	Penicillin G	A tetracycline [8]; streptomycin
V. cholerae (cholera) [29]	A tetracycline [8]	Trimethoprim-sulfamethoxazole [9]
Y. pestis (plague)	Streptomycin	A tetracycline [8]; chloramphenicol [5]
ACID FAST BACILLI		
M. tuberculosis [30]	Isoniazid with rifampin [31]	Ethambutol, streptomycin [5]; para-aminosalicylic acid (PAS); pyrazinamide [5]; cycloserine [5]; ethionamide [5]; kanamycin [5]; capreomycin [5]
M. kansaii [30]	Isoniazid with rifampin [9] with or without ethambutol	Streptomycin [5]; an erythromycin; ethionamide [5]; cycloserine [5]; amikacin [5]
M. avium-intracellulare complex [30]	Isoniazid, rifampin,[9] ethambutol and streptomycin [5]	Amikacin [5]; ethionamide [5]; cycloserine [5]
M. fortuitum [30]	Amikacin [5,9]	Rifampin [9]; doxycycline [9]
M. scrofulaceum	See footnote 32	
M. marinum (balnei) [33]	Minocycline [9]	Rifampin [9]
M. leprae (leprosy)	Dapsone [5] with or without rifampin [9]	Acedapsone [5,34]; rifampin [9]; clofazimine [34]
ACTINOMYCETES		
A. israelii (actinomycosis)	Penicillin G	A tetracycline [8]
Nocardia	Trisulfapyrimidines	Trimethoprim-sulfamethoxazole [9]; trisulfapyrimidines with minocycline [9] or ampicillin [9] or erthromycin [9]; cycloserine [5,9]
CHLAMYDIA		
C. psittaci (psittacosis; ornithosis)	A tetracycline [8]	Chloramphenicol [5]
C. trachomatis		
Trachoma	A tetracycline [8] (topical plus oral)	A sulfonamide (topical plus oral)
Inclusion conjunctivitis	An erythromycin	A tetracycline [8]; a sulfonamide
Pneumonia	An erythromycin	A sulfonamide
Urethritis	A tetracycline [8]	An erythromycin
L. venereum	A tetracycline [8]	An erythromycin; a sulfonamide
FUNGI		
Aspergillus	Amphotericin B [5]	No dependable alternative
Blastomyces dermatidis	Amphotericin B [5]	Hydroxystilbamidine [5]
* *Candida species* [35]	Amphotericin B[5] with or without flucytosine [5,36]	Nystatin (oral or topical); miconazole (topical); clotrimazole (topical)
Chromomycosis	Flucytosine [5]	No dependable alternative
C. immitis	Amphotericin B [5]	Miconazole
C. neoformans	Amphotericin B [5,37] with or without flucytosine [5,36]	No dependable alternative
Dermatophytes (tinea)	Clotrimazole (topical) or miconazole (topical)	Tolnaftate (topical); haloprogin (topical); griseofulvin [5]
H. capsulatum	Amphotericin B [5]	No dependable alternative
Mucor	Amphotericin B [5]	No dependable alternative

(continued)

TABLE 18-2. ***(cont.)***

Infecting Organism	Drug of First Choice	Alternative Drugs
P. brasiliensis	Amphotericin B [5]	A sulfonamide; miconazole
S. schenckii	An iodide [38]	Amphotericin B [5]
MYCOPLASMA		
M. pneumoniae	An erythromycin or a tetracycline [8]	
PNEUMOCYSTIS CARINII	Trimethoprim-sulfamethoxazole	Pentamidine [5,34]
RICKETTSIA—Rocky Mountain spotted fever; endemic typhus (murine); tick bite fever; typhus, scrub typhus; Q fever	A tetracycline [8]	Chloramphenicol [5]
SPIROCHETES		
Borrelia recurrentis (relapsing fever)	A tetracycline [8]	Penicillin G
Leptospira	Penicillin G	A tetracycline [8]
T. pallidum (syphilis)	Penicillin G [1]	A tetracycline [8]; an erythromycin
T. pertenue (yaws)	Penicillin G	A tetracycline
VIRUSES		
Herpes simplex (keratitis)	Vidarabine (topical)	Idoxuridine (topical)
Herpes simplex (encephalitis)	Vidarabine	No alternative
Influenza A [39]	Amantadine	No alternative
Vaccinia	Methisazone [34] with or without vaccinia immune globulin	No alternative

1. Penicillin V is preferred for oral treatment of infections caused by non-penicillinase-producing staphylococci and other gram-positive cocci but is ineffective for gonorrhea. For initial therapy of severe infections, crystalline penicillin G, administered parenterally, is first choice. For somewhat longer action in less severe infections due to group A streptococci, pneumococci, gonococci, or *T. pallidum,* procaine penicillin G, an intramuscular formulation, is administered once or twice daily. Benzathine pencillin G, a slowly absorbed intramuscular preparation, is usually given in a single monthly injection for prophylaxis of rheumatic fever, once for treatment of group A streptococcal pharyngitis, and once or more for treatment of syphilis.
2. The cephalosporins have been used as alternatives to penicillins in patients allergic to penicillins, but such patients may also have allergic reactions to cephalosporins. Currently available cephalosporins are not recommended for treatment of meningitis.
3. For oral use against penicillinase-producing staphylococci, cloxacillin or dicloxacillin is preferred; for severe infections, a parenteral formulation of methicillin, nafcillin, or oxacillin should be used. Ampicillin, amoxicillin, carbenicillin, or ticarcillin are not effective against penicillinase-producing staphylococci. Occasional strains (about 1 to 2 percent) of coagulase-positive staphylococci may be resistant to penicillinase-resistant penicillins, and these strains are usually also resistant to cephalosporins; infections due to these resistant strains are treated with vancomycin, with or without either rifampin or gentamicin.
4. Occasional strains of group A streptococci and pneumococci may be resistant to erythromycins.
5. Because of the frequency of serious adverse effects, this drug should be used only for severe infections when less hazardous drugs are ineffective.
6. In endocarditis, disk sensitivity testing may not provide adequate information; dilution tests for susceptibility should be used to assess bactericidal as well as inhibitory end points. Peak bactericidal activity of the serum against the patient's own organism should be present at a serum dilution of at least 1:8.
7. Routine antimicrobial susceptibility tests may be misleading. Ampicillin is often effective in urinary tract infections, while streptomycin, kanamycin, or gentamicin alone are not.
8. Tetracycline hydrochloride is preferred for most indications. Doxycycline is recommended for uremic patients with infections outside the urinary tract for which a tetracycline is indicated. Tetracyclines are generally not recommended for pregnant women, infants, or children 8 years old or younger.
9. Not approved for this indication by the U.S. Food and Drug Administration.
10. In patients allergic to penicillin, an erythromycin is preferred for respiratory infections, and chloramphenicol is recommended for meningitis. Rare strains of *S. pneumoniae* may be resistant to penicillin; these strains are susceptible to vancomycin.
11. Since many strains of gonococci are relatively resistant to penicillin G, ampicillin, or amoxicillin, large doses together with probenecid are prescribed for single-dose treatment of uncomplicated infection; pelvic inflammatory disease and disseminated gonococcal infection are treated with multiple doses (*Medical Letter* 21:66, 1979). Some strains of gonococci produce penicillinase and are totally resistant to penicillin G, ampicillin, or amoxicillin; these strains may also be resistant to tetracycline, and should be treated with spectinomycin or cefoxitin. Penicillin V, benzathine penicillin G, and penicillinase-resistant penicillins should not be used for gonococcal infection.
12. Rifampin is recommended for prophylaxis in close contacts of patients infected by sulfonamide-resistant organisms. Minocycline may also be effective for such prophylaxis but frequently causes vomiting and vertigo. An oral sulfonamide is recommended for prophylaxis in close contacts of patients known to be infected by sulfonamide-sensitive organisms.
13. Sulfonamide-resistant strains are frequent in the United States, and sulfonamides should be used only when susceptibility is established by susceptibility tests.

(continued)

TABLE 18-2. *(cont.)*

14. Debridement is primary. Large doses of penicillin G are required. Hyperbaric oxygen therapy may be a useful adjunct to surgical debridement in management of the spreading, necrotic type.
15. For prophylaxis, tetanus toxoid and, in some patients, tetanus immune globulin (human) are required.
16. Antitoxin is primary; antimicrobials are used only to halt further toxin production and to prevent the carrier state.
17. Chloramphenicol is recommended when clindamycin is ineffective or infection is in the central nervous system.
18. In severely ill patients, some *Medical Letter* consultants would add carbenicillin or ticarcillin, but see footnote 27.
19. For an acute, uncomplicated urinary tract infection, before the infecting organism is known, the drug of first choice is one of the oral soluble sulfonamides, such as sulfisoxazole, ampicillin, or amoxicillin.
20. In severely ill patients, some *Medical Letter* consultants would add ampicillin, carbenicillin (or ticarcillin), or a cephalosporin, but see footnote 27.
21. In severely ill patients, some *Medical Letter* consultants would add a cephalosporin.
22. Large doses (6 gm or more daily) are usually necessary for systemic infections. In severely ill patients, some *Medical Letter* consultants would add gentamicin or tobramycin.
23. Ampicillin or amoxicillin may be effective in milder cases. Ampicillin is the drug of choice for *S. typhi* carriers.
24. Most cases of *Salmonella* gastroenteritis subside spontaneously without antimicrobial therapy.
25. Some strains of *H. influenzae* are resistant to ampicillin, and rare strains are resistant to chloramphenicol. Chloramphenicol (100 mg/kg/day IV) plus ampicillin should be used for initial treatment of meningitis or epiglottitis in children more than 2 months old until the organism is identified and its antimicrobial susceptibility is determined. Ampicillin is preferred by most *Medical Letter* consultants for treatment of organisms known to be susceptible.
26. Rifampin should be added only for patients who do not respond to erythromycin alone.
27. Neither gentamicin, tobramycin nor amikacin should be mixed in the same bottle with carbenicillin or ticarcilin for intravenous administration.
28. Seriously ill patients should be treated with both tetracycline and chloramphenicol.
29. Antibiotic therapy is an adjunct to and not a substitute for prompt fluid and electrolyte replacement.
30. Susceptibility tests should be performed by appropriate reference laboratories. Antituberculosis drugs may be effective in vivo even when in vitro tests show resistance; some isolates may require vigorous chemotherapy using multiple drugs.
31. Rifampin should be used concurrently with other drugs to prevent emergence of resistance. It is always included in treatment regimens for isoniazid-resistant organisms and is generally used together with isoniazid in the treatment of cavitary and for advanced pulmonary tuberculosis as well as for extrapulmonary tuberculosis. Concurrent use of rifampin and isoniazid can, however, cause adverse hepatic reactions, particularly in older patients.
32. Cervical adenitis in children should be treated by surgical excision and not with drugs.
33. Most infections are self-limited without drug treatment.
34. An investigational drug in the United States.
35. Amphotericin B administered intravenously is first choice for systemic candidal infections, although some *Medical Letter* consultants recommend concurrent use of flucytosine and amphotericin B; for gastrointestinal infections, oral nystatin may be sufficient. Topical miconazole, clotrimazole, or nystatin can be used for skin or vaginal infections.
36. Some strains may be resistant to flucytosine, or resistance may emerge during treatment.
37. In some patients with meningitis who do not respond to intravenous amphotericin B, intraventricular or intrathecal administration of amphotericin B may be helpful.
38. Lymphocutaneous form only.
39. Uncomplicated influenza usually needs no treatment.

From Abramowicz M (ed): *Handbook of Antimicrobial Therapy.* New Rochelle, *Medical Letter,* 1980, p 17.

antibiotic regimen should not be prematurely abandoned because the initial culture results fail to confirm the isolation of a slow-growing organism within the first few days. This admonition is of particular importance in the treatment of mixed bacterial infections.

Antibiotic Sensitivity Testing

A sensitive organism is said to be one whose growth is inhibited in vitro by an antibiotic at concentrations normally obtained in the blood or at the infected site after the usual dose. This premise has been of great use clinically, although there are important exceptions.

The disk-diffusion method provides qualitative, or at best semiquantitative, data about the susceptibility of an organism to a given agent. Quantitative data require serial dilutions of the antimicrobial agents in media. The lowest concentration of the agent that prevents visible growth after an 18- to 24-hour incubation period is known as the minimum inhibitory concentration (MIC). The minimal bactericidal concentration (MBC) or minimal lethal concentration (MLC) can be determined by subculturing on antibiotic-free media those containers that show no growth in the determination of the minimum inhibitory concentration.[2]

It is not necessary to routinely determine the antibiotic susceptibility of every organism; some organisms (Table 18-6)[3] have constant antibiotic susceptibility patterns. In contrast, the sensitivity patterns of other organisms are so unpredictable that susceptibility tests should virtually always be performed. Table 18-6 is a general guide to the need for sensitivity testing of the various organisms. Be aware, however, that resistant strains of all bacteria (even pneumococci) are constantly emerging.

There are a number of common errors in the interpretation of sensitivity results from hospital laboratories: (1) using drugs intended mainly for treatment of urinary tract infections for systemic infections instead (eg, nitrofurantoin, methenamine mandelate, nalidixic acid), because the laboratory indicated the organism was sensitive; (2) failing to use some nontoxic antibiotics for urinary tract infections (eg, ampicillin, cephalothin) because the laboratory reported the organism as resistant when in fact the high urinary concentration of these antibiotics would make them suitable (some knowledge of the degree of "resistance" should be available before using the antibiotic to which the organism is resistant); (3) in endocarditis, using an antibiotic to which the organism is sensitive by disc test but which is bacteriostatic and therefore unsuitable for this infection (eg, tetracycline, chloramphenicol); and (4) using drugs for the treatment of central nervous system infections which do not penetrate the blood-brain barrier (eg, aminoglycosides).

TREATMENT FAILURE AND ITS PREVENTION

Although failure of a bacterial infection to respond to a particular antibiotic is commonly regarded as evidence that the wrong antibiotic was selected, the other factors listed in Table 18-7[3] are usually responsible. Most cases of treatment failure call for continuation of the same antibiotic, with either a change in the way the antibiotic is being used or the addition of an adjuvant (or subtraction of an antagonistic) substance or procedure. Because most of these causes have different remedies, it is important to determine which one is guilty. Surgeons are sometimes the last to recognize that a septic focus requiring drainage, debridement, or excision is responsible for antibiotic failure—a delay compounded whenever infection complicates a procedure performed by the surgeons themselves.

Enhancing the Activity of Antibiotics

In some special situations, the conventional activity of an antibiotic may be increased or decreased. For example, in urinary tract infections, the pH of the urine can easily be changed. The aminoglycosides and erythromycins are much more active in an alkaline medium, whereas others are more active in acidic medium (tetracyclines, mandelamine, nitrofurantoin). NH_4Cl or ascorbic acid (usually 4–8 gm per day) can be given to acidify the urine, or $NaHCO_3$ (8–18 gm per day) or acetazolamide (0.5–2.0 gm per day) to alkalinize the urine. The activity of the antibiotic may frequently be increased 100-fold, and in some instances 500-fold.[4] Obviously, evaluation of the patient's overall condition must be made to determine whether administration of these acidifying or alkalinizing agents would be contraindicated. With these techniques, erythromycin plus alkali can be as effective as conventional therapy in urinary tract infections caused by gram-negative bacilli,[5] or the dose of potentially toxic agents (eg, gentamicin) can be drastically reduced if the urine is made alkalinic.[4]

A second technique for enhancing antibacterial activity is to combine antibiotics for a synergistic effect, such as treating enterococcal or staphylococcal endocarditis with a penicillin plus an aminoglycoside. A similar synergistic effect is achieved by carbenicillin plus gentamicin against *P. aeruginosa*.[6]

A third technique for increasing the activity of a given dose of antibiotic is to delay its excretion. By administering probenecid, 0.5 gm, every 6 hours to an average-weight adult, the peak serum concentrations of most penicillins and cephalosporins can be doubled, and the duration of effective serum antibiotic concentrations can be prolonged. Probenecid competes with the penicillins for the active transport mechanism in the renal tubules, which are responsible for 80 percent of the excretion. We usually prescribe probenecid along with benzylpenicillin for adults with normal renal function in whom 10 million or more units of benzylpenicillin per day, (or comparable amounts of other penicillins or cephalosporins) are recommended.

A fourth method for increasing the activity of a given antibiotic is to increase its dose. Excretion of some antibiotics is highly variable. For example, the aminoglycoside excretion in septic hyperdynamic patients, who have increased renal blood flow and elevated aminoglycoside clearance, results in inadequate blood levels even when nomograms based on standard average excretory patterns are used. Conversely, it is easy to overdose a patient who has diminished renal function. For these reasons, antimicrobial agents must be assayed in the blood to determine whether appropriate levels have been achieved; the dose must then be adjusted.

Increasing the dose of the cephalosporins, for example, which after standard doses achieve levels of 50–100 μg per ml in the blood, have greatly augmented their spectrum, especially with respect to *B. fragilis*. While cephamandole has little activity at normal dose levels against *B. fragilis*, many more strains are sensitive at higher serum levels. Doses of many nontoxic drugs can be safely increased—especially the penicillins and cephalosporins.

An additional method of increasing the total dose is to prolong the therapy. Effective therapy should not be arbitrarily discontinued unless the infection is under control. By similar reasoning, systemic intravenous therapy should not be prematurely changed to oral therapy with its resultant lower serum levels. Determining the point of discontinuation of therapy is difficult—the lack of a febrile reponse does not necessarily indicate a cure.

Continuing therapy for arbitrarily prolonged periods may sometimes be necessary to prevent relapse of fungal or more chronic infections. Unfortunately, rigid data on the proper duration of therapy is lacking.

Responses to appropriate antibiotics may be improved by changing the route of administration. Oral administration is seldom sufficient in patients with serious deep tissue infections. Intramuscular therapy may fail to achieve adequate serum levels in patients with unstable hemodynamic responses. Intravenous therapy should, therefore, be used in patients with severe life-threatening infections, and maintained until the patient is clearly improved.

Local or topical therapy will seldom control any but the most superficial pyoderma or infected wound surface. However, the high local concentrations that can be achieved by topical administration may be useful in prevention of infection in recently contaminated wounds or

TABLE 18-3. SUSCEPTIBILITY OF GRAM-NEGATIVE RODS ISOLATED AT THE UNIVERSITY OF MINNESOTA

	Acineto-bacter	Citro-bacter diversus	Citro-bacter freundii	E. coli	Entero. aerogenes	Entero. cloacae
	%	%	%	%	%	%
Amikacin	100	100	100	98	98	98
Ampicillin	10	5	25	74	10	6
Carbenicillin	71	0	75	73	47	69
Cefamandole	7	100	80	95	83	83
Cephalothin	20	94	19	78	16	4
Chloramphenicol	30	94	84	91	74	82
Gentamicin	90	100	100	99	100	100
Kanamycin	100	94	88	88	98	86
Nitrofurantoin	40	83	100	98	83	50
Tetracycline	90	100	78	76	80	86
Tobramycin	90	100	100	99	100	98
Trimeth/Sulfa	100	100	94	95	100	94

% = susceptible strains; NT = not tested.
For susceptibilities of more infrequently isolated organisms, please call the laboratory.

Data courtesy of Donna J. Blazevic, MPH; Henry H. Balfour, Jr, MD; Grace Mary Ederer, MPH; Stephen C. Marker, MD; Marcia L. Weber, MS; Clinical Microbiology Laboratory, University of Minnesota Hospitals.

TABLE 18-4. SUSCEPTIBILITY OF ANAEROBES ISOLATED AT THE UNIVERSITY OF MINNESOTA (1975–79)*

Anaerobe	Chloro	Clinda	Erythro	Pen	Tetra
B. fragilis	100	99	71	3	50
Bacteroides spp.	100	100	98	54	80
Bifido spp.	100	86	86	100	72
Clostridium spp.	99	88	82	87	75
Eubacterium spp.	100	89	89	89	70
Fusobacterium spp.	100	100	36	92	96
Peptococcus	100	100	84	96	80
Peptostreptococcus	100	90	80	90	77
Streptococcus spp.	100	100	100	100	94
Veillonella	100	100	42	92	80

* Percentages of susceptible strains.

Data courtesy of Donna J. Blazevic, MPH; Henry H. Balfour Jr., MD; Grace Mary Ederer, MPH; Stephen C. Marker, MD; Marcia L. Weber, MS. Clinical Microbiology Laboratory, University of Minnesota Hospitals.

on serosal surfaces to which organisms have not yet become adherent or invasive. This would seem to be their principal use.

TISSUE PENETRATION BY ANTIBIOTICS

Treatment of localized infections with systemic antimicrobial agents demands that an adequate concentration of drug be delivered to the site. Ideally, the tissue concentration of antibiotics should exceed the minimum inhibitory concentration even though there is evidence that subinhibitory concentrations of antimicrobials may occasionally result in clinical cure (eg, subinhibitory concentrations of some penicillins enhance the phagocytosis of *S. aureus*).

Tissue penetration appears to depend in part on antibiotic protein binding. Only the unbound form of antibiotic will pass the capillary wall in vivo[7] or act to inhibit bacterial growth in vitro. The penetration of antibiotics into fibrin clots—an important factor in the capacity of antimicrobial agents to penetrate areas of tissue injury—depends on the concentration of free antibiotics. Therapeutic outcome, on the other hand, seems not to correlate with protein affinity, presumably because protein binding is easily reversible.

The lipid solubility of an antibiotic is an important factor in its tissue penetration. It determines its capacity to pass through membranes by nonionic diffusion or into wounds, bone, cerebrospinal fluid, aqueous and vitreous humor of the eye, endolymph of the ear, or into the vegetations of bacterial endocarditis, abscesses, and other areas of devitalized tissue. Prolonged high-dose systemic therapy or even local therapy is required for antibiotics with

Kleb. oxytoca	Kleb. pneumo.	Morganella morganii	Proteus mirabilis	Providencia	Pseudo. aerug.	Serratia species	Haem. infl.
%	%	%	%	%	%	%	%
100	100	100	96	100	94	94	NT
0	3	5	86	36	2	2	93
0	2	97	83	83	71	37	NT
NT	95	79	89	100	3	15	NT
83	88	0	83	8	1	0	NT
94	77	69	79	96	94	96	100
100	99	100	98	76	94	96	NT
97	87	98	94	100	21	76	NT
78	86	25	3	4	2	5	NT
98	86	60	7	4	23	32	NT
100	100	100	98	92	96	87	NT
97	95	98	98	64	29	94	98

TABLE 18-5. SUSCEPTIBILITY OF GRAM-POSITIVE COCCI ISOLATED AT THE UNIVERSITY OF MINNESOTA

	Coag + Staphylococcus	Coag − Staphylococcus	Enterococcus
	%	%	%
Ampicillin	NT	NT	97
Cephalothin	99.7	94	6
Chloramphenicol	94	76	92
Clindamycin	95	49	9
Erythromycin	93	39	62
Gentamicin	94	80	14
Methicillin	98	68	NT
Nitrofurantoin	NT	NT	97
Penicillin	11	12	9
Tetracycline	93	61	22
Trimeth/Sulfa	99	79	97

NT = not tested.
% = percent of isolates tested.

Data courtesy of Donna J. Blazevic, MPH; Henry H. Balfour, Jr, MD; Grace Mary Ederer, MPH; Stephen C. Marker, MD; Marcia L. Weber, MS; Clinical Microbiology Laboratory, University of Minnesota Hospitals.

poor penetration into the infected areas. Table 18-8 [7] lists the factors thought to be important in the tissue penetration of a hypothetical antibiotic agent.

Even when therapeutic concentrations are achieved at the sites of tissue infections, local factors may influence the antimicrobial activity. For example, aminoglycosides and polymyxins are inactivated by purulent material, whereas carbenicillin does not lose activity in pus. For this as well as other reasons, drainage of purulent secretions is sometimes necessary. It is also important to recognize that infections caused by mixed species, one of which produces beta-lactamase, will render the hydrolyzable penicillins ineffective against even sensitive organisms within the infection. Penicillins and tetracyclines are also bound by hemoglobin and may be less effective in the presence of hematomas.[8] Similarly, *P. aeruginosa* is protected from the action of aminoglycosides by high concentrations of calcium and magnesium in the culture medium.[9] Local decreases in oxygen tension, such as occur within abscesses, will render certain antimicrobial agents less effective. For example, aminoglycosides are much less effective in anaerobic environments because oxygen is required for transport of these agents into the bacterial cell. Similarly, phagocytic and killing cellular mechanisms are inhibited in an anaerobic environment, so that bacteriostatic agents are also less effective.[10]

TABLE 18-6. ORGANISMS ON WHICH ANTIBIOTIC SENSITIVITY TESTS SHOULD BE PERFORMED

Organism	Virtually Never	Almost Always	Always
GRAM-POSITIVE COCCI			
Staphylococci			X
S. pneumoniae	X		
Streptococcus excepting enterococcus	X*6		
Enterococcus	X*†		
GRAM-NEGATIVE COCCI			
N. gonorrhoeae	X		
N. meningitidis	X		
GRAM-POSITIVE BACILLI			
B. anthracis		X	
C. perfringens	X		
C. tetani	X		
Other *Clostridium* species			X
C. diphtheriae	X		
Other *Corynebacterium* species			X
Listeria	X		
ENTERIC GRAM-NEGATIVE BACILLI			
E. coli, Klebsiella, Enterobacter, Providencia, Serratia			X
Pseudomonads			X
Other gram-negative bacilli			X
Salmonella, Shigella, Acinetobacter, Campylobacter			X
H. influenzae			X
ACID-FAST BACILLI			
M. tuberculosis	X		
Atypical *Mycobacteria* species			X
SPIROCHETES	X		
ACTINOMYCETES *(Actinomyces, Nocardia)*	X		
RICKETTSIA	X		
CHLAMYDIA	X		
MYCOPLASMA	X		
FUNGI	X		

*Susceptibility (minimum bactericidal concentration, MBC) should be determined in endocarditis.

† In endocarditis, a simple test is to determine if patient's organism can be inhibited by 500 μg/ml streptomycin, kanamycin, or gentamicin. If not inhibited, that drug is not suitable for use with ampicillin or penicillin.

Modified from Sabath LD: Use of antibiotics in obstetrics. In Charles D, Finland M (eds): *Obstetric and Perinatal Infections.* Philadelphia, Lea & Febiger, 1973, p 581.

Tissue Distribution of Antibiotics [7]

Blood

The concentration of an antibiotic in the blood or any other compartment is the difference between what has entered and what has left or been inactivated. The rapidity of excretion is therefore an important clinical consideration. Nitrofurantoin is excreted so rapidly that no antimicrobial effect can be achieved in the blood. In contrast, cefazolin is excreted slowly, and higher blood levels are obtained than with an equivalent dose of cephalosporins, which are excreted more rapidly.

Urine

Most antibiotics in common use (sulfonamides, penicillins, cephalosporins, aminoglycosides, vancomycin, the tetracyclines, polymyxins, nitrofurans, flucytosine) are excreted appreciably, if not principally, in urine. Prominent exceptions are erythromycin and chloramphenicol. Many antimicrobial substances used for treating urinary tract infections usually appear in the urine at 50 to 200 times the concentration at which they are found in blood. Indeed, their efficacy is often dependent on that special body distribution; consequently, in severe renal disease, treatment of infection within the urinary tract becomes more difficult.

Central Nervous System

Distribution of antimicrobial compounds in cerebrospinal fluid is related not only to the nature of the antimicrobial

TABLE 18-7. POSSIBLE CAUSES OF ANTIBIOTIC TREATMENT FAILURE

A. INAPPROPRIATE ANTIBIOTIC
   1. Organism not susceptible to antibiotic at concentrations achievable in focus of infection.
   2. Superinfection (or erroneous initial diagnosis).
   3. New, unrelated infection elsewhere in body.
   4. Failure of drug to reach site of infection (eg, because of shock or poor penetration of drug into appropriate body compartment as gentamicin and polymyxin not passing into central nervous system and cerebrospinal fluid).
   5. Bacteria in a dormant state or present as wall-deficient form when growth of cell wall must be present for antibiotic action.

B. APPROPRIATE ANTIBIOTIC BUT INSUFFICIENT TREATMENT
   6. Too small a dose of drug given or dose given too infrequently (aminoglycosides, penicillin).
   7. Course of therapy too short.
   8. Drug administered by inappropriate route (eg, orally rather than intravenously).
   9. Wrong preparation of appropriate drug (eg, procaine benzylpenicillin, which yields very low blood levels, rather than aqueous crystalline penicillin, which yields very high serum levels, when high levels are required).

C. APPROPRIATE ANTIBIOTIC BUT OTHER THERAPY REQUIRED
   10. Failure to institute appropriate measures in addition to prescribing antibiotics (eg, surgical drainage, debridement, replace blood volume, correct metabolic disorders).
   11. Failure to prescribe necessary adjuvant medication (eg, acidifying or alkalinizing medication in certain instances of urinary tract infections).
   12. Presence of substances (indigenous or prescribed) that antagonize the antibacterial activity of the drug being used.
   13. Impaired host defenses (cellular, humoral, or nutritional, naturally occurring or secondary to physical or chemical injury).
   14. Treatment started too late, ie, after changes had been initiated that cannot be stopped or reversed by effective chemotherapy.

Modified from Sabath LD: Use of antibiotics in obstetrics. In Charles D, Finland M (eds.): *Obstetric and Perinatal Infections.* Philadelphia, Lea and Febiger, 1973, pp 563–623.

agent but also to the extent of inflammation. Table 18-9[7] summarizes the facility with which various antimicrobial agents enter the cerebrospinal fluid.

The most important practical matter is that the lipid-soluble agents chloramphenicol, isoniazid, rifampin, sulfonamides, and flucytosine enter the cerebrospinal fluid especially well, the aminoglycosides and polymyxins enter with great difficulty, and amphotericin B does not enter at all. Therefore, when amphotericin B must be used for infection of the central nervous system, it must usually be administered directly into the cerebrospinal fluid (*Cryptococcus* meningitis does not require direct amphotericin B instillation). Of the tetracyclines, doxycycline and minocycline enter most readily because of their lipid solubility.

Interstitial Fluid

In general, high prolonged blood levels and freedom from protein binding favor diffusion of antibiotic into extravascular tissues. Absolute levels in a particular tissue may not accurately represent the therapeutic potential of the drug, however, because the drug may be so tightly bound to the tissue that it is not available for binding to bacteria.

Bile

Only urine and bile regularly contain higher concentrations of antibiotic than does serum. Table 18-10 [11] lists the concentration factors (bile concentration–blood concentration) for a variety of antibiotics. Nafcillin and rifampin may reach concentrations in bile 500 times their serum concentrations. The penicillins, cephalosporins, tetracyclines, and clindamycin are also concentrated in bile to varying degrees. Chloramphenicol, although not concentrated in bile, readily enters bile and has been frequently used successfully in biliary tree infections. Aminoglycoside antibiotics enter the bile less well, especially when liver disease is present (Table 18-10).

Bone

Tetracyclines and clindamycins bind readily to bone. They have been used successfully in osteomyelitis, as have many other antibiotics that do not bind as well. Thus, present data do not permit a judgment that this binding is a distinct advantage. Table 18-11 lists the concentration factors (bone-serum concentration) for a variety of antibiotics.

Prostate, Seminal Vesicles, and Epididymis

Using a split ejaculate technique, and measuring zinc content (which indicates prostate origin), pH, and antibiotic, investigators have found that the ampicillin, erythromycin, and doxycycline present in ejaculate primarily originate from the prostate and seminal vesicle in about equal concentrations. Some variation in results has been noted with both sulfonamides and metronidazole, although the latter appears to enter mainly via the prostate.[7]

Eye

With the exception of chloramphenicol and flucytosine (and possibly rifampin), most antibiotics do not easily enter the vitreous humor, even after subtenon injection. Direct injection (at the time of intraocular operation) of appropriate concentration of antibiotic (about ten times the desired concentration needed to inhibit the organism) may be the preferable means of getting these other antibiotics into the eye, when this is needed. Once in, it is as difficult for the antibiotics to leave as it was for them to enter. Retention of the drug is desirable in delivering antibiotic into the eye.[7]

TABLE 18-8. IMPORTANT FACTORS IN TISSUE PENETRATION BY ANTIBIOTICS

1. Maximum level of concentration in the blood
2. Duration of that maximum blood level
3. Serum protein binding
4. Serum factors that influence protein binding
5. Active transport mechanisms and secretory organs (especially kidney and liver)
6. Electrical charge on the antibiotic
7. Lipid solubility
8. Urine pH
9. Barriers to diffusion
10. Biotransformation of antibiotic
11. Circulating or local antibiotic inactivators
12. Tissue binding of antibiotic

From Sabath LD: Body distribution of antibiotics. J Surg Pract 8:56, 1979.

TABLE 18-9. ENTRY OF ANTIMICROBIAL AGENTS INTO CEREBROSPINAL FLUID

Antimicrobial Agent or Class	Ability to Enter
Chloramphenicol	Excellent
Flucytosine	Excellent
Sulfonamides	Excellent
Isoniazid	Excellent
Rifampin	Excellent
Tetracyclines (minocycline best)	Good
Vancomycin	Good
Penicillins	Poor; better with inflammation
Erythromycin	Poor; better with inflammation
Cephalosporins	Poor, even with inflammation (except for cephaloridine and [?] cephradine)
Clindamycin	Poor
Aminoglycosides	Poor
Polymyxin	Poor
Amphotericin B	Essentially not at all

Modified from Sabath LD: Body distribution of antibiotics. J Surg Prac 8:56, 1979.

Abscesses

There are only few data of clinical relevance concerning the distribution of antibiotics into abscesses. Clearly, however, the generalization that antibiotics do not penetrate abscesses is untrue. The penicillins and cephalosporins seem to penetrate mature abscess cavities poorly[12,13] whereas metronidazole, chloramphenicol, and clindamycin can achieve inhibitory concentrations.[14,15]

TABLE 18-10. BILIARY CONCENTRATION FACTORS (BILE LEVEL/BLOOD LEVEL) FOR ANTIBIOTICS USED IN INFECTIONS OF THE BILIARY TREE

Antibiotic	Bile Level/ Blood Level Ratio
Penicillin G	0.5
Ampicillin	3.6
Rifampin	100
Nafcillin	594
Gentamicin	0.6–0.96
Cephalothin	22
Erythromycin	4
Lincomycin	8–15
Clindamycin	6–15
Chloramphenicol	2
Chlortetracycline	3.5

Modified from Sabath LD: Pharmacology of antibiotics used in infection of the biliary tree. International Workshop, Biliary Infections. Darmstadt, Dietrich Steinkopff Verlag, 1977.

TABLE 18-11. CONCENTRATION OF VARIOUS ANTIBIOTICS IN BONE AFTER PARENTERAL ADMINISTRATION

Antibiotic	Approximate Bone/Serum Concentration Ratio
PENICILLINS	
Penicillin G	Not evaluable
Methicillin	0.2
Oxacillin	<0.1
Carbenicillin	0.12
Dicloxacillin	0.15
CEPHALOSPORINS	
Cephalothin	0.3(0–100)
Cefazolin	0.2–0.4
Cephradine	0.5
LINCOMYCIN	0.15
CLINDAMYCIN	0.2–0.4
AMINOGLYCOSIDES	
Gentamicin	0.2
OTHER ANTIBIOTICS	
Rifampin	0.15

Adapted from Waldvogel FA, Vasey H: Osteomyelitis: the past decade. *N Engl J Med* 303:360, 1980.

A separate problem is whether, after penetration and concentration, an antibiotic can retain antimicrobial efficacy under the conditions of pH and low redox potential and high concentration of both microbial and mammalian tissue products. Metronidazole and clindamycin both penetrate and retain antimicrobial potency in such environments.[15] The apparent failure of the penicillins and cephalosporins to penetrate may be related to the concurrent presence within the abscess of beta-lactamase, which inactivates the antibiotic. The newer beta-lactamase-resistant cephalosporins (cefoxitin and moxalactam) appear not to penetrate but are effective in sterilizing abscesses.[16] Chloramphenicol can penetrate an abscess [17] but can be inactivated in vivo by organisms (eg, *B. fragilis*) which are usually sensitive to it, so that treatment failure is common.

It is possible that the ability of antibiotics to penetrate and be concentrated in abscesses is related to their ability to be concentrated in leukocytes. Rifampin has the ability to be concentrated in neutrophils, and clindamycin becomes concentrated in alveolar macrophages.[18]

Using Topical Antibiotics to Achieve High Local Concentrations in Tissue

The unpredictability of antibiotic penetration into injured or inflamed tissues has led to the use of antibiotics and antiseptics topically in both fresh and inflamed wounds. In the former circumstance, topical antibiotics have been shown to be highly effective agents in the prophylaxis of experimental wound infection.[19] There are also a few randomized controlled studies to support their use in contaminated wounds. Brokenbrough and Moylan [20] found that local application of kanamycin significantly reduced wound infections in emergency exploratory laparotomies. Rickett and Jackson [21] showed similar results for topical ampicillin powder in appendicitis. The aminoglycosides have the advantage of prompt bactericidal activity, but their toxicity is a severe limitation to their topical use. The beta-lactam antibiotics are quite safe, but require prolonged contact; thus, they should be used topically throughout the operation rather than at its termination. Topical antiseptics, including povidone-iodine, are probably too tissue-toxic to be used routinely. The local and systemic prophylactic use of antibiotics is discussed in Chapter 23. No direct comparison between topical and systemic drug use has been made.[19] Topical prophylaxis should have the theoretical advantage of high local concentration (with its expansion of spectrum), low systemic toxicity, and minimal pressure for the development of microbial resistance.

In deep infections, however, topical antibiotics can generally provide only surface decontamination because penetration is poor. The exceptions include the special formulation of sulfanomides which are known to penetrate burn eschar.

USE OF ANTIBIOTICS IN COMBINATION

The indications for the simultaneous use of two or more antibiotics are listed in Table 18-12.[3] In general surgical practice, the major reasons to consider the combinations are mixed infections or fulminating infections, caused by unknown organisms, which will require empiric treatment before definitive identification of the causative bacteria. The most common circumstance exists when a mucosal barrier has been breached to cause soft tissue or intra-abdominal infections with mixtures of bacteria from the alimentary tract or female genital tract. Under these circumstances, anaerobic organisms are frequently present in combination with facultative gram-positive cocci and gram-negative bacilli. Although newer cephalosporin and penicillin derivatives may encompass the entire spectrum, combinations are frequently selected for breadth of spectrum. Table 18-13 lists the gaps in the antimicrobial spectrum of combinations that are frequently used by surgeons

TABLE 18-12. POSSIBLE INDICATIONS FOR USE OF ANTIBIOTICS IN COMBINATION

1. Mixed infection by two or more organisms not susceptible to a single antibiotic
2. Two different infections not treatable by a single antibiotic
3. Fulminating infection, but organism or its sensitivity not known
4. Delay emergence of resistant organisms
5. Achieve additive or synergistic effect required for adequate therapy
6. Reduce possibility of toxicity (by using lower dosage of components with different modes of toxicity)

Adapted from Sabath LD: Use of antibiotics in obstetrics. In Charles D, Finland M (eds.): *Obstetric and Perinatal Infections.* Philadelphia, Lea and Febiger, 1973, pp 563–623.

TABLE 18-13. ANTIMICROBIAL "GAPS" IN ANTIBIOTIC COMBINATIONS

Combination	Organisms Not Adequately Covered
Penicillin, chloramphenicol	*Pseudomonas,* some staphylococci
Penicillin, aminoglycoside	Some *Pseudomonas, B. fragilis*
Carbenicillin, aminoglycoside	Enterococci
Cephalothin, chloramphenicol	*Pseudomonas,* Enterococci
Cephalothin, aminoglycoside	Enterococci, *B. fragilis*
Ampicillin, aminoglycoside	*B. fragilis*
Ampicillin, clindamycin	Many gram-negative enteric, *Pseudomonas, Serratia*
Cefoxitin, clindamycin	Some gram-negative enteric, *Pseudomonas*
Clindamycin, aminoglycoside	Enterococci, some *Clostridium* spp.
Cephalothin, aminoglycoside, clindamycin	Enterococci
Ampicillin, aminoglycoside, clindamycin	Rare gaps

before they receive culture results. Because of these gaps, most of these combinations are poor empiric choices for serious intraperitoneal or pelvic sepsis.

The rationale of the first three indications for the use of antibiotics in combination (Table 18-12) is obvious. The fourth reason—to prevent the emergence of resistant organisms—has its greatest application in the treatment of active tuberculosis, for which a single drug should never be used. Similarly, neither rifampin nor flucytosine should be used alone, because resistant organisms readily arise.

Synergy and Antagonism in Antibiotic Combinations

Antibiotic combinations are often used to achieve an additive or synergistic effect in the treatment of a severe infection. In truth, there is evidence in favor of synergism in only a few infections (Table 18-14).[22] The traditional example is treatment of endocarditis, especially that due to group D streptococci (enterococci). Penicillin seems to enhance the uptake of aminoglycosides by enterococci, resulting in enhanced killing. More recently, a combination of trimethoprim plus sulfamethoxazole has proved to be synergistic against many gram-positive and gram-negative organisms by interfering at different points in the folic acid metabolic pathway.[23]

Jawetz law is only a crude guide to thinking about the effect of antibiotic combinations: (1) bacteriostatic plus bacteriostatic drugs are usually additive; (2) bactericidal plus bactericidal drugs *may* be synergistic; and (3) bactericidal plus bacteriostatic drugs *may* be antagonistic (Table 18-15). One exception to these rules is the finding that two bactericidal drugs, carbenicillin and aminoglycosides, may be antagonistic, with the former chemically inactivating the latter.[24] This fact has little clinical importance, however, and such combinations actually show synergistic activity against *P. aeruginosa.* Although it is easy to show in the laboratory that a bacteriostatic drug (such as chloramphenicol) can antagonize the bactericidal effect of a penicillin, such an effect is less easily demonstrable in people. Similarly, in vitro antagonism between chloramphenicol and the aminoglycosides (because of their competition for ribosome binding sites) is rarely of clinical importance. Nevertheless, the fact that the combined use of antibiotics may result in antagonism should always be kept in mind (Table 18-15).

TABLE 18-14. ANTIBIOTIC COMBINATIONS CLAIMED TO BE CLINICALLY ADDITIVE OR SYNERGISTIC

Useful Combinations	Additive or Synergistic Against
Penicillin plus aminoglycoside	Synergy against enterococcal endocarditis, *S. viridans, S. aureus, L. monocytogenes,* and gram-negative bacilli
Carbenicillin plus gentamicin or tobramycin	*Pseudomonas aeruginosa*
Ampicillin plus gentamicin	Enterococcus, *Listeria*
Nafcillin plus gentamicin	*Staphylococcus,* Enterococcus
Penicillin plus clavulanic acid	Some penicillinase-producing bacteria
Penicillin plus clindamycin	*Clostridium*
Penicillins plus rifampin	*Staphylococcus*
Rifampin plus co-trimoxazole	Resistant urinary tract pathogens
Amphotericin B plus flucytosine	*Cryptococcus, Candida*
Trimethoprim plus sulfamethoxazole	Synergistic by inhibiting sequential steps in folic acid metabolism
Trimethoprim plus sulfamethoxazole plus polymyxin B	Synergy against gram-negative bacilli

Modified from Rahal JJ Jr: Antibiotic combinations: the clinical relevance of synergy and antagonism. *Medicine* 57:179, 1978.

TABLE 18-15. ANTIBIOTIC COMBINATIONS CLAIMED TO BE ANTAGONISTIC

Antibiotic Combinations	Against
Aminoglycosides plus tetracycline or chloramphenicol	Antagonism of the aminoglycoside against gram-negative bacilli. Most pronounced in neutropenia. Mechanism: inhibition of cellular penetration by aminoglycoside
Erythromycin plus chloramphenicol	Antagonism of activity against staphylococci and streptococci
Penicillin plus tetracycline	Antagonism of penicillin in streptococcal and pneumococcal infections
Penicillin plus chloramphenicol	Antagonism of penicillin effect on pneumococcus, *Streptococcus, Klebsiella.* No antagonism occurs when penicillin concentrations are high. No antagonism when ampicillin and chloramphenicol are combined to treat *Hemophilus* and pneumococcal meningitis, or brain abscess

Modified from Rahal JJ Jr: Antibiotic combinations: the clinical relevance of synergy and antagonism. *Medicine* 57:179, 1978.

Various combinations of antibiotics seem to be more effective in treating sepsis in immunocompromised patients—especially those with neutropenia produced by cytotoxic cancer chemotherapy. Combinations were first used in these patients primarily because neither the organism nor its sensitivity was known. There is evidence, however, that combinations of bactericidal drugs are more effective in inhibiting bacteria sensitive to both.[25]

Reduction of Toxicity

Theoretically, it would be an excellent idea to use antibiotics A and B together at half their usual doses if their actions were additive and their toxicities were for different organs (Table 18-12). The rationale for the use of triple sulfas (a combination of equal amounts) was essentially that—their antibacterial actions were additive, and the major toxicity of each was crystalluria caused by the relative insolubility of each component and its products. By using one-third the usual dose of each, it was possible to get the desired antibacterial effect with a much smaller chance of exceeding the solubility of each (which did not interfere with the solubility of the others). The introduction of highly soluble sulfonamides (eg, sulfisoxazole) has made it unnecessary to use triple sulfas in urinary tract infections. Triple sulfas are still preferred, however, to sulfisoxazole for tissue infections.

USE OF ANTIBIOTICS FOR PROPHYLAXIS

There is enormous controversy over many of the prophylactic uses of antibacterial agents.[26] The most common use is essentially unchallenged—the instillation of 1 percent silver nitrate (or more rarely, an antigonococcal antibiotic) into the eye of the newborn to prevent gonococcal ophthalmia neonatorum.

The concept of using essentially harmless drugs for a few days to prevent enormous morbidity or even mortality seems attractive enough, and the belief that it is easier to treat an incipient disease than a well-established one seems sound. Unfortunately, the potential harm—sometimes substantial—that may result from the use of any drug must be recognized.

In general, there are two major objections to antibiotic prophylaxis: (1) evidence of real benefit is often lacking, and (2) no regimen eradicates all organisms. Almost all regimens alter the host flora to the extent that the infections that eventually occur are caused by organisms that are much more difficult to treat because they are resistant not only to the antibiotics used for prophylaxis but usually to many others as well.

The conservative advice is: (1) to use antibiotics for prophylaxis only when they are known to be of value, (2) not to initiate prophylaxis too far in advance of the event (eg, operation) for which prophylaxis is desired (1 to several hours is usually plenty of time) to avoid replacing the normal flora with a resistant flora, (3) not to continue prophylaxis for longer than necessary, and (4) to use appropriate doses when prophylaxis has been decided upon (the most common error is to use too small a dose). The prophylactic use of antibiotics against the danger of wound infections is discussed in Chapter 23. A list of situations for which the prophylactic use of antibiotics has been widely accepted appears in Table 18-16.[25] Newer indications are appearing almost daily.

THE USE OF ANTIBIOTICS IN PATIENTS WITH HEPATIC AND RENAL FAILURE

Hepatic Failure

Although numerous antibiotics are partially excreted via the hepatobiliary system (Table 18-10), and some are primarily metabolized by the liver (tetracycline, chloramphenicol, sulfonamides, p-aminosulfonic acid, isoniazid), there are few data about how these antibiotics should be used—or avoided—in patients with abnormalities of the hepatobiliary system. A summary of reasonable practices appears in Table 18-17. Because penicillins, cephalosporins, and aminoglycosides are excreted mainly by the kidneys and have low direct toxicity, there is no reason to decrease their dosage in patients with liver disease. Although one would expect that chloramphenicol, lincomycin, clindamycin, and erythromycin would accumulate in patients with obstructive or hepatocellular disease, the evidence is lacking. Initially, therefore, it would seem advisable to use normal doses of these antibiotics in such patients (if reasonable alternative antibiotics are not likely to be effective), but to measure serum or plasma concentrations every 3 to 7 days, and to reduce doses if excessive concentrations are present.

TABLE 18-16. PROVED INDICATIONS FOR SYSTEMIC ANTIMICROBIAL PROPHYLAXIS

	Agent
SURGICAL OPERATION	
Vaginal hysterectomy	Cephalosporin
Abdominal hysterectomy	Cephalosporin
High-risk cesarean section	Cephalosporin
Elective colorectal surgery	Cephalosporin (parenteral), erythromycin-neomycin or kanamycin-metronidazole (oral)
Coronary bypass surgery	Penicillinase-resistant penicillin
Vascular prosthetic grafts	Cephalosporin
Cardiac prosthetic implants	Cephalosporin
Total hip replacement	Cephalosporin
Head and neck cancer surgery	Cephalosporin
High-risk gastric and biliary surgery	Cephalosporin
After splenectomy	Penicillin
MEDICAL INDICATIONS	
Travelers' diarrhea	Doxyclycline
Pneumocystis carinii infection	Trimethoprim-sulfamethoxazole
Recurrent urinary tract infections in women	Trimethoprim-sulfamethoxazole
Dental manipulation in patients with valvular heart disease	Penicillin plus aminoglycoside
Rheumatic fever	Penicillin
Malaria (chloroquine sensitive)	Chloroquine
Tuberculosis in PPD converters	Isoniazid

TABLE 18-17. USE OF ANTIBIOTICS IN PATIENTS WITH SEVERE HEPATIC FAILURE OR CHOLESTASIS

Avoid, if possible
- Sulfonamides
- Novobiocin
- Pyrazinamide
- Tetracycline

Reduce dosage if prolonged (> 3 days) use necessary
- Lincomycin (perhaps half normal dose after 2–3 days)
- Clindamycin (perhaps half normal dose after 2–3 days)
- Chloramphenicol (probably no more than 2 gm/day)
- Erythromycin * (perhaps half normal dose after 2–3 days)

No change in normal dosage

Penicillins	Amphotericin B
Polymyxin B	p-aminosulforic acid
Colistin	Isoniazid †
Vancomycin	Cycloserine
Nitrofurantoin	Ethambutal
	Rifampin †

* Some advocate avoiding estolate in hepatic disease, but evidence is lacking unless the hepatic disease is estolate-induced allergic hepatitis.

† Can worsen liver problems.

Adapted from Sabath LD: Use of antibiotics in obstetrics. In Charles D, Finland M (eds.): *Obstetric and Perinatal Infections.* Philadelphia, Lea and Febiger, 1973, pp 563–623.

Renal Failure

Antibiotics normally excreted primarily by the kidneys accumulate in the sera of patients with impaired renal function. The dosage should, therefore, be reduced or the interval between doses should be lengthened. There are many schedules that detail how to estimate dosage of antibiotics normally excreted by the kidneys [27] but all such compendia, including that shown in Table 18-18, are unreliable. One must not use the data in Table 18-18 without frequently obtaining direct measurements of serum or plasma antibiotic concentrations to verify that the appropriate doses are being administered. The obvious dangers to the patient of too little antibiotic (leaving the infection virtually untreated) or too much (possibly resulting in toxicity to the kidneys, and often to the 8th nerve) are much greater than the cost of obtaining frequent antibiotic determinations.

The general approach to antibiotic usage in patients with renal failure is to give a first dose of 80 to 100 percent the usual amount and then to estimate the timing and amount of the second dose according to the schedule in Table 18-18. Peak levels (1½ to 2 hours after the second intramuscular dose or immediately at the end of the second intravenous dose) should be taken, and the third dose can be adjusted (regarding timing and amount) on the basis of the results. In patients with severe infections and rapidly changing renal function, it may be advisable to assay peak serum concentrations once daily after injection of an antibiotic. In less severely ill patients, or in those with stable renal function, only one or two assays may be required. Trough concentrations may help detect incipient toxicity.

Anuric patients or those in whom the creatinine clearance is less than 10 ml per minute will invariably have toxic serum or plasma levels of aminoglycosides if they continue to receive average doses for 24 hours; the second dose must be tailored to individual requirements. Although such patients can usually be prevented from receiving toxic concentrations of antibiotic by being given half the usual dose every half-life of the antibiotic, patients with long antibiotic half-lives (greater than 24 hours) should receive somewhat smaller doses more frequently to keep serum or plasma concentrations above required inhibitory levels. This is especially desirable if there is a life-threatening infection, when it would seem inadvisable to have the patient go many hours with antibiotic concentrations well below the concentration required to inhibit the infecting organism.

Recently, a computer-assisted pharmacokinetic technique has been developed for determining the proper dose of the aminoglycosides in patients with compromised renal function. This technique requires three levels—peak, trough, and a value intermediate in time—to graph the elimination of the agent and predict the next dose. Use of this technique should permit precise dosages, which ensure adequate therapeutic levels without toxicity.[28]

Table 18-19 [27] lists those antibiotics which are cleared by peritoneal dialysis or hemodialysis. One cannot empha-

TABLE 18-18. A GUIDE TO USE OF ANTIBIOTICS IN PATIENTS WITH RENAL FAILURE *

Antibiotic	Serum Creatinine <1.5 mg%	Creatinine Clearance 10–35 ml/min. Serum Creatinine 1.5–10 mg %	Creatinine Clearance <10 ml/min. Serum Creatinine >10 mg%
NO REDUCTION (or minimal)			
Chloramphenicol			
Erythromycin			
Clindamycin			
Lincomycin			
Isoniazid			
Doxyclycline			
Nalidixic acid			
Rifampin			
Amphotericin B			
Nafcillin			
MAJOR REDUCTION *			
Demethylchlortetracycline	0.3 gm q6h po	0.15 gm q12–24h	0.15 gm q36–48h
Gentamicin or tobramycin †	1.0–1.6 mg/kg q8h IM, IV	0.8 mg/kg q16–36h	0.8 mg/kg q36–48h
Kanamycin or amikacin †	7.5 mg/kg q12h IM, IV	4 mg/kg q18–48h	7.5 mg/kg q2–4d
Streptomycin	0.5 gm q6–12h IM	0.5 gm q36–48h or 0.25 gm q18–24h	0.5 gm q72h or 0.25 gm q36h
Tetracycline	0.5 gm q6h po 8 mg/kg q6h IV	0.5 gm q24–48h or 0.25 gm q12–24h	0.5 gm q3–4d 0.25 gm q36–48h
Vancomycin	7 mg/kg q6h IV 14 mg/kg q12h IV	7 mg/kg q24–48h	7 mg/kg q3–4d or 3.5 mg/kg q36–48h
MODERATE REDUCTION			
Carbenicillin and ticarcillin	1.0–1.25 gm/hr IV	1.0 gm q2–4h	2.0 gm q8–12h
Cephalothin (and other cephalosporins)	0.5–2.0 gm/4 hr IV	0.5–2 gm q6–8h	0.5–2.0 gm q24h
Benzylpenicillin	to 1–4 Mu/2 hr IV	to 1–4 Mu q5–12h	to 1–4 Mu q24h
AVOID (in renal failure)			
Cephaloridine			
Bacitracin			
Chlortetracycline			
Nitrofurantoin			
Methenamine			
Para-aminosalicyclic acid			
Long-acting sulfonamides			

* Recommended Dosage for Adult (70 kg).
† Frequent assay of serum or plasma antibiotic concentration is recommended in all patients with serious infections when reduced doses are contemplated. First dose should always be 80 to 100% normal dose, regardless of renal function; subsequent doses are determined by schedule and on basis of assay data.

Adapted from Sabath LD: Use of antibiotics in obstetrics. In Charles D, Finland M (eds.): *Obstetric and Perinatal Infections.* Philadelphia, Lea and Febiger, 1973, pp 563–623; and Sabath LD: Body distribution of antibiotics. *J Surg Prac* 8:56, 1979.

size too vigorously the admonition that patients can be managed only by frequent determination of their serum drug levels.

ALLERGY TO ANTIBACTERIAL AGENTS

All antibiotics have been accused of initiating allergic reactions. Persistence or recurrence of fever in a patient whose infection has been controlled as indicated by all other clinical criteria should always be considered a possible manifestation of allergy to the antibiotics. The problem is obviously complicated in patients who are receiving multiple drugs if several are common causes of allergic reactions. In such circumstances, all drugs should be stopped if the condition permits. After the putative allergic signs or symptoms have subsided, the drugs are instituted (over a period of days) one at a time until the offending agent is identified (unless the possible consequences are unacceptable).

It is far better to avoid an allergic reaction than to encounter it. Avoidance is best done by eliciting a medical history of previous adverse reactions. Obviously, the primary allergic response cannot be anticipated by history taking.

A safe test, which would help detect the allergy-prone patient before the antibiotic is used, is obviously desirable. Despite encouraging early reports that in vivo or in vitro tests would identify patients allergic to penicillin, no reliable clinically applicable test is currently available. Many experts in infectious diseases use only the patient's statement as a means of detecting penicillin allergy.

TABLE 18-19. ANTIMICROBIAL AGENTS REMOVED BY HEMODIALYSIS OR PERITONEAL DIALYSIS

Antifungal Agents	Hemodialysis	Peritoneal Dialysis
Amphotericin B	No	No
Aminoglycosides (all)	Yes	Yes
Cephalosporins (all)	Yes	Yes
Chloramphenicol	Yes	No
Clindamycin	No	No
Erythromycin	No	No
Flucytosine	Yes	Yes
Metronidazole	Yes	No
Penicillins		
Penicillin G	Yes	No
Ampicillin-amoxacillin	Yes	No
Carbenicillin-ticarcillin	Yes	Yes
Beta-lactamase-resistant penicillins	No	No
Sulfonamides (including co-trimoxazole)	Yes	Yes
Tetracyclines	No	No
Vancomycin	No	No

Adapted from Bennett WM, Mutner RS, Parker RA, Feig P, Morrison G, Golper TA, Singer I: Drug therapy in renal failure: dosing guideline for adults. *Ann Intern Med* 93:62, 1980.

Penicillin Allergy

Penicillin allergy occurs in about 3 percent of the population, and is most commonly of the delayed type (fever, erythema, urticaria, rash, arthritis), which rarely causes significant morbidity or mortality. A majority of patients with documented histories of previous delayed reactions to penicillin G can receive it again without any adverse response, and it is rare for such patients to develop immediate anaphylactic-type reactions. Nonetheless, patients with previous delayed reactions should receive therapy with unrelated compounds whenever possible. Erythromycin is adequate for many infections of moderate severity (pneumococcal pneumonia or streptococcal pharyngitis) but not for life-threatening infections (eg, endocarditis), which require bactericidal drugs. The use of (1) a completely unrelated antibiotic (eg, vancomycin), (2) a cephalosporin (our usual custom, except in enterococcal endocarditis), and (3) penicillin have been successful. Although antihistamines plus steroids are sometimes required to suppress the allergy, there is usually no adverse effect. Although delayed allergy to penicillin is almost never fatal, inadequately treated endocarditis always is.

After there has been an immediate (anaphylactic) reaction to a penicillin, all penicillins and cephalosporins must be avoided. Although the matter of "cross allergenicity" between penicillins and cephalosporins is unsettled, most investigators agree that there is cross allergenicity among the penicillins.

Ampicillin appears to be in a class by itself. Rashes that appear after its use occur much more frequently than after benzylpenicillin [29]—in some series at a frequency greater than 20 percent.[30] There appears to be some relationship between dose of ampicillin and frequency of rashes—more rashes occur after the administration of larger doses.[30] Some think that these reactions are not true reflections of penicillin allergy.

If penicillin or cephalosporin is to be given to someone who has had a previous adverse reaction, 1:1000 aqueous epinephrine should be drawn into a syringe, and a tourniquet should be available at the bedside when the first dose is given. The treatment of anaphylaxis for any other drug includes the following procedures.

1. Inject (deep IM, or IV over 15–30 seconds) 0.5 ml of a 1:1000 dilution of aqueous epinephrine, and repeat with 0.25 ml 3–5 minutes later if immediate improvement does not occur.
2. Be sure there is adequate pulmonary ventilation. Insert an endotracheal tube, if available, or perform an emergency tracheotomy if laryngospasm occurs. Assist respiration, if necessary, with bag breathing, respirator, or mouth-to-mouth breathing if other equipment is not at hand. A mouth gag should be available.
3. Follow blood pressure. With the patient lying down, elevate feet if the blood pressure falls.
4. If arterial pulses disappear, perform closed heart massage.
5. Do not give steroids and antihistamines. Although they are often given, they probably have no effect until well after the true emergency is over.[31]
6. Inform the patient of the event, and conspicuously label his or her records. Most patients will recover.

Chloramphenicol Reactions

Although penicillin allergy is the most frequent antibiotic allergy, it is rarely a catastrophe. In contrast, allergic or idiosyncratic reactions to chloramphenicol may lead to irreversibly fatal aplastic anemia. Fortunately, the incidence is only one per 30,000 or more courses of therapy.

Other Allergies

Two other characteristic allergic reactions to antimicrobial agents are (1) bullous eruptions (fortunately rare) following the use of sulfonamides, which can develop to a fatal Stevens-Johnson syndrome, and (2) cholestatic jaundice associated with use of the esters of erythromycin, which is reversible after stopping use of the drug.[32] Sometimes, there is also right upper quadrant tenderness and fever, which simulate acute cholecystitis.[32]

Any of the antibiotics is capable of producing fever or rashes, neither of which is diagnostic.

SPECIAL PROBLEMS IN ANTIBIOTIC ADMINISTRATION

Age

Penicillin Absorption

The gastrointestinal absorption of antimicrobial agents partly depends on their acid stability in the stomach. The oral absorption of penicillin G is reduced by gastric acid, but adequate levels can be achieved in children and in elderly patients who have reduced gastric acid secretion. Penicillin V is not necessary in these patients.

Renal Function

The serum half-lives of drugs primarily excreted by the kidneys are increased in neonates and the elderly. The doses of many antimicrobial agents must therefore be altered (Table 18-18). Failure to take these facts into consideration will increase antimicrobial toxicity.

Both nephrotoxic reactions and true hypersensitivity reactions to these drugs are more common in the elderly. In part, these reactions are due to declining renal function in the elderly, which is aggravated by secondary drug-induced nephrotoxicity. Prior exposure may sensitize older patients to previously received antibiotics.

Hepatic Function in the Neonate

The neonatal liver is underdeveloped. Chloramphenicol is normally conjugated to the inactive glucuronide form in the liver, but neonatal hepatic levels of glucuronyl transferase are insufficient. High levels of unconjugated chloramphenicol can produce shock, cardiovascular collapse, and death (the gray syndrome).[33] For this reason, chloramphenicol can be safely administered only in reduced dosage.[33]

Sulfonamides should not be given to neonates, because the sulfonamides compete with bilirubin for binding sites on serum albumin. Kernicterus can be induced by increased serum levels of unbound bilirubin. A similar problem may follow the use of novobiocin, which inhibits hepatic glucuronyl transferase, which normally conjugates bilirubin.

Hepatic toxicity caused by isoniazid increases with age, apparently the result of poorly defined abnormalities in the livers of older patients. For this reason, prophylactic isoniazid should not be given to patients older than 35 who have had positive tuberculin test results, unless they have recently converted.[34]

Tetracyclines should be avoided in young children because the tetracyclines bind to developing teeth (resulting in stained teeth) and bone.

Pregnancy

Tetracycline should also be avoided in pregnancy, not only because of its adverse effects on fetal dentition, but also because pregnant women appear to be vulnerable to the hepatotoxic effects.[35]

Pregnancy poses certain problems for the administration of any drug. For example, all suspected teratogenic drugs should be avoided. Metronidazole and ticarcillin are teratogenic in rodents, and the teratogenic potential of many other antibiotics has not been ruled out.

It is possible that antimicrobial clearance is greater during pregnancy, so that the doses may need to be revised upward. Although this is clear for ampicillin, data on other antimicrobial agents is not available.

Most antimicrobial agents appear in breast milk in low concentration. Sulfonamides in breast milk may be dangerous to premature babies, because they predispose the child to kernicterus. Nalidixic acid and the sulfonamides in breast milk can cause hemolysis in infants with glucose-6 phosphate-dehydrogenase deficiency.[36]

DRUG INCOMPATIBILITIES

Antibiotics should not be mixed with other drugs in syringes or intravenous bottles. Some incompatible drug combinations form insoluble precipitates, which inactivate the antibiotic—other combinations inactivate one another without forming a distinctive precipitate. In other instances, one drug may antagonize the action of a second, or prolong or shorten the duration of the activity, leading to serious problems of apparent over- or underdosage.

Another important problem is drug instability in solution. This most commonly occurs with penicillins, which are shipped as dry powders for parenteral use. If the drug is dissolved many hours in advance, there may be significant deterioration of activity before or during administration—if given over many hours. Instability is a well-documented problem for methicillin (which is unstable in acidic fluids) dissolved in saline or other unbuffered fluids with low pH, and most penicillins in fluids that contain carbohydrate. Most of these problems can be avoided by dissolving the penicillin immediately before use, and making up no more than will be given over the next 1 to 2 hours. The pH of fluids that contain methicillin should be checked and adjusted to approximately 7.0 with sterile $NaHCO_3$. Table 18-20 is a list of the more important antibiotic drug incompatibilities.[37] Of particular note are the increased toxicity of drugs normally metabolized in the liver (warfarin, barbiturates, tolbutamide, phenytoin) when combined with antibiotics that are also metabolized in the liver (chloramphenicol, sulfonamides, INH, rifampin). Alternatively, these drugs may induce microsomal enzymes (tolbutamide, oral contraceptives), which then reduce the effectiveness of the drug by accelerating its metabolism.

ANTIBACTERIAL AGENTS

PENICILLINS

Chemistry

Benzylpenicillin (penicillin G) is produced by strains of *Aspergillus* and *Penicillium* (particularly *P. notatum* and *P. chrysogenum*). Fleming first isolated penicillin in 1929, but not until 1941 did it come into clinical use. Chemical modification of the basic penicillin structure has dramatically altered the pharmacokinetic and antibacterial properties (Fig. 18-1).

Pharmacology

Penicillin V, ampicillin, amoxicillin, and cyclacillin are well absorbed from the gastrointestinal tract, whereas the other penicillins are degraded by the acidic environment of the stomach. Penicillins given intravenously immediately reach high blood levels and are distributed quickly to most body compartments, including interstitial fluid, bone, and placenta. Ampicillin penetrates best into the cerebrospinal fluid, achieving about 50 percent of the blood level when the meninges are inflamed. Because the penicillins are excreted unchanged by rapid glomerular filtration and tubular secretion (average half-life of 0.5–1.5 hours), they

TABLE 18-20. COMMON ANTIBIOTIC-DRUG INTERACTIONS

Antimicrobial Agent	Interacting Drug	Comment
Aminoglycosides	Neuromuscular blockers (ie, tubocurarine, pancuronium)	Additive blockade
	Ototoxins (ie, ethacrynic acid, furosemide)	Increased incidence of reactions
	Nephrotoxins (ie, amphotericin B, vancomycin)	Increased incidence of reactions
	Carbenicillin/ticarcillin (other penicillins or cephalosporins)	Acid-base reaction when mixed
Ampicillin/amoxicillin	Allopurinol	Skin rash
Chloramphenicol	Warfarin	Decreased warfarin metabolism and inhibition of vitamin K-producing gut bacteria, thus increased prothrombin time
	Phenytoin	Decreased phenytoin metabolism (levels increase)
Isoniazid	Warfarin, phenytoin	Increased risk of toxicity by decreased drug metabolism
	Rifampin, PAS	Additive hepatotoxicity
	Oral contraceptives	Decreased contraceptive effect
Metronidazole	Alcohol	Disulfiram-like reaction (nausea, vomiting)
Rifampin	Warfarin, phenytoin	Increased risk of toxicity by decreasing drug metabolism
	Isoniazid, PAS	Additive hepatotoxicity
	Oral contraceptives	Decreased contraceptive effect
Sulfonamides	Warfarin, phenytoin	Displaces drugs from protein-binding sites causing increased warfarin and phenytoin effects
Tetracyclines	Antacids, oral iron	Interferes with absorption

Modified from Hansten P: *Drug Interactions*. Philadelphia, Lea & Febiger, 4th ed, 1979.

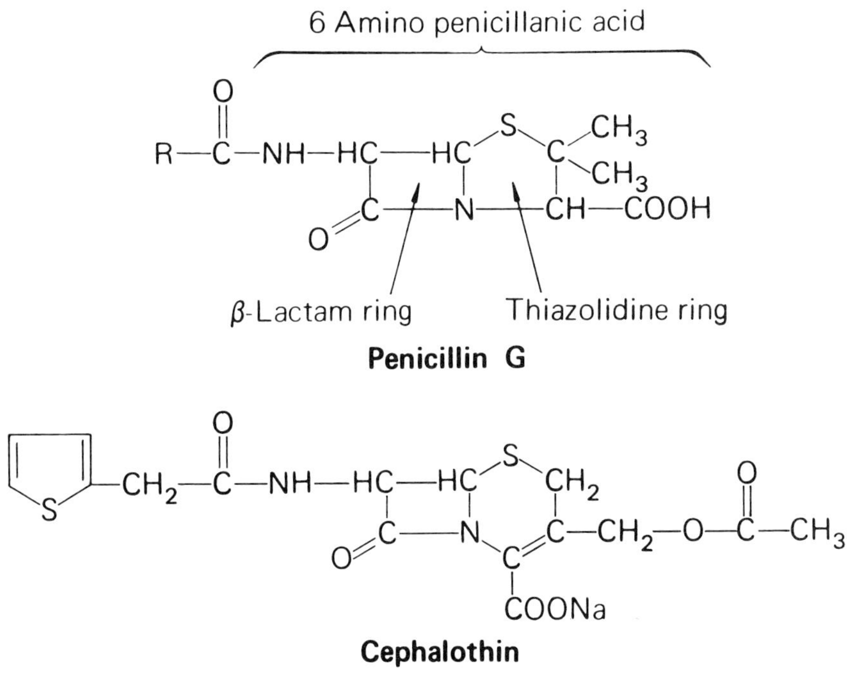

6 Amino penicillanic acid

β-Lactam ring

Thiazolidine ring

Penicillin G

Cephalothin

Fig. 18-1. Structure of beta-lactam antibiotics. (From Pratt WB: The inhibitors of cell wall synthesis. In Pratt WB: *Chemotherapy of Infection*. New York, Oxford Univ. Press, 1977, p 22.)

TABLE 18-21. ANTIMICROBIAL SPECTRUM OF THE PENICILLINS

Organism	"Natural" Penicillins: Penicillin G, Penicillin V	Penicillinase Resistant: Methicillin, Nafcillin, Oxacillin, Cloxacillin, Dicloxacillin	"Broad-Spectrum" Penicillins — Aminopenicillins: Ampicillin, Amoxicillin	"Broad-Spectrum" Penicillins — Carbenicillin, Ticarcillin
GRAM-POSITIVE COCCI				
S. aureus (penicillin-sensitive)	+++	+++	+++	+++
S. aureus (penicillin resistant)	−	+++	−	−
S. epidermidis	−	++	−	−
S. pyogenes	+++	++	+++	+++
Pneumococcus	+++	++	+++	+++
Enterococcus	+	±	++	±
GRAM-NEGATIVE COCCI				
Meningococcus	+++	+	+++	+++
Gonococcus	+++ (not pen V+)	+	+++	++
GRAM-POSITIVE RODS				
C. diphtheriae	+++	?	+++	?
GRAM-NEGATIVE RODS				
E. coli	±	−	++	++
Klebsiella	−	−	−	−
Enterobacter	−	−	−	±
P. mirabilis	+/++	−	+++	+++
Other *Proteus*	−	−	−	±
Pseudomonas	−	−	−	++
Serratia	−	−	−	−
H. influenzae	+	±	++	++
ANAEROBES				
B. fragilis	±	−	−	++
Clostridium	+++	++	+++	+++
Anaerobic cocci	+++	++	+++	+++
Listeria	++	?	++	++

+++ = highly susceptible; ++ = moderately susceptible; + = weakly susceptible; minus sign = resistant.

Adapted from Barza M, Weinstein L: Pharmacokinetics of the penicillins in man. *Clin Pharmacokinet* 1:297, 1976.

must be administered every 4 to 6 hours to maintain effective blood levels. Dosage of all penicillins, except nafcillin, should be somewhat decreased in patients with impaired renal function—nafcillin is cleared by the liver (Table 18-18). Most penicillins are secreted into bile in amounts exceeding serum concentrations. Nafcillin achieves greater than 100 times the serum level in bile, and penicillin G and ampicillin as much as ten times.[38] When penicillin G is given intramuscularly as a procaine or benzathine suspension, low peak levels are achieved but with sustained antibacterial activity (48 hours and 2 to 4 weeks respectively).

Antimicrobial Spectrum and Clinical Uses

The penicillins have antibacterial activity against most gram-positive, gram-negative, and anaerobic organisms. Table 18-21 lists the usual spectrum for each of the penicillins. Sensitivity is so variable, however, that it is important to know the antibiotic sensitivity pattern for each organism in one's own institution and area of practice.

Table 18-22 [39] summarizes the specific infections for which penicillins should be used, either alone or in combination with other agents. Structural changes in the cephalosporins have made these agents as active as many penicillins, but with broader spectrums of antibacterial coverage. This must be considered when selecting antibiotic therapy, especially for surgical patients, who often have mixed infections that require a broader spectrum.

Penicillin G and V have limited bacterial coverage compared to the semisynthetic agents. The penicillinase-resistant penicillins are useful only in proved *S. aureus* infections, although they are moderately active against streptococci, pneumococci, and anaerobic cocci. All the penicillinase-resistant penicillins are similar; methicillin should be avoided, because it is likely to cause interstitial nephritis.

Ampicillin is active against most gram-positive cocci including enterococcus, except those *S. aureus* strains that produce penicillinase. Ampicillin kills three common

TABLE 18-22. MAJOR USES FOR THE PENICILLINS *

THERAPY OF CHOICE	PENICILLIN TYPE
Pneumococcal infections	Penicillin G
Staphylococcal infections	Penicillinase-resistant penicillin
Streptococcal infections	Penicillin G
S. viridans Endocarditis	Penicillin G with aminoglycoside
Enterococcal endocarditis	Penicillin G with aminoglycoside
Meningococcal infections	Penicillin G
Gonorrhea Uncomplicated genital	Penicillin G (or ampicillin)
Diphtheria	Penicillin G
Clostridial infections	Penicillin G
Actinomycosis	Penicillin G
Listeria infections	Penicillin G (or ampicillin)
Anthrax	Penicillin G
Shigellosis	Ampicillin
P. multocida	Penicillin G
Syphilis	Penicillin G
Aspiration pneumonia and lung abscess; oropharyngeal anaerobic infection	Penicillin G
EFFECTIVE ALTERNATIVE THERAPY	
Typhoid fever and other salmonellosis	Amoxacillin or ampicillin
H. influenzae infection	Ampicillin or amoxacillin
Pseudomonas infections	Ticarcillin or carbenicillin with aminoglycoside
PROPHYLAXIS	
Rheumatic fever	Penicillin V
Bacterial endocarditis	Penicillin G plus aminoglycoside

* See Table 18-2 for other less common penicillin indications.

Adapted from Barza M, Weinstein L: Pharmacokinetics of the penicillins in man. *Clin Pharmacokinetics* 1:297, 1976.

gram-negative rods—*H. influenzae, E. coli,* and *P. mirabilis*—but the rest are usually resistant.

Carbenicillin and ticarcillin have the broadest gram-positive antibacterial activity of the penicillins, killing most organisms except for penicillinase-producing staphylococcus and enterococcus. Carbenicillin and ticarcillin are also active against many gram-negative rods, including *Pseudomonas,* although *Klebsiella* and *Serratia* tend to be resistant. Anaerobic bacteria including *B. fragilis* and *Clostridium* are generally sensitive to either of these agents when large doses are given.

The newer investigational acylureido-penicillins, piperacillin, pirbenicillin, mezlocillin, aplocillin, and azlocillin are similar to carbenicillin and ticarcillin in antibacterial spectrum. They have greater antibacterial activity at similar dosage, especially against *P. aeruginosa,* but are still beta-lactamase sensitive.[40] Mecillinam and pivmecillinam are investigational amidopenicillins, which are similar to ampicillin and have potent activity against most gram-negative bacilli, with the important exception of *P. aeruginosa.* They are also less active against enterococcus.[41] Both are beta-lactamase sensitive.

Clavulanic acid, an inhibitor of most beta-lactamases, is being investigated in combination with penicillin for the treatment of infections by organisms that produce beta-lactamase. This important advance has application in both gram-positive and gram-negative infections.[42]

Adverse Reactions

Many adverse reactions to the penicillins have occurred, but they are rare considering the number of patients who receive these agents. Immediate anaphylactic reactions occur in less than 0.04 percent of penicillin-treated patients. Local reactions are the most common, including rash, swelling at injection site, gastritis, and diarrhea. Table 18-23 [43] summarizes the reported reactions to penicillins, including common (ie, diarrhea) and rare (ie, vasculitis).

Mechanisms of Antibacterial Action

Penicillins and cephalosporins appear to have similar mechanisms of antibacterial action—they alter bacterial cell wall synthesis. Specifically, they block multiple bacterial enzymes that the organism uses to build peptidoglycan polymers. They also block endopeptidase and glycosidase—enzymes that are needed to open free ends on the mucopeptide structure for further cell growth. Other actions have been described elsewhere.[44]

Mechanisms of Antibacterial Resistance

The synthesis of beta-lactamase by bacteria, which opens the beta-lactam ring, is the major mechanism of bacterial resistance. Bacteria also alter the cell wall enzymes to disrupt the effective interaction of the penicillins (see subsequent section on cephalosporin).

TABLE 18-23. REPORTED ADVERSE REACTIONS TO PENICILLINS

Reactions	Agent
Immediate anaphylaxis	All penicillins
Serum sickness	All penicillins
Rash (to exfolitive dermatitis)	All penicillins
Diarrhea (to antibiotic colitis)	All penicillins; more common with ampicillin
Hepatitis	Oxacillin, carbenicillin
Nephritis	All (methicillin)
Coomb positive hemolytic anemia	All
Pancytopenia	All
Thrombophlebitis	All
CNS changes (convulsions)	All
Platelet dysfunction	Carbenicillin, ticarcillin
Vasculitis	All
Superinfections	All
Hypokalemia	Carbenicillin, ticarcillin
Hypernatremia	Carbenicillin, ticarcillin
Hyperkalemia	Potassium penicillin G (1.7 mEq K^+/1 MU)

Modified from Kucers A, Bennett N: *The Use of Antibiotics. A Comprehensive Review with Clinical Emphasis,* 3rd ed. London, Heinemann, 1979.

By changing the cell wall structure, bacteria can block antibiotic penetration to the site of antibacterial action. Most resistant strains of gonococci appear to be developing resistance by this mechanism.[45]

Preparations and Doses

Table 18-24 lists the usual doses of the penicillins. The low toxicity of these drugs permits higher doses to be given in appropriate circumstances.

CEPHALOSPORINS

Chemistry

Most cephalosporins are derivatives of the fungus *Cephalosporium acremonium,* and the cephalomycins are derived from *Streptomyces* species. Cephalosporin C, the basic compound, resembles penicillin with a beta-lactam structure in which the five-member thiazolidine ring (characteristic of penicillin) is replaced by a six-member dihydrothiazine ring (Fig. 18-1). The antibacterial activity of this compound can be modified by substitutions at position 7 of the beta-lactam ring. Changes in pharmacokinetics and metabolic parameters are achieved by substitution at position 3 of the dehydrothiazine ring.[46]

Pharmacology

Table 18-25 lists the cephalosporins. All the oral agents are similar in pharmacology to cephalexin. Only one agent, cephradine, is effective by both parenteral and oral routes; most cephalosporins require parenteral administration. Except for moxalactam, none penetrate cerebrospinal fluid and all are excreted, usually unchanged, by the kidneys. Dosages should be altered in patients with renal insufficiency (Table 18-18). High concentrations are achieved in the fetus and in synovial, pericardial, pleural, and peritoneal cavities. Bile levels are usually high, with cephazolin and cefamandole being excreted in the bowel.[47]

ANTIMICROBIAL SPECTRUM AND CLINICAL USES

The cephalosporins are active against many gram-positive and gram-negative organisms.[48] In general, most streptococci, staphylococci, *E. coli, Klebsiella,* and *P. mirabilis* are sensitive, as are most anaerobes. There are, however, important exceptions to this rule; enterococci, methicillin-resistant staphylococci, *Enterobacter* species, indole-positive *Proteus* species, *Providencia, Serratia,* and the pseudomonads are resistant to most of the older cephalosporins. Among the anaerobes, *B. fragilis* is an important resistant organism.

Of the newer (second generation) cephalosporins, cefamandole has activity against *Enterobacter* species, indole-positive *Proteus,* and *H. influenzae.*[49] Unfortunately, it is slightly less active against gram-positive organisms. Cefoxitin is especially active against indole-positive *Proteus* species, *Serratia,* and *B. fragilis.*[50] Newer (so-called third generation) cephalosporin antibiotics are emerging, which are designed to have activity against: (1) pseudomonads, (2) the beta-lactamase producers, and (3) *B. fragilis* (Table 18-25). Such broad-spectrum antibiotics should be useful in the treatment of the mixed aerobic-anaerobic infections so troublesome to surgeons.[50a]

Clinical Uses

Cephalosporins are effective against a broad range of infections. They were formerly characterized as another penicillin, but now their spectrum is so wide, and clinical usefulness so apparent, that they are appropriate second-choice drugs in many circumstances and are becoming first-choice drugs in others. Their use as perioperative prophylaxis before elective contaminated operations is discussed in Chapter 23 and shown in Table 18-16.

Cephalosporins are probably the drugs of choice for staphylococcal infections in patients who are allergic to penicillin. Most *Klebsiella* infections will respond. Cefamandole is useful as a suitable single therapeutic agent for the majority of community-acquired bacterial pneumonias because of its activity against staphylococci, pneumococcus, *Klebsiella,* and *H. influenzae.* A cephalosporin has frequently been used for the treatment of mixed infections of the peritoneal cavity or soft tissues in combination with an aminoglycoside. Except when cefoxitin is used, the combination in normal doses lacks activity against many strains of *B. fragilis,* so that the combination of an aminoglycoside plus clindamycin is a better first choice for mixed enteric bacterial infections.

Of the parenteral cephalosporins, cephalothin or cephapirin are the drugs of choice in severe staphylococcal infections.

Cefazolin is more active against *E. coli* and *Klebsiella* species than cephalothin, and its serum levels are higher after parenteral administration than those of either cephaloridine or cephalothin. Its half-life is 1.8 hours, as compared with 0.5 hours for cephalothin, because its renal

TABLE 18-24. PENICILLIN PREPARATIONS AND DOSES

Generic Name	Preparations	Usual Dose: Pediatric	Usual Dose: Adult
NATURAL PENICILLINS			
Penicillin G	Tablets: 125, 250, 500 mg Parenteral Vials: 1, 5, 10, 20 million units (K^+ or Na^+) Procaine salt: 300,000 or 600,000 μ/ml Benzathine salt: same as Procaine	25,000–3,000,000 units/kg/day in 4–6 doses IV	2 to 24 million units in 6 doses
Penicillin V	Tablets: 125, 250, 500 mg Suspension: 125 or 250 mg/5 ml	125–250 mg/day in 4 doses; 50 mg/kg/day in 3 doses	250 mg–2 gm in 4 doses
PENICILLINASE-RESISTANT PENICILLINS			
Methicillin	Parenteral Vials: 1, 4, 6 gm	50–200 mg/kg/day in 4–6 doses IV, IM	4–12 gm in 4–6 doses IV or IM
Nafcillin	Capsules: 250 and 500 mg Solution: 250 mg/5 ml (with 2% alcohol in 80 ml bottle)	50–200 mg/kg day in 4 doses	1–6 gm/day in 4 doses
	Parenteral Vials: 500 mg; 1, 2, 4 gm	25–100 mg/kg/day in 4 doses IV	0.5 to 6 gm in 4 doses IV maximum dose 12 gm/day)
Oxacillin	Capsules: 125, 250 and 500 mg Liquid: 250 mg/5 ml	50–150 mg/kg/day in 4 doses	1–6 gm/day in 4 doses
	Parenteral Vials: 500 mg, 1 and 2 gm	50–300 mg/kg/day in 6 doses IM, IV	4–12 gm in 6 doses IV
Dicloxacillin	Capsules: 125, 250 and 500 mg Suspension: 62.5 mg/5 ml	25–100 mg/kg/day in 4 doses	500 mg to 4 gm/day in 4 doses
Cloxacillin	Capsules: 250 and 500 mg Suspension: 125 mg/5 ml	25–100 mg/kg/day in 4 doses	1–4 gm/day in 4 doses po in 4 doses
BROAD-SPECTRUM PENICILLINS			
Ampicillin	Capsules: 250 and 500 mg Suspension: 125 and 250 mg/5 ml	75–300 mg/kg/day in 4 doses po	2–12 gm/day in 4 doses
	Parenteral Vials: 125, 250, 500 mg and 1, 2 gm	75–300 mg/kg/day in 4 doses IV, IM	2–12 gm/day in 4 doses, IV, IM
Amoxicillin	Capsules: 250 and 500 mg Liquid: 125, 250 mg/5 ml	20–100 mg/kg/day in 4 doses	1–4 gm/day in 4 doses
Carbenicillin	Parenteral Vials: 1, 2, 10 gm	400–600 mg/kg/day in 4 or 6 doses IV	4–30 gm/day in 4 or 6 doses IV
Indanyl carbenicillin	Tablets: 382 mg of carbenicillin (or 500 mg of the indanyl sodium salt)	10–30 mg/kg/day in 4 doses	1–2 tablets q6h
Ticarcillin	Parenteral Vials: 1, 2, and 5 gm	100–300 mg/kg/day in 4 or 6 doses	4–24 gm/day in 4 or 6 doses
INVESTIGATIONAL PENICILLINS			
Piperacillin	Parenteral Investigational	50–300 mg/kg/day in 4 or 6 doses	4–24 gm/day in 4 or 6 doses
Mecillinam	Parenteral Investigational	Unknown	2–12 gm/day in 4 doses IV
Pivmecillinam	Oral Investigational	800–1600 mg/day in 4 doses	2–12 gm/day in 4 doses
Mezlocillin	Parenteral Investigational	Unknown	4–24 gm/day in 4 doses IV
BETA-LACTAMASE INHIBITOR			
Clavulanic Acid	125 mg tablet	Unknown	125–250 mg q8h

TABLE 18-25. CEPHALOSPORINS

Generic Name	Special Features	Usual Dose	
		Pediatric	**Adult**
PARENTERAL CEPHALOSPORINS			
Cephalothin	Most active against gram-positive organisms	100–200 mg/kg/day in 4 doses	0.5–2.0 gm q4–6h IV
Cephaparin	Like cephalothin	—	0.5–2.0 gm q4–6h IV
Cephaloradine	Most nephrotoxic	—	0.5–1.0 gm q8h IV
Cefazolin	Most active against gram-positive cocci	25–50 mg/kg/day	0.25–1.0 gm q6–12h
Cephradine	Both parenteral and oral forms available	—	0.5–2.0 gm q4–6h IV
Cefamandole	Extended spectrum against aerobic gram-negative rods Most active against *H. influenzae* and *Enterobacter* spp.	25–100 mg/kg/day in 4 doses IV	0.5–2.0 gm q4–6h
Cefoxitin	Extended spectrum against *B. fragilis,* indole-positive *Proteus* spp, *Serratia* spp.	25–100 mg/kg/day in 4 doses IV	1.0–2.0 gm q4–6h
THIRD-GENERATION DRUGS			
Moxalactam	Extended gram-negative spectrum including indole-positive *Proteus, Pseudomonas* Most active of cephalosporins against *B. fragilis.*	—	500 mg–6 gm/day in 4 doses IV
Cefotaxime	Similar to moxalactam; less active against *B. fragilis.*	—	500 mg–6 gm/day in 4 doses IV
Cefaperazone	Similar to moxalactam; less active against indole-positive *Proteus* and *B. fragilis*	—	500 mg–6 gm/day in 4 doses IV
Cefuroxime	Like cephalothin with slightly increased gram-negative spectrum not including most *Proteus* or *Pseudomonas*	—	500 mg–8 gm/day in 4 doses IV
Cefsulodin	Not active against gram-negative bacteria except *P. aeruginosa*	—	500 mg–8 gm/day in 4 doses IV
ORAL CEPHALOSPORINS			
Cephalexin	High urine concentration	25–100 mg/kg/day in 4 doses	250 mg q6h
Cephradine	Similar to cephalexin	25–100 mg/kg/day in 4 doses	250 mg q6h
Cefaclor	Increased activity against *H. influenzae,* gram-negative aerobes	25–100 mg/kg/day in 4 doses	250–500 mg q8h
Cefadroxil	Like cephalexin, longer half-life	—	500 mg q12h

excretion is lower and its volume of distribution smaller. These properties, and the fact that it is well tolerated by intramuscular injection, make it an excellent parenteral prophylactic agent during intestinal operations (Chapter 23).

Cefoxitin is highly resistant to beta-lactamases and more active than cephalothin against certain gram-negative organisms, although less active than cephamandole against *Enterobacter* species and *H. influenzae.* It has a special role because of its increased activity against *B. fragilis.* It may be a good choice in mixed infections of the pelvis or peritoneum.[50a] Cefotaxime and moxalactam are two investigational cephalosporin derivatives with broad antimicrobial activity against gram-negative organisms, including *P. aeruginosa* and *B. fragilis.* Clinical experience is limited, but these drugs may be useful in treatment of mixed bacterial infections. The appropriate doses of all the cephalosporins are shown in Tables 18-18 and 18-25.

Mechanisms of Antimicrobial Action

Until recently, all beta-lactam antibiotics were thought to have the same mechanism of action—interference with cell wall structure by disruption of the cross-linking of the peptidoglycan polymer. Now it is known that beta-lactam antibiotics block enzymes that govern important steps in the biosynthesis of peptidoglycan. In addition, beta-lactam antibiotics may also inhibit the inhibitor of a bacterial autolysin, which is then free to damage the bacterial cell itself.[44]

Mechanisms of Bacterial Resistance

The most important mode of bacterial resistance to the cephalosporins is the hydrolysis of the beta-lactam ring by bacterial beta-lactamases. Whereas most gram-positive organisms secrete their beta-lactamase into the environment, gram-negative organisms retain most beta-lactamase within the cell and are therefore far more effective in resisting cephalosporins.[51] In general, however, cephalosporins are all relatively more resistant to beta-lactamases than the penicillins.

Additional modes of resistance include: (1) poor penetration of beta-lactam antibiotics through gram-negative cell walls; gram-positive bacteria, by contrast, have accessible sites of antibiotic binding; (2) genetic resistance is un-

TABLE 18-26. AMINOGLYCOSIDE DOSES AND SAFE SERUM LEVELS

Aminoglycoside	Serum Levels μg/ml		Usual Dose/Day*	
	Peak†	*Trough*‡	*Pediatric*	*Adult*
Streptomycin	25–30	?	20–40 mg/kg in 4 doses IM	IM, 1–2 gm
Kanamycin	20–25	<5	6–15 mg/kg in 3 doses IM	IM, 15 mg/kg
Amikacin	15–25	<5	15–22.5 mg/kg in 3 doses IM, IV	IM, IV 15 mg/kg
Gentamicin	6–10	<2	3–7.5 mg/kg in 3 doses IM, IV	IM, IV 3–5 mg/kg
Tobramycin	6–10	<2	3–7.5 mg/kg in 3 doses IM, IV	IM, IV 3–5 mg/kg
Netilmicin	6–10	<2	3–5 mg/kg in 3 doses IM, IV	IM, IV 6 mg/kg
Sisomicin	6–10	<2	3–4 mg/kg in 3 doses IM, IV	IM, 4 mg/kg
Neomycin	—	—	50–100 mg/kg/day in 4 doses po for *E. coli* Tablet 500 mg Liquid 125 mg/5 ml Ampoule 500 mg	40 mg/kg/day in 6 doses po prior to bowel surgery 50–100 mg/kg/day po in 4 doses po for hepatic coma

* The aminoglycoside doses are suggested starting points and often need to be modified to achieve desirable serum levels.
† Peak level is defined as antibiotic concentration achieved 60 minutes after intramuscular injection or at the termination of intravenous infusion over 60 minutes.
‡ Trough level is defined as antibiotic concentration just before the next dose.

usual—beta-lactam antibiotics bind to multiple enzymatic sites so that resistance would require several simultaneous mutations; (3) tolerance defined as dissociation of inhibitory and killing actions. The mechanism may be related to the deficiency of autolytic enzymes in the cells, so that the antibiotic becomes bacteriostatic rather than bactericidal.[52]

Adverse Reactions

The cephalosporins are among the safest of drugs, although thrombophlebitis frequently occurs after intravenous administration. The most common side effects are delayed allergic reactions (anaphylaxis and bronchospasm are relatively rare), such as a maculopapular rash which appears after several days of therapy. Although immunologic cross-reactivity with penicillin is found in 20 percent of penicillin-allergic patients, clinical cross-reactivity occurs in only 5 to 10 percent of patients. Patients with a history of a recent severe and immediate reaction to penicillin should not be given cephalosporins. Rare adverse reactions include hemolysis, granulocytopenia, thrombocytopenia, and defects in platelet aggregation.

More controversial are the reports that cephalosporins are potentially nephrotoxic, which is true of cephaloridine. There is some evidence that the combination of cephalothin plus gentamicin or tobramycin is synergistically nephrotoxic,[53] especially in older patients or patients with other causes for renal insufficiency. A moderate dose reduction is necessary in patients with renal insufficiency, and an increase in dose is required during dialysis (Table 18-18).

AMINOGLYCOSIDES

The aminoglycoside antibiotics (Table 18-26)[54–56] share many pharmacologic and antimicrobial properties. All are primarily useful in the treatment of aerobic gram-negative enteric bacteria and can be used in combination with other antimicrobial agents in the treatment of staphylococcal and enterococcal infections. In addition, all except tobramycin and sisomicin are active against mycobacterial species, including tuberculosis. The gram-positive organisms, except for staphylococci, are generally resistant, and anaerobic organisms are almost all resistant. The differences in spelling between "mycin" or "micin" depends on whether these compounds were isolated from *Streptomyces* or *Mycomonosporum* species, respectively.[54]

Chemistry

Aminoglycoside antibiotics contain at least two aminosugars joined by glycosidic linkage to a central hexose (streptidine or deoxystreptidine). Aminocyclitols are related compounds.

Pharmacology

None of the aminoglycosides can be absorbed from the gastrointestinal tract and all must be administered parenterally. All are excreted, unchanged, in the urine, so that doses must be modified in patients with renal functional impairment (Table 18-18). Although they are not absorbed from the gastrointestinal tract in large quantities, their absorption in patients with renal failure can produce toxic levels. Absorption from the peritoneal cavity and other tissue sites is complete, so that toxic levels can be achieved easily after topical use.

Penetration into the cerebrospinal fluid, eye, biliary tree, and tracheal-bronchial secretions is poor after systemic administration. An intrathecal or subconjunctival injection yields high levels in cerebrospinal fluid and aqueous fluid respectively.[57] Penetration into serous cavities yields levels equal to one-half the peak plasma level.

Antimicrobial Spectrum and Clinical Uses

Aminoglycoside antibiotics are active against aerobic gram-negative bacilli and *S. aureus.* They are virtually inactive against anaerobes. Sensitivity is defined as inhibition by easily achievable serum concentrations, ie, less than 4 μg per ml for gentamicin, tobramycin, and netilmicin, and less than 16 μg per ml for amikacin and kanamycin. Certain differences in antimicrobial spectrum between the aminoglycosides should be emphasized. Tobramycin and gentamicin, the most commonly useful antimicrobial agents, have similar spectra, except that tobramycin is more active against strains of *Proteus* and especially *P. aeruginosa.* Kanamycin and streptomycin are no longer clinically useful parenteral antibiotics for the treatment of gram-negative aerobic infections except in isolated circumstances (ie, streptomycin for tularemia, plague, brucellosis, and mycobacterial infections). Sisomicin and netilmicin are similar to gentamicin except that they show almost no activity against *Serratia,* and netilmicin is poorly active against *Proteus* species.

All the aminoglycosides can be useful for staphylococcal infections, but not for other gram-positive organisms. Enterococci are relatively resistant, but gentamicin is a useful synergising agent for enterococcal endocarditis in combination with penicillin.

Tuberculosis is highly sensitive to streptomycin, gentamicin, and kanamycin, but these agents are not useful for atypical mycobacteria. Amikacin is active against both tuberculosis and the atypical mycobacteria. Tobramycin and sisomicin are inactive against *Mycobacteria.*

Antimicrobial Combinations. Aminoglycosides are rarely used alone except for urinary infections. The betalactam antibiotics act synergistically or additively with aminoglycosides against staphylococci, enterococci, the enteric bacteria, and pseudomonads (Tables 18-12 to 18-14). Carbenicillin (or ticarcillin) plus tobramycin is a particularly useful combination against *P. aeruginosa,*[58] but one must not mix them in the same infusion since carbenicillin can inactivate the aminoglycoside.[59] Vancomycin and aminoglycosides are also a powerful, but nephrotoxic, combination.

Neomycin is too toxic for parenteral use, and the toxic serum levels that can occur after peritoneal instillation, wound irrigation, or cutaneous application seriously restrict this indication.[60] Neomycin should be restricted to oral use for the suppression of intestinal flora in preoperative preparation of the colon, and in the treatment of hepatic failure.

Kanamycin is no longer indicated for the initial treatment of suspected gram-negative infections because resistance is common. It is still useful in the reduction of bacterial flora in the bowel before intestinal operations and in patients with hepatic coma, but neomycin is cheaper.

Amikacin has a broad spectrum of activity against gram-negative bacilli including *Serratia,* indole-positive *Proteus, Pseudomonas,* and *Providencia.* It is not susceptible to bacterial enzymes which inactivate other aminoglycosides and consequently is useful against gentamicin and tobramycin resistant strains of enteric bacteria.[61] Resistance to amikacin seldom occurs. Most authorities advocate the restriction of amikacin use to specific indications, in order to minimize the emergence of resistant mutants.

Spectinomycin is an aminocyclitol with pharmacologic activities similar to aminoglycosides. Its only use is the treatment of uncomplicated gonococcal urethritis, cervicitis, or proctitis in patients unresponsive or allergic to penicillin (a single 2 gm dose IM). It is not useful for pharyngeal gonococcal infections because it is not secreted into saliva.[62] In doses of 2–4 gm per day for 5 days it may be useful for the treatment of pelvic inflammatory disease.

The incidence of postgonococcal urethritis will be higher after spectinomycin treatment than with penicillin because spectinomycin is inactive against *Chlamydiae.* It is also inactive against *T. pallidum,* so that serologic tests for syphilis should be performed at the initial examination and 3 months later in all patients treated with spectinomycin for gonococcal infections.

Use of Aminoglycosides in Renal Failure. When renal function is impaired, the doses of all aminoglycosides must be modified (Table 18-18). No theoretical method is totally satisfactory, despite the widespread availability of dosage nomograms that have been devised, including those shown in Table 18-18. The most accurate guide to therapy is the determination of serum aminoglycoside levels. Both peak levels and trough levels should be obtained to assure adequate blood levels and to minimize the possibility of toxicity. Serum antibiotic concentrations should be monitored frequently and at least once 24 hours after any change of dose scheduling.

Aminoglycosides are easily removed both by peritoneal dialysis and hemodialysis. Approximately one-half the initial loading dose should reestablish adequate serum concentration after an efficient hemodialysis run. During peritoneal dialysis, it is best to add the desired serum level of aminoglycoside to the peritoneal dialysis fluid to maintain the serum levels.

Mechanism of Antimicrobial Action

Aminoglycosides are bactericidal antibiotics because they interfere with the synthesis of essential proteins. They bind irreversibly to the 30S subunit of bacterial ribosomes, which leads to a misreading of mRNA codons. A nonsense sequence of amino acids results in an abnormal protein.[54]

Mechanisms of Bacterial Resistance to Aminoglycosides

Three mechanisms are responsible for the resistance of bacteria to aminoglycoside antibiotics. The most common type is due to extranuclear plasmids, which code for enzymes which can acetylate, adenylate, or phosphorylate hydroxyl, or amino groups on the aminoglycoside molecule. The modified aminoglycoside does not penetrate the microbe or bind to the ribosome in sufficient quantity. Resistance to kanamycin and streptomycin have made these antibiotics obsolete for parenteral administration. Gentamicin and tobramycin cross-resistance is common, except that some gentamicin-resistant strains of *Pseudomonas* are still susceptible to tobramycin. Amikacin has so few sites for enzyme modification that resistant strains are relatively infrequent.

The second mechanism of bacterial resistance to aminoglycosides is the emergence of bacterial mutants, which prevent aminoglycoside transport into bacteria. Most instances of amikacin resistance are the result of such mutants.

A rare cause of bacterial resistance is the emergence of bacterial chromosomal mutants, which are deficient in binding sites.[54]

Adverse Effects

There are three major adverse effects of the aminoglycoside antibiotics.

Ototoxicity. Permanent and irreversible deafness can appear without warning, and nystagmus, vertigo, nausea, vomiting, and acute Menière's syndrome can also occur. Audiograms and electronystagmograms suggest a high rate of subclinical nerve damage—especially high-frequency tone loss. The risk is increased with increasing age, duration of therapy, total dose, preexisting renal impairment with high serum antibiotic concentration, preexposure to other aminoglycosides, and concurrent administration of other ototoxic agents, particularly furosemide.

Renal Toxicity. Neomycin is the most nephrotoxic agent, and streptomycin the least. The true incidence is difficult to determine because infection, hypotension, and other effects on renal function are difficult to assess.[63] All levels of nephrotoxicity can be observed—oliguric or nonoliguric renal failure, proteinuria, cylindruria, and hematuria.

Neuromuscular Blockade. Flaccid paralysis of skeletal muscle sometimes follows local irrigation with large doses of aminoglycosides during the use of anesthesia. Respiratory arrest has been reported. The paralytic effects can be reversed by anticholinesterases (neostigmine) and calcium.[64]

Other toxic reactions include local pain, erythema, and occasionally hypersensitivity rashes. Prolonged oral administration of poorly absorbed antimicrobial agents can precipitate or aggravate the development of pseudomembranous enterocolitis, as can almost any antibiotic.

TETRACYCLINES

Tetracyclines are broad-spectrum bacteriostatic antibiotics, listed in Table 18-27.

Chemistry

The chemical structure of tetracycline and its analogues are shown in Figure 18-2.[65] The basic structure consists of the hydronaphthacene nucleus, which contains four fused rings.

Pharmacology

Because the longer-acting tetracyclines are more readily absorbed from the gastrointestinal tract, lower doses are required. Food impairs the absorption of the tetracyclines, especially by complexing with divalent and trivalent cations—calcium, magnesium, and aluminum. Milk, iron, or antacids should not be administered with tetracyclines. Intravenous preparations are available, but thrombophlebitis is a common complication.

Penetration of most tissues is excellent, but cerebrospinal fluid levels are low. The tetracyclines cross the placenta and are incorporated into fetal bone and teeth. Because they are excreted in the milk, they should not be given during pregnancy or lactation. The drug concentrates in the bile and urinary levels are sufficient for the treatment of susceptible organisms within the urinary tract.[65]

Only one tetracycline, doxycycline, can be used in patients with renal failure, because it can be excreted via the gastrointestinal tract under these circumstances.[66]

Antimicrobial Spectrum and Clinical Uses

All tetracyclines share a similar antimicrobial spectrum, and a tetracycline disk is used for susceptibility testing. Minocycline and doxycycline are the most active analogues. Most gram-positive and gram-negative aerobic and anaerobic organisms are susceptible to the tetracyclines, including *S. aureus, S. pyogenes, S. pneumoniae, H. influenzae,* and the gram-negative enterics. The tetracyclines find few indications in the treatment of serious life-threatening surgical diseases because of the gaps in the spectrum (Tables 18-3 to 18-5). For this reason, tetracyclines can rarely be presumed to be effective therapy for common bacterial infections until sensitivity testing is done. The exceptions include gonococci and meningococci, which are extremely susceptible, and pneumococci and many *H. influenzae* organisms, which cause sinusitis and bronchitis. Table 18-28 lists the infections for which tetracyclines are useful.

Because tetracycline is active against *B. fragilis,* the combination of neomycin and tetracycline or doxycycline alone can be used as an oral, preoperative bowel preparation.[67]

Mechanism of Antimicrobial Action

The tetracyclines inhibit protein synthesis by binding to the 30S ribosomal subunit, which interferes with the addition of amino acids to the growing peptide chain.[65]

Mechanism of Resistance

The principal mechanism of resistance is the development of impermeability of a bacteria to the antibiotic. Enteric organisms become resistant by means of R factors.[65]

Adverse Reactions

The principal adverse reactions are the irritative effects on the upper gastrointestinal tract—esophageal ulcerations, nausea, vomiting, epigastric distress. Diarrhea is caused by alteration of enteric flora, and pseudomembranous colitis has been reported.

Incorporation of tetracycline into teeth and bones during the deposition of tooth enamel (ie, in children up to

TABLE 18-27. TETRACYCLINES: PREPARATIONS AND DOSES

Drug	Preparations	Usual Dose	
		Pediatric *	*Adult*
SHORT-ACTING			
Tetracycline	Capsules: 100, 250, 500 mg Syrup: 125 mg/5 ml	25–50 mg/kg/day in 3 doses po	250 mg–1.0 gm/q6h po
	Vials: 100, 250, 500 mg	10–20 mg/kg/day in 2 doses IV (IM painful)	500 mg q6h IV
Chlortetracycline	Capsules: 250 mg Vials: 100, 250, 500 mg	25–50 mg/kg/day in 3 doses po	500 mg q6h po 25–50 mg/kg/day in 3 doses po
Oxytetracycline	Capsules: 100, 125, 250 mg Vials: 100, 250, 500 mg	25–50 mg/kg/day in 3 doses po	500 mg q6h po 25–50 mg/kg/day in 3 doses po
INTERMEDIATE ACTING			
Methacycline	Capsules: 150, 300 mg Suspension: 75 mg/5 ml	7–13 mg/kg/day in 2–4 doses po	300 mg q12h po
Demeclocycline	Capsules: 150 mg Tablets: 75, 150 mg	7–13 mg/kg/day in 2–4 doses po	300 mg q12h po
LONG-LASTING			
Doxycycline	Capsules (hyclate): 50 mg, 100 mg Syrup (calcium): 50 mg/5 ml Suspension (monohydrate): 25 mg/5 ml	5 mg/kg/day in 2 doses po	100–200 mg q12h po
Minocycline	Capsules: 50, 100 mg Syrup: 50 mg/5 ml	4 mg/kg/day in 2 doses po	100 mg q12h po

* Tetracyclines have only selected indications in infancy and childhood because of their accumulation in bone and teeth and their potential to interfere with growth. Their use should be avoided if possible until 8–10 years of age to avoid discoloring and pitting of tooth enamel. They may cause increased intracranial pressure in infants (pseudotumor cerebri).

Modified from Mandell GL, Douglas RG Jr, Bennett JE (eds): *Principles and Practice of Diseases.* New York, Wiley, 1979; and Nelson JD, Grassi C (eds): *Current Chemotherapy and Infectious Disease,* Vol 11. Proceedings 11th ICC and 19th ICCAC Meeting. Washington, D.C., American Society for Microbiology, 1980.

age 8) will result in permanent discoloration of the teeth. Hypersensitivity reactions are unusual. Tetracycline can aggravate the azotemia of renal failure by inhibiting protein synthesis, but doxycycline is safe in renal failure.

Vertigo, a unique side effect of minocycline, is so common in women (70 percent) that it has seriously limited the use of this drug.

Effectiveness of the tetracyclines is reduced by concurrent administration of diphenylhydantoin and barbiturates, which induce enzymes capable of metabolizing the drug.[68,69]

CHLORAMPHENICOL

Chloramphenicol is an extremely useful antibiotic in seriously ill patients despite the rare, tragic appearance of irreversible aplastic anemia.

Chemistry

The chemical structure of chloramphenicol is shown in Figure 18-3. Although it was originally derived from *Streptomyces venezuelae,* it is now synthesized.

Pharmacology

Oral administration results in higher levels than intravenous administration because (1) the drug is almost totally absorbed in active form and (2) intravenous chloramphenicol succinate must be hydrolized to biologically active chloramphenicol.[70] The intramuscular route results in even lower levels and is not recommended. Adequate therapeutic levels are found in all tissues and body fluids, including the brain and cerebrospinal fluid.

Chloramphenicol is metabolized in the liver, where it is conjugated with glucuronic acid and excreted in the kidneys. Newborn infants require half the recommended adult dose (Table 18-29) because they metabolize it slowly. Renal excretion of the unchanged drug is low, and no alteration is necessary in renal insufficiency, although metabolites continue to accumulate in the blood. The dose must be reduced for patients with hepatic failure to avoid suppression of the bone marrow.

Antimicrobial Activity and Clinical Uses

Chloramphenicol is active against bacteria, spirochetes, *Rickettsia, Chlamydiae,* and *Mycoplasmas.* The indica-

TETRACYCLINE

SHORT ACTING — CHLORTETRACYCLINE, OXYTETRACYCLINE

INTERMEDIATE — DEMECLOCYCLINE, METHACYCLINE

LONG ACTING — MINOCYCLINE, DOXYCYCLINE

Fig. 18-2. The chemical structure of the tetracyclines. The analogues differ from tetracycline at the fifth, sixth, or seventh position as indicated by the arrows. (From Standiford HC: Tetracyclines and chloramphenicol. In Mandell GL, Douglas RB Jr, Bennett JE (eds.): *Principles and Practice of Infectious Disease.* New York, Wiley, 1979, p 273.)

TABLE 18-28. MAJOR THERAPEUTIC INDICATIONS FOR THE TETRACYCLINES *

Therapy of Choice	Effective Alternative Therapy
Brucellosis (with streptomycin in seriously ill patients)	Acne (the preferred antibiotic when systemic antimicrobials are indicated)
Chancroid	Actinomycosis of the mandible
Chlamydial infections	Anthrax
Nonspecific urethritis	Chronic bronchitis (acute exacerbations)
Ornithosis	Gonococcal urethritis
	Nocardiosis (minocycline)
Trachoma	Pelvic inflammatory disease
Cholera	Rat bite fever
Lymphogranuloma venereum	*(Spirillum minus)*
Granuloma inguinale	Sinusitis
Mycoplasma pneumoniae (some prefer erythromycin)	Syphilis
	Vincent infection
Melioidosis (with chloramphenicol in seriously ill patients)	Whipple disease
	Yaws, nasopalatal
Relapsing fever (Borrelia recurrentis)	*Yersinia enterocolytica*
	Alternative prophylaxis
Rickettsial infections (some prefer chloramphenicol)	Oral bowel prep for intestinal surgery (tetracycline in combination with neomycin or doxycycline alone)
	Meningococcal disease (only minocycline)
Prophylaxis of choice:	
None	

* Preferred analogue, unless specified otherwise.

Adapted from Mandell GL, Douglas RG Jr, Bennett JE (eds): *Principles and Practice of Diseases.* New York, Wiley, 1979.

tions for its use are listed in Table 18-30.[65] Almost all gram-positive and gram-negative bacteria, whether aerobes or anaerobes, are susceptible. The notable exceptions are most of the methicillin-resistant *S. aureus, P. aeuruginosa, S. marcescens,* and indole-positive *Proteus* organisms; many *Enterobacter* species are also resistant. Many more active and less toxic therapeutic agents are available for the pathogens that are susceptible to chloramphenicol. Despite its broad spectrum, chloramphenicol is the best drug in a relatively narrow set of indications (Table 18-30). It is, however, effective alternative therapy in many mixed infections of gram-positive and gram-negative organisms, and in selected patients with bacteria proved to be susceptible by susceptibility testing studies.

Because of its high penetration into cerebrospinal fluid and cerebral tissue, it is the drug of choice for many central nervous system infections, including the three most common causes of meningitis in childhood (*H. influenzae, S. pneumoniae,* and *N. meningititis*).[71] Because of its activity against *B. fragilis,* chloramphenicol is a good second choice in the treatment of mixed aerobic and anaerobic

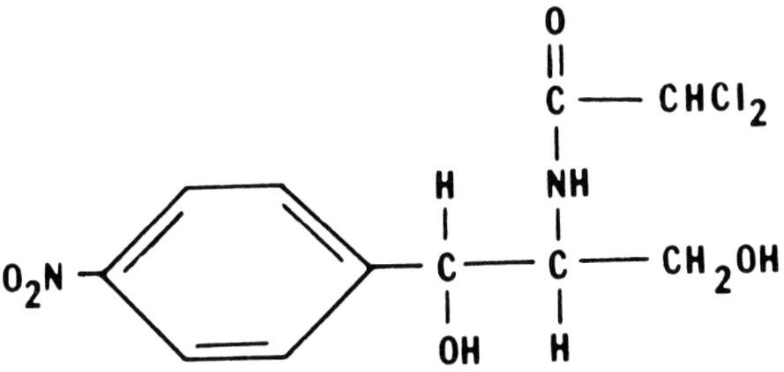

Fig. 18-3. The chemical structure of chloramphenicol. (From Standiford HC: Tetracycline and chloramphenicol. In Mandell GL, Douglas RB Jr, Bennett JE (eds.): *Principles and Practice of Infectious Disease.* New York, Wiley, 1979, p 273.)

TABLE 18-29. CHLORAMPHENICOL PREPARATION AND DOSES

Drug	Preparation	Usual Dose	
		Pediatric *	*Adult*
Chloramphenicol			
Oral	Capsules 50, 100, 250 mg Suspension 150 mg/5 ml	25–100 mg/kg/day in 4 doses po, 25 mg/kg/day for premature infants and newborns; 100 mg/kg/day for meningitis	2–8 gm/day in 3–4 doses po
Parenteral	Vial: 1 gm powder	25–100 mg/kg/day in 4 doses IV: 25 mg/kg/day for premature infants and newborns; 100 mg/kg/day for meningitis	2–8 gm/day in 3–4 doses IV

* Newborn infants are susceptible to developing the gray-baby syndrome.

enteric infections, such as peritonitis, or the soft tissue infections caused by fecal contamination (necrotizing fasciitis). It is commonly used in conjunction with penicillin for the treatment of clostridial infections.

Mechanism of Antimicrobial Action
Chloramphenicol inhibits protein synthesis and is bacteriostatic. The drug binds to the 50S ribosomal subunit that interferes with peptide formation.

Mechanisms of Microbial Resistance
Bacteria become resistant to chloramphenicol by becoming impermeable to the drug or by R factors capable of inducing an enzyme which degrades the antibiotic to the inactive derivative.[72]

TABLE 18-30. INDICATIONS FOR CHLORAMPHENICOL

Indication	Comment
THERAPY OF CHOICE	
Brain abscess	Used with a penicillin
Meningitis	
H. Influenzae	
Gram-negative aerobic rods	Often used initially with intrathecal plus parenteral aminoglycoside
Typhoid fever and salmonellosis (invasive)	Some strains may be chloramphenicol-resistant Not used for gastroenteritis or carrier state
EFFECTIVE ALTERNATIVE THERAPY	
B. fragilis infections	With aminoglycoside in intestinal perforations
Meningitis	For penicillin-allergic patients
S. pneumoniae	
N. meningitidis	
Rickettsial infections	Preferred drug when patients require parenteral therapy

Modified from Mandell, GL, Douglas RG Jr, Bennett JE (eds): *Principles and Practice of Diseases.* New York, J Wiley, 1979.

Adverse Reactions
The principal adverse reaction is suppression of the bone marrow, which can take one of two forms; (1) a reversible, dose-related, bone marrow depression caused by an inhibition of protein synthesis, and (2) an idiosyncratic, irreversible, generally fatal aplastic anemia unrelated to dose.[73] Irreversible, fatal aplastic anemia can occur either during or after therapy. A few cases have been reported after parenteral administration.[74] Leukocyte counts should be carried out in all patients who receive chloramphenicol, and the drug should be stopped if levels below 2,500 mm^3 are found.

Hemolytic anemias occasionally occur in patients with a severe form of glucose-6-phosphate dehydrogenase (G6-P-D) deficiency.

Other toxic manifestations include the gray syndrome in neonates—abdominal distension, vomiting, flaccidity, cyanosis, circulatory collapse, and death—the result of the incapacity of neonates to detoxify chloramphenicol.

Coumadin toxicity can be induced by the concurrent dose of chloramphenicol, which can inhibit hepatic metabolism of this and other drugs (Table 18-20). Chloramphenicol is a bacteriostatic agent and, theoretically, should antagonize bactericidal activity of the penicillins, cephalosporins, or the aminoglycoside antibiotics. This has doubtful clinical significance. Bacteriostatic agents should not be used, however, in granulocytopenic and other immunodepressed subjects.[75]

ERYTHROMYCIN

Erthyromycin is an extremely safe antibiotic which, in addition to its usefulness as an alternative to penicillin G, has important primary indications.[76]

Chemistry
The structure of erythromycin (Fig. 18-4) consists of a macrocyclic lactone ring attached to two sugars.

Pharmacology
Erythromycin is rapidly inactivated by gastric acid and must be protected during oral administration. Gastrointes-

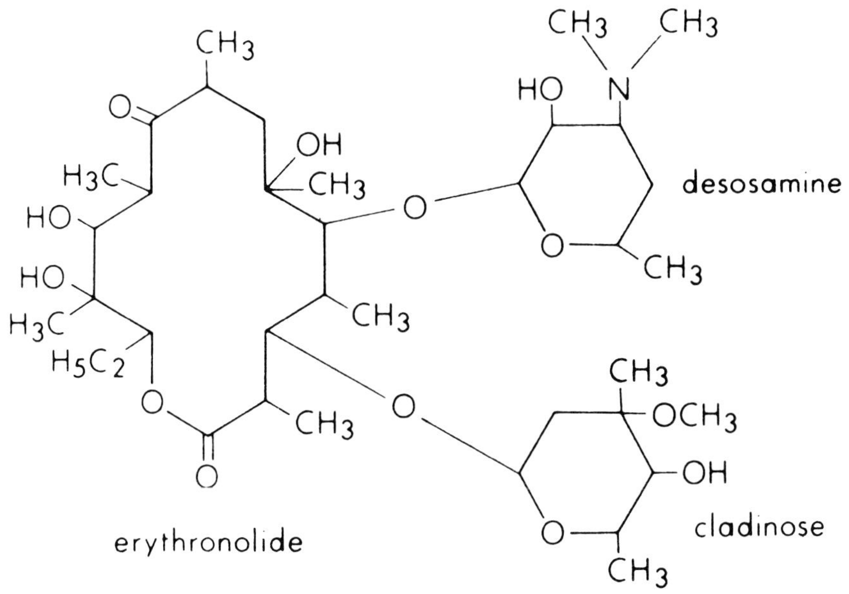

Fig. 18-4. **Erythromycin base. (From Steigbigel NH: Erythromycin, lincomycin, and clindamycin. In Mandell GL, Douglas RB Jr, Bennett JE (eds.): *Principles and Practice of Infectious Disease.* New York, Wiley, 1979, p 290.)**

tinal absorption of all oral preparations (Table 18-31)[55] is good, but much higher levels can be obtained by intravenous administration. Tissue distribution is excellent everywhere except in the cerebrospinal fluid, middle ear, and synovial fluid. Urine concentrations are variable. Erythromycin is concentrated in the liver and excreted in the bile; fecal excretion can be high. Erythromycin base and neomycin are a popular and effective antimicrobial bowel preparation because the erythromycin base is only partially absorbed. In such high concentrations, it exerts a potent antianaerobic effect on the gut flora. The preparations and doses available are listed in Table 18-31.

Antimicrobial Spectrum and Clinical Uses

Table 18-32 lists the major uses of erythromycin. It has a broad spectrum against gram-positive bacteria and is active in vitro against *Actinomyces, Mycobacterium, Treponema, Mycoplasma, Chlamydiae,* and *Rickettsia.* It is bactericidal in high concentration and under circumstances of rapid bacterial growth. Its activity in urine is

TABLE 18-31. ERYTHROMYCIN: PREPARATIONS AND DOSES

		Usual Dose	
	Preparations	***Pediatric***	***Adult***
ORAL			
Base	Tablets: 250, 500 mg	30–50 mg/kg/day in 4 doses po	2–4 gm/day in 4 doses
Stearate	Tablets: 125, 250, 500 mg Vials: 100, 500 mg	30–50 mg/kg/day in 4 doses po	1–4 gm/day in 4 doses
Ethylsuccinate	Tablets: 200, 400 mg Suspension: 200, 400 mg/ml	30–50 mg/kg/day in 4 doses po	1–4 gm/day in 4 doses
Estolate	Tablets, capsules: 125, 250 mg Suspension: 125, 250 mg/5 ml	30–50 mg/kg/day in 4 doses po	1–4 gm/day in 4 doses (hepatotoxic—avoid)
PARENTERAL			
Lactobionate	Vials: 500 mg, 1 gm/ vials for IV use	15–20 mg/kg/day in 4 doses IV	1–4 gm/day in 4 doses IV
Gluceptate	Vials: 500 mg, 1 gm	15–20 mg/kg/day in 4 doses IV	1–4 gm/day in 4 doses IV
Ethylsuccinate	Vials: 2, 10 ml as 50 mg/ml for IM use	15–20 mg/kg/day in 4 doses IM	0.5–2 gm/day in 2–4 doses IM only

Modified from Nelson WE: Appendix. In Nelson WE (ed): *Textbook of Pediatrics,* 11th ed. Philadelphia, Saunders, 1979, p. 2056.

TABLE 18-32. MAJOR USES OF ERYTHROMYCIN

Indication	Alternative Drug
THERAPY OF CHOICE	
M. pneumoniae infections	Tetracycline
Legionnaires' disease	Rifampin + erythromycin
Diphtheria	Penicillin G
Pertussis	Ampicillin
C. trachomatis	Tetracycline
EFFECTIVE ALTERNATIVE THERAPY	DRUG OF FIRST CHOICE
Groups A, B, C, G streptococci	Penicillin G
S. pneumoniae	Penicillin G
Gonorrhea	Penicillin G
Syphilis	Penicillin G
Bronchopulmonary anaerobic infections	Penicillin G
Urinary tract infections	Many agents
PROPHYLAXIS	
Rheumatic fever prophylaxis	Penicillin G
Prevention of bacterial endocarditis	Penicillin G
With neomycin for presurgical bowel preparation	

accelerated by increasing the pH into the alkaline range of 8.5.[77] At that level, it is active even against Enterobacteriaceae, which are otherwise quite resistant. Unfortunately, the enterococcus, *S. aureus, S. epidermidis, C. perfringens, H. influenzae,* and *B. fragilis* have unpredictable susceptibility at achievable serum concentrations, so that erythromycin cannot be used as empiric therapy of infections that are frequently caused by these organisms until sensitivity testing is done. Infections for which erythromycin can occasionally be used are *Actinomyces israelii, Mycobacterium scrofulaceum, M. kansasii,*[78] and combined with ampicillin against *N. asteroides.*[79]

Mechanisms of Antimicrobial Action. Erythromycin is a bacteriostatic drug, which inhibits RNA-dependent protein synthesis by binding to the 50S ribosomal subunit.[76]

Mechanisms of Bacterial Resistance. Resistance to erythromycin is sometimes due to (1) decreased permeability of the cell wall (gram-negative enterics), (2) alteration of the 50S ribosomal protein receptor site (chromosomal mutation), or (3) alteration in the 23S ribosomal RNA of the 50S ribosomal subunit by methylation of adenine. This resistance is mediated by a plasmid. Cross-resistance with lincomycin and clindamycin is common.[76]

Adverse Reactions. Erythromycin is one of the safest antibiotics, although gastrointestinal irritation, occasional allergic reactions, and superinfection have been reported. Cholestatic hepatitis is rare and reversible. Transient hearing losses have been reported with large intravenous doses of drug, especially if other ototoxic drugs are in concurrent use (eg, aminoglycosides).

LINCOMYCIN AND CLINDAMYCIN

The lincosamide antibiotics are chemically unrelated to erythromycin but share pharmacologic and antimicrobial properties.[76]

Chemistry

The basic structure of lincosamide antibiotics is shown in Figure 18-5.[76]

Pharmacology

Adequate serum and tissue levels are reached with the usual doses (Table 18-33). The cerebrospinal fluid has inadequate concentrations, and most of the absorbed drug is metabolized in the liver. The dose need not be reduced in renal failure; the drug is not dialyzed (Table 18-18).

Antimicrobial Spectrum

Clindamycin and lincomycin have a broad spectrum of activity against the gram-positive cocci, especially streptococci and pneumococci. Most strains of staphylococci are sensitive, but enterococci, gonococci, and meningococci are resistant. Almost all anaerobic organisms, including most clostridial species and *B. fragilis,* are susceptible—clindamycin is more active than lincomycin. Gram-negative enteric organisms are resistant. Clindamycin is the most active antibiotic available against *B. fragilis,* and resistant strains are rare. Of the anaerobes, a few peptococcus and clostridial species [80] are resistant to clindamycin. Consequently, resistant strains of *C. difficile* can induce pseudomembranous enterocolitis after clindamycin therapy.[81]

Most authorities agree that clindamycin should be limited in its indications [1] to only those infections which are likely to involve *B. fragilis,* and which are outside the central nervous system. It is an extremely useful drug in combination with an aminoglycoside for the treatment of mixed intra-abdominal, gynecologic, or gangrenous soft tissue infections caused by facultative and anaerobic gram-negative and gram-positive bacteria. Oral lincomycin is commonly prescribed by British surgeons for the adjunctive treatment of subcutaneous abscesses which contain both aerobic and anaerobic gram-positive cocci (Chapters 8 and 25).

Clindamycin is occasionally useful as an alternative to penicillin G for anaerobic necrotizing pulmonary infections.[82] Clindamycin is also useful as an alternative to, or in combination with, penicillin in the treatment of *C. perfringens* infections. Although high concentrations of clindamycin are achieved in bone, no clinical advantage of clindamycin for the treatment of osteomyelitis has been established.

Mechanisms of Action

The lincosamide antibiotics bind to 50S ribosomal binding sites as do the macrolides and chloramphenicol. Protein synthesis is thereby inhibited.[76]

Mechanisms of Resistance

Failure of clindamycin, like erythromycin, to penetrate the gram-negative organisms results in resistance. Some

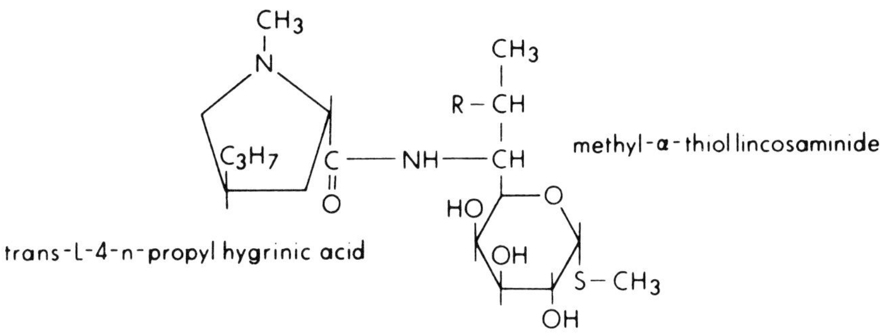

Fig. 18-5. **The lincosamide antibiotics: lincomycin (R = OH), clindamycin (R = Cl). (From Steigbigel NH: Erythromycin, lincomycin, and clindamycin. In Mandell GL, Douglas RB Jr, Bennett JE (eds.): *Principles and Practice of Infectious Disease.* New York, Wiley, 1979, p 290.)**

TABLE 18-33. MAJOR THERAPEUTIC INDICATIONS AND DOSES FOR CLINDAMYCIN

	Usual Dose	
	Pediatric	***Adult***
THERAPY OF CHOICE		
Suspected or proven *B. fragilis* infections outside the central nervous system	8–20 mg/kg/day in 4 doses po, IV, or IM	1–3 gm/day in 4 doses po, IV, or IM
EFFECTIVE ALTERNATIVE THERAPY		
Clostridial infections (alternative or in combination with penicillin)		
Many gram-positive infections		

resistant bacteria are mutants with changes in the binding site on the 50S ribosomal protein.

Adverse Reactions

Minor adverse reactions of the allergic type and mild hepatotoxicity have been noted; however, the principal toxic effect of lincosamide antibiotics is diarrhea. Most evidence supports the idea that clindamycin-associated diarrhea is usually caused by an enterotoxin elaborated by colonic *C. difficile.* In the more severe cases, a true pseudomembranous enterocolitis is produced. True pseudomembranous enterocolitis has been reported in up to 10 percent of clindamycin recipients followed prospectively,[83] but a much lower incidence of this complication has been reported after parenteral administration. Pseudomembranous enterocolitis, its pathogenesis and treatment, is discussed extensively in Chapter 39. Whenever possible, the appearance of antibiotic-associated diarrhea should prompt discontinuation of the responsible antibiotic—most cases are mild and will resolve spontaneously. The most severe cases of pseudomembranous enterocolitis will respond to oral vancomycin, even though relapses after treatment occasionally occur. Cholestyramine, which can bind the *C. difficile* toxin, has been suggested as well.

BACITRACIN

Bacitracin was originally isolated from *Bacillus licheniformis (subtilis)* and was formally used for the treatment of severe staphylococcal infections. Because of its nephrotoxicity, it is rarely administered systemically but it can be used, without serious side effects, as a topical antibiotic. Toxicity due to systemic absorption has not been reported even when used in large doses to irrigate the peritoneal cavity.[83a] The best bacitracin is a peptide antibiotic composed of peptide-linked aminoacids. It is highly active against most gram-positive bacteria including *S. pyogenes,* group A beta hemolytic streptococci, and C and G beta hemolytic streptococci. Group B streptococci are usually resistant, however, as are gram-negative bacilli. Other pyogenic cocci such as the *Neisseria* are sensitive. Acquired bacterial resistance is unusual although some resistant *S. pyogenes* strains have been found.[83b]

Bacitracin interferes with bacterial cell wall synthesis by inhibiting the dephosphorylation of a lipid pyrophosphate. In addition, it damages the bacterial cytoplasmic membrane and is active against protoplast.

Bacitracin is most often used topically as creams, ointments, antibiotic sprays and powders, and in solutions for wound irrigation or bladder instillation. Most commonly, it is combined with both neomycin and polymyxin B to provide an effective cover for gram-negative bacilli and *Pseudomonas,* in addition to its own activity against gram-positive cocci.[83c]

POLYMYXINS

Polymyxins are cyclic basic polypeptides that are much too toxic for routine clinical use. Only polymyxin B and E (colistin) are available.

Pharmacology

Polymyxin is not absorbed from the gastrointestinal tract, and intramuscular injections are painful. Topical preparations (0.1 percent polymyxin) in combination with other antibiotics (bacitracin, neomycin) have been found useful in the prophylaxis of wound infections and in the treatment of superficial infections of skin and mucous membranes. Continuous irrigation of serous or wound cavities is contraindicated, because absorption can produce nephrotoxicity and apnea.

Antimicrobial Spectrum and Clinical Uses

Polymyxins are only active against gram-negative bacilli, especially *Pseudomonas,* and they are used intravenously, almost exclusively, for serious life-threatening *Pseudomonas* infection when other drugs cannot be used (1.5–2.5 mg per kg per day by continuous intravenous infusion).

Even so, the polymyxins are poor drugs for the treatment of deep-seated infections and immunocompromised patients. The best results have been obtained in urinary tract infections or in cases of septicemia that arise from the urinary tract. Intrathecal administration is necessary for the treatment of meningitis.

Polymyxins are of principal clinical use in the topical treatment of superficial infections, eg, external otitis or corneal ulcers. Bladder infections can be treated by continuous irrigation with a solution of neomycin (40 mg per liter) and polymyxin B (20 mg per liter).[84]

Combinations of the polymyxins with sulfamethoxazole and trimethoprim are said to be synergistic in the treatment of serious infections with multiple drug-resistant *Serratia, P. cepacia, P. maltophilia,* or *P. aeuruginosa.*[85] A combination of polymyxin B and rifampin has been used to treat patients with *Serratia* infections.[86] Experience with both combinations is limited.

Adverse Reactions

The two important side effects of the polymyxins, nephrotoxicity and neurotoxicity, are reversible and can be reduced by reducing the dosage. Neurotoxicity manifests itself as paresthesias with flushing, dizziness, vertigo, ataxia, slurred speech, drowsiness, or confusion. In addition, the polymyxins have a curare-like action on striated muscles and block neuromuscular transmission. If apnea occurs, it can be treated with intravenous calcium chloride.[87]

VANCOMYCIN

Chemistry

Vancomycin is a complex glycopolypeptide unrelated to any other antibiotic.[88]

Pharmacology

It is usually given intravenously, because it is not absorbed by mouth and is painful on intramuscular injection. It is excreted almost exclusively by the kidney. Organisms susceptible to less than 10 μg per ml (the peak serum concentration after intravenous administration of a 500 mg dose) are considered susceptible. There is some penetration into the cerebrospinal fluid of patients with meningitis, but penetration through uninflamed meninges is poor. It is irritating in serous cavities. Because it is excreted in the kidney, the dose must be reduced in patients with renal malfunction—hemodialysis does not adequately remove it. It is best to monitor the serum levels in uremic patients to prevent excessive accumulation in the serum, even though formulas for reduction of dose are available.

TABLE 18-34. MAJOR THERAPEUTIC USES OF VANCOMYCIN

THERAPY OF CHOICE
- Serious infections with methicillin and cephalosporin-resistant staphylococci
- Enterococcal endocarditis in patients allergic to penicillin (in combination with aminoglycoside)
- Prosthetic valve endocarditis due to penicillin-resistant *Corynebacterium* spp
- Antibiotic-associated colitis secondary to *C. difficile*

ALTERNATIVE THERAPY
- Serious gram-positive infections in patients allergic to penicillin or for organisms resistant to cephalosporins and penicillins

Antimicrobial Spectrum and Clinical Uses

Gram-positive organisms (*S. aureus, S. epidermidis, S. pyogenes, S. pneumoniae,* anaerobic streptococci, *N. gonorrheae*), *Clostridium, B. anthracis, Actinomyces,* and *C. diphtheriae* are usually susceptible. *S. viridans, S. bovis,* and *S. faecalis,* although inhibited, resist killing. Vancomycin plus an aminoglycoside may be synergistic against *S. faecalis.* Gram-negative bacilli, *Mycobacterium, Bacteroides,* and fungi are not susceptible. The development of resistance is rare during treatment.[89]

The clinical uses of vancomycin are listed in Table 18-34. Because of its toxicity, vancomycin is prescribed only for the treatment of serious gram-positive infections in patients who are allergic to penicillin or for organisms not susceptible to penicillin or cephalosporins. Appropriate doses are listed in Table 18-35.[56]

Vancomycin is the drug of choice for pseudomembranous enterocolitis, whether caused by staphylococci or toxigenic clostridia, and is best given by mouth.[90]

Adverse Reactions

The most common side effects of its parenteral administration are fever, chills, and thrombophlebitis. Shock, leukopenia, and rashes are rare complications. The most

TABLE 18-35. VANCOMYCIN: USUAL DOSES

	Usual Dose	
Drug	***Pediatric***	***Adult***
Vancomycin		
Oral	40 mg/kg/day in 2–4 doses po	0.125–0.5 gm q6h
Parenteral	25–40 mg/kg/day in 2–4 doses IV	0.5 mg–2 gm/day in 2–4 doses IV

Adapted from Fekety R: Vancomycin. In Mandell GL, Douglas RG Jr, Bennett JE (eds.): *Principles and Practice of Infectious Diseases.* New York, Wiley, 1979, p. 304; and Gellis SS, Kagan BM: *Current Pediatric Therapy,* Vol 9. Philadelphia, Saunders, 1980, pp 531.

important adverse reaction is neurotoxicity as manifested by auditory nerve damage and hearing loss. Nephrotoxicity is now unusual,[91] since the impurities in the preparation have been removed. The major "toxicity" of oral administration is its disagreeable taste.

SULFONAMIDES

Chemistry and Classification

The sulfonamides have a structure similar to that of para-aminobenzoic acid (PABA), a factor necessary for bacterial folic acid synthesis (Fig. 18-6).[92] Substitutions of the 4-amino group result in decreased gastrointestinal absorption. Substitutions at the SO_2NH_2 group alter the pharmacologic properties of the drug, but the antimicrobial spectrum remains the same. Zinner[92] has classified the sulfonamides into: (1) short- or medium-acting sulfonamides useful for urinary tract infections, (2) long-acting sulfonamides (sulfamethoxypyridazine and sulfameter), (3) sulfonamides limited to the gastrointestinal tract (sulfaguanidine, sulfathalidine, salicylazosulfapyridine), and (4) topical sulfonamides (mafenide acetate, silver sulfadiazine). Topical preparations applied to extensive burns are absorbed.

Pharmacology

Intravenous administration of sulfadiazine, sulfisoxazole, and co-trimoxazole is possible, but most sulfonamides are administered orally or topically. After absorption from the gastrointestinal tract, they are distributed throughout the body, including the cerebrospinal fluid and serous cavities. The drugs undergo acetylation and glucuronidation in the liver, and both free and metabolized drugs are excreted in the urine. The usual doses are listed in Table 18-36. The doses should be reduced during renal failure (Table 18-18).

Antimicrobial Spectrum and Clinical Uses

Sulfonamides are active in vitro against a broad spectrum of gram-positive and gram-negative aerobic bacteria plus *Actinomyces, Chlamydiae, Plasmodium,* and *Toxoplasma* (Tables 18-3 to 18-5). But the activity is irregular, and certain organisms, *S. marcescens, P. aeruginosa,* enterococci, and anaerobes, are frequently resistant at serum levels which can easily be obtained after oral administration. The clinical uses of the sulfonamides are listed in Table 18-37.

Antimicrobial Resistance

Susceptible organisms may develop resistance by mutations, which result in overproduction of para-aminobenzoic acid, or a structural change in folic acid synthesizing enzyme so that it has lower affinity for sulfonamide.[93] The resistance can be mediated by R factors.

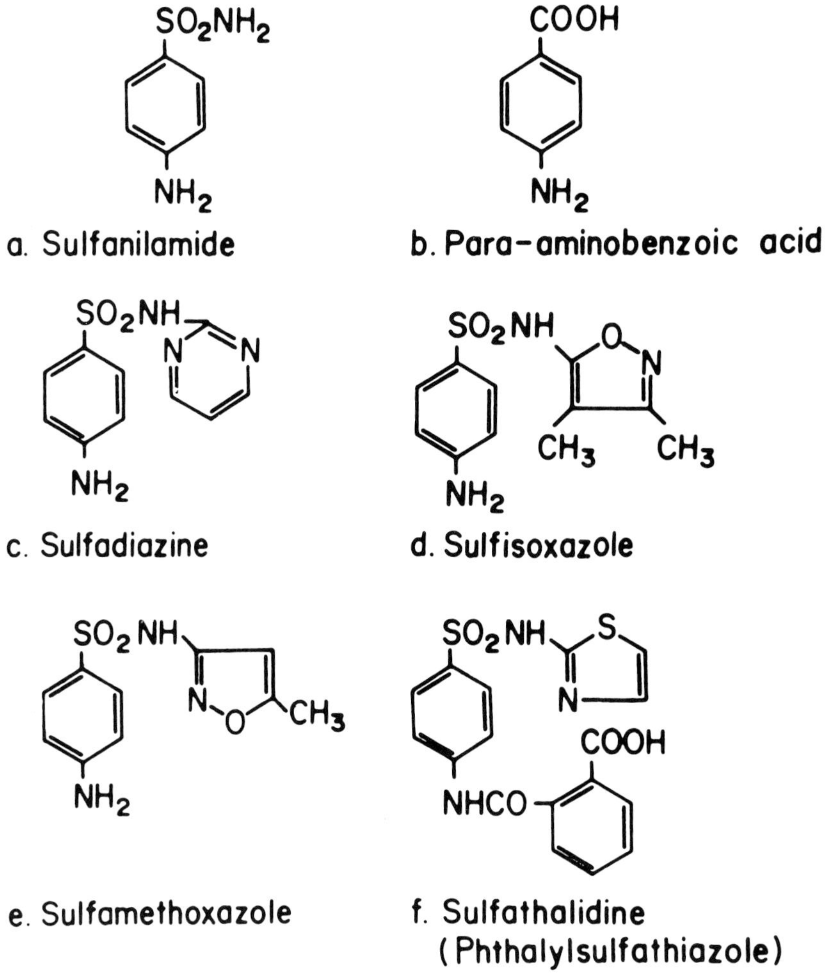

a. Sulfanilamide

b. Para-aminobenzoic acid

c. Sulfadiazine

d. Sulfisoxazole

e. Sulfamethoxazole

f. Sulfathalidine (Phthalylsulfathiazole)

Fig. 18-6. **Structural formulas of selected sulfonamides. (From Zinner SH: Sulfonamides and trimethoprim. In Mandell GL, Douglas RB Jr, Bennett JE (eds.): *Principles and Practice of Infectious Disease.* New York, Wiley, 1979, p 308.)**

TABLE 18-36. SULFONAMIDE PREPARATIONS AND USUAL DOSES

		Usual Dose	
Drug	**Preparation**	***Pediatric***	***Adult***
Co-trimoxazole (trimethoprim/ sulfamethoxazole)	Oral: tablets 80/ 400 mg and 160/ 800 mg Suspension 40/200 mg/5 ml Parenteral: 80 mg/400 mg per 5 ml ampule investigational	20/100 mg/kg/day in 2–4 dose po	2–4 tablets daily po (for urinary tract infections and prophylaxis) 20/100 mg/kg/day in 4 doses IV, po
Sulfisoxazole	Tablets: 500 mg Liquid: 500 mg/5 ml Ampules: 400 mg/ml in 5–10 ml	120–150 mg/kg/day in 4–6 doses po or IV	4 gm/day in 4 doses po, IV
Sulfamethoxazole	Tablets: 500 mg Liquid: 500 mg/5 ml	50–60 mg/kg/day in 2 doses	1 to 8 gm/day in 2–4 doses po
Sulfadiazine	Tablets: 325, 500 mg	150 mg/kg/day in 4 doses (6 gm max)	2–4 gm/day in 4 doses

TABLE 18-37. MAJOR CLINICAL USES OF THE SULFONAMIDES

THERAPY OF CHOICE
- Acute urinary tract infections caused by susceptible bacteria
- *Nocardia* infections
- Chancroid
- Topical therapy of burns

EFFECTIVE ALTERNATIVE THERAPY
- *Chlamydia* infections including nongonococcal urethritis
- Lymphogranuloma venereum
- Toxoplasmosis (with pyrimethamine)
- Melioidosis
- Dermatitis herpetiformis
- *Pneumocystis carinii* infections (with trimethoprim)

EFFECTIVE PROPHYLAXIS
- Rheumatic fever (group A *S. pyogenes*)
- *N. meningitidis* infections
- Recurrent urinary tract infections in women (with trimethoprim)
- Topical use on burns
- *P. carinii* infections (with trimethoprim)

Adverse Reactions

Sulfonamides are known to cause nausea, vomiting, diarrhea, rash, fever, headache, depression, jaundice, hepatic necrosis, and a serum sickness–like syndrome. Soluble sulfonamides rarely produce crystalluria anymore. Acute hemolytic anemia (associated with glucose-6-phosphate dehydrogenase deficiency), aplastic anemia, agranulocytosis, thrombocytopenia, and leukopenia have all been reported. Serious hypersensitivity reactions (ie, erythema nodosum, erythema multiforme) are more common in children. Because the sulfonamides compete with bilirubin-binding sites on plasma albumin, they may increase the chances of kernicterus and therefore should not be administered during the last month of pregnancy.

Sulfonamides interact with many other drugs. They increase the effect of activity of warfarin by displacing it from albumin-binding sites; anticoagulant dosage should be reduced during sulfonamide therapy. Numerous other drug interactions have been described by Zinsser.[92]

TRIMETHOPRIM AND CO-TRIMOXAZOLE

The sulfonamides act in synergy with trimethoprim, and a fixed drug combination is available (co-trimoxazole). Trimethoprim itself is useful in the treatment of urinary tract infections.

Chemistry

The structure of trimethoprim is noted in Figure 18-7. Trimethoprim inhibits bacterial dihydrofolate reductase, the enzymatic step that follows the step in bacterial folic acid metabolism–inhibited sulfonamides. Because both drugs block the same biosynthetic pathway at different sites, their combination acts synergistically against a wide spectrum of microorganisms. Since mammals do not synthesize folic acid, purine synthesis is not affected significantly.

Pharmacology

Trimethoprim plus sulfamethoxazole (co-trimoxazole) in a ratio of 1:5 is available for oral use (Table 18-36) and an intravenous preparation will probably soon be available. Trimethoprim (like sulfamethoxazole) is readily absorbed from the gastrointestinal tract, and after the usual dose (160 mg trimethoprim, 800 mg sulfamethoxazole), the serum levels are 1.6–3.2 μg per ml (Table 18-36). It is widely distributed in tissues, and the levels reached in the cerebrospinal fluid are therapeutic. Trimethoprim is concentrated in prostatic fluid. It is excreted by the kidney, and its half-life is prolonged by renal insufficiency. The concentrations in the urine are usually far in excess of the maximum inhibitory concentration for most urinary pathogens.[94] In severe uremia, a loading dose followed by half the dose once or twice daily has been recommended.

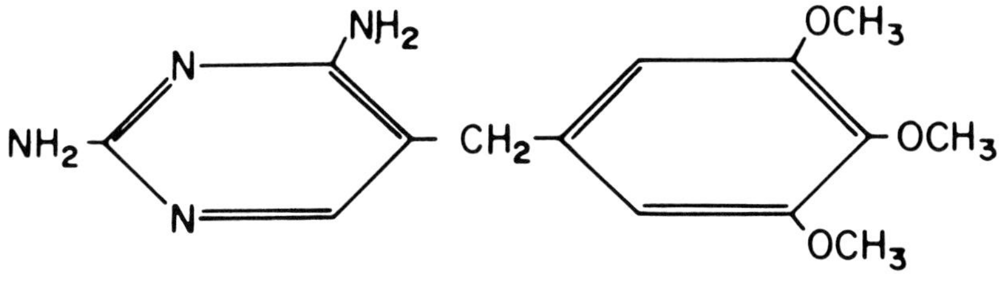

TRIMETHOPRIM

(2,4-diamino-5-(3',4',5'-trimethoxybenzyl)pyrimidine)

Fig. 18-7. Chemical structure of Trimethoprim [2,4-diamino-5-(3', 4', 5'-trimethoxybenzyl) pyrimidine]. (From Zinner SH: Sulfonamides and trimethoprim. In Mandell GL, Douglas RB Jr, Bennett JE (eds.): *Principles and Practice of Infectious Disease.* New York, Wiley, 1979, p 308.)

Antimicrobial Spectrum and Clinical Uses

Most gram-positive cocci and most gram-negative rods, except *P. aeruginosa* and *Bacteorides* species, are susceptible. Synergy with sulfamethoxazole (Tables 18-3 to 18-5) and with the polymyxins and the aminoglycosides has been reported.[95,96] The optimal ratio for in vitro synergy of trimethoprim and sulfamethoxazole in combination is 1:20. Even strains resistant to sulfamethoxazole will become sensitive to the combination in many cases, although this cannot be universally predicted.[97] The proved clinical uses of co-trimoxazole are listed in Table 18-38.

The principal clinical use of trimethoprim is in combination with sulfamethoxazole (co-trimoxazole) for the treatment of acute and chronic urinary tract infections. This combination is also useful for long-term suppressive therapy of recurrent or chronic urinary tract infections—it can control bacteria in vaginal secretions and in stool flora.[98,99]

Co-trimoxazole is useful in the treatment of pneumonia or bronchitis caused by sensitive organisms, but parenteral therapy with other agents is currently preferred. It may also be useful in the prophylaxis of acute exacerbations in patients with chronic bronchitis. Prophylaxis against *P. carinii* pneumonia in cancer patients and other immunosuppressed patients can be achieved by long-term, daily therapy with 150 mg per m^2 of trimethoprim and 750 mg per m^2 of sulfamethoxazole.[100] Co-trimoxazole is useful in reducing the incidence of gram-negative rod bacteremia in neutropenic patients (two tablets twice a day, or more, until stools are free of enteric organisms). Gastrointestinal anaerobes are not affected by this prophylaxis, so that the aerobes are seldom replaced by resistant organisms.[101]

TABLE 18-38. CLINICAL USES OF CO-TRIMOXAZOLE *

THERAPY OF CHOICE
Recurrent or chronic urinary tract infections due to susceptible organisms
P. carinii infections
ALTERNATIVE THERAPY
Prostatitis
Otitis media
Bronchitis and pneumonitis due to sensitive organisms
Typhoid fever and chronic *Salmonella* carriage
Shigellosis resistant to ampicillin
Brucellosis
Nocardiosis
Gonorrhea
PROPHYLAXIS
P. carinii (in immunosuppressed patients)
Bacteremia in neutropenic patients
Urinary tract infections in renal transplant patients

* Sulfamethoxazole-trimethoprim

Adverse Reactions

The adverse reactions of the sulfonamides are seen with the use of co-trimoxazole—a megaloblastic marrow with hypersegmented polymorphonuclear leukocytes, leukopenia, thrombocytopenia, and granulocytopenia can result. The administration of folic acid usually prevents or treats the side effects, and the antibacterial efficacies (except possibly against enterococci) are not impaired by such prophylaxis.

METRONIDAZOLE

Chemistry and Pharmacology

Metronidazole is a nitroimidazole derivative that is rapidly absorbed orally, with peak levels occurring 1 to 3 hours after ingestion. A parenteral form is now available. Two-thirds of the drug is executed unchanged in the urine, with only trace quantities identifiable in the feces. Tissue penetration is excellent and therapeutic levels are found in the cerebrospinal fluid.

Antimicrobial Spectrum and Uses

Metronidazole is active against the protozoa *Trichomonas vaginalis, Giardia lamblia,* and *Entamoeba histolytica.* It is the drug of choice for trichomoniases and of use in intestinal amebiasis and amebic liver abscess. Metronidazole shows marked activity against almost all anaerobic bacteria, especially *B. fragilis.* It appears to be the clinical equal of clindamycin in this regard.

Metronidazole is effective in the treatment of antibiotic-associated colitis caused by *C. difficile.* The potent antianaerobic bacterial activity makes this agent effective in reducing wound infections when given in combination with neomycin for preparation of the bowel before colorectal surgery (Chapter 39).[102]

Adverse Effects
Gastrointestinal distress with symptoms of anorexia, nausea, diarrhea, and abdominal cramps are common complaints. Less common side effects are skin rashes, leukopenia, and central nervous system symptoms (dizziness, vertigo, ataxia tremor). Darkening of the urine to a reddish-brown color is of no significance. Patients should not drink alcohol while taking metronidazole, because this agent has disulfiram-like properties and will cause flushing, vomiting, and abdominal cramping.

Studies in animals suggest that metronidazole has an oncogenic potential. The human significance of this finding has yet to be determined.

Dosage
The clinical uses and appropriate doses are listed in Table 18-39.

RIFAMPIN

Chemistry
The rifamycins are a group of antibacterial agents isolated from cultures of *Streptomyces mediterranei.* Rifamycin B is the active parent compound, which yields rifamide and rifampin after chemical modification.

Pharmacology
Rifampin is lipid soluble and is rapidly absorbed orally with peak serum levels of 5–10 μg per ml after a 600 mg oral dose 1 to 3 hours before. Rifampin penetrates liver, lung, placenta, bone, ascitic fluid, pleural exudates, and other intracellular and extracellular spaces in concentrations equal to or greater than that in the serum. The cerebrospinal fluid concentrations are greatest when the meninges are inflamed. Eighty percent of the drug is protein bound in plasma, and deacetylation takes place in the liver with 60 percent excretion in the feces. Bile concentrations of rifampin are about 100 times that of simultaneous serum levels. Urine concentrations are about ten times those in the serum.[43]

Spectrum
Gram-positive bacteria are usually sensitive to rifampin, including *Staphylococcus* strains (penicillin- and methicillin-resistant strains), pneumococcus, most *Streptococcus* (enterococcus is moderately sensitive), and *Clostridium.* Many gram-negative organisms are also sensitive including gonococci, meningococci, *H. influenza, E. coli, Enterobacter, Klebsiella, Proteus, P. aeruginosa, Salmonella, Shigella,* and *Bacteroides* species. *M. tuberculosis, M. kansasii, M. ulcerans, M. marinum, M. phlei,* and *M. leprae* are usually sensitive but *M. avium-intracellulare, M. smegmatis,* and *M. fortuitum* are resistant. Rifampin shows in vitro activity against *Chlamydiae* and some viruses, including cytomegalovirus, vaccinia, and adenoviruses.

Clinical Uses
Rifampin is a first-line agent, in combination with others, for the treatment of tuberculosis and asymptomatic pharyngeal carriers of *N. meningitidis.* In general, rifampin should not be used alone, because resistance develops rapidly.[103] Because of its broad spectrum, however, it is becoming increasingly useful in combination with other antibiotics (trimethoprim, nafcillin) for the treatment of resistant staphylococci (Table 18-40).

Mechanism of Action
RNA synthesis is blocked by rifampin by inhibiting DNA-dependent RNA polymerase. The human RNA polymerase is much less sensitive than the bacteria and thus is unaffected.

Adverse Effects
Flushing, itching, and rash of the face can occur after taking large doses of rifampin. Liver damage is the most serious effect. Thrombocytopenia has also been reported. Rifampin colors the urine red, as it does other body fluids.

Dose
The usual doses are listed in Table 18-40. A parenteral preparation is only available for investigational use.

URINARY TRACT ANTISEPTICS

Urinary tract antiseptics (Table 18-41) are drugs that are concentrated in the urine but are not useful for the treatment of systemic infections.[104] Nalidixic acid, oxolinic acid, and nitrofurantoin are useful for acute or recurrent infections and methenamine for chronic urinary tract suppression.

TABLE 18-39. CLINICAL USES AND USUAL DOSES FOR METRONIDAZOLE

	Usual Adult Dose
THERAPY OF CHOICE	
Trichomonas vaginalis	250 mg po tid × 7 days (female)
	250 mg po bid × 7 days (male partners)
Entamoeba histolytica	500–750 mg po tid × 5–7 days
EFFECTIVE ALTERNATIVE THERAPY	
Giardia lambnia	250–500 mg po tid × 5–7 days
Anaerobic infections including *B. fragilis*	1 gm q6h po
	30 mg/kg/day in 4 doses IV
PROPHYLAXIS	
Colorectal surgery	250 mg po tid × 2 days

TABLE 18-40. RIFAMPIN: USES, PREPARATIONS, AND DOSES

	Preparation	Usual Dose	
		Pediatric	*Adult*
THERAPY OF CHOICE			
Tuberculosis	300 mg capsules	10–20 mg/kg/day in one dose po	600 mg daily po
ALTERNATIVE THERAPY			
Leprosy	300 mg capsules	10–20 mg/kg/day in one dose po	600 mg daily po
Methicillin-resistant staphylococci (with other antistaphylococcal drugs)			
PROPHYLAXIS			
N. meningitidis contacts		10–20 mg/kg/day in one dose po for 4 days	300 mg bid for 4 days

TABLE 18-41. URINARY TRACT ANTISEPTICS

Agent Useful for Treatment	Therapeutic Dose for Acute and Recurrent Urinary Tract Infections	Suppressive Dose
Nalidixic acid	Adults: 1 gm qid for 1–2 weeks; thereafter, if needed, 0.5 gm qid for periods longer than 2 weeks Children: 55 mg/kg in 4 doses po	1 gm per day in single dose
Oxolinic acid	Adults: 750 mg bid for 2 weeks Children: Not recommended	Not useful as chronic suppressive
Nitrofurantoin	Adults: 50 or 100 g qid for 1–2 weeks Children: 1.25–1.75 mg/kg qid for 1–2 weeks	50–100 mgm in single dose (1 mg/kg bid in children)
Methenamine	Not useful in acute infection	Adults: 0.5–2 gm (usually 1 gm) qid or bid Children: 15 mg/kg qid Only when urine pH is 5.5 or less
Methenamine mandelate	Not useful in acute infection	Adults: 1 gm qid Children: 15 mg/kg qid Only when urine pH is 5.5 or less
Methenamine hippurate	Not useful in acute infection	Adults: 1 gm bid Children age 6–12 years: 0.5–1 gm bid Only when urine pH is 5.5 or less

Adapted from Andriole VT: Urinary tract agents: nalidixic acid, oxolinic acid, nitrofurantoin, and methenamine. In Mandell GL, Douglas RG Jr, Bennett JE (eds): *Principles and Practice of Infectious Diseases.* New York, Wiley, 1979, p 317.

Nalidixic Acid and Oxolinic Acid

These compounds are chemically related and have similar pharmacologic characteristics and clinical uses. Both inhibit DNA synthesis in bacterial cells and have a broad spectrum against gram-negative bacteria, but *Pseudomonas* species and gram-positive bacteria are resistant. Cross-resistance has been demonstrated between the two agents.

Both drugs are absorbed after oral administration and are excreted primarily by the kidneys. Both can be used in moderate or advanced renal failure,[105] although metabolites may accumulate in the blood.

Most adverse reactions are minor and disappear with discontinuation of the drug. These include gastrointestinal side effects, dermatologic reactions, and occasional visual abnormalities. Central nervous system reactions with excitation, headache, restlessness, insomnia, and dizziness have been observed with both drugs. The usual doses are listed in Table 18-41.

Nitrofurantoin

Nitrofurantoin is a useful drug in the treatment of acute urinary tract infections because it inhibits multiple enzymes within bacterial cells. It is effective against most strains of *E. coli* and other enteric gram-negative rods, but many *Klebsiella, Enterobacter,* and *Proteus* strains are resistant—*Pseudomonas* is almost always resistant. Gram-positive cocci including enterococci are generally sensitive.

Nitrofurantoin is administered orally and is rapidly absorbed from the gastrointestinal tract and excreted in the urine after some metabolic changes. Secretion into the urine of patients with renal malfunction is decreased so that it is not useful in patients with renal failure.

The common adverse reactions are minor, and most are reversed by cessation of drug therapy. Gastrointestinal irritation is the most common side effect; hypersensitivity reactions, and dermatologic allergic manifestations are generally mild and infrequent. Acute or chronic hypersensitivity and interstitial pneumonitis [106] occur in elderly patients and may require steroid therapy. The most serious side effects of nitrofurantoin therapy are neurologic reactions, especially polyneuritis which occurs primarily in patients with renal failure and patients who receive prolonged therapeutic courses. Demyelination and degeneration of both sensory and motor nerves occur. Use of the drug should be stopped at the earliest signs of paresthesias.[107]

Methenamine

Methenamine has no antibacterial action by itself but is metabolized in acid pH to formaldehyde. The normal urine pH is sufficient for this transformation although various attempts to increase the acidity of urine have been tried using mandelic acid, hippuric acid, ascorbic acid, or cranberry juice. Methenamine is virtually useless, therefore, for the treatment of urea splitting organisms such as *Proteus* species. All gram-positive and gram-negative bacteria and fungi are equally susceptible to formaldehyde at concentrations of 20 mg per liter.[108]

Although the drug is rapidly absorbed from the gastrointestinal tract, it is inactive until excreted into acid urine. Only bladder urine contains adequate levels of formaldehyde. For this reason, the only toxic effects are upper gastrointestinal distress and bladder irritation. Methenamine is useful primarily as a chronic suppressive agent and is not useful for acute upper or lower urinary tract infections.

Of the four agents (Table 18-41), nitrofurantoin is the most versatile, since it is effective in treating both upper and lower urinary tract infections and recurrent bacteriuria. It can also be used as a long-term suppressive agent in children and pregnant women.

ANTIMYCOBACTERIAL AGENTS

FIRST-LINE ANTITUBERCULOSIS DRUGS (Table 18-42) [109]

Isoniazid

Isoniazid is a bactericidal drug that is active against growing *M. tuberculosis* but static against resting organisms. Resistance to the drug develops rapidly when it is administered alone. It is absorbed after oral or intramuscular administration and distributed through the body, and achieves adequate cerebrospinal fluid levels. It is acetylated in the body with acetylation affected by the genetic status of the recipient (ie, a fast acetylation or a slow acetylator). Dosage modification is not necessary in hepatic or renal failure unless the patient is a slow acetylator.

Isoniazid is a safe drug, except that the acetylhydrazine metabolite sometimes causes hepatitis, especially in the elderly. No longer is routine isoniazid prophylaxis advised for adult PPD skin test converters.

The second toxic reaction is a peripheral neuropathy, which can be ameliorated and prevented by concurrent pyridoxine administration. Other hypersensitivity phenomena are unusual. Liver toxicity is increased when rifampin is concurrently used, and isoniazid serum levels are increased by concurrent para-aminosalicyclic acid administration (Table 18-42).

Ethambutol

Ethambutol is tuberculostatic through an action on RNA synthesis. It is absorbed through the gastrointestinal tract and distributed into the cerebrospinal fluid, as well as other tissues, in patients with meningitis. Since it is excreted in the urine, dosage must be reduced in patients with renal malfunction. Resistance is unusual.

The principal toxicity of ethambutol is a retrobulbar neuritis with impairment of visual acuity or color vision and constriction of visual fields. Those changes are reversible on drug cessation. Other toxicities are unusual. Ethambutol has replaced para-aminosalicylic acid as a companion drug for isoniazid (Table 18-42).

Rifampin

The pharmacology and spectrum of rifampin are discussed in a preceding section. Rifampin is a potent tuberculocidal drug, which is excreted primarily in bile and consequently does not require dosage reduction in renal failure (Table

TABLE 18-42. FIRST-LINE ANTITUBERCULOUS DRUGS: PREPARATIONS AND DOSES

	Preparations	Usual Dosage: *Pediatric*	Usual Dosage: *Adult*
Isoniazid (INH) *	Tablets: 100, 300 mg Capsules: 300 mg Liquid: 10 mg/ml Vial: 100 mg/ml (for IV or IM use)	10–15 mg/kg/day (up to 300 mg) in single dose po, IV, IM	300 mg/day in single dose po, IV, IM
Ethambutol	Tablets: 100, 400 mg	15–20 mg/kg/day †	15–25 mg/kg/day
Rifampin	Capsules: 300 mg	10–20 mg/kg/day in single dose po	600 mg/day in single dose po
Streptomycin	Ampules: 0.5 gm/ml in 2-ml or 10-ml vials	20–40 mg/kg/day in 2 IM doses	1–2 gm/day in 2 IM doses

* Given with 10–50 mg po of pyroxidine.
† Not recommended for children under 13 years of age.

18-42). Resistance to *M. tuberculosis* develops fairly frequently.[110] The only serious adverse reaction is its additive hepatic toxicity to isoniazid and its intrinsic mild hepatotoxicity with other hepatotoxic drugs. In addition, it is mildly immunosuppressive and colors all body secretions orange, including urine, serum, semen, saliva, feces, and cerebrospinal fluid—patients should be warned.

Streptomycin

Streptomycin and amikacin are tuberculocidal aminoglycosides.[111] Streptomycin is used as part of multiple drug therapy for *M. tuberculosis* infections. Combination regimens delay development of resistance to streptomycin, which would otherwise develop rapidly. The doses are listed in Table 18-42. The other properties of the aminoglycosides are discussed in a preceding section.

SECOND LINE ANTITUBERCULOUS DRUGS

Para-aminosalicylic Acid (PAS)

This compound is administered orally and excreted after metabolism in the urine. It interferes with mycobacterial growth by impairing folate synthesis. Its principal toxic effect is gastrointestinal pain and nausea. Hypersensitivity phenomena are common, and its administration along with streptomycin can lead to hypersensitivity to those drugs. Because PAS inhibits isoniazid acetylation, increased toxicity of isoniazid may be associated with PAS therapy. The sodium salt may lead to congestive symptoms in patients with cardiorenal insufficiency.

Currently, PAS is not used in the United States in combination with isoniazids because ethambutol is a better combinant. Its low cost indicates its use in less developed countries in combination therapy (adult dose: 8 to 12 gm per day in three divided oral doses).[109]

Cycloserine

Cycloserine is a broad-spectrum antibiotic which is one of several drugs used to treat resistant, or retreat previously treated, recurrent tuberculosis. It is absorbed from the gastrointestinal tract and penetrates the cerebrospinal fluid. Its principal side effect is peripheral neuropathy with central nervous system disorders (adult dose: 500 mg per day in two oral doses).[109]

Ethionamide

Ethionamide is a tuberculostatic derivative of isonicotinic acid, which is absorbed orally, penetrates the cerebrospinal fluid, and inhibits isoniazid acetylation. Severe gastrointestinal intolerance may necessitate a gradual increase in dose from 250 mg twice a day to the peak dose of 500 mg–1 gm per day. In addition, it has central nervous system and peripheral neuropathic symptoms, which may be alleviated by administration of pyridoxine or nicotinamide.[109]

Pyrazinamide

Pyrazinamide is a tuberculostatic drug which is absorbed from the gastrointestinal tract and achieves therapeutic levels in the cerebrospinal fluid when the meninges are inflamed. Its high incidence of severe hepatotoxicity has severely limited its use in the United States to the treatment of resistant disease. However, because it is a cheap, effective agent and can be administered in once-weekly doses (90 mg per kg) it has been useful in developing countries (usual adult dose: 20–35 mg per kg per day by mouth in two to three doses).[109]

Other Second-Line Drugs

Five other second-line drugs can be used for the treatment of tuberculosis. These include the aminoglycosides (kanamycin, amikacin) and the polypeptide antibiotics viomycin and capreomycin. These four have ototoxicity and nephrotoxicity and should never be used in combination with one another or with streptomycin. All are administered intramuscularly, usually in hospitalized patients. Daily treatment should be used only for a short time, as in the case of streptomycin.[109]

Amithiozone is a first-line drug in East Africa. It has

gastrointestinal toxicity, marrow suppression, and hepatotoxicity, and is not available in the United States. It is useful only in combination with other drugs, because resistance develops rapidly in recipients of the single drug.[109]

DRUGS FOR THE TREATMENT OF ATYPICAL MYCOBACTERIAL INFECTIONS

The difficulties with the treatment of atypical mycobacterial infections and the selection of drugs has been described in Chapter 7. There is limited clinical experience, and in vitro sensitivity data are meager. Surgical therapy of atypical mycobacterial infections is frequently required to achieve total therapeutic success with antimicrobial agents.

In general, antituberculous drugs cannot be considered a priori active against atypical mycobacteria, and drugs ineffective against tuberculosis are sometimes highly efficacious against atypical mycobacteria. Generally, combinations of agents are required.[112] Table 18-43 [109] lists the antimicrobial agents that are likely to be effective against certain atypical *Mycobacterium*.[113] Individual sensitivity studies should be performed in all isolated atypical mycobacterial infections.

ANTIFUNGAL AGENTS

Amphotericin B

Chemistry

Amphotericin is a polyene macrolide antibiotic obtained from *Streptomyces nodosus*. Amphotericin B exerts its action by its ability to combine with cytoplasmic membrane sterols, principally ergosterol in fungi. Resistant mutants with abnormal membrane sterols are rare in clinical practice.[114]

Pharmacology

Amphotericin B is poorly soluble in water at neutral pH, so that a colloidal suspension in 5 percent glucose is used intravenously. The infusion bottle does not have to be shielded from the light. Saline solutions cause the colloid to aggregate, resulting in suboptimal therapeutic effects. Even without aggregation, the colloidal solution is partially retained by a 0.22 micron membrane filter.

Following intravenous infusion, more than 95 percent of the drug is bound to beta-lipoproteins, presumably as a result of the cholesterol carried on this protein. The majority of the drug then promptly leaves the circulation. The reservoir of the drug is unknown, but it slowly reenters the circulation. It is apparently degraded in situ, and only a small amount is excreted in the bile or urine. Blood levels are not influenced by renal function or hemodialysis. The amphotericin B concentrations and fluids obtained from an inflamed area, such as the pleuroperitoneum or joint and aqueous humor, are approximately two-thirds of the serum levels. Amphotericin B cannot, however, penetrate into the cerebrospinal fluid, vitreous humor, or amniotic fluid. Therefore, to treat fungal meningitis, intrathecal or intercisternal administration is recommended. The peak serum concentrations with the usual intravenous administration are 1.2–2.0 μg per ml, but these concentrations rapidly fall to a plateau of approximately 0.5 μg per ml.[115]

TABLE 18-43. ANTIMICROBIALS FOR ATYPICAL MYCOBACTERIA: LIKELIHOOD OF IN VITRO SENSITIVITIES BEING WITHIN RANGE OF ACHIEVABLE SERUM LEVELS

Runyon Group	Mycobacterial Species	Likelihood of Antimicrobial Sensitivity
I. Photochromogens	*M. kansasii*	Erythromycin (4+), ethionamide (4+), rifampin (4+), streptomycin (4+), amikacin (3+), cycloserine (3+), ethambutol (3+), viomycin (3+), INH (2+)
	M. marinum	Rifampin (4+)
II. Scotochromogens	*M. scrofulaceum*	Amikacin (4+), erythromycin (4+), kanamycin (4+), streptomycin (4+), rifampin (3+), ethionamide (2+), INH (+), PAS (±)
III. Nonchromogens	*M. avium-intracellulare* (Battey)	Amikacin (4+), ethionamide (2+), rifampin (2+), streptomycin (2+), kanamycin (1+), viomycin (1+), erythromycin (1+)
IV. Rapid growers	*M. fortuitum* complex	Tetracycline (3+), amikacin (2+), capreomycin (1+), ethionamide (1+), gentamicin (1+), kanamycin (1+), viomycin (1+), erythromycin (±), streptomycin (±)
	M. ulcerans	Rifampin (4+), streptomycin (4+)

Adapted from Alford RH: Antimycobacterial agents. In Mandell GL, Douglas RG Jr, Bennett JE (eds): *Principles and Practice of Infectious Diseases.* New York, Wiley, 1979, p 338.

Antimicrobial Spectrum

Amphotericin B is useful for infection with almost all fungal pathogens, including *C. neoformans, C. albicans, B. dermatiditis, S. schenckii, P. brasiliensis, H. capsulatum, C. imitis, Aspergillus* species, *Torulopsis glabrata,* and *Phycomycetes,* which cause mucormycosis (Chapter 9).

Adverse Effects

The toxicity of amphotericin B represents the most serious limitation to its use. These toxic effects are so notorious that inexperienced physicians, who fear the toxicity more than the infection, frequently withold it from needy patients. Despite the fact that some toxic effects are almost inevitable, almost all patients can complete a conventional course of therapy.

Fever (sometimes with shaking chills), headache, nausea and vomiting, anorexia, malaise, and muscle and joint pains are frequent problems at the onset of therapy. Therapy should not be curtailed, however, because these effects usually abate as therapy progresses. Hydrocortisone, diphenhydramine, and salicylates are frequently used to control the side effects. Because of these potentially grave constitutional symptoms, therapy is begun slowly (see subsequent section), and increased by daily increments to maintenance doses. Tolerance to the febrile reactions develop with time, allowing diminution in the hydrocortisone and diphenhydramine. Frequently, they can be discontinued altogether. Patients who are already receiving steroid therapy, such as renal transplant recipients, get little benefit from additional steroids.[115,116]

Renal toxicity is the most serious problem associated with amphotericin B therapy. A dose-related decrease in renal blood flow and glomerular filtration occurs, and changes in the glomerular basement membranes and tubules are produced. Hypokalemia may require potassium supplementation, and a mild renal tubular acidosis can be produced. Renal function improves when amphotericin B is stopped, but permanent deterioration of clearance occurs in patients who receive extremely high doses. The hope that mannitol or alkali infusion could reduce nephrotoxicity has not been borne out. Administration of amphotericin B on alternate days, rather than daily, will reduce nephrotoxicity, but only if the cumulative rate of administration is halved.

The other toxic reactions associated with amphotericin B include thrombophlebitis and local pain at the injection site, normocytic anemia usually accompanied by a normal bone marrow, and hypokalemia. Less frequent side effects are cardiovascular toxicity including arrhythmias, hypertension, thrombocytopenia, leukopenia, and burning sensations on the soles of the feet. These side effects, which disappear slowly during the first 3 months after therapy, reflect slow catabolism of the drug.

The dosage schedule of amphotericin administration has been manipulated in an attempt to reduce its toxicity. To obviate the nausea, vomiting, fever, and chills, the infusion can be given over a longer period than the usual 6 hours. Some patients have fewer reactions if the dose is given during 2 hours, and others have shown that the drug can be given safely with no increase in side effects over 45 minutes or even 10 minutes. Short-term infusion has been reported to decrease the incidence of nausea and chills, to reduce the premedication needed, and to shorten the length of clinic visits for outpatients who are receiving amphotericin B.[116]

Preparations and Doses

The available preparations are listed in Table 18-44. The usual daily maintenance dose ranges from 0.4 to 0.6 mg per kg. These doses are decreased somewhat from the previously recommended daily dose of 1 to 1.5 mg per kg. Therapy is usually begun with test doses, such as 1 mg, to determine whether or not the patient will develop a fever. The doses then increase by 5 mg increments daily up to the full therapeutic dose. In patients with rapidly progressing infections, the second dose can be increased to 0.3 mg per kg. The dose is then advanced to 0.5 mg per kg per day by the third to fifth day. The duration of therapy is usually 6 to 12 weeks, with a total adult dose equaling 1 to 3 gm depending on the mycosis treated, but no reliable guidelines for duration of therapy exist. After initially treating patients in the hospital and establishing their tolerance to the drug, one can treat them as outpatients if their clinical status permits. These rather arbitrary dose schedules appear to be necessary for the eradication of chronic histoplasmosis and cryptococcal meningitis. Such prolonged high-dose therapy is probably not necessary in cases of infected wounds, empyema, or fungal peritonitis, in which cases short courses of therapy (total dose approximately 6 to 8 mg per kg) are probably adequate.[116a]

Cerebrospinal fluid levels are inadequate, and intrathecal or intracisternal injections via Omaya reservoirs are occasionally used in patients with fungal meningitis. When given intrathecally, the lumbar injections may cause temporary radicular pain and loss of motor function in the legs, rectum, and bladder. Use of 10 percent glucose as a diluent, and positioning the patient during injection to permit hyperbaric flow toward the brain, may decrease this local myopathy. Bladder irrigations with amphotericin 50 μg per ml in distilled water have been used in *Candida* cystitis. The cornea may be bathed with a solution containing 1 mg per ml of amphotericin. The solution is irritating but is beneficial in keratomycosis. Local infusion into joints and other body cavities has been useful.[114]

Amphotericin B in Combination with Other Drugs

Amphotericin B has been used in combination with other antifungal agents in an effort to reduce its toxicity and increase its therapeutic effect. Because amphotericin B combines with the cell membranes of fungi and increases permeability, these other agents are able to gain entrance into the fungal cell in larger quantities. For this reason, antibiotics such as tetracycline and rifampin appear to have an amphotericin-sparing effect,[117] but clinical experience is limited.

Flucytosine has increased antifungal activity against *Candida* and *Cryptococcus* when combined with amphotericin. Flucytosine should not be administered alone because of the rapid emergence of resistant organisms.

Some new antifungal agents have also been tried in combination with amphotericin B. Clotrimazole enhances the effectiveness of amphotericin B against *Candida* spe-

TABLE 18-44. ANTIFUNGAL AGENTS: PREPARATIONS AND DOSES

	Preparations	Pediatrics	Adult
Amphotericin B	50 mg powder dilute 1 mg to 10 ml D_5W	Increase gradually to 0.3–0.7 mg/kg/day	Increase gradually * to 0.3–0.7 mg/kg/day
Nystatin	Vaginal tablet: 100,000 units/tablet Tablets: 500,000 units Liquid: 100,000 units/ml in 60-ml bottles with calibrated dropper. Also available as cream and ointment	5–10 ml swished and swallowed every 4 hours (increased as necessary) Vaginal tablets qid × 2 weeks	51–10 ml swished and swallowed every 4 hours (increased as necessary) Vaginal tablets bid-qid × 2 weeks
Flucytosine	250 and 500 mg capsules (injectable under investigation)	50–150 mg/kg/day in 4 doses po	100–150 mg/kg/day in 4 doses po
Miconazole	2% cream (topical and vaginal) Ampule 200 mg in 20 ml	—	0.6–1.0 gm q8h IV
Ketoconazole (investigational)	200 mg tablets	—	200–400 mg po in single daily dose
Griseofulvin	Tablets and capsules: 125, 250, 500 mg Liquid: 125 mg/5 ml	10 mg/kg/day in single dose	0.5–1.0 gm/day in single dose

* Treatment of acute life-threatening infections may require use of full therapeutic doses.

cies in vitro, but it is antagonistic against *Torulopsis* in vitro. Similarly, miconazole is antagonistic with amphotericin B against *Candida.*

Nystatin

Nystatin is a polyene macrolide antibiotic, which is both fungistatic and fungicidal, like amphotericin B. Because of its toxicity after parenteral administration, it is used only topically and orally. It is not absorbed from the gastrointestinal tract and is currently used most often for the prophylaxis and therapy of esophageal, gastrointestinal, vaginal, or cutaneous candidiasis. Its efficacy is proportional to its concentration and dose. The available preparations and commonly used doses are listed in Table 18-44. Higher doses (up to 1 million units) have been recommended for prophylaxis of oral candidiasis in severely immunodepressed patients. Even higher doses (4 million units every 4 hours) have prevented *Candida* sepsis in neutropenic children during leukemia chemotherapy. Theoretically, candidemia in such patients originates in gastrointestinal overgrowth and persorption of the yeasts through the intestinal wall. Reduction of the yeast count in the intestine by high-dose nystatin may prevent this complication. There is as yet, however, no evidence to support this concept in general surgical patients, on broad-spectrum antibiotics, who have high *Candida* counts in their gastrointestinal tract, even though the practice is common.

Flucytosine

Flucytosine (5-fluorocytosine) was first synthesized as a cytosine antimetabolite for the treatment of leukemia. The drug proved ineffective for this purpose but was found to be effective as an antifungal agent.[118]

Pharmacology

Flucytosine is absorbed from the gastrointestinal tract, and peak serum levels are reached in 2 to 6 hours. Because it is excreted unchanged by glomerular filtration, the dose must be reduced in patients with renal failure. The appropriate dose is best monitored by measuring the drug in serum 2 hours after the last dose and immediately before the next dose. These values should range between 50 and 100 μg per ml. The drug is removed by hemodialysis. In patients on hemodialysis, therapeutic nontoxic serum levels of flucytosine can usually be maintained by administering a single dose (25–50 mg per kg) after each dialysis.

5-Fluorocytosine is well distributed in body tissues and fluids, including the cerebrospinal fluid.

Antifungal Properties and Clinical Uses

Flucytosine is currently recommended for cryptococcosis, candidiasis, torulopsis, and chromoblastomycosis. Because of the tendency of resistant strains to emerge, and the greater efficacy when combined with amphotericin, it is never used as a sole agent.

Mechanisms of Action

Flucytosine enters a cell by way of permease enzymes located on the cell membrane and is believed to exert its effect by deamination in the fungal cells to the antimetabolite 5-fluorouracil. Resistance of fungi to 5-fluorocytosine may be due to a change in their plasma membrane which prevents penetration of the drug into the cell. The synergistic effect of 5-fluorocytosine and amphotericin B against some fungi probably results from the action of amphotericin B, which permits more flucytosine to enter the cell.

Adverse Effects

Flucytosine has relatively few toxic side effects. Nausea and diarrhea can occur but are uncommon. Skin rashes have also occasionally been seen. Because so many of the patients who receive flucytosine have underlying hematopoietic disorders and have also been receiving amphotericin B, its toxicity on the bone marrow alone is difficult to assess, but individual reports of bone marrow depression and aplastic anemia have been reported. Anemia, neutropenia, thrombocytopenia, and eosinophilia have also been described. Transient liver enlargement associated with elevated transaminase levels has been noted in a few patients. Nephrotoxicity has not been ascribed to 5-fluorocytosine.

Miconazole

Miconazole is a synthetic imidazole antifungal compound that is chemically related to the nitroimidazoles, such as the antiparasitic agents metronidazole and mebendazole. Topical treatment has long been available. After intravenous infusion, penetration into the cerebrospinal fluid is poor, and urine concentrations are too low to treat mycosis of the urinary tract.

The mode of action of miconazole appears to be due to its ability to damage the fungal plasma membrane by its interference with ergosterol metabolism or synthesis. The fungal cytoplastic membrane becomes more permeable, causing leakage of cytoplasmic contents. Although cytoplasmic membrane damage is also the effect of amphotericin B, no synergism occurs between miconazole and amphotericin B, and antagonism has been reported.

Toxic reactions include anorexia, nausea, diarrhea, hyponatremia, phlebitis, drowsiness, arthralgias, acute psychosis, hyperlipidemia, and an elevation in liver function test results. This drug may also potentiate the anticoagulant effect of coumarin drugs such as warfarin.[114]

Intravenous miconazole has some therapeutic effect in patients with coccidioidomycosis, paracoccidioidomycosis, and petriellidosis,[119] but the failure and relapse rate is high for coccidioidomycosis. Although it is approved for cryptococcosis and candidasis, there is no convincing evidence that it is effective. The available preparations and dosages are listed in Table 18-44.

Clotrimazole

Clotrimazole is an effective topical agent for *Candida* or dermatophyte infections, but is not useful for systemic infections.

Ketoconazole

Ketoconazole is another imidazole derivative, which has undergone recent clinical trials. This agent is slightly less active than miconazole in vitro, but oral absorption is much better.

Ketoconazole is an investigational antifungal agent that inhibits the growth of most fungi in low concentrations. Limited clinical studies have suggested it is active against many species of fungi, including paracoccidioidomycosis, coccidioidomycosis, candidiasis, cryptococcosis, and histoplasmosis. Ketoconazole is administered orally and is distributed to most organs including liver, kidney, bone marrow, brain, and lung. Excretion is primarily by liver metabolism, although the unchanged drug is also present in stool and urine.

Ketoconazole acts by inhibiting fungal ergosterol biosynthesis leading to increased membrane permeability and cell lysis. Nausea has been reported as the only common side effect, but experience is far too limited to know the long-term effects. The current suggested dose is 200 mg orally once daily [120,120a]

Griseofulvin

In 1939 griseofulvin was isolated from a culture of *Penicillium griseofulvium.* It is only active against dermatophytes; no activity has been demonstrated against bacteria, yeasts, or filamentous fungi. Its use is thus limited to the treatment of Microsporum, Epidermophyton, and Trichophyton infections of the skin, hair, and nails. Skin infections respond to 2 to 3 weeks of therapy, although palms and soles take 4 to 8 weeks, and the nails 6 to 12 months for cure. The usual dose of griseofulvin in these situations is 10 mg per kg for children and 0.5 to 1 gm daily for adults (Table 18-44), given either as a single dose or in 2 to 4 divided doses per day. Side effects, although rare, include headache, gastritis, leukopenia (WBC counts should be done weekly), erythematous rash, estrogen-like effects and elevations in liver enzyme levels.

ANTIVIRAL AGENTS

Because viruses use the metabolic machinery of the host mammalian cells for their essential synthetic activities, it has been difficult to develop antiviral agents that specifically attack the virus. Many putative antiviral agents are toxic for the host's cells as well as the virus. In contrast, the unique structural and metabolic machinery of bacteria has allowed the antibiotics to be both toxic to these organisms and safe for humans.

In recent years, intracellular processes unique to virus replication have been identified. These processes can serve as specific targets for chemotherapeutic attack. Other new antiviral agents affect the viral envelope before the virus can enter the mammalian cell. In addition, the newer diagnostic tests that permit the rapid diagnosis of viral disease have permitted the administration of these agents at an earlier time. Because some agents are only effective if given prior to infection of the cell by virus, some viral infections can now be treated within hours of obtaining appropriate specimens (Chapter 12). Despite this optimism, it is still early in the development of antiviral agents, and only a few proved effective agents are available for a small number of viral diseases.[121,137]

Amantadine and Rimantadine

Amantadine (1-adamantanamine hydrochloride) is a tricyclide amine. It was originally used as prophylaxis against influenza-A virus, but it is only licensed for use in Asian influenza (H_2N_2). Rimantadine is a similar but unlicensed drug.

Antiviral Activity

In cell cultures, amantadine prevents infection with RNA viruses of several groups (myxovirus, paramyxoviruses, togaviruses). Its only clinical application is against influenza A viruses. Many influenza A virus strains are sensitive to less than 0.4 μg per ml. Resistance can be induced in vitro, however, by serial passage of influenza A virus strains in low concentrations of amantadine. Much higher and more toxic concentrations of amantadine (25–50 μg per ml) are inhibitory for some other viruses.

The mechanism of the antiviral activity is not fully appreciated. Amantidine interferes with successful penetration of the cell by influenza virus, and it blocks uncoating of the virus and release of the viral nucleic acid into the cell.[121] It does not directly inactivate the virus, nor does it inhibit the viral neuramidinase. When added 1.5 hours after virus inoculation, amantadine no longer inhibits virus multiplication.

Pharmacology and Toxicity

Amantadine is rapidly absorbed from the gastrointestinal tract, and peak serum levels of approximately 0.3 μg per ml are achieved 2 to 4 hours after a dose of 2.5 mg per kg body weight. The half-life in serum is approximately 20 hours. With the usual adult dose of 100 mg every 12 hours, 48 hours are required to reach maximum tissue concentration. Approximately all the drug is excreted unchanged in the urine, so that if renal function is compromised, the dose must be reduced. Most side effects occur in patients with compromised renal function.

Side effects occur in 3 to 7 percent of healthy adults and usually include insomnia and difficulty in concentration. Confusion, hallucinations, convulsions, anxiety, and coma have also been reported. Symptoms of toxicity usually occur shortly after amantadine is begun, as peak blood levels are reached, and the effects are reversible when the drug is discontinued. Insomnia may be minimized by giving the full daily dose of 200 mg in the morning rather than 100 mg every 12 hours.

Clinical Indications

The prophylactic efficacy of amantadine has been clearly demonstrated. The drug reduced morbidity by 50 percent during an epidemic of influenza As/Hong Kong, and 100 percent in an epidemic of a H_3N_2 strain (80 percent reduction in seroconversion). Amantadine is effective against H_2N_2, H_3N_2, and H_1N_1 subtypes of influenza A in doses of 200 mg per day. Dose-response curves have not been established in clinical studies. When deciding on its use, however, one must remember that influenza A virus attack rates are only 10 to 20 percent, so therefore amantadine given to 100 persons will prevent influenza in only seven to 16 of them; at the same time, it will cause minor central nervous system side effects in five or six people who would not be expected to contract the disease. Other problems with the use of prophylactic administration of amantadine has been the lack of virologic facilities to find the cause of many outbreaks of respiratory illnesses in scattered communities and the inability to rapidly distribute amantadine among the population.[122]

When given therapeutically in controlled studies, amantadine causes a decrease in fever and a shortening of the illness.[123]

Amantadine is approved for use in the United States for both prevention and treatment of influenza A virus infections. Prophylactic use is appropriate in certain circumstances, only if there is virologic epidemiologic confirmation of an outbreak of influenza A and if vaccination cannot be carried out. Prophylaxis is then indicated for unvaccinated persons at high risk of serious complications because of underlying immunodeficiency, pulmonary, metabolic, or cardiovascular disease. In addition, older persons who have not received influenza vaccine and unimmunized adults whose activity is essential to the community should be vaccinated. Prophylaxis should be begun as soon as influenza is identified in the region, and it should be continued throughout the risk period because any beneficial effect ceases within 48 hours after the drug is discontinued. Since amantadine does not interfere with immunogenicity of an inactivated vaccine, the drug can be started in conjunction with immunization and continued for 2 weeks until protective antibody develops.

For amantadine to be effective therapeutically, it must be administered within the first 24 to 48 hours of the onset of symptoms. Patients for whom such therapy should be considered are those at high risk for developing serious problems from influenza, such as the elderly, those with immunodeficiency disorders, and those with pulmonary disease.

Vidarabine

Vidarabine (adenine arabinoside) is one of several nucleoside derivatives that are effective against the herpesvirus family. This agent is currently approved in the United States for treatment of herpes simplex encephalitis and herpes simplex catarrhal conjunctivitis.

Antiviral Activity

Vidarabine has activity against the herpes group viruses, pox viruses, and even possibly hepatitis B viruses. Vidarabine and its less active metabolic product arabinosyl hypoxanthine are converted within the cell to monophosphates, diphosphates, and triphosphates, which may in turn selectively and competitively inhibit the activity of the herpesvirus DNA polymerase. The phosphorylated drug is then incorporated into both cellular and viral DNA. Incorporated viral vidarabine has been reported to act as a chain terminator for newly synthesized herpes simplex DNA strains. Antiviral activity is greatest against herpes simplex virus types I and II, cytomegalovirus, varicella zoster virus, vaccinia, and variola virus.[124] Other DNA viruses, such as adenoviruses and papovaviruses, are not inhibited, apparently because they lack a DNA polymerase.

Pharmacology and Toxicity

The plasma half-life of vidarabine is approximately 4 hours in adults, and nearly 60 percent of the dose is recovered in the urine, principally as hypoxanthine arabinoside. It must be given in reduced doses to patients with decreased renal function. Administration to patients with compromised renal function is further complicated by its poor solubility, which requires that it be diluted in large fluid volumes.

Little toxicity is seen at doses of 5–15 mg per kg per day given by 12-hour intravenous infusion. Nausea, vomiting, and diarrhea have been observed in a small percentage of patients. Large doses, 20 mg per kg, cause tremors, weight loss, and bone marrow megaloblastosis. Other adverse reactions include anorexia, nausea, vomiting, diarrhea, skin rash, thrombophlebitis at the intravenous site, and weakness. Central nervous system side effects include tremor, dizziness, hallucinations, psychosis, ataxias, and electroencephalogram changes. Rapid mental deterioration with agitation, tremulousness, facial grimacing, and eventual coma and death occurred in four renal transplant patients who each received 10 mg per kg vidarabine per day for cytomegalovirus infections.[125]

Clinical Indications

In a randomized crossover study vidarabine was effective treatment for 87 immunocompromised patients with zoster. Vidarabine is also as effective as idoxuridine against herpes simplex catarrhal conjunctivitis, even in patients who cannot take idoxuridine because of allergy, toxicity, or drug resistance.

In a double-blind treatment study of 28 biopsy-proven cases of herpes simplex encephalitis, the mortality was reduced from 70 to 28 percent. Survival in patients with herpes simplex encephalitis who were treated with vidarabine was enhanced if the patient (1) had a minimally altered level of consciousness at the start of therapy, (2) was under 40 years of age, or (3) had low virus titers in the brain. Although neurologic sequelae often occur in survivors, about 40 percent of these patients resumed normal activity after vidarabine therapy. However, patients who are already in a coma at the onset of drug therapy did not benefit from the drug.[126]

Other controlled studies show that vidarabine was not effective for smallpox or for cytomegalovirus infections in renal transplant recipients. Uncontrolled studies with patients with congenital cytomegalovirus and the cytomegalovirus mononucleosis syndrome, however, showed that vidarabine transiently suppressed virus excretion in the urine. Similarly, serum DNA polymerase activity was suppressed in two patients with chronic active hepatitis.[127]

Vidarabine is presently recommended only for the treatment of biopsy-proven herpes simplex encephalitis (15 mg per kg per day for 10 days by slow infusion) and for herpes simplex catarrhal conjunctivitis (a 3 percent ophthalmic ointment applied every 3 hours). Culture-proven disseminated or central nervous system herpes simplex infection will also respond to a 10-day course of intravenous vidarabine, although this indication has not yet been formally approved by the Food and Drug Administration.

Idoxuridine

Antiviral Activity

Idoxuridine (5-iodo-2-deoxyuridine, IUdR) was the first clinically effective antiviral nucleoside. It is a halogenated pyrimidine, the structure of which resembles thymidine. It is phosphorylated in cells, and the triphosphate derivative is incorporated into both viral and whole cellular DNA replacing thymidine. This results in a mismatch during DNA replication and transcription. Idoxuridine has activity against a variety of DNA viruses, especially the herpesvirus family and the poxviruses at concentrations of less than 10 μg per ml. Viral DNA synthesis can be inhibited at much lower dosage than that needed to affect normal mammalian cells.

Pharmacology and Toxicity

Systemic idoxuridine has a low therapeutic index[128] and is not approved for systemic therapy.

Clinical Indications

Currently, idoxuridine is effective only for the topical treatment of herpes simplex keratitis. It is not effective for recurrent herpes labialis or localized herpes zoster. It is available as a 0.1 percent ophthalmic solution in distilled water (1 drop each hour during the day; every 2 hours at night) and as a 0.5 percent ophthalmic ointment in petrolatum base (use every 4 hours).

Acyclovir

Acyclovir (acycloguanosine) is a nucleoside derivative with great therapeutic promise, although it is currently available only for investigational use. It is a potent antiviral agent in vitro and in the treatment of animals with herpesvirus infections.[129]

Antiviral Activity

Acyclovir is effective in vitro against herpes simplex, varicella zoster, and to a much lesser extent Epstein-Barr virus and cytomegalovirus. Herpes virus coat-enzyme, thimidine kinase, converts the nucleoside analogue to acycloguanosine monophosphate, which in turn is further phosphorylated by other kinases to acycloguanosine triphosphate, which in turn inhibits herpesvirus DNA polymerase. The apparently high therapeutic index results from the viral specificity of the thymidine kinase and the fact that the triphosphate derivative of the drug is only a weak inhibitor of mammalian DNA polymerase.[129] In tissue culture, acyclovir is many times more active against herpes simplex type I than are vidarabine or idoxuridine.[130]

Pharmacology and Toxicity

Over 95 percent of acyclovir is excreted in the urine in unaltered form and toxicity is minimal in animals. The only toxicity observed among 23 patients with herpes simplex and zoster infections was a mild increase in the blood urea nitrogen levels of a few. Whether this renal impairment was related to underlying illness or to acyclovir is unclear, but it improved before completion of the 5-day treatment course. Most observers have noted few side effects.[131]

Clinical Uses

The therapeutic efficacy of acyclovir has been evaluated almost exclusively in experimental animals—it is very effective. In herpes simplex–induced skin infections of mice, early topical application prevents both skin lesions and latent infections in sensory ganglia. In herpes simplex keratitis in rabbits, acyclovir ointment was more effective than vidarabine or idoxuridine; healing of the epithelial ulcers and elimination of the virus were more rapid. In a small group of patients with herpes dendritic corneal ulcers, topical treatment prevented the early recurrence of lesions observed in the patients treated with placebo. In an uncontrolled study of 23 patients with underlying neoplastic disease or recent bone marrow transplantation, intravenous therapy arrested cutaneous or systemic zoster or herpes simplex virus infections.

Interferon

Antiviral Activity

The interferons are a family of cellular glycoproteins which act mainly on the species of animal cells, by which they are produced, to render these cells resistant to subsequent virus infection. They are not virus-specific; they are capable of interfering with a wide variety of viruses. Infection by most human viral pathogens can be inhibited by achievable levels of circulating interferon. Virus-induced human interferon (type I) differs from the interferon produced by leukocytes (type II) during the immune response in vivo or blast transformation in vitro in several properties, ie, host range, pH, and heat stability. Although immune type II interferon is an important lymphokine and mediator of cellular immunity, it has not yet been produced in sufficient quantities to evaluate its antiviral activity. Type I interferons can be induced by viral infection or by a variety of stimuli, including double-stranded RNA, endotoxin, polyriboinosinicpolyribocytodylic (poly I: poly C) polymers, certain arylpyrimidines, and a variety of intracellular pathogens *(L. monocytogenes, Rickettsia,* and protozoa). Production of interferon requires double-stranded RNA and protein synthesis. Interferons are not themselves antiviral. Rather, they seem to elicit by derepression the synthesis of an antiviral protein that allows the cell to resist virus infections.[132]

As antiviral agents, interferons act indirectly by first binding to specific cell surface receptors and inducing the production of cellular enzymes that subsequently block viral reproduction by inhibiting the translation of viral messenger RNA to viral protein.

Pharmacology and Toxicity

Difficulties in production and purification of large quantities of human interferon has limited knowledge of the pharmacology and toxicity of interferon. Most human leukocyte interferon used by clinical testing has been made in the laboratory of Cantrell in Finland. Human leukocyte interferon has been administered by the intravenous, subcutaneous, and intramuscular routes. The intramuscular route is usually used because of the ease of its administration and the presence of interferon in the serum is prolonged (the half-life is 4 to 6 hours). On the other hand, human fibroblast interferon is readily inactivated in muscle tissue and should be given intravenously. Little is known about the metabolism of interferons in people. Body fluids (ie, urine, saliva, serum, bile, stool, cerebrospinal) readily inactivate interferon at 37C, and the interferons do not penetrate the cerebrospinal fluid easily.

Topical administration of interferon intranasally or into the eye has not been associated with serious side effects, and the toxicity of parenteral leukocyte interferon has been reduced by increasing purity. Fever, nausea, vomiting, local erythema, and pain have been reported after intramuscular injection of leukocyte interferon. Leukopenia and thrombocytopenia have also been reported.

Clinical Indications

Clinical and experimental trials have used both human leukocyte interferon and interferon inducers. Some of these interferon inducers, however (such as poly I: poly C), are too toxic for clinical use.

In randomized controlled studies, human leukocyte interferon has been shown to: [133] (1) reduce the incidence of visceral complications of varicella in immunodepressed children,[134] (2) reduce the incidence of herpes simplex reactivation after trigeminal nerve decompression,[135] and (3) shorten the period of cytomegalovirus and Epstein-Barr virus shedding in renal transplant patients.[116] Several studies have been carried out to investigate the effect of human leukocyte interferon against chronic hepatitis B virus infection. Some investigators have noted diminution in laboratory markers such as hepatitis B surface antigen and DNA polymerase; others have found no activity.

Leukocyte interferon administered by intranasal spray reduced the clinical symptoms of viral shedding in a controlled trial of rhinovirus 4 infection. In similar studies, fibroblast interferon had no effect.[136]

Newer methods of producing human leukocyte interferon have resulted in a much greater supply at a much lower cost. Recombinant DNA has been used to permit bacterial production of human interferon. No doubt such improvements in the future will result in interferon's becoming readily available. It is an especially promising antiviral agent for clinical use.

Methisazone

Antiviral Activity

Methisazone is an inhibitor of viral protein synthesis and possibly virus assembly. Although some activity has been reported against adenoviruses, its greatest activity is against poxviruses. Its activity appears to be a result of its selective inhibition of late viral mRNA. Clinical trials have reported effectiveness against alastrim in Brazil and smallpox in India, but these trials were poorly controlled and have not yet been confirmed.[137]

Other Compounds

A variety of other compounds, including ribavarin, inosiplex, rifampin, phosphonoacidic acid, and other agents have been extensively studied in vitro and in vivo, but have not been proved to be safe or effective antiviral agents. Other treatments, such as ether, BCG vaccine, photodynamic inactivation, and vitamin C, have been discredited by controlled trials.

GERMICIDES, ANTISEPTICS, DISINFECTANTS

A germicide is a general term for any agent that destroys microorganisms. Germicides may be further divided according to their antimicrobial spectrum—bactericides, fungicides, virucides—or use.

An antiseptic is a germicide that is usually applied to living tissue, and disinfectant is usually applied to inanimate objects. Such agents tend to denature protein and are not licensed for use in body cavities or wounds.

DESIRABLE PROPERTIES OF ANTISEPTICS AND DISINFECTANTS

Antiseptics

One of the most important properties of antiseptics, of course, is germicidal potency. An agent that is lethal to microorganisms is superior to one that merely inhibits growth. A broad antimicrobial spectrum is essential, especially for microorganisms that inhabit the skin or wounds. Bactericidal and fungicidal properties are much more important than virucidal or protozoacidal actions. Antiseptics should spread over the skin or wound surfaces and therefore should have a low surface tension. These agents should also retain their potency in the presence of inflammatory exudates in infected regions. The action of antiseptics should be both rapid and sustained, so that bacteria and fungi are killed rapidly during hand washing or skin preparation, to minimize the time required for these activities, and yet continue to exert their antimicrobial effect throughout an operation. They should not be inactivated by soaps used for cleansing the skin. Antiseptic agents should not cause irritation of skin or tissues and should not interfere with mechanisms of healing and tissue repair. They also should not cause hypersensitivity reactions and should not be systemically absorbed.

Disinfectants

Disinfectants should also have high germicidal efficacy, a wide antimicrobial spectrum, rapid action, and the ability to penetrate into crevices and cavities and beneath films of organic matter. It is essential that lethal concentrations of the agent can be obtained in the presence of organic matter such as blood, sputum, pus, and fecal matter. Disinfectants should be compatible with soaps and other chemical substances that are likely to be present on the material to be disinfected. The disinfecting agent should be stable for prolonged periods and should not corrode surgical instruments or injure other materials. Other important considerations in choosing a disinfectant include odor, staining qualities, and cost.

LEVELS OF DISINFECTION

Different materials require different levels of disinfection, depending on their intended use. For instance, some surgical instruments and prosthetic devices must be sterile but cannot be autoclaved. Four high-level germicides that will ensure destruction of all bacteria and spores are 20 percent formalin, 2 percent alkalinized aqueous glutaraldehyde, gaseous ethylene chloride, and a 10 to 20 percent stabilized aqueous solution of hydrogen peroxide.

Intermediate-level disinfectants include those which are not sporicidal but do kill tubercle bacilli, fungi, and non-lipid-containing viruses. Low-level disinfectants do not kill tubercle bacilli or resistant non-lipid-containing viruses. They do, however, kill vegetative forms of bacteria, many fungi, and the more susceptible viruses.

The level of disinfection required also varies according to what the item is to be used for. Internal prosthetic devices must be sterile. For endoscopes, contaminated by mucosal surfaces, on the other hand, the level of disinfection should only be high enough to destroy viruses, fungi, and bacteria, but spores need not be killed. Other items can be contaminated with nonpathogenic bacteria and fungi, and hence only a low level of disinfection is required.

COMMONLY USED ANTISEPTICS AND DISINFECTANTS

Phenols and Phenol Derivatives

Phenol (carbolic acid) was first used by Lister in 1867. Phenol is also of historical interest because in 1903 Rideal and Walker[138] developed the phenol coefficient test, which allowed the comparison of various germicides to the standard phenol in their ability to kill selected bacteria. Because of its toxicity, however, it is rarely used today. Instead, less toxic and more bactericidal derivatives of phenol are in use. Phenol causes leakage of essential intracellular metabolites through the cell wall and also inactivates many intracellular enzymes.

Hexachlorophene

The chlorine-substituted bis-phenol, hexachlorophene, is the most commonly used phenol derivative. It is more effective against gram-positive than against gram-negative organisms. Hexachlorophene is highly bacteriostatic, but prolonged contact is required to kill microorganisms. The growth of pathogenic fungi is also inhibited by this agent.

Organic matter such as pus and serum reduces its efficiency, but it does not lose potency in the presence of soap. Three percent hexachlorophene is a synthetic detergent vehicle. Hexachlorophene Liquid Soap, USP, and other hexachlorophene preparations are frequently used as operative scrubs and as germicidal soaps for hand washing. Maximal reduction of skin flora is attained only after several days of hand washing because the chemical only gradually builds up on the skin and reaches optimal concentrations. To gain this thin film of hexachlorophene on the skin with its continuous degerming action, it is necessary to wash the hands with hexachlorophene exclusively and frequently.[139] Because repeated use of hexachlorophene is required for maximal efficiency, it is less effective as an antiseptic for the operative site.

Hexachlorophene has been incorporated into bar and liquid soap to control staphylococcal skin abscess in hospital nurseries, to reduce the incidence of mastitis, and to aid in the treatment of acne and aczematous dermatoses.[140]

Alcohols

Alcohols are bactericidal, cheap, have a cleansing action, and evaporate readily. They are colorless, but dyes can easily be added when required. Their bactericidal activity increases with molecular weight, but only ethyl and isopropyl alcohol are extensively used clinically.

Alcohols are believed to exert their antibacterial action by denaturing proteins. Proteins are not as easily denatured in the absence of water as when water is present, which explains why absolute ethyl alcohol is less bactericidal than mixtures of alcohol and water. Alcohol in a 0.41 molar concentration also interferes with bacterial metabolism and may account for some of the bacteriostatic action of alcohols.[141] Ethyl alcohol also exerts substantial fungicidal and virucidal activity.

Ethyl Alcohol

Ethyl alcohol is widely used as an antiseptic before venipuncture, hypodermic injections, and finger pricks. It is also used before operation for degerming the operative site and hands after washing, although it is currently being used much less frequently for these purposes. For skin degerming, alcohol concentrations between 70 and 92 percent by weight are equally effective.[142]

Alcohol is also an effective disinfectant when killing spores is not required, but it is not completely reliable.[140] *C. tetani* and *C. perfringens* are not killed after an exposure of 18 hours.[140] Alcohol is useful, however, for disinfecting instruments such as clinical thermometers, where sterilization is not required.

Isopropyl Alcohol

The alcohol most commonly used clinically is isopropyl alcohol. It is the highest molecular weight alcohol miscible with water in all proportions, and it is not subject to the legal restrictions and taxation of ethyl alcohol. Isopropyl alcohol is nonpotable and does not have to be denatured. It is more bactericidal than ethanol, but like ethyl alcohol, has no effect on spores. It has no harmful effects on human skin, although its vapors can be absorbed through the lungs and produce toxic side effects—usually narcosis in children. For skin degerming, solutions of 70 percent or more are recommended. The bactericidal action of isopropyl alcohol increases with its concentration.

Iodine

Iodine is one of the oldest antiseptics. Tincture of iodine was used as an antiseptic by a French surgeon as early as 1839 and for treating battle wounds in the Civil War.

Elemental iodine is bactericidal and sporicidal over a wide pH range against bacteria, fungi, viruses, and protozoa. Acid solutions markedly increase germicidal efficiency. It kills extremely rapidly. A 1:20,000 solution of iodine kills almost all bacteria within 1 minute; 15 minutes is required to kill spores with this concentration.

Because toxicity of iodine is extremely low in relation to its germicidal capacity, it is a safe antiseptic agent. Strong iodine solutions (above 5 percent iodine), however, can cause burns if placed on large areas of the skin.

Iodine Preparations Containing Free Iodine

The 2 percent iodine tincture, USP, contains 2 percent iodine and 2 percent sodium iodide in 44 to 55 percent ethyl alcohol. Using 70 percent alcohol instead may provide a superior solution; it spreads evenly, dries slowly, does not burn the skin, and rarely causes any patient discomfort. Iodine is also an effective antiseptic and disinfectant in aqueous solution. An iodide salt must be added to solubilize the iodine. Iodine solution, NF, contains 2 gm iodine and 2.4 gm sodium iodide dissolved in distilled water to make a 100 ml solution. The use of this solution avoids alcohol in cases where it may harm the object to be disinfected.

Stronger iodine solutions, such as Lugol solution, which contains 5 percent iodine, and strong tincture of iodine, NF, which contains 16.5 percent iodine, are used occasionally to prepare solutions with lower concentrations of free iodine for antiseptic purposes.

Iodophors

An iodophor is the combination of iodine and a solubilizing agent or carrier that liberates free iodine in solution. Povidone-iodine is a complex of iodine and polyvinylpyrrolidone. The compound slowly releases free iodine when dissolved in water. It is claimed that povidone-iodine is more effective and less toxic than aqueous or alcoholic solutions of free iodine when dissolved in water. It is claimed that povidone-iodine is more effective and less toxic than aqueous or alcoholic solutions of free iodine, but definite proof is lacking. Blatt and Maloney [143] found that the germicidal properties of three different iodophors were similar to those of iodine solutions of equivalent iodine content. King and Price,[144] however, showed that 1 percent iodine in 70 percent alcohol was superior as a skin antiseptic to any of five iodophors tested, including povidone-iodine. Iodophors produce less pain when applied around wounds and abrasions. There is also no allergic response to iodine even in sensitive individuals when applied in the form of an iodophor.

Iodophors have broad-spectrum antimicrobial activity. They are nonirritating to the eyes, skin, nose, mouth, vaginal mucosa. They are marketed in a variety of forms—solutions, ointments, aerosol sprays, skin cleansers, swabsticks, gauze pads, surgical scrubs, douches, and other disposable forms. In dilutions, they do not permanently stain skin or natural fabrics. Their stability permits easy storage. A variety of solubilizing agents other than povidone are also used.

Chlorine

Chlorine is widely used in treating municipal water supplies, swimming pool water, utensils and equipment in dairy and food processing industries, and in sewage and waste water treatment. It is used considerably less in the hospital setting. Dakin's solution, a buffered solution of sodium hypochlorite, was introduced in World War I as an antiseptic irrigant for wounds. It is injurious to tissues. Modified Dakin's solution contains 0.5 percent instead of

5 percent sodium hypochlorite and is much less injurious to tissues. As a disinfectant in hospitals, chlorine has limited use. Yet sodium hypochlorite solution is still one of the best germicides for spot disinfection. It is a particularly effective germicide for spills contaminated with hepatitis B virus.

Chlorine appears to exert its antibacterial action in the form of undissociated hypochlorous acid. Chlorine combines with water to form HOCl and dissociated HCl. HOCl is undissociated in neutral or acid solutions and exerts a strong bactericidal effect. In alkaline solutions, it dissociates, and the hypochlorite ion is much less effective.

Quaternary Ammonium Compounds

Quaternary ammonium compounds were for many years the most popular disinfectants because of their blandness and low cost. Unfortunately, however, they are relatively inactive against gram-negative bacteria. They are rapidly inactivated by traces of soap that may be left on the skin or inanimate objects by regular washing, and they form a thin film on the skin under which bacteria can remain viable. They can become contaminated by *Pseudomonas* if allowed to stand, and have been the source of some hospital-acquired infections.[145]

Commonly used commercial preparations include benzalkonium chloride (Zephiran) and cetylpyridium chloride (Ceepryn). Tincture of benzalkonium chloride is more effective than an aqueous solution; indeed, a considerable portion of the benefit is attributed to the alcohol-acetone solvent. A 1:1000 tincture is recommended for degerming the unbroken skin. A 1:10,000 to 1:2000 aqueous concentration is used for denuded skin and mucous membranes. A 1:20,000 aqueous concentration is used for bladder irrigation and a 1:40,000 concentration for retention lavage.

Heavy Metals and Their Salts

Mercurials

Inorganic mercury compounds were among the earliest antiseptics used. Mercurials—both organic and inorganic—are bacteriostatic compounds, which combine with sulfhydryl groups on enzymes either on the cell wall or in the cytoplasm. Growth of mercury-inhibited bacteria can be reactivated by exposing the bacteria to sulfhydryl groups. Because numerous sulfhydryl groups are readily available in the body, organisms inhibited by mercury can become reactivated when introduced into the body. Because mercury also inactivates enzymes in tissues, mercurials are toxic and have a low therapeutic index.

Organic mercurial compounds are more bacteriostatic, less irritating, and less toxic than the inorganic mercurial salts. Mebronin (mercurochrome) is a fluorescein derivative. It is only feebly active—its bacteriostatic activity is greatly reduced by organic matter, and it is relatively inactive at the pH of body fluids. Thirmerosal (merthiolate) is commonly applied to cuts and abrasions. Tinctures of organic mercurials are more effective than aqueous solutions but not as effective as 70 percent ethyl alcohol.

Mercurials should not be used to prepare the skin or as disinfectants for instruments, because more effective agents are available.

Silver

Silver, like mercury, appears to exert its antimicrobial activity by inhibiting cellular enzymes. It also binds to DNA and blocks replication. Silver compounds are bactericidal in high (10 percent) concentrations but only bacteriostatic in lower concentrations. Silver nitrate solutions are applied as antiseptics to mucous membranes for ulcers of the mouth. Weak (0.5 percent) solutions were formerly applied to second- and third-degree burns to protect against contamination of the burn wound by gram-negative bacteria. One percent silver nitrate is used as eyedrops at birth to prevent opththalmia neonatorum.

Currently, silver sulfadiazine, administered as 1 percent cream, is applied to burns to prevent bacterial infections (Chapter 48). This compound is bactericidal and is easier to work with than silver nitrate. Rooms do not become stained black because of spilling the silver nitrate and subsequent precipitation of silver salts during use. Silver sulfadizine is painful (burns) when it is applied to third-degree burns. Furthermore, it is a carbonic anhydrase inhibitor and can cause a metabolic acidosis.

Other silver salts of acetate, citrate, and lactate are used for eye lotion, treating burn wounds, and dusting on wounds. Silver proteinates are colloidal preparations of silver. They are used for eyedrops, urethral irrigations, throat and nose sprays, and vaginal and rectal suppositories.

OTHER ANTISEPTICS AND DETERGENTS

Soaps

Soap is a poor antiseptic. While a bar of soap will quickly sterilize itself after it has been used, it is relatively ineffective in degerming skin. Its value lies in its ability to remove gross dirt, grease and oils, and other surface debris that might contain microorganisms. Soap can be used as an initial skin cleanser but cannot be relied on to remove the bacteria on the skin.

Organic Agents

Organic agents such as ether, acetone, chloroform, and xylene have also been used to degerm the skin but are somewhat injurious, and especially drying, to skin. In addition, because ether and acetone are extremely flammable, they are banned from many operating rooms, because flammable agents are no longer used.

Formalin

Formalin is a solution of formaldehyde gas dissolved in water. Eight percent formaldehyde dissolved in water makes a solution of 20 percent formalin. It is a high-level germicide. A combination of 20 percent formalin and 65 to 70 percent isoprophyl alcohol is rapidly bactericidal and even kills tubercule bacilli. It is also sporicidal, but the time required may be 24 hours or more. Formalin is extremely toxic to tissues, so disinfected materials must be thoroughly rinsed before use.

Glutaraldehyde

Glutaraldehyde is a high-level bactericidal disinfectant. When combined with alcohol, it is also tuberculocidal. At the present time, aqueous buffered glutaraldehyde is the only highly effective chemical sterilant recommended by the Center for Disease Control for disinfecting respiratory therapy equipment.

Hydrogen Peroxide

Hydrogen peroxide has long been used as an antiseptic and disinfectant. It is frequently used in granulating and other open wounds to reduce bacterial contamination. Low concentrations of unstable preparations, however, are usually applied to tissues, and these are rapidly inactivated by catalase in the tissues. Consequently, numerous bubbles of oxygen gas are formed when the hydrogen peroxide is placed into open tissues, which makes the physician and the patient think the agent is extremely active. The bubbles, however, only signify rapid inactivation of the hydrogen peroxide. It is almost totally ineffective as an antiseptic, and has been generally abandoned.

Recently, hydrogen peroxide has been available in pure stabilized preparations with a long shelf-life. Experimental tests have shown it to be an extremely effective germicide, but it has not achieved widespread use. It has been used to some degree to sterilize drinking water, but has not received wide attention in hospital settings. Still, hydrogen peroxide in relatively high (10 to 25 percent) concentrations is a promising sporicidal agent. It has been recommended for the disinfection of acrylic resin sections used as surgical implants. It is also used for disinfection of hydrophil soft contact lenses.

BIBLIOGRAPHY

Abramowicz M (ed): Handbook of Antimicrobial Therapy. New Rochelle, Medical Letter, 1980.

Block SS: Disinfection, Sterilization, and Preservation, 2nd ed. Philadelphia, Lea and Febiger, 1977.

Eisenberg MS, Furukawa C, Ray CG: Manual of Antimicrobial Therapy and Infectious Diseases. Philadelphia, Saunders, 1980.

Galasso GJ, Merigan TC, Buchanan RA: Antiviral Agent and Viral Diseases in Man. New York, Raven, 1979.

Gilman AG, Goodman LS, Gilman A (eds): Goodman and Gilman's The Parmacological Basis of Therapeutics (6th ed). New York, Macmillan, 1980.

Hayden FG, Douglas RG Jr (eds): Antiviral agents. In Mandell GL, Douglas RG Jr, Bennett JE (eds): Principles and Practice of Infectious Diseases. New York, Wiley, 1979, p 353.

Kucers A, Bennett N (eds): The Use of Antibiotics, 3rd ed. London, Heineman, 1979.

Mandell GL, Douglas RG Jr, Bennett JE (eds): Principles and Practice of Infectious Diseases. New York, Wiley, 1979.

Nelson JD, Grassi C (eds): Current Chemotherapy and Infectious Disease, Vol 1. Proceedings 11th ICC and 19th ICCAC Meeting. Washington, D.C., American Society for Microbiology, 1980.

Pratt WB: Chemotherapy of Infection. New York, Oxford Univ. Press, 1977.

REFERENCES

1. Abramowicz M (ed): Handbook of Antimicrobial Therapy. New Rochelle, Medical Letter, 1980.
2. Sabath LD, Anholt JP: Assay of antimicrobics. In Lenette EH, Balows A, Housler WJ, Truant JP (eds): Manual of Clinical Microbiology (3rd ed). Washington, D.C., American Society for Microbiology, 1980, p 486.
3. Sabath LD: Use of Antibiotics in Obstetrics. In Charles D, Finland M (eds): Obstetric and Perinatal Infections. Philadelphia, Lea and Febiger, 1973, pp 563–623.
4. Sabath LD, Gerstein DA, Leaf CD, Finland M: Increasing the usefulness of antibiotics: treatment of infections caused by gram-negative bacilli. Clin Pharmacol Ther 11:161, 1970.
5. Klastersky J, Debusscher L, Daneau D: Effectiveness of erythromycin plus alkalinization and nitrofurantoin in the treatment of urinary tract infections. Curr Ther Res 13:427, 1971.
6. Brumfitt W, Percival A, Leigh DA: Clinical and laboratory studies with carbenicillin. A new penicillin active against Pseudomonas pyocyanea. Lancet 1:1289, 1967.
7. Sabath LD: Body distribution of antibiotics. J Surg Prac 8:56, 1979.
8. Craig WA, Kunin CM: Significance of serum protein and tissue binding of antimicrobial agents. Ann Rev Med 27:287, 1976.
9. Zimelis VM, Jackson GG: Activity of aminoglycoside antibiotics against *Pseudomonas aeruginosa:* specificity and site of calcium and magnesium antagonism. J Infect Dis 127:663, 1973.
10. Bryan LE, Van DenElzen HM: Streptomycin accumulation in susceptible and resistant strains of *Escherichia coli* and *Pseudomonas aeruginosa.* Antimicrob Agent Chemother 9:928, 1976.
11. Sabath LD: Pharmacology of antibiotics used in infection of the biliary tree. International Workshop, Biliary Infections. Darmstadt, Dietrich Steinkopff Verlag, 1977.
12. Louie T, Onderdonk AB, Bartlett JG, Gorbach SL: Failure of penicillin in experimental intra-abdominal sepsis. Interscience Conference on Antimicrobial Agents and Chemotherapy, Abstract #62, 1975.
13. Louie T, Onderdonk AB, Bartlett JG, Gorbach SL: Failure of penicillin in experimental *Bacteroides fragilis* infections. Clin Res 23(3):307A, 1975.
14. Lewis C, Stern KF, Zurenko GE: A comparison in mice of blood and *Bacteroides fragilis*–induced abscess levels of antibiotics. 80th Annual Meeting, American Society Microbiology. Abstract #A-18, 1980.
15. Joiner K, Lowe B, Dzink J, Tally F, Bartlett J: Antibiotic levels and efficacy in mouse abscess model. 80th Annual Meeting, American Society Microbiology. Abstract #A-19, 1980.
16. O'Keefe JP, Tally FP, Barza M, Gorbach SL: Penetration of cephalothin and cefoxitin into experimental infections with *Bacteroides fragilis.* Rev Infect Dis 106, 1979.
17. Thadepalli H, Gorbach SL, Bartlett JG: Apparent failure of chloramphenicol in the treatment of anaerobic infections. Curr Ther Res 22:421, 1977.
18. Francis JB, Corwin RW, Johnson JD, Hand WL: Antibiotic uptake by alveolar macrophages. Clin Res 26:394A, 1978.
19. Moylan JA: The proper use of local antimicrobial agents in wound. World J Surg 4:433, 1980.
20. Brokenbrough EC, Moylan, JA: Treatment of contaminated surgical wounds with a topical antibiotic: a double-blind study of 240 patients. Am Surg 35:789, 1969.
21. Rickett JWS, Jackson BT: Topical ampicillin in the appendectomy wound: report of double-blind trial. Br Med J 4:206, 1969.
22. Rahal JJ Jr: Antibiotic combinations: the clinical relevance of synergy and antagonism. Medicine 57:179, 1978.
23. Hitchings GH: Species differences among dihydrofolate reductases as a basis for chemotherapy. Postgrad Med J 45 (suppl):7, 1969.
24. McLaughlin JE, Reeves DS: Clinical and laboratory evidence for inactivation of gentamicin by carbenicillin. Lancet 1:261, 1971.

25. Klastersky J, Hensgens C, Meunier-Carpentier F: Comparative effectiveness of combinations of amikacin with penicillin G and amikacin with carbenicillin in gram-negative septicemia: double-blind clinical trial. J Infect Dis 134(S):S433, 1976.
26. Hirshmann JV, Inui TS: Antimicrobial propholaxis: a critique of recent trials. Rev Infect Dis 2:1, 1980.
27. Bennett WM, Mutner RS, Parker RA, Feig P, Morrison G, Golper TA, Singer I: Drug therapy in renal failure: dosing guidelines for adults. Ann Intern Med 93:62, 1980.
28. Zaske DE, Cipolle RJ, Strate RJ: Gentamicin dosage requirements: wide interpatient variations in 242 surgery patients with normal renal function. Surgery 87:164, 1980.
29. Shapiro S, Slone D, Siskind V, Lewis GP, Jick H: Drug rash with ampicillin and other penicillins. Lancet 2:969, 1969.
30. Sleet RA, Sangster G, Murdoch JM: Comparison of ampicillin and chloramphenicol in treatment of paratyphoid fever. Br Med J 1:148, 1964.
31. Cluff LE: Serum sickness and related disorders. In Wintrobe MM, Thorn GW, Adams RD, Bennett IL Jr, Braunwald E, Isselbacher KJ, Petersdorf RG (eds): Harrison's Principles of Internal Medicine (6th ed.), New York, McGraw-Hill, 1970, p 374.
32. Kohlstaedt KG: Propionyl erythromycin ester lauryl sulfate and jaundice. JAMA 178:89, 1961.
33. McCracken GH Jr: Pharmacological basis for antimicrobial therapy in newborn infants. Am J Dis Child 128:407, 1974.
34. Moellering RC Jr: Factors influencing the clinical use of antimicrobial agents in elderly patients. Geriatrics 33:83, 1978.
35. Weinstein L, Dalton AC: Host determinants of response to antimicrobial agents. N Engl J Med 279:467, 1968.
36. Vorherr H: Drug excretion in breast milk. Postgrad Med 56:97, 1974.
37. Hansten P: Drug Interactions, 4th ed. Philadelphia, Lea and Febiger, 1979.

ANTIBACTERIAL AGENTS

Penicillins

38. Barza M, Weinstein L: Phaarmacokinetics of the penicillins in man. Clin Pharmacokinet 1:297, 1976.
39. Barza M: Antimicrobial spectrum, pharmacology and therapeutic use of antibiotics, Part 2. Penicillins. In Miller RR, Greenblatt DJ (eds): Drug Therapy Reviews, Vol. 2. New York, Elsevier, 1979.
40. Spicehandler JR, Bernhardt L, Simberkoff MS, Rahal JJ Jr: Mezlocillin and piperacillin: a comparative clinical evaluation. In Nelson JD, Grassi C (eds): Current Chemotherapy and Infectious Disease, Vol I. Washington, D.C., American Society for Microbiology, 1980, pp 293–294.
41. Cleeland R, DeLorenzo W, Beskid G, Titsworth E, Chistenson J, Grunberg E: Correlation of in vitro and in vitro synergistic responses of Enterobacteriaceae to Mecillinan combined with ampicillin, carbenicillin, and cephalothin. In Nelson JD, Grassi C (eds): Current Chemotherapy and Infectious Disease, Vol I. Washington, D.C., American Society for Microbiology, 1980, p 310.
42. Ball AP, Davey PG, Geddes AM, Farrell ID, Brookes GR: Clavulanic acid and amoxycillin: a clinical, bacteriological, and pharmacological study. Lancet 1:620, 1980.
43. Kucers A, Bennett N: The use of antibiotics. A comprehensive review with clinical emphasis, 3rd ed. London, Heineman, 1979.
44. Tomasz A, Holtje J: Murein hydrolases and the lytic and killing action of penicillin. In Schlesinger D (ed): *Microbiology.* Washington, D.C., ASM, 1977, p 209.
45. Neu HC: Penicillins. In Mandell GL, Douglas RG Jr, Bennett JE (eds): Principles and Practice of Infectious Diseases. New York, Wiley, 1979, p 218.

Cephalosporins

46. Abraham EP, Loder PB: Cephalosporin C. In Flynn EH (ed): Cephalosporins and Penicillins. Chemistry and Biology. New York, Academic, 1972, p 2.
47. Mandell GL: Cephalosporins. In Mandell GL, Douglas RG Jr, Bennett JE (eds): Principles and Practice of Infectious Diseases. New York, Wiley, 1979, p 238.
48. Washington JA II: The in vitro spectrum of the cephalosporins. Mayo Clin Proc 51:237, 1976.
49. Neu HC: Cefamandole, a cephalosporin antibiotic with an unusually wide spectrum of activity. Antimicrob Agents Chemother 9:994, 1976.
50. Eickhoff TC, Ehret JM: In vitro comparison of cefoxitin, cefamandole, cephalexin, and cephalothin. Antimicrob Agents Chemother 9:994, 1976.
50a. Tally FP, McGowan K, Kellum JM, Gorbach SL, O'Donnell TF: A randomized comparison with or without amikacin and clindamycin plus amikacin in surgical sepsis. Ann Surg 193:318, 1981.
51. Richmond MH, Sykes RB: The beta-lactamases of gram-negative bacteria and their possible physiological role. Adv Microb Physiol 9:31, 1973.
52. Sabath LD, Wheeler N, Laverdiere M, Blazevic D, Wilkinson BJ: A new type of penicillin resistance of *Staphylococcus aureus.* Lancet 1:443, 1977.
53. Wade JC, Petty BG, Conrad G, Smith CR, Lipsky JJ, Ellner J, Leitman PS: Cephalothin plus an aminoglycoside is more nephrotoxic than methicillin plus an aminoglycoside. Lancet 2:604, 1978.

Aminoglycosides

54. Koreniowski OM, Hook EW: Aminocyclitols: aminoglycosides and spectinomycin. In Mandell GL, Douglas RG Jr, Bennett JE (eds): Principles and Practice of Infectious Diseases. New York, Wiley, 1979, p 249.
55. Nelson WE, Vaughan VC III, McKay RJ Jr, Behrman RE (eds): Nelson Textbook of Pediatrics, 11th ed. Philadelphia, Saunders, 1979, p 2052.
56. Gellis SS, Kagan BM: Current Pediatric Therapy, Vol 9. Philadelphia, Saunders, 1980, pp 531–536.
57. Kaiser AB, McGee ZA: Aminoglycoside therapy of gram-negative bacillary meningitis. N Engl J Med 293:1215, 1975.
58. Kluge RM, Standiford HC, Tatem B, Young VM, Schimpff SC, Greene WH, Calia FM, Hornick RB: Carbenicillin-gentamicin combination against *Psuedomonas aeuruginosa.* Correlation of effect with gentamicin sensitivity. Ann Intern Med 81:584, 1974.
59. Riff LJ, Jackson GG: Laboratory and clinical conditions for gentamicin inactivation by carbenicillin. Arch Intern Med 130:887, 1972.
60. Trimble GX: Neomycin ototoxicity: dossier and doses. N Engl J Med 281:219, 1969.
61. Yu VL, Rhame FS, Pesanti EL, Axline SG: Amikacin therapy: use against infections caused by gentamicin- and tobramycin-resistant organisms. JAMA 238:943, 1977.
62. Schroeder AL, Raynolds GH, Holmes KK et al: Spectinomycin in the treatment of gonorrhea. J Am Vener Dis Assoc 1:139, 1975.
63. Wilfert J, Burke J, Bloomer HA, Smith CB: Renal insufficiency associated with gentamicin therapy. J Infect Dis 124(S):S148, 1971.
64. Pittinger CB, Eryasa Y, Adamson R: Antibiotic-induced paralysis. Anesth Analg 49:487, 1970.

Tetracyclines

65. Standiford HC: Tetracyclines and chloramphenicol. In Mandell GL, Douglas RB Jr, Bennett JE (eds): Principles and Practice of Infectious Disease. New York, Wiley, 1979, pp 273–289.
66. Whelton A: Tetracyclines in renal insufficiency: resolution of a therapeutic dilemma. Bull NY Acad Med 54:223, 1978.
67. Washington JA II, Dearing WH, Judd ES, Elveback LR: Effect of preoperative antibiotic regimen on development of infection after intestinal surgery: prospective, randomized, double-blind study. Ann Surg 180:567, 1974.
68. Neu HC: A symposium on the tetracyclines: a major appraisal. Introduction. Bull NY Acad Med 54:141, 1978.
69. Pratt WB: Bacteriostatic inhibitors of protein synthesis. In Pratt WB: Chemotherapy of Infection. New York, Oxford Univ. Press, 1977, p 127.

Chloramphenicol

70. McCrumb FR, Snyder MJ, Hicken WJ: The use of chloramphenicol acid succinate in the treatment of acute infections. Antibiotics Annual. New York, Medical Encyclopedia, 1958, p 837.
71. Sabath LD, Stumpf LL, Wallace SJ, Finland M: Susceptibility of *Diplococcus pneumoniae, Haemophilus influenzae,* and *Neisseria meningitidis* to 23 antibiotics. In Hobby GL (ed): Antimicrobial Agents and Chemotherapy, 1970. Proceedings of the 10th Interscience Conference on Antimicrobial Agents and Chemotherapy. Bethesda, American Society for Microbiology, 1971, p 53.
72. Okamoto S, Mizuno D: Mechanism of chloramphenicol and tetracycline resistance in *Escherichia coli.* J Gen Microbiol 35:125, 1964.
73. Best WR: Chloramphenicol-associated blood dyscrasias. A review of cases submitted to the American Medical Association Registry. JAMA 201:181, 1967.
74. Polin HB, Plaut ME: Chloramphenicol. NY State J Med 77:378, 1977.
75. Braude AI: Antimicrobial Drug Therapy. Philadelphia, Saunders, 1976, p 82.

Erythromycin

76. Steigbigel NH: Erythromycin, lincomycin, and clindamycin. In Mandell GL, Douglas RG Jr, Bennett JE (eds): Principles and Practice of Infectious Diseases. New York, Wiley, 1979, p 290.
77. Sabath LD, Gerstein DA, Loder PB, Finland M: Excretion of erythromycin and its enhanced activity in urine against gram-negative bacilli with alkalinization. J Lab Clin Med 72:916, 1968.
78. Molavi A, Weinstein L: In vitro activity of erythromycin against atypical mycobacteria. J Infect Dis 123:216, 1971.
79. Finland M, Bach MC, Garner C, Gold O: Synergistic action of ampicillin and erythromycin against *Nocardia asteroides:* effect of time incubation. Antimicrob Agents Chemother 5:344, 1974.

Lincomycin and Clindamycin

80. Sutter VL: In vitro susceptibility of anaerobes: comparison of clindamycin and other antimicrobial agents. J Infect Dis 135(S):S7, 1977.
81. Nastro LJ, Finegold SM: Bactericidal activity of five antimicrobial agents against *Bacteroides fragilis.* J Infect Dis 126:104, 1972.
82. Bartlett JG, Gorbach SL: Treatment of aspiration pneumonia and primary lung abscess: penicillin G vs. clindamycin. JAMA 234:935, 1975.
83. Tedesco FJ: Clindamycin and colitis: a review. J Infect Dis 135(S):S95, 1977.
83a. Noon GB, Beall AC, Jordan GL, Riggs S, DeBakey ME: Clinical evaluation of peritoneal irrigation with antibiotic solution. Surgery 62:73–78, 1967.
83b. Rountree PM, Beard MA: The spread of neomycin-resistant staphylococci in a hospital. Med J Aust 1:498–502, 1965.
83c. Kucers A, Bennett NM: The Use of Antibiotics. London, William Heineman Medical Books, 1979.

Polymyxins

84. Martin CM, Brookrajian EN: Bacteriuria prevention after indwelling urinary catheterization. Arch Intern Med 110: 703, 1962.
85. Thomas FE Jr, Leonard JM, Alford RH: Sulfamethoxazole-trimethoprim-polymyxin therapy of serious multiply drug-resistant *serratia* infections. Antimicrob Agents Chemother 9:201, 1976.
86. Ostenson RC, Fields BT, Nolan CM: Polymyxin B and rifampin: new regimen for multiresistant *Serratia marcescens* infections. Antimicrob Agents Chemother 12:655, 1977.
87. Fekety R: Polymyxins. In Mandell GL, Douglas RG Jr, Bennett JE (eds): Principles and Practice of Infectious Diseases. New York, Wiley, 1979, p 300.

Vancomycin

88. Fekety R: Vancomycin. In Mandell GL, Douglas RG Jr, Bennett JE (eds). Principles and Practice of Infectious Diseases. New York, Wiley, 1979, p 304.
89. Geraci JE: Vancomycin. Mayo Clin Proc 52:631, 1977.
90. Rifkin GD, Fekety FR, Silva J Jr, Sack RB: Antibiotic-induced colitis implication of a toxin neutralised by *Clostridium sordellii* antitoxin. Lancet 2:1103, 1977.
91. Appel GB, Neu HC: The nephrotoxicity of antimicrobial agents (second of three parts). N Engl J Med 296:722, 1977.

Sulfonamides and Trimethoprim

92. Zinner SH: Sulfonamides and trimethoprim. In Mandell GL, Douglas RG Jr, Bennett JE (eds): Principles and Practice of Infectious Diseases. New York, Wiley, 1979, p 308.
93. Wolf B, Hotchkiss RD: Genetically modified folic acid synthesizing enzymes of *Pneumococcus.* Biochemistry (Washington) 2:145, 1963.
94. Craig WA, Kunin CM: Trimethhoprim-sulfamethoxazole: pharmacodynamic effects of urinary pH and impaired renal function. Ann Intern Med 78:491, 1973.
95. Simmons NA: Colistin, sulphamethoxazole, and trimethoprim in synergy against gram-negative bacteria. J Clin Pathol 23:757, 1970.
96. Parsley TL, Provonchee RB, Glicksman C, Zinner SH: Synergistic activity of trimethoprim and amikacin against gram-negative bacilli. Antimicrob Agents Chemother 12:349, 1977.
97. Bach MC, Finland M, Gold O, Wilcox C: Susceptibility of recently isolated pathogenic bacteria to trimethoprim and sulfamethoxazole separately and combined. J Infect Dis 128:S508, 1973.
98. Harding GKH, Ronald AR: A controlled study of antimicrobial prophylaxis of recurrent urinary infections in women. N Engl J Med 291:597, 1974.
99. Stamey TA, Condy M, Mihara G: Prophylactic efficacy of nitrofurantoin macrocrystals and trimethoprim-sulfamethoxazole in urinary infections. N Engl J Med 296:780, 1977.

100. Hughes WT, Kuhn S, Chaudhary S, Feldman S, Verzosa M, Auri RJA, Pratt C, George SL: Successful chemoprophylaxis for *Pneumocystis carinii* pneumonitis. N Engl J Med 297:1419, 1977.
101. Gurwith MJ, Brunton JL, Lank BA, Harding GKM, Ronald AR: A prospective controlled investigation of prophylactic trimethoprim/sulfamethaxazole in hospitalized granulocytopenic patients. Am J Med 66:248, 1979.
102. Matheson DM, Arabi Y, Baxter-Smith D, Alexander-Williams J, Keighley MRB: Randomized multicentre trial of oral bowel preparation and antimicrobials for elective colorectal operations. Br J Surg 65:597, 1978.
103. Kunin C, Brandt D, Wood H: Bacteriologic studies of rifampin, a new semisynthetic antibiotic. J Infect Dis 119:132, 1969.

Urinary Tract Antiseptics

104. Andriole VT: Urinary tract agents: nalidixic acid, oxolinic acid, nitrofurantoin, and methenamine. In Mandell GL, Douglas RG Jr, Bennett JE (eds): Principles and Practice of Infectious Diseases. New York, Wiley, 1979, p 317.
105. Stamey TA, Nemoy NJ, Higgins M: The clinical use of nalidixic acid. A review of some observations. Invest Urol 6:582, 1969.
106. Dawson RB Jr: Pulmonary reactions to nitrofurantoin. N Engl J Med 274:522, 1966.
107. Ellis FG: Acute polyneuritis after nitrofurantoin therapy. Lancet 2:1136, 1962.
108. Stamey TA (ed): Urinary Infections. Baltimore, Williams and Wilkins, 1980.

ANTIMYCOBACTERIAL AGENTS

109. Alford RH: Antimycobacterial agents. In Mandell GL, Douglas RG Jr, Bennett JE (eds): Principles and Practice of Infectious Diseases. New York, Wiley, 1979, p 328.
110. Stottmeier KD: Emergence of rifampin-resistant *Mycobacterium tuberculosis* in Massachusetts. J Infect Dis 133:88, 1976.
111. Sanders WE Jr, Cacciatore R, Valdez H, Schneider N, Hartwig C: Activity of amikacin against mycobacteria in vitro and in experimental infections with *M. tuberculosis*. Am Rev Respir Dis 113:59, 1976.
112. Hobby GL, Redmond WB, Runyon EH, Schaefer WB, Wayne LG, Wichelhausen RH: A study of pulmonary disease associated with mycobacteria other than *Mycobacterium tuberculosis:* identification and characterization of the mycobacteria. XViii. A report of the Veterans Administration-Armed Forces Cooperative Study. Am Rev Respir Dis 95:954, 1967.
113. Sanders WE Jr, Hartwig EC, Schneider NJ, Cacciatore R, Valdez H: Susceptibility of organisms in the *Mycobacterium fortuitum* complex to antituberculous and other antimicrobial agents. Antimicrob Agents Chemother 12:295, 1977.

ANTIFUNGAL AGENTS

114. Bennet JE: Antifungal agents. In Mandell GL, Douglas RG Jr, Bennet JE (eds): Principles and Practice of Infectious Diseases. New York, Wiley, 1979, p 343.
115. Atkinson AJ Jr, Bennet JE: Amphotericin B pharmacokinetics in humans. Antimicrob Agents Chemother 13:271, 1978.
116. Medoff G, Kobayashi GS: Strategies in the treatment of systemic fungal infections. N Engl J Med 302:145, 1980.
116a. Solomkin JS, Simmons RL: Candida infections in surgical patients. World J Surg 4:381, 1980.
117. Arroyo J, Medoff G, Kobayashi GS: Therapy of murine aspergillosis with amphotericin B in combination with rifampin or 5-fluorocytosine. Antimicrob Agents Chemother 11:21, 1977.
118. Bennett JE: Flucytosine. Ann Intern Med 86:319, 1977.
119. Stevens DA: Miconazole in the treatment of systemic fungal infections. Am Rev Respir Dis 116:801, 1977.
120. Borelli D, Bran JL, Fuentes J, Legendre R, Leiderman E, Levine HB, Restrepo MA, Stevens DA: Ketoconazole, an oral antifungal: laboratory and clinical assessment of imidazole drugs. Postgrad Med 55:657, 1979.
120a. Restrepo A, Stevens DA, Utz JP (eds): First International Symposium on Ketoconazole. Rev Infect Dis 2:519, 1980.

ANTIVIRAL AGENTS

121. Hirsch MS, Swartz MN: Antiviral agents (2 parts). N Engl J Med 302:903, 949, 1980.
122. Monto AS, Gunn RA, Bandyk MG, King CL: Prevention of Russian influenza by amantadine. JAMA 241:1003, 1979.
123. Little JW, Hall WJ, Douglas RG Jr, Mudholkar GS, Speers DM, Patel K: Airway hyperreactivity and peripheral dysfunction in influenza A infection. Am Rev Respir Dis 118:295, 1978.
124. Champney K, Lauter CB, Bailey EJ, Lerner AM: Antiherpesvirus activity in human sera and urines after administration of adenine arabinoside. In vitro and in vivo synergy of adenine arabinoside and arabinosylhpoxanthine in combination. J Clin Invest 62:1142, 1978.
125. Marker SC, Howard RJ, Groth KE, Mastri A, Simmons RL, Balfour HH: A trial of vidarabine for cytomegalovirus infection in renal transplant patient. Arch Intern Med 140:1441, 1980.
126. Whitley RJ, Soong SJ, Dolin R, Gallasso GJ, Chien LT, Alford CA, and the Collaborative Study Group: Adenine arabinoside therapy of biopsy-proved herpes simplex encephalitis. National Institute of Allergy and Infectious Diseases Collaborative Antiviral Study. N Engl J Med 297:289, 1977.
127. Hayden FG, Douglas RG Jr: Antiviral agents. In Mandell GL, Douglas RG Jr, Bennett JE (eds): Principles and Practice of Infectious Diseases. New York, Wiley, 1979, p 353.
128. Failure of high dose 5-iodo-2-deoxyuridine in the therapy of herpes simplex virus encephalitis: evidence of unacceptable toxicity. Boston Interhospital Virus Study Group and the NIAID-sponsored Cooperative Antiviral Clinical Study. N Engl J Med 292:599, 1975.
129. Schaeffer HJ, Beauchamp L, Miranda P, Elion GB, Bauer DJ, Collins P: 9-(2-hydroxyethoxymethyl) guanine activity against viruses of the herpes group. Nature 272:583, 1978.
130. Furman PA, St. Clair MH, Fyfe JA, Rideout JL, Keller PM, Elion GB: Inhibition of herpes simplex virus–induced DNA polymerase activity and viral DNA replication by 9-(2-hydroxyethoxymethyl) guanine and its triphosphate. J Virol 32:72, 1979.
131. Spector SA, Hintz M, Quinn RP, Keeney RE, Connor JD: Single-dose pharmacokinetic and toxic properties of acyclovir. In Nelson JD, Grassi C (eds): Current Chemotherapy and Infectious Disease, Vol II. Washington, D.C., American Society for Microbiology, 1980, p 1390.
132. Ball A: Molecular biology of the production and action of interferons. In Nelson JD, Grassi C (eds): Current Chemotherapy and Infectious Disease, Vol II. Washington, D.C., American Society for Microbiology, 1980, p 1419.
133. Merigan TC, Rand KH, Pollard RB, Abdallah PS, Jordan GW, Fried RP: Human leukocyte interferon for the treatment of herpes zoster in patients with cancer. N Engl J Med 298:981, 1978.

134. Arvin AM, Feldman S, Merigan TC: Human leukocyte interferon in the treatment of varicella in children with cancer: a preliminary controlled trial. Antimicrob Agents Chemother 13:605, 1978.
135. Pazin GJ, Lam MT, Armstrong JA, et al: Interferon prevention of HSV reaction. 19th Interscience Conference on Antimicrobial Agents and Chemotherapy. Abstract #265, 1978.
136. Borden E: Antiviral therapy and some antitumor trials in man. In Nelson JD, Grassi C (eds): Current Chemotherapy and Infectious Disease Vol II. Washington D.C., American Society for Microbiology, 1980, p 1423.
137. Hayden FG, Douglas RG Jr: Antiviral agents. In Mandell GL, Douglas RG Jr, Bennett JE (eds): Principles and Practice of Infectious Diseases. New York, Wiley, 1979, p 353.

GERMICIDES, ANTISEPTICS, DISINFECTANTS

138. Rideal S, Walker JTA: Standardization of disinfectants. JR Sanit Inst 24:424, 1903.
139. Price PB: Fallacy of a current surgical fad—the three-minute preoperative scrub with hexachlorophene soap. Ann Surg 134:476, 1951.
140. Block SS: Disinfection, Sterilization and preservation, 2nd ed. Philadelphia, Lea and Febiger, 1977.
141. Dagley S, Dawes EA, Morrison GA: Inhibition and growth of *Aerobacter aerogenes:* the mode of action of phenols, alcohols, acetone, and ethyl acetate. J Bacteriol 60:369, 1950.
142. Price PB: Ethyl alcohol as a germicide. Arch Surg 38:528, 1939.
143. Blatt R, Maloney JV Jr: Evaluation of the iodophor compounds as surgical germicides. Surg Gynecol Obstet 113:699, 1961.
144. King TC, Price PB: An evaluation of iodophors as skin antiseptics. Surg Gynecol Obstet 116:361, 1963.
145. Sanford JP: Disinfectants that don't. Ann Intern Med 72:282, 1970.

CHAPTER 19

Immunotherapeutic Approaches to the Treatment of Infection in the Surgical Patient

J. Wesley Alexander and J. Dwight Stinnett

In some respects, it is remarkable that man and other animals continue to exist since they are constantly exposed to an unending and varied assault by potentially pathogenic microbes. They survive only because epithelial barriers exclude the majority of microbes and because microbes that penetrate this initial defense are met by an extremely effective inflammatory response, involving opsonins and phagocytic cells. Specific immunologic adaptive responses to invading organisms may play a subsequent role in their clearance. It is now clear that resistance to infection is extremely complex (Chapter 13).[1]

In surgical patients, defective chemotaxis of neutrophils, impaired inflammatory responses, deficient antibacterial function of neutrophils, and other cellular abnormalities have been associated with an increased incidence of infection. Deficiencies in opsonins appear to play a minor role in the development of infection compared to abnormalities of cellular defense.[2] More important, it has been possible to prevent or correct some of these deficiencies, with improved resistance to infection and improved survival.[3,4] These favorable results indicate that the next major advance in the control of surgical infection will come from immunotherapeutic approaches that prevent, correct, and potentiate host defense against infectious agents.

REPAIR OF IMMUNOLOGIC ABNORMALITIES BY A NUTRITIONAL APPROACH

There has always been a close association between malnutrition and infection[5,6] both in underdeveloped areas and in highly industrialized countries.[7] Indeed, infection itself can contribute to malnutrition, since when appetite and food intake are reduced, catabolism is increased and selected organ involvement (ie, liver) can further contribute to deranged nutrition.[6,8] Malnutrition commonly accompanies a variety of other illnesses, ie, trauma, burns, cirrhosis, gastrointestinal fistulas, cancer, and hypermetabolic states like hyperthyroidism.[9,10] Surgical patients are often starved for several days in the perioperative period. In fact, it has been estimated that half the patients on surgical services of large city hospitals or patients hospitalized for longer than 1 week have evidence of malnutrition.[7]

DEFECTS ASSOCIATED WITH MALNUTRITION

A state of malnutrition may be characterized in terms of its cause, the missing nutrient(s), and its degree. Primary malnutrition is caused by an inadequate or improper diet. Secondary malnutrition may arise from inadequacies of ingestion, absorption, or utilization, or from increased requirements or excessive excretion. Both primary and secondary malnutrition may occur concomitantly. Although there is a complex interplay of nutritional components, and single deficiencies rarely occur, relatively pure deficiencies will be discussed for simplicity.

Starvation and Protein Deficiency

It is difficult to distinguish clearly between the clinical effects of total starvation and protein deficiency. Protein provides the amino acids essential for tissue repair and growth. If the energy consumed is more than the intake, catabolism of body tissue, including protein, will exceed synthesis. If caloric intake is adequate but lacks protein, a pure protein deficiency will result. In practice, varying degrees of energy and protein deficiency usually occur in combination. Dietary deficiency of energy and protein results in a spectrum of disease termed protein-energy malnutrition. Severe cases may be classified by clinical and biochemical findings into marasmus, due mainly to energy (calorie) deficiency, and kwashiorkor, in which protein deficiency predominates. Intermediate forms with mixed etiology and symptomatology exist.

Patients with kwashiorkor have defects in the phagocytic capability, the glycolytic pathway, and the intracellular killing of bacteria by neutrophils.[11] Lymphocytes from patients with protein-calorie malnutrition respond poorly to phytomitogens, and patients who die display atrophy of the thymus and peripheral lymphoid tissues, affecting T cell–dependent more than B cell–dependent areas.[12] In addition, both classical and alternative complement pathway components and siderophilin levels are decreased in malnourished children.[13,14] Some confusion exists with respect to immunoglobulin levels in malnourished patients. Several reports have described normal or elevated rather than low immunoglobulin levels. At least part of this discrepancy appears to depend on whether or not the individuals are chronically or repeatedly infected.[15] Similarly, there are conflicting reports concerning T-cell functions. Both depressed [14] and normal [15] function has been described.

In order to clarify discrepancies such as these, animal models have been developed to mimic the human disease state. Both acute and chronic starvation result in a progressive decrease in the phagocytic index of isolated leukocytes.[16]

Malnutrition sometimes depresses nonspecific serum opsonins and antibody titers. However, antibody production on a per cell basis was not diminished in protein-depleted animals, suggesting that reduced antibody titers are due to fewer clones of cells producing antibody.[17] Addition of normal syngeneic thymocytes would restore the immune response, implying that depressed immunity in malnutrition may be partly a result of disturbance in thymic function.[18]

Vitamin Deficiency

The early report of Blackberg [19] was one of the first adequately controlled experimental investigations regarding vitamin deficiency and immunity. In this investigation, killed typhoid bacilli or small doses of live bacilli injected into rats deficient in vitamins A, D, and the B complex, resulted in lower titers of agglutinin and bacteriolysin than in control animals. Since then, the elegant studies of Axelrod [20] have greatly expanded our understanding of vitamin deficiency and immune function.

Vitamin A Deficiency

Vitamin A (retinol) deficiency is associated with higher susceptibility to and severity of infection.[6] Vitamin A is a fat-soluble vitamin, which is stored in the liver as retinyl palmitate. It is released into the circulation as retinol, bound to retinol-binding protein or tryptophan-rich prealbumin. Vitamin A deficiency is common in marasmus or kwashiorkor not only because the diet is deficient, but also because storage and transport are defective.

Unfortunately, the precise defects in host defense associated with retinol deficiency have not been clearly defined. Since retinol is required for maintenance of epithelial layers, the loss of integrity of these exposed surfaces probably contributes to microbial invasion. In addition, phagocytic function is depressed in deficient animals.[21] The relatively mild effects of vitamin A deficiency on serum opsonins may be of some importance as well.

Vitamin B_6 Deficiency

Vitamin B_6 comprises a group of closely related compounds—pyridoxine, pyridoxal, and pyridoxamine—which function as coenzymes in many reactions including decarboxylation and transamination of amino acids, the deamination of hydroxyamino acids and cysteine, the conversion of tryptophan to niacin, and the metabolism of fatty acids. Primary deficiency is rare, but secondary deficiencies can result from malabsorption, inactivation by drugs, excessive loss, and increased metabolic activity.

Vitamin B_6 deficiency severely impairs antibody responses to a variety of antigens.[22] In addition, delayed cutaneous hypersensitivity reactions are depressed, skin allograft rejection is delayed, and numbers of lymphocytes are reduced. Some of these defects may be due to impaired T-lymphocyte differentation since B_6 deficiency has been shown to affect thymic epithelial cell function.[23] In addition, phagocytes from pyridoxine-deficient animals are defective in their ability to ingest and kill bacteria.[24] This defect seems to correlate with the decreased myeloperoxidase content of the phagocytes. The prosthetic group of myeloperoxidase is derived from protoporphyrin IX, and the initial reaction in the biosynthetic pathway of protoporphyrin IX is pyridoxalphosphate dependent.

Vitamin C

In recent years, vitamin C (ascorbic acid) has probably received more public attention than any other nutrient. It is a strong reducing agent and is reversibly oxidized and reduced readily in the body. Vitamin C is essential for collagen formation and helps to maintain the integrity of tissue of mesenchymal origin. Although the value of high doses of vitamin C for preventing infection is hotly contested, a deficiency in vitamin C does result in a striking predeliction for infection. As early as 1948, it was reported that vitamin C deficiency depresses phagocytosis by neutrophils. Moreover, the number of peritoneal macrophages in vitamin-deficient guinea pigs is reduced, and the random migration of these phagocytes in vitro is considerably depressed.[25] In contrast, continuing studies using defined diets in guinea pigs do not show any effect of ascorbic acid depletion on neutrophil function or serum opsonins.

By far the major controversy surrounding vitamin C is the prophylactic value of high doses in the prevention of colds.[26] The most recent double-blind study, involving 674 marine recruits, failed to show any prophylactic value of 2 gm of vitamin C per day.[26]

Other Vitamins

Other vitamins have not been as completely studied as these. A deficiency in pantothenic acid impairs specific antibody induction. There is no evidence for a defect in antigen processing or protein synthesis per se. Consequently, Axelrod [20] has proposed that the defect rests in the secretory mechanism of the antibody-producing cells. Riboflavin deficiency is also associated with a moderate depression of antibody formation and may aggravate infection. Vitamin D and B_{12} deficiencies seem to have little effect on antibody synthesis. Thiamine deficiency results in increased susceptibility to bacterial infection.

Mineral Deficiencies

The role of the trace metals in susceptibility to infection is unclear. During infection, most of the intracellular minerals (ie, K, Mg, Zn, Se, P) are lost in proportion to the loss of body nitrogen. Serum levels of zinc fall during infection, and there may be a correlation between the zinc content of phagocytes and their bactericidal activity.[28]

Iron appears to be a two-edged sword—deficiencies may contribute to susceptibility, but high levels of iron seem to enhance the growth of infecting organisms.[14,27] In many instances, repletion of the iron-depleted individual who is infected will worsen the infection. Also, vitamin E and selenium may aid conversion of Fe^{+++} to the metabolically active Fe^{++} [29]

NUTRITIONAL REPLETION AND HOST RESISTANCE

The defect in killing of bacteria by neutrophils in patients with kwashiokor can be corrected by dietary protein and caloric intake. Similarly, immune competence as measured by delayed skin reactivity can be improved by intravenous hyperalimentation in malnourished surgical patients as can lymphocyte counts, response to phytohemagglutinin, immunoglobulin levels, neutrophil migration, and serum levels of C3.[13,30] We observed that the institution of oral hyperalimentation regimens in seriously burned children was accompanied by a dramatic reduction in death from sepsis and that this reduction in mortality was associated with an improvement in neutrophil function.[4] Wholesale nutritional repletion therefore restores immune function, but except for specific vitamin and mineral deficiencies,[31] exactly which component(s) of the diet are essential for restoration is unclear. Moreover, total restoration may require 30 to 60 days of nutritional repletion,[32] although most variables are corrected within 2 weeks. Daly et al [34] found that depressed cell-mediated immunity in protein-calorie malnourished rats could not be restored by synthetic amino acid diets without concomitant calorie repletion. In contrast, our continuing studies in guinea pigs have shown that minimal amounts of essential amino acids will restore immune function within 2 weeks, but nonessential amino acids will not suffice. Such high protein diets have been recommended in infected patients in order to spare body protein reserves [35] because a septic patient may require a 40 percent or greater increase in nitrogen intake to maintain equilibrium.[36] Similar or even greater requirements accompany trauma.

Because of our favorable experience with aggressive nutritional support in burned children, we recently initiated a clinical study to investigate the value of elevated protein intake. Patients in one group are receiving a caloric intake equal to resting metabolic expenditure (RME = basal × 1.3) for weight, height, and age plus 1 percent of the RME for each percentage of body surface area burned with approximately 15 percent of the calories given as protein. Patients in the second group are receiving an equivalent amount of calories, but the diet is altered to contain 25 percent of the calories as protein supplement. The carbohydrate-fat ratio in the two diets is identical. Early results from this study show a clear improvement of neutrophil function in recipients of the higher protein diet. We anticipate such diet modification may be of significant advantage in the treatment of many hypercatabolic, high-risk patients.

MODES AND RATIONALE OF NUTRITIONAL REPLETION

Clearly, the correction of nutritional deficiencies can result in restoration of immunologic competence. Of the several means available to correct malnutrition,[4,37] the best is the ingestion of an adequate normal meal. When that is not possible but the gastrointestinal tract is functioning (eg, coma), tube feeding should be used. When the gastrointestinal tract cannot be used, parenteral alimentation will suffice.

Protein requirements for parenteral nutrition can be met in the form of protein hydrolysate of amino acids, but caloric requirements cannot be met by the usual 5 percent dextrose solution since the fluid volume would be excessive. When using a peripheral vein, a concentrated energy source such as a fat emulsion may be preferred. On the other hand, fat is not well utilized for energy in hypermetabolic septic patients, where the preferred energy source is dextrose. Concentrated dextrose solutions (20 to 50 perent) are safe if administered by superior vena cava catheter. Unfortunately, there are numerous problems associated with this route of administration. Some inadvertent deficiencies of certain nutrients may occur, nutritional unbalance may ensue, and the frequency of infection associated with indwelling lines is high.[38] Care must also be taken to adequately meet all nutritional requirements as well as caloric needs of the patient. Certain conditions (ie, burns, severe trauma) result in metabolic demands that require supranormal caloric intake.

Some guidelines are useful in determining the need for nutritional supplementation (hyperalimentation) in surgical patients to prevent or correct immunologic defects.[31,39]

1. Supplemental oral hyperalimentation is preferred. Intravenous hyperalimentation should be reserved for patients who are unable to take nourishment by mouth.
2. Intravenous hyperalimentation should be instituted in anyone who is expected to be unable to take oral nutrition for longer than 5 to 7 days.
3. Whenever possible, patients with preexisting malnutrition should have the nutritional defects corrected before therapy, which may aggravate the nutritional problem, is begun. This includes elective operations.
4. Patients with severe infections that do not respond promptly to therapy should have supplemental hyperalimentation.
5. The hyperalimentation regimen should ensure adequate caloric intake for the basal metabolic needs, plus the estimated needs imposed by a hypercatabolic state where more proteins or amino acids are required.
6. Supplementation with vitamins for individuals not previously vitamin deficient should be in the range of two

to three times recommended daily allowance. For hypermetabolic patients, a daily dose of 500–1000 mg of vitamin C is recommended.

7. The requirements for metals during infection have not been clearly identified, although they are probably important. Oral hyperalimentation programs contain enough trace metals to ensure against deficiencies, but they must be added to intravenous regimens. Free iron should be avoided during acute infections.

8. Nutritional repletion may worsen some infections in chronically undernourished patients, notably those caused by many viruses and certain other intracellular pathogens, including malaria.

SPECIFIC ACTIVE AND PASSIVE IMMUNIZATION

Vaccination to improve resistance to a specific infection has been practiced since the pioneering discovery by Jenner in 1798 that infection with the cowpox virus would cause subsequent immunity to smallpox. Later, Pasteur showed that chicken cholera, animal anthrax, and rabies in humans could be prevented by vaccination. Killed bacterial vaccines were introduced by Solman and Smith in 1886. In 1888, Roux and Yersin discovered diphtheria exotoxin and found it could be neutralized by antitoxin. Two years later, von Behring and Kitasato actively immunized animals against the toxins of diphtheria and tetanus, and demonstrated passive immunity by serum transfer. In 1894, Roux produced tetanus antitoxin in horses; similar preparations were used in man until only recently. Unfortunately, the discovery of antimicrobial agents resulted in apathy toward the immunologic control of infections. Only in the last decade or so has interest in this approach risen again. Vaccination will prevent a variety of infections, many of which are surgically important.

Tetanus

In some parts of the world, including the United States, tetanus has almost been eradicated by the routine vaccination of preschool children with tetanus toxoid. Nevertheless, unless there is proof of vaccination, all patients with fresh open wounds should be treated as though they were unvaccinated. Several recommendations can be made regarding tetanus prophylaxis (Chapter 46): [40]

1. All injuries causing skin penetration should be considered as a potential portal of entry for tetanus.

2. In many patients with a previous full course of vaccination, immunity is long lasting, perhaps for a lifetime. However, a booster shot of toxoid should be given if more than 1 to 2 years have passed since the last booster. Routine boosters are recommended every 10 years.

3. In patients without prior immunization, 250 to 500 units human tetanus antitoxin should be administered intramuscularly depending on severity and age of the injury. At a separate site, the first immunizing dose of tetanus should be given, followed by a full course of active immunization.

Gas Gangrene

Even though exotoxins of *Clostridium* play a role in gas gangrene, there is little evidence that either active or passive therapy is beneficial.

Pneumococcal Infections

Most infections caused by *S. pneumoniae* seldom require operation. However, a prior splenectomy slightly increases the incidence and greatly increases the severity of pneumococcal infections, especially in infants and children (Chapter 36). Because of this increased risk, splenic repair for traumatic injury is advocated to preserve the spleen whenever technically possible. When splenectomy is necessary, at any age, patients should be actively immunized with multivalent pneumococcal vaccine. Patients who are splenectomized in childhood may also have an increased risk of infection caused by encapsulated extracellular bacteria.

Staphylococcal Infections

Vaccines to prevent staphylococcal infections have generally been ineffective because of the diversity of antigenic specificity among the staphylococci. Chronic or recurrent staphylococcal infections are sometimes improved by the use of autogenous vaccines.

Pseudomonas Infections

P. aeruginosa has a limited number of immunotypes. Highly purified polysaccharide antigens from seven of these will induce protection against about 90 percent of isolates causing infections in surgical patients, and active immunization with a polyvalent vaccine will result in significant protection of susceptible populations.[41,42] Likewise, an anti-pseudomonas hyperimmune globulin preparation appears to be protective for active infections.[43] Unfortunately, neither the vaccine nor the hyperimmune globulin is commercially available.

Infections with Other Gram-Negative Bacteria

Vaccines against the common gram-negative enteric pathogens are not yet available, but antigenic analysis of the structures of these bacteria shows some common antigens.[44] How protective these antigens and their corresponding antisera will be for protection against infection in man remains to be determined.

NONSPECIFIC PASSIVE IMMUNOTHERAPY

PASSIVE THERAPY WITH CELLULAR COMPONENTS

Granulocyte Transfusion

Cytotoxic and other chemotherapeutic agents frequently cause severe leukopenia. While transient lymphopenia causes few adverse consequences, marked neutropenia may be associated with severe and often fatal infections. Transfusions with granulocytes are usually recommended for patients in whom recovery of bone marrow function is anticipated when their peripheral blood count is less than 500 granulocytes per mm^3 in the absence of infection, and less than 1,000 granulocytes per mm^3 during infection.[45] Most commonly, the procedure is used for patients who have bone marrow suppression after receiving intensive chemotherapy for cancer. Granulocyte transfusions have no proven benefit in patients who have abnormal granulocyte function with normal numbers, or in patients who have bone marrow suppression caused by sepsis. At best, the benefit from granulocyte transfusions is short-lived (about 1 day) and expensive. The results may be better if the cells are harvested from HLA identical donors.[45a]

Transfer Factor

Transfer factor is a low molecular weight (dializable) extract of lymphocytes. Considerable controversy centers about the immunologic specificity of the agent, but its administration has caused apparent benefit in leprosy, mucocutaneous candidiasis, and a few viral and fungal diseases.[46] Its place in therapy of surgical infections remains to be determined.

PASSIVE THERAPY WITH HUMORAL COMPONENTS

While both antibody and nonspecific opsonins of the complement system are absolutely essential for normal resistance to infection by most extracellular bacterial pathogens, a considerable in vivo reserve exists. In a recent prospective study in highly susceptible surgical patients, we showed that low levels of serum opsonins (IgG, C3, properdin, factor B) were not associated with bacteremic episodes unless abnormal phagocytic function was also present.[2] In another controlled study in patients with large burns, the routine administration of plasma resulted in no difference in levels of opsonic proteins late in the burn course, and there was no statistically significant benefit.[47] Plasma should be administered, therefore, only to patients who are expected to be deficient in blood opsonins, ie, severely malnourished or hypermetabolic patients who have sepsis that is responding poorly to conventional antibiotic therapy. A prerequisite, of course, is that surgically correctable sites of localized infection have been treated appropriately.

Our investigations of the opsonophagocytic requirements for *P. aeruginosa* have shown that nearly all of the isolates we have tested have an absolute requirement for specific antibody. We also showed that active infection of burn wounds with *P. aeruginosa* can cause selective consumption of the specific protective antibody for the patient's serum.[43] For these reasons, pooled gammaglobulin might confer benefit in highly selected patients. Overall, however, passive gammaglobulin probably produces little benefit in patients with normal levels of IgG (greater than 500 mg per dl) because only a few patients in our bacteremic study had reduction of opsonic activity against the infecting organism during the bacteremic episode, and most organisms exhibited an intrinsic relative resistance to opsonization by both patient and pooled normal human sera.

NONSPECIFIC ACTIVE IMMUNOTHERAPY: IMMUNOMODULATORS

Drugs affecting immunologic responses were formerly termed adjuvants, immunoadjuvants, immunosuppressors, and immunopotentiators. Immunomodulator is a more descriptive term, and a new field, immunopharmacology, is emerging specifically for the study of these agents. The generality implied by immunomodulation is necessitated by the complexity of the immune system and the pleiotropic effects of any one agent on that system. Obviously, any attempt to fully describe the interactions of immunomodulators with all aspects of immune function is beyond the scope of this chapter, which will instead be limited to those aspects that appear to offer promise in the areas of infection control in surgical patients.

Many means are available to augment the immune response and host defense. Some agents have paradoxical effects, stimulating one activity while suppressing another. This seemed inexplicable, but many agents affect macrophages, and macrophages, which were first recognized for their phagocytic activity, play an integral role in almost every phase of host defense. Macrophages are essential for the induction of specific immune responses at both T and B cell level,[48] are involved in the regulation of those responses, and synthesize at least some complements.[49] In view of these multiple activities of a single cell type, it is not surprising that any modification of that cell's function by drugs or other means could have far-reaching impact on the entire system. With this in mind, we will examine the effects of selected agents on host defense mechanisms.

IMMUNOPHARMACOLOGIC AGENTS

Endotoxin

Endotoxins are heat-stable, high molecular weight lipopolysaccharides (LPS) whose basic chemical structure is shown in Figure 2-15. They form part of the cell wall of most gram-negative bacilli but all endotoxins, regardless of their source, produce a similar syndrome when given to experimental animals.[50]

Immediately following injection of large doses of LPS, a period of increased susceptibility to infection (negative phase) has been observed.[50] The appearance and duration depend primarily on the dose of endotoxin challenge, and result from a number of immediate responses—a transient decrease in serum complement levels, impairment of leukocyte migration, granulocytopenia (36 hours), and diminished tissue perfusion.[51] The increased susceptibility is short-lived, eg, mice injected with endotoxin initially show a marked susceptibility to *E. coli* infection but become resistant to a challenge that was delayed for 24 hours.[52] Now it is clear that injections of modest doses of LPS enhance the resistance of laboratory animals to a variety of unrelated organisms, including many bacteria, fungi, viruses, and parasites.[50] The rapidity with which increased resistance appears (as early as 4 hours) makes it unlikely that the induction of antibodies is totally responsible. It is more likely that the mechanism involves the prompt synthesis of properdin, C-reactive protein, C3, lysozyme, and interferon.[53] After an initial phase of granulocytopenia, a more sustained granulocytosis may also be an important mechanism of increased resistance.

The lipid A component of LPS is also a potent polyclonal activator of B cells.[54] This ability of gram-negative bacilli to enhance antibody levels has been of significant importance in mixed vaccines such as those involving typhoid bacilli and tetanus toxoid.

Endotoxin has direct effect on macrophages. For example, in vitro exposure to LPS stimulates macrophages to produce C2 and C4.[55] In addition, endotoxin promotes differentiation of the macrophage into an "activated" state.[56] Activation is accompanied by complex metabolic alterations in the macrophage and the acquisition of enhanced microbicidal and tumoricidal properties. No clear pathway of differentiation has yet been discerned, but it is known that some stimuli produce the metabolic changes without necessarily producing a functional state of enhanced tumor cytotoxicity.

Surprisingly, although LPS increases antibody production and enhances host resistance, it depresses T-cell function as measured by delayed hypersensitivity responses.[57] Part of this depression may be due to activated macrophages, which also participate in other adjuvant systems.

To summarize, LPS administration ultimately leads to elevated responsiveness of B cells, macrophage activation, depression of selected T-cell functions, increased serum complement levels, and granulocytosis. Quite possibly, many of the effects on macrophages could be attributed to a direct effect of lipid A on B cells, which produce lymphokines to activate macrophages which in turn, regulate T-cell functions, and increase their output of complement components. Other protective effects appear to result from complement activation.

Products of Mycobacteria

Freund's Adjuvant

Freund's adjuvant is a classic, oil emulsion–based adjuvant, which may or may not include bacteria or bacterial products. Most commonly, Freund's complete adjuvant (FCA) includes mycobacteria. FCA apparently does not potentiate immune responses to thymus-independent antigens, but is known for its promotion of high levels of avid antibody and high, persisting levels of cell-mediated immunity to protein antigens. On the other hand, use of the incomplete mixture (lacking mycobacteria) stimulates antibody, but only a transient form of delayed type cutaneous reactivity. Current interpretation of the effects of FCA is that the adjuvant does not directly affect the biosynthesis of antibody, but subverts the normal feedback inhibition mechanism(s), allowing a new phase of biosynthesis.[58] FCA seems to augment helper T-cell function as well, while suppressing cytotoxic T-cell functions.[59] The inclusion of mycobacteria into the emulsion also affects the kind of antibody produced. For example, ovalbumin in Freund's incomplete adjuvant (FIA) elicits only IgG_1 in guinea pigs. When mycobacteria are added to the emulsion, IgG_2 is also seen.[60]

Mycobacterium Bovis (Strain BCG)

Mycobacteria of the strain Bacillus-Calmette-Guerin (BCG) have quite different effects from those of water in oil emulsions with added mycobacteria such as FCA. Originally developed as a tuberculosis vaccine, BCG has found revival in cancer immunotherapy. This live, attenuated vaccine is a potent stimulant of the reticuloendothelial system (RES), enhances resistance to tumors, accelerates rejection of tissue allografts, and enhances resistance to infection.[61] Infection of experimental animals with BCG stimulates resistance to a wide variety of infectious diseases, especially those caused by intracellular pathogens (*Salmonella*,[62] *Herpesviruses, Babesia, Plasmodium, Schistosoma, Trypanosoma*, and *Trichinella*[63] species). Resistance to a variety of other agents has been reported including *S. aureus, C. albicans*, and endotoxin.[62] Isoniazid treatment will lessen or sometimes abolish the enhanced resistance. As might be expected, the mechanism of action of BCG is complex. BCG activates lymphocytes and macrophages in vitro[64] and in vivo so that the augmentation of host defense could involve heightened antibody production, better lymphocyte function, and elevated phagocyte activity. All these effects could in turn be mediated directly or indirectly by the effects of macrophages. It has been suggested that enhanced interferon production is an important aspect of protection. Ruitenberg et al[65] have shown that BCG failed to enhance *Listeria* clearance in nude mice lacking a thymus, indicating that the effect of BCG was T-cell dependent. The protective effect against *S. aureus* and *C. albicans* was reduced, but not abolished, in animals treated with a large dose of cyclophosphamide.[62] Unfortunately, BCG preparations from different sources vary considerably both in their chemical components and in their systemic effect. The chemical nature of the active component of mycobacteria and similar microorganisms has been pursued exhaustively. Only the wax D fractions derived from certain strains of mycobacteria are active. Wax D is a peptidoglycolipid combined with glucolipid. The main difference between active and inactive wax D is the presence of a peptide moiety in the former, namely n-acetylmuramyl-L-alanyl-D-isolglutamine (muramyl dipeptide of MDP). MDP has been synthesized, which will allow more discrete analysis of mechanism of action.[66]

Corynebacterium parvum

A systematic search for a bacterium with properties similar to mycobacteria uncovered *C. parvum*.[67] One strain, *C. parvum* 936B, was an unusually potent stimulant of the RES. There is considerable strain variability with respect to effects on the immune system, and the taxonomy is not entirely clear. McBride et al[68] compared various strains of anaerobic coryneforms and closely related propionibacteria and found that all strains enhanced colloidal carbon clearance but only certain strains had antitumor activity. Vaccines that have in vivo antitumor activity, produced splenomegaly, elicited activated (tumoricidal) macrophages, and induced activated macrophage cell surface antigen are *Propionibacterium* strains. We will continue the usage of the historical *C. parvum,* because most individuals are more familiar with that designation.

Pretreatment of mice with *C. parvum* increases resistance to infection with *B. abortus, B. pertussis, S. typhi, S. enteritidis, S. aureus, C. albicans, Herpesvirus,* and malaria.[69] Similarly, *C. parvum* is effective against *Listeria monocytogenes* and *S. aureus* infections in mice on chronic, high dose cortisone regimens.[70] Ruitenberg et al [65] have shown that *Listeria* clearance is enhanced in nude mice treated with *C. parvum,* suggesting that the effect is not under T-cell control. A variety of models for virus infections in animals have been studied using *C. parvum* with somewhat varying results.[71,72] Animals treated 7 to 10 days before inoculation were protected against lethal infection with *Herpesvirus hominis* type 2, encephalomyocarditis virus, murine cytomegalovirus, or Semliki Forest virus.[72] On the other hand, Budzko [71] reported that *C. parvum* injected before infection with Junin virus infection was ineffective, but significant protection was afforded when *C. parvum* was administered simultaneously with the virus or shortly thereafter. Most research with *C. parvum* has centered on its antitumor properties.[69]

The macrophage appears to be the primary target, and the tumoricidal properties of activated macrophages from *C. parvum*-treated animals appear similar to those activated by other agents. Peritoneal as well as pulmonary macrophages from vaccine-treated mice inhibit growth and DNA synthesis of tumor cells and are selectively cytotoxic for tumor cells in a cell contact–dependent mechanism.[73]

There appear to be at least two mechanisms involved in macrophage activation by *C. parvum.*[74] Naive, resident peritoneal macrophages can be activated when incubated with *C. parvum*–immune lymphocytes in the presence of *C. parvum,* and inflammatory macrophages (oil-induced) can be activated directly by *C. parvum.* The first mechanism is probably a classical lymphokine-mediated activation, and the second is a phenomenon that has been observed by others. We found that *C. parvum* would activate macrophages in congenitally athymic (nude) mice, indicating a T-independent mechanism for macrophage activation in vivo. However, some of the histologic characteristics and the extent of macrophage mobilization were quite different in nude animals when compared to normal animals.[75] This observation supports other studies, which showed that *C. parvum* was an effective antitumor agent in T-deprived animals.

Like other immunomodulators, *C. parvum* has a multiplicity of other effects on the immune system. Animals treated with *C. parvum* exhibit heightened antibody responses to both T-dependent and T-independent antigens,[67] depressed delayed type hypersensitivity and in vitro T-lymphocyte mitogenic responses, and decreased graft versus host reactions.[76] Most data suggest activated macrophages are responsible for the suppression of many T-lymphocyte functions.[77] Several studies have concluded that macrophages are also directly involved in the adjuvant effects of *C. parvum.*[78] In addition, *C. parvum* causes shifts in antibody class like FCA.[79] Lest one's sensibilities are insulted by assigning so many activities to macrophages, Lee and Berry [80] have found considerable functional heterogeneity among macrophage subpopulations.

In addition, *C. parvum* activates complement,[81] increases bone marrow macrophage colony production,[82] induces interferon production by T lymphocytes,[83] and is a chemoattractant for monocytes and neutrophils.[84] As with the mycobacteria, attempts have been made to identify the active principle of *C. parvum.* Both lipid components and water-soluble fractions have activity.[85] Adlam et al [85] concluded that the backbone component of the cell wall is responsible for the immunomodulating properties of *C. parvum.* It will be interesting to see if the molecular structure of this component is similar to the MDP essential for BCG activity (see previous section).

Pyran

Pyran is a synthetic anionic copolymer of divinyl ether and ethylene maleic anhydride. Although there is some batch variability due to molecular weight classes resulting from the polymerization, pyran, in general, is a potent adjuvant, induces interferon, has a broad spectrum of antiviral activity,[86] is an effective antitumor agent,[87] and protects against lethal bacterial and fungal infections.[88]

Because pyran is a potent interferon inducer, it is effective in protecting against herpesvirus infections,[89] even in thymectomized animals.[90] Pyran is also capable of increasing resistance to infection by *K. pneumoniae, S. aureus,* or *L. monocytogenes.*[70] The protective effect starts to diminish by 21 days.

Most evidence suggests that pyran's antitumor effect is mediated by activated macrophages independent of T cells. Moreover, pyran will activate macrophages and protect against infection in mice receiving chronic, high doses of cortisone.[70] Pyran also enhances a secondary response, suggesting that the adjuvant acts to expand the number of antibody-producing B cells or memory helper T cells.[91] Baird and Kaplan [91] concluded that the site of action of pyran, with respect to antibody responses, is the T lymphocyte, even though lymphocyte blastogenesis was inhibited by activated macrophages. Pyran in the presence of serum is chemotactic for both neutrophils and monocytes.[75] The evidence suggested that pyran might activate the complement sequence.

A comparison of various molecular weight species of pyran found variations in each activity.[92] Pyran fractions of lower molecular weights appear to maintain antitumor activity with better therapeutic index. Moreover, these small molecules had higher antiviral activity and did not sensitize to endotoxin.

Levamisole

Initially developed as an antihelminthic drug, levamisole (and its d-enantiomer, tetramisole) has been shown to potentiate immune responses both in vitro and in vivo.[93,94] Almost all functions associated with cell-mediated immune reactions are affected. Most of the levamisole seems to restore function in a compromised host, with little effect on a normal host. Levamisole increases phagocytosis by both PMNs and macrophages and corrects defective PMN chemotactic responses. Delayed hypersensitivity responses and the number of antibody-producing cells are both augmented.[95] One possible mechanism of levamisole action is to enhance the maturation of cells to a normally responsive state.[96] Although some protection against herpetic eye reinfection has been demonstrated [97] few animal studies have evaluated the effect of levamisole on infection.

STUDIES OF IMMUNOMODULATORS IN HUMANS

Endotoxin

Deliberate administration of high doses of LPS in order to enhance resistance to infection cannot be considered ethical today. There has been some experience in this area for tumor therapy; however, that is of historical interest. In the late nineteenth century, Coley [98] noted that an inoperable lymphosarcoma of the neck had regressed after an attack of erysipelas. Beginning in April 1891, Coley unsuccessfully attempted to produce erysipelas, as a therapeutic measure, in ten patients with inoperable malignant tumors. Subsequently, he learned of the investigations of Roger on *B. prodigiosus (Serratia marcescens)* in combination with other organisms.[99] Various mixtures of these organisms, known as Coley's toxin, were developed and a commercial preparation, Parke-Davis Type IX, was available from 1899 until 1907, but the extreme variability and uncontrollability from batch to batch discouraged investigation.

Beebe and Tracy [100] later utilized mixtures of *S. marcescens, S. pyogenes, S. aureus,* and *E. coli* in the so-called Huntington Research Fund Preparations (Tracy's X and XI). As they reported: "The results . . . certainly demonstrated the destructive action . . . on tumor cells of this type by bacterial toxins. Such action, while chiefly local, is at the same time something more than this, for it is repeatedly observed that tumors at a distance . . . undergo regression simultaneously with those inoculated, while in one instance the entire treatment was by inoculation remote from tumor." As a result of these studies, Tracy evolved the first stable but most potent preparation of Coley's mixed toxins. Commercial preparations, however, proved less reliable, and interest waned. Another contributing factor was no doubt the terrifying responses of many patients to the repeated administration of these LPS preparations. Coley's toxin eventually led to agents such as BCG and *C. parvum* in cancer immunotherapy.

Mycobacterium bovis BCG

BCG has been given to more than 500 million people as a vaccination for tuberculosis. In 1959, Old et al [101] reported the efficacy of BCG in treating tumors in animals. Since that time there has been widespread interest in BCG as an antitumor agent. It has not been seriously considered for the nonspecific treatment of infection, primarily because of the serious complications that often accompany its administration.[102]

Corynebacterium parvum

Since *C parvum* was first used in the treatment of human malignancy in the early 1970s,[103] approximately 2,500 patients have been treated with some 20,000 doses (Burroughs-Wellcome, personal communication). The relationship between dose and toxicity has been variously reported. Adverse reactions (chills, fever, and vomiting) occur in more than half the recipients, and a small number of life-threatening complications have occurred. The serious reactions are limited to patients with cachexia, severe underlying cardiovascular disease, and intracranial tumors. As might be expected, the clinical efficacy in cancer therapy has varied. Nonetheless, it has been reported [104] that the survival of patients with oat cell carcinoma of the lung, sarcomas, metastatic breast cancer, and melanoma receiving chemotherapy and *C. parvum* is significantly greater than those receiving chemotherapy alone. Although the previously described animal studies would also suggest the use of *C. parvum* to prevent or treat certain infections, we are not aware of systematic clinical study in that area at this time.

Levamisole

Levamisole is a synthetic substance of low molecular weight that will correct altered immunologic function and has no serious side effects. It has been applied in a broad spectrum of human disease where an imbalance of immune homeostasis was known or at least postulated. So far, clinical experience with 3,046 patients has been reported in 132 studies.[94] Treatment has been given daily or intermittently, and the longest treatment was two consecutive days every week for 3 years. Nausea was reported in 167 of the cases, and granulocytopenia, the most serious side effect, occurred in 23 patients. There is no evidence of nephrotoxicity, hepatotoxicity, or bone marrow toxicity in humans.[94]

To our knowledge, only levamisole has been studied systematically in humans in regard to its ability to induce resistance to microbial infections. Bierman [105] performed a double-blind cross-over study in 40 patients with dermic, recurrent herpes progenitalis and found no improvement in the treated group. Meakins et al [3] have recently performed a double-blind study using levamisole to prevent infection in high-risk patients who were anergic or relatively anergic to delayed hypersensitivity antigens. Levamisole recipients had significantly fewer septic complications. Chemotaxis of neutrophils and skin reactivity were also improved but not to a significant degree.

A dramatic example of the clinical use of this drug in infection was also described by Oettgen et al.[104] A six-year-old girl presented with a history of multiple, recurrent staphylococcal abscesses, extensive mycotic and bacterial skin infections, and chronic bronchial infection. Lymphocyte response to PHA was normal, but skin tests were negative. Total hemolytic complement, C2, C4, IgM, IgG, and IgA were normal, but serum would not support the phagocytosis of yeast by neutrophils. Following a course of levamisole therapy (2.5 mg per kg, orally, 3 consecutive days every 2 weeks for 1 month), all manifestations of disease disappeared, skin tests became normal, and serum supported phagocytosis. A literature review has revealed [106] that of nine defined immunodeficiency diseases treated, only chronic mucocutaneous candidiasis was not corrected by levamisole.

Zymosan

Zymosan is a three-micron yeast cell wall preparation derived from *Saccharomyces cerevisiae,* composed of protein, lipid, ash, and a complex of polysaccharides, namely 18 percent mannan and 58 percent glucan. Glucan comprises the inner cell wall, mannan the outer.

Benacerraf and Sebestyen [107] were the first to demonstrate zymosan's ability to stimulate the RES. Treated animals manifested increased phagocytic capacity, increased rate of intracellular degradation of phagocytized particles, increased resistance to infection, increased properdin levels, enhanced humoral immunity, and inhibition or regression of various experimental tumors.

Glucan has not proved to be protective in infection. In fact, glucan pretreatment leads to increased susceptibility to endotoxin in animals.[108] The component responsible for zymosan's effectiveness in RES stimulation and immunologic protection remains unidentified.

A single intravenous injection of zymosan (40 mg per kg) is followed by a rapid decrease in the number of circulating platelets and a biphasic increase in the rate of clearance of injected colloidal carbon with peaks at two and 72 hours after zymosan injection. The circulating platelets return to normal levels after 14 days. Antibody production in the rat is stimulated, and zymosan-induced tolerance to drum trauma can be transferred by serum or spleen cells.[109] Zymosan stimulation is not accompanied by any measurable change in plasma or blood volume, nor any alteration in pressor responses to exogenous catecholamines; thus, it appears unlikely that the shock-protective action of zymosan is mediated either through an adrenergic circulatory blockage or through expansion of plasma volume.[110]

Zymosan has been shown in vitro to increase β-glucuronidase and cathepsin D release from cultured mouse peritoneal macrophages during the process of phagocytosis,[111] but zymosan-protected animals release smaller amounts of laposomal enzymes during hemologic shock.[112]

A standard, empirical, experimental protocol for RES stimulation has been to administer a zymosan dose of 10 mg per kg intravenously each day for 3 days prior to inducing shock. However, the intravenous route results in RES hyperplasia and hypertrophy (increased liver, lung, and spleen weights). While these are reversible, it would be more desirable to induce a local protection without the systemic RES effects. Joyce et al [113,114] have demonstrated that zymosan given intraperitoneally does induce local (and to a lesser degree, systemic) resistance to *E. coli* peritonitis in the rat. Intraperitoneal zymosan gave no significant alteration in liver, lung, and spleen weights or in RES phagocytic clearance activity.[113] Local resistance in the dog to an ischemic closed intestinal loop model and to an *E. coli*–induced cholecystitis septic shock model have also been demonstrated.[114] There is no experience in humans.

BIBLIOGRAPHY

Ascher MS, Gottlieb AA, Kirkpatrick CH: Transfer Factor. Basic Properties and Clinical Applications. New York, Academic, 1976.

Chandra RK, Newberns PM: Nutrition, Immunity and Infection. Mechanisms of Interactions. New York, Plenum, 1977.

Halpern B (ed.): *Corynebacterium parvum:* Applications in Experimental and Clinical Oncology. New York, Plenum, 1975.

Horstmann DM: Viral vaccines and their ways. Rev. Infect. Dis. 1: 502, 1979.

Richards JR, Kinney JM (eds.): Nutritional Aspects of Care in the Critically Ill. New York, Churchill Livingston, 1977.

Wolstenholme GEW, Knight J (eds.): Immunopotentiation. Amsterdam, Elsevier, Scientific Publishers, 1973.

REFERENCES

1. Alexander JW, Good RA: Fundamentals of Clinical Immunology. Philadelphia, Saunders, 1977.
2. Alexander JW, Stinnett JD, Ogle CK, Ogle JD, Morris MJ: A comparison of immunologic profiles and their influence on bacteremia in surgical patients with a high risk of infection. Surgery 86:94, 1979.
3. Meakins JL, Christou NV, Shizgal HM, MacLean LD: Therapeutic approaches to anergy in surgical patients: surgery and levamisole. Ann Surg 190:285, 1979.
4. Lennard ES, Alexander JW, Craycraft TK, MacMillan BG: Association in burn patients of improved antibacterial defense with nutritional support by the oral route. Burns 1:98, 1975.

NUTRITIONAL APPROACHES

5. McNeill WH: Plagues and Peoples. Garden City, New York, Anchor, 1977.
6. Chandra RK, Newberns PM: Nutrition, Immunity and Infection. Mechanisms of Interactions. New York, Plenum, 1977.
7. Hill GL, Pickford I, Schorah CJ, Blackett RL, Burkinshaw L, Warren JV, Morgan DB: Malnutrition in surgical patients: an unrecognized problem. Lancet 3:689, 1977.
8. Beisel WR: Malnutrition as a consequence of stress. In Suskind RM (ed): Malnutrition and the Immune Response. New York, Raven, 1977, p 21.
9. Kinney JM: The metabolic response to injury. In Richards JR, Kinney JM (eds): Nutritional Aspects of Care in the Critically Ill. New York, Churchill Livingston, 1977, p 95.
10. Richards JR: Metabolic responses to injury, infection and starvation: an overview. In Richards JR, Kinney JM (eds): Nutritional Aspects of Care in the Critically Ill. New York, Churchill Livingston, 1977, p 273.
11. Schopfer K, Douglas SD: Neutrophil function in children with kwashiorkor. J Lab Clin Med 88:450, 1976.
12. Smythe RM: Thymolymophatic deficiency and depression of cell-mediated immunity in protein-calorie malnutrition. Lancet 2:939, 1971.
13. Sirisinha S, Edelman R, Suskind R, Charupatana C, Olson RE: Complement and C3-proactivator levels in children

with protein-calorie malnutrition and effect of dietary treatment. Lancet 1:1016, 1973.
14. Chandra RK: Iron and immunocompetence. Nutrition Rev 34:129, 1976.
15. Rafii M, Hashemi S, Nahani J, Mohagheghpour N: Immune responses in malnourished children. Clin Immunol Immunopathol 8:1, 1977.
16. Wunder JA, Stinnett JD, Alexander JW: The effects of malnutrition on variables of host defense in the guinea pig. Surgery 84:542, 1978.
17. Kenney MA, Roderuck CE, Arnrich L, Piedad F: Effect of protein deficiency on the spleen and antibody formation in rats. J Nutr 95:173, 1968.
18. Mathur M, Ramalingaswami V, Deo MG: Influence of protein deficiency on 19S antibody-forming cells in rats and mice. J Nutr 102:841, 1974.
19. Blackberg SM: Effect of the immunity mechanism of various avitaminoses. Proc Soc Exp Biol Med 25:770, 1927.
20. Axelrod AE: Immune processes in vitamin deficiency states. Am J Clin Nutr 24:265, 1971.
21. Krishan S, Krishan AD, Mustafa AS, Talwar GP, Ramalingaswami V: Effect of vitamin A and undernutrition on the susceptibility of rodents to malarial parasite *Plasmodium berghei.* J Nutr 106:784, 1976.
22. Axelrod AE, Hojper S: Effects of pantothenic acid, pyridoxine and thiamine deficiencies upon antibody formation to influenza virus PR-8 in rats. J Nutr 72:325, 1960.
23. Willis-Carr HF, St Pierre RL: Effects of vitamin B_6 deficiency in thymic epithelial cells and T lymphocyte differentiation. J Immunol 120:1153, 1978.
24. Van Bijsterveld OP: The digestive capacity of pyridoxine-deficient phagocytes in vitro. J Med Microbiol 4:337, 1971.
25. Ganguly R, Durieux MF, Waldman RH: Macrophage function in vitamin C deficient guinea pigs. Am J Clin Nutr 29:762, 1976.
26. Pitt HA, Castrini AM: Vitamin C prophylaxis in marine recruits. JAMA 241:908, 1979.
27. Weinberg ED: Iron and susceptibility to infectious disease. Science 184:952, 1974.
28. Lennard EA, Bjornson AB, Petering HG, Alexander JW: An immunologic and nutritional evaluation of burn neutrophil function. J Surg Res 16:286, 1974.
29. Murray J, Murray A: Suppression of infection by famine—a paradox? Perspect Biol Med 20:471, 1977.
30. Dionigi R, Zonta A, Diminioni L, Gres F, Ballabio A: The effects of total parenteral nutrition on immunodepression due to malnutrition. Ann Surg 185:467, 1977.
31. Stinnett JD, Alexander JW: Nutrition as related to host defense and infection. In Richards JR, Kinney JM (eds): Nutritional Aspects of Care in the Critically Ill. New York, Churchill Livingston, 1977, p 557.
32. Copeland EM: Effect of intravenous hyperalimentation. Ann Surg 184:60, 1976.
33. Edelman R, Suskind R, Olson RE, Sirisinha S: Mechanisms of definitive delayed cutaneous hypersensitivity in children with protein-calorie malnutrition. Lancet 1:506, 1973.
34. Daly JM, Dudrick SJ, Copeland EM: Effects of protein depletion and repletion on cell-mediated immunity in experimental animals. Ann Surg 188:791, 1978.
35. Blackburn GL, Flatt JP, Clowes GHA, O'Donnell TF, Hensle TE: Protein sparing therapy during periods of starvation with sepsis or trauma. Ann Surg 177:588, 1973.
36. Long CL, Crosby F, Geiger JW, Kinney JM: Parenteral nutrition in the septic patient: nitrogen balance, limiting plasma amino acids and calorie to nitrogen ratios. Am J Clin Nutr 29:380, 1976.
37. Wilmore DW, McDougal WS, Peterson JP: Newer products and formulas for alimentation. Am J Clin Nutr 30:1498, 1977.
38. Parkinson RS, Kern LB, Bowring AC. Intravenous alimentation in the neonate and infant. Med J Aust 1:1182, 1972.
39. Alexander JW: Nutrition and surgical infections. In Ballinger W (ed): Manual on Nutrition. Philadelphia, Saunders, 1975, p 386.

IMMUNIZATION

40. Furste W, Skudder PA, Hampton OP Jr: The evolution of prophylaxis against tetanus from the Civil War to the present. Bull Am Coll Surg, Sept/Oct, 1967.
41. Alexander JW, Fisher MW: Immunization against *Pseudomonas* infection after thermal injury. J Infect Dis 130 (Supp):S152, 1974.
42. Jones RJ, Roe EA: Low mortality in burned patients in a *Pseudomonas* vaccine trial. Lancet 2:401, 1978.
43. Jones CE, Alexander JW, Fisher MW: Clinical evaluation of *Pseudomonas* hyperimmune globulin. J Surg Res 14:87, 1973.
44. Alexander JW, Stinnett JD: Emerging concepts in the control of surgical infections: a reappraisal. In de Boer HHM (ed): Intra-abdominal sepsis. Utrecht, Bunge Scientific Publishers, 1979.

PASSIVE IMMUNOTHERAPY

45. Boggs DR: Transfusion of neutrophils as prevention or treatment of infection in patients with neutropenia. N Engl J Med 290:1055, 1974.
45a. Wright DG: Leukocyte transfusion. In Verhoef J, Peterson PK, Quie PG: Infections in the Immunocompromised Host—Pathogenesis, Prevention and Therapy. North Holland, Elsevier, 1980, p 261.
46. Ascher MS, Gottlieb AA, Kirkpatrick CH: Transfer Factor. Basic Properties and Clinical Applications. New York, Academic, 1976.
47. Alexander JW, Ogle CK, Stinnett JD, White M, MacMillan BG, Edwards BK: Fresh frozen plasma vs plasma protein derivative as adjunctive therapy for patients with massive burns. J Trauma 19:502, 1979.

NONSPECIFIC ACTIVE IMMUNOTHERAPY

48. Thomas DW: Genetic control of T lymphocyte responses by in vitro sensitization with macrophage-bound antigens. J Immunol 121:61, 1978.
49. Bentley C, Fries W, Brode V: Synthesis of factors D, B and P of the alternative pathway of complement activation, as well as C3, by guinea pig peritoneal macrophages in vitro. Immunology 35:971, 1978.
50. Landy M: Increase in resistance following administration of bacterial lipopolysaccharides. Ann NY Acad Sci 66:292, 1956.
51. Cluff LE: Effects of endotoxins on susceptibility to infections. J Infect Dis 122:205, 1970.
52. Rowley D: Endotoxin induced changes in susceptibility to infection. In Landy M, Braun W (eds): Bacterial Endotoxins. New Jersey, Rutgers Univ. Press, 1964, p 359.
53. Landy M, Pillemer L: Increased resistance to infection and accompanying alteration in properdin levels following administration of bacterial lipopolysaccharides. J Exp Med 104:383, 1956.
54. Andersson J, Sjoberg O, Moller G: Induction of immunoglobulin and antibody synthesis in vitro by lipopolysaccharides. Eur J Immunol 2:349, 1972.
55. Colten HR: Biosynthesis of serum complement. In Brent

L, Holborow J (eds): Proceedings of the Second International Congress of Immunology. Amsterdam, North-Holland, 1974, Vol 1, p 183.
56. Cohn ZA: The activation of mononuclear phagocytes: fact, fancy and future. J Immunol 21:813, 1978.
57. Lagrange PH, Mackaness GB, Miller TE, Pardon P: Effects of bacterial lipopolysaccharide on the induction and expression of cell-mediated immunity. I. Depression of the afferent arc. J Immunol 114:442, 1975.
58. White RG: The adjuvant effect of microbial products on the immune response. Ann Rev Microbiol 30:579, 1976.
59. Reinisch CL, Gleiner NA, Schlossman SF: Adjuvant regulation of T-cell function. J Immunol 116:710, 1976.
60. White RG, Jenkins GC, Wilkinson PC: The production of skin-sensitizing antibody in the guinea pig. Int Arch Allergy Appl Immunol 22:156, 1963.
61. Ratzan KR, Musher DM, Keusch GT, Weinstein L: Correlations of increased metabolic activity, resistance to infection, enhanced phagocytosis and inhibition of bacterial growth by macrophages from Listeria and BCG-infected mice. Infect Immun 5:499, 1972.
62. Sher NA, Chaparas SD, Greenberg LE, Bernard S: Effects of BCG, *Corynebacterium parvum* and methanol-extraction residue in the reduction of mortality from *Staphylococcus aureus* and *Candida albicans* infections in immunosuppressed mice. Infect Immun 12:1325, 1975.
63. Grove DI, Civil RH: Trichinella spiralis: effects on the host-parasite relationship in mice of BCG (attenuated *Mycobacterium bovis*). Exp Parisitol 44:181, 1978.
64. Mokyr MB, Mitchell MB: Activation of lymphoid cells by BCG in vitro. Cell Immunol 15:264, 1975.
65. Ruitenberg EJ, Steerenberg PA, van Noorle Jansen LM: Effect of BCG and *C. parvum* on in vivo Listeria clearance and tumor growth. Comparative studies in normal and congenitally athymic (nude) mice. Dev Biol Standard 38:103, 1978.
66. Parant M, Damais C, Audibert F, Parant F, Chedid F, Sache L, Lefransier E, Choay P, Lederer E: In vivo and in vitro stimulation of nonspecific immunity by the B-D-p-aminophenyl glycoside of N-acetylmuramyl-L-alanyl-D-isoglutamine and an oligomer prepared by cross-linking with gluteraldehyde. J Infect Dis 138:378, 1978.
67. Howard JG, Christie GH, Scott MT: Biological effects of *Corynebacterium parvum* IV. Adjuvant and inhibitory activities on B lymphocytes. Cell Immunol 7:290, 1973.
68. McBride WH, Dawes J, Dunbar N, Ghaffar A, Woodruff MFA: A comparative study of anaerobic coryneforms. Immunology 28:49, 1975.
69. Halpern B: *Corynebacterium parvum:* applications in experimental and clinical oncology. New York, Plenum, 1975.
70. Stinnett JD, Morris MJ, Alexander JW: Macrophage activation and increased resistance to infection in immunosuppressed mice treated with *Corynebacterium parvum* or pyran copolymer. J Reticuloendothel Soc 25:525, 1979.
71. Budzko DB, Casals J, Waksman BH: Enhanced resistance against junin virus infection induced by *Corynebacterium parvum*. Infect Immun 19:893, 1978.
72. Geniteau M, Quero AM, German A: Action of *Corynebacterium parvum* on different viral infections in the mouse. Ann Pharm Fr 35:181, 1977.
73. Ghaffar A, Cullen RT, Woodruff MFA: Further analysis of the anti-tumour effect in vitro of peritoneal exudate cells from mice treated with *Corynebacterium parvum*. Br J Cancer 31:15, 1975.
74. Bomford R, Christie GH: Mechanisms of macrophage activation by *Corynebacterium parvum* II. In vivo experiments. Cell Immunol 17:150, 1975.
75. Stinnett JD, Majeski JA: Macrophage activation and mobilization in nude mice by *Corynebacterium parvum* and pyran: a functional and histologic study. Cancer Res (submitted).
76. Scott MT: Biological adjuvant *Corynebacterium parvum* I. Inhibition of PHA, mixed lymphocyte and GVH reactivity. Cell Immunol 5:459, 1972.
77. Bash JA: Suppression of rat T cell proliferation by *Corynebacterium parvum:* T cell requirement for induction. J Reticuloendothel Soc 23:63, 1978.
78. Sljivic VA, Brown CA, Watson SR: Further studies on the enhancement of the antibody response in vitro by *C. parvum*. Dev Biol Standard 38:147, 1978.
79. James K: Antibody responses, antitumor antibodies and Ig class and subclass levels in *C. parvum* treated mice. Dev Biol Standard 38:173, 1978.
80. Lee K-C, Berry D: Functional heterogeneity in macrophages activated by *Corynebacterium parvum:* characterization of subpopulations with different activities in promoting immune responses and suppressing tumor cell growth. J Immunol 118:1530, 1977.
81. Biran H, Moake JZ, Reed R, Freireich EJ: Complement activation during immunotherapy with *Corynebacterium parvum*. Clin Res 23:409A, 1975.
82. Wolmark N, Fisher B: The effect of a single and repeated administration of *Corynebacterium parvum* on bone marrow macrophage colony production in syngeneic tumor-bearing mice. Cancer Res 34:2869, 1974.
83. Sugiyama M, Epstein LB: Effect of *Corynebacterium parvum* on human T-lymphocyte interferon production and T-lymphocyte proliferation in vitro. Cancer Res 38:4467, 1978.
84. Stinnett JD, Majeski JA: Chemoattractant properties of *Corynebacterium parvum* and pyran copolymer for human monocytes and neutrophils. J Natl Cancer Inst 58:781, 1977.
85. Adlam C, Reid DE, Tarkington P: The nature of the active principle of *Corynebacterium parvum*. In Halpern B (ed): Corynebacterium parvum: Application in Experimental and Clinical Oncology. New York, Plenum, 1975, p 40.
86. Morahan PS, Regelson W, Munson AE: Pyran and polyribonucleotides: differences in biological activities. Antimicrob Agents Chemother 2:16, 1972.
87. Hirsch MS, Black PH, Wood ML, Monaco AP: Effects of pyran copolymer on oncogenic virus infections in immunosuppressed hosts. J Immunol 108:1312, 1972.
88. Regelson W, Munson AE: The reticuloendothelial effects of interferon inducers: polyanionic and nonpolyanionic phylaxis against microorganisms. Ann NY Acad Sci 173:831, 1970.
89. Morahan PS, Kern ER, Glasgow LA: Immunomodulator-induced resistance against herpes simplex virus (39730). Proc Soc Exp Biol Med 154:615, 1977.
90. Morahan PS, McCord RS: Resistance to herpes simplex type 2 virus induced by an immunopotentiator (pyran) in immunosuppressed mice. J Immunol 115:311, 1975.
91. Baird LG, Kaplan AM: Immunoadjuvant activity of pyran copolymer. I. Evidence for direct stimulation of T-lymphocytes and macrophages. Cell Immunol 20:167, 1975.
92. Regelson W, Morahan P, Kaplan AM, Baird LG, Munson JA: Synthetic polyanions: molecular weight, macrophage activation and immunologic response. In Wagner WH, Hahn H, Evans R (eds): Activation of Macrophages. New York, American Elsevier, 1974.
93. Tripodi D, Parks LC, Brugmans J: Drug-induced restoration of cutaneous delayed hypersensitivity in anergic patients with cancer. N Engl J Med 289:354, 1973.
94. Symoens J, Rosenthal M: Levamisole in the modulation of the immune response: the current experimental and clinical state. J Reticuloendothel Soc 21:175, 1977.

95. Flannery GR, Rolland JM, Nairn RC: Levamisole. Lancet 1:750, 1975.
96. Amery WK: A hypothesis. The mechanism of action of levamisole: immune restoration through enhanced cell maturation. J Reticuloendothel Soc 24:187, 1978.
97. Friedlaender MH, Smolin G, Okumoto M: The treatment of herpetic reinfection with levamisole. Am J Ophthalmol 86:245, 1978.
98. Coley WB: Contribution to the knowledge of sarcoma. Ann Surg 14:199, 1891.
99. Roger H: Contribution a l'etude experimentale du streptocoque de l'erysipele. Rev de Med (Paris) 12:929, 1892.
100. Beebe SP, Tracy M: The treatment of experimental tumors with bacterial toxins. JAMA 49:1493, 1907.
101. Old LJ, Benacerraf B, Clarke DA, Carswell FA, Stockert A: Effect of bacillus Calmette-Guerin infection in transplanted tumors in the mouse. Nature 184:291, 1959.
102. Sparks FC, Silverstein MF, Hunt JS, Haskell CM, Pilch YH, Morton DL: Complications of BCG immunotherapy in patients with cancer. N Engl J Med 289:827, 1973.
103. Halpern B, Israel L: Study of the action of an immunostimulin associated with *Corynebacteria* anerobes in human and experimental neoplasms. CR Acad Sc Paris 273:2186, 1971.
104. Oettgen HF, Pinsky CM, Delmonte L: Treatment of cancer with immunomodulators. *Corynebacterium parvum* and levamisole. Med Clin North Am 60:511, 1976.
105. Bierman SM: Double-blind cross-over study of levamisole as immunoprophylaxis for recurrent herpes progenitalis. Cutis 21:352, 1978.
106. Brugmans J: Levamisole in infectious diseases—a review of the literature. J Rheumatol 5(Suppl 4):115, 1978.
107. Benacerraf B, Sebestyen MM: Effects of bacterial endotoxins on susceptibility to infection with gram-positive and acid-fast bacteria. Fed Proc 16:860, 1957.
108. Trejo RA, Crafton CG, DiLuzio NR: Influence of RE functional alterations on mortality patterns in endotoxin and tourniquet shock. J Reticuloendothel Soc 9:299, 1971.
109. Reichard SM: RES stimulation and transfer of protection against shock. J Reticuloendothel Soc 12:604, 1972.
110. Kampine JP, Banaszak EF, Smith JJ: Alteration of RES activity and circulatory responsiveness in the dog. J Reticuloendothel Soc 2:172, 1965.
111. Ringrose PS, Parr MA, McLaren M: Effects of anti-inflammatory and other compounds on the release of lysosomal enzymes from macrophages. Biochem Pharm 24:607, 1975.
112. Lentz PE, Smith JJ: Effect of reticuloendothelial stimulation on plasma acid hydrolase activity in hemorrhagic shock. Proc Soc Exp Biol Med 124:1243, 1967.
113. Joyce LD, Hau T, Hoffman R, Simmons RL, Lillehei RC: Evaluation of the mechanism of zymosan-induced resistance to experimental peritonitis. Surgery 83:717, 1978.
114. Joyce LD, Mauer HG, Smith JM, Lillehei RC: Resistance to experimental peritonitis induced by local nonspecific stimulation of the reticuloendothelial system. Adv Shock Res 4:49, 1980.

PART VI: WOUND INFECTIONS AND THEIR PREVENTION

CHAPTER 20
Wound Infections: Epidemiology and Clinical Characteristics

PETER J. E. CRUSE

HISTORY

THE history of wound infection is discussed in Chapter 1. Paré discovered the safeguarding of the local resistance of the wound. Semmelweis realized that infection was transmitted directly, and Lister instituted surgical antisepsis. Despite the advances made by these pioneers, the misery and mortality of "hospital gangrene" continued until the 1890s. In 1874, Von Nussbaum deplored that wound sepsis "gnawing like a wild beast, slew or permanently crippled 80 out of every hundred" of his surgical patients.[1] Indeed, he had 100 percent mortality with 34 consecutive through the knee amputations during the Franco Prussian War of 1870. On the French side during this war, 13,173 amputations of all kinds, including digits, were performed, with 10,006 deaths.

Kocher of Berne, Switzerland, introduced meticulous bloodless surgical technique, and by 1899 was able to report a 2.3 percent infection rate in clean cases. In the United States, Halsted became a champion of asepsis and Kocher's technique.

Wound infections are still common. Disability, delayed healing, deformity, or death can result. In addition, the quality of life, both physical and psychologic, has often been affected or permanently altered.

INCIDENCE

In 1963, approximately 25,000,000 patients were admitted to hospitals in the United States. More than 1,000,000 developed postoperative or hospital-acquired infections (Table 20-1). The overall wound infection rate of 7.4 percent is based on the incidence in five American university centers.[2,3] The type of operation helps determine the incidence of infection. Based on the common definitions (Table 20-2) of clean, clean-contaminated, contaminated, and dirty operations, the incidence of wound infection in these hospitals is listed in Table 20-3. In addition, the incidence of infection varies with the type of operation (Table 20-4). The incidence of postoperative wound infection was increased three- to fivefold whenever a viscus was opened during a planned elective operation (Table 20-4).

MONETARY COST OF HOSPITAL INFECTIONS

One of the most comprehensive studies of the cost of hospital infections was made by Swartz at the University of Virginia.[4] During a period of 1 year (1968–69), 1,115 surgical patients were carefully observed by a nurse epidemiologist who found 48 patients with wound infection (4.3 percent), of whom four died. Swartz then calculated costs in three categories—direct, indirect, and intangible. No price tag could be placed on the cost of pain, discomfort, isolation, and various incalculable expenses the patient otherwise would not have had—the intangible costs. Indirect costs were calculated on the basis of salary lost because of prolonged illness or death. Direct costs included hospital room, physicians' charges, and infection control costs.

For the 48 infected patients the direct cost was $114,576. This was computed on the basis of a cost of $100 per day for the 23.87 additional (average) hospital days for each patient. The noninfected population had a mean length of stay of 11.61 days; patients with wound infections had a mean stay of 35.48 days.

The estimated sum of all the direct and indirect costs ranged from $6,700 to $9,500 per patient. The estimated

TABLE 20-1. HOSPITAL INFECTIONS IN THE UNITED STATES: 1967

Estimated Incidence	
Hospital admissions	31,600,000
Surgical procedures performed in the operating room	18,800,000
Estimated number of postoperative wound infections for all types of operations (7.4 percent of operations)	1,391,200
Estimated number of hospital-acquired infections	2,101,037

Altemeier WA, Burke JF, Pruitt BA Jr, Sandusky WR (eds): Incidence and cost of infection. In *Manual on Control of Infection in Surgical Patients.* Philadelphia, Lippincott, 1976, p 6.

overall cost for wound infections in the United States in 1967 was approximately $9.8 billion (estimated 1,400,000 wound infections). Since hospital costs have escalated approximately three times since 1967, the enormous societal expense can be seen. In the Foothills Hospital study, a wound infection delayed a patient's discharge by 10.1 days which, at the $200-a-day rate, amounts to $2,000 for hospitalization alone.

FOOTHILLS HOSPITAL WOUND STUDY

In 1967, we began a 10-year prospective study of all surgical wounds at Foothills Hospital with four aims in mind: (1) to obtain an accurate monthly infection figure to be used as the guide to the efficient functioning of the operating rooms, surgical wards, and the surgeons; (2) to obtain a 10-year bank of wound statistics with which future variables could be compared; (3) to determine the factors that influence our infection rate; and (4) to reduce our infection rate.

Our 10-year goal was achieved in 1977 with the accumulation and study of 62,939 wounds. We now compare our yearly wound statistics with our 10-year yardstick to show trends and to single out changes in etiologic factors.

A full-time surgical surveillance nurse, R. Foord, RN, personally observed all wounds throughout each patient's hospital stay. Telephone follow-up continued for a total of 28 days. We excluded oral, rectal, and vaginal operations, burns, and circumcisions from our study. Details of the operation and the patient's progress were recorded, and the information was stored in a computer.

DEFINITIONS

We used the definitions from the 1964 National Research Council Study on wound infection and the influence of ultraviolet light [3] so that our results could be compared.[5]

WOUND CATEGORIES

Wounds are classified as: (1) clean, (2) clean-contaminated, (3) contaminated, or (4) dirty, based on a clinical estimate of contamination made by the circulating nurse in the operating room. Our criteria were slightly modified from those of the National Research Council (Table 20-2).

Clean wounds included those in which the gastrointestinal or respiratory tract was not entered, no apparent inflammation was encountered, and no break in aseptic technique occurred. Cholecystectomy, incidental appendectomy, and hysterectomy were included in this category if no acute inflammation was present. We combined the National Research Council categories of refined clean and other clean.

TABLE 20-2. NATIONAL RESEARCH COUNCIL CLASSIFICATION OF OPERATIVE WOUNDS IN RELATION TO CONTAMINATION AND INCREASING RISK OF INFECTION

CLEAN
- Nontraumatic
- No inflammation encountered
- No break in technique
- Respiratory, alimentary, genitourinary tracts not entered

CLEAN-CONTAMINATED
- Gastrointestinal or respiratory tracts entered without significant spillage
- Appendectomy
- Oropharynx entered
- Vagina entered
- Genitourinary tract entered in absence of infected urine
- Biliary tract entered in absence of infected bile
- Minor break in technique

CONTAMINATED
- Major break in technique
- Gross spillage from gastrointestinal tract
- Traumatic wound, fresh
- Entrance of genitourinary or biliary tracts in presence of infected urine or bile

DIRTY AND INFECTED
- Acute bacterial inflammation encountered, without pus
- Transection of "clean" tissue for the purpose of surgical access to a collection of pus
- Traumatic wound with retained devitalized tissue, foreign bodies, fecal contamination and/or delayed treatment, or from dirty source

Adapted from Altemeier WA, Burke JF, Pruitt BA Jr, Sandusky WR (eds): Definitions and classifications of surgical infections. In *Manual on Control of Infection in Surgical Patients.* Philadelphia, Lippincott, 1976, p 20.

TABLE 20-3. INCIDENCE OF INFECTION FOR OPERATIVE WOUNDS DURING A TWO AND ONE-HALF YEAR COLLABORATIVE STUDY IN FIVE UNIVERSITY HOSPITALS

Type of Operative Wound	Incidence of Infection		
	No.	*No.*	*Percent*
Clean	11,690	594	5.1
Clean-contaminated	2,589	280	10.8
Contaminated and dirty	1,262	277	21.9
Not reported	72	6	8.3

Adapted from Altemeier WA, Burke JF, Pruitt BA Jr, Sandusky WR (eds): Incidence and cost of infection. In *Manual on Control of Infection in Surgical Patients.* Philadelphia, Lippincott, 1976, p 6.

TABLE 20-4. INCIDENCE OF INFECTION FOLLOWING SELECTED, COMMONLY PERFORMED OPERATIVE PROCEDURES

Operative Procedure	Number of Procedures	Incidence of Infection (percent)
Herniorrhaphy*	1,312	1.9
Thyroidectomy	406	2.2
Hysterectomy	628	6.1
Cholecystectomy	756	6.9
Partial colectomy	220	10.0
Subtotal gastrectomy	288	10.1
Appendectomy	551	11.4
Nephrectomy	127	17.3
Radical mastectomy	227	18.9

*Including inguinal, femoral, and epigastric; excluding incisional and ventral.

Adapted from Altemeier WA, Burke JF, Pruitt BA Jr, Sandusky WR (eds): Incidence and cost of infection. In *Manual on Control of Infection in Surgical Patients.* Philadelphia, Lippincott, 1976, p 10.

Clean-contaminated included clean operations that entered the gastrointestinal tract or respiratory tract but in which there was no significant spillage.

Contaminated included operations in which acute inflammation (without pus formation) was encountered, or in which gross spillage from a hollow viscus occurred. Fresh, traumatic wounds and operations in which a major break in aseptic technique occurred were included in this category.

Dirty included operations in which pus was encountered or in which a perforated viscus was found. Old, traumatic wounds were also included in this group.

DEFINITION OF WOUND INFECTIONS

Wound infections are difficult to define.[6] Discharges may be reported sterile when cultured, even from wounds definitely infected. Conversely, bacteria can be recovered from wounds that are healing without infection. Unfortunately, classification based solely on clinical judgment is subjective and biased. Most investigators, including ourselves, have agreed on uniform clinical criteria.[7] Surgical wounds are considered *uninfected* if they heal per primum without discharge. They are *definitely infected* if pus is discharged, even if organisms are not cultured from the purulent material. Wounds that are inflamed without discharge and wounds that drain culture-positive serous fluid are considered *possibly infected.* Stitch abscesses are excluded from definite or possible if (1) inflammation and discharge are minimal and confined to points of suture penetration or (2) the incision heals per primum without drainage.

RESULTS OF THE FOOTHILLS HOSPITAL STUDY

The overall infection rate of 62,939 wounds in our study was 4.7 percent (Table 20-5). (Compare with Table 20-

TABLE 20-5. TEN-YEAR PROSPECTIVE STUDY: ANALYSIS OF INFECTION RATES RELATED TO WOUND TYPES AT THE FOOTHILLS HOSPITAL (1967–77)

	Number	Infected	Percent
Clean	47,054	732	1.5
Clean-contaminated	9,370	720	7.7
Contaminated	442	676	15.2
Dirty	2,093	832	40.0
Overall	62,939	2,960	4.7

3.) Ten percent of infected wounds became evident only after the patient had left the hospital—an aspect of infection that is commonly ignored in surveys.

There is such a wide variation of overall infection rate in different hospitals [8] that overall infection rate has limited epidemiologic value. If mostly clean cases are done (eg, hernias), the overall infection rate of the institution will be much lower than if many bowel operations are performed (Tables 20-3, 20-4, and 20-5). The clean wound infection rate is a much more definitive figure and is therefore one of the most valuable reflections of the quality of surgical care in any hospital. Endogenous bacterial contamination is at a minimum in these wounds, and the influence of other procedures related to exogenous contamination, eg, hand scrub, skin preparation, and other factors such as age and obesity, can be accurately assessed. Further, it allows for comparison between the various surgical departments and between surgeons (Figs. 20-1, 20-2). Whereas the overall infection rates vary between departments, the differences in the clean wound infection rates are not large (Fig. 20-1). Using the same wound criteria, Altemeier's General Surgical Service at Cincinnati General Hospital achieved a clean wound infection rate of 1.2 percent during a 14-month period,[9] and a number of Foothills' surgeons have, over a 10-year period, achieved a clean wound infection rate of less than 1 percent. A clean wound infection rate of less than 1 percent is exem-

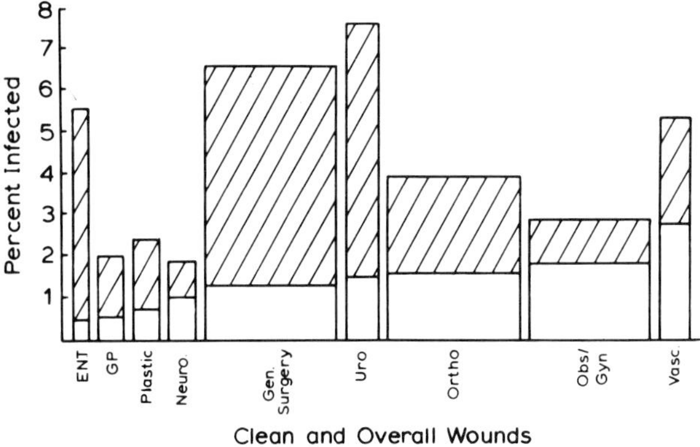

Fig. 20-1. **Department infection rates—1967–77 (white area, clean wound infection rates; shaded area, overall rate). (Figures 20-1 to 20-7 from Cruse PJE, Foord R: Epidemiology of wound infection. Surg. Clin N Am, 60:27, 1980.)**

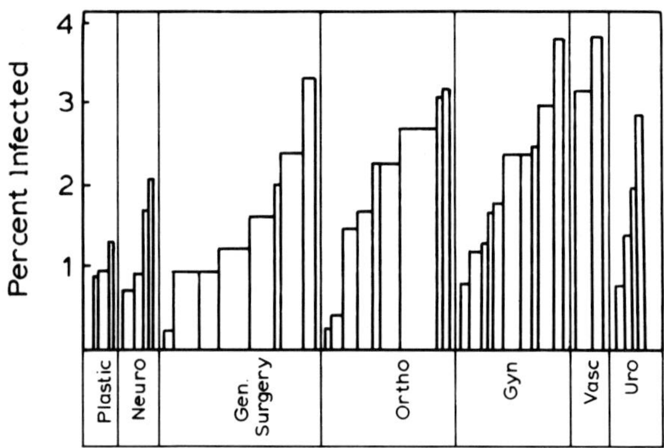

Fig. 20-2. **Clean wound infection rates of various surgeons within various departments.**

plary, 1 percent to 2 percent is acceptable, and more than 2 percent is a cause for concern.

Since surgeons in each discipline do the same operations and use the same operating rooms and wards, the variation in clean wound infection rate must be ascribed to differences in operating technique. Those surgeons with a low clean wound infection rate pride themselves on this achievement, take pains to reduce contamination, and adhere to the meticulous Halstedian principles of wound care. The clean wound infection rate is the standard discussed in this hospital at the monthly department of surgery business meetings. The generation of a friendly competitive atmosphere among staff surgeons encourages perfection of technique. In fact, surveillance itself reduced the infection rate during the second 6-month period of study.

EXOGENOUS FACTORS INFLUENCING THE INFECTION RATE

To have an infection requires a contaminated wound, and an array of vectors have come under scrutiny.

THE SURGEON'S HANDS

Semmelweis, in 1847, identified the hands of doctors and students as the carriers of infection in puerperal sepsis. He reduced the mortality of puerperal sepsis by insisting on hand washing in hypochlorite solution. It is ironic that Semmelweis died of a wound infection the day after Lister applied carbolic acid to the compound fracture of little James Greenlees at the Glasgow Royal Infirmary (August 13, 1865).

Lister cleansed his hands before an operation by soaking them in a 1 in 20 carbolic lotion and suffered severe cracks in his skin and nails. He said that he could always recognize a fellow-Listerian on first shaking because the skin was hard and cracked and the nails were brittle.[10] Halsted developed the surgical glove because his operating room nurse developed sensitivity to the bichloride of mercury he used.

The gloves must cover the fingers and hands and extend over the wristlets of the gown. At the proximal end, a thickened band of rubber discourages the wrist of the glove from rolling back. A flat wide band is more efficient than a small round one. The majority of gloves currently in use are disposable, but reusable gloves are still available. All gloves are packaged with the cuff turned back so that they can be handled by the exposed part of the inside of the glove.

The purpose of scrubbing and disinfecting the hands prior to operation is to reduce the bacterial population to the vanishing point with reasonable assurance that it will remain minuscule during the operation. If a hole should develop in the glove, bacterial contamination of the wound should, therefore, be minimal.

In 1939, Devenish and Miles [11] observed that some 30 percent of gloves develop perforations during the course of an operation, and various studies since then have confirmed the finding.[12] Using a sophisticated electronic circuit, we found leaks in 11.6 percent of gloves after operation, but none of the wounds became infected.

Skin Antiseptics

Decontamination of the surgeon's hands appears to be more important than gloves.[13] Price showed that scrubbing with soap and water for 6 minutes reduced the skin flora by only one-half. The transient, more pathogenic flora were more readily eliminated. However, bacteria always remain, and the regeneration time of scrubbed skin covered with rubber gloves is quite short.

Several skin disinfectants are effective in reducing resident organisms on hands,[14,16] but none can satisfactorily degerm the nails.[13a] Hexachlorophene has the disadvantage of acting slowly but, because a residue stays on the skin, the skin flora are further reduced after an hour. To achieve its greatest efficacy, hexachlorophene should be used repeatedly and consistently. Butcher et al,[15] however, showed that hexachlorophene is absorbed with hand scrubs and can be detected in the blood. Because of its potential for cumulative toxicity, hexachlorophene has been replaced in some hospitals.

Povidone-iodine surgical scrub has a greater immediate effect than a single application of hexachlorophene. However, unlike hexachlorophene, this preparation has no prolonged further action inside the glove,[16] where the moisture fosters bacterial proliferation.

Rinsing the hands in aqueous or alcoholic solution of chlorhexidine is also very efficacious in reducing the bacterial counts. The counts are further decreased with repeated use of this rinse. Lowbury, Lilly, and Bull [16] found that the addition of alcoholic chlorhexidine rinse after repeated use of hexachlorophene reduced the bacterial count in hand washings to zero in four out of nine subjects.

In our study, we compared the incidence of wound sepsis in clean wounds when the surgeon used an iodophor preparation (Betadine) or hexachlorophene (PhisoHex). The clean wound infection rate was unaffected. Many surgeons now use a chlorhexidine scrub (Hibitane) because it combines the benefits of iodophor and hexachlorophene. It is effective against both gram-negative and gram-positive organisms, and a residue film remains on the skin.

Scrub Time

Dineen[17] studied bacterial counts on surgeons' hands at the end of 2-hour operations. He found no difference between 5- and 10-minute surgical scrubs provided povidone-iodine or hexachlorophene was used. Indeed, his in vitro tests indicate that 1 minute of scrub time should be adequate. Galle et al[18] pointed out that a 10-minute scrub consumes 50 gallons of water. The savings in reducing the conventional 10-minute scrub are obvious. Most surgeons in our institution now brush-scrub with one of the detergent antiseptics for only 3 to 5 minutes for the first operation and for 2 to 3 minutes with a sponge between cases. This practice has not been associated with an increase in clean wound infection rates.

PREPARATION OF THE PATIENT'S SKIN

Preoperative Shower

A preoperative shower with hexachlorophene appears to be of value in reducing wound infection.[7] The infection rate was 2.3 percent if the patient did not shower and 2.1 percent if a shower with ordinary bath soap was done before operation. If an antiseptic detergent containing hexachlorophene was used, the infection rate fell to 1.3 percent.

Shaving the Operation Site

In patients who were shaved more than 2 hours before operation, the clean infection rate was 2.3 percent; in patients who had no shave but had only their body hair clipped, the infection rate fell to 1.7 percent; and in patients who had no shave or clipping, the infection rate was 0.9 percent. This rather surprising finding agrees with the findings of Seropian and Reynolds,[19] who reported on 406 patients and found that in those shaved, the infection rate was 5.6 percent, and in those not shaved, 0.6 percent. Further, in patients on whom a depilatory cream was used instead of shaving, the infection rate was also 0.6 percent. Altemeier and Seropian and Reynolds have stressed the importance of shaving immediately before operation to prevent bacterial growth in razor nicks. Despite this well-documented fact, shaving is still performed in most hospitals the night before operation.

Preparation of Operative Area on the Patient's Skin

The preparation of the operative area should be done by someone who is knowledgeable and specially trained for this purpose. Sterile gloves should be worn during this procedure and sterile supplies used. Initial cleansing by soap or a nonirritating detergent solution or a fat solvent should be carried out. A degerming agent should then be applied. The antiseptics available for skin degerming are discussed in Chapter 18.

Lowbury, Lilly, and Bull[16] found 1 percent iodine in 70 percent alcohol and 0.5 percent chlorhexidine in 70 percent alcohol to be the most effective skin antiseptics, significantly better than povidone-iodine, in reducing the resident skin flora. Because of this work, the committee on aseptic methods in the operating suite advocates the use of either 1 percent iodine in 70 percent alcohol or 0.5 percent chlorhexidine in 70 percent alcohol applied with friction for 2 minutes as a preoperative skin preparation.

From 1967 to 1971, green soap and alcohol were used in the operating rooms for the skin preparation. During those years, the clean infection rate was 2 percent (251 out of 12,849). In 1972, the routine was changed so that a few hours before operation, each patient was washed with a povidone-iodine scrub sponge on the ward, and in the operating room, the skin was painted with tincture of chlorhexidine (Hibitane). The clean infection rate is now 1.6 percent. Numerous other protocols for skin degerming have been described.[20]

Draping

Appropriate draping is important as a means of demarcating, maintaining, and protecting a limited area prepared for the operation by cleansing and degerming techniques. Uniform drape design and application are timesaving, neat, reduce contamination, decrease costs, and facilitate the planning of ordering supplies. Each hospital should develop standard draping techniques. The types of drapes currently in use include: (1) the conventional double thickness linen towels and sheets (288-thread count) modified for use in various types of operations, (2) disposable prefabricated drapes, and (3) plastic adhesive skin drapes. Disposable plastic adhesive skin drapes are thought to be particularly useful in excluding contamination from sinuses, fistulas, colostomies, and other contaminated or infected drainage tracts.

In routine practice, however, the use of adhesive plastic skin drapes was not associated with a reduction in wound infection. With the usual cloth drapes, the infection rate was 1.5 percent (405 out of 26,303); with plastic drapes, 2.3 percent (214 out of 9,252). Paskin and Lerner[21] also found the incidence of wound infection was doubled with the use of adherent plastic drapes. As a consequence, adhesive plastic drapes are not used routinely in the Foothills Hospital—a considerable economy.

Plastic adhesive drapes have several disadvantages: (1) skin occlusion permits bacterial proliferation under the drape, (2) the antiseptic solution applied to the skin must be removed to get the drapes to stick, and (3) the edges loosen with time so that even greater numbers of bacteria are released into the wound. Plastic adhesive drapes with povidone-iodine incorporated into the adhesive may reduce bacterial proliferation under the drape.

If fluid-impermeable drapes are not used, it is important to avoid wetting linen drapes because this permits bacteria to penetrate. Certain commercial disposable drapes also permit wet strike-through and should be avoided (Chapter 21).

ENVIRONMENTAL FACTORS IN THE EPIDEMIOLOGY OF CLEAN WOUND INFECTION

Preoperative Hospitalization

The longer the patient stays in the hospital before an operation, the more likely he is to develop a wound infection (Fig. 20-3). With a 1-day preoperative stay, the infection

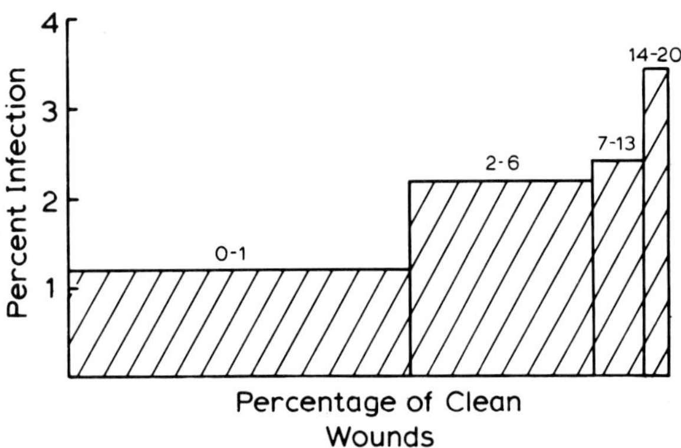

Fig. 20-3. **Effect of preoperative hospital stay on clean wound infection rate.**

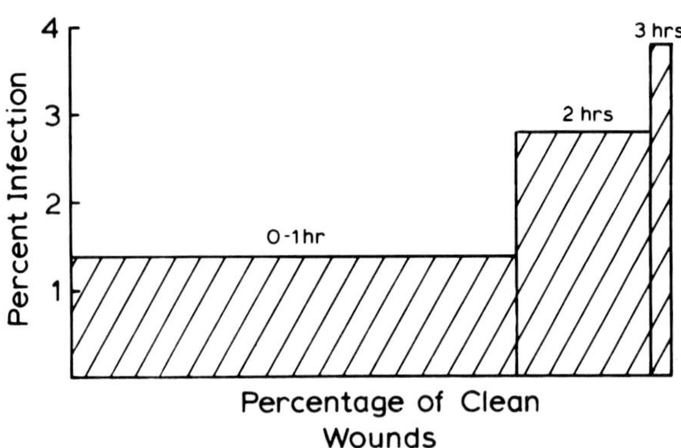

Fig. 20-4. **Effect of duration of operation on clean wound infection rate.**

rate is 1.2 percent; with a 1-week preoperative stay, 2.1 percent; and if he stays in for more than 2 weeks, 3.4 percent.[7]

Theaters and Anesthetists

There is no difference in the clean wound infection rate in various operating theaters; further, there is no difference in the clean infection rate involving individual anesthetists. Obviously, an occasional medical attendant will be the reservoir for a wound infection epidemic, but it is rare. Personnel with known staphylococcal infections should be excluded. In general, the fewer people, less talk, shorter hair, and less movement, the greater will be the margin of safety (Chapter 21).

Duration and Time of Operation

There is a direct relation between length of operating time and infection rate. The clean rate roughly doubles with every hour (Fig. 20-4). Other studies have also shown a rise in the infection rate associated with prolongation of operating time.[3,8] There are four possible explanations: (1) dosage of bacterial contamination increases with time, (2) wound cells are damaged by drying and retractors, (3) increased amounts of suture and electrocoagulation may reduce the local resistance of the wound, and (4) longer procedures are more likely to be associated with blood loss and shock, thereby reducing the general resistance of the patient.[22]

Surgical Wards

The clean wound infection rate did not differ in the four general surgical wards. During the first 5 years of this study, each of the eight general surgeons admitted patients to each of the four wards. The same dressing and isolation techniques were used. However, the clean wound infection rate of the individual surgeons differed significantly (Fig. 20-2). We concluded that the surgeon was responsible for his clean wound infection rate, that the groundwork for succeeding wound infection was laid in the operating room, and that the ward care did not play a significant role in the development of wound infection. As a consequence, hospital regulations were relaxed during the second 5 years. Nurses do not wear gloves or masks during the performance of wound dressings, clean wounds are exposed after 48 hours, and the septic wound isolation technique was simplified. These steps saved much effort and expense and were not associated with any increase in the clean wound infection rate.

RESISTANCE OF THE PATIENT TO WOUND INFECTION

It is paradoxical that many heavily contaminated wounds heal without complication, while some wounds become infected. This implies that sepsis will occur only when host defense mechanisms are insufficient to keep bacterial proliferation under control. These host factors can be classified into systemic and local factors.

SYSTEMIC FACTORS

Age

All studies show that there is an increase in wound infection rate with advancing years.[3,8,23] Figure 20-5 indicates the increase in wound infection rate in clean wounds with advancing age.

Sex

The clean infection rate is the same in male and female.

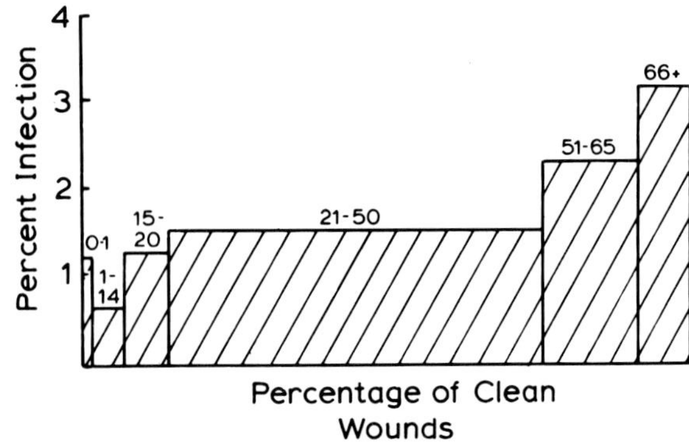

Fig. 20-5. **Effect of age on clean wound infection rate.**

Malnutrition

Malnutrition was associated with a clean wound infection rate of 16 percent. A higher clean wound infection rate was also encountered in patients with diabetes (7.8 percent) and in patients with extreme obesity (6.9 percent). A similar effect of malnutrition was noted by the National Research Council.[3]

THE LOCAL RESISTANCE OF THE WOUND TO INFECTION

Surgical Technique

The local resistance of the wound is much more important than the general resistance of the patient, and the importance of proper technique in the prevention of wound infection is discussed in Chapter 22. Kocher and Von Bergman first showed that meticulous hemostasis and gentle handling of tissue were associated with a lower wound sepsis rate. Halsted adopted these views and stressed meticulous attention to operative detail with his principles of complete hemostasis, adequate blood supply, removal of devitalized tissue, obliteration of dead space, use of fine, nonabsorbable suture material, and wound closure without tension.

The experimental demonstration of these principles waited almost 50 years. Elek and Conen [8a] demonstrated that only 100 *S. aureus* organisms were required to produce a pustule in volunteers if the bacteria were introduced into the skin on a silk suture. If the silk was omitted, several million were required. They concluded that the bacteria could multiply in the interstices of the suture while being protected from the tissue defenses in the wound, but Edlich and his colleagues have demonstrated similar effects with monofilament suture (Chapter 22). Howe and Marston [24] showed the infective dose could be even further reduced if tissue was included within the ligated suture.

Local blood supply seems essential for local host defenses. In experimental animals, the induction of shock to the point of impaired skin perfusion reduced the minimal dose of bacteria necessary to initiate infection 10,000-fold.[22] Distant trauma increased the susceptibility of the wound to infection, probably by decreasing the blood flow to the wound.[25] Sonneland [26] demonstrated that patients who developed infections after gastric and colonic operations had lost more blood and received more transfusions than nonseptic patients.

Although fastidious surgical technique is easily recognized, it is difficult to measure. In the Foothills Hospital series, the surgeons with a clean wound infection rate below 1 percent were also those with punctilious technique. Hematoma in the operative area is the biggest problem in reducing local resistance, but how hematoma formation is avoided is also important to the pathogenesis of clean wound infection. In preventing hematoma formation, consider the influence of the electrosurgical unit and drains. For example, in 1967, electrosurgical units were scarce, and surgeons used them to cut tissue or coagulate tissue grasped in hemostats. At this time, we noted a doubling in the clean infection rate whenever a Bovie unit was used. With more experience, and especially with the use of fine, smooth-tipped tissue forceps (McIndoe) to grasp the bleeding vessels, the amount of coagulated tissue was decreased. There is now no difference in the clean infection rate whether or not the electrosurgical unit is used for hemostasis.

Drains were originally designed to evacuate hematomas, but a wound drained with a Penrose drain is associated with a higher infection rate.[3,27] Nora showed that bacteria can migrate from the exterior to the depths of a wound along a nonsuction drainage tube.[28] The closed-suction drain has been a great advance; the tip of the catheter remains sterile, and the stagnant wound fluid, deficient in complement, is removed, allowing fresh wound fluid with opsonins to enter the wound.[29] Indeed, there is a decrease in the infection rate when the subcutaneous layer of wounds are drained with closed-suction drains (Tables 20-6 and 20-7).

The closed-suction drain has the further advantage of requiring less nursing time. It takes a student nurse 5 minutes to empty and measure a closed-suction drain as opposed to 35 minutes for dressing the stab wound with a Penrose drain. The increased risk of bringing the Penrose drain through the wound itself is shown in Table 20-7.

OTHER IMPORTANT ASPECTS OF THE PREVENTION OF WOUND INFECTION

DISSEMINATION OF WOUND INFECTION INFORMATION

If the staff is acquainted with the wound infection statistics, the clean wound infection rate can be kept lower. Four steps are useful: (1) A graph indicating the clean wound infection rate and the overall infection rate is posted in the operating room and in all the surgical and gynecologic wards (Fig. 20-6). (2) A detailed analysis of the wounds that became infected during the previous month is published and displayed on notice boards in the hospital and

TABLE 20-6. EFFECT OF DRAINAGE TECHNIQUE ON THE INCIDENCE OF WOUND INFECTION AFTER CHOLECYSTECTOMY

	Percent
Closed suction	1.2
Penrose stab	1.8
None	2.9
Penrose through wound	7.4

TABLE 20-7. EFFECT OF CLOSED SUCTION DRAINS ON THE INCIDENCE OF WOUND INFECTION AFTER SPINAL FUSIONS

	No Drain	Closed Suction
Wounds	125	408
Infection	6	4
Percent	4.8	1.0

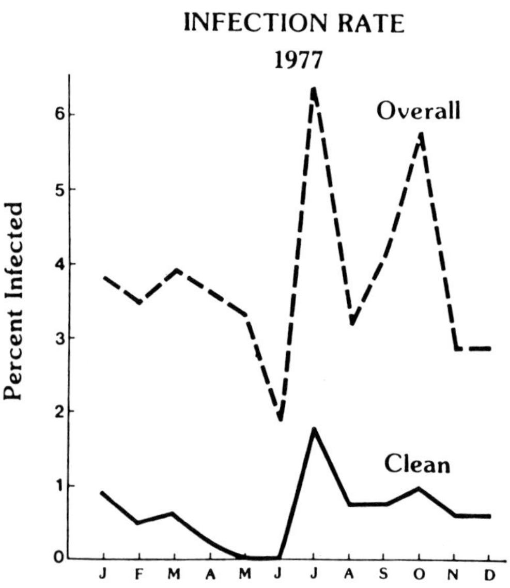

Fig. 20-6. **Clean wound and overall wound infection rate per month in 1977. (This graph is posted in the operating room and in the surgical wards as a reminder that the rate can be reduced.)**

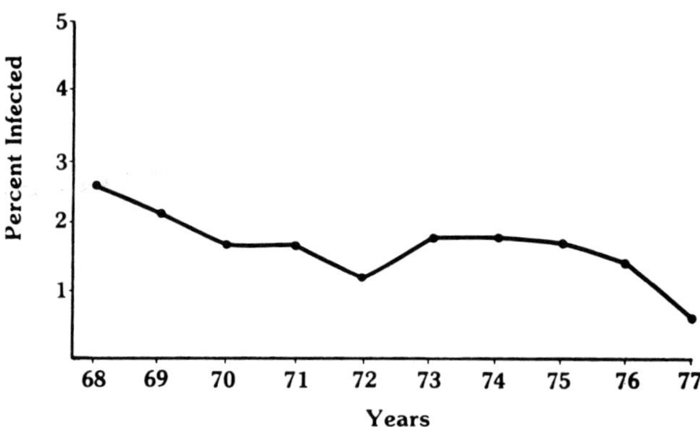

Fig. 20-7. **The clean wound infection rate shows a steady decline with time.**

discussed at the infection control committee meeting. (3) The wound infection rates for the various departments are discussed at the monthly departmental business meeting. (4) Every surgeon receives a yearly computerized report listing the operations he had performed and stating his own clean wound infection rate as well as the average clean wound infection rates of his peers. These steps produced a steady reduction in the clean wound infection rate (Fig. 20-7).

RESTORING HOST DEFENSES

Before Admission to Hospital

Obesity

Every attempt must be made to get the patient to ideal weight before an elective operation. Indeed, the operation may well be the motivation the patient requires to reduce weight. Obesity is associated with a high risk of wound infection and pulmonary complications. Weight reduction is particularly desirable before a repair of incisional hernia or hiatus hernia.

Nutrition

Malnutrition is also associated with an increased risk of wound infection,[3,7] and should be corrected, if necessary by total parenteral nutrition to restore the general resistance to infection.

Remote Infections

The risk of wound infections is increased by the concurrent presence of remote infections. Asymptomatic infections are particularly hazardous because they are so easily overlooked and can triple the clean wound infection rate.[30] A search should be made for infection, especially heralded by an elevated white count or an abnormality on urinalysis. Acute respiratory infections, chronic ear infections, furuncles, draining sinuses, etc., are strong indications to postpone elective operations.[31]

Other Diseases

Diabetes, uremia, and cirrhosis require particular efforts to restore the patient's physiology as far as possible for the operation. Patients with chronic pulmonary disease should ideally be seen by a respirologist to assess respiratory status and institute a preoperative regime of physiotherapy with emphasis on inspiratory maneuvers and encouragement of maximal inflation. The patient should stop smoking for at least 4 weeks before the operation.

DECREASING ENDOGENOUS BACTERIAL CONTAMINATION OF THE WOUND

Mechanical Bowel Preparation

The usual mechanical bowel preparation consists of laxatives, a low-residue diet, and repeated enemas for 3 days. Whole-gut lavage (WHOGULA) promises to provide better mechanical cleansing with considerably less distress in nonobstructed patients.[32-33] The technique is simple and can be carried out on any ward. A nasogastric tube is passed and isotonic saline containing KCl, 4 mEq per liter, is infused at the rate of 3 liters per hour. Defecation commences after approximately half an hour. The infusion is continued until the effluent is clear, which usually takes about 3 hours. Patients who have had the classic bowel preparation at one time and WHOGULA at another much prefer the latter method.

Oral Antibiotics to Reduce Bowel Organisms

The feasibility of gut "sterilization" has been argued since the introduction of the sulphonamides in the 1930s. At present, the neomycin and erythromycin regime described by Nichols et al [34] is the most popular. After mechanical bowel preparation, Nichols administers three doses of neomycin 1 gm and erythromycin base 1 gm by mouth at 1 P.M., 2 P.M., and 11 P.M. for operations scheduled at 8 A.M the next day. Wound infections after elective colonic surgery are substantially reduced by this preoperative regimen.[34]

Prophylactic Antibiotics

Antibiotics enhance the ability of a wound to withstand contamination but, as Miles et al[35] showed in 1957, for antibiotics to be effective, they must be present in the wound fluid within 3 hours of bacterial contamination. Alexander et al[36] demonstrated that after intravenous injection, ampicillin achieved peak wound levels within 1 hour, cephalosporin between 1 and 2 hours, and clindamycin after 2 hours. The effectiveness of prophylactic antibiotics in preventing wound infection was shown by Polk and Lopez-Meyer[37] and more recently, by Stone et al[38] in elegant double-blind studies (Chapter 23). Similarly, Ledger has shown the advantages in gynecologic surgery.[39] It seems reasonable to administer prophylactic antibiotics before any operation in which contamination is expected,[6] or in which infection would be catastrophic (eg, with vascular or orthopedic prosthetic implants). As with all drugs, the dangers of antibiotic administration must be weighed against the potential advantages.

DELAYED PRIMARY CLOSURE

John Hunter's method of delayed primary closure is still the best to treat heavily contaminated wounds. Once healthy granulation tissue is present, usually after 4 to 6 days, wound edges can be pulled together with adhesive strips. Some authorities recommend delayed primary closure for all large bowel surgery, but we have not found this necessary at the Foothills Hospital. A wound treated with delayed primary closure is more uncomfortable than one closed primarily.

POSTOPERATIVE CARE

Ward care does not play a significant role in the development of wound infection. All dressings can be safely removed from closed wounds after 48 hours. This benefits the patient psychologically, saves nursing time, and allows for easy wound surveillance.

CLINICAL CHARACTERISTICS OF WOUND INFECTION

The preceding section describes an epidemiologic approach to the prevention of wound infection which has been successful. Nevertheless, wounds still become infected after planned and emergency operations. A broad range of clinical characteristics are seen—abscess, cellulitis, and any of the gangrenous infections described in Chapter 25 (Table 25-20). Only brief consideration of the more general aspects of infected incised wounds are presented here. We must stress the fact that infections in the skin and subcutaneous tissues of incised wounds may reflect deeper or more extensive infection. Failure to respond to drainage and debridement should prompt a search for other sources of infection.

Etiology

Table 20-8 lists the postoperative wound pathogens reported by the National Nosocomial Infections Study carried out between January 1970 and August 1973. Although many investigators have reported a decrease in *S. aureus* wound infections, these are still among the two most common infecting organisms isolated. The high incidence of *E. coli*, *P. aeruginosa*, and *P. mirabilis* and the growing incidence of *B. fragilis* further support the impression that endogenous infection has replaced skin contamination as the principal source of infecting organisms. Altemeier has pointed out that the incidence of anaerobic pathogens such as *C. perfringens*, *B. fragilis*, and *Peptostreptococcus* probably underestimates their actual frequency because of the problems of anaerobic cultivation and identification that prevail in many hospitals.[40]

It must be stressed that the pathogenic organism will vary considerably with the site of surgery and the operation performed. Fungal[40a] and viral wound infections have been reported but are relatively uncommon as primary pathogens. They are discussed in detail in Chapter 25.

Clinical Manifestations

Clinical manifestations of infection depend in large part on the infecting organism and the tissue infected. A comprehensive survey of the many types of soft tissue, and therefore wound infections, and their many clinical varieties is discussed in Chapter 25. The most common wound infections should be mentioned here.

Staphylococcal Wound Infections

The incubation period is usually 4 to 6 days, and the infections tend to be localized; an initial area of erythema, edema, and pain is followed by abscess formation. The pus is usually thick, creamy, and odorless, sometimes with a yellowish tinge. Spread to lymph nodes is unusual, but septicemia is common. Fever and leukocytosis are usually present.

Such infections are normally caused by strains of *S. aureus* colonizing the patient.[41] Occasional epidemics have derived, of course, from members of the operating room staff who have active clinical staphylococcal disease or who are asymptomatic disseminating carriers.

The treatment of staphylococcal wound infections depends on early recognition and the opening of the infected portion or of the entire length of the infected wound. The general principles of infection treatment—immobilization, heat, and elevation—should be instituted but may have no beneficial result. Infected sutured wounds should first be reopened by removing a few skin sutures, and the hemostat should be inserted into the point of maximum pain, swelling, or fluctuation. The opening can then be enlarged to the size of the cavity. The cavity is gently irrigated with saline solution and loosely packed open with fine mesh gauge. If pus and necrotic material are present, their removal should be complete.

In general, antibiotics are not considered necessary for well-localized staphylococcal wound infections. If manipulation of the wound is contemplated in an attempt to debride it and evacuate the pus, or if spreading cellulitis, lymphangitis, lymphadenitis, or septicemia are present, antibiotics should be given prior to wound manipulation. A penicillinase-resistant penicillin or cephalosporin should be utilized. Erythromycin, lincomycin, clindamycin, and vancomycin are also effective. It is important to remove all devitalized tissue, pus, and foreign bodies that limit the efficaciousness of antibiotic therapy.

***S. epidermidis* Wound Infections.** *S. epidermidis* has long been considered to be nonpathogenic. Wound infections caused by this normal component of patient skin flora are being reported with increasing frequency. Such infections are most commonly mild, without extensive invasion or necrosis and may appear many days after the patient has left the hospital. Their appearance in wounds that contain prosthetic devices are the principal cause for concern.[41a]

Gram-Negative Bacillary Wound Infections

Wound infections caused by aerobic gram-negative bacilli are increasing in relative frequency in recent years, primarily because of the increased incidence of operative procedures in elderly, debilitated patients with chronic diseases. Incisional wound infections caused by *E. coli, Enterobacter, Klebsiella, Proteus,* or *Pseudomonas* are commonly accompanied by anaerobic streptococci and *B. fragilis,* since these infections result from contamination with enteric contents. The incubation period appears longer than staphylococcal or streptococcal infections (7 to 14 days), and many such patients have been discharged prior to the discovery of infection. In patients who receive antibiotics, the incubation period is even longer. There is usually less cellulitis, edema, erythema, and pain than in staphylococcal infections. Instead, many such infections present with cryptogenic fever, tachycardia, and other signs of systemic sepsis. Bacteremia may even be discovered before the local inflammation. As noted in Chapter 16, the classic features of "endotoxin shock" are not seen in such patients. Instead, they may manifest hyperglycemia, hypertriglyceridemia, and the hyperdynamic state more often than hypotension and vasoconstriction.

Whatever their clinical manifestations or their need for systemic therapy (Chapter 16), the wound should be opened, the necrotic tissue debrided, pus evacuated, and systemic antibiotic therapy maintained until granulations are healthy. If Gram stain of the smeared purulent material reveal mixed gram-negative and gram-positive organisms, and if the preceding surgical procedure produced wound contamination with enteric flora, a combination of aminoglycoside and clindamycin (with or without ampicillin to eliminate enterococci) is required.[42]

Persistence of septic manifestations for more than a few days after drainage of the subcutaneous wound should suggest that the superficial wound manifestations may only reflect a deeper subfascial or intra-abdominal source for the infection.

Group A Streptococcal Infections

Infections with group A streptococci run a fulminant course. A diffuse cellulitis, lymphangitis, and lymphadenitis with a large blood-filled local blebs around the primary focus is seen. There is little tendency to form abscesses, but local breakdown, gangrene, or necrotizing fascitis can occur in untreated infections. A thin, watery, purulent exudate is characteristic, and septicemia is common. These manifestations of acute streptococcal cellulitis (Chapter 25) usually appear within the first few days of the wounding. Chills, fever, tachycardia, sweats, prostration, and other signs of toxemia are common. Surgical scarlet fever has been reported.

Wound erysipelas, although now rare, usually appears within 1 to 3 days of wounding. It does not differ from spontaneous erysipelas except in location. The advancing border is sharp, red, irregular, and elevated.

Streptococcal wound infections can sometimes be treated with high dose parenteral penicillin alone. Erythromycin, lincomycin, and cephalothin are alternatives. However, if there is any accumulation of pus or necrotic tissue, or if the wound becomes undermined or gangrenous, the wound should be opened and debrided. Skin grafting may even be ultimately required for coverage.

Prevention of Group A Streptococcal Infections. Streptococci may derive from endogenous sources (upper respiratory tract, draining infected sinuses, other infected wounds, or contaminated instruments or dressings). They rarely come from airborne bacteria. Carriers working in the operating room can be asymptomatic. Epidemics have been traced to fecal carriers, pharyngeal carriers, or attendants with infected skin. Oral lincomycin is effective in eliminating the fecal carrier state, and treatment of infected attendants with penicillin usually eradicates the organisms from the pharynx or skin. Attendants who are known to be infected should exclude themselves from the operating room until rid of the bacteria.

Enterococci. Enterococcal infections (ie, those due to *S. faecalis* or other group D streptococci) are far less invasive than group A streptococci and appear in conjunction with mixed enteric gram-negative organisms. Enterococci should be treated with ampicillin and, because enteric gram-negative organisms are almost always present, aminoglycosides should be added.

Microaerophilic and Anaerobic Streptococcal Infections. The microaerophilic streptococcal infections usually occur in combination with *S. aureus* or *Proteus* species and act in synergism. Meleney's progressive cutaneous gangrene is very rare today (Chapter 25). Such wound infections most commonly follow the drainage of an empyema or abdominal abscess. The incubation period is 10 to 14 days after operation. The wound and surrounding skin become tender, red, and edematous, particularly around stay sutures. A massive cellulitis develops over a few days, and the central area gradually assumes a purplish color and ulcerates. This results in the characteristic appearance of the lesion, which consists of the central, enlarging area of ulceration bordered by a purplish-black narrow margin of gangrenous skin and a large area of spreading cellulitis. Pain and tenderness in the violaceous region occurs. These infections were formerly chronic and resistant to treatment. Currently, however, excision of the gangrenous tissue, institution of a penicillinase-resistant penicillin, cephalosporin or other staphylococcal antibiotic, permits ready skin grafting and healing. Zinc peroxide cream or ointment was formerly applied and may be useful in the deeper reaches and less antibiotic-penetrated areas of the wound.

Anaerobic Steptococcal Infections. Peptostreptococci are reported to produce a variety of severe postoperative infections with or without bacteremia, particularly after operative procedures upon the genital, intestinal, or respiratory tracts. It is a frequent bacterial component of many infections seen in incisional wounds and deep abscesses. The pus is characteristically thick and greyish and has a fetid anaerobic odor. Surgical drainage of abscesses is appropriate and antibiotic therapy with penicillin G should suffice.[43]

Surgical Diphtheria

Wound infections due to contamination of the wound by *C. diphtheriae* are extremely rare. The diagnosis will be difficult, since only "diphtheroids are seen on smear," and the true pathogenic nature of these organisms is not suspected. The infection presents as a chronic indolent ulcer covered with a grey membrane. The bacterium itself will not grow except on special media. Consequently, any patient with acute ulceration and cellulitis with infiltration of the skin and subcutaneous tissues around the wound should be suspected of having such an infection.

Mixed or Synergistic Infection

Many wound infections that complicate surgical operations or trauma are caused by mixed bacterial flora with aerobic and anaerobic, gram-negative and gram-positive organisms whose origin most often is a lesion or perforation of the gastrointestinal, respiratory, or genitourinary tracts. There may be synergism in their interaction. All clinical manifestations can be seen: cellulitis, abscess formation, thrombosis, necrosis, gangrene, and crepitus. The varieties of descriptive terms for these infections are listed in Table 25-20.

Gas Gangrene and Clostridial Cellulitis

Clostridial infections occasionally occur in clean wounds but most often follow traumatic wounds that still contain devitalized muscle, impaired blood supply, and are grossly contaminated by dirt, other foreign bodies, or feces. The most common elective operation that precedes a clostridial infection is an amputation of a gangrenous lower extremity. The onset of the infection is usually spectacular and mortality is high (Chapter 25). The most important organism is *C. perfringens*,[44,45] but other clostridia are also found. Not all clostridia are susceptible to penicillin, chloramphenicol, or clindamycin. For this reason, combinations should be used in conjunction with radical debridement (Chapter 25).

Clostridial infections may manifest themselves as a spreading crepitant or noncrepitant cellulitis without the systemic manifestations of the gas gangrene syndrome. Whereas gas gangrene is primarily an infection of skeletal muscles, which spreads rapidly, clostridial cellulitis is a far more benign disease of the superficial fascia and subcutaneous tissues. It should be treated as a form of necrotizing fasciitis. The tissue should be opened widely and debrided free of all necrotic tissue under antibiotic coverage.

The prevention of clostridial infections in traumatic wounds is discussed in Chapter 25. Early adequate debridement of infected wounds with removal of contaminated foreign bodies and devitalized tissue is essential. Hyperbaric oxygen treatment is supportive and of equivocal value. It is important that hypovolemia be corrected by the administration of blood, plasma, and crystalloid solutions.

Rare Causes of Wound Infection

Numerous rare infections can occur under special circumstances (Chapter 25). For example, tuberculosis of the wound can occur after operation on tuberculous lesions without antimicrobial coverage. Actinomycotic infections result from operating on wounds contaminated with *A. israeli* after esophageal gastric, thoracic, or colonic surgery. Mycotic infections of wounds are common, especially

TABLE 20-8. POSTOPERATIVE WOUND PATHOGENS REPORTED BY NATIONAL NOSOCOMIAL INFECTIONS STUDY

	Service							
Pathogen	*Surg.*	*Gyn.*	*Med.*	*Obst.*	*Ped.*	*Newborn*	Total	Percent
Escherichia coli	4,899	850	183	226	53	24	6,235	18.7
Staphylococcus aureus	5,300	347	345	104	90	43	6,229	18.6
Pseudomonas aeruginosa	2,612	105	166	18	46	4	2,951	8.8
Proteus mirabilis	1,461	247	65	72	9	2	1,856	5.6
Bacteroides	986	203	35	55	7	0	1,286	3.8
Proteus species *	794	172	55	43	6	2	1,072	3.2
Hemolytic streptococci †	400	95	20	26	4	3	548	1.6
Group A streptococci	261	29	24	8	8	0	330	1.0
Clostridium perfringens	324	8	14	7	2	0	355	1.0
Other pathogens	9,963	1,342	579	495	104	63	12,546	37.6
Totals	27,000	3,398	1,486	1,054	329	141	33,408	99.9

* Species unknown
† Group unknown
From National Nosocomial Infections Study (NNIS), January 1970–August 1973.

Adapted from Altemeier WA: Surgical infections: Incisional wounds. In Bennett JV, Brachman PS (eds): *Hospital Infections.* Boston, Little, Brown, 1979, p 287.

as secondary invaders or in areas previously infected. *Candida* superinfections are particularly common in open granulating wounds or fistulous tracts. Most represent surface contamination. The finding of mycelial elements, however, in addition to yeast fragments in biopsy specimens, strongly suggests that invasive candidiasis is present. Topical therapy may be useful in preventing invasion. Long-term therapy with amphotericin B is recommended for control of superficial infections, but short courses are highly effective in sterilizing the wound.

BIBLIOGRAPHY

Altemeier WA, Burke JF, Pruitt BA Jr, Sandusky WR (eds): Manual on Control of Infection in Surgical Patients. Philadelphia: Lippincott, 1976.

REFERENCES

1. Von Nussbaum JN: Quoted by Lindes F: The control of wound infection in wound healing. Symposium based upon the Lister Centenary Scientific meeting, Glasgow, 1965. Illingworth C (ed). London: Churchill, p 148, 1966.
2. Altemeier WA, Burke JF, Pruitt BA Jr, Sandusky WR (eds): Incidence and cost of infection. In Manual on Control of Infection in Surgical Patients. Philadelphia, Lippincott, 1976, p 6.
3. National Research Council Division of Medical Sciences, Ad Hoc Committee of the Committee of Trauma: Postoperative wound infections: The influence of ultraviolet irradiation of the operating room and various other factors. Ann Surg 160 (Suppl 2):1, 1964.
4. Atlemeier WA, Burke JF, Pruitt BA Jr, Sandusky WR (eds): Incidence and cost of infection. In Manual on Control of Infection in Surgical Patients. Philadelphia: Lippincott, 1976, p 11.
5. Cruse, PJE: Incidence of wound infection on the surgical services. Surg Clin North Am 55:1269, 1975.
6. Altemeier WA, Burke JF, Pruitt BA Jr, Sandusky WR (eds): Definitions and classifications of surgical infections. In Manual on Control of Infection in Surgical Patients. Philadelphia, Lippincott, 1976, p 20.
7. Cruse PJE, Foord R: A five-year prospective study of 23,649 surgical wounds. Arch Surg 107:206, 1973.
8. Incidence of surgical wound infection in England and Wales. A report of the Public Health Laboratory Service. Lancet 2:659, 1960.
8a. Elek SD, Conen PE: The virulence of Staphylococcus pyogenes for man. A study of the problems of wound infection. Br J Exp Pathol 38:573, 1957.
9. Culbertson WR, Altemeier WA, Gonzalez LL, Hill EO: Studies on the epidemiology of postoperative infection of clean operative wounds. Ann Surg 154(Suppl 2):599, 1961.
10. Cartwright FF: Lister—The man. Lister Centenary Conference April 1967. Br J Surg 54:405, 1967.
11. Devonish EA, Miles AA: Control of *Staphylococcus aureus* in an operating theatre. Lancet 1:1088, 1939.
12. Taylor FW: An experimental evaluation of operative wound irrigation. Surg Gynecol Obstet 113:465, 1961.
13. Price PB: The bacteriology of normal skin; a new quantitative test applied to a study of the bacterial flora and the disinfectant action of mechanical cleansing. J Infect Dis 63:301, 1938.
13a. Gross A, Cutright DE, D'Alessandra SM: Effect of surgical scrub on microbial population under the fingernails. Amer J Surg 138:463, 1979.
14. Lowbury EJL, Lilly HA: Disinfection of the hands of surgeons and nurses. Br Med J 1:1445, 1960.
15. Butcher HR, Ballinger WF, Gravens DL, Dewar NE, Ledlie EF, Barthel WF: Hexachlorophene concentrations in the blood of operating room personnel. Arch Surg 107:70, 1973.
16. Lowbury EJL, Lilly HA, Bull JP: Methods for disinfection of hands and operation sites. Br Med J 2:531, 1964.
17. Dineen P: An evaluation of the duration of the surgical scrub. Surg Gynecol Obstet 129:1181, 1969.
18. Galle PC, Homesley HD, Rhyne AL: Reassessment of the surgical scrub. Surg Gynecol Obstet 147:214, 1978.
19. Seropian R, Reynolds BM: Wound infections after preoperative depilatory versus razor preparation. Am J Surg 121:251, 1971.
20. Altemeier WA, Burke JF, Pruitt BA Jr, Sandusky WR (eds): Preoperative preparation of the patient. In Manual on Control of Infection in Surgical Patients. Philadelphia, Lippincott, 1976, p 68.
21. Paskin DL, Lerner HJ: A prospective study of wound infections. Am Surg 35:627, 1969.
22. Miles AA, Niven JSF: The enhancement of infection during shock produced by bacterial toxins and other agents. Br J Exp Pathol 31:73, 1950.
23. Barnes BA, Behringer GE, Wheelock FC, Wilkins EW: Surgical sepsis: analysis of factors associated with sepsis following appendectomy (1937–1959). Ann Surg 156:703, 1962.
24. Howe CW, Marston AT: A study on sources of postoperative staphylococcal infection. Surg Gynecol Obstet 115:266, 1962.
25. Conolly WB, Hunt TK, Sonne M, Dunphy JE: Influence of distant trauma on local wound infection. Surg Gynecol Obstet 128:713, 1969.
26. Sonneland J: Postoperative infection. II. Etiological factors. Pacific Med Surg 74:165, 1966.
27. Lidwell OM: Sepsis in surgical wounds: Multiple regression analysis applied to records of postoperative hospital sepsis. J Hyg (Lond) 59:259, 1961.
28. In discussion of Cruse PJE, Foord R: A five-year prospective study of 23,649 wounds. Arch Surg 107:206, 1973.
29. Alexander JW, Korelitz J, Alexander NS: Prevention of wound infections—A case for closed suction drainage to remove wound fluids deficient in opsonic proteins. Am J Surg 132:59, 1976.
30. Zwick R, Cruse PJE: Unpublished data.
31. Edwards LD: The epidemiology of 2056 remote site infections and 1966 surgical wound infections occurring in 1865 patients: A four year study of 40,923 operations at Rush-Presbyterian-St. Luke's Hospital, Chicago. Ann Surg 184:758, 1976.
32. Cruse PJE, McPhedran NT: Complications of surgery. In Beahrs O (ed): General Surgery. New York, Houghton Mifflin, 1978, p 14–1.
33. Crapp AR, Powis SJA, Tillotson P, Cooke WT, Alexander-Williams J: Preparation of the bowel by whole-gut irrigation. Lancet 2:1239, 1975.
34. Nichols RL, Condon RE, Gorbach SL, Nyhus LM: Efficacy of preoperative antimicrobial preparations of the bowel. Ann Surg 176:227, 1972.
35. Miles AA, Miles EM, Burke J: The value and duration of defense reactions of the skin to the primary lodgement of bacteria. Br J Exp Path 38:79, 1957.
36. Alexander JW, Sykes NS, Mitchell MM, Fisher MW: Concentration of selected intravenously administered antibiotics in experimental surgical wounds. J Trauma 13:423, 1973.
37. Polk HC Jr, Lopez-Mayor JF: Postoperative wound infection: A prospective study of determinant factors and prevention. Surgery 66:97, 1969.

38. Stone HH, Haney BB, Kolb LD, Geneber CE, Hooper CA: Prophylactic and preventive antibiotic therapy. Ann Surg 189:691, 1979.
39. Ledger WJ: Infections in the Female. Philadelphia, Lea & Febiger, 1977.
40. Altemeier WA, Burke JF, Pruitt BA Jr, Sandusky WR (eds): Sterilization. In Manual on Control of Infection in Surgical Patients. Philadelphia, Lippincott, 1976, p 252.
40a. Codish SD, Sheridan ID, Monaco AP: Hycotic wound infections: A new challenge for the surgeon. Arch Surg 114:831, 1979.
41. Smith G: Primary postoperative wound infection due to *Staphylococcus pyogenes*. Curr Probl Surg 16:1, 1979.
42. Altemeier WA, Todd JC, Inge WW: Gram-negative septicemia: a growing threat. Ann Surg 166:530, 1967.
43. Altemeier WA: Surgical infections: incisional wounds. In Bennett JV, Brachman PS (eds): Hospital Infections. Boston, Little, Brown, 1979, p 287.
44. MacClennan JD: Anaerobic infections in tripolitania and tunisia. Lancet 1:203, 1944.
45. Altemeier WA, Fullen WD: Prevention and treatment of gas gangrene. JAMA 217:806, 1971.

CHAPTER 21
Environmental Aspects of the Prevention of Wound Infection

HAROLD LAUFMAN

DESIGN plays an important role in the overall efficiency of an operating suite. It affects utilization patterns, materials handling, traffic and commerce in and around the suite, and to a certain extent the effectiveness of people, machines, and air handling. The relationships among design, efficiency, traffic patterns, and human behavior can affect the incidence of surgical infection. There are two interdependent aspects of an operating room—how the suite is designed and how it is used. Attempts to demonstrate a direct effect of operating room design on the incidence of surgical infection have been frustrating, largely because of the multitude of factors involved. Perhaps for this reason more than any other, architects have had to rely on indirect evidence, deductive reasoning, and related but not necessarily relevant information for proof of the effectiveness of their designs.

In the search for operating room designs that will reduce the likelihood of infection, one is faced with so many factors one hardly knows which to tackle first. Prominent among these are two sets of problems: (1) traffic and movement of equipment in and out of the suite and (2) the clean area of the suite itself.

The operating room should be (1) accessible for delivery of patients and supplies, (2) secluded from main corridor thoroughfares in the hospital, and (3) close or accessible to the emergency department, laboratories, and radiology department. The architectural and engineering design should consider all hazards, including that of contamination. When planning for the expansion or renovation of an inadequate surgical suite, the four systems to consider are the environment, traffic and commerce, communication, and management.[1] Although cost is a constraint to such decisions, an equally important issue is hazard-free patient care.

An appropriate traffic pattern between the surgical suite and the outside world is a unique problem among hospital departments. The goal is to bring people, patients, and materials from a "dirty environment," such as a common hospital corridor or even the street, to the clean environment of the operating room with a minimum of contamination.

VESTIBULE PLAN

One way people and material can get from the public corridors of the hospital to the surgical suite is via a generously proportioned vestibular area, which has an entrance to the suite with a double set of doors separating the suite from the outside. This design serves a number of purposes related to infection control. It permits an area for outside unfiltered air, which contains high bioparticle counts, to be diluted with filtered air, which is constantly being delivered to all areas within the suite. If the pressure of the air is higher inside the suite than it is in hospital corridors, the direction of airflow will be toward the outside.

One can enter locker rooms, offices, and mixed or "grey" spaces from the vestibular area. In turn, the clean area of the surgical suite can be entered from the locker rooms or offices only after "scrub" clothes and shoe covers are put on. Thus, locker rooms and offices opening from the vestibule serve as airlocks between the outside and inside. An advantage of the vestibular plan, at least from the standpoint of security, is that it calls for one main entrance to the surgical suite. A separate entrance can be designed for supplies.

MULTIPLE ENTRANCE PLAN

An alternative is individual entrances to locker rooms and offices from common corridors. This design uses each of these areas as its own airlock. A disadvantage of this design is poor security. Multiple entrances are difficult to guard, especially in off-hours. When doors are locked, there is the inconvenience of key distribution and other problems that attend middle of the night emergencies.

TRAFFIC OF PERSONNEL

In a survey of old and new surgical suites,[2] the most common defect in design was a confused traffic pattern, especially associated with the clean-dirty or inside-outside movements of personnel.

The entrances to the operating suite in relation to the operating rooms made it necessary to walk past the entrances of active operating rooms, while still in street clothes and shoes, to reach the lockers. Personnel who were wearing scrub clothes and shoe covers had to walk over the same floors that were traversed by people who had recently come in from the outside. In addition, the sedated, anxious patients who were lying on carts in the hallway outside the operating rooms, waiting to be wheeled into the room, were in the direct line of traffic of the personnel in street clothes.

The location of the supervisor's office or booking office in the suite made it necessary for the clean traffic of circulating nurses or technicians to cross and mix with outside traffic, such as drug and equipment salesmen and surgeons in street clothes who come in to schedule future operations.

Personnel lounges and refreshment areas permitted surgeons in scrub clothes to mix with physicians in street clothes and have coffee (and often cigarettes) together. All too often, surgeons and house staff members went directly from the lounge to scrub for the next operation, still wearing the same shoe covers and reusing the same mask that they wore under their chin in the lounge area.

Locker rooms for surgeons, nurses, and other personnel were improperly located across a shared hospital corridor from the operating room or on another floor. In either case, shoe covers were often put on before leaving the locker room so that they were worn to walk across a dirty hall, or to use a stairway. The problem of a stairway can be overcome by dedicating it to clean traffic only, an inside "clean stairway" between locker rooms and surgical suite. Shoe covers should be put on when entering the clean area and discarded when leaving it.

The preceding examples, of course, related more to the aberrations of personal behavior and lack of hygienic discipline than they do to errors in architecture. Undoubtedly, more hygienic personal behavior can be encouraged by more appropriate architectural design.

Designers of operating rooms must have a clear idea of the importance of separating clean from dirty traffic and realize that outside bacteria can reach the operative field by being carried into the operating room on scrub clothing. Precise predesign programming of movement of personnel, patients, and supplies can prevent the cross-traffic between people in street clothes and people in scrub clothes. Provision for a holding area for patients awaiting entry into an operating room obviates the necessity of people in street clothes walking by apprehensive patients lying on carts. In the absence of a holding area, such as in surgical suites built more than 20 years ago, preoperative patients should be held in inside corridors of the surgical suite, away from the hubbub of front door traffic.

Location of supervisors' offices or booking offices within the suite must also be done with good traffic programming. In many hospitals where salesmen, vendors, surgeons, housekeeping personnel, and nurses intermingle in the offices located inside the surgical suite, the error can be corrected by reallocation of spaces and minor renovations. Attempts to separate the traffic by painting dividing lines or placing tapes on the floor seldom work. Potential for contamination from the outside depends not only on underfoot pathways, but equally on contact with outside garments and inadequate or inappropriate air movement and air dilution.

Much of the problem of mixed traffic in surgeons' lounges can be corrected by the surgeons themselves, as much as by the architects. Surgeons could bar nonsurgeons from their lounges, yet such communication is useful. Surgeons should shed their disposable shoe covers as they leave the clean area of the surgical suite, making it necessary to don a new pair of shoe covers upon reentering the suite. The placement of the shoe cover bin, as well as the receptacle for used shoe covers, and a bench or stool for comfortable changing would make the practice easier to follow. Cross-over benches by means of which street shoes touch the ground on one side and covered shoes on the other side only, are being used in more and more hospitals. Surgeons should not walk around the hospital in scrub greens or used shoe covers but should change their clothes on leaving the surgical suite.

There are a variety of commercial efforts to solve this theoretical problem of tracking in "dirt" from the hospital to the operating room. One company manufactures a tacky floor mat, which is placed at the main entrance to the surgical suite. The tacky surface is to be replaced once or twice per day. We found that although the total number of bacteria on shoe soles or wheels traversing the mat may be moderately reduced, when the mat had previously been traversed the next set of wheels or shoes picked up bacteria deposited during the preceding trip.[3] Also the frame of these mats often accumulates a rim of "mud" at the contact line with the floor.

Other devices designed for similar duty consist of sponge rubber or sponge plastic mats, or a patch of carpeting soaked with a strong antiseptic solution. These devices may be self-sterilizing, but they definitely do not have a significant effect on the bacterial content of cartwheels or shoe soles. Since the most powerful antiseptic solutions (quaternary ammonium compounds and phenolic compounds) require a contact time of at least 30 seconds to kill most bacteria, walking a few steps over a soaked or chemically treated mat will do little to control bacteria. It could, however, cause a person to slip on the wet floor. In short, we do not recommend such mats. There is no better way to keep floors clean than to wet-clean them with an effective phenolic detergent solution several times a day.

PATIENT TRAFFIC

A vestibular area serves as a convenient place to transfer patients from hospital carts to operating room carts. In some hospitals, it is standard practice to wheel the patient from any area in the hospital directly to the operating table. In other hospitals, the patient is transferred to a "clean" operating room cart in a vestibular exchange area located immediately inside the doors of the surgical suite. This is done on the premise that bacteria may be tracked into the operating room on the wheels of the cart. Although this possibility seems plausible, there is no evidence that supports this practice as a way of reducing surgical infection.

One architect[4] has described the patient on a cart as a "bundle of infection" coming into the operating room. To counteract this invasion, he advocated a separate preoperative department within the clean area, a kind of glamorized holding area, to which the patient would be brought the evening before operation for prepping. This rather ingenuous and naive solution to the endogenous etiology of surgical infection has never been put into widespread practice.

If one uses the inside cart system, it is necessary to make provision for a cart cleaning area in which carts can be wiped down with detergent solution or 70 percent alcohol between uses. This system does not obviate the need for additional space to store carts while they are not in use.

Many hospitals use the recovery room mobile bed as the clean patient cart. If this is the case, a system must be devised for returning the patient to his room from the clean recovery area. If this is done with the mobile bed, the bed must be thoroughly cleaned before being returned to the recovery room. If the return is made with a separate, outside cart, the cart that breaches the clean area when it picks up the patient in the recovery area must be properly cleaned before it is used.

The design of new surgical suites should include a corridor cart alcove outside each operating room for storage. Even though this design has gone far to decongest the corridors of the surgical suite, adequate cart storage and cleaning facilities must be provided elsewhere.

A number of methods of transferring patients from outside to inside environment are available.

1. Most hospitals wheel the patient directly to the operating table on the outside cart. This method has nothing to recommend it.

2. The oldest and simplest method of patient transfer is to bring the side of an outside cart to a line on the floor, or a barrier resembling a fence, and have the patient shift over to the inside cart on the other side of the barrier.

3. A commercial system of stretcher carts with removable tops is available. The patient, together with the cart top, is transferred from an outside set of wheels to an inside set of wheels. Only one lift or patient shift to the operating table from the inside cart is necessary.

4. A pass-through, mechanically operated hatchway is available to carry the patient from the outside to the inside on a padded platform, which becomes the operating table top when attached to a stationary base.

MATERIALS TRAFFIC IN AND OUT OF THE OPERATIVE SUITE

Materials traffic, like people traffic, has two sets of movement problems related to a surgical suite—those of in-and-out movement and those of inside-the-suite movement. In the design of an efficient suite, one must consider the type of materials being used (reusable, disposable), the required conveyance (cartage, mechanical, mechanically assisted, manual), and the system and location of operations for recycling, disposal, and maintenance of materials. The design of the facilities in which these functions are to take place has obvious implications for their efficiency and economy, and hence for control of infection.

If the instruments are to be sterilized in a remote central supply department, an efficient system of delivery must exist to and from the suite. The containment of sterile packs must be dependable, and there must be an adequate supply of instruments so that an operation is not interrupted for want of sterile instruments. The design of the entire system must function economically.

Curiously, remote instrument processing is being recommended on the basis that one processing plant for the entire hospital is more economical than one devoted to surgical instruments. This is not true. Automated delivery systems are extremely costly to build, uneconomical to operate, and inefficient in supplying surgeons with the instruments they need when they need them.[4] Contrary to many enthusiastic recommendations, the safest, most efficient, and economical design for instrument cycling (especially for large surgical suites with more than eight operating rooms) is to provide for processing in, or close to, the suite. The remote cycling system encourages maldistribution of instruments to other parts of the hospital, damage, pilferage, and contamination.

Another common functional error in materials handling is the delivery of goods in cartons to the clean area. Often these cartons come directly from trucks, often with street dirt still clinging to them. These outer cartons should be removed in a primary or secondary storage area outside the suite before the supplies are delivered for on-site storage.

There are usually two types of storage within the surgical suite, regional storage near the operating rooms and inside-the-room cabinets. Operating room cabinets should have perforated or wire shelving and clean air circulation from a vented ceiling. This type of cabinet reduces dust accumulation and the emission of particles into the room when the cabinet is opened. Storage spaces must also be organized and kept as dust-free as possible. Wire or perforated shelving helps to minimize dust accumulation in these areas as well.[1]

TRAFFIC INSIDE THE SURGICAL SUITE

A number of architectural configurations have been devised to separate clean from dirty traffic *within* the surgical suite. One of them is the "clean core race track" design, in which a clean central working space surrounded by operating rooms is in turn encircled by a peripheral corridor. Alternatively, the peripheral corridor can separate the central core from the ring of rooms. These designs have certain shortcomings, including uneconomic use of space, lack of essential storage and other working areas, a rather dirty "clean" central core, and violations of the originally planned traffic pattern.[3] A much better plan for large surgical suites consists of four or six operating rooms, together with properly located support facilities. This utilizes horizontal space most efficiently, provides a sensible interior traffic pattern, and is extremely functional.[5]

Rather than design for an unrealistic division of one type of clean traffic from another it would be more practical simply to make sure that:

1. People in scrub clothes do not mingle with people in street clothes.
2. All used instruments and disposable materials are packaged before they leave the operating room.
3. Used gowns, gloves, and drapes are left inside the operating room and not worn outside the clean area.
4. Clean storage areas are so located that clean materials distribution inside the suite is facilitated.
5. There are enough well-placed, interior janitorial closets and other cleaning facilities (wet vacuum outlets, cleaning equipment storage space, etc.).

If these principles are followed, it is unnecessary to design separate corridors to segregate postoperative from preoperative patients and materials. A popular European design of separate intubation and extubation rooms for each operating room, as well as a peripheral corridor for the collection of used surgical instruments and supplies, wastes space and money. Using this plan, one part of the clean traffic (the patient before operation) is segregated from another part of the clean traffic (the patient after operation). To justify the added construction costs, the claim is made that down-time between operations is shortened. Our studies do not substantiate this claim unless duplicate anesthesia staffs are available. The main contributor to down-time is cleaning and setting up of the room, followed closely by availability of anesthesia service. The presence of a holding area should obviate the need for a preparatory room, provided the anesthesiologists do not object to inducing in the operating room. The induction of anesthesia on a patient lying on the operating room table has no known effect on the incidence of infection. The need for an extubation room is likewise questionable.

SURFACES

In general, harder and less porous surfaces are more bacteria-resistant and easier to clean. The new smooth grouting materials make ceramic tile now suitable for the operating room. Other suitable surface materials include laminated polyesters with an epoxy finish and hard vinyl coverings, which can be heat-sealed and leave no seams.

Floors also should be as nonporous as possible. Terrazzo floors have stood the test of time as an easy to clean, relatively nonporous surface, but plastic terrazzo tends to dry with small holes. A variety of hard, seamless plastics are less expensive than terrazzo and withstand heavy traffic for many years. Wet vacuuming between operations is the most desirable method of cleaning floors.

RECOVERY ROOMS

Most recovery rooms and surgical intensive care units are conducive to cross-infection.[7] Beds are often as close as 2 feet from each other, and the air is often poorly circulated. Attendants and nurses often go from patient to patient without always washing their hands. Many recovery rooms close late in the afternoon, so emergency patients or others operated on late in the day must be taken directly to an intensive care unit. This unit is usually located at some distance from the operating room and frequently has no separation of patients, thus exposing the vulnerable postoperative patient to cross-infection. Recovery rooms are now being designed as an important component of the clean surgical suite with individual cubicles for each bed. Adequate space is being allocated to permit the enclosure of every bed with glass and metal walls and a foldaway front. Hand sinks are located for easy use between beds. The cubicle design permits isolation precautions to be practiced without depriving patients of special care. The ventilation should be as high in quality as that of the operating rooms.

FAMILY WAITING ROOM

A family waiting room near the surgical suite, although useful for surgeon-family communication, can threaten good hygiene. Surgeons wearing operating clothes and leaving the suite to talk to the family often do not change into fresh surgical garb when they return to the operating room. If the waiting room were more remote, the surgeon would have to change his clothes or talk with the family through telephone or video communication.

AIR HANDLING SYSTEMS

Operating rooms should be ventilated with bag or high-efficiency particulate air filtering. Such operating rooms are as clean as those having costly, special chambers.[8] The role of airborne contamination in wound infection has gone through several cycles of argument. Today's consensus holds that airborne organisms are important in causing wound infection only when a properly designed and installed air handling system is abused, or during procedures in which a large foreign body is implanted.

Leaving a corridor door open during operative procedures, permitting unrestricted opening and closing of operating room doors as people come and go, failure to cover long hair, sideburns, or beards, and allowing personnel in short-sleeved shirts to circulate in and out of operating rooms, can render the best ventilation system ineffective. No matter how particulate-free the air blown into a room, the quantity of bioparticulate matter circulated around the room is inevitably directly proportionate to the number of people in the room and the area of hair and skin exposed. Shed particles mount exponentially with excessive numbers of improperly covered visitors and unnecessary activity such as the flapping of drapes, towels, and gowns and other maneuvers that may unsettle previously shed particles from horizontal surfaces.

Public Health Service and National Fire Protection Association (NFPA) requirements call for a minimum of 12 changes of operating room air per hour in existing facilities and a minimum of 25 changes per hour in new facilities, positive pressure compared to corridors, relative humidity between 50 and 55 percent, temperatures between 23.6 and 18.2C, and, depending on the locality, up to 80 percent recirculation with effective filtering. Some states still require 100 percent outside air with no recirculation.

Although Code 56A of the NFPA permits air to be circulated into an operating room either from the ceiling or from distributors high on the walls, a center ceiling grill is considered more in keeping with unidirectional flow of clean air originating from the center of the ceiling and exhausted low on the walls or corners of the room.

Air in the corridors of a surgical suite should be as clean as air in the operating room; indeed, we believe that air in the entire surgical suite—including closets, storage areas, personnel areas, and recovery rooms—should be as well-filtered and ventilated as air in the operating room.

LAMINAR FLOW

The term "laminar" is usually applied to any unidirectional air-blowing systems, ranging from virtually any ceiling or wall diffuser to a variety of air systems producing a curtain effect. So-called laminar flow can be delivered in a horizontal or a vertical direction, although neither direction has been shown to be superior to the other or, indeed, to nonlaminar flow. The British surgeon Charnley promoted laminar flow chambers by attributing to them his reduction in wound infections from 9 to 1 percent after hip replacement operations.[9] Charnley's critics point out that the improvement could have been the cumulative result of several changes in his technique, such as including a coverall surgical gown.

A number of American orthopedic surgeons have performed thousands of hip replacement operations in conventional operating rooms without laminar flow chambers and report a combined 2-year infection rate of 0.45 percent, a rate equivalent to, or lower than, that reported by surgeons who performed comparable numbers of operations in laminar flow chambers.[8] Moreover, the bacteria cultured from wound infections following hip replacement surgery differ from those found in the air of the room or chamber.[10]

Air filtering is often confused with laminar air flow; one is a filtering capability, the other a method of diffusing air into a space in a somewhat unidirectional manner. Laminar flow may be imparted to either filtered or unfiltered air, and air can be delivered by any type or size of diffusing method: laminar or nonlaminar, high speed or low speed. HEPA filtering produces air that is almost particle-free as it first leaves the diffuser and enters the room; particles produced in the room will not be removed until the air is filtered again.

Although large-volume, unidirectional airflow can reduce bacterial counts, no evidence suggests that this type of flow alone affects the incidence of operative wound infections or that unidirectional flow is superior to a well-functioning, properly installed, unabused conventional nonlaminar system. Ultraviolet light is as effective as special air handling in the control of airborne contamination despite drawbacks related to the need to protect skin from the rays.[11]

OPERATING ROOM APPAREL

People are the major source of bioparticles in the operating room. If personnel are sufficiently covered, they will shed desquamated skin containing bacteria into the environment. When hair or skin are inadequately covered or covered with permeable materials, the number of bioparticles entering the environment is directly proportional to the shedding potential of the people involved.[12] Some people are "shedders" and release up to 100 times the number of particles of nonshedders. The amount of dry shedding is related to the amount of contamination of the covered scrub suit or skin and to the tightness of the weave or mesh of the barrier garment.[13] However, this source of contamination is relatively minor compared to that produced by "moist bacterial strike-through" of surgical materials, by means of which direct passage of bacteria takes place from unsterile skin or garment to sterile field.[14]

Traditional garb consists of gowns, caps, masks, and shoe covers of woven, launderable material, or nonwoven, disposable material. Impermeability to moisture is important in any barrier material because a wicklike effect tends to transmit bacteria. Surgical gowns reinforced on the front with sleeves with a tightly woven material treated with waterproofing (Barbac or Liquishield) have demonstrated impermeability at reinforced areas for up to 100 launderings.[15] Unless they are reinforced with plastic film, however, very few nonwoven materials will withstand the stresses of repeated operating room use without becoming permeable to moist contaminants.[16]

Coverall hoods with plastic masks or helmets and gowns that cover the entire head and body will prevent bioparticulate shedding. Because of the discomfort of heat retained by such outfits, however, vacuum exhaust of the space between the wearer and the uniform is necessary. All hair must be covered in the operating room because hair acquires and sheds bacterial particles.[17] Hoods rather than caps, therefore, are recommended for all personnel.

Nonwoven shoe covers are disposable, easy to put on, and equipped with a conductive strip and should be put on every time a person enters the suite from the outside. Shoe covers are recommended because the usual white shoes, with dried secretions on the leather, are unsanitary for a number of reasons, including the tendency for flakes to come off with motion.

BIBLIOGRAPHY

Altemeier WA, Burke JF, Pruitt BA Jr, Sandusky WR (eds.): Manual on Control of Infection in Surgical Patients. Philadelphia, Lippincott, 1976.

REFERENCES

1. Laufman H: Surgical hazard control: effect of architecture and engineering. Arch Surg 107:552, 1973.
2. Laufman H: What's wrong with our operating rooms? Am J Surg 122:332, 1971.
3. Laufman H: The surgeon's environment. In Preston FW (ed): Practice of Surgery. Hagerstown, Harper & Row, 1975.

4. Jacobs RH Jr: The surgical center: a proposal for the reorganization of the surgical service. Am Inst Architects J, November, 1962.
5. Laufman H: Space and Facility Program for a Surgical Center. Montefiore Hospital and Medical Center. Private printing, 1967.
6. Laufman H: Conductive footwear in the operating room in absence of flammable anesthetics. Reply to questions and answers. JAMA 237:1263, 1977.
7a. Northey D, Adess ML, Hartsuck JM, Rhoades ER: Microbial surveillance in a surgical intensive care unit. Surg Gynecol Obstet 139:321, 1974.
7b. Laufman H: The infection hazard of intensive care. Surg Gynecol Obstet 139:413, 1974.
8. Laufman H: Current status of special air handling systems in operating rooms. Med Instrum 7:7, 1973.
9. Charnley J: A clean air operating enclosure. Br J Surg 51:202, 1964.
10. Irvine R, Johnson BL Jr, Amstutz H: The relationship of genitourinary tract procedures and deep sepsis after total hip replacement. Surg Gynecol Obstet 139:701, 1974.
11. Goldner JL, Gaines RW, Higgins M: Ultraviolet light in the orthopaedic operating room at Duke University—37 years experience, 1937–74. National Research Council Workshop on Control of Operating Room Airborne Bacteria. Washington, DC, 1976, p 104.
12. Blowers R, Hill J, Howell A: Shedding of *Staphylococcus aureus* by human carriers. In Hers JFP, Winkler KC: Airborne Transmission and Airborne Infection. New York, Wiley, 1973, p 432.
13. Moylan JA Jr, Balish E, Chan J: Intraoperative bacterial transmission. Surg Gynecol Obstet 141:731, 1975.
14. Laufman H, Eudy WW, Vandernoot AM, Liu D, Harris CA: Strike-through of moist contamination by woven and nonwoven surgical materials. Ann Surg 181:857, 1975.
15. Laufman H, Siegal JD, Edberg SC: Moist bacterial strike-through of surgical materials: confirmatory tests. Ann Surg 189:68, 1979.
16. Laufman H, Montefusco C, Siegal JD, Edberg SC: Scanning electron microscopy of moist bacterial strike-through of surgical materials. Surg Gynecol Obstet, 150:165, 1980.
17. Dineen P, Drusin L: Epidemics of postoperative wound infections associated with hair carriers. Lancet 2:1157, 1973.

CHAPTER 22
Technical Factors in the Prevention of Wound Infections

RICHARD F. EDLICH, GEORGE T. RODEHEAVER AND JOHN G. THACKER

THE ultimate goal of the surgeon is to restore the physical integrity and function of injured or diseased tissue.

Whether the tissue injury will be limited to the initial wound depends on the outcome of the interaction between the microbial contaminants and the traumatized tissue. A catastrophic outcome can be averted by the implementation of well-devised surgical care in both the making of an operative wound and in the treatment of an accidental one. The major focus of this chapter is on the traumatic soft tissue wound, but the principles are applicable to all wounds.

MECHANISM OF INJURY

The outcome of both accidental and operative injury can be predicted by applying the physical concepts of power, work, and force. Surgery simply employs various principles of energy transfer in a planned procedure. The traumatic injury is caused by the same energy sources even though the incident is uncontrolled. If the surgeon does not control the sources of energy used, an operation becomes an assault similar to a traumatic injury. The surgeon must also be aware of the consequences of uncontrolled amounts of energy on tissues, as occurs in accidental injury, and treat the resultant wound appropriately. Wounded tissue is more susceptible to infection than unwounded tissue.[1] The magnitude of this enfeebled resistance to infection will vary with the mechanism of wounding.

MECHANICAL ENERGY

Shear

Three mechanical forces can lead to soft tissue injury—shear, tension, and compression. To divide tissue with scissors or scalpel, the surgeon applies a carefully controlled shearing force of equal magnitude, in opposite directions, in two adjacent parallel planes separated by a small distance. Because the volume of tissue contacted is extremely small, little total energy is required to produce tissue failure.

Scalpel Design and Use

When cutting tissues, the surgeon must use a scalpel that divides tissue with the least trauma. The sharpness of the blade is dependent on the radius of curvature of its ultimate ground edge (Fig. 22-1). The sharpest blades are ground by a rotary grinding process. With equivalent applied force, blades ground by the rotary process can cut to a greater depth than blades ground by other techniques.

A ritual practice in surgery has been to discard the sharp blade following its use on skin, in the fear that it introduces skin contaminants into the depths of the wound. Jacobs[2] reported that scalpels subsequent to cutting skin are almost always sterile and need not be discarded.

Despite all the technical advances in scalpel design, the ultimate performance of the scalpel rests with the surgeon's skill. The experienced surgeon can cut to the desired depth with one sweep of the blade—10^6 or more bacteria are necessary to elicit infection in such a wound.[3] This level of host resistance is comparable to that encountered in nearly 80 percent of traumatic soft tissue injuries. Such injuries are due to a piece of metal or glass and are recognized by their characteristic linear configuration. Wounds made with multiple strokes of the knife damage a greater volume of tissue, impair local defenses, and invite infection with much smaller microbial inocula.

Tension and Compression

When a wound is caused by a collision of two bodies, the mechanisms of injury are predominantly compression or tension, or both, rather than shear. In either case, two forces of equal magnitude are applied in opposite directions. Unlike shear forces, compression and tension forces act in the same plane. The injury is caused by tension force when a flat body hits soft tissue not supported by

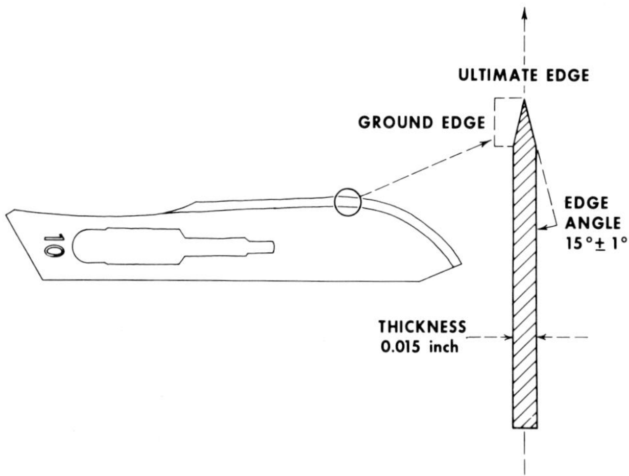

Fig. 22-1. **Physical design of the scalpel blade. (Figs. 1-3, 5-10, 12 are from Hunt TK, Dunphy JE: Fundamentals of Wound Management. New York, Appleton-Century-Crofts, 1979.)**

underlying bone. Compressive forces are operative when a flat body hits soft tissue overlying bone.

The energy requirement for tissue failure as a result of these forces is considerably greater than for shear forces because the energy is distributed over a larger volume of tissue. The amount of energy absorbed by tissue during an impact can be calculated by the following equation:

$$T = \frac{MV^2}{2}$$

Where T equals kinetic energy (joules), M equals mass of impacting object (kg), V equals relative velocity between the impacting object and tissue (m/sec). Obviously, changes in the relative velocity of the object that impacts has a greater influence on the level of kinetic energy than do variations in the mass of the object.

Blunt Trauma

When the mechanism of injury is compression, tissue failure occurs at energy levels of 2.52 joules per cm,[4] which is comparable to the energy encountered when a car going 8 km per hour strikes a tree. The momentum of the collision causes the victim's head, weighing approximately 4 kg, to hit the dashboard with an area of impact approximately 8 cm^2. This absorbed level of energy disrupts the skin, resulting in a characteristic stellate laceration. In addition, the wound edges are damaged and rendered relatively ischemic. Wounds caused by impact injuries are 100-fold more susceptible to infection than wounds caused by shear forces, and immediate antibiotic treatment is warranted to suppress the growth of the bacterial contaminants. Even then, antibiotic efficacy is substantially less than in contaminated wounds caused by shear forces.

Missile Injury

A collision between a missile and the human body represents a considerably higher level of energy absorption per unit volume of tissue than that encountered in automobile accidents. The interaction of missile and man combines shear, tensile, and compressive forces. The severity of the injury is directly proportional to the amount of kinetic injury lost by the missile in the tissue. Because $T = MV^2/2$, doubling the weight of the missile doubles its kinetic energy, while doubling its velocity quadruples its kinetic energy.

The velocities of missiles are divided into two groups. Pistol bullets and 0.22-inch rimfire rifle bullets with velocities less than 300 meters per second are called low-velocity missiles.[5] They leave a deep narrow tract within tissue, with the injury confined to its immediate pathway. High-velocity rifles and newer fragmentation devices release missiles with muzzle velocities exceeding 1000 meters per second. When high-velocity projectiles strike the human body, initial shock waves with pressure up to 100 to 200 atmospheres are created in both forward and lateral directions. As a result of the lateral explosive force, a large space, known as a temporary cavity is created, which attains its maximum volume 2 to 4 milliseconds after missile impact. The tissue then rebounds, narrowing the cavity. Depending on the tissue, the compressive forces creating the temporary cavity may cause damage at a distance from the permanent missile tract. Such forces are sufficient to fracture bones, rupture organs, and lacerate vessels adjacent to the tract but not directly struck by the missile. The magnitude of this tissue destruction is extensive and difficult to ascertain accurately soon after injury.

The density and character of the tissue itself have considerable influence on the magnitude of the injury. Amato et al[6] found that the size of the temporary cavity is proportional to the specific gravity of the injured tissue(s) and directly related to the ultimate severity of the injury. Following passage of high-velocity missiles through lung parenchyma (specific gravity 0.4 to 0.5), the tissue rapidly absorbs the energy and then recoils to leave an almost imperceptible tract. Because larger permanent wound tracts develop in tissues with high specific gravities (liver—1.01 to 1.02; muscle—1.02 to 1.04; bone—1.11 or greater), the temporary cavity and resultant wound tract in the liver would be larger than in the lung, even though the identical energies were absorbed.

The construction and configuration of the missile has an important influence on the magnitude of injury.[7] Increase in missile mass will increase the energy absorbed by the tissue. In comparison to streamlined bullets, blunt nose and hollow bullets tend to expand, flatten, and lose greater amounts of kinetic energy per unit volume of tissue. Expanding bullets used for hunting create a permanent wound tract much larger than that produced by a standard military bullet. The wound volumes resulting from the expanding bullets may be forty times that caused by the nonexpanding type.

Shotgun pellets progress from the muzzle in a cone-like fashion at a relatively low velocity (335 to 396 meters per second).[8] In hunting, the effective range is from about 20 to 40 meters. In people, the most serious shotgun wounds are inflicted at distances considerably less (2 meters) than effective hunting range. The pellets impact as a single mass of metal, causing extensive destruction of tissue.

In treating a gunshot injury, the victim or witnesses

should be questioned regarding the weapon used and the circumstances of injury (ie, muzzle distance from wound). The appearance and location of the wound must be described and recorded as accurately as possible and should include information about the presence of powder soot, strippling, or grains. If the wound has an unusual appearance such as a stellate or muscle imprint, this should also be noted. An attempt should be made to obtain the firearm as well as a sample of the cartridge. These data can be useful in estimating the degree of tissue destruction induced.

ELECTRICAL ENERGY

Electricity is the flow of electrons from one atom to another, and electrons set in motion by electric force (voltage) collide with each other and generate heat. The amount of heat developed by a conductor varies directly with its resistance. The magnitude of resistance to electron flow varies widely in different tissues, eg, the high resistance of skin and low resistance of muscle to electron flow. The control and localization of the heating effect of electric current comprises the fundamental basis for electrosurgery.

Electric power is usually generated with a continuous reversal of the direction of electric pressure (voltage). The pressure in the conductor first pushes and then pulls electrons (AC). The frequency of the current in hertz (Hz) or cycles per second is the time in which the complete cycle of positive and negative pressure occurs. The usual wall outlet in the United States provides a current with 120 reversals of the direction of flow occurring each second. Passage of 60 cycles of alternating current through a patient can induce ventricular fibrillation as well as muscle contractions. Involuntary spasmodic contractions of muscle in response to a low-frequency electrical stimulus subside as the frequency of the applied current is increased above 60 Hz. At frequencies greater than 10,000 Hz, no muscle response is noted. In addition, high-frequency current can flow along paths that virtually block the 60-cycle current.

The frequency of the current generated in electrosurgery is 250,000 to 2,000,000 Hz, and its ability to damage tissue depends on its concentration or density. As the current density increases, its heating effect becomes more pronounced. For example, the size of the active monopolar electrode is deliberately kept small so that concentrated heating will occur at its point of contact with tissue. Following contact, the current is dispersed to the return (ground) electrode, which encounters low current density and no tissue heating. The distribution of the current can be more carefully controlled by making the active electrode bipolar, usually in the form of forceps so that the tissue through which the current will pass is precisely delineated. An equivalent current passed through a monopolar electrode causes approximately three times as much necrosis of the surrounding tissue as the use of bipolar coagulation.[9]

When undamped high-frequency currents are passed through tissue, the active electrode acts as a bloodless knife (Fig. 22-2). The cells at the edge of the resultant wound literally disintegrate. Away from the plane of cutting one can see elongated tissue cells as well as histologic evidence of a mild thermal injury. Blood vessels at the wound edge are usually thrombosed, accounting for the hemostatic effect of the high-frequency current. This histologic evidence of tissue damage is also associated with an increased susceptibility to infection. Wounds made by electrosurgery are approximately three times more susceptible to infection than wounds made with the stainless steel scalpel (Fig. 22-3). In a prospective clinical study by Cruse and Foord,[10] the use of electrosurgery almost doubled the infection rates of operative wounds. The increased susceptibility of such wounds to infection mitigates against the use of electrosurgery for cutting skin and subcutaneous tissue.

In massive excisional operations (eg, large soft tissue tumors, debridement of third-degree burns), the threat of blood loss frequently outweighs the potential problems of subsequent infection. Levine et al [11] reported that blood loss and operating time were halved during electrosurgical excision of burn wounds when compared to scalpel excision.

When the oscillations are damped (Fig. 22-2), hemostasis is achieved without cutting. This type of current causes a rapid dehydration of living cells and the affected tissue is fused into a hyalinized mass. We prefer pinpoint electrosurgical coagulation of small bleeding vessels to suture ligation, but the power should be kept to the absolute minimum needed for vessel thrombosis.

Electrocoagulation will not control bleeding from cut ends of large vessels over 2 mm in diameter. Hemostasis can be achieved easily with a suture ligature of nonreactive materials. The intact vessel should be isolated over a short length and clamped with small hemostats applied contiguously. Alternatively the isolated vessel can be divided between the ligatures. Either technique is preferred over cutting the vessel first and then clamping the retracted vessel along with the contiguous bloodstained tissue. In the latter case, Ferguson [12] reported that the amount of strangulated tissue was about five times as much as with the vessel-isolating technique.

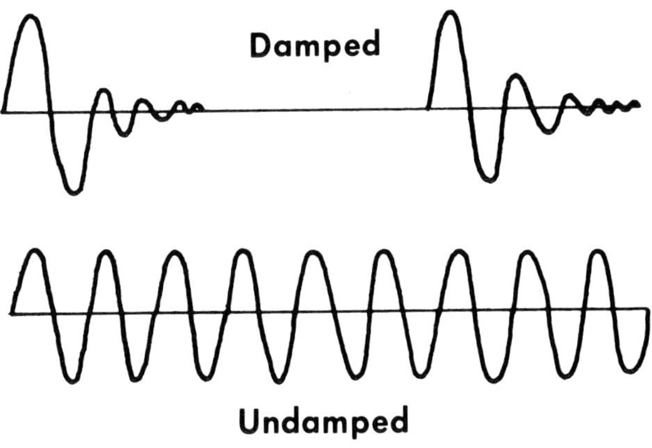

Fig. 22-2. Schematic representation of damped and undamped electrical currents. Undamped high-frequency current acts as a bloodless knife, while damped current exhibits a hemostatic effect without cutting.

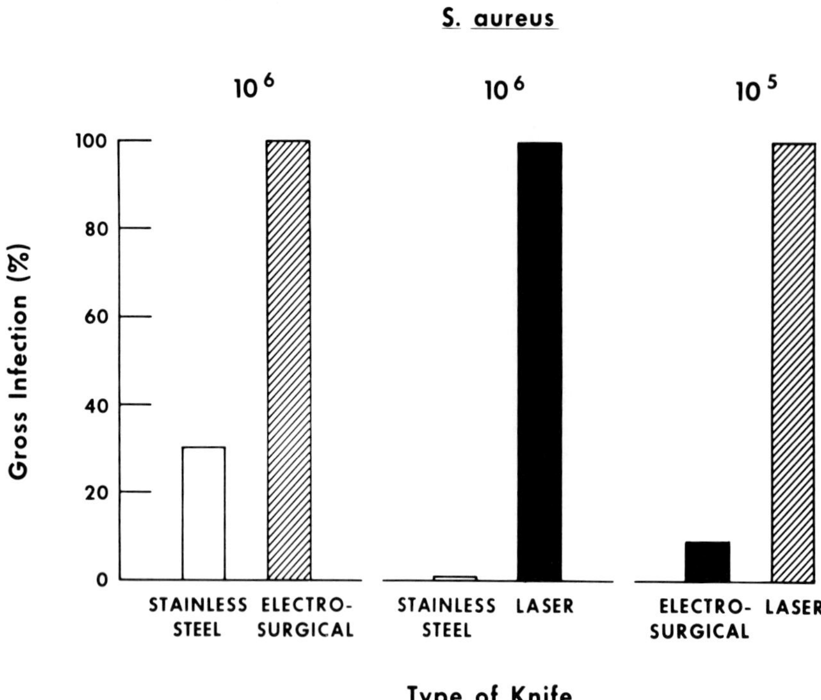

Fig. 22-3. **Standardized wounds made by either a stainless steel, electrosurgical, or laser knife were contaminated with a specified dose of *S. aureus.* Four days later, the incidence of gross infection was significantly greater in wounds made by the bloodless knives than those made by the stainless steel scalpel.**

Hemostasis must be accomplished with the least amount of electrocoagulation and suture material. The best method to control oozing and minor bleeding is to gently exert continual pressure on the bleeding surface with sponges moistened with cool saline. Rubbing or abrading the tissue will dislodge thrombi and can cause further bleeding. Furthermore, hot (150F), wet sponges should never be used for hemostasis. In animals, this treatment causes hyperthermic injury to tissue and potentiates the development of infection.[13]

An accidental acute electrical injury is a result of the reciprocal transformation of electricity into heat generated by the electrical current, and the results can be disastrous.[14] Accidental electrical injuries differ from electrosurgical wounds only in the relative frequency and voltage of the current delivered to the tissues.

RADIANT ENERGY

Radiant or electromagnetic energy can be employed as a scalpel. This energy consists of photons that are both waves and particles. Once absorbed by tissue, radiant energy is converted into heat which, applied to a small volume of tissue, divides it bloodlessly.

The concept of light as a source of energy is realized in lasers. Light waves emitted from lasers are coherent and are so nearly parallel that they can travel for miles in a straight line without spreading apart or converging. This coherent light provides tremendous pulses of power that do not diminish over great distances.

Lasers used in surgery get their energy from rotation and vibration of electrons in the CO_2 molecule. The resultant emission of light has a wavelength of 10.6 microns. These infrared waves are directed along an articulated arm and into a handpiece by means of mirrors located in precision rotary joints. A lens in the handpiece focuses the energy to a point less than 1 mm in diameter. This high concentration of energy at the focal point allows the beam to cut through skin and soft tissue. Despite this technologic advance, laser surgery is limited in usefulness by the cumbersome design of the surgical arm, as well as an insufficient level of power.

The hemostatic effect of the laser scalpel makes it especially suitable for massive excisions. Blood loss encountered by scalpel excisions is nearly 3.3 times greater than the blood loss following the use of laser energy. Electrosurgical excision has 1.67 times the blood loss of laser excision. The superior hemostatic effect of the laser over that of electrosurgery is associated with increased damage to the tissue defenses. Experimental wounds made by a laser are approximately tenfold more susceptible to infection than those made by electrosurgery (Fig. 22-3).[12] Fortunately, the tissue damage resulting from either electrosurgery or the laser does not interfere with the take of either autografts or homografts on wound beds with low bacterial counts ($< 10^5$ bacteria per gram of tissue).

BIOLOGY OF TISSUE INFECTION

The development of infection is a function of the interaction of several factors—the nature and degree of local contamination and both local and general resistance of the patient to infection.[15] The term infected refers to a wound that exhibits the classic signs of inflammation (calor, rubor, tumor, dolor) as a result of microbial contamination. In contrast, contamination refers only to the viable and nonviable foreign bodies within the wound that have as yet failed to elicit inflammation.

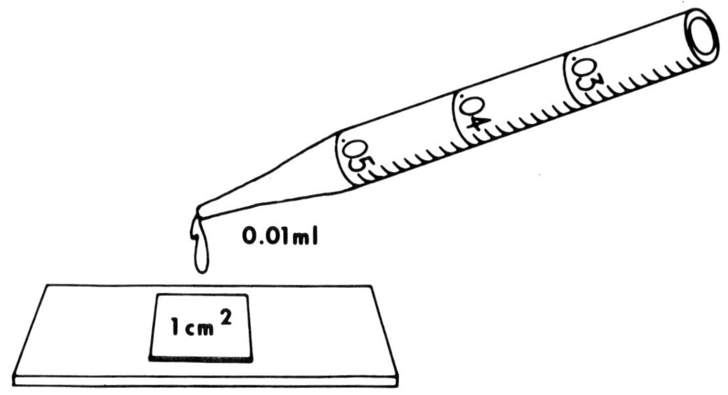

A.
$$\frac{\text{No. Bacteria in 10 fields}}{10} = \frac{\text{No. bacteria}}{\text{1 field}}$$

B.
$$\frac{\text{No. Bacteria}}{\text{1 field}} \times \frac{\text{4000 fields}}{1\ \text{cm}^2} = \frac{\text{No. bacteria}}{1\ \text{cm}^2}$$
where 1 field $= 0.025\ \text{mm}^2$

C.
$$\frac{\text{No. Bacteria}}{1\ \text{cm}^2} \times \frac{\text{homogenate volume (ml.)}}{\text{0.01 ml.}} \times \frac{1}{\text{Sample wt. (gm.)}} = \frac{\text{bacteria}}{\text{gm. tissue}}$$

Fig. 22-4. **Rapid bacterial quantitation technique.**

INFLUENCE OF BACTERIAL NUMBER

In experimental animals, the critical infective dose of a pure culture of obligate and facultative aerobic bacteria in wounds is 10^6 bacteria, or greater, per gram of tissue; below this level, wounds heal without infection.[3] This remarkable resistance to infection has been identified in all soft tissues tested.[3] The type of aerobic bacteria contaminating a wound surface is less important in the development of infection than the number of bacteria. Apparent clinical differences in virulence may be based on ecologic advantages possessed by the pathogens and may not reflect specific differences in the host-parasite relationship. The critical number of anaerobic bacteria that will elicit soft tissue infection has not been documented. Unless quantitative microbiologic techniques are performed under strict anaerobic conditions (rarely achieved in hospital laboratories), the presence and number of these organisms can not be appreciated.

This relationship between bacterial counts and clinical wound infection has been a stimulus for the development of quantitative tissue bacteriologic techniques.[16,17] These measurements are initiated by excising a $2 \times 1 \times 0.5$ cm sample of tissue, which weighs approximately 0.5 gm. The biopsy is weighed on an analytical balance and homogenized in a measured amount of 0.9 percent saline. Direct microscopic examination measures the total number of living and dead bacteria in the suspension. The major advantage of this technique is the speed with which the results are available to the surgeon, within 20 minutes after biopsy. In this measurement, a designated amount (0.01 ml) of the undiluted suspension, homogenate, or a serial dilution or both are spread uniformly over a delineated 1-cm² area of a glass slide, which is then placed on a warmer to dry (Fig. 22-4). The smear is then subjected to the Gram stain technique developed in our laboratory.[18] Ten separate fields of each smear are examined and the average number of bacteria per field is recorded (Fig. 22-4). Appropriate calculations are performed to determine the number of bacteria per gram of tissue (Fig. 22-4).

The rapid slide technique gives accurate and reliable measurement when 400 or more bacteria are in the 0.01 ml suspension delivered to the slide ($> 2.5 \times 10^5$ organisms per gram of tissue). When less than this number of bacteria is added to the slide, bacteria are not detectable on microscopic examination. This technique does not replace quantitative serial dilution and plating techniques, which are always performed concomitantly because they allow speciation of the pathogen and antibiotic sensitivity testing. Quantitative bacteriology, consisting of rapid slide technique as well as serial dilution and plating, is now used routinely by surgeons in our medical center to predict the safety of wound closure (both primary and delayed primary),[16] to determine graft bed receptivity, and to diagnose the onset of burn wound sepsis.[17]

An infective dose of bacteria may be derived from an exogenous source (eg, wounding instrument) or from the endogenous microflora of the patient which are discussed in Chapter 3. Table 22-1 emphasizes the great quantitative variation in endogenous flora which exist from place to place in the body. The surgeon must focus attention on the regions of the healthy human body that contain concentrations of organisms sufficient to elicit infection of tissue (also see Table 25-1).[3] When planning operations at these sites, preoperative suppression of the microbiota is essential.

TABLE 22-1. THE NORMAL MICROFLORA ON SKIN AND MUCOUS MEMBRANES

	Total Bacterial Concentrations	Ratio Anaerobe:aerobe
Skin		
Moister areas (axillae, perineum, etc.)	10^4–10^6 *	1:10
Drier areas (trunk, upper arms and legs)	10^1–10^3	1:5–10
Exposed areas (head, face, feet) †	10^4–10^6	1:5–10
Respiratory system		
Nasal cavity	10^2 *	1:1
Paranasal sinuses	0	0
Trachea	0	0
Bronchi	0	0
Digestive system		
Saliva	10^6 ‡	3–5:1
Tooth surface	10^{11}	1:1
Gingival crevice	10^{11}	100–1,000:1
Stomach	0–10^5	1:1
Proximal small bowel	10^2–10^4	1:1
Ileum	10^5–10^8	1:1
Colon	10^9–10^{11}	100–1,000:1
Urogenital system		
Male urethra	10^2–10^3 ‡	Aerobes
Female urethra	10^2–10^3	Aerobes
Endocervix	10^8–10^9	5–10:1
Vagina	10^8–10^9	5–10:1

* per cm^2 of tissue
† Anaerobes may outnumber aerobe in the skin of the cheeks, upper back, and presternum.
‡ per gm of exudate

SYSTEMIC HOST FACTORS IN THE RESISTANCE TO INFECTION

The quantitative relationship between the host's resistance to infection and the number of bacteria can be upset by both systemic and local factors. Of the systemic factors, advancing age appears to be one of the most important in increasing infection rate. Infection rates are reported to be higher in patients with diabetes mellitus, obesity, malnutrition, or on steroid therapy. Shock, remote trauma, or distant infection also enhance wound infection. In addition, rare immunologic deficiencies, both primary and secondary, contribute to a diminished host's resistance (Chapter 13).

LOCAL FACTORS IN RESISTANCE TO INFECTION

Local factors are especially important in determining the outcome of the interaction between the host and bacteria. Whether present by accident or intention, any foreign body in the wound damages the local tissue's defenses and invites infection. The magnitude of this damage appears to be related to the chemical reactivity of the foreign body. Soil and dirt are frequent contaminants in traumatic injuries. Although it has been recognized for centuries that severe bacterial infection often develops in wounds containing dirt and soil, only recently has their role been clarified.[19] Specific infection-potentiating fractions have now been identified in soil, which include its organic components as well as inorganic clay fractions. For wounds contaminated by these fractions, only 100 bacteria per gram of tissue will elicit infection. The ability of these fractions to enhance the incidence of infection appears to be related to their damage to host defense:

1. In the presence of these fractions, leukocytes are not able to ingest and kill bacteria [20]—a result of a direct interaction between the highly charged soil particles and white blood cells.

2. Soil infection-potentiating fractions also eliminate the nonspecific bactericidal activity in serum.

3. These highly charged anionic particles also react chemically with amphoteric and basic antibiotics, limiting their activity in contaminated wounds.

The concentration of these fractions in soil can be correlated with their location. Environmental conditions in swamps and marshes encourage the production of soil with as much as 98 percent organic infection-potentiating fractions. The major inorganic infection-potentiating particles are the clay fractions, which reside in heaviest concentration in the subsoil rather than in topsoil. Hence, traumatic soft tissue injuries that occur in swamps or excavations run a high risk of being contaminated by these fractions, which predispose the wound to serious infection.

A corollary to these observations is that some soil contaminants, like sand grains, are relatively innocuous. This fraction, which has a large particle size and a low level of chemical reactivity, exerts considerably less damage to tissue defenses. Surprisingly, the black dirt on the surface of highways appears to have minimal chemical reactivity.

TECHNICAL FACTORS IN THE PREVENTION OF WOUND INFECTION

When caring for a traumatic wound, the surgeon must make judgments that frequently tip the balance in favor of either infection or healing per primum. The following specific recommendations regarding the management of the surgical wound are based on the best currently available clinical and experimental studies.

LOCAL ANESTHESIA

Cleansing of bacteria, soil, and other debris from traumatic injuries and debridement cannot be accomplished without anesthesia. The ideal anesthetic agent should have rapid onset of local action and should not impair the wound's ability to resist infection. The effect of the local anesthetic agent on the viability of microorganisms is another important consideration. For infected wounds, an agent that displays antimicrobial activity may kill the pathogen and interfere with its identification.

Lidocaine hydrochloride does not exhibit amtimicrobial activity or damage the local wound defenses. Its clinical usefulness can sometimes be enhanced by adding the vasoconstrictor epinephrine, which slows the clearance of lidocaine, thereby prolonging the duration of anesthesia. Epinephrine will also damage the local wound defenses. The infection-potentiating effect of this powerful local vasoconstrictor is proportional to its concentration and results from its vasoactivity.[21] This damage to tissue defenses mitigates against the use of epinephrine in potentially heavily contaminated wounds.

The majority of traumatic lacerations can be anesthetized by using infiltration anesthesia. The subcutaneous branches of the sensory nerves to the wound are anesthetized by injecting 1 percent lidocaine into intact skin at the periphery of the wound. Injections by inserting the needle through the cut edge of the wound may be less painful but will disseminate bacteria. In clean straight lacerations in children, however, the reduced pain outweighs the risk of infection. Pain of injection can also be reduced by employing a No. 27 or 29 needle rather than a larger gauge needle.

Regional nerve block is a valuable clinical tool, which permits better wound cleansing and more thorough debridement in the prevention of infection without danger of bacterial dissemination. Its clinical value is greatest when anesthetizing the palm and the sole, which are exquisitely sensitive to local infiltration.

HAIR REMOVAL

Shaving had become a routine part of preoperative preparation until it was clearly shown to increase wound infection rates (Chapter 20).[22] The increased incidence of infection after razor shaves is probably related to the trauma inflicted by the razor. A safety razor consists of a blade held in a fixed geometry by the head. The exposure of the blade with respect to the razor head is the most important determinant of the blade's performance. The exposure of the surgical prep razor blade is so great that the infundibulum of the hair follicle is transected, so that the wounded hair follicles provide access and substrate for bacteria. In addition, the impermeable corneal layer is damaged and the exudate provides a moist field for bacterial proliferation. Inoculation of shaved skin results in dermatitis. In contrast, skin shaved with a recessed blade is refractory to bacterial contamination.

On the basis of these findings, hair removal should be used only when that hair would substantially interfere with performance of the operation. In these cases, clipping the hair with scissors or shaving the skin with a razor containing a recessed blade is recommended.

ANTISEPSIS

The term antisepsis refers to the use of antimicrobial chemicals on human tissue, while disinfection applies to the use of these agents on inanimate objects. In addition to an antiseptic agent, surgical scrub solutions contain a detergent or surface active agent, which facilitates removal of the surface contaminants.

The clinical efficacy of an antiseptic agent can be evaluated by several parameters including: (1) the effect of storage, (2) its spectrum of activity, (3) its duration of antimicrobial activity, (4) the degree of local and systemic damage to the host, and (5) the influence of the carrier on the performance of the agent. First, if it is rapidly inactivated during storage, the antiseptic agent must be freshly prepared before each use. Second, the antiseptic agent should exhibit antimicrobial activity against a broad spectrum of organisms. If active against gram-positive organisms alone, topical treatment of contaminated tissue may result in a potentially harmful shift of the normal flora. The widespread use of antimicrobials that act only against gram-positive organisms is associated with a tremendous increase in infections caused by gram-negative organisms in hospitals. Third, the antimicrobial activity should be fast-acting and substantive. A substantive effect is due to the retention of the agent by binding to a tissue (eg, stratum corneum) after rinsing. The bound antiseptic agent limits the proliferation of the residual bacteria. Fourth, the degree to which the agent damages the host, both locally and systemically, must also be known. Finally, the influence of the vehicle or carrier (ie, surfactant or detergent) on the performance of the antiseptic agent is of great importance to the surgeon. The inactivation of cationic surface active agents by anionic surface agents is a case in point.

Not all antiseptic agents are used for the same purpose, nor should the requirements for their effectiveness be identical. Specific definitions for the antimicrobial product categories were established in a report by the advisory review panel on over-the-counter antimicrobial drug products for repeated daily use.[23] This report provides detailed information regarding patient preoperative skin preparations, hand washing, and surgical wound cleansers.

Patient Preoperative Skin Preparation

The ideal agent for preoperative skin disinfection must be a safe, fast-acting, broad-spectrum antimicrobial preparation which significantly reduces the number of microorganisms on intact skin, usually following a single application. The most commonly employed antimicrobial agents for wound cleansing are iodophors. These compounds are composed of complexes of iodine, which are more stable than iodine in aqueous solution. Iodine is recognized to be a broad-spectrum antimicrobial agent with activity against fungi, viruses, and gram-positive and gram-negative bacteria.

There are three general categories of iodophors in clinical use: (1) solubilized inorganic elemental iodine, such as tincture of iodine, (2) iodine complexed with various surfactant compounds, and (3) iodine complexed with different nonsurfactant compounds like polyvinylpyrrolidone (PVP). In tincture of iodine, all the iodine is in the free form and is available for instantaneous reaction with both bacteria and other proteinaceous material. If the iodine solution does not eliminate all the bacteria within these first few seconds, no further significant bacterial kill will be observed since there is no residual activity. This instantaneous availability of iodine accounts for the skin irritation occasionally encountered after topical treatment. The local toxicity necessitates limiting its use to painting intact skin at the operative site. It should not be used on open wounds.

Highly complexed iodine compounds are stable, do not stain, have no odor, and are considerably less irritating to tissues than tincture of iodine.[24] Although the level of free iodine is low, it is still highly effective in killing bacteria. On skin, such complexes release iodine slowly, resulting in prolonged activity (Fig. 22-5). Release of iodine occurs only when the steady level of free iodine is depleted by the reaction with the contaminating substance. The parameters of greatest importance to this reaction are concentration of surfactant, amount of iodine, concentration of iodide, and pH of the final solution.

In developing a highly complexed iodophor, the selection of the protein or surfactant to solubilize the iodine is critical. The use of Pluronic polyol F-68 has many distinct advantages. It is a nonionic surfactant without tissue toxicity. Stable soluble complexes with elemental iodine possess antimicrobicidal activity and the chemical structure of Pluronic polyol F-68 remains unchanged.

The most popular preoperative skin preparation agent is povidone iodine (PVP-I). Polyvinylpyrrolidone (PVP) reacts with iodine to form stable, nonreversible carbon-iodine bonds, the toxicity of which has not been determined. PVP, once used as a plasma expander, is incompletely excreted because molecular weight fractions of PVP greater than 40,000 daltons cannot be excreted. Several clinical reports have noted the formation of cutaneous lesions after the administration of PVP.[25,26] Because some of the commercially available PVP iodophors, like Betadine, do contain molecular weight fractions greater than 40,000, it would seem prudent to restrict their use to topical applications on intact skin. The evidence for possible tissue toxicity of PVP-I when used as a wound irrigant is discussed in a subsequent section.

Hand Washing

Hands are the leading vector of pathogenic bacteria to the wound. Hands can transmit an infective dose of bacteria during any patient care activity (shaving, marking, lifting) conducted before and after the operation or through punctured gloves during the procedure. Glove punctures are found after 5–60 percent of all operations.[27]

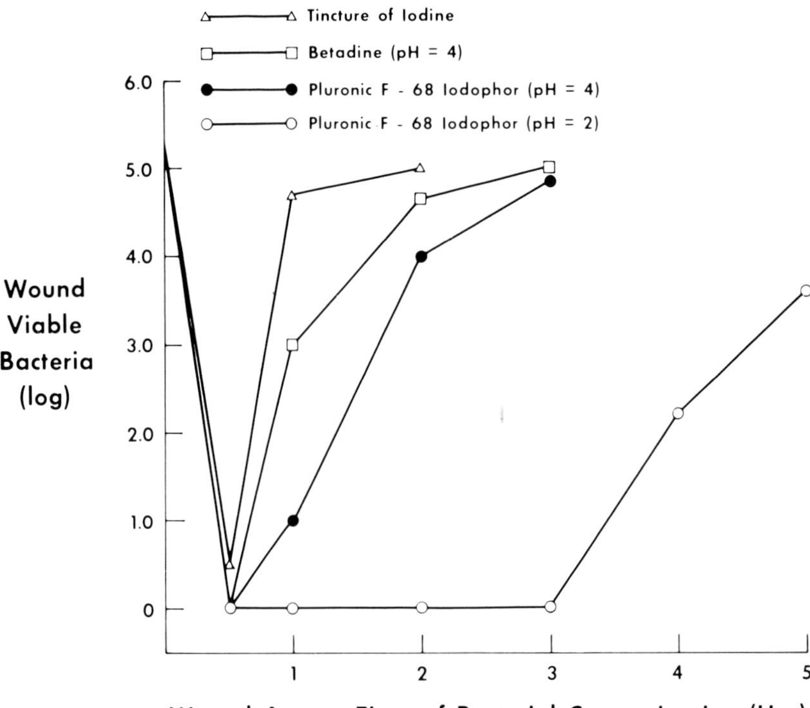

Fig. 22-5. **Antiseptic activity of iodine solutions in wounds. Standardized experimental wounds were subjected to a topical treatment with different antiseptic agents. At specified times after treatment, the wounds were subjected to repetitive bacterial challenges, after which the wound was recultured. The tincture and aqueous iodine solutions were inactivated within 60 minutes, thus losing their antibacterial activity. The antiseptic activity of Pluronic polyol F-68 iodophor persisted the longest.**

Normally, the organisms are quite sparse on the palms and dorsa of the hands, numbering in the hundreds per cm^2. The majority of organisms (10,000 to 100,000) on the hands reside beneath the distal end of the nail plate or adjacent to the proximal or lateral nail folds. These recesses frustrate efforts to disinfect the hands.

Before and after patient contact, hand washing is mandatory even though the risk of acquiring an infective dose of bacteria from patients during routine physical examination would seem to be negligible. Washing one's hands for 15 seconds with any of a variety of agents, including tap water, removes large numbers of bacteria and significantly reduces the bacterial count.[28] The hands should be rinsed and then dried. Because rings and chipped nail polish make removal of organisms more difficult,[29] operating room personnel should wear neither.

Repeated use of an antiseptic agent before and after patient contact appear to be unwarranted and may occasionally lead to the development of dermatitis.[30] Ordinary bar soap appears to be an excellent alternative to antiseptic agents for routine hand washing as long as the bars are small and kept on drainage racks between uses.

We favor antiseptic agents for special circumstances in which invasive procedures will be performed.[30] Hand washing with antiseptic agents should last at least 15 seconds, while surgical procedures require the greatest degree of hand antisepsis.

A variety of agents can be employed. Semmelweis in 1861 [31] decreased the incidence of puerperal fever by ordering the medical students to wash their hands in chlorinated lime. Lister degermed his hands in a 1:20 solution of carbolic acid. Until the 1950s, tincture of green soap followed by an alcohol rinse was used. Currently, three antiseptic agents have been advocated for hand washing before operation as well as preoperative patient skin preparation—hexachlorophene, iodophor, and chlorhexidine. Surgical scrubs of hands and forearms of adults, five times a day, with a 3 percent hexachlorophene preparation leaves blood levels of 0.5 mg per ml or higher in selected individuals after 10 days.[32] Because these levels are potentially toxic, hexachlorophene should not be used routinely by operating room personnel, and should be dispensed only by prescription. Fortunately, both other solutions appear to be safe.[33,34] Following hand wash with iodophor or chlorhexidine solutions, the bacterial counts of the skin are suppressed and the buildup of microbial counts under the occlusive surgical glove is limited. Neither agent is superior to the other.

The surgical hand wash should begin by cleaning the fingernails with a plastic stick. The hands should then be scrubbed with a sponge or brush for 5 minutes with a chlorhexidine or iodophor solution. The sponge causes less irritation to the skin.[35,36]

Dermatitis from any cause, including washing, results in a high concentration of skin bacteria.[37] Afflicted personnel who are members of the operating team should be limited to patient care not directly related to the operative procedure. During patient contact, personnel with dermatitis should wear gloves. The best treatment of this condition is to refrain from using an antiseptic agent or wearing gloves for longer than 5 minutes.

Skin Wound Cleansers

Skin wound cleansers are designed to aid in the removal of bacterial and other contaminants from superficial wounds, and may or may not contain an antimicrobial agent. While cleansing the wound, the agent must not damage the wound or systemic defenses, or deter healing.

Dilute solutions (1:750) of quaternary ammonium salts (quats) satisfy many of these requirements. These compounds are cationic surface-active agents, which are basically organically substituted ammonium compounds. Although they affect cell membrane potential, the consequences are clinically apparent only at concentrations higher than those recommended for clinical use.

Gram-positive microorganisms are generally more susceptible to quats than gram-negative bacteria. The gram-negative *Pseudomonas* species are usually resistant and even proliferate in the stored solution, accounting for occasional serious nosocomial outbreaks of gram-negative infection.

In contrast, the commercially available surgical scrub solutions containing iodophors and hexachlorophene are not safe for use in surgical wounds. These solutions contain toxic anionic detergents that damage the tissue defenses and potentiate the development of infection.[38] Until this observation was made, detergents and surfactants in surgical scrub solutions were considered by many to be innocuous ingredients.

Pluronic polyol F-68, a nonionic surfactant, is an excellent substitute for toxic detergents. It belongs to a family of surfactants made of a series of block copolymers with a water-soluble polyoxyethylene group at both ends of a water-insoluble polyoxypropylene chain.[39] It has a molecular weight of 8,350 and contains 80 percent ethylene oxide. Long-term toxicity studies in animals and people reveal it to be safe for intravenous use. Concentrated solutions containing as much as 40 percent Pluronic polyol F-68, when applied topically to the wound, do not damage resistance to infection. This surfactant also has negligible effect on bacterial viability. While Pluronic polyol F-68 has no intrinsic antibacterial activity, it forms stable soluble complexes with elemental iodine that possess antimicrobial capability,[24] but such complexes might be expected to release elemental iodine into wounded tissue and their local safety in open wounds needs to be determined.

Pluronic polyol F-68 has been approved by the Food and Drug Administration as a skin wound cleanser.[23] Unlike all other commercial scrub solutions, this surfactant is so innocuous that it "does not bring tears to a baby's eye." Patients with painful, partial-thickness burns, or abrasions washed with it find it soothing. In our emergency medical service, this agent has completely replaced all other surgical scrub solutions for use in traumatic wounds.

Topical iodophors, even without addition of a surfactant, would seem to be poor choices for skin wound antiseptics. Application over a large surface area often results in a substantial elevation of serum free-iodide.[40] Unexplained abnormalities have occurred in some patients, including renal failure, metabolic acidosis, and elevation of serum glutamic oxaloacetic transaminase. It is conceivable that large iodide loads were, at least in part, responsible for these abnormalities. Iodophors and many other antiseptics depend on an oxidative reaction between the antiseptic and the organism. But iodine reacts as easily with mammalian as bacterial cells and within seconds after instillation of a lethal dose of iodophor into the sterile peritoneal cavity, the titratable iodine is undetectable, having all reacted with the normal tissues.[41] In the heavily contaminated peritoneal cavity, bacterial counts are rapidly reduced by iodophors, but not all bacteria are killed.[42] The iodine can react with normal mesothelium and cause a chemical peritonitis, which is fatal in experimental animals even in the absence of bacteria. Repeated treatment of an open wound with this iodophor may delay healing.

Povidone-iodine is cytocidal to human neutrophils at commercially available concentrations (1 percent titratable iodine). Even dilutions of 1:100 result in irreversible loss of a neutrophil's ability to respond to chemotactic stimuli. Local antibiotics have a broad spectrum of activity without toxicity to mammalial tissue and continue to kill bacteria for prolonged periods. They appear to be safer agents for wound irrigation than most antiseptics.

Unaware of these potential toxic manifestations of PVP-I complexes, many surgeons have continued to apply these agents to contaminated wounds with surprisingly good results. Gilmore and Martin[43] have made well controlled studies of the efficacy of PVP-I powders in the treatment of contaminated wounds. In a series of 451 consecutive cases of appendectomy, topical PVP-I treatment reduced the wound infection rate and was found to be superior to an antiseptic spray. These beneficial effects of PVP-I in the treatment of contaminated wounds were later reported by Stokes and his associates[44] in a prospective randomized study of abdominal surgical patients. When topical prophylactic PVP-I was compared with topical cephaloridine in another series, however, antibiotic treated wounds escaped infection far more often than those treated with the antiseptic (Chapter 23).[44a]

SURGICAL DEBRIDEMENT

Debridement is probably the most important single factor in the management of the contaminated wound.[45] First, it removes tissue heavily contaminated by soil infection-potentiating factors and bacteria, protecting the patient from invasive infection. Second, it removes permanently devitalized soft tissues that, if left in a wound, would damage its defenses and encourage the development of infection.[46] The capacity of devitalized fat, muscle, and skin to enhance bacterial infection is comparable. The infection-potentiating effect of skin is further enhanced by exposing it to a dry thermal injury. This change in the capacity of skin to damage the wound's defenses may be related to the development of a burn toxin. This observation is consistent with the experimental findings of Allgöwer et al,[47] who identified a toxin in skin that was subjected to dry heat. This toxin appears to be generated by a polymeric dehydration of a substance(s) that occurs naturally in the skin.

There are at least three mechanisms by which devitalized soft tissue enhances infection: (1) it acts as a culture medium promoting bacterial growth, (2) it inhibits leukocyte phagocytosis and subsequent bacterial kill, and (3) the anaerobic environment within devitalized tissue must also limit leukocyte function. (At low oxygen tension, the killing of certain bacteria by leukocytes is impaired.[48]) While the need for debridement of devitalized tissue is undisputed, identification of the exact limits of devitalized tissue in wounds remains a challenging problem, especially in muscle. Traditionally, the viability of muscle is determined by its contractility, vascularity, color, and consistency. The best criterion is its capacity to contract after being stimulated,[49] but all clinical indicators are more accurate when the wound is examined 4 to 5 days after the initial operation.

The viability of skin is considerably easier to judge than that of muscle. At 24 hours after injury, a sharp line of demarcation is often apparent between the devitalized and viable skin. In fresh skin wounds in which this demarcation is not precise, the distribution of an intravenously injected fluorescein dye within the tissues may prove helpful.[50] Early staining of the injured tissue by fluorescein is evidence of tissue viability. At times, active bleeding from the distal dermal margin may be present and indicates viability.

In some anatomic sites, like the trunk, debridement is best accomplished by a more liberal excision of the skin and deep tissues. The soft tissue here is relatively free of tissues (eg, nerves or tendons) that perform important physical functions, and cosmetic considerations are less important.

The adequacy of debridement may be monitored by forcibly packing the wound with gauze or by coloring the wound surface with a vital dye. Flooding the field with a mixture of methylene blue and peroxide will encourage deep penetration of the dye into distant cavities. Complete excision of the wound, back to a margin of normal tissue, is judged by dissecting in a plane that will not expose the gauze or the blue dye. Suturing the skin edges of the wound prior to excision may further minimize mechanical spread of the wound contaminants into uninjured tissue.

When a heavily contaminated wound contains specialized tissues, such as nerves or tendons, complete excision is often not feasible. In such cases, high-pressure irrigation, followed by excision of all fragments of tissue that are not clearly viable, is indicated. In a compound wound of the hand, selective debridement of nonviable fascia, tendon, and fat is tedious but essential as the site constitutes a favorable environment for bacterial growth.

One must not debride certain specialized tissues that perform important physical functions, regardless of their viability.[51] Tissues like dura, fascia, and tendon may survive as free grafts without living cells if immediately covered by healthy pedicle flaps. If these tissues can be rendered surgically clean, they should be left in the wound. Retraction of the wound edges during debridement is best accomplished by hooks. Kocher clamps or bulldog forceps should contact the wound only when the piece of tissue grasped is destined to be removed. Similarly, compressive retractors should be avoided; for prolonged exposure of the wound, its edges can be retracted by stay sutures placed in the dermis.

Following debridement, the surgeon's ultimate selection of wound closure technique is dependent on the level of wound contamination and the amount of residual devitalized tissue (see subsequent section).

MECHANICAL CLEANSING

The surgeon commonly employs mechanical forces to rid the wound of surface bacteria and other particulate matter retained by adhesive forces. Because these forces must exceed the adhesive forces of the contaminants, the two basic modes used are hydraulic forces and direct contact.

In irrigation, the hydraulic forces of the irrigating stream act on particulate matter in the wound. The total force component exerted on the particle by the moving stream is defined as drag. The total drag due to the fluid pressure and stress is expressed by the following equation:

$$\text{Drag} = \text{CAp}\frac{V^2}{2}$$

where C is an experimentally derived drag coefficient dependent in part on the configuration of the particle; A is the projected area of the particle on a plane perpendicular to flow, p is the density of the fluid, and V is the relative velocity of the fluid with respect to the particle. It takes significantly smaller hydraulic pressures to rid the wound of large foreign bodies than it does to remove bacteria.

Irrigation will be most efficient if the velocity of the irrigating stream is raised by increasing the pressure and enlarging the internal diameter of the needle. The pressure exerted by fluid delivered through a 19 gauge needle by a 35 ml syringe is 8 psi.[52] Such high-pressure irrigation (≥8 psi) successfully cleanses the wound of small particulate matter, bacteria, and soil infection-potentiating factors, thereby reducing the infection rate of experimentally contaminated wounds (Fig. 22-6). In contrast, low-pressure syringe irrigation (as with a bulb syringe), even with large volumes of fluid, removes neither small nor large particulate matter.

Despite the advantages of high-pressure irrigation, several objections have been raised against its routine use. One commonly expressed concern is that foreign bodies on the surface of the wound may be disseminated more deeply into the wound as a result of high-pressure irrigation, although experimental studies indicate that this fear is unfounded.[53] Consequent to high-pressure irrigation, the bacteria remain at the surface of the wound even though the irrigant solution may disseminate deeply into the tissues. The tissue penetration of a high-pressure irrigating stream is predominantly lateral, similar to a jet parenteral injection.

The concern that high-pressure irrigation can damage tissue defenses, however, appears to be justified. Pulsatile or syringe irrigation results in trauma to the tissues, which makes the wound more susceptible to experimental infection. High-pressure irrigation, therefore, should not be performed indiscriminately but should be reserved for use in heavily contaminated wounds.

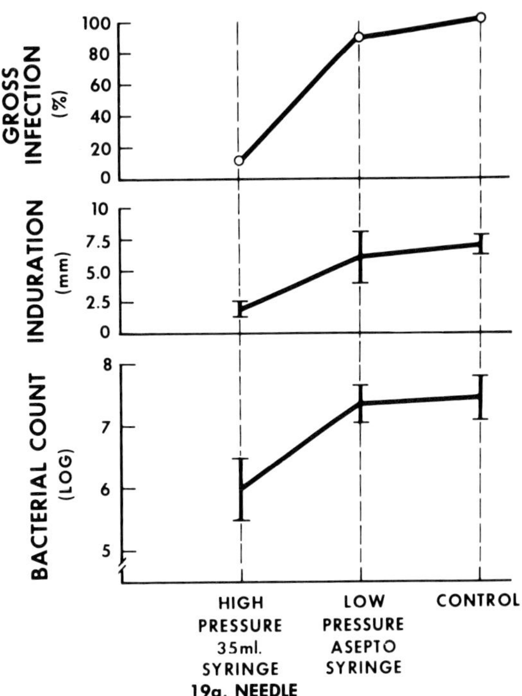

Fig. 22-6. **Effect of pressurized irrigation on experimental wound infection. Standardized contaminated wounds were subjected to either high- or low-pressure irrigation or no treatment prior to closure. Four days later, the inflammatory responses (gross infection, induration) of wounds subjected to high-pressure irrigation were significantly less than those of the control wounds or of wounds treated by low-pressure irrigation.**

In the clinical setting, high-pressure irrigation is accomplished with an inexpensive disposable irrigation assembly consisting of a 19-gauge plastic needle attached to a 35-ml syringe (Fig. 22-7). Sterile electrolyte solution (250 ml of 0.9 percent sodium chloride) is delivered through a one-way valve attached to the syringe barrel via standard intravenous plastic tubing. The tip of the needle, fastened to the syringe filled with saline, is placed perpendicular, and as close as possible, to the surface of the wound; then the surgeon exerts maximal force to the syringe plunger delivering the irrigant to the wound.

Another force to cleanse a wound is direct mechanical contact. An example is scrubbing a dirty wound with a sponge. Although this technique removes bacteria from wounds, it does not decrease the incidence of infection. Also, trauma to the tissue, inflicted by the sponge, impairs the wound's ability to resist infection and allows the residual bacteria to elicit an inflammatory response.[54] The magnitude of the damage to the local tissue resistance is correlated with the porosity of the sponge—the less porous sponges are more abrasive and cause more damage to the wound. The addition of a nontoxic surfactant, such as Pluronic polyol F-68, to a sponge minimizes the tissue damage it inflicts while maintaining the bacterial removal efficiency of mechanical cleansing. Consequently, the use of a surfactant-soaked sponge reduces the incidence of infection in contaminated wounds in experimental animals.

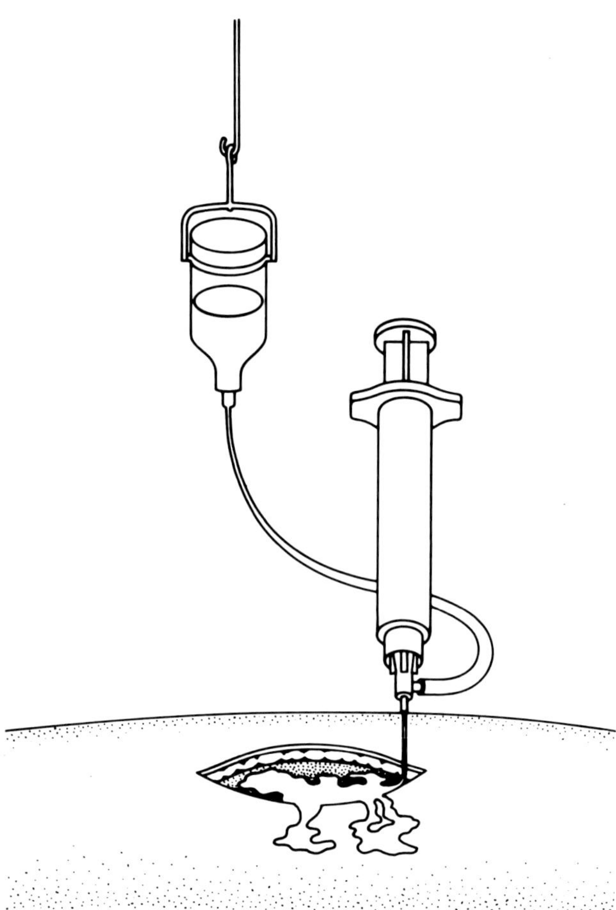

Fig. 22-7. **High-pressure syringe irrigation assembly. The needle is held as close as possible and perpendicular to the irrigated wound.**

ANTIBIOTICS

Systemic Administration of Antibiotics

The relative success of antibiotic therapy in the prevention of traumatic wound infection appears to be influenced by several factors. The timing of administration influences the success of such therapy. In laboratory and clinical studies, antibiotic therapy is significantly more effective when the drug is initiated preoperatively rather than at any other time. Delay consistently diminishes its therapeutic merit.

When there is an unavoidable delay, a sequence of events occurs that substantially limits the therapeutic value of antibiotics.[55] The wound capillaries become thrombosed, and antibiotics do not reach the wound bacteria. In addition, there is evidence that bacteria adhere to the resulting fibrinous coagulum so that they are isolated from contact with the antibiotic.[56] Paradoxically, the fibrinous wound coagulum which limits the effectiveness of antibiotics may be a crucial positive factor in the host's defense against infection. The coagulum may serve as a plug in the open mouths of lymphatics, preventing dissemination of bacteria. Occlusion of lymphatics by the coagulum then becomes an obstacle to the invasion of bacteria and accounts in part for the resistance of an open wound to systemic sepsis.

The surface coagulum may be disrupted by a variety of procedures. Gentle scrubbing of the surface of the wound with a gauze sponge allows an antibiotic to gain intimate contact with the bacteria.[57] Consequently, the therapeutic effectiveness of systemic antibiotics is measurably enhanced by this treatment. Enzymatic digestion is a less traumatic and more selective means of disrupting the coagulum.[58,59] The in vitro fibrinolytic capacity of certain enzymes provides an accurate measure of their ability to potentiate antimicrobial activity. Travase (a proteolytic enzyme produced by *B. subtilis,* the most potent fibrinolytic agent in vitro) is the most effective enzymatic adjunct to antibiotic treatment. Hydrolysis of the protein coagulum can be accomplished within 30 minutes by the topical application of an appropriate solution of this proteolytic enzyme. Such a brief exposure does not damage the wound's defenses or its healing capacity.

The bacterial count of the wound can influence the outcome of antibiotic treatment. When the wound is contaminated by exceedingly large numbers of organisms (greater than 10^9), infection will develop despite systemic antibiotic treatment (Fig. 22-8). This circumstance is encountered when the wound surface is contacted by either pus or feces.

The indications for systemic antibiotic treatment are dependent on the mechanisms of injury, the age of the wound, the total bacterial count, and the presence of soil infection-potentiating fractions. An antibiotic should be administered to all patients with impact injuries.[4] In these wounds, the weakened local tissue defenses make them susceptible to a relatively small inoculum of bacteria (10^4 per gram of tissue). It is fortuitous that systemically administered antibiotics can gain contact with pathogens in the ischemic tissue of impact injuries.

Another indication for antibiotic treatment is a laceration in which treatment has been delayed for 3 or more hours. During this time, bacteria can proliferate to a level that will result in infection. Concurrently, a thick fibrinous exudate appears on the wound surface, which becomes a protective barrier against topically or systemically administered antibiotics.

Antibiotic treatment is also mandatory in wounds containing pus, feces, saliva, or vaginal secretions. While antibiotic treatment significantly reduces these levels of heavy contamination, residual viable bacteria are often sufficient to elicit infection after primary closure. Consequently, open wound management of these heavily contaminated wounds should supplement antibiotic treatment.

The presence of soil infection-potentiating fractions in wounds also has considerable influence on the efficacy of specific antibiotics. The basic (eg, gentamicin) and amphoteric (eg, tetracycline) antibiotics are inactivated by these negatively charged fractions. The acidic antibiotics, like cephalosporins and penicillin, do not bind with these fractions and exert their antibacterial effect in contaminated wounds.

Finally, antibiotics must be administered to patients with wounds in which the magnitude of tissue injury is

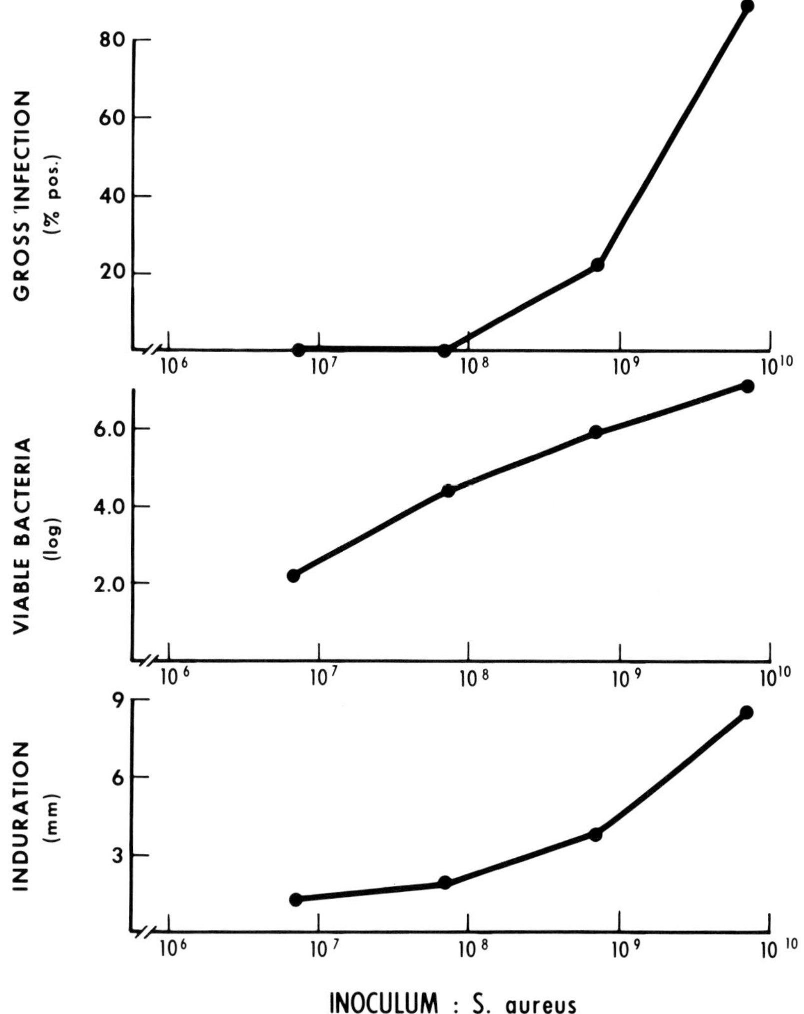

Fig. 22-8. **Effect of bacterial inoculum size on the efficacy of systemic antibiotics. Graded doses of a penicillin-sensitive strain of *S. aureus* were injected into the dermis of experimental animals. Immediately after inoculation, each animal received an intraperitoneal injection of benzylpenicillin (1,000,000 units). Four days later, the inflammatory responses of the wounds and their bacterial counts were measured. The therapeutic value of antibiotic treatment decreased as the dose of inocula increased.**

extensive and difficult to ascertain accurately soon after injury. In such cases, open management of the wound is the best treatment, with subsequent additional debridement, as dictated by its appearance. It must be emphasized that antibiotic therapy is an adjunct to debridement, not a replacement.

The immediate selection of the specific antimicrobial agent is based on consideration of the results of direct microscopic examination of a wound biopsy, the normal bacterial flora harbored in different parts of the body, and the pathogens usually encountered in various diseases or conditions. Later, the results of immediate antibiotic sensitivity testing can also influence the surgeon's choice of antibiotic. In our laboratory, antibiotic sensitivity testing is performed under aerobic conditions directly on the bacterial suspension prepared from the wound biopsy specimen rather than on strains isolated from the tissue.[60]

Performing the antibiotic sensitivity test directly on the tissue sample allows the surgeon to receive the test results 7 hours after submitting the specimen, rather than 38 to 52 hours later, as required with the conventional technique. Use of this modification does not alter most of the standards recommended by the Food and Drug Administration because there is no inclusive change in the medium, agar depth, or antibiotic sensitivity disc.[61]

Aliquots of the bacterial suspensions are streaked in three directions onto the surface of Mueller-Hinton agar plates (5 × 150 mm) using sterile cotton swabs. After a 3-minute delay, antibiotic discs are applied to the surface of the agar with an automatic dispenser and pressed onto the surface with sterile forceps. After incubation at 37C for 7 and 18 hours, the zone of inhibition around each disc is measured with a ruler. The zone diameters as recommended by the Food and Drug Administration are used to interpret the susceptibility of the bacteria to the antibiotic.

In clinical and experimental studies, the changes in the test necessitated by using the clinical suspension did not significantly alter the interpretation of the antibiotic susceptibility.[60] Even when larger numbers of bacteria (10^6 to 10^9) were present in the suspension, variation in the inoculum size did not appreciably change the results of the antibiotic susceptibility tests. Reducing the standard Kirby-Bauer antibiotic susceptibility test to 7 hours also did not limit accuracy.

As expected, the variable most difficult to standardize is the heterogeneous inoculum containing large numbers (10^7) of different organisms. A zone of inhibition interpreted as sensitive with one organism was occasionally masked by the presence of the confluent growth of another with a resistant zone of inhibition. We did not encounter the circumstances in which a number of sensitive species gave reactions interpreted as resistant when tested in combination. However, even in these cases it is possible that the results of mixed culture sensitivities may provide the most valid information for treating mixed infections, because they most closely simulate the clinical situation. The merit of direct antibiotic sensitivity testing of clinical specimens must await further experimental and clinical studies. The results of this proposed sensitivity test will have to show some correspondence with the clinical response to treatment.

DEAD SPACE

The importance of dead space in the potentiation of wound infection has long been recognized and can be demonstrated experimentally.[62,63] (See Fig. 22-9A).

Although dead space is bad, suture closure of dead space is worse (Fig. 22-9B).[62,63] The mechanism by which dead space potentiates the infectivity of a subinfective bacterial inoculum is not clear. One possibility is that even a bloodless exudate potentiates wound infection. Wood et al[64] demonstrated that phagocytosis of bacteria suspended in a fluid medium is difficult unless the bacteria have been opsonized. In the same way, Ahrenholz[65] demonstrated that sterile saline aggravated experimental peritonitis unless the bacteria were preopsonized. Alexander et al[66] have demonstrated that wound exudates are depleted of opsonins. Suspension of contaminating bacteria in opsonin-depleted exudate may well interfere with antibacterial phagocytosis. The presence of the suture material appears to potentiate the development of infection (Fig. 22-9C). The harmful effects of suture closure of dead space in experimental animals also occur in surgical incisions not involving muscle (Fig. 22-9D). Obliteration of the potential space between the cut edges of adipose tissue by sutures potentiated the incidence of infection.

These studies, combined with clinical observations, form the basis for the recommendation that suture closure of dead space should be avoided in contaminated wounds. Although dead spaces in wounds should definitely be avoided, the collapse of such space can be achieved by physiologic methods such as relaxing incisions, rotation of distal flaps, and splinting dressings that may provide gentle surface pressure. The closure of dead space by sutures produces localized areas of wound ischemia and necrosis, and the presence of additional suture material adds further danger of wound complication. Whether suction drainage will achieve the effect of obliterating dead space without realizing the known effect of drains to potentiate infection is unknown.[66]

SKIN WOUND CLOSURE

The technique of wound closure selected depends on the type of wound. There are essentially two types of wounds—either with or without a loss of tissue. In the latter, primary closure can be accomplished simply by reapproximating the divided wound edges. For wounds with associated tissue loss, grafts or flaps are often required to close the defect.

Timing of Skin Closure

The timing of the closure is also critical. A decision must be made as to whether the closure should be immediate or delayed. Immediate closure should be reserved for (1) wounds resulting from elective procedures classified as being either clean, refined-clean, or clean-contaminated, and (2) traumatic wounds that have not been contacted by feces, saliva, purulent exudate, or soil infection-potentiating fractions. Immediate approximation of the skin edges of this group of wounds should be accompanied by an extremely low infection rate (less than 5 percent, regardless of the closure technique employed). Highly contaminated wounds should be treated with delayed closure.

The fundamental bases for delayed closure are the experience of military surgeons,[67] who learned repeatedly over the centuries that immediate closure of battle wounds frequently resulted in infection. These wounds are best left open until delayed closure can be undertaken. All wounds resulting from high velocity missile injuries, regardless of their appearance, are also candidates for delayed primary closure. In such cases, the magnitude of residual devitalized tissue is more accurately ascertained 4 days after wounding. Wounds contacted by feces or saliva, as well as those in which treatment is delayed longer than 6 hours, should also be considered for open wound management. A delay longer than that is often associated with the development of infection. Quantitative bacterial counts on the wound edges can help make the decision.[16]

The rationale for delayed primary closure is that the healing open wound will gain resistance to infection and permit an uncomplicated closure (Fig. 22-10). The reparative process of open wounds associated with this developing resistance to infection in the open wound undergoing primary closure is associated with accelerated healing.

In a group of patients with contaminated battle wounds in Vietnam, Surgeon General Heaton reported an astoundingly low 2.5 percent incidence of infection.[67] Using experimental models, we have confirmed the superiority of delayed closure in the treatment of contaminated wounds.[68] The optimal time for closure of the contaminated wound is on, or after, the fourth postwounding day (Fig. 22-10).

Open wound management prior to delayed primary closure is accomplished by packing the wound with sterile fine meshed gauze (type I), which is then covered by sterile dressing. The wound should not be disturbed for the first 4 postoperative days unless the patient develops an unexplained fever. Unnecessary inspection during this period increases the risk of contamination and subsequent infection. On or after the fourth day, the wound margins can be approximated with minimal risk of infection. The selection of the technique for delayed primary closure will be based on the same considerations as used in primary closure. If percutaneous sutures are selected for wound closure, they should be passed through the wound edges at

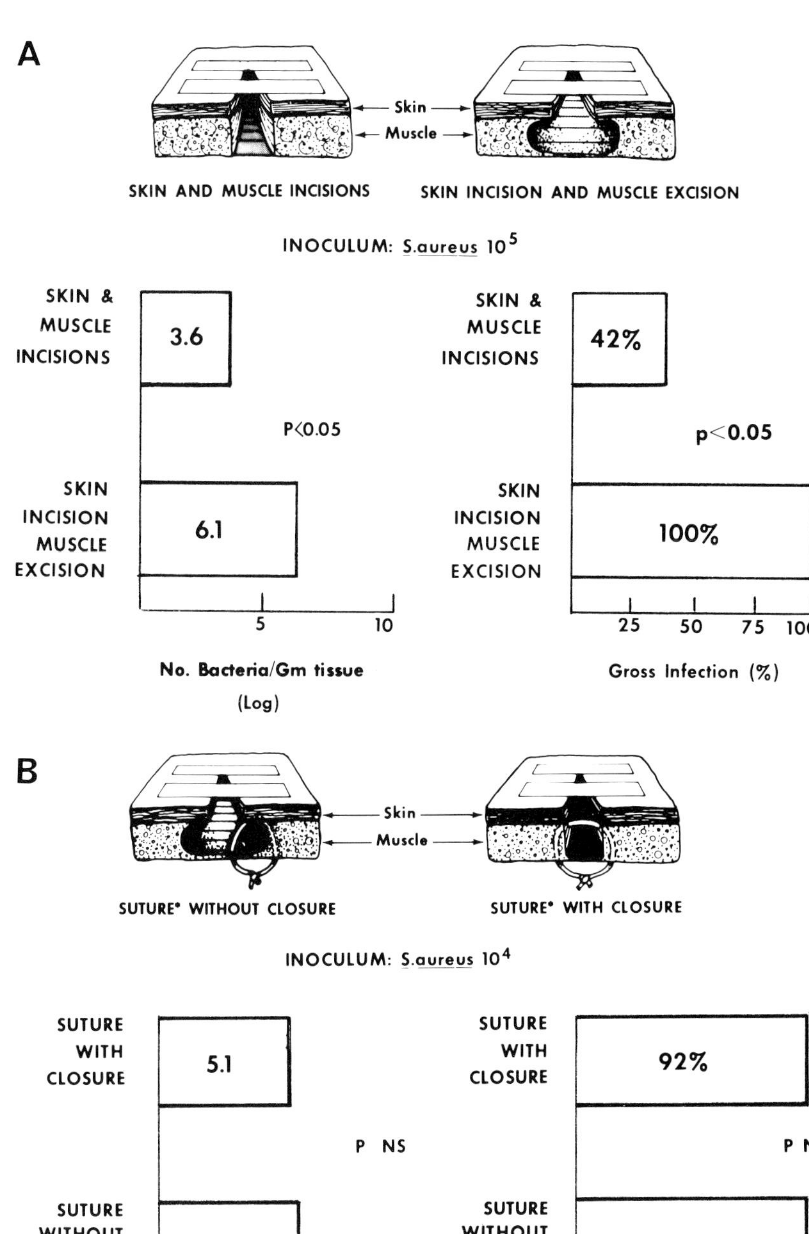

Fig. 22-9. **A. In experimental contaminated wounds, dead space was created by excising muscle adjacent to the wound edge. Four days later, the incidence of infection and the number of viable bacteria were significantly greater in wounds containing dead space than in wounds without muscle excision. B. Suture closure of the excised dead space did not eliminate the infection-potentiating effect of dead space. The infection rate of wounds and their viable bacteria following suture closure of dead space was comparable to that of wounds without dead space closure but containing the same quantity of suture.**

the end of the initial operation and left untied until the time of delayed primary closure. This step spares the patient an additional local or general anesthetic agent, which is required for sutural closure. The occasional wound that is destined to develop infection after delayed closure can be identified by using quantitative microbiology. When the bacterial count of the tissue is less than 10^5 organisms per gram of tissue, delayed closure can be accomplished without infection.[16] With the proven merit of open wound management, it is inconceivable that some surgeons resort to primary closure of contaminated and dirty wounds and risk life-threatening consequences.

Technique of Skin Wound Closure

There are several different methods to provide an accurate and secure approximation of the skin edges—tissue adhesives, sutures, tapes, or staples. Ideally, the choice should

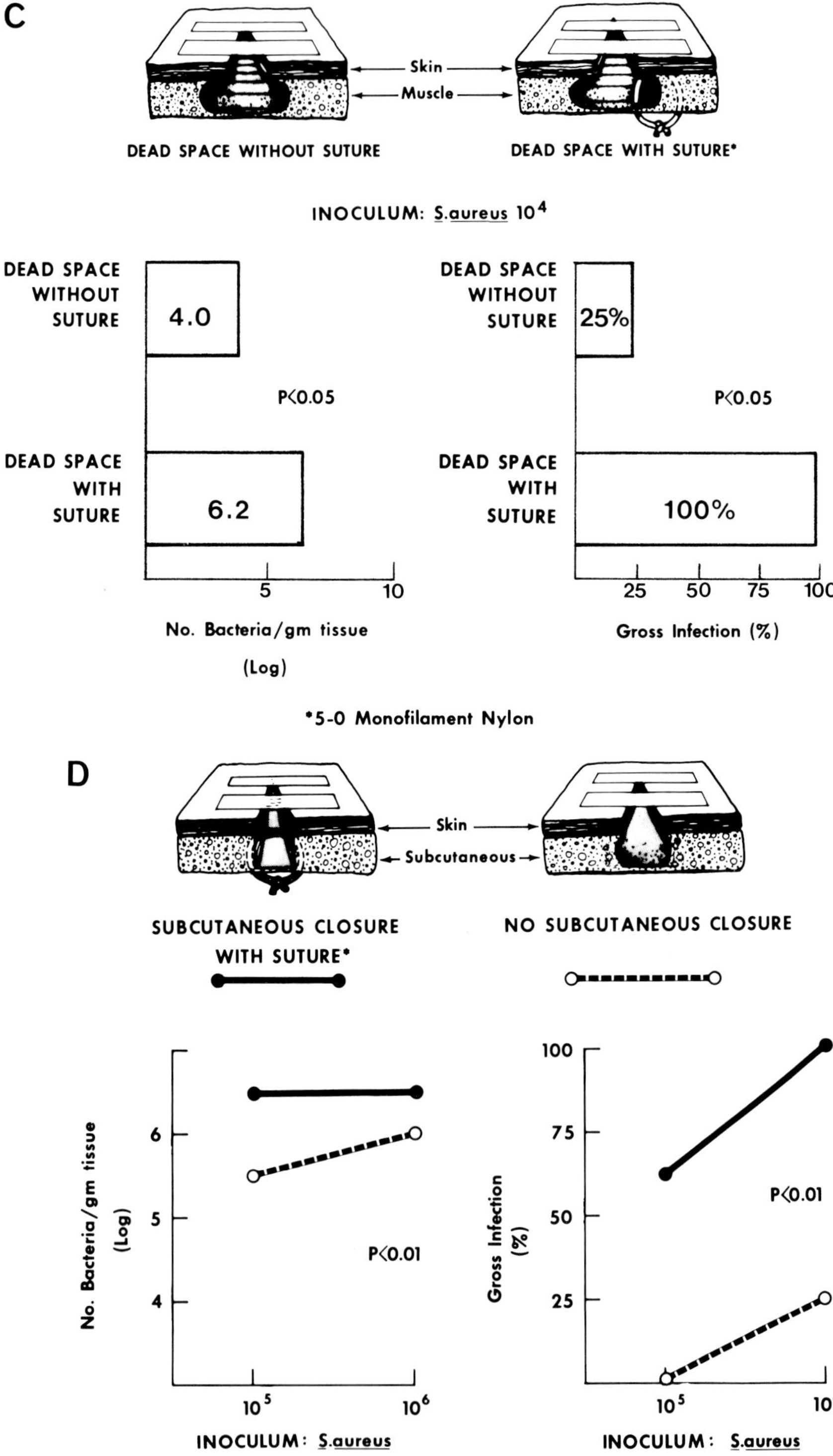

Fig. 22-9 (Cont.) C. The incidence of infection and level of bacterial contamination in wounds following suture closure of dead space was higher than that in wounds without dead space closure. D. The gross infection rate and the number of bacteria in taped skin wounds subjected to suture closure of subcutaneous tissue were higher than that in wounds without suture closure.

be based on the biologic interaction of the materials employed, the tissue configuration, and the biomechanical properties of the wound. The tissue should be held in apposition until the tensile strength of the wound is sufficient to withstand stress. A common theme of the few reportable investigations is that all biomaterials placed within the tissue damage the host defenses and invite infection.

Tissue Adhesives

Cyanoacrylate tissue adhesives have been advocated for repair of organs, or as hemostatic agents in emergency or mass combat casualty situations. Their use, however, is not indicated for skin closure.[69] The polymer acts as a barrier between the growing edges of the wound, which delays healing and increases susceptibility to infection.

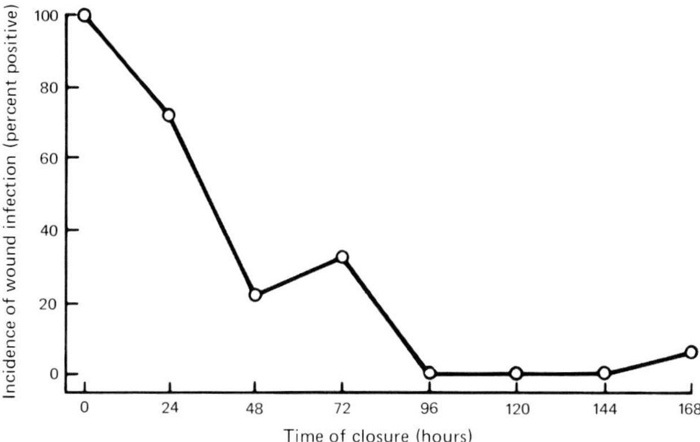

Fig 22-10. **Optimal time for delayed primary closure. Experimental wounds were contaminated with an infective dose of bacteria and closed immediately, or after a specified delay. Only delayed primary closure 96 hours (4 days) or more after wounding was associated with negligible infection.**

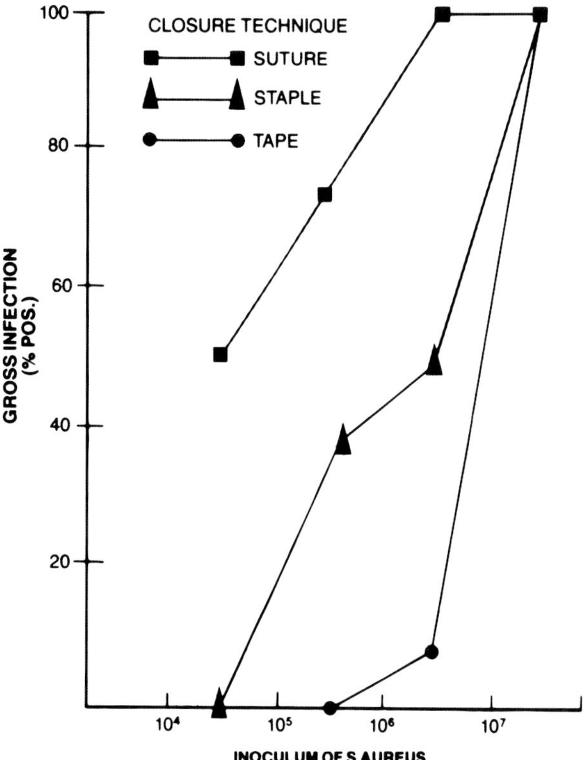

Fig. 22-11. **Effect of closure technique on wound infection. Standardized experimental wounds were subjected to graded doses of bacterial inocula prior to closure by either tape skin closures, staples, or nylon sutures. Four days later, the taped wounds displayed the least infection followed by stapled wounds and then the sutured wounds.**

Clips and Staples

Metal clips have been used for closure of skin wounds for many years, primarily for the head and neck. While skin clips are rapidly applied, wounds closed with clips are significantly weaker, have a lower modulus of elasticity, and are able to absorb less energy than similar wounds closed with monofilament nylon sutures in the same animal.[70]

Skin closure can be accomplished quickly and economically with disposable stapling devices. Furthermore, staples show a low level of tissue reactivity, and stapled skin wounds are more resistant to infection than the least reactive suture, monofilament nylon (Fig. 22-11). Wounds approximated by tape skin closure still demonstrated a superior resistance to infection when compared to the stapled wounds.

Sutures

Sutures remain the most common method of approximating the divided edges of skin. Selection of a suture material is based on its biologic interaction with the wound as well as its mechanical performance in vivo and in vitro.

Measurements of the in vivo degradation of sutures separate them into two general classes.[71] Sutures that undergo rapid degradation in tissues, losing their tensile strength within 60 days, are considered absorbable sutures. Those that maintain their tensile strength for longer than 60 days are called nonabsorbable sutures. This terminology is somewhat misleading, because even nonabsorbable sutures (eg, silk, cotton, and nylon) lose their tensile strength rapidly after the second month and by the sixth month have either disintegrated or are so weak they have little or no effect in reinforcing the tissue.

The absorbable sutures are gut (derived from sheep submucosa or beef serosa) and the synthetics , polyglycolic acid (PGA) and polyglactin (a copolymer of glycolide and lactide). Treatment of gut with chromium salts, a cross-linking agent, prolongs retention of the suture's tensile strength and increases its resistance to absorption by enzymatic action of the body.

The nonabsorbable sutures are classified according to their origin: natural (silk, cotton, and linen), metallic (stainless steel), and synthetic (nylon, Dacron, polyethylene, polypropylene). Sutures may also be characterized by their physical configuration. Those constructed from one filament are called monofilament. Multiple fibers braided together are called multifilament sutures. Only nylon and stainless steel sutures are available in both monofilament and multifilament constructions; all others are available in only one physical configuration.

All sutures damage the local tissue defenses to infection, and several mechanisms are implicated:

1. The trauma of inserting a needle is sufficient to cause an inflammatory response.

2. The surgeon's suturing technique is crucially important. Sutures tied too tightly impair blood and cause tissue necrosis.[72]

3. Sutures that penetrate the intact skin provide an avenue for wound contamination via the perisutural cuff.

4. The presence of the suture material itself increases the tissue's susceptibility to infection. The magnitude of this local injury to defenses is related to the quantity of suture within the wound (eg, diameter, length) and to its chemical composition.

The infection-potentiating effects of suture materials are listed in Table 22-2. Polyglycolic and polyglactin sutures elicit the least inflammatory response of the absorbable sutures, followed by plain gut and then chromic gut.

TABLE 22-2. EFFECT OF CHEMICAL COMPOSITION ON INFECTION-POTENTIATING EFFECT OF SURGICAL SUTURES *

Absorbable	Nonabsorbable
Polyglycolic = polyglactin =	Nylon = polypropylene
Plain gut	Dacron (coated = noncoated)
Chromic gut	Metal
	Silk = cotton

* The least reactive sutures are listed first.

Of the nonabsorbable sutures, nylon and polypropylene are the least reactive.

The relatively high infection rates encountered with either monofilament or multifilament stainless steel sutures may be the result of their chemical or physical configuration. Stainless steel is not generally as inert as pure polymers and undergoes degradation in vivo. In addition, metallic sutures are so stiff that movement induces tissue damage and impairs the wound's ability to resist infection.

Sutures made of natural fibers potentiate infection more than any other nonabsorbable sutures, which correlates with the tissue's reaction to these sutures in clean wounds.[73] It would appear from these experimental studies that the use of silk and cotton should be avoided in wounds having known gross bacterial contamination.

Surprisingly, our studies indicate that the physical configuration of the suture has a relatively unimportant role in the development of infection. Although the incidence of infection in contaminated tissue containing monofilament sutures was lower than in those containing multifilament sutures, these differences were not statistically significant.

It is relevant to give some thought to proper selection and placement of sutures because failure of the suture itself, or the tissue through which it passes, will permit the wound to reopen. An extensive series of recent investigations that reevaluate suture-tying techniques should be consulted.[74-76]

In general, the techniques of sutural closure of skin can be divided into two types: percutaneous sutures and dermal (subcuticular) sutures. The selection of the technique for closure is influenced by the wound's configuration and biochemical properties as well as other special circumstances.

Percutaneous sutures of monofilament nylon or polypropylene are excellent for the immediate closure of clean, refined-clean, and clean-contaminated skin wounds. These suture materials exert the least damage to the wound's defenses and can elongate without breaking during the postoperative period when there is considerable swelling of the wound edges.[76] Sutures with less extensibility like polyester or silk will frequently lacerate or necrose the encircled tissue, thereby increasing susceptibility to infection. Percutaneous sutures must be removed before the eighth postwounding day to prevent the development of needle puncture scars. Immediately thereafter, the wound edges should be reinforced with tape skin closures to prevent wound dehiscence. During approximation of the wound, the skin edges should not be grasped or crushed.

Dermal sutures can be used alone or as an adjunct to the percutaneous sutures in lacerations subjected to high skin tensions, to serve as an added precaution against disruption of the wound. Because the magnitude of the suture's damage to the local tissue defenses is related to the quantity of the suture within the wound (eg, diameter, length) we use the most narrow-diameter suture (5–0 or 6–0) whose strength is sufficient to resist disruption of the skin wound. Dermal sutures do not improve the cosmetic appearance of the scar.[77]

In special circumstances, percutaneous sutures should be totally avoided in favor of a continuous dermal suture: (1) in infants frightened at the prospects of suture removal, (2) when follow-up appointments are difficult to keep, (3) when wounds are covered by casts, and (4) in patients prone to the development of keloids. When dermal closure alone is used, it is advisable to immediately apply tape skin closures to the wound edges to provide a more accurate approximation of the epidermis.

The most severe limitation of dermal skin closure is that it potentiates the susceptibility to infection in clean-contaminated and contaminated wounds more than do percutaneous sutures.[78] This increased rate appears to be related to the large quantity of suture material required for a continuous dermal skin closure. After infection develops, the collecting purulent exudate spreads preferentially between the divided edges of fat rather than penetrating the tightly sutured skin edges. By the time the infection becomes clinically apparent, it has involved the entire extent of the wound. This circumstance is distinct from the localized collections of purulent discharge encountered in infected taped closed wounds. In the latter instances, the purulent discharge first exits between its wound edges before spreading between the divided layers of adipose tissue.

Tape Skin Closure

Taped wounds demonstrate far superior resistance to infection when compared to sutured wounds.[79] The ease with which wounds can be closed by tape varies according to the anatomic and biomechanical properties of the wound site. Linear wounds in skin subjected to minimal static and dynamic tensions are easily approximated by tape. The relatively lax skin of the face and abdomen makes it amenable to wound closure by tapes. Contrary to the usual expectation, approximation and eversion of skin edges with tape is easily accomplished in obese patients. The taut skin of the extremities, subjected to frequent dynamic joint movements, requires that tape skin closures be supplemented with dermal sutures. The copious secretions from the skin of the axilla, palms, and soles also discourage tape adherence.

There are numerous advantages to tape closure at linear wounds subjected to weak skin tensions: (1) the cosmetic results are excellent, (2) the discomfort of suture removal is avoided, (3) suture puncture scars are eliminated, and (4) no local anesthetic agent is required for suturing. This closure technique is being used on approximately 10 percent of the patients with lacerations seen in our emergency medical service.

During the last decade, a new sterile, reinforced surgical tape with an aggressive adhesive has been specifically developed for wound closure.

Even this new tape will not adhere to excessively wet skin. An adhesive adjunct such as compound benzoin tincture if applied to the skin prior to tape application reduces the chance for dislodgement. Inadvertent spillage of this adjunct will impair the wound's ability to resist infection.[80] To minimize the chance of contamination, the adhesive adjunct is applied with applicator sticks in a thin film at the wound edge.

WOUND DRAINAGE

Use of surgical drainage requires a delicate weighing of potential benefits and harmful effects. The obvious beneficial effect of drainage is its ability to evacuate or at least provide tracts for the elimination of potentially harmful collections of certain fluids like pus, blood, bile, gastric and pancreatic juices from wounds or body cavities. Pus is detrimental to the healing of wounds. Even sterile pus injected under the skin impairs healing of a distant wound.[81,82] Smith and Enquist[83] reported that subacute experimental staphylococcal wound infection in animals initiated profound gross, histologic, and biochemical changes in local and distant tissue. Pus within a wound or body cavity exerts many deleterious effects on the host and should be removed whenever a localized collection can be drained.

Sterile collections of blood per se are not major irritants to tissues, but hematomas enhance bacterial virulence.[84,85] Krizek and Davis[85] found that when red blood cells were injected into the same subcutaneous tissue site as *E. coli*, a fatal infection often occurred, whereas the injection of bacteria alone was relatively innocuous. The precise mechanisms are unknown, but crude hemoglobin preparations impair leukocyte function[86] and hemoglobin may provide iron essential for bacterial proliferation.[84]

Fibrin clot has a paradoxical role in tissue infection, preventing the systemic dissemination of wound bacteria, on the one hand, and isolating it from phagocytic defense mechanisms, on the other. A case can be made for the use of drains to eliminate some collections, but in instances where no definite localized collection of fluid exists, drainage must be considered prophylactic. In these circumstances, its potentially harmful effects become more important. Drains act as retrograde conduits through which skin contaminants gain entrance into the wound. Cerise et al[87] performed a splenectomy in rabbits and innoculated the skin around the drain tract with type 6 *Streptococcus*, taking care not to innoculate the drain. Twenty percent of the animals had positive intraperitoneal cultures at 24 hours, and 56 percent at 72 hours, compared to positive culture results in only 5 percent of the undrained animals.

Nora et al[88] performed laparotomies in dogs and inserted Penrose drains separately into the splenic fossa and in Morison's pouch. Gross intra-abdominal infection was detected in nine of the ten dogs with drains in the splenic fossa. No infections occurred in the undrained dogs. In a clinical study, the same investigators detected skin contaminants on the intra-abdominal portion of drainage tubes in 17 of 50 patients. *S. epidermis*, a skin contaminant, was found in 14 of the 17 cases. Of the 17 infected patients, 12 had minimal egress of fluid from the drain tract, and neither the gastrointestinal nor genitourinary tract had been opened at operation. Morris[89] showed significantly less infection when closed suction was used in 53 patients undergoing radical mastectomy, as compared to the use of standard Penrose drainage—retrograde contamination might be minimized by the use of a closed suction system. Meticulous postoperative aseptic care of the skin at the drain exit has much to do with low infection rates.

The air vent within a sump tube provides another potential conduit for organisms. Baker and Borchardt[90] demonstrated that the degree of contamination is proportional to the degree of suction used. When continuous suction is employed at 10 psi, airborne contamination occurs, but it can be eliminated by lowering the vacuum pressure attached to the suction. Plugging the vents with cotton or gauze, and using a synthetic air filter, provide the same benefit.

The presence of drains impairs the resistance of tissues to infection. Drains placed within experimental wounds exposed to subinfective innoculations of bacteria enhanced the rate of wound infection (Fig. 22-12A).[91] Both silastic and Penrose drains dramatically enhance the infection rate of soft tissue wounds in guinea pigs. The rate of infection when the drain was brought out through the wound was similar to the rate when the drain lay entirely within the wound, suggesting a deleterious effect of the drain (Fig. 22-12B).

Studies of the impairment of wound healing in the presence of drains have been performed with intestinal anastomoses. Berliner et al[92] performed proximal and distal intestinal anastomoses in dogs, draining one anastomosis in each dog. Three of the 20 undrained anastomoses leaked compared to 11 of 20 drained anastomoses; of these 11, anastomotic disruption proved fatal in four cases. Manz et al[93] confirmed the damaging effects of drains on colonic anastomoses in dogs. Of 20 dogs with Penrose drainage at their anastomoses, nine died of anastomotic disruption and peritonitis, and the remainder had extensive adhesions, as well as varying degrees of stricture formation. All dogs with drainage had evidence of bacterial contamination at the site of the anastomosis; the control animals had only filmy adhesions and no stricture formation.

It has been postulated that an adjacent drain may block the desquamated mesothelial cells from contacting the anastomosis, thereby interfering with its healing. The drain may also act as a retrograde conduit for bacteria that then contaminate the anastomotic site, thereby predisposing to infection and leakage.

POSTOPERATIVE WOUND CARE

Postoperative wound care should optimize healing and should be tailored to the type of wound. Unfortunately, a 10-minute discussion of technical aspects of postoperative care should probably include 9 minutes of silence, because the literature dealing with this aspect of wound management deals more with testimonials than with scientific fact.

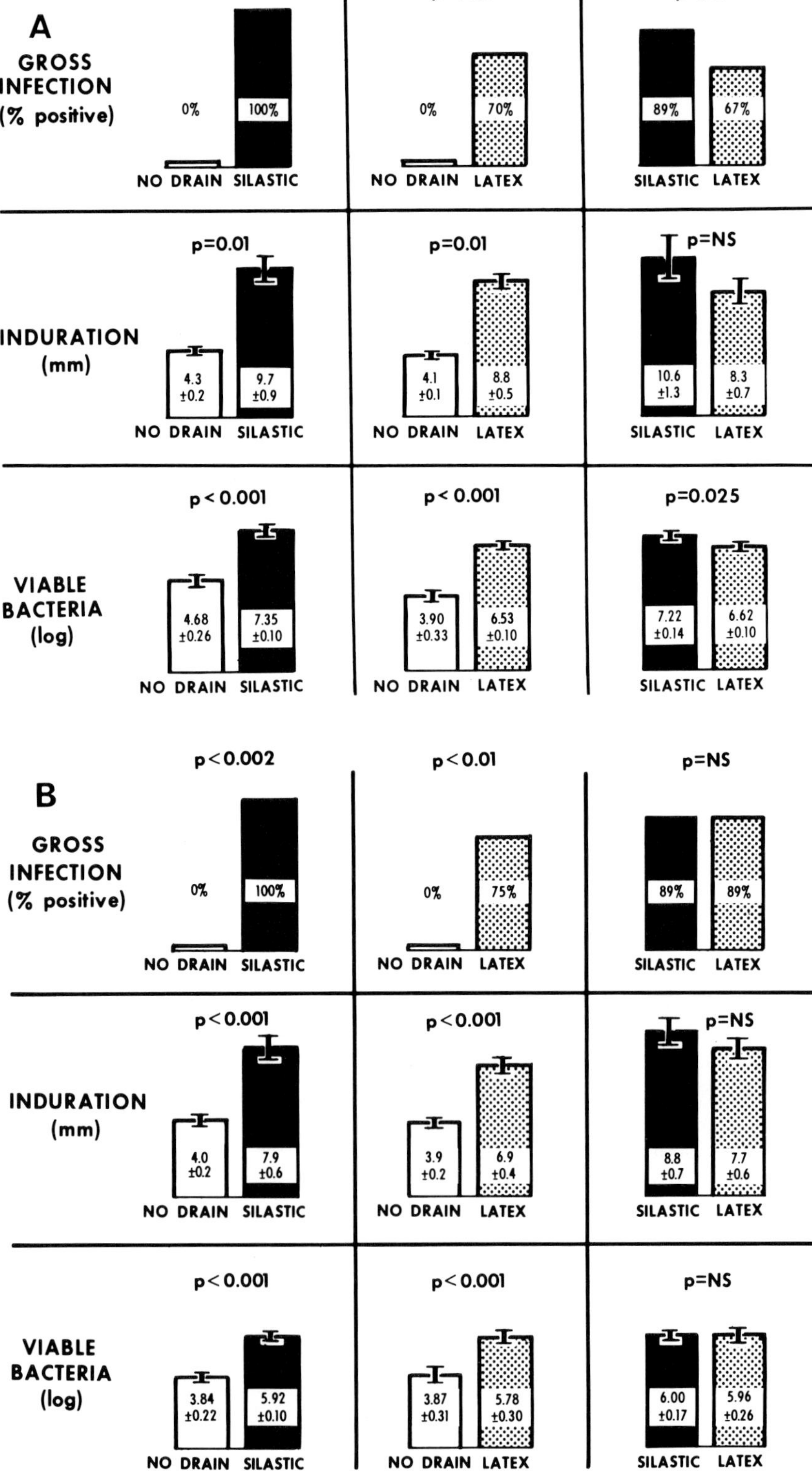

Fig. 22-12. **A. Influence of surgical drains on postoperative infection. Experimental wounds were contaminated with subinfective doses of *S. aureus.* Prior to closure, drains were placed in the wounds and allowed to exit between the wound edges. In contralateral wounds, closure was accomplished without drains. Four days later, the inflammatory responses and bacterial counts of wounds containing drains were significantly greater than those without drains. B. Influence of drain material on wound infection. The deleterious effect of drains was related to the presence of the foreign body. When drain material was placed entirely within a closed wound, its inflammatory response and bacterial count remained significantly higher than a wound closed without a drain.**

Wound Dressings (Table 22-3)

The manner in which a dressing functions is determined by its physical and chemical composition.[94] There are eight types of absorbent cotton gauze, each type defined by the number of warp and woof threads per square inch. The degree of dressing adherence to a wound is directly related to the size of dressing interstices.[95] The larger the interstice size, the greater the chance that the dressing will be penetrated by the granulation tissue. If debridement is the objective, the surgeon should use the dressing with greater interstice size, at least larger than type I. Absorption of wound exudates is another important function of a dressing. The beneficial effects of absorbency

TABLE 22-3. TYPES OF GAUZE DRESSINGS

Type	Threads per Inch²	
	Warp	Woof
I	41–47	33–39
II	30–34	26–30
III	26–30	22–26
IV	22–26	18–22
V	20–24	16–20
VI	18–22	14–18
VII	18–22	10–14
VIII	12–16	8–12

are: (1) the bacteria contained within the absorbed fluid are removed, (2) the exudate itself is removed, depleting the wound of bacterial nutrients, and (3) tissue maceration is prevented. Absorption is due to the capillary forces of attraction exerted by the capillary spaces between the dressing fibers. The magnitude of the capillary forces depends on the surface tension of the aqueous solution, as well as the chemical bonds that form between the molecules of the exudate and dressing. The rate and amount of fluid absorbed are easily measurable parameters of the absorbency of a dressing. The sinking test described in the British Pharmaceutical Code is a standardized measurement, which records the rate of absorbency of dressings. High absorbency is incompatible with nonadhesion because the serous exudate forms a powerful and coherent glue as it dries. Removal of the absorbent dressing disrupts the fibrinous scab and any granulation tissue that has become entrapped in the dressing. Absorbent dressings are therefore useful for the debridement of open wounds.

In primarily closed wounds, the surgical dressing acts as a barrier against exogenous bacteria. Soaking dressings with serum permits passage of bacteria through the dressing.[96,97] Saturation of a dressing with fluid, which wets both inner and outer surfaces of the dressing, is called fluid strike-through. As long as its outer surface remains dry, however, a dressing will remain an effective barrier to bacterial contamination.

The length of time that dry dressings should cover the closed wound is based on knowledge of the period during which the wound is susceptible to bacterial penetration. Warren [98] reports that the wound edges seal rapidly with a coagulum, thereby eliminating the need for dressings on primarily closed wounds. Other surgeons recommend that the dressing remain undisturbed, as long as it is dry, until the sutures or staples are ready for removal.

Sutured wounds, as they heal, become increasingly resistant to the development of infection following surface contamination.[99] Swabbing the surface of the wound with either *S. aureus* or *E. coli* during the first 48 hours after closure caused localized gross infections. Contamination after the third postoperative day did not produce gross infection in the sutured wound. Thus barrier dressings are useful to protect the fresh incision from surface contamination in the first few days. Thereafter, removal of the dressing permits daily inspection and palpation of the wound.

Wounds closed with tape have a greater capacity to resist infection than do sutured wounds. Even immediate contamination seldom caused infection in any taped wounds. This resistance to infection of taped wounds after surface contamination reduces the need for protective dressings during the postoperative period in wounds free of sutures. In a real sense, the skin suture has the objectionable features of a small drain.

Another important purpose of some dressings is to exert pressure on the underlying tissues. A pressure dressing minimizes the accumulation of the intercellular fluid and limits the dead space. The application of pressure dressings is easiest on convex surfaces (ie, skull, extremity). Maximal pressure should be applied to the wound site, as well as distal to it. Proximal to the wound, the pressure applied is decreased to minimize any chance of compromising the venous or lymphatic return.

Immobilization

A pressure dressing, by the very nature of its bulk, will immobilize what it covers. Immobilization of the site of injury is of great value—lymphatic flow is reduced, thereby minimizing the spread of the wound microflora. Furthermore, immobilized tissue demonstrates the best resistance to the growth of bacteria.[100] Whenever possible, the site of injury should be elevated above the patient's heart, to limit the accumulation of fluid in the wound interstitial spaces.

Most importantly, dressings must provide a physiologic environment that is conducive to epithelial migration from the wound edges across the surface of the fresh wound. When an area of epidermis is lost, water vapor begins at once to evaporate from the exposed dermal tissue. The exudate on the surface dries and becomes the outer layer of the scab, which does not prevent water from evaporating from the dermis underneath. The surface of the dermis itself progressively dries (within 18 hours). This dry scab and dried dermis resist migration of epidermal cells, which must seek the underlying fibrous tissue of the upper reticular layer of dermis where enough moisture remains to support cellular viability.[101]

When the wound is covered by a dressing that prevents or delays evaporation of water from the wound surface, the scab and underlying dermis remain moist. Epidermal cells can easily migrate through the moist scab over the surface of the dermis. Under such dressings, epithelialization is more rapid, and no dry dermis is sacrificed.

The totally occlusive dressing would seem to be ideal for coverage of primarily closed wounds, and has been usefully employed in the treatment of donor sites, mesh grafts, and dermabraded skin.[102] Unfortunately, excessive exudate may make it difficult to keep the fully occlusive dressing in place, and the moist exudate, which provides an ideal medium for epidermal repair, is also a suitable culture medium for the multiplication of microorganisms. Consequently, Scales [94] suggested that an ideal wound dressing would be a compromise between occlusion and nonocclusion.

Many dressings are commercially available for wound coverage. Unfortunately, their performance has not been documented by scientific studies, so that selection must be based on testimonials. In our clinical service, primarily closed wounds (with the exception of those located on the face) are covered by nonwoven microporous polypropylene dressings, which are attached to surrounding skin by wide strips of microporous tape with no reinforcing fibers.

In facial lacerations the development of blood clots between the edges of the sutured wounds are of more concern than the potential dangers of surface contamination. These clots will be replaced by a healing scar that can be easily avoided by swabbing the wound with half-strength hydrogen peroxide every six hours until the wound edge is free of blood. The sutures will lose their color and can be easily removed before the eighth day after closure.

In abraided skin this method of suture line care is ineffective. Despite washing the wound with hydrogen peroxide, a scab develops which makes suture removal tedious and often painful to the patient. In such cases, we swab the wound and its adjacent edges with a water soluble ointment, such as polyethylene glycol, which becomes dissolved by wound exudates, thereby encouraging their exodus from the wound. These sutures also must be removed before the eighth postoperative day because needle puncture scars can develop. The wound edges then should be supported by sterile, reinforced, microporous tape skin closures until their adhesive bond weakens.

A whole new host of synthetic dressing materials are now available. Op-site is an adhesive drape that is based upon either Hydron (polyhydroxyethylmethacrylate) or an elastomeric polyurethane with an adhesive backing for attachment to the adjacent dry skin.[103] Because of its hydrophilic nature, it is permeable to water vapor, making it suitable for use on abrasions and donor sites. Op-site is impermeable to bacteria and thereby prevents exogenous contamination. Unfortunately, the water vapor permeability rate is low and fluid build-up beneath the dressing can eventually cause wound maceration and detachment of the dressing.[104,105] A more permeable film with similar mechanical characteristics would be of interest to the surgeon.

Polyhydroxyethylmethacrylate has also been incorporated into a two-component system with a solvent, polyethylene glycol 400 (PEG) to form a spray-on gel.[106] The dressing is built up in two to three layers, and after application, the "polymer-solvent" mixture takes about 30 minutes to form a solid film. It attaches directly to the wound and follows its surface contours. A shortcoming is that movement results in cracking of the dressing. This disadvantage may be obviated by other systems, such as the Pluronic range of copolymers.[107] A particular form of this polymer can form a gel, which follows all the contours of the body, enclosing it from the environment.

BIBLIOGRAPHY

Edlich RF, Rodeheaver GT, Thacker JG, Edgerton MT: Fundamentals of Wound Management in Surgery: Technical Factors in Wound Management. South Plainfield, New Jersey, Chirurgecom, 1977.

Cruse PJE, Foord R: A five-year prospective study of 23,649 surgical wounds. Arch Surg 107:206, 1973.

Hunt TK: Wound Healing and Wound Infection: Theory and Surgical Practice. New York, Appleton-Century-Crofts, 1980.

Hunt TK, Dunphy JE: Fundamentals of Wound Management. New York, Appleton-Century-Crofts, 1979.

Peacock EE, Van Winkle W: Repair of skin wounds. In Surgery and Biology of Wound Repair. Philadelphia, Saunders, 1970.

REFERENCES

MECHANISM OF INJURY

1. Edlich RF, Rodeheaver GT, Thacker JG, Edgerton MT: Fundamentals of Wound Management in Surgery: Technical Factors in Wound Management. South Plainfield, New Jersey, Chirurgecom, 1977.
2. Jacobs HB: Skin knife-deep knife: the ritual and practice of skin incisions. Ann Surg 179:102, 1974.
3. Roettinger W, Edgerton MT, Kurtz LD, Prusak M, Edlich RF: Role of inoculation site as a determinant of infection in soft tissue wounds. Am J Surg 126:354, 1973.
4. Cardany CR, Rodeheaver GT, Thacker JG, Edgerton MT, Edlich RF: The crush injury: a high risk wound. J Am Coll Emerg Phys 5:965, 1976.
5. Charters AC III, Charters AC: Wounding mechanism of very high velocity projectiles. J Trauma 16:464, 1976.
6. Amato JJ, Billy LT, Lawson NS, Rich NM: High velocity missile injury: an experimental study of the retentive forces of tissue. Am J Surg 127:454, 1974.
7. DeMuth WE Jr: Bullet velocity and design as determinants of wounding capability: an experimental study. J Trauma 6:222, 1966.
8. DeMuth WE Jr: The mechanism of shotgun wounds. J Trauma 11:219, 1971.
9. Madden JE, Edlich RF, Custer JR, Panek PH, Thul J, Wangensteen OH: Studies in the management of the contaminated wound. IV. Resistance to infection of surgical wounds made by knife, electrosurgery, and laser. Am J Surg 119:222, 1970.
10. Cruse PJE, Foord R: A five-year prospective study of 23,649 surgical wounds. Arch Surg 107:206, 1973.
11. Levine NS, Peterson HD, Hugh D, Salisbury RE, Pruitt BA Jr: Laser, scalpel, electrosurgical and tangential excisions of third degree burns. A preliminary report. Plast Reconstr Surg 56:286, 1975.
12. Ferguson DJ: Advances in the management of surgical wounds. Surg Clin North Am 51:49, 1971.
13. McDowell AJ: Wound infections resulting from the use of hot sponges. Plast Reconstr Surg 23:168, 1959.
14. Hunt JL, Mason AD Jr, Masterson TS, Pruitt BA Jr: The pathophysiology of acute electric injuries. J Trauma 16:335, 1976.
15. Robson MC, Krizek TJ, Heggers JP: Biology of surgical infection. Curr Probl Surg 10:1, 1973.
16. Robson MC, Lea CE, Dalton JB, Heggers JP: Quantitative bacteriology and delayed wound closure. Surg Forum 19:501, 1968.
17. Edlich RF, Rodeheaver GT, Spengler M, Herbert J, Edgerton MT: Practical bacteriologic monitoring of the burn victim. Clin Plast Surg 4:561, 1977.
18. Magee CM, Rodeheaver GT, Edgerton MT, Edlich RF: A more reliable gram staining technique for diagnosis of surgical infections. Am J Surg 130:341, 1975.

BIOLOGY OF TISSUE INFECTION

19. Rodeheaver GT, Pettry D, Turnbull V, Edgerton MT, Edlich RF: Identification of the wound infection-potentiating factors in soil. Am J Surg 128:8, 1974.

20. Haury BB, Rodeheaver GT, Pettry D, Edgerton MT, Edlich RF: Inhibition of nonspecific defenses by soil infection potentiating factors. Surg Gynecol Obstet 144:19, 1977.

TECHNICAL FACTORS IN THE PREVENTION OF WOUND INFECTION

21. Stevenson TR, Rodeheaver GT, Golden GT, Edgerton MT, Wells JH, Edlich RF: Damage to tissue defenses by vasoconstrictors. J Am Coll Emerg Phys 4:532, 1975.
22. Seropian R, Reynolds BM: Wound infections after preoperative depilatory versus razor preparation. Am J Surg 121:251, 1971.
23. Department of Health, Education, and Welfare, Food and Drug Administration. OTC topical antimicrobial Products. Fed Reg 43:1210, 1978.
24. Rodeheaver GT, Turnbull V, Edgerton MT, Kurtz L, Edlich RF: Pharmacokinetics of a new skin wound cleanser. Am J Surg 132:67, 1976.
25. Dupont A, Lachapelle JM: Dermite due à un dépot médicamenteux au cours du traitement d'un diabète insipide. Bull Soc Fr Dermatol Syphiligr 71:508, 1964.
26. Lachapelle JM: Thésaurismose cutanée par polyvinylpyrrolidone. Dermatologica 132:476, 1966.
27. Walter CW, Kundsin RB: The bacteriologic study of surgical gloves from 250 operations. Surg Gynecol Obstet 129:949, 1969.
28. Sprunt K, Redman W, Leidy G: Antibacterial effectiveness of routine hand washing. Pediatrics 52:264, 1973.
29. A Report to the Medical Research Council by the Subcommittee on Aseptic Methods in Operating Theatres of their Committee on Hospital Infection: Aseptic methods in the operating suite. Lancet 1:705, 1968.
30. Steere AC, Mallison GF: Handwashing practices for the prevention of nosocomial infections. Ann Intern Med 83:683, 1975.
31. Slaughter FG: Immortal Magyar: Semmelweis, Conqueror of Child-bed Fever. New York, Schuman, 1950, p. 3.
32. US General Services Administration O-T-C topical antimicrobial products and drug and cosmetic products. Fed Reg 39(179):33118, 1974.
33. Smylie HG, Logie JRC, Smith G: From Phisohex to Hibiscrub. Br Med J 4:586, 1973.
34. Lowbury EJL, Lilly HA: Use of 4% chlorhexidine detergent solution (Hibiscrub) and other methods of skin disinfection. Br Med J 1:510, 1973.
35. Bornside GH, Crowder VH Jr, Cohn I Jr: A bacteriological evaluation of surgical scrubbing with disposable iodophor-soap impregnated polyurethane scrub sponges. Surgery 64:743, 1968.
36. Michaud RN, McGrath MB, Goss WA: Improved experimental model for measuring skin degerming activity on the human hand. Antimicrob Agents Chemother 2:8, 1972.
37. Walter CW: Disinfection of hands. Am J Surg 109:691, 1965.
38. Custer J, Edlich RF, Prusak M, Madden J, Panek P, Wangensteen OH: Studies in the management of the contaminated wound. V. An assessment of the effectiveness of pHisoHex and Betadine surgical scrub solutions. Am J Surg 121:572, 1971.
39. Edlich RF, Schmolka IR, Prusak MP, Edgerton MT: The molecular basis for the toxicity of surfactants in surgical wounds. I. EO:PO block polymers. J Surg Res 14:277, 1973.
40. Lavelle KJ, Doedens DJ, Kleit SA, Forney RB: Iodine absorption in burn patients treated topically with povidone-iodine. Clin Pharmacol Ther 17:355, 1975.
41. Ahrenholz D, Simmons RL: Povidone iodine in peritonitis. I. Adverse effects of local instillation in experimental *E. coli* peritonitis. J Surg Res 26:458, 1979.
42. Bolton JS, Bornside GH, Cohn I Jr: Intraperitoneal povidone-iodine in experimental canine and murine peritonitis. Am J Surg 137:780, 1979.
43. Gilmore OJA, Martin TDM: Aetiology and prevention of wound infection in appendicectomy. Br J Surg 61:281, 1974.
44. Stokes EJ, Howard E, Peters JL, Hackworthy CA, Milne SE, Witherow RO: Comparison of antibiotic and antiseptic prophylaxis of wound infection in acute abdominal surgery. World J Surg 1:777, 1977.
44a. Pollock AV, Evans M: Povidone-iodine for the control of surgical wound infection: a controlled clinical trial against cephaloridine. Br J Surg 62:292, 1975.
45. Jones RC, Shires GT: Principles in the management of wounds. In Schwartz SI (ed): Principles of Surgery. New York, McGraw-Hill, 1974, p 204.
46. Haury B, Rodeheaver G, Vensko J, Edgerton MT, Edlich RF: Debridement: an essential component of traumatic wound care. Am J Surg 135:238, 1978.
47. Allgöwer M, Cueni LB, Städtler K, Schoenenberger GA: Burn toxin in mouse skin. J Trauma 13:95, 1973.
48. Mandell GL: Bactericidal activity of aerobic and anaerobic polymorphonuclear neutrophils. Infect Immun 9:337, 1974.
49. Scully RE, Artz CP, Sako Y: The criteria for determining the viability of muscle in war wounds. In Battle Wounds, Vol 3. Surgical Research Team, Army Medical Service Graduate School, Washington, DC, 1956.
50. Myers MB: Prediction and prevention of skin sloughs in radical cancer surgery. Pacific Med Surg 75:315, 1967.
51. Peacock EE, Van Winkle W: Repair of skin wounds. In Surgery and Biology of Wound Repair. Philadelphia, Saunders, 1970, p 71.
52. Stevenson TR, Thacker JG, Rodeheaver GT, Bacchetta C, Edgerton MT, Edlich RF: Cleansing the traumatic wound by high pressure syringe irrigation. J Am Coll Emerg Phys 5:17, 1976.
53. Wheeler CB, Rodeheaver GT, Thacker JG, Edgerton MT, Edlich RF: Side-effects of high pressure irrigation. Surg Gynecol Obstet 143:775, 1976.
54. Rodeheaver GT, Smith SL, Thacker JG, Edgerton MT, Edlich RF: Mechanical cleansing of contaminated wounds with a surfactant. Am J Surg 129:241, 1975.
55. Edlich RF, Smith QT, Edgerton MT: Resistance of the surgical wound to antimicrobial prophylaxis and its mechanisms of development. Am J Surg 126:583, 1973.
56. Arenholz D, Simmons RL: Fibrin in peritonitis. I. Beneficial and adverse effects of fibrin in experimental *E. coli* peritonitis. Surgery, 88:41, 1980.
57. Edlich RF, Madden JE, Prusak M, Panek P, Thul J, Wangensteen OH: Studies in the management of contaminated wounds. VI. The therapeutic value of gentle scrubbing in prolonging the limited period of effectiveness of antibiotics in contaminated wounds. Am J Surg 121:668, 1971.
58. Rodeheaver GT, Edgerton MT, Elliott MB, Kurtz LD, Edlich RF: Proteolytic enzymes as adjuncts to antibiotic prophylaxis of surgical wounds. Am J Surg 127:564, 1974.
59. Rodeheaver GT, Marsh D, Edgerton MT, Edlich RF: Proteolytic enzymes as adjuncts to antimicrobial prophylaxis of contaminated wounds. Am J Surg 129:537, 1975.
60. Verklin R, Rodeheaver GT, Hudson R, Edgerton MT, Edlich RF: Rapid antibiotic disk sensitivities of burn eschar and infected wounds. Surg Gynecol Obstet 144:507, 1977.
61. Bauer A, Kirby W, Sherris J, Turck M: Antibiotic susceptibility testing by a standardized single disk method. Am J Clin Path 45:493, 1966.
62. Ferguson DJ: Clinical application of experimental relations between technique and wound infection. Surgery 63:377, 1968.

63. deHoll D, Rodeheaver G, Edgerton MT, Edlich RF: Potentiation of infection by suture closure of dead space. Am J Surg 127:716, 1974.
64. Wood WB Jr, Smith MR, Perry WD, Berry JW: Studies on the cellular immunology of active bacteremia. I. Intravascular leukocytic reaction and surface phagocytosis. J Exp Med 94:521, 1951.
65. Ahrenholz DH: Effect of intraperitoneal fluid on mortality of *Escherichia coli* peritonitis. Surg Forum 30:483, 1979.
66. Alexander JW, Korelitz J, Alexander NS: Prevention of wound infection: a case for closed suction drainage to remove wound fluids deficient in opsonic proteins. Am J Surg 132:59, 1976.
67. Heaton LD, Hughes CW, Rosegay H, Fisher GW, Feighny RE: Military surgical practices of the United States Army in Viet Nam. Curr Probl Surg, November 1966, p 19.
68. Edlich RF, Rogers W, Kasper G, Kaufman D, Tsung MS, Wangensteen OH: Studies in the management of the contaminated wound. I. Optimal time for closure of contaminated open wounds. II. Comparison of the resistance to infection of open and closed wounds during healing. Am J Surg 117:323, 1969.
69. Edlich RF, Thul J, Prusak M, Panek P, Madden J, Wangensteen OH: Studies in the management of the contaminated wound. VIII. Assessment of tissue adhesives for repair of contaminated tissue. Am J Surg 122:394, 1971.
70. Harrison ID, Williams DF, Cuschieri A: The effect of metal clips on the tensile properties of healing skin wounds. Br J Surg 62:945, 1975.
71. Edlich RF, Panek PH, Rodeheaver GT, Turnbull VG, Kurtz LD, Edgerton MT: Physical and chemical configuration of sutures in the development of surgical infection. Ann Surg 177:679, 1973.
72. Edlich RF, Tsung MS, Rogers W, Rogers P, Wangensteen OH: Studies in management of the contaminated wound. I. Technique of closure of such wounds together with a note on a reproducible model. J Surg Res 8:585, 1968.
73. Postlethwait RW: Long-term comparative study of nonabsorbable sutures. Ann Surg 171:892, 1970.
74. Thacker JG, Rodeheaver GT, Kurtz L, Edgerton MT, Edlich RF: Mechanical performance of sutures in surgery. Am J Surg 133:713, 1977.
75. Tera H, Aberg C: Tensile strengths of twelve types of knot employed in surgery, using different suture materials. Acta Chir Scand 142:1, 1976.
76. Holmlund DEW: Knot properties of surgical suture materials. A model study. Acta Chir Scand 140:355, 1974.
77. Winn HR, Jane JA, Rodeheaver G, Edgerton MT, Edlich RF: Influence of subcuticular sutures on scar formation. Am J Surg 133:257, 1977.
78. Foster GE, Hardy EG, Hardcastle JD: Subcuticular suturing after appendicectomy. Lancet 1:1128, 1977.
79. Edlich RF, Rodeheaver G, Kuphal J, deHoll JD, Smith SL, Bacchetta C, Edgerton MT: Technique of closure: contaminated wounds. JACEP 3:375, 1974.
80. Panek PH, Prusak MP, Bolt D, Edlich RF: Potentiation of wound infection by adhesive adjuncts. Amer Surgeon 38:343, 1972.
81. Carrel A, Hartmann A: Cicatrization of wounds. I. The relation between the size of a wound and the rate of its cicatrization. J Exp Med 24:429, 1916.
82. Carrel A: Cicatrization of wounds. XII. Factors initiating regeneration. J Exp Med 34:425, 1921.
83. Smith M, Enquist IF: A quantitative study of impaired healing resulting from infection. Surg Gynecol Obstet 125:965, 1967.
84. Lee JT Jr, Ahrenholz DH, Nelson RD, Simmons RL: Mechanisms of the adjuvant effect of hemoglobin in experimental peritonitis. V. The significance of the coordinated iron component. Surgery 86:41, 1979.
85. Krizek TJ, Davis JH: The role of the red cell in subcutaneous infection. J Trauma 5:85, 1965.
86. Hau T, Nelson RD, Fiegel VD, Levenson R, Simmons RL: Mechanisms of the adjuvant action of hemoglobin in experimental peritonitis. 2. Influence of hemoglobin on human leukocyte chemotaxis in vitro. J Surg Res 22:174, 1977.
87. Cerise EJ, Pierce WA, Diamond DL: Abdominal drains: their role as a source of infection following splenectomy. Ann Surg 171:764, 1970.
88. Nora PF, Vanecko RM, Bransfield JJ: Prophylactic abdominal drains. Arch Surg 105:173, 1972.
89. Morris AM: A controlled trial of closed wound suction. Drainage in radical mastectomy. Br J Surg 60:357, 1973.
90. Baker BH, Borchardt KA: Sump drains and airborne bacteria as a cause of wound infections. J Surg Res 17:407, 1974.
91. Magee C, Rodeheaver GT, Golden GT, Fox J, Edgerton MT, Edlich RF: Potentiation of wound infection by surgical drains. Am J Surg 131:547, 1976.
92. Berliner SD, Burson LC, Lear PE: Use and abuse of intraperitoneal drains in colon surgery. Arch Surg 89:686, 1964.
93. Manz CW, LaTendresse C, Sako Y: The detrimental effects of drains on colonic anastomoses: an experimental study. Dis Colon Rectum 13:17, 1970.
94. Scales JT: Wound healing and the dressing. Br J Indust Med 20:82, 1963.
95. Noe JM, Kalish S: The problem of adherence in dressed wounds. Surg Gynecol Obstet 147:185, 1978.
96. Colebrook L, Hood AM: Infection through soaked dressings. Lancet 2:682, 1948.
97. Lowbury EJL, Hood AM: A disinfectant barrier in dressings applied to burns. Lancet 1:899, 1952.
98. Warren R: Surgery. Philadelphia, Saunders 1963, p 43.
99. Schauerhamer RA, Edlich RF, Panek P, Thul J, Prusak M, Wangensteen OH: Studies in the management of the contaminated wound. VII. Susceptibility of surgical wounds to postoperative surface contamination. Am J Surg 122:74, 1971.
100. Futrell S, Rust RS, Rodeheaver GT, Edlich RF: Regional factors in lymphatic localization of wound contamination. J Surg Res, in press, 1981.
101. Winter GD: Formation of the scab and the rate of epithelization of superficial wounds in the skin of the young domestic pig. Nature 193:293, 1962.
102. Rovee DT, Kurowsky CA, Labun J, Downes AM: Effect of local wound environment on epidermal healing. In Maibach HI, Rovee DT (eds): Epidermal Wound Healing. Chicago, Yearbook Medical Publishers, 1972, p 159.
103. Seymour DE, DaCosta NM, Hodgson ME, Dow J: British patent. #1, 280, 631.
104. Lamke LO, Nilsson GE, Reithner HL: The evaporative water loss from burns and the watervapor permeability of grafts and artificial membranes used in the treatment of burns. Burns 3:159, 1977.
105. James JH, Watson ACH: The use of Opsite, a vapour permeable dressing, on skin graft donor sites. Br J Plast Surg 28:107, 1975.
106. Nathan P, Law EJ, MacMillian BG, Murphy DF, Ronel SH, D'Andrea MJ, Abrahams RA: A new biomaterial for the control of infection in the burn wound. Trans Amer Soc Artif Intern Organs 22:30, 1976.
107. Nalbandian RM, Henry RL, Wilks HS: Artificial skin. II. Pluronic F-127, silver nitrate or silver lactate gel in the treatment of thermal burns. J Biomed Mater Res 6:583, 1972.

CHAPTER 23
Chemoprophylaxis of Wound Infections

HIRAM C. POLK, JR. AND MICHAEL P. FINN

CHEMOPROPHYLAXIS

FEW techniques of clinical surgery have excited as much controversy and produced as much conflicting data as the use of antimicrobial drugs to prevent incisional infection. Nevertheless, the effectiveness of chemoprophylaxis for some procedures is well documented, and the indications for and techniques of appropriate use are well defined. Three methods of chemoprophylaxis—local or topical therapy, systemic prophylaxis, and intestinal antisepsis with orally administered, poorly absorbed antibiotics—will be discussed.

TOPICAL PROPHYLAXIS

Virtually all antibiotic agents have been used at one time or another for direct application to wounds and body cavities. While enthusiasm for such use has waxed and waned, there is a sound body of experimental and clinical data demonstrating effectiveness for some agents. The rationale for topical antibiotic use in incisional and intraperitoneal infections is that concentrated antibacterial activity can be delivered directly to the site of actual or potential contamination in a concentration that is greater at that site than could be safely achieved by systemic administration alone. The properties of an ideal topical antimicrobial agent are delineated in Table 23-1.[1,2]

One of the brightest chapters of near optimum application of these principles is topical chemotherapy for the burn patient. While not within the realm of this chapter, the regular use of effective surface antimicrobials has significantly increased survival of patients sustaining large burns[3,4] (Chapter 48).

Local Use in the Surgical Wound

Experimental Studies

Consistently favorable reductions in wound infections have been reported in experimentally contaminated wounds. Gray and Kidd[1] reported excellent results when Neosporin powder was used in wounds contaminated with *Staphylococcus, Pseudomonas pyocyaneus, Clostridium welchii,* or *E. Coli* and *Proteus vulgaris.* Hopson et al[5] and Singleton[6] reported significant reductions in the rate of experimental wound infection treated with neomycin (1 percent) or kanamycin (1 percent) solutions. Cephalothin powder was effective when used by Waterman[7] for infections due to *S. aureus, S. pyogenes,* and *E. coli.* Hopson et al,[5] however, found that cephalothin solution (1 percent) was less effective than kanamycin solution (1 percent) in preventing staphylococcal infections in animals. DiGiglia et al[8] used kanamycin and bacitracin in combination in experimental wounds containing arterial prostheses, and found reductions in wound infections, graft infections, and graft failures. The temporal relationship of antibiotic administration and prophylactic effectiveness is important in both systemic and antibacterial therapy. Howes[9] found that a streptomycin-mafenide combination protected crushed contaminated wounds when applied during contamination. If drug application was delayed more than 3 hours, no protection was effected unless precise wound debridement was also employed, an effect noted by others when hexachlorophene or neomycin solution was used.[6,10,11] Obviously, the concept of the decisive period applies to all local wound manipulations, whether via systemic or topical routes.[12]

Clinical Studies

Topical prophylaxis with single agents or antibiotic combinations used in the form of sprays, solutions, or powders have been used in a variety of clinical settings (Table 23-2). Studies involving potentially contaminated or contaminated wounds have shown that topically applied Neosporin, neomycin, kanamycin, and cephaloridine are effective in reducing rates of wound infection. Stone[11,13] found that Neosporin spray and primary wound closure produced as good a result as delayed primary closure, a well-established procedure for dealing with contaminated emergency celiotomy incisions. Pollack and associates[14-16] found that topically applied cephaloridine reduced rates of wound sepsis in high-risk colorectal procedures and in obese patients more effectively than ampicillin or povidone-iodine.[14-16] The extensive studies of Cohn et al[17,18] consistently documented the effectiveness of topically applied kanamycin. Clinical studies employing cephalothin as a wound irrigant have produced conflicting results. Wound irrigation with the combination of cephalothin and kanamycin significantly reduces infections in clean vascu-

TABLE 23-1. PROPERTIES OF AN IDEAL TOPICAL ANTIMICROBIAL AGENT

Wide range of antimicrobial effect
Minimal local tissue irritation
Minimal systemic toxic effect
Minimal systemic absorption if toxicity is a hazard
Minimal allergenicity
Infrequent emergence of resistant microbial forms

Adapted from Gray FT, Kidd E [1] and Poth EJ.[2]

lar wounds; [19] however, the contribution of each of the agents is unclear, particularly if systemic antibiotics are also used.

Penicillin and ampicillin have occasionally been advocated for topical therapy,[20,21] such as Andersen's [21] studies on the effect of topical ampicillin powder on infection associated with colorectal procedures. In patients *not* receiving intestinal antiseptics, topical ampicillin resulted in a 6 percent incidence of wound infection compared with a 35 percent incidence in the control group.[21] Predictably, if one examines only those patients receiving intestinal antiseptics, no statistically significant additional benefit could be attributed to the use of topical ampicillin powder.

Povidone-iodine allows use of a nonantibiotic antiseptic with a wide antimicrobial spectrum.[14,16,22,23] Early reports suggested a high degree of efficacy when this was used as a degerming agent [24] and as a topical antiseptic on granulating wounds.[25] Povidone-iodine spray yielding 0.5 percent available iodine was found to reduce wound infection rates significantly when compared with the propellant alone.[26] However, in a carefully controlled, well-designed clinical study of high-risk colorectal procedures, povidone-iodine was no better than saline wound irrigation and was less effective than topical cephaloridine.[14] Povidone-iodine was shown to have no protective effect in low-risk abdominal procedures or in clean surgical wounds.[14-16] Povidone-iodine spray (0.5 percent) was compared to systemic tobramycin and lincomycin in 113 heterogeneous patients undergoing abdominal (including emergency) operations. The spray was no more effective than no treatment at all, whereas parenteral lincomycin-tobramycin was associated with a significant reduction in wound infection.[22]

Neither Stone [11] nor Pollock [15] observed benefit when neomycin or Neosporin were applied to clean wounds. Existing data suggest that the use of topical antimicrobial agents in clean wounds is not justified,[14-16,27] although a few reports contradict this seemingly sound thesis,[19,20] especially when vascular prostheses may be present.[20a]

Intraperitoneal Use

The use of antimicrobial agents in the peritoneal cavity to treat peritonitis and to prevent septic complications has also enjoyed periods of favor and disfavor. Cohn [17] has detailed succinctly the history of intraperitoneal antibiotic use. Because sulfonamides, tetracyclines, and streptomycin have produced potentially severe toxic local and systemic side effects in animals, their use cannot be recommended. Emphasis in both experimental and clinical studies has been on agents effective against gram-negative bacteria. The aminoglycosides and neomycin and kanamycin, cephalothin, bacitracin (usually in combination with an aminoglycoside), and povidone-iodine may be useful in treating or preventing intraperitoneal infectious complications (Chapter 34).

Experimental

In the early 1950s, Poth [2] demonstrated that intraperitoneally administered neomycin protected the murine peritoneum from the lethal effects of fecal soiling. Intraperitoneal kanamycin reduced the 24-hour mortality rate in a canine cecal ligation model of experimental appendicitis. Cohn suggested that kanamycin is less toxic than neomycin and is associated with a lower risk of drug-induced respiratory depression.[17,18] Instillation of kanamycin (500 mg) intraperitoneally has produced elevated intraperitoneal and serum kanamycin levels. When kanamycin was given as a single intraperitoneal dose, peritoneal fluid and serum kanamycin levels were sustained for only about 4 hours, and the agent was eliminated within 12 hours. Therefore, multiple intraperitoneal doses of kanamycin should be used.[18]

TABLE 23-2. CLASSIFICATION AND INDICATIONS FOR TOPICALLY APPLIED AGENTS AFTER POTENTIALLY CONTAMINATED OR CONTAMINATED OPERATIONS

Drug	Effective Dose	Controversial Drug
Neomycin *	1% solution as wound irrigant; avoid intraperitoneal use	Ampicillin
Kanamycin †	0.5%–1% solution for wound or intraperitoneal irrigation	Povidone-iodine
Neosporin	Powder or spray in subcutaneous wounds	Cephalothin
Cephaloridine	1% solution for wound irrigation	Penicillin
Kanamycin-bacitracin *	1 gm–50,000 units in saline for wound irrigation	

* Aminoglycosides *are* absorbed from subcutaneous wounds; observe for potential ototoxic and/or nephrotoxic effects.

† Intraperitoneal aminoglycosides may produce respiratory depression.

Intraperitoneal cephalothin has been studied experimentally.[28,29] Dogs with gangrenous bowel segments that were treated with multiple peritoneal instillations of cephalothin (56 mg per kg) lived longer than either those treated with intravenous cephalothin or intraperitoneal saline. Cephalothin was administered through a transperitoneal catheter during a 28-hour period in 2 to 5 doses. The 69 percent survival of intraperitoneally treated animals was significantly better than saline-treated controls. Intraperitoneal kanamycin was compared to intraperitoneal cephalothin in experimental canine appendicitis.[29] A five-dose regimen of cephalothin (1.5 mg per dose) was at least as effective as a five-dose regimen of kanamycin (0.5 gm per dose) in reducing mortality. Although no difference in infection rate was noted between the two antibiotic groups, they were significantly more effective than saline.

The effectiveness of intraperitoneal povidone-iodine was first studied in the rat model.[30] Doses not exceeding 2.5 ml per kg of 10 percent povidone-iodine aqueous solution were uniformly nontoxic. A single intraperitoneal injection (2.5 ml per kg) protected rats inoculated with a lethal intraperitoneal challenge of *E. coli*. Povidone-iodine was effective only if given within 1 hour of microbial inoculation. Animals receiving the agent at 2 hours exhibited no improvement in survival when compared to controls. Further, povidone-iodine (2.5 ml per kg) was as effective as single intraperitoneal doses of cephalothin or kanamycin when given 1 hour after bacterial challenge.

LaGarde et al [31] administered povidone-iodine intraperitoneally to dogs with induced appendicitis. In preliminary studies, doses of 10 percent povidone-iodine exceeding 2.0 ml per kg were uniformly toxic. When animals were treated with 2.0 ml per kg of 10 percent povidone-iodine 24 hours after cecal ligation, mortality in the treated animals exceeded that of controls. Intraperitoneal administration of 10 percent povidone-iodine (2 ml per kg) 2 hours after intraperitoneal *E. coli* inoculation did not improve survival.

Flint et al [32] recently studied the effectiveness of povidone-iodine in polymicrobial rat peritonitis. Ten percent povidone-iodine (2.5 ml per kg) as a single instillation failed to improve survival when given 2 hours after fecal soiling of the peritoneal cavity. Interestingly, lavage with 1.5 percent povidone-iodine in saline (600 ml per kg) resulted in significant reductions in 24-hour mortality when compared with animals treated with sham operation alone. Peritoneal lavage 2 hours postinoculation with cephalothin in saline was also quite effective. The failure of 10 percent povidone-iodine to reduce mortality did not appear to be the result of povidone-iodine toxicity. Peritoneal fluid cultures revealed that povidone-iodine 10 percent or 1.5 percent reduced bacterial counts, but the effect persisted only 3 hours; rapid intraperitoneal bacterial proliferation was noted by 6 hours. Povidone-iodine probably failed to control systemic infection—there was an improvement in survival if a single delayed intravenous dose of cephalothin (200 mg per kg) was given 1 hour after intraperitoneal administration of povidone-iodine. Thus, povidone-iodine 10 percent used alone does not effectively treat established experimental peritonitis.

Dilute povidone-iodine solutions (0.075 and 0.1 percent) were used in mouse and rat *E. coli* peritonitis.[33] The agent was administered 1 minute after bacterial inoculation with 7.5×10^9 bacteria per kg body weight. In both models studied, the dilute povidone-iodine given intraperitoneally exhibited a significant protective effect. These findings suggest that dilute intraperitoneal povidone-iodine may be a useful preventive adjunct in patients undergoing elective alimentary tract operation if given before peritonitis becomes established.

The problem with povidone iodine is that it damages host tissues, so that if bacteria survive, their subsequent proliferation may be unopposed.[33a]

Clinical Studies

Experimental studies [2,26] led to the successful clinical use of intraperitoneally administered neomycin. Initial enthusiasm for intraperitoneal neomycin waned in 1956 when Pridgen [34] reported four instances of respiratory arrest. Neomycin as well as other aminoglycosides possess a nondepolarizing, postganglionic, neuromuscular blocking effect, which appeared to be enhanced by the concomitant presence of ether or neuromuscular blocking agents, such as curare. Consequently, the intraperitoneal use of neomycin has been abandoned in favor of less toxic agents. Neomycin continues to be used topically in nonabdominal surgical wounds, but because it is absorbed, the potential for systemic toxic effect must be considered.

Significant amounts of neomycin (1 percent) can be absorbed via open hip wounds when it is used alone as a topical irrigant for wounds.[35] Serum concentrations of neomycin as high as 7–10 μg per ml were observed. Although no adverse effects were seen, the potential exists for systemic nephrotoxicity or ototoxicity, as well as drug-induced respiratory depression resulting from potentiation of anesthetic ganglionic blockade.

Kanamycin has been used extensively as an intraperitoneal topical agent [17,33,36-39] and has been alleged to cause less respiratory depression,[17,18] although sporadic reports of death or respiratory insufficiency have appeared.[40,41] Clinical experiences suggest that intraperitoneal kanamycin is effective in reducing mortality from established peritonitis as well as the incidence of septic complications. Prigot [40] treated 30 patients with single intraperitoneal instillation of 500 mg of kanamycin in saline. Of the 30, 18 patients with established peritonitis recovered without complications. Of 12 patients with peritoneal contamination, 10 recovered without incident and 2 died. One of the deaths may have been the result of kanamycin-induced respiratory depression.

Cohn and associates have studied both single and multiple dose regimens of kanamycin.[17,36,38,39] Multiple intraperitoneal instillation of kanamycin, 0.5 mg per dose, during a 72-hour intraoperative and postoperative period significantly reduced the incidence of infectious complications.[17] Wound infections were observed in only 8.5 percent of these patients with established peritonitis. Patients who received single dose instillation of kanamycin, however, exhibited a 27 percent incidence of wound infection.

Noon et al [37] compared intraperitoneal kanamycin-bacitracin in combination (1 gm and 50,000 units, respectively) to saline irrigation in 404 individuals with spontaneous or traumatic perforative lesions of the gastrointestinal tract. Postoperative infectious complications occurred less frequently in patients treated with kanamycin-bacitracin than in those treated with saline irrigation (12 percent versus 24 percent). However, recent data confirm the systemic absorption and distribution of bacitracin, an agent long recognized to possess significant nephrotoxic potential.[42]

Intraperitoneal cephalothin has also been popular, although objective assessment of its effect is difficult to make. McMullan and Barnett[43] treated a heterogeneous group of 32 patients undergoing abdominal operations. Most of these patients received multiple dose cephalothin via an intraperitoneal catheter postoperatively, and only three infectious complications resulted. Cephalothin, as a single-dose intraperitoneal irrigation in 24 patients with contaminated peritoneal cavities, provided no more protection than saline alone.[44] Despite initial enthusiasm for intraperitoneal cephalothin based on experimental studies, Cohn[45] has abandoned its use because of the lack of protective effectiveness in clinical trials.

The effectiveness of intraperitoneal povidone-iodine has not been studied in a controlled clinical trial. We used intraperitoneal povidone-iodine, however, in patients with severe peritonitis or massive peritoneal contamination secondary to trauma. Our impressions of benefit are just that, impressions, but its clinical safety is quite clear.

The experimental data to support the use of topical agents is largely well founded and clear cut. However, because most clinical studies include the uncontrolled, concomitant use of powerful systemic or intestinal prophylactic regimens, the contention that topical antibiotics or povidone-iodine results in significant reductions in wound infection rates cannot be substantiated. Systemic and intestinal prophylactic regimens are associated with infection rates of 4 to 7 percent in well-designed, controlled, prospective, randomized, double-blind series. In no instance has topical prophylaxis been shown to be equivalent, or superior, to these methods when used alone. The small additional reduction in infection rates when cephaloridine[16] or ampicillin[21] have been used in combination with intestinal antisepsis does not appear to be significant, nor does it obviate the additional potential danger of unnecessary antibiotic exposure. A recent report from the University of Sydney provides new clinical evidence in favor of a multiple drug attack upon organisms responsible for severe peritonitis.[46] There are some problems, as noted above as well as in study design; however, the data are impressive.[47]

Poorly absorbed agents (Neosporin, neomycin, kanamycin) may have value, however, when delay in treatment is expected, such as in mass casualties or in combat wounds. The question that remains unanswered is whether local wound therapy is safer and more effective than systemic prophylaxis or, in the case of elective intestinal procedures, whether it is better than oral administration of poorly absorbed antibiotics. Furthermore, one cannot determine with certainty whether such methods may be additive; preliminary data suggest they are not. There is the additional fear that endorsement of topical prophylaxis may lead to a slackening of operative technique and the reliance upon topical therapy to "cover" otherwise preventable technical errors.

SYSTEMIC PROPHYLAXIS

The merit of specific antibacterial activity present within the tissues at the time of bacterial contamination is based on experimental data. The goal of systemic prophylaxis is to augment local incisional defense mechanisms by the suffusion of the wound with effective antibiotic concentrations (Table 23-3).

Clinical evaluation of the efficacy of systemic prophylaxis has failed to consistently agree with experimental findings. Many early studies indicated that systemic antibiotic prophylaxis had no protective effect, and some even claimed that attempted prophylaxis increased wound infection rates. Of 131 systemic prophylaxis studies (from 1960 to 1976) reviewed, 107 (82 percent) were either inadequately designed or well designed but not evaluable.[48] In the remaining 24 studies, the prophylactic antibiotics were probably effective in only a limited group of abdominal and refined-clean procedures.

The innate resistance of the operative wound to bacterial colonization and proliferation is the critical factor. Theoretically, this resistance may be enhanced by adequate antibiotic wound levels. The presence of bacteria within a wound does not necessarily lead to infection, as indicated by the 7 percent infection rate among patients initially surviving nonsterile thoracotomy for open cardiac massage.[49]

Experimental Studies

The natural host defense mechanisms are the most important factors in determining the outcome of wound contamination. To understand more fully the relationship of host defense and bacterial lodgment, Miles and associates[27,50] examined the effect of modifiers of host resistance on experimentally contaminated wounds (Fig. 23-1). Local wound ischemia was effected by dehydration or by the local use of epinephrine at various times after contamination. Such impairment of wound blood supply resulted in test lesions of greater size than controls, indicating reduced defense against contaminants. Similarly, blockade of complement activity with Liquoid resulted in increased lesion size. The temporal relationship between inhibition of host defenses and size of test lesions clearly showed that there was a "decisive period" during which enhancement of the size of lesions could be achieved. Inhibition of defense mecha-

TABLE 23-3. PRINCIPLES OF SYSTEMIC PROPHYLAXIS

Safe agent with low systemic toxicity
Activity against expected pathogens
Administer immediately preoperatively
Short course of 2 or 3 doses postoperatively
Use appropriate when
infection frequent
infection unusually severe

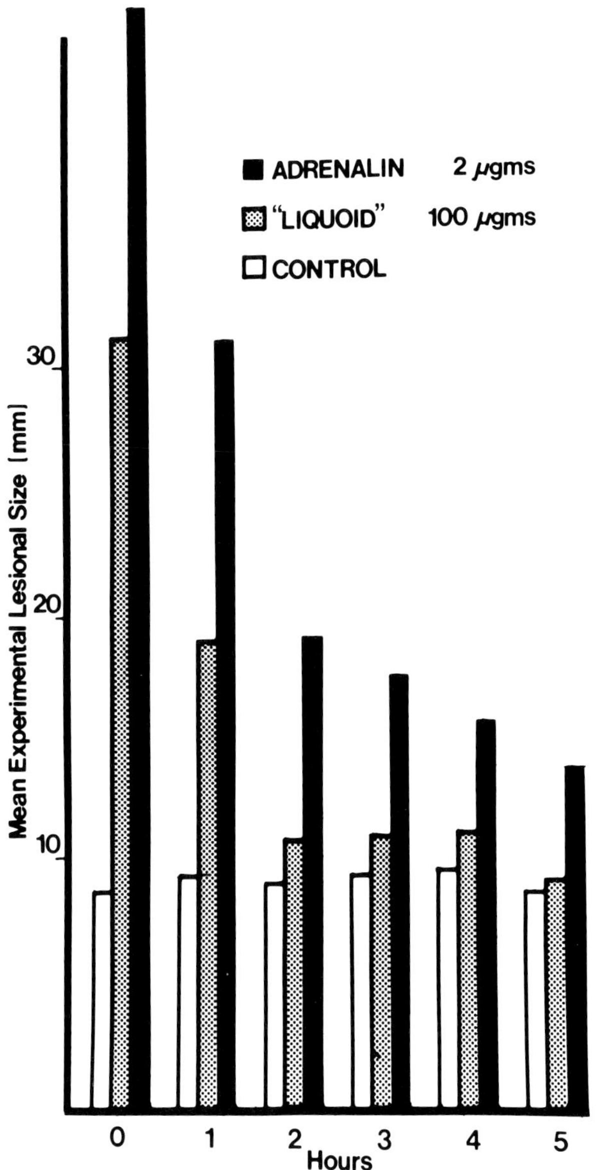

Fig. 23-1. **Time-dependent enhancement of lesional size by several modifiers of host resistance.**

nisms accomplished 0 to 1.5 hours after contamination resulted in maximal increase of lesion size. If ischemia or complement blockade was produced more than 1.5 hours after contamination, progressively less enhancing effect was noted, so that at 5 hours, no increase of lesion size resulted. In other test wounds, the parenteral administration of an antibiotic reduced the maximal size of lesions most effectively if given before contamination; if antibiotic was given later, progressively less effect was noted until 4 hours, when none existed (Fig. 23-2). Indeed, if antibiotic was given before contamination, the effect was the same as that produced by the injection of autoclaved bacteria.

The effectiveness of systemic antibiotics is so time-dependent that antibiotics given 2 to 3 hours after staphylococcal wound contamination are ineffective.[51] These studies explain the virtually routine failure of postoperative systemic prophylaxis. To be most effective, systemic prophylaxis must be administered before microbial wound contamination. Similarly, the drug selected must be appropriate for the most likely contaminating organisms.

Clinical Studies

The first clinical study to confirm these experimental data was the report by Bernard and Cole.[52] A regimen of penicillin G, methicillin, and chloramphenicol was administered preoperatively, intraoperatively, and 5 days postoperatively in a randomized trial in 145 patients undergoing potentially contaminated abdominal operations. Eight percent of the patients receiving antibiotic developed postoperative infections, whereas 27 percent of patients receiving the placebo became infected. A surprising reduction in nonwound postoperative infectious complications (eg, pneumonia, urinary tract infection) was also observed. Unfortunately, additional antibiotics were also used in 27 patients, leaving the results of this trial subject to question.

Polk and Lopez-Mayor [53] reported a series of 199 consecutive, potentially contaminated alimentary tract operations treated in a prospective, randomized, doubleblind fashion with perioperative cephaloridine; biliary and pancreatic operations were excluded. No patient received oral intestinal antibiotics or other preoperative or postoperative antibiotic therapy. A three-dose regimen of cephaloridine, 1 gm intramuscularly, given on call to the operating room, and at 5 to 12 hours postoperatively was used. Wound cultures and serum and wound antibiotic levels were obtained. The group of patients receiving the systemic antibiotic had a 7 percent incidence of infection, while 29 percent of the patients receiving a placebo developed infections. The findings were highly significant in any and all combinations, and the drug and placebo groups were similar. Furthermore, nonwound complications were similar between the groups.

The effective systemic prophylactic agents are shown in Table 23-4. Chetlin and Elliott [54] evaluated the same preoperative regimen of intramuscular cephaloridine in individuals at high risk for postoperative infection after biliary tract operations (older than 70 years, acute cholecystitis, obstructive jaundice, choledocholithiasis without jaundice). Such individuals have a significantly increased frequency of infected bile and are expected to have increased infectious complications. In a randomized, but not blind, study of 84 patients, the incidence of postoperative infectious complications was 4 percent in the group treated with cephaloridine and 27 percent in those not receiving antibiotics. Regular intraoperative bile cultures done in all patients disclosed that the drug used had no effect in altering cultures in either treated or untreated groups. The significance of this study resides equally in the demonstration of the effectiveness of prophylactic systemic antibiotics and in the identification of a genuinely high-risk group of patients undergoing cholecystectomy. About 90 percent of these high-risk patients can be identified preoperatively, so that the groups most likely to benefit from prophylactic antibiotic therapy can be selected.

McLeish et al [55] have used intraoperative Gram stains

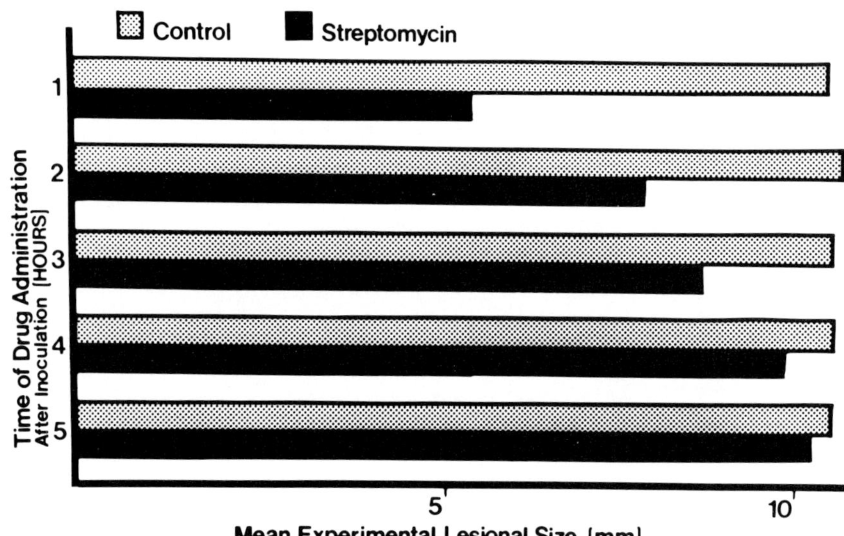

Fig. 23-2. Decreasing susceptibility of experimental infectious lesions. Note that after 3 hours virtually no reduction in lesional size occurs despite intravenous antibiotic.

TABLE 23-4. EFFECTIVE SYSTEMIC PROPHYLACTIC AGENTS

Agent	Dose Regimen
Cephaloridine	1 gm, 3 doses perioperatively
Cefazolin	1 gm, 3 doses perioperatively
Tobramycin-lincomycin	160 gm/600 gm, 1 or 2 doses perioperatively

to determine risk for postoperative infection. A significant reduction of postoperative wound infection was observed in patients treated with intraoperative systemic antibiotic therapy when Gram stains were positive. Patients were not classified, however, according to the stages of their illnesses. This scheme loses the advantages of pretreatment and has modest (3 percent) false-negative results. This practice has now been discontinued in their hospital.[56] The reliability of the criteria of Chetlin and Elliott[54] has repeatedly been shown to be clinically useful.

In a study of premenopausal women undergoing vaginal hysterectomy, Ledger and associates[57] used a perioperative regimen of intramuscular cephaloridine in a prospective, double-blind, randomized fashion. Significantly fewer patients treated with cephaloridine had postoperative pelvic infection, and all infectious morbidity was reduced. "Low-dose" carbenicillin was judged protective in a blind, prospective study of abdominal and vaginal hysterectomy without distinction of menopausal status,[58] and a retrospective study supported the effectiveness of a single dose of cephalothin before vaginal hysterectomy.[59] (See also chapter 44).

More recently, Stone and associates[60] studied the effectiveness of cefazolin used perioperatively in potentially contaminated gastrointestinal procedures. Wound infection following gastric (4 percent), biliary (2 percent), and colonic (6 percent) operations was significantly reduced compared to placebo-treated patients. However, in patients undergoing colonic operations, oral, poorly absorbed antibiotics were permitted, which makes these results subject to query. The initiation of antibiotic prophylaxis postoperatively resulted in identical infection rates in both treated and placebo groups. Other recent studies have shown similar effectiveness of perioperative cefazolin in potentially contaminated operations. Holman et al[61] found cefazolin an effective prophylaxis in premenopausal women subjected to vaginal or abdominal hysterectomy but of no benefit to postmenopausal women. Strachan et al[62] reported that a single preoperative dose of cefazolin was highly effective in preventing postoperative wound infection in patients undergoing cholecystectomy.

The benefit of systemic prophylaxis in noncardiac thoracic operations cannot be determined from the available studies, which are conceptually or technically flawed. The field warrants much better definition.[63-65]

Individuals who sustain penetrating wounds to the abdomen have a significantly increased incidence of infectious complications. A retrospective series of 295 patients were divided into those who received prophylactic penicillin-tetracycline or penicillin-chloramphenicol preoperatively, intraoperatively, and postoperatively.[66] The average delay from injury to operation was 105 minutes. These investigators observed a significant reduction in total infectious complications and wound infections when antibiotic therapy was received preoperatively (in the emergency room). No protective effect could be detected if the antibiotic administration was delayed until the intraoperative or postoperative phase. The rate of infection did not correlate with the number of organs injured, the presence of shock, or improvements in technique over the 13-year study. When examined separately, injury to the colon was associated with an 11 percent incidence of infection when antibiotic was administered preoperatively. When prophylaxis was delayed until the intraoperative or postoperative periods, the incidence of infection rose to 50 percent and 70 percent respectively. While this study was retrospective, the results lend indirect support to the contention that individuals with penetrating trauma to the abdomen benefit significantly from the administration of preoperative prophylactic antibiotic therapy.

Systemic prophylaxis is generally not appropriate in

clean operations (Chapter 20). Because the risk of wound infection is sufficiently small, large numbers of patients need not receive unnecessary antibiotics. The risk of antibiotic side effects in such cases may be greater than the risk of infection. Nevertheless, in some clean and refined clean operations a wound infection can lead to unusually severe complications, particularly in procedures where large foreign bodies are implanted. The potentially disastrous consequences of prosthetic infection may outweigh the inherent risk of the antimicrobial agent. Ericson [67] demonstrated a significant benefit from prophylactic cloxicillin in patients undergoing prosthetic hip replacement. Nafcillin has been shown to be of prophylactic benefit in hip nailing procedures.[68] The effectiveness of cefazolin (1 gm intravenously) before operation and 4 doses after operation was studied in 462 patients undergoing peripheral vascular and abdominal aortic reconstructive procedures.[69] Among the 225 patients who received cefazolin, 2 infections occurred (0.8 percent). In the placebo (saline) group, 16 infections occurred (6.7 percent). The difference between these two groups is highly significant. No emergence of microbial resistance to the drug was noted. Graft infection occurred in 4 patients in the placebo group. In intrathoracic vascular procedures, no benefit from the use of cefazolin was shown, presumably because of the low infection rate in the placebo group. The effectiveness of either topical or systemic prophylactic cephalosporins in clean vascular surgery is now established.[20a]

The growing awareness of the possible role for anaerobic organisms in abdominal infections has led to recommendations for the use of appropriate systemic agents.[21,69-72] Galland and associates [22] found that high-dose systemic tobramycin-lincomycin was effective in preventing not only wound infection after colonic procedures but also, specifically, infections that result from anaerobic organisms. Similarly, in several double-blind, randomized, prospective series,[70,71] one- or two-dose regimens of tobramycin-lincomycin given preoperatively and immediately after operation were protective. No emergence of microbial resistance was noted, and no patient developed pseudomembranous enterocolitis during these short-course regimens. Infections caused by colonic aerobes and anaerobes were significantly reduced when compared to controls. In the studies reporting the effectiveness of cephaloridine and cefazolin, anaerobic organisms were seldom encountered as causes of postoperative wound infection, even when sought diligently.

The significance of intraperitoneal anaerobic bacteria has recently been studied by Stone and associates [74] in a series of 512 consecutive patients subjected to emergency celiotomy. After initial trials, 300 patients were randomly selected to receive intravenous cephalothin or clindamycin as preoperative, systemic prophylaxis. Aerobic and anaerobic culture examinations were performed after the abdomen was opened, sequentially through the procedure, and at wound closure. All discharges or exudates encountered postoperatively were also subjected to culture examination. Anaerobic organisms uniformly contaminated the peritoneal cavity whenever distal or obstructed intestine had been perforated. Two-thirds of the 123 wound and intra-abdominal infections contained one or more different anaerobic species, which were always associated with aerobic organisms. No significant difference in the incidence of postoperative infection or in the type of infecting bacteria could be found with respect to the antibiotic administered. One antibiotic was totally ineffective against anaerobes, and the other was specifically chosen for its activity in that sphere. When anaerobic infection occurs, it usually does so in conjunction with aerobic bacterial proliferation. The aerobic bacteria elaborate metabolic products, which produce significant reductions in oxidation-reduction potential. Stone suggested that the effective use of antimicrobial agents directed toward aerobes alone results in the disruption of these synergistic relationships, creating an environment where anaerobic bacteria cannot survive.[74] He observed that the duration of bacterial exposure to atmospheric oxygen was the most critical factor in recovering anaerobic organisms.

ENTERAL PROPHYLAXIS

Operative procedures that require opening the colon have long been associated with a high risk of wound infection. Mechanical cleansing, while an important part of preparing the colon for operation, does not eliminate bacteria. Therefore, residual colonic bacterial concentration is only slightly altered.[75] Large numbers of both aerobic and anaerobic bacteria exist in the normal and mechanically cleansed colon. Numerous attempts have been made to "sterilize" the colon with oral antibiotics. Sterilization is a pathetic misnomer and is usually accomplished only in an autoclave. Optimum oral antimicrobial therapy produces a 100- to 1000-fold reduction in colonic bacterial concentration but regularly leaves bacterial densities of 10^5 to 10^6 organisms per gram of feces. The goal of intestinal antisepsis is, then, to reduce the flora in the lumen, expecting ultimately to reduce proportionately the number of organisms that reach the incision. Numerous agents have been used singly or in combination in an attempt to protect the operative wound (Chapter 39).

Poth [2] originally characterized the ideal intestinal antiseptic (Table 23-5). Studies in the early 1940s suggested a possible role for sulfa derivatives. Enteral administration of succinylsulfathiazole was found by Sarnoff and Poth [76] to exert a protective effect in a canine model of peritonitis. Clinical application based on this work far exceeded their observations. They found significant protection from intraluminal sulfonamides only when blood supply was impaired. From these limited observations, far-reaching applications were suggested and widely practiced. Sulfonamides were subsequently shown to have variable effects on colonic aerobes and no effect on anaerobes.[75] Although tetracycline suppresses colonic anaerobes, its effects on aerobic organisms varies.

Poth [2] found that orally administered neomycin, given every 4 hours in 1-gm doses for 3 days preoperatively, suppressed all the easily cultured aerobic fecal organisms. He therefore advocated this drug for the preoperative preparation of the colon. The subsequent observation of overgrowth of *Aerobacter aerogenes* in 10 percent of patients so treated led to a recommendation of the addition of sulfathalidine. Dearing and Needham [77] demonstrated

TABLE 23-5. PROPERTIES OF AN IDEAL INTESTINAL ANTISEPTIC

Broad antibacterial spectrum *
Minimal local and systemic toxicity
Chemical stability in the presence of digestive ferments
Capacity to prevent overgrowth of resistant bacterial variants *
Rapidity of action *
Minimal systemic absorption *
Activity in the presence of food or other foreign substances
Aid in mechanical cleansing of the bowel without causing dehydration
Nonirritant to gastrointestinal mucosa
Noninterference with tissue growth and repair
Low dosage requirement
Solubility in water
Palatability
Inhibitive activity on excessive growth of fungi
Restricted use as intestinal antiseptic only

* Because no single agent can meet these formidable criteria, characteristics that are of greatest value are indicated.

that neomycin effectively reduced aerobic bacterial concentration but failed to reduce the numbers of anaerobic organisms recovered, particularly *Bacteroides* species.

The advantages of neomycin are rapid onset of action, broad-spectrum effectiveness against fecal aerobic organisms, and the need for administration only during the 24-hour period before operation. However, the lack of significant effectiveness against the predominantly anaerobic flora of the colon, in theory, precluded its use as the sole agent for intestinal antibiotic preparation.

Other single agent regimens have been tried. The tetracyclines, while effective against anaerobes, have been associated with alleged outbreaks of staphylococcal enterocolitis. Streptomycin has also been associated with the overgrowth of resistant bacterial forms. Kanamycin is virtually ineffective against anaerobic organisms.

In the period from 1945 to 1975, antibiotic preparation of the colon was employed extensively. The popularization of these agents was based, however, on poorly designed and largely uncontrolled studies, in which concomitant systemic antibiotic therapy frequently occurred. Such studies contributed little to genuine insight into the role of preoperative antibiotic preparation of the colon. Excessively prolonged preoperative oral therapy or concomitant systemic therapy may help explain the sporadic appearance of pseudomembranous enterocolitis. Until relatively recently, no controlled or randomized trials had demonstrated the clear effectiveness and safety of these regimens in preventing operative wound infection, nor had there been careful determination of which agents have the lowest incidence of systemic toxicity or emergence of resistant organisms.

In 1974, the first well-designed, prospective, randomized, double-blind series was published, in which oral antibiotic preparation of the colon was compared to mechanical cleansing alone.[78] Neomycin alone, neomycin and tetracycline in combination, and placebo were compared in patients undergoing elective colon procedures. The combined use of neomycin-tetracycline was associated with a significantly reduced incidence of infectious complications. Neomycin alone, however, did not significantly reduce the incidence of operative wound infection or other infectious complications. Altemeier[79] and others have suggested that the benefits observed are largely the result of absorption of the tetracycline and consequent systemic activity.

Nichols et al[80] proposed the use of neomycin and erythromycin base, because each agent is allegedly poorly absorbed, and benefit was demonstrated in a pilot trial. This combination, which effectively depresses both aerobic and anaerobic organisms, has recently been shown to be better than placebo in reducing the rate of overall systemic and abdominal wound infectious complications after elective colonic surgery.[81] All patients underwent mechanical preparation. The placebo group had a 43 percent incidence of septic complications and a 35 percent incidence of wound infections. The antibiotic-treated group exhibited 9 percent wound infections, which constituted all their infectious complications. Anaerobic infection was observed in five placebo-treated patients and only 1 antibiotic-treated patient. Quantitative cultures of colonic content showed a 10,000- to 100,000-fold decrease in the concentration of both aerobic and anaerobic organisms in the antibiotic group when compared to the group treated with placebo.

Metronidazole is quite effective against anaerobic organisms and against *Bacteroides* species in particular.[82] The successful clinical management of anaerobic infections with this agent has also been reported.[83] The use of metronidazole is advocated for the preoperative preparation of the colon for elective operation.[84-86]

Goldring et al[84] evaluated the effect of a 3-day preoperative regimen of kanamycin (1 gm) and metronidazole (200 mg) administered every 6 hours in conjunction with mechanical cleansing. No other preoperative, intraoperative, or postoperative antibiotics were given. Fifty patients undergoing elective colon operations were divided into two groups, those treated with kanamycin-metronidazole and those receiving purgative alone. There was a highly significant difference in postoperative infectious complications. In the group receiving the antibiotics, two patients developed staphylococcal infections. Eleven of the patients treated with mechanical cleansing alone developed postoperative infections, which were generally caused by coliforms. Two deaths occurred in this group; one patient had *Bacteroides* septicemia.

Willis and associates[85] recently reported a double-blind, prospective, randomized study of 46 patients undergoing elective colon procedures in which metronidazole was the sole oral agent used for antibiotic colon preparation. All patients underwent mechanical cleansing; unfortunately, for purposes of analysis, all patients also received 80 mg of intramuscular gentamicin on call to the operating room. Metronidazole or placebo administered orally or by suppository was continued until the seventh postoperative day. Eight percent of the patients treated with metronidazole developed infections caused by aerobic organisms. In contrast, 58 percent of placebo-treated patients developed anaerobic infections and one patient developed aerobic infection.

The double-blind, prospective, randomized series of 70 patients reported by Brass et al [86] had either neomycin-erythromycin base or neomycin-metronidazole as oral preparation for elective colon surgery. All patients received mechanical cleansing. Metronidazole was given in 750-mg doses three times a day for 2 days before operation. Erythromycin base and neomycin were given three times a day in 1-gm doses, each during a 24-hour period preoperatively. In addition, all patients received a three-dose perioperative regimen of 1-gm doses of cephalothin intravenously. Ordinarily, the use of systemic drugs would fatally flaw such a study; however, data presented later in this chapter indicate that systemic cephalothin achieves surprisingly low wound antibiotic levels and appears to exert minimal, if any, effect on the overall results of this study. All of the 10 infections in the neomycin-erythromycin group of 40 patients were associated with coliform organisms. The two infections in the group treated with metronidazole were due to staphylococcal organisms; no coliform organisms were observed.

While these studies clearly demonstrate the effectiveness of metronidazole in suppressing anaerobic flora, a comparison with the report by Clarke and associates [81] is difficult to make because of the certain absorption and therefore concomitant systemic activity of both metronidazole and erythromycin. The perioperative use of cephalothin, an agent with probable low systemic prophylactic effectiveness, contributes another major difference from the study by Clarke.

Höjer and Wetterfors [87] used oral doxycycline, a tetracycline derivative, for oral prophylaxis in patients undergoing colonic operations. Doxycycline possesses antibacterial activity against both aerobes and anaerobes and has a high affinity for intestinal tissue. In a double-blind, prospective, randomized study, 58 patients received doxycycline and 60 patients received placebo. Doxycycline was administered as a 200-mg oral loading dose during the 24-hour preoperative period and was continued parenterally for 5 days postoperatively at 100 mg per day. Abdominal wound sepsis occurred in 8 percent of patients receiving the doxycycline and 41 percent of those receiving placebo. Mean serum doxycycline levels were often *exceeded* by doxycycline levels in intestinal mucosa. Eighty-three percent of anaerobes and 71 percent of aerobes were classified as being sensitive to this agent. However, overall aerobic resistance to doxycycline increased from 22 percent in the controls to 50 percent in the experimental group.

Both systemic prophylaxis and enteral prophylaxis appear to reduce the rate of infectious complications following operation upon the colon. A randomized study by Lewis et al [88] compared these two regimens in patients undergoing elective colon operation. Systemic therapy was accomplished by using perioperative cephaloridine, and enteral prophylaxis was completed using neomycin-erythromycin base. The patient populations in both groups were well matched. In the total group of 79 patients, no significant difference was observed in the rate of infectious complications after elective colon operation. The distribution of anaerobic organisms in stool culture specimens was essentially the same, and each group had one episode of anaerobic wound infection. Edmondson has informed us of a similar outcome in an as yet unpublished, careful trial of the same regimens. It appears that systemic prophylaxis and enteral prophylaxis are nearly equally protective in preventing infectious complications in patients undergoing elective operation upon the colon.[89]

Jones et al [90] evaluated an "instant preparation" of the colon using either povidone-iodine or a neomycin-erythromycin base. In dogs, 10-minute exposure of colonic contents to povidone-iodine resulted in a significant reduction in aerobic growth. Povidone-iodine was also significantly better than neomycin-erythromycin in the elimination of anaerobic organisms grown from stool culture. In an in vivo study in dogs undergoing resection and primary anastomosis of unprepared sigmoid colon, povidone-iodine was used as an intraoperative agent by intracolonic injection. Mean total bacterial counts after treatment were compared with the use of saline. A highly significant reduction in the concentration of aerobic and anaerobic organisms after intraoperative treatment with 10 percent povidone-iodine was observed. This instant preparation may be of value in patients requiring emergency operation on the colon, when time does not permit the use of standard intestinal preparation.

CHEMOPROPHYLAXIS: PRINCIPLES AND PRACTICE

For success, chemoprophylaxis must take place before or at the time of contamination. Various studies [12,27,50,91-95] have established that no grace period exists after contamination of the wound. Prophylactic antibiotic therapy is not indicated, nor will it be beneficial in *all* surgical wounds. In most clean operative wounds (eg, herniorrhaphy, thyroidectomy), the risk of infection approaches 1 percent. It is, at best, questionable whether the routine use of systemic or topical chemoprophylaxis can successfully reduce this rate further. The risks of drug reactions and the tendency toward selection of resistant organisms outweigh the potential benefit of topical or systemic antibiotics in low risk patients. Many studies have disclosed no benefit associated with the use of topical or systemic agents in clean operative wounds.[11,13-16,22,47] The major exception is in clean procedures in which prosthetic devices are implanted where infection introduces the risk of unusually severe complication.[19,20a,48,66,68] The primary indication for prophylactic agents is in cases associated with a high frequency of, or unusually severe, sequelae of infection. Genuine high-risk situations may appear in variable forms [52-55] (Table 23-6 and Table 18-16).

The selection of an antimicrobial agent must be based on the sensitivity of the expected flora. In operations on the alimentary tract, agents with broad gram-negative coverage are required, usually with some activity against the traditional *Staphylococcus*. Cephaloridine and cefazolin are the only systemically administered antibiotics whose use is supported by well controlled clinical trials. Topical aminoglycoside antibiotics, Neosporin, and cephaloridine are also effective (Table 23-2).

Topical therapy allows the use of poorly absorbed, more toxic agents in higher local concentrations than can

TABLE 23-6. SOUND INDICATIONS FOR SYSTEMIC PROPHYLAXIS

Elective alimentary tract operations
High-risk biliary operation
Premenopausal vaginal hysterectomy
Prosthetic implants
Arterial reconstruction in abdomen or extremity
Total hip replacement
Penetrating abdominal trauma

be safely achieved by systemic administration alone. In addition, local therapy has been advocated because there may be less antibiotic-induced alterations in granulocyte function, a concern of as yet undetermined clinical significance. No studies show that topical therapy fully obviates the problem of systemic absorption; topical neomycin is absorbed in significant quantities.[87] Curiously, no studies appear to have compared topical therapy in a controlled fashion to either systemic or intestinal prophylactic methods. Aminoglycosides are absorbed from the peritoneal cavity and the use of intraperitoneal antibiotics, while probably effective, requires that precautions be taken to prevent respiratory complications or nephrotoxic or ototoxic effects. Effective topical agents are delineated in Table 23-2.

Whether prophylactic regimens should include antibiotics directed against anaerobic bacteria is not completely resolved, but there are indications that successful management of the aerobic component of the more common, mixed aerobic-anaerobic synergistic infection will alter the wound environment sufficiently to interfere with the growth requirements of anaerobic organisms.[74] This implies that inclusion of antibiotics directed toward anaerobic bacteria may be unnecessary in peritoneal infections, which can be fully exposed to ambient oxygen and mechanically cleansed.

A major determining factor in successful systemic prophylaxis is the ability of parenterally administered agents to penetrate the tissues in sufficiently high concentrations to exceed the minimal inhibitory concentration of expected contaminating flora. Experimental and clinical determination of antibiotic levels [93-95] have demonstrated that cephaloridine and cefazolin rapidly penetrate interstitial fluid. Bagley et al [95] found that cefazolin achieved rapid penetrance with sustained levels. Two hours after a 1-gm intravenous dose, wound levels reached 28 μg per ml and were 41 μg per ml at 3 hours. In a similar fashion, 1 gm of cephaloridine administered intravenously produced sustained wound levels in excess of 10 μg per ml up to 3 hours. In earlier studies, Polk [53,98] found that intramuscular administration of 1 gm of cephaloridine resulted in consistent wound levels of 10 μg per ml in wound fluid. Relative differences in protein binding between cefazolin and cephaloridine are such that even at these levels cephaloridine produces and maintains higher levels of free, active antibiotic.

Cephalothin is so rapidly excreted that its tissue levels cannot be maintained without frequent readministration. After a 1-gm intravenous dose, the wound level of cephalothin was below 10 μg per ml 1 to 3 hours later.[95] After a 2-gm intravenous dose, wound fluid levels were consistently below 10 μg per ml after 1 hour and were significantly below levels achieved by 1 gm of parenteral cephaloridine.[95]

The modest peak and rapid disappearance of cephalothin in wounds may help explain the relatively high frequency of prophylactic failures with cephalothin, as contrasted with the other two cephalosporins, which effect higher levels for much longer periods (Fig. 23-3).

It is clear that cephalothin achieves much lower and shorter lasting wound levels than either cefazolin or cephaloridine. Condon et al [96] have recently reported a double-blind, prospective, randomized trial of intravenously administered preoperative cephalothin. The use of this regimen was associated with a 30 percent incidence of operative wound infection compared to only 6 percent in those patients receiving oral erythromycin-neomycin with concomitant cephalothin. On this basis, the use of cephalothin as a prophylactic agent should be discontinued in favor of cefazolin or cephaloridine; their wound kinetics appear to be consistent and are the probable basis of their consistent efficacy in properly controlled trials.

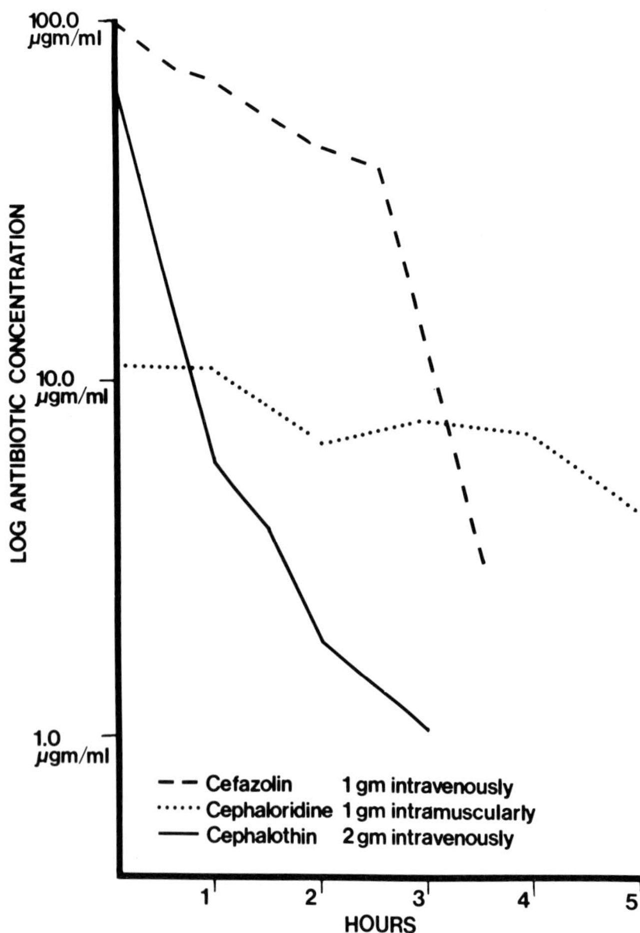

Fig. 23-3. Antibiotic wound levels. Antibiotic wound activity was measured at timed intervals in surgical wounds. Note the impressively low cephalothin levels after 1 hour.

While some orally administered intestinal antibiotics are effective in reducing infectious complications after colon operation,[78,81] no clear benefit from their use is apparent when compared to systemic prophylaxis.[88] A potential risk of intestinal antibiotics includes a low incidence of staphylococcal enterocolitis.[75] Although most patients are relatively asymptomatic or have only mild diarrhea, severe enterocolitis has been associated with several deaths. Children and infants are unusually susceptible to overgrowth with *Candida* species,[75] posing an additional risk in this age group. In such pediatric groups an antifungal agent may be needed in addition to other prophylactic intestinal agents.[75] Systemic prophylactic antibiotics are not always helpful, however; Altemeier and associates [97] observed an increased incidence of postoperative infection in patients receiving preoperative intestinal antibiotic preparation with neomycin and postoperative systemic antibiotics.[97] The benefit of systemic prophylaxis in patients receiving thorough intestinal mechanical preparation is well documented. Resistant strains have not emerged, and the incidence of anaerobic infections is extremely low.

In view of the effectiveness of these methods in reducing infectious complications, the question of the appropriateness of combination prophylaxis warrants discussion. At this point, well-conceived and well-conducted studies, either experimental or clinical, are few and far between. Pitt et al [20a] found no benefit when topical drug use was added to systemic administration, or vice versa; they did, however, confirm the advantages of one or the other over untreated control vascular operations. Similarly, Dion et al [99] found no clinical difference between oral and parenteral use of metronidazole in colon operations, but did show an antimicrobial effect upon bacteria in the colon following systemic therapy.

While more may be better for antibiotic dosages, the same is not unequivocally true for addition of antibiotic regimens. In this regard, we feel that preoperative manipulation of patients' host defense mechanisms via immunomodulating techniques may serve as a more valuable and productive route of inquiry than further refinements in antibiotic manipulation (Chapter 19).

ERRORS IN THE CHEMOPROPHYLAXIS OF WOUND INFECTION

Antimicrobial prophylaxis is clearly useful in some circumstances, and the principles (Table 23-3) are clear. Two recent studies have highlighted the errors in the use of prophylactic antibiotics.[100,101] All the principles are commonly violated, but unnecessary, prolonged preoperative use, improper timing of the perioperative dose, and prolonged postoperative administration were the most common. These habits are both expensive and potentially dangerous.

BIBLIOGRAPHY

Hirshmann JV, Inui TS: Antimicrobial prophylaxis: A critique of recent trials. Rev Infect Dis 2:1, 1980.

Burke JF: Preventing bacterial infection by coordinating antibiotic and host activity: A time dependent activity. Southern Medical Journal, Birmingham (suppl) 1:24, 1977.

Barza M, Butler T: The penetration of penicillins and cephalosporins into selected sites of clinical interest. In Weinstein L, and Fields BN (eds.): Seminars in Infectious Disease, Vol III. New York, Thieme-Stratton, 1980.

REFERENCES

TOPICAL PROPHYLAXIS

1. Gray FJ, Kidd E: Topical chemotherapy in prevention of wound infection. Surgery 54:891, 1963.
2. Poth EJ: Intestinal antisepsis in surgery. JAMA 153:1516, 1953.
3. Polk HC Jr, Stone HH (eds): Contemporary Burn Management. Boston, Little, Brown, 1971, pp 171–244.
4. Polk HC Jr, Monafo WW, Moyer CA: Human burn survival: Study of efficacy of 0.5 percent aqueous silver nitrate. Arch Surg 98:262, 1969.
5. Hopson WB Jr, Britt LG, Sherman RT, Ledes CP: The use of topical antibiotic in the prevention of experimental wound infection. J Surg Res 8:261, 1968.
6. Singleton AO, Julian J: An experimental evaluation of methods used to prevent infection in wounds which have been contaminated with feces. Ann Surg 151:912, 1960.
7. Waterman NG, Howell RS, Babich M: The effect of a prophylactic topical antibiotic (cephalothin) on the incidence of wound infection. Arch Surg 97:365, 1968.
8. DiGiglia JW, Leonard GL, Ochsner JL: Local irrigation with an antibiotic solution in the prevention of infection in vascular prostheses. Surgery 67:836, 1970.
9. Howes EL: Topical use of streptomycin in wounds. Am J Med 2:449, 1947.
10. Gingrass RP, Close AS, Ellison EH: The effect of various topical and parenteral agents on the prevention of infection in experimental contaminated wounds. J Trauma 4:763, 1964.
11. Stone HH, Hester TR Jr: Incisional and peritoneal infection after emergency celiotomy. Ann Surg 177:699, 1973.
12. Polk HC Jr, Miles AA: The decisive period in the primary infection of muscle by *Escherichia coli.* Br J Exp Pathol 54:99, 1973.
13. Stone HH, Hester TR Jr: Topical antibiotic and delayed primary closure in the management of contaminated surgical incisions. J Surg Res 12:70, 1972.
14. Pollock AV, Froome K, Evans M: The bacteriology of primary wound sepsis in potentially contaminated abdominal operations: the effect of irrigation, povidone-iodine and cephaloridine on the sepsis rate assessed in a clinical trial. Br J Surg 65:76, 1978.
15. Pollock AV, Leaper DJ, Evans M: Single dose intra-incisional antibiotic prophylaxis of surgical wound sepsis: a controlled trial of cephaloridine and ampicillin. Br J Surg 64:322, 1977.
16. Pollock AV, Evans M: Povidone-iodine for the control of surgical wound infection: a controlled clinical trial against cephaloridine. Br J Surg 62:292, 1975.
17. Cohn I Jr: Intraperitoneal antibiotic administration. Surg Gynecol Obstet 114:309, 1962.
18. DiVincenti FC, Cohn I Jr: Intraperitoneal kanamycin in advanced peritonitis. Am J Surg 111:147, 1966.
19. Lord JW Jr, Rossi G, Daliana M: Intraoperative antibiotic wound lavage: an attempt to eliminate postoperative infec-

tion in arterial and clean general surgical procedures. Ann Surg 185:634, 1977.
20. Casten DF, Nach RJ, Spinzia J: An experimental and clinical study of the effectiveness of antibiotic wound irrigation in preventing infection. Surg Gynecol Obstet 118:783, 1964.
20a. Pitt HA, Postier RG, MaGowan WAL, Frank LW, Surmak AJ, Sitzman JV, Bouchier-Hayes D: Prophylactic antibiotics in vascular surgery. Ann Surg 192:356, 1980.
21. Andersen B, Korner B, Ostergaard AH: Topical ampicillin against wound infection after colorectal surgery. Ann Surg 176:129, 1972.
22. Galland RB, Saunders JH, Mosley JG, Darrell JH: Prevention of wound infection in abdominal operations by perioperative antibiotics or povidone-iodine: a controlled trial. Lancet 2:1043, 1977.
23. Gilmore OJ, Martin TD: Aetiology and prevention of wound infection in appendicectomy. Br J Surg 61:281, 1974.
24. Polk HC Jr, Ehrenkranz NJ (eds): Therapeutic Advances and New Clinical Implications: Medical and Surgical Antisepsis with Betadine Microbicides. New York, Purdue Frederick, 1972.
25. Connell JF Jr, Rousselot LM: Povidone-iodine. Extensive surgical evaluation of a new antiseptic agent. Am J Surg 108:849, 1964.
26. Gilmore OJ, Sanderson PJ: Prophylactic interparietal povidone-iodine in abdominal surgery. Br J Surg 62:792, 1975.
27. Polk HC Jr, Miles AA: Enhancement of bacterial infection by ferric iron: kinetics, mechanisms, and surgical significance. Surgery 70:71, 1971.
28. Barnett WO, Oliver RI, Elliott RL: Elimination of the lethal properties of gangrenous bowel segments. Ann Surg 167:912, 1968.
29. Crook JN, Cotlar AM, Bornside GH, Cohn I Jr: Intraperitoneal cephalothin in the treatment of experimental appendiceal peritonitis. Am Surg 34:736, 1968.
30. Lavigne JE, Brown CS, Machiedo GW, Blackwood JM, Rush BF Jr: The treatment of experimental peritonitis with intraperitoneal Betadine solution. J Surg Res 16:307, 1974.
31. Lagarde MC, Bolton JS, Cohn I Jr: Intraperitoneal povidone-iodine in experimental peritonitis. Ann Surg 187:613, 1978.
32. Flint LM Jr, Beasley DJ, Richardson JD, Polk HC Jr: Topical povidone-iodine reduces mortality from bacterial peritonitis. J Surg Res 26:280, 1979.
33. Gilmore OJA, Reid C, Houang ET, Shaw EJ: Prophylactic intraperitoneal povidone-iodine in alimentary tract surgery. Am J Surg 135:156, 1978.
34. Pridgen A: Respiratory arrest thought to be due to intraperitoneal neomycin. Surgery 40:571, 1956.
35. Weinstein AJ, McHenry MC, Gavan TL: Systemic absorption of neomycin irrigating solution. JAMA 238:152, 1977.
36. Nelson JL, Kuzman JH, Cohn I Jr: Intraperitoneal lavage and kanamycin for the contaminated abdomen. Surg Clin North Am 55:1391, 1975.
37. Noon GP, Beall AC Jr, Jordan GL Jr, Riggs S, DeBakey M: Clinical evaluation of peritoneal irrigation with antibiotic solution. Surgery 62:73, 1967.
38. DiVincenti FC, Cohn I Jr: Prolonged administration of intraperitoneal kanamycin in the treatment of peritonitis. Am Surg 37:177, 1971.
39. Cohn I Jr, Cotlar AM, Richard L Jr: Intraperitoneal kanamycin—clinical experience. Am Surg 29:756, 1963.
40. Prigot A, Shidlovsky BA, Campbell EA: Intraperitoneal use of kanamycin as an adjunct in the therapy of established peritonitis and peritoneal contamination. Ann NY Acad Sci 76:204, 1958.
41. Mullett RD, Keats AS: Apnea and respiratory insufficiency after intraperitoneal administration of kanamycin. Surgery 49:530, 1961.
42. Ericsson CD, Duke JH Jr, Pickering LK, Qadri SMH: Systemic absorption of bacitracin after peritoneal lavage. Am J Surg 137:65, 1979.
43. McMullan MH, Barnett WO: The clinical use of intraperitoneal cephalothin. Surgery 67:432, 1970.
44. Rambo M: Irrigation of the peritoneal cavity with cephalothin. Am J Surg 123:192, 1972.
45. Cohn I Jr: Discussion of Rambo WM: Irrigation of the peritoneal cavity with cephalothin. Am J Surg 123:192, 1972.
46. Stephen M, Loewenthal J: Generalized infective peritonitis. Surg Gynecol Obstet, in press. 1981.
47. Polk HC Jr: Editorial: Generalized peritonitis: a continuing challenge. Surgery 86:77–78, 1979.

SYSTEMIC PROPHYLAXIS

48. Chodak GW, Plaut ME: Use of systemic antibiotics for prophylaxis in surgery: a critical review. Arch Surg 112:326, 1977.
49. Altemeier WA, Todd J: Studies on the incidence of infection following open chest cardiac massage for cardiac arrest. Ann Surg 158:596, 1963.
50. Miles AA, Miles EM, Burke J: The value and duration of defence reactions of the skin to the primary lodgement of bacteria. Br J Exp Pathol 38:79, 1957.
51. Burke JF: The effective period of preventive antibiotic action in experimental incisions and dermal lesions. Surgery 50:161, 1961.
52. Bernard HR, Cole WR: The prophylaxis of surgical infection: the effect of prophylactic antimicrobial drugs on the incidence of infection following potentially contaminated operations. Surgery 56:151, 1964.
53. Polk HC Jr, Lopez-Mayor JF: Postoperative wound infection: a prospective study of determinant factors and prevention. Surgery 66:97, 1969.
54. Chetlin SH, Elliott DW: Preoperative antibiotics in biliary surgery. Arch Surg 107:319, 1973.
55. McLeish AR, Keighley MR, Bishop HM, Burdon DW, Quoraishi AH, Dorricott NJ, Oates GD, Alexander-Williams J: Selecting patients requiring antibiotics in biliary surgery by immediate Gram stains of bile at operation. Surgery 81:473, 1977.
56. Alexander-Williams J: Personal communication, 1979.
57. Ledger WJ, Sweet RL, Headington JT: Prophylactic cephaloridine in the prevention of postoperative pelvic infections in premenopausal women undergoing vaginal hysterectomy. Am J Obstet Gynecol 115:766, 1973.
58. Roberts JM, Homesley HD: Low dose carbenicillin prophylaxis for vaginal and abdominal hysterectomy. Obstet Gynecol 52:83, 1978.
59. Lander JL, Steigrad SJ: Single dose preoperative prophylactic antibiotic in vaginal hysterectomy. Aust NZ J Obstet Gynecol 18:73, 1978.
60. Stone HH, Hooper CA, Kolb LD, Geheber CE, Dawkins EJ: Antibiotic prophylaxis in gastric, biliary, and colonic surgery. Ann Surg 184:443, 1976.
61. Holman JF, McGowan JE, Thompson JD: Perioperative antibiotics in major elective gynecologic surgery. South Med J 71:417, 1978.
62. Strachan CJ, Black J, Powis SJ, Waterworth TA, Wise R, Wilkinson AR, Burdon DW, Severn M, Mitra B, Norcott H: Prophylactic use of cephazolin against wound sepsis after cholecystectomy. Br Med J 1:1254, 1977.
63. Bryant LR, Dillon ML, Mobin-Uddin K: Prophylactic antibiotics in noncardiac thoracic operations. Ann Thorac Surg 19:670, 1975.
64. Kvale PA, Ranga V, Kopacz M, Cox F, Magilligan DJ, Davila JC: Pulmonary resection. South Med J 70(suppl 1):64, 1977.

65. Truesdale R, D'Alessandri R, Manuel V, Daicoff G, Kluge RM: Antimicrobial vs. placebo prophylaxis in noncardiac thoracic surgery. JAMA 241:1254, 1979.
66. Fullen WD, Hunt J, Altemeier WA: Prophylactic antibiotics in penetrating wounds of the abdomen. J Trauma 12:282, 1972.
67. Ericson C, Lidgren L, Lindberg L: Cloxacillin in prophylaxis of postoperative infections of the hip. J Bone Joint Surg (Am) 55(1):808, 1973.
68. Boyd RJ, Burke JF, Colton T: A double blind clinical trial of prophylactic antibiotics in hip fractures. J Bone Joint Surg (Am) 55:1251, 1973.
69. Kaiser AB, Clayson KR, Mulherin JL, Roach AC, Allen TR, Edwards WH, Dale WA: Antibiotic prophylaxis in vascular surgery. Ann Surg 188:283, 1978.
70. Griffiths DA, Simpson RA, Shorey BA, Speller DE: Single dose preoperative antibiotic prophylaxis in gastrointestinal surgery. Lancet 2:325, 1976.
71. Stokes EJ, Waterworth PM, Franks V, Watson B, Clark CG: Short term routine antibiotic prophylaxis in surgery. Br J Surg 61:739, 1974.
72. Keighley MR, Crapp AR, Burdon DW, Cooke WT, Alexander-Williams J: Prophylaxis against anaerobic sepsis in bowel surgery. Br J Surg 63:538, 1976.
73. Leigh DA: Wound infections due to *Bacteroides fragilis* following intestinal surgery. Br J Surg 62:375, 1975.
74. Stone HH, Kolb LD, Geheber CE: Incidence and significance of intraperitoneal anaerobic bacteria. Ann Surg 181:705, 1975.
75. Nichols RL, Condon RE: Preoperative preparation of the colon. Surg Gynecol Obstet 132:323, 1971.
76. Sarnoff SJ, Poth EJ: Intestinal obstruction: I. The protective action of succinylsulfathiazole following simple venous occlusion. Surgery 16:927, 1944.
77. Dearing WH, Needham GM: The effect of oral administration of neomycin on intestinal bacterial flora of man. Proc Mayo Clin 28:502, 1953.
78. Washington JA II, Dearing WH, Judd ES, Elvebach LR: Effect of preoperative antibiotic regimen on development of infection after intestinal surgery: prospective, randomized, double-blind study. Ann Surg 180:567, 1974.
79. Altemeier WA: Discussion of Whelan JP, Hale JH: Bactericidal activity of metronidazole against *Bacteroides fragilis*. J Clin Pathol 26:393, 1973.
80. Nichols RL, Broido P, Condon RE, Gorbach SL, Nyhus LM: Effect of preoperative neomycin-erythromycin intestinal preparation on the incidence of infectious complications following colon surgery. Ann Surg 178:453, 1973.
81. Clarke JS, Condon RE, Bartlett JG, Gorbach SL, Nichols RL, Ochi S: Preoperative oral antibiotics reduce septic complications of colon operations: results of prospective, randomized, double-blind clinical study. Ann Surg 186:251, 1977.
82. Whelan JP, Hale JH: Bactericidal activity of metronidazole against *Bacteroides fragilis*. J Clin Pathol 26:393, 1973.
83. Ingham HR, Rich GE, Selkon JB, Hale JH, Roxby CM, Betty MJ, Johnston RWG, Uldall PR: Treatment with metronidazole of three patients with serious infections due to *Bacteroides fragilis*. J Antimicrob Chemother 1:235, 1975.
84. Goldring J, McNaught W, Scott A, Gillespie G: Prophylactic oral antimicrobial agents in elective colonic surgery: a controlled trial. Lancet 2:997, 1975.
85. Willis AT, Ferguson IR, Jones PH, Phillips KD, Tearle PV, Fiddian RV, Graham DF, Harland DH, Hughes DF, Knight D, Mee WM, Pashby N, Rothwell-Jackson RL, Sachdeva AK, Sutch I, Kilbey C, Edwards D: Metronidazole in prevention and treatment of *Bacteroides* infections in elective colonic surgery. Br Med J 1:607, 1977.
86. Brass C, Richards GK, Ruedy J, Prentis J, Hinchey EJ: The effect of metronidazole on the incidence of postoperative wound infection in elective colon surgery. Am J Surg 135:91, 1978.
87. Höjer H, Wetterfors J: Systemic prophylaxis with doxycycline in surgery of the colon and rectum. Ann Surg 187:362, 1978.
88. Lewis RT, Allan CM, Goodall RG, Lloyd-Smith WC, Marien B, Wiegand F: Antibiotics in surgery of the colon. Can J Surg 21:339, 1978.
89. Edmondson HT: Personal communications, 1979.
90. Jones FE, DeCosse JJ, Condon RE: Evaluation of "instant" preparation of the colon with povidone-iodine. Ann Surg 184:74, 1976.
91. Burke JF: Preventing bacterial infection by coordinating antibiotic and host activity: a time-dependent relationship. South Med J (suppl)1:24, 1977.
92. Burke J: The effective period of preventive antibiotic action in experimental incisions and dermal lesions. Surgery 50:161, 1961.
93. Waterman NG, Raff MJ, Scharfenberger L, Barnwell P: Antibiotic concentrations in hepatic interstitial and wound fluid. Surg Gynecol Obstet 142:235, 1976.
94. Waterman NG, Raff MJ, Scharfenberger L, Barnwell P: Protein binding and concentrations of cephaloridine and cefazolin in serum and interstitial fluid of dogs. J Infect Dis 133:642, 1976.
95. Bagley DH, MacLowry J, Beazley RM, Gorschboth C, Ketcham AS: Antibiotic concentration in human wound fluid after intravenous administration. Ann Surg 188:202, 1978.
96. Condon RE, Bartlett JG, Nichols RL, Schulte WJ, Gorbach SL, Ochi S: Preoperative prophylactic cephalothin fails to control septic complications of colorectal operations: results of controlled clinical trial: a Veterans Administration cooperative study. Am J Surg 137:68, 1979.
97. Altemeier WA, Hummel RP, Hill EO: Prevention of infection in colon surgery. Arch Surg 93:226. 1966.
98. Polk HC Jr, Pearlstein L, Jones CE: Operating-room acquired infection: its epidemiology and prevention. Surg Ann 9:83, 1977.
99. Dion YM, Richards GK, Prentis FML, Hinchey EJ: The influence of oral versus parenteral preoperative metronidazole on sepsis following colon surgery. Ann Surg 192:221, 1980.
100. Weiner JP, Gibson G, Munster AM: Use of prophylactic antibiotics in surgical procedures: Peer review guidelines as a method for quality assurance. Amer J Surg 139:348, 1980.
101. Crossley K, Gardner LC: Antimicrobial prophylaxis in surgical patients. JAMA 245:722, 1981.

CHAPTER 24
Nosocomial Infections in Surgical Patients

Richard J. Howard

Nosocomial or hospital-acquired infections are infections that develop within a hospital or are caused by microorganisms acquired within a hospital. While the patient population is the center of interest, nosocomial infections can also affect the hospital staff, visitors, workmen, salesmen, and delivery personnel. Nosocomial infections occur in every hospital in the country. Hospitals which report extraordinarily low rates of nosocomial infections most likely have no or poor surveillance techniques. Nosocomial infections are expensive both in terms of the pain and suffering and even death they can cause the patient and his family, and in terms of the economic costs of the increased hospital stay and time lost from work.

INCIDENCE OF NOSOCOMIAL INFECTIONS

The National Nosocomial Infections Study, carried out by the Center for Disease Control, surveys numerous hospitals throughout the country for nosocomial infections. The most recently published report covers hospital infections occurring in 79 hospitals in 31 states during 1977.[1] These hospitals reported 43,774 nosocomial infections occurring in 1,281,009 patients hospitalized and discharged during the year. The mean nosocomial infection rate was 3.4 percent of acute-care patients discharged. The nosocomial infection data were summarized in two parts, January through June and July through December. The summary for the first six months is presented in Table 24-1. The surgical services had a higher rate of hospital infections than did other services (Table 24-2), but this higher rate largely reflects surgical wound infections, most of which were precluded on other services. Urinary tract infections occurred most commonly (179.5 per 10,000 patients discharged), followed by wound infections (142.9 per 10,000 patients discharged) and lower respiratory tract infections (74.1 per 10,000 patients discharged). The common use of invasive diagnostic and therapeutic modalities, such as operations, urinary catheters, intravenous catheters, arterial catheters, respirators, and total parenteral nutrition, no doubt contributes to the high rate of nosocomial infections in surgical patients.

Escherichia coli is the pathogen most commonly cultured (Table 24-3). In the 1950s and early 1960s, *Staphylococcus aureus* and other gram-positive cocci caused most of the nosocomial infections. In the 1970s, the gram-negative bacteria have come to account for the majority of nosocomial infections.

Other studies have estimated the nosocomial infection rate to be as high as 15 percent of all hospital admissions, with a rate of 24 percent in the newborn intensive care unit in one study.[2-4] Because surgical patients account for 40–65 percent of the patients in general hospitals, reducing their rate of hospital-acquired infections would greatly diminish the nosocomial infection rate in the hospital. The highest rates of nosocomial infections occur in the surgical services.[1,3]

There have not been any significant changes in the incidence of wound infections since 1974, but infections are generally decreasing (Fig. 24-1).

COST OF NOSOCOMIAL INFECTIONS

The direct in-hospital costs of nosocomial infections have varied widely depending on the methods used to calculate costs. Bennett[5] estimated that in 1976 there were 2,035,100 nosocomial infections that resulted in 150,000 deaths in the United States. With an average direct cost per infection of 550 dollars, the total cost for the year was 1,119,305,000 dollars.

Haley et al[6] reviewed 16 studies that were reported between 1933 and 1975 and found that surgical nosocomial infections resulted in an average of 5–26.3 extra days of hosptialization, with extra direct hospital costs ranging from 669 to 2,387 dollars. Surgical wound infections alone result in an average of 7.4 extra days in the hospital, with a range of 0–68 days, and in an average additional cost of 839 dollars to the patient's bill, with a range of 0–7,900 dollars.

Green and Wenzel[7] compared the extra costs and additional stay as a result of wound infections for specific operations and used matched controls for comparison (Table 24-4). The direct cost attributable to wound infection ranged from 527.50 dollars for caesarean section to 2,602.68 dollars for coronary artery bypass graft.

Because of inflation and increases in the cost of hospitalization, these estimated costs of nosocomial infections

TABLE 24-1. NOSOCOMIAL INFECTION SUMMARY, NNIS HOSPITALS, BY HOSPITAL CATEGORY, JANUARY–JUNE 1977

	Community	Community–Teaching	Federal	Municipal or County	University	All Hospitals
Number of hospitals	36	23	3	5	12	79
Number of discharges	240,425	214,055	12,568	50,174	120,085	637,307
Number of infections	5,766	7,386	613	2,285	4,827	20,877
Infection rate/100 discharges	2.4	3.5	4.9	4.6	4.0	3.3
Percent infections cultured	90.3	93.2	97.4	85.1	89.9	90.0
Percent infections causing death	0.6	0.3	0.8	1.8	0.4	0.6
Percent infections contributing to death	2.2	2.0	2.1	5.3	1.3	2.3
Median infection rate	2.2	3.3	5.2	4.3	4.1	2.9
Range of Infection Rates: Low	1.0	1.7	4.4	3.2	1.2	1.0
High	5.8	5.4	5.2	10.8	10.0	10.8

From Center for Disease Control: National Nosocomial Infections Study Report, 1977 (6-month summaries). November 1979.

would be even higher today. Furthermore, the estimates of the number of nosocomial infections are conservative because they are based on surveillance data, which give only the minimum number of infections. Even a 65 percent efficiency would be generous in the extreme. In addition, the above estimates are direct hospital costs and do not include such indirect items as lost wages, the cost of death, and cost to the general population of increased insurance premiums. It also does not include the costs of infections that spread from patients to community contacts outside the hospital.

Alexander [2] calculated the total economic loss at 7,000 dollars per infection in 1973 in the United States. With an estimated 18,000,000 operations per year and 7.4 percent incidence of wound infections, the estimated yearly economic loss of all wound infections in the United States was 9.4 billion dollars. In current dollars, the cost would be substantially greater.

SURVEILLANCE

Surveillance, when applied to disease, may be defined as "the systematic, active, ongoing observation of the occurrence and distribution of disease within a population and of the events or conditions that increase or decrease the

TABLE 24-2. NOSOCOMIAL INFECTION RATES * BY SERVICE AND SITE OF INFECTION, JANUARY–JUNE 1977

	Medicine	Surgery	Obstetrics	Gynecology	Pediatrics	Newborn Nursery	All Services
Primary bacteremia	20.3	17.1	2.8	2.5	9.7	13.2	14.6
Surgical wound	7.9	142.9	93.7	109.6	12.0	6.9	73.5
Upper respiratory	5.8	3.8	1.4	2.5	6.5	3.9	4.2
Lower respiratory	75.7	74.0	4.2	11.5	14.7	20.7	53.5
Cardiovascular	5.8	3.9	0.1	0.9	2.7	1.8	3.6
Gastrointestinal	0.5	1.0	0.0	0.2	3.2	3.9	1.1
Intraabdominal	3.7	2.6	0.0	0.0	1.7	2.6	2.4
Urinary tract	178.2	179.5	45.2	148.4	13.2	5.1	134.7
Gynecologic	2.4	2.3	33.9	8.5	0.2	0.0	5.9
Central nervous system	0.5	2.1	0.1	0.0	0.7	2.6	1.2
Burn wound	0.3	5.9	0.0	0.0	0.5	0.0	2.2
Cutaneous	16.0	19.0	4.8	3.6	16.5	51.4	18.4
Other sites	16.1	11.8	0.6	1.6	10.0	23.3	12.1
ALL SITES	333.2	465.9	186.8	289.3	91.6	135.4	327.4
Secondary bacteremia	14.2	19.6	8.1	2.7	4.2	6.9	13.3

From Center for Disease Control: National Nosocomial Infections Study Report, 1977 (6-month summaries). November 1979.

* Per 10,000 patients discharged.

TABLE 24-3. RATE * AND RELATIVE FREQUENCY † OF SELECTED PATHOGENS CAUSING NOSOCOMIAL INFECTIONS, BY SITE OF INFECTION, JANUARY–JUNE 1977

	Primary Bacteremia	Surgical Wound	Lower Respiratory	Urinary Tract	Cutaneous	Other	All Sites
S. aureus	2.4 *(14.9)*	15.9 *(14.6)*	7.2 *(10.8)*	3.2 *(2.0)*	6.9 *(29.6)*	6.3 *(15.1)*	41.9 *(10.1)*
S. epidermidis	1.3 *(7.9)*	5.3 *(4.8)*	0.5 *(0.8)*	6.0 *(3.8)*	1.3 *(5.5)*	1.4 *(3.4)*	15.8 *(3.8)*
S. pneumoniae	0.1 *(0.9)*	0.1 *(0.1)*	2.5 *(3.7)*	‡ *(–)* §	‡ *(0.1)*	0.1 *(0.3)*	2.9 *(0.7)*
Streptococcus, group A	0.1 *(0.4)*	0.8 *(0.8)*	0.2 *(0.3)*	0.2 *(0.1)*	0.3 *(1.1)*	0.5 *(1.3)*	2.1 *(0.5)*
Streptococcus, group B	0.4 *(2.7)*	2.0 *(1.8)*	0.3 *(0.5)*	1.5 *(0.9)*	0.2 *(0.8)*	0.7 *(1.6)*	5.1 *(1.2)*
Streptococcus, group D	1.2 *(7.5)*	10.8 *(9.9)*	0.9 *(1.3)*	23.0 *(14.6)*	1.7 *(7.3)*	2.4 *(5.7)*	40.0 *(9.6)*
E. coli	2.6 *(16.0)*	16.6 *(15.2)*	4.8 *(7.1)*	50.9 *(32.3)*	1.7 *(7.1)*	3.7 *(8.8)*	80.3 *(19.3)*
Klebsiella sp	1.6 *(10.3)*	5.3 *(4.8)*	7.0 *(10.5)*	13.2 *(8.4)*	1.1 *(4.8)*	2.0 *(4.8)*	30.2 *(7.3)*
Enterobacter sp	0.7 *(4.5)*	3.8 *(3.4)*	3.7 *(5.5)*	5.6 *(3.5)*	0.5 *(2.1)*	0.8 *(2.0)*	15.0 *(3.6)*
Proteus-Providencia sp	0.5 *(3.4)*	7.5 *(6.9)*	4.1 *(6.1)*	15.2 *(9.6)*	1.4 *(6.0)*	1.8 *(4.2)*	30.5 *(7.4)*
Pseudomonas aeruginosa	1.0 *(6.2)*	4.4 *(4.0)*	4.8 *(7.2)*	13.7 *(8.7)*	1.1 *(4.8)*	1.8 *(4.4)*	26.9 *(6.5)*
Pseudomonas, other sp	0.3 *(1.6)*	1.3 *(1.2)*	1.3 *(2.0)*	3.6 *(2.3)*	0.2 *(1.0)*	0.8 *(1.8)*	7.5 *(1.8)*
Serratia sp	0.4 *(2.6)*	0.9 *(0.8)*	1.8 *(2.7)*	3.0 *(1.9)*	0.2 *(0.9)*	0.4 *(0.9)*	6.7 *(1.6)*
Bacteroides fragilis	0.6 *(3.7)*	3.9 *(3.5)*	‡ *(0.1)*	‡ *(–)* §	0.3 *(1.1)*	0.6 *(1.5)*	5.4 *(1.3)*
Candida sp	0.5 *(3.1)*	1.1 *(1.0)*	2.3 *(3.5)*	6.9 *(4.4)*	0.7 *(3.0)*	3.5 *(8.4)*	15.0 *(3.6)*
Other fungi	0.1 *(0.7)*	0.3 *(0.3)*	0.3 *(0.4)*	3.2 *(2.0)*	0.2 *(0.7)*	0.5 *(1.3)*	4.6 *(1.1)*
Other pathogens	1.9 *(12.0)*	14.4 *(13.2)*	5.7 *(8.5)*	5.4 *(3.4)*	1.7 *(7.3)*	4.7 *(11.3)*	33.8 *(8.2)*
No culture: no pathogen ‖	0.3 *(1.7)*	14.9 *(13.7)*	19.5 *(29.0)*	3.1 *(2.0)*	3.9 *(16.6)*	9.6 *(23.0)*	51.2 *(12.4)*
ALL PATHOGENS #	15.9 *(100.0)*	109.2 *(100.0)*	67.1 *(100.0)*	157.5 *(100.0)*	23.3 *(100.0)*	41.5 *(100.0)*	414.5 *(100.0)*
Secondary Bacteremia	NA *(–)* §	3.3 *(3.0)*	2.4 *(3.6)*	3.4 *(2.1)*	0.7 *(3.2)*	3.6 *(8.6)*	13.3 *(3.2)*

* Rate is number of isolates reported per 10,000 patients discharged; up to 4 isolates may be reported per infection.
† Relative frequency (in parentheses) is expressed as percent of all isolates from each site.
‡ Incidence is <0.1 per 10,000 discharges.
§ Relative frequency is <0.1% of all isolates from that site.
‖ No culture: no pathogen includes infections for which no culture was obtained or from which no pathogen was isolated or identified.
\# Relative rates differ from those in other tables because more than one pathogen may be isolated from a single site.

From Center for Disease Control: National Infections Study Report, 1977 (6-month summaries). November 1979.

risk of such disease occurrence."[8] Surveillance of disease includes the selection, recording, analyzing, and dissemination of data about that disease.

Although surveillance is different from control of hospital-acquired infections, it is an important part of infection control. It facilitates the early detection of outbreaks of infection, especially when an uncommon source is at fault, something that would be difficult in the absence of baseline surveillance data. The effectiveness of old and newly instituted infection control measures can only be assessed if adequate surveillance data are available. Surveillance data are also useful for detecting problems within the hospital that contribute to nosocomial infections, and which departments or what part of a patient's hospital stay is most likely to result in a nosocomial infection. Surveillance is required for determining baseline information about nosocomial infections so that deviations can be recognized. It can also be used as a continuing reminder to

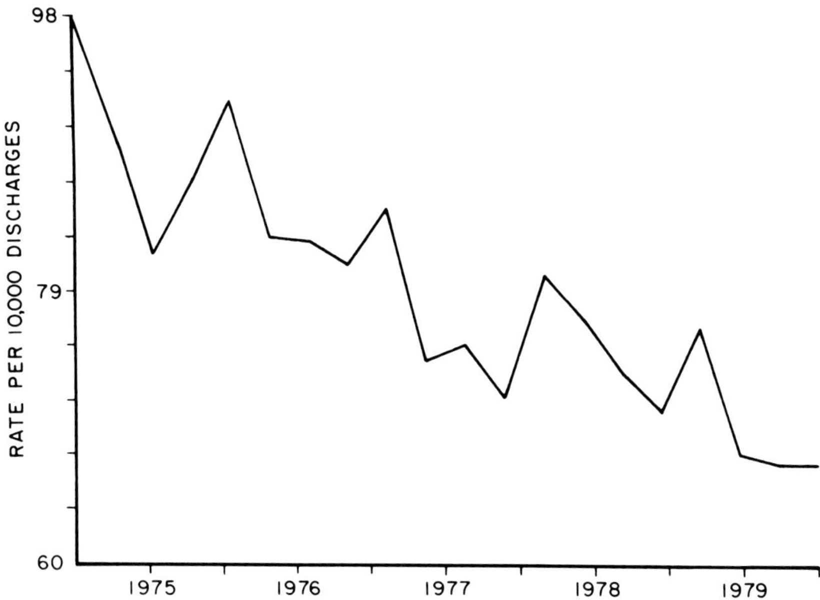

Fig. 24-1. Surgically related infection rates have gradually decreased since 1974. The rate per 10,000 discharges refers to all discharges from the hospital, not just discharges of surgical patients. (Derived from the National Nosocomial Infections Study. Reproduced with permission from Brachman PS, Dan BB, Haley RW, Hooton TM, Garner JS, Allen JR: Surg Clin North Am 60:15, 1980.)

medical and nursing personnel of the importance of adhering to good infection control practices.[8] For these reasons, the Joint Commission on Accreditation of Hospitals requires that each hospital have a practical surveillance system carried out under the direction of an infection control committee.

Surveillance data are only as reliable as the concepts and figures on which they are based. The population to be studied must first be defined. For nosocomial infections, the patients must obviously be surveyed, but ancillary personnel, such as the hospital staff, visitors, delivery men, salesmen, and service personnel, should also be included.

The events to be surveyed must also be defined. It is important to decide prior to beginning surveillance just what constitutes an infection so that the criteria can be applied consistently and uniformly. This job is not always as easy as it might seem. For instance, everyone will agree that a wound infection is present if a surgical wound drains purulent material and bacteria are cultured from the drainage fluid. But what if a wound drains clear, serous fluid and no bacteria are cultured? Or what if the wound margins become erythematous and inflammation seems to be present, but no fluid drains and no microorganisms are cultured? Should wound infections be diagnosed in these two instances? Similarly, what should be the criterion of a urinary tract infection? The usual criterion is 10^5 bacteria per milliliter of urine or 10^2 organisms per milliliter from a specimen obtained by suprapubic puncture. If a urinary catheter is in place, the urine may not reside in the bladder long enough for the bacteria to divide sufficiently to reach a concentration of 10^5 organisms per milliliter. In this case, what concentration of bacteria constitutes an infection? Even what constitutes urinary catheterization must be defined. If the skin around an intravenous catheter becomes inflamed, does this constitute an intravenous catheter infection even if no bacteria

TABLE 24-4. INCREASED HOSPITAL STAY AND DIRECT COST OF HOSPITALIZATION ATTRIBUTABLE TO POSTOPERATIVE WOUND INFECTION

	Patients with Wound Infection (per Case)		Controls (per Case)		Attributable to Wound Infection (per Case)	
Operations	*Postoperative Stay (Days)*	*Cost*	*Postoperative Stay (Days)*	*Cost*	*Postoperative Stay (Days)*	*Cost*
Appendectomy	12.3	$1,394.48	6.3	$ 705.51	6.0	$ 688.97
Cholecystectomy	18.5	2,582.13	11.4	2,139.12	7.1	443.01
Colon resection	26	4,417.77	12.2	2,823.58	13.8	1,594.19
Hysterectomy	13.3	1,885.29	6.8	1,096.44	6.5	788.85
Low transverse caesarean section	11.5	1,302.80	5.7	775.30	5.8	527.50
Coronary arterial bypass graft	26	7,542.50	14.6	4,939.82	11.4	2,602.68

From Green JW, Wenzel RP: Ann Surg 185:264, 1977.

are cultured from the bloodstream or from the catheter? Or should catheter sepsis be diagnosed if a patient has a central venous catheter and develops bacteremia but no bacteria are cultured from the catheter tip and yet the bacteremia does not recur after the catheter is removed.

A wide variety of sources must be used to gather data about nosocomial infections both within and outside of the hospital. Sources of nosocomial infection information include: reports from the microbiology laboratory; rounds made by the infection control nurse or other surveillance personnel on patients, with particular attention to those having fevers, surgical wounds, other high-risk procedures, and those receiving antibiotics; X-ray reports for diagnosis of pneumonia; autopsy reports for undetected or unsuspected infections; postdischarge follow-up of selected patients, such as surgical patients whose wound infections may not be detected until after discharge or neonates whose infections may not show up until discharge; verbal reports by physicians and other nurses; the pharmacy for information regarding distribution of antibiotics; and the outpatient clinic. Other sources for information about nosocomial infections include employee health clinics, local public health officials regarding community outbreaks, and the admissions office. Obviously, getting as much information as possible from a variety of sources will provide the surveillance team with only the minimum number of nosocomial infections, since one can never be sure of gathering data about each and every hospital infection that occurs.

A study reported by Mulholland et al [4] demonstrates that the nosocomial infection rate is directly related to surveillance. The nosocomial infection rate was 1.3 infections per 100 admissions when physicians reported infections. When a part-time (75 percent) infection control nurse was employed, the nosocomial infection rate increased to 10.8 infections per 100 admissions. It increased to 13.2 per 100 admissions with a full-time infection control nurse and to 16.7 per 100 admissions when the infection control nurse had a part-time assistant. When a prevalence study was carried out, the rate was 14.4 infections per 100 admissions. Thus, the more seriously nosocomial infections are sought, and the more personnel devoted to the search, the more nosocomial infections are detected.

THE INFECTION CONTROL COMMITTEE

The Joint Commission on the Accreditation of Hospitals has published guidelines and standards for infection prevention, control, surveillance, and reporting.[9] The American Hospital Association [10] and the Committee on Control of Surgical Infections of the Pre- and Postoperative Care Committee of the American College of Surgeons [11] agree with the guidelines and standards. Each hospital should provide (1) the appointment of an infection control committee, (2) procedures and techniques for meeting established sanitation and asepsis standards that are evaluated and revised on a continuing basis, (3) a practical surveillance system for reporting, evaluating, and keeping records of infections among patients and personnel, (4) policies and procedures for isolation of infected patients, (5) the development of written standards for hospital sanitation and medical asepsis and proper instruction of hospital personnel in medical and surgical asepsis, (6) an adequate microbiology service, (7) adequate measures against contamination of food, and (8) periodic review of antibiotic usage.[11]

The infection control committee should have a physician as permanent chairman and should have representatives from surgery, internal medicine, pediatrics, obstetrics, microbiology (pathology), nursing, and hospital administration. The infection control nurse and hospital epidemiologist, if there is one, should also attend the meetings. Representatives of other hospital departments, such as the operating room, radiology, dietary service, housekeeping, pharmacy, central supply service, and maintenance can be regular members of the committee or may only be invited to attend meetings when needed. The committee should have regularly scheduled meetings and should hold additional meetings when necessary. All activities relating to infection control should be carried out under the guidance of the infection control committee. The committee should have responsibility for developing procedures and policies relating to infection control and for carrying out an effective surveillance system.

THE INFECTION CONTROL NURSE

The infection control nurse (nurse epidemiologist) is usually the only hospital employee whose full-time activity is devoted to infection control. While most hospitals have one infection control nurse, a large, active surgical service may justify a full-time surgical infection control nurse. The major responsibility of the infection control nurse is to carry out hospital surveillance of nosocomial infections. The nurse should detect and record data about nosocomial infections in a systematic and current manner, analyze such data, and prepare monthly reports for the infection control committee. In order to detect the greatest number of nosocomial infections, the infection control nurse should check daily with the microbiology laboratory for culture reports that might represent infections, and should also make regular ward rounds looking for clues of infections (fevers, isolation, use of antibiotics). If the time and personnel are available, it is also helpful if the infection control nurse actually looks at each wound, both in the hospital and in the outpatient clinic after discharge.

The infection control nurse should interpret hospital policy on the isolation and disposition of patients who have infections, assist in the development and implementation of improved infection control measure, and assist with employee orientation and in-service training programs related to infection prevention and control.

DETERMINANTS OF NOSOCOMIAL INFECTIONS

The development of nosocomial infections is determined by several factors, among which are the source of infection, the microbial agent, the route of transmission, the susceptibility of the host, and the environment.

SOURCES OF INFECTION

The sources of microorganisms in the hospital are persons, inanimate objects, food, animals, and arthropods. All persons in the hospital whether they are patients, hospital personnel, or visitors are potential sources of infection. Many patients who develop wound infections or intraabdominal abscesses after intestinal surgery are themselves the sources of infection. Their own endogenous organisms frequently cause wound infections or other postoperative infections.

Inanimate objects (fomites) other than food, such as anesthesia equipment, nebulizers, intravenous catheters and solutions, furniture, and linen supplies, can also be sources of nosocomial infections. Occasionally, food and water may be contaminated with bacteria—especially *Clostridium* and *Salmonella*—and may also be sources of nosocomial infections. Infrequently, animals, such as rats and other vermin, and insects are important sources of infections in hospitals.

THE MICROBIAL AGENT

Patients may be exposed to many types of pathogens during hospitalization. The likelihood of infection depends on several microbe-determined factors: the type of pathogen, its virulence or disease-producing ability (Chapter 2), and the numbers introduced into the patient. Many microbes normally of low virulence can cause infections if the patient is a compromised host (Chapter 47), if sufficient numbers are introduced into the patient, and if they are introduced by the correct route.

ROUTE OF TRANSMISSION

Microorganisms can be transmitted within the hospital by four routes: contact, a common vehicle, air, or a vector. More than one route may be operative for a given pathogen.

Contact Transmission

Contact transmission occurs when the patient acquires the infection by contact with the source. Contact-spread infection is either direct, indirect, or by droplets. Direct contact occurs when there is actual physical contact between the person or object harboring the infectious agent and the patient. Infections (wound infections, abscesses) in which the patient is the source of the bacteria are direct autogenous infections. Hepatitis A, gonorrhea, and syphilis also occur by direct contact spread.

Indirect contact spread occurs when the patient comes in contact with an intermediate object, usually inanimate, from which there is transfer of an infectious agent. Hepatitis B can be spread in this manner by contaminated needles and syringes. Contact contamination can occur from virtually any inanimate object, for example, endoscopes, cystoscopes, dialyzers, nebulizers, anesthesia equipment, thermometers, venous arterial catheters, pressure transducers, antiseptics, suction equipment, bedpans, urinals, and barium enema equipment. Medicine, blood, food, and water are additional sources, and there are numerous other sources as well.

Droplet spread refers to brief spread of the infectious agent through the air in contaminated droplets when the source and victim are relatively near each other. Talking, sneezing, and coughing can result in droplet spread of streptococcal pharyngitis and measles.

Common-Vehicle Transmission

In common-vehicle spread infection, multiple cases of the same infection are transmitted from a common source. Medicine, blood and blood products, food, and water are the most common sources of common-vehicle spread. Other sources, such as intravenous fluids, contaminated eye drops, diagnostic dyes, cosmetics, and bronchodilators, have been responsible for common-vehicle spread of nosocomial infections.

Airborne Transmission

Airborne spread refers to transmission of microorganisms through the air for more than the several feet between source and victim. The organisms are contained in droplet nuclei or dust particles whose small size (less than 5 μm) permit them to remain suspended in the air for a prolonged time. Examples of nosocomial infections that can be transmitted by airborne spread include chickenpox, tuberculosis, and influenza. Dust from a variety of sources can also cause nosocomial infections. *Aspergillus* infections have been attributed to fireproofing materials in a new hospital,[12] and an outbreak of salmonellosis occurred due to contaminated dust in a vacuum cleaner bag. Each time the vacuum cleaner was used, the dust was resuspended.[13]

Vectorborne Transmission

Vectorborne spread of nosocomial infections no longer occurs in the United States, but spread by flies or cockroaches, which are frequently found in hospitals, theoretically could occur.

HOST SUSCEPTIBILITY

More and more surgeons are dealing with compromised hosts (Chapters 13 and 47). Patients at the extremes of age and patients with certain diseases, especially leukemia, lymphoma, and other types of cancers, uremia, and diabetes mellitus, and those receiving immunosuppressive therapy, radiation therapy, and chemotherapy have decreased resistance to infection. Anesthesia and surgery themselves inhibit a host's immune response.[14]

THE ENVIRONMENT

The environment is yet another factor that can affect infection. Overcrowding of patients, especially in intensive care units, favors patient-to-patient spread of infections. The humidity and temperature can affect the persistance of a microbe at its source, its transmission through the air, and the effectiveness of the host's mucous membranes. Routinely taking cultures from environmental sources (walls, floors, furniture) is not helpful in reducing hospital-acquired infections.

NOSOCOMIAL INFECTIONS RELATED TO DIFFERENT HOSPITAL DEPARTMENTS

Each department within the hospital is a potential source of nosocomial infection, frequently of a specific type. While many departments, such as the food preparation service, laundry service, and pharmacy, are a potential source of hospital-acquired infection to all patients within the hospital, some departments, such as the operating room, intensive care ward, and dialysis unit, are of particular concern to surgical patients.

THE OPERATING ROOM

Since bacterial contamination of host tissues most often occurs in the operating room, infection control practices in this area are of great importance. Many wound infections are due to contamination of the wound with the patient's own bacteria, frequently from the intestine during gastrointestinal or gynecologic procedures. Few operating room infection control practices can alter this type of wound contamination, but certain techniques of patient preparation (Chapter 20), operative care (Chapter 22), and antibiotic use (Chapter 23) can help. Infection control measures in the operating room can reduce nosocomial infections due to environmental contamination (Chapter 21).

Many sites in the operating room are potential sources of nosocomial infections. Operating room personnel are one potential source. Small holes in surgeons' gloves develop commonly during operative procedures, and the wound infection rate is higher where such punctures occur. The contamination comes from the hands of the surgeon. Even the soap that the surgeon uses to wash his or her hands can be contaminated with bacteria.

Personnel who are nasal carriers of *Staphylococcus aureus* can disseminate these organisms into the operating room air so that they cause wound infections, even if they are not standing directly at the operating table.[15]

The inanimate objects in the operating room, blood and blood products, intravenous catheters and solutions, urinary catheters, and anesthesia equipment are also potential sources of nosocomial infections. Inanimate objects, such as oxygenators used for open heart surgery, surgical instruments, cystoscopes, drapes and linens, sutures, gloves, and sponges, may not be sterile. Blood, blood products, and intravenous fluids may be contaminated with bacteria or hepatitis virus. Anesthesia equipment and anesthesia can give rise to bacteremia and aspiration. There is a 16 percent incidence of bacteremia following nasotracheal intubation compared to no bacteremia with orotracheal intubation.[16] The organisms isolated were oral and nasal bacteria, such as α-hemolytic streptococci. Aspiration of gastric contents occurs in as many as 16.3 percent of anesthetized patients, and half of them are not clinically recognized and are detected only when actively looked for.[17] Wound infections are not the only types of nosocomial infections that can originate in the operating room!

THE INTENSIVE CARE UNIT

Intensive care units are designed to give special care to critically ill patients and to certain patients with special needs. Infection control measures should be adequately stressed. In most community hospitals, surgical intensive care units admit all postsurgical and injured patients requiring special care. In many larger hospitals, intensive care units are specialized into general surgery units, cardiac surgery units, burn units, respiratory units, neurosurgery units, coronary-care units, oncology units, transplantation units, and neonatal units.

The intensive care unit brings together many patients in close proximity who are highly susceptible to infection. Their illnesses, operations, burns, and trauma suppress their host defenses.[14] They are frequently treated with antibiotics, thus favoring the emergence of resistant bacteria, and they have a variety of invasive procedures in addition to operations, such as central nervous system catheters, arterial catheters, Swan-Ganz catheters, chest tubes, tracheostomies, endotracheal tubes, and urinary catheters. Many times, these invasive procedures must be done in the intensive care ward during a medical emergency, and proper sterile precautions are compromised.

There have been a variety of recommendations to reduce the frequency of nosocomial infections: flexible and transparent enclosures to separate patients, traffic control, proper introduction and removal of material, air-conditioning, and ultraviolet light. Some of these methods are helpful but expensive; others, such as ultraviolet lights, probably are not useful.

Partial separation of patients can be important in suppressing cross infection. Single rooms can provide barriers between patients, but observing patients closely can be difficult, even with remote monitoring devices, especially if there is a nursing shortage. Physical barriers can also be placed between patients so that they are separated on three sides. Such a system retards cross infection but still allows close observation. United States government standards require at least 7 feet between beds and a clear area of 120 square feet around each bed.[18]

Placement of patients in a unit can also be important. In some intensive care units, it is common practice to place patients with similar problems (ie, endotracheal tubes, tracheostomies, or urinary catheters) near each other, but the risk of transmission of microbes on the hands of personnel is increased if patients with similar tubes or catheters are placed near one another. Rather than grouping patients, they should be spread out as much as possible.

Contact transmission is the most likely method of spread of most nosocomial infections within intensive care facilities. Organisms are spread from patient to patient on the hands of hospital personnel. The most effective method of preventing such spread is diligent handwashing between patient contacts. To encourage hand washing, sinks must be readily available. Multiple bed units should have one sink for every six beds, and every isolation room should have its own sink.[18] Wearing gloves is more effective than hand washing. Personnel should be encouraged to wear gloves when handling intravenous or arterial catheters, wounds, dressings, and urinary catheters. Wearing gloves should be required when handling or suctioning tracheostomies or endotracheal tubes.

DIALYSIS UNIT

There are approximately 50,000 people on chronic hemodialysis in the United States, and the number is increasing yearly. Surgeons are frequently called on to perform vascular access procedures and other operations on uremic patients. Nonuremic patients can develop renal failure after operations or trauma and might require temporary dialysis and thus come in contact with chronic dialysis patients.

Dialysis patients are subject to nosocomial bacterial and viral infections. Kaslow and Zellner [19] surveyed five dialysis units and found that there were 5.6 to 7.6 infections, exluding hepatitis, per 100 patient-months. There were 3.5 shunt infections per 100 patient-months, and these infections accounted for 33 to 67 percent of all infections. Shunt infection rates are usually 2.5 to 3.5 per 100 patient-months, but infection rates as high as 26.6 per 100 patient-months have occurred. Most shunt infections are due to *S. aureus*, which is not sensitive to penicillin G. Bacterial endocarditis occurs infrequently in dialysis patients but has been reported in up to 2.7 percent of all patients. It usually follows shunt infections. Bacteremia accounts for 4 to 30 percent of bacterial infections.[19] Most bacteremia is due to *S. aureus* from infections of vascular access sites, and there is a 19 percent mortality rate. Most gram-negative bacteremias occur in patients with acute renal failure, and the organisms originate in the lungs and gastrointestinal tract.[20] It is believed that these organisms frequently enter the blood from water in the dialysate bath that enters the blood through tiny breaks in the membrane of the dialyzer.

Viral infections, especially hepatitis B, are an even more serious problem in dialysis units. Many hemodialysis units have reported the frequent occurrence of hepatitis B in patients and staff, sometimes in epidemic proportions.[21,22] The hepatitis B attack rate was 6.2 percent of patients and 5.8 percent of staff in hemodialysis units.[21] Ninety percent of patients who became hepatitis B surface antigen (HBsAg)-positive remained so. Eighty percent of dialysis centers have had hepatitis in patients or staff.[22] While hepatitis B virus is the common source of hepatitis in dialysis patients, cytomegalovirus and Epstein-Barr virus can also cause hepatitis in these patients.

Obviously, control of hepatitis B is of major concern in dialysis units because of risk to both patients and staff. Some dialysis centers are no longer accepting HBsAg-positive patients, making it extremely difficult to find a center that will dialyze them. The advent of a new hepatitis B vaccine (Chapter 10) should eliminate the danger to uninfected patients and staff members.

Hepatitis can be introduced into a hemodialysis unit by admission of patients or staff infected with hepatitis B virus, by patients already on dialysis becoming infected elsewhere and bringing the infection into the unit, by administration of blood and blood products contaminated with hepatitis B virus, and through transplantation of a kidney from an infected patient.

Once the virus is introduced into a unit, spread to other patients and staff is likely because of the frequency of exposure to the patients' blood from needle puncture or aerosolization of the blood. Very frequently, contamination is not recognized.

Surveillance of patients and staff should be done regularly. They should be watched for clinical indications of hepatitis. Blood samples should be obtained for determination of HBsAg, antibody to HBsAg, and serum glutamicoxalic transaminase. Patients or staff who become HBsAg-positive should be isolated. Many dialysis units now have special sections for HBsAg-positive patients who are cared for by staff who are HBsAg-positive or who have serum antibody to HBsAg. Antigen-negative patients and staff are not permitted to enter this area. Other units encourage HBsAg-positive patients to dialyze at home.

Dialysis personnel should practice a high level of personal hygiene. They should change uniforms when entering the dialysis unit and should not eat or smoke there. Separate toilet facilities for staff and patients should be available, and strict hand washing practices should be observed. Gloves should be worn when coming in contact with blood, body fluids, urine, or feces.

It is desirable that each patient have a separate dialysis machine, but this is often not practical. HBsAg-positive patients should never share dialysis machines with HBsAg-negative patients. Patients should never share dialyzers with others. Dialyzers are often used two or three times. Between uses, dialyzers are filled with formaldehyde (16 percent), which will kill the hepatitis virus. Commonly used monitoring equipment and rooms where machines and dialyzers are cleaned and stored are also potential areas of cross contamination, and special care is needed in these areas.

Other Departments

Nosocomial infections in surgical patients can originate in other hospital departments as well.

Admitting and Outpatient Departments

Frequently, the admitting office and outpatient departments are overlooked in the infection control policies of a hospital because they are frequently not regarded as intergral parts of the hospital itself. Insofar as infection control is concerned, the admitting office and outpatient facilities should be considered as inpatient facilities. An attempt should be made in both of these departments to judiciously separate infected patients from uninfected patients, especially those whose infections might be spread through the air to other persons. Infected patients should perhaps bypass the admissions office and should not be allowed to come into close contact with uninfected patients or with those who are going to have surgical procedures during their hospital admission. Appropriate hospital personnel, such as the infection control nurse, should make known the special needs of infected patients to personnel in the admitting office.

Similarly, the infection control nurse should devote the time necessary to carry on surveillance activities in the admitting office and especially in the outpatient department. Many of these patients will have been previously discharged from the hospital, and their nosocomial infection, eg, wound infections and postransfusion hepatitis, may only be detected by follow-up in these departments after discharge from the hospital.

Laundry

Linens from both hospital wards and the operating room frequently are contaminated by infectious materials, and diseases can be transmitted by soiled linens. *Salmonella typhimurium* and Q fever have been transmitted to hospital employees handling soiled linens.[23]

All soiled linen should be bagged and placed into covered carts where they should remain until transmitted to the laundry. In the laundry, linen should be washed in hot water in order to kill contaminating microorganisms. Water temperatures above 71C for 25 minutes kill almost all microorganisms except spores. Even with the potential for transmission of pathogens, nosocomial infections related to linen supplies are extremely rare.

Central Supply Service

The central supply service is responsible for processing, storing, and dispensing supplies and equipment required for all aspects of patient care, diagnosis, and treatment. The central supply service is thus responsible for cleaning and disinfecting contaminated reusable items, such as endoscopic equipment, thermometers, bedpans, urinals, respiratory therapy equipment, anesthesia supplies, and procedure trays used for cutdowns on the wards. They are also responsible for cleaning diagnostic equipment, such as sigmoidoscopes, anoscopes, vaginal speculums, and laryngoscopy instruments.

Hospitals have found it economically advantageous to have all reusable supplies and equipment requiring specialized cleaning, disinfection, and sterilization to be handled by the central supply service whenever possible. Therefore, a lot of equipment passes through the central supply service that could be a potential source of transmitting infections. It is, therefore, essential that the central supply service have adequate facilities for decontaminating items that have been used by hospital patients, for washing and cleaning this equipment, and finally for disinfecting it or sterilizing it and packaging it for reuse. In addition, the central supply service should have adequate storage areas for equipment. These areas should be ventilated with at least two air changes per hour, and the temperature should be maintained between 18 and 25C.

Pharmacy

The pharmacy is frequently not thought of as a potential source of disseminating infection within the hospital. However, pharmacies are currently responsible for mixing solutions for total parenteral nutrition therapy. These solutions are easily contaminated with bacteria and provide growth media for many kinds of organisms. Because hyperalimentation solutions do not come prepared from the manufacturer but have to be mixed in the pharmacy, contamination can occur. In addition, some medications purchased from commercial sources have been found to be contaminated with such potential pathogens as *E. coli, Pseudomonas, Proteus,* and *Salmonella.* These drugs have included digitalis alkaloids, barbiturates, and oral tranquilizers. The hospital pharmacy is also a good place for surveillance for antimicrobial usage within the hospital.

Food Service

The food service has the task of providing attractively prepared, wholesome, appetizing food that is safe to eat. Because such a high percentage of patients and staff eat hospital food, the food service is a potential source of widespread nosocomial infections.

Foodborne illnesses have been caused by staphylococcal enterotoxins, *Clostridium perfringens, Salmonella, Shigella,* and hepatitis A.[24] The most common responsible agents are *C. perfringens* and *Salmonella,*[25] and these types of illnesses can be responsible for patient death, especially in old and frail patients. The major factors leading to outbreaks of foodborne illnesses are inadequate refrigeration (46 percent of outbreaks), preparing food far in advance of planned service (22 percent), handling of food by infected persons who practice poor personal hygiene (21 percent), inadequate cooking or heat processing (19 percent), holding food in warming devices at bacteria-incubation temperatures (16 percent), uncooked foods contaminated by raw ingredients (12 percent), and inadequate reheating (9 percent).[24]

Hospital food can become contaminated before, during, and after preparation. Meat and poultry are frequently contaminated with *C. perfringens* and *Salmonella* at the time of purchase; up to 50 percent of poultry is contaminated by *Salmonella.* The external surface of unprocessed eggs can be contaminated with fecal matter containing *Salmonella.* Raw fish can be contaminated with *C. perfringens* and *Vibrio parahaemolyticus.*

Prevention of foodborne transmission involves proper handling of food and personal hygiene by foodhandlers. Food must be adequately cleaned, refrigerated or stored, and adequately cooked. Prepared foods and foods that are to be reused must also be adequately stored, stored at cold enough temperatures, and adequately reheated prior to use.

Foodhandlers and kitchen personnel should be instructed in infection control measures. Hand washing facilities should be convenient, since the hands are probably the chief mode of transmission of nosocomial infections by foodhandlers.

ISOLATION PROCEDURES

Isolation procedures are designed to prevent the spread of microorganisms among patients, hospital personnel, and visitors. Because microorganisms and host factors are difficult to control, isolation procedures are directed at the chain of transmission in order to interrupt the chain of infection. Isolation procedures are difficult, time consuming, and costly, and they should be suited to both the patient and to the infection to be controlled. Furthermore, isolation makes frequent visits by physicians, nurses, and other hospital personnel inconvenient and may discourage the hospital from giving the best possible care. In addition, the requirement for a private room might necessitate using space designed to accommodate additional patients, thus causing an economic loss for the hospital. Thus, isolation procedures should not be used when not required.

The infection control committee is responsible for developing isolation policies and procedures. The policies and procedures should be reviewed from time to time and modified as necessary. The infection control nurse should be knowledgeable about isolation procedures and should serve as a consultant on isolation policies and procedures. The Center for Disease Control publishes *Isolation Techniques for Use in Hospitals*,[26] which details isolation procedures that can be used in small community hospitals and in large metropolitan hospitals as well. These isolation procedures are easily adapted by virtually any hospital.

TYPES OF ISOLATION

The Center for Disease Control[26] recommends seven types of isolation: (1) strict isolation, (2) wound and skin precautions, (3) respiratory isolation, (4) enteric precautions, (5) discharge precautions, (6) blood precautions, and (7) protective isolation. The term "isolation" is used when a private room is indicated, and the term "precaution" is used when a private room is not required. These categories differ in whether a private room is required and in the barriers (ie, gown, gloves, mask) placed between the patient and hospital personnel and visitors (Table 24-5).

Strict Isolation

The purpose of strict isolation is to prevent transmission of a highly communicable disease, frequently fatal, that is easily spread by direct contact transmission, by indirect contact transmission with inanimate objects that have come in contact with the infected patient, and by the airborne route.

Wound and Skin Precautions

This category is designed to prevent patients and personnel from acquiring infection from direct contact with wounds and heavily contaminated articles contaminated with wound or skin secretions. Wound infections caused by gram-positive organisms have usually caused more concern than those due to gram-negative organisms, but gram-negative organisms can be transmitted by contact and can cause wound infections.

Respiratory Isolation

This category is designed to prevent transmission of microorganisms by the airborne route or by droplets that are coughed, sneezed, or breathed into the environment. Some diseases (measles and rubella) requiring respiratory isolation are infrequently spread by indirect contact with freshly contaminated articles. Hands are usually not a mode of transmission, but should be washed appropriately.

Enteric Precautions

The purpose of this category of precautions is to prevent diseases that can be transmitted through direct or indirect contact with the feces and, in some cases, with heavily contaminated articles. Transmission of the pathogen depends on ingestion of the pathogen. Careful hand washing after any patient contact is the best method of preventing these types of diseases. Viral hepatitis (including hepatitis A and hepatitis B) is included in this category because of the difficulty of distinguishing between the various types on clinical grounds.

Discharge Precautions

The purpose of discharge precautions is to prevent the direct spread of infection by oral, fecal, or lesion discharges. The likelihood of cross infection with these diseases is very slight. Patients requiring discharge precautions need to be treated separately only when handling their potentially infectious discharges. Discharge precautions only are required for small wounds with minimal drainage; they employ a no-touch dressing technique when changing dressings on these lesions.

Blood Precautions

This category is designed to prevent acquisition of infection by patients and personnel from contact with blood or items contaminated with blood. These precautions primarily involve handling needles and syringes contaminated with blood with extreme care.

Protective Isolation

Protective isolation prevents contact between uninfected patients who have compromised host defenses and persons potentially carrying pathogens. Whereas other types of isolation and precaution are designed to prevent spread of an infectious agent from an infected patient to uninfected patients and hospital personnel, protective isolation or reverse isolation protects an uncontaminated patient from exposure to pathogenic agents in the environment around him and to other patients, personnel, and visitors. Patients with neutropenia, extensive uninfected burns, bone marrow transplants, and in late stages of leukemia and lymphoma require protective isolation.

Card System of Isolation

Many hospitals use a card system of isolation. A color-coded card that can be attached to each patients' door or bed is available for each type of isolation. The card system is designed to give concise information for specific communicable diseases on the front. On the back of the card can be listed the diseases listed in the specific category. These cards are available from the US Government Printing Office.[26]

FACILITIES FOR ISOLATION

The facilities required for isolation will vary from one hospital to another. In some hospitals, a separate and special ward may be used for patients requiring different kinds of isolation. In other hospitals, special rooms may be situated in different areas for special isolation procedures. In still others, a private room may be used only as required.

TABLE 24-5. RECOMMENDED ISOLATION FOR SURGICALLY RELATED INFECTIONS

	Private Room	Mask	Gown	Gloves	Excreta and Excreta-soiled Articles	Blood	Secreta and Secreta-soiled Articles
STRICT ISOLATION							
Burn, skin, or wound infection with *S. aureus* or group A streptococcus that is not covered by a dressing or that has copious purulent drainage	X	X	⊗	⊗			X
Pneumonia—*S. aureus* and group A streptococcus	X	X	⊗	⊗			X
Varicella (chickenpox), disseminated herpes zoster	X	X *	X	X		X	
WOUND AND SKIN PRECAUTIONS							
Burns, skin or wound infections, limited, including infections with *S. aureus* or group A streptococcus, that are covered by and the discharge adequately contained by a dressing	D	⊗	⊗	⊗			X
Burn, skin, or wound infections, major (except *S. aureus* and group A streptococcus, see strict isolation) that are not covered by a dressing that have copious purulent discharge	D		X	X			X
Gas gangrene (due to *C. perfringens*)	D			⊗			X
Cellulitis, impetigo, erysipelas, furunculosis	D			⊗			X
If draining: closed cavity infection, empyema, lung abscess (nontuberculous), peritonitis	D	⊗	⊗	⊗			X
Localized herpes zoster	D	X *	X	X			X
RESPIRATORY ISOLATION							
Pulmonary tuberculosis, measles, mumps, rubella	X	X *					X
ENTERIC PRECAUTIONS							
Viral hepatitis, types A, B, or unspecified	D				X	X	X
Gastroenteritis due to enteropathogenic or enterotoxic *E. coli, Salmonella, Shigella,* or *Yersinia enterocolitica*	D		⊗	⊗	X		
DISCHARGE PRECAUTIONS							
Oral and lesion secretions (minor skin lesions, syphilis, gonorrhea, minor wound infections, draining lesions due to actinomycosis, brucellosis, candidiasis, coccidioidomycosis, nocardiosis, tuberculosis, granuloma inguinale, herpes simplex, lymphogranuloma venereum, bacterial pneumonia)							X
Excretions (amebiasis, *C. perfringens* food poisoning, enterobiasis, giardiasis, staphylococcal food poisoning, tapeworm disease)					X		
BLOOD PRECAUTIONS							
Viral hepatitis, type A, B, or unspecified, malaria						X	
PROTECTIVE ISOLATION							
Agranulocytosis, extensive, noninfected burns in certain patients, lymphomas and leukemias in certain patients, immunosuppressed patients (ie, bone marrow transplant recipients), severe noninfected vesicular, bullous, or eczematous disease	X	X	X	⊗			

X, recommend at all times; ⊗, with direct contact; X *, for susceptibles; D, desirable but optional. No isolation is required if abscesses, empyemas, peritonitis, closed cavity infections are not draining.

Modified from Center for Disease Control: Isolation Techniques for Use in Hospitals. Washington, DC, US Government Printing Office, DHEW Publication No. (CDC) 76–8314, 1975.

Isolation Area

A private room or area set aside for patients requiring isolation should contain hand washing, bathing, and toilet facilities. There should be no crosscirculation or recirculation of air between the isolation area and other areas of the hospital.[11] Air movement should be from the hall into the isolation unit, except in rooms for patients requiring protective isolation.

Isolation Equipment

Gowns, gloves, and masks should be readily available when indicated. They should be placed conveniently outside each patient's room so as not to discourage the hospital staff from entering the room. The single most important factor in any isolation procedure is hand washing before and after contact with the patient whether gloves are used or not. Sterile gowns should be used with patients in protective isolation. Otherwise, clean, freshly laundered, or disposable gowns can be used. Needles, syringes, dishes, and utensils for patients requiring isolation should be disposable. Other patient care items, such as stethoscopes and sphygmomanometers, should be kept in the patient's room and should be properly disinfected when the patient leaves the hospital.

Disposable items, dressings, and tissue contaminated by wound drainage, secretions, or excretions (depending on the type of isolation) should be placed in an impermeable, disposable bag in the patient's room. This bag should be placed in a second bag or container (double-bagged) when removed from the room and incinerated or autoclaved.

TYPES OF NOSOCOMIAL INFECTIONS IN SURGICAL PATIENTS

Most surgical patients are not more susceptible to nosocomial infections than the rest of the hospital population, but some important differences do exist. The great majority of surgical patients have operative procedures that subject them to wound infections that patients who have not had operations cannot get. In addition, patients with extensive trauma or burns, who have severely compromised host defenses, are almost always housed on surgical services. Finally, in addition to their operations, surgical patients frequently are subjected to invasive diagnostic and therapeutic procedures, such as tracheostomies, endotracheal tubes, intravenous catheters, cutdowns, arterial catheters, and urinary catheters.

Nosocomial infections in surgical patients are dealt with throughout this book, since postoperative complications are often associated with infections. Infections in prosthetic devices (cardiac valves, pacemakers, vascular prostheses, artificial hips and other orthopedic prostheses, ventriculoatrial shunts) are frequently associated with disastrous complications and are also discussed throughout this book.

RESPIRATORY TRACT INFECTIONS

According to the National Nosocomial Infections Study for 1977, lower respiratory tract infections are the third most common nosocomial infection occurring in surgical patients, next to urinary tract infections and wound infections, with a rate of 74.0 per 10,000 discharges (Table 24-2). Respiratory tract infections are more common in surgical services than in most other services.

Criteria of Respiratory Tract Infection

The criteria for definition of lower respiratory tract infections differ with various investigators. The Hospital Infections Branch of the Center for Disease Control, which monitors the National Nosocomials Infections Study, requires that in adults there must be onset of purulent sputum production more than 48 hours after admission in a patient with no preceding pulmonary infection, or increased production of purulent sputum with evidence of fever in a patient admitted with pulmonary disease. In addition, the patient must either have an infiltrate seen on chest roentgenogram or characteristic physical findings of pneumonia or cough, fever, and pleuritic chest pain. The diagnosis of pneumonia in a child can be made in the absence of purulent sputum if an infiltrate is seen on the chest roentgenogram and the child has cough, fever, and pleuritic chest pain. A diagnosis of pneumonia by an attending physician is accepted even when the above criteria are not completely fulfilled. Johanson et al,[27] on the other hand, have used more stringent criteria and classified lower respiratory tract infections as definite if the patient had all four of the following indications: (1) radiographic appearance of a new or progressive pulmonary infiltrate, (2) fever, (3) leukocytosis, and (4) purulent tracheobronchial discharge. The diagnosis is only probable if only the first three criteria are met. Note that in neither the Center for Disease Control or in the criteria in Johanson et al [27] are the culture results necessary for making a diagnosis of lower respiratory tract infections. Some pneumonias, such as viral and fungal pneumonias in severely compromised hosts, may not be accompanied by any sputum production, especially in the early phases.

Sputum is a poor source of cultures for determining the etiology of the lower respiratory infection. All sputum must come through the mouth and is, therefore, contaminated by the oropharyngeal flora, which may not be representative of the cause of pneumonia. Only organisms isolated from blood, pleural fluid, lung biopsy specimens, or transtracheal aspirates in patients with clinical evidence of pneumonia have been considered as being etiologic in the cause of the pneumonia. While the tracheobronchial tree below the vocal cords is sterile in most patients, the upper trachea can become contaminated with bacteria in patients who have been hospitalized. Thus, even transtracheal aspirates potentially can give a misleading bacteriologic diagnosis of lower respiratory tract infections.

Susceptibility to Lower Respiratory Tract Infections in Surgical Patients

While the lower respiratory tract has a variety of defense mechanisms that protect the lungs from infections (Chapter 30), many of these defense mechanisms are compromised in surgical patients by their basic disease, metabolic status, or surgical operations. Preexisting pulmonary disease and bronchitis further predispose to postoperative respiratory infections. Anesthesia, alcohol, and operations on the head and neck can interfere with the normal protective cough reflex and may permit aspiration of infected material. The pain associated with trauma or operations to the chest and upper abdomen may also interfere with coughing and breathing and thus allow accumulation of secretions within the tracheobronchial tree. This pain can interfere with deep breathing and normal alveolar expansion, leading to atelectasis of the lungs, a condition that predisposes to pulmonary infections. Trauma or operations involving any site on the body may interfere with movement and with deep breathing and normal alveolar expansion. The basic disease processes and the aftereffects of any operation frequently lead to a depressed central nervous system that also interferes with deep breathing and predisposes to aspiration of infected material.

Pulmonary edema resulting from injudicious use of intravenous fluids, cardiac failure, chest injuries, bacterial sepsis, renal failure, or inhalation of hot or irritant gases by burn patients also leads to pulmonary infection. The fluid that accumulates in the alveoli prevents normal phagocytic activity of alveolar macrophages. On the other hand, if patients are dehydrated or are on a respirator and receive the normal anhydrous oxygen as it comes out of most lines without adequate humidification, the cilia and the tracheobronchial tree do not function normally to clear bronchial secretions.

Spread of Microbes to the Lower Respiratory Tract

Microbes may invade the lower respiratory tract by one of four routes: (1) aspiration from the oropharynx, (2) direct entrance through tracheostomies, (3) suspension in inhaled gases, and (4) from the blood.

Aspiration from the Oropharynx

Only 2 to 6 percent of physiologically normal subjects have gram-negative bacteria in their oropharynxes. Johanson et al [28] found that gram-negative bacteria can be cultured from the oropharynxes of 35 percent of moderately ill patients and 73 percent of moribund patients. The prevalence of gram-negative bacteria was not related to the duration of hospitalization. In a subsequent study, these authors prospectively examined 213 patients.[27] Twenty-two percent became colonized on the first hospital day and 45 percent became colonized sometime during their hospital stay. On the first hospital day, there was colonization of 76 percent of the patients who became persistently colonized, and 12.2 percent of these patients developed nosocomial respiratory infections. Patients were predisposed to develop gram-negative colonization if they had coma, hypotension, sputum production, tracheal intubation, acidosis, azotemia, abnormal white blood cell counts, or received antimicrobial drugs. Glover and Jolly [29] reported a 40 to 63.2 percent gram-negative bacterial colonization rate of the respiratory tract of hospitalized patients, depending on the number of cultures taken.

Surgical patients periodically aspirate small but unrecognized quantities of material from the oropharynx and gastrointestinal tract that are contaminated with microorganisms. Probably this unrecognized aspiration occurs much more frequently than gross aspiration of gastrointestinal contents that occurs occasionally with vomiting episodes. Culver et al [17] placed Evans blue dye into the stomach of 300 surgical patients before induction of anesthesia. After completion of anesthesia, the mouth, pharynx, larynx, trachea, and main bronchi were examined by laryngoscopy and bronchoscopy. Regurgitation (dye detected in the pharynx) occurred in 26.3 percent of the patients, and 16.3 percent aspirated (dye detected below the vocal cords). Unsuspected aspiration (no vomiting) occurred in 8.3 percent of patients. Aspiration was more common when nasogastric tubes were not used (23.9 percent of cases) than when they were used (5.6 percent). Aspiration occurred with all anesthetics used.

Thus, the oropharynxes of surgical patients are frequently contaminated by gram-negative bacteria, and aspiration occurs during anesthesia and surgery—both conditions favoring the development of nosocomial respiratory infections.

Entrance of Microorganisms through a Tracheostomy

Respiratory infections occur in 5 to 26 percent of patients following tracheostomy, and pneumonia is frequently the cause of death.[30] The use of mechanical ventilation does not seem to increase the incidence of pneumonia. Tracheostomy leads to drying of the tracheal mucosa because the inhaled air bypasses the humidification provided by the nasal mucosa. Drying leads to decreased ciliary movement, with increased likelihood of colonization. Tracheostomy also prevents the buildup of airway pressure required for effective coughing. Finally, the microorganisms colonizing the skin and tracheostomy wound have direct access to the bronchial tree. All of these factors favor respiratory tract infections.

Suspension of Microorganisms in Inhaled Gases

Coughing, sneezing, and talking can aerosolize microorganisms. It is estimated that particles generated by these activities range from 1 μm to more than 20 μm in diameter. It is estimated also that 50 percent of particles 1 to 2 μm in diameter are able to reach the terminal bronchioles. Thus, a small percentage of organisms aerosolized by sneezing, talking, and coughing are able to reach the terminal bronchioles and even the alveoli. Probably direct aerosolization of microorganisms by these activities is of minor importance as a cause of nosocomial pneumonia in the modern hospital setting.

Although tuberculosis and some other bacterial pneumonias can be spread this way, most airborne spread of infection probably occurs with the use of respirators and the necessity for having nebulizers to humidify the air. Gases delivered directly to the respirator have low or no water vapor. Therefore, it is necessary for humidification devices or nebulization devices to be attached to the respirator. Nebulizers are able to generate particles in the range of 1 to 2 μm in diameter and are used to ensure humidification of the inhaled air. Currently, they are also being used to deliver such medications as antibiotics to the lower respiratory tree. Humidifiers saturate gases with water vapor by having the gases bubble through the liquid, usually water, contained in the humidification devices. Because the water in the humidifier evaporates into the gas being bubbled through it, no aerosolization should occur, and, hence, the gas should not become contaminated with bacteria that grow in the water used in the humidification device. However, with vigorous bubbling of the gas through the humidifier, suspension of potentially bacteria-laden droplets can occur.

On the other hand, nebulizers saturate the gas with water vapor by dispersing aerosols or droplets into the gas by means of the Venturi principle. Any bacteria that grow in the nebulization device can become dispersed into the inhalation gas and will reach the alveoli. Even sterile water placed into nebulization devices can support the growth of *Pseudomonas aeruginosa*.[31] Nebulizers have been shown to be the source of bacteria that contaminate the distal bronchial alveolar tree. In addition, water from the nebulizer or from other sources that finds its way into the lines that are used for inhalation gases can become static and also can support the growth of microorganisms, which can lead to aerosolization of bacteria into the inhaled gas. For these reasons, it is essential that all nebulization equipment be cleaned daily and filled with sterile water and that all lines through which gases flow from the respirator to the patient be changed daily. While the respirator nebulizer is the most common potential source for bacterial contamination, any site in the respirator can potentially lead to aerosolization of microbes and lower respiratory tract infections. Aerosolization can occur from other sources as well. Tubin et al [32] reported Legionnaires' disease occurring in a renal transplant unit. The source was traced to water in a shower. Droplets containing *Legionella pneumophila* were probably aerosolized during showering and inhaled by the patients.

Hematogenous Spread

Invasion of the lungs via the bloodstream is a theoretical cause of pneumonia. It can occur when there is bacteremia, and this may lead to pneumonia, but it is probably an uncommon source. Septic thrombophlebitis can also lead to a septic pulmonary embolism that might lead to septic infarct and pulmonary abscess. Septic thrombophlebitis especially may occur with the use of indwelling venous catheters. *P. aeruginosa* pneumonia may occur via hematogenous spread from burn wounds.

URINARY TRACT INFECTIONS

Infections of the urinary tract are the most common nosocomial infections that occur in both the general hospital population and surgical patients. According to the National Nosocomial Infections Study, the rate of urinary tract infections on surgical services for the first six months of 1977 was 179.5 per 10,000 discharges (Table 24-2).[1] Others have shown that up to 12 percent of hospital patients develop a urinary tract infection sometime during their hospital course.[33]

Urinary tract infections in surgical patients occur most commonly because of instrumentation. Mulholland and Bruun [33] found that 67 percent of patients with hospital-acquired urinary tract infections have had an operation on the lower urinary tract, instrumentation of the bladder, or catheterization.

Virtually every urinary tract infection is associated with a colony count of 10^5 organisms per milliliter or more. There are very few exceptions to this rule (Chapter 45). If the urine is obtained directly from the bladder by suprapubic bladder puncture, a colony count of 10^2 bacteria per milliliter is considered sufficient for diagnosing a urinary tract infection. In addition, large numbers of bacteria and neutrophils found in the microscopic examination of the urinary sediment are considered presumptive evidence of a urinary tract infection. Culture of the tip of the urinary catheter has been advocated, but studies show that most patients with positive catheter tip cultures do not have significant bacteriuria.

ORGANISMS CAUSING URINARY TRACT INFECTIONS

Most urinary tract infections are due to gram-negative aerobic bacteria found in the gastrointestinal tract. The most common organisms found to cause urinary tract infections in the National Nosocomial Infections Study were *E. coli*, enterococcus, *Klebsiella*, *Proteus*, *Pseudomonas*, *Candida*, and *Enterobacter* (Table 24-3). No doubt the high frequency of infection with fecal flora is due to the close approximation of the urethra and anus and the likely contamination of the nearby skin by fecal organisms.

RISKS OF CATHETERIZATION

Most nosocomial urinary tract infections in surgical patients are due to the use of indwelling urinary catheters. Bacteriuria is seen in 1–5 percent of patients after a single, short-term catheterization.[34] The risk is higher in pregnant females, elderly or debilitated patients, and patients with urologic abnormalities.[35] Single catheterizations are done to relieve overdistention of the bladder or temporary obstruction that might occur after an operative procedure, to obtain roentgenographic studies of the bladder and urethra, to determine residual urine, or to obtain a clean specimen for culture.

Urinary tract infections are much more common following the use of indwelling catheters, which are used commonly on surgical wards to prevent overdistention of the bladder and to monitor urinary output. They are required for patients having urologic procedures, especially operations on the urethra to facilitate repair, and for operations on the rectum. They are also used for severely injured patients who cannot void, burn patients, patients with fractures who may have difficulty voiding, and neurologically injured patients who cannot void because of the neurologic injury.

Patients with a normal lower urinary tract are usually able to rid themselves of the infection spontaneously following removal of the urinary catheter. Many, however, remain infected. In these patients and in patients who have continued need for urinary catheterization there is always the risk of sepsis, shock, and death. Furthermore, the costs and possible side effects of antimicrobial therapy and the costs of hospitalization required all add to the cost of unnecessary urinary catheterization. One study showed that only 8–10 percent of patients on catheter drainage for two to seven days had significant bacteriuria once the catheter was removed, and only 0.7 percent had subsequent clinical infections after removing the catheter.[36] Nevertheless, because of the large number of patients who have urinary catheters sometime during their hospital course and because of the large number of patients on surgical wards and in hospitals, the number of patients with significant bacteriuria attributed to catheter use (an estimated 300,000 to 760,000 cases per year) and the consequent costs in terms of increased hospital stay, further diagnostic tests, and antimicrobial therapy, as well as such effects as bacteremia, shock, and death are substantial. The risk of developing a urinary tract infection increases with the duration of catheterization, and the risk of developing bacteriuria is 5–10 percent for each day of catheterization.[35]

MODES OF CONTAMINATION OF BLADDER IN PATIENTS WITH URINARY CATHETERS

Prior to the use of closed drainage systems, patients with indwelling catheters had open drainage systems in which the catheter was merely drained into a bottle or other receptacle. With such open drainage systems, 90–95 percent of patients with indwelling catheters had bacteriuria within three to four days. The advent of closed drainage systems has greatly reduced the incidence of bacteriuria in catheterized patients. Nevertheless, there are many routes by which bacteria can still find their way into the urine. First, the periurethral area in the male and introitus and periurethral area in the female may not be adequately prepared prior to insertion of the catheters. These areas, especially that of the female, are frequently contaminated by the fecal flora. Poor aseptic technique in introducing catheters or other instruments introduced into the urethra or inadequate cleaning of these instruments may also lead to bacteriuria. Bacteria can also enter the bladder from the urethral meatus, going up the urethra around the outside of the urinary catheter. This problem is usually not seen until late and is more common in females. The urinary tract can also become contaminated at any site where there is a break in the closed drainage system. Thus, contamination of the end of the urinary catheter where it connects to the drainage tube can also lead to urinary tract infections. Contamination of the collection vessel lower down may also lead to retrograde infection via the urinary stream. Irrigation of the bladder with contaminated irrigating solutions also is a source of potential urinary tract infections.

Condom catheter drainages and suprapubic catheters can be used to try to reduce the incidence of urinary tract infections. These are especially appropriate where prolonged urinary catheterization would be required, such as in comatose patients, incontinent males, or spine-injured patients. The condom and its attached collection tube should be changed daily, and the penis should be carefully cleaned and dried to avoid maceration. Suprapubic drainage is becoming more popular because it does not lead to obstruction of the urethral glands by the urethral catheter. This type of drainage has been mostly used for patients having gynecologic surgery, but it could also be used for other surgical and general medical patients as well. Preliminary results have shown a delayed onset of infection and a reduced incidence of infection in patients with suprapubic urinary catheters.

The correct placement of urinary catheters is discussed in Chapter 45.

NOSOCOMIAL INFECTIONS DUE TO INTRAVASCULAR INFUSIONS

Up to 12 percent of hospital patients have some type of intravascular infusion catheter. This rate is much higher in surgical patients, since every patient having a general or spinal anesthetic requires an intravenous cannula. Intravenous catheters are used for the administration of intravenous fluids, drugs, blood and blood products, and total parenteral nutrition. Most intravenous catheters are left in place for only a few days, but some may be left in place indefinitely for prolonged administration of total parenteral nutrition or chemotherapeutic agents. In addition, arterial catheters are used for blood pressure monitoring, and Swan-Ganz catheters are used for hemodynamic measurements in seriously ill patients.

INCIDENCE OF INTRAVENOUS CANNULA-ASSOCIATED INFECTIONS

Reports vary widely on the incidence of positive cultures from intravenous cannulas, all the way from 4 to 64 percent.[37] The incidence varies according to the type of cannula (Table 24-6). Steel needle or scalp intravenous catheters have the lowest incidence of cannula-tipped contamination (14.6 percent), whereas subclavian catheters have the highest incidence (26.3 percent).[38] Data in this table are not strictly comparable, however, because plastic catheters are the ones most often inserted in emergency

TABLE 24-6. INFECTIONS ASSOCIATED WITH INTRAVENOUS CANNULAS

	Percent of Contaminated Cannula Tips	Percent of Cannula-associated Septicemia
Plastic cannulas		
Percutaneous	17.9	0.5
Peripheral	17.9	0.5
Subclavian	26.3	3.8
Umbilical	23.3	6.5
Cutdowns	24.2	6.5
Steel needles	14.6	0.2

From Rhame FS, Maki DG, Bennett JV: In Bennett JV, Brachman PS (eds): Hospital Infections, 1979. Courtesy of Little, Brown and Company.

situations and are inserted by physicians rather than by trained intravenous teams. Furthermore, they tend to remain in place longer than steel needles and are more likely to be used in sicker patients. The rate of septicemia from intravenous cannulas is much lower, however, generally from 0.5 to 7 percent.[37]

For certain groups of patients, the infection rate associated with intravenous catheters is higher. When central venous catheters are used for total parenteral nutrition, the rate of catheter-associated sepsis is 27 percent.[39] Most septic episodes are due to *Candida albicans.* Suppurative thrombophlebitis associated with intravenous cannulas is seen almost exclusively in burn patients and is associated with a virtual 100 percent mortality rate unless the infected vein is entirely excised.[40]

The definition of intravenous catheter-associated infection may vary from one study to another. It is clear that when purulent thrombophlebitis occurs in a vein that has an intravenous catheter, there is a catheter-associated infection, but when inflammation only occurs around the site of the intravenous catheter or when a thick cord develops or thrombophlebitis develops, it is more difficult to say that there is an intravenous catheter-associated infection.

Microbiologic Criteria of Catheter Contamination

Formerly, catheter tips were cultured by placing them in broth culture. One problem with this technique is that even one bacterium could possibly cause growth and lead to a diagnosis of catheter contamination. Recently, semiquantitative cultures have been used by rolling the catheter on Petri plates containing a nonselective nutrient agar.[41] Using this technique, the plates that show 15 or more colonies are considered to be positive semiquantitative cultures. Most positive semiquantitative cultures show confluent growth. This technique may also be used for steel needles after removing them from the hub by repeated bending with a sterile clamp.

Infections Relating to Intravenous Infusion

Septicemic episodes may also be caused by microbial contamination of infused fluids. Contamination of the intravenous fluid itself has been due to inadequate sterilization by the manufacturer, contamination of the rubber dam around the administration site, punctures in plastic containers, contamination due to additives, and nonsterile addition of drugs or electrolytes to the intravenous fluid by piggyback infusions that are not appropriately kept free of contaminating microbes. Stopcocks and other junctions may also become sites where bacteria can reside and enter the intravenous infusion. Injections into the intravenous infusion line can also potentially lead to contamination of the intravenous infusions and catheter.

There have been scattered reports of septicemia traced to intravenous fluid contamination.[42] This problem received great publicity in the United States in 1971 when a nationwide epidemic of septicemia occurred.[43] It was attributable to the contamination of rubber dams on the tops of intravenous infusion bottles due to inadequate sterilization and condensation of the steam on the inside of the cap. These episodes of contamination of manufactured fluids are generally attributed to a breakdown in the sterilization process.

PREVENTING NOSOCOMIAL INTRAVENOUS CATHETER-ASSOCIATED INFECTIONS

Cutdown should be avoided insofar as possible because of the higher risk of sepsis. Steel needles rather than indwelling plastic cannulas should be used when short-term intravenous therapy is to be used. Intravenous catheters should be placed above the waist, and the saphenous vein or femoral vessels should be used only in emergency situations and the catheter should be removed as soon as the emergency is over. The skin should be thoroughly cleansed with an iodine-containing disinfectant or 70 percent ethanol. Sterile gloves and drapes should be used when the cannula will be a central venous catheter, when it will be used for total parenteral therapy, or when the catheter is placed in an immunosuppressed patient. All cutdowns should be done in the operating room unless there is an emergency. Where cannulas have been inserted with suboptimal asepsis, they should be removed and replaced as soon as possible. Antimicrobial ointments applied at the skin cannula junction at the time of insertion and every 24 hours thereafter can significantly reduce the incidence of intravenous cannula-associated sepsis.[38]

Any evidence of thrombophlebitis or cellulitis or suspicion of septic complications due to intravenous cannulas should generally lead to prompt removal of the cannula. Catheters should be replaced every 48–72 hours because the incidence of catheter-associated sepsis increases markedly thereafter. Frequently, central venous cannulas, especially the newer silastic cannulas, are used long-term for the administration of chemotherapy and total parenteral nutrition in patients who are compromised hosts, with lymphoreticular malignancies and low white counts. These patients frequently have fevers and septic episodes. More often than not the fever is not due to the cannula. Because only a limited number of sites are available for insertion of such cannulas and because they are so valuable for the therapy of the patient, a judicious search should be made for all other sites of infection. If, finally, no infection stemming from any other site can be identified, these cannulas probably then should be removed.

Because contamination can occur at virtually every point in an intravenous infusion system, addition of medications to the intravenous fluid container, injections into the tubing, piggyback administration catheters, and introduction of stopcock manometers and other devices into the lines should be kept to an absolute minimum. Changes in bottles, administration sets, and irrigation of clotted catheters all increase the risk of contamination.

Nosocomial infections stemming from infection or contamination of the intravenous fluid is most frequently seen with total parenteral nutrition therapy. These nosocomial infections can be reduced by changing all bottles and intravenous infusion lines daily and by having a micropore filter in line with the intravenous fluids so that the total parenteral nutrition fluid is filtered prior to administration to the patient. Total parenteral nutrition fluid has a contamination rate as high as 38 percent.[44]

INFECTIONS ASSOCIATED WITH BLOOD TRANSFUSIONS

Hepatitis

Viral hepatitis is the most common infection associated with blood transfusion. Before testing for HBsAg was started, the incidence of hepatitis was 0.06 cases per 100 units of blood transfused.[45] It was estimated that 6.5 million units of blood were transfused in the United States in 1971, and from these transfusions there were an estimated 120,000 instances of jaundice and 14,000 deaths.[46] The number of cases of posttransfusion hepatitis is a minimum, since many cases may not be detected until the patient leaves the hospital and may go unreported. Furthermore, most cases of infection with hepatitis B virus are anicteric and most likely are never detected. The estimated number of anicteric cases ranges from 75 percent to 99 percent.[47] The incidence of posttransfusion hepatitis varies with the vigor with which it is sought by routine screening. Most carriers of hepatitis B virus can be detected by routine screening of blood donors for HBsAg,[46] and screening has reduced the incidence of transfusion-associated hepatitis B. Currently, 95 percent of posttransfusion hepatitis is caused by a virus which is neither A nor B (non-A, non-B hepatitis).[48]

The incidence of transfusion-associated hepatitis is higher when commercial donors are used than when volunteer donors are used. Early reports suggested transfusion-associated hepatitis B was extremely low with frozen red cells or washed red cells. However, more recent studies report that transfusion-associated hepatitis is not prevented by using frozen or washed red cells. Adding gamma globulin to blood before transfusion can reduce the incidence of posttransfusion hepatitis.[49] Pooled blood products, such as antihemophilic factor (factor VIII concentrates), increase the likelihood of hepatitis transmission.

At present, the best ways of reducing transfusion-associated hepatitis include (1) improved tests for hepatitis carriers, (2) use of volunteer blood donors, (3) antiviral blood additives, (4) new forms of antiviral agents, and (5) active immunization against hepatitis.

Surgeons are at high risk for hepatitis B viral infection. In a recent study among 224 Danish surgeons, 23 percent had anti-HBsAg antibody in their sera, but only 14 (6 percent) had clinical hepatitis, from which they recovered.[50] None became carriers of HBsAg. The rate of antibody-positive surgeons increased with age, and it was five times that of age-matched controls. The high rate of anti-HBsAg antibody positivity among surgeons no doubt reflects that they encounter patients who are carriers of HBsAg commonly in their practices. These include immunocompromised hosts and dialysis patients. The risk to surgeons can be reduced by taking measures to protect patients and staff, such as HBsAg screening of blood transfusions, surveillance of such high-risk patients as hemodialysis patients, and passive immunization of staff after accidental exposure, and vaccination (Chapter 10). While the study among Danish surgeons failed to detect any carriers of HBsAg and there were no fatalities, other studies show that chronic hepatitis may develop in 5–10 percent of infected patients, and perhaps 1 in 100 acute attacks ends fatally.[51]

Cytomegalovirus

Cytomegalovirus infection can also be transfusion-associated. It is a herpesvirus that exists in a latent form in the white blood cells (Chapter 10). Posttransfusion cytomegaloviral infection is most frequently seen after open heart procedures with extracorporeal perfusion. A syndrome resembling infectious mononucleosis and characterized by fever, erythematous rash, hepatomegaly, splenomegaly, eosinophilia, and atypical lymphocytosis appears three to five weeks after operation. It is variously called the postperfusion syndrome, the postpump syndrome, and the posttransfusion syndrome. The disease is almost always self-limited. It is unusual in adults but can affect 10 percent of children and young adults.

The postperfusion syndrome has been attributed to both cytomegalovirus and to Epstein-Barr virus. Most cases have been attributed to cytomegalovirus, and the transfused blood is almost certainly the source of the virus.[52]

Other Transfusion-associated Infections

Other transfusion-associated infections occur only sporadically. Bacteremia, especially with gram-negative bacteria, can occur from contaminated blood but fortunately is rare.

Plasmodia that cause malaria can be found in red blood cells years after infection in some cases. Therefore, transmission of this disease by transfusion is a possibility. The likelihood is very small in the United States, but because of worldwide travel and the increased incidence found in servicemen returning from Vietnam, the number of cases of transfusion-associated malaria increased from one case per year before 1966 to five to nine cases per year from 1968 to 1971.[53]

In Central and South America, the trypanosomes causing Chagas' disease have been transmitted with transfused blood and have caused disease in the recipient. On rare occasions, brucellosis has been transmitted to a patient by a donor.

Transmission of syphilis hardly ever occurs anymore since the advent of routine serologic screening of all blood and the abandonment of direct transfusion. Treponemes do not survive storage at refrigerator temperatures for more than a few days, further contributing to the rarity of transmission of syphilis by transfusion.

BIBLIOGRAPHY

Alexander JW: Nosocomial infections. Curr Probl Surg 10:1, 1973.

American Hospital Association, Committee on Infections Within Hospitals: Infection Control in the Hospital, 4th ed. Chicago, American Hospital Association, 1979.

Bennett JV, Brachman PS: Hospital Infections. Boston, Little, Brown, 1979.

REFERENCES

THE ENVIRONMENT AND THE HOST

1. Center for Disease Control: National Nosocomial Infections Study Report, 1977 (6-month summaries), November 1979.
2. Alexander JW: Nosocomial infections. Curr Probl Surg 10:1, 1973.
3. Wenzel RP, Osterman CA, Hunting KJ: Hospital-acquired infections. II. Infection rates by site, service and common procedures in a university hospital. Am J Epidemiol 104:645, 1976.
4. Mulholland SG, Creed J, Dierauf LA, Bruun JN, Blakemore WS: Analysis and significance of nosocomial infection rates. Ann Surg 180:827, 1974.
5. Bennett JV: Human infections: Economic implications and prevention. Ann Intern Med 89:761, 1978.
6. Haley RW, Schaberg DR, Von Allmen SD, McGowan JE Jr: Estimating extra charges and prolongation of hospitalization due to nosocomial infections: A comparison of methods. J Infect Dis 141:248, 1980.
7. Green JW, Wenzel RP: Postoperative wound infection: A controlled study of the increased duration of hospital stay and direct cost of hospitalization. Ann Surg 185:264, 1977.
8. Aber RC, Bennett JV: Surveillance of nosocomial infections. In Bennett JV, Brachman PS: Hospital Infections. Boston, Little, Brown, 1979, p 53.
9. Joint Commission on Accreditation of Hospitals. Accreditation Manual for Hospitals. Chicago, Joint Commission on Accreditation of Hospitals, 1979.
10. American Hospital Association. Committee on Infections within Hospitals. Infection Control in the Hospital, 4th ed. Chicago, American Hospital Association, 1979.
11. Altemeier WA, Burke JF, Pruitt BA Jr, Sandusky WR (eds): Manual on Control of Infection in Surgical Patients. Philadelphia, Lippincott, 1976.
12. Aisner J, Schimpff SC, Bennett JE, Young VM, Wiernik PH: *Aspergillus* infections in cancer patients. Association with fireproofing materials in a new hospital. JAMA 235:411, 1976.
13. Bate JG, James U: *Salmonella typhimurium* infection dustborne in a children's ward. Lancet 2:713, 1958.
14. Howard RJ: Host defense against infection. Part I. Curr Probl Surg 17:267, 1980.
15. Dineen P, Drusin L: Epidemics of postoperative wound infections associated with hair carriers. Lancet 2:1157, 1973.
16. Berry FA Jr, Blankenbaker WL, Ball CG: A comparison of bacteremia occurring with nasotracheal and orotracheal intubation. Anesth Analg 52:873, 1973.
17. Culver GA, Makel HP, Beecher HK: Frequency of aspiration of gastric contents by the lungs during anesthesia and surgery. Ann Surg 133:289, 1951.
18. US Department of Health Education and Welfare: Minimum Requirements of Construction and Equipment for Hospital and Medical Facilities. Washington, DC, US Government Printing Office, DHEW Publication No. (HRA) 74–4000, 1974.
19. Kaslow RA, Zellner SR: Infections in patients on maintenance hemodialysis. Lancet 2:117, 1972.
20. Editorial: Septicaemia in dialysis patients. Lancet 1:521, 1980.
21. Snydman DR, Bregman D, Bryan JA: Hemodialysis-associated hepatitis in the United States, 1974. J Infect Dis 135:687, 1977.
22. Garibaldi RA, Bryan JA, Forrest JF, Hanson BF, Dismukes WE: Hemodialysis-associated hepatitis. JAMA 225:384, 1973.
23. Steere AC, Craven PJ, Hall WJ III, Leotsakis N, Wells JG, Farmer JJ III, Gangarosa EJ: Person-to-person spread of *Salmonella typhimurium* after a hospital common-source outbreak. Lancet 1:319, 1975.
24. Bryan FL: Status of food borne disease in the United States. J Environ Health 38:74, 1975.
25. Editorial: Food poisoning in hospitals. Lancet 1:576, 1980.

ISOLATION PROCEDURES

26. Center for Disease Control: Isolation Techniques for Use in Hospitals, 2nd ed. Washington, DC, US Government Printing Office. DHEW Publication No. (CDC) 76–8314, 1975.

RESPIRATORY INFECTIONS

27. Johanson WG Jr, Pierce AK, Sanford JP, Thomas GD: Nosocomial respiratory infections with gram-negative bacilli: The significance of colonization of the respiratory tract. Ann Intern Med 77:701, 1972.
28. Johanson WG Jr, Pierce AK, Sanford JP: Changing pharyngeal bacterial flora of hospitalized patients. Emergence of gram-negative bacilli. N Engl J Med 281:1137, 1969.
29. Glover JL, Jolly L: Colonization of the respiratory tract by gram-negative bacilli in hospitalized patients. Exp Med Surg 29:114, 1971.
30. Bryant LR, Trinkle JK, Mobin-Uddin K, Baker J, Griffen WO Jr: Bacterial colonization profile with tracheal intubation and mechanical ventilation. Arch Surg 104:647, 1972.
31. Grieble HG, Colton FR, Bind TJ, Toigo A, Griffith LG: Fine-particle humidifiers. Source of *Pseudomonas aeruginosa* infections in a respiratory-disease unit. N Engl J Med 282:531, 1970.
32. Tubin TO, Beare J, Dunhill MS, Fisher-Hoch S, French M, Mitchell RG, Morris PJ, Muers MF: Legionnaires' disease in a transplant unit: Isolation of the causative agent from shower baths. Lancet 2:118, 1980.

URINARY TRACT INFECTIONS

33. Mulholland SG, Bruun JA: A study of urinary tract infections. J Urol 110:245, 1973.
34. Stamm WE: Guidelines for prevention of catheter-associated urinary tract infections. Ann Int Med 82:386, 1975.
35. Kunin CM: Detection, Prevention and Management of Urinary Tract Infections. Philadelphia, Lea & Febiger, 1972.
36. Guinan PD, Bayley BC, Metzger WI, Shoemaker WC, Bush IM: The case against "The case against the catheter": Initial report. J Urol 101:909, 1969.

INTRAVASCULAR INFECTIONS

37. Maki DG, Goldmann DA, Rhame FS: Infection control in intravenous therapy. Ann Intern Med 79:867, 1973.
38. Rhame FS, Maki DG, Bennett JV: Intravenous cannula-associated infections. In Bennet JV, Brachman PS (eds): Hospital Infections. Boston, Little, Brown, 1979, p 433.
39. Curry CR, Quie PG: Fungal septicemia in patients receiving parenteral hyperalimentation. N Engl J Med 285:1221, 1971.
40. Pruitt BA Jr, McManus WF, Kim SH, Treat RC: Diagnosis and treatment of cannula-related intravenous sepsis in burn patients. Ann Surg 191:546, 1980.
41. Maki DG, Weise CE, Sarafin HW: A semiquantitative culture method for identifying intravenous-catheter-related infection. N Engl J Med 296:1305, 1977.
42. Duma RJ, Warner JF, Dalton HP: Septicemia from intravenous infusions. N Engl J Med 284:257, 1971.
43. Maki DG, Rhame FS, Mackel DC, Bennett JV: Nationwide epidemic of septicemia caused by contaminated intravenous products. I. Epidemiologic and clinical features. Am J Med 60:471, 1976.

44. Deeb EN, Natsios CA: Contamination of intravenous fluids by bacteria and fungi during preparation and administration. Am J Hosp Pharm 28:764, 1971.

INFECTIONS ASSOCIATED WITH BLOOD TRANSFUSIONS

45. Grady GF, Chalmers TC, Boston Inter-hospital Liver Group: Risk of post-transfusion viral hepatitis. N Engl J Med 271:337, 1964.
46. Holzbach RT, Leon MA: Posttransfusion viral hepatitis and the hepatitis-associated antigen (HAA). Ohio State Med J 67:329, 1971.
47. Hampers CL, Prager D, Senior JR: Post-transfusion anicteric hepatitis. N Engl J Med 271:747, 1964.
48. Conrad ME, Knodell RG, Bradley EL Jr, Flannery EP, Ginsberg AL: Risk factors in transmission of non-A, non-B post-transfusion hepatitis. The role of hepatitis B antibody in donor blood. Transfusion 17:579, 1977.
49. Katz R, Rodrigueq J, Ward R: Post-transfusion hepatitis: Effect of modified gamma globulin added to blood in vitro. N Engl J Med 285:925, 1971.
50. Hardt F, Aldershville J, Dietrichson O: Hepatitis B virus infections among Danish surgeons. J Infect Dis 140:972, 1975.
51. Editorial: Hepatitis B virus infection among surgeons. Lancet 2:300, 1980.
52. Howard RJ, Balfour HH Jr, Simmons RL: The surgical significance of viruses. Curr Probl Surg 14:5, 1977.
53. Hvestis DW, Bove JR, Busch S (eds): Practical Blood Transfusions, 2nd ed. Boston, Little, Brown, 1976, p 275.

PART VII: REGIONAL SURGICAL INFECTIONS

CHAPTER 25
Infections of the Skin and Soft Tissues

RICHARD L. SIMMONS AND DAVID H. AHRENHOLZ

THE PATHOBIOLOGY OF INFECTIONS OF THE SKIN AND SOFT TISSUES

ANATOMY OF THE SKIN, FASCIAE, AND MUSCLE

The skin is a two-layered membrane consisting of an outer ectodermal layer, the epidermis, and an inner mesodermal layer, the dermis. The latter is subdivided into two regions, the papillary dermis lying between the epidermal papillae of the skin, and the reticular dermis deep to the papillae. Both consist principally of collagen fibers, although the papillary layer has a finer texture. The epidermis and dermis are firmly cemented together to form a cohesive membrane, which varies in thickness over the surface of the body from 1.5 to 4 mm (Fig. 25-1). The skin resides on subcutaneous tissue (hypodermis or tela subcutaneum), which is superficial fascia.

Skin Appendages

Sweat glands, hair follicles, sebaceous glands, apocrine glands, and nails constitute the skin appendages. They extend into the hypodermis so that infections of these structures can readily spread into adjacent subcutaneous tissue (Fig. 25-2).

Vascular Supply of the Skin

The epidermis lacks nerves, blood vessels, or lymphatics, so that its superficial layers are relatively isolated from humoral or cellular host defenses. The skin vessels and nerves lie within the dermis. The arterial supply to the skin arises as a flat network near the junction of the superficial fascia and dermis (Fig. 25-3) originating from branches of larger arteries running more deeply in the superficial fascia. Branches pass outward from the deep plexus to form another flat network of small vessels (Fig. 25-3) just below the papillary dermis. From this plexus, arcades of capillaries loop into the papillae and periadnexal dermis. Venules accompany the arteries, forming arteriovenous shunts surrounded by aggregates of smooth muscle cells called glomus cells. These regulate skin temperature by altering tissue perfusion.

The lymphatics of the skin follow the arterioles. One plexus resides in the outermost superficial fascia and contains a few valves, while the superficial plexus in the dermis lacks valves. Blind-ended lymphatics in the papillae drain the epidermis. Any infectious focus in the skin can result in circumferentially spreading erythema, edema, and cellulitis because the superficial blood and lymphatic plexuses lack valves. Thrombosis of the superficial vascular plexus can result in foci of cutaneous gangrene, which appear as small ulcers. Deep infections, which spread within the fascial cleft between the subcutaneous tissue and the deep fascia (necrotizing fasciitis), result in more extensive areas of gangrene only when the infection spreads superficially and causes thrombosis of the deep plexus. For this reason, extensive undermining can occur without gangrene if the infection stays in the cleft deep to the subcutaneous tissues where vessels are few.

The Subcutaneous Tissues and Fasciae

All fibrous connective tissue within the body is called fasciae except for the specifically organized structures like tendons, aponeuroses, and ligaments. There are three principal subdivisions of the fascial system: the superficial fascia, the deep fascia, and a subserous fascia. Surgeons generally regard the deep fascia overlying and separating muscle groups as the fascia, which deters the spread of infections from superficial layers to the muscular compartments. On the face and scalp, the deep fascia is missing; subcutaneous or submucosal infections meet no deep fascial barrier and readily extend to other tissue planes.

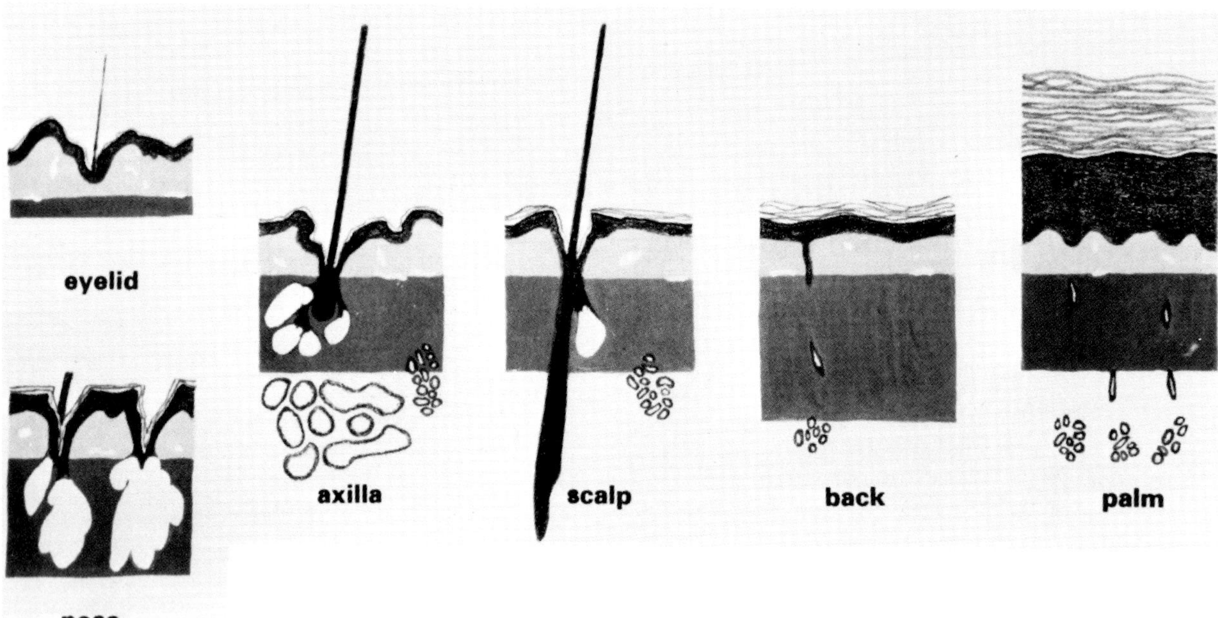

Fig. 25-1. Schematic cross-sections of skin in various regions, representing the varying thicknesses of the epidermis and dermis. The epidermis is thickest on palms and soles. The dermis is thinnest on eyelids and thickest on the back. In many regions the skin appendages reach the subcutaneous tissues. (From Ackerman AB: Structure and function of the skin. I. Development, morphology and physiology. In Moschella SL, Pillsbury DM, Hurley HJ Jr: *Dermatology,* Philadelphia, Saunders, 1975, p 1.)

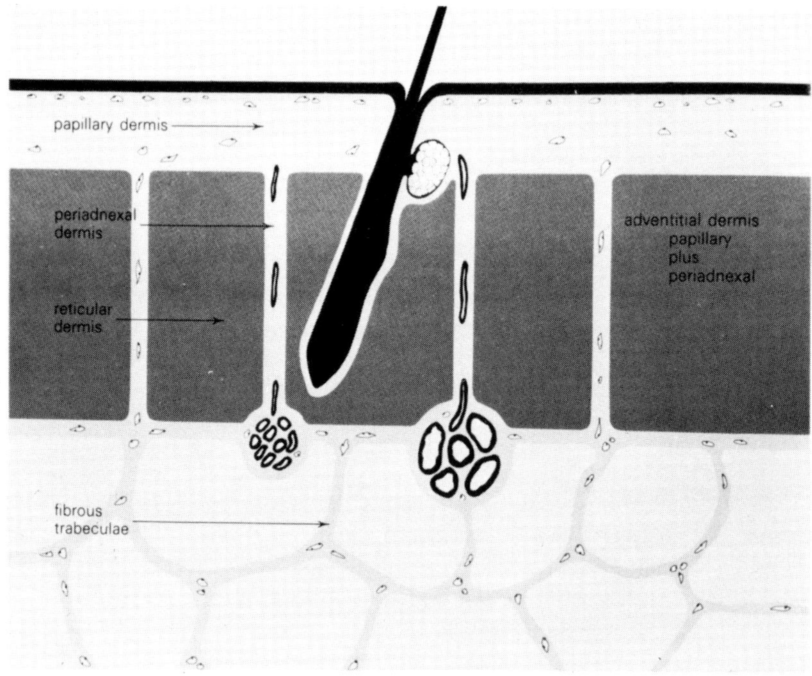

Fig. 25-2. The connective tissue of the papillary and periadnexal dermis, which together are called the adventitial dermis, are similar. The fibrous trabeculae of the subcutaneous fat are analogues of the adventitial dermis. (From Ackerman AB: Structure and function of the skin. I. Development, morphology, and physiology. In Moschella SL, Pillsbury DM, Hurley HJ Jr (eds): *Dermatology.* Philadelphia, Saunders, 1975, p 1.)

Most soft tissue infection (wound infections, cellulitis, subcutaneous abscesses, lymphangitis, and superficial thrombophlebitis) occur within the superficial fascia, ie, the subcutaneous layer between the deep fascia and skin. Within this superficial fascia lie the superficial nerves, arteries, veins, lymphatics, as well as mammary glands and muscles of the face.

In most areas, the subcutaneous tissue can easily be separated from the deep fascia. These potential spaces are called fascial clefts, and infection can spread readily along these planes. The spread of infection is limited wherever the fascia become adherent, ie, over bony prominences. Infections of the fascial cleft frequently spare the blood supply of the skin until direct involvement of the superficial fascial vessels occurs. The fascia of the scrotum is tightly adherent to the skin, so infections in the perianal region cause gangrene of the scrotal skin (Fournier gangrene).

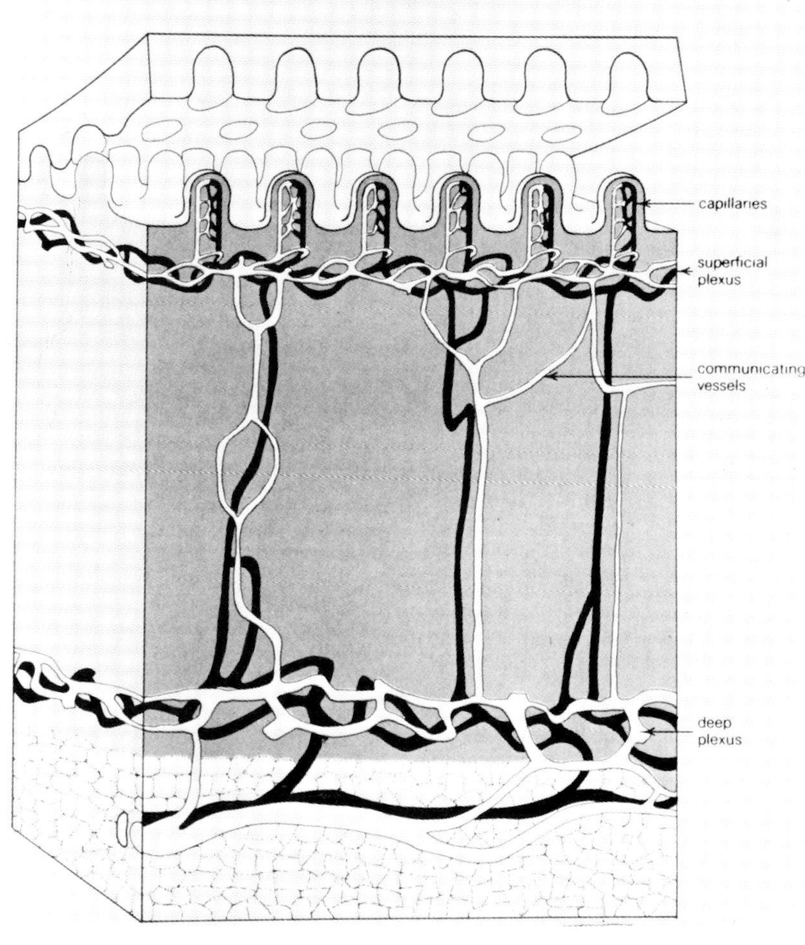

Fig. 25-3. The dermal vasculature consists of a three-dimensional network of two plexuses that parallel the skin surface; one in the lower reticular dermis (deep plexus), the other beneath the papillary dermis (superficial plexus). Perpendicularly oriented communicating blood vessels connect the deep and superficial plexuses. The rich capillary supply of the adventitial dermis constitutes a microcirculation, in contrast to the relatively straight, large conduits of the two parallel plexuses and their communicating vessels. (From Ackerman AB: Structure and function of the skin. I. Development, morphology, and physiology. In Moschella SL, Pillsbury DM, Hurley HJ Jr: *Dermatology.* Philadelphia, Saunders, 1975, p 1.)

Skeletal Muscle

Striated muscle is made up of long multinucleate fibrillar cells enclosed in an acellular sarcolemma. Bundles of cells are encased in a connective tissue epimysium containing the nerves and vessels. The blood supply is rich—several capillaries may abut on each muscle fiber. Unlike cardiac muscle, which has lymphatics in the endomysium, the lymphatics of skeletal muscle are confined to major connective tissue elements. The highly effective defenses of muscle against infection are presumed due to its good blood supply, although some experiments have failed to demonstrate an exceptional resistance to infection.[1]

MICROBIAL ECOLOGY OF THE SKIN

Anatomic and Physiologic Factors

The epidermis is a relatively dry stratified squamous epithelium whose regenerative layers rest on the dermis. The proliferating cells are pushed outward, and cellular degeneration results in a surface composed of closely packed keratin scales called the stratum corneum. The thick stratum corneum provides the major barrier against infection, since it is virtually impermeable to bacteria, undergoes a constant slow desquamation which removes bacteria, and provides a barrier to fluid transudation from the moist tissue below. The normal skin bacteria reside in the chinks in this keratin armor. Scanning electron microscopy reveals that the bacteria lie between the desquamating loosely adherent cells to a depth of 2 or 3 cell layers.[2]

The various skin appendages affect cutaneous microbial colonization. Eccrine sweat glands (Fig. 25-2) are found everywhere on the skin but are highly variable in number. The secretory portion lies at the dermal-subcutaneous junction, with a duct leading straight to the skin surface. Eccrine sweat is a hypotonic saline solution containing small concentrations of amino acids, ammonia, urea, and lactic acid, which slightly acidify the skin and have minimal nutrient value for bacteria. Because the eccrine sweat glands have straight ducts and a watery secretion, they are rarely the source of primary skin or subcutaneous infections. However, miliaria of the eccrine glands may be clinically misdiagnosed as folliculitis.

Sebaceous glands are found everywhere on the skin except the palms and both surfaces of the feet. Sebaceous glands discharge their contents into almost every hair follicle on the body. Because the secretory cell dies during secretion, sebaceous glands are called holocrine glands. They produce sebum, a complex mixture of lipids including triglycerides, wax esters, squalene, cholesterol esters, and cholesterol, which are inhibitory to staphylococci, streptococci, and gram-negative organisms but stimulate diphtheroid growth. The diphtheroids, in turn, competitively inhibit the growth of pathogenic organisms. Electron micrographs show the resident bacteria aggregated into microcolonies at the openings of hair follicles, usually adherent to clumps of sebum.[2]

Apocrine secretory glands are under endocrine control and do not function until puberty. They also drain into hair follicles but are found only around the areolae, axillae, and anogenital regions. Modified apocrine glands form the ceruminous glands of the ear, Moll glands of the eyelid, and the mammary glands. These are mesodermal holocrine glands, which rest in the subcutaneous tissue with relatively straight ducts through to hair follicles. Hidradenitis suppurativa is an infection of these apocrine glands.

Hair follicles are found over most of the skin surface. Their openings appear to provide crevices in which bacterial colonization occurs. The hair itself can become infected by dermatophytes, and the hairy pubic and axillary regions appear more suceptible to many infections, although the responsible factors have not been determined.

Other factors affect the skin microflora. At birth, the skin pH is 7 but decreases to 5.5 within the first year of life. Excreted lactate, glutamate, and aspartate acidify the environment; fatty and amino acids contribute little. The temperature is usually about 5C below the internal temperature, but varies from region to region. The surface of the skin has a 90 percent relative humidity rising to 100 percent only in intertriginous areas.[2]

Many factors limit the normal flora of the skin. A minimal skin flora is maintained by: (1) a dry surface, (2) constant desquamation of the superficial keratin layers, (3) the presence of an inhibitory normal bacterial flora, (4) a deficient nutrient supply, (5) an acidic and lipid-rich surface inhibitory to bacteria, and (6) a cool temperature. Any changes in these factors can increase the density of surface pathogenic and nonpathogenic bacteria.

Normal Cutaneous Microflora (See Chapter 3)

There are huge variations in the skin bacterial counts reported by different investigators. In 1965, Williamson[3] recorded mean surface bacterial counts of 2.4×10^6 per cm^2 in the axillae and 2×10^5 per cm^2 on the forehead, while Ulrick[4] reported values of 106 per cm^2 and 348 per cm^2 at the same sites. Most of the reported discrepancies are due to differences in sampling methods. A comparison of aerobic bacterial counts derived by washing techniques is shown in Table 25-1. There is an enormous individual range of counts depending upon individual hygiene, environmental exposure, endocrine changes, and anatomic site. In general, the lowest bacterial counts are found on exposed, dry, cool skin surfaces such as the arms and face. Certain spaces such as the axillae, perineum, toewebs, and anterior nares have a higher temperature and higher relative humidity, which result in more frequent colonization by all types of bacteria.

Skin has resident and transient microbial flora. Transients are bacteria collected from the environment and are of infinite variety. The bacteria lie free on the skin and are loosely attached by grease or dirt. They are easily lost, however, with the passage of time. The resident flora, by contrast, is a relatively stable population both in size and composition, consisting mostly of diphtheroids and staphylococci. These organisms reproduce within the relatively protected skin crevices and follicle openings and are resistant to removal.

Diphtheroids (genus *Corynebacterium*) are gram-positive, nonmotile, catalase-positive, pleomorphic rods which have a beaded appearance on Gram stain. The organisms may be aerobic, microaerophilic, or anaerobic. Aerobes predominate except around sebaceous glands, where anaerobic diphtheroids (especially *C. acnes*) are numerous. Diphtheroids flourish in a lipid environment and break down sebum to produce free fatty acids, which inhibit the growth of other bacteria. *C. diphtheriae,* the cause of diphtheria, is not a member of the normal skin flora, although it may infect the skin. Only a few skin diphtheroid species are pathogens, causing such superficial skin infections as trichomycosis axillaris, erythrasma, pitted keratolysis, and possibly acne. They occasionally produce systemic infection including endocarditis, lymphadenitis, vaginitis, neonatal sepsis, bacteremia, hepatitis, liver abscess, and brain abscess. They are frequent contaminants in blood culture bottles and in mixed infections of the skin and soft tissues, but usually play a minor role in the pathogenesis of infection.

TABLE 25-1. MEAN AND RANGE QUANTITATIVE AEROBIC COUNTS ON SKIN OBTAINED BY SCRUBBING ON 22 HEALTHY INDIVIDUALS

Site	Arithmetic Mean	Geometric Mean	Range
Forehead	1.6×10^5	1.1×10^4	2.6×10–2.9×10^6
Sternum	1.5×10^4	2.1×10^3	6.6×10–1.4×10^5
Periumbilicus	2.7×10^3	1.4×10^3	17.9×10–8.0×10^4
Thigh, upper front	2.3×10^3	7.7×10^2	9.9×10–2.0×10^4
Dorsum of foot	8.6×10^2	3.6×10^2	3.3×10–5.4×10^3
Back, upper center	1.2×10^4	1.1×10^3	7–8.2×10^4
Calf	2.4×10^3	3.1×10^2	<7–1.5×10^4
Sole of foot	2.1×10^5	1.6×10^4	7.2×10–1.6×10^4
Axilla, lower margin	4.1×10^4	8.7×10^2	1.3×10–2.8×10^5
Palm of hand	9.8×10^2	4.4×10^2	6.6×10–5.6×10^3

Modified from Noble WC, Somerville DA (eds): Cutaneous populations. In *Microbiology of Human Skin.* London, Saunders, 1974, p 50.

Micrococcaceae, including the genera *Staphylococcus*, *Micrococccus*, and *Sarcina*, are the other major components of the human skin flora (Chapter 4). Aside from the diphtheroids, *S. epidermidis* is the most common bacterial resident on the skin. *S. aureus* is not usually considered a resident organism, although colonization is common, especially in the nose, axillae, perineum, and toewebs. Nasal carriage is found in 10 to 40 percent of the normal adult population, but in 100 percent of recently discharged hospital patients. The *S. aureus* is the most common pathogenic organism found on the skin and the most frequent single infecting agent in soft tissue infections. *S. epidermidis* and other micrococci are less frequent primary pathogens in soft tissue infections, but can cause infections of surgical prostheses, septicemia, and urinary tract infections. Streptococci are not part of the normal skin flora.[2]

Gram-negative bacilli are comparatively rare on normal skin, with the exception of the *Acinetobacter (Mima, Herellea)* genus which may be part of the normal flora of the axillae, groin, and toewebs. *Proteus* species rarely colonize the skin, but are surprisingly frequent agents in subcutaneous abscesses of the upper body.[5] The other gram-negative rods are only occasionally found in quantity in moist areas like the axillae, groin, and toewebs. On glabrous skin, fecal coliforms disappear rapidly, presumably as a result of dessication, although they may persist long enough on the hands to be a problem to food handlers or on the surgical wards.

Both the filamentous and yeast form fungi are frequently isolated from the skin, but it is difficult to determine whether they are transients acquired from the environment or true inhabitants (Table 25-2). *Pityrosporum orbiculare,* which causes pityriasis versicolor, is a member of the normal flora in 75 percent of people.

C. albicans, although frequently found in the vagina and mouth, is a rare cutaneous isolate except in the groin, axillae, and toewebs. These infections are more common in tropical countries. The normal bacterial skin flora inhibits the growth of *C. albicans,* but the use of local antibiotics may permit unrestrained yeast overgrowth. Dermatophytes frequently colonize the feet and other skin areas and are not always associated with dermatophytic infection.

Viruses are rarely recovered from the skin in the absence of viral disease. Of the skin fauna, only two can be regarded as normal, the mite *Demodex folliculorum* and the flagellate *Trichomonas vaginalis.*[2]

Although the flora of the normal skin is sparse, many skin diseases decrease its ability to inhibit microbial colonization. A variety of skin conditions result in massive bacterial overgrowth.

TABLE 25-2. YEAST COMMONLY ISOLATED FROM HEALTHY SKIN

Candida parapsilosis
C. guilliermondii
C. pseudotropicalis
C. tropicalis
C. zeylanoides
Debrayomyces hansenii
D. kloeckeri
Torulopsis glabrata
T. famata
Rhodotorula spp.
Cladosporium spp.
Trichosporon cutaneum
Cryptococcus spp.
(other than *C. neoformans*)
Saccharomyces spp.
Geotrichum candidum

From Nobel WC, Somerville DA (eds): The fungal flora. In *Microbiology of Human Skin.* London, Saunders, 1974, p 206.

PATHOGENESIS OF SOFT TISSUE INFECTIONS

Experimental Skin Infections

Normal skin is extremely resistant to infection, and few pathogenic organisms are capable of penetrating and invading intact epidermis. Topical application of even high concentrations of pathogenic bacteria does not result in infection.[6] The requirements to produce infection include: (1) a high concentration of microorganisms, (2) occlusion, which both prevents desquamation and provides a moist environment in which the bacteria can proliferate, (3) nutrients in the area, and (4) sufficient damage to the corneal layer for the organisms to penetrate. Corneal layer damage can be achieved by repeated stripping of the skin with cellophane tape, by plucking hair, by incision, or by occlusive dressings which result in skin maceration. In addition, a foreign body within the skin will potentiate most infections and is required for the production of infections from a small inoculum. Experimental folliculitis or impetigo results when *Staphylococcus, Streptococcus,* or *Candida* is applied in combination with these factors. In this sense, skin infections are usually opportunistic, ie, caused by normal skin flora, transient residents, or environmental contaminants, which have low pathogenic potential in themselves but can colonize and infect tissue with impaired local host defenses.

Susceptibility of Soft Tissues to Infection

Subcutaneous and soft tissue infections most often arise from breaks in local (and less often systemic) host defenses. Soft tissue infections, however, are not the natural consequence of simple microbial innoculation into tissue. Large numbers of bacteria are necessary to produce suppuration in intact tissue. Roettinger et al[1] found that 3×10^6 *S. aureus* was noninfective when injected into the soft tissues of guinea pigs; 2×10^9 *S. aureus* were required to produce infections consistently. With *E. coli,* 3×10^6 organisms were required to infect more than half the sites. The site of innoculation (tongue, subcutaneous fat, skin, or skeletal muscle) did not influence the rate of infection.

The resistance to infection of intact tissue has not been thoroughly studied. Duncan et al[6] noted that the infection rate after standardized lesions of the skin were exposed to a mixture of staphylococci and streptococci was dependent on the skin site—15 percent of arm lesions and 38 percent of leg lesions became infected. They hypothesized that these differences were due to the decreased cutaneous blood flow to the lower extremity, which delayed appropriate responses by natural defense mechanisms.

Differences in the infection rates at different sites is more likely related to the inherent pathogenicity of the local bacteria, the susceptibility of the tissue to trauma, and the size of the inoculum rather than to different degrees of local immunity. In men performing manual labor, the hands and arms are the most frequently infected sites, presumably owing to the high incidence of trauma.[5] In women, the axillae and submammary regions are frequently infected—minor trauma in both areas results in exposure to a relatively large bacterial inoculum growing in moist intertriginous areas.[5]

Differences in blood supply or tissue pO_2 may be additional factors in regional differences in infection.[6] Ischemic limbs and areas affected by radiation vasculitis and fibrosis are prone to infection. The local injection of epinephrine increases the experimental infection rates for a given bacterial inoculum.[1]

It is also possible that such differences in susceptibility are not due to decreases in arterial supply but may represent differences in lymphatic drainage of various areas; the lymphatics are thought to remove bacteria from the site of inoculation. Delong and Simmons (unpublished observation, 1981), however, have recently shown that bacteria are minimally cleared during the first 6 hours after subcutaneous inoculation, even though lymphatic function is normal. Areas of lymphedema and venous stasis are prone to infection even if the regional nodes are intact.

Role of Trauma in Soft Tissue Infection

Trauma not only inoculates the bacteria into the soft tissue, but also impairs host defenses. The degree of tissue damage is probably the most important factor in the pathogenesis of soft tissue infections.[7] For this reason, the nature and velocity of the wounding agent is a critical factor in the development of infection after soft tissue trauma (Chapter 22).

Foreign Bodies

Foreign bodies have long been recognized as important adjuvant factors in the production of infection. Cotton dust [8] and suture material are classic adjuvants increasing the infectivity of small bacterial inocula. Environmental contaminants (eg, soil) have also been implicated,[9] and devitalized endogenous tissue may play such a foreign body role.

Not all foreign bodies potentiate infection.[10,11] Injection of a liquid silicone or a local anesthetic does not stimulate the development of experimental staphylococcal infections. Different suture materials enhance the development of infection to varying degrees (Chapter 22). Other adjuvant agents are adhesive adjuncts, such as compound tincture of benzoin, ace adherent, Vi-drape adhesive, and aerozoin (Chapter 22).

EPIDEMIOLOGY OF SOFT TISSUE INFECTIONS

Most infectious diseases of the skin are the result of traumatic breaks of the skin with inoculation of ambient microbes. The kind of clinical infection produced depends not only on the species of microbe inoculated but also on the depth of inoculation. Intracutaneous inocula yield pyoderma, impetigo folliculitis, and erysipelas; subcutaneous inocula yield cellulitis and subcutaneous abscesses. If the fascial cleft between superficial and deep fascia is reached, the barriers to lateral spread are weak and dissemination within this plane can occur; a spreading fasciitis may result. Finally, if the inoculum reaches muscle and bone, myositis and contiguous osteomyelitis are produced.

Most inocula, however, encounter intact local and systemic defenses. The infection is aborted or limited in extent. A large inoculum or damage to local defenses will permit infection to persist. Few of these minor infections are recorded as occupational diseases. In fact, in California in 1966, only 14,030 occupational dermatoses were due to infections. In four other states, only 9 of 1,319 skin illnesses related to occupation were infections. Table 25-3 lists the commonly cited occupational infections of the soft tissues, and Table 25-4 lists those occupations in which the more common pyogenic or more exotic skin infections are seen.

Some rare infections are the result of contact with animal reservoirs of certain microbes. Table 25-5 lists those soft tissue infections in which animal reservoirs are known. Table 25-6 lists those soft tissue infections with known insect vectors. Omitted from this table are the numerous infections caused by the contamination of the traumatic breaks in the skin induced by insect bites themselves, or the scratching that frequently ensues.

CLINICAL MANIFESTATIONS AND DIFFERENTIAL DIAGNOSIS OF SOFT TISSUE INFECTIONS

Dermatologists and other clinicians recognize that many soft tissue infections can be diagnosed by the appearance of the cutaneous lesions they produce. In addition, the distribution and physical characteristics of the lesions usually indicate the definitive diagnostic maneuver, ie, the decision to smear, culture, biopsy, order special stains, perform serologic studies or skin tests, or delay diagnostic maneuvers and await spontaneous resolution. Many lesions are so common and their appearance so typical that the diagnosis of rare diseases that mimic them is overlooked. The following discussion and Tables 25-7 to 25-16 present the characteristic presentations of cutaneous soft tissue infections and the differential diagnostic considerations. The individual diseases are discussed in later sections.

It is useful to define a few terms that describe cutaneous diseases. A *macule* is a circumscribed area of abnormal skin color without elevation or depression. The pigment may be the result of melanin or hemosiderin, extravasation of blood, or vascular proliferation or dilation. A *papule* is a solid lesion less than 1 cm in diameter elevated above

TABLE 25-3. COMMONLY REPORTED OCCUPATIONAL INFECTIONS OF THE SKIN AND SOFT TISSUES

Disease	Occupation
BACTERIA	
Anthrax	Animal product-associated industries (wool, ivory)
Brucellosis	Meat packer, livestock grazers, veterinarians, contact with domestic animals, especially cattle
Erysipelas	Fishermen, butchers, handlers of raw fish, poultry, and meat products
Glanders	Contact with horses
Tularemia	Hunters, trappers, furriers
Leptospirosis	Farmers, hunters, abbatoir workers (domestic animals) and wild animals (squirrels, rats)
Verruca necrogenica (tuberculosis)	Postmortem attendants, pathologists, laundry workers, butchers (butchers' tubercle)
Syphilis	Glassblowers, sharing blowpipes
Trachoma	Sharers of towels
FUNGI	
Ringworm	Handlers of horses, cattle, cats, and birds
Sporotrichosis	Gardeners
VIRUSES	
Orf	Sheep handlers
Epidemic keratoconjunctivitis (shipyard conjunctivitis)	Shipyard workers

Modified from Hunter D: *The Diseases of Occupations.* Boston, Little Brown, 1978.

TABLE 25-4. SKIN INFECTIONS ARE MOST LIKELY TO OCCUR IN THE FOLLOWING OCCUPATIONS

Animal handlers (bacteria and fungi)	Felt hat makers
Bakers (fungi)	Fish dressers (erysipeloid)
Barbers and hairdressers	Flour mill workers (fungi)
Bartenders (candidiasis)	Fur processers (zoonoses)
Basket weavers (fungi)	Gardeners (sporotrichosis)
Broom and brush makers (fungi and bacteria)	Janitors
	Nurses
Butchers (zoonoses)	Physicians
Button makers (erysipelas)	Pathologists
Canners	Slaughterhouse and packing house workers
Demolition workers	
Dairy workers (zoonoses)	Stockyard workers
Dishwashers (candidiasis)	Taxidermists (parasites, zoonoses)
Dock workers	
Embalmers	Upholsterers
Farmers	Veterinarians

Modified from Pittelkow R: Occupational dermatoses. In Zenz C (ed): *Occupations Medicine.* Chicago, Yearbook Medical Publishers, 1975.

the surrounding skin. Papules may be the result of epidermal or dermal hyperplasia, local infiltrations, or vegetations. A number of infectious exanthems present as maculopapular eruptions (Table 25-7). Most do not require drainage or debridement and are clearly nonsurgical diseases. A few may require biopsy to differentiate them from similar lesions of a noninfectious origin.

Special forms of maculae include purpura, petechiae, or ecchymosis—all signs of extravasated red cells. Embolic infections (eg, endocarditis, meningococcemia) can present in this way. Infarcts or gangrenous patches are, strictly speaking, forms of maculae as well but are discussed in a subsequent section.

A warty or *verrucous* lesion is a type of papule consisting of multiple closely packed elevations, which may be dry and keratotic or soft and smooth. Infectious causes include warts, orf, milker's nodules, epidermodysplasia, verruciformis, as well as tuberculosis, leprosy, nocardiosis, and the cutaneous fungi.

A *vesicle* (less than 0.5 cm) or *bulla* (more than 0.5 cm) is a circumscribed elevated lesion containing serum, lymph, or blood. Vesicles and bullae arise from a cleavage between skin layers (intraepidermal) or at the epidermal-dermal interface (subepidermal). A subcorneal vesicle characterizes impetigo; intraepidermal vesication may appear as a nodule as in delayed hypersensitivity reactions. Viruses cause degeneration of epidermal cells and produce the vesicles of the viral exanthems, which often have depressed (umbilicated) centers. Trauma from mechanical, thermal, or chemical agents can cause bullae, as can a variety of diseases with unknown etiology (pemphigus and pemphigoid). A *pustule* is a vesicle containing pus or a very superficial abscess of the skin. Not all pustules have an infectious etiology (rosacea, pustular psoriasis). The generalized vesiculopustular exanthems are listed in Table 25-7.

When vesicles or pustules rupture, the exudative lesions produce *crusts* as they dry on the skin surface. The crusts can be serous (yellow), purulent (green or yellow-green), or hemorrhagic (brown). *Ecthyma* refers to a shallow ulcerative disease of the epidermis with thick, adherent crusts. Table 25-8 lists regional infections that typically present as vesicles, bullae, or crusting lesions.

TABLE 25-5. ANIMAL RESERVOIRS FOR INFECTIONS OF THE SKIN AND SOFT TISSUES

Disease	Microbial organism	Reservoir
BACTERIA		
Erysipeloid	*Erysipelothrix insidiosa*	Swine, fish, shellfish, poultry
Anthrax	*Bacillus anthracis*	Sheep, goats, many others
Tularemia	*Francisella tularensis*	Rabbit and other rodents, foxes
Pet bite infection	*Pasturella multocida*	Dogs, cats, many others
Plague	*Yersinia pestis*	Rodents, prairie dogs
Brucellosis	*Brucella* species *B. abortus; B. suis*	Domestic animals, cattle
Rat bite fever	*Streptobacillus moniliformis*	Rodents
Leptospirosis (Weil disease)	*Leptospira icterohaemorrhagiae*	Domestic animals, wild rodents
Glanders	*Pseudomonas mallei*	Horses
PROTOZOA		
African trypanosomiasis	*Trypanasoma gambiensis*	
American trypanosomiasis	*T. cruzi*	Dogs, cats, monkeys, pigs, rodents
Leishmaniasis	*Leishmania donovani, L. braziliensis, L. tropica*	Dogs, rodents
HELMINTHS		
Schistosomiasis	*Schistosoma haematobium* *S. mansoni* *S. japonicum*	Snails
Larva migrans	*Ancylostoma braziliensis* *A. caninum* *B. unostomasum phlebotamus*	Dogs, cattle
Trichinosis	*Trichinella spirilis*	Swine
Sparganosis	*Spirometra mansonoides*	Snakes, birds, pigs, frogs, dogs, cats, mammals
Cysticercosis	*Taenia solium*	Swine
Echinococcosis	*E. granulosis* *E. multilocularis*	Dogs, sheep, cattle Wild animals
VIRUS		
Cowpox	Pox virus	Cattle
Cat scratch disease	Unknown	Domestic animals
Ecthyma contagiosum	Pox virus	Sheep
Milker's nodules	Paravaccinia	Cattle
Orf	Paravaccinia	Sheep
Vaccinia	Vaccinia	Formerly cattle—now in laboratory

TABLE 25-6. INSECT VECTORS FOR INFECTIONS OF SKIN AND SOFT TISSUES

Disease	Microbial organism	Insect vector
BACTERIA		
Bartonellosis	*Bartonella bacilliformis*	Sandfly *(Lutzomyia)*
Plague	*Yersinia pestis*	Flea
Tularemia	*Francisella tularensis*	Deerfly, tick
Rickettsioses	*Rickettsia* species	Tick, mite, louse, flea
PROTOZOA		
African trypanosomiasis	*Trypanasoma gambiensis*	Tse tse fly
American trypanosomiasis	*T. cruzi*	Kissing bugs (triatomids)
Leishmaniasis (kala azar)	*Leishmania donovani*	Mosquito *(Phlebotomus)*
Mucocutaneous leishmaniasis	*L. braziliensis*	
HELMINTHS		
Cutaneous loiasis	*Loa Loa*	Fly *(Chrysops)*
Onchocerciasis	*Onchocerca volvulus*	Black fly *(Simuliidae)*

TABLE 25-7. DIFFERENTIAL DIAGNOSIS OF GENERALIZED EXANTHEMS

Vesiculopustules	Maculopapules	Urticaria	Petechiae
Drug eruption	Drug eruption	Varicella (urticaria around vesicle)	Drug eruption
Herpes simplex	Secondary syphilis	Coxsackie A5, A9	Bacterial endocarditis
Variola	Scarlet fever	Infectious hepatitis	ECHO 9
Vaccinia	ECHO 9, 16	Mononucleosis	Coxsackie A5, A9
Varicella	Coxsackie A5, A9, A16, B5	*Mycoplasma pneumoniae*	Mononucleosis
Generalized zoster	Reovirus 2	Hepatitis	Rubella
Rickettsialpox	Erythema infectiosum		Thrombocytopenia with many acute infections
Coxsackie A and B	Gianotti-Crosti syndrome		
Reovirus 2	Rubella		
Mycoplasma pneumoniae	Rubeola		
ECHO 4	Hepatitis		
Orf	Infectious mononucleosis		
	Arbovirus (dengue)		
	Rickettsioses		

From Burnett JW, Crutcher WA: Viral and rickettsial infections. In Moschella SL, Pillsbury DM, Hurley HJ Jr (eds): *Dermatology,* Vol 1. Philadelphia, Saunders, 1975, p 558.

TABLE 25-8. DIFFERENTIAL DIAGNOSIS OF REGIONAL VESICLES, BULLAE, OR CRUSTS

BACTERIA
- Impetigo
- Bullous impetigo
- Folliculitis, furunculosis

VIRUSES
- Herpes simplex
- Zoster
- Molluscum contageosum (pustular type)
- Vesicular stomatitis virus
- Kaposi varicelliform eruption
- Ecthyma contagiosum (orf)
- Cat scratch disease

FUNGI
- Kerion reactions to dermatophytoses
- Vesicular ringworm
- Dermatophytid reactions

PARASITES
- Flea bites

NONINFECTIOUS CAUSES
- Acne
- Pustular psoriasis
- Drug sensitivities especially to halides
- Erythema multiforme
- Pemphigus

A *wheal* (hive) is a special type of pale papule—usually sharply circumscribed (eg, a mosquito bite) but sometimes extensive (angioneurotic edema). Wheals simply represent edema of the epidermis and dermis sometimes seen at the edges of erysipelas or cellulitis. Some infections with protozoa or helminths will elicit wheals, eg, Chagas disease due to *Trypanasoma cruzi* or schistosomiasis.

Scales are accumulations of desquamated stratum corneum. Any epithelial inflammatory process, including a superficial infection, can induce scaling. Scales can be the only sign of some noninflammatory dermatophytoses.

SUBCUTANEOUS MANIFESTATIONS

Cellulitis is an acute red, tender, swollen area of inflammation within the dermis and subcutaneous tissues, which is frequently part of any infection of these tissues. Acute lymphangitis can be part of the picture in classical group A streptococcal infections (see subsequent section on lymphangitis). Almost any microbe can be responsible for cellulitis.

A *nodule* is a palpable solid lesion lying principally within the dermis or subcutaneous tissue. Nodules are typical manifestations of granulomatous infections, which sometimes progress to ulceration *(ulceronodular disease)* or even to suppuration or sinus formation. There may be considerable undermining or heaping up of the ulcer margin, and the base may be clean, covered with a membrane, or thick with granulation tissue. If biopsies are performed, a portion of excised tissue should routinely be homogenized and cultured for fungi as well as aerobic and anaerobic bacteria. In addition, special stains (Giemsa, PAS, mucicarmine, methenamine silver) should be requested for the histopathologic diagnosis of fungal or viral infection. The differential diagnosis of nodular and ulceronodular infectious diseases are listed in Table 25-9.

Ulcers are the result of destructive processes that remove the epidermis and varying amounts of underlying tissue. Nodular infectious lesions which ulcerate secondarily have already been listed in Table 25-9. Table 25-10 lists infections that commonly appear as ulcers without prior nodular lesions. Some are part of a *chancroid complex* in which a primary infection is associated with regional adenopathy—the primary chancre of syphilis, primary tuberculosis, and the rare primary cutaneous infections with the dimorphic fungi. In other diseases that present with a chancroid complex, the regional adenopathy predominates and the primary ulcer may be almost invisible, eg, plague, glanders, meliodosis, rat bite fever (see subsequent section on lymphadenitis and lymphadenopathy). In undermining infections such as necrotizing fasciitis, multiple contiguous ulcers provide an important

TABLE 25-9. NODULAR AND ULCERONODULAR INFECTIONS OF SKIN AND SUBCUTANEOUS TISSUES

BACTERIA
- Pyogenic bacteria
  - Cutaneous abscesses
  - Botryomycosis
  - Hidradenitis suppurativa
  - Acne conglobata
  - Infected epidermal inclusions
    - Sebaceous cyst
    - Pilonidal cyst
- Treponemal infections
  - Benign tertiary syphilis (gumma)
  - Yaws
  - Pinta
- Mycobacterial lesions
  - Leprosy
  - Tuberculosis
    - Lupus vulgaris
    - Tuberculous gumma
- Atypical mycobacteria
  - Swimming pool granuloma
  - Cutaneous atypical mycobacteria
- Sexually transmitted diseases
  - Granuloma inguinale
  - Lymphogranuloma venereum

FUNGI
- Inflammatory reactions to dermatophytes
- *Candida* granuloma
- Subcutaneous mycoses
  - Chromoblastomycosis
  - Mycetoma
  - Phaeosporotrichosis
  - Rhinosporidiosis
- Systemic mycoses
  - Coccidioidomycosis
  - Blastomycosis
  - Paracoccidioidomycosis
  - Histoplasmosis
  - Cryptococcosis
- Sporotrichosis
- Phycomycosis
- Aspergillosis

VIRUSES
- Warts
- Mollusum contagiosum
- Cowpox
- Milker's nodule

PROTOZOA AND HELMINTHS
- Leishmaniasis
- Cutaneous filarids
  - Onchocerca volvulus
  - Loa loa
  - Dracunculus medinensis

INSECT BITES
- Furuncular myiasis
- Trombiculosis

ALGAE
- Protothecosis

TABLE 25-10. PRIMARY INFECTIOUS ULCERS OF THE SKIN WITHOUT PROMINENT UNDERLYING NODULES

BACTERIA
- Anthrax
- Diphtheria
- Ecthyma
- Glanders
- Tropical ulcer
- Gangrenous bacterial infections
  - Streptococcal gangrene
  - Necrotizing fasciitis
  - Meleney ulcer
  - Gas gangrene
- Treponemes
  - Primary syphilis
  - Yaws
- Mycobacteria
  - Primary cutaneous tuberculosis
  - Atypical mycobacteria
  - *M. ulcerans*
  - Leprosy
- Chancroid
- Nocardiosis

FUNGI
- Primary fungal infections
  - Coccidioidomycosis
  - Blastomycosis
  - Histoplasmosis
- Phycomycosis
- Chromoblastomycosis
- Sporotrichosis

VIRUSES
- Ulcerated vesicular diseases
  - Herpes simplex
  - Zoster
  - Vaccinia necrosum

PROTOZOA AND HELMINTHS
- Amebiasis
- Leishmaniasis
  - Cutaneous
  - Mucocutaneous
  - Kala azar
- Schistosoma cutis

clue to the progressive nature of the disease. Most cutaneous ulcers, however, are not the result of primary microbial infections but of noninfectious necrotizing processes which become infected secondarily by ambient bacteria (Table 25-11).

A special form of nodular ulcerative disease is associated with granulomatous infections—most notably sporotrichosis. A primary lesion forms at the site of injury to the skin—a nodule, ulcer, or infiltrated plaque. Weeks to months later, new nodular-ulcerative lesions appear along lymphatic pathways. Pus may exude when the lesions break down, and the areas can become secondarily infected with ambient bacteria. The lymphatics between nodules become palpably thickened, but lymph node involvement is unusual. Table 25-12 lists some of the ulceronodular diseases that sometimes manifest this clinical *sporotrichoid pattern*.

TABLE 25-11. NONINFECTIOUS CAUSES OF LEG ULCERS

TRAUMATIC: Mechanical, physical, chemical, irradiative, heat, cold

VASCULAR
Small vessels
Vasculitis: allergic and necrotizing angiitis, those associated with connective tissue diseases, malignant atrophic papulosis
Embolism: infections (subacute bacterial endocarditis), tumor
Livedo reticularis
Chronic pernio
Hypertensive ischemic leg ulcer
Atrophie blanche
Raynaud's disease
Large vessels
Thromboangiitis obliterans
Arteriosclerosis obliterans
Chronic venous insufficiency (stasis ulcer)
Periarteritis nodosa with or without granuloma
Arteriovenous fistula

HEMATOLOGIC DISEASES OR STATES
Hemoglobinopathies: sickle cell anemia (30 to 50 percent), hereditary spherocytosis, thalassemia (major and minor)
Dysglobulinemias (hypogammaglobulinemia, cryoglobulinemia, macroglobulinemia)
Thrombocythemia, polycythemia vera
Felty syndrome
Coagulation disorders
Microthrombotic angiopathy

METABOLIC STATES
Diabetes mellitus: necrobiosis lipoidica diabeticorum, diabetic dermopathy, peripheral neuropathy
Porphyria cutanea tarda
Calcinosis cutis
Tophaceous gout
Gaucher disease

NEUROLOGIC DISEASES
Tabes dorsalis
Syringomyelia
Spina bifida
Hereditary sensory radicular neuropathy
Primary amyloidosis (especially familial)
Congenital indifference to pain

DRUG-INDUCED
Ergotism
Halogenoderma
Barbiturate intoxication
Methotrexate

NEOPLASMS
Epithelioma: melanoma, squamous cell carcinoma, basal cell cancer, complications of Marjolin ulcer
Cutaneous lymphoma (mycosis fungoides, lymphosarcoma)
Kaposi sarcoma
Metastatic carcinoma
Lymphangioendothelioma and lymphangiosarcoma

MISCELLANEOUS
Lichen planus
Pyoderma gangrenosum
Panniculitides (primary and secondary)
Epidermolysis bullosa
Werner syndrome
Acrodermatitis chronica atrophicans

Modified from Moschella SL: Diseases of the peripheral vessels and their contents. In Moschella SL, Pillsbury DM, Hurley HF Jr (eds): *Dermatology,* Vol I. Philadelphia, Saunders, 1975, p 837.

An *abscess* is a localized accumulation of purulent material situated in the dermis or subcutaneous tissue. Pus is not visible through the intact skin. Most abscesses are caused by pyogenic bacteria, but any agent (infectious or otherwise) that elicits necrosis and the influx of polymorphonuclear cells can be etiologic. Palpation classically produces fluid shifts within the cavity (fluctuance), but this is an unreliable clinical sign. Rupture or surface necrosis results in purulent drainage. If the abscess is relatively deep in the tissue, the drainage tract from skin to abscess is called a *sinus.* Extensive tissue infections can drain through more than one sinus tract. Table 25-13 lists diseases that characteristically present with abscesses or sinus tracts. Curettings of the tissue, rather than cotton swabs, should be used to obtain cultures, because superficial colonization by ambient bacteria can occur whatever the true etiology of the abscess.

Cysts are sacs containing liquid or semisolid material. In contrast to abscesses, they are resilient rather than fluctuant to palpation. Most cysts are epidermal cysts lined with squamous epithelium and are filled with keratinous material. Sebaceous cysts are of pilar origin. Cysts can become infected without changing character—some erythema may be evident, and tenderness is prominent. A few deep infections appear as cysts—cystic chromoblastomycosis, the early manifestations of mycetoma, ecchinococcosis, trichinosis, cryptococcosis.

TABLE 25-12. CAUSES OF A SPOROTRICHOID PATTERN OF INFECTION

Sporotrichosis
Tuberculosis
Atypical mycobacteria
Tularemia
Scopulariopsis spp.
Mycetomas *(N. braziliensis)*
Syphilis
Yaws
Cutaneous leishmaniasis
Primary coccidioidomycosis

LYMPHANGITIS AND LYMPHADENITIS

Lymphangitis refers to inflammation of lymphatic tissue channels usually in the subcutaneous tissues which present, in cases of bacterial infections, as visibile red streaks. Acute lymphangitis is most often associated with group

TABLE 25-13. INFECTIOUS CAUSES OF PERSISTENT DRAINING SINUSES ON SKIN

BACTERIA
Pyogenic infection with associated foreign body
Inadequately drained abscess
Carbuncle
Infected branchial cleft cyst
Infected pilonidal cyst
Dental sinus
Scrofula or scrofuloderma
Hidradenitis suppurativa
Acne conglobata
Actinomycosis
Nocardiosis
Necrotizing fasciitis (See Table 25-20)
Gas gangrene
Fistulas to rectum in Crohn disease
Enterocutaneous fistulas
FUNGI
Kerion
Mycetoma
Cystic chromomycosis
PROTOZOA
Amebiasis

A streptococcal cellulitis but can be caused by *S. aureus*, *Spirillum minus* (rat bite fever), or certain filaria. Chronic lymphangitis leads to a sporotrichoid pattern. Both acute and chronic lymphangitis can produce permanent lymphedema of the distal tissues, which are then more susceptible to subsequent infection.

Lymphadenitis occurs when microbial agents reach the lymph nodes and precipitate an inflammatory reaction. Lymphadenitis can be restricted to a solitary node, to a localized group of nodes (regional lymphadenitis), or can be generalized. Infections that cause regional lymphadenitis in the course of a typical infection are listed in Table 25-14 and those associated with generalized lymphadenitis in Table 25-15. The latter infections seldom come to the attention of the surgeon, since suppuration or an ulceroglandular syndrome are seldom part of the picture. In regional lymphadenitis, the gross features may be those of nonsuppurative, suppurative, or caseous inflammation depending on whether the infecting microorganism is viral or bacterial or induces granulomas. Biopsy of nonsuppurative lymphadenitis reveals swelling and hyperplasia of the sinusoidal lining cells and infiltration of leukocytes. This may progress to abscess formation. In granulomatous infections, stellate abscesses become surrounded by palisading epithelioid cells (granulomatous abscess) and caseous necrosis can be seen. Biopsy specimens should not only be cultured for common and rare etiologic agents, but imprints of the cut surface of the node should be stained for fungi, acid-fast organisms, protozoa, and bacteria. The pathologic diagnosis is usually made before cultural isolation of the etiologic agent.

Certain clinical patterns of regional lymphadenopathy are worthy of note. Acute regional lymphadenitis due to pyogenic bacteria are much more common in children than adults and are usually due to *S. aureus* rather than the previously common group A streptococci. Pharyngitis and tonsilitis are common precursor diseases of cervical lymphadenitis. Cellulitis and infection of the hand usually produce subpectoral or axillary lymphadenitis. The epitrochlear nodes are sometimes found associated with hand infections. Suppurative iliac lymphadenitis due to infection of leg, perineum, or abdominal wall can lead to psoas space abscesses.

Ocular glandular syndromes can be caused by conjunctival infection with mycobacteria, tularemia, cat scratch disease, listeriosis, lymphogranuloma, or epidermic keratoconjunctivitis. *Ulceroglandular syndromes* are those in which a small wound of entrance (perhaps an ulcer) is overshadowed by a prominent, sometimes suppurative lymphadenitis as in tularemia, plague, rat bite fever, and anthrax. Inguinal lymphadenitis (bubo formation) is characteristic of primary infections with syphilis, chancroid, lymphogranuloma venereum, and the primary mycoses. Suppuration is unusual, although spontaneous rupture of the buboes of lymphogranuloma venereum and chancroid can occur so that such lesions appear to be primary ulcerations.

GANGRENOUS MANIFESTATIONS

The *gangrenous infections* are characterized by more extensive necrosis of subcutaneous tissue, fascia, and muscle. Group A streptococci, *Clostridia*, and polymicrobial aerobic and anaerobic organisms are the common etiologic agents. Cutaneous gangrene with blue-black changes in the skin may or may not be part of the clinical picture, depending on whether the blood supply to the skin is affected. The clinical differential diagnosis is discussed in a subsequent section (Tables 25-16 and 25-20).

Crepitus in the soft tissues is due to accumulated gas. It is not necessarily indicative of clostridial myonecrosis (gas gangrene) but may be gas-derived from traumatic injury, perforation of a gas-containing viscus (lung, esophagus, bowel), or a sign of anaerobic bacterial metabolism resulting in the production of insoluble gases (H_2, N_2, methane).[12] Many facultative as well as obligate anaerobic organisms can produce gas in tissue. The differential diagnosis of tissue crepitus is presented in Table 26-16.

COMMON PYOGENIC BACTERIAL INFECTIONS

Microbial organisms within a cutaneous lesion are not pathognomonic of infection. Some infections, clearly arising in skin that appears healthy and related to a single organism with well-defined morphologic features, are called primary skin infections (eg, impetigo, ecthyma, furuncle). In secondary infections, the microflora do not initiate the disease, but may be important in its protracted or complicated course (eg, infections following trauma). Primary infection seldom requires surgical therapy and has a predictable course; secondary infections may require surgical therapy and have an unpredictable outcome. In secondary infections, it is frequently difficult to distinguish the infect-

TABLE 25-14. INFECTIOUS CAUSES OF REGIONAL LYMPHADENITIS

Disease	Infecting Organism	Regional	Regional with Suppuration (or Caseation)	Inguinal Bubo Formation	Ulcero-glandular
BACTERIA					
Pyogenic	Group A strep; *S. aureus*	+	+		
Scarlet fever	Group A strep	+	+		
Diphtheria	*C. diphtheriae*	+			
Fusospirochetal angina	*B. melaninogenicus;* pepto streptococci, etc.	+			
Scrofula	*M. tuberculosis*	+	+		
	M. scrofulaceum	+	+		
Syphilis	*T. pallidum*	+			
Chancroid	*H. ducreyi*			+	
Plague	*Y. pestis*	+	+	+	
Tularemia	*F. tularensis*		+		+
Rat bite fever	*Streptobacillus moniliformis or Spirillum minus*	+			+
Anthrax	*B. anthracis*	+			+
Melioidosis	*P. pseudomallei*	+	+		
Glanders	*P. mallei*	+	+		
FUNGI					
Histoplasmosis	*H. capsulatum*				
	H. capsulatum var. *duboisii*	+			
Paracoccidioidomycosis	*P. brasiliensis*	+			
RICKETTSIA					
Boutonneuse fever, etc.	*R. conori*				+
Scrub typhus	*R. tsutsugamushi*	+			
Rickettsialpox	*R. akari*	+			
CHLAMYDIA					
Lymphogranuloma venereum	*C. trachomatis*			+	
VIRUSES					
Genital herpes infection	HSV-type 2	+			
Pharyngoconjunctival fever	Adenovirus (types 3 & 7)	+			
Cat scratch disease	?	+	+		+
Postvaccinial lymphadenitis	*Vaccinia* virus	+			
PROTOZOA					
African trypanosomiasis	*T. brucei*	+			

Modified from Swartz MN: Lymphadenitis and lymphangitis. In Mandell GL, Douglas RG Jr, Bennett JE (eds): *Principles and Practice of Infectious Diseases,* Vol 1. New York, Wiley, 1979, p 825.

ing organism from one that is simply colonizing the wound. Both primary and secondary infections are of importance to the surgeon, and arbitrary separation is impossible. For the surgeon, it is better to separate infections due to common pyogenic bacteria from the more exotic and rare infections. This system is used here.

COMMON PYOGENIC BACTERIAL INFECTIONS OF THE SKIN AND ITS APPENDAGES

Most of the following infections are caused by common pyogenic bacteria and involve the skin itself (pyoderma) or its appendages. Some extend into the subcutaneous tissues but will be discussed here.

Impetigo

Impetigo exists in two separate clinical forms: (1) bullous impetigo, consisting of large intraepidermal blebs which rupture leaving thin crusts, and (2) an epidemic form, which progresses from transient vesicles to thick encrustations.[13]

Etiology

The etiology of impetigo has been the subject of much debate. Bullous impetigo is clearly due to *S. aureus,* usually phage type II-71. The more common form of epidemic

TABLE 25-15. INFECTIOUS CAUSES OF GENERALIZED LYMPHADENITIS

BACTERIA
- Scarlet fever
- Miliary tuberculosis
- Brucellosis
- Leptospirosis
- Syphilis
- Melioidosis
- Glanders

FUNGUS
- Histoplasmosis

RICKETTSIA
- Scrub typhus

CHLAMYDIA
- Lymphogranuloma venerum

VIRUSES
- Measles
- Rubella
- Infectious mononucleosis
- CMV mononucleosis
- Dengue fever
- West Nile fever
- Epidemic (Far Eastern) hemorrhagic fevers
- Lassa fever

PROTOZOA
- Kala-azar
- African trypanosomiasis
- Chagas disease
- Toxoplasmosis

HELMINTHS
- Filariasis

Modified from Swartz MN: Lymphadenitis and lymphangitis. In Mandell GL, Douglas RG Jr, Bennett JE (eds): *Principles and Practice of Infectious Diseases,* Vol 1. New York, Wiley, 1979, p 825.

impetigo is thought to be a primary group A streptococcal infection with rapid *S. aureus* superinfection.

Epidemiology

S. aureus is a frequent contaminant of human skin and is a resident in the anterior nares of many children and about 20 to 30 percent of adults. Many epidemics have been associated with individual nasal or perineal carriers.

Streptococcal pyoderma and impetigo appear primarily in infants and young children during the warm humid months. Predisposing conditions include minor trauma, insect bites, poor hygiene, and preexisting skin disease. Spread within families is common by direct contact with infected material or by insects that either damage the skin directly or induce scratching.

Pathogenesis and Pathology

Certain strains of *S. pyogenes* can colonize and survive on normal skin, although minor trauma is necessary to initiate infection. The pathogenetic factors of the streptococci are discussed in Chapter 4. The streptococci causing impetigo are not different from those that cause erysipelas or wound infections. The initial lesion of impetigo is a vesicle in the superficial epidermis. Acute inflammation with polymorphonuclear cell infiltration follows, and the pustule ruptures leaving an ulcer crater; angiitis, or rarely cellulitis, may follow. Bacteremia is uncommon. Scarring is seldom seen with epidermal lesions alone.

Bullous impetigo produces large superficial skin blebs, which may be extensive in neonates (pemphigus neonatorum). *S. aureus,* phage group II produces an exfoliative toxin—streptococci are rarely found. Cellulitis and lymphangitis are uncommon.

Clinical Manifestations

Impetigo begins as a small red macule, progressing to a vesicle which ruptures leaving a honey-colored crust—the hallmark lesion (Fig. 25-4A, B). Perioral and nasal lesions are most characteristic, but satellite lesions may develop anywhere, occasionally appearing as annular lesions with central healing. The process may last for months, and glomerulonephritis is a feared complication, especially with certain serotypes.

Bullous impetigo presents as vesicles progressing to easily ruptured bullae without erythema (Fig. 25-5).

Diagnosis

Isolation of the responsible organism from an unruptured vesicle confirms the diagnosis. Gram stains showing *S. aureus* or streptococcal morphology plus the clinical picture strongly suggest the diagnosis. Culture of vesicular fluid or the raw surface is critical, since a variety of skin lesions may simulate one phase or another of impetigo or bullous impetigo. Embolic pustular lesions occur in septicemic patients with *P. aeruginosa* and *S. aureus,* but these have a characteristic appearance. A variety of serologic tests are available to confirm the diagnosis of staphylococcal or streptococcal infections (Chapter 4).

Prognosis

Recurrence in the same patient and transmission to family members is common. Most suppurative complications with lymphadenitis, soft tissue infection, and cellulitis are self-limited or easily treated. Epidemic nephritis has been found in children following epidemics of impetigo. Although 95 percent of such patients recover, progressive renal failure occasionally follows streptococcal pyoderma.

Treatment

Good hygiene with rupture of vesicles and bullae, and removal of crusts with soap and water, are essential. Washing must be repeated frequently. Topical gentamycin or neomycin-bacitracin should be rubbed in thoroughly three times daily for several days after new lesions appear. Systemic penicillin in streptococcal epidemics reduces the incidence of nephritis. Penicillin may not eradicate the streptococci if mixed infections with penicillinase-producing staphylococci are present and erythromycin has proved useful. Antibiotic sensitivities of staphylococci should be obtained in order to guide therapy if initial empirical therapy is unsuccessful. Bullous impetigo should be treated with penicillinase-resistant penicillin.

TABLE 25-16. DIFFERENTIAL DIAGNOSIS OF CREPITANT SOFT TISSUE WOUNDS

	Clostridial Cellulitis	Nonclostridial Anaerobic Cellulitis	Gas Gangrene	Streptococcal Myositis	Necrotizing Fasciitis *	Infected Vascular Gangrene	Noninfectious Causes of Gas in Tissues
PREDISPOSING CONDITIONS	Local trauma or operation	Diabetes mellitus; preexisting localized infection	Local trauma or surgery	Local trauma	Diabetes mellitus abdominal surgery, perineal infection, drug addiction	Peripheral arterial insufficiency	Mechanical effects of penetrating trauma; injuries involving use of compressed air; entrapment of air under loosely sutured wounds or under ulcers; irrigation of wounds with hydrogen peroxide; intravenous catheter placement
SWELLING	Moderate	Moderate	Marked	Moderate	Marked	Moderate or marked	Slight or absent
SKIN APPEARANCE	Minimal discoloration	Minimal discoloration	Yellow-bronze; dark bullae; green-black patches of necrosis	Erythema	Erythematous cellulitis	Discolored or black	Only those due to initiating trauma
EXUDATE	Thin, dark	Dark pus	Serosanguinous	Abundant seropurulent	Seropurulent	0	0
GAS	++++	++++	++	±	++	+++	Variable but present; does not extend
ODOR	Sometimes foul	Foul	Variable; slightly foul or peculiar sweet	Slight; "sour"	Foul	Foul	0
SYSTEMIC TOXICITY	Minimal	Moderate	Marked	Only late in course	Moderate or marked	Minimal	0
MUSCLE INVOLVEMENT	0	0	++++	+++	0	Dead	0

* The term "necrotizing fasciitis" is employed here to designate forms of this syndrome exclusive of streptococcal gangrene.

Modified from Swartz MN: Subcutaneous tissue infections and abscesses. In Mandell GL, Douglas RG Jr, Bennett JE: Principles and Practice of Infectious Diseases. New York, John Wiley & Sons, 1979, p 813.

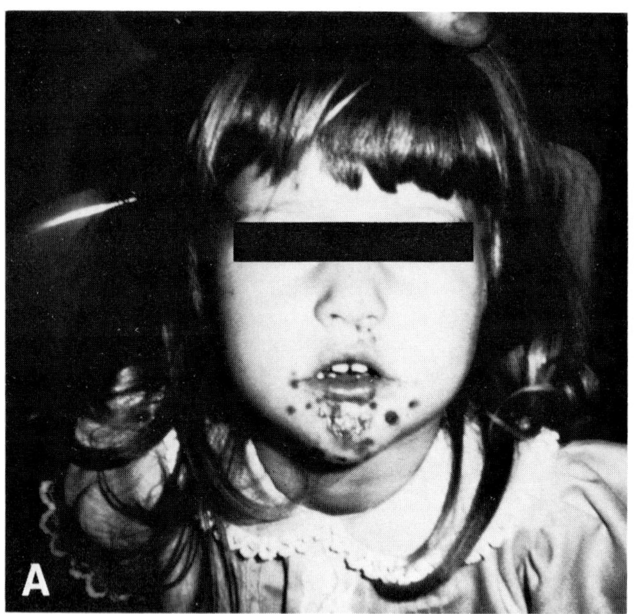

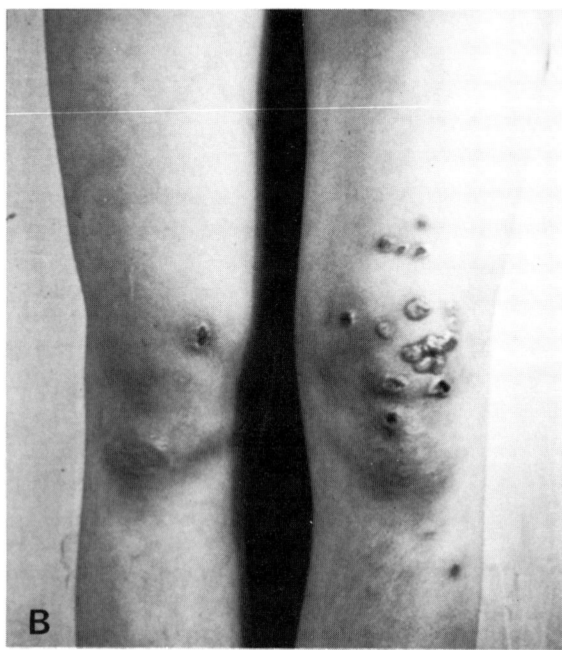

Fig. 25-4. **Impetigo. A. Crusted perioral lesions are characteristic of epidemic impetigo in children. B. Ecthyma characterized by punched-out ulcerated nodules is a rare manifestation of streptococcal impetigo. (Courtesy of Robert W. Goltz, MD, professor and head, Department of Dermatology, University of Minnesota, Minneapolis, Minnesota.)**

Prevention

Both contamination and minor skin trauma are difficult to control in socioeconomic circumstances where skin hygiene is neglected. Streptococcal vaccines are not helpful, and elimination of the nasal or perineal staphylococcal reservoir is difficult. Public health measures to reduce the number of insects is important. Strict skin hygiene and the occasional use of systemic antibiotic chemoprophylaxis (penicillin V) may be useful in limiting spread to contacts while the index case is being treated.

To counter staphylococcal epidemics in newborn nurseries, recolonization with a less virulent strain (strain 502A) has been tried after topical gentamycin or administration of a systemic antistaphylococcal agent.

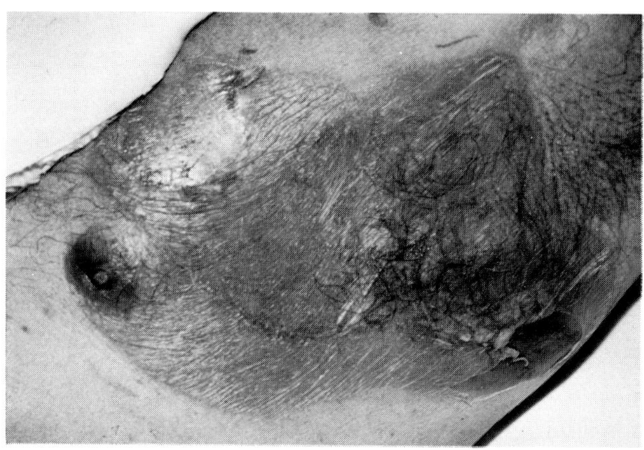

Fig. 25-5. **Bullus impetigo is caused almost exclusively by staphylococci, usually phage type 71. (Courtesy of Robert W. Goltz, MD, professor and head, Department of Dermatology, University of Minnesota, Minneapolis, Minnesota.)**

Ecthyma

Ecthyma is essentially a deeper form of impetigo which begins as a vesicle and progresses to a punched-out ulcer surrounded by a violaceous border covered with a firm eschar (Fig. 25-4B). The legs of children are most commonly affected, and the pathogenesis involves the infection of areas of minor trauma, pediculosis, eczema, etc. Beta-hemolytic streptococci are most often recovered. The crust should be removed, and local warm wet compresses applied to remove debris so that local antibiotics can penetrate. Systemic antibiotics are needed only for widespread diseases or compromised hosts.

Similar lesions sometimes arise from the hematogenous dissemination of *S. aureus* or *aeruginosa* in patients with seriously compromised defenses. Systemic therapy of the primary infecting agent is always required in these cases, and the prognosis is poor.

Chancriform Pyoderma

This disease is rare and of importance only because of its resemblance to a primary syphilitic chancre. Most often, a papulopustule appears on the face near the eyes and progresses to an ulcer 1–4 cm in diameter. Regional lymphadenopathy is present, and the disease resolves in 4 to 8 weeks. *S. aureus* is found, and the results of serologic tests for syphilis are negative. Antistaphylococcal antibiotics hasten resolution.

Scarlet Fever and the Scalded Skin Syndrome

Scarlet fever is a diffuse erythematous eruption caused by an erythrogenic toxin produced during group A streptococcal pharyngeal or tissue infection. Only bacteria infected with a lysogenic bacteriophage produce the toxin. Delayed hypersensitivity to the toxin may also be necessary for the rash, which involves the whole body, blanches on pressure, and has a sandpaper quality. Immunity to the toxin prevents recurrence. Treatment with penicillin is curative.

Phage group II *S. aureus* produces an exfoliative exotoxin which results in widespread bullae and exfoliation, especially in the newborn-scalded skin syndrome.[14] A toxic epidermal necrolysis (TEN) characterized by superficial epidermal bulla formation without local inflammation results. The infection is elsewhere—not within the affected skin. The diagnosis of a staphylococcal infection may or may not already be apparent when sudden fever, skin tenderness, and a scarlatiniform rash appear (staphylococcal scarlet fever). Bullae form, rupture, and a red denuded skin surface result.[14] Toxic shock syndrome (Chapters 4 and 44) is probably caused in a similar way.

Therapy should consist of a penicillinase-resistant penicillin and fluid replacement for increased insensible losses. Topical or systemic steroids are contraindicated for TEN with an *S. aureus* etiology.

Erysipelas

Etiology

This characteristic superficial cellulitis of the skin with extensive lymphatic involvement is almost always due to *Streptococcus pyogenes,* Lancefield group A. Other streptococcal groups (B, C, G in the newborn) and *S. aureus* can also be etiologic agents.

Epidemiology

Infants, children, and the elderly are most commonly afflicted. Patients with nephrotic syndrome are particularly susceptible. Streptococcal pharyngitis or an infection in the umbilical stump can precede the frank disease. Preexisting lymphatic obstruction or edema due to regional nodal dissection or prior episode of lymphangitis predispose to these infections.

Clinical Manifestations

The lesion is painful, edematous, indurated, and sharply circumscribed by an advancing border (Fig. 25-6). Fever and leukocytosis are common, but the infection seldom spreads beneath the dermis. A common form involves the bridge of the nose and the cheeks, but the infection can occur anywhere and recurring infections can lead to an elephantiasis-like syndrome with persistent swelling secondary to lymphatic stasis.

Diagnosis

Diagnosis is based on the typical appearance of the lesion, although other types of cellulitis, dermatitis, or giant urticaria may have a similar appearance. Streptococci can sometimes be aspirated from the edge of the advancing lesion.

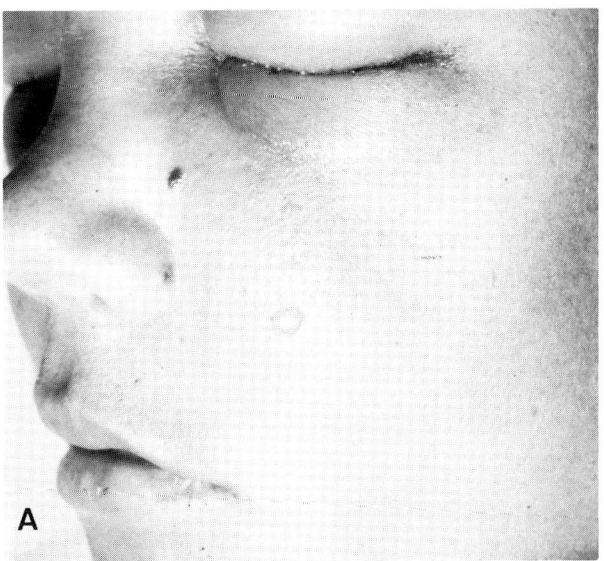

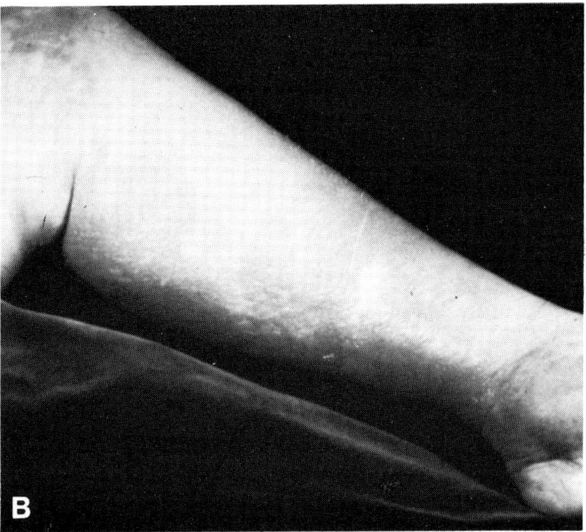

Fig. 25-6. **Erysipelas edema, a superficial infection, is characterized by induration and a sharply circumscribed border. The most common form extends from (A) the bridge of the nose to the cheeks, (B) but infection can occur anywhere.**

Therapy

Therapy should be instituted as soon as the diagnosis is considered; intramuscular penicillin G (or erythromycin for allergic patients) is usually sufficient. Extensive erysipelas should be treated in the hospital with parenteral aqueous penicillin G.

Erythrasma

This superficial skin disease is of almost no surgical significance except that incisions through involved areas should be avoided. *Corynebacterium minutissimum*, a nonmotile gram-positive rod normally found in toe folds, can induce dry, scaly, slight pink to brown lesions in the groin, pubic, axillary, or intergluteal and inframammary folds. The disease is quite common in patients with diabetes and may coexist with taenia versicolor and cutaneous candidiasis, which generally induces more erythema. The diagnosis is usually made by Wood light—a coral red fluorescence is diagnostic, but the responsible porphyrin pigment can be washed off. Gram stain smears and cultures of scrapings should be performed to rule out other or concurrent infections. Treatment with an antibacterial soap is usually effective, but erythromycin used for a week controls more extensive disease.

Erysipeloid

Erysipeloid is an acute slowly developing self-limited infection of the skin, caused by *Erysipelothrix insidiosa (rhusiopathiae)*, a gram-positive rod which lives in soil and decomposed organic matter. Infection in humans occurs in patients who have handled dead animal matter, meat, fish, or shells. After inoculation into the skin, intense inflammation appears in the dermis. The bacilli are located deep in the corium scattered around the capillaries. A purplish-red nonvesiculated lesion defined by an irregular raised border is usually seen on the fingers. The lesions itch and burn without lymphangitis or lymphadenitis. Erysipelas, by contrast, typically affects the face and scalp with a bright red-hot tender lesion that spreads relatively rapidly with regional adenopathy and a systemic illness. Diagnosis depends on a full thickness biopsy of the skin for culture, although aspiration after injection of saline into the periphery of an advancing lesion, or abrasion of the lesion with culture of the exudate may permit adequate culture. It is important to differentiate this organism from the diphtheroids. Erysipeloid may rarely spread and produce a systemic illness with endocarditis and arthritis. The treatment is pencillin or erythromycin.[15]

Folliculitis, Furunculosis, and Carbuncle

Folliculitis originates within a hair follicle, usually as a consequence of *S. aureus* infection. When host defenses are impaired, other organisms including normal skin flora may be involved. *Furunculosis* is an infection of several hair follicles within a relatively limited area. A *carbuncle* (boil) is a confluent infection of multiple contiguous follicles in which the infection is limited to the subcutaneous tissue by thick overlying skin and dense subcutaneous fascia.

Etiology

Almost all of these infections are due to *S. aureus*. The intrinsic pathogenetic factors associated with this organism are discussed in Chapter 4. *P. aeruginosa* folliculitis may arise from contaminated swimming pools or whirlpools. Gram-negative infections appear in patients on antibiotics, and *Candida* has been reported.[16]

Epidemiology and Pathogenesis

S. aureus is frequently found in the anterior nares or perineum, especially in chronic carriers or hospitalized patients. If assiduously sought, it can be found transiently on the skin of most persons. Patients with recurrent folliculitis usually have large numbers of *S. aureus* on their normal skin as well.

Most cases of folliculitis in healthy persons are minor and self-limited. Certain patients, however, seem especially prone to serious or recurrent infections: (1) patients with congenital or acquired hypogammaglobulinemia, (2) patients with diabetes mellitus, (3) patients with cancer or organ transplants receiving immunosuppressive drugs (with adequate skin hygiene, primary bacterial skin infections are uncommon even in these patients), (4) patients with Job syndrome (Hill-Quie syndrome). This disease consists of eczema, recurrent boils, eosinophilia, and elevated plasma levels of IgE antibodies to staphylococci. Influx of neutrophils in this condition may be inhibited by IgE-triggered release of histamine locally.[17] (5) Chronic granulomatous disease; these patients have a defect of host defenses characterized by recurrent cutaneous and visceral abscesses. Their neutrophils lack the ability to kill catalase-positive organisms (Chapter 13).[18] A number of other conditions sometimes underlie the recurrent appearance of furunculosis: poor hygiene, pediculosis, scabies, excoriations, hyperhidrosis, obesity, hematologic disorders, seborrhea, malnutrition, occupational trauma, exposure of skin to hydrocarbons, and pyogenic infections in the family.

Experimental infection of a hair follicle is difficult. Although the normal skin microflora are most concentrated in the sebum within the follicular orifice, the deeper reaches of the hair follicle are sterile. *S. epidermidis* and diphtheroids, common in sebum, seldom cause folliculitis. Experimentally, Duncan et al[6] found that local trauma, such as plucking the hair and contaminating the skin with *S. aureus*, produced folliculitis in humans. The trauma to the stratum corneum of hair follicle sustained in shaving results in the frequent appearance of folliculitis of the beard (sycosis barbae). The hair follicle, once damaged, is relatively isolated from host defenses, and edema at the orifice results in obstruction so that contaminated sebaceous secretions accumulate and infection may result.

Clinical Manifestations

Folliculitis progresses from a small red papule to a vesicle which spontaneously ruptures and resolves with some degree of scarring depending on the depth of destruction (Fig. 25-7). Furunculosis consists of crops or areas of folliculitis, especially in traumatized or macerated areas. Certain patients without discernible predisposing causes have repeated episodes of furunculosis over a period of years.

Carbuncles begin as furuncles on the back of the neck, axilla, or pubic regions (Fig. 25-8). Contiguous spread into adjacent follicles and penetration to the subcutaneous space results in a subcutaneous abscess with multiple tracts; a red, painful, tender mass under the tough skin of the back of the neck with multiple draining sites is diagnostic. Fever and systemic toxicity are common.

There are superficial and deep forms of folliculitis.

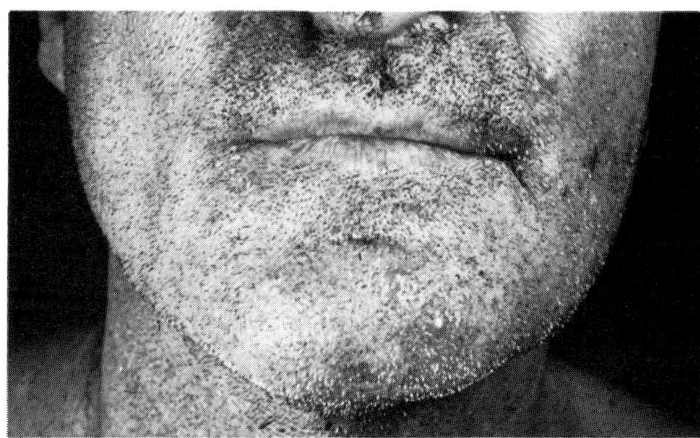

Fig. 25-7. **Folliculitis of the bearded region.**

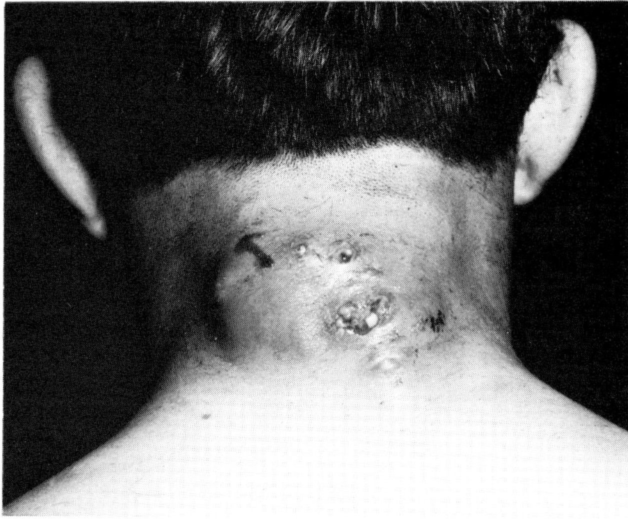

Fig. 25-8. **The carbuncle in this patient involves the entire back of the neck, with a complex of abscesses with multiple draining sinuses and interconnecting tracts. (From Armed Forces Institute of Pathology, Neg. No. DET B477–4.)**

The superficial form may progress to the deeper form and produce subcutaneous abscesses. Most superficial staphylococcal folliculitis occurs in the scalp, beard, and extremities, especially in macerated areas near wounds and discharges. Elimination of occupational exposure to cutting oils or of occlusive dressings is often curative. Gram-negative folliculitis occurs in acne-prone areas such as the nose in patients treated with antibiotics.[16] *Propionibacterium acnes* scalp infection looks like chronic recurrent folliculitis of the scalp. Cultures are usually sterile, so that Gram stain of purulent smears makes the diagnosis. Acne necrotica miliaris is similar but has a necrotic element.

Distinct forms of deep folliculitis have been described. Sycosis barbae (barber's itch) is a pustular folliculitis on the beard area, usually in unshaven parts. Pseudosycosis barbae is a noninfective inflammation due to ingrown hairs exclusively in shaved areas, especially in Negros. Lupoid sycosis is a chronic scarring form of folliculitis. A sty (hordeolum) involves the cilia of the lid margin.

Perforating folliculitis of the nose begins as a pustule of the nasal vibrissae, which is normally self-limited. In the severe form, it penetrates and forms an abscess under the skin. Treatment of the skin lesion alone is not effective.

Diagnosis

All these infections can be diagnosed clinically. Drainage followed by Gram stain should reveal gram-positive cocci in clumps in all except those due to gram-negative organisms.

A variety of other vesicular or pustular diseases may simulate furunculosis (Table 25-8). Aspiration of the vesicular fluid with Gram stain should rule them out. Rarely, skin infiltration with neoplastic cells mimics furunculosis. Sporotrichosis may resemble furunculosis if the pattern of deep lymphatic infiltration is not recognized.

Treatment

Most small furuncles recede with minimal therapy. Warm skin compresses and good hygiene, such as frequent washing with antiseptic soaps (povidone-iodine), are usually sufficient. Abrasion and maceration should be avoided in order to minimize opportunities for autoinoculation. Predisposing conditions should be sought and eliminated. Systemic antibiotics are usually not necessary unless lesions are widespread with fever and leukocytosis or there is evidence for impaired host defenses. A penicillinase-resistant penicillin is the preferred choice (erythromycin or clindamycin for the allergic). Incision and drainage is required only for fluctuant or confluent necrotic lesions. If drainage (spontaneous or iatrogenic) occurs, local antibiotics around the lesion may prevent autoinoculation.

Carbuncles should always be treated with antibiotics in addition to incision and drainage. Extensive cruciate incisions and undermining of the flaps are necessary to obtain adequate drainage. This is a painful procedure even with local anesthesia. Carbuncles may recur years after otherwise successful therapy.

Prevention

Prevention of staphylococcal skin infections consists primarily of good skin hygiene and avoidance of trauma. Plucking eyebrows or upper lip hair should be discouraged. Shaving instruments should be sterilized and replaced as they become dull. The temporary use of intranasal antibiotic creams (especially gentamycin) may eliminate the nasal carrier state in certain high-risk patients with recurrent furunculosis. Long-term antibiotic prophylaxis may be essential (see preceding section on impetigo). Predisposing factors should be eradicated. Table 25-17 lists useful advice to patients with recurrent disease. Vaccines or inoculation with less pathogenic *S. aureus* strain 502A is rarely useful.

Acne Vulgaris and Its Variants

Acne vulgaris is a disease of the sebaceous follicles characterized by comedones, papules, pustules, nodules, and cysts. Later, these active lesions are replaced by pits and scars. It is not per se an infectious disease—the primary defect is the plugging of follicles with keratinous debris.

TABLE 25-17. ADVICE FOR PATIENTS WITH RECURRENT FURUNCULOSIS

General skin care: Soap and water should be used to reduce the numbers of *S. aureus* on the body surface and careful handwashing should be performed after contact with lesions. A separate towel and washcloth (carefully washed in hot water before reuse) should be reserved for the patient. Some physicians prefer hexachlorophene, chlorhexidine, or povidone-iodine to soap.

Care of clothing: Sheets and underclothing should be laundered at high temperatures and should be changed daily in problem patients.

Care of dressings: Draining lesions should be covered at all times with sterile dressings to prevent autoinoculation, and the dressings should be wrapped and promptly disposed after removal.

From Swartz MN: Cellulitis and superficial infections. In Mandell GL, Douglas RG Jr, Bennett JE (eds): *Principles and Practice of Infectious Diseases,* Vol 1, New York, Wiley, 1979, p 797.

Sebum sometimes escapes into the tissues, where a reactive inflammation occurs especially in response to free fatty acids. All bacteria contain lipases, which can break down the fats in sebum to free fatty acids. The anaerobic diphtheroid, *Corynebacterium (Proprionobacterium) acnes* is the most abundant organism in sebaceous glands and is the most lipolytic.

The diagnosis of acne is seldom confused with true infections. The classic appearance at adolescence of comedones (blackheads or whiteheads) on the face, back, and shoulders is diagnostic. The inflammatory lesions arise from the closed comedones (whiteheads) and vary from small papules with a red areola to pustules, fluctuant nodules and cysts (Fig. 25-9A). Pits and scars are remnants of prior inflammation deep in the dermis.

The treatment of uncomplicated acne is detailed in dermatology texts. Cleanliness, topical benzoyl peroxide, and topical antibiotics (tetracycline, erythromycin, clindamycin) are a common treatment combination. Various types of surgical therapy, ultraviolet light, x-ray, and intralesional steroid have been successful.

The oral administration of tetracycline (500 mg–1 gm per day) will reduce free fatty acid production but takes several weeks to be effective. Treatment is usually continued for months but should not be given to infants with neonatal acne, or to pregnant women, because of its affinity for mineralized tissue. An increasingly frequent complication is gram-negative folliculitis *(Klebsiella, Enterobacter,* or *Proteus* sp.). Flare-up of the inflammatory lesions should suggest the diagnosis. Surgeons have also noted that the course of some acute abdominal conditions, most notably appendicitis, is modified by tetracycline therapy for acne.

Acne Conglobata

The many forms of inflammatory acne make it an important consideration in the differential diagnosis of folliculitis and its variants. Of greatest importance to surgeons is the condition called acne conglobata. This is an inflammatory disease with comedones, pustules, nodules, and abscesses.

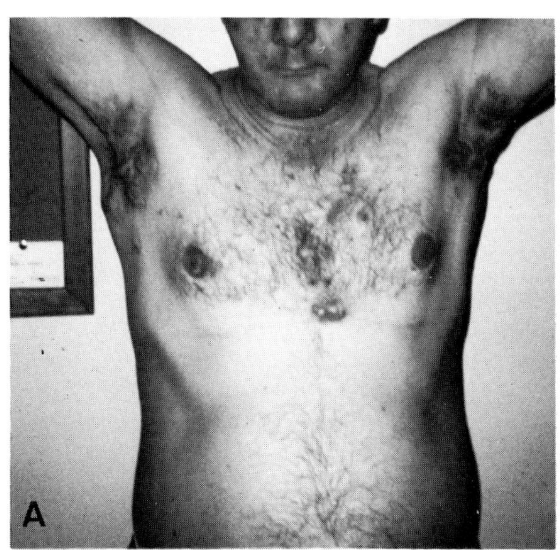

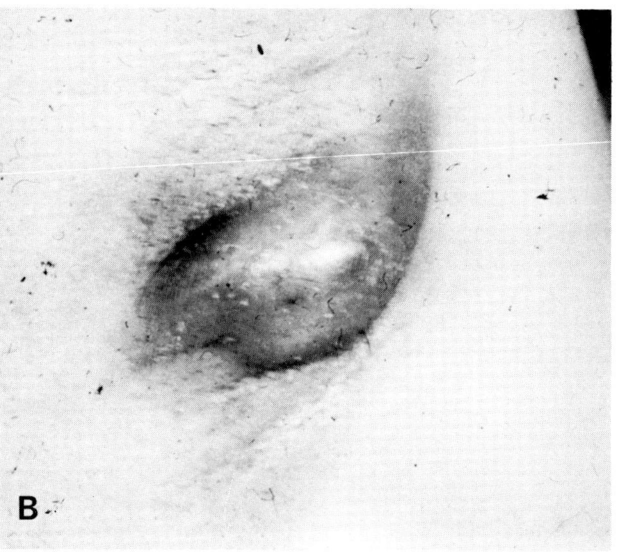

Fig. 25-9. **Hidradenitis suppurativa of the axilla. A. Bilateral axillary involvement in an adult male with acne of his face and acne conglobata of his anterior thorax. B. A tender, red swelling with multiple sinus tracts. (Courtesy of Robert W. Goltz MD, professor and head, Department of Dermatology, University of Minnesota, Minneapolis, Minnesota.)**

Subcutaneous undermining can result in multiple draining sinus tracts. The pus may be foul-smelling and mucopurulent. Healing involves extensive scarring and keloid formation. Adult males rather than adolescents are affected and the trunk, back, shoulders, and buttocks are most often involved. Hidradenitis suppurativa may be present simultaneously (Fig. 25-9A). *S. aureus* and *S. pyogenes* group A have both been isolated, but the etiology has not been established.

Treatment is unsatisfactory. Systemic antibiotics may be necessary to control the infection. Incision, excision, and debridement may be required. Systemic and local injections of steroids are helpful, but cessation of therapy leads to recurrence.

Acne Fulminans

Acne fulminans is similar to acne conglobata, but the acute inflammatory ulcers, leukocytosis, and fever affect the backs of adolescent males. Antibiotic therapy must be intensive.

Hidradenitis Suppurativa

Etiology

Hidradenitis suppurativa is a chronic recurrent infection of obstructed apocrine glands in the axillary, perianal, and genital regions. *S. aureus* is the most frequent isolate, but *Proteus* species and other enteric gram-negative bacilli and pseudomonads are also found.

Epidemiology

The disease is more common in the axillae of women and the perianal region of men. It never occurs before puberty when these glands begin to function. People with acne and acne conglobata seem especially susceptible.

Pathogenesis

The apocrine glands almost never become infected unless they are first obstructed with keratinous debris. Skin bacteria can then multiply within the gland and produce microabscesses. The gland ruptures and infects adjacent glands, along with the surrounding dermal and subcutaneous spaces. Drainage is established spontaneously through multiple sinus tracts to the skin, and a carbuncle of grouped apocrine glands is produced.[19] The role of shaving, depilatories, deodorants, and antiperspirants is unknown.

Clinical Manifestations

A tender red swelling appears in previously healthy persons who may have a history of acne or obesity. If untreated, the boil ruptures and is followed at intervals of weeks to months by sequential infections in the same or other areas of apocrine secretion. Sinus tracts gradually appear with scarring, which can become so severe that motion of the arm is restricted (Fig. 25-9). "Bridge" scars spanning old areas of inflammation are characteristic. In the perianal region, scarring can affect the anus and rectum.

Diagnosis

Any abscess in the apocrine gland region should be suspect, but carbuncles, lymphadenitis, or other perineal infections must be ruled out. The disease may be confused with the more exotic granulomatous diseases like tuberculosis, actinomycosis, and the sexually transmitted granulomatous diseases.

Treatment

Treatment must be varied depending on the stage of disease. In the early stages, antibiotics should suffice. Incision and drainage, which may cause sinus formation, should be avoided. Antibiotics (penicillinase-resistant penicillin, erythromycin, or lincomycin) should be given until the disease has resolved. Some authorities [19] recommend parenteral therapy followed by oral treatment for 2 weeks. Steroids have also been recommended—either systemically (40–60 mg prednisone per day for 7 to 10 days) or intralesionally (5–15 mg per ml triamcinalone suspension).

After successful treatment of the early lesion, subsequent lesions can be prevented by avoiding shaving, depilatories, or deodorants, and substituting application of an antibiotic ointment in a hydrophilic base (neosporin or gentamycin) and povidone-iodine baths.

Surgical treatment is required in advanced, recurrent, or scarred cases. Piecemeal excisions or repeated incision and drainage is contraindicated. If the process is clearly restricted to one area, it can be excised. In extensive cases, complete full thickness excision of the entire axillary skin may be required, using skin graft or rotation flaps for closure.[19a]

Pyodermas in Immunodepressed Patients—*P. aeruginosa* Pyoderma

Septicemia due to *P. aeruginosa* is common in immunodepressed patients (see subsequent section). In addition, pyodermas of the nails, toewebs, skin, and external auditory canal occur in immunodepressed patients.[20]

The bacteriology and pathogenesis of pseudomonad infections are discussed in Chapter 5. Chronically macerated areas of skin such as the toewebs, external auditory canal, the paronychial regions of the nails, open wounds, burns, or areas of dermatitis are especially vulnerable.

Several clinical presentations are typical:

1. *Paronychia.* Patients with chronic immersion of hands in water, soaps, and detergents develop painful paronychial lesions with or without characteristic green or blue discoloration of the nails.
2. *Web space infections.* Persistent soreness and scaling of the web tissues occur in patients with hyperhydrosis of the feet or who work in areas of high humidity.
3. *Folliculitis.* This has been reported in individuals who use public whirlpool facilities.
4. *External otitis* (Chapter 27). A swollen, macerated appearance of the external canal without involvement of the drum is characteristic. In diabetic patients, the mortality can be as high as 50 percent.
5. *Superficial pyoderma. Pseudomonas pyoderma* is characterized by irregular, superficial pustular lesions with a greenish-blue purulent exudate (pyocyanin). The pigmented exudate and grapelike odor (trimarethylamine) are distinctive. Mixed infections with other gram-negative rods or with *Candida* may be observed. Some strains produce a yellow-green fluorescein, which fluoresces under a Wood ultraviolet lamp.

Superficial pseudomonas infections are best treated by topical antibiotic therapy (polymyxin B, colistin sulfate) and by drying of the infected area. Systemic antibiotics are required for malignant external otitis as well as drainage of the pinna (Chapter 27). For local infection, acetic acid, silver nitrate, or gentian violet compresses applied intermittently with long periods of drying are very useful. Paronychia respond to surgical drainage, nail trimming, and 4 percent thymol in chloroform. Acetic acid in 50 percent ethyl alcohol, polymixin (0.1 percent) in acetic acid, or corticosteroids with neomycin are effective for otitis externa. A 5 percent solution of acetic acid used topically is most effective on chronic ulcers.[20]

COMMON PYOGENIC BACTERIAL INFECTIONS OF THE SUBCUTANEOUS TISSUES

Although descriptive terminology has traditionally been used to separate suppurative and nonsuppurative infections, they are often part of a continuous spectrum of disease—erysipelas can become cellulitis and thereafter acute streptococcal gangrene. Folliculitis and hidradenitis suppurativa readily become subcutaneous abscesses. Despite this continuity, we will continue to describe these entities separately, because a patient's presentation may more closely resemble one than the other.

Cellulitis

Definition and Etiology

Cellulitis is an acute expanding infection of the skin and subcutaneous tissues characterized by heat, erythema, and edema. It may begin as an erysipelas and advance to necrosis, suppuration, lymphangitis, and lymphadenitis. It is not a single disease entity but a collection of clinical manifestations which can accompany any inflammation of the skin and subcutaneous tissues—both bacterial and nonbacterial.

Classical cellulitis caused by *S. pyogenes* Lancefield group A (beta-hemolytic streptococcus) appears in unbroken skin and suppuration is absent. Other gram-positive pyogenic cocci such as *S. aureus, S. pneumoniae,* and many other streptococci (group B in newborns, *S. milleri,* group C,F,G,L) can be involved. Typical cellulitis has been seen with *Erysipelothrix insidiosa* (see erysipeloid section)[15] or mixed gram-negative bacilli.[20] A special form similar to erysipeloid occurs in patients exposed to *Aeromonas hydrophila* during fresh water swimming.[21] *H. influenzae* can cause cellulitis of the face in children—less often in adults. These special forms are discussed in subsequent sections.

Pathology and Pathogenesis

Cellulitis is a clinical diagnosis characterized by heat, erythema, and edema of the skin surface secondary to local vasodilation and interstitial edema. All layers of skin and subcutaneous tissue are acutely inflamed and infiltrated with polymorphonuclear leukocytes, typically without necrosis or suppuration. Bacteria may be abundant both within and without phagocytes.

The most common predisposing conditions are minor trauma or an underlying skin lesion. Although in this sense the infection is always "secondary," classically there is no obvious break in the skin surface. On the other hand, cellulitis may occur as a postoperative wound infection, as a result of perforation of a viscus into the soft tissues, or it may overlay any other suppurative or gangrenous infection of soft tissue or bone. Cellulitis of the incised wound can be caused by any organism, but most fulminant and rapidly spreading lesions are due to *S. pyogenes* or *C. perfringens.*

Clinical Manifestations

There may or may not be evidence of previous damage to the skin. Local tenderness, pain, and erythema rapidly progress to a red-hot swollen lesion associated with malaise, fever, and chills. Unlike erysipelas, the margins are indistinct. The area expands rapidly, and in streptococcal infections lymphangitis with regional adenopathy and bacteremia is common. Local areas of subcutaneous necrosis, crepitation, and skin breakdown may develop, and abscesses are common sequelae. When skin necrosis occurs, superinfection with other environmental microbes is common (see subsequent section on streptococcal gangrene).

Diagnosis

The presumptive diagnosis of *S. pyogenes* infection is frequently made erroneously and penicillin therapy instituted without laboratory diagnostic studies. A Gram stain of a smear obtained by the injection and aspiration of a small volume (0.1–1.0 ml) of saline into the advancing edge of the erythematous margin is said to help make a specific etiologic diagnosis, but is most often of no diagnostic value because no bacteria are retrieved.

Any purulent material should be cultured for aerobic and anaerobic organisms, preferably by aspirating pus or obtaining a small tissue biopsy, especially if there is a poor response to empiric penicillin treatment. Crepitus is not seen with streptococcal infections (Table 25-16).

Presumptive Therapy

Early cellulitis is usually of streptococcal origin in the absence of a break in the skin and should be treated with parenteral penicillin G. Erythromycin is the usual alternative in allergic patients. A mixed bacterial infection with gram-positive cocci and gram-negative aerobic and anaerobic bacilli cause most cellulitis of the lower extremity and trunk around chronic ulcers, such as those seen in diabetic patients with ischemic gangrene or chronic venous insufficiency. Anaerobes are almost always found in such infections.[22] Many such infections will respond to penicillin alone, since most anaerobes except *B. fragilis* are sensitive to penicillin. Infections due to *S. aureus* respond to penicillinase-resistant penicillin, a cephalosporin, or in serious cases, vancomycin. In patients who manifest signs of systemic toxicity, hospitalization, Gram stain, culture of aspirate and blood are all required. When the Gram stain of the smear demonstrates a mixture of gram-negative and gram-positive organisms, a combination of a cephalosporin, an aminoglycoside, and clindamycin is required pending definitive culture and sensitivity results (see subsequent section on gram-negative cellulitis).

Local care of cellulitis includes immobilization and elevation of the infected part to reduce swelling. Warm, moist dressings are useful to reduce local pain, though such treatment probably does not help to localize the infection. In general, incision and drainage is contraindicated in the absence of local necrosis and suppuration; judicious needle aspiration may be required to detect areas of necrosis. Failure to achieve a prompt clinical response to antibiotic therapy is a far more reliable early sign of suppuration than is fluctuance. The major mistake made by inexperienced clinicians is to delay drainage until skin necrosis develops. Perineal infections can be fatal if drainage is delayed.

Prognosis

Most patients with cellulitis promptly treated with parenteral antibiotics are cured rapidly in the absence of underlying local or systemic host compromise. Rapid progression in areas of local compromise such as chronic edema or ischemia may lead to loss of limb or life. Failure to respond to the presumptive therapy may indicate systemic illnesses, unsuspected foreign bodies, osteomyelitis, or subcutaneous pus.

Hemophilus influenzae Cellulitis

Etiology

H. influenzae causes a purple-red cellulitis of the face, neck, or upper extremities of young children. The bacteriology and pathogenic aspects of *H. influenzae* are discussed in Chapter 7.

Pathogenesis

An upper respiratory tract infection precedes most cases of facial cellulitis, and the ear or respiratory tract probably provides the primary septic focus in children. Most adults have bactericidal and anticapsular antibody to *H. influenzae* and are less often afflicted.

Clinical Manifestations

Typically, a young infant or child develops an area of swelling, induration, and purplish discoloration of the face or arm following several days of coryza and fever. The cellulitis can occur in conjunction with otitis media, sinusitis, or epiglottitis and pneumonia. Fever, leukocytosis, and positive blood cultures are common. In children aged 3 to 24 months, this disease must be distinguished from streptococcal, staphylococcal, pneumococcal cellulitis, or erysipelas. Aspiration, Gram stain, and culture of the margin of cellulitis reveal the organisms in about half the cases.

Treatment

Ampicillin (150–250 mg per kg per day intravenously in four to six divided doses) is effective in most children. With the recent emergence of R factor–mediated (beta-lactamase-producing) ampicillin-resistant strains, alternative regimens have been recommended, including chloramphenicol (50–100 mg per kg daily in children above the age of 3 months) alone, or in combination with ampicillin. Cefamandole, a cephalosporin derivative, is useful against ampicillin-sensitive and resistant strains. Cotrimoxazole or the combination of sulfisoxazole and streptomycin can also be used.[20]

Gram-Negative Cellulitis

Cellulitis caused by gram-negative organisms,[20] especially *E. coli, Proteus, Klebsiella, Enterobacter, Serratia,* or *Bacteroides* species, usually follows contamination of adjacent tissues by bowel contents or a breakdown in the skin. Patients present: (1) after bowel perforation due to appendicitis, neoplasm, diverticulitis, or rectal mucosal tear, (2) after colon surgery, (3) with a history of peripheral edema, (4) with vascular insufficiency, (5) with decubitus, diabetic or venous insufficiency ulcers, (6) percutaneous lines, or (7) superficial perineal dermatitis including diaper rash. These patients may also have poorly controlled diabetes or alterations in host defense mechanisms, eg, granulocytopenia and poor nutrition. Gas-forming strains of bacteria cause crepitant, gas-containing cellulitis, especially in patients with poorly controlled diabetes; *Bacteroides* species or anaerobic streptococci are common copathogens (see subsequent sections on the gangrenous soft tissue infections).[23-25]

Clinical Manifestations

The typical findings of cellulitis with warmth, redness, and brawny edema are found progressing to areas of gangrene in some cases. Palpable tenderness and crepitus can define the extent of the process. Needle aspiration of mixed aerobes and anaerobes confirms the diagnosis.

Treatment

Immediate antibiotic therapy guided by Gram stain smears of the exudate and surgical drainage are essential although extensive debridement is usually unnecessary and hyperbaric oxygen is not indicated. The existence of a feeding source of contamination should be sought, eg, from a ruptured appendix, diverticulum, or rectal tear. If a lower bowel perforation is found, a diverting colostomy should be performed in addition to local drainage and debridement. Decubitus ulcers must be carefully evaluated for undermining necrosis, abscess formation, and cellulitis. The antibiotics chosen should be directed toward gram-negative enteric organisms, anaerobic gram-negative organisms, and anaerobic streptococci, all of which may be present. For this reason, the combination of an aminoglycoside with clindamycin is ideal, since it provides coverage for staphylococci, streptococci, gram-negative enterics, and *B. fragilis.* Chloramphenicol or cefoxitin may also be useful.

Subcutaneous Abscesses

Many infections of the skin and soft tissues present as abscesses in the subcutaneous tissue, especially following folliculitis, cellulitis, or trauma.

Incidence

Localized cutaneous abscesses are a common inducement to visit a physician. At the University of Chicago, approximately 2.5 percent of all adult outpatient visits are for evaluation of such abscesses.[5]

Etiology

The bacteria isolated from 135 subcutaneous abscesses by Meislin et al[5] in otherwise healthy persons are listed in Table 25-18 and Table 25-19.

S. aureus was the organism most commonly found oc-

TABLE 25-18. FREQUENCY OF ISOLATION OF AEROBES FROM 135 OUTPATIENT ABSCESSES

Anatomic Area	Staphylococcus aureus	Staphylococcus epidermidis	Beta-Hemolytic Streptococcus (Group A and B)	Alpha and Nonhemolytic Streptococcus	Corynebacterium species (Diphtheroids)	Proteus mirabilis	Enterobacteriaceae (other than P. mirabilis)
Head and neck	16 *	24	4	8	8	12	12
Trunk	18	18	0	9	0	36	0
Axilla	50	9	0	9	5	31	9
Extremity	38	6	6	6	13	6	13
Hand	25	38	38	0	0	13	13
Inguinal	29	0	0	14	0	0	14
Vulvovaginal	8	0	8	21	0	0	8
Buttock	33	0	8	17	25	0	0
Perirectal	0	5	5	48	10	0	10

* Numbers indicate percentage of abscesses containing these organisms.

Modified from Meislin HW, Lerner SA, Graves MH, McGehee MD, Kocka FE, Morello JA, Rosen P: Cutaneous abscesses: Anaerobic and aerobic bacteriology and outpatient management. *Ann Intern Med* 87:145, 1977.

curring in one-quarter of all abscesses. It was isolated in pure culture 90 percent of the time and accounted for 70 percent of all pure cultures. It was most often found in abscesses of the upper torso, and rarely from the perineum, and was almost always resistant to penicillin G.

The majority of subcutaneous abscesses contain mixed bacteria,[5] a finding contrary to traditional teaching. The organisms isolated from untreated abscesses depend to a large degree on the site of the infection. Anaerobes are commonly isolated from abscesses of the perineal, inguinal, and buttock region. An average of 3 to 5 anaerobic species are found in each abscess. Single species of obligate anaerobic organisms rarely cause suppurative infections. Clostridia species, though common in feces and soil, are only rarely cultured from cutaneous abscesses. The presence of gas within an abscess implies anaerobic metabolism by facultative or anaerobic bacteria. *B. fragilis* was not found as often as other *Bacteroides* species, although its well-known resistance to penicillin G makes it an important finding in perineal infections (Table 25-19). Almost all the other anaerobes found in subcutaneous abscesses are sensitive to the penicillins.

Nonperineal infections are most often caused by mixed aerobes (Table 25-18). *S. epidermidis* and enteric gram-negative bacteria were isolated almost exclusively from nonperineal areas. *P. mirabilus,* the most common

TABLE 25-19. FREQUENCY OF ISOLATION OF ANAEROBES FROM 135 OUTPATIENT ABSCESSES

Anatomic Area	Peptococcus species	Peptostreptococcus species	Clostridium species	Eubacterium species	Propionibacterium species	Lactobacillus species	Bacteroides melaninogenicus	Bacteroides corrodens	Bacteroides fragilis	Other Bacteroides species	Fusobacterium species
Head and neck	56 *	0	0	0	28	0	8	8	4	8	0
Trunk	36	9	0	0	36	0	18	9	9	9	9
Axilla	31	9	0	5	14	0	5	0	5	0	0
Extremity	19	6	19 †	6	0	6	6	13	0	13	0
Hand	13	0	0	0	0	0	0	0	0	0	0
Inguinal	57	57	0	0	0	29	57	29	0	29	14
Vulvovaginal	46	62	8	15	8	23	39	31	23	23	46
Buttock	50	25	8	0	0	25	58	33	17	25	25
Perirectal	67	57	10	29	5	14	81	57	47	29	43

* Numbers represent percentage of abscesses containing these organisms.
† These isolates were all *Clostridium perfringens.*

Modified Meislin HW, Lerner SA, Graves MH, McGehee MD, Kocka FE, Morello JA, Rosen P: Cutaneous abscesses: Anaerobic and aerobic bacteriology and outpatient management. *Ann Intern Med* 87:145, 1977.

gram-negative aerobe found, was more common than all the other Enterobacteriaciae combined. Surprisingly, *Proteus* is rarely isolated from the perineal region and is seen in cutaneous abscesses of the upper torso where it is not a normal inhibitant. *E. coli* is rarely found, and only from perineal abscesses.

Subcutaneous abscesses are seldom found to be sterile unless antibiotics have been started or the material has been collected improperly for both aerobic and anaerobic culture. Truly sterile abscesses most often arise from the injection of sterile foreign material by drug addicts or in psychologically disturbed paramedical personnel (see subsequent section on factitious soft tissue infections).

Pathogenesis and Pathology

Cutaneous abscesses occur everywhere on the body. Any break in the integrity of the skin permits invasion by the normal flora of the skin and adjacent mucous membranes. The traumatizing instrument is a major source of contamination. Abscesses in the perineum, axilla, and head and neck may arise from infections in apocrine or sebaceous glands. Such abscesses are seen mostly in adults, because these glands become active only after puberty (see preceding section on hidradenitis suppurativa).

Perirectal abscesses commonly arise from anal crypts. Pilonidal abscesses result from secondary infection of pilonidal cysts. Vulvovaginal abscesses usually begin in obstructed Bartholin glands but, contrary to common belief, are rarely due to *N. gonorrheae.* Any hair follicle infection can extend into the subcutaneous tissues, but infections originating in sweat glands are rare. In general, men present with head and neck, perirectal and extremity abscesses, while women suffer axillary, vulvovaginal, and perirectal abscesses. The congenital immunodeficiencies and leukocyte abnormalities discussed in Chapter 13 should be suspected and ruled out in infants and children with recurrent abscesses.

Clinical Manifestations

Patients most frequently complain of recent localized pain and swelling around the infected site. Systemic toxicity is unusual, although mild fever and slight tachycardia are common. Induration, cellulitis, lymphedema, lymphangitis, and regional adenopathy may be present. Fluctuance is easy to detect when it overlies firm nonfatty tissue, but it is a late sign of suppuration. It is common to underestimate the amount of pus a subcutaneous abscess contains, especially in perineal and extremity abscesses where induration without fluctuance may be the only clue to the presence of underlying pus. If there is any doubt, needle aspiration through the sterilized skin should be attempted. Any amount of aspirated pus is significant, because aspiration of thick pus is difficult through a needle, and incision will almost always reveal more.

Treatment

The traditional treatment for localized cutaneous abscess in the otherwise healthy, nontoxic patient is incision and drainage alone.[26]

Incision and Drainage. Incision and drainage is most often carried out without admitting the patient to the hospital. Local anesthesia along the roof of the abscess decreases incisional pain, but the evacuation of the abscess and its packing may still be painful. Deep infiltration of local anesthetic agents is thought to spread the infection into deeper normal tissues. General anesthesia is frequently required for extensive abscess drainage, such as perirectal abscesses, and postoperative analgesia is always required. In the emergency room, small abscesses can be drained under local anesthesia, but premedication with opiates may be necessary.

Careful positioning to allow complete visualization of the abscess site is essential. For example, vulvovaginal abscesses are easily treated with a patient in the lithotomy position, but perirectal and pilonidal abscesses are best treated with the patient in the knee-chest, Sim's, or prone position. Wide adhesive tape extending from buttock to the table edge may be used to retract the buttocks to ensure adequate exposure.

The site should be widely scrubbed with povidone-iodine and surgically draped. Infiltration with a 1 percent lidocaine or spray with ethyl chloride may help reduce superficial incisional pain. An initial small incision permits the surgeon to judge the extent of the cavity by introducing the gloved finger. Probing a wound with instruments is avoided because the abscess wall may easily be perforated, spreading bacteria into sterile tissue planes. Bartholin abscesses should be incised through the mucosal rather than the cutaneous surface, and all the incisions should be placed in the natural skin folds. Most abscesses are not spherical but possess radial extensions of loculated granulation tissue and pus along the planes of least resistance. Hence, the cavity should be digitally probed in all directions to break up loculated pockets and thoroughly irrigated with saline until all pus and necrotic debris have been removed. Irrigation with antibiotics is probably unnecessary. Irrigation with antiseptics of any kind is probably harmful to host tissue.

After debridement, the abscess should be loosely packed from the skin to its depth with a plain gauze wick to obtain hemostasis, and a dry absorbent dressing applied. The perineal area is an especially difficult region in which to maintain an adequate dressing, but a sanitary napkin seems to work well. If the gauze packing dislodges, the patient should be instructed not to replace it but to begin warm water soaks or sitz baths for 20 to 30 minutes four times daily. Prolonged soaking will macerate the wound, and careful drying of the skin around the wound after soaking is essential.

All abscesses are rechecked in 48 hours except facial abscesses, which are rechecked in 24 hours. The packing is removed and warm soaks begun. Deep abscess cavities will require irrigation and debridement from time to time. Insertion of rubber drains either at the primary drainage procedure or after removal of packing may be indicated to keep the skin open until healing by secondary intention has taken place. Packs remaining in place more than 48 hours may impede drainage.

A variety of packs, drains, and other local treatments have been suggested as alternative methods of evacuating the contents of abscesses. For example, Philip[27] utilizes a Petzer catheter inserted into the abscess cavity and left in place from 5 to 10 days. Continuous irrigation with antibiotic (or less likely, antiseptic) solutions may have some benefit in poorly localized deep-seated infections in conjunction with systemic antibiotics, but it is not required in most subcutaneous abscesses. There are no well-controlled studies evaluating these procedures. Irrigation washes out necrotic debris and bacteria, which may be the greatest benefit of this therapy. Secondary infections with *Candida, Pseudomonas,* or *Serratia* are common in macerated wounds irrigated for prolonged periods.

Robson et al [28] perform occasional quantitative bacteriology in large abscess cavities. When the bacterial counts of cavity wall fall below 10^5 organisms per gram of tissue, the cavity can be closed secondarily. This technique shortens the course considerably.

Alternative Methods of Therapy. An alternative method of therapy of small acute abscesses in an outpatient setting is incision, curettage, and primary suture under antibiotic cover. This technique has gained popularity in the United Kingdom, and a recent review demonstrates that it is not statistically inferior to incision and drainage without antibiotics although recurrence is somewhat more common. [26] Jones and Wilson [29] use the following technique. Lincomycin (600 mg) is given intramuscularly before incision, and clindamycin, 150 mg, orally every 6 hours, is continued for 4 days postoperatively. The abscess is incised under general anesthesia, and the wall of the cavity is systematically broken down by curettage, filling the cavity with antibiotic-laden blood. After the abscess wall has been completely removed, the clot is evacuated and the cavity obliterated with mattress sutures and a compression dressing. The patient is checked at 5 days, and the sutures are usually removed 2 or 3 days later. Optimal results are obtained if the incision is made before the abscess points and is less successful if skin necrosis has taken place. The second principle is the use of a safe antibiotic effective against the infecting organisms, such as lincomycin and clindamycin for short periods. Jones and Wilson [29] report 22,000 prescriptions for clindamycin without a single case of pseudomembranous colitis. Other data suggest, however, that such promiscuous use is dangerous (Chapter 39).

A prospective clinical trial by Macfie and Harvey [26] demonstrated that the mean healing time following incision, curettage, and primary suture with antibiotic cover was 9 days, but that 11.7 percent of such patients had recurrence. In contrast, there were no recurrences in 57 abscesses treated by incision and open drainage with antibiotic cover, and 7.3 percent of patients treated with incision and open drainage without antibiotic coverage had recurrences. Either technique will cure the majority of minor abscesses. Deep infections or infections in compromised hosts, however, should be treated with continual drainage.

Antibiotics. The vast majority of abscesses that have been correctly incised and drained will resolve without antibiotics. Parenteral antibiotics are definitely indicated in: (1) the clinically septic patient with significant tachycardia and fever, (2) the patient with an abscess in certain critical areas, ie, mastoid area or central triangle of the face drained by the emissary veins to the cavernous sinus, (3) the patient at risk due to preexisting systemic disease, eg, rheumatic heart disease, Hodgkin disease, and (4) patients on immunosuppressive drugs or chemotherapy. Some surgeons prefer to use antibiotics briefly when draining any large multiloculated abscess to prevent toxicity secondary to bacteremia induced by surgical trauma. The abscess recurrence rate is slightly but not statistically smaller if antibiotics are used in conjunction with traditional incision and drainage.[26] If drainage is adequate, antibiotics need not be administered for the prolonged periods required for systemic infections.

The choice of antibiotic can be based on certain clinical and laboratory findings. For example, infections of the trunk and hands of working men are frequently caused by *S. aureus* alone; those of the axilla and trunk of women frequently contain *Proteus,* and perineal abscesses contain mixed aerobes and anaerobes (Tables 25-18 and 19). Foul-smelling pus is presumptive evidence of anaerobic infection. A Gram-stained smear of the aspirate will correctly identify sterile abscesses, mixed gram-positive and gram-negative abscesses, and abscesses infected with pure *S. aureus* even before operation. Once tentative bacteriologic identification is made, the most appropriate antibiotic can be chosen—for *S. aureus* a penicillinase-resistant penicillin or cephalosporin, and for gram-negative aerobic organisms an aminoglycoside. *Bacteroides* infections common in the perineum respond to clindamycin, which is a good choice for staphylococci and anaerobic cocci, which are frequent co-pathogens.

Page and Freeman [29a] have studied the antibiotic sensitivities of aerobes obtained from superficial abscesses in an outpatient clinic. They recommend cloxacilin or lincomycin to treat abscesses in which *S. aureus* is predominant, but an orally administered cephalosporin may be a better choice. For perineal infections in which aerobic gram-negative bacilli and anaerobes are both expected, they recommend a combination of ampicillin and clindamycin, which can be given either parenterally or orally. Antibiotics are rarely necessary for more than a few days for a properly drained abscess in an individual with normal host defenses. Arbitrary courses of 7 to 10 days are not necessary. As soon as the wound is granulating (usually 4 to 5 days), antibiotics can be discontinued.

In the compromised patient, hospitalization and parenteral administration of antibiotics are indicated; the choices are more varied and the need for prolonged therapy more common. Because staphylococci, gram-negative enteric organisms, and anaerobes are frequently seen on Gram stain, we prefer to use an aminoglycoside and clindamycin in combination, until the pathogens have been isolated and sensitivities determined.

Botryomycosis (Actinophytosis)

This rare disease is in essence a small cutaneous or subcutaneous abscess the pus from which appears to contain granules—similar to those seen in mycetoma or actinomycosis. The abscesses are usually single, located in the genital region, and associated with a foreign body. Incision and

TABLE 25-20. DIFFERENTIAL DIAGNOSIS OF GANGRENOUS INFECTIONS OF SUBCUTANEOUS TISSUES AND SKIN

	Bacterial Synergistic Gangrene	Necrotizing Fasciitis	Streptococcal Gangrene	Gas Gangrene	Necrotizing Cutaneous Mucormycosis	Bacteremia Gangrenous Cellulitis	Pyoderma Gangrenosum
Predisposing conditions	Wound infection; draining sinus	Wound infection; perineal infections; diabetes; drug addiction	Occasionally diabetes or myxedema; after abdominal surgery	Local trauma to deep soft tissues	Diabetes; corticosteroid therapy	Burns; immunosuppression; cancer chemotherapy	Ulcerative colitis, rheumatoid arthritis
Pain	Severe	Variable	Severe	Severe	Minimal	Minimal	Moderate
Toxicity	Minimal	Marked	Marked	Very marked	Variable	Marked	Minimal
Fever	Minimal or absent	Moderate	High	Moderate or high	Low	High	Low
Crepitus	Absent	Frequent	Absent	Frequent	Absent	Absent	Absent
Appearance	Central shaggy necrotic ulcer surrounded by dusky margin and erythematous periphery	Drainage from single or multiple areas of skin necrosis; extensive undermining of skin along fascial plane	Extensive undermining of subcutaneous tissue; bullae and necrotic "burned" appearance of overlying skin	Marked swelling; yellow-bronzed discoloration of skin; brown bullae, green-black patches of necrosis; serosanguineous discharge	A central black necrotic area with purple raised margin	A sharply demarcated necrotic area with black eschar and surrounding erythema, resembling a decubitus ulcer; may evolve from initial hemorrhagic bullae	Begin as bullae, pustules, or erythematous nodules that ulcerate deeply; often multiple; large and coalescent; usually on lower extremities or abdomen
Etiology	Microaerophilic streptococcus plus *S. aureus* (or *Proteus*)	Usually a mixture of aerobic and anaerobic organisms	Primarily group A streptococci	*C. perfringens* (occasionally other clostridia)	*Rhizopus, Mucor, Absidia*	*P. aeruginosa* *S. aureus*	Not a primary infection; secondary by polymicrobial flora

Modified from Wilson CB, Siber GR, O'Brien TF, Morgan AP: Phycomycotic gangrenous cellulitis. *Arch Surg* 111:532, 1976.

drainage is curative. The granules consist of clumped *S. aureus* organisms.

Self-Induced Subcutaneous Infections

Self-induced subcutaneous infection is part of a greater problem of factitious illness. A recent review by Aduan et al[30] describes 32 patients with factitious fever, of whom 11 had recurrent skin infections—three had recurrent polymicrobial bacteremia, and one endocarditis. Most admitted intravenous or subcutaneous inoculation of foreign bodies (dirt, saliva, laboratory bacterial cultures, milk), self-induced excoriation of mucous membranes or skin, as well as thermometer manipulation. Females with medical or paramedical occupations predominated (nurse, student nurse, pharmacist, laboratory technologist, navy corpsman, former medical student). These patients manifested the typical characteristics of Munchausen syndrome. The underlying psychopathology is varied, and the psychodynamics are discussed by Aduan et al.[30]

Numerous other cases of similar self-induced infections have been reported. In general, polymicrobial bacteremia in a normal host without underlying malignancy, gastrointestinal, biliary tract, or urinary tract obstruction, or previous cardiac surgery must be viewed with suspicion. Fortunately, the normal patient usually clears such bacteremia readily and without sequelae. One clue is that patients have bacteremia with multiple different organisms. This pattern is so unusual that when it occurs, factitious illnesses should be suspected in patients with subcutaneous infections.

These patients have real illnesses, although they are

self-inflicted, and they may confuse the picture with thermometer manipulation and other devices. The surgeon seeing patients with recurrent subcutaneous infections should bear this syndrome in mind. In general, the localized infections and episodes of bacteremia must be treated as if they were spontaneous. Unfortunately, local tissue infections may appear to be unresponsive, because these patients continue to manipulate and contaminate the wounds.

Blunt confrontation of the patient with the factitious nature of his or her disease may precipitate self-destructive behavior or flight. Confrontation, therefore, must not be made until a plan of social-psychiatric care, as described by Wedel[30a] can be arranged.

Infected Bites

Infected bites produce infections that do not differ in essentials from other pyogenic infections of the skin and soft tissues that follow trauma. Certain peculiarities require emphasis, however.

Infected Human Bites

These injuries can occur in the form of bites or blows to the teeth. The injury itself is usually minor, but subsequent infection can be tragic. The first injury induces a special wound—the obvious injury to the skin of the knuckle plus a hidden injury to the extensor tendon and the metacarpophalangeal joint capsule. When the hand is opened, the tendons retract so that the deeper parts of the wound are sealed. The anaerobes of the mouth are free to proliferate in the avascular tendon tissues.

Human dental plaque is made up of both aerobic and anerobic microorganisms (Chapter 3). These include *S. aureus,* anaerobic streptococci, *B. melaninogenicus, Fusobacterium,* spirochetes, *S. viridans,* and *Actinomyces.* All these organisms can be found in human bite infections.

If prophylactic treatment is delayed, a mixed infection of the soft tissue, tendon, joint, or bone results. This may present as abscess, cellulitis, lymphangitis, necrotizing fasciitis, osteomyelitis, or septicemia (Chapter 43).

The treatment of established human bite infections can require drainage of the abscesses, opening of areas of necrotizing fasciitis, and debridement of nonviable tissue. Through-and-through drainage and continuous antimicrobial irrigation may be necessary to avoid progression. Loss of a digit, hand, or life has been reported. All patients with established infections should be hospitalized and treated with heat, elevation, splinting, and systemic parenteral antimicrobial agents. Penicillin G should control most infections due to bites, but cultures and sensitivity testing must be performed. Cephalosporins and erythromycin are good alternatives.

Most human bite infections can be prevented. The principles of the prevention of infection in traumatic wounds are discussed in Chapter 22. Devitalized tissue must be excised, foreign particles removed, and blood supply reestablished. Superficial wounds should be left open, unless joints, bone, or tendon are exposed. If the injury is seen early following wounding, divided tendons, nerves, and blood vessels can be repaired—a recommendation that was once controversial.[31] Hospitalization for minor wounds is not required if surgical repair of vital structures is not necessary. However, the part should be placed at rest, splinted if possible, and antibiotic prophylaxis administered. Oral penicillin or an oral cephalosporin are highly effective prophylactic agents. If treatment has been delayed or grossly neglected, such patients should be admitted and treated as if clinical infection was already established. Tetanus prophylaxis must be given to all patients, and follow-up examinations must be continued in order to ensure against missed injuries to the hand or more indolent infections.

The patients who suffer bites to the closed fist may not comply with admonitions to take prophylactic antibiotic therapy. The seriousness of the resulting illness must be stressed.

Animal Bites

Dog bites and other animal bites should be treated to prevent wound infection, rabies, and tetanus as well as to correct any anatomical injury. Rabies is discussed in Chapter 10, and tetanus is discussed in Chapter 46. Although dog bites are said to be frequently infected,[32] they are less often infected than human bites.

Pasteurella Multocida Infections. *P. multocida* is a small, ovoid, gram-negative rod (Chapter 7). The organism is found in the upper respiratory tract of healthy cats, dogs, rats, and mice but can cause hemorrhagic septicemia in these animals. The most common disease in humans is a local infection at the site of an animal bite with redness, swelling, ulceration, and a small amount of seropurulent drainage. A rapidly spreading cellulitis with associated lymphangitis and lymphadenopathy may progress to local necrosis and abscess formation. Fever is usually absent, and leukocytosis is present. The disease must be distinguished from cat scratch disease, ulceroglandular tularemia, and other innoculation infections (Table 25-5). Isolation of the organism is diagnostic.

Most strains are susceptible to penicillin, which should be administered in doses of 2 to 4 million units intramuscularly daily until the lesion is well healed to avert possible osteomyelitis. Tetracycline is an alternative, but susceptibility testing must be performed. Abscesses should be surgically drained.

Rat bite fever. Rat bite fever, caused by *Streptobacillus moniliformis* or *Spirillum minus* (Chapter 7), usually follows the bite or scratch of a rat but may follow ingestion of contaminated food. (Haverhill fever was a milk-borne outbreak in 1926.) The rat bite has usually healed by the time the systemic illness begins several days later. Fever, chills, headache, and malaise are associated with an erythematous macular or papular rash. A serious arthritis can involve the large joints, and regional adenopathy is common. A small abscess may develop at the bite site. *S. minus* has a lower incidence of arthritis and a slower healing bite wound. The differential diagnosis should include meningococcemia, gonococcemia, viral exanthems, and Rocky Mountain spotted fever. Treatment is penicillin 600,000 units intramuscularly every 6 hours for 10 to 12 days. Tetracycline or streptomycin are alternatives in the penicillin-allergic patient. Rarely, endocarditis complicates the illness.

Cat scratch disease is discussed in a subsequent section on viral disorders.

SECONDARY BACTERIAL INFECTIONS IN NONINFECTIOUS ULCERS

Table 23-11 lists many of the causes of noninfective skin ulceration. All these ulcers can become secondarily infected and produce cellulitis, subcutaneous abscesses, osteomyelitis, or can progress to the gangrenous infections discussed in a subsequent section.[24,34,35] The secondary infections can be caused by any ambient pathogen, but mixed aerobic and anaerobic infections are most common. In fact, the agents that cause necrotizing fasciitis (see subsequent section) are those most often found in chronic ulcers with superinfection. Two ulcer types exemplify these lesions—decubitus ulcers and ulcers in the feet of diabetics.

Infections in Decubitus Ulcers

Decubitus ulcers are commonly located in proximity to the anus, and anaerobic conditions are present because of tissue necrosis and undermining. In addition, patients with decubitus ulcers are typically debilitated, bedridden, and soiled with feces.

Mitchell[36] reported 24 cases of decubitus ulcers yielding enteric gram-negative facultative organisms, staphylococci, aerobic and anaerobic streptococci, and gram-negative anaerobes—especially *Bacteroides*.

Galpin et al[24] reported 21 patients with systemic sepsis that had begun within a decubitus ulcer. In all, the edges of the ulcer were undermined. Infection had spread in the fascial cleft beneath apparently normal skin (see subsequent section on necrotizing fasciitis). Ten of the 21 patients died in spite of antibiotic treatment and surgical debridement.[24] The undermining and necrosis must be recognized before systemic sepsis supervenes.

Local care includes reducing maceration and fecal contamination and avoiding pressure. Excision and primary closure is sometimes effective if bony prominences are eliminated, and thick normal tissue can be used for coverage. The principal mistake in management is the failure to recognize that the margins of the ulcer are undermined with synergistic mixed aerobic and anaerobic infections spreading under apparently normal skin. The presence of multiple contiguous skin ulcers is a simple clue to the undermining.[25] Osteomyelitis is a common complication and impairs chances of local cure.

Infections of the Diabetic Foot

Pathogenesis

The foot of the diabetic patient is particularly prone to primary soft tissue infections and to ischemic or neuropathic ulceration with secondary infections.[35]

Diabetic patients suffer both large and small vessel disease. Thrombosis of large vessels results in gangrene of a large segment of the leg, which can become secondarily infected. Occlusion of the smaller vessels results in small or patchy areas of gangrene, especially of the toes. Small vessel disease also leads to atrophic skin changes that, after minor trauma, may ulcerate and become infected. An additional type of vascular disease is caused by cholesterol-rich emboli to the small peripheral vessels from atheromata in the larger vessels.[35]

Although the ischemic changes associated with angiopathy are important, neuropathy is ultimately responsible for most diabetic foot problems that lead to infection. Loss of pain and temperature sensation permits painless trauma of the ischemic foot leading to ulceration. If uncontrolled infection develops in these ulcers, local infections compromise the vascular system further and enlarge the process. Loss of sensation also produces bone changes such as Charcot's joint or osteolysis, which in turn cause the foot to become deformed. Foot deformities also occur because of muscle atrophy secondary to motor nerve neuropathy. With changes in the configuration of the foot, the gait is altered and new pressure points are created, resulting in ulceration of these points.

Involvement of the autonomic nervous system also plays a role in the pathogenesis of foot infections. The most important factor is the absence of sweating, which leads to a dry, cracked skin that may become secondarily infected. Orthostatic hypotension, a complication of autonomic neuropathy, can lead to a decrease in perfusion of these vessels, impairing healing and permitting infection to take hold.

The last local characteristic that seems to impair the defenses against local infection in the diabetic are the dermatologic lesions. Diabetics have a variety of dermatologic problems, including eruptive xanthoma, diabetic dermopathy, xanthochromia, necrobiosis lipoidica diabeticorum, bullous diabeticorum, and pruritus. The last three can be associated with cutaneous trauma and ulceration, which subsequently lead to infection.

Diabetics also tend to develop cardiac and renal failure. Peripheral edema due to either will complicate existing foot problems and may impair healing and increase susceptibility of the foot to infection.

Although the diabetic patient is subject to minor unperceived trauma that leads directly to ulceration of the ischemic foot, the cutaneous fungi and bacteria ultimately lead to infection. There are few differences in the skin flora of diabetics and nondiabetics. Diabetics do not carry pathogenic organisms or yeasts more frequently on the normal skin. Erythrasma, however, occurs more frequently in the diabetic than in normal young adults, and in some studies dermatophytosis of the interdigital areas of the feet are more common in diabetics.

Serious infections are often preceded by minor infections of the toenails, nail beds, and adjacent structures. The fungus invades the distal nail first and subsequently disrupts the normal nail plate–nail bed attachment, permitting air to collect under the nail. As the disease progresses, the fungus invades along the stratum corneum of the nail bed and the excessive horn produced elevates the nail plate. Secondary bacterial invasion by *Pseudomonas* and *Proteus* species is common.

There is little evidence for systemic defects in host defense in the well-controlled diabetic.[37] Hyperglycemia and acidosis do interfere with neutrophil function, but most evidence supports the integrity of host defense—except at the local level, where blood supply and sensation is impaired. It is important to understand the relationship between infection and gangrene in diabetes. Regional infections increase tissue turgor and metabolic rate of the local tissues. Tissue demand for oxygen is thus increased in the face of relative ischemia. Infection further increases extravascular tissue tension and attracts neutrophils, which release tissue-destructive enzymes. Local thrombosis of small vessels then occurs, perpetuating the vicious cycle.

Etiology

Anaerobic bacteria play an important role in the pathogenesis of diabetic foot infections. Vascular insufficiency creates anaerobic conditions within neuropathic ulcers. Gas in the infected tissues is common. Louie et al [22] cultured the foot ulcers of 20 diabetic patients. Each ulcer yielded an average of 5.8 species per specimen (3.2 aerobes and 2.6 anaerobes). The principal isolates were *Bacteroides* species (17), peptococci (16), *Proteus* species (11), enterococci (9), *S. aureus* (7), clostridia (7), and *E. coli* (6). *S. aureus* were found in only 7 of the 20 patients and never in pure culture. Cultures and sensitivity tests should always be done, preferably utilizing biopsy material, especially if bone is involved. The choice of antibiotics should obviously be broad enough to cover this extensive array of organisms.

Clinical Manifestations

Superficial Infections (Fig. 25-10). The initial event in diabetic foot infections is a break in the skin followed by penetration of bacteria. Certain lesions are typical:

1. The initial break in the skin frequently originates near nails deformed by trauma, fungus infection, or systemic disease in the neuropathic foot. Neglect allows the nails to grow too long, and a nail may gouge the skin of the neighboring toe. In the elderly, the nail grows too long, curves, and partially encircles the distal nail bed. Stubbing the toe can break the skin. With fungal infections, excess keratin and debris accumulate under the nail and in the nail folds, permitting the nail to encircle the distal toe. Infections beginning in the nail bed typically spread on the dorsal and lateral aspects of the toes, the infections being prohibited from reaching the pad of the toe by fibrous septa that extend from dermis to periostium. Relief of infections near the nail may require removal of the nail, which must be done cautiously.

2. Toe deformities caused by neurologic imbalances produce characteristic ulcers at the apex of the cock-up deformity or on the callus overlying hammer toes. Infection can spread along the muscles of the great toe to infect the midplantar space.

3. Web infections are particularly hazardous, since they may occur without preexisting anatomic deformity. Infections in the interdigital webs frequently involve the digital arteries and can spread via the lumbrical tendons to deeper structures of the foot.

4. Mal perforans is a chronic indolent ulcer of the sole of the foot, usually over the head of the first, second, and third metatarsal. The tendon, joint, and bone are soon infected because the lesion is painless and the patient does not get off his feet.

5. Infections of the middle foot occur only after painless injury by penetrating objects, since the middle foot is not normally subject to pressure. Infection here spreads directly to the central plantar space.

6. Infections of the heel occur over the bony prominences of the calcaneus. When ulceration and gangrene occur in the heel, amputation is required.

Deep Infections. Major infections of the foot are of three types (Fig. 25-10): (1) abscesses in the deep spaces of the foot especially in the central plantar space, (2) nonsuppurative phlegmon of the dorsum of the foot, and (3) mal perforans ulcer foot. The deep plantar space may become infected in several ways: direct penetration by foreign bodies in the insensate foot, web space infections extending to the bursa of the lumbrical tendons and following the tendons into the central plantar space, or extension from involvement of the flexor tendon sheath into the central plantar space. Once the infection is established in the plantar space, the characteristic signs of plantar abscess appear—loss of the longitudinal arch convexity and bulging of the area. The sole of the foot becomes edematous. After a few days, edema of the dorsum of the foot appears, along with fever, malaise, loss of diabetic control, and ketoacidosis. The infection then spreads to the leg along the flexor tendons of the toes. Thrombotic obliteration of small vessels may occur and produce necrosis of the foot. This is first seen in the middle toes, since the plantar digital arteries of the second, third, and fourth toe arise from the plantar arch.

Paronchia or ulcerated calluses on hammer toes produce infections, which spread easily to the dorsum of the foot via lymphatics. A dorsal foot phlegmon is produced. In the insensate foot, the infection is aggravated by the dependent position and continued activity. An infective vasculitis then produces necrosis of the skin overlying the phlegmon. Amputation is frequently required.

Osteomyelitis. Osteomyelitis frequently affects the toes and small bones of the feet in diabetic patients. Systemic manifestations are few but pain, swelling, erythema, and indolent ulcers are seen. Both clinically and roentgenographically, it is difficult to distinguish between osteomyelitis and the osseous lesions of the foot that occur in severe diabetic peripheral neuropathy.[38] Most cases of osteomyelitis of the foot and lower leg of these patients begin as chronic perforating ulcers, which may heal and recur repeatedly for years because the predisposing factors resist treatment. In an unhealing ulcer, bacterial invasion may progress at the base of a lesion by spreading along fascia planes or by penetrating fascia and soft tissues to reach the periostium (Fig. 25-10).

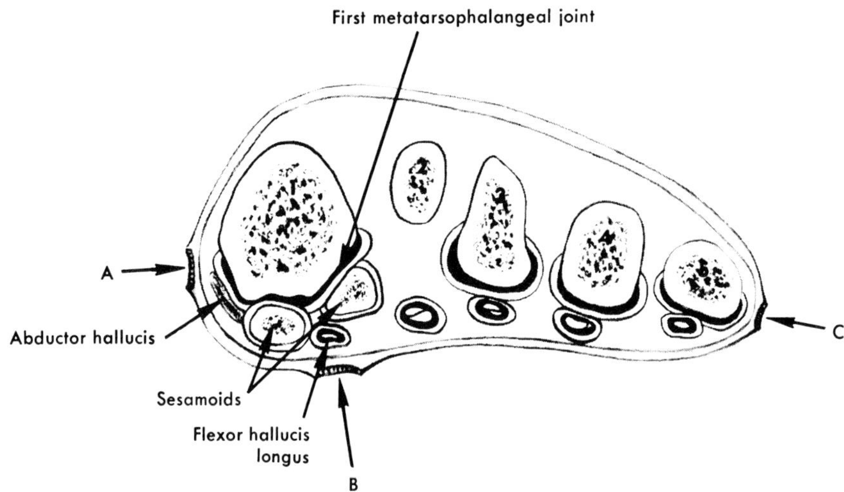

Fig. 25-10. **Common modes of spread of infection in distal diabetic foot. A. Infection from an ulcerated bunion may enter the lateral plantar space or the first metatarsophalangeal joint fairly easily. The joint infection can then penetrate into the central plantar space. B. Mal perforans fixes flexor tendons. With progression of infection the plantar space, or a joint, may be entered. C. Ulcerated tailor's bunion finds meager tissue barrier to entry into the fifth metatarsophalangeal joint. (From O'Neal LW: Surgical pathology of the foot and clinicopathologic correlations. In Levin ME, O'Neal LW: *The Diabetic Foot.* St. Louis, 1977, p 108.)**

Treatment

Cellulitis should be treated with broad-spectrum antibiotics (cephamandole, cefoxitin, gentamicin plus clindamycin), although penicillin is often effective. The foot should be elevated and the diabetes controlled. Abscesses must be drained and necrotic tissue debrided. If the blood supply of the foot is intact or can be restored, the ulcer may heal. Amputation should be avoided because it subjects the opposite foot to further pressure, which can ultimately lead to a second amputation.[35]

Prevention

Many of the abnormalities in the diabetic foot will ultimately lead to infection as neuropathy progresses and vascular flow is further impaired. Good podiatric treatment and follow-up can avoid many of these problems without reconstructive surgery. Whenever vascular supply is good and healing prompt, correction of the basic deformity should be considered. Ingrown nails, incurving nails, bunions, calluses, and hammer toes do not improve spontaneously.

GANGRENOUS INFECTIONS OF SUBCUTANEOUS TISSUE DUE TO COMMON PYOGENIC BACTERIA

Meleney[39] coined the term "infectious gangrene" to describe infections that cause extensive necrosis of the subcutaneous tissues (superficial fascia) and may cause gangrene of the overlying skin. Table 25-20 lists a number of these infections, which have been described as separate clinical entities over the past century. Attempts to discriminate one from the other on clinical grounds alone are hopeless, since the pattern of infection is basically similar in all. The manifestations depend on the etiologic agents, predisposing conditions, and anatomic location of the infection. Almost all forms of infectious gangrene involve a greater or lesser degree of necrosis of the subcutaneous tissues, with hemorrhage, vasculitis, and thrombosis of small arteries and veins and infiltration by polymorphonuclear leukocytes. In clostridial cellulitis and gangrene, leukocytes are notably absent and gas is abundant. The presence of gas in tissue, long considered pathognomonic of clostridial infections, simply means that anaerobic bacterial metabolism has produced insoluble gases such as hydrogen, nitrogen, and methane. Both facultative and obligate anaerobes are capable of such a metabolic activity. Trapped air disseminated by muscular activity can also lead to a similar picture (Table 25-16).

In most clinical situations, infectious gangrene results after inoculation of the infecting organisms into the tissues. The precipitating event is usually obvious—an area of crush injury, an operative incision, enterotomy stoma, or a secondarily infected cutaneous ulcer. Perineal fistulas are less visible but common sources of infection. More rarely, rupture of a viscus into the subcutaneus tissues of the abdomen, perineum, or thigh can occur, or infectious gangrene can begin at a site of metastatic hematogenous infection in immunodepressed patients.

The extent of skin gangrene is variable. Necrotizing faciitis due to mixed aerobes and anaerobes typically spreads in the fascial cleft between the subcutaneous tissue and deep fascia, sparing the major vessels within the subcutaneous tissue and preserving extensive areas of skin. Debridement can frequently be carried out without removing all the skin. In contrast, streptococcal gangrene leads to relatively early necrosis of the overlying skin.

STREPTOCOCCAL GANGRENE

Etiology

Acute streptococcal gangrene is a form of necrotizing faciitis caused by *S. pyogenes*, Lancefield group A (beta-hemolytic streptococci). Although Meleney first described the condition and its treatment in 1924,[39] this disease was probably the "hospital gangrene" of the Civil War, and is also known as "necrotizing erysipelas."

Incidence and Epidemiology

Acute streptococcal gangrene is currently a rare disease, which appears in occasional literature case reports. Typically, a surgical wound of an extremity is affected, but any region can be infected with or without antecedent trauma.

Pathogenesis

Basically, it is a fulminant type of necrotizing fasciitis with extensive skin necrosis. The gangrene results from thrombosis of the blood vessels that supply the skin within the superficial fascia. Destruction of cutaneous nerves may produce late anesthesia. Meleney first believed this disease was an allergic or Shwartzman type of reaction, but it is more likely that the gangrene is due to a tendency of the streptococcus organism to affect vascular structures of all types (Chapter 4).

Clinical Manifestations

The clinical course is fulminating. The affected skin is hot, red, swollen, and extremely painful at first. Fever, chills, tachycardia, and prostration are also present. Within 2 to 4 days, the skin overlying the infection develops dusky, irregular patches and large bullae containing bacteria and a dark exudate (Fig. 25-11). Without treatment, these areas progress to frank cutaneous gangrene and a burnlike eschar. Muscle and bone are generally spared. If the untreated patient survives, the slough separates from the underlying tissue in 2 to 3 weeks. The essential undermining nature of the infection is best recognized by passing a probe through a skin incision along the fascial cleft overlying the deep fasciitis without resistance (Fig. 25-12). The edema that accompanies these infections can be so extensive that hypovolemia is produced. Extension through deep fascia can produce myonecrosis and compartmental hypertension. Fasciotomy may be required even if the muscle is not affected.

Diagnosis

The differential diagnosis must include gas gangrene caused by *C. perfringens*, erysipelas, and cellulitis. The blister fluid will frequently show gram-positive streptococci on smear. Gas and odor are notably absent. Lymphangitis is uncommon.

Treatment

High-dose parenteral penicillin G is the treatment of choice, but always in conjunction with surgical debridement within a few hours. An incision along the entire length of the undermined area should be carried down to the muscles (Fig. 25-12). All the necrotic tissue is excised, but viable skin is not removed even though undermined. Some authors spare patent blood vessels to minimize more extensive gangrene.

After incision and debridement through the superficial fascia, the wound is treated by rest, elevation, and frequent dressing changes, which aid in the mechanical debridement. If gangrene progresses, repeated debridement may be necessary. Skin grafting can be carried out in denuded areas when a granulating base has been established.

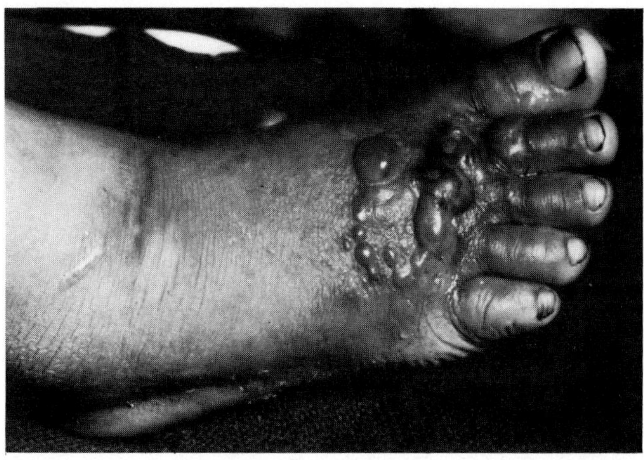

Fig. 25-11. **Clostridial cellulitis of the foot. Bullae, full of black bacteria-laden fluid, are present in the skin. The infection is spreading in the fascial cleft that overlies the tendons of the foot. This is essentially a necrotizing fasciitis, and it appears clinically identical to some cases of streptococcal gangrene. (From Baxter CR: Surgical management of soft tissue infection. *Surg Clin North Am* 52:1483, 1972.)**

NECROTIZING FASCIITIS

Definition

Although the term necrotizing fasciitis originally described streptococcal gangrene, currently it more commonly means mixed bacterial infections. Necrotizing fasciitis, clostridial cellulitis, nonclostridial anaerobic cellulitis, anaerobic cutaneous gangrene, Fournier gangrene, and synergistic necrotizing cellulitis all have a similar pathogenesis, treatment, and prognosis. Each is essentially an infection of the subcutaneous tissues (ie, the superficial fascia), which spreads in the fascial clefts overlying deep fascia and sparing the skin. Skin gangrene results only after the vessels to the skin thrombose. Each of these syndromes was originally described separately, and new terminology is constantly appearing in the literature (Table 25-20).

Etiology

A variety of organisms have been reported as predominant in these infections, including beta-hemolytic streptococcus,[39] the hemolytic staphylococcus, and gram-negative organisms,[25] in addition to gram-positive cocci. Rea and Wyrick [40] confirmed that mixtures of bacteria were typical and claimed that inadequate collection or laboratory bacteriology techniques were responsible for failure to document the mixed etiology of this infection.

Most available data now suggest that necrotizing fasciitis is most often a synergistic bacterial surgical infection, produced by the combination of gram-positive cocci and gram-negative bacilli. Both aerobes and anaerobes are typically found. Modern bacteriologic techniques have clarified the etiology to some degree: Tables 25-21 and 25-22 list the bacteria cultured from 16 patients with necrotizing fasciitis by Guiliano et al.[41] A total of 75 bacterial species were identified in the 16 patients (Table 25-21). At least one facultative *Streptococcus* was recovered from 15

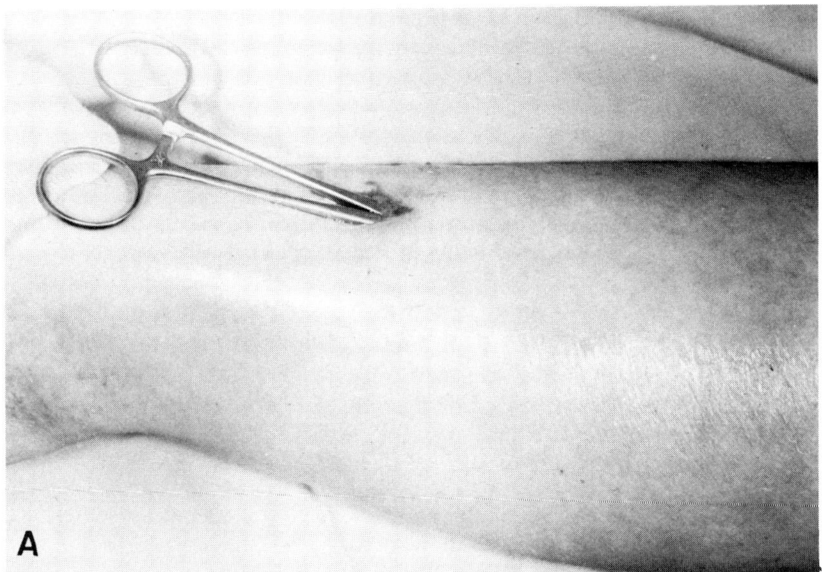

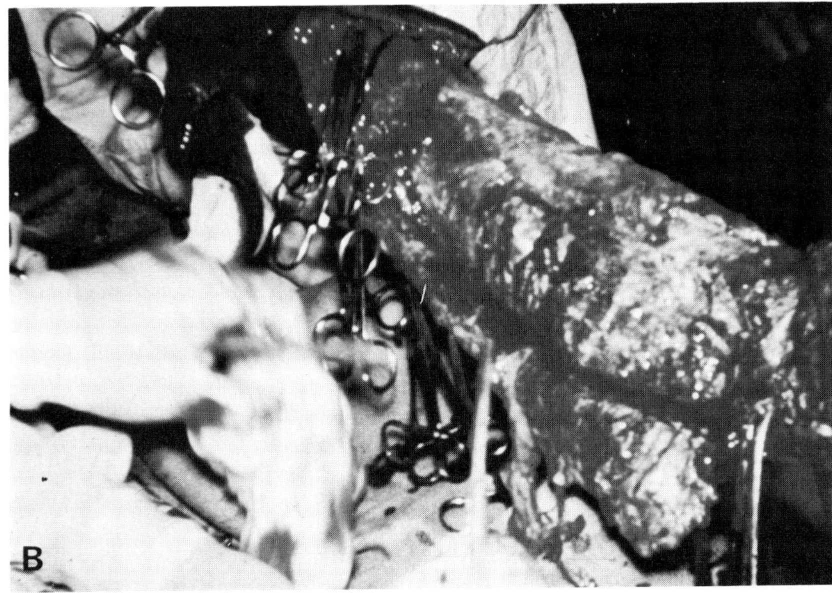

Fig. 25-12. Necrotizing fasciitis. A. A probe can be passed along the fascial cleft between the subcutaneous tissue and deep fascia in a patient in whom only a small draining tract is visible. (From Baxter CR: Surgical management of soft tissue infection. *Surg Clin North Am* 52:1483, 1972.) B. Incision reveals extensive necrosis of subcutaneous tissue and fascia (Courtesy of P. William Curreri, MD, New York Hospital, Cornell Medical Center, New York, NY.)

patients, a *Bacteroides* species was recovered from 10, and a *Peptostreptococcus* from eight. Giuliano et al conclude that there are two types of necrotizing fasciitis. Most commonly anaerobic bacteria and facultative bacteria (Enterobacteriaceae and streptococci other than group A) act in combination; anaerobes are rarely cultured alone. In the second group, group *A Streptococcus* was isolated alone or in combination with *S. aureus* or *S. epidermidis* representing classical streptococcal gangrene (see preceding section).

The organisms cultured by Stone and Martin [25] were different in many regards. Giuliano's patients [41] were primarily drug addicts with infections of the upper extremities, trunk, and shoulders, whereas the patients of Stone and Martin were debilitated bedridden patients, frequently with diabetes, with infections of the lower extremities, trunk, and perineal regions. No beta-hemolytic streptococci were found, but there was a higher incidence of facultative (aerobic) gram-negative bacilli (62 percent) and enterococcus (19 percent) in combination with anaerobic *Streptococcus* (51 percent) and *Bacteroides* species (24 percent).[25] Both sets of investigators speculate that synergism between aerobic and anaerobic organisms is taking place.[25,41]

Pathogenesis and Pathology

The infection is almost always introduced through a break in the skin—the subcutaneous or intravenous injection of illicit drugs, an incised wound, an enterostomy, a decubitus ulcer, perineal fistula, or diabetic foot. Of the 63 patients studied by Stone and Martin,[25] 47 had diabetes, 33 cardiovascular and renal disease, and 54 were either starved or obese. In drug addicts, extremity infections are most common; in other patients, infections of the trunk, perineum, buttocks, and thighs represent spread of infection

TABLE 25-21. BACTERIA CULTURED FROM NECROTIZING FASCIITIS

	Total no. of Isolates
ANAEROBIC BACTERIA (GRAM-POSITIVE)	
Peptostreptococcus species	8
Peptococcus species	4
Eubacterium species	1
Propionibacterium species	4
Clostridium perfringens	3
Clostridium (not perfringens)	1
ANAEROBIC BACTERIA (GRAM-NEGATIVE)	
Bacteroides (total)	15
B. melaninogenicus	5
B. fragilis	2
B. corrodens	2
B. species	6
Fusobacterium necrophorum	1
FACULTATIVE BACTERIA	
Streptococcus (total)	22
S. pyogenes (group A)	3
S. agalactiae (group B)	1
Streptococcus (group D)	
enterococcus	4
S. bovis	2
S. angiosus (group F)	1
Streptococcus, beta-hemolytic (not group A, B, or F)	3
S. intermedius	1
Streptococcus, alpha-hemolytic (not group D)	7
Staphylococcus aureus	0
S. epidermidis	1
Enterobacteriaceae (total)	12
Escherichia coli	4
Citrobacter freundii	1
Klebsiella pneumoniae	2
Enterobacter cloacae	2
Serratia marcescens	2
Proteus mirabilis	1
AEROBIC BACTERIA	
Pseudomonas aeruginosa	2

All bacteria isolated from each specimen are counted in this table. Individual patient's cultures may contain more than one *Bacteroides,* Enterobacteriaceae, or other group.

From Giuliano A, Lewis F Jr, Hadley K, Blaisdell FW: Bacteriology of necrotizing fasciitis. *Am J Surg* 134:52, 1977.

from previously infected sites that had been overlooked or ignored. Phycomycotic gangrene must be considered in all such infections (Table 25-20).

The role of synergism in mixed bacterial infections has been discussed in Chapter 8. Little is known about synergistic infections of the soft tissues. It is assumed that facultative bacteria assist the growth of anaerobes by utilizing oxygen, diminishing the redox potential, or supplying catalase which detoxifies H_2O_2. Proof of bacterial synergism in these infections is lacking. *S. pyogenes,* group A, is capable of producing a necrotizing fasciitis either alone or in the presence of staphylococcus.

Clinical Manifestations

The course of necrotizing fasciitis is variable (Table 25-20). Usually the portal of entry is obvious—the site of trauma, postoperative wound infection, or extension from a previous site of primary infection, ie, perirectal abscess, infected decubitus ulcer, infected diabetic ulcer. It may remain an indolent undermining infection or may become suddenly fulminant and rapidly progress to gangrene and death, in a manner similar to acute streptococcal gangrene.

In the chronic progressive type, cellulitis, rather than gangrene, predominates. Multiple skin ulcers drain a thin, reddish-brown, foul-smelling fluid characterized by Stone and Martin [25] as "dishwater pus." The telltale signs are multiple ulcers, which communicate beneath superficially normal, but extensively undermined, intervening skin. Superficial gangrene is limited. Crepitance in the soft tissues is frequent, and sensation may range from exquisite local tenderness to anesthesia.

The diagnosis is easily made by passing a probing instrument through the area of necrosis and determining that undermining exists between the subcutaneous tissue and deep fascia (Fig. 25-12). In simple cellulitis or abscess, such a probing instrument cannot be passed laterally into the fascial cleft parallel to the skin surface.

Frank pus is an unusual finding despite widespread necrosis. Thus, the extent of the necrosis is frequently overlooked until sudden systemic toxicity supervenes. In fact, most patients are admitted with symptoms and signs of septicemia. At that time, blood cultures are frequently positive, and hypercalcemia may occur when necrosis of the subcutaneous tissues is extensive. Only then are the rather insignificant ulcerating lesions recognized as the septic source. In short, the classic clinical picture is a manifestation of neglect. Without question, the undermining infection takes a long time to develop. The factors which foster a septicemic rather than indolent outcome are unknown—but diabetes, anemia, and renal failure are commonly found.[25]

At the other clinical extreme, a picture identical with acute streptococcal gangrene can be seen in which clinical attention is immediately focused on extensive areas of cutaneous gangrene involving the skin, with patchy areas of dusky necrosis progressing to frank eschar formation or bullae (Fig. 25-11). These patients also demonstrate fever, chills, and shock, but the local process is obvious.

Numerous terms have been applied to these subcutaneous necrotizing infections (Table 25-20). Some deserve special comment:

1. *Clostridial anaerobic cellulitis* is a necrotizing clostridial infection of devitalized subcutaneous tissues without involvement of deep fascia or muscle. Gas formation is often extensive. Clostridial species, usually *C. perfringens* or *C. septicum,* can be seen on Gram stain and culture. The infection is usually found at the sites of dirty or inadequately debrided traumatic wounds, especially around the perineum, abdominal wall, buttocks, and lower extremities, ie, areas contaminated with fecal flora. The clinical picture is similar to necrotizing fasciitis (Table 25-20) but has few of the features of gas gangrene. A dark foul-smelling drainage, often containing fat globules, has been described; frank crepitus seems to extend widely beyond

TABLE 25-22. BACTERIAL ASSOCIATIONS OBSERVED IN 16 CASES OF NECROTIZING FASCIITIS

	Frequency	All Str, Not Group D	Group D Str	aH Str Not Group D	Group A Str	S	E	B	C	P	PS
FREQUENCY		12	4	6	3	2	9	10	4	4	8
Bacteroides (B)	10	10	4	6	0	0	6	—	2	4	7
Fusobacterium	1	1	1	1	0	0	1	1	1	1	1
Clostridium (C)	4	3	3	1	0	0	4	2	—	0	1
Propionibacterium	4	4	1	3	0	0	2	3	0	2	4
Peptococcus (P)	4	4	1	3	0	0	2	4	0	—	4
Peptostreptococcus (PS)	8	8	2	5	0	0	5	7	1	4	—

When more than one organism of a genus or group is isolated from one specimen, it is counted only once in this table. Str = streptococcus; aH = alpha-hemolytic; S = staphylococcus; E = Enterobacteriaceae.

From Giuliano A, Lewis F Jr, Hadley K, Blaisdell FW: Bacteriology of necrotizing fasciitis. *Am J Surg* 134:52, 1977.

the areas of active infection. Roentgenograms of soft tissue show abundant gas. Sometimes, the clostridia are present in mixed culture with facultative organisms. The operative treatment is identical to necrotizing fasciitis.

2. *Nonclostridial anaerobic cellulitis* presents a picture similar to that of clostridial anaerobic cellulitis. The syndrome is essentially identical to necrotizing fasciitis, but mixed anaerobic flora predominate.

3. *Synergistic necrotizing cellulitis* refers to a variant of necrotizing fasciitis with systemic toxicity and bacteremia occurring in patients with diabetes mellitus, obesity, advanced age, and cardiorenal disease.[25] Most infections are located on the lower extremities or near the perineum. Bacteremia and death are common.

4. *Fornier's gangrene*[42] occurs about the male genitals (idiopathic gangrene of the scrotum, streptococcal scrotal gangrene, perineal phlegmon) (Fig. 25-13). It may involve the scrotum and surrounding perineum, penis and abdominal wall in patients with diabetes, local trauma, paraphimosis, periurethral extravasation of urine, perirectal or perineal infections, and may follow operation in the area. The extensive gangrene of the skin is due to interruption of the blood supply to the scrotum and is readily involved by spreading perineal necrotizing fasciitis. The organisms are those seen in necrotizing fasciitis in this region, including facultative enteric organisms (*E. coli, Klebsiella,* enterococci) and anaerobes (*Bacteroides, Fusobacterium,* clostridia, anaerobic peptostreptococci) (Chapter 45).

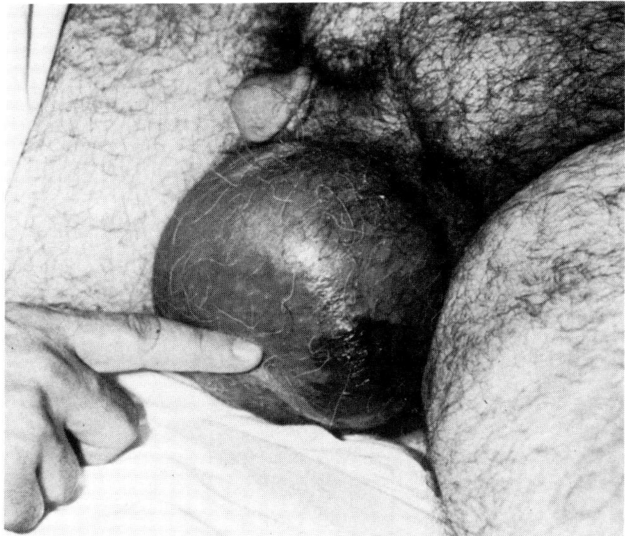

Fig. 25-13. **Fournier's gangrene is necrotizing fasciitis of the scrotum and perineum with a patch of skin gangrene. (From Charles A. Kallick MD, Cook County Hospital, Chicago.)**

Diagnosis

The etiologic diagnosis is readily made on Gram stain of exudate. Most often mixed gram-positive and gram-negative organisms are found except in patients with streptococcal or clostridial gangrene. Phycomycotic infections may have a similar presentation, but the diagnosis is best made on the basis of the histopathologic picture.[43] Other aspects of the differential diagnosis of gangrenous infections are listed in Table 25-20. The differential diagnosis of crepitant soft tissue is listed in Table 25-16.

Treatment

Infections of the trunk, perineum, perirectal area, periurethral area, buttock, and thigh frequently involve four types of organisms: Enterobacteriaceae, enterococci, anaerobic streptococci, and *Bacteroides.* It would seem appropriate in these potentially fatal infections to begin triple drug therapy, including ampicillin (for enterococci and anaerobic peptostreptococci), an aminoglycoside for the Enterobacteriaceae, and clindamycin for *B. fragilis* and peptostreptococci. The new broad-spectrum cephalosporin antibiotics, such as cefoxitin, moxalactam, or cefotaxime have not yet been evaluated for these mixed infections. Other antibiotic combinations, such as carbenicillin and tobramycin, may be effective but remain second choices. Cloramphenicol with its broad spectrum and efficacy in vitro against *B. fragilis* is a useful alternative, but because it is bacteriostatic, potentially toxic, and occasionally ineffective against *B. fragilis,* it is not recommended as a first choice. Penicillin G is effective for clostridial or beta-hemolytic streptococcal necrotizing fasciitis.

Blood culture results are frequently positive in patients with necrotizing fasciitis, and one might choose an antibiotic based on these results. Stone and Martin [25] found the blood cultures were positive for gram-negative rods in more than one-third of the cases, and an anaerobe could be isolated from the blood in 20 percent. Mixed bacteria were only isolated from the blood cultures in six of 63 patients, but mixed infections were always present in the wounds. Antibiotic therapy should not be based only on blood cultures but on the presumptive bacteria in the wound. Frequently, clinical laboratories fail to culture the anaerobic organisms in mixed infections, so that the clinician is tempted to prematurely discontinue those agents directed at presumptive anaerobes.

The primary therapy of necrotizing fasciitis is radical debridement. The incision should extend beyond the outermost extent of the fascial involvement in all planes. The dead material is resected, although the skin can frequently be preserved after removal of the necrotic underlying fat. The wounds are packed loosely open with fine mesh gauze, and several small catheters are placed in the wound for constant delivery of local antibiotics (Fig. 25-12). Baxter [44] recommends a solution containing 100 mg of neomycin and 100 mg of polymixin B per liter of normal saline. Other workers would prefer less toxic antibiotics (eg, carbenicillin).

The fine mesh gauze should be changed frequently during the first days after the operation. These dressing changes aid in superficial debridement of the wound and permit examination to determine whether additional surgical debridement is necessary.

Repeated culturing of the wound is necessary as secondary inoculation with *Pseudomonas, Serratia,* and *Candida* occurs. Fascial porcine heterografts can be used to cover the wound, as in burns. The porcine heterografts can be left in place until there is complete adherence of the biologic dressing. When the wound is ready (less than 10^5 organisms per gram of tissue) under the biologic cover, the large skin flaps may be replaced, and any remaining open areas grafted with split thickness skin grafts. A meshed graft is advantageous for covering these large wounds. Sulfamylon or silver sulfadiazine can be applied to the open wounds, as in treatment for burns, to retard secondary infection.

Prognosis

The prognosis is grave and depends in part on the underlying disease, the physiologic condition of the patient, delay in treatment, the site of infection, and the bacteriology of the wound. In young drug addicts with mixed gram-positive aerobic and anaerobic infections, amputation is occasionally necessary for infections of the distal extremity. In the series of Giuliano et al,[41] only two of 16 patients died. In the more chronically debilitated patients treated by Stone and Martin,[25] the overall mortality was 76 percent and almost 50 percent of the patients died within a week after admission. All surviving patients had considerable residual morbidity and a prolonged hospital course.

Patients with severe renal disease almost never survive, and diabetes mellitus significantly worsens the prognosis (85 percent mortality). One of the most decisive influences on survival was the area of involvement. When the infection developed within an extremity, radical debridement by either amputation or disarticulation was usually practical. All patients with deep infections of the pelvis and neck died, and there were only two survivors of the 24 patients with extension from a perirectal origin, whereas infections of the buttock and distal extremities had a lower mortality. If these progressive lesions had been recognized before the onset of systemic sepsis, survival results certainly would have been better.

BACTERIAL SYNERGISTIC GANGRENE

Bacterial synergistic gangrene (progressive synergistic gangrene, Meleney synergistic gangrene) is an infection primarily of the subcutaneous tissue, which rarely spreads in the fascial planes, although it is caused by the same organisms found in aerobic and anaerobic cellulitis, subcutaneous abscesses, and necrotizing fasciitis.

Etiology

The classic etiology is the combination of a microaerophilic nonhemolytic streptococcus that is found primarily in the spreading periphery of the lesion, and *S. aureus* in the zone of gangrene. The microaerophilic streptococcus has been found to be *S. evolutus.*[45] The *Streptococcus* can be an obligate anaerobe, and a wide variety of other organisms can be seen instead of or in addition to the *Staphylococcus; Proteus, Enterobacter, Pseudomonas,* and *Clostridium* species have been isolated. The microaerophilic streptococcus may be difficult to isolate in culture.

Clinical Manifestations

Bacterial synergistic gangrene (Table 25-20) develops most often following abdominal or thoracic surgery or drainage of a peritoneal abscess or thoracic empyema. Sometimes, it develops around a colostomy or ileostomy site or following a trivial accidental wound. The major symptom is severe pain and tenderness. The lesion first appears about 2 weeks after wounding, in an area around the foreign body suture or wound closure. A purple central area of induration becomes surrounded by a zone of erythema. Tenderness is pronounced. As the lesion progresses, three zones become demarcated: (1) the outer zone is fiery red, (2) the middle zone is purple and tender, and (3) the central portion of the purplish area becomes frankly gangrenous, the color changing to a dirty gray-brown or a yellow-green with a typical suede leather appearance. As the lesion spreads outward, the inner margin of the gangrenous zone becomes undermined and melts away. Eventually, the center of the lesion becomes a granulating ulcer, and epithelium may be seen to generate here (Fig. 25-14). The progression is slow but unremitting. The depth is usually limited to the upper third of the subcutaneous

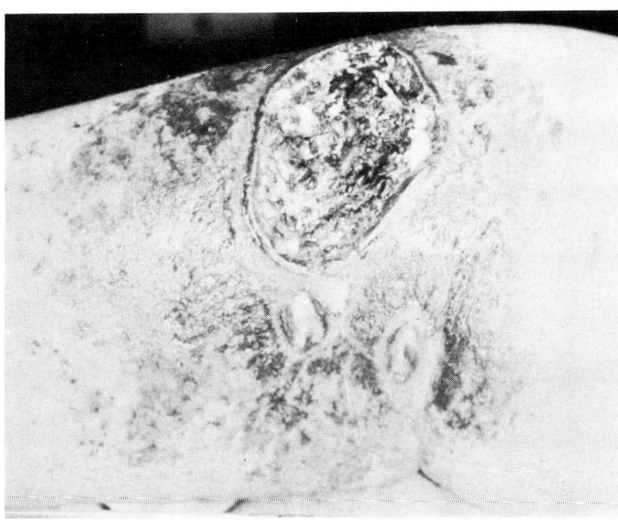

Fig. 25-14. **Bacterial synergistic gangrene. Central necrosis with undermining edges, a purple irregular border, and an outer zone of redness. Satellite lesions surround the ulcer. (From Baxter CR: Surgical management of soft tissue infection. *Surg Clin North Am* 52:1483, 1972.)**

fat and rarely extends deep to fascia. Satellite lesions may surface as the infection tunnels through the fat. Fever is minimal, but anemia and malnutrition are common.

Chronic undermining ulcer or Meleney ulcer is probably the same disease. In this form, the satellite lesions attract attention, and multiple ulcers and sinuses may develop at a distance from the original ulcer with undermining of the intervening skin.

Treatment

Initially, wide excision alone with zinc peroxide ointment was considered necessary for cure. However, antimicrobial therapy alone may suffice to prevent spread, and debridement will then effect cure. The progress of this disease is slow, and zealous excision is no longer required. The fact that two cases of antibiotic control followed by local steroid treatment have resulted in cure suggests that part of the process may be delayed hypersensitivity response.[45]

GANGRENOUS INFECTIONS OF THE SOFT TISSUES INVOLVING MUSCLE

GAS GANGRENE (CLOSTRIDIAL MYONECROSIS)

Gas gangrene is a rapidly progressive, life-threatening, toxemic infection of skeletal muscles due to *Clostridium* species (principally *C. perfringens*). It usually follows the contamination by animal or human feces of severe crushing muscle injury. It may be part of clostridial cellulitis, but in its classical form, muscle is principally involved.

Etiology

C. perfringens is isolated from 80 to 95 percent of the cases. *C. novyi* is found in 10 to 40 percent, *C. septicum* in 5 to 20 percent, and *C. bifermentans, C. histolyticum,* and *C. phallax* have all been implicated. Other aerobes and facultative organisms are also usually isolated. The clinical syndromes produced are all similar. *C. novyi* is supposed to produce toxemia and massive gelatinous edema with little gas. *C. septicum* is most often associated with colon carcinoma.[45] All *Clostridium* species sporulate, producing potentially lethal organisms resistant to almost all physical and many chemical agents.

Epidemiology and Pathogenesis

C. perfringens and other histotoxic clostridial species are essential for true gas gangrene. They can be inoculated by accidental traumatic or high-velocity wounds, which severely impair muscle viability. Compound fractures are said to be particularly susceptible because of local calcium salts which favor clostridial growth. In addition, they are sometimes seen in wounds after large bowel or biliary tract surgery or in the presence of ischemic impairment of a muscular region, especially after amputations of the lower extremity for ischemic gangrene. Cases have followed contaminated injections, especially of vasospastic agents, such as epinephrine in oil. Three factors are usually present: (1) contamination of wounds with clostridia (eg, fecal contamination), (2) devitalized tissue creating an anaerobic environment, and (3) foreign bodies. Debridement and delayed primary closure of war wounds substantially reduces the incidence. Primary carcinomas of the colon, with or without penetration or perforation, have been associated with gas gangrene. Immunocompromised patients have a high risk even in the presence of minor trauma.

Clinical Manifestations

Table 25-20 compares the clinical manifestations of several gangrenous infections. The incubation period of clostridial myonecrosis is much shorter than for most pyogenic infections; the full-blown picture may be present within 1 to 3 days of wounding. Only group A streptococci or clostridial infections are normally so fulminant. The onset is usually acute—a pain so severe that a vascular catastrophe must be suspected. No other soft tissue infection produces a comparable degree of pain.

The local lesion becomes rapidly edematous, cool, and exquisitely tender. Swollen muscle may herniate through an open wound, and a serosanguinous dirty appearing discharge, which contains numerous organisms but few leukocytes, escapes. The wound has a peculiar sweet but foul odor; gas bubbles may be visible in the discharge. Crepitus, if present, is not as prominent as in other anaerobic soft tissue infections. The skin adjacent to the wound is initially swollen and pale, but rapidly takes on a yellowish or bronze discoloration. Tense blebs containing thick, dark fluid develop in the overlying skin, and areas of green-black cutaneous necrosis appear (Fig. 25-15).

Toxemia is usually severe long before cutaneous gangrene appears. Although the systemic signs are nonspecific, they are a prominent part of the clinical picture. The patient is severely ill, pale, sweaty, and apprehensive. Delirium may follow. Tachycardia, hypotension, shock, and renal failure follow in rapid succession. Fever is gener-

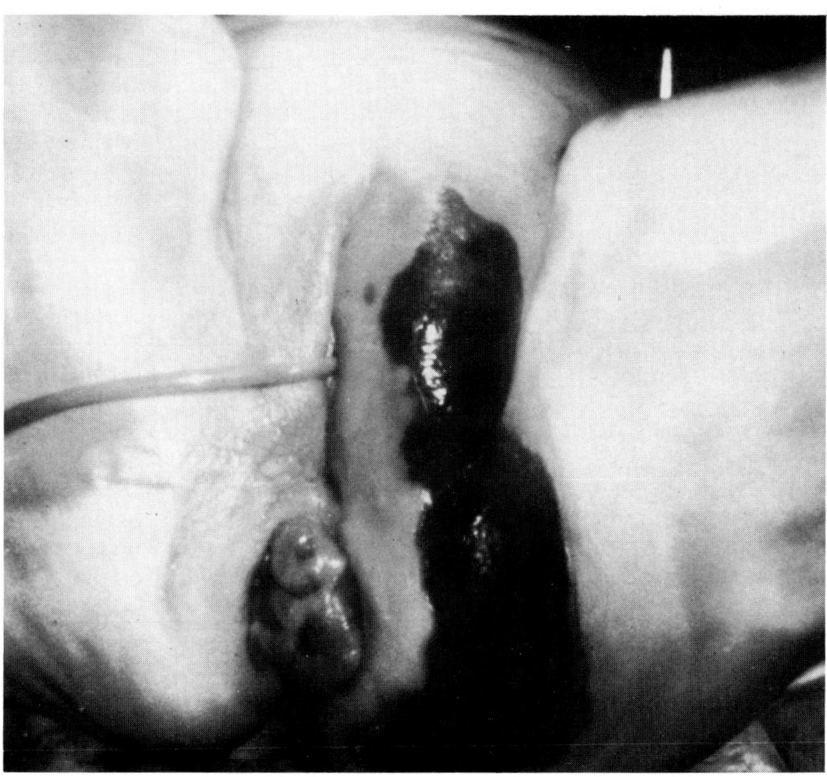

Fig. 25-15. Gas gangrene of perianal region and vulva. The lesion is painful and the skin is bronzed. The central necrotic area overlies a much more extensive area of necrotizing fasciitis and myonecrosis. (Courtesy of Claude R. Hitchcock, MD, chief of surgery, Hennepin County Medical Center, Minneapolis, Minnesota.)

ally not too high, and hypothermia is associated with terminal shock, as is jaundice.

Diagnosis

Operative exploration must be carried out on suspicion. Bacteremia with *C. perfringens* occurs in only 15 percent of the patients with gas gangrene, but hemolysis, presumably associated with bacteremia, is a common complication, especially after intrauterine infections.

Gram-stained smears of the wound exudate or an aspirate from one of the blebs reveals large gram-positive bacilli with blunt ends but few polymorphonuclear leukocytes. Spores are usually not evident. Other gram-positive and gram-negative bacteria may be present, particularly in grossly contaminated wounds, so that the diagnosis can be overlooked if only bacteriologic diagnosis is sought.

Roentgenograms of the involved areas show extensive and progressive gaseous dissection of muscle and fascial planes.

The differential diagnosis is outlined in Table 25-20 and the differential diagnosis of crepitant wound infections in Table 25-16. The degree of toxemia, the rather limited crepitance usually masked by edema, the severe degree of local pain, and the characteristic skin lesions with bronzing, dark blebs, and gross ischemic necrosis differentiate this disease from nonclostridial crepitant myositis and cellulitis. The absence of leukocytes and the presence of clostridia on smear are helpful diagnostic signs, although clostridia can be part of mixed bacterial crepitant and noncrepitant infections such as necrotizing fasciitis.

At exploration, the infected muscle itself may be unimpressive; it may exhibit only pallid edema and elasticity, fail to contract on stimulation, and not bleed from a cut surface. Later, it becomes discolored to a reddish purple before becoming black and friable.

Treatment

Treatment includes emergency operation to define the nature and extent of the gangrenous process, directly examine the muscles at the site of infection, and widely excise the infected tissue. Gram stains of the infected muscle should be carried out during debridement. Only when resected muscle is free of bacteria should debridement be stopped. Some surgeons irrigate the wound in the postoperative period with H_2O_2; others pack the wound with zinc peroxide. All infected or possibly infected muscles should be excised, and fasciiotomies performed to decompress and drain the swollen or potentially swollen fascial compartments of adjacent uninfected muscle groups. Amputation is a highly effective treatment of distal infections and should be carried out promptly in any patient with clostridial myonecrosis who manifests systemic toxicity. For this reason, the mortality is much higher for truncal and perineal gas gangrene than for limb infections. All wounds should be left to close by secondary intention. Repeated inspection of the wound in the operating room is necessary at frequent intervals after primary debridement to determine if further excision is required.

Antibiotic Therapy. Antibiotic therapy is essential. Penicillin G is administered intravenously in a dosage of 1 to 2 million units every 2 to 3 hours. Most authorities advocate a second antibiotic (chloramphenicol for mixed infections or an aminoglycoside).[46] Chloramphenicol is a good alternative drug in the penicillin-allergic patient. A few strains of *Clostridium* are resistant to tetracycline and clindamycin.

Ancillary Surgical Therapy. If autogenous fecal contamination is responsible for the infection, diversion of the fecal stream will be required. Skin grafting and other reconstructive procedures are almost always required in survivors.

Hyperbaric Oxygen Therapy. Hyperbaric oxygen therapy has been advocated as an additive treatment, particularly for patients with diffuse spreading infections.[47] Until controlled clinical trials are completed, it may be useful in the management of patients with extensive involvement of the trunk or perineum where adequate surgical debridement is impossible. It is not a substitute for debridement or antibiotics.

General Maintenance. Attention to fluid and electrolyte balance and nutrition is essential in the management of these patients. Renal failure and secondary organ failure syndromes are common.

Antitoxin. A polyvalent gas gangrene antitoxin is no longer available, and its usefulness was controversial. Before the ready availability of penicillin, military surgeons were convinced of its value,[45] though the mechanism of action was unclear. Finegold strongly advocates its use when there is evidence of hemolysis.[45]

Prevention

The disease in wartime is more rare than in civilian practice. The military medical policy of wide debridement of all fresh wounds with delayed (4-day) primary closure has effectively reduced the incidence. Prophylactic antibiotics for wounded patients may be useful adjuncts, but prophylactic excision of all devitalized tissue is the principal prophylactic maneuver. Only 22 cases occurred in 139,000 casualties in Vietnam, where this policy was generally followed. There were 27 cases in Miami in a recent 10-year period, suggesting that the policy is not followed in civilian practice.[48]

NONCLOSTRIDIAL INFECTIOUS MYONECROSIS

Myonecrosis can be caused by organisms other than *Clostridium*—most prominent among them is the anaerobic *Streptococcus.*

Anaerobic Streptococcal Myonecrosis

Anaerobic streptococcal myonecrosis is a rare disease even in wartime. The anaerobic streptococci are usually accompanied by *S. aureus* or group A streptococci. The predisposing causes are the same as for clostridial myonecrosis, but the incubation period is longer (3 to 4 days) and the course less fulminating. The wounded area is edematous, and seropurulent drainage is seen. Pain is not the initial symptom but can become severe. Gas is present but not extensive. The odor may be sour. Toxemia is a later and preterminal sign. When *S. pyogenes* or *S. aureus* are present, the wound takes on some of the clinical characteristics of infections with these organisms. Treatment with wide debridement and penicillin is appropriate. Penicillinase-resistant penicillins or cephalosporins should be added for *S. aureus.*

Synergistic Nonclostridial Anaerobic Myonecrosis

The disease is similar to necrotizing cellulitis or necrotizing cutaneous myositis,[44] in which the skin, subcutaneous tissue, fascia, and muscle are all involved. As in necrotizing fasciitis, many patients have diabetes or other debilitating conditions. *B. fragilis* is the key pathogen, in combination with aerobic or anaerobic streptococci and facultative gram-negative enteric organisms. Basically, this disease is necrotizing fasciitis with muscular involvement. Combination antibiotics (aminoglycoside plus clindamycin) are required as adjuncts to wide debridement.

Infected Vascular Gangrene

Infected vascular gangrene is simply secondary infection of a dead extremity in which amputation has been delayed. A variety of organisms have been reported, and true gas gangrene also occurs.

PRIMARY PYOGENIC BACTERIAL INFECTION OF SKELETAL MUSCLE

Skeletal muscle infection (infectious myositis) is rare. Bacteria, viruses, and parasitic agents can each be responsible. Bacteria can invade muscle either from contiguous sites or by hematogenous spread. Swartz [49] has characterized infectious myositis on the basis of clinical manifestations (Table 25-23). Nonpyogenic myositis will not be discussed here.

PYOMYOSITIS

Pyomyositis is a primary acute bacterial infection of skeletal muscle, usually due to *S. aureus* in the absence of apparent predisposing conditions. Blood cultures are usually negative, and disseminated staphylococcal sepsis is rarely associated with pyomyositis.

Tropical pyomyositis accounts for 1 to 4 percent of hospital admissions in some tropical areas, but in the United States pyomyositis occurs rarely, except in persons who have recently immigrated from the tropics. In some cases, recent trauma to the involved areas suggests that local muscle damage predisposes to infection by transient staphylococcal bacteremia.

Etiology

The disease is usually due to *S. aureus,* with rare cases due to *S. pneumoniae* and *E. coli.* A fulminant form due

TABLE 25-23. CLASSIFICATION OF INFECTIOUS MYOSITIS

Type of Process	Clinical Pattern	Principal Specific Etiologies
Pyogenic and predominantly localized (spreading by contiguity)	Pyomyositis	*S. aureus;* group A streptococcus (rarely);
	Gas gangrene	*C. perfringens;* occasionally other histotoxic clostridial species
	Nonclostridial (crepitant myositis) anaerobic streptococcal gangrene	*Peptostreptococcus* (plus group A streptococci or *S. aureus*
		Mixed infections: *Bacteroides* and other anaerobic non-spore-forming gram-negative bacilli; *Peptostreptococcus* and various streptococci; *E. coli; Klebsiella; Enterobacter*
	Infected vascular gangrene	Same as for synergistic nonclostridial anaerobic myonecrosis
	Psoas abscess	Gram-negative bacilli; *S. aureus* mixed infections; *M. tuberculosis*
Nonpyogenic and predominantly generalized	Myalgias	Viral infections (eg, influenza, dengue); infective endocarditis; bacteremias (eg, meningococcemia); rickettsioses (eg, Rocky Mountain spotted fever); toxoplasmosis
	Pleurodynia syndromes	*Coxsackievirus B*
	Myalgias with eosinophilia	
	Trichinosis	*Trichinella spiralis*
	Cysticercosis (also subcutaneous nodules)	*Taenia solium*
	Muscle degeneration and destruction associated with infections elsewhere	
	Acute rhabdomyolysis	Viral influenza
	Zenker degeneration	*S. typhi*

From Swartz MN: Myositis. In Mandell GL, Douglas RG Jr, Bennett JE (eds): *Principles and Practices of Infectious Diseases,* Vol 1. New York, Wiley, 1979, p 818.

to group A streptococci [50] has been reported with an associated high mortality.

Clinical Manifestations

In the typical case, there is gradual development over several days of localized muscle pain, swelling, and tenderness. Fever generally follows the appearance of local findings, although an acute onset appears in some circumstances.

The muscles of the lower limb and trunk are most frequently affected, and a single muscle group is usually involved. The initial local swelling is diffuse and only moderately tender. Erythema and heat appear only when the infection dissects into the subcutaneous tissues. Leukocytosis and elevation of serum muscle enzyme levels are common. Eosinophilia has been reported but may simply reflect the prevalence of concurrent parasitic infestation in patients from tropical areas.

Treatment

The abscesses should be incised and evacuated. Excision is not necessary, but drainage until the granulating cavity is clean is essential.

Initial antibiotic therapy should be a beta-lactamase–resistant penicillin or cephalosporin to treat the presumptive *S. aureus.* Failure to improve after drainage and antibiotic therapy suggests the presence of other sites.

INFECTIONS OF MUSCLE SHEATHS

Although experimental studies do not demonstrate that skeletal muscle is more resistant to a standard innoculum of bacteria than fat,[1] infections of viable muscle with pyogenic organisms are rare. Muscle sheaths, on the other hand, can become infected secondary to contiguous infection. Two such sheath infections are relatively common—psoas abscess and rectus sheath abscess.

Psoas Abscess

Psoas abscess is an infection confined within the psoas fascia usually secondary to contiguous infections. Since the fascial envelope extends into the groin, the infection may point in the inguinal region. The classic cause is pyogenic or tuberculous osteomyelitis, but now it is more commonly the result of the direct extension of intra-abdominal infections, ie, diverticulitis, appendicitis, Crohn disease, carcinoma of the colon. A perinephric abscess or secondary infection of a retroperitoneal hematoma are also predisposing causes. *S. aureus* is the most common cause of psoas abscess secondary to vertebral osteomyelitis, and mixed infections arrive from perinephric or intraintestinal infections.

The clinical manifestations include fever, lower abdominal back pain, pain referred to the hip or knee, and associated limp. Flexion of the hip may develop from reflex spasm, suggesting septic arthritis of the hip. The psoas sign is evident, ie, pain on passive extension of the hip. Sometimes, a tender mass can be palpated in the groin, and gas may be present on roentgenograms of the abdomen. Calcification of the psoas abscess suggests a tuberculous etiology. The abscess cavity can be evacuated and drained through the groin or through a retroperitoneal approach through the flank. Antibiotic therapy and correction of the principal intraperitoneal cause are essential.

Rectus Sheath Abscess

A rectus sheath abscess is usually secondary to a transabdominal operation in which the rectus sheath has been opened—paramedian or transverse incision. Almost invariably, such infections are the result of extension of intra-abdominal infection or an early manifestation of a visceral-cutaneous fistula. Contiguous sites of sepsis should always be sought.

CONTIGUOUS OSTEOMYELITIS

Virtually any soft tissue infection can lead to osteomyelitis of underlying bone (Chapter 42). Usually, however, such diseases have had a protracted chronic course because intact bone is relatively resistant to a direct invasion. This is in contrast to hematogenous spread to which intact bone is extremely sensitive. Contiguous osteomyelitis should be suspected in any chronic soft tissue infection that does not respond to antimicrobial therapy and local soft tissue debridement. Staphylococci, *Pseudomonas*, and mixed enteric organisms are frequently isolated. The patients may present with a chronic draining sinus tract or old decubitus ulcer.

Clinically this is a difficult diagnosis. Bone scans only detect hyperemia of the bone, which may be due to surrounding tissue reaction or even a fracture. Plain radiographs acutely show a slight haziness and loss of definition in the bone structure which may progress to a radiolucency or increased radiodensity with the formation of a sequestrum.

The diagnosis is definitively made upon bone biopsy which shows boney involvement with the infection. Culture of the biopsy specimen is necessary to make an etiologic diagnosis because the soft tissue may be contaminated. Mixed aerobic and anaerobic organisms are common. Finegold [45] has suggested that anaerobic growth is facilitated in bone because the mineral components neutralize the fatty acids which are the end products of anaerobic bacterial metabolism. This allows continued growth of the bacteria which otherwise would be inhibited by these end products.

Treatment of this condition is rather difficult. Debridement of devitalized tissue is essential with removal of any sequestrum and grossly infected overlying tissue. Extremities are immobilized and the patient is treated with high dose long-term parenteral antibiotics. In extreme cases, amputation may be necessary for cure (Chapter 42).

UNUSUAL BACTERIAL INFECTIONS OF THE SKIN NOT USUALLY REQUIRING SURGICAL THERAPY

Cutaneous Anthrax

Anthrax is a zoonotic disease which affects the skin, lungs, and gastrointestinal tract in humans.[51] The cutaneous form accounts for 95 percent of the cases seen in the United States. Meningitis and septicemia are common complications of the pulmonary form.

Etiology

Bacillus anthracis is a gram-positive nonmotile encapsulated bacillus producing spores (Chapter 7).

Epidemiology

The disease is limited to workers in contact with raw wool and hides in agriculture and industry.[52] Consumers are rarely afflicted.

Pathogenesis and Pathology

Anthrax spores are inoculated into skin, eaten, or inhaled. The spores germinate, multiply locally, and produce a toxin which induces regional edema, capillary thrombosis, and tissue necrosis. Pulmonary capillary thrombosis is a major cause of respiratory failure. Gastrointestinal anthrax results in ulceration, edema, and mucosal necrosis with hemorrhagic diarrhea.

Clinical Manifestations

Two to five days after inoculation, a small papule appears, which vesiculates. A small ring of vesicles coalesces to form a single large vesicle (malignant pustule) with central ulceration and peripheral erythema and edema. In a few days, the clear vesicular fluid becomes black; rupture reveals a depressed ulcer crater with black eschar. Fever, malaise, lymphangitis, and lymphadenopathy may occur, but progression to general toxemia is rare. Usually, the eschar sloughs off and slow healing takes place.

A disease called malignant edema is used to describe cutaneous anthrax associated with significant local reactions such as multiple bulli, extensive edema, induration, and systemic toxemia. Meningitis complicating cutaneous anthrax can be fatal.

Diagnosis

The diagnosis is suspected when a nontender, pruritic papule on an exposed part of the body vesiculates and forms a black depressed eschar. *B. anthracis* can be recovered from vesicular fluid or from the ulcer exudate. Staphylococcal skin lesions, tularemia, plague, milker's nodules, and contagious pustular dermatitis (ecthyma contagiosum or orf) must be considered in the differential diagnosis. Serologic testing on paired serum specimens confirms the diagnosis. In anthrax meningitis, the organism can be recovered from the cerebrospinal fluid.

Therapy

Cultures should be taken before therapy, since penicillin inhibits bacterial recovery. Parenteral penicillin G is required for severe cases, but oral penicillin G cures the mild ones. Erythromycin, tetracycline, and chloramphenicol are also effective. Antibiotic ointments have no effect. Steroids may counter malignant edema.

Prevention

Workers exposed to wool can be immunized. To prevent spread, lesions should be kept covered and soiled dressings should be incinerated.

Prognosis

Untreated cutaneous anthrax is lethal in 10 to 20 percent of cases; fewer than 1 percent of patients die with effective antimicrobial therapy. Cutaneous lesions progress to a black eschar regardless of therapy. Protective immunity results. Antibody increases are found in employees of goat hair mills with no history of anthrax, suggesting that subclinical infections occur.[51,52]

Cutaneous Diphtheria

Diphtheria is primarily a systemic illness caused by diphtherial toxin, an extracellular protein elaborated by toxogenic strains of *C. diphtheriae*[53] (Chapter 7). Primary pharyngeal infections are classic, but cutaneous infection occurs after inoculation into the skin. Systemic toxicity and postdiphtheritic complications of myocarditis and polyneuritis are rare after cutaneous disease.

Etiology and Epidemiology

The characteristics of *C. diphtheriae* and its toxin are discussed in Chapter 7. This organism should be carefully distinguished from other *Corynebacterium* species, including the skin saprophytes. Poor hygiene, especially in tropical areas, predisposes to the cutaneous disease in unimmunized persons. Patients with cutaneous disease are important reservoirs in epidemics.[53]

Pathogenesis and Pathology

Diphtheria toxin is systemically absorbed from the local site of infection and primarily affects myocardial, renal tubular, and central nervous cells. It is internalized by endocytosis, blocks protein synthesis, and kills affected cells. At the site of local infection, a fibrinopurulent membrane forms, but deep erosion is not seen.

Clinical Manifestations

Three types of skin disease are described: (1) wound diphtheria—a membrane partially covers the wound, which is surrounded by edema and erythema; (2) primary cutaneous diphtheria begins as a tender pustule, which ruptures to reveal an oval punched-out ulcer with a grey membrane at the base. The ulcer has edematous, rolled, bluish margins; and (3) superinfection of eczematoid skin. Myocarditis is a rare complication, but neurologic symptoms (blurred vision, diplopia, numbness of tongue, palatal paralysis, and the Guillain-Barré syndrome) have been described in 3 to 5 percent of patients with cutaneous diphtheria.

Diagnosis

C. diphtheriae are visible in methylene blue or toluidine blue-stained smears of the membrane and are isolated on selective media (Loeffler or tellurite agar). Demonstration of toxin production in vitro confirms the diagnosis.

Treatment

Diphtheria antitoxin (20,000–40,000 units intramuscularly or intravenously) is essential after skin testing and desensitization because neurologic complications can occur even in cutaneous disease. Antibiotics (procaine penicillin 2 million units per day for 7 to 10 days, or erythromycin) and debridement of necrotic tissue may help eliminate the carrier state. Active immunization is also necessary in convalescent patients.[54]

Prevention

Active immunization using toxoid (formalin detoxified diphtheria toxin) prevents the complications of diphtheria but not the infection itself and is routine in children receiving diphtheria-pertussis-tetanus (DPT) shots. Immunity lasts only 10 years, so virtually the whole adult population is unprotected. The Schick test is a test of antitoxin immunity using a minute amount of diphtherial toxin injected intradermally, which causes an inflammatory reaction in 4 to 7 days in the absence of immunity (Schick-positive). The presence of circulating antitoxin blocks the response, indicating immunity (Shick-negative). Reimmunization with highly purified toxoid is advisable in combination with tetanus toxoid immunization.

THE TREPONEMATOSES—SYPHILIS

Etiology

Treponema pallidum is discussed in Chapter 7. *T. pallidum* can produce virtually every manifestation of disease seen in the skin and mucous membranes. In the past, massive textbooks were produced to illustrate these presentations. Disease can be transmitted by placental transmission from the mother resulting in congenital syphilis, but other infections are usually acquired by sexual activity.[55]

Clinical Manifestations

Primary syphilis is characterized by a chancre which appears approximately 3 weeks after inoculation. The chancre is painless, slightly tender, and has a relatively clean base, without undermining or raised edges (Fig. 25–16). A nontender, nonfluctuant, rather firm regional lymphadenopathy (bubo) may accompany the chancre (chancre complex). Healing takes 3 to 6 weeks. Any other sexually transmitted disease can coexist and last longer. Secondary

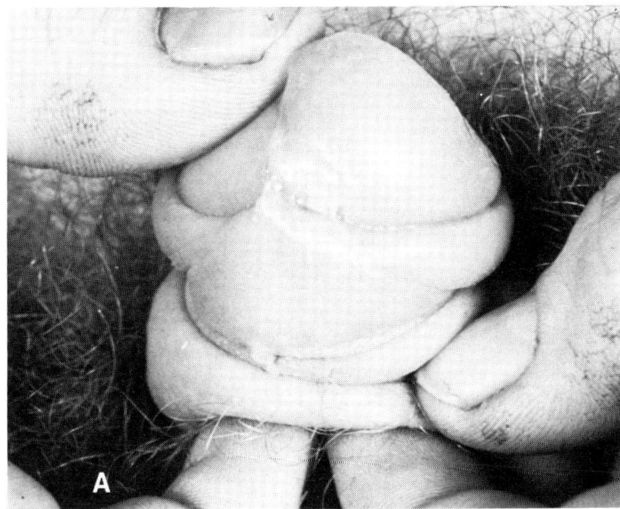

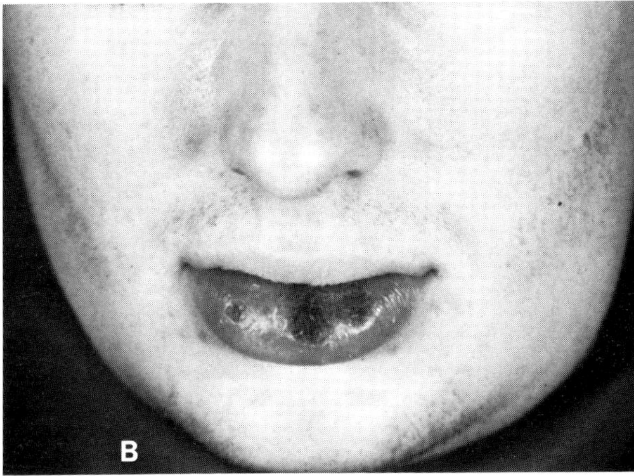

Fig. 25-16. **A primary syphilis chancre of the (A) glans penis, and (B) lip. (Courtesy of Robert W. Goltz, MD, professor and head, Department of Dermatology, University of Minnesota, Minneapolis, Minnesota.)**

bacterial infection may produce local pain. Extragenital chancres on the lip, mouth, fingers, breasts, or anus are usually associated with an enlarged unilateral lymph node. Chancres in females commonly go unnoticed because of an internal location.

The secondary cutaneous lesions, appearing within a few weeks after healing the chancre, are usually dry, macular, or papular, and involve any skin surface. They can mimic any dermatosis, but lesions of the palms and soles suggest the diagnosis. Pustules may occur and lead to surgical consultation; frankly vesicular or bullous lesions are absent. In intertriginous areas or on mucous membranes, the papules may coalesce and erode to produce moist grey or red plaques (condyloma lata), which teem with spirochetes. The secondary skin manifestations can be accompanied by low-grade fever, malaise, leukocytosis, laryngitis, arthralgias, and generalized adenopathy. Arthritis, glomerulonephritis, and hepatitis are rare. Relapses can occur, especially within 2 years of the primary infection.

Soft Tissue Lesions in Late Syphilis. Tertiary syphilis may present as destructive granulomas called gummas (late benign syphilis), most often of subcutaneous tissues but also of bone and any other organ. In the tissues, the nodules are usually single but may be grouped or multiple. Breakdown of the skin may result in a punched-out lesion with a scalloped border. Coalescence of the lesions produces arsiniform and serpiginous outlines, which are characteristic (Fig. 25-17). The lesions may persist for years, with gradual extension at one border and healing in other areas. Lesions of the mucous membranes of the nose and throat may produce extensive destructive changes, including perforation of the palate (which is pathognomonic in the absence of injury), malignant tumor, or lead poisoning. Treponemes are not demonstrable in the nodules.

Patients with tabes dorsalis or locomotor ataxia may develop indolent pressure ulcers of the toes and feet, or destruction of weight-bearing joints and adjacent bones (Charcot joints), which can become secondarily infected.[55]

Diagnosis

The laboratory diagnosis of syphilis is discussed in Chapter 7. Demonstration of *T. pallidum* with a dark-field microscope requires skill and experience. The material is scraped or aspirated from the deep portion of the primary or secondary lesion. The serologic tests for syphilis are obtained and repeated weekly and monthly if they remain negative.

Treatment

Penicillin is the drug of choice in the nonallergic patient for all stages of syphilis. A single intramuscular injection of 2.4 million units of benzathine penicillin G is curative in most cases of primary or secondary syphilis. The gummatous lesions are very susceptible to low-dose penicillin, but other forms of tertiary syphilis should be treated with 2.4 million units of benzathine penicillin per week for 3

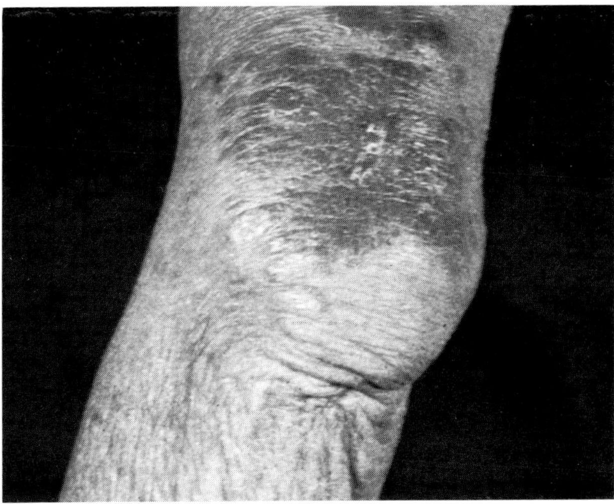

Fig. 25-17. **Gumma in tertiary syphilis. Several lesions have coalesced but no ulceration is present. (Courtesy of Robert W. Goltz, MD, professor and head, Department of Dermatology, University of Minnesota, Minneapolis, Minnesota.)**

weeks (total dose 7.2 million units). Differing recommendations exist for active neurosyphilis and congenital syphilis. Tetracycline, erythromycin, chloramphenicol, and the cephalosporins are effective alternative drugs. Detailed guides to dosages are readily available.

THE ENDEMIC TREPONEMATOSES

Yaws, pinta, and bejel are endemic, communicable diseases caused by the treponemes confined to tropical, economically underdeveloped countries.[56] They are transmitted by nonvenereal contact before puberty, are susceptible to penicillin, and are best controlled by improved hygiene. All yield positive serologic tests for syphilis and have some degree of reciprocal immunity.[55]

Yaws

Yaws (frambesia, pian, buba, bouba) is characterized by early nondestructive skin lesions, a period of latency, and late destructive lesions of skin and bone.

Pathogenesis and Pathology

The organism, *T. pertenue,* is probably inoculated through traumatic breaks in the skin. Bloodstream invasion rapidly occurs, and the course parallels that of syphilis. The early lesions are not destructive and usually heal. A latent period is followed by granulomatous destructive lesions of bones and skin free of bacteria. Hypertrophic periostitis, gummatous periostitis, osteitis, and osteomyelitis affect the bones of limbs, hands, feet, and skull.

Clinical Manifestations

In primary yaws, skin papules appear on exposed skin (usually of the leg), become papillomatous, ulcerate, and heal spontaneously in about 6 months. In secondary yaws, a general eruption of widely dispersed papillomas is accompanied by lymphadenopathy and some malaise. In several months, the eruption heals. Several relapses of secondary lesions may occur over the years and may be accompanied by periostitis, osteitis, and osteomyelitis particularly involving the shafts of the long bones, fingers, or maxilla. Polydactylitis is frequent.

In tertiary yaws, after an asymptomatic period of 3 or more years, papillomatous lesions of the hands and feet appear, which are now destructive and solitary. Plantar and palmar hyperkeratoses with painful fissures (crab yaws) are the most common late lesions. The late bone lesions of the limbs, hands, and skull may ulcerate through the skin at bony prominences. Impressive destructive ulceration of the nose and palate may occur (gangosa mutilans).

Diagnosis

The diagnosis is difficult in nonendemic areas, yet travel has made the disease worldwide. Dark-field examination of primary or secondary lesions by experts can make the diagnosis. The late lesions are dark-field-negative. Serologic syphilis tests are positive.

Prognosis

Yaws may undergo spontaneous resolution, but most cases progress to late lesions with disfigurement, contractures of the hands, and periarticular ulcers. Secondary bacterial infection leading to osteomyelitis can occur. Infection and cure leads to lifelong immunity.

Therapy

A single injection of 600,000 units of procaine penicillin in aluminum monosterate 2 percent (PAM) is curative. Tetracycline and chloramphenicol are also effective.[56]

Surgical Significance

To the surgeon dealing with local manifestations of obscure diseases, the appearance of gangrenous ulcerative single lesions may be confusing, especially if secondarily infected. Young adults from endemic areas with lesions not responding to local therapy should be suspect. Surgical therapy should be discontinued and penicillin administered.

Pinta

Etiology

Pinta is caused by the gram-negative spirochete *Treponema carateum.*

Epidemiology

Pinta is chronic, contagious, nonvenereal treponematosis usually affecting adolescents and young adults, limited to tropical Central and South America. Intimate contact with infected persons transmits the disease.[56]

Clinical Manifestations

The changes in pinta are restricted to the skin, especially the epidermis. In the early stages, small erythematous papules gradually enlarge to 1–3 cm in diameter, coalesce, and develop satellites, which may persist or disappear. Most characteristic is the variety of colors that may be seen. The early lesions are red and violaceous; later lesions in the face and neck may be blue, slate-grey, or black. Dark blue lesions of the face and neck are said to be striking. The tertiary or late stage results in the development of depigmented areas of the skin. Destructive or gangrenous lesions are not seen.[56]

Diagnosis

The diagnosis depends on clinical suspicion and evidence of *T. carateum* by dark-field examination of primary and secondary, but not tertiary, lesions. The serologic tests for syphilis are positive. The prognosis of the disease is good, but disfiguring lesions may cause social ostracism.

Therapy

Penicillin G in doses of 1.2 million units of long-acting penicillin is adequate. Tetracyclines and chloramphenicol are also effective. The clinical response may take 6 to 12 months, and repigmentation of tertiary lesions does not occur.[55]

Bejel (Endemic Syphilis)

Bejel is a nonvenereal treponematosis acquired in childhood caused by *T. pallidum II* (var. endemic syphilis).[55,56] It is spread predominantly by household contact to prepubertal children among rural populations with poor personal hygiene. The manifestations are those of syphilis. The primary lesion is usually missed, and secondary lesions on mucous membranes produce anogenital condylomas on the lips, tongue, or angular stomatitis of the palate and larynx. The late manifestations are similar to those of venereal syphilis, but the severe cardiovascular and neural lesions are rare. Gummas of the nasopharyngeal area may produce focal disfigurement. Cutaneous gummas often extend laterally, with marked ulceration. The diagnosis is difficult or impossible outside the endemic setting. Serologic test results for syphilis are positive. The best treatment is 1.2 million units in a single dose of benzathine penicillin G.

CUTANEOUS MYCOBACTERIAL INFECTIONS

Tuberculosis of the Skin

Table 25-24 lists the clinical expressions of cutaneous tuberculosis. The general aspects of tuberculosis are discussed in Chapter 7. Primary and reactivation infections produce different types of cutaneous responses.

Primary Cutaneous Tuberculosis

The primary inoculation of *M. tuberculosis* into the skin of a previously unsensitized person induces a tuberculous chancre. It is especially common among physicians. A local cutaneous inflammatory response is induced with a predominance of polymorphonuclear leukocytes and lymphocytes. Areas of necrosis with numerous bacilli are first seen; later, typical tubercles develop, from which acid-fast bacilli are difficult to isolate.

The most common lesion is the chancre, a nodule that evolves into an indolent, firm, nontender, sharply delimited ulcer with regional adenopathy. Other lesions are the impetiginous lesion, a superficial small ulceration with a loose crust, and the ecthymatous form, with heaped-up margins surrounding a central ulceration. There may be lymphangitis between the primary chancre and the enlarged node which completes the formation of the primary complex. The ulcer slowly involutes and heals with scarring.

Early, the acid-fast organisms are easily recovered from currettings or biopsies of the ulcer and adjacent lymph nodes. The differential diagnosis includes granuloma pyogenicum, luetic chancre, sporotrichosis, subacute

TABLE 25-24. CLASSIFICATION OF TUBERCULOSIS OF THE SKIN

Types	Mode of Infection or Spread	Bacilli Demonstrable	State of Immunity	Tuberculin Sensitivity	Histologic Caseation
TRUE CUTANEOUS TUBERCULOSIS					
Primary Tuberculosis					
Tuberculous chancre	Inoculation	+++	+++	0 (initially)— + (late)	+++
Miliary	Hematogenous	++	0	0 (terminal anergy)	+++
Secondary Tuberculosis					
Lupus vulgaris	Inoculation	± (with difficulty)	+++	+++	+
Tuberculosis verrucosa cutis	Inoculation	+	+++	+++	++
Scrofuloderma	Local extension	++	+++	+++	+++
Tuberculous gumma	Hematogenous	++	+	+	+++
Tuberculous cutis orificialis	Local extension	++	+	0 (terminal anergy or +++)	+++
TUBERCULIDS					
Papular Forms					
Lupus miliaris disseminatus facei	Hematogenous	0	+++	+++	++
Papulonecrotic tuberculid	Hematogenous	0	+++	+++	+++
Lichen scrofulosorum	Hematogenous	0	+++	+++	0
Nodular					
Erythema induratum	Hematogenous	± (sometimes)	+++	+++	+++

0 = absent; + = slight; ++ = moderate; +++ = considerable.

From Moschella SL: Benign reticuloendothelial diseases. In Moschella SL, Pillsbury DM, Hurley HJ (eds): *Dermatology*, Vol 1. Philadelphia, Saunders, 1975, p 751.

tularemia, cat scratch disease, swimming pool granuloma, and an epithelioma with metastasis to regional lymph nodes.

Treatment with antituberculous drugs discussed in Chapters 7 and 18 should be effective. Before the advent of adequate chemotherapy, complete surgical excision of the primary lesion and involved regional lymph nodes was a satisfactory method of treatment. Local excision of fluctuant nodes may still be useful.[57]

Skin Manifestations of Disseminated Primary Tuberculosis

Other forms of tuberculosis of the skin are listed in Table 25-24. Miliary tuberculosis can be primary or secondary. The skin lesion usually consists of malculopapular rash with occasional vesicular changes. Sometimes, however, chronic miliary tuberculosis produces a systemic febrile wasting syndrome, especially in malnourished children. The lesions present as subcutaneous nodules that become fluctuant and drain with undermined ulceration and sinus formation. Histopathologic examination reveals tuberculous granulomata with acid-fast bacilli in the pus (tuberculosis colliquativa).

Secondary Tuberculosis

Lupus Vulgaris. Lupus vulgaris is the most common cutaneous manifestation of tuberculosis and usually affects the face. It may result from inoculation of infected secretions or hematogenous or lymphatic spread.[57] It may appear as ulcers, nodules, hypertrophic verrucous or vegetative plaques, sclerotic masses, papillomatous overgrowths, and edematous thickenings (Fig. 25-18). Ulceration appears secondary to the underlying vegetative lesions. Tissue destruction can be extensive, and when the lesions resolve, scarring, keloid formation, lymphedema, and functional impairment due to contractures remain. The diagnosis depends on biopsy, which reveals typical tuberculoid granulomas, except that caseous necrosis is slight and the tubercle bacilli are difficult to demonstrate on culture (Table 25-24).

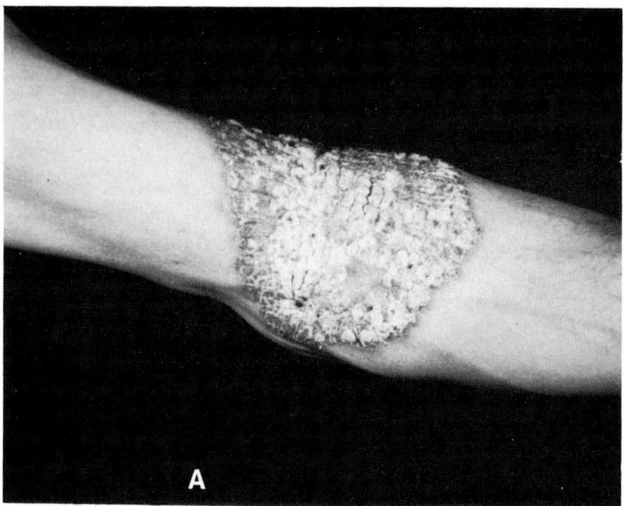

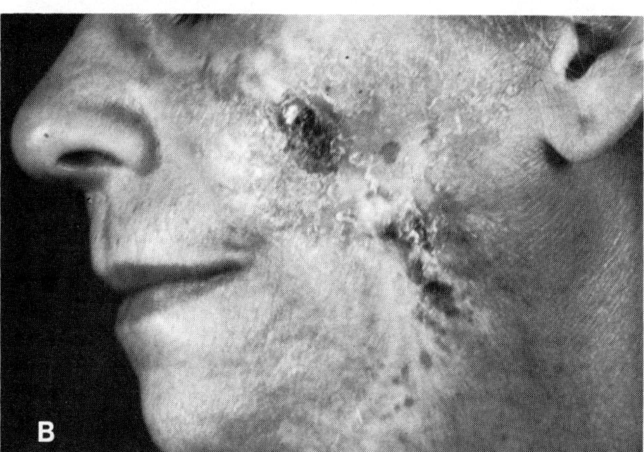

Fig. 25-18. **Tuberculosis of the skin: (A) lupus vulgaris, (B) lupus vulgaris with carcinoma. (Courtesy of Robert W. Goltz, MD, professor and head, Department of Dermatology, University of Minnesota, Minneapolis, Minnesota.)**

Tuberculosis Verrucosa Cutis. Tuberculosis verrucosa cutis is a warty growth resulting from an inoculation injury in an immune individual.[57] Occupational inoculation of pathologists, surgeons, and morgue attendants leads to verrucoid lesions called verucca necrogenica on exposed areas, particularly fingers and hands. The lesion begins as a deep-seated, dull red papule or pustule, which becomes verrucoid and sometimes crushed with exudate. Although it can be mutilating and destructive, most often the lesion gradually involutes and heals.

Scrofuloderma

Scrofuloderma classically results from the breakdown of cervical nodes with fistula and sinus formation in the overlying skin.[57] The disease formerly predominated in children with bovine tuberculosis, tonsillar involvement, and cervical adenitis, but is now seen in pulmonary tuberculosis. Painless swellings appear in the neck from a single or a matted group of nodes (Fig. 25-19). Suppuration results in sinus and ulcer formation in the skin. Fungating tumors may result from granulation tissue overgrowth. Neither excision nor drainage is necessary; antituberculous therapy is effective.

Anorectal Tuberculosis

Tuberculous ischiorectal abscess and fistula-in-ano is an extension of intestinal tuberculosis.

Tuberculids

Tuberculids were once said to be skin lesions resulting from delayed hypersensitivity reactions to tuberculosis elsewhere in the body. Their pathogenesis is currently not clear. The various types are listed in Table 25-24. Although a variety of shapes and forms are taken, the papular or nodular lesions appear in clusters or crops and can undergo spontaneous necrosis and healing. By definition, acid-fast bacteria cannot be isolated.

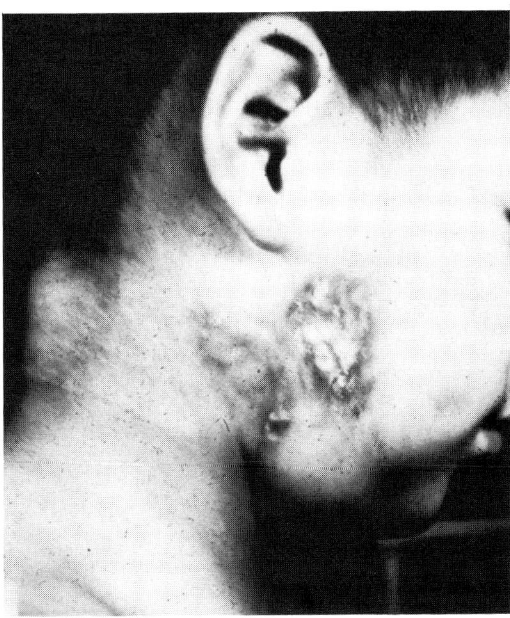

Fig. 25-19. **Scrofuloderma. (Courtesy of Robert W. Goltz MD, professor and head, Department of Dermatology, University of Minnesota, Minneapolis, Minnesota.)**

Atypical Mycobacteria

The pecularities of mycobacteria groups I–IV have been described in Chapter 7, and newer classifications are emerging.[58] These mycobacteria may produce pulmonary disease, cervical adenitis, osteomyelitis, miliary tuberculosis, and skin infections (cutaneous granulomas, ulcers, and abscesses). All infections with groups I–IV mycobacteria produce histologic pictures similar to *M. tuberculosis* except group IV, which does not produce characteristic caseating granulomatous disease. PPD skin antigens for each of the major groups are available, but cross-reactivity is common.

Group II mycobacteria, especially *M. scrofulaceum,* tend to cause cervical lymphadenitis in children 1 to 3 years of age (Table 25-14). The oropharynx is thought to be the portal of entry when children put foreign bodies in their mouths. The submandibular nodes are involved, rather than the anterior cervical nodes characteristic of scrofula. The disease also progresses fairly rapidly and suppurates earlier than tuberculous adenitis. Fever and leukocytosis are absent, the chest roentgenogram is usually negative, and the PPD test results can be negative. Treatment of lymphadenitis is surgical excision. Drug therapy yields equivocal results. Sensitivities are variable. *M. kansasii* and *M. avium intracellulare* can both cause lymphadenitis. Although excision may be useful, drug therapy is also important for these organisms.[58]

Group I (*M. kansasii, M. marinum*) and group IV *Mycobacteria* tend to produce a subcutaneous lymphatic sporotrichoid form of infection. The infections listed in Table 25-12 must be ruled out.

Most group IV mycobacteria are saprophytes, but *M. fortuitum* and *M. chelonei* can produce deep, painful nodules with indefinite margins that may suppurate, drain, and produce fairly large ulcers after accidental inoculation. Debridement is essential. Effective drug combinations have not been defined. *M. fortuitum* has been found contaminating Elastoplast dressings and in wound infections.[58]

Atypical mycobacteria are difficult to eradicate. They have variable in vitro sensitivity to antituberculous drugs, and usually a combination of two or three drugs is required (Table 18-43 and Chapter 7). The organisms are rarely susceptible to isoniazid.

Swimming Pool Granuloma. This is a chronic granulomatous infection at sites of trauma incurred while swimming or cleaning fish tanks. *M. marinum* (group I) and perhaps other unclassified mycobacteria are responsible. Histologically, a tuberculous-like granulomatous infection is seen with Langhans giant cells but without caseation necrosis. Red papules or pustules that can grow to the size of a pea follow abrasion of elbows (70 percent), knees, dorsa of hands, feet, or nose. Some of the lesions break down and develop brownish crusts. The lesions tend to be solitary but can ascend proximally in a sporotrichoid fashion. Regional lymphangitis and lymphadenopathy have not been described. Healing takes place spontaneously in a few months to several years.

The organisms are susceptible to streptomycin but are resistant to isoniazid, PAS, and thiacetazone. Surgical excision commonly results in recurrence unless accompanied by chemotherapy. Disinfecting pools and excluding infected individuals from swimming areas are useful preventive measures.

Mycobacterial Phagedenic Ulceration. *M. ulcerans* (group III) can lead to inoculation infections of scratches and abrasions in tropical areas of Africa, Australia, and Mexico. The initial papule ulcerates and progresses to a large deep undermined ulcer with a necrotic base. The spreading ulcerative granulomatous process often destroys subcutaneous tissue, including fascia and muscle (Buruli ulcers). The legs are most commonly infected, but lymphadenopathy and systemic illness do not occur. The ulcers are teeming with organisms. Histologically, there is necrosis of the skin and tuberculoid reaction. Spontaneous healing may take place after months. *M. ulcerans* is resistant to current antituberculous agents. The only effective therapy presently available is wide surgical excision and skin grafting.

Leprosy

Leprosy (Hansen disease) is a common chronic intracellular nonfatal infectious disease, with many cutaneous manifestations. The diagnosis is made by skin biopsy. Surgical reconstruction of musculoskeletal and cosmetic defects may be required.

Etiology

M. leprae is an acid-fast obligate intracellular parasite capable of invading nerves. It fails to grow in culture, but splenectomized mice and rats develop systemic infection following inoculation.

Epidemiology

Leprosy is a common disease in tropical and subtropical regions and is endemic in Texas, Hawaii, California, Louisiana, Puerto Rico, Cuba, Mexico, and Vietnam. Immigration has made it more common in other parts of the United States as well. Transmission is thought to involve human–human contact through breaks in skin, but skin lesions shed relatively few organisms. Nasal secretions and breast milk from infected persons are rich in bacteria. The incubation period is 3 to 5 years.

Pathogenesis and Pathology

Leprosy usually first involves the skin in association with hair follicles and sebaceous glands. It spreads to contiguous skin areas especially along the nerves, dermal appendages, and blood vessels. Lymphohematogenous dissemination occurs early, and spread along the sensory nerves impairs motor fibers within their trunks. The central nervous system is not affected. Pathologically, the granulomatous reaction destroys nerves and dermal appendages, but the epidermis is not invaded. With progression from the tuberculoid to the lepromatous form, the infiltrating lymphocytes in the granulomas are replaced by foamy histiocytes and bacteria.

Involvement of the lymphoid tissues results in general impairment of cellular immunity with normal or enhanced humoral antibody responses.

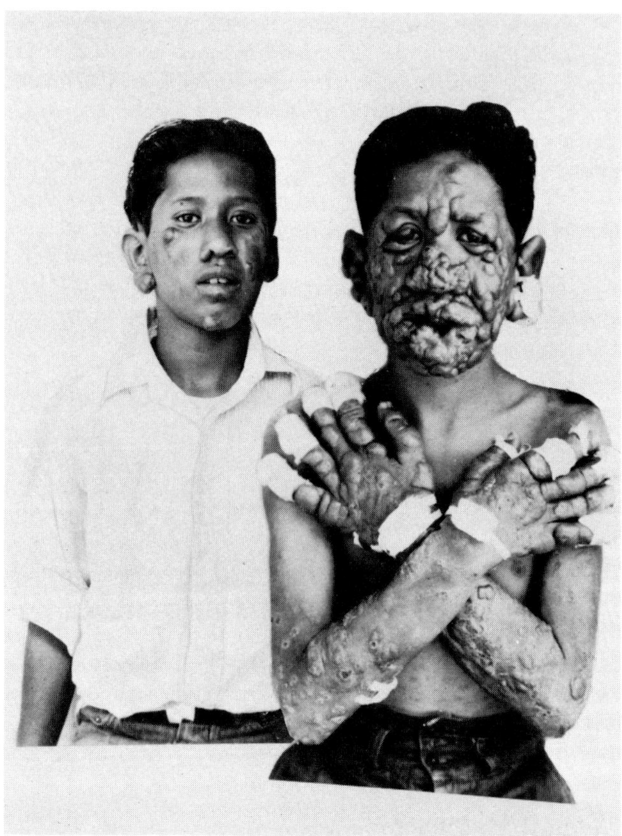

Fig. 25-20. **Early and late lepromatous leprosy. (From Armed Forces Institute of Pathology, Neg. No. 75–2479–2.)**

Clinical Manifestations

Leprosy produces a spectrum of disease, which progresses from one form to another as the patient's immunologic response changes. Ridley and Joplin[59] have described a spectrum from the most limited form to the most generalized disease as follows: TT—full tuberculoid, BT—borderline tuberculoid, BB—borderline, BL—borderline lepromatous, and LL—full lepromatous. The ends of the spectrum are stable forms of disease; the intermediary stages are clinically unstable.

Indeterminate (borderline) leprosy begins as a flat ill-defined skin lesion on the face and trunk, with minimal sensory changes. There may be a history of contact with a leprosy patient but skin biopsy is the only way to make the diagnosis at this stage. If punch biopsies are taken at the advancing margin in the earlier phases, only the acid-fast bacilli in nerves suggest the diagnosis. Tuberculoid leprosy occurs when a large erythematous plaque, with clear sharp outer margins, fades centrally to a flattened clear zone of healing that is rough, anhydrotic, hairless, hypopigmented, and anesthetic. This is a response to the development of cell-mediated immunity to the organism.

Lepromatous leprosy (Fig. 25-20) lies at the other end of the spectrum and consists of diffuse vascular infiltration which coarsens the skin. This appears if effective cell-mediated immunity fails to develop. There may be more than 10^9 organisms per gram of tissue with continuous bacteremia and seeding to multiple organs. On the skin, symmetrically distributed macules, papules, plaques, and nodules (lepromas) are common, with loss of hair (except on the scalp) and edema of the extremities.

The feature common to all forms of leprosy is nerve infection, with denervation of tissue and resultant deformities. Ulnar nerve denervation leads to clawing of the fourth and fifth fingers and wasting of intrinsic hand musculature. Posterior tibial denervation leads to clawing of the toes and plantar anesthesia. Superficial peroneal nerve denervation leads to foot drop; median nerve destruction produces thenar wasting, loss of thumb opposition, and palmar anesthesia. Radial nerve destruction produces wrist drop, and facial nerve involvement produces inability to close the eye with anesthesia of the cornea and conjunctiva. Secondary neuropathic ulcers can result. The anesthetic anterior eye can result in corneal ulceration and blindness. Other deformities result from destruction of the nasal cartilages with septal perforation.

One form of LL leprosy, erythema nodosum leprosum, often leads to diffuse nodular skin lesions during chemotherapy. A high fever, necrosis of the nodules, and neuritis can progress to glomerulonephritis and even death. An Arthus-like reaction is seen in nodule biopsies. Rarely, Lucio phenomenon, erythema necroticans, leads to a necrotizing vasculitis with ulceration and sloughing of large areas of skin.

Diagnosis

The diagnosis depends on a properly performed skin biopsy. Biopsies should include both central and peripheral lesions, and must be deep enough to include fat. An elliptical excisional biopsy 12–15 mm long is better than a punch biopsy. The differential diagnosis includes the entire range of granulomatous skin diseases. Acid-fast stains of tissue must be requested in any granulomatous skin biopsy (Table 25-9).

A lepromin skin test contains a standard suspension of killed leprosy bacilli. A delayed hypersensitivity response is positive. It has no diagnostic value, but in patients with documented leprosy a positive skin test denotes tuberculoid leprosy and a negative result carries a prognosis of lepromatous leprosy if the patient is not treated.

Prognosis

Most indeterminate leprosy is self-limited, but it may evolve into tuberculoid form with severe local damage before infection is arrested. Lepromatous leprosy follows a relentless course to deformity and blindness when neglected. Death is rare except when systemic amyloidosis appears. Tuberculosis and pyogenic infection may also terminate the course.

Therapy

Most *M. leprae* are killed in 3 to 6 months of therapy, but treatment should continue until all *M. leprae* have disappeared from the skin, a matter of at least 5 years with occasional lifelong chemotherapy necessary. Dapsone (DDS 50–100 mg by mouth per day) should cure TT and BT disease. Treatment for BB-LL should include other drugs (3 to 6 months) as well as DDS, because resistance to DDS develops when it is used alone. Clofazimine is used (100 mg orally twice weekly) to prevent ENL reactions. Rifampin (600 mg per day) is a good choice for early treatment of BB-LL, since it is bactericidal for *M. leprae.* ENL reactions, if they appear, will require steroids or thalidomide for control. Bullock has recently summarized the therapeutic approach in detail.[59a]

Prevention

BCG immunization may be protective. Prophylactic therapy with DDS may be useful in children.

Surgical Treatment of Leprosy Complications

The surgical complications of untreated or neglected leprosy are now receiving much attention.[60] Orthopedic and plastic procedures may be indicated, including operations for wrist drop, flail foot, tendon transfers in the hand, and sling operations on the eyelids for lag ophthalamous. Longitudinal incision of the nerve sheaths is sometimes indicated for relief of severe nerve pain. Plastic operations are useful for deformed noses, gynecomastia, madarosis, sagging face, unsightly ear lobes, wasted thumb webs, persistently enlarged and visible great auricular nerves, etc. Orthopedic shoes (molded microcellular rubber insoles on a rigid sole) are required to prevent plantar ulceration. Various appliances and artificial limbs have been designed to relieve the secondary deformities. Physiotherapy and vocational training are an essential part of the treatment of leprosy.

GLANDERS

Glanders is a disease of horses, caused by the bacterium *Pseudomonas mallei,* which is rarely transmitted to humans. The clinical picture takes one of two forms: (1) an acute febrile disseminated infection whose entire course may encompass 10 to 30 days; (2) an indolent, relapsing, chronic infection of the skin with multiple cutaneous and subcutaneous abscesses and draining sinuses. "Farcy" is the name given to the disease in horses and refers to the nodular subcutaneous abscesses occurring along the course of lymphatics.[54]

Etiology

The pseudomonads are discussed in Chapter 5. Humans are infected by direct contact with horses, but the disease has been almost eradicated in the United States. The organisms gain entry through abrasions in the skin, via the conjunctivae, by inhalation, or by ingestion.

Clinical Manifestations

In the acute fulminating form, an incubation period of 2 to 5 days is followed by an abrupt febrile illness with headache, malaise, chills, nausea, and vomiting. The more chronic form has similar manifestations over a longer period of time. Only several weeks later do the typical cutaneous and subcutaneous nodules, abscesses, and draining sinuses develop.

Cutaneous Lesions. In acute glanders, a nodule or cellulitis appears at the site of inoculation. Local swelling and suppuration occur, and the lesion ulcerates. The ulcer is painful and has irregular edges with a grey-yellow base. Nodular sores rapidly develop along the lymphatics and ulcerate, forming draining sinuses. Regional adenopathy is present. Widespread dissemination may follow, with multiple nodular necrotic abscesses in subcutaneous tissues and muscle. Lesions frequently coalesce into gangrenous areas. Bacteremic spread produces a generalized eruption or one that is localized to the face and neck consisting of papules, bullae, and pustules in crops. Lesions of the nasal mucosa lead to mucopurulent bloody nasal discharge, and infection may spread to the peranasal sinuses, pharynx, and lungs.

In chronic glanders, cutaneous and subcutaneous nodules appear on the extremities and occasionally on the face. The lesions ulcerate, and draining sinuses develop. Repeated cycles of healing and breakdown may continue for weeks or months. Pneumonia, empyema, meningitis, septic arthritis, or osteomyelitis are common complications. The leukocyte count is usually normal or only slightly elevated. Skin biopsy shows suppurative necrosis containing numerous intracellular and extracellular bacteria. In the chronic form, a granulomatous process with few giant cells suggestive of tuberculosis is seen. The lymphatic nodules resemble the lesion of sporotrichosis, but in acute disease, miliary TB, typhoid, staphylococcal mycotic infections, or melioidosis must be ruled out.

Treatment

Patients should be isolated. Sulfonamides have been used successfully (sulfadiazine 100 mg per kg daily in divided doses), and a combination of intramuscular streptomycin with tetracycline has been recommended. Acute glanders formerly had a mortality rate of over 90 percent. Chronic glanders is more successfully treated.[54]

MELIOIDOSIS

Melioidosis is caused by the gram-negative bacillus *Pseudomonas pseudomallei* which, although rare in the United States, is endemic in Southeast Asia [61] (Chapter 5). Its clinical manifestations are similar to those of glanders, but it is transmitted by contamination of abraded skin with infected soil. Two clinical forms are seen: (1) acute melioidosis with pneumonia or septicemia, and (2) chronic melioidosis producing unresolved pneumonia or a cavitary lesion. Both forms can be accompanied by skin lesions with abscesses, sinus development, and localized suppurative infections of bones, joints, liver, spleen.

The acute pneumonic form may not be accompanied by any skin lesion but appear abruptly with chills, fever, cough, dyspnea, and chest pain. The acute septicemic form usually starts with an ulceration at the site of inoculation, lymphangitis, and regional lymphadenitis. Chronic melioidosis may follow the acute disease, usually as an indolent pulmonary infection with multiple superficial abscesses. Late recrudescence of a previous infection may be precipitated by various illnesses, including thermal burns, diabetic ketoacidosis, or pneumonia.[61] The cutaneous manifestations are nonspecific.

In chronic melioidosis, subcutaneous abscesses and draining sinuses from bone or lymph nodes are common features and may occur even in the absence of fever. Sharply circumscribed abscesses are found in many organs and in the subcutaneous tissues.

The disease may imitate typhoid fever, staphylococcal pneumonia, mycotic infections, pulmonary tuberculosis, nocardiosis, fungal infections, and lung abscess.

Treatment

Chloramphenicol is the preferred treatment, with tetracycline and sulfisoxazole as alternatives. Abscesses should be drained.[61]

BARTONELLOSIS (CARRION DISEASE)

Bartonella bacilliformis, a gram-negative coccobacillus transmitted by sandflies, causes a disease restricted to the valley regions of the Andes Mountains, particularly in Colombia, Ecuador, and Peru.[62] Because the incubation period is 19 to 30 days, visitors have usually returned to their homes before the onset of symptoms, and after the fly bite has been forgotten.

In the first stage, intermittent fever, malaise, myalgias, headache, gastrointestinal irritability, and finally symptoms due to increasingly severe hemolytic anemia appear (Oroya fever). Splenomegaly, pallor, and icterus are characteristic. In the second stage of the disease, verruga peruana, miliary erythematous macules, and papules appear on the face and extensor surfaces of the extremities. In addition, subcutaneous nodules 1–2 cm in diameter appear in crops on the extremities and may ulcerate and bleed. In the acute phase, the bacilli are easily seen in Giemsa-stained blood smears. Phagocytized *Bartonella* can be seen in the endothelial and histiocytic cells of verrugas if the diagnosis is suspected, but a histopathologic picture resembling a neoplasm has been noted. Blood culture results may be positive even during the cutaneous phase.

Penicillin, streptomycin, tetracycline, and chloramphenicol have all been used successfully. Patients are predisposed to secondary *Salmonella* infections, as are patients with any kind of hemolytic anemias.[62]

LEPTOSPIROSIS

Leptospirosis is caused by the spirochete *Leptospira interrogans,* which can be cultured on special (Fletcher semisolid) media. The disease is a septicemia derived directly from farm, domestic, or wild animals or indirectly through contaminated water or soil.[63] Organisms enter through a break in the skin, mouth, or conjunctiva, but no local skin lesion appears. After an incubation period of 7 to 14 days, a biphasic infection results, with headache, fever, chills, nausea, vomiting, and myalgias followed by defervescence and a second febrile illness, often with meningitis. Skin lesions are most often produced by *L. icterohaemorrhagiae,* with jaundice, azotemia, and hemorrhagic manifestations in the skin. Surgical implications are negligible. Antibiotics may or may not be useful. Penicillin G or tetracycline are the drugs of choice. In jaundiced patients, the mortality rate may be as high as 40 percent.

RICKETTSIAL DISEASE

The *Rickettsiae* are discussed in Chapter 7, because diseases caused by them are rarely encountered by surgeons. The organisms are transmitted through the skin by arthropods and usually produce acute systemic infections of varying severity, characterized by fever, headache, and rash. A surgeon may be asked to treat the primary lesion of scrub typhus or one of the spotted fever groups. The lesion is usually a vesicle which ruptures to form an eschar or, on occasion, a suppurative or necrotic lesion (Table 7-4). The appearance of the eschar usually precedes the systemic manifestations, so that the diagnosis is not clear. A generalized rash is a common manifestation of the vasculitis associated with systemic rickettsiosis, and diffuse gangrene of the skin due to ischemic vasculitis can appear.

TULAREMIA

Human infection with *Pasteurella (Francisella) tularensis* is discussed in Chapter 7. The ulceroglandular type of tularemia is the most common expression of the disease, but oculoglandular, typhoidal, and pulmonary forms are seen.

Inoculation occurs through the bite of infected ticks and flies or contact with infected animals, particularly wild rabbits and hares. Hunters, trappers, and furriers are most often infected. Tick-borne lesions affect the lower extremities; contact-acquired infections affect the upper body.

After an incubation period of 1 to 10 days, fever, sweats, chills, and myalgias are sometimes followed by stupor and coma. Only then does the primary skin lesion develop as a painful papule at the site of a minor injury or insect bite. The papule enlarges rapidly and undergoes necrosis, producing an indolent ulcer with raised edges and a necrotic base. The lesion is usually on an exposed extremity, and regional adenopathy develops after the appearance of the chancre-like primary lesion, usually without lymphangitis (Table 25-14). In a few patients, tender nodules develop along the course of lymphatic channels, similar to sporotrichosis (Table 25-12). The enlarged nodes may suppurate (Fig. 25-21).

The systemic and febrile infection lasts 2 to 4 weeks with constant bacteremia. In the oculoglandular type, the primary lesion is a purulent conjunctivitis. The constitutional symptoms are so profound that the primary cutaneous lesion and the diagnosis may be missed. However, 90 percent of untreated patients survive, and with treatment cure is almost universal. The differential diagnosis must include plague, cat scratch disease, melioidosis, or glanders. Since most laboratories are reluctant to isolate the highly contagious organism, serologic diagnosis is preferred. Tularemia agglutination titers become positive in the second week of the illness and remain positive for life. Fluorescent antibody staining may identify the organisms in biopsies or currettings.

An attenuated vaccine administered intradermally by multiple puncture technique is available from the Centers for Disease Control, Atlanta, Georgia. Streptomycin is the preferred treatment (15–20 mg per kg per day intramuscularly for 7 to 10 days). Tetracycline or chloramphenicol are effective, but relapses occur more frequently. Aspiration or incision and drainage of fluctuant lymph nodes may be required but is best delayed until antibiotic therapy is well advanced.

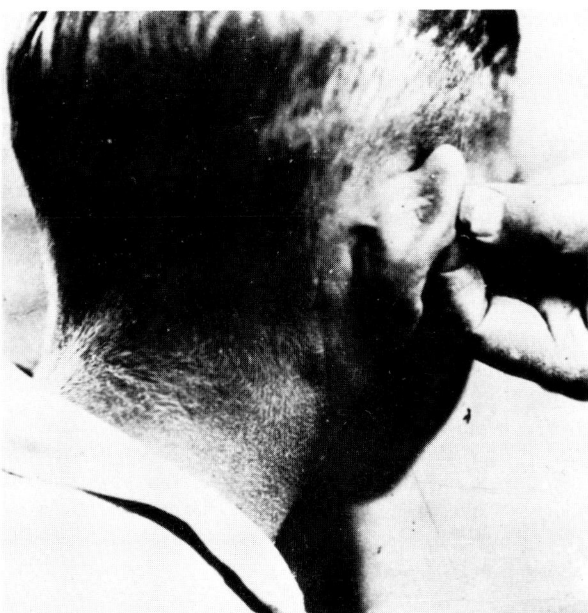

Fig. 25-21. **Tularemia, caused by a fly bite on the ear, with an enlarged posterior auricular node. (From Armed Forces Institute of Pathology. Neg. No. 68–5644.)**

PLAGUE

Plague *(Yersinia pestis)* is an acute, febrile, fatal disease characterized by inflammation of the lymphatics, septicemia, and diffuse hemorrhages into the skin and subcutaneous tissues. Suppurative lymphadenitis with bubo formation is characteristic. Plague is presently endemic in the western United States.

Etiology

Yersinia pestis is a short, nonmotile, gram-negative, bipolar-staining bacillus, which exhibits marked pleomorphism and is often encapsulated. A potent endotoxin is produced. A more complete discussion is available in Chapter 7.

Plague is a disease of rats and other rodents, transmitted incidentally to man by the bite of a rat flea. It occurs in three forms: bubonic, primary septicemic, and primary pneumonic.

Clinical Manifestations

Most plague presents in the bubonic form, ie, an ulceroglandular process with the portal of entry on an extremity. The incubation period is 2 to 10 days, and the onset of the disease is sudden. The bite mark may or may not be noted, but the hallmark is the bubo (Fig. 25-22), a large, painful, tender, fixed, matted mass of lymph nodes with overlying skin erythema and a gelatinous consistency. A carbuncle may form near the bubo and resemble the malignant pustule of anthrax. Complications include septicemia, disseminated intravascular coagulation, pneumonia, and meningitis.[64] The differential diagnosis includes sta-

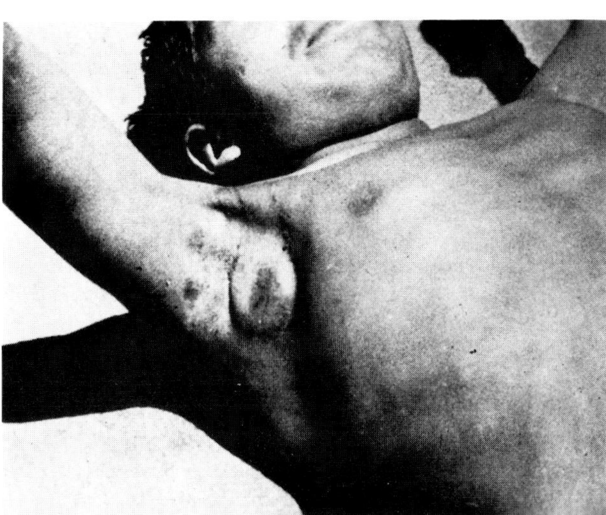

Fig. 25-22. **The hallmark of plague is an axillary or inguinal bubo. (From the Armed Forces Institute of Pathology. Neg. No. 219 900–7–B.)**

phylococcal or streptococcal lymphadenitis, tularemia, cat scratch fever, incarcerated hernia, and acute appendicitis (Table 25-14). Any ulceroglandular process should be considered.

Diagnosis

A Gram stain and culture of material aspirated from affected lymph nodes should be performed on all patients with suspected plague. A fluorescent antibody test, performed by the Center for Disease Control, is a rapid, specific means of making the diagnosis from various clinical specimens, including bubo aspirates. Acute and convalescent serum specimens should be obtained from all patients to detect hemagglutinating antibodies, which appear 8 to 14 days after onset of the disease.

Treatment

Hospitalization and isolation are recommended. Streptomycin (tetracycline or sulphonamides) are effective. Streptomycin, 30 mg per kg per day in divided doses, or tetracycline, 30–50 mg per kg per day in divided doses, should be given for 10 days. Chloramphenicol is necessary for meningitis.

Prevention

Chemoprophylaxis (tetracycline or sulphonamide) is recommended for all contacts. An effective formalin-killed vaccine is available for persons in high-risk occupations in plague endemic areas.

NOCARDIA

The etiologic agent and pathogenesis of *Nocardia* infections are discussed in Chapter 7. Soft tissue involvement with *N. asteroides* is usually secondary to hematogenous dissemination from a pulmonary focus in immunodepressed patients. Primary infections of the soft tissues are uncommon. *N. brasiliensis* frequently involves the skin and subcutaneous tissues in tropical regions and is one of the more common causes of mycetoma in tropical regions [65] (see subsequent section on cutaneous fungal infections).

Both *N. asteroides* and *N. brasiliensis* can produce suppurative infections of traumatic wounds contaminated with soil organisms. Cellulitis, subcutaneous abscess, pustules, pyoderma, and lymphadenopathy develop. Debridement and drainage may be adequate therapy but should be combined with sulphonamides. Gram stain of purulent drainage shows polymorphonuclear cells and beaded gram-positive branching organisms consistent with *Nocardia.* Rarely, a sulfur granule is seen in a skin biopsy. *Nocardia* takes 2 to 5 days for the colonies to become visible on blood agar plates, and the laboratory diagnosis may be missed. Wound cultures should be maintained for at least a week before being discarded.

Although dissemination of locally inoculated *Nocardia* is rare, undertreatment can result in the dissemination of the organism to visceral foci if the more invasive chronic lymphocutaneous infection develops.[65]

Cutaneous manifestations of pulmonary nocardiosis are usually part of a disseminated miliary syndrome with diffuse organ abscesses. Subcutaneous abscesses may be single or multiple, more firm than fluctuant, and do not form fistulas. The disease is usually identified at autopsy. Treatment is described in Chapter 7.

ACTINOMYCOSIS

Actinomycosis is a chronic suppurative infection that forms external sinuses, which discharge characteristic sulfur granules and spreads across anatomic barriers whenever endogenous oral commensals invade tissues of the face and neck, lungs, and ileocecal regions. *A. israelii* is most commonly isolated, but other bacteria are frequently found, especially *Actinobacillus actinomycetemcomitans, Hemophilus* species, *Fusobacterium,* anaerobic and other streptococci, micrococci, staphlococci, and oral *Bacteroides* accompany the cervicofacial, nervous system and thoracic infections. Coliforms and intestinal anaerobes are often associated with abdominal actinomycosis. The etiologic agent and pathogenesis of these infections is discussed in Chapter 6.

Pathogenesis

The endogenous actinomycoses enter damaged tissues after infection, trauma, or surgical manipulation such as dental extraction. The soft tissues are usually involved before the skin, although mycetoma (see subsequent section) can be caused by the actinomycetes via primary inoculation from contaminated soil. Although antecedent disease or operation usually predisposes to infection, no antecedent event, even dental trauma, precedes many infections.

Clinical Manifestations

The cervicofacial form resembles an acute pyogenic infection along the mandible, or even a cold pseudotumor. Either spontaneous or operative drainage leads to a persistent cutaneous fistula (Fig. 25-23). Adenopathy is not common, though dental roentgenograms may reveal lytic bone lesions. Antibiotics may modify this course.

Thoracic infections are the result of aspiration, esophageal penetration, or extension into the mediastinal lymph nodes from the neck or up from the abdomen. Although usually pulmonary disease is manifest, fistulization of the skin and subcutaneous tissues may be the presenting sign (Fig. 25-23). Disseminated infection may occur from pulmonary disease with subcutaneous abscesses and chronic fistulas. Thoracic actinomycosis is suspected when pulmonary lesions extend directly through the chest wall with bony involvement of vertebra, ribs, or even extension from lobe to lobe within the lung.

Abdominal or pelvic actinomycosis is the result of prior surgery for inflammatory bowel disease or perforation of chronic diverticulitis, duodenal ulcer, or abdominal gunshot wound. The diagnosis and therapy are discussed in detail in Chapters 6, 27, 30, and 34.

Noma

Noma (gangrenous stomatitis, cancrum oris) is a term used by Finegold [45] to designate all forms of spontaneous gan-

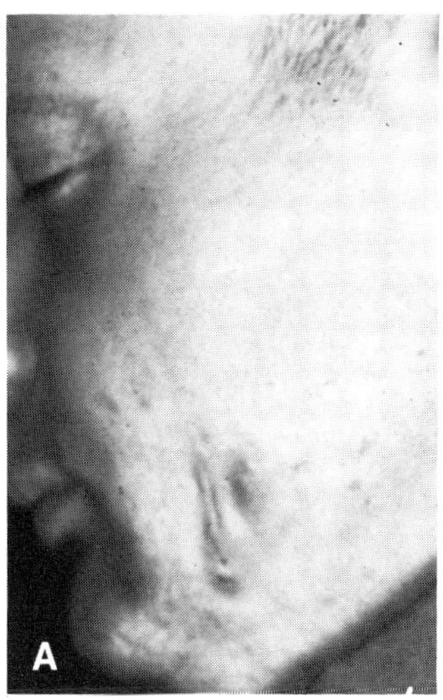

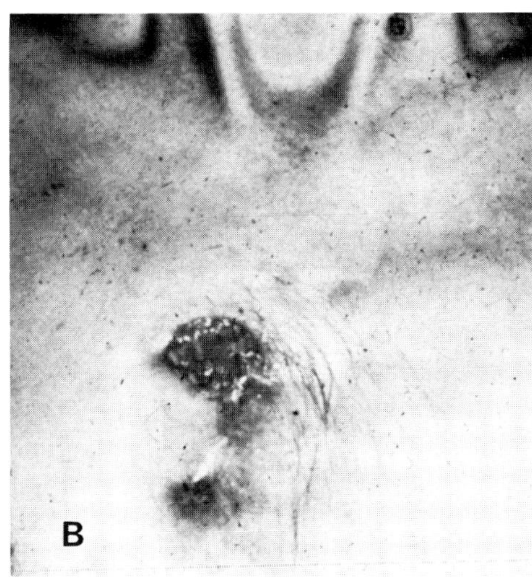

Fig. 25-23. **A. Cervicofacial and (B) thoracic actinomycosis. The findings of a fistula draining a ulceronodular lesion are classic.**

grene involving mucous membranes or mucocutaneous orifices. Although it occurs most frequently about the mouth, it may also affect the nose, auditory canal, vulva, prepuce, or anus.

Etiology
Fusiform bacillae and spirochetes are found together. *B. melaninogenicus* can be isolated from some specimens, and Emslie [66] has suggested that this organism may be a key pathogen in mixed fusospirochete-anaerobic infections.

Pathogenesis
Children with predisposing systemic disease, malnutrition, poor oral hygiene, measles, smallpox, malaria, and parasitic infection are most often affected. Herpetic gingivostomatitis may predispose to acute ulcerative gingivitis and then to noma. Adults in concentration camps or with oral carcinomas are occasionally afflicted.[45]

Clinical Manifestations
The constitutional symptoms are mild at first, but as development occurs, the symptoms become suddenly severe with fever, apathy, weakness, and prostration. The odor of the breath or dull red spots on the cheek may be the first indication of the disease. Inspection of the mouth will reveal a dark greenish-black area on the gum or at the inside of the adjacent cheek. The surrounding tissues are reddened and swollen to two or three times normal size. There is an extremely offensive odor. The destructive process progresses with great rapidity, attacking the periosteum and the underlying bone. The gums are destroyed, and the teeth fall out (Fig. 25-24). Large bony sequestra form and then come away. In untreated cases, the process may extend to the other cheek, into the nose, and may result in almost complete destruction of the face before death. The usual duration of the disease without therapy is 5 to 10 days. There is little or no pain, and children sometimes push their fingers through the necrotic areas of the cheek. Hemorrhage is rare because of thrombosis of this area. After treatment, the affected tissue is ultimately sloughed.[45]

Prognosis
Before antimicrobial therapy, the mortality was 70 to 100 percent, and patients who survived had virtually irreparable defects.

Treatment
Intensive penicillin therapy is the best treatment.[66]

Tropical Ulcer

Tropical ulcer is a chronic sloughing ulcer, which may take on a more invasive character and which seldom heals spontaneously.[45] The disease is found in all tropical and subtropical regions of Africa, Asia, and America.

Etiology
The fusiform bacilli (an anaerobic gram-negative rod) and a spirochete, morphologically identical to *Treponema (Bor-*

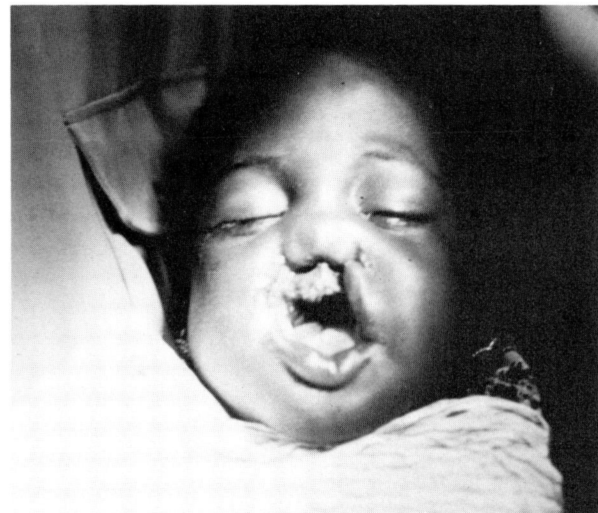

Fig. 25-24. **Noma (gangrenous stomatitis) of the mouth of an infant. (From the Armed Forces Institute of Pathology, Neg. No. 68–741–3.)**

relia) vincentii apparently play an important role, but secondary bacterial infection is so common that the exact role played by each is unknown.

Clinical Manifestations

Tropical ulcer generally affects the lower limbs, particularly the lower third of the leg, ankle, and dorsum of the foot. A small painful papule surrounded by a deeply infiltrated dusky red zone soon progresses to a pustule and then to an ulcer, which enlarges in depth and breadth (5–10 cm). The margins of the ulcer are flat, and undermining is not prominent, but the base is necrotic, purulent, and foul-smelling. The surrounding areas are edematous, but tenderness is minimal. Left untreated, the ulcer may assume a real phagedenic character involving a large area and extending into the deeper structures to destroy muscle, tendon, and periosteum. Untreated lesions commonly reach a diameter of 5–10 cm and may persist for years without endangering life.[45]

Diagnosis

Fusiform bacilli and spirochetes are abundant in the superficial base of the ulcer, but secondary colonization by ambient bacteria confuses the picture. One should rule out cutaneous diphtheria, *M. ulcerans,* and cutaneous leishmaniasis.

Treatment

Topical therapy, including tyrothricin and combinations of streptomycin, bacitracin, and polymixin, is said to be effective. Systemic penicillin, tetracycline, chloramphenicol, and metronidazole are all very effective.[68] Bed rest, elevation, conservative debridement, plus antibiotic therapy will heal small ulcers and permit skin grafting of larger ones.

BLOOD-BORNE BACTERIAL SOFT TISSUE INFECTIONS

Many infections cause rash. The following section will briefly discuss infections that metastasize through the bloodstream to the soft tissues.

Meningococcemia

Primary meningococcal suppurative lesions of the soft tissues are rarely seen, but skin lesions are often the most dramatic manifestations of meningococcemia.

Etiology

Neisseria meningitidis is one of the pyogenic cocci discussed in Chapter 4.

Pathogenesis and Pathology

The skin lesions associated with meningococcemia result from damage to small dermal blood vessels. Bacteria become pinocytosed by endothelial cells as well as by polymorphonuclear leukocytes, leading to local endothelial damage, thrombosis, and necrosis of the vessel walls. Edema, infarction of overlying skin, and extravasation of red blood cells are responsible for the characteristic progression from macular to hemorrhagic necrotic lesions. The potent endotoxin of *N. meningitidis* may precipitate a dermal Shwartzman reaction. The shock-like states associated with meningococcemia may also be due to the Shwartzman reaction or to an endotoxin shocklike state.

Most adults possess bactericidal antibody of both IgM and IgG classes to *N. meningitidis.* Consequently, most cases occur in children under conditions of close contact with carriers within the family or in child care centers. Crowding of susceptible individuals, as in army camps, can also lead to outbreaks.

Clinical Manifestations

Patients usually become systemically ill, with fever, obtundation, and other manifestations of meningitis. In fulminant meningococcemia, vomiting, stupor, hemorrhagic rash, and hypotension follow. The skin lesions are primarily petechial and most commonly located on the extremities and trunk. Sometimes, hemorrhagic lesions develop, and gangrenous hemorrhagic areas of the advanced disease are indistinguishable from pupura fulminans (Fig. 25-25). Septic foci in joints, pericardium, endocardium, and lung have been reported. Biopsy reveals organisms in swollen endothelial cells and polymorphonuclear leukocytes in the inflammatory reaction, entrapped by fibrin thrombi in vessels.

Treatment and Prognosis

Meningitis usually responds well to therapy, with recovery in 90 percent of patients, but severe meningococcemia with extensive cutaneous lesions is almost always fatal. Penicillin G (adult dose of 2 million units intravenously every 2 hours) is required. In chronic meningococcemia, lesser doses are effective. Chloramphenicol can be used in penicillin-allergic patients. Some strains are still sulfonamide-sensitive.

Prevention

Chemoprophylaxis is effective in contacts. A single dose of rifampin (600 mg orally for 4 days) is best. Vaccines for groups A and C serotypes have been developed and are useful in certain populations, ie, army inductees.

Pseudomonas Septicemia

Etiology and Pathogenesis

The bacteriology and pathogenesis of pseudomonad infections are discussed in Chapter 5. *Pseudomonas* septicemia occurs primarily in premature infants, especially those with omphalitis, diarrhea, or urinary tract infection complicating congenital lesions (eg, extrophy of the bladder). Adults who are treated with immunosuppressive drugs or long-term antibiotics, or who require indwelling venous catheters, are also susceptible. The distinctive lesion is a necrotizing vasculitis, in which the walls of small arteries and veins are invaded by myriads of bacteria. The endothelial surface is intact, and thrombosis is unusual. The occlusion of the vessel by the perivasculitis leads to the formation of cutaneous lesions. The skin is then invaded

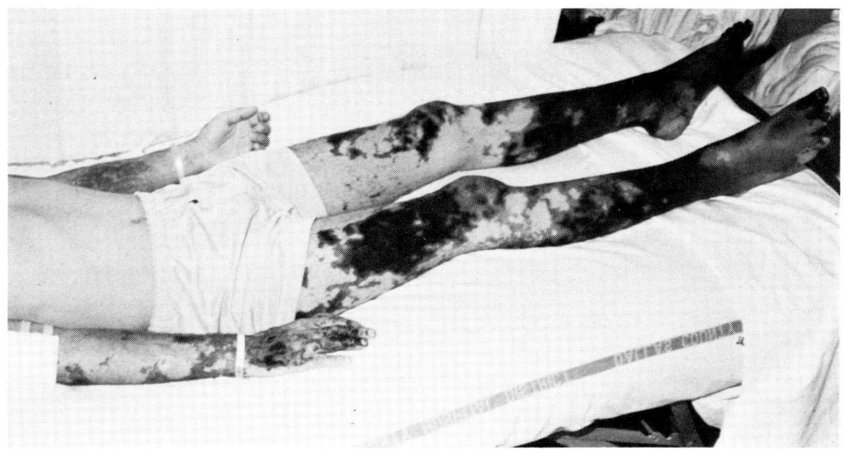

Fig. 25-25. **The hemorrhagic, advanced stage of meningococcemia. Dry gangrene of the toes and forefeet and full thickness necrosis of skin is present over 40 percent of the body surface. (Courtesy of P. William Curreri, MD, New York Hospital, Cornell Medical Center, New York, NY.)**

by bacteria directly. Other organs may be involved in multiple discreet nodular necrotic lesions.

Clinical Manifestation

Sudden worsening of the course of an immunodepressed patient may be the signal that *Pseudomonas* superinfection has occurred. Although hemorrhagic manifestations similar to meningococcemia can occur, *Pseudomonas* usually produces other kinds of skin lesions—vesicles, bulli, macules, papules, or nodular lesions. Several other more deeply situated lesions may prompt surgical consultation in these debilitated patients (Chapter 47).

The typical lesions are of three types:

1. A round, indurated, ulcerated, painless area with central black eschar, surrounded by erythema (necrotic vesicle). These lesions are most often found in the anal, genital, or axillary region.
2. Gangrenous cellulitis is a sharply demarcated, superficial, painless, necrotic lesion that may resemble a decubitus ulcer but is not located in a pressure area.
3. Nodular cellulitis has red, warm, nodular lesions situated too deep to feel fluctuant. Incision or aspiration reveals pus, and *P. aeruginosa* can be cultured.

Diagnosis

Aspiration of skin lesions with Gram stain of the smear and culture will reveal the organisms. Blood cultures are frequently positive as well.

Prognosis

Pseudomonas septicemia is frequently the terminal event in a complex illness. Antibiotic therapy can sometimes be effective, as can the elimination of the underlying cause, such as removal of intravascular catheters.

Treatment

Pseudomonas septicemia will require an aminoglycoside (gentamycin, tobramycin, or amikacin) in combination with carbenicillin or ticarcillin. Aminoglycoside levels should be monitored (Chapter 18). Carbenicillin dosage is about 30 gm daily, intravenously administered as aliquots every 2 to 4 hours. The nodular and pustular lesions benefit from incision, drainage, and debridement.

A polyvalent vaccine has been developed against *P. aeruginosa* for use in patients with thermal burns or cystic fibrosis. The results are encouraging in immunocompetent patients but are less impressive in impaired hosts.[20]

SEXUALLY TRANSMITTED BACTERIA: CAUSES OF SKIN ULCERATION

Lymphogranuloma Venereum

Etiology

Lymphogranuloma venereum is a venereal disease characterized by suppurative inguinal adenitis. The causative agent is a strain of *Chlamydia trachomatis.* Like all *Chlamydia,* it exists in two forms—the infective nondividing elementary body, which is extracellular, and the intracellular noninfective reticulate body (Chapter 7).

Incidence and Epidemiology

Lymphogranuloma venereum (LGV) is endemic in tropical areas of Asia, Africa, and South America, but an increasing number of cases have been found in the United States since the war in Vietnam. It is reported three times as frequently in men as in women and is especially common in patients returning from endemic regions, in male homosexuals, and in the lower socioeconomic classes living in the southeastern United States. Nonsexual transmission has also been reported.[69]

Pathogenesis

After sexual transmission, the extracellular elementary body becomes attached to phagocytes and undergoes endocytosis. It then forms the reticulate body, which grows by binary fission. *Chlamydia* lack the ability to generate energy and must utilize the cell's nucleoside triphosphates. After phagocytosis, the *Chlamydia* can grow within the phagosome without causing lysosomal fusion. Intracellular *C. trachomatis* can then lead to cell death.

Clinical Manifestations

Several days to 3 weeks after exposure, a painless vesicle or papule will sometimes develop on the penis or vulva. The lesion heals quickly without a scar. In homosexuals, a primary anorectal infection may occur manifested by diarrhea, tenesmus, and a rectal discharge.

Two to six weeks after the initial exposure, a painful regional lymphadenopathy develops adjacent to the site of initial infection. For perineal sites, this involves the inguinal and femoral lymph nodes; with anorectal infection, the hypogastric and deep iliac nodes; and with vaginal or cervical infection, the obturator and iliac nodes. The nodes become matted, small abscesses form, coalesce, become necrotic, and ultimately break through the skin to form fistulas. The tracts heal over a period of months, but the scars remain. Systemic manifestations include fever, chills, anorexia, headache, and myalgias. There is a leukocytosis with elevated sedimentation rate and frequently abnormal liver function tests. Approximately 5 percent of men will develop chronic disease, with persistent fistulas or urethral or rectal strictures.

Diagnosis

The definitive diagnosis is established by isolation of the organism from a bubo, although these cultures are positive in only about 30 percent of cases. A complement-fixation test with a titer of greater than 1:64 is suggestive. The Frei test, formerly thought to be quite specific, is now rarely used because of low sensitivity and uncertain specificity.

The differential diagnosis includes syphilis, genital herpes, and chancroid. Clinically, LGV differs from chancroid in that the ulcer is more prominent and systemic symptoms are rare in the latter. Herpes simplex has painful tender vesicles with nonsuppurative regional lymphadenopathy. Syphilis is differentiated from LGV by its positive serologic test as well as secondary rash and nontender inguinal lymphadenopathy.

Treatment

Fluctuant lymph nodes are aspirated to prevent rupture. Dark-field examination is done on genital lesions to rule out syphilis. LGV is sensitive to sulfomanides, 1 gm per day for 21 days, or tetracycline, 500 mg per day for 21 days. These help resolve the constitutional symptoms, but the bubos heal slowly. Surgical procedures may be required for strictures, fistulas, or local elephantiasis.

Chancroid

Etiology

Chancroid or soft chancre is a sexually transmitted disease caused by *Haemophilus ducreyi.* These are small pleomorphic gram-negative coccobacilli, which are slow growing and strict parasites. They require hemin, nicotinamide adenine dinucleotide (NAD), or both for growth in culture (Chapter 7).

Incidence and Epidemiology

Chancroid occurs worldwide, especially where hygiene is poor. It is most common among nonwhite uncircumcised males; only about 10 percent of cases occur in women, who may be asymptomatic carriers.

Clinical Manifestations

After an incubation period of 2 to 5 days, genital or perianal papules, with surrounding erythema, appear. Erosion leads to a soft, undermined, painful, nonindurated ulcer which bleeds easily, and may be covered by a necrotic exudate. Multiple ulcerations sometimes appear, which can coalesce and, after superinfection (especially fusospirochetal), destroy the genitalia. Painful, unilateral, inguinal lymphadenitis is characteristic. Like LGV, spontaneous rupture of the abscessed node and fistula formation can occur.

Diagnosis

The differential diagnosis includes primary syphilis, herpes, and lymphogranuloma venereum. The diagnosis is confirmed by the demonstration of *Haemophilus ducreyi* on smear and culture of the lesion. The ulcers are cleaned with sterile saline and dried, and exudate from the ulcer border is inoculated into chocolate agar containing isovitalex and vancomycin. A Gram stain may reveal large numbers of gram-negative coccobacilli usually in chains or "school of fish" patterns. Approximately 10 percent of chancroid patients have primarily syphilis, so dark-field examination to rule out syphilis is required. If these study results are negative, serologic studies for 3 months have been suggested.

Treatment

The treatment of choice is oral sulfisoxazole, 1 gm orally every 6 hours for 1 to 2 weeks. Tetracycline has also been successfully used. In Southeast Asia, resistance to these agents has been reported, but kanamyacin has been successfully used. Bubos should be aspirated to prevent rupture and fistula formation.[70]

Granuloma Inguinale

Etiology

The causative agent is *Calymmatobacterium (Donovania) granulomatis,* a gram-negative bacterium that usually lives within histiocytes (Chapter 7). The organisms are encapsulated with small filamentous projections resembling pili.

Incidence and Epidemiology

Granuloma inguinale is common in India, Central Australia, New Guinea, and the Carribean. Fewer than 100 cases are reported annually in the United States. Most likely it is a mildly contagious sexually transmitted disease, which requires repeated exposure for transmission.

Pathology and Clinical Manifestations

The primary genital lesion is a nodule which appears 8 to 80 days after exposure and erodes to form a granulomatous heaped-up ulcer. This progresses slowly, and pathologic examination shows a dense dermal infiltrate of plasma cells and histiocytes, many containing intracellular organisms. The pathognomonic feature is a large infected mononuclear cell, 25 to 90 microns in diameter containing intracytoplasmic cysts filled with deeply staining organisms. The patients appear to have bubos but in fact have subcutaneous granulomas. Secondary infection may cause tissue destruction and subsequent scarring. Metastatic spread to bone, joints, and liver may occur.

Diagnosis

The diagnosis is readily confirmed by a Wright- or Giemsa-stained imprint granulation tissue. The diagnostic Donovan bodies appear as clusters of blue or black staining organisms, which look like safety pins because of chromatin condensation at the poles. Histologic examination of the fixed lesions rarely shows the Donovan bodies.

Treatment

Three-week courses of gentamicin or chloramphenicol are most effective. Tetracycline and ampicillin have been used, but failures are high. Clinical response to therapy is indicated by shrinking and decreasing redness of the lesions within 1 week, but medication should be continued until the lesions disappear. The lesions will heal even if drugs are stopped early, but recurrence will be frequent.[70a]

FUNGAL INFECTIONS

These diseases are of greater interest to dermatologists than surgeons. A few require operation to either diagnose or treat, and many frequently masquerade as suppurative or malignant lesions.

SUPERFICIAL FUNGAL INFECTIONS

Dermatophytosis (Tineas, Ringworms)

These diseases are caused by the dermatophytes and other fungi that infect the skin and its appendages. They are of little importance per se to the surgeon because they are restricted to the cornified layer of the skin, hair, and nails. Unfortunately, they are sometimes important in the pathogenesis of deeper local or systemic infections by bacteria or more invasive fungi. Furthermore, the inflammatory manifestations of some of them can be confused with abscesses and cellulitis.

Etiology

Table 25-25 lists some of the more common dermatophytic fungi and the other species that infect the cornified layers of the skin. Fungi that infect only the hair are omitted. These diseases are usually classified by anatomic region rather than by etiology.

Pathogenesis, Pathology, and General Clinical Manifestations

These fungi invade only dead, cornified layers of the skin, hair, and nails. Only a few organisms are necessary to in-

TABLE 25-25. ETIOLOGIC AGENTS OF THE SUPERFICIAL FUNGUS INFECTIONS OF THE SKIN

	Tinea Capitis	Tinea Barbae	Tinea Cruris	Tinea Pedis	Tinea Unguium	Tinea Versicolor	Tinea Nigra	Tinea Corporis
Dermatophytes								
MICROSPORUM SPECIES								
M. audouinii	Noninflammatory ++++							+
M. canis	++ inflammatory	+ inflammatory						+
M. nanum	+ inflammatory							
M. gypseum	+ inflammatory							+
M. fulvum	+ inflammatory							
EPIDERMOPHYTON SPECIES								
E. floccosum			++	++	+			+
TRICHOPHYTON SPECIES								
T. mentagrophytes	+ inflammatory	+++ inflammatory	+++	+++	+++			+
T. rubrum		+ superficial	+++	++	+++			+
T. tonsurans	+ black dot							+
T. schoenleini	+ favus							
T. concentricum								+
T. furrugineum	+							+
T. violaceum	+ black dot	+ inflammatory			+			+
T. verrucosum	+ inflammatory	+++ inflammatory			+			+
T. megninii	+ inflammatory	+ inflammatory						
T. gallinae	+ favus							
Nondermatophytes								
PITYROSPORUM ORBICULARE (MALASSEZIA FURFUR)						+		
CANDIDA SPECIES							+	
CLADOSPORIUM WERNECKII							+	

+++ Very common; + Rare

Modified from Jones HE, Harrell ER: Superficial fungus infections of the skin. In Hoeprich PD (ed): *Infectious Diseases: A Modern Treatise of Infectious Processes,* (2nd ed.), Hagerstown, Harper & Row, 1977, p 836.

duce an infection, but trauma or occlusion are necessary predisposing conditions. Dermatophytes grow in filamentous form within the stratum corneum. The downward extension of these hyphae is restricted because certain nutrients, principally iron, are not available in the deeper tissues of the skin. Consequently, lateral invasion from the focus of inoculation occurs leading to the annular pattern seen on the skin surface.

The dermatophytes do not directly damage skin, but a delayed hypersensitivity reaction may appear at the lateral borders of the growing fungi after the host becomes sensitized to soluble fungal antigens. The inflammatory response results in a circinate pattern of erythema and edema, followed by exudation. Invasion of hair follicles results in inflamed nodules, deep-seated pustules, and abscesses. In addition, inflammation accelerates shedding of the stratum corneum and the invading fungi. The skin becomes inflamed only after cell-mediated immunity to the dermatophyte develops. In its absence, only a dry, erythematous, scaly, pruritic, fissured, and cracked skin results. Two basic types of dermatophyte infection can result: (1) the acute or inflammatory type of infection, associated with cell-mediated immunity to the fungus, which generally heals spontaneously or responds readily to treatment, and (2) the noninflammatory type which is difficult to eradicate (Table 25-25).

Hairy regions are particularly favorable for dermatophyte growth, since the hair is composed solely of nonliving keratin. Within the hair strand, the organisms are isolated from cellular defenses so that areas with almost continuous active hair growth like the scalp are particularly difficult to cure.

Clinical Manifestations

Tinea Capitis. Ringworm of the scalp ordinarily produces round or oval areas with broken hairs (partial alopecia) in children. The first patch is the largest and the last to disappear. The borders of the round areas are slightly elevated. The central area shows scaling but fungal elements are absent. Itching may be the only symptom. *M. audouini* or *M. canis* fluoresce a bright blue-green under a Wood lamp, but culture is necessary for species identification.

Tinea capitis due to *M. audouini* is characteristically noninflammatory, but other forms may produce exudative folliculopustules. Permanent alopecia results only when severe secondary bacterial infection supervenes. The inflammatory changes (kerions) signal spontaneous cure, although hair regrowth may be slow. Incision and drainage of lesions is almost never necessary.

Tinea Barbae. Ringworm of the beard often presents as a highly inflammatory kerion—a boggy, nodular, exudative circumscribed tumefaction studded with pustules. Suppuration and secondary bacterial invasion are common, but a noninflammatory form also occurs. Differentiation from bacterial folliculitis may be difficult, except that bacterial infections do not produce alopecia.

Tinea Pedis (Athlete's Foot). Athlete's foot is the most common type of ringworm. It occurs primarily in young males who wear shoes, and hygienic measures within locker rooms are virtually useless. Three principal forms are described, but gradations occur frequently:

1. The intertriginous form produces maceration, weeping, scaling, and fissuring in the interdigital spaces, with accompanying malodor and pruritus. Scaling differentiates it from the many other forms of intertrigo. Warm weather and hyperhidrosis aggravate the condition. Secondary bacterial infection is a serious complication, especially in diabetics.

2. The vesicular form occurs primarily on the instep and may represent a dermatophid (sensitization reaction in the absence of fungi).

3. Squamous ringworm is most frequently caused by *T. rubrum*, a noninflammatory organism which produces diffuse scaling which makes the foot appear excessively dry. The first two forms tend to be inflammatory and recurrent. The third is comparatively noninflammatory and extraordinarily persistent.

Tinea Corporis. Ringworm of glabrous skin can produce vesicles, scaling, eczematous lesions, or massive granulomas, which may be mistaken for skin cancer. Tropical climates appear to predispose; most lesions tend to remain localized except in patients suffering from systemic diseases such as diabetes and leukemia. A variety of other dermatoses can be mimicked, and the diagnosis requires examination of scrapings from the border of the lesion.

Tinea Cruris. Groin ringworm is extremely common in males and uncommon in females except those habitually wearing tight-fitting slacks or panty hose. It is essentially an intertriginous infection starting in the moist crural or perineal folds with extensions onto the thighs. Bilateral involvement is common with half moon–shaped circinate lesions on each upper inner thigh with or without central clearing. Scaling is not a prominent feature. A Woods lamp helps make the diagnosis. Recurrence is due to high environmental temperatures, poor hygiene, and intertriginous moisture.

Tinea Unguium. Superficial fungal infections of the toenails are common in people wearing shoes and may be caused by fungi not classified as dermatophytes. They are frequent in patients with athlete's foot or the chronic squamous type of foot ringworm caused by *T. rubrum.* The distal nail becomes discolored and thickened by subungual hyperkeratosis, which ultimately leads to separation from the nail bed and considerable cosmetic distortion.

Tinea Versicolor. This is an infection of the stratum corneum caused by a nondermatophyte fungus, *Pityrosporum orbiculare (P. furfur, Malassezia furfur).* It produces asymptomatic hyperpigmented scaling lesions of no surgical importance.

Diagnosis

Microscopic examination of potassium hydroxide–treated scrapings from the afflicted areas reveals the characteristic hyphal growths. The organisms can be identified by their growth on simple or more complex agars if necessary.

Treatment

The details of treatment are best reviewed in dermatology texts. The principles are exemplified in the treatment of athlete's foot. Drying the skin is essential for treatment and prevention. The areas are washed, gently abraded to remove scales and macerated skin, and dried carefully. Leaving the areas open to the air (eg, going barefoot) is useful. Dusting powder and cotton inserts are useful if frequently changed and not permitted to become wet. Affected nails can be removed, but this will not cure the disease.

Severe cases necessitate the administration of griseofulvin (Chapter 18). Topical application of an imidazole (miconazole or clotrimazole) as a cream or solution may cure mild cases. Tinea capitus will respond to x-ray depilation, which should only be used in patients allergic to griseofulvin. Tinea versicolor is easily cured with a 1 percent selenium sulfide–based shampoo.

Superficial Candidiasis (Moniliasis)

The cutaneous manifestations of candidiasis are commonly seen in dermatologic practice, and as a nosocomial infection in surgical patients whose skin becomes chronically wet or macerated around open wounds or enterostomy sites.

The etiology, pathogenesis, and diagnosis of *Candida* infections are discussed in Chapter 9. The diagnosis of superficial candidiasis is made by microscopic demonstration of the organism in scrapings of the lesion. Cultural isolation of such a common commensal organism from a superficial lesion is not diagnostic. Although superficial candidiasis is not amenable to surgical therapy, extensive mucocutaneous candidiasis frequently precedes or accompanies systemic candidiasis in surgical patients in intensive care units.

Mucocutaneous Candidiasis

Thrush. Thrush is the most common candidal infection and is frequently seen in patients on antibiotics in whom the normal oropharyngeal flora has been altered. It is easily suppressed in such patients by oral nystatin swished around the mouth and swallowed.

The characteristic lesions are white patches on the mucous membranes of the mouth, usually sparing the pharynx. The patches are soft, creamy or crumbly, and poorly adherent, revealing a red base when removed. In extensive cases, the patches may extend into the trachea, upper bronchi, or even the esophagus. Perleche (cracks and fissues at the corners of the mouth) may be caused by *C. albicans*. On microscopic examination, the white crumbly material is comprised predominantly of pathognomonic budding cells and filaments.

Vulvovaginal Candidiasis. *Candida* is a normal resident of the vagina. Candidiasis occurs more frequently in pregnancy, diabetes, and in women taking oral contraceptives or antibiotics. A white or yellow curdy discharge containing dense masses of budding cells and filaments is diagnostic of vaginal candidiasis. The vagina is red, and curdy flakes can be seen attached to the vaginal wall. Itching of the vulva is a constant complaint, and the vulva may become red and swollen, secondary to the discharge. Candida intertrigo progresses to a macerated, eroded, red, weeping dermatitis. Debilitated nonambulatory women receiving antibiotics or immunosuppressive therapy are common victims (Chapter 44).

Cutaneous Candidiasis. Many varieties of this illness occur:

1. *Candida* intertrigo (diagnosed by the demonstration of large quantities of fungus in scrapings) causes lesions in the groin, axilla, intergluteal cleft, and the inframammary region as a dermatitis.
2. *Candida* paronychia is associated with physical trauma to the nail or frequent immersion of the hands in water. *C. albicans* has no keratinolytic enzymes and does not disorganize nail substance, but produces nail plate defects by damage to the matrix as does any type of chronic paronychia. The paronychial tissue is swollen and red, but relatively nontender and nonfluctuant although a drop of pus may be expressed from under the nail fold. Several fingers are usually involved. It is not clear whether *C. albicans* is a primary or a secondary invader.
3. Generalized cutaneous candidiasis is a rare generalized eruption.
4. Folliculitis, balanitis, and nodular and granulomatous manifestations are occasionally seen.

Chronic Mucocutaneous Candidiasis. This progressive candidal infection of mucous membranes, skin, and its appendages is usually found in patients with an inability to respond effectively to *Candida* antigens, which are present in high titers. The T cells of many patients are responsive to other antigens and to *Candida*. The mucous membranes are covered with thrush, and the skin with candidal paronychia or intertrigo. A generalized hyperkeratotic crusted dermatosis can result in disfiguring granulomas. Scarring and loss of hair are common. Secondary bacterial infection can occur, but candidal dissemination is rare. The disease appears to respond temporarily to systemic amphotericin B therapy but recurs promptly when the drugs are stopped. Ketoconazole controls the disease. Immunostimulation with various experimental preparations (such as levamisole, transfer factor) has been tried. An acquired endocrine (parathyroid, adrenal) disorder has been reported.

Treatment of Superficial Candidiasis

The polyene antibiotics nystatin and amphotericin B are effective, but amphotericin B is rarely required for mucocutaneous candidiasis. Thrush can be prevented by oral nystatin, 500,000 units (5 ml) four times daily. Patients who are immunosuppressed or on high-dose antibiotics may require higher doses. Similarly, nystatin can be administered as a vaginal tablet, and the gastrointestinal reservoir of *C. albicans* can be suppressed by oral nystatin tablets in doses of 1 to 3 million units taken several times a day. Ketoconazole is highly effective for both treatment and prophylaxis but is still under investigation.

The treatment of candidal intertrigo involves removing the predisposing macerating factors. Ointments must be avoided, since they can perpetuate the predisposing causes. Amphotericin, miconazole, and clotrimazole creams may be helpful.

THE SUBCUTANEOUS MYCOSES AND MYCETOMAS

The subcutaneous mycoses (chromomycosis, sporotrichosis) and the mycetomas are the result of traumatic implantation of the fungus into the skin and subcutaneous tissues. The ensuing disease generally remains localized to this area or slowly spreads to the surrounding tissue. In some diseases, slow extension via lymphatic channels is characteristic (sporotrichosis), but in others, either hematogenous or lymphatic dissemination is possible (chromomycosis). The etiologic agents are soil saprophytes, which are quite heterogeneous—their only common feature is the type of local disease produced.

Chromomycosis

Chromomycosis includes four clinical entities caused by pigmented fungi: (1) chromoblastomycosis or verrucous dermatitis is the classic form of the disease—a chronic granulomatous infection characterized by warty nodules and plaques which may ulcerate,[71] (2) the brain abscess syndrome (cladosporiosis), (3) a cystic subcutaneous form,[72] and (4) possibly a systemic form.[72]

Etiology

The disease is caused by a wide variety of closely related pigmented fungi, which produce black or brown thick-walled spores in tissue. *Phialophora verrucosa, Fonsecaea pedrosoi, F. compactum, F. dermatitidis,* and *Cladosporium carrionii* are the most common causes of chromoblastomycosis. Other less pathogenic species of these three genera produce cystic chromomycosis, especially *P. gougerotii.*[71]

Epidemiology

Most cases occur in male agricultural workers from humid tropical regions. The spores of soil fungi are implanted at sites of trauma on the feet and legs. Children exposed to the same conditions rarely develop the disease, suggesting that spores can lie dormant for prolonged periods. The cystic form is the result of mycelial growth in deep puncture wounds.

Pathology

The verrucous lesion shows a pseudoepitheliomatous hyperplasia of the surface epithelium and microabscesses containing neutrophils in the underlying dermis surrounded by epithelioid and giant cell granulomas. Brown yeast cells may be seen in and around the foreign body and Langhans giant cells. Fibrosis may be a feature in long-standing cases. The cystic lesion is essentially a mycelial ball surrounded by a thick fibrous capsule.

Clinical Manifestations

Chromoblastomycosis. This is the classic form of chromomycosis. A small pink scaly papule appears at the site of skin trauma (usually on the foot) and enlarges to a warty tumor, which may persist or spread out to form a plaque. The plaques may be verrucous with central scarring (tuberculoid), extensively scarred with a serpiginous border (syphiloid), scaly (psoriasiform), or indurated with draining sinuses (mycetomatoid). There is no invasion of muscle or bone, but tendon contractures, muscle atrophy, and osteoporosis may occur. Secondary ulceration from trauma or superinfection can lead to gross lymphedema and elephantiasis. Progress is slow, and satellite lesions along lymphatics may spread to involve a whole limb over 10 to 15 years. Although patients may seek medical assistance early because the disease is cosmetically unacceptable, most wait until they are disabled by lymphedema. Rarely, haematogenous spread and metastases occur to uninvolved areas of the body and the brain. Lymphatic spread is frequent after treatment by cautery and curettage, and biopsies can cause local spread.[71,72]

The differential diagnosis of this form includes blastomycosis, sporotrichosis, mycetoma, tuberculous verrucosa cutis, candidiasis, leishmaniasis, tertiary syphilis, and yaws. The diagnosis of chromomycosis is confirmed by culture of the organisms, by microscopic visualization of the thick-walled dark spores in 20 percent KOH-treated scrapings from the lesions, or by histologic examination of a biopsy showing the granulomatous reaction and spores.[71]

Cystic and Nonspecific Chromomycosis (including Phaeosporotrichosis). A puncture wound can inoculate the fungi deep into the subcutaneous tissues; single or multiple deep cysts containing masses of brown pigmented fungi of varied morphology result. The clinical designation phaeosporotrichosis is unfortunate, because the disease does not resemble sporotrichosis and the etiologic agents are not related. Phaeomycotic cyst is probably the best name.

The most common clinical presentation is a cutaneous, subcutaneous, or intramuscular abscess, which evolves into a hard cyst several centimeters in diameter, covered by a raised, thickened epidermis. Occasionally, the cyst may ulcerate and extrude pus containing brown hyphae and sclerotic cells. The regional lymph nodes are not involved, and dissemination is rare. Aspiration of the lesions sometimes results in a chronic fistula.

The differential diagnosis of this form of the disease includes the gumma of tertiary syphilis, sebaceous cyst, foreign body granuloma, tendon sheath ganglion, and sporotrichosis. Demonstration of pigmented fungi in material from lesions and their isolation in culture establish the diagnosis.

Treatment

Traditionally, chromoblastomycosis has been resistant to treatment. In the early verrucous lesion, wide and deep excision and grafting give good results. Curettage and cautery may cause dissemination of infection with lymphatic spread. Systemic amphotericin B is not useful, since fungicidal levels cannot be obtained in vivo. The most promising results have been with the antihelminthic thiabendazole orally (25 mg per kg per day) for 3 to 22 months, or 5-fluorocytosine (100 to 200 mg per kg per day) until healing is complete. Cystic chromomycosis should be excised. Contamination of the surrounding tissue can lead to recurrence.[71]

Sporotrichosis

Sporotrichosis is caused by the fungus *Sporothrix (Sporotrichum) schenckii.* As in all the subcutaneous mycoses, traumatic implantation of the fungus produces a chronic, benign-looking, cutaneous-lymphatic disease. A systemic infection characterized by polyarthritis and pneumonia can occur without the distinctive skin lesions.

Etiology

S. schenckii is a fungus which grows in tissues as a round or cigar-shaped yeast form. Its mycologic properties are discussed in Chapter 9.

Epidemiology

The fungus is found worldwide in soil, decaying vegetation, and gardening supplies and is introduced by accidental cutaneous implantation by a thorn (rose gardener's disease) or other minor trauma. Most cases are reported from Africa, France, Mexico, and the southern United States, especially in persons handling plants.

Pathogenesis and Pathology

After an injury, a small ulcer or subcutaneous nodule appears with erythema and fluctuance. Secondary nodules develop to mark the intermittent course of lymphatic spread. The nodular lesions consist of central necrotic tissue with a few neutrophils, eosinophils, and monocytes surrounded by epithelioid cells and occasional Langhans giant cells. Microabscesses are surrounded by lymphocytes and plasma cells. The asteroid body, amorphous eosinophilic material that radiates from a central fungal cell, is often seen in sporotrichosis as well as coccidioidomycosis and aspergillosis.

Clinical Manifestations

The ulcerating nodular lesions begin in the extremity at a site of injury with centripital spread marked by multiple subcutaneous nodules along the course of the draining lymphatics (Fig. 25-26). Little pain or disability results unlike bacterial cellulitis and lymphangitis. A pulmonary [73]

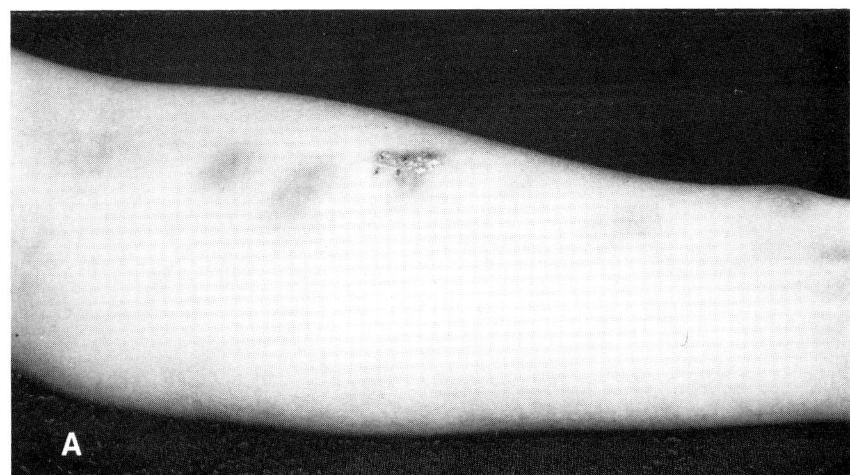

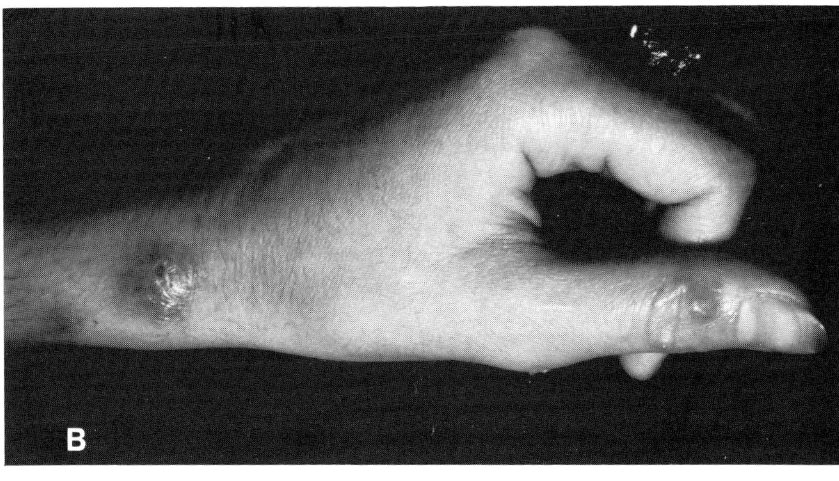

Fig. 25-26. **Sporotrichosis is an ulceronodular lesion with nodules that form along the course of lymphatic vessels. (Courtesy of Robert W. Goltz MD, professor and head, Department of Dermatology, University of Minnesota, Minneapolis, Minnesota.)**

and a disseminated form have also been described. The latter produces multifocal lesions in skin, synovia, or bone especially in metacarpal, phalangeal, or tibial bones.

Diagnosis

Isolation of the fungus is pathognomonic, since it is never a saprophyte in man. Histologic diagnosis is difficult, since visible fungi or asteroid bodies in tissue are rare and secondary bacterial infections are common. Many other chronic granulomatous infections can give an identical clinical picture (Table 25-12).

Therapy

The cutaneous-lymphatic form responds rapidly to treatment with a saturated solution of potassium iodide (1 gm per ml given in a dosage of 9–12 gm per day in three divided doses). Amphotericin B, to a total dose of 1.5–2.5 gm, has been employed (Chapter 9). Mortality and relapses are rare after adequate treatment.

The Mycetomas

A mycetoma is a chronic, granulomatous pseudotumor of the subcutaneous tissues, frequently extending into bone, characterized by abscess formation, sinuses, and fistulas which intermittently drain.[74,75] Fungi and aerobic actinomycetes introduced into the skin by trauma are the causal agents. Although clinically and pathologically identical to mycetomas, cervicofacial actinomycosis due to anaerobic actinomycetes and botryomycosis due to some eubacteria are not usually categorized as such (Table 25-26). The lesions most often occur on the foot as Madura foot, but the disease may occur on any part of the body.

Etiology

The organisms causing mycetomas belong to two groups, fungi and actinomycetes. The mycetomas are consequently divided into two groups, the mycotic mycetomas (eumycetomas or true maduromycoses) and the actinomycotic mycetomas, although the clinical pictures are identical. Almost 90 percent of mycetomas in North and Central America are due to *N. brasiliensis*, but even dermatophytes can cause mycetomas of the scalp and neck. A useful classification is based on the characteristic color of the grossly visible mycetomic grains found in pus or biopsy material (Table 25-26).

Epidemiology

Mycetomas are common in the tropical and hot temperate zones, especially in tropical North America (Mexico), Central America (except Costa Rica), India, and Africa. They also exist to a lesser extent in the southern United States, southern Europe, and the Near East. Alternating dry and wet seasons favor the disease. Mycetomas develop following a minor injury in subjects (mostly barefoot) who are in contact with contaminated material (field laborers, farmers, herdsmen, fishermen). Scalp and back mycetomas affect laborers carrying contaminated material on their heads or over the shoulder.

TABLE 25-26. ETIOLOGIC CLASSIFICATION OF MYCETOMAS

MYCOTIC MYCETOMAS
Caused by eumycetes (branched filaments, 3–4 μm or more in diameter)
Black grain
Madurella mycetomi
M. grisea
Pyrenochaeta romeroi
Phialophora jeanselmei
Leptosphaeria senegalensis
L. tompkinsii
Whiteish to yellowish grain
Allescheria boydii-Monosporium apiospermum (Petriellidium boydii)
Cephalosporium sp. *(C. recifei, C. falciforme)*
Fusarium sp.
Neotestudina rosatii
Aspergillus nidulans
ACTINOMYCOTIC MYCETOMAS
Caused by aerobic actinomycetes (branched filaments, 1 μm or less in diameter)
Whiteish to yellowish grain
Actinomadura madurae
Streptomyces somaliensis
Red grain
Actinomadura pelletieri
Small grain (grains invisible to the naked eye)
Nocardia brasiliensis
N. asteroides
N. caviae
ACTINOMYCOSIS *(SENSU STRICTO)*
Caused by anaerobic or microaerophilic actinomycetes (short filaments, 1 μm in diameter)
Yellow grains
Actinomyces israelii
A. bovis
BOTRYOMYCOSIS
Caused by *eubacteria* (cocci or short rods)
Yellow grains
Actinobacillus lignieresii
Staphylococcus sp.
Streptococcus sp.

From Mariat F, Destombes P, Segretain G: The mycetomas: clinical features, pathology, etiology and epidemiology. *Contrib Microbiol Immunol* 4:1, 1977.

Pathology and Pathogenesis

A typical mycetoma consists of large granulomatous tumor with a purulent center surrounded by a thick fibrotic reaction. Communicating, draining sinuses extend along fascial planes and through the skin. The central suppurative zone is in contact with the grain, surrounded by a ring of histiocytes often arranged in palisade fashion and frequently appearing as foreign body giant cells. In a third concentric zone, a subacute nonspecific granuloma is observed containing new capillaries, edema, histiocytes, plasma cells, mast cells, and eosinophils. Lymphocytes are generally localized in a more peripheral zone, sometimes embedded in the fibrotic tissue.

The central grain is an agglomeration of fungal or actinomycotic filaments with a diagnostic shape, composition, and color. Other organisms can cause grain formation, including actinomycosis *(A. israelii)*, lumpy jaw *(A. bovis)*, botryomycosis (*Staphylococcus* and other bacteria), and cryptic tonsillitis *(Leptothrix)*.[74]

Clinical Manifestations

After inoculation, there is a delay before onset of symptoms. The patient first notes a feeling of discomfort at the point of inoculation, accompanied by a small subcutaneous nodule adhering to the skin and sometimes to deeper tissues. The primary lesion subsequently opens to the skin, and grains may be extruded (Fig. 25-27A). New nodules then form around the initial abscesses. The mycetoma develops slowly, invading along fascial planes, forming fistulas and abscesses in the midst of the inflammatory tumor. Involvement of bone is common. In the foot, for instance, small cavities are formed in the bone, appearing as osseous "geodes," 2–10 mm in diameter. The medullary canal and epiphyses can also be invaded. Destruction of bone and the formation of osteophytes can give rise to a complete remodeling or destruction of the bone (Fig. 25-27B). At this stage of the disease, radiography is of great value, and in some typical cases the diagnosis and prognosis can be made on the basis of roentgenographic examination.

During the late phase, all the tissues may be involved. When this occurs, secondary bacterial infections supervene and cultures obscure the diagnosis. Visceral metastases via lymphatics from primary subcutaneous foci can be observed. Pulmonary metastases from primary thoracic mycetomas and abdominal and visceral metastases from mycetomas of the legs, thigh, and perineum have been reported, especially with *Nocardia* and *A. pelletieri*, perhaps because the small grains of these species can pass easily through the lymphatic vessels.[74,75]

Foot lesions (Madura foot) (Fig. 25-27B) are most often encountered. The destruction of the metatarsal bones with widespread plantar fibrosis and scarring of tendons give the foot a characteristic shortened and raised appearance.

Mycetomas develop slowly, spreading over a period of even 25 years or more. Sinuses may heal, only to open again in another area. The patient frequently has a long delay in medical therapy because of the absence of pain and the fear of amputation. Although cranial mycetoma can be rapidly fatal, most mycetomas are indolent and compatible with long life.

Diagnosis

Mycetoma must be differentiated from all the other diseases that cause persistent draining sinuses (Table 25-13), including some cancers (sarcoma, Kaposi disease). The etiologic agent can frequently be identified by the morphology of the grain in tissue sections stained with hemotoxylin and eosin. Grains removed from deep biopsies are cultured, but bacterial contamination is common. Immunologic methods of diagnosis can also be used.

Treatment

Amputation of the destroyed part is necessary in advanced cases. Debridement is not curative, and amputation must be extensive to avoid relapse. Chemotherapy has not been successful, except for sulfonamides for *Nocardia* species.[75]

CUTANEOUS AND SOFT TISSUE INFECTIONS WITH SYSTEMIC FUNGI

The biology, the clinical aspects, and the treatment of systemic infections with *Aspergillus*, the *Zygomycetes*, *Cryptococcus*, *Histoplasma*, *Blastomyces*, *Coccidioides*, and *Paracoccidiodes* have been discussed in Chapter 9. All these fungi can produce both primary and metastatic infection of the skin and soft tissues.

Cutaneous Aspergillosis

Aspergillosis is a disease caused by allergic phenomenon, simple colonization, or true tissue invasion (Chapters 9

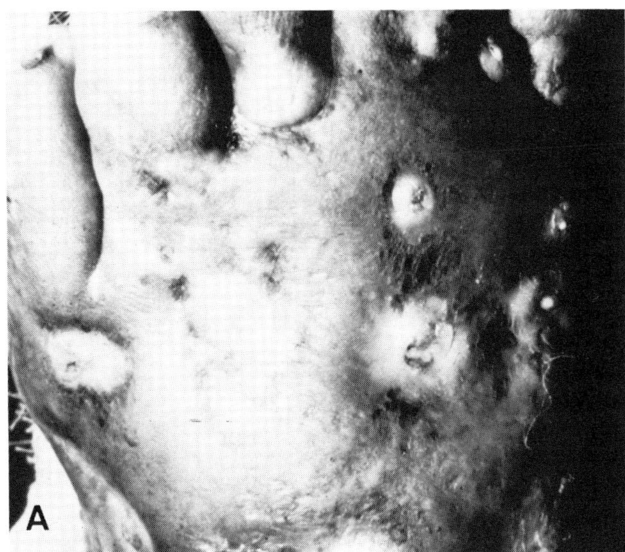

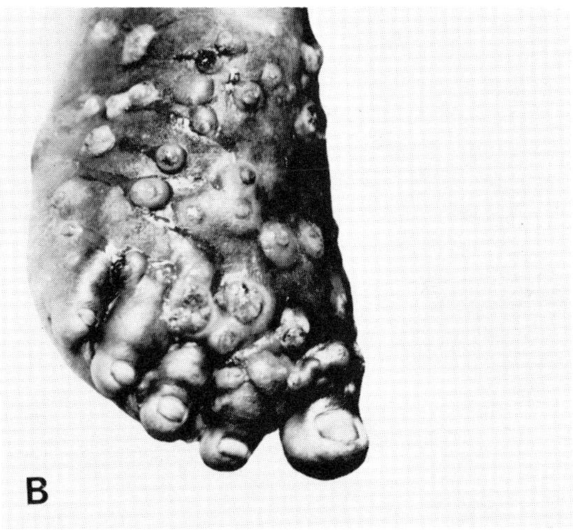

Fig. 25-27. **A. A moderately advanced lesion of mycetoma and even later, (B) a Madura foot. (From the Armed Forces Institute of Pathology, Neg. No. N-39280 (6490).)**

and 47). A number of *Aspergillus* species have been implicated, but most invasive infections are due to *A. fumigatus*.

Invasive infections are rarely seen in immunocompetent hosts. Immunosuppressed patients sometimes develop necrotic skin ulcers with black eschars at sites of minor trauma, but most infections originate in the lungs. Transpleural extension to bone or soft tissue is rare, as is hematogenous dissemination to soft tissue or bone. Chronic infections of the paranasal sinus may erode into adjacent tissues including the brain. The diagnosis depends on cultural isolation and the demonstration of hyphae in tissue specimens. Dissemination from a primary cutaneous infection is unusual.

Cutaneous and wound infections usually begin with blisters or pustules, which progress to hemorrhagic vesicles and progressive gangrene. The tendency of these organisms to thrombose blood vessels leads to necrosis, which spreads circumferentially. Smears reveal gram-positive organisms suggesting staphylococci, but histopathologic study demonstrates fungi with broad nonseptate hyphae in the necrotic debris. Drug therapy with amphotericin B is ineffective in the presence of necrotic tissue. Wound infections require wide debridement combined with systemic amphotericin B and topical antifungal therapy to prevent reinfection.

Cutaneous Zygomycosis

Zygomycosis (mucormycosis, phycomycosis) due to organisms of the genera *Mucor, Absidia,* and *Rhizopus* have been reported mostly in immunosuppressed or debilitated patients (diabetes mellitus, leukemia, lymphoma, renal failure, malnutrition and malignancy) (Fig. 25-28 A and B). In Uganda, primary subcutaneous infections with zygomycetes are not uncommon even in normal persons, particularly with *Entomophthora* and *Basidiobolus*.[77] The more common rhinocerebral and pulmonary infections in immunosuppressed patients have been discussed in Chapters 9, 27, and 30.

Direct inoculation into the skin accounts for the skin infections, since these fungi are ubiquitous in soil. Burned tissue is susceptible.[76]

It is important to recognize these fungi as a component of mixed gangrenous infections. Their clinical differentiating features are listed in Table 25-20. Diabetic or immunosuppressed patients with recent wounds or operations are usually affected. The lesion begins innocently as a necrotic ulcer or blister in the edge of the wound. Pain is minimal, fever is low grade, and crepitus is absent. The ulcerating lesion progressively expands and invades the skin and soft tissue so that progressive synergistic gangrene or necrotizing fasciitis is suspected. Wide debridement and systemic amphotericin B are required for control.[77] Histopathologic examination of the debrided tissue edges is necessary to be assured that debridement is sufficient.

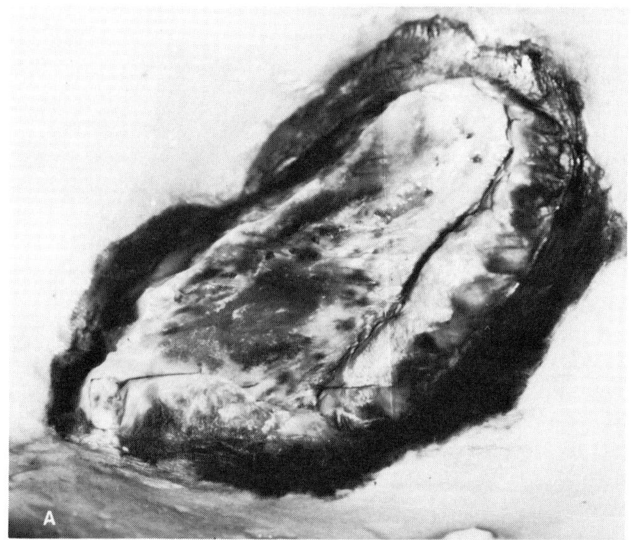

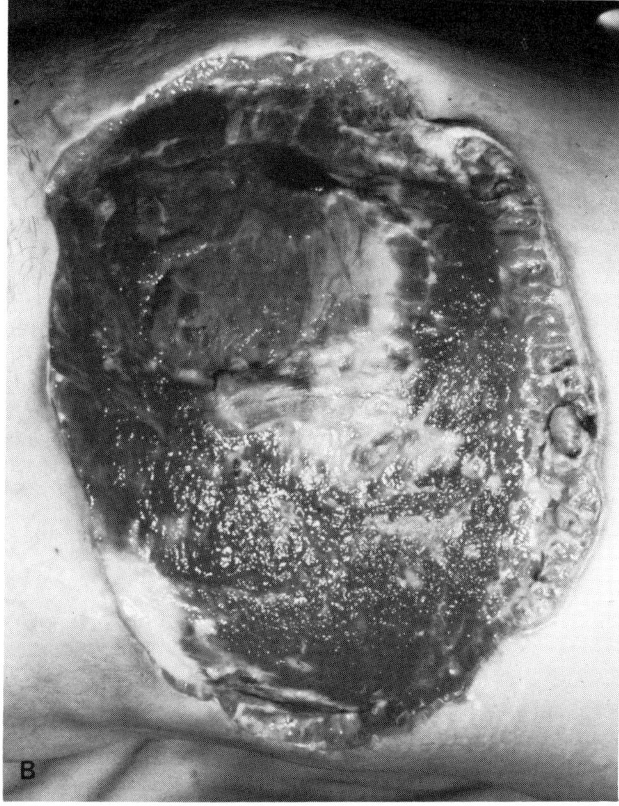

Fig. 25-28. **This cutaneous zygomycotic ulcer (A) is surrounded by black necrotic tissue, but debridement must include tissue outside the area of obvious necrosis. B. Progressive debridement required to treat this zygomycotic ulcer in the abdominal wall of a renal transplant recipient. There is still a rim of progressive gangrene at the top right of the picture. (Courtesy of William Sterling, MD, University of New Mexico.)**

Cutaneous Coccidioidomycosis

Etiology and Pathogenesis

The diagnosis and treatment of coccidioidomycosis has been discussed in Chapter 9. Extrapulmonary extension from an active, but perhaps asymptomatic, pulmonary focus is more common in blacks and Filipinos; the skin is especially favored. The lesions are granulomas and have few identifying characteristics. Chronic necrotic ulcers or abscesses draining a thick mucoid pus result from necrosis of subcutaneous granulomas. Multiple lesions can fuse, producing extensive ulcerations which ultimately develop veruccous or papillomatous changes. Neoplastic transformation can supervene.

In addition to the systemic cutaneous form, a rare primary cutaneous coccidioidomycosis produces a chancreform syndrome with regional adenopathy. Multiple draining nodules may form along the course of the lymphatics in a sporotrichoid pattern (Table 25-13). This is a self-limited disease quite different from the localized coccidiocidal granuloma produced by hematogenous dissemination.

The diagnosis and treatment of disseminated coccidioidomycosis are discussed in Chapter 9. The coccidioidin skin test is diagnostic in limited disease, but patients with disseminated disease become anergic; a rising complement-fixation titer signals progression and dissemination.

The diagnosis is made by demonstrating the characteristic endosporulating spherules on smears of sputum or biopsy specimens or by culture of the fungus. Disseminated disease is treated with amphotericin B.

Cutaneous Blastomycosis

The etiology, pathogenesis, diagnosis, and treatment of blastomycosis is discussed in Chapter 9. Eighty percent of the patients with systemic infections will develop skin lesions, which are the initial manifestations 25 to 40 percent of the time. The lesions begin as a papule or nodule, which ulcerates and discharges purulent material. Usually, there is a single lesion on the face, wrist, hands, or feet, but any site can be affected (Fig. 25-29). The lesion enlarges eccentrically and clears centrally, leaving a dense scar. Progression is slow but relentless, with an arciform or serpiginous, sharply elevated, verrucous, violaceous border (Fig. 25-29). Miliary abscesses contain organisms and are always found within the abruptly sloping border. Multiple abscesses may be present in disseminated blastomycosis. Accidental inoculation in physicians and laboratory workers leads to a chancreform syndrome with a localized cutaneous plaque and regional adenopathy. The primary lesion heals spontaneously, and the disease involutes.

The diagnosis and treatment of blastomycosis has been discussed in Chapter 9. Biopsy samples should be obtained from the border of the lesions, but the demonstration of round, budding organisms in a potassium hydroxide mount is difficult because organisms are sparse. The organism is best cultured by aspirating unruptured subcutaneous nodules. The blastomycin skin reaction has presumptive diagnostic value, and a primary pulmonary source should be sought. Cutaneous blastomycosis must be differentiated from tuberculosis, neoplasm blastomycosis, drug eruptions, syphilis, granuloma inguinale, and other deep-seated fungal infections. Chronic granulomatous pyoderma may be a particular source of confusion.

Treatment, using amphotericin B, has been discussed in Chapter 9. Excision or debridement is usually contraindicated.

Cutaneous Paracoccidioidomycosis

The etiology and pathogenesis of paracoccidioidomycosis has been discussed in Chapter 9. The most common type of disseminated paracoccidioidomycosis is first seen as lymph node enlargement. The skin may be the site of numerous granulomatous ulcerative lesions originating in the mucous membranes of the mouth, tongue, gum, palate, cheek, lips, and occasionally nasal, mucosa. A smooth, firm ulcer dotted with punctate hemorrhages rapidly enlarges to produce a hard brawny mass. New ulcers arise in the mouth and also extend rapidly, destroying most of the mucosal surface and spreading out onto the skin around the lips and nose. The lymph nodes of the neck and other sites enlarge massively and necrose to form draining sinuses. Spread to the lung resembles tuberculosis, and occurs in over 70 percent of the cases, but is seldom seen without associated mucocutaneous and lymphatic involvement. Visceral extension with hepatosplenomegaly is frequently fatal. The thick-walled yeast-like organisms with their diagnostic multiple buds are readily found in biopsy specimens, pus aspirated from lymph nodes, or currettings from mucous membrane lesions (Chapter 9).

Lobo Disease (Keloidal Blastomycosis)

This chronic localized disease occurs in the northern and Caribbean part of South America and overlaps the en-

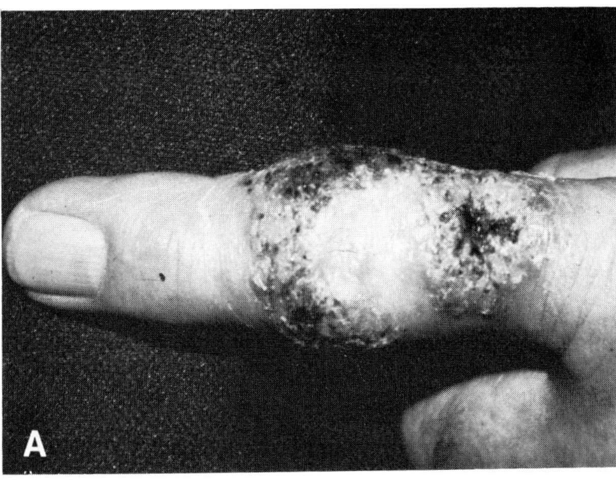

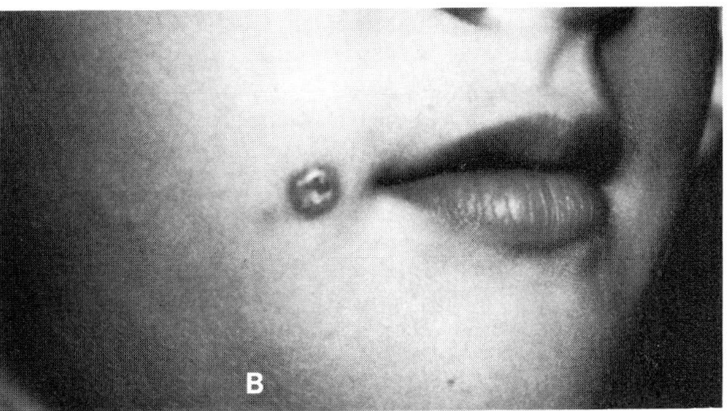

Fig. 25-29. **Cutaneous blastomycosis: A. extensive ulceronodular involvement of the finger; and B. an early facial lesion. (Courtesy of Robert W. Goltz MD, professor and head, Department of Dermatology, University of Minnesota, Minneapolis, Minnesota.)**

demic area of paracoccidioidomycosis. Lesions may be localized, beginning as intracutaneous nodules which become verrucous and crusted, spreading slowly by peripheral extension or autoinoculation. Lymphatic and visceral involvement is not seen. Excision of localized nodules may be curative. The causative organism *Loboa loboi* is probably a variant of paracoccidioidomycosis or a separate species.

Cutaneous Histoplasmosis

Primary histoplasmosis of the skin usually occurs in laboratory or autopsy workers. It produces the typical chancreform syndrome, with a chancre at the site of entry and regional lymphadenopathy. These infections are usually self-limited and seldom result in disseminated disease. Isolated, circumscribed, persistent lesions occasionally occur on the skin and the mucous membranes of the mouth and penis without evidence of disease elsewhere. The lesions are benign expressions of the disease, analogous to the circumscribed pulmonary lesions, and the prognosis is generally good.

Most cutaneous lesions are associated with the progressive form of histoplasmosis. The lesions are not distinctive but usually appear as a persistent punched-out or granulomatous ulcer. Other cutaneous manifestations (purpura, crops of papules, chronic abscesses, impetiginous dermatitis, and furunculoid and vegetating lesions) are also seen. Lesions of mucous membranes often appear as persistent ulcerative granulomas, which suggest that disseminated disease may enter through the gastrointestinal tract rather than the lung. In immunodepressed patients, either chronic or rapidly progressive disseminated disease can occur.

Diagnosis of the disseminated form, particularly in immunodepressed patients, can be difficult, requiring serologic tests, bone marrow biopsy, and aspiration (Chapter 9).

African histoplasmosis, caused by *H. duboisii*, usually presents with multiple subcutaneous and cold osseous abscesses rather than pulmonary disease. Pathologic fractures are common. The endemic area encompasses a wide band that extends across the African continent between the Sahara desert to the north and the Kalahari desert to the south.

Cutaneous Crytococcosis

Cutaneous lesions are almost always due to hematogenous spread of the organism *(C. neoformans)*. Immunodepressed patients (eg, renal transplant recipients) may have cutaneous lesions but no other symptoms of pulmonary or meningeal disease. Blood and cerebrospinal fluid culture results are frequently positive under these circumstances. The skin lesions can take many forms, including subcutaneous granulomas, papules, nodules, ulcers, or granulating sores. Cutaneous disease should prompt a search for cryptic pulmonary, blood, or meningeal disease. Treatment with amphotericin B and 5-fluorocytosine is effective without excision or debridement.

Cutaneous *Allescheria* Infections

Allescheria boydii is a small saprophyte, which behaves like *Aspergillus*. Infections of the paranasal sinuses and lung are most common. Like many soil saprophytes (see preceding section on mycetoma), inoculation into the skin will lead to localized granulomatous infection especially in the immunodepressed patient.[78] Surgical debridement combined with amphotericin B is frequently necessary for cure.

Rhinosporidiosis

Rhinosporidium seeberi is thought to be a fungus which forms cysts 10–200 μm in diameter in the submucosa of the nose, pharynx, or conjunctiva. Males are more often afflicted. The lesion is painless but enlarges to form a friable pedunculated mass. Excision is curative.

CUTANEOUS ALGAL INFECTIONS

Protothecosis

Prototheca are unicellular achloric alga-like organisms, which rarely cause human disease but can enter the body after skin trauma to cause a papulonodular lesion which drains intermittently. Wound infections have been reported. Dissemination in humans is rare. *P. wickerhamii* is the most common isolate. The diagnosis requires histopathologic examination of Gomori methanamine silver or PAS stained biopsy specimens. The organisms can be cultured on Saboroud agar. Excision of early lesions may be curative, and response to amphotericin B therapy is reported.

VIRAL DISEASES OF THE SKIN

Surgeons are rarely consulted for viral skin infections, but viral infections increasingly complicate treatment of surgical patients. A few require operation for diagnosis or cure.

SUPERFICIAL VIRAL INFECTIONS OF THE SKIN

Herpes Simplex

The herpes viruses are discussed as a group in Chapter 10. Their interest for the surgeon resides in their appearance in immunodepressed surgical patients and their occasional tendency to become necrotic and require surgical care.

Etiology

Two types of herpes simplex virus (HSV) are recognized: HSV type 1 is classically associated with nongenital (usually oral) lesions, and type 2 with genital lesions, although changing sexual behavior is altering the sites of infection. The two types can only be distinguished by serologic tests and their effects on cells in tissue culture.

Clinical Manifestations

Cutaneous herpes may present as primary or recurrent disease. Either type 1 or type 2 herpes simplex virus can manifest in any of the clinical forms.

Primary Herpes Simplex Infection. Although most primary infections with either virus are subclinical, two classical presentations are described: primary gingivostomatitis (HSV-1) in children aged 2 to 5, and primary vulvovaginitis in adolescents (HSV-2), characterized by a sudden development of painful mucosal lesions, high fever, regional adenopathy, and malaise. The painful vesicles and white plaques appear on the mucosa of mouth, pharynx, gingiva, or vagina, with surrounding erythema and edema (Fig. 25-30A). Spontaneous resolution takes about 2 weeks, but adenopathy can persist. Recurrence is common with all herpetic lesions.[79]

Primary herpes simplex virus infections can occur in any area as a localized vesicular eruption with regional adenopathy. Primary venereal (usually HSV-2) disease can appear on the penis, vulva, perineum, cervix, or anus (especially in male homosexuals). The exquisitely tender vesicles may rupture and ulcerate. An accompanying sacral radiculomeningitis can produce urinary retention and obstipation. Other veneral diseases must be ruled out.

A herpetic whitlow on a finger following slight trauma and contact with an infected patient is an occasional presentation, especially in medical or dental personnel (Fig. 25-30C). Recurrent herpetic whitlow may be mistaken for bacterial cellulitis because of the surrounding edema and erythema. The grouped, discrete vesicles at the margin of the lesion suggest the diagnosis. Incision and drainage is contraindicated.[79]

Surgical wounds have also been reported as sites of primary herpetic infections. Infection normally subsides but may recur in this site later. Kaposi varicelliform eruption (eczema herpeticum) is a form of primary herpes simplex which can be fatal in infants with eczema and in patients of any age with burns. In eczematous children, fever and umbilicated varicelliform lesions appear over areas of atopic dermatitis. The vesicles, which become hemorrhagic and pustular and may persist for several days to a week, are accompanied by severe adenopathy and local edema. A similar disease occurs in burned patients, and may convert second degree burn areas to third degree; bacterial superinfection is common. Visceral extension has been reported. Because burn patients are already covered with crusts, secondary viral superinfection is difficult to appreciate. The diagnosis is suggested by vesiculation of the margins of the burn wound, followed by an increase in the extent of third degree burn with patches of bacterial infection and by high fever which does not respond to antibiotics (Chapter 48). Biopsy of burn wound margins shows viral inclusion bodies; surviving patients develop a fourfold or greater rise in herpes neutralizing antibody titers.

Recurrent Herpes Simplex. Most adults show herpes neutralizing antibodies in their serum, which indicates prior infections. Recurrent lesions often develop after some form of stress such as high fever, prolonged illness,

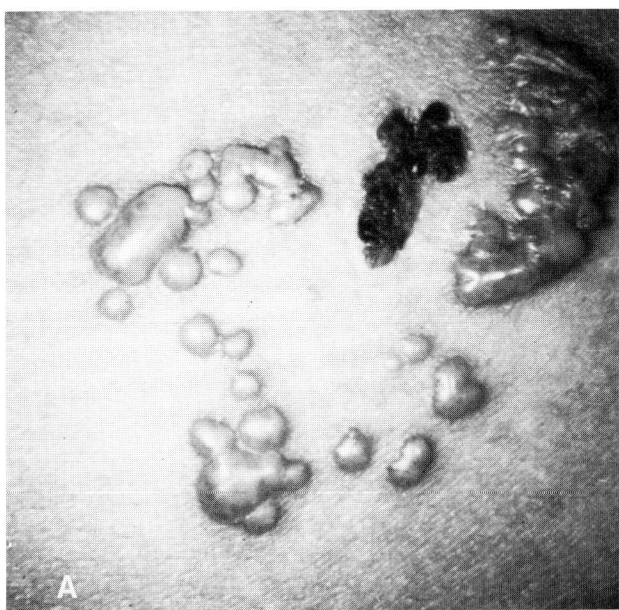

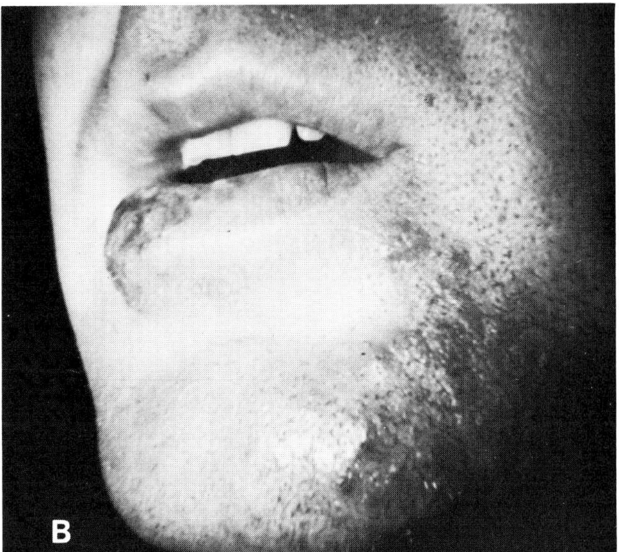

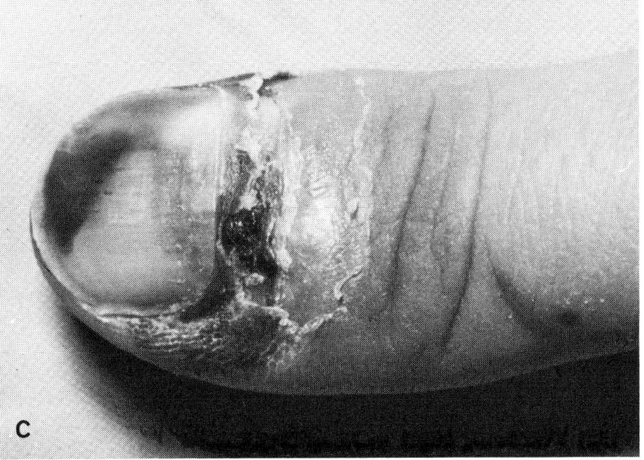

Fig. 25-30. **A. Painful vesicles of primary herpes simplex infection. B. Recurrent herpetic lesions of the lips. C. Herpetic whitlow in a renal transplant recipient who bites her fingernails.**

immunosuppression, or exposure to sunlight. The development of painful vesicles grouped on an erythematous base is usually preceded by a local tingling or burning sensation for several hours to days. The lesions usually persist for only a few days without much exudation and are most frequent about the lips, perioral, or genital region (Fig. 25-30B). A dangerous form of recurrent herpes affects the eye. The eyelids and palpebral conjunctivae are typically affected, but a dendritic keratitis can develop and progress to include the stroma. Prevention of bacterial superinfection by using a broad-spectrum antibiotic ophthalmic solution is critical (Chapter 26).

Lesions of the lip, pharynx, and esophagus are sometimes seen in immunodepressed patients. Dissemination of recurrent disease is rare, but occasionally occurs without typical cutaneous manifestations in immunosuppressed children. Operative division of the sensory nerve for trigeminal neuralgia is frequently followed by herpetic vesicles, and there is evidence that the herpes virus may remain latent within the trigeminal ganglion.

Diagnosis

The diagnosis of classical primary or secondary infections is simple. Scraping the roof or floor of a vesicle or ulcer with a blade, fixing the smear with alcohol on a glass slide, and staining with Giemsa stain to demonstrate the multinucleate giant cells confirms the viral etiology. This Tzanck preparation is positive for herpes simplex as well as varicella-zoster; by contrast, vaccinia produces intracytoplasmic inclusions. The viruses are identified by demonstration of a cytopathogenic effect in tissue culture and appropriate serologic tests (Chapter 10).

Treatment

No effective specific antiviral treatment of recurrent or primary cutaneous herpes is currently available in the United States. Photoinactivation of herpesviruses can be demonstrated in vitro and may be efficacious in vivo, but the oncogenicity of the virus may be reactivated. Ocular herpes responds to topical idoxuridine or adenine arabinoside (Ara A). Systemic Ara A has some efficacy in disseminated disease, but may be dangerous to central nervous function in immunosuppressed patients.[80] Acyclovir has been highly effective in clinical trials as an early treatment of herpes simplex and varicella zoster. Because of the low toxicity, this drug will almost certainly prove to be a useful antiherpetic drug (Chapter 18).

Varicella Zoster

The etiology and pathogenesis of varicella-zoster infections have been discussed in Chapter 10.

Varicella

Clinical chicken pox has little surgical significance, although occasional episodes of primary or even secondary disseminated varicella infections occur in immunodepressed children.[81] Superimposed bacterial pyoderma frequently complicates the course of such patients. Bleeding can occur from vesicles in the bladder or nose. Laryngeal edema rarely requires tracheostomy; a fatal purpura fulminans and even intestinal gangrene have been reported.[82] Immunosuppressed children who have not had chicken pox should receive zoster immune globulin, to abort the disease, as soon as they are exposed to it.

Zoster

Shingles is a recrudescence of varicella-zoster virus infection in an "immune" patient. The disease is associated with Hodgkin disease and other lymphomas, radiotherapy, chemotherapy, and organ transplantation, and may signal an occult malignancy. Zoster produces necrotizing ganglionitis of the nerve root and posterior ganglion. Loss of neurofibrils occurs early in affected skin, so that pain and paresthesias precede the cutaneous lesions. Grouped vesicles appear on an erythematous base in a unilateral dermatomal pattern within 1 to 7 days after onset of pain and hyperesthesia (Fig. 25-31A and B). The eruption usually clears in about 2 to 3 weeks, but secondary bacterial infection or gangrenous changes can prolong the healing time. Regional lymphadenopathy, malaise, and low-grade fever are common, and persistence in the form of intractable neuralgia is a feared complication. The most frequently affected dermatomes are thoracic, but any segment can be involved. *H. zoster* affects the eye less often than *H. simplex*. The eye is most in danger when the nasociliary branch of the ophthalmic branch of the trigeminal nerve is affected (Fig. 25-31A).

The Ramsay-Hunt syndrome is *H. zoster* of the geniculate ganglion, ie, the 7th cranial nerve that inervates deep facial tissues. Painful vesicles along the uvula, palate, anterior tongue, auricle, and posterior auricular areas may be accompanied by paresis of the face. Glossopharyngeal zoster produces pain in the ear and pharynx with vesiculoulcerative lesions of the soft palate and vesicles of the ear. Vagal zoster may cause paresis of the larynx and pharynx as well as cardiac and epigastric distress. There may be vesicles on the base of the tongue, epiglottis, and arytenoids. C2 to C4 phrenic involvement may paralyze the ipsilateral diaphragm. With thoracic zoster (Fig. 25-31B), pleural friction rubs may be heard near the involved skin, and at times electrocardiogram changes occur. Lumbosacral involvement mimics renal colic and may result in urinary retention. Generalized zoster is potentially lethal in patients with Hodgkin disease, lymphoma, leukemia, or severely immunodepressed patients.

The diagnosis depends on finding multinucleate giant cells on a Tzanck preparation and serologic tests.

Adenine arabinoside may be effective in disseminated disease, but its potential toxicity precludes its use in regional zoster.[80] There is no other effective specific therapy currently available in the United States. Interferon is experimental. Acyclovir has been highly effective in clinical trials in immunodepressed patients, and will probably prove useful (Chapter 18). Currently, however, intractable pain may require neurosurgical intervention. Immunoglobulin from convalescent zoster serum, although useful in the prevention of primary varicella infections, is useless in the prevention and treatment of zoster itself. An experimental vaccine has been developed for patients at high risk for chicken pox,[83] but its value in the prevention of zoster is unknown.

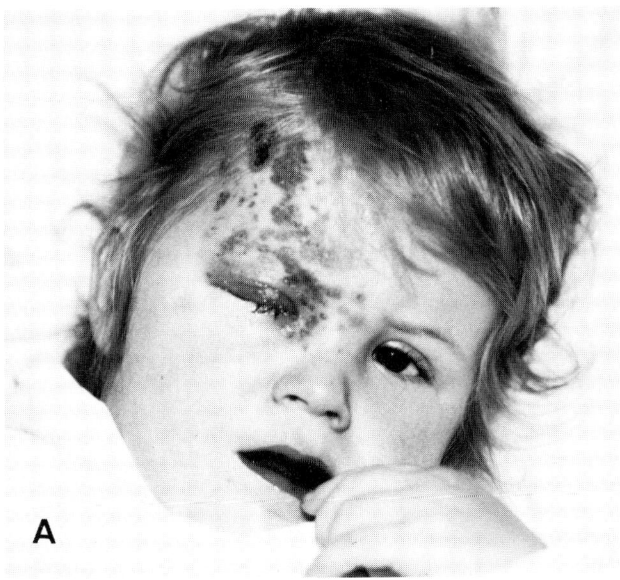

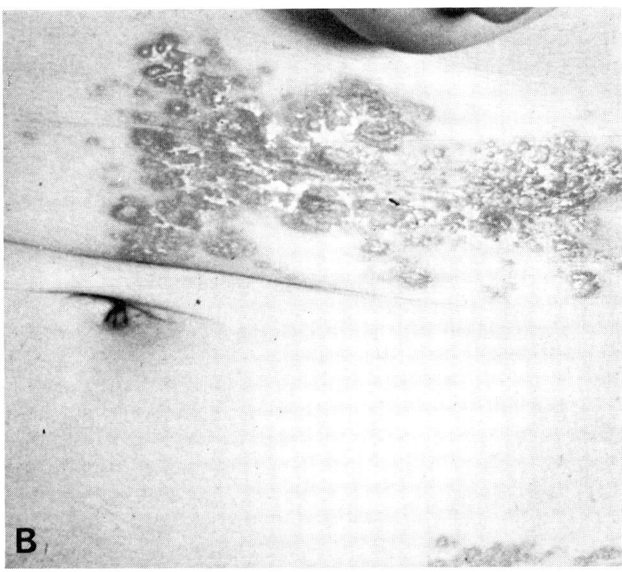

Fig. 25-31. Zoster (A) face of a child and (B) thoracic zoster in an immunosuppressed adult. (Courtesy of Robert W. Goltz MD, professor and head, Department of Dermatology, University of Minnesota, Minneapolis, Minnesota.)

Warts

Warts, or verrucae, are extremely common viral skin infections characterized by an unpredictable clinical course. Warts are called ectotropic because they affect only the skin and the mucous membranes adjacent to mucocutaneous junctions. Although they are principally an infection of childhood and young adult life, they may be incurable.[84]

Etiology

Warts are probably caused by a filterable infectious agent, a DNA human papilloma virus (HPV). This conclusion is derived primarily from evidence for their autoinoculation, and transmission from person to person, although the virus has not been cultivated.

Pathogenesis and Pathology

The virus is apparently inoculated through breaks in the skin and stimulates epithelial cell hyperplasia with hyperkeratosis and areas of parakeratosis and papillomatosis. In young verrucae, large vacuolated cells appear in the stratum malpighii and in the granular layer with rounded, deeply basophilic nuclei, which contain aggregates of virus particles on electron microscopy.

Clinical Manifestations

Warts present various morphologic forms. Sessile lesions with a rough gray surface are usually seen on the extremities. Filiform or digitate warts resembling cutaneous horns or nevoid skin tags are commonly encountered on the face and neck. Plantar warts occur where pressure prevents verrucous elevation, especially on the sole where they are often exquisitely painful. The callouslike lesions demonstrate diagnostic obliteration of the skin lines. The wart is usually discernible if the surface of the lesion is shaved off. Plantar warts may be single, multiple, or grouped together in a mosaic fashion. Hyperhidrosis may aid dissemination and seeding of the lesions on the feet. Flat warts, which resemble lightly pigmented nevi, are usually seen in children, especially on the face or forehead.

In moist intertriginous areas, the wart virus causes anogenital warts (condyloma acuminata), which may be so large and painful that coitus or defecation is avoided (Fig. 25-32). The lesions are pink or white with a strawberry-like surface and may be sexually transmitted. Differentiation from the highly infectious syphilitic condyloma lata is important. Malignant transformation is commonly reported.[85]

In addition to their varied morphologic pattern, warts have an unpredictable course, undergoing capricious spontaneous disappearance, dissemination, or stubborn persistence. In general, warts disappear with age but will commonly recur in immunosuppressed patients.[84]

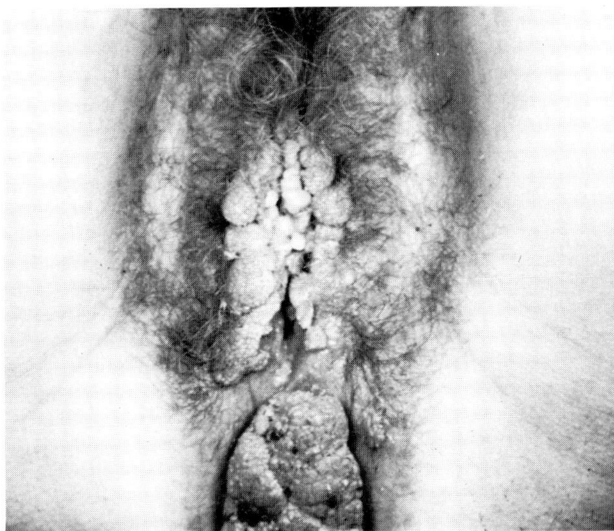

Fig. 25-32. Anogenital warts (condyloma accuminata). (Courtesy of Robert W. Goltz, MD, professor and head, Department of Dermatology, University of Minnesota, Minneapolis, Minnesota.)

Treatment

Dermatologists usually treat warts,[84] but surgeons must recognize two principles: (1) the diagnosis must be clear to avoid treating painful calluses or hyperkeratotic pressure points as warts, and (2) extensive full-thickness resection is unnecessary because the wart is an entirely intraepidermal tumor.

Scarring from excessive operation may cause a significant permanent disability. The preferred treatment for sessile warts is electrodesiccation or cryosurgery with liquid nitrogen. The top of the wart is shaved, lightly electrocoagulated until it softens, then curretted and the bleeding points cauterized. Undue coagulation of the base of the lesion will retard healing and produce excessive scarring without improving the chances of cure. Cryosurgery is performed cautiously to avoid freezing digital vessels and nerves with consequent permanent paresthesias.

Although most warts need not be removed, periungual warts (those on either the nail fold or under the distal margin of the nail plate) should always be removed immediately before the inevitable extension occurs. Local chemotherapy with 10 to 25 percent glutaraldehyde solution, 10 percent formalin ointment, or 0.7 percent cantharidin in acetone, and flexible collodion under tape occlusion is preferred to cryosurgery or electrodesiccation. Repeated application of these agents after paring away the white macerated tissue is necessary, but irritant reactions to the medications may limit usefulness.

Flat warts are amenable to psychotherapy in children, reinforced by lotions such as those used to treat acne. Electrodesiccation or freezing is useful for warts of the scalp or bearded areas, but recurrence is common.

Plantar warts pose the most serious therapeutic challenge. Irreversible painful scarring on pressure points must be avoided. A wide variety of cauterant chemicals that require repeated application can be used. Repeated nightly applications of 5 to 20 percent formalin solution produce hardening and drying of the skin surface, which may allow the warts to be shelled out. Phenolnitric acid–salicylic acid is useful when only a few warts are being treated. The keratotic surface of the wart is first shaved off, and fuming nitric acid is applied to the wart tissue only. Then phenol is applied, which results in a brown eschar. A salicylic acid plaster (30 percent salicylic acid paste coated with a protective moleskin or leather ring and firm adhesive dressing) cut to fit the entire hyperkeratotic area is firmly applied. In a day or two, pain may result from liquifaction of the base of the wart, and the entire wart may then drop out. If this does not occur, it is worthwhile to repeat the treatment at intervals of 2 weeks for a total of 6 to 8 sessions.

Podophyllin is effective against warts in moist areas but is ineffective on dry warts. Plantar warts can be treated if maceration is first produced. After paring down the wart, a 20 percent solution of podophyllin in compound tincture of benzoin is applied and overlain with nonporous adhesive tape to increase maceration. This is repeated at intervals of 48 to 72 hours. Electrodesiccation is not useful in plantar warts because painful scarring may result.

Warts occurring in moist intertriginous areas frequently become numerous and exuberant. A 20 percent solution of podophyllin in compound tincture of benzoin is applied, allowed to dry, and the site powdered lightly with talc. The patient is instructed to wash the area thoroughly in 5 to 6 hours. Sitz baths are helpful in relieving subsequent discomfort. Failure to remove the agent may result in excruciating pain by the following morning. The treatment is repeated every week or two, and scarring is minimal. Sexual partners should be examined and treated to avoid reinfection. Resistant condyloma are excised or electrodesiccated, but excessive scarring can produce strictures in the perianal, periurethral or vaginal areas. Biopsies will exclude exuberant squamous cell carcinoma.[85]

Molluscum Contagiosum

Molluscum contagiosum is a common pox virus infection of the skin and occasionally causes conjunctivitis in children. Spread occurs by direct contact. Pathologically, the epidermis grows into the dermis to form saccules, which contain clusters of intracytoplasmic virus. Clinically, scattered discrete lesions are found, each a slightly umbilicated, cone-shaped, hard, shiny, pale papule 2–5 mm or larger in diameter. Caseous material, which contains the microscopically visible molluscum bodies, can be expressed. In children, the trunk, face, extremities, and conjunctiva are favored sites, but in adults the pubic, genital, and perineal areas are usually affected. Shelling out the inclusions with a currette is curative; light electrocautery or freezing is also effective. The lesions are benign, and wide excision is discouraged.[86]

Viral Exanthems

Many viral illnesses are accompanied by symmetric, erythematous eruptions of the skin (and mucous membranes) called exanthems—measles, atypical measles, rubella, roseola, fifth disease, variola (smallpox), vaccinia, and enteroviral exanthems (Table 25-7). Rarely is surgical consultation required for either diagnosis or therapy of these diseases, even in immunodepressed patients.

Epidermodysplasia Verruciformis

Epidermodysplasia verruciformis is a rare warty viral disease of childhood or adolescence sometimes associated with parental consanguinity and mental retardation. The lesions, unlike warts, persist indefinitely. Many lesions progress to invasive malignancy for which excision is required. Radiotherapy is thought to be contraindicated.

SUPERFICIAL VIRAL INFECTIONS OF THE SKIN CONTRACTED FROM ANIMALS

Cat Scratch Disease

Etiology

The infecting organism of cat scratch disease[87] is unknown, though both chlamydial and viral etiologies have been postulated.

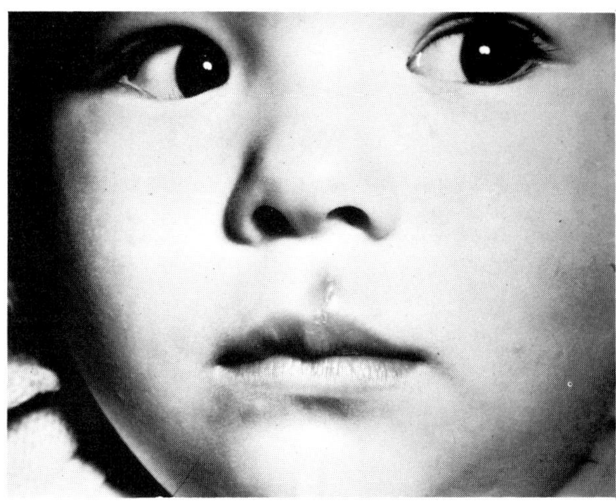

Fig. 25-33. **Pustule of cat scratch disease at site of inoculation. (From Armed Forces Institute of Pathology, Neg. No. 56–12797.)**

Clinical Manifestations

The disease is most common in children and adolescents, especially during the winter months. It may arise from a bite or scratch from any pet or from a splinter. After 3 to 30 days, an inflamed papule or pustule appears at the site of inoculation and persists for several weeks (Fig. 25-33). Regional lymphadenopathy which may suppurate and drain develops without intervening lymphangitis. Fever and malaise are common, but systemic dissemination is unusual.

Diagnosis

Exposure to a pet, the clinical symptoms, and failure to isolate an organism from aspirated pus help establish a presumptive diagnosis. The histologic picture of stellate abscesses surrounded by epithelioid cells is suggestive, and a positive delayed hypersensitivity response to intradermal skin test (Hanger-Rose test) with an easily prepared antigen is diagnostic. All the causes of a local skin lesion with regional adenopathy must be considered in the differential diagnosis (Table 25-14).

There is no specific treatment; the disease is usually self-limited, although adenopathy may persist. Fluctuant nodes are aspirated with an 18 or 19 gauge needle, and repeat aspiration may be necessary. Surgical drainage sometimes results in sinus tract formation.

Ecthyma Contagiosum

This pox virus infection produces vesicular and pustular eruptions of the mucocutaneous regions in sheep. Humans are occasionally infected after direct contact with sheep and less often after handling contaminated lumber or clothing. Lesions develop on the hands, to progress from an erythematous macule to a papule and finally an eczematous nodular disease. Lymphadenitis is uncommon. The differential diagnosis includes vaccinia, cutaneous malignancy, verruca, orf, and an infected keratoanthoma. Serologic diagnosis is possible but rarely used.

Milker's nodules

The paravaccinia virus, a pox virus that infects cow teats or calf muzzles, is sometimes transmitted to the hands of humans. It produces single or multiple firm, nonfixed, sometimes ulcerated and crusted red papules or nodules, 0.5–1.5 cm in diameter. The lesions heal in about 6 weeks. Regional adenopathy is common. The virus may be the same as that which causes ecthyma contagiosum. For definitive diagnosis, electronmicroscopic examination of crusts from the lesions reveal the cigar-shaped virus, 310 nm long and 140 nm wide, in the cytoplasm of infected cells.

Orf

The paravaccinia virus, which causes contagious pustular dermatitis (orf) in sheep, can spread to persons employed in the wool or meat industries. It is similar in other respects to milker's nodule, which is caused by a similar paravaccinia virus. A self-limited hyperplastic nodular mass results, and electron microscopy reveals long ovoid viral particles.

PROTOZOAN AND HELMINTH INFECTIONS OF THE SKIN AND SOFT TISSUES

The protozoan and helminth infections of interest to surgeons are discussed in Chapter 11. Several of these produce characteristic or severe infections of the skin and soft tissues. Table 11-5 lists the subcutaneous filariads.

PROTOZOAN

Cutaneous Amebiasis

Amebiasis is discussed in Chapter 11; its colonic and hepatic manifestations are discussed in Chapters 39 and 36. Cutaneous amebiasis usually occurs as a direct extension from, or after operation on, diseased viscera. Autoinoculation of the perianal region, buttocks, vulva, and face occur in patients with colitis. Venereal spread is possible, and penile lesions have been described. The skin lesions spread rapidly and cause death in young patients with dysentery. The lesion consists of a painful ulcerating granuloma (ameboma) containing a purulent exudate with raised erythematous borders and undermined edges. Regional lymphadenopathy is present. The diagnosis is confirmed by finding trophozoites in the fresh material from the edge of the ulcer. Repeated stool examinations should be made even if there is no evidence of dysentery. Both systemic and enteric therapy, as described in Chapter 11, are required. Surgical debridement is contraindicted unless fistulas persist after successful chemotherapy.[88]

Trypanosomiasis

Trypanosomiasis is discussed in Chapter 11. African trypanosomiasis is a systemic infection; the only cutaneous manifestation is a red nodule with lymphangitis and lymphadenopathy at the site of the tsetse fly bite.

American trypanosomiasis (Chagas disease) caused by *T. cruzi* produces a tumorlike edematous mass (Romana sign) at the site of inoculation. The lymphatics and draining lymph nodes become enlarged within 4 to 5 days, followed by hepatosplenomegaly. Myocarditis and meningoencephalitis can be fatal complications of the acute disease. The chronic form of disease is characterized by chronic heart failure and megaesophagus and megacolon, without soft tissue manifestations. There is no known treatment for the chronic degenerative form of the disease (Chapter 11).

Leishmaniasis

Infections with *Leishmania* organisms produce either a systemic infection involving the reticuloendothelial system or a localized cutaneous infection without systemic involvement. There are also mucocutaneous infections characterized by cutaneous and metastatic mucous membrane infections. Three species of *Leishmania* have been designated, but they may represent the same organism—*L. donovani* causes kala-azar, *L. brasilliensis* causes the mucocutaneous form, and *L. tropica* causes cutaneous leishmaniasis.

Clinical Manifestations

Kala-azar. Kala-azar (black death) is a visceral disease, which produces fever, emaciation, edema, splenomegaly, and pigmentation of temples and perioral regions.

Mucocutaneous leishmaniasis (American leishmaniasis). Mucocutaneous leishmaniasis is found from Mexico to Argentina, where its vector is the phlebotomus fly. The initial lesion, a hard nodule, appears 2 weeks to 2 months after the fly bite (Table 25-9). The lesion increases in size (3–12 cm), and becomes secondarily infected. A sporotrichoid pattern appears along the lymphatics (Table 25-12).

The metastatic mucosal involvement is delayed for 3 to 10 years, producing ulcerated granulomatous lesions at the mucocutaneous junctions of the nose or mouth to destroy the nose (Fig. 25-34), or spread to the pharynx, palate, and larynx. Malnutrition and respiratory complications can be fatal.

The diagnosis depends on identification of the organism in smears, cultures, or tissue sections; the leishmanian skin test is almost always diagnostic. Pyoderma, sporotrichosis, syphilis, yaws, chromoblastomycosis, leprosy, and carcinoma must be ruled out.

Treatment has traditionally been with the pentavalent antimonials (stibosan, stibamine), but amphotericin B is also effective.[89]

Cutaneous leishmaniasis. Oriental sore is a specific granuloma of the skin caused by *L. tropica* in tropical areas of the Eastern Hemisphere. The sand fly (phlebotomus) is the main vector. Most patients are children because the infection produces permanent immunity. A granuloma appears weeks or months after inoculation, grows to 2 cm in size, and ulcerates (Table 25-9). Secondary bacterial

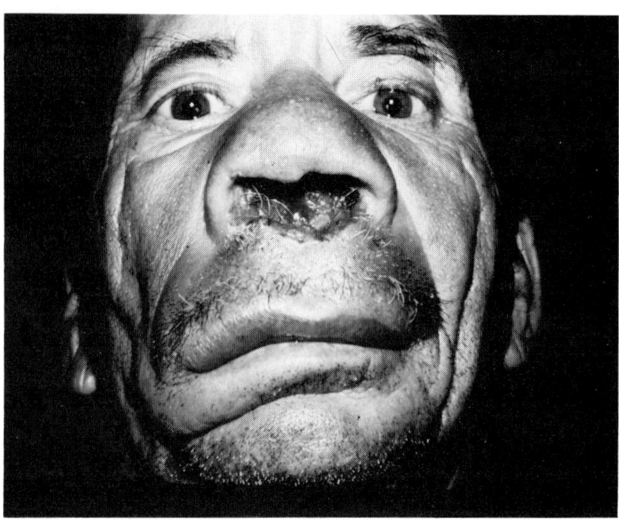

Fig. 25-34. **Mucocutaneous leishmaniasis of the nose has destroyed the nasal septum and collapsed the nose. (From Armed Forces Institute of Pathology, Neg. No. 74–8873–1.)**

infection is common, but healing is spontaneous. Multiple ulcers are caused by autoinoculation or multiple bites.

The diagnosis depends on demonstration of the parasite in stained currettings or aspirates from the ulcer edges. The ulcer surface does not show the parasite.

Surgical excision is not recommended; cryosurgery is useful for some chronic lesions. Pentavalent antimonials such as glucantime (methylglucamine antimoniate) and antimalarials (chloroquine, quinacrine) are the agents most commonly used.[89] Antimony sodium stibogluconate and Neostibosan are useful for systemic therapy.[89a]

HELMINTH INFECTIONS

Platyhelminths (Flatworms)

Schistosomiasis

There are several cutaneous lesions associated with schistosomiasis, a parasitic worm which resides in the portal venous system (Chapter 11). The surgeon is most likely to see the paragenital granulomas which commonly occur in the Middle East where *S. haematobium* is endemic. Granulomatous lesions involve the vaginal area, perineum, and buttocks and are usually associated with extensive communicating fistulas and sinuses. Ectopic cutaneous schistosomiasis produces cutaneous plaques secondary to the hematogenous spread of the worms. Skin or rectal biopsies reveal presence of the ova in both cases. Treatment is described in Chapter 11 (Table 11-4).

Sparganosis

Sparganosis has a worldwide distribution but occurs mostly in the Orient. The disease is caused by the procercoid larva (sparganum) of *Spirometra mansonides* and *S. mansoni* tapeworms. The definitive tapeworm hosts are dogs and cats; people are intermediate hosts after ingesting the ova. The larva penetrates the intestine and develops into a spargoma in the subcutaneous tissue or muscle causing edematous, painful areas. The worm usually dies and produces intense inflammatory tissue destruction and eosinophilia. Incision and drainage with removal of the worm is the preferred therapy. Arsenicals (neoarsphenamine) are said to produce a good response (Chapter 11).[90]

Cysticercosis

Taenia solium (the pork tapeworm) infects the human intestine after the ingestion of infected incompletely cooked pork. The larval form invades the subcutaneous tissues to produce cysticercosis, manifested by round, rubbery, painless subcutaneous cysts (Fig. 25-35 A and B). The diagnosis is made on histopathologic examination of excised cysts. Niclosamide eliminates the adult intestinal worm, but the cysts must be excised (Table 11-3).

Echinococcosis

The larval form of the dog tapeworms *E. granulosus* and *E. multilocularis* penetrates the intestine and invades various tissues (including liver, lung, and bone) producing soft, painless, fluctuant subcutaneous cysts of various sizes, which calcify or are resorbed. Bouts of urticaria may accompany echinococcosis of various sites. The diagnosis is made on roentgenographic findings of calcified cysts and serologic skin tests. Excision of the cysts is diagnostic and therapeutic (Chapter 11).

Nematodes

Cutaneous Larva Migrans (Chapter 11, Table 11-5)

The surgical significance of cutaneous larva migrans is limited to the need for occasional diagnostic biopsy. Creeping eruption is caused by the infectious larval form of several hookworm species, especially *Ancylostoma braziliense.* The larvae can penetrate the intact skin and migrate beneath the epidermis at 1–2 cm per day. The hands, feet, buttocks, and genital areas become marked by serpiginous tracts, 2–3 mm wide, with advancing margins and local inflammation caused by a hypersensitivity reaction of the host (Fig. 25-36 A and B). Itching and scratching can lead to eczematization or secondary bacterial infection. The diagnosis is suspected by the location and the appearance of the lesions; biopsy samples taken at the advancing edge demonstrate the infecting larva. The infection is self-limited but may be chronic—no protective immunity develops.

In the case of autoinfection, systemic thiabendazole by mouth (50 mg per kg body weight per day, in two equal portions, for 2 days, with a maximum daily dose of 3 gm) is effective. Adverse reactions to the drug include nausea, vomiting, drowsiness, and hematuria. Local treatment with dry ice or ethyl chloride spray applied to the advancing edge of the burrow blisters the epidermis, and the larva is shed.

Larva currens is caused by the larval form of the human hookworm *Strongyloides stercoralis* which penetrates the perianal skin. Its migration is rapid and is accompanied by an intense itching urticarial or papulovesicular rash. The larvae then invade the deeper tissues, and the rash fades. Treatment is identical to larva migrans.[91]

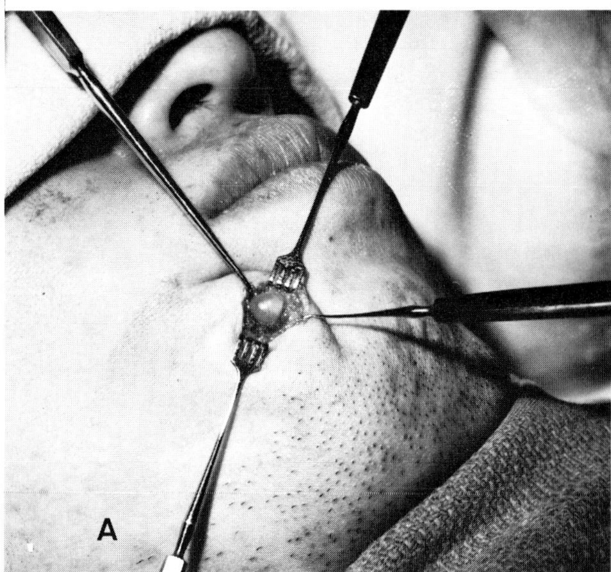

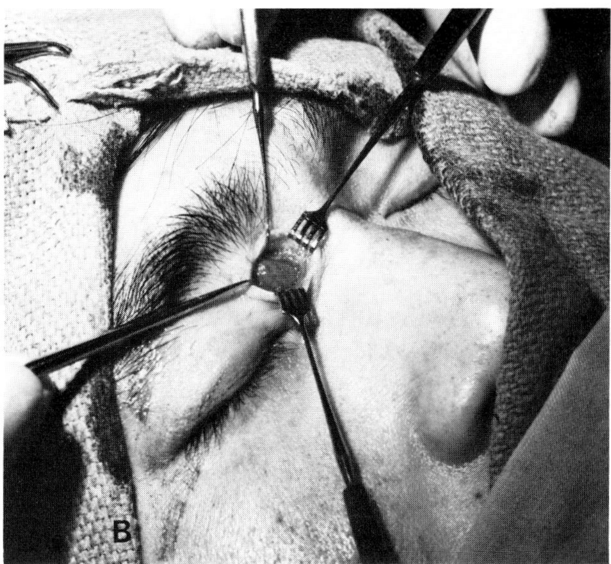

Fig. 25-35. **Subcutaneous cystecercosis. The larval form of taenia soluim (pork tapeworm) in two subcutaneous locations (A and B) in one patient. (From the Armed Forces Institute of Pathology, Neg. No. 69–2890–3–4.)**

Cutaneous Filariasis

Three agents cause the disease: *Dracunculus medinensis* and the true filariae *Onchocerca volvulus* and *Loa loa.* All three come to the attention of surgeons in the tropics, although none are endemic to the United States (Table 11-5).

Onchocerciasis. *Onchocerca volvulus* is spread by the bite of female black flies, genus *Simulium,* found along the west coast of Africa and from Central America to

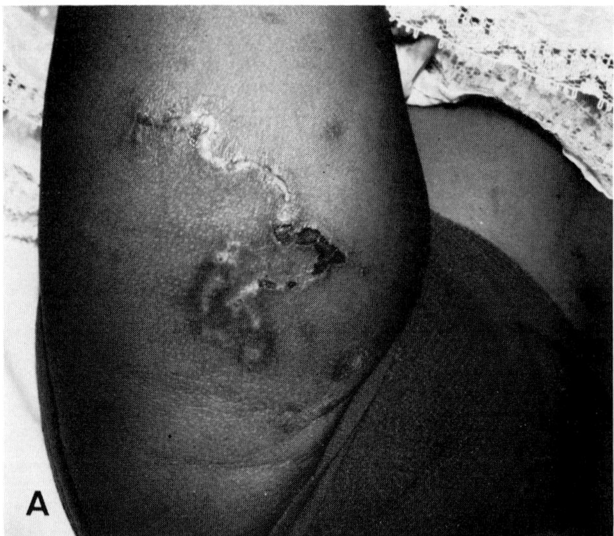

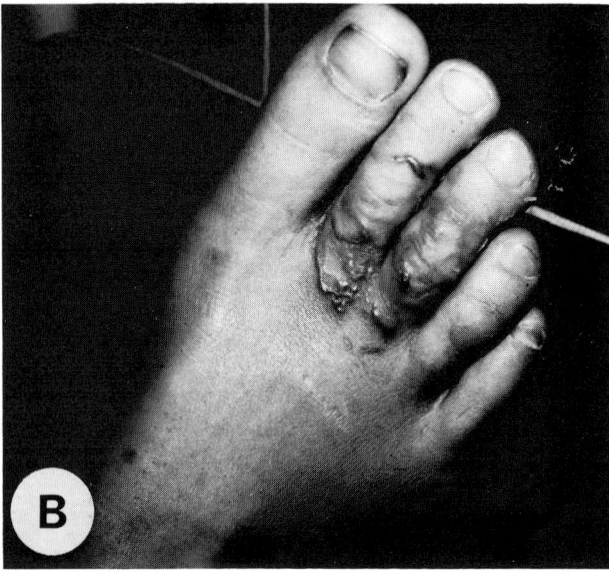

Fig. 25-36. **Cutaneous larva migrans of the (A) arm, (B) foot. (From Armed Forces Institute of Pathology. Neg. Nos. 74–8291–2 and 74–8291–1.)**

northern South America. Africans bear lesions on the legs, and in Central America the nodules occur on the head, reflecting the different biting habits of the vectors involved.

The adult worm is long-lived (7 to 15 years), but takes a year or so to develop from the larvae injected by the fly. A foreign body granulomatous reaction to the adult worm is produced, which leads to cutaneous nodules. Abscesses may form because the worms occasionally degenerate. The microfilariae laid by the adult worm spread out in the tissues thickening the epidermis with a low-grade inflammatory reaction, which produces the clinical manifestations of persistent itching, skin rash, and subcutaneous nodules. When the cornea is involved, blindness may result. The nodules vary greatly in size, from 1 to 8 cm, especially over body prominences (Fig. 11-17).

The diagnosis depends on the finding of microfilariae in bloodless biopsy specimens of superficial skin taken with a razor blade. The material is teased apart to reveal the swimming microfilariae. The results of a filarial complement-fixation test may be positive. Scabies and superficial mycoses must be ruled out.

Systemic suramin kills adult worms when given as six weekly intravenous injections of 17 mg per kg body weight in each dose. Diethylcarbamazine is effective in killing microfilariae but not adult worms. Where practical, all nodules should be excised to reduce the load of adult worms.

The black fly larvae and pupae are sensitive to DDT in river water; this is the most effective form of control for the insect vector.

Loaiasis. Infection with *Loa loa* is characterized by transient, inflamed, edematous swellings of the skin called Calabar swellings, thought to be the migration sites of adult worms in the subcutaneous tissue. The erythematous swellings, 5–10 cm in size, usually affect the upper limbs. The disease, limited to the west coast of Africa, is transmitted by biting deerflies of the genus *Chrysops.* The swellings result from hypersensitivity to the adult worm or its byproducts, and roentgenograms may reveal calcified worms in tissue. Biopsy is not indicated, and the swellings never suppurate. The worms can be excised. Blood drawn during the day may reveal eosinophilia, sheathed microfilariae, and a positive filarial complement-fixation test. The disease is of little consequence except when the eye, a peripheral nerve, or the central nervous system is involved.

Diethylcarbamazine kills both adults and microfilariae in doses of 12 mg per kg per day in three divided doses, by mouth for 14 days.

Dracunculiasis (Guinea Worm Infection). People become infected after ingesting infected water fleas which bear the larvae of the guinea worm *Dracuncula medinensis,* which is edemic in the Middle East, North Africa, and the Caribbean. The larvae invade the intestine and mate. When ready to discharge their larvae, the pregnant female adults migrate to the surface of the skin, possibly selecting regions in humans that are likely to be immersed in cold water. As the adult female worm approaches the skin, a blister is followed by an ulcer several centimeters wide (Figs. 11-14 and 11-15). The anterior end of the worm then extrudes to discharge the microfilariae. Superinfection of the ulcer with a resultant cellulitis is common, although eosinophils are found locally. The lesion usually occurs on the lower leg but may be found elsewhere including the joints. Observing the protruding worm is diagnostic. The worm may die and calcify in tissues to produce a characteristic roentgenographic picture. Cellulitis and secondary infection often occur if the gravid worm dies in situ or is broken during extraction. Septicemia or tetanus are reported complications.

It is important to extract the worm slowly to avoid breaking it. Gradually winding the worm out of the ulcer by turning on a stick a few centimeters a day is common practice. Surgical extraction has been practiced. Niridazole has been reported to be lethal to the adult worm in a dose of 25 mg per kg body weight per day by mouth for 7 days; the worm can then be easily withdrawn.[92]

Filariasis

The adult filaria, *Wuchereria bancrofti, Brugia malayi,* and other species of the superfamily Filaroides live in the lymphatics of the extremities and external genitalia proximal to the lymph nodes. Numerous mosquitoes can serve as vectors. Elephantiasis takes several years to develop. There are multiple episodes of lymphadenitis or lymphangitis. Ultimately, fibrosis and obstruction of the lymphatics produces thick, dry, course swellings of legs and genitalia (Fig. 25-37). The skin may crack, become secondarily infected, and develop chronic ulcers.

Early diagnosis in endemic areas can be made by nodal biopsy or an intradermal skin test. During the acute symptomatic phase, the filaria can be seen in thick blood smears.

Treatment of the acute disease with diethylcartamigene (Banocide) 4–6 mg per kg for 2 weeks kills the microfilariae, but the adult worm is resistant so recurrence requires retreatment. Operation may be necessary to reduce the massive elephantiasis.

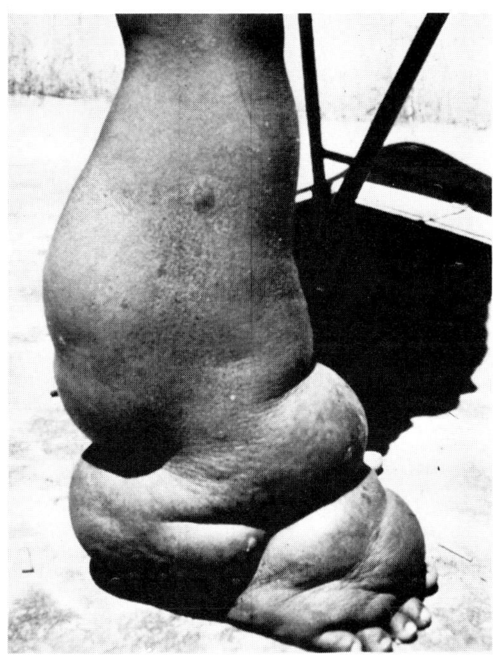

Fig. 25-37. **Elephantiasis (filariasis) of the leg. (From Armed Forces Institute of Pathology, Neg. No. 74–6426–2.)**

BIBLIOGRAPHY

Baxter CR: Surgical management of soft tissue infection. Surg Clin N Amer 52:1483, 1972.

Levin ME, O'Neal LW: The Diabetic Foot. St. Louis, Mosby, 1977.

Moschella SL, Pillsbury DM, Hurley HJ Jr (eds): Bacterial infections. In Dermatology Vol I. Philadelphia, Saunders, 1975, pp 482–557.

Emmons CW, Binford CH, Utz JP, Kwon-Chung KJ: Medical Mycology (3rd ed), Philadelphia, Lea & Febiger, 1977.

Fitzpatrick TB, Eisen AZ, Wolff K, Freedberg IM, Austen KF (eds): Disorders due to microbial agents. In Dermatology in General Medicine, (2nd ed), New York, McGraw-Hill, 1979, pp 1415–1749.

Swartz MN: Skin and soft tissue infections (Section 1). In Mandell GL, Douglas RG Jr, Bennett JE (eds): Principles and Practices of Infectious Diseases, Vol 1. New York, Wiley, 1979, pp 797–834.

Mandell GL, Douglas RG Jr, Bennett JE (eds): Infections related to trauma. In Principles and Practice of Infectious Diseases, Vol 1. New York, Wiley, 1979, pp 835–845.

Noble WC, Somerville DA (eds): Microbiology of Human Skin. London, Saunders, 1974.

Finegold SM: Anaerobic Bacteria in Human Disease, New York, Academic, 1977.

REFERENCES

PATHOBIOLOGY

1. Roettinger W, Edgerton MT, Kurtz LD, Prusak M, Edlich RF: Role of inoculation site as a determinant of infection in soft tissue wounds. Am J Surg 126:354, 1973.
2. Noble WC, Somerville DA (eds): *Microbiology of Human Skin.* London, Saunders, 1974.
3. Williamson P.: Quantitative estimation of cutaneous flora. In Maibach HI, Hildick-Smith G, (eds): Skin Bacteria and their Role in Infection. New York, McGraw-Hill, 1965, p 3.
4. Ulrich JA: Dynamics of bacterial skin populations. In Maibach HI, Hildick-Smith G (eds): Skin Bacteria and Their Role in Infection. New York, McGraw-Hill, 1965, p 219.
5. Meislin HW, Lerner SA, Graves MH, McGehee MD, Kocka FE, Morello JA, Rosen P: Cutaneous abscesses: anaerobic and aerobic bacteriology and outpatient management. Ann Intern Med 87:145, 1977.
6. Duncan WC, McBride ME, Knox JM: Experimental production of infections in humans. J Invest Dermatol 54:319, 1970.
7. Madden JE, Edlich RF, Custer JR, Panek PH, Thul J, Wangensteen OH: Studies in the management of the contaminated wound. IV. Resistance to infection of surgical wounds made by knife, electrosurgery, and laser. Am J Surg 119:222, 1970.
8. Agarwal DS: Subcutaneous staphylococcal infection in mice. I. The role of cotton-dust in enhancing infection. Br J Exp Pathol 48:436, 1967.
9. Haury BB, Rodeheaver GT, Pettry D, Edgerton MT, Edlich RF: Inhibition of nonspecific defenses by soil infection potentiating factors. Surg Gynecol Obstet 144:19, 1977.
10. Edlich RF, Schmolka IR, Prusak MP, Edgerton MT: The molecular basis for toxicity of surfactants in surgical wounds. I. EO:PO block polymers. J Surg Res 14:277, 1973.

DIFFERENTIAL DIAGNOSIS

11. Burnett JW, Crutcher WA: Viral and rickettsial infections. In Meschella SL, Pillsbury DM, Hurley HJ Jr (eds): Dermatology, Vol 1. Philadelphia, Saunders, 1975, p 558.
12. Nichols RL, Smith JW: Modern approach to the diagnosis of anaerobic surgical sepsis. Surg Clin North Amer 55:21, 1975.

COMMON BACTERIAL INFECTIONS OF THE SKIN

13. White A, Brook GF: Furunculosis, pyoderma, and impetigo. In Hoeprich PD (ed): Infectious Diseases, 2nd ed. Hagerstown, Harper and Row, 1977, p 785.

14. Dajani AS: The scalded skin syndrome: relationship to phage II staphylococci. J Infect Dis 125:548, 1972.
15. Grieco MH, Sheldon C: Erysipelothrix rhusiopathiae. Ann NY Acad Sci 174:523, 1970.
16. Leyden JJ, Marples RR, Mills OH, Jr, Kligman AM: Gram-negative folliculitis—a complication of antibiotic therapy in acne vulgaris. Br J Dermatol 88:533, 1973.
17. Hill HR, Estensen RD, Hogan NA, Quie PG: Severe staphylococcal disease associated with allergic manifestations, hyperimmunoglobulinemia E, and defective neutrophil chemotaxis. J Lab Clin Med 88:796, 1976.
18. Good RA, Quie PG, Windhorst DB, Page AR, Rodey GE, White J, Wolfson JJ, Holmes BH: Fatal (chronic) granulomatous diseases of childhood: a hereditary defect of leukocyte function. Seminars Hematol 5:215, 1968.
19. Hurley HJ Jr: Apocrine glands. In Fitzpatrick TB, Eisen AZ, Wolff K, Freedberg IM, Austen KF (eds): Dermatology in General Medicine, 2nd ed., New York, McGraw-Hill, 1979, p 473.
19a. Hyland WT, Neale HW: Surgical management of chronic hidradenitis suppurativa of the perineum. South Med J 69:1002, 1976.
20. Weinberg AN, Swartz MN: Gram-negative coccal and bacillary infections. In Fitzpatrick TB, Eisen AZ, Wolff K, Freedberg IM, Austen KF (eds): Dermatology in General Medicine, 2nd ed., New York, McGraw-Hill, 1979, p 1445.

INFECTIONS OF THE SUBCUTANEOUS TISSUE

21. Davis WA, Kane J, Garagush V: Human *Aeoromonas* infections. Medicine 57:267, 1978.
22. Louie TJ, Bartlett JG, Tally FP, Gorbach SL: Aerobic and anaerobic bacteria in diabetic foot ulcers. Ann Intern Med 85:461, 1976.
23. Culbertson WR: Acute nonclostridial crepitant cellulitis. Arch Surg 77:462, 1958.
24. Galpin JE, Chow AW, Bayer AS, Guz LB: Sepsis associated with decubitus ulcer. Am J Med 61:346, 1976.
25. Stone HH, Martin JD Jr: Synergistic necrotizing cellulitis. Ann Surg 175:702, 1972.
26. Macfie J, Harvey J: The treatment of acute superficial abscesses: a prospective clinical trial. Br J Surg 64:264, 1977.
27. Philip RS: A simplified method for the incision and drainage of abscesses. Am J Surg 135:721, 1978.
28. Robson MC, Shaw RC, Heggers JP: The reclosure of postoperative incisional absesses based on bacterial quantification of the wound. Ann Surg 171:279, 1970.
29. Jones NAG, Wilson DH: The treatment of acute abscesses by incision, curettage and primary suture under antibiotic cover. Br J Surg 63:499, 1976.
29a. Page RE, Freeman R: Superficial sepsis: the antibiotic of choice for blind treatment. Br J Surg 64:281, 1977.
30. Aduan RP, Fauci AS, Dale DC, Herzberg JH, Wolff SM: Factitious fever and self-induced infection: a report of 32 cases and review of the literature. Ann Intern Med 90:230, 1979.
30a. Wedel KR: A therapeutic confrontation approach to treating patients with factitious illness. Soc Work 16:69, 1971.
31. Malinowski RW, Strate RG, Perry JF, Jr, Fischer RP: The management of human bite injuries of the hand. J Trauma 19:655, 1979.
32. Chambers GH, Payne JF: Treatment of dog bite wounds. Minn Med 52:427, 1969.
33. Blattner RJ: Rat-bite fever. J Pediatr 67:884, 1965.
34. Manson MH: Pathogenic gas-producing anaerobic bacilli in chronic ulcers. Arch Surg 24:752, 1932.
35. Levin ME, O'Neal LW (eds): The Diabetic Foot, 2nd ed., St. Louis, Mosby, 1977.
36. Mitchell AAB: Incidence and isolation of bacteroides species from clinical material and their sensitivity to antibiotics. J Clin Pathol 26:738, 1973.
37. Gocke TM: Infection complicating diabetes mellitus. In Grieco MH (ed): Infections in the Abnormal Host. New York, Yorke Medical Books, 1980, p 585.
38. Friedman SA, Rakow RB: Osseous lesions of the foot in diabetic neuropathy. Diabetes J 20:302, 1971.

GANGRENOUS INFECTIONS

39. Meleney FL: Hemolytic streptococcus gangrene. Arch Surg 9:317, 1924.
40. Rea WJ, Wyrick WJ Jr: Necrotizing fasciitis. Ann Surg 172:957, 1970.
41. Giuliano A, Lewis F, Jr, Hadley K, Blaisdell FW: Bacteriology of necrotizing fasciitis. Am J Surg 134:52, 1977.
42. Rudolph R, Soloway M, DePalma RG, Persky L: Fournier's syndrome: synergistic gangrene of the scrotum. Am J Surg 129:591, 1975.
43. Wilson CB, Siber GR, O'Brien TF, Morgan AP: Phycomycotic gangrenous cellulitis. Arch Surg 111:532, 1976.
44. Baxter CR: Surgical management of soft tissue infections. Surg Clin North Am 52:1483, 1972.
45. Finegold SM (ed): Infections of the skin, soft tissue, and muscle. In Anaerobic Bacteria in Human Disease. New York, Academic, 1977, p 386.

MYOSITIS

46. Burbrick MP, Hitchcock CR: Necrotizing anorectal and perineal infections. Surgery 86:655. 1979.
47. Roding B, Groenveld PHA, Borema I: Ten years of experience in the treatment of gas gangrene with hyperbaric oxygen. Surg Gynecol Obstet 134:579, 1972.
48. Brown PW, Kinman PB: Gas gangrene in a metropolitan community. J Bone Joint Surg 56A:1445, 1974.
49. Swartz MN: Myositis. In Mandell GL, Douglas RG Jr, Bennett JE (eds): In Principles and Practice of Infectious Diseases, New York, Wiley, 1979, p 818.
50. Svane S: Peracute spontaneous streptococcal myositis. A report on 2 fatal cases with review of literature. Acta Chir Scand 137:155, 1971.

UNUSUAL BACTERIAL INFECTIONS OF THE SKIN

51. Brachman PS: Anthrax. In Hoeprich PD (ed): Infectious Diseases, 2nd ed. Hagerstown, Harper and Row, 1977, p 807.
52. Brachman PS, Fekety FR: Industrial anthrax. Ann NY Acad Sci 70:574, 1958.
53. Koopman JS, Campbell J: The role of cutaneous diptheria infection in a diptheria epidemic. J Infect Dis 131:239, 1975.
54. Swartz MN, Weinberg AN: Miscellaneous bacterial infections with cutaneous manifestations. In Fitzpatrick TB, Eisen AZ, Wolff K, Freedberg IM, Austen KF (eds): Dermatology in General Medicine, 2nd ed. New York, McGraw-Hill, 1979, p 1459.
55. Rhodes AR, Luger AFH: Syphilis and other treponematoses. In Fitzpatrick TB, Eisen AZ, Wolff K, Freedberg IM, Austen KF (eds): Dermatology in General Medicine, 2nd ed. New York, McGraw-Hill, 1979, p 1677.
56. Demis DJ: Nonsyphilitic treponematoses. In Hoeprich PD (ed): Infectious Diseases, 2nd ed. Hagerstown, Harper and Row, 1977, p 823.

57. Wolff K: Mycobacterial diseases: Tuberculosis. In Fitzpatrick TB, Eisen AZ, Wolff K, Freedberg IM, Austen KF: Dermatology in General Medicine, 2nd ed. New York, McGraw-Hill, 1979, p 1473.
58. Johnson RA: Atypical mycobacteria. In Fitzpatrick TB, Eisen AZ, Wolff K, Freedberg IM, Austen KF: Dermatology in General Medicine, 2nd ed. New York, McGraw-Hill, 1979, p 1505.
59. Ridley DS, Joplin WH: Classification of leprosy according to immunity: a five-group system. Int J Lepr 34:255, 1966.
59a. Bullock WE: Mycobacterium leprae (leprosy). In Mandell GL, Douglas RG Jr, Bennett JE (eds): Principles and Practice of Infectious Diseases, Vol. 2. New York: Wiley, 1979, p 1943.
60. Fritschi EP: Reconstructive Surgery in Leprosy. England, Wright, 1971.
61. Sanford JP, Moore WL Jr: Recrudescent melioidosis: a Southeastern Asia legacy. Am Rev Respir Dis 104:452, 1971.
62. Herrer A: Bartonellosis. In Hunter GW III, Swartzwelder JC, Clyde DF (eds): Tropical Medicine, 5th ed. Philadelphia, Saunders, 1976, p 256.
63. Heath CW Jr, Alexander AD, Galton MM: Leptospirosis in the United States: analysis on 483 cases in man, 1946–61. N Engl J Med 273:857, 915, 1965.
64. Butler T, Bell WR, Linh NN, Tiep ND, Arnold K: *Yersinia pestius* infection in Vietnam. I. Clinical and hematologic aspects. J Infect Dis 129:S78, 1974.
65. Zecler E, Gilboa Y, Elkina L, Atlan G, Sompolinsky D: Lymphocutaneous nocardiosis due to *Nocardia brasiliensis*. Arch Dermatol 113:642, 1977.
66. Emslie RD: Cancrum oris. Dent Pract 13:481, 1963.
67. O'Brien JP: Tropical ulcer. In Hunter GW III, Swartzwelder JC, Clyde DF (eds): Tropical Medicine, 5th ed. Philadelphia, Saunders, 1976, p 666.
68. Lindner RR, Adeniyi-Jones C: The effects of metronidazole on tropical ulcers. Trans Soc Trop Med Hyg 62:712, 1968.
69. Richmond SJ, Sparling PF: Genital chlamydial infections. Am J Epidemiol 103:428, 1976.
70. Marmar JL: The management of resistant chancroid in Vietnam. J Urol 107:807, 1972.
70a. Hart G: Chancroid, donovanosis, lymphogranuloma venereum. US Department of HEW Publication No. (CDC) 75–8302, 1975.

FUNGAL INFECTIONS OF THE SOFT TISSUE

71. Vollum DI: Chromomycosis: a review. Br J Dermatol 96:454, 1977.
72. Carrion AL: Chromoblastomycosis and related infections. New concepts, differential diagnosis, nomenclatorial implications. Int J Dermatol 14:27, 1975.
73. Brook CJ, Ravikrishnan KP, Weg JG: Pulmonary and articular sporotrichosis. Am Rev Respir Dis 116:141, 1977.
74. Mariat F, Destombes P, Segretain G: The mycetomas: clinical features, pathology, etiology and epidemiology. Contrib Microbiol Immunol 4:1, 1977.
75. Emmons CW, Binford CH, Utz JP, Kwon-Chung KJ: The mycetomas. In Medical Mycology, 3rd ed. Philadelphia, Lea & Febiger, 1977, p 437.
76. Bruck HM, Nash G, Foley FD, Pruitt BA Jr: Opportunistic fungal infection of the burn wound with phycomycetes and *Aspergillus*. Arch Surg 102:476, 1971.
77. Gartenberg G, Bottone EJ, Keusch FT, Weitzman I: Hospital-acquired mucormycosis *(Rhizopus rhizopodiformis)* of skin and subcutaneous tissue. Epidemiology, mycology and treatment. Med Intell 299:1115, 1978.
78. Halpern AA, Nagel DA, Schurman DJ: *Allescheria boydii* osteomyelitis following multiple steroid injections and surgery. Clin Orthoped 126:232, 1977.

VIRAL INFECTIONS OF THE SKIN

79. Nahmias AJ, Roizman B: Infection with herpes-simplex virus 1 and 2. N Engl J Med 289:667, 719, 781, 1973.
80. Marker SC, Howard RJ, Groth KE, Mastri A, Simmons RL, Najarian JS, Balfour HH Jr: A trial of vidarabine for cytomegalovirus infection in renal transplant patients. Arch Intern Med 140:1441, 1980.
81. Feldhoff CM, Balfour HH Jr, Simmons RL, Najarian JS, Mauer SM: Varicella in children with renal transplants. J Pediatr 98:25, 1981.
82. Simmons RL, Balfour HH Jr: Complication of disseminated varicella zoster infection (editorial). Surgery 83:486, 1978.
83. Izawa T, Ihara T, Hattori A, Iwasa T, Kamiya H, Sakurai M, Takahashi M: Application of live varicella vaccine in children with acute leukemia or other malignant diseases. Pediatrics 60:805, 1977.
84. Pass F: Warts. Biology and current therapy. Minn Med 57:844, 1974.
85. Kovi J, Tillman RL, Lee SM: Malignant transformation of condyloma accuminatum. J Clin Pathol 61:702, 1974.
86. Hewitt J, Haguenau F: Warts and molluscum contagiosum. In Debre R, Celers J (eds): Clinical Virology. Philadelphia, Saunders, 1970, p 474.
87. Carithers HA, Carithers, CM, Edwards RO Jr: Cat-scratch disease (its natural history). JAMA 207:312, 1969.

PROTOZOAN AND HELMINTH INFECTIONS OF THE SOFT TISSUES

88. Sunarwan I: A case of cutaneous amoebiasis. Dermatologica 151:253, 1975.
89. Rocha H: *Leishmania* species (kala-azar). In Mandell GL, Douglas RG Jr, Bennett JE (eds): Principles and Practice of Infectious Disease, Vol 2. New York, Wiley, 1979, p 2110.
89a. Chemotherapy of Parasitic Diseases (Section XI). In Gilman AG, Goodman LS, Gilman A (eds): The Pharmacological Basis of Therapeutics, 6th ed. New York, Macmillan, 1980, pp 1013–1079.
90. Taylor RL: Sparganosis in the United States: report of a case. Am J Clin Pathol 66:560, 1976.
91. Katz R, Ziegler J, Blank H: The natural course of creeping eruption and treatment with thiabendazole. Arch Dermatol 91:420, 1965.
92. Muller R: Dracunculus and dracunculiasis. Adv Parasitol 9:73, 1971.

CHAPTER 26
Ocular Infections

STEPHEN R. WALTMAN

THE physician may be required to diagnose and initiate therapy for certain ocular infections. These can occur independently of a patient's systemic disease or may be the ocular component of systemic infections that occur in compromised hosts. Indeed, ocular changes may be the initial indication of a systemic infection. This chapter will review the diagnosis and therapy of infections of the eye and its surrounding structures that may be of concern to the general surgeon.

ANATOMY AND PHYSIOLOGY

EYE

The eye is almost spherical, with a diameter of approximately 24 mm. The delicate intraocular structures, which are the photosensitive elements of the eye and which regulate intraocular pressure and accommodation, are enveloped in a tough collagenous coat. The anterior part of this limiting coat is the cornea, a transparent structure approximately 0.6 mm thick, lined on its anterior and posterior surfaces with living cells. The outer surface is covered by an epithelial layer five to six cell layers thick, which is resistant to penetration by most microorganisms. The inner surface is lined by a single cell layer of endothelium. Both of these layers are important for preventing hydration of the cornea and maintaining its clarity. The stroma is composed of interlacing collagen fibers with a rich mucopolysaccharide ground substance between the regularly spaced and arranged fibrils. The cornea is approximately 12 mm in diameter and merges gradually at the limbus into the opaque white sclera. The sclera is a direct extension of the cornea and is also made up of collagen fibrils, but they are arranged in a relatively disorderly fashion with minimal ground substance between them. This tough, resistant outer coat, composed of the cornea and sclera, prevents most intraocular infections from spreading outward and prevents orbital and periocular infections from spreading inward. The outer layer is also resistant to rupture.

The anterior chamber is directly behind the cornea and is approximately 3.5 mm deep. It contains aqueous humor, an extracellular fluid with a low protein content, which nourishes the anterior segment of the eye. The iris forms the posterior border of the anterior chamber, and immediately behind this is the lens. The vitreous is immediately behind the lens and comprises two-thirds of the ocular volume. It is an avascular, gelatinous substance with a high hyaluronic acid content.

The retina and choroid line the sclera and separate it from the vitreous. The retina lies immediately adjacent to the vitreous and is composed of ten layers. It contains the photosensitive elements of the eye. This nerve tissue is a direct extension of the brain, connected to it by the optic nerve. The optic nerve is composed of the ganglion cells that have their origin in the inner retinal layers. The retina is highly vascular, a fact that may explain why metastatic infections may lodge here. Interposed between the retina and sclera is the choroid, a vascular layer of mesodermal origin, which provides nutrients to the outer retinal layers. Because they are contiguous and are so closely associated, inflammations or infections originating in either the choroid or the retina frequently involve the other layer. If isolated, the infection is called choroiditis or retinitis, or chorioretinitis if both layers are involved.

ORBIT

The globe is enclosed within the bony orbit, which is a four-sided pyramid. It is open anteriorly, and its posterior apex communicates through several openings with the middle cranial fossa. The nerves to the extraocular muscles come through these openings, as does the optic nerve. The nerve and blood supplies to the extraocular muscles and the globe itself are encased in orbital fat within the bony contents. The bony orbit protects the globe from all but direct anterior blows. Three of the four orbital walls are contiguous with the facial sinuses. The roof of the orbit is contiguous with the frontal sinus; the floor of the orbit forms the top wall of the maxillary sinus, and the ethmoid sinus runs along the medial aspect of the orbit. Therefore, infections of the sinuses have a direct route to the periocular orbital structures.

LIDS

The lids are complex structures, lined on one side by skin and on the other by conjunctiva. A cartilaginous tarsal plate, located between these two surfaces, helps support and gives form to both upper and lower lids. Meibomian glands are partially embedded within the tarsal plates.

Medial and lateral canthal ligaments attach the tarsal plate and lids to the bony orbital walls. Extending from the superior border of the upper tarsus and the inferior border of the lower tarsus is the orbital septum, a diaphanous connective tissue that extends to the orbital rim and keeps the orbital fat in place. Conjunctiva lines the inner surface of the lid and is continuous in the fornices with the conjunctiva lining the globe. Accessory lacrimal glands and goblet cells provide secretion and lubrication of these surfaces, allowing the eye free movement beneath the lids. Cilia are present along the mucocutaneous border of both lids. Associated with these cilia are the glands of Zeiss (sebaceous glands) and the glands of Moll (accessory sweat glands). The lids provide a natural barrier against foreign bodies coming in contact with the globe. They are blinked approximately 15 to 20 times a minute, and in so doing wash away bacteria and other products of the external environment that may come in contact with the globe.

LACRIMAL SYSTEM

The lacrimal system has both secretory and excretory components. It provides a constant flow of tears, which lubricates the ocular surfaces and dilutes and washes away accumulated toxins. Secretion occurs from the main and accessory lacrimal glands. The main lacrimal gland is located in the upper temporal quadrant of the orbit in a depression in the superior orbital wall. This gland secretes tears in response to foreign bodies, conjunctivitis, or emotions. Normal ocular lubrication occurs in its absence. The basal aqueous lacrimal secretion comes from the accessory lacrimal glands, which are richly distributed throughout the conjunctiva. Numerous conjunctival goblet cells secrete mucus, which wets the normally hydrophobic anterior corneal surface and allows it to be bathed by the aqueous tears secreted by the lacrimal glands. Lysozyme and IgA are secreted locally and serve as part of the natural defense mechanisms of the eye. These macromolecules, along with constant blinking which further washes away outside intruders, provide natural barriers to infection.

Patients with rheumatoid arthritis and certain collagen vascular diseases may have a deficiency of aqueous tear production. This deficiency in lubrication leads to epithelial corneal irregularities, filamentary keratitis, and a decrease in the natural ocular defenses against infection. These patients are therefore prone to develop external ocular infections, especially corneal ulcers, and require close supervision and constant tear replacement.

The lacrimal excretory system consists of openings called puncta, located at the medial aspect of the upper and lower lids. Canniculi extend from the puncta approximately 12 mm to the lacrimal sac, which is located in a depression along the anterior aspect of the medial orbital wall. The nasolacrimal duct extends from the inferior portion of the lacrimal sac and opens under the inferior turbinate within the nose. Tears constantly drain along this route, and substances placed in the conjunctival fornices frequently find their way into the nose. From here they may be swallowed or absorbed systemically. It is important that physicians be aware of the possible distant systemic effects of these topically applied, yet systemically absorbed, medications. Obstruction in the excretory lacrimal system usually leads to infection, with distension of the lacrimal sac and purulent discharge through the canniculi and puncta.

NORMAL FLORA OF THE EYE

Nonpathogenic bacteria can frequently be cultured from the normal conjunctival epithelium, since this surface is exposed to the environment (Table 26-1).[1] Approximately 10 to 20 percent of normal individuals have pathogenic bacteria present on routine conjunctival cultures, but these are not of clinical significance in most cases.

INFECTIONS OF THE LID

BLEPHARITIS

Blepharitis is usually a low-grade, chronic infection involving the cilia of the lids and their associated glands. Crusting occurs at the base of the cilia with erythema, telangiectasia, and thickening of the lid margins. The cilia and glands are frequently colonized with staphylococci, which secrete toxic products. These products accumulate at the lid margins, producing symptoms of burning and conjunctival redness. Since blinking is absent during sleep, the toxins accumulate during the night, and symptoms are frequently worse in the morning. Therapy is directed at local hygiene, including mechanical removal of the desqua-

TABLE 26-1. INDIGENOUS MICROBIOTA OF THE EYES

Species or Group	Conjunctiva
Bacteria	
Gram-positive cocci	
Staphylococcus epidermidis	37–94 *
S. aureus	0–30
Streptococcus mitis; undifferentiated α and γ streptococci	0.3–1
S. pyogenes (usually group A unless noted)	0.3–2.5
S. pneumoniae	0–5
Gram-negative cocci	
Neisseria catarrhalis; other nonpathogenic *Neisseria* sp.	2.3
Gram-positive bacilli	
Lactobacillus sp.	3–83
Aerobic *Corynebacterium* sp.	
Aerobic gram-negative bacilli	
Enterobacteriaceae	2.1
Klebsiella sp.	0.1
Proteus mirabilis, other *Proteus* sp.	0.4
Alcaligenes faecalis	±
Moraxella lacunata	±
Acinetobacter calcoaceticus	±
Haemophilus influenzae	0.4–25

±—irregular or uncertain (may be only pathologic).
* Range of incidence in percent, rounded, in different surveys.

From Hoeprich PD (ed): Infectious Diseases (2nd ed). New York, Harper and Row, 1977, p 1164.

mated epithelium at the lid margin. A combination antibiotic-corticosteroid product may also be used. The antibiotic reduces the bacterial count, and the corticosteroid provides symptomatic relief from the toxic bacterial products. Occasionally, systemic antibiotic therapy is needed for persistent infections.

HORDEOLUM

Hordeolum, or stye, is a blocked, acutely infected gland of the eyelid, more frequent on the lower lid and usually pointing externally. Treatment is by local application of heat. If close to the medial aspect of the lids, systemic antibiotics are used because of the proximity of the angular vein. Bacteria can pass into the cavernous and other venous sinuses of the brain through the angular vein. Resolution usually occurs within a few days and may be accompanied by pointing and spontaneous drainage. If spontaneous drainage does not occur, the area may be incised with a small horizontal incision parallel to the lid folds. The stye will drain, frequently without significant scarring.

CHALAZION

Chalazion is a chronic granuloma, usually involving the meibomian glands of the tarsal plates. There is diffuse swelling and erythema. Application of heat, occasionally with a topical antibiotic preparation to prevent reinfection, frequently leads to resolution of this lesion. Many weeks of treatment may be required, and if the chalazion does not completely resolve, a cosmetic deformity may result. A chalazion may be curettaged from the internal conjunctival surface after removing a small piece of the tarsal plate to allow for continuous drainage of the area. The conjunctiva is not closed, and no external scar results.

INFECTIONS OF THE CONJUNCTIVA

Redness, discomfort, photophobia, a sensation of something on the eye, and a mucoid or mucopurulent discharge are the signs and symptoms of conjunctivitis. Bacteria and viruses cause most infective conjunctivitis; fungal infections are extremely rare.

VIRAL CONJUNCTIVITIS

Viral conjunctivitis is usually a bilateral disease and often accompanies an upper respiratory infection. It may be associated with signs and symptoms of a systemic viral illness and is frequently caused by an adenovirus. The discharge is mucoid and watery without purulence. The conjunctiva is moderately injected and has a pale, edematous appearance and a follicular type response. A large, tender preauricular node is frequently present. This node is located over the ramus of the mandible just anterior to the ear. It is a hallmark of viral infections and occurs infrequently with bacterial conjunctivitis.

Patients with viral conjunctivitis may be treated symptomatically with vasoconstrictors and ocular lubricants.

BACTERIAL CONJUNCTIVITIS

Bacterial conjunctivitis is associated with a velvety, intensely red, papillary conjunctival response with mucopurulent discharge without adenopathy. In the morning, photophobia and the sensation of foreign matter are more intense, and the lids may be stuck shut. Conjunctival cultures may be difficult to interpret, because 10 to 20 percent of normal people harbor pathogenic bacteria. When bacterial conjunctivitis occurs, signs of obstruction of the lacrimal system or predisposing factors along the lid margin should be sought.

Patients with bacterial conjunctivitis are treated with topical, broad-spectrum antibiotics. There is no need for systemic therapy. Topical sulfonamides or a combination of neomycin, polymyxin, and gramacidin are frequently used. Eyedrops are used during the day to wash away the accumulated bacterial products, and ointment is applied at bedtime. The tremendously high concentration of antibiotics thus attained in the tear film may help eliminate bacteria that would not ordinarily be susceptible to serum concentrations. Vigorous treatment of conjunctivitis is necessary to prevent further ocular complications such as corneal ulcers (Table 26-2).[2]

OPHTHALMIA NEONATORUM

Conjunctivitis in newborns, called ophthalmia neonatorum, has been largely prevented by the use of the Credé prophylactic procedure (instillation of 1 percent silver nitrate onto the conjunctiva) at birth. Laboratory studies are mandatory in the infants who develop conjunctivitis because of the possibility of gonococcal conjunctivitis. Untreated, this type of conjunctivitis can rapidly progress to severe ocular involvement and corneal perforation with eventual loss of the eye. The laboratory studies include Gram stain of conjunctival smears for identification of bacteria, and Wright or Giemsa stain for cellular morphology. Cultures are done on blood agar, thioglycolate, Sabouraud agar (when fungal etiology is suspected), and on chocolate agar for identification of gonococci. Smears will initially identify the suspected organism prior to confirmation from cultures. In adults, laboratory studies are done primarily for a hyperacute, possible gonococcal conjunctivitis.

LACRIMAL GLAND INFECTIONS

Acute dacryoadenitis, or inflammation of the main lacrimal glands, is rare. It may occur following direct trauma with introduction of microorganisms into the glands, but it is more frequently part of a generalized viral infection. Typical signs and symptoms include pain, ptosis, and an S-shaped swelling of the upper lid, which eventually closes completely. Observation of the lacrimal gland from the conjunctival side reveals localized chemosis and erythema in the upper, outer quadrant of the conjunctiva. Spontaneous resolution usually occurs in 1 to 2 weeks. Metastatic gonococcal dacryoadenitis can occur and is usually associated with other signs of systemic infection. It is an acute bilateral condition, which may go on to suppuration and

TABLE 26-2. MOST FREQUENT ORGANISMS IN BACTERIAL CONJUNCTIVITIS AND CORNEAL ULCERS

Organism	Conjunctivitis Percent	Corneal Ulcer Percent
Staphylococcus aureus	21	50
Diplococcus pneumoniae	36	35
Pseudomonas	—	5.5
Hemophilus influenzae	31	—
Neisseria gonorrhoeae	6	—

From Gutierrez E: Bacterial infections of the eye. In Locatcher-Khorazo D, Seegal BC (eds): Microbiology of the Eye. St. Louis, Mosby, 1972, pp 64–69.

spontaneous drainage. Mumps may also cause acute bilateral dacryoadenitis, which may precede or follow the parotid swelling. It resolves spontaneously, usually without drainage. The local application of heat may speed resolution of the process and make the patient more comfortable. Infectious mononucleosis may also cause a unilateral or bilateral acute dacryoadenitis.

INFECTIONS OF LACRIMAL EXCRETORY SYSTEM

Dacryocystitis, or acute infection and inflammation of the lacrimal sac, is much more common than dacryoadenitis. It is the result of a localized obstruction in the drainage system, with stagnation and infection. Congenital obstructions of the nasolacrimal duct occur at its nasal end near the inferior turbinate. Infection results with a localized swelling and redness of the sac along the medial canthal area (Fig. 26-1). The sac is indurated, distended, and acutely tender. Gentle pressure on the sac causes regurgitation of purulent material through the upper and lower puncta. This condition is treated with topical and systemic

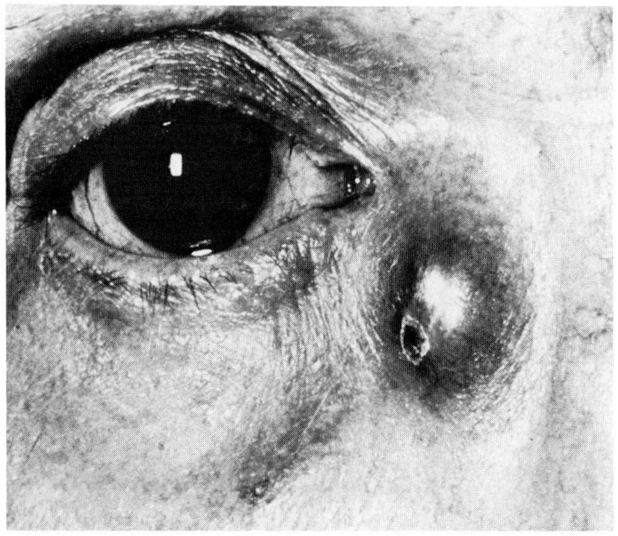

Fig. 26-1. **Dacryocystitis with swelling and induration below the medial canthus.**

antibiotics and analgesics. In children, probing of the nasolacrimal duct may relieve the obstruction after the process is resolved. In adults, obstruction of the lacrimal drainage system frequently occurs at the upper end of the nasolacrimal duct where it joins the sac, making probing much less successful. Dacryocystitis may also follow trauma, when the nasolacrimal duct is injured and permanently closes. If simple probing does not relieve the obstruction, a dacryocystorhinostomy is performed in the quiescent period after infection to allow for complete drainage of the excretory system and prevention of reinfection.

INFECTION OF THE ORBIT

Orbital cellulitis is much more serious than dacryocystitis and is frequently associated with systemic signs and symptoms including fever, malaise, and positive blood cultures.[3] Edema and erythema of the orbital region occur, frequently with fever and constitutional symptoms (Fig. 26-2). There may be considerable pain and diminished ocular rotations. The bony orbit prevents spread of the infection, but it may make the local consequences worse because of the localized ischemia and pressure that may occur. The infectious agent may enter from the paranasal sinuses or trauma, or it may be hematogenous. Serious ocular sequelae occur in 20 to 25 percent of cases. Evidence of sinusitis is available clinically and radiologically in half the patients over the age of 3 years. The bony orbit prevents posterior spread of the infection, so proptosis and anterior displacement of the globe frequently occur. Serious complications include intracranial abscesses, cavernous sinus thrombosis, persistent ophthalmoplegia, persistent proptosis, and optic atrophy.

S. aureus occurs in half the cases where the etiology of orbital cellulitis can be documented. *H. influenzae* and *S. pneumoniae* are frequent causes of this disease in children under the age of 3 years; antibiotic choice should be based on these considerations. Because of the serious nature of the condition, patients should be hospitalized and given systemic antibiotics. Topical antibiotic therapy is not sufficient for this deep-seated infection.

Subacute orbital cellulitis with proptosis, chemosis, and edema may occur in adult patients with diabetes mellitus. Phycomycosis may be the etiologic agent, and the prognosis is guarded. (See Chapter 27.)

CORNEAL INFECTIONS

The cornea is partially protected from external infections by the normal blink mechanism of the lids. Blinking washes away foreign particles and bathes the eye with tears. Tears contain IgA and lysozyme, which aid the physical defense mechanisms of the external eye. The normal corneal epithelium is resistant to invasion by most bacteria. Corneal ulcers can occur when a virulent virus or bacterium overcomes the normal defenses, or when these defenses are weakened by immunosuppression, decreased tear secretion, or lack of a normal protective blink mechanism

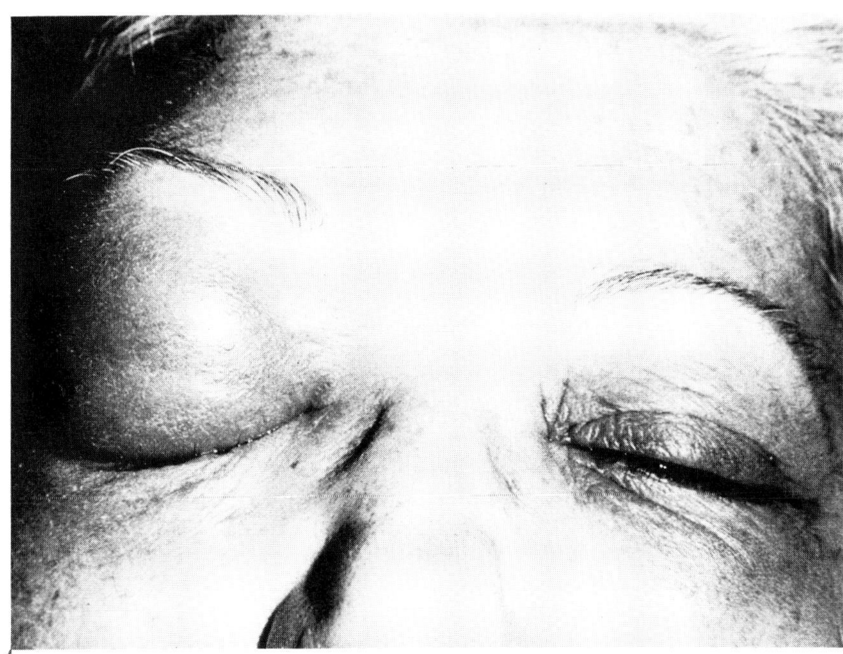

Fig. 26-2. Orbital cellulitis.

in comatose patients. Trauma that would normally be insignificant may lead to breakdown of the corneal epithelium and allow invasion of the cornea by microorganisms. Therefore, suitable precautions must be taken in unresponsive patients to prevent corneal exposure.

Corneal ulcers are breaks in the epithelium with infiltration or loss of the underlying corneal stroma. Ulcers are associated with pain, redness, discharge, decreased vision, and yellow or white infiltrates in the normally clear cornea. These ulcers are usually bacterial or viral; bacterial ulcers predominate after trauma. Fungal corneal ulcers are rare except in the warmer climates of the United States, where they usually follow trauma with twigs, thorns, and branches.

Bacterial corneal ulcers may be caused by staphylococci, streptococci, pneumococci, *Pseudomonas,* or a variety of other organisms. Smear specimens for initial diagnosis and therapy and cultures for confirmation are mandatory. Failure to institute appropriate therapy results in progressive loss of corneal stroma, perforation, intraocular spread of the infection, and possible loss of the eye. After laboratory studies are initiated, topical and subconjunctival antibiotics are instituted. Systemic antibiotic therapy is used depending on the depth of the ulcer and the amount of anterior chamber reaction. Topical drops are used hourly to deliver a high concentration of antibiotic and wash away the debris. Broad-spectrum coverage includes hourly topical medications using gentamicin and neomycin-polymyxin-gramicidin. Subconjunctival methicillin and gentamicin may be added, and when indicated, intravenous methicillin, gentamicin, and penicillin are used. After the offending organism has been identified and sensitivity tests run, therapy can be changed. Initial therapy depends on the sensitivities of local prevailing organisms.

Herpes simplex virus corneal infections are common and may be more frequent in immunosuppressed patients. The major complaint of the patient is usually decreased vision, caused by an irregular corneal surface, a result of epithelial breakdown. There is usually only slight discomfort, redness, and discharge. A typical branching, stellate, dendritic-like pattern occurs in the corneal epithelium. Diagnosis can be confirmed after topical installation of fluorescein, which outlines the areas of epithelial loss caused by the virus. Therapy consists of antiviral ointments, either idoxuridine or adenine arabinoside, five times a day until the epithelial lesion is completely healed.

Varicella-zoster virus may also lead to ocular complications. Corneal and intraocular inflammation or incomplete lid closure may occur because of induration and stiffness of the lids. This may lead to corneal exposure and possible perforation. The globe is frequently involved when the tip of the nose is involved because of the distribution of the nasociliary nerve, which innervates both areas. Therapy is directed at reducing inflammation by the use of topical cycloplegic and corticosteroid drops. The globe is protected by assuring that there is complete lid closure or by the use of ointments or patching to prevent exposure and drying.

CHORIORETINITIS

Infections of the choroid or retina are potentially devastating and may rapidly lead to loss of sight. Because of the small amount of tissue involved, spread from the initial nidus of infection may destroy most of the photosensitive elements of the eye within a short time. Furthermore, since the retinal elements are contained in a tough, inelastic outer coat (sclera), the infection frequently spreads laterally and is confined to the intraocular contents, with extensive destruction. The infection may start in the retina or choroid, but usually spreads rapidly to the outer layer, unless the infecting organism has a predilection for either tissue. Further spread into the avascular vitreous may occur by direct continuity. There are no lymphatics in the eye, and the defense mechanisms for control of intraocular infection are not potent. The infection may be exogenous from trauma or intraocular surgery or endogenous from a metastatic focus. Even if from a metastatic focus, the ocular signs may be the first signs. Patients who are immunologically compromised (eg, kidney transplant recipients) and patients who have long-term indwelling intravenous catheters may develop ocular infections, which are the initial signs and may be the most serious signs of the systemic infection.

CYTOMEGALOVIRUS RETINITIS

Cytomegalovirus (CMV) infection is common in immunosuppressed patients, and may present as a necrotizing retinitis.[4] The retinitis may not occur until a patient has been on immunosuppressive therapy for several years. The symptoms are blurred vision, detectable scotomas or defects in the visual field, and reduced visual acuity. If the central retinal macular area is not involved, patients may be asymptomatic despite extensive peripheral retinitis. The condition may be unilateral or bilateral.

Ophthalmologic findings are vessel sheathing, retinal edema, and scattered hemorrhages and yellow exudates along an area of retinal vasculature. These findings initially resemble a localized retinal vascular occlusion. Extension may occur from a focal process to generalized involvement with confluent edema and extensive intraretinal hemorrhage. Pigment epithelial atrophy and scarring frequently occur. Because necrotizing retinitis destroys the retinal receptors, control of this disease usually does not lead to significant visual improvement, although it may prevent progressive visual loss. It is therefore important that the retinitis be diagnosed as early as possible. Early diagnosis requires that patients who are receiving chronic immunosuppression be aware of the early symptoms and receive regular ocular examinations. The available therapeutic alternatives in patients with cytomegalovirus retinitis include reduction of immunosuppression, antiviral therapy, and perhaps the use of transfer factor. If possible, host antiviral defense mechanism should be allowed to recover by reduction or discontinuation of immunosuppressive therapy. The retinitis may still not respond to this form of therapy because of the firmly established, localized intraocular infection. The problems associated with the reduction of immunosuppressive agents must be balanced against the potential hazards of unchecked cytomegalovirus retinitis and possible generalized infection.

CANDIDA CHORIORETINITIS

Hematogenous Candida endophthalmitis occurs most often in patients during prolonged intravenous feeding with or without immunosuppressive drugs, and in drug addicts.[5] *Candida* chorioretinitis and subsequent endophthalmitis frequently follow bacteremia. Patients complain of sudden or gradual visual impairment, frequently bilateral. Spots or floaters are frequent, and pain occurs in and around the eye in approximately half the patients. Single or multiple discrete, fluffy, white lesions occur in the retina with overlying vitreous reaction and sometimes anterior chamber reaction (Fig. 26-3). The lesions initially appear like white mounds on the surface of the retina, resembling similar *Candida* lesions on blood agar plates. Frank intravitreal extension with haziness of the vitreous overlying the involved retina occurs in untreated cases. The lesions are sufficiently distinct to be differentiated from other types of metastatic endophthalmitis, such as occur following subacute bacterial endocarditis. Here Roths spots occur—hemorrhages in the retinal layers with small, round, central white spots.

Therapy consists of systemic amphotericin B and 5-flucytosine when appropriate. Topical ocular medications consist of cycloplegic agents such as atropine to reduce the anterior segment inflammation and make the patient more comfortable. Retinal lesions without overlying vitreal involvement may regress within a relatively short time after the administration of amphotericin B. After 6 to 12 weeks, the original lesions may be replaced by translucent, gray-white, gliotic scars. Clearing of the vitreous may lead to improvement of visual acuity if the central macular region has not been scarred. Patients are often asymptomatic, at least initially, when therapy is most effective. Therefore, frequent eye examinations are indicated in those patients with positive *Candida* blood cultures or those prone to develop them.

BACTERIAL ENDOPHTHALMITIS

Metastatic bacterial endophthalmitis can also occur in immunosuppressed hosts, especially if they have had previous

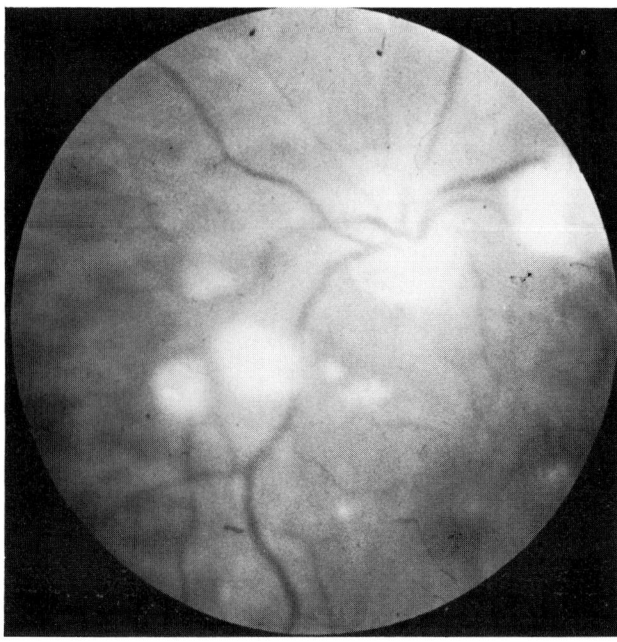

Fig. 26-3. ***Candida*** **chorioretinitis.**

septicemia. The aqueous humor and vitreous of eyes taken from cadavers who have had septic episodes may contain bacteria.[6] This occurs despite the lack of ocular symptoms in these eye donors premortem. Patients on maintenance hemodialysis, who have been treated for staphylococcal septicemia, may develop a low-grade endophthalmitis several months after cessation of their systemic antimicrobial therapy.[7] This endophthalmitis is frequently indolent and usually responds to systemic antibiotics. Perhaps the uremic state has modified the host responses to the intraocular infection. All patients on dialysis who have ocular complaints should be examined regularly. Furthermore, those patients who have an episode of systemic sepsis should also be examined frequently, even if they are initially asymptomatic.

Although patients with renal failure, both before and after kidney transplantation, may develop a red eye syndrome thought to be the result of soft tissue calcification, repeated ocular examinations are mandatory to eliminate infection as a cause of the inflammation.[8]

POSTOPERATIVE ENDOPHTHALMITIS

Postoperative endophthalmitis is a dreaded, devastating infection that occurs after intraocular surgery. Fortunately, it is rare, with an incidence of less than one in a few hundred cases. It is caused by apparent bacterial contamination during operation, or a leaking wound or tract. It may also be metastatic from a distant focus. Most cases of postoperative endophthalmitis are associated with cataract operations, primarily because they are the most frequent intraocular procedures performed. Endophthalmitis is an infectious inflammatory process that involves the ocular cavities and adjacent retinal and uveal tissue.

Clinical Manifestation

The signs and symptoms usually appear 1 to 5 days postoperatively, depending on whether prophylactic subconjunctival and systemic antibiotics have been used. The interval between operation and the appearance of endophthalmitis also depends on the virulence of the infecting organisms. There is usually increasing pain after an initial pain-free period, increasing redness, reactive ptosis and edema of the upper lid, and chemosis or swelling of the conjunctiva. Visual acuity is often reduced to light perception. A hypopyon (layering out of white cells in the anterior chamber) occurs, along with vitreous haze and a yellow or dark fundus reflex. If the condition is not diagnosed and treated rapidly, destruction of the intraocular contents, including the retina and ciliary body, may lead to irreversible loss of light perception and a soft, phthisical eye. Sometimes a severe sterile postoperative inflammatory reaction may be confused with endophthalmitis, but it is imperative that the appropriate diagnostic and therapeutic steps be taken to rule out an infection.

Diagnosis

In the case of suspected endophthalmitis, an extensive microbial workup is necessary. The wound and lid margins are cultured, and anterior chamber and vitreous taps are done with fine, sharp needles, especially in the aphakic patient. In the patient who still has the lens in place, vitreous taps should be done in the operating room through the pars plana. Immediate smear is done, and cultures are plated on appropriate media, including fungal media. Less than half the cases of endophthalmitis reveal positive anterior chamber cultures, but slightly more reveal positive vitreous cultures. Anterior chamber taps can be done at the bedside using topical cocaine or other suitable anesthesia. A sharp 27-gauge needle on a tuberculin syringe can be inserted into the anterior chamber. Approximately 0.2 ml of fluid may be aspirated.

Treatment

Antibiotics are selected depending on the organism seen on smear, and therapy is appropriately altered as the cultures are reported. If no organisms are seen, broad-spectrum antibiotic coverage against gram-positive and gram-negative organisms is mandatory. Appropriate antibiotics for initial treatment are determined in part by the resistance of the organism cultured in the hospital where the infection occurred. Antibiotics are given by topical, subconjunctival, and systemic routes, usually intravenously.

Topical, subconjunctival, and systemic corticosteroids are often used after initial antibiotic therapy for 12 to 24 hours. This is done in an attempt to preserve the integrity and transparency of the ocular structures and the functioning of the photosensitive layers. Extensive scarring and destruction of the delicate intraocular elements with loss of function can occur despite sterilization of the infection. Therefore, corticosteroids are instituted early in the course, and indeed some advocate giving them at the time of initial antibiotic therapy.

Recently, the use of intravitreal antibiotics and corticosteroids has been advocated as effective therapy for postoperative endophthalmitis.[9] The series reported to date have been rather small, but at least in the experimental animal the results are encouraging.

Infection of the vitreous can lead to progressive opacification and organization of this structure. Because the vitreous provides an excellent culture medium for growing organisms, some have advocated immediate vitrectomy to remove the large nidus of bacteria and toxic products that are capable of destroying the delicate intraocular structures. As long as the peripheral retina can be seen and the vitreous abscess remains central, vitrectomy may not be necessary. If, however, the vitreous fills with organisms and white blood cells, an attempt should be made to remove the central aspects of the vitreous to decompress and drain the abscess and to lessen the toxic load presented to the retina. Great care must be taken not to attempt to remove all of the vitreous, because the peripheral cortical vitreous may be intimately involved with the retina in an infection.

With the institution of appropriate diagnostic and therapeutic procedures, many eyes that were previously lost are now saved and may retain useful vision of 20/400, which is sufficient for walking and normal daily activities. While this degree of acuity is not sufficient for reading and fine visual tasks, it does provide a patient with vision sufficient to remain independent.

Fungal endophthalmitis is a much rarer condition, which usually occurs 1 to 4 weeks after surgery in a much more indolent, low-grade fashion. Fluff balls appear on the vitreous face and anterior vitreous with eventual hypopyon. The eye is not nearly as red, and the onset and resulting visual loss is quite gradual. Diagnosis can be made by finding the organisms in the anterior chamber or vitreous, and appropriate antifungal therapy can be instituted. Because the condition is usually monocular, and antifungal therapy has more morbidity associated with it than antibacterial therapy, the decision as to whether or not to treat the infection with long-term systemic antifungal agents requires consideration and consultation. Amphotericin B, given over a 6-week course, or flucytosine are the appropriate drugs. Newer antifungal agents may be used if the organism appears to be sensitive to them. Fortunately, fungal endophthalmitis is rare, as the therapeutic efficacy of the drugs has not been encouraging.

BIBLIOGRAPHY

Locatcher-Khorazo D, Seegal BC (eds.): Microbiology of the Eye. St. Louis, Mosby, 1972.

REFERENCES

1. Hoeprich PD (ed): Infectious Diseases, 2nd ed. New York, Harper and Row, 1977, p 1164.
2. Gutierrez E: Bacterial infections of the eye. In Locatcher-Khorazo D, Seegal BC (eds): Microbiology of the Eye. St Louis, Mosby, 1972, pp 64–69.
3. Robie G, O'Neal R, Kelsey DS: Periorbital cellulitis. J Ped Ophth 14:354, 1977.
4. Murray HW, Knox DL, Green WR, Susel RM: Cytomegalovirus retinitis in adults: a manifestation of disseminated viral infection. Am J Med 63:574, 1977.
5. Fishman LS, Griffin JR, Sapico FL, Hecht R: Hematogenous candida endophthalmitis—a complication of candidemia. N Engl J Med 286:675, 1972.
6. Keates RH, Michler KE, Reidinger D: Bacterial contamination of donor eyes. Am J Ophthalmol 84:617, 1977.
7. Bloomfield SE, David DS, Cheigh JS, Kim Y, White RP, Stenzel KH, Rubin AL: Endophthalmitis following staphylococcal sepsis in renal failure patients. Arch Intern Med 138:706, 1978.
8. Berlyne GM, Shaw AB: Red eyes in renal failure. Lancet 1:4, 1967.
9. Baum JL, Peyman GA: Viewpoint—antibiotic administration in the treatment of bacterial endophthalmitis. Surv Ophthalmol 21:332, 1977.

CHAPTER 27
Infections of the Head and Neck

George L. Adams

Although most texts on infectious disease devote considerable space to viral infections of the upper respiratory tract and ear, the emphasis here will be on the complications for which otolaryngologists are most commonly consulted.

ANATOMIC CHARACTERISTICS OF INFECTIONS OF THE HEAD AND NECK

Infections of the head or neck are unique for a variety of reasons. A rich vascular supply derives primarily from divisions of the external carotid artery system. This blood supply probably promotes rapid healing after surgery or trauma and permits rapid mobilization of host defenses. Conversely, the coexisting rich venous drainage permits the spread of embolic infection throughout the body. Retrograde venous flow along the ophthalmic vein to the cavernous sinus and along the mastoid emissary vein to the petrosal vein permits the extension of infection to the meninges and the central nervous system (Fig. 27-1). The predictable pattern of lymphatic channels and lymph nodes provides known routes for the extension of infection .

The mastoids and sinuses are unique air-filled cavities within the head. The sinuses, mastoid cavity, eustachian tube, middle ear, and the respiratory portion of the pharynx are lined by respiratory (pseudostratified, columnar, ciliated) epithelium, the condition of which is affected by continuous environmental changes, such as humidity and temperature. The clearance of secretions and contaminants is dependent on ciliary activity, which in turn is easily affected by medications, hydration, and disease, especially upper respiratory viral infection. A constantly renewable mucous blanket coats this respiratory epithelium, and it flows continuously toward the pharynx, cleansing the area of foreign material and bacteria. The maxillary sinuses lie in close proximity to the roots of the upper teeth so that dental infections can extend into the sinuses.

The investing fascia of the neck (superficial layer of the deep cervical fascia), acts like a cylinder to surround the important muscles. A separate deeper layer of fascia surrounds the important viscera of the neck, including the pharynx, trachea, and major salivary glands (Fig. 27-2). These fasciae communicate along the region of the carotid sheath. Thus, infections are initially confined to specific areas within the neck, and a pattern is established for their extension. Unfortunately, these fascial spaces communicate with similar spaces that extend into the mediastinum.

DEVELOPMENTAL CHANGES

Infections in children can be more serious and have a different clinical course than similar infections with the same organism in an adult. For example, the newborn child has only rudimentary maxillary and ethmoid sinuses, with virtually no development of the frontal sinuses or sphenoid sinus. Thus, sinus infections in children are primarily confined to the ethmoid sinuses. Problems in both the frontal and sphenoid sinuses are more likely in the young adult. Although present at birth, the maxillary sinuses continue to increase in size as the contour of the face changes.

The mastoid system is poorly developed in the newborn and develops over the first few years of life. Its development depends on proper eustachian tube function, which in turn depends on structural alterations and defects present in the child. For example, the eustachian tube of the child lies on a more horizontal plane than the adult and is wider and shorter. Its function is directly dependent on the musculature of the pharynx, primarily of the tensor veli palatini and levator veli palatini. Loss of function in this muscular system, such as occurs in a child with a cleft palate, affects the eustachian tube function, which in turn affects mastoid and middle ear development and physiology.

Structures in the pharynx and nasopharynx also undergo changes related to age. The adenoid mass hypertrophies through early childhood years and can cause nasal and eustachian tube obstruction. Tonsils similarly undergo hypertrophy during this same period and begin to undergo involution in adolescence. Because childhood infections coincide with tonsillar hypertrophy, a causal relationship has been postulated.

The larynx of a newborn, as compared to that of an adult, is disproportionately small among the other structures in the head and neck. Its cartilaginous skeleton is less firm, and the soft tissues are more subject to swelling

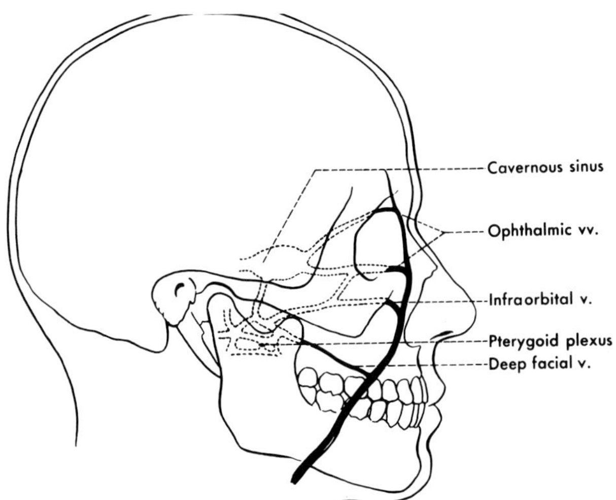

Fig. 27-1. **Chief connections of the facial vein to the cavernous sinus. (From Hollinshead HW (ed): The face. In *Anatomy for Surgeons. Vol 1, The Head and Neck,* 2nd ed. Hagerstown, Harper & Row, 1968, p 331.)**

and edema. The larynx is also located higher in the neck and descends with growth. The disproportionately small size of the upper airway of the child permits airway obstruction to occur with only minimal inflammatory swelling.

THE CARTILAGINOUS SUPPORT

A large number of appendages and structures in the head and neck are formed from cartilage, rather than bone. Cartilage has no direct blood supply and derives its nutrition entirely from the surrounding perichondrium. Infectious injury to this perichondrium frequently results in dissolution of the cartilage and loss of its structure. Fibrous tissue, which replaces cartilage, lacks a functional shape. Thus, infections that extend into the perichondrium of the ear or nasal septum are not only difficult to control with systemic antibiotics but leave permanent cosmetic damage when they finally resolve. Perichondritis in the larynx, epiglottis, or trachea is uncommon, but does occasionally appear after prolonged intubation, trauma, or irradiation. Tracheomalacia with asphyxiation or residual stricture formation are two of the more serious consequences.

ETIOLOGIC AGENTS

VIRUS

Infections of the head and neck are in many instances sequelae of upper respiratory infections, which commonly include infections of the nose, paranasal sinuses, middle ear, pharynx, and pharyngeal lymphoid tissue. As a group, these colds and sore throats are the most common infections seen by physicians. Most are benign, self-limited processes without residual adverse consequences. Ninety percent are caused by viruses. The most important causes of upper respiratory infections are the rhinoviruses. Descriptions of these agents are given in Chapter 10, and more details are available in standard texts of medical virology.[1] Their interest to the surgeon primarily lies in the predisposition of the virally infected mucosa to edema and obstruction of the orifices of sinuses and eustachian

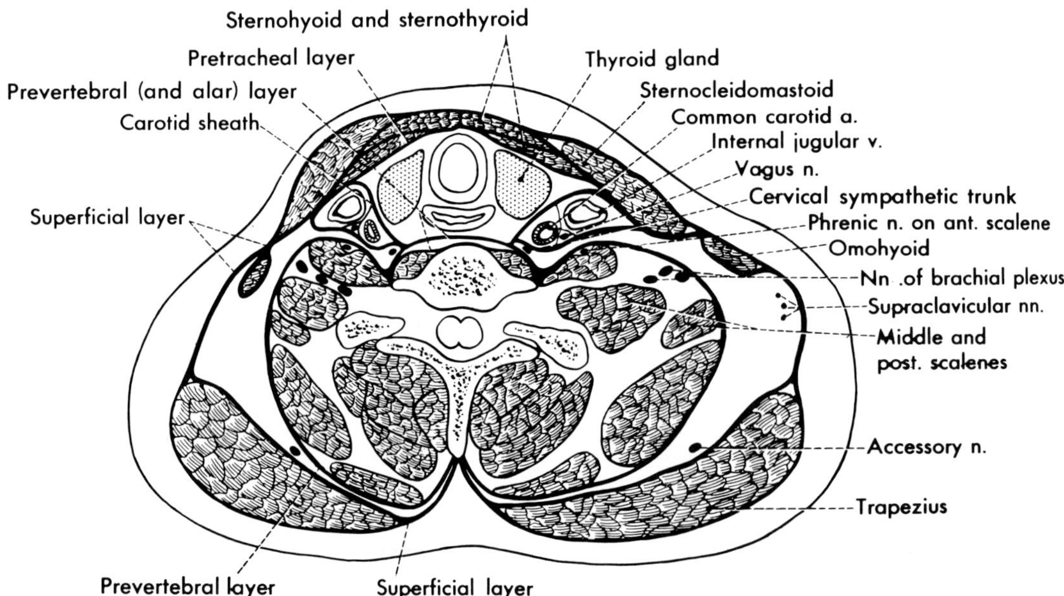

Fig. 27-2. **The deep cervical fascia is itself divided into superficial and deep layers, which encompass trapezuis and sternocleidomastoid muscles. The prevertebral layer surrounds the deeper muscles of the neck. The visceral (pretracheal) layer surrounds the trachea, thyroid, and pharyngoesophagus. The visceral and prevertebral layers communicate with the mediastinal fascia. (From Hollinshead HW (ed): Fascia and fascial spaces. In *Anatomy for Surgeons. Vol 1, The Head and Neck,* 2nd ed. Hagerstown, Harper & Row, 1968, p 306.)**

tubes, which produce conditions favorable for secondary bacterial infection. Occasionally the virus itself is the cause of important surgically correctable lesions, ie, serous otitis or acute laryngotracheitis in children.

BACTERIA

Normal Microbial Flora

Chapter 3 (Tables 3-6 to 3-8) lists the microorganisms commonly found in the mouth, nasal passages, nasopharynx, and oropharynx. In the nose, staphylococci (*S. aureus, S. epidermidis,* and diphtheroids are the most common). The streptococci (*S. pyogenes* group A and *S. pneumoniae*), *Haemophilus influenzae,* and other gram-negative bacteria are far less common. The oropharynx contains the same organisms plus the prominent addition of the *S. viridans* species and the nonpathogenic *Branhamella Neisseria catarrhalis.* The alpha-hemolytic streptococci have an inhibitory effect on colonization by group A streptococci, pneumococci, *S. aureus,* and the gram-negative bacilli. The latter organisms therefore appear in hospitalized, debilitated patients who are receiving antibiotics.

The normal microbial flora of the mouth are more complex and depend to a large extent on the condition of the teeth (Table 3-8). Some bacteria have receptors for tooth surfaces *(S. sanguis, S. mutans)* or mouth epithelium *(S. salivarius).* These organisms grow in dental plaque and provide an anaerobic environment for *Bacteroides melaninogenicus, B. oralis, Veillonella alcalescens,* or *S. mutans,* which is associated with caries. Caries themselves provide a favorable environment for treponemes and other anaerobes.

The only common fungus is *Candida albicans.* Some mycoplasmas and protozoa *(Entamoeba gingivitis, Trichomonas tenax)* inhabit the oropharynx.

Common Bacterial Pathogens

It is important to distinguish between infections in which no obvious preceding breakdown in the local or systemic defenses has occurred and those in which there is necrotic tissue, tumor, chronic obstruction, or systemic debilitation. Acute infections of this region without associated trauma, surgery, or preexisting disease are most often caused by *S. pyogenes, S. pneumoniae, S. aureus,* or *H. influenzae.* Because all can be members of the normal flora, their presence in culture is not diagnostic of infection. These organisms (plus *C. diphtheriae*) can infect outwardly normal tissues because they all appear to have receptors for adherence to mucosal surfaces. Thus attached, the mechanical sweeping action of the cilia is less effective, and the bacteria may proliferate, invade, or secrete their toxins.

A different situation exists when the mucosal integrity has been breached by trauma, surgery, or preexisting disease (ie, dental caries). In these circumstances, all the indigenous mixed aerobic and anaerobic flora of the region have access to the soft tissues. The factors governing the progress of soft tissue infection (discussed in Chapter 25) are then brought into play. Consequently, an array of pathogenic and nonpathogenic organisms has been found in such diseases as chronic sinusitis, parotitis, and otitis. Careful Gram stains, preparations, and aerobic and anaerobic cultures must be performed in any cavitary infection that does not respond promptly to antibiotics chosen empirically.

INFECTIOUS DISEASES OF THE ORAL CAVITY AND PHARYNX

Most infections of the oral cavity and pharynx can be identified in the course of a routine history and physical examination, with the assistance of appropriate cultures. Certain types of infections have a predilection to extend into the nasopharynx and sinuses, eustachian tube, and mastoid. Treatment and recognition of the pharyngeal problem is therefore important, not only to treat the problem in the oral cavity and pharynx but also to prevent its extension. Patients who have acute infections generally have pain while chewing or swallowing, fever, and cervical lymphadenopathy. Chronic infections may show only erythema, local tenderness, and nontender cervical adenopathy. For many of the acute infections, culture (as taken for suspected beta-hemolytic streptococcal pharyngitis) must be incubated for 24 hours before the organism can be identified. A culture is frequently less informative in the chronic sore throat and chronic oral cavity diseases. If there is a suspicion of infection, a culture should be obtained but a biopsy of the ulceration or whitish plaque tissue may be more revealing. A fungal infection, such as candidiasis, may be present. KOH smear findings along with clinical signs of a thick, whitish exudate may be sufficient to make the diagnosis.

LEUKOPLAKIA AND ULCERS

White patches and shallow ulcers are common in the mouth and pharynx. Any ulcer that persists for 2 weeks or longer should be evaluated histologically. Other important factors in the patient's history include smoking, denture irritation, alcohol abuse, poor dietary habits, and poor oral hygiene. Medical treatment should include not only the appropriate antibiotics, but also instructions on the improvement of oral care, such as sodium chloride and sodium bicarbonate mouthwash, correct care of the teeth, and removal of dentures at night.

PHARYNGITIS AND TONSILLITIS

Pharyngitis and tonsillitis are inflammatory diseases of microbial etiology—usually viral or group A streptococci. Both are usually self-limited, but the latter can produce suppurative or nonsuppurative complications.

Viral pharyngitis is most often caused by the adenoviruses (named for adenoid tissue from which they were first isolated) and the coxsackie viruses (types A2, 4, 5, 6, 8, 10), which cause herpangina and acute lymphonodular pharyngitis in children. Herpes simplex virus can cause an ulcerative pharyngitis.

The group A *Streptococcus* is most commonly associated with pharyngitis and rheumatic fever. The streptococci are discussed as a group in Chapter 4. Classically, pharyngitis and rheumatic fever are associated with each other. Glomerulonephritis rarely follows pharyngitis, but is most often associated with streptococcal pyoderma.

Viral pharyngitis is a disease of the mucosal cells with superficial necrosis. Extension to the adjacent paranasal sinuses, eustachian tube and middle ear can be associated with obstruction and suppurative complications of these cavities; cervical adenitis and dissemination to lungs are common. Bacteremia can cause metastatic infections. The surgeon's role in treatment is to recognize the disease and to perform a biopsy when indicated.

Tonsillitis

Acute, recurrent, tonsillar pharyngitis occurs in children and particularly young adults. The tonsils become hypertrophic and scarred, and crypt formations associated with chronic sore throat may occur. In others, recurrent episodes of acute tonsillitis with swelling, edema, inflammation, and pain may occur. Beta-hemolytic *Streptococcus*, group A, is the most common cause of this infection; however, adenovirus and Epstein-Barr virus have also been identified. Acute streptococcal tonsillitis should be treated with appropriate antibiotics.

The indications for tonsillectomy have not even now been established. There is general agreement that children younger than 10 who have more than three episodes of culture-documented streptococcal pharyngitis per year for at least 2 years would benefit from tonsillectomy. The benefit is no longer obvious after the children reach age 10.[2,3] Consideration for tonsillectomy and adenoidectomy should be made separately—they are two specific operations and do not need to be performed at the same time. The indications for each procedure should be separately noted. A child with recurrent episodes of acute otitis media with nasal obstruction from hypertrophied adenoids may benefit from an adenoidectomy. Recurrent streptococcal tonsillitis is an indication for tonsillectomy, not adenoidectomy.

Adults occasionally require tonsillectomy, despite an increased incidence of bleeding and postoperative pain. Current indications include: (1) peritonsillar abscess, (2) nasopharyngeal airway obstruction with cor pulmonale, (3) airway obstruction with sleep apnea syndrome, secondary to tonsillar hypertrophy, (4) suspicion of malignancy (lymphoma), and, most controversially, (5) repeated documented episodes of beta-hemolytic streptococcal pharyngitis.

Peritonsillar Abscess

One of the most serious and frequent complications of tonsillitis is a peritonsillar abscess. This usually occurs 3 days after an acute tonsillitis episode, even though the tonsillitis may already be controlled by antibiotics. Symptoms include severe trismus, difficulty in swallowing, severe throat pain, and ipsilateral cervical adenopathy. The process is almost always unilateral but can occur bilaterally. When the patient is finally coaxed to open his mouth, the tonsil is seen to be pushed across the midline but may no longer be inflamed. Instead, the swelling is usually evident in the area of the soft palate and lateral to the tonsil (Fig. 27-3). Infection has extended through the tonsillar capsule and is trapped between the superior pharyngeal constrictor and the tonsil. The possibility of a parapharyngeal abscess (Figs. 27-2, 27-4, 27-5, 27-6) occurring as a direct extension of a peritonsillar abscess should always be considered. In fact, a parapharyngeal abscess in a patient who has had a previous tonsillectomy can resemble a peritonsillar abscess. It is important to make this differential diagnosis, because a parapharyngeal abscess is best drained through an external or lateral neck approach (Fig. 27-6), but a peritonsillar abscess is drained through an intraoral approach. Cultures for aerobic and anaerobic bacteria are obtained as well as for Gram stain. If the patient has already been on a high dosage of penicillin, the cultures may show no growth. Usually, the responsible organism

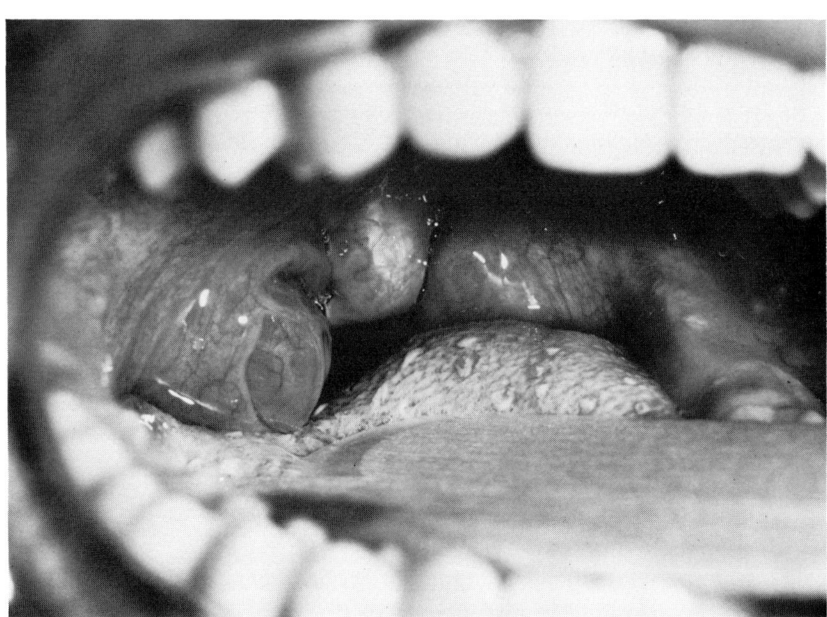

Fig. 27-3. **Acute right peritonsillar abscess. The tonsil is pushed medially by the abscess. The tonsil may appear enlarged but not infected.**

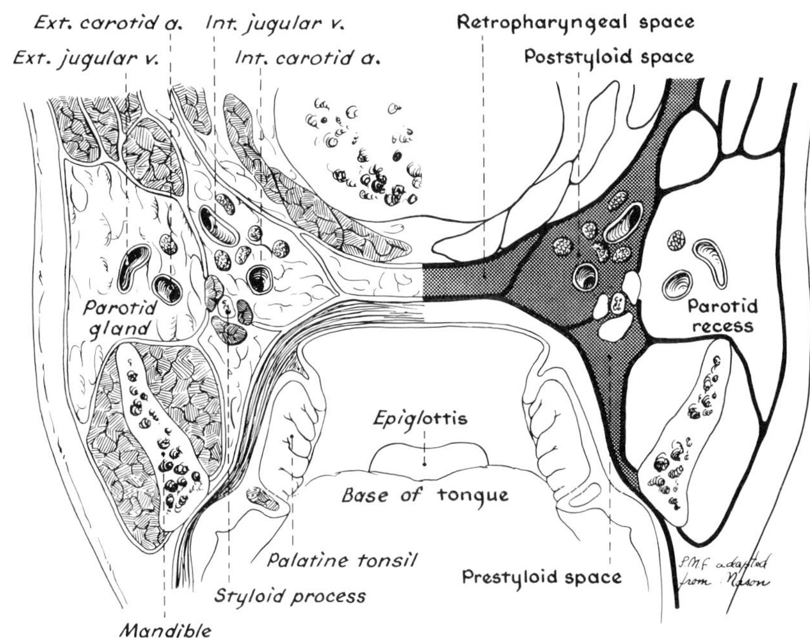

Fig. 27-4. Important fascial spaces of the neck: The parapharyngeal (pharyngomaxillary) space is divided into an anterior (prestyloid) and a posterior (poststyloid) space by the styloid process and its attached ligament. (From Adams G: Special examinations in otolaryngology. In Adams G, Boies LR Jr, Paparella MM (eds): *Boies's Fundamentals of Otolaryngology,* 5th ed. Philadelphia, Saunders, 1978, p 28.)

is *S. pyogenes,* but anaerobic infection has been demonstrated.[4]

There are two approaches to the management of patients with acute peritonsillar abscess. First, an anesthetic can be applied topically to the area of infection. With the patient sitting upright, an incision is made just through the mucosa (Fig. 27-7). Using a blunt instrument, such as a hemostat, the incision is widened and spread into the area of the abscess. Culture samples are obtained and suction applied to remove the thick, frequently foul-smelling pus. The patient is concurrently given intravenous antibiotics and fluids until he is again able to swallow. Frequent irrigations with warm salt water provide comfort and seem to speed resolution of the swelling. Systemic

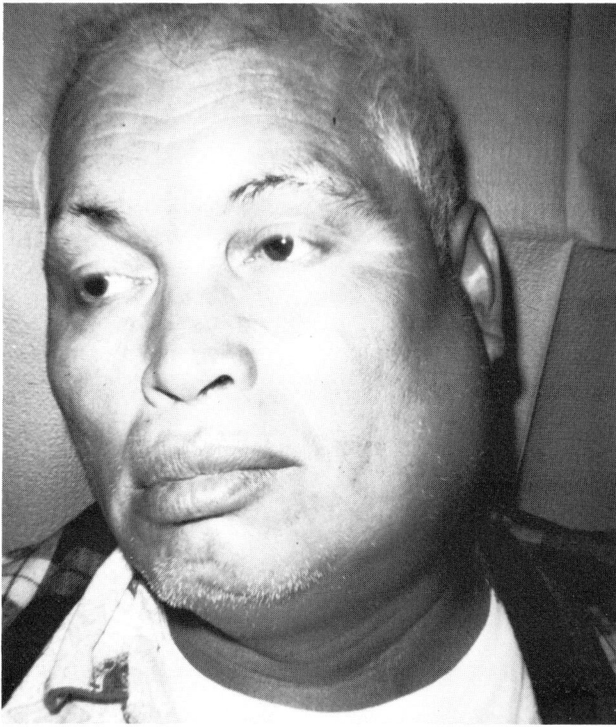

Fig. 27-5. Left parapharyngeal space (pharyngomaxillary space) abscess. The left neck and parotid area are diffusely swollen. The angle of the mandible is obliterated.

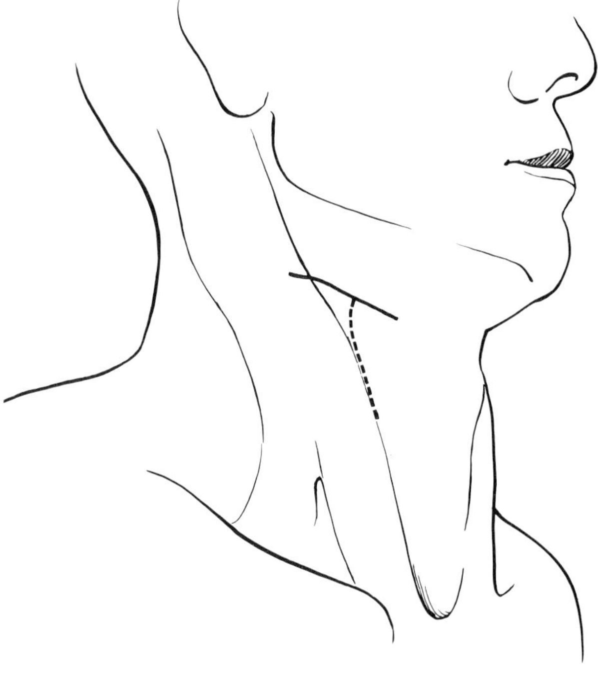

Fig. 27-6. Incision described by Mosher to drain a parapharyngeal space abscess. Dotted line indicates possible incision to control extension of infection along the carotid sheath. This same incision can be used to drain infections of the submandibular space and retropharyngeal space.

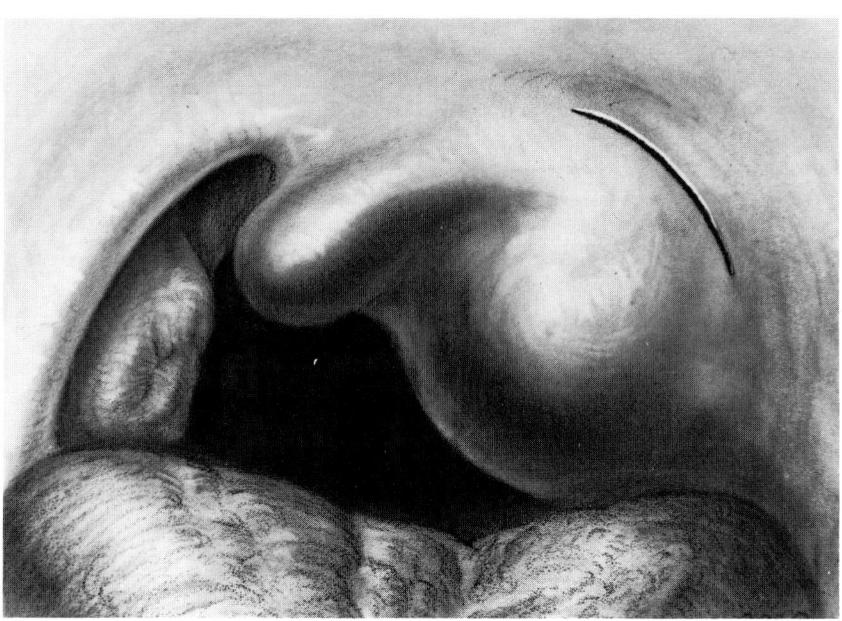

Fig. 27-7. **Location of incision for drainage of peritonsillar abscess. (From Adams G: Special examinations in otolaryngology. In Adams G, Boies LR Jr, Paparella MM (eds): *Boies's Fundamentals of Otolaryngology,* 5th ed. Philadelphia, Saunders, 1978, p 28.)**

oral antibiotics are used for at least 10 days. Four to 6 weeks later, the patient should undergo a routine tonsillectomy.

A second approach, which has become more popular recently, is to perform an immediate emergency tonsillectomy under general anesthesia. Because the pus has already done the dissection, the tonsil is easily removed. The opposite tonsil is removed at the same time. Immediate abscess tonsillectomy is preferred by some because it cures the abscess, prevents a second hospital stay for the patient, and in some cases is technically easier.[5,6] Intravenous penicillin should be begun before operation and continued for 48 hours. Physicians who favor the delayed tonsillectomy prefer not to operate when the patient is septic, has had poor oral intake, or has a compromised airway. They also feel that increased bleeding can occur with an acute tonsillectomy in association with an abscess.

Infectious Mononucleosis

Infectious mononucleosis is an important cause of acute pharyngitis with enlarged tonsils. This infection is probably one of the many diseases caused by the Epstein-Barr virus.[7] The patient has a prodromal syndrome of lethargy and pharyngitis. The tonsils can enlarge and actually obstruct the airway. A membranous exudate is present over the tonsil, and in 30 percent of the cases a culture will reveal an associated beta-hemolytic streptococcus. Cervical adenopathy, particularly of the posterior cervical nodes, becomes evident. The patient may also develop other symptoms, including neurologic disturbances and liver or spleen enlargement. Although enlargement of Waldeyer's ring can cause airway obstruction and cyanosis, tracheostomy is seldom necessary in such patients when 40 mg per day of prednisone is initiated. This drug usually rapidly reduces the size of the lymphoid tissue. The diagnosis is made by examining the peripheral blood smear for leukocytoid lymphocytes, and by a mononucleosis spot test, which is a hemoagglutination test. In addition, immunologic studies are available to ascertain the presence of infectious mononucleosis (heterophile antibody titer 1:160 or higher). Such patients, if their oral intake is satisfactory and their pain is not sufficient to require hospitalization, may be treated at home with rest. Certainly, they should not return to their usual activities for 2 weeks or more, and then only after the disease and particularly spleen enlargement have resolved. There have been reports of splenic rupture when young athletes prematurely return to their sports. In a few cases, the tonsils remain hypertrophied after a bout of mononucleosis. If they do not return to normal size in 6 months, tonsillectomy is considered by some otolaryngologists.

DENTAL INFECTION

The normal oral flora have been discussed in Chapter 3, but individuals actually develop their own normal flora dependent on their general and local dental health, use of antibiotics, and previous irradiation therapy. For example, the oral flora of patients in an intensive care unit will show many gram-negative organisms not ordinarily found in the oral cavity. Sprinkle and Veltri [8] have shown that the oral cavity of a child after repeated episodes of tonsillitis and pharyngitis, and repeated administration of antibiotics, can be restored to a normal flora only after a tonsillectomy. The predominance of anaerobic organisms in the oral cavity is difficult to explain. Many anaerobes have a predilection to certain microenvironments. For example, some occur at the junction of the gingiva and teeth, others are found in the gingival-buccal folds. In these regions the oxidation-reduction potential of the tissues supports anaerobic organisms. The oxygen pressure (Po_2) in these areas is usually less than 1 percent. It is important to remember that bacteremia with the seeding of many metastatic sites (brain, liver, heart valve, prosthesis, etc.) is a common consequence of dental procedures. Appropriate chemoprophylaxis is required in all patients at high risk for such complications (Chapters 31 and 33).

Most of the dental infections discussed in this section are caused by mixed aerobic and anaerobic normal flora of the mouth. Almost all the organisms are sensitive to penicillin. However, penicillin-resistant organisms, especially *B. fragilis*, are found often enough to require culture to be performed in every case not responding promptly to appropriate operative therapy and penicillin. An extensive literature on dentoalveolar infections is cited by Finegold.[4]

Gingivitis and Periodontitis

Two organisms found only in the oral cavity, which live in symbiosis, include the *Borrelia vincenti* and the *Bacillus fusiformis*. *B. vincenti* cannot be grown on an artificial medium, and it must be identified on Gram stain. These two bacteria may lead to an infection of the gingiva known as Vincent disease. The gingiva is usually foul-smelling and ulcerated. Treatment in severe cases includes a systemic antibiotic, usually penicillin, given for 5 days, and improved oral hygiene, including the use of a peroxide mouthwash. *Fusobacterium* and *B. melaninogenicus* and anaerobic gram-negative rods are commonly identified with these infections and are probably the responsible organisms. With extension of the infection, the periodontal ligament becomes involved and acute periodontitis can develop. Besides the gingiva and periodontal ligament, the adjacent alveolar bone becomes infected, with eventual loss of teeth.

Periapical Abscess

Extension of infection up the root canal causes first pulpitis and then a periapical abscess. The patient complains of fever, and percussion of the affected tooth causes pain. In chronic cases, a periodontal pocket develops, which may eventually communicate with the maxillary sinus. Depending on the involved tooth, the apical abscess can perforate either the maxillary or mandibular bone on either the lingual or buccal suture. The abscess with granulation tissue is referred to as a gum boil. The incisor and canine teeth of the mandible are in the middle of the bone and have a thin alveolar plate so that an abscess can perforate either the lingual or buccal alveolar plate. Because the apex of the roots of the 2nd and 3rd mandibular molars extend well below the mylohyoid line, infections from these two teeth may extend directly into the deep neck and into the area of the submandibular lymph node. These two teeth are then most responsible for dental causes of deep neck abscess. Infection of the more anterior teeth will remain confined by the mylohyoid muscle to the anterior floor of the mouth.

Treatment of acute periapical abscesses requires drainage through a root canal. At a later stage, a root canal filling is made. If the infection has extended through the alveolar plate, this area must also be incised and drained. The decision for a root canal procedure or extraction is up to the dentist. Generally, if a 2nd or 3rd molar is involved and has caused the infection, extraction is preferred, particularly if the molar is dead. The location of the tooth is important in determining whether a root canal drainage should be performed.

Oroantral Fistula

The maxillary premolar and molar teeth are in close relationship to the sinus. In fact, when these teeth are extracted, no effort should be made to probe the depths of the extraction cavity because only a thin membrane of periosteum may be separating the tooth socket from the maxillary antrum. If the membrane is perforated, the hole should be closed and the area cleansed immediately and packed to prevent the formation of an oroantral fistula. If a fistula develops, a palatal buccal flap is devised, the osteitic bone in the area removed, and the wound closed primarily. It should be emphasized that if a fistula develops, sinusitis also develops. The otolaryngologist must institute drainage, via nasoantral windows, or even antrostomies to reestablish a noninfected sinus. Only then will the fistula close.

Alveolar Osteitis

Alveolar osteitis (dry socket) is a common and feared complication after extraction. Basically, there is a loss of the clot formed at the site of the extraction, and a localized osteitis develops with exposure of the underlying alveolar bone, most commonly after mandibular extractions. A characteristic foul odor develops. Treatment includes cleansing with a warm saline solution to remove the necrotic debris in the socket. Then, some type of antiseptic material is applied to the socket, such as iodoform packing or Eugenol. This treatment may have to be repeated over a period of days. If there is fever with the infection, a systemic antibiotic such as penicillin is used.

Differential Diagnosis of Sinusitis versus Dental Pain

Approximately 10 to 12 percent of sinusitis is associated with underlying dental disorders. Sometimes, it is difficult to determine whether the patient's pain is secondary to gingivitis, apical abscess, or sinusitis. Dental film, such as panorex, can be helpful in making the differential diagnosis. The most important test for determining pulpitis or periapical abscess is percussion of the suspected teeth. An upright Water's view of the sinuses will aid in determining whether an underlying sinusitis is present. Infection related to the maxillary molars is the most frequent dental cause of sinusitis. In addition, many benign dental tumors appear as bony erosion or an expanding cyst as seen on dental films, panorex, or maxillary sinus films. Diagnosis includes differentiating cysts from an acute infection. Following extraction, the cyst lining should be removed for histologic diagnosis.

INFECTIOUS DISEASES OF THE MAJOR AND MINOR SALIVARY GLANDS

ANATOMIC AND PHYSIOLOGIC PREDISPOSING FACTORS

The major and minor salivary glands combine to produce between 1 to 1.5 liters of saliva per day. Saliva is essential for the protection of the teeth and the mucous membrane of the oral cavity and pharynx. Saliva contains enzymes (eg, ptylin, amylase), which help initiate digestion, and certain electrolytes (primarily sodium phosphate, calcium chloride, and bicarbonate and phosphate buffers). IgA that is formed by the plasma cells lining the acini of the parotid gland combines with saliva to form soluble IgA, which inhibits adherence of bacteria to mucosal cells. Ninety percent of the saliva is produced by the parotid and submandibular glands. The parotid, a primarily serous salivary gland, emits a thin, watery secretion, the production of which is vastly increased by chewing and acid (particularly ascorbic acid) in the mouth. The submandibular glands are mixed serous and mucous glands, and produce a more viscous saliva. There is a constant flow of saliva from the submandibular glands, and it too is increased when food is present in the mouth.

The minor salivary glands and sublingual glands produce the remaining 10 percent of saliva. The sublingual glands are primarily mucous glands, located anteriorly in the floor of the mouth, deep to the mylohyoid muscle, just anterior to the submandibular gland. Additional minor salivary glands are located on the lips, buccal mucosa, and along the anterior tonsillar pillar. They are most concentrated at the junction of the hard and soft palate.

The parotid gland is incompletely encapsulated by splitting of superficial layers of the deep cervical fascia. In addition, septa of this fascia extend vertically into the gland, dividing it into many septated smaller sections. The divisions of the facial nerve run through the midportion of the gland, artificially dividing the gland into its more lateral (superficial) lobe and the deep lobe. Approximately 20 lymph nodes are located within the parotid region. These nodes are both extraglandular (lying over the capsular surface of the gland) and deep. The extracapsular nodes receive the lymph from the region of the face, eyelids, scalp, and preauricular areas (such as the tragus). Deep lymph nodes drain the paranasal sinuses, pharynx, and particularly the deeper aspects of the inner ear canal.

The submandibular gland lies inferior to the lower margin of the mandible, but the anteriormost portion of this gland projects medially into the floor of the mouth, through an opening along the lateral border of the mylohyoid muscle. The submandibular duct (Wharton's duct) is 5 to 6 cm long. It passes along the floor of the mouth just deep to the mucosa to enter the oral cavity through a papilla near the lingual frenulum. Thick secretions in this duct are subject to stasis, obstruction, or stone formation.

GENERAL PATHOGENETIC FACTORS

Infections within the major salivary glands occur as the result of three problems: (1) decreased salivary flow, possibly secondary to drugs, dehydration, or radiation, (2) formation of viscous saliva, either caused by abnormal formation of saliva from generalized systemic disease or drugs, and (3) obstruction to salivary flow by stones in the duct, stricture, or retrograde infection from the oral cavity.

Table 27-1 lists possible effects of systemic medications on the major salivary glands. In addition to the systemic effects, local irritations from dehydration, smoking, oral irritants and astringents, or poor oral hygiene establish an environment in which ascending infection is possible. Systemic diseases that cause parotid enlargement and changes in the salivary flow rate include: (1) cystic fibrosis, (2) primary aldosteronism, (3) Addison's disease, (4) Cushing's disease, (5) cirrhosis, (6) diabetes mellitus, and (7) gouty parotitis.

TABLE 27-1. DRUGS AFFECTING SALIVARY GLANDS

Decrease salivary flow
Parasympathomimeter (atrophic)
Sympathomimeter
Digitalis
Sialadenitis
Heavy metals
Mercury
Bismuth
Enlargement
Iodine
Phenothiazine

ACUTE SUPPURATIVE SIALADENITIS

Parotitis

Acute suppurative parotitis most often occurs in the dehydrated postoperative patient, debilitated by disease, with poor oral hygiene. Salivary flow decreases disproportionately with dehydration; even minor degrees of dehydration cause immediate major decrease in salivary flow. Infection usually ascends along the parotid duct. The organism responsible in over 90 percent of the cases is *S. aureus*, but *Streptococcus viridans* and *S. pyogenes* can also be responsible. Because the parotid is divided by multiple septa, localized fluctuation and suppuration cannot be demonstrated. Instead, diffuse parotid enlargement with tenderness and redness over the involved gland and side of the face are seen. Treatment includes hydration both orally (if possible) and with intravenous fluids, correction of electrolyte disturbances, and administration of intravenous antibiotics, preferably methicillin or cephalosporin derivatives. Improved oral hygiene is also important. Heat applied to the gland (in the form of warm moist packs) may provide some symptomatic relief. If there is no evidence of improvement, some physicians recommend between 400 to 600 rads of cobalt irradiation over a period of 2 to 3 days. This treatment is most effective when initiated within the first 48 hours. The radiation decreases the saliva formation and decreases the inflammatory response. If there is no improvement in 4 to 5 days, surgical drainage becomes necessary. A modified Blair or lazy S incision is used. Skin is elevated and a series of incisions are made through the capsule of the parotid gland in multiple areas, being careful to place the incisions parallel to the divisions of the facial nerve. Penrose drains are placed, and the wound is allowed to heal by secondary intention.

Another variant of acute suppurative parotitis—again caused by *S. aureus*—can occur within the first year of life in children. Treatment with systemic antibiotics is usually successful, but failure to respond may necessitate operative drainage as described for the adult.

Submandibular Gland Sialadenitis

Acute infection in the submandibular gland is usually the result of ductal stricture or stone. Antistaphylococcal antibiotics are used prior to manipulation. Stones felt on bimanual palpation along the course of the duct in the floor of the mouth can be removed by an intraoral incision over the stone. The incision must follow the longitudinal axis of the duct to prevent fistula formation. Stones deep in the hilum of the gland should be removed by a submandibular approach. If there has been an associated, recurrent episode of swelling and a sialadenitis because of the stone, it is worthwhile to remove the entire gland during a quiescent interlude.

CHRONIC RECURRENT SIALADENITIS

Chronic sialadenitis is manifested by recurrent acute episodes of sialadenitis, especially of the parotid and submandibular glands. During the quiescent phase, with no evidence of any acute inflammation, sialography may be helpful. The orifice of the duct is anesthetized (4 percent topical cocaine), gently dilated with a lacrimal duct probe (start with size 00 and dilate to No. 2) and polyethylene tubing (PE-90 or PE-60) inserted 1–2 cm. A contrast medium (1.5–2 ml Pantopaque) is carefully injected with fluoroscopic control to fill the entire ductal system. Should the patient develop pain, no further contrast material is injected. After completing the first series of roentgenograms, the patient can be given concentrated lemon juice. Normally, all contrast material will be discharged from the duct system within 10 minutes, and a repeat film at this time that shows large amounts of contrast present means either an obstruction or a dysfunction of the gland.

Sialography should demonstrate any area of obstruction in the duct, either extrinsic or intrinsic, stone or stricture. Certain forms of chronic sialadenitis have typical sialographic appearance. Sialectasia shows ectasia of the ductal system similar to the appearance of bronchiectasis on a bronchogram. There may be saccular dilatations and areas of obstruction throughout the duct system, primarily in the region of the small duct lobules. Punctate sialectasis is a term used to describe an end-stage of sialadenitis. Spotty collections of contrast throughout the entire glandular system are noted. This appearance is characteristic of Sjögren's disease or benign lymphoepithelial disease.

Chronic Nonobstructive Sialadenitis

This disease most commonly affects the parotid gland. Recurrent enlargement and pain are the most frequent symptoms, but there are no calculi. External pressure expresses very viscous saliva from the duct. A sialogram demonstrates tubular changes in the duct, and the roentgenogram is similar to that seen in tubular bronchiectasis. Treatment involves the use of sialagogues, eg, lemon juice, chewing gum, and increased fluid intake. With increasing symptoms and continuous enlargement that no longer responds to antibiotics and sialagogues, three possible surgical treatments exist. An indirect approach is tympanic neurectomy, ie, sectioning Jacobson's nerve over the promontory of the middle ear. This interrupts the parasympathetic nerve supply to the parotid gland, thus causing a decrease in the salivary flow and atrophy of the glandular tissue. The second indirect method of treatment is ligation of the parotid duct through an intraoral approach. This surgical treatment requires that a certain amount of parotid function still be present, as the atrophy of the gland depends on the back pressure of the salivary flow to destroy the remaining glandular elements. The third and most effective treatment is total parotidectomy, with preservation of the facial nerve. This resection is performed in a manner similar to the procedure for small benign parotid tumors; however, there is increased risk to the facial nerve. Total rather than superficial parotidectomy is necessary, because the gland is diffusely abnormal with possible small microabscesses and increased fibrosis.

Kasmaul's Disease

Kasmaul's disease is a specific form of chronic parotitis, similar to the already described types. It is characterized by stringy, thick parotid secretions when pressure is applied to the gland. Treatment is similar to that mentioned above.

BENIGN LYMPHOEPITHELIAL DISEASE AND SJÖGREN SYNDROME

Benign lymphoepithelial disease can affect both major and minor benign glands and be associated with chronic sialadenitis. The origin of this disease is not established, but a viral etiology has been suggested. There is a diffuse lymphocytic infiltrate within the involved glands. When confined to the parotid gland, there is chronic recurring enlargement with a typical sialographic appearance of punctate sialectasis (Mikulicz's disease). When it becomes associated with decreased lacrimal gland flow, and with a collagen disorder (especially rheumatoid arthritis, lupus erythematosis, or sclerodoma), it is called Sjögren syndrome. The pathologic features of Sjögren syndrome include diffuse atrophy of the salivary gland, lymphocyte infiltration, and myoepithelial islands of lymphocytes surrounding the tubular acini. Hypergammaglobulinemia (primarily of the IgM fraction) is common. A systemic lymphoma and other lymphoproliferative disorder's are a common sequela, especially histiocytic lymphoma, Hodgkin's disease, and Waldenstrom's macroglobulinemia. The early rise in IgM associated with lymphoproliferative phases of the disease is then followed by a drop in the serum IgM levels. This drop has been suggested to indicate malignant changes in the lymphoproliferative process. The verification of the diagnosis of a lymphoproliferative disorder or benign lymphoepithelial disease requires sialogram and an open biopsy of the involved parotid gland. Biopsy of the lip near the vermillion border or of the salivary glands at the junction of the hard and soft palate is likely to demonstrate the same pathologic features as demonstrated in the parotid gland. Surgery may become necessary when the associated swelling and enlargement of the parotid gland with repeated infections becomes intractable. Biopsy may be necessary to recognize other possible causes of parotid enlargement. Before any surgical treatment, thorough medical evaluation is necessary. This may include laboratory evaluations for antinuclear antibody, rheumatoid factor, serum protein electrophoresis and immunoelectrophoresis, and urine analysis.

GRANULOMATOUS DISEASES OF THE SALIVARY GLANDS

Tuberculosis

Chronic granulomatous diseases can involve the major salivary glands and again, most frequently, the parotid gland. Tuberculosis can present as a silent, enlarging mass within the parotid gland. Pulmonary involvement is almost always present, and parotid disease may simply be a cervical form of tuberculosis which occurs most commonly in the age group 20 to 40. It may be encapsulated and, should surgery be undertaken for a parotid mass, excision is preferable to a drainage procedure. The preferred treatment, however, is antituberculous chemotherapy (Chapter 18).

Sarcoidosis

Sarcoidosis is not clearly an infectious process. Between 6 and 10 percent of diffuse enlargements of the parotid gland are caused by this granulomatous process, which may present with facial nerve paralysis. There are almost always other manifestations of sarcoidosis, hilar adenopathy, hypercalcemia, splenomegaly, and uveitis. The combination of fever, parotid enlargement of one or both glands, and uveitis is called uveoparotid fever. A needle biopsy is indicated if the diagnosis is in doubt, and systemic steroids are the most effective treatment.

DIFFERENTIAL DIAGNOSIS OF SALIVARY GLAND ENLARGEMENT

It is not always easy to distinguish a chronic inflammation from an underlying parotid tumor because both produce parotid swelling. In addition, cystic masses within the parotid gland, such as a type I or type II pharyngeal cleft cyst, can cause recurrent episodes of parotid swelling. In a type I pharyngeal cleft cyst, there may be cartilaginous duplication of the external ear canal, and the fistulous tract generally exists in the postauricular crease. In a type II pharyngeal cleft cyst, a fistulous tract often enters the upper neck just below the angle of the mandible. Because the tract can pass either medial or lateral to the facial nerve before entering the external ear canal, excision of such a fistulous tract should be performed only after culture, and after antibiotic treatment has removed the acute infection.

A firm nontender mass in the parotid gland which does not fluctuate in size suggests a primary tumor (80 percent are benign pleomorphic adenoma). The diagnosis cannot be established by roentgenogram techniques (such as sialography), and biopsy is necessary. Needle biopsies are used only in select cases and in centers in which pathologists are accustomed to interpreting such specimens. Most pathologists prefer to examine a larger specimen, and a superficial parotidectomy is recommended for biopsy of suspicious parotid masses.

INFECTIONS OF THE NOSE AND PARANASAL SINUSES

Serious infections of the nose and paranasal sinuses develop only when the normal physiologic activities of these structures are altered. Normally, the nose acts to cleanse, warm, and humidify inspired air. Most foreign material is deposited on the anterior portion of the middle turbinate. Ciliary activity and the overlying mucous blanket carry the particulate debris posteriorly into the nasopharynx. For this to occur normally, the pH of the nose must be neutral. Any of the following events can disrupt these important physiologic activities: (1) an allergic response can cause edema and excess secretion, (2) upper respiratory viral infections severely impair ciliary activity because thick mucous retards ciliary movement, and (3) some medications, both systemic and topical, can interfere with normal ciliary activity. Certain gross anatomic abnormalities—a deviated nasal septum, nasal polyp, tumor, or foreign body—can also obstruct the sinusoidal ostium. Any obstruction, functional or morphologic, impedes the drainage of mucus so that microbial proliferation can occur. The resulting mucosal edema and death of mucosal cells further impedes drainage by aggravating the obstruction and abrogating cilial motion. Mucosal regeneration is rapid if obstruction is promptly relieved. If not relieved, the epithelium is permanently damaged; polyps and mucoceles can develop, and chronic sinusitis results. Almost 10 percent of maxillary sinusitis is associated with preexisting dental infection.

Etiology

The most common bacterial organisms to cause acute sinusitis are pneumococci, streptococci, staphylococci, and *H. influenzae.* Cultures of the nasal secretions are unreliable in determining the responsible organisms.

Chronic sinusitis and maxillary sinusitis associated with dental infections are more commonly anaerobic because the cavities lose their air content and the increased intrasinusoidal pressure impairs mucosal blood flow. Such infections generally contain large volumes of fetid secretion. Almost all oral, nasal, or pharyngeal anaerobic flora have been found—especially *Peptostreptococcus, Peptococcus, Bacteroides, Veillonella,* and *Actinomyces.* Many anaerobic infections probably result in sterile cultures, because bacteria are seen on smear but no growth is found.[9]

General Clinical Manifestations

Pain, headache, fever, and tenderness over the involved area with swelling and redness are common manifestations of acute sinusitis. During chronic infection the symptoms and signs are much more subtle—congestion, blockage, and chronic nasal discharge. Careful physical examination includes evaluation of the nasal mucosa, search for obstruction by edema or nasal polyps, and examination of nasal secretions. Roentgenograms of the paranasal sinuses, particularly the upright Water's view of the maxillary and ethmoid sinuses, are necessary. The Caldwell view provides the best information about the frontal sinus. The lateral view is helpful for examination of the ethmoid and frontal sinuses, and essential for evaluation of the sphenoid sinus (Fig. 27-8).

General Aspects of Treatment

Acute sinusitis should respond promptly without operation. A vasoconstrictor (aqueous 0.25 to 0.50 percent phenylephrine) should be applied as nosedrops every 4 to 6 hours to decrease edema; hot packs or high humidity may provide symptomatic relief. Antibiotics may not be necessary in most cases, but if fever, pain, and leukocytosis are present, penicillin G, ampicillin, or erythromycin should be given for at least 3 to 4 days after clinical resolution. The anaerobic organisms in the sinuses are almost always sensitive to these drugs. *B. fragilis* infections are rare. Rational choice of antibiotic is empirical because reliable noninvasive culture techniques do not exist. Aspiration and puncture techniques of obtaining truly diagnostic specimens from each sinus are described in subsequent sections. An operation is almost never necessary in acute sinusitis.

SPECIAL FORMS OF SINUSITIS

Acute Maxillary Sinusitis

The maxillary sinuses are present at birth and are the most common sinuses to become infected in adults. The maxillary ostium drains into the middle nasal meatus. Infection generally occurs with obstruction of this ostium, whether from a bacterial, viral, or allergic cause. Ten percent result from preexisting dental disease. A roentgenogram of the sinuses that shows an air fluid level will verify the diagnosis of sinusitis (Fig 27-9).

If the use of empirical antibiotics and decongestants does not help after 10 days, or if the symptoms are worsening, antral puncture is indicated. One of three common techniques is used. The first technique requires application of a topical anesthetic, such as 4 percent cocaine, to the inferior nasal meatus. With the patient seated, a trocar is pushed through the lateral nasal wall, as high as possible, yet still beneath the inferior turbinate. The trocar is aimed upward toward the lateral canthus of the eye. With gentle pressure, the trocar passes through the thin bone and enters the maxillary cavity. Aspiration with a syringe will permit removal of purulent material for smear, Gram stain, KOH preparations, and aerobic and anaerobic culture. An anaerobic infection should be suspected, especially when purulent foul-smelling material is obtained and none of the common organisms can be isolated.

The second antral puncture technique uses cannulation of the natural orifice above the middle meatus. Again, a cocaine topical anesthesia is used, not only for its anesthetic effect but for its vasoconstrictor effect. A specially curved cannula is inserted into the natural ostium, and the sinus is aspirated and culture material obtained.

A third method uses an anterior approach over the canine fossa. Here, injectable local anesthesia (2 percent xylocaine with epinephrine) is used. By lifting the upper lip, the trocar can be placed directly into the maxillary sinus. The bone is thicker here and greater pressure must be applied. This approach can be done using direct visualization, and it can be used in patients with underlying blood dyscrasias. Its main disadvantage is increased discomfort to the patient.

Chronic Maxillary Sinusitis

Chronic maxillary sinusitis occurs when there is obstruction of the normal drainage through the maxillary ostium. At first, there may be episodes of recurrent acute infections, which resolve with antibiotics and decongestants. Eventually, however, the patient has an almost continuous sinus infection. Roentgenograms may no longer reveal a fluid level; instead, an opacified sinus or thickened mucosal lining can be seen. Mucosa thicker than 2 mm is consistent

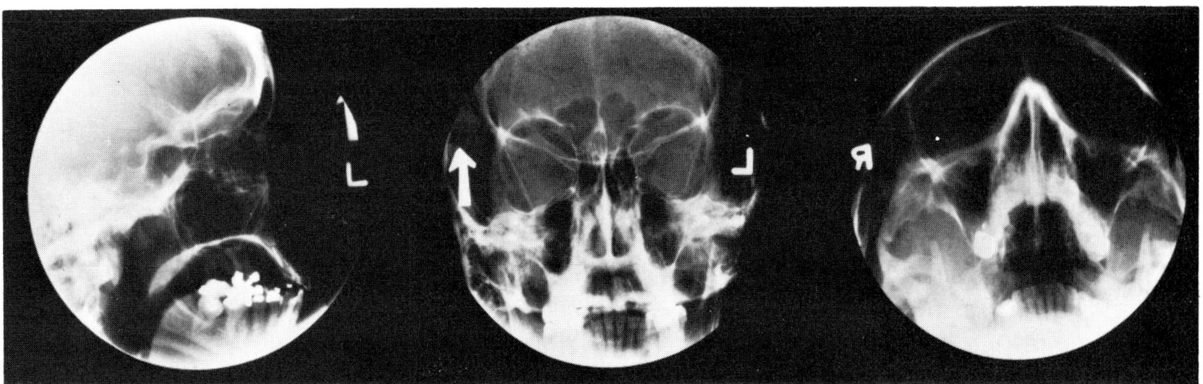

Fig. 27-8. **A. Lateral, B. Caldwell's, and C. Water's views of normal paranasal sinuses. (Courtesy of Frick M, Department of Radiology, University of Minnesota.)**

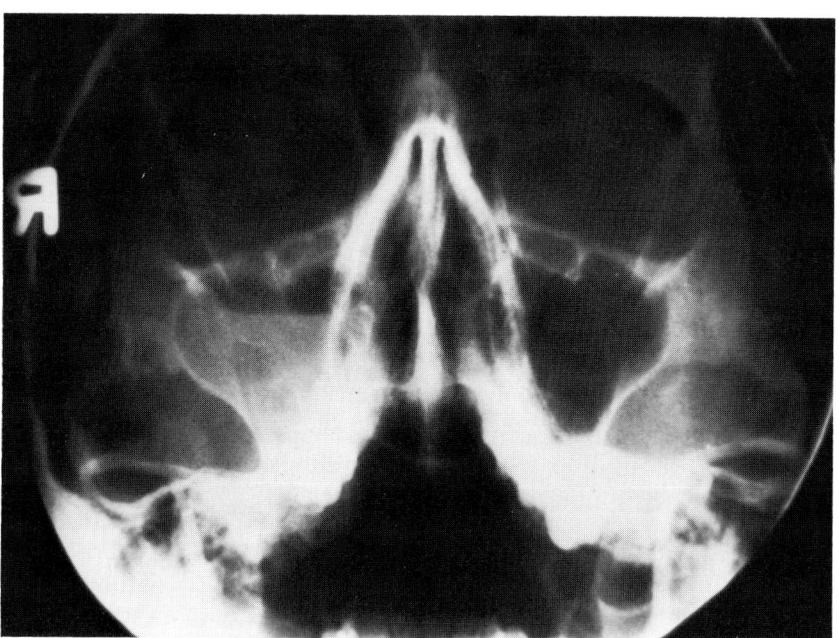

Fig. 27-9. **Air fluid level in the right maxillary sinus seen in an upright Water's view of the maxillary sinus.**

with the diagnosis of chronic sinusitis (but may mean something else). Rather than perform repeated antral puncture, with or without repeated lavage of the sinus, a permanent intranasal antrotomy (NA window) may be performed. The inferior turbinate is fractured upward and a mucoperiosteal flap elevated in the inferior meatus. The lateral nasal wall is punctured and enlarged. An opening of at least 2 cm × 2 cm provides excellent drainage. The mucoperiosteal flap from the lateral nasal wall is now laid into the sinus. Cultures and irrigations can be performed at the same time. The examiner may be able to examine the entire sinus through this newly created opening or even the natural ostium by means of recently developed flexible fiberoptic scopes.

When it is necessary to have more information about the maxillary sinus, a Caldwell- Luc procedure (or radical antrostomy) is preferred. Under either local or general anesthesia, an incision is made through the mucoperiostium over the canine fossa. An opening is created into the maxillary sinus. Bacterial cultures and examinations of the sinus are then made, and the chronically infected mucosa is removed. A nasal antral window is then created from the antral side. Since the floor of the antrum lies 0.5 cm lower than the nasal floor, this approach permits a lower position to be selected for long-term dependent drainage than does the transnasal route. After a nasal antral window is created, the mucoperiosteum of the anterior antral wall is closed. The advantage of this procedure is better visualization and drainage. In addition, mucosa and polypoid tissue can be removed for study. Its disadvantage is that it is a more extensive procedure and can potentially cause denervation of maxillary teeth.

Acute Frontal Sinusitis

Frontal sinuses seldom create a clinical problem until they develop in the teen years. Acute infection causes fever and severe pain over the sinus and periorbital region. Pressure on the orbital roof will cause exquisite tenderness. Intranasal examination will show congestion, and after application of a topical vasoconstrictor, purulent material can be seen draining from the duct area high in the middle meatus. Infections in this region are more serious than maxillary infections because of the proximity of intracranial structures. In addition, the posterior wall of the frontal sinus is thin and an osteitis of this wall can cause an extradural or subdural abscess.

Hospitalization may be necessary for surveillance. Treatment of acute frontal sinusitis requires systemic antibiotics and topical decongestants. If there is no improvement after 48 hours, an external drainage or trephine procedure should be considered (Fig. 27-10). It is certainly indicated whenever any impending intracranial complication is suspected. An orbital incision is made above the inner canthus. The roof of the orbit is exposed, and a drill is used to remove a small amount of bone from the sinus floor. This area is selected because it provides dependent drainage, and because the cortical bone in this region is relatively resistant to osteomyelitis. A catheter is inserted through the trephine opening and sutured into position. Daily irrigations with antibiotic solutions or saline can be administered. After the acute infection has resolved, the nasofrontal duct should again become patent. This can be ascertained by injecting a small amount of dye into the sinus through the tube and checking the nose for the presence of dye. When the duct is patent, the tube is removed. The wound will close spontaneously or with closure by a few sutures. The cosmetic result is acceptable.

Chronic Frontal Sinusitis

Chronic frontal sinusitis may require definitive operation either to establish a drainage path, to replace the occluded nasofrontal duct, or to obliterate the frontal sinus entirely.

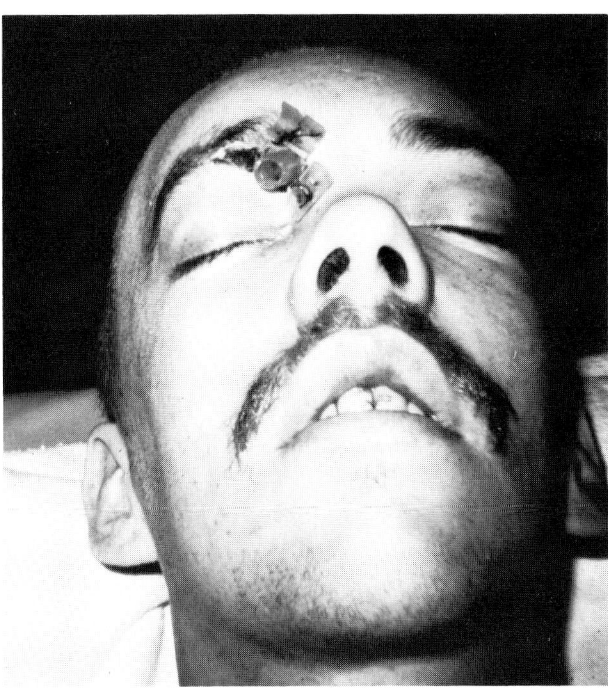

Fig. 27-10. **Trephine of the frontal sinus for acute suppurative frontal sinusitis. This sinus is entered through the orbital roof. A portion of a #24 silastic chest tube is sewn in place to serve as a drain.**

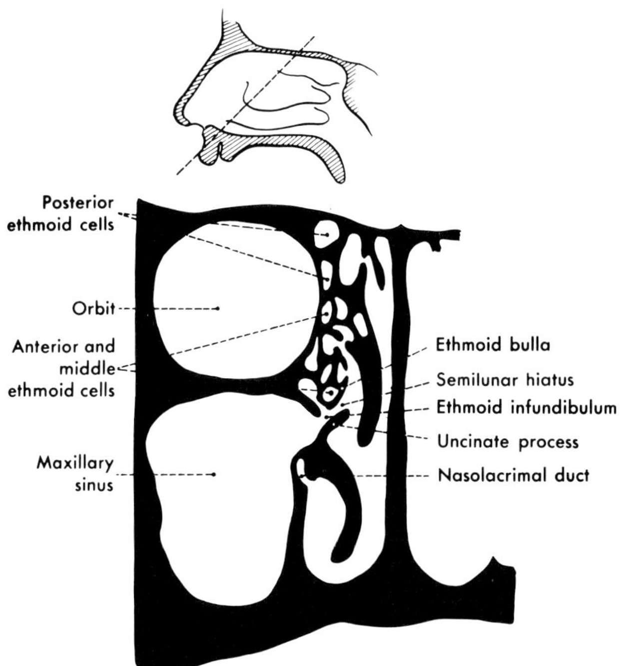

Fig. 27-11. **The ethmoid air cells, together constituting the ethmoid sinus, are shown in this hypothetical section through the lateral nasal wall. The section represents the slant indicated in the inset. (From Hollingshead HW (ed): The nose and paranasal sinuses. In *Anatomy for Surgeons. Vol 1, The Head and Neck,* 2nd ed. Hagerstown, Harper & Row, 1968, p 253.)**

Boyden-Sewall Procedure

The Boyden-Sewall procedure establishes a new, larger patent frontal duct, permitting the infection to resolve. A curvilinear incision is made on the inner aspect of the orbit and is extended down along the lateral nasal dorsum. With a drill, the cortical bone from the lateral wall of the nose is removed. This exposes the superior portion of the nasal septum. Additional bone is removed to identify the floor of the frontal sinus and the diseased sinus mucosa is curetted out. Access is available to the ethmoid cells if this area is also chronically infected (Fig. 27-11). A mucosal flap is developed from the nasal septum and rotated up into the frontal sinus. Stenting with tubed silastic sheeting is now done through the nose. The wound is closed, and the stent remains in place up to 6 weeks while the patient is treated with systemic antibiotics.

Frontal Sinus Obliteration

Since the sinus has little physiologic function, obliteration is a logical alternative. The approach can be by a Killian incision in the brow or by a coronal exposure. A template of the frontal sinus is cut out from a Caldwell view roentgenogram and placed on the forehead to guide the construction of a bone flap composed of the entire anterior sinus wall. The entire frontal sinus is thus laid open and the entire mucosa of the sinus is removed using an operating microscope. Not only is it important to get all the mucosa, but the entire inner table of this bone must be obliterated using a drill. It is only by removing this bone that total mucosal destruction can be accomplished, because the sinus mucosa has peglike extensions into the tiniest bony crevices. In addition, this best prepares the frontal sinus to accept a fat graft; autogenous subcutaneous fat is packed into the sinus. The frontal duct is obstructed by infolding its lining and packing the lumen with fascia. The bone flap is replaced, and the periosteum is carefully sutured. The skin flap is then resewn. Montgomery[10] reports excellent results, particularly when a mucocele or pyocele complicates the sinusitis.

Ethmoid Sinusitis

The ethmoid sinuses are actually composed of a series of cells (Fig. 27-11). There are about eight large ethmoid cells, divided into anterior and posterior groups on each side. The anterior group of cells are most closely associated with the anterior portion of the nasal cavity, while the posterior cells extend backward to the region of the sphenoid sinus. They are present at birth, and acute ethmoiditis is most often seen in children or when nasal polyps obstruct the ethmoid ostia. It usually presents as orbital cellulitis (Fig. 27-12). Acute ethmoiditis requires systemic antibiotics and nasal decongestants for treatment.

Chronic ethmoiditis is treated by removing the infected and often polypoid tissue within the ethmoid cells. There are basically three approaches that can be used. The first and perhaps most common approach is an intranasal ethmoidectomy, which is frequently combined with a nasal polypectomy and can be done under topical anesthesia. Frequently, only the anterior cells can be totally

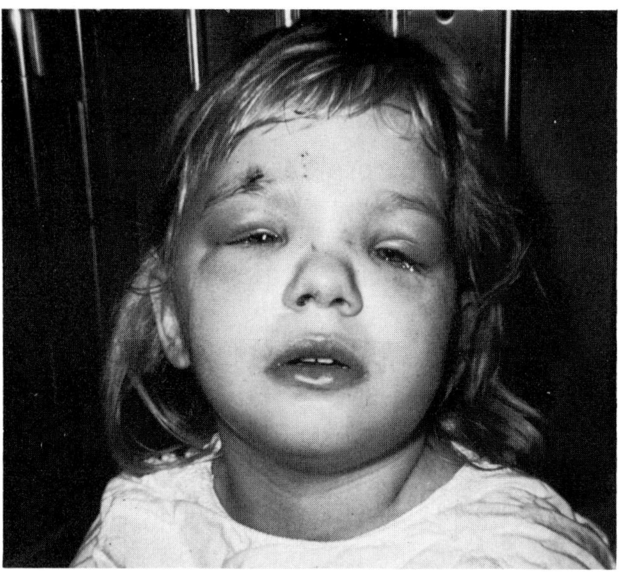

Fig. 27-12. **Bilateral orbital cellulitis in a child with acute ethmoiditis.**

removed with this method. Because of the close association of the ethmoid cells with the optic nerve and the cribiform plate, this technique requires great familiarity with the ethmoid anatomy. The roof of the ethmoid cells is higher than the cribiform plate, so that the medial attachment of the middle turbinate is maintained as a landmark to avoid perforating the cribiform plate to cause a subsequent leak of cerebrospinal fluid.

The second approach to the ethmoid cells is transantral ethmoidectomy. The maxillary sinus is opened via a Caldwell-Luc approach, and the ethmoids are exposed and excised through the medial portion of the maxillary sinus. This approach does not allow access to the more anterior ethmoid cells.

The third approach, external ethmoidectomy, is used most commonly for severe or complicated chronic ethmoidal infections. A curvilinear incision is made along the medial canthus and extended along the lateral nasal dorsum. The lacrimal bone, lacrimal sac, and tendon of the superior oblique muscle are identified and preserved. The lamina papyracea of the ethmoid is then perforated and the opening into the ethmoids is enlarged. The anterior ethmoid artery is generally ligated. Although this approach will leave a scar, it is probably the most effective and safest method of eliminating all chronic diseased tissue in the ethmoid labyrinth.

Sphenoid Sinusitis

The sphenoid sinus is not present at birth and becomes important only in adults. There is close association of the most posterior ethmoid cells to intracranial structures, the optic nerve, ophthalmic division of the 5th nerve, 3rd, 4th, and 6th cranial nerves, and the cavernous sinus. Sphenoid sinusitis is generally associated with infection of all the sinuses. Pain is felt in the midportion of the head or may be referred to the occipital area. Treatment of acute sphenoid infection is dependent on antibiotics and decongestants. If these modalities are unsuccessful, direct puncture of the anterior wall of the sphenoid sinus may be indicated. It is usually easier to directly puncture the anterior wall than to find the natural ostium for culture and irrigation. Chronic sinusitis may actually require removal of the anterior wall of the sinus, creating a single large cavity opening directly into the posterior nasal cavity and nasopharynx. For complicated cases, the sphenoid sinus is best approached via an external ethmoidectomy because the most posterior ethmoid cells are immediately adjacent to the sphenoid.

Sinusitis in Children

During the first 2 years of life, the ethmoid sinuses are the only ones that are completely developed and consequently the only ones to become infected. Infection is usually associated with an acute or chronic rhinitis and involves the entire ethmoid labyrinth. A common complication is unilateral or bilateral orbital cellulitis characterized by inflammation and swelling in the periorbital area (Fig. 27-12). Treatment with systemic antibiotics and decongestants is usually sufficient. Surgical drainage is rarely indicated. While viral inflammatory processes may be the inciting cause, secondary bacterial infection follows. The organism responsible is generally of the same group of organisms that causes acute sinusitis in adults. However, in children, *H. influenzae* infection is more frequent.

During the first year of life, the maxillary sinuses are small and only after the second year, when the teeth are developing, do they begin to play a role. Surgical drainage is seldom necessary in children; however, an antral puncture is occasionally required. The Caldwell approach is rarely used in children because the sinus is much smaller and located higher in the maxilla, and because the anterior approach threatens the developing teeth. Preferable to repeated antral punctures is placing a catheter into the sinus and taping it to the side of the face. This permits repeated irrigations with either saline or antibiotic solutions.

The frontal sinus develops after the age of 9 and reaches its adult size at approximately age 15. Acute sinusitis in young adults has been associated with swimming and diving. The treatment is similar to that of adults.

With recurrent viral rhinitis and sinusitis, the search for the cause of the repeated infections is necessary. Immunologic deficiencies should be considered, but most cases are due to allergy with its attendant nasal polyps, chronic mucoid drainage, and obstruction. When polyps are present in children, the possibility of cystic fibrosis must also be considered, and sweat chloride tests should be performed.

COMPLICATIONS OF SINUSITIS

Complications of sinusitis occurring with both the acute and chronic forms of the disease can be gradual or sudden in onset. The complications can best be divided into intracranial and extracranial forms.

Extracranial Orbital Complications

Periorbital Cellulitis and Subperiosteal Orbital Abscess

The most common extracranial complications of sinusitis are those which involve the orbit. Extension of infection through the thin, lamina papyracea of the ethmoid sinus or from the frontal sinus to the orbit cause first a periorbital cellulitis (Fig. 27-12). When the infection is not controlled, it may advance to form a subperiosteal abscess, accumulating pus between the loosely attached periorbita of the globe and the lamina papyracea. In certain patients, the lamina papyracea is so thin that areas of it may actually be dehiscent. Visual disturbances predominate; ophthalmoplegia of the 3rd nerve leads to diplopia, and increased pressure results in changes in the visual field size and diminished visual acuity. Emergency drainage of the orbit is required along with intravenous antibiotics. An ophthalmologist must measure visual acuity several times a day. Evidence of obstruction of the venous drainage of the eye should suggest the possibility of a cavernous sinus thrombosis.

An incision similar to that described for the external surgical approach to chronic ethmoiditis is utilized.

Orbital Abscess

Extension of the infection through the orbital periosteum into the region posterior to the globe can occur. This space is filled with fat and loose connective tissue. Infection soon leads to fat necrosis. Exophthalmos develops because of increased pressure within the orbit. Increased orbital pressure causes decreased venous drainage and visual loss. The combination of increased venous pressure, inflammation, and possible optic neuritis can lead to blindness.

An orbital abscess can be demonstrated by an orbital axial computerized tomography scan. It is essential to differentiate the abscess from a cavernous sinus thrombosis, which may present a clinically similar picture.

The responsible bacterial organisms are *S. pneumoniae* and *S. pyogenes. H. influenzae* is the most common organism in children. Blood cultures may be positive and are more likely than nasal smears to reveal the causative organism. The periorbita should be elevated and the abscess drained under antibiotic coverage. It may be noted at this time that the abscess extends over the roof of the globe, yet within the orbit and far more laterally than was recognized. Penrose drains are inserted and gradually advanced daily. Appropriate cultures are obtained. Vision usually returns to normal.

Complications of Frontal Sinusitis

Mucocele and Pyocele. Complete obstruction of the frontal sinus duct permits development of a cystic-type lesion, which gradually expands as fluids accumulate within it. The eye is pushed downward and forward by the enlarging contents of the frontal sinus. The walls of the sinus remain intact but are gradually pushed away over a period of months or years by the enlarging mucocele. The onset has been reported as late as 20 years after trauma to the frontal duct. Infection that develops within the mucocele makes this a pyocele. The symptoms of infection, rather than gradual enlargement, become more evident. The diagnosis of a frontal sinus mucocele must be considered in evaluation of any patient with a unilateral exophthalmus. Obliteration of the frontal sinus is the best treatment.

Frontal Bone Osteomyelitis. Pott's puffy tumor describes a subperiosteal accumulation of pus, which develops from an underlying osteomyelitis of the anterior wall of the frontal sinus (Fig. 27-13). Swelling and edema of the upper eyelid occurs, and the eye appears to be pushed downward and forward. The abscess is tender and requires drainage. Usually, a trephine procedure of the frontal sinuses is performed to treat the underlying frontal sinusitis and apparent obstruction of the frontal sinus duct at the same time.

Intracranial Complications of Sinusitis

Epidural Abscess and Meningitis

The intracranial complications of sinusitis occur more as a result of infection in the frontal sinus than the other sinuses. The infection may extend to the meninges directly by osteomyelitis of the posterior wall of the frontal sinus, or indirectly by the development of frontal vein phlebitis, extending along the venous drainage and eventually leading to the cavernous or sagittal sinus (Fig. 27-1). The intracranial complication is heralded by the onset of severe headache and nausea secondary to the increased cerebrospinal fluid pressure. Ophthalmologic examination will demonstrate papilledema, and the pupil on the infected side may remain dilated. More advanced disease can lead to hemiparesis. Neurosurgical consultation should be obtained immediately, and an emergency CAT scan and angiogram are required to define the extent of central nervous system involvement. Headache is the primary symptom if the infection is limited to the area adjacent

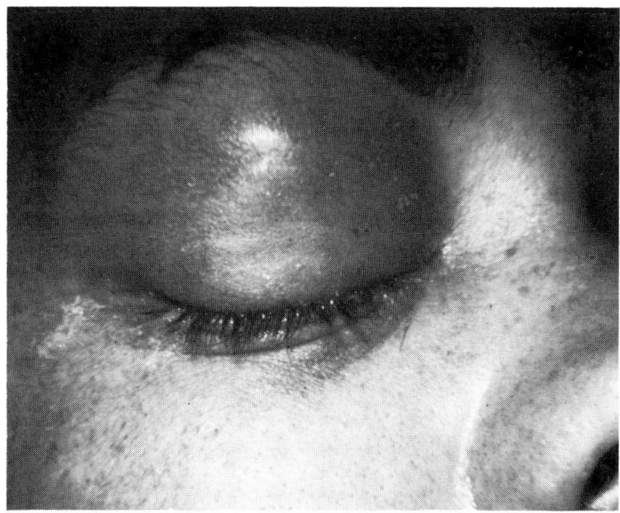

Fig. 27-13. **Swelling of the upper lid and subperiosteal abscess is a complication of acute frontal sinusitis (Pott's puffy tumor).**

to the posterior plate of the frontal sinus, and an epidural abscess develops. Drainage via a neurosurgical approach rather than a frontal one is required. If the infection extends along the emissary veins, the meningitis develops and meningismus suggests the need for a lumbar puncture. This should be performed with care and only after it is certain that the CSF pressure is not elevated as evidenced by the eye examination and absent papilledema.

Brain Abscess

Brain abscess occurs most commonly in the area between the white and gray matter, which has the poorest blood supply. When an abscess develops as a complication of sinusitis or mastoiditis, it is usually located directly over the region of the infected sinus or mastoid. Most brain abscesses caused by sinusitis contain anaerobic organisms, particularly anaerobic streptococci, *B. fragilis, Fusobacterium, Veillonella,* and other *Bacteroides* species. At the same time, the cultures from acute and chronic sinusitis demonstrate aerobes—*Staphylococcus, Streptococcus, H. influenzae,* and *E. coli.* Thus, the treatment of the developing brain abscess will require different antibiotics. High intravenous doses (30 to 40 million units per day) of penicillin are frequently effective, but chloramphenicol is more effective against *B. fragilis.* Clindamycin has poor penetration into brain abscesses. Metronidazole may prove to be useful. The indications for neurosurgical operation are discussed in Chapter 28. The underlying sinus problem should be treated as previously described.

Cavernous Sinus Thrombosis

The venous drainage from the ethmoid and frontal area extends posteriorly and into a complex of the dural sinuses, referred to as the cavernous sinus (Fig. 27-1). The veins of the mid one-third of the face have no valves, so the blood can flow in either direction. Through the cavernous sinus pass the optic nerves, the 3rd, 4th, and 6th cranial nerves, and the ophthalmic division of the 5th cranial nerve. Clinical symptoms of a cavernous sinus thrombosis are manifested by loss in visual acuity, headache, fever, meningitis, proptosis, and development of ophthalmoplegia. Because the cavernous sinuses adjoin each other, the symptoms soon become bilateral, which is the clinical key in the diagnosis. Treatment consists of intravenous penicillin and chloramphenicol. The question of anticoagulation is controversial. Its advantage is possible prevention of an extension of the thrombosis posteriorly to the petrosal veins. The disadvantage of anticoagulation is that thrombi might help to limit the infection to the cavernous sinus. The rarity of this most severe complication with its associated blindness, and death, has prevented any controlled clinical trials.

UNUSUAL SOFT TISSUE INFECTIONS OF THE FACE

RHINOCEREBRAL PHYCOMYCOSIS (MUCORMYCOSIS, ZYGOMYCOSIS)

The mucormycoses have been discussed in Chapter 9. This particular form generally begins in the nose and maxillary sinus and has a 50 percent mortality. Most patients are diabetics with ketoacidosis, but cancer patients who are undergoing chemotherapy and debilitated patients with malnutrition are also susceptible. Black crusts, which resemble a recent bloody discharge, initially appear on the turbinates and the nasal septum. Septal perforation can appear later. An acute maxillary sinusitis develops with facial cellulitis, and the overlying skin of the sinus may become necrotic. The orbit and ethmoid sinus are soon involved, so that proptosis and ophthalmoplegia develop. As the mycotic infection extends directly into this region, blindness ensues with thrombosis of the central retinal artery. Acute infection can extend directly into the brain along venous pathways, for these organisms tend to invade and thrombose vessels. Thus, it may extend along the angular vein to the ethmoid vein and then enter the cranium through the superior orbital fissure. Direct extension can occur along the carotid artery or through the cribiform plate. It should be differentiated from the cavernous sinus thrombosis by its rapid progression to an orbital apex syndrome and retinal artery occlusion. In cavernous sinus thrombosis, the bacterial infection extends along the veins and the posterior portion of the orbit may be spared, orbital pain is less, and blindness occurs later.

The progression of the disease along the internal carotid artery soon leads to hemiparesis. The 5th and 7th cranial nerves can also be involved. Differential diagnosis includes other problems such as tuberculosis, syphilis, lethal midline granuloma, squamous cell carcinoma, and aspergillosis. The diagnosis is made by biopsy and histologic demonstration of the organism invading the tissue. The presence of the organism on culture is not sufficient to establish its invasive quality.

Treatment requires control of the diabetes, the use of amphotericin B, and surgical debridement of the destroyed tissue. This is generally in the form of a Caldwell-Luc procedure with extensive drainage of all infected sinuses. The use of heparin must also be considered. Mortality has been reduced from 80 to 90 percent in the 1950s to 50 percent today. Those patients who survive, however, have residual morbidity.

FACIAL CELLULITIS

Facial cellulitis can develop and spread rapidly over the face from numerous sources. An abscess of the maxillary teeth can cause facial cellulitis and periorbital cellulitis. The symptoms of maxillary sinusitis can include inflammation, swelling, and redness over the cheek.

Cellulitis of the nasal tip is associated with a vestibulitis or inflammation of the vestibule or skin of the nose. There is frequently a history of manipulation of the small vibrisae in the nose. Dryness and cracking of the nasal vestibular skin can contribute to the infection. Cellulitis beginning in the nasal vestibule extends to the tip, causing inflammation. *S. aureus* is the organism most frequently isolated from the nasal vestibule.

Facial cellulitis can develop after trauma to the region or from manipulation of a furuncle. An abscess can form and can be localized within the cheek. Drainage through a small external incision is preferred. Facial cellulitis should be distinguished from the herpetic lesions seen in varicella zoster ophthalmicus. In zoster, typical vesicules develop over the distribution of the sensory divisions of the 5th nerve. Because of possible corneal involvement, ophthalmologic examination is mandatory. The veins in this region permit the infection to extend retrograde toward the cavernous sinus. Thus, all areas of cellulitis in the middle one-third of the face are considered potentially serious. Hospitalization and the use of intravenous antibiotics should be considered in every patient with an area of facial or nasal cellulitis. Facial cellulitis in infants and children is often caused by *H. influenzae* and should be treated with ampicillin, chloramphenicol, or cefamandole.

INFECTIONS OF THE NECK

ANATOMY OF THE CERVICAL FASCIAL SPACES

There are basically four important layers of cervical fascia which circumferentially divide the neck into compartments (Fig. 27-2).

The superficial layer is the outermost layer, which completely surrounds the neck like a cylinder. Anteriorly, it lies just beneath the skin and divides to surround the platysma muscle. (This is not shown in Fig. 27-2.) The deep cervical fascia is itself divided into a superficial layer and a deep layer. The superficial component of the deep cervical fascia completely encases the neck. Anteriorly, it splits to cover the sternocleidomastoid and trapezius muscles, the parotid, and submandibular glands. It is attached firmly to the hyoid bone, which in turn separates it into superior and inferior compartments. Superiorly, it is attached to the lower border of the mandible, and above the parotid it is attached to the zygoma. The deep layer of the deep cervical fascia partially encloses the deep portion of the parotid gland and is attached to the styloid and mastoid processes. A thickening of this layer between the styloid and mandible is called the stylomandibular ligament.

The deepest layer of the deep cervical fascia does not encompass the entire neck, rather it surrounds the muscles associated with the vertebral column, so that it is also called the prevertebral layer. It is important because it extends inferiorly into the mediastinum.

One additional layer of cervical fascia encloses the pharynx, esophagus, larynx, and trachea, and thus is referred to as the visceral layer. Anteriorly, where it is closely adherent to the trachea, it is referred to as the pretracheal fascia (Fig. 27-2). This fascia plane also provides potential access for extension of infection into the mediastinum.

PHARYNGOMAXILLARY (PARAPHARYNGEAL) SPACE INFECTIONS

The most common potential deep cervical space to become infected is the pharyngomaxillary or parapharyngeal space (Fig. 27-4). It is a pyramid-shaped space with its base along the base of the skull extending inferiorly to its apex at the hyoid bone. It lies just lateral to the superior constrictor muscle and medial to the parotid gland. It is most often infected as an extension from the pharynx or tonsillar region. Abscesses at the petrous apex, however, can extend into this space. Posteriorly, it is adjacent to the retropharyngeal space, and anteriorly it is closely associated with the submaxillary space (Fig. 27-4). Infections from the parotid can also extend into the pharyngomaxillary space because the fascia is not complete in the region of the parotid gland. During an infection, the space expands and fills with pus. The close association with the parotid gland causes edema to occur within the gland, and the swelling of the gland then becomes evident in the neck (Fig. 27-5). Intraoral examination shows the lateral pharyngeal wall in the region of the tonsil to be pushed medially, but the tonsil itself should appear normal. Because many infections in this space will resolve with appropriate intravenous antibiotics, at least 72 hours of intravenous antibiotics is indicated. Immediate surgical drainage is indicated if no response is seen or if the infection worsens. The strongest indication for immediate surgical drainage is bleeding from the ear, which suggests that either one of the tributaries of the jugular vein or the branches of the carotid arteries are infected.

The external approach to drainage is mandatory. In no case should the abscess be approached intraorally, because a pseudoaneurysm of the carotid artery can rupture and there will be no access to control the hemorrhage. The technique described by Mosher[11] in the 1920s is still the most effective. A transverse incision is made anterior to the sternocleidomastoid muscle two finger-breadths below the margin of the mandible (Fig. 27-6). The anterior border of the sternocleidomastoid muscle is retracted posteriorly. The fascia overlying the submandibular gland is identified and traced posteriorly and medially, until the space is entered. Next, a finger is passed up and the styloid process palpated. It may be necessary to divide the ligament between the styloid process and the mandible, which is formed by a thickening of the deep cervical fascia. Further, the styloid process itself divides the pharyngeal space into an anterior and posterior compartment. It is almost always the anterior compartment that is infected. This is apparent by the trismus, which develops because of the intimate relationship to the medial pterygoid muscle. The posterior compartment of this space contains primarily the last four cranial nerves, the jugular vein, and the carotid artery. When these structures become infected, the symptoms are usually caused by vascular problems. Soft rubber drains are inserted into the parapharyngeal space and withdrawn gradually over a period of days. Aerobic and anaerobic cultures should be obtained as well as Gram stain. Intravenous antibiotics are continued until the patients symptoms subside. The wound is allowed to heal by secondary intention.

RETROPHARYNGEAL SPACE INFECTIONS

The retropharyngeal space lies posterior to the superior and middle constrictor muscles of the pharynx (Fig. 27-4). It is divided into a left and right side by the median raphe. This space is only a potential space. In children under age 2 years, it contains a few lymph nodes. Suppuration and breakdown of these nodes with adenoid infections in early childhood can result in retropharyngeal space abscesses. In adults, infection of the retropharyngeal space is usually associated with trauma (Fig. 27-14). This includes instrumentation in the pharynx and particularly traumatic passage of some type of endoscopic equipment. Rarely, tuberculosis will spread into this space from the cervical spine.

Because the retropharyngeal space can communicate with the prevertebral space, retropharyngeal abscesses can extend into the mediastinum. Immediate drainage with intravenous antibiotic coverage is therefore the best treatment. The preferred approach in children is transpharyngeal with the child in a Rose or head-down position and suction apparatus immediately available to prevent aspiration. A midline incision is then made, the pus aspirated, and appropriate Gram stains and cultures obtained (Fig. 27-15). In certain cases, a chronic lymphadenitis is found in this space rather than a frank abscess. Alternative approaches include a lateral neck incision anterior or posterior to the sternocleidomastoid muscle. The lateral incision is preferred in adults after endoscopic trauma (Fig. 27-14).

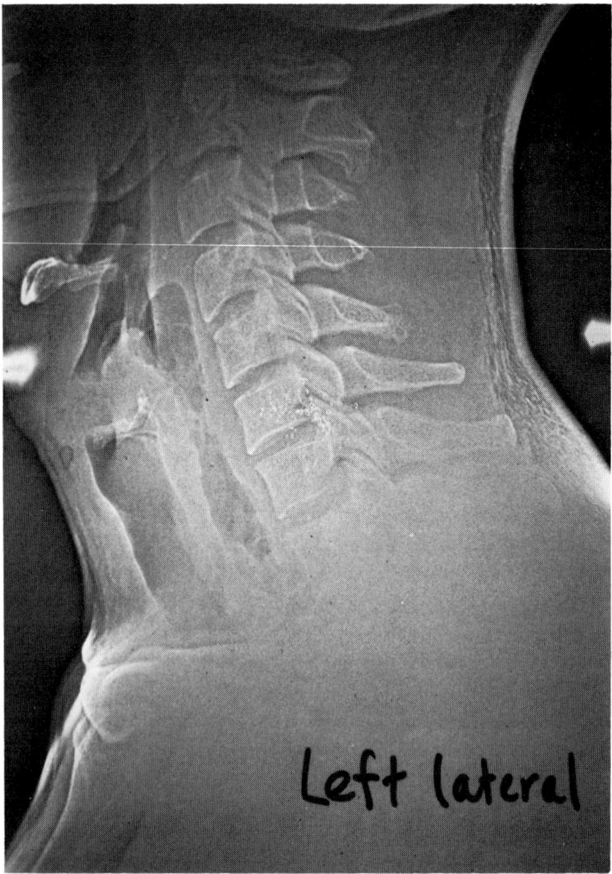

Fig. 27-14. **Free air in the retropharyngeal space following bullet wound to the neck. A large retropharyngeal space abscess was drained through an external approach.**

SUPRAHYOID SPACE INFECTIONS

The deep cervical fascia attaches firmly to the hyoid bone, thereby confining infection extending from the oral cavity to this suprahyoid space. The anterior belly of the digastric muscle further divides the space into the submental and the submandibular space. Infections from the oral cavity and floor of the mouth, particularly those associated with dental disease or fracture of the mandible, will initially remain between the mucosa of the floor of the mouth and the mylohyoid muscle. As the abscess increases in size and swelling occurs, the tongue is pushed upward and posteriorly so that airway obstruction becomes a threat. Ludwig's angina is a phlegmon of this area characterized by edema rather than suppuration. Incision and release of the tension of the myelohyoid is sometimes necessary to prevent airway obstruction. Tracheostomy should be considered prior to incision and drainage (Fig. 27-16). The organisms responsible are the aerobic and anaerobic bacteria associated with dental disease and are generally sensitive to penicillin.

Infections in the submandibular space are associated with infections in the gland itself or direct extensions from the floor of the mouth. Another area where there is a lack of fascial closure and a potential pathway for the rapid spread of infection from the oral cavity to the neck is along the anterior portion of the submandibular gland as it curves around the posterior border of the myelohyoid muscle. Drainage is secured through an incision similar to the one described previously.

INFECTIONS OF MASTICATOR SPACE

The masticator space is formed by the splitting of the superficial layer of the deep cervical fascia to enclose the temporalis, masseter, and medial pterygoid muscles. This space abuts the pharyngomaxillary space, submandibular space, and the parotid gland. These infections almost always originate in the mandible as a result of dental infection and tend to respond to antibiotic treatment. A 7-day course of antibiotics is generally tried before drainage needs to be considered. When the abscess points into the floor of the mouth or laterally into the gingival sulcus, drainage is indicated. External drainage through the neck is also possible. Should the infection extend upward, a separate incision is made posteriolateral to the lateral canthus of the eye above the zygoma. When there is a prolonged indolent infection not responding to the above regimen, actinomycosis or chronic osteomyelitis of the mandible must be considered.

CERVICAL ADENITIS

The lymph nodes of the neck are most easily classified by their relationship to major cervical landmarks: (1) the jugular chain along the jugular vein (subdivided into high, middle, and low), (2) the supraclavicular lymph nodes falling within the triangle formed by the clavicle, anterior sternocleidomastoid muscle, and shoulder, (3) the accessory chain following the accessory nerve and running between the posterior border of the sternocleidomastoid

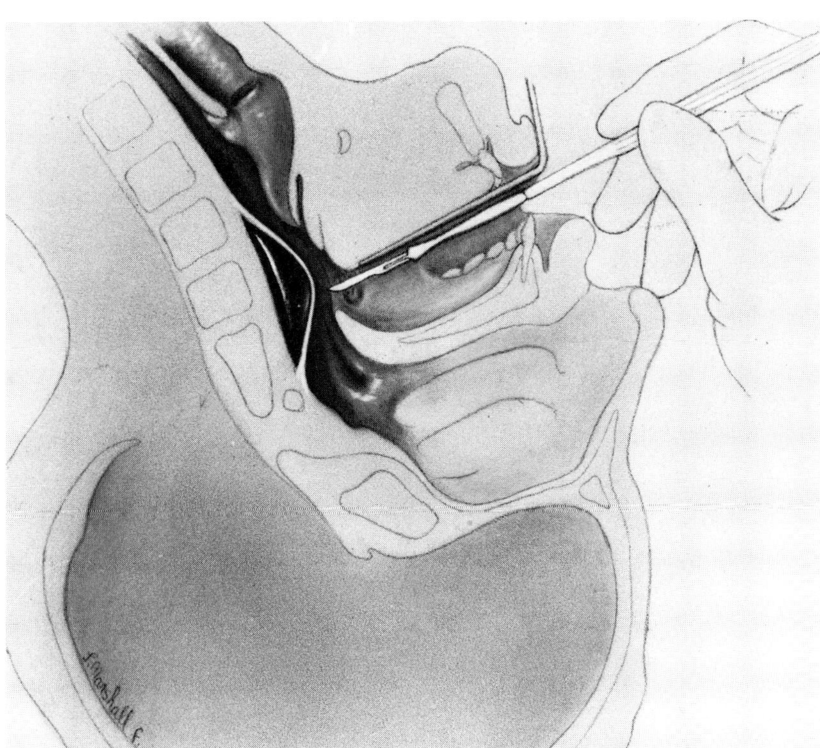

Fig. 27-15. Drainage of retropharyngeal space. (From Adams G: Special examinations in otolaryngology. In Adams G, Boies LR Jr, Paparella MM (eds): *Boies's Fundamentals of Otolaryngology*, 5th ed. Philadelphia, Saunders, 1978, p 28.)

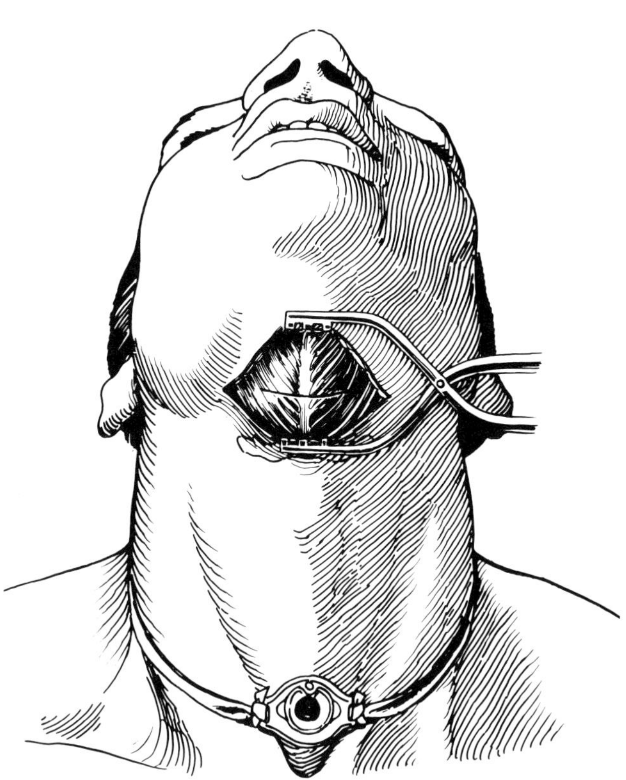

Fig. 27-16. Incision and drainage used in Ludwig's angina. The mylohyoid muscle is incised. This patient required a tracheostomy for airway protection prior to the drainage procedure.

muscle and the anterior margin of the trapezius muscle, (4) the submental nodes in the submental triangle, (5) the submandibular nodes adjacent to the submandibular glands, (6) the parotid nodes next to and within the gland substance, and (7) the retropharyngeal lymph nodes not normally palpable, even when enlarged, which are associated with the posterior lateral aspect of the pharynx.[12]

Tuberculous Cervical Adenitis

The most common form of extrapulmonary tuberculosis is cervical tuberculous lymphadenitis. Any of the Mycobacteria discussed in Chapter 7 can be etiologic, but *M. tuberculosis* is most common. The PPD skin test results are positive. Patients present with solitary, enlarged nontender lymph nodes containing caseating granulomas. After excluding the diagnosis of regional or systemic malignancy, the node should be excised. The diagnosis is a histologic one, and incisional biopsy may cause a continuously draining fistulous tract. Antituberculosis therapy is described in Chapter 18. It is not known why some individuals develop extrapulmonary tuberculosis. Young black adults appear to have the highest incidence. Scrofuloderma is a distinct form of atypical mycobacterial cervical lymphadenitis, usually occuring in children, caused by *M. scrofulaceum.* Excision of the infected node is adequate therapy and drug treatment is often not required (Chapter 25).

Cat Scratch Fever (Benign Inoculation Lymphoreticulosis)

This form of cervical adenitis is diagnosed by history and biopsy. Because of its associated systemic symptoms, it is probably caused by a virus although no virus has been isolated. There is no effective treatment, and the disease is self-limited. Biopsy is not necessary for treatment, but it is necessary to distinguish this from other causes of cervical adenopathy, and excision may be required to eliminate persistent nodes. In one-fourth of the patients, purulent drainage will occur from the node but cultures are usually sterile.

Toxoplasmosis

Cervical lymphadenopathy is the most frequent manifestation of acquired toxoplasmosis. The responsible organism, *Toxoplasma gondii,* is an intracellular parasite in which the final host is the cat. Humans most likely become infected by ingestion of the oocysts after cleaning the litter box of their pet cats and not washing their hands thoroughly afterward. The congenital form of this disorder has received far more attention because of its manifestations of deafness, retardation, blindness, microcephaly, and cerebrocalcification. Patients presenting with the cervical form may complain of fatigue, low-grade fever, and muscle weakness. The disease usually runs a benign course with enlarged, mildly tender cervical lymph nodes as the major complaint. However, in extreme cases, the patient becomes acutely ill and can develop splenomegaly, loss of visual acuity, and other neurologic symptoms. Diagnosis is made by history of exposure and by indirect fluorescent antibody test. A titer of greater than 1:1024 is considered evidence of recent exposure. Biopsy becomes necessary to distinguish this disease from the similar clinical findings in lymphoma. Histologic examination of the lymph nodes shows a well-preserved node structure with large follicles which is suggestive, rather than diagnostic, of the disease.

Treatment is unnecessary when cervical lymphadenopathy is the only manifestation of the disease and the fluorescent antibody titer level continues to fall. In the unusual acute form with abdominal and neurologic manifestations, sulfonamide and pyrimethamine are used.

Cervical-Facial Actinomycosis

Actinomycosis is discussed in Chapter 6. The most common presentation of this disease is cervical-facial actinomycosis, or lumpy jaw. This infection usually appears at the angle of the mandible but has also been seen over the lateral neck or even in the midline. The thyroid, deep cervical tissues, and maxillary sinus can all be affected. Acute, painful swelling or swelling and multiple draining fistulas can indicate the infection. Culture can be obtained by biopsy or by direct aspiration of the mass. Yellow particles (sulfur granules), which are actually aggregated bacteria, can sometimes be identified on the dressing. When an abscess suspected of harboring actinomyces is excised, portions should be submitted to both the microbiology and pathology laboratories for evaluation. Gram stains and acid-fast stains should make the diagnosis, since cultures may take 2 weeks for identification.

Actinomycosis responds readily to penicillin (2 to 20 million units per day, intravenous for 2 weeks, followed by oral therapy for 2 months). Tetracycline, clindamycin, and cephalosporins have been used in penicillin-sensitive persons.

INFECTED EMBRYOLOGIC DEFORMITIES

There are three distinct embryologic abnormalities that can present with infection in the neck: (1) cystic hygroma (or lymphangioma), (2) pharyngeal and branchial cleft cysts and fistulas, and (3) thyroglossal duct cysts.

Cystic Hygroma

This diffuse, cystic, tumor mass is usually evident within the first 2 years of life. It commonly involves the lower aspects of the neck but can appear anywhere in the cervical region. It is probably an abnormal development of lymph vessels from the jugular lymphatic sacs. Sudden enlargement by infection or hemorrhage into a lymphangioma can cause obstruction of the upper airway. During an acute inflammation, it is better to initially treat the patient with broad-spectrum antibiotics until there is resolution of the acute process. Total excision should then be performed to prevent recurrence or further enlargement. The first procedure should be as complete as possible, as all subsequent procedures are more difficult, less likely to remove all lymphangiomatous elements, and more likely to cause damage to underlying cervical structures.

Pharyngeal Cleft Cysts

A pharyngeal cleft cyst can develop from the 1st, 2nd, or 3rd pharyngeal clefts; the 2nd is most common. During development, both 2nd and 3rd cleft cysts actually develop from the sinus of Hiss. They usually present in childhood as fistulas or masses just posterior to the angle of the mandible along the anterior border of the sternocleidomastoid muscle. Second pharyngeal cleft cysts have a tract leading beneath the digastric muscle above the hypoglossal nerve between the internal and external carotid arteries to the region of the posterior tonsillar pillar. Tracts from the first pharyngeal cleft pass either medial or lateral to the facial nerve and enter the anterior floor of the external ear canal at the junction of the bony and cartilaginous canals. The mass can fluctuate in size and enlargement can be associated with upper respiratory infection. Acute inflammation should be treated with a broad-spectrum antibiotic before resection. The diagnosis can be confirmed, and the pathway of the fistulous tract outlined by injection of a radioopaque dye. Treatment is resection. A cyst lying low in the neck may require two transverse or horizontal incisions which heal with superior cosmetic results, compared to an incision along the anterior border of the sternocleidomastoid muscle. The entire tract should be excised to prevent recurrence. If there is an opening into the pharynx, it should be oversewn, but sometimes the tract is atrophic and does not reach the pharynx.

Thyroglossal Duct Cysts

The thyroid gland originates from the foramen cecum of the tongue and descends through the body of the hyoid bone into the anterior neck. Any residual secretory lining may give rise to a thyroglossal duct cyst, which presents as a midline cystic structure. It can cause respiratory obstruction or a fistula only if infected. Treatment requires resection, preferably during a quiescent period. The preferred operation (the Sistrunk procedure) removes the cyst and its tract to the base of the tongue including the middle one-third of the hyoid bone.

INFECTIONS OF THE EAR

INFECTIONS OF THE EXTERNAL EAR

Acute External Otitis

Bacterial and fungal infections of the external ear and auricle are common, particularly in summer when external otitis is sometimes called swimmer's ear. Acute external otitis is usually caused by *P. aeruginosa*, *S. aureus*, or *E. coli*, and the major predisposing factor is persistent moisture from any cause. A low-grade infection ensues and is aggravated by the patient's efforts to scratch or clear the canal. The auricle can become red and tender, and the tenderness can extend into the neck. In advanced cases there is preauricular and occipital adenopathy. Treatment requires cleaning the debris from the canal, insertion of a cotton wick into the canal to enable the medication to penetrate, and the administration of drops into the wick. There are two common types of eardrops available. One type includes topical antibiotics, such as neomycin or colistin, and polymyxin B, combined with a topical steroid. A second contains an acetic acid preparation combined with a steroid in an effort to diminish bacterial growth by reducing the pH of the canal.

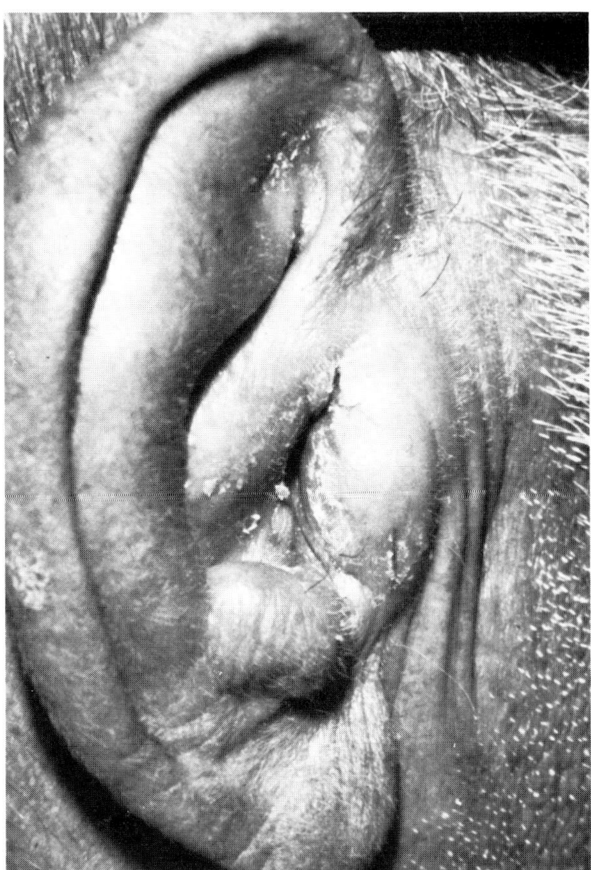

Fig. 27-17. **Chronic external otitis. Placement of a cotton wick into the external canal will aid in reduction of the chronic inflammation.**

Chronic External Otitis

This is a superficial infection superimposed on an underlying dermatitis (eczema, psoriasis) and aggravated by the patient's scratching (Fig. 27-17). In long-standing infections, *Aspergillus* and *Candida* superinfection can occur.

Malignant External Otitis

A particularly severe form of external otitis caused by *P. aeruginosa* was initially described by Chandler.[13] He noted that external otitis was not limited to the canal in certain elderly diabetic patients but included the surrounding area. Intravenous antibiotics are required because the usual treatment is not effective in these patients. The current regimen includes carbenicillin or ticarcillin combined with gentamicin or tobramycin. The two antibiotics should not be mixed. Debridement of the chronic osteomyelitis in the mastoid and canal may also be necessary, and the surrounding soft tissue beneath the temporal bone may have to be excised in advanced cases. Debridement is never undertaken without prior high-dose combination antibiotic therapy, and the antibiotics are continued for at least 7 days after resolution.

Perichondritis of the Ear

In certain cases, external otitis will extend into the perichondrium of the pinna. The auricle becomes inflamed, swollen, and tender. If the pinna takes on a leathery characteristic, systemic antibiotic treatment is needed in addition to local treatment. This perichondritis can become an actual chondritis. When the blood supply of the perichondrium is interrupted, destruction of the cartilage ensues and resection of cartilage may be needed. Stroud[14] recommends resection of the overlying skin as well as the cartilage.

Various methods have been developed to save as much cartilage as possible and thereby preserve the cosmetic appearance of the auricle (Fig. 27-18A–E). These methods include debridement of the underlying cartilage, placement of tubes or drains through and through the auricle, with frequent irrigations with acetic acid or gentamicin solutions. A deformed auricle and a prolonged course of treatment are to be expected.

VIRAL INFECTIONS OF THE EXTERNAL EAR

Bullous Myringitis

Certain viral infections have a propensity for the external canal, pinna, or tympanic membrane. Bullous myringitis is a viral infection of the tympanic membrane. Because it is preceded by an upper respiratory viral infection and has occasionally been associated with pneumonia, influenza A virus has been incriminated but not definitely es-

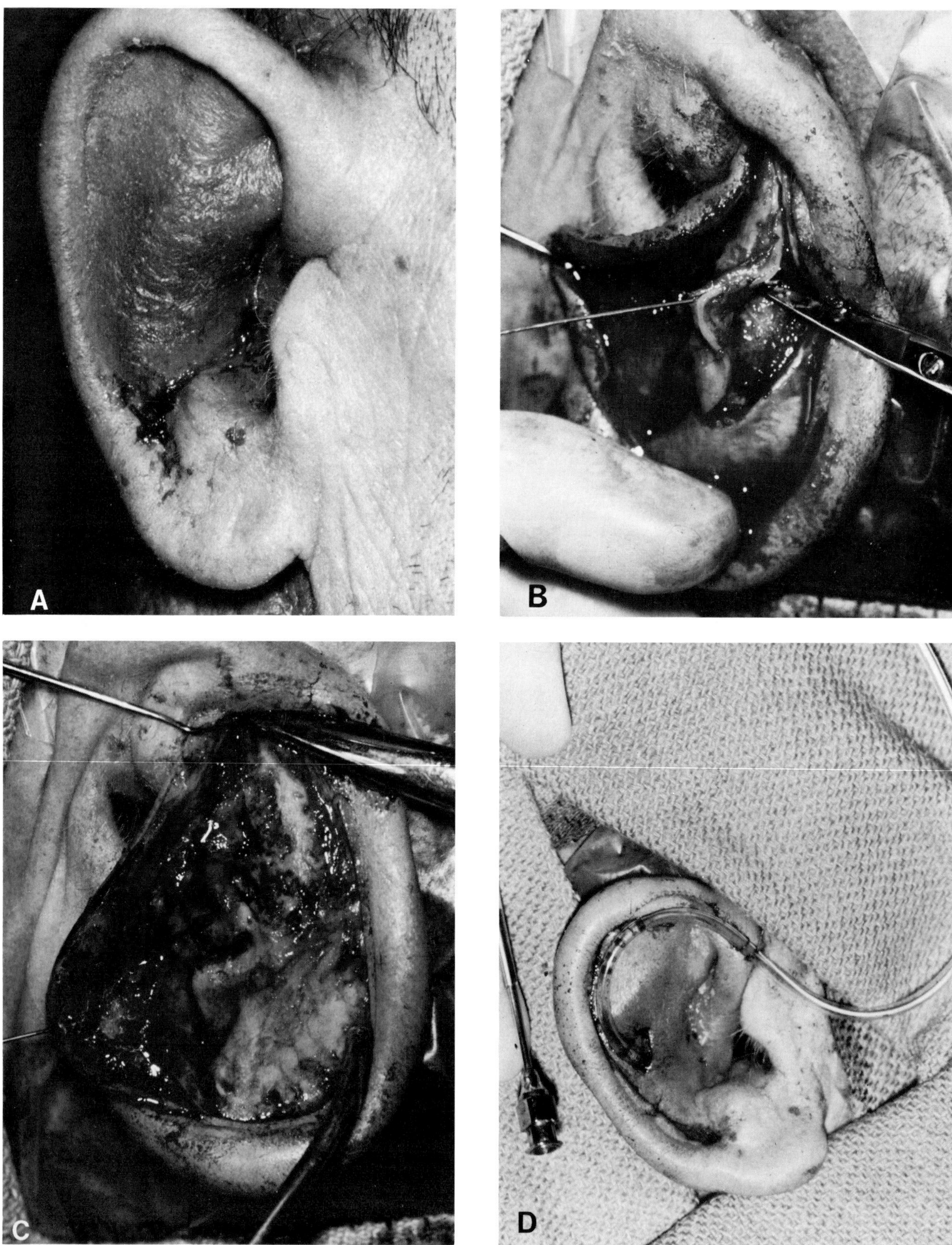

Fig. 27-18. A. Postoperative acute chondritis of the auricle. B. Incision and exposure of infected cartilage. C. Removal of all involved cartilage. D. Catheter irrigation postoperatively.

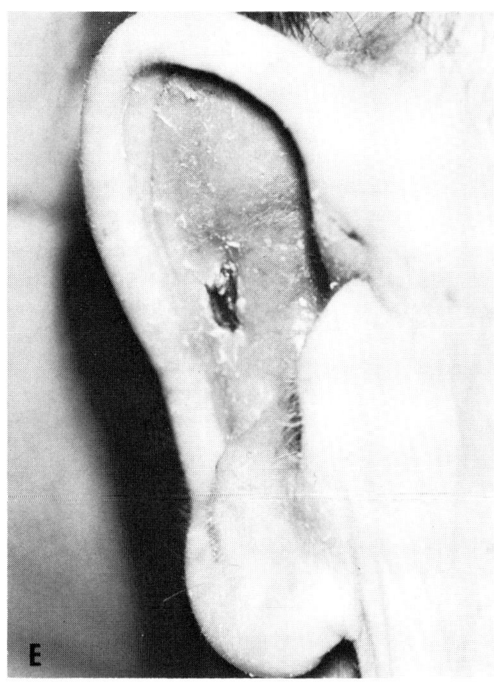

Fig. 27-18 (Cont.) **E. Thirteen days after removal of cartilage.**

tablished as a cause. The bacterium *Mycoplasma* has also been implicated. Large, painful blebs form on the tympanic membrane and skin of the ear canal. Although some authors have advocated the use of erythromycin, the disease resolves spontaneously in 5 to 7 days. There are usually no adverse long-lasting effects, although some patients have developed sensorineural hearing loss. Secondary bacterial otitis media can develop, requiring systemic antibiotics.

Herpes Zoster Otitis

The varicella-zoster virus can cause painful vesicles over the distribution of the sensory division of the 7th nerve around the pinna and external canal. The sensory fibers of the 7th nerve supply the posterior superior portion of the external canal and a small area around the conchal region of the auricle. Because the herpetic lesions can occur diffusely over the auricle and the mastoid area, some of the other sensory fibers, such as the 2nd and 3rd cervical divisions of the 5th cranial nerve, must sometimes be affected. Infection of the motor division of the 7th nerve can lead to facial paralysis. The complex of pain, facial palsy, and hearing loss was first described in 1907 by Ramsay Hunt, and the syndrome bears his name. Persistent facial paralysis associated with denervation of the facial muscles has led several authors to advocate immediate facial nerve decompression. Since it is a viral illness, others feel that return of function can be expected. Decompression of the 7th nerve all the way to the internal auditory meatus has been recommended because the viral infection probably infects primarily the 7th nerve medial to the geniculate ganglion. Clinically, it is manifested by decreased tearing on the side of the infection, due to involvement of the superior petrosal nerve which supplies the lacrimal glands. Failure of return of function after 4 weeks and evidence on electromyographic and galvanic-faradic stimulation of nerve degeneration are indications for decompression of the nerve. Decompression requires microscopic removal of surrounding bone to permit the nerve to swell freely, because its blood supply is diminished by the compression within a confined bony canal. In a few patients with Ramsay Hunt syndrome, there is also involvement of the 8th nerve with decreased sensorineural hearing. The morbidity of such an infection is further aggravated by prolonged neuralgic pain over the distribution of the occipital division of the 5th and 7th nerves. Acute pain can be relieved by analgesics and, in many cases, by systemic steroids. Topical steroids applied to the auricle also provide some relief. Steroids are not recommended if there is coexisting herpetic involvement of the ophthalmic nerve.

INFECTIONS OF THE MIDDLE EAR AND MASTOID

Acute Suppurative Otitis Media

Otitis media is most often seen in preschool age children with eustachian tube dysfunction secondary to infections in the oropharynx, nasopharynx, sinuses, and nose. The infection can initially be caused by a virus, but bacterial infection supervenes, especially with repeated infections. The causative organisms are the pneumococcus, *Streptococcus, Staphylococcus,* and in children under 6 years of age *H. influenzae.* The patient develops fever and otalgia. The tympanic membrane is red and inflamed, and it bulges. Myringotomy was commonly practiced in the past to relieve the pressure and is sometimes still indicated to relieve pain or to obtain an aspirate for culture. Antibiotic treatment usually suffices, however.

Complications of Suppurative Otitis Media

Facial Nerve Paralysis. When facial nerve paralysis is a complication of acute suppurative otitis media (Fig. 27-19), a wide myringotomy (smile) incision is needed. Cultures should be obtained and intravenous antibiotics started. The facial paralysis usually resolves within 1 to 2 weeks. However, if the paralysis persists or denervation is suspected, a mastoidectomy is urgently indicated. The osteitic bone around the facial nerve is removed only if it is obviously infected. Otherwise, a complete mastoidectomy with preservation of the posterior canal wall should suffice. The operation also provides an opportunity to rule out any other mastoid or middle ear pathology responsible for paralysis.

Acute Mastoiditis. Before the advent of penicillin, acute suppurative otitis media led to acute suppurative mastoiditis (Fig. 27-20). This latter disease is uncommon today, but sometimes occurs in a patient who is undergoing cancer chemotherapy. Myringotomy should be performed

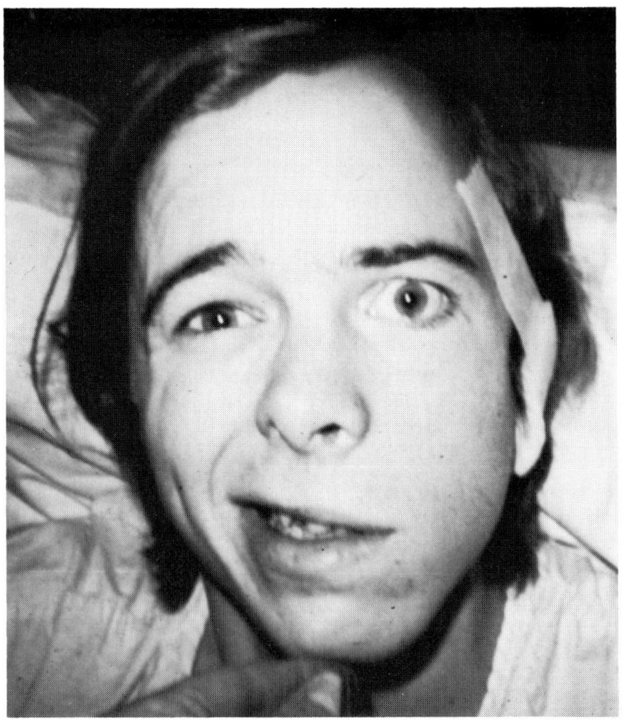

Fig. 27-19. **Left complete peripheral facial nerve paralysis during acute suppurative otitis media. A wide myringotomy was performed for culture and drainage.**

with the use of systemic antibiotics. Mastoid decompression is indicated only in cases that do not respond to this conservative regimen, if the pain becomes too severe or if there is a threat of intracranial complications.

Acute mastoiditis usually occurs in young children. The onset may be sudden in a well-pneumatized temporal bone. The patient has a fever and appears acutely ill. The tympanic membrane loses the usual landmarks. There is bulging of the anterior and superior canal wall. Subperiosteal swelling, redness, and tenderness to firm palpation can develop in the postauricular area.

Blood cultures and cultures from a myringotomy will identify the organism, most often *H. influenzae* and *S. pneumoniae.* Failure to show improvement after 4 days of antibiotic therapy is sufficient indication for an emergency mastoidectomy.

Development of a subperiosteal abscess is a sign of coalescent mastoiditis. Should the abscess protrude anteriorly, it becomes evident at the zygoma adjacent to the temporalis muscle. Pus that ruptures medial to the cells of the mastoid tip into the digastric groove is called Bezold's abscess. This abscess can extend directly into the retropharyngeal space.

The presence of any of these abscesses is an indication for immediate complete mastoidectomy. It is more difficult to determine whether operation is necessary in "masked" mastoiditis. Antibiotic therapy may be sufficient to eliminate the classical signs of mastoiditis such as pain, fever, and tenderness over the mastoid. However, there may be a recurrence after the antibiotics have been discontinued. Recurrence of pain and drainage along with roentgenographic evidence of mastoiditis requires a complete mastoidectomy.

Tuberculous Otitis Media

An unusual form of otitis media, which can lead to chronic mastoiditis, is caused by *M. tuberculosis*—it occurs in only 1 percent of patients with tuberculosis. Initially, there may be a series of perforations of the tympanic membrane with painless drainage. Later, these perforations coalesce into a single large perforation. If suspected, smears and culture for tuberculosis are obtained and the PPD test performed. Treatment is usually medical (Chapter 18). Indications for mastoidectomy are the same as for other causes of chronic suppurative otomastoiditis, but it preferably follows initiation of a chemotherapeutic regimen.

Chronic Otitis Media

Chronic Serous Otitis Media

Far more common in the otologist's practice than the acute form of otitis media are the various forms of chronic otitis media. Meyerhoff et al [15] differentiate purulent otitis media, serous otitis media, and mucous otitis media, depending on the appearance of the middle ear fluid at the time

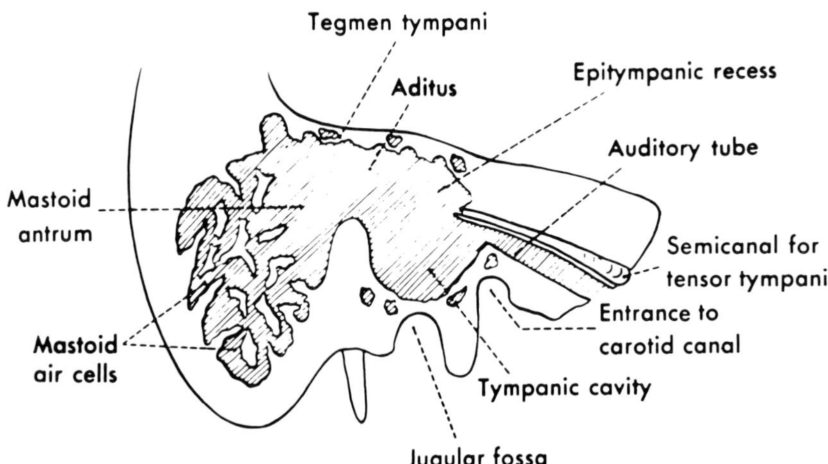

Fig. 27-20. **Diagram of the middle ear cavity and its connecting air spaces, in a sagittal section. (From Hollingshead HW (ed): The ear. In *Anatomy for Surgeons. Vol 1, The Head and Neck,* 2nd ed. Hagerstown, Harper & Row, 1968, p 183.)**

of myringotomy. Otitis media is the most common cause of hearing loss in school-age children; other symptoms include fullness and pressure in the ear. Sometimes, the onset is gradual, and the teacher is the first to notice hearing loss in a child who is not attentive in class.

Chronic diseases of the middle ear and mastoid are directly related to obstruction of the eustachian (auditory) tube (Fig. 27-20), which normally opens during swallowing, yawning, or sneezing so that the atmospheric pressure remains equal on both sides of the tympanic membrane. Inflammation, whether of bacterial, viral, or allergic origin, can induce edema and obstruction of the tube. Air in the mastoid and middle ear is then absorbed, a negative pressure is established within the middle ear cleft, and an effusion forms within the middle ear and mastoid. Return of normal eustachian tube function and patency is essential in the treatment of both acute and chronic diseases of the middle ear and mastoid, although temporary relief can be achieved by myringotomy.

There are many causes of eustachian tube obstruction: allergy, sinusitis, chronic nasopharyngitis, as well as hypertrophied adenoids. Children with a cleft palate deformity have a much higher incidence of tubal dysfunction and serous otitis media. In adults, there may be other underlying causes, such as tubal blockage caused by a rapid airplane descent or a nasopharyngeal tumor. Chronic serous otitis media may also occur after resection of the maxillary and ethmoid sinuses or the soft palate for cancer.

In serous otitis media, the middle ear fluid is an exudate not a transudate, and the appearance does not help determine whether bacteria are present. The clear, thin fluid may be just as likely to harbor bacteria as the thick mucoid variety. Changes in the middle ear mucosa also occur in chronic serous otitis media. There are metaplastic changes from low cuboidal epithelium to columnar epithelium with an increased number of goblet cells. In longstanding serous otitis media, fibrosis and diffuse adhesions can occur.

Adenoidectomy is never recommended for longstanding cases of chronic otitis media until a conservative medical approach has been tried.[16] Medical therapy usually involves systemic and nasal decongestants, and antibiotics when there is a chronic, underlying infection.

The most frequently used procedure to keep the pressure across the tympanic membrane equal is myringotomy with insertion of a ventilating tube shaped like a collar button. With relief of the negative pressure in the middle ear, the drumhead returns to its normal position and the fluid resolves. The tube may remain in position for 3 to 6 months and will be extruded.

Chronic Otomastoiditis

While acute suppurative otomastoiditis is no longer a common disease, various forms of chronic otomastoiditis are more prevalent today than in the preantibiotic era. Chronic otomastoiditis is generally characterized by a perforated tympanic membrane and intermittent drainage. The aural discharge may occur after upper respiratory infections or after the ear canal has been accidently immersed in water. The organisms associated with this chronic form of disease are entirely different than those seen in the acute phase. They are generally species of *Staphylococcus, P. aeruginosa, Proteus,* and other gram-negative organisms. In addition, anaerobic species including *B. melaninogenicus, B. fragilis,* and peptostreptococci have been found. Treatment of the recurring episodes includes systemic antibiotics and eardrops. Drops containing a combination of neomycin, colistin, or polymyxin B are most often used. Roentgenograms of the mastoid are necessary to determine the extent of the destruction in the bone.

Perforations of the tympanic membrane have been categorized into safe and unsafe. A safe perforation refers to one in the midportion of the tympanic membrane. It usually occurs in the anterior-inferior or posterior-inferior quadrants. Drainage associated with an upper respiratory infection responds to antibiotics and stops after the acute stage is resolved. Unsafe perforations occur in the posterior superior quadrant of the tympanic membrane and along the margin. Such perforations are usually associated with underlying mastoid disease, especially cholesteatoma. Cholesteatoma is a collection of encapsulated keratinizing squamous epithelium, somewhat like a dermoid cyst that, when entrapped in bone, expands and causes gradual destruction of the surrounding structures. The ossicles, the horizontal semicircular canal, and the facial nerve can be destroyed by a cholesteatoma. Eventually, such destruction can include the tegmen tympani (Fig. 27-20) and tegmen mastoideum. Such exposure of the dura leads to extracranial and intracranial complications.

Equally often, chronic perforations have been associated with a form of temporal bone infection referred to as chronic granulation tissue mastoiditis. The mastoid cells become filled with chronically infected granulation tissue that is as destructive as cholesteatoma.[15] Topical antibiotic drops with steroids and systemic antibiotics are used to temporarily stop the infection. When these medications are discontinued, drainage and suppuration can recur.

A third form of chronic otitis media and mastoiditis is known as cholesterin granuloma. This infection is related to chronic granulation tissue mastoiditis and is the result of a breakdown product of cholesterol crystals.

Treatment of Chronic Otomastoiditis. The objectives of surgical treatment of otomastoiditis are: (1) to remove all infected tissue, (2) to establish a mastoid and middle ear cavity which will no longer be susceptible to repeated infections, and (3) to reestablish the ossicular chain and provide the best hearing possible in an already damaged ear. The operations for establishing an intact tympanic membrane and ossicular chain are referred to as tympanoplasty.

Mastoidectomy is performed when the middle ear is still intact. The incision follows the postauricular crease. Fascia may be obtained from the temporalis muscle to be used later as a graft for possible tympanic membrane repair. The muscles and periosteum are elevated from the mastoid bowl. Incisions are made within the external canal so that the auricle may be folded forward. Using a mastoid type burr, the mastoid cells are carefully exenterated and the antrum of the mastoid cavity is identified. The posterior ear canal wall is preserved if possible, although it is thinned to make certain that all the air cells overlying the facial nerve are also removed. Healthy normal-appearing bone should be identified up to the sigmoid sinus and the sinodural angle, and abnormalities should be looked for in the middle ear. Upon completion, the ear canal is packed and the postauricular incision is closed, usually without a drain.

A radical mastoidectomy entails complete exenteration of the mastoid cells, middle ear contents, and tympanic membrane, converting it all into one large, clean cavity.

The classical radical mastoidectomy as originally described is now used only for extensive cholesteatoma, a malignant external otitis, or with tumors. Both the posterior canal wall and the lateral attic wall are removed. The floor of the ear canal is lowered to the level of the hypotympanum. The eustachian tube is either plugged with bone chips or muscle or allowed to remain open.

The modified radical mastoidectomy is designed to preserve the middle ear while eradicating all infection from the mastoid process. In contrast to a radical mastoidectomy, a less extensive cholesteatoma has been found. This cholesteatoma needs to be completely exposed and removed. To provide adequate visualization, the entire posterior canal wall may need to be lowered to the level of the facial nerve, thus creating a single cavity between the external ear canal and the mastoid. Tympanoplasty can be combined with this procedure to reconstruct middle ear structures. When the posterior canal wall is removed, the mastoid bowl can always be checked for recurrence of infection. The disadvantage of such a cavity is a lifelong need to have it cleaned by a physician.

INTRACRANIAL AND EXTRACRANIAL COMPLICATIONS OF MIDDLE EAR AND MASTOID DISEASE

Extracranial Complications

Horizontal Canal Fistula

Erosion of the lateral semicircular canal by cholesteatoma can lead to the formation of fistulas between the middle ear and the semicircular canal. Nystagmus, vertigo, and sensorineural hearing loss result. Treatment is by modified radical mastoidectomy with removal of all chronically infected tissue. While the vertigo may eventually subside, no improvement of the hearing loss can be anticipated.

Facial Nerve Paralysis

Infection of the facial nerve can lead to a complete peripheral facial paralysis. In 25 percent of patients, there is an area of dehiscence of the facial nerve close to the region of the oval window without erosion of the bone. When facial paralysis complicates an existing chronic otomastoiditis, immediate mastoidectomy and facial nerve decompression are indicated.

Petrositis

Pneumatization of the petrous portion of the temporal bone is present in 30 percent of adult temporal bones and is usually symmetrical. There are two groups of air cells extending to the petrous tip. One group is posterior, passing from the region of the antrum and semicircular canals to the petrous apex. The second group is anterior and inferior, extending from the region of the hypotympanum and the eustachian tube to the petrous tip.

Infection extends from cell to cell within the pneumatized temporal bone. Osteomyelitis can develop if there is incomplete pneumatization of the petrous portion. In addition, the bony labyrinth acts as an obstruction to drainage from the petrous apex into the rest of the mastoid.

Even though the infection in the mastoid can be resolved by antibiotics or operation, an abscess can be overlooked in the petrous tip so that drainage persists after mastoidectomy. Retro-orbital headache and 6th nerve paralysis (Gradenigo's syndrome) is pathognomonic for this condition, which may respond to high-dose intravenous antibiotic therapy. Drainage is required if there is no improvement after 24 hours of intravenous therapy, or if symptoms or drainage recur or if petrositis develops in combination with chronic otomastoiditis. Complete mastoidectomy is first performed, and the anterior and posterior petrous cell tracts are identified. They are used as landmarks and followed to the petrous apex. In the absence of these cell tracts, the method described by Lempert is used. The approach is anterior to the cochlea. The eustachian tube orifice and tensor tympanii muscles are identified, and the carotid artery is followed to the apex. As long as the infection remains within the petrous portion of the temporal bone, no meningeal or spinal fluid abnormalities can be demonstrated. This type of abscess can also rupture into the superior portion of the parapharyngeal space.

Lateral Sinus Thrombosis

Direct extension of infection through the thin layer of cortical bone which overlies the lateral sinus as it makes its sigmoid curve to the jugular vein has been associated with chronic otomastoiditis. In the preantibiotic era, an infected thrombus within the sigmoid sinus was associated with a hectic febrile course, during which septic emboli could pass through the venous drainage system of the brain. Today, this classical picture is unusual and the signs are far more subtle. In fact, thrombosis of the sigmoid sinus may first be recognized at the time of mastoidectomy for chronic otomastoiditis. Removal of the infected clot and packing off of the sinus are necessary. High-dose systemic antibiotics are administered. A lumbar puncture is performed if the preoperative diagnosis is lateral sinus thrombosis. The pressure is measured and compression is applied to each jugular vein in sequence. When compression of one jugular vein causes an elevation in the spinal pressure, the opposite sigmoid sinus is probably blocked by a thrombus. While this test theoretically appears important, it is not dependable.

Suppurative Labyrinthitis

Middle ear infection can cross through the thin round window to include the sensitive membranous labyrinth. The mere presence of a contiguous infection or cholesteatoma can produce vertigo and sensorineural hearing loss and is referred to as serous labyrinthitis. An adjacent infection is sufficient to affect the composition of the perilymph with subsequent deterioration of hearing and balance. Should the infection actually extend into this region, the membranous labyrinth is quickly destroyed. Surgical procedures on the mastoid under this circumstance require opening, draining, and destroying the labyrinth. Fortunately, this complication is rare and such radical treatment is seldom the initial procedure. The surgeon instead removes the infection in the middle ear and mastoid and hopes for a serous labyrinthitis instead. Histopathology reviews in the temporal bone collections have demonstrated total destruction of the membranous labyrinth following infection, deposition of new bone within the otic capsule, and complete calcification of the labyrinthine structures.

Intracranial Complications of Middle Ear and Mastoid Infections

Any of the preceding temporal bone complications of mastoiditis and acute and chronic otitis media can lead to an intracranial complication (Chapter 28). Pathways of extension include bone erosion of the tegmen of the middle ear or mastoid and thrombophlebitis of the emissary veins draining directly from the mastoid to the dura.

Extradural Abscess

The collection of pus over the middle ear or mastoid tegmen, but outside the dura, establishes an extradural abscess. The patient complains of otalgia and headache. Such an abscess can be an incidental finding during mastoid operation. Drainage is accomplished through the mastoid with removal of the osteitic bone. Postoperative antibiotics are indicated, and the outlook is usually excellent.

Subdural Abscess (Empyema)

The patient becomes acutely ill with headache (first localized, then generalized) and high fever during the course of chronic, purulent otitis media or mastoiditis. Neurologic symptoms progress to include seizure (frequently Jacksonian), contralateral hemiplegia, and loss of consciousness. The organism isolated is the same as in the infected ear.

Treatment requires a neurosurgical approach. Drainage is accomplished by multiple burr holes with placement of drains and irrigation of the subdural space. Multiple brain abscesses may develop. Even today, the mortality rate is 30 percent and patients commonly develop neurologic sequelae (Chapter 28).

Meningitis

The most common intracranial complication of acute otomastoiditis is meningitis. There is frequently preexisting (acute or chronic) otitis media. Patients develop fever, stiffness of the neck, headache, and eventually nausea with vomiting. Symptoms can progress to coma. Lumbar puncture is essential for diagnosis and to determine the responsible organism, and treatment is by intravenous antibiotics. While waiting for a culture report, the Gram stain of the spinal fluid can be of some help in the selection of the appropriate antibiotics. In addition, it is helpful to differentiate chronic otomastoiditis (associated with cholesteatoma) from the acute meningitis that follows acute otitis media. The organisms most commonly responsible for these different types of infections have been previously discussed. If there is associated chronic otitis media, mastoidectomy to eliminate the source of infection is indicated when the patient is stable and the meningitis has resolved.

Brain Abscess

Otogenic brain abscess is usually a complication of chronic otitis or otomastoiditis. Two forms occur: (1) in the temporal lobe of the middle cranial fossa and (2) in the cerebellum (posterior fossa). An abscess in the posterior fossa can result from extension from the sigmoid sinus directly into the cerebellum. An abscess in the temporal lobe can have its origin in the tegmen of the mastoid or middle ear. The course of a cerebellar abscess is more sudden than with an abscess of the middle cranial fossa. A cerebellar abscess is associated with such neurologic signs as ataxia, tremor, and dysdiadochokinisia. Temporal lobe infection can produce headache, seizures, and aphasia. Abscess at either site shows signs of increased intracranial pressure (such as vomiting, fever, and lethargy). The CAT scan is useful in the diagnosis. Treatment is drainage or excision accompanied by a course of intensive intravenous antibiotic therapy (Chapter 28). When the intracranial abscess has been resolved, elimination of the source of infection from the mastoid is indicated.

Recurrent Bacterial Meningitis

Thirty percent of the cases of meningitis originate in an otogenic or sinus source and all patients require a thorough otolaryngologic examination including roentgenograms of the mastoids and sinuses. While the mortality rate has decreased because of effective chemotherapy, the morbidity remains high. *H. influenzae* is the most common cause in children, but *S. pneumoniae* is associated with the highest number of complications in adults. When the ear appears to be the source of trouble, tympanograms and tympanocentesis for bacterial culture are useful.

If the infection appears to arise from a contiguous mastoid bone or paranasal sinus, drainage is required. The operation should usually be limited to drainage, and reconstructive efforts should be avoided. Exenterative procedures should be delayed until recovery from the meningitis. When no immediate source of the infection is evident, patients with recurrent meningitis should be evaluated for a cerebrospinal fluid leak, which in turn might be caused by unrecognized trauma, nasal or ear surgery, or even a congenital bony dehiscence. For example, trauma to the frontal-ethmoid region can cause a tear in the dura at the cribriform plate. A complaint of a salty fluid dripping from the nose while in a head-down position suggests a leak in the region of the cribriform plate, but similar symptoms can arise from a leak from the middle or posterior cranial fossa into the mastoid or middle ear cavity communicating with the pharynx via the eustachian tube.

There are basically three methods available to identify

cerebrospinal leaks: (1) roentgenographic studies, (2) injection of intrathecal radioactive materials (eg, radioactive albumin), and (3) injection of intrathecal dyes (Evan's blue, fluorescein). Whichever of the latter two techniques is selected, pledgets should be placed (1) in the middle meatus, in the area of drainage of the nasal frontal duct, (2) high near the cribriform plate, and (3) just below the eustachian tube orifice.[17] Pledgets should be changed at least every 30 minutes, depending on the extent of the leak.

Chemical studies for cerebrospinal fluid rhinorrhea such as glucose determinations can be misleading. Tears and nasal secretions can confuse the results.

An effective way of determining an otogenic cerebrospinal fluid leak is with intrathecal fluorescein. When the drumhead is perforated or contains a ventilating tube, the green color of the dye can readily be observed in the middle ear with the help of a Wood's light (ultraviolet light). Examination should be performed within 15 minutes of the injection of the intrathecal dye, because spread of this dye throughout tissues of the body can give misleading results. Intrathecal fluorescein is injected slowly using 5 percent fluorescein solution diluted with 5–10 ml of cerebrospinal fluid.

When the source of the spinal fluid leakage has been found, one should wait at least 3 weeks after a known traumatic incident for spontaneous closure. During this period, it helps to keep the patient in a sitting position to reduce the cerebrospinal fluid pressure. During the wait, avoid the use of repeated otoscopic examination to reduce the risk of contamination. After closed head injury, increased cerebrospinal fluid pressure with internal hydrocephalus can result. This increased pressure can activate a leak, which closes spontaneously only to reopen. Control of the spinal fluid leakage can be resolved by a shunting procedure, such as a lumbar-peritoneal shunt. Shunts are available with valves that can be opened or closed without additional operations.

To close such leaks, a neurosurgical approach is often more effective than the extracranial route. The brain and underlying dura can be more readily inspected and the fistula repaired with a fascia graft. A leak into the sphenoid requires a direct procedure by a transsphenoid approach for effective control and more direct access to the source of the leakage. Rhinorrhea after extensive ethmoid sinus or nasal operation can be repaired by a transnasal-transethmoid approach. A middle fossa craniotomy provides a good access to leaks over the tegmen mastoideum.

INFECTIONS OF THE LARYNX AND TRACHEA

ACUTE SUPRAGLOTTITIS (EPIGLOTTITIS)

Supraglottic laryngitis refers to an acute inflammation of the supraglottic structures, which include the epiglottis, the false cords, and the aryepiglottic folds. It is usually caused by *H. influenzae* type B, but streptococci and staphylococci have also been isolated. Cultures can be obtained from the larynx and blood. Epiglottitis usually occurs in children about 6 years of age, but it occasionally affects younger children, and rarely, adults. The onset is marked by severe dysphagia, followed rapidly by refusal to swallow saliva and respiratory distress. The child can be well in the morning, develop increasing respiratory distress and painful swelling in the afternoon, and be hospitalized and require emergency tracheostomy by dinnertime. The soft and resilient laryngeal tissues in a child permit easy and rapid swelling so that the massive edema of the epiglottis causes airway obstruction. In fact, downward pressure on the posterior tongue can cause the swollen epiglottis to completely obstruct the upper airway. The child appears acutely ill, with the head extended forward in an effort to maintain an open airway. As it becomes too painful to swallow, the child will begin to drool. Examination is best performed in the operating room, so that if the swollen epiglottis is seen, an airway can be established. In a child less severely ill, a soft tissue lateral roentgenogram of the neck and chest are obtained to eliminate the possible presence of a foreign body or pneumonia, which have similar symptoms.

Ampicillin is the preferred antibiotic, and chloramphenicol is a good second choice, since *H. influenzae* is almost always the cause. The etiology can be confirmed by laryngeal Gram stain and culture or blood culture, because streptococci and staphylococci can cause a similar clinical picture. The major concern, however, is the compromised airway. The current recommendation is examination in the operating room by personnel skilled at bronchoscopy, intubation, and tracheostomy. If the disease is in the advanced stages, it is hazardous to attempt passage of a soft, flexible endotracheal tube through inflamed edematous firm tissues. Under these circumstances, a pediatric bronchoscope should be inserted and a tracheostomy performed. With less edema and inflammation, it may be possible to insert an endotracheal tube, but the more conservative approach remains tracheostomy.

ACUTE LARYNGOTRACHEOBRONCHITIS (CROUP)

Acute laryngotracheobronchitis (LTB) should be distinguished from acute supraglottic laryngitis. LTB occurs in a younger age group, generally around 2 years of age. The name croup refers to the typical seal-like barking cough. It is generally caused by parainfluenza viruses type I and II and influenza viruses. However, superimposed bacterial infections (*Streptococcus, Staphylococcus,* or *H. influenzae*) can occur. The major site of the obstruction is the subglottic area (Fig. 27-21). It is here that the tissues are most susceptible to swelling and inflammation. Secretions build up within the trachea, and if they become thick the child is unable to raise them.

The child usually has a 2- to 3-day history of an upper respiratory infection with gradually increasing respiratory stridor. As airway obstruction progresses, use of the accessory muscles of respiration become more and more active, and mild cyanosis can appear. There is a low-grade fever and a mild leukocytosis.

Ampicillin is generally the antibiotic of choice. With the compromised airway, these children need high humid-

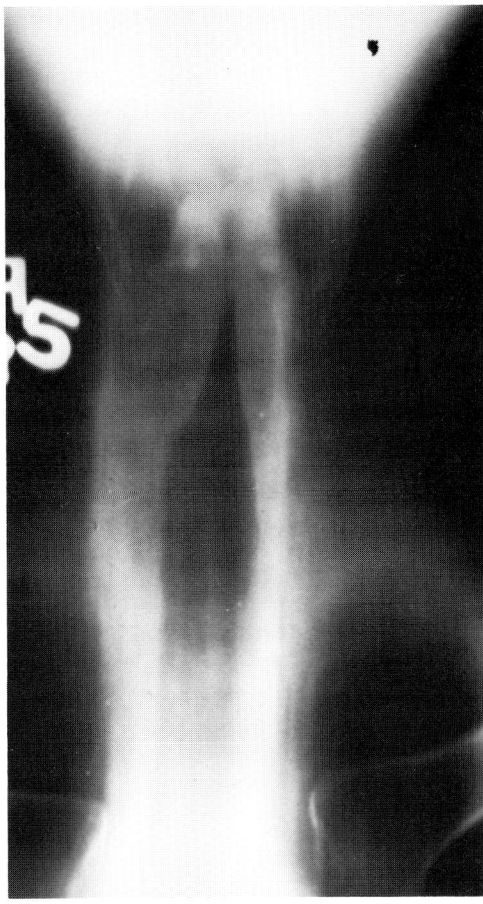

Fig. 27-21. **Acute laryngotracheobronchitis: massive subglottic swelling is demonstrated on a laryngeal tomogram in an atypical adult case.**

ity (to liquefy the secretions and avoid the crusting that occurs in the trachea). Aerosolized racemic epinephrine administered by mask has been demonstrated to cause relief of laryngeal edema. Intramuscular steroids have been advocated to reduce the subglottic edema.

Increasing respiratory distress with a pulse rate greater than 160 and respiratory rate greater than 60 per minute suggest the need for an artificial airway. Both endotracheal intubation and tracheostomy have been used, but the preferred method is tracheostomy. Placing an endotracheal tube through an acutely inflamed subglottic larynx invites complications. Less than 1 percent of children with acute laryngotracheobronchitis require tracheostomy if proper medical treatment is provided.

OTHER CAUSES OF LARYNGITIS

Diphtheria (Chapter 7) can create a gray, shaggy membrane over the larynx. Immunizations have virtually eliminated this disease in the United States.

Other infections of the larynx include fungal infections (such as histoplasmosis, blastomycoses, and *Candida* infection) and tuberculosis. Such infections are usually associated with pulmonary involvement with the same organism. Constant cough will cause the infection to spread from the lungs to the larynx. The treatment is the same as required for the pulmonary tissue. Tracheostomy and intubation are not needed in most instances. Other causes of acute laryngeal inflammation can be related to allergic disorders.

TRACHEOSTOMY

The advent of disposable endotracheal tubes and the increased use of intensive care units for patients who require prolonged intubation has lowered the need for tracheostomy. When an endotracheal tube is in place for prolonged periods (over 72 hours in the adult, or over 2 weeks in the infant), tracheostomy may be necessary. Tracheostomy is frequently necessary preceding an extensive head and neck operation and to maintain an airway after maxillofacial or neck trauma.

Similarly, in the advanced stages of tetanus—Guillain-Barré syndrome (ascending paralysis)—and in other subacute or chronic neurologic disorders, tracheostomy is preferred to prolonged endotracheal intubation, which must later be converted to a tracheostomy.

There are numerous complications associated with tracheostomy. (1) Mediastinal air collections and (2) pneumothorax are most common in children because of the high location of the dome of the pleura. A pneumothorax occurs readily if one deviates even slightly from the midline. Other complications include: (3) postoperative bleeding from the tracheostomy site, (4) infection around the tracheostomy tube, (5) dryness of the tracheal mucosa with an associated tracheobronchitis, (6) stenosis developing as the result of localized pressure by the tube or its cuff, (7) difficult recannulation, particularly in children, (8) subcutaneous emphysema, (9) erosion of the inominate artery with massive hemorrhage, (10) pneumonia from aspiration, and (11) injury to the recurrent laryngeal nerve.

The incidence of many of these complications is decreased by properly performing the tracheostomy. It helps, for instance, to operate in an operating room under a good light and with an endotracheal tube or bronchoscope in place. The cricoid cartilage should be identified and the tracheal opening made well below it (usually in the third tracheal ring). Either a small window of cartilage is removed or a flap of cartilage can be created. A vertical incision through two cartilages is preferred in children under age 2, thus avoiding removal of tissue. It is important that the tracheal rings actually be identified and counted to make certain that the tracheostomy tube is in the third and fourth ring in the child and the third ring of the adult. If the placement of the tube is too low, it can cause the inflated cuff to rub up and down on the tracheal wall and eventually erode directly into the inominate artery. Positioning the tracheostomy too high places the tracheotomy site into the conus elasticus region, which is more subject to edema and swelling and can cause delayed stricture. Staying in the midline avoids injury to large vessels and recurrent laryngeal nerves. The thyroid isthmus may have to be identified and ligated to provide better access.

Accidental decannulation and subsequent difficulty of replacing the tube can be avoided by proper tracheostomy tube placement. Two 3–0 silk sutures, placed on either side of the remaining cartilage and brought out and taped to the neck, will act as guides to the tracheostomy site should accidental decannulation occur. The tracheostomy tube should never be forced back into the wound, as it may create a false passageway. This makes subsequent attempts to replace the tube even more difficult. If the tract cannot be identified, an endotracheal tube can be immediately placed as a precaution. Then, with the airway reestablished, a search for the tracheal lumen through the tracheostomy site can continue.

Infection occurs at the tracheostomy site more frequently when a cuffed tube is used. A patient requires respiratory care because of the loss of ability to cough and clear secretions. Frequent suctioning becomes necessary. Sterile technique is mandatory, and the suction catheter should be placed only 1 to 2 cm beyond the lower level of the tracheostomy tube. If deeper suctioning is required, it should be performed by a physician. Passing the cannula repeatedly into the major bronchi can cause more irritation and increased secretions. Because the 80 to 90 percent humidity provided by the nose has been bypassed, continuous humidity should be given to the tracheotomy opening. Dry crusts form on the tracheal wall and increase the risk of infection. Tracheostomy wounds should be left opened to avoid subcutaneous emphysema. Sterile porous dressings should be applied to the site and changed frequently. If infectiion occurs, cultures and Gram stains are indicated. Organisms most frequently encountered are *S. aureus, P. aeruginosa,* and other gram-negative rods. Systemic antibiotics should be given, in addition to local care.

Frequent changes of 0.5 percent of acetic acid solution–soaked dressings are useful in reducing *P. aeruginosa* contamination. The tracheostomy tube itself will have to be changed more frequently and careful attention paid to the inner cannula. It, too, requires more frequent cleaning and removal of thick mucus.

A variety of tracheostomy tubes are available, including metal tubes with a silver coating, Portex nylon, and plastic. Some cuffs have cut-off valves, which can limit the amount of air pressure to avoid erosion of the tracheal wall. Twenty-five to 28 mm Hg pressure is generally all that is needed. Ideally, there should be a slight leak around the cuff after it has been inflated, and the air should be periodically released. The tracheostomy tube should be large enough to fill one-half to one-third of the trachea. In children or neonates, the tube may have to be relatively larger. With tubes of such small caliber, secretions and suctioning can become a problem. Cuffs are not used on tubes smaller than size 2.

When the tracheostomy is no longer necessary, the cuffed tube is replaced by a smaller, noncuffed tube. Tubes of gradually smaller size are inserted and finally the tube is plugged. If the patient tolerates the plugged tube for 24 to 48 hours without respiratory distress, the tube can be removed. After prolonged intubation or tracheostomy, the patient's larnyx and trachea should be examined before removing the tracheostomy tube. Granulation tissue at the site of the tracheostomy may be found and should be removed.

INFECTIONS ASSOCIATED WITH SURGERY AND RADIATION THERAPY OF THE HEAD AND NECK

PREVENTION

Tumors of the head and neck are frequently treated by a combination of radiation therapy and operation. Radiation is felt to be more effective when used prior to operation. The disadvantage is that the surgeon must operate in an irradiated field. The early effects of radiation are generally mucositis and skin changes. These effects can be limited by careful control of the radiation field and of the daily dosage. Later effects include a proliferative vasculitis with compromise of the blood supply of the treated areas. Ideally, operations should be performed after the early effects have subsided and before the delayed effects of radiation occur. Thus, the ideal time for surgery is 4 to 6 weeks after the cessation of radiation. Postoperative radiation therapy is frequently used when microscopic cervical metastases are found at operation or when an inadequate margin of normal tissue was resected around the tumor. It has also been used in areas where the overall cure rate for operation is low, such as in the base of the tongue, hypopharynx, or pyriform sinus. The advantage of postoperative radiation therapy is that the tissues are healed before the irradiation is initiated. Although infectious complications occur after operations and radiation therapy, several precautions can decrease their incidence, eg, ensuring that the patient is in the best nutritional status possible, that other diseases such as diabetes are under the best possible control, that preexisting infections have been resolved, and that the operation and all incisions are properly planned.

The blood supply to the neck generally runs in a vertical direction. The poorest blood supply to the neck is across the midline of the neck; therefore, the most popular flap design for composite resections or laryngectomy is a single or half H. The vertical limb of the incision is mostly posterior to the carotid artery and crosses the artery in only one location. If necrosis of the flap should occur, it is unlikely to expose the carotid artery.

In heavily irradiated tissue, such as in a patient who is undergoing a salvage operation when irradiation fails and the oral cavity or pharynx is entered, a controlled fistula pharyngostome should be considered. Closed suction drains should be used to decrease fluid accumulation under the flap. The carotid artery can be protected by using muscle flaps or dermal grafts. Heavily irradiated skin may have to be excised and replaced with cervical or chest flaps. Regional flaps to be brought into the area should be delayed, if time permits. Dental extractions should be performed before radiation therapy and good oral and dental hygiene maintained.

PHARYNGOCUTANEOUS FISTULAS

Pharyngocutaneous fistulas are common complications after ablative head and neck surgery. Infections are primarily caused by *Staphylococcius* or *Pseudomonas.* Cultures should be obtained and the appropriate antibiotics given, but proper local wound care is equally important. The management of wound infections depends on early recognition and treatment. A patient who develops a low-grade fever and some redness and swelling in the skin flaps should be checked carefully for a fistula. If this occurs, the flaps must be opened widely and immediately drained. It is important that this be done early to direct the salivary flow away from the carotid artery and from the tracheostomy site or laryngostome if one is present. The more conservative approach is immediate, wide drainage and debridement, rather than reliance only on intravenous antibiotics. As soon as possible, either horizontal chest flaps (Bakanjian), nape of neck, or forehead flaps should be delayed or swung, to make certain that the carotid artery is protected.

A fistula in the midline of the neck can be treated by local wound care and replacement of the nasogastric tube. If the fistula persists, the possibility of persistent cancer or stricture of the esophagus must be considered.

OSTEONECROSIS OF THE MANDIBLE

The blood supply of the mandible can be adversely affected by the combination of operation and radiation. Subsequent bacterial infection leads to a smoldering osteomyelitis (osteonecrosis). Table 27-2 lists the many factors that affect the development of this serious complication. Proliferative vasculitis can actually lead to thrombosis of the vessels and subsequent sclerosis. Sequestra form, which have to be excised. Should an oral cutaneous fistula develop, and medical management fail, resection of the involved segment of the mandible may be necessary. Before operation, a thorough effort should be made to control the infection with broad-spectrum antibiotics, such as tetracycline and clindamycin. Frequent oral irrigation and removal of sequestered or exposed bone are required. Particular importance is given to any remaining teeth, and appropriate dental care should be delivered.

Recently, hyperbaric oxygen, delivered at 2 atmospheres pressure for periods of up to 40 hours, has allowed osteonecrosis of the mandible to heal without the need for partial mandibulectomy.

Osteonecrosis can be prevented by removing any teeth in the potential field of radiation which are not in excellent condition and supported by normal, healthy bone. Patients undergoing radiation therapy should be given fluoride treatments and instructed to practice good oral hygiene (Table 27-3). At the time of extraction, the alveolar rim should be smoothed and a primary mucoperiosteal closure obtained. Radiation should not be started until the bone has healed properly, usually within 1 week to 10 days. The development of new infection, particularly *C. albicans*, must be guarded against. The saliva flow diminishes after only a few treatments of radiation therapy. The mucosa becomes less able to defend against infection, and a mild mucositis can develop. The use of artificial saliva preparations is often helpful. Some patients lose their appetite and need encouragement to eat.

TABLE 27-2. FACTORS INFLUENCING THE DEVELOPMENT OF OSTEORADIONECROSIS

Tumor factors
Tumor overlaying or invading bone (especially floor of mouth)
Large primary
Dental or surgical treatment factors
Elective extractions
Inadequate delay after extractions
Trauma (dentures, surgical salvage)
Patient factors
Poor oral care (poor patient education or poor compliance with instructions)
Poor nutritional status preventing healing
Radiation factors
Salivary suppression
Radical treatment (high dose, high fraction size)
Large volume (decreased collaterals)
Interstitial radiation overlaying bone (especially floor of mouth and base of tongue)
Orthovoltage radiation (should never be used externally, ie, only intraoral treatment acceptable with orthovoltage)

Courtesy Dr. Robert E. Haselow, Department of Therapeutic Radiology, University of Minnesota.

CHONDRITIS

High doses of radiation administered to the larynx can result in radionecrosis of the laryngeal cartilage. As the blood supply to the perichondrium diminishes, a chondritis occurs. The thyroid cartilage can become infected and actually dissolve. There is intense pain in the area of skin overlying the cartilages, and fistulas can form. There is swelling and edema, and loss of the normal architectural landmarks of the larynx. Treatment is primarily intensive, intravenous antibiotics.[18] Prolonged trials of antibiotic therapy along with wound debridement and cleansing is indicated. Laryngectomy is needed only when complete loss of the skeletal support structures of the larynx or breakdown of overlying skin with fistula formation or intractible pain occur. Again, hyperbaric oxygen has been helpful.

WOUND INFECTION WITH EXPOSURE OF THE CAROTID ARTERY

Pharyngo- or orocutaneous fistulas with breakdown of the cervical flaps in the region of the carotid artery expose the vessel, and infection with oral organisms ensues. This problem usually occurs only when there has been an extensive resection in combination with intensive radiation therapy for advanced disease. Because the normal oral flora have been altered by radiation and operation, the infecting organisms are frequently *Pseudomonas*, *Staphylococcus*, and other gram-negative organisms. Cultures and Gram stains should be obtained. Intravenous antibiotics are administered, and immediate plans are made for protection of the carotid artery system. The dilemma is complex: the longer the artery remains exposed, the greater the risk of rupture; at the same time, placement of a flap over frank necrosis only hides the impending carotid artery rupture. The vessel must therefore be kept moist with an antibiotic solution or dilute povidone iodine.[19] The area

TABLE 27-3. ORAL AND DENTAL HYGIENE IN HEAD AND NECK CARCINOMA PATIENTS UNDERGOING RADIATION

Goals
- Decrease incidence and severity of osteonecrosis
- Improve oral hygiene
- Nutritional support
- Reduce incidence and severity of postradiation tooth decay

Preradiation dental evaluation
- Cleaning, prophylaxis all dentulous patients
- Restoration, root canals as indicated
- Extractions if teeth are nonsalvagable or if the patient is unreliable—wait 2 weeks after extractions for oral cavity, oropharyngeal, or nasopharyngeal radiation
- If extractions done, need to have smooth alveolar surface (to avoid pressure points and bone spicules) for later dentures
- Primary closure for full mouth extractions

During radiation
- Dentulous—daily flouride treatment
- All patients need to maintain oral hygiene. Oral salt and soda irrigations—½ tsp. table salt and ½ tsp. baking soda in 1 quart water—irrigate mouth qid
- Artificial saliva, few drops on tongue prn (Xerolube, First Texas Pharmaceutical, Dallas, Texas)
- Dietary counseling: soft, bland, high-calorie, high-protein diet with food supplementation. Avoid mouth washes, citrus juices, hot or spicy foods
- IVs and NG tube feedings as needed
- Educate patients to the need for continued oral hygiene and prophylaxis every 3 to 4 months
- Oral analgesia
  - Viscous xylocaine (may mix with water to decrease viscosity) best for oral cavity symptoms. Swallow no more than 15 ml qid

Milk of Magnesia or Maalox	240 ml
Benadryl elixir, 12.5 mg/5 ml	160 ml
Mycostatin (15 cc orally qid)	40 ml
	440 ml

- Antifungal agent as needed

Post radiation
- Because of the change in the gingiva following radiation, dental prostheses should be delayed for at least 6 months. Soft liners should be used
- Periodic reinforcement of dental hygiene with fluoride treatments and cleaning every 3 to 4 months
- Continue artificial saliva
- Management of dental failures
  - Silver filling for caries
  - If severely decayed, smooth tooth to avoid sharp irritating edges. The mere existence of a decayed tooth in the mandible is *not* a reason for extraction
  - Try to avoid oral surgical procedure as long as possible. If it is necessary, an adequate alveoplasty should be performed with generous wound irrigation, watertight soft tissue closure, and antibiotic coverage
  - Small areas of exposed bone should be treated conservatively by maintaining meticulous oral hygiene. Spicules of bone should be removed gently

Courtesy Dr. Robert E. Haselow, Department of Therapeutic Radiology, University of Minnesota.

must be debrided, and a horizontal cervical chest flap can be delayed or swung immediately to protect the carotid artery. Cross-matched blood must always be available until healing is complete.

A slight blood loss from an area of eschar over the vessel means rupture is impending (sentinal bleed). There is no time to wait for epithelium to form, and the artery must be ligated in the operating room. If the vessel actually ruptures, pressure is applied over the vessel and a blood transfusion started. Stroke inevitably follows if the vessel is ligated while the patient is in shock, but the incidence can be reduced to 30 percent if the blood volume is restored prior to ligation.

To prevent exposure of the carotid should postoperative infection occur, a split thickness skin graft of 0.013 to 0.014 inch is first elevated from the thigh, and a second graft of 0.013 inch is taken of the underlying dermis. The split thickness skin graft is then laid back and sutured into position, and the dermal graft is spread over the carotid artery and sutured down to the cervical fascia. An exposed dermal graft can undergo epithelialization.

PROPHYLACTIC ANTIBIOTICS IN MAJOR HEAD AND NECK SURGERY

There is still controversy over the use of antibiotics as a prophylactic measure at the time of operation. Poor risk patients, those in a poor nutritional state, or those who have undergone heavy irradiation have an increased incidence of postoperative wound infection and postoperative fistula. In an effort to offset these disabilities, antibiotics have been given immediately before, during, and for a short period after operation. The rationale has been that communication with the oral cavity or pharynx allows the normal oral flora to extend into the structures of the neck. Infections that develop when antibiotics are withheld are usually not caused by normal oral flora. *S. aureus* is still the most frequent organism responsible for infections in nonirradiated patients, but irradiated patients are frequently infected with gram-negative rods, particularly *P. aeruginosa* and *E. coli.* Cultures of hemovac drain exudate [20] may help predict the potentially infecting organisms. Patients who receive more than 6,800 rads prior to operation have especially high infection rates. Seagle et al [21] have demonstrated the efficacy of prophylatic cefazolin (Chapter 23).

INFECTION ASSOCIATED WITH TRAUMA

TRAUMA TO THE EXTERNAL EAR

Avulsion

Trauma to the ear varies from a clean laceration to an avulsion of a portion of the auricle to a potentially septic infection (as occurs from a dog or human bite). In the case of a clean laceration or avulsion, all effort is made to protect the cartilage—minimal amounts of tissue are debrided to cover and protect the exposed cartilage and perichondrium. It is even possible to reapproximate an avulsed, clean segment. An antistaphylococcal antibiotic is administered. With a carefully placed external stent, the avulsed segment has a chance to survive. The cartilage is seldom salvageable in cases of avulsion caused by a dog bite. If several hours have elapsed since the injury, it is not worthwhile to attempt reanastomosis of the avulsed segment. Instead, the cartilage can be buried beneath the skin over the mastoid process for later secondary reconstruction. Again, antibiotics are recommended for 5 days. Infection that develops secondarily is treated after appropriate culture and sensitivity studies.

Thermal Injury

Most frostbite injuries are superficial, involving the helix, and should be treated by immediate rapid rewarming with saline-soaked sponges or cotton to a temperature of 38.3 to 42.2C. Broad-spectrum antibiotics are administered only to patients in whom a deep injury is suspected. Silver nitrate (0.5 percent) dressings are carefully applied to the auricle. No debridement is undertaken initially. It is important to prevent secondary infection. Large blebs must neither be opened nor aspirated. If they rupture, they must be cleaned daily with antiseptic solutions. When delineation of the devitalized tissues becomes evident, conservative debridement is undertaken.

Burns of the head and neck usually occur in association with other burn injuries and may not be evident initially. More severe injuries will take priority. Again, care should be taken to prevent the spread of infection to the cartilage of the ear. *P. aeruginosa* is the most common organism found in this form of smoldering perichondritis. When actual chondritis develops, it is treated like perichondritis, discussed earlier in this chapter.

TRAUMATIC PERFORATION OF THE TYMPANIC MEMBRANE

Perforation of the tympanic membrane can result when foreign objects are introduced into the ear canal and from concussion, such as a slap to the ear. These wounds are generally not associated with infection. Treatment includes protection of the ear from introduction of any foreign material, including water. A baseline audiogram is obtained to rule out damage to the ossicles. The margins of the perforation when examined with the microscope are usually curled medially under the drumhead and can be retrieved with a small pick. A small patch is applied to the drumhead to maintain them in position. Antibiotics are administered only if infection develops.

Perforations that occur when diving, water skiing, or surfing, however, are almost always associated with an immediate onset of a purulent otitis media. The responsible organisms are initially gram-positive, but soon the gram-negative rods predominate. In addition to systemic antibiotics, a topical antibiotic-steroid ear drop may be helpful. These perforations should not be closed while there is an active infection.

If there is any suspicion that the stapes is dislocated and could be pushed medially into the inner ear, immediate operation is indicated. As a result of such a displacement, the patient has hearing loss as well as vertigo. An emergency stapedectomy may be necessary to save the hearing.

TEMPORAL BONE FRACTURE

Severe falls and motor vehicle accidents can cause basal skull fractures and associated temporal bone trauma. Three types of temporal bone fractures—longitudinal, transverse, and mixed—can be distinguished by clinical presentation and direction of the fracture.

In the longitudinal variety, the most common, the fracture line extends along the longitudinal axis of the temporal bone from the petrous pyramid to the mastoid region. It usually begins in the middle cranial fossa near the foramen spinosum, follows along the carotid canal anteriorly across the middle ear and out onto the squamosa portion of the temporal bone. Although it usually does not include the firm labyrinthine bone, this fracture causes injury to the middle ear, a disrupted ossicular chain, a tear in the tympanic membrane, and often a laceration in the postsuperior quadrant of the ear canal. Facial nerve paralysis occurs in 20 to 25 percent of such fractures, and the nerve injury is usually distal to the geniculate ganglion.

Transverse fractures are less common and are associated with injuries to the frontal or occipital region of the skull. The fracture line extends transversely across the petrous line. There is an associated injury to the labyrinthine capsule, with resultant deafness and loss of vestibular function. Because there is no laceration of the tympanic membrane, a hemotympanum results without bleeding into the external canal. Trauma to the facial nerve with facial paralysis occurs in 50 percent of patients, and the injury to the facial nerve is proximal to the geniculate ganglion. With an intact tympanic membrane, cerebrospinal fluid otorrhea may drain down the eustachian tube and present as rhinorrhea.

Mixed fractures are common in more severe trauma and are a combination of the previous two types. Polytomographic examination of the temporal bone will help determine the extent of these injuries. The possibility of a fracture to the opposite side of the skull must always be considered, and special roentgenograms of that side should be taken. If the patient's condition permits, complete audiologic evaluation is needed for clinical and medicolegal reasons. Such patients are usually admitted to the hospital by the neurosurgical service.

Otolaryngologic consultation is indicated to assess the extent of injury to the ear and facial nerve, especially if there is bleeding from the external ear canal. A postauricular area of ecchymosis developing over the mastoid region is referred to as Battle's sign and is pathogenomonic of temporal bone fracture. Primary care of the patient usually rests in the hands of the neurosurgeon who treats the more threatening intracranial injury. It is best to postpone exact assessment of the ear injury while there is copious bleeding from the ear canal, because attempts to remove the blood clot may introduce microbes. The combination of hemorrhage from the ear, hearing loss, and facial nerve palsy make up the diagnosis of basilar skull fracture. Detailed information about the tympanic membrane in this acute stage is not necessary. The only similar injury that can cause such ear hemorrhage is a direct blow to the symphysis of the mandible, forcing the condyle of the mandible through the anterior aspects of the ear canal, with resultant skin laceration. This can usually be ruled out by the lack of associated mandibular fracture. Later, when the patient's condition stabilizes and there is no longer active bleeding, crusted blood is removed from the ear canal under aseptic conditions and the extent of the ear injury is determined. A dark blue tympanic membrane indicates that there is hematoma present in the middle ear, and a conductive hearing loss is found either because of discontinuity of the ossicles or because this collection of blood prevents ossicular movement. Lacerations of the ear canal usually need no specific treatment and will heal spontaneously. Patients with cerebrospinal fluid otorrhea must be watched until their general condition has stabilized. Daily examination of facial nerve function is made. When nerve function is present initially and later decreases, the paralysis will usually recover spontaneously. A facial nerve that is absent immediately after the trauma is not likely to recover. Such nerve injuries should be explored as soon as the patient's general condition permits.

Spinal fluid otorrhea usually ceases spontaneously within 1 week. Failure to stop requires a combined neurosurgical and otolaryngologic approach to the mastoid region for closure of this leak. During the time there is active hemorrhage from the canal or a spinal fluid leakage, the patient should be treated with an antibiotic effective against gram-positive organisms. Early infections are most commonly caused by *S. pneumonia, S. aureus,* and *H. influenzae.* With persistent otorrhea, repeated cultures must be obtained, because the gram-negative rod organisms have a more dominant role as the cause of later infections.

NASAL TRAUMA

Nasal trauma is the most common of all facial injuries. Obvious deformity of the nasal dorsum with deflection to the side and epistaxis bring the patient to the emergency room. In the acute phase when there is significant swelling and the patient is apprehensive, ice packs and analgesics are the best treatment until the swelling subsides. The nasal septum must then be examined because hematomas that develop between the septum and mucoperichrondrium will continue to increase in size, and complete nasal obstruction will eventually occur (Fig. 27-22). If present, bilateral nasal packing is inserted and the patient is started on an antistaphylococcal penicillin, because nasal packs have been firmly placed bilaterally. This is important, since an undrained hematoma almost always leads to abscess, which in turn leads to dissolution of the cartilaginous tissues. In an effort to preserve the physiologic functions and cosmetic appearance of the nose, it will be necessary to replace the missing septal cartilage with autogenous cartilage after the infection is cleared. Correction of the nasal bony deformity can be performed under local or general anesthesia on the third or fourth postinjury day. Early repair is important in children because their fractures show signs of healing within that time. It is still possible to mobilize the fracture fragments of adults at 7 days. Stenting, both externally and internally, is then necessary.

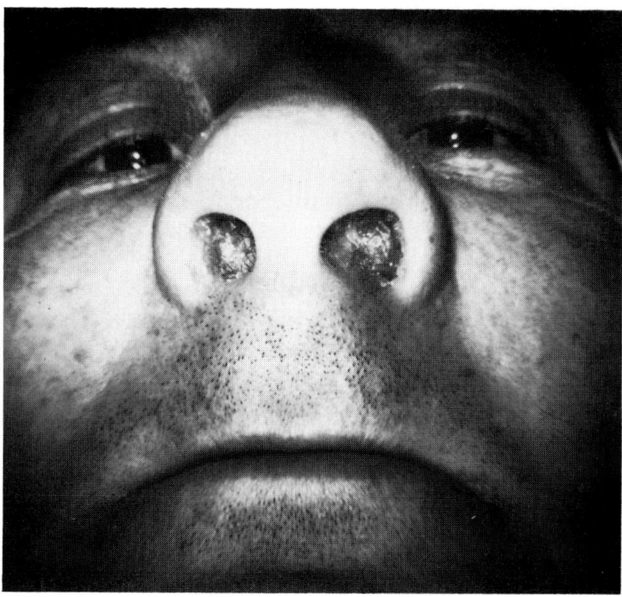

Fig. 27-22. **Septal hematoma completely obstructs both nares after blunt nasal trauma.**

MAXILLOFACIAL TRAUMA

Automobile and motorcycle accidents cause the most severe maxillofacial trauma. Although injuries from fist fights and athletic mishaps are more common, they are usually less severe. Any fracture line extending through the tooth-bearing areas of the mandible or maxilla causes an associated laceration of the tightly associated gingiva and must be considered as a compound fracture. Treatment is aimed not only at correcting the fracture, but also at prevention of infection and subsequent osteomyelitis.

To prevent large gaps at the fracture sites and avoid exposure of bare bone surfaces, early fragment stabilization is required. This may involve temporary placement of wire ligatures (ivy loops) or the application of portions of arch bars to immobilize the jaw fragments. By stabilizing the mandible, the tongue is also stabilized and the airway protected. Clots of blood and other foreign material need to be removed from the oral cavity.

Loose fragments of bone with attached alveolar mucoperiosteum should not be debrided unless they are definitely dead. Suturing of the mucoperiosteum frequently prevents loss of bone and provides a better opportunity for later reconstruction by the oral surgeon or the prosthodontist.

Tracheostomy and inflated cuffed tracheostomy tubes will keep the severely injured patient from aspirating blood and other foreign materials.

Injury to the maxilla usually exposes the sinus cavity. Fractures through the maxillary and ethmoid sinus cavities tend to develop infection. These sinus cavities need adequate drainage. Obviously, devitalized fragments of bone and soft tissue must be removed. Fractures extending across the frontoethmoid region may displace and obstruct the nasofrontal duct. Such fractures can result in acute frontal or ethmoid sinusitis and can lead to mucocele and pyocele many (10 to 20) years later. For this reason, some physicians advocate the immediate obliteration of the frontal sinus when the duct has been damaged.[10] Others will attempt to reconstruct the duct or perform a trephine to maintain drainage of the sinus while the mucosal reaction subsides and the duct becomes patent again.

Severe epistaxis may be associated with maxillofacial trauma. Anterior packs control some hemorrhages, but more frequently, when the hemorrhage is severe, a posterior nasal pack is also necessary. The posterior pack is pulled firmly into the posterior choana. This will prevent obstruction of the eustachian tube orifice and resultant otitis media. An antibiotic ointment, such as Bacitracin, on the pack reduces the local infection and the associated foul odor. Because obstruction of several sinus ostia occurs when the nasal pack is in position, a systemic antibiotic (such as penicillin) should also be administered. The packs remain in place for 3 to 5 days. Twenty-four hours after removal, antibiotics may be discontinued. Simultaneous occurrence of epistaxis and cerebrospinal fluid otorrhea should be treated with packs to control the hemorrhage, and with systemic antibiotic to prevent meningitis. Persistent cerebrospinal fluid rhinorrhea alone is not a contraindication to reducing a frontoethmoid fracture. In fact, the rhinorrhea may be stopped by reduction of the fracture. When the posterior plate of the frontal sinus is fractured, the cerebrospinal fluid rhinorrhea cannot be expected to stop spontaneously. An open approach can be used to repair the dura and obliterate the sinus. Such procedures are safely undertaken only with simultaneous administration of antibiotics, especially those effective against *S. aureus*.

SHOTGUN WOUNDS OF THE HEAD AND NECK

Shotgun wounds, usually self-inflicted, can cause massive loss of soft tissue, severe hemorrhage, airway obstruction, and later general infection of the exposed tissues. Treatment in the case of face wounds includes: (1) establishment of a safe airway by immediate tracheostomy with a cuffed endotracheal tube, (2) control of hemorrhage by wide exposure of the involved area in the operating room, (3) systemic antibiotics, (4) removal of all obviously devitalized soft tissue and bone, (5) establishment of sinus drainage if sinuses have been entered, (6) identification of severed nerves, particularly the facial nerve with metallic suture for a delayed repair on the twenty-first day. Massive wounds with loss of soft tissue have an almost 100 percent incidence of infection, and immediate nerve graft repair is seldom effective. Later on, when the wound is closing and healthy granulation tissue appears, the facial and other cranial nerves can be repaired or grafted, and (7) repair of any pharyngeal lacerations with wide and adequate drainage. Later, chest flap, cervical flap, or forehead flap can be used to replace the extensive soft tissue loss. Eye injuries, which are common under these circumstances, are treated by the ophtalmologist and frequently may include exenteration.

The loss of mandibular bone is best treated in stages. In the first stage, healthy soft tissue coverage is established. Later, reconstructive techniques, such as placement of mesh graft filled with bone marrow, rib, and cortical bone, are tried. It is essential that there be no evidence of infection, orocutaneous fistula, or osteomyelitis at the time of attempted reconstruction, which may be delayed for up to 6 months to 1 year. Maintenance of the mandibular position is ensured by wire pin (Kirschner wires) placement to prevent soft tissue fibrosis and distortion. External fixation devices such as biphase plates are excellent to maintain the stability of the mandibular segments during healing.

BLUNT LARYNGEAL TRAUMA

Blunt injuries to the larynx or trachea will present with subcutaneous emphysema, loss of voice, airway obstruction, and pain and tenderness over the involved cartilage. Tracheostomy is frequently necessary as an emergency procedure. As soon as the patient's condition permits, within the first 24 to 48 hours if possible, an endoscopic evaluation and open reduction of any fractures of the larynx and trachea should be carried out in the operating room. Delay inevitably results in infection with loss of cartilaginous support. Prior to endoscopy, the recurrent laryngeal nerve function should be evaluated. A lateral soft tissue roentgenogram and esophogram should be performed to diagnose a ruptured viscus. All wounds of the esophagus, pharynx, and larynx must be drained and systemic antibiotics administered. Injuries to the larynx and trachea require splinting by either prefashioned endotracheal tubes or silastic or foam rubber stents. These stents are usually held in position with wire sutures brought out through the neck, tied over a button, and maintained in position for 6 to 8 weeks. Associated injuries to the major vessels include the common carotid artery or jugular vein, and if suspected, require contrast studies and immediate exploration. The jugular vein may be resected, but the carotid artery is preserved or a saphenous vein graft substituted for a severely injured vessel.

In all instances in which massive wounds occur, the patient is treated with an antibiotic that is effective against *S. aureus*. Repeat cultures are performed on any wounds that continue to remain infected, because more resistant and gram-negative organisms show up with time. Tetanus prophylaxis, in the form of tetanus toxoid, is also given to all these trauma patients.

BIBLIOGRAPHY

Adams G, Nelms C: Complicated mandibular fractures. Otolaryngol Clin North Am 9:453, 1976.

Bartlett J, Gorbach S: Anaerobic infections of the head and neck. Otolaryngol Clin North Am 9:655, 1976.

Bean SF: Oral cicatricial pemphigoid (immunoflorescent studies). Trans Am Acad Ophthalmol Otolaryngol 84:530, May–June 1977.

Becker GD, Parell GJ, Busch DF, Finegold SM, Acquarelli MJ: Anaerobic and aerobic bacteriology in head and neck cancer surgery. Arch Otolaryngol 104:591, 1978.

Beck AL: Deep neck infections. In English GM (ed): Otolaryngology, Vol IV. Hagerstown, Prior, 1978.

Bluestone CD, Cantekin EI, Beery QC: Certain effects of adenoidectomy on eustachian tube ventilatory function. Laryngoscope 85:113, 1975.

Bluestone CDD, Steiner RE: Intracranial complications of acute frontal sinusitis. South Med J 58:1, 1965.

Calcaterra TC, Stein F, Ward PH: Dilemma of delayed radiation injury to the larynx. Ann Otolaryngol Rhinolaryngol 81:501, 1972.

Cantrell RW, Jensen JH, Reid D: Diagnosis and management of tuberculous cervical adenitis. Arch Otolaryngol 101:53, 1975.

Davison FW: Acute laryngeal obstruction in children: a fifty-year review. Ann Otolaryngol 87:606, 1978.

Deegan MJ: Immunologic diseases of the salivary glands. Otolaryngol Clin North Am 10:351, 1977.

Emmett JR, Fischer ND, Biggers WP: Tuberculous mastoiditis. Laryngoscope 87:1157, 1977.

Harker LA, Koontz FP: Bacteriology of cholesteatoma: clinical significance. Trans Am Acad Ophthalmol Otolaryngol 84:683, July–August 1977.

Jaffe B, Strome M, Khaw K, Schwachman H: Nasal polypectomy and sinus surgery for cystic fibrosis—a 10-year review. Otolaryngol Clin North Am 10:81, 1977.

Kashima HK, Holliday MJ, Hyams J: Laryngeal chondronecrosis: clinical variations and comments on recognization and management. Trans Am Acad Ophthal Otolaryngol 84:878, Sept–Oct 1977.

Keim RJ: Meningitis: the influence of routine otolaryngologic consultation on morbidity and mortality in 290 cases. Laryngoscope 88:1, Feb 1978.

LeMay DR: Penetrating wounds of the larynx and cervical trachea. Arch Otolaryngol 94:558, 1971.

Page RC, Engel LD, Narayanan AS, Clagett JA: Chronic inflammatory gingival and peridontal disease. JAMA 240:545, 1978.

Roydhouse N: A controlled study of adenotonsillectomy. Arch Otolaryngol 92:611, 1970.

Sessions DG, Stallings JO, Mills WJ, Beal DD: Frostbite of the ear. Laryngoscope 81:1223, 1971.

Thorn GW, Adams RD, Braunwald E, Isselbacher KJ, Petersdorf RG: Harrison's Principles of Internal Medicine, 8th ed. New York, McGraw-Hill, 1977.

REFERENCES

1. DeBré R, Celers J: Clinical Virology. Philadelphia, Saunders, 1970.
2. Mawson SR, Adlington P, Evans M: A controlled study evaluation of adeno-tonsillectomy in children. J Laryngol Otolaryngol 81:777, 1967.
3. McKee WJE: A controlled study of the effects of tonsillectomy and adenoidectomy in children. Br J Prev Soc Med 17:49, 1963.
4. Finegold SM: Anaerobic Bacteria in Human Disease. New York, Academic, 1977, p 140.
5. Bonding P: Routine abscess tonsillectomy: late results. Laryngoscope 86:286, 1976.
6. Yung AK, Cantrell RW: Quinsy tonsillectomy. Laryngoscope 86:1714, 1976.
7. Goldstein JC: Grand rounds: Epstein-Barr virus—the ravager. Ann Otolaryngol Rhinolaryngol 87:729, 1978.
8. Sprinkle PM, Veltri RW: The tonsil and adenoid dilemma: medical or surgical treatment? Otolaryngol Clin North Am 7:909, 1974.
9. Frederick J, Braude AL: Anaerobic infection of the paranasal sinuses. N Engl J Med 290:135, 1974.
10. Montgomery WW: Surgery of the Upper Respiratory System, Vol 1. Philadelphia, Lea & Febiger, 1971.
11. Mosher HP: President's address: submaxillary fossa approach to deep pus in neck. Trans Am Acad Ophthalmol Otolaryngol (34th Annual Meeting), 1929, p 19.
12. Feind CR: The head and neck. In Haagensen CD, Feind CR, Herter FP, Slanetz CA Jr, Weinberg JA (eds): The Lymphatics in Cancer. Philadelphia, Saunders, 1972, p 60.
13. Chandler JR: Malignant external otitis: further considerations. Ann Otolaryngol 86:417, 1977.
14. Stroud MH: Treatment of suppurative perichondritis. Laryngoscope 88:176, 1978.
15. Meyerhoff WL, Kim CS, Paparella MM: Pathology of chronic otitis media. Ann Otolaryngol 87:749, 1978.
16. Bluestone CDD, Wittel RA, Paradise JL, Felder H: Eustachian tube function as related to adenoidectomy for otitis media. Trans Am Acad Ophthalmol Otolaryngol 76:1325, 1972.
17. Duckert LG, Mathog RH: Diagnosis in persistent cerebrospinal fluid fistulas. Laryngoscope 87:18, 1977.
18. McGovern FH, Fitz-Hugh JS, Constable W: Post radiation perichondritis and cartilage necrosis of the larynx. Laryngoscope 83:808, 1973.
19. Dedo DD, Alonso WA, Ogura JH: Povidone-iodine: an adjunct in the treatment of wound infections, dehiscences and fistulas in head and neck surgery. Trans Am Acad Ophthalmol Otolaryngol 84:68, Jan–Feb 1977.
20. Yoder MG, Silva J: Anaerobic isolates in hemovac lines. Laryngoscope 87:63, 1977.
21. Seagle MB, Duberstein LE, Gross CW, Fletcher JL, Mustafa AQ: Efficacy of Cefazolin as a prophylactic antibiotic in head and neck surgery. Otolaryngology 86:568, 1978.

CHAPTER 28
Neurosurgical Infections

MICHAEL E. CAREY

THE central nervous system (CNS) can be involved directly by infection, or it may be affected by infection located in contiguous structures. Vertebral body osteomyelitis, for instance, can cause spinal cord compression and result in paraplegia. Nervous system infections are caused by bacteria, viruses, fungi, or parasites that can cause diffuse or localized disease. This chapter will deal primarily with focal infections of the nervous system and surrounding structures that are amenable to operation. Both spontaneously occurring and postoperative infections will be considered.

The brain, spinal cord, and cauda equina are completely enveloped by dura mater except where various cranial and somatic nerves exit. Although bacteria will occasionally penetrate it, the dura is an extremely good barrier against infection. Even when cranial bone flaps become infected postoperatively and the epidural space is full of pus, intracranial extension through the dura is rare. The excellent natural defense of the dura, however, can be circumvented in several ways (Fig. 28-1). Fractures of the skull that lacerate the dura can lead to meningitis and local brain infection. Bacteria can also reach the brain through the arteries that supply it, by way of scalp veins that drain into skull diploic spaces and then into emissary veins that pierce the dura and enter the subdural and subarachnoid spaces. Where cranial and somatic nerves penetrate the dura, they are ensheathed in arachnoid, which becomes continuous with the neurolemma of the distal nerve. This anatomic arrangement affords an entry to the central nervous system for bacteria from a contiguous focus of infection (eg, a diseased mastoid bone). Organisms can spread retrograde along the cranial nerve and subarachnoid sheath to infect the intracranial compartment.

The brain itself is quite resistant to infection—it is difficult to infect it even by direct bacterial inoculation. Usually, in order to produce an experimental abscess, it is necessary to inject simultaneously bacteria plus a foreign substance, such as blood agar.[1-3] Even using this technique, however, Falçoner et al [2] initiated brain infections in only 98 of 132 rabbits. Rabbits injected with bacteria alone into the carotid artery developed meningitis but not a brain abscess.[4] Molinari [5] had to use a bacteria-coated arterial embolus to create a hematogenous abscess in dogs.

INTRACRANIAL INFECTIONS

PYOGENIC BRAIN ABSCESS

Pyogenic brain abscesses can follow trauma if a comminuted, depressed fracture tears the dura and exposes the brain. They can also result from an adjacent infection, such as osteomyelitis of the skull, a suppurative infection of a boney sinus, or meningitis. Hematogenous (metastatic) brain abscesses arise when bacteria from elsewhere in the body enter cerebral blood vessels and lodge in the brain. Pyogenic brain abscess can also occur as a complication after neurosurgery.

Incidence

In underdeveloped countries brain abscess accounts for a large part of neurosurgical practice. Bhatia et al [6] from India, reported that 8 percent of all intracranial space-masses seen from 1965 to 1970 were caused by brain abscesses. In more economically advanced countries, pyogenic brain abscesses account for a much smaller portion of neurosurgical cases. Any large general hospital in the United States can expect to encounter approximately four patients per year with a brain abscess.[7,8] The autopsy incidence of this disease ranges from 0.2 to 0.7 percent.[9]

Pathogenesis of Various Types of Brain Abscess

Posttraumatic Brain Abscess. Infection that follows a basal skull fracture usually takes the form of meningitis, but central nervous system infection after a compound comminuted fracture of the cranial vault more often results in brain abscess. Jennett and Miller [10] found a 10.6 percent brain infection rate in a series of 359 depressed, open vault fractures. Joubert and Stephanov,[11] reporting from South Africa in 1977, observed that 10 of the 23 brain abscesses in their series followed trauma. These infections most often occur when the initial wound has been inadequately cleansed and debrided. In areas where neurosurgical care is readily available, posttraumatic abscesses should comprise a rather small proportion of all intracerebral pyogenic abscesses.[7,8]

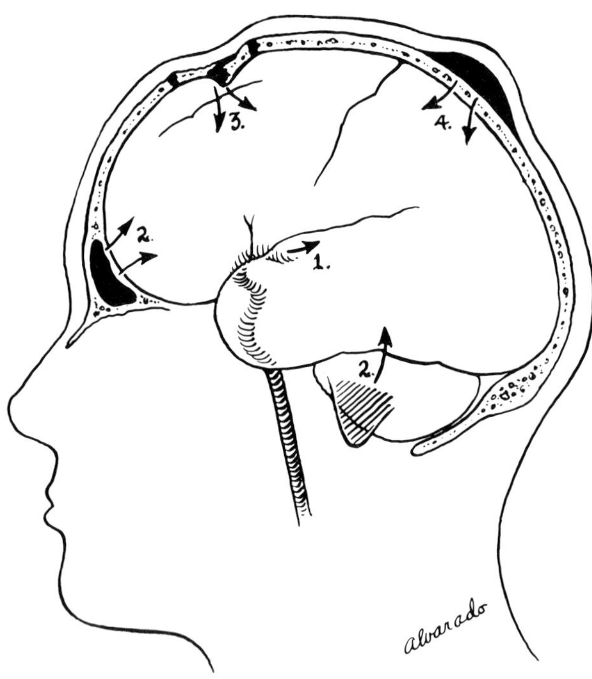

Fig. 28-1. **Bacteria may gain access to the brain in several ways. (1) They may spread to the brain from distant foci of infection (so-called hematogenous or metastatic abscesses). These abscesses often lie in the distribution of the middle cerebral artery. Individuals with right-to-left cardiac or pulmonary shunts are particularly prone to these abscesses. (2) Paranasal sinus infection may also spread intracranially. (3) Open skull fractures may allow direct bacterial implantation within the brain. (4) Overlying scalp and skull infections may allow bacteria to enter the skull and/or brain either by direct extension or by the diploic spaces and emissary veins.**

Abscesses Secondary to Adjacent Infection. Suppuration of paranasal or mastoid sinuses may lead to a brain abscess. Bacteria from the infected sinus can reach the brain by spread through the inner sinus wall and by penetrating the dura and infecting the brain. Bacteria can also invade intact or thrombosed venous channels that drain the sinus and enter the intracranial compartment through emissary veins. A brain abscess secondary to a paranasal sinus infection usually involves the frontal lobe. Middle ear mastoid infection can result in either a temporal lobe or cerebellar abscess. The former is more common, however, because the roof of the middle ear is much thinner than the posterior wall.

Osteomyelitis of the skull can result from paranasal sinus suppuration, from open skull fracture, from hematogenous spread from another infective focus, or from a postoperative infection of the craniotomy flap. Bacteria from the area of osteomyelitis may spread into the epidural and subdural spaces or the brain itself directly or through vascular channels.

Brain abscesses sometimes follow meningitis, possibly as a sequel to cortical vein thrombosis. The resulting infarcted and edematous brain provides fertile territory for colonization by bacteria from the subarachnoid space.

Hematogenous or Metastatic Brain Abscesses. These abscesses usually occur in the posterior frontal and parietal lobes, which are perfused by the middle cerebral artery. Chronic pulmonary infections, especially bronchiectasis, have been common antecedent infective sources, but skin, pelvis, mouth, and long bones are other frequent primary foci. Many patients have no obvious infective focus, but it must be assumed that bacteria enter the bloodstream and spread to the brain from some occult source or from mucosal trauma.

Hematogenous abscesses tend to occur initially at the gray-white junction where blood flow in the capillary bed is slowest. What actually causes an organism to adhere to and penetrate a brain capillary is unknown. Experimentally,[5] bacteria plus encephalomalacia are required for formation of metastatic abscesses.

Normally, bacteria are present intermittently in venous blood, but most are effectively cleared by the pulmonary capillary bed. Patients with right-to-left cardiac shunts have approximately 10 times more risk of brain abscess formation than the general population because bacteria present in venous blood circumvent the lung capillaries and pass directly to the arterial system to enter the brain. Patients with congenital cyanotic heart disease, ie, tetralogy of Fallot and transposition of the great vessels, have the highest incidence of brain abscess. Such patients not only have right-to-left shunts but also have increased blood viscosity and reduced blood flow, which can lead to an area of encephalomalacia that can be colonized by bacteria. Reduced blood Po_2 in cyanotic individuals also enhances the growth of certain bacteria within the brain.[9]

In the preantibiotic era, the mortality for hematogenous brain abscesses approached 100 percent,[12] often as a result of the underlying cardiac or pulmonary disease. Even at this time, the mortality for metastatic brain abscesses may be more than 50 percent.[7,13]

The different types of brain abscess vary in relative frequency from series to series,[7,8,11,14,15] depending upon the patient population served by the medical center.

Pathology

Infectious bacteria within the brain cause edema and an inflammatory reaction with polymorphonuclear cells around the infected area. The surrounding astrocytes and microglia proliferate, and the nearby blood vessels undergo reticuloendothelial hyperplasia. Nearby veins may be thrombosed by fibrin. If this acute state of cerebritis is not reversed, necrosis and liquefaction of the infected brain will follow. The subacute phase occurs within the first several weeks after the onset of infection. During this time, the vascular hyperplasia that surrounds the infective nidus intensifies and forms a limiting wall of granulation tissue. As the abscess becomes chronic, collagenous connective tissue gradually replaces the granulation tissue, and the surrounding astrocytes undergo a pronounced gliosis. Hence, a well-developed brain abscess is comprised of three defined layers: (1) an inner layer of degenerated leukocytic debris and bacteria, (2) an intermediate layer of collagen fibers associated with vascular hyperplasia and neovascularization, and (3) an outer layer of inflammation with glial hyperplasia. Varying degrees of cerebral edema extend peripherally from the abscess capsule and may account for much of the lesions's mass effect. The separation of brain abscess evolution into acute, subacute, and chronic stages is arbitrary because, as the infection proceeds, both destructive (acute) and reparative (subacute or chronic) processes can occur simultaneously in different parts of the abscess.

Encapsulation is more likely to occur in the highly vascular cortex than in the less vascular white matter. Hence, a brain abscess usually extends in the white matter, where encapsulation is deficient. If inward extension remains unchecked, ventricular rupture and ventriculitis will occur.

Whatever their underlying etiology, pyogenic brain abscesses can be single or multiple, they can contain a single cavity, or they can be multilocular. Fortunately, abscesses of surgical significance tend more often to be single. Many patients who are dying as a result of overwhelming septicemia or septic endocarditis have a myriad of minute brain abscesses that are not treatable by operation.

Etiology

Before antibiotics, the gram-positive cocci *Staphylococcus, Streptococcus,* and *Streptococcus pneumoniae* were the three most prevalent organisms cultured from brain abscesses. In the antibiotic era, *S. pneumoniae* is rare, and gram-negative rods, such as *Haemophilus* or *Proteus,* or mixtures of gram-positive cocci and gram-negative rods are commonly cultured. In the past, substantial numbers of sterile brain abscesses were reported, and investigators often reasoned that previously administered antibiotics had sterilized them. Heineman and Braude,[16] however, were able to culture anaerobic bacteria from 16 of 18 brain abscesses by using meticulous anaerobic culture techniques. Subsequent investigators have also ascertained that many brain abscesses contain anaerobic or microaerophilic streptococci, diphtheroids, fusiforms, or *Bacteroides* alone or in association with aerobic bacteria. In a recent cooperative study, de Louvois et al [17] succeeded in culturing bacteria from 46 brain abscesses. No sterile cultures were obtained, and *Bacteroides* was recovered from 11 of 43 aspirates (Table 28-1). Streptococci were isolated from abscesses of all types and in all locations, while staphylococci predominated in traumatic or postoperative abscesses. Enterobacteriacae and *Bacteroides* were isolated in mixed cultures, principally from temporal lobe abscesses associated with middle ear infections. The importance of *Bacteroides* in these latter infections has also been shown by Ingham et al.[18,19]

Opportunistic Infections. Ubiquitous, saprophytic commensals rarely cause infections in healthy people but may cause disease in those with compromised defense mechanisms.[20,21] In developed countries, the following underlying factors commonly predispose to opportunistic infections: diabetes mellitis, uremia, collagen disease, cancer, immunosuppression, and transplantation. Malnutrition, which can be prevalent in underdeveloped areas, also predisposes to opportunistic infection. Opportunistic organisms that are found in brain abscesses include *Pseudomonas, Klebsiella, Escherichia coli, Listeria, Cryptococcus,* varicella-zoster virus, herpes simplex virus, *Pneumocystis, Mycobacterium, Herellea, Serratia, Candida, Actinomyces, Aspergillus, Mucor, Nocardia,* diphtheroids, *Bacteroides, Proteus, Clostridium,* and *Torulopsis.*

Clinical Manifestations

Symptoms and signs can arise both from the systemic infection and from the space-occupying brain lesion. Local manifestations can be particularly prominent with brain abscesses secondary to sinus-mastoid infection or cranial osteomyelitis. In addition to having fever, patients so infected can have local pain and tenderness about the involved sinus or bone, as well as nuchal rigidity if the insertions of cervical muscles are locally inflamed. Later, as the abscess progresses, symptoms and signs of cerebral infection appear—generalized headache, nausea, vomiting, localized motor or sensory deficits, cerebellar signs, papilledema, mental aberrations, lethargy, and coma. The clinical picture will vary tremendously depending upon abscess type, location, size, and chronicity. When an abscess becomes quite large or is associated with widespread edema, localizing findings become less prominent, while diminished levels of consciousness or other signs of generalized increased pressure caused by brain stem dysfunction supervene (Fig. 28-2A). Occasionally, fairly subtle and

TABLE 28-1. LOCALIZATION AND NUMBER OF ISOLATES IN PYOGENIC BRAIN ABSCESS

	Location and Number of Abscesses					
Organism	***Temporal***	***Frontal***	***Cerebral***	***Other***	***Extra or Subdural***	***Total***
Number of patients	(13)	(11)	(6)	(5)	(8)	(43)
Streptococcus	7	10	3	3	6	29
Staphylococcus aureus	1	2	—	1	—	4
Bacteroides	6	3	—	1	1	11
Proteus	6	—	—	1	—	7
Enterobacter aerogenes	1	—	—	—	—	1
Haemophilus aphrophilus	—	1	—	—	—	1

From de Louvois J, Gortvai P, Hurley R.[17] Bacteriology of abscesses of the central nervous system: A multicentre prospective study. *Br Med J 92:981,* 1977.

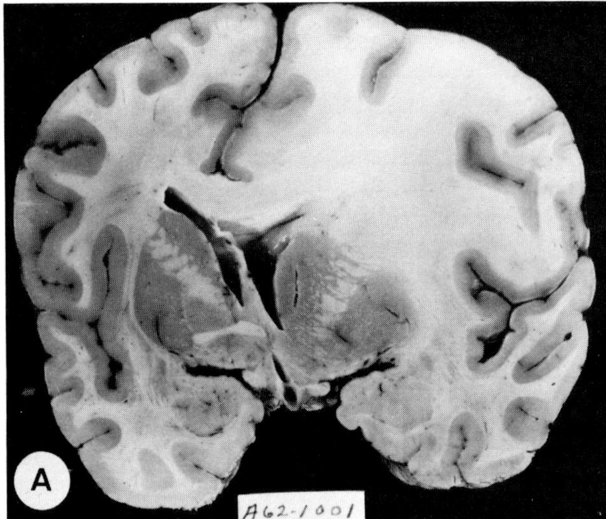

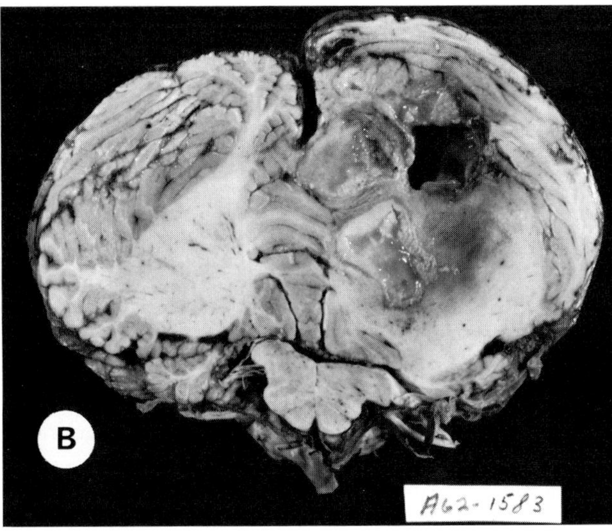

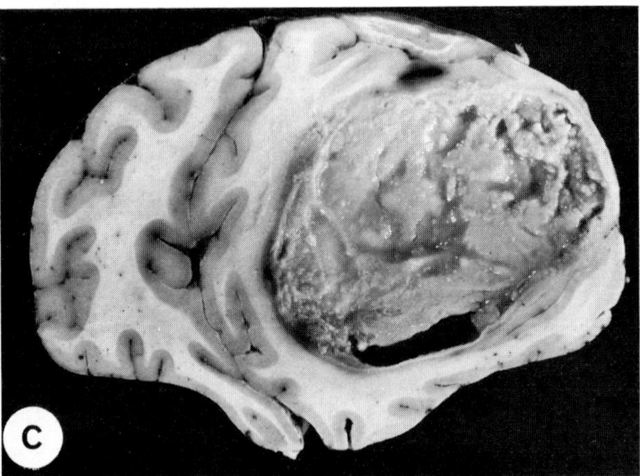

Fig. 28-2. **A. Edema associated with frontal lobe abscess. Brain surrounding an abscess is often very edematous, and, in this case, the edema has caused significant ventricular displacement and herniation of the cingulate gyrus under the falx. The mass effect associated with abscesses may cause temporal lobe and brainstem herniations and lead to death. Herniation is a far more frequent cause of death from a brain abscess than is ventriculitis or meningitis. B. Cerebellar abscess. This cerebellar abscess is associated with much cerebellar edema, and the cerebellar mass is compressing the medulla. Many people with treated cerebellar abscesses survive and have relatively normal neurologic function. C. Frontal lobe abscess. This massive abscess has caused a major herniation of the involved frontal lobe across the midline. (Courtesy of Carlos Garcia, MD, State University Medical School, New Orleans, Louisiana.)**

unexplained changes in behavior may be the only manifestation of a frontal lobe abscess. Cerebellar abscesses occur within the relatively confined space of the posterior fossa and may obstruct cerebrospinal fluid flow or may apply direct pressure to the brain stem. Either of these mechanisms can cause sudden death. Often, a seizure or signs of generalized increased pressure herald the presence of a huge abscess that otherwise would have been expected to cause focal findings. Presumably, an expanding abscess pushes aside but does not destroy much of the surrounding brain parenchyma. Seizures are more prone to occur with hematogenous abscesses in the motor strip than with frontal abscesses caused by frontal sinusitis or with posteriorly situated temporal lobe abscesses consequent to mastoid disease.

The peripheral blood count usually shows only a mild degree of leukocytosis, 11,000–12,000 per mm^3. The erythrocyte sedimentation rate, however, is frequently elevated. Patients who have brain abscesses consequent to cyanotic congenital heart disease usually will not have an elevated sedimentation rate because of the associated polycythemia.

Diagnosis

A high index of suspicion is crucial for the expeditious diagnosis of a brain abscess because the associated symptoms and signs can be extremely atypical and misleading. This is particularly true for hematogenous brain abscesses, which can be unsuspected prior to death or surgery. *Delay in diagnosis is a major factor contributing to the persistently high mortality associated with brain abscesses.*

Skull Roentgenograms. Roentgenograms of the skull should be made because paranasal sinus and mastoid infection or osteomyelitis of the skull can readily be demonstrated and may lead directly to the diagnosis of abscess. When sinus or bone infection is suspected, detailed radiographic views of that part of the skull should be obtained. If the pineal gland or choroid plexus is calcified and shifted, a mass lesion within the brain is indicated. If the patient exhibits any evidence of infection, such as mild fever, slight leukocytosis, or elevated sedimentation rate, the mass lesion can be presumed to be an abscess. Occasionally, gas associated with an intracranial abscess will be seen on plain skull films.

Computerized Axial Tomography. Computerized axial tomographic (CAT) scans have simplified the process of correctly diagnosing brain abscesses. Both plain and postcontrast infusion scans should be obtained.[22] When an abscess is present, plain CAT scans reveal extensive areas of diminished absorption, associated with density measurements indicative of edema (Fig. 28-3). Mass effect with ventricular displacement also is usually evident. After contrast infusion, a dense rim around the abscess becomes evident in almost all cases.[23,24] This ring of enhancement may be 3–6 mm thick, or it may be uniform in thickness, or there may be evidence of thinning on the medial aspect. The inner margins of the abscess rim are usually smooth, while the outer border is surrounded by irregular areas of low absorption, representing surrounding edema. The use of steroids can diminish the contrast enhancement of the abscess capsule.[25] Multilocular lesions are commonly demonstrated. Glioblastomas,[26] metastases,[27] and occasionally infarcts [22] may all show rings on contrast-enhanced CAT scans. Therefore, clinical information is paramount in the CAT scan diagnosis of brain abscess. Gas can occasionally be seen within the abscess.

Computerized axial tomography has been able to diagnose up to 100 percent of brain abscesses.[22-25] Diagnostic failures are often caused by technically inadequate studies. Despite occasional failures, at this time the noninvasive technique of CAT must be considered the primary diagnostic study for the diagnosis of brain abscesses.

Cerebral Angiography. A cerebral angiogram demonstrates the mass effect of an abscess by vascular displacement (Fig. 28-4). In about half the cases a "ring sign" represents the contrast media within the highly vascular abscess capsule. A chronic abscess is more likely to demon-

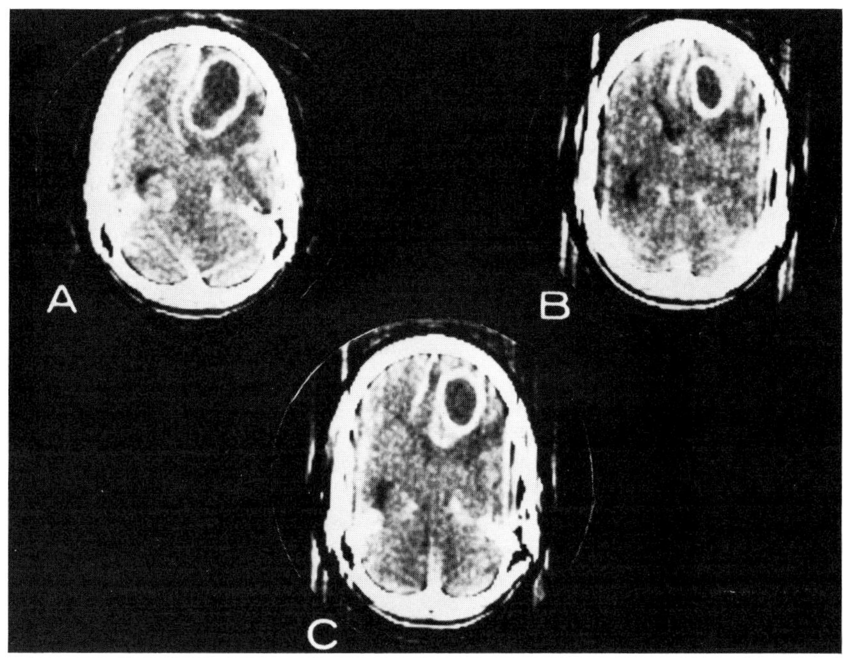

Fig. 28-3. Large frontal abscess. CAT scan of the brain after contrast enhancement shows mass in left frontal lobe with low dense center, thick irregular capsule, and surrounding edema. Note marked midline shift. (Courtesy of Lawrence H. A. Gold, MD, and Mathis P. Frick, MD, University of Minnesota.)

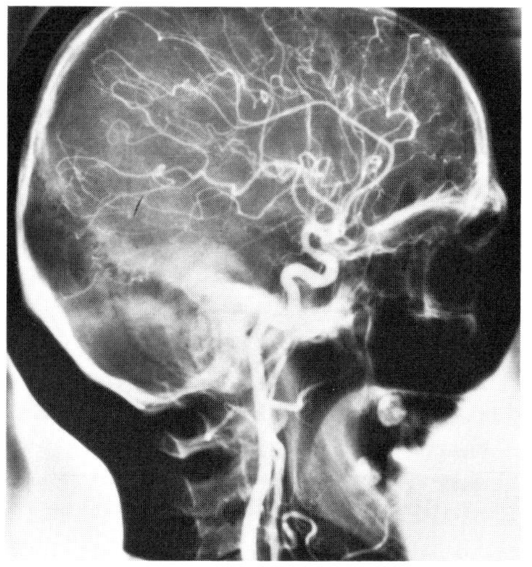

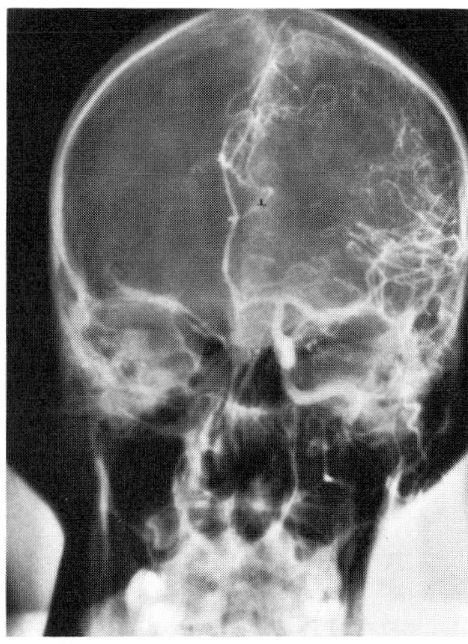

Fig. 28-4. Carotid angiogram of left parietal abscess, arterial phase. Parietal mass effect causing midline shift of anterior cerebral arteries and forward and downward displacement of the sylvian triangle. (Courtesy of Lawrence H. A. Gold MD, and Mathis P. Frick, MD, University of Minnesota.)

strate this sign than is an acute one. Kaufman and Leeds [23] feel that angiography provides no additional information on the location of diagnosed brain abscess over CAT scanning, but angiography might be expected to provide additional information (as neovascularity) and, occasionally, to help differentiate abscess from neoplasm.

Radioisotopic Brain Scan. Isotopic brain scanning helps locate approximately 90 percent of all supratentorial abscesses, but posterior fossa abscesses are sometimes missed because the overlying suboccipital muscles, which also take up the isotope, can obscure the abscess. The radioactive isotope is concentrated in the pus as well as in the abscess capsule and surrounding brain because of a breakdown in the blood-brain barrier.[28] The isotopic ring, or doughnut sign, is occasionally present and indicates that the lesion could be an abscess. This sign consists of a curvilinear dense uptake surrounding a clearer central area. Presumably, the isotope is taken up in the abscess capsule or surrounding edematous brain more than in the pus itself. Although this sign is nonspecific and also occurs with brain tumors or infarcts,[29] abscess should be suspected if the ring is seen in conjunction with inflammatory disease.

Lumbar Puncture. The dangers and inadequacy of lumbar puncture for the diagnosis of brain abscess have been repeatedly stressed.[7,9,30,31] This procedure is dangerous because a brain abscess acts principally as an expanding mass lesion. After withdrawal of spinal fluid from the lumbar subarachnoid space, intracranial hydrodynamics may be altered and cause the temporal lobe on the infected side to shift into the tentorial opening and the brain stem to shift rostrally. This can result in fatal cerebral herniation.

The spinal tap was once thought to be useful as an aid in the diagnosis of brain abscess. Because of this, one series [7] analyzed the possible diagnostic benefits of lumbar puncture in 62 patients with proven brain abscess. The opening pressure and cerebrospinal fluid protein were normal in one third of the patients, while cerebrospinal fluid glucose was normal in two thirds of the patients. Surprisingly, one third of the cerebrospinal fluid specimens showed 10 or fewer white blood cells per mm^2. Only a few Gram stains of cerebrospinal fluid were positive, and these had poor morphologic correlation with subsequently cultured brain abscess flora. Less than 15 percent of the cerebrospinal fluid culture results were positive. These data indicate that the possible diagnostic yield from lumbar puncture in cases of brain abscess is small and that some of the negative results are misleading. In the above series, 8 deaths were probably precipitated by spinal tap. *Lumbar puncture has no place in the diagnosis of brain abscess.*

Electroencephalography (EEG). In the era of CAT scanning, use of EEG seems somewhat anachronistic, but this technique is available in some areas where CAT scans are not. In reality, EEG is highly reliable in locating brain abscesses. The most consistant EEG finding is a focal delta wave with a frequency as low as 0.5 cycles per second. In one report,[27] 11 of 12 supratentorial brain abscesses were located and the remaining abscess lateralized by EEG. A cerebellar abscess was missed. In the same series, 5 of 6 radioisotopic brain scans and 6 of 7 arteriograms correctly localized brain abscesses.

Air Studies. Pneumoencephalography and ventriculography have been virtually outmoded by CAT scanning. Pneumoencephalography requires a spinal puncture and, therefore, is a dangerous procedure. Ventriculography can lead to upward herniation or cause the abscess to rupture into the ventricle. Should the brain cannula pass through the abscess into the ventricle, ventriculitis may result. It must be noted, however, that in the past ventriculography quite successfully localized abscesses and occasionally inadvertently drained them!

Treatment

Drug Penetration into Brain Abscess. The blood level of a drug depends upon dose, frequency, and route of administration, plus its breakdown or excretion. Free entry of a drug into brain and rapid equilibration between blood and brain occur with substances showing a high degree of lipid solubility, low ionization at physiologic pH, and lack of plasma protein binding. Slow brain entry and lack of equilibration occur with substances that are poorly soluble in lipids, those that are ionized at physiologic pH, and those bound to plasma proteins.

Sulfonamides, for instance, may be ionized when in plasma, and their ionic form may be bound to plasma proteins. The degree of sulfonamide ionization can be altered as plasma pH changes, and this can change the degree of plasma binding. Alterations in plasma pH can, therefore, change the amount of unbound sulfonamide available for entry into cerebral compartments. The degree to which a number of drugs bind to plasma proteins will be modified by other drugs which compete for the same binding sites—sulfinpyrazone effectively displaces several sulfonamides from plasma albumin, while probenecid competes with penicillin for binding to serum proteins.[32]

Entry of drug into cerebrospinal fluid is largely determined by the ability of the drug to pass through the choroid plexus, while entry into brain depends upon passage through the blood-brain barrier associated with brain capillaries.

The optimal pharmacologic data on the penetration of drugs into brain abscesses would be obtained by measuring plasma and brain or cerebrospinal fluid drug levels at specific time intervals, so that a drug transfer constant could be established.[33] Such ideal data are not currently available either experimentally or clinically. Consequently, widely divergent brain abscess:blood ratios have been observed. Sometimes, the abscess:blood ratio has been greater than unity, probably indicating that the drug had been cleared from the blood at the time the specimen was drawn rather than that there was uphill transport of drug into the abscess cavity.

Black et al [34] obtained the most comprehensive initial data on antibiotic penetration into brain abscesses, and their work suggested that, given high enough blood levels, chloramphenical, methicillin, and penicillin will penetrate a brain abscess in amounts greater than minimal inhibitory concentrations. More recently, however, de Louvois and associates[35,36] have provided an extensive study relative to antibiotic penetration into brain abscesses. It was concluded that penicillin penetrates abscesses reasonably well, but other beta-lactam antibiotics do not. The penetration of chloramphenicol was deemed erratic, and aminoglycosides penetrate poorly. Lincomycin and fusidic acid penetrate brain abscesses well. Ingham et al[18,19] demonstrated that oral or intravenous metronidazole resulted in high drug concentrations within otogenic cerebral abscesses.

To be effective, not only must an antibiotic penetrate the blood-brain barrier and abscess capsule, but it must also retain its antibacterial properties. Black et al[34] ascertained that viable bacteria could be cultured from all abscesses even though antibiotics were present within the abscess in amounts greater than minimal inhibitory concentrations. It was unclear whether antibiotic failure was secondary to their inactivation or diminished host resistance. It has subsequently been shown that some microorganisms produce enzymes capable of destroying a wide range of beta-lactam antibiotics, and even in the absence of beta-lactamase-producing bacteria, some purulent exudates are able to inactivate beta-lactam antibiotics.[36]

Initial Medical Treatment. Treatment of brain abscess requires eradication of infection and elimination of the increased intracranial pressure caused by the abscess and the surrounding edema. Antibiotic treatment should begin as soon as brain abscess is suspected, even before either Gram stain or culture and sensitivity data are available. Antimicrobial agents that cover a wide range of organisms should be used first, until the specific organisms have been identified. On the basis of his recent study[17] of brain abscess flora, de Louvois proposes the following initial treatment scheme[35] (Table 28-2):

1. *Abscesses of sinusitic origin* are most often caused by penicillin-sensitive streptococci, and mixed infections are unusual. Therefore, penicillin 16 to 24 million units per day is indicated.

2. *Abscesses of otitic origin* are usually caused by a mixture of aerobic and anaerobic bacteria. A combination of broad-spectrum antibiotics should therefore be used, such as chloramphenicol and metronidazole with or without the addition of penicillin, ampicillin, or cotrimoxazole.

3. *Metastatic (or cryptogenic) abscesses* can be streptococcal or can be caused by a mixture of bacteria. Broad-spectrum antibiotics (penicillin, chloramphenicol) should be used until specific bacteriologic data are available.

4. *Spinal and posttraumatic intracranial abscesses* are usually caused by *Staphylococcus aureus*. Fusidic acid is the drug of first choice.

The elegant data of de Louvois and his conclusions notwithstanding, I feel that the combination of agents—penicillin, methicillin, and chloramphenicol—capable of dealing with both gram-positive and gram-negative bacteria, aerobes and anaerobes should be used as initial medical treatment for any abscess. Regardless of the statistical probability of encountering a specific organism, abscesses can be caused by unusual or unsuspected organisms that must be treated as early as possible. An incorrect selection even based on the soundest available data can be disastrous for the patient.

Glucocorticoids are commonly used to treat cerebral edema associated with brain abscess. Because steroids decrease the host inflammatory response and can retard other host defense mechanisms, including abscess encapsulation, theoretical arguments may be raised against the use of steroids in patients with brain abscesses. Long and Meacham[37] found that steroids did not significantly inhibit abscess encapsulation in dogs, but Quartey et al[38] showed that dexamethasone diminished both edema and abscess encapsulation. Furthermore, infecting bacteria were eliminated from the brain in rabbits treated with antibiotics alone but remained in those treated with antibiotics plus steroid.

Unfortunately, death from a brain abscess is usually caused by brain swelling, increased intracranial pressure, and brain stem herniation, so that amelioration of cerebral edema must remain a paramount aim of medical therapy. The beneficial effects of steroids on cerebral edema may make their use imperative in certain cases. Concomitant administration of large doses of antibiotics will usually control the infection while the patient is being prepared for operation.

As long as a patient with a brain abscess remains alert and neurologically intact with antibiotics and steroid administration, the work-up and treatment can proceed expeditiously but not necessarily as an emergency. If any neurologic deterioration occurs, however, operation should be undertaken promptly. If neurologic and brain stem function have been jeopardized seriously prior to definitive operation, such osmotic agents as mannitol or urea can be used to remove water from the brain, reduce intracranial pressure, and provide time for operative decompression.

TABLE 28-2. PERCENTAGE OF CULTURED BACTERIA SENSITIVE TO ANTIBIOTICS USED IN TREATMENT

	Penicillin	Chloramphenicol	Cephaloradine	Cotrimoxazole	Aminoglycoside
Streptococcus	94	100	94	96	—
Staphylococcus	—	100	100	100	100
Enterobacteriaceae	—	88	25	88	100
Bacteroides	36	100	66	100	—
H. aphrophilus	100	100	100	100	100

From de Louvois J, Gortvai P, Hurley R: Antibiotic treatment of abscesses of the central nervous system. *Brit Med J 2:985,* 1977.

Occasionally, lesions that were thought to have been brain abscesses have resolved on antibiotic therapy alone.[39,40] The resolution can be followed with serial CAT scans.[24,41] While several cases of brain abscess cured by antibiotics alone have been reported, in general the best treatment is still surgical.

Surgical Treatment. Three forms of operative treatment are available: excision, drainage, and aspiration. Often initial drainage or aspiration is used in conjunction with eventual excision.

Total Excision. After the diagnosis of a mass lesion is made, the ideal treatment is obviously a complete extirpation of the mass. With one stroke, the intracranial pressure will be relieved and the infection eradicated. For this purpose, a craniotomy is performed with the patient under general anesthesia. The dura is opened, and the abscess is located by using a probing brain needle. The capsule is usually near the cortical surface. Often it is possible to dissect around the capsule with a suction apparatus while the brain is being retracted, thus isolating and removing the abscess in toto. This excludes contamination of the operative field by the pus. If intracranial pressure is high or if the abscess is too large, this technique may require excessive brain retraction or resection. Under such circumstances, it is safer to aspirate as much pus as possible to reduce the pressure and shrink the mass. This latter technique increases the possibility of spreading infection, but with antibiotic coverage in addition to care and protection of the surrounding brain by pledgets, the collapsed abscess can be extirpated without causing cerebritis or meningitis.

While excision effectively removes the infection, it does have the following limitations:

1. If the abscess is poorly encapsulated and is in the sensorimotor area or if it is deep within the brain, radical removal can produce or increase a neurologic deficit.

2. Abscesses in patients with cyanotic congenital heart disease can be extremely large, with well-formed vascular capsules. In addition, these patients often have a coagulopathy. Abscess excision in these individuals may result in operative or postoperative hemorrhage, severe neurologic deficit, or death.

3. Patients who are seriously ill may not tolerate the extensive craniotomy required for excision.

4. Abscesses can recur after excision as well as after drainage or aspiration, and excision does not lessen the incidence of postoperative seizures.[7]

Drainage. An alternative method of treatment is to drain the abscess without excising the capsule. A burr hole or small craniectomy over the suspected site is made under either general or local anesthesia. After the dura is opened, the abscess is located by probing with a brain needle, and the pus is partially but not completely drained. The brain needle is then withdrawn after the depth and angulation required to reach the abscess have been ascertained. A rubber drain of appropriate size is then inserted along the needle path into the abscess cavity, which is held open by the residual pus. A large drain, No. 18 or 20 French is necessary if the pus is highly viscous. The drain should not be placed so deeply as to penetrate the medial wall of the capsule next to the ventricle, since this may lead to ventriculitis. The drain is secured to the scalp by sutures and is then cut off 0.5 cm above the skin. The abscess cavity is emptied of pus by irrigating through the drain with a small volume of isotonic saline solution containing diluted bacitracin or a penicillin-chloramphenicol solution until the returning fluid is free of debris. Dressings should be applied so that lying on the drain site will not cause the drain to be forced further into the brain. The dressings should be changed frequently, and drain patency should be checked if the dressing is dry. As a rule, only minimal drainage occurs postoperatively. As drainage stops and the patient is improving, the drain can be gradually removed. Appropriate antibiotics should be continued for at least several weeks following removal of the drain. The use of contrast agents (eg, thorium dioxide or micropaque barium) to assess the evolution of the abscess cavity is no longer necessary. Regression can be followed satisfactorily by CAT scanning.

The obvious disadvantages of drainage are that pus may reaccumulate and that a multiloculated abscess may be incompletely drained. Fortunately, frequent post-drainage CAT scans can be used to monitor the adequacy of abscess drainage. If the abscess has been incompletely drained a decision will have to be made whether to redrain or to excise the abscess. Despite this drawback to drainage, the mortality and morbidity associated with this form of therapy are usually comparable to that associated with excision [7,8,42] in spite of the fact that patients treated by drainage are often in a much more neurologically deteriorated state than those treated by craniotomy and excision. The incidence of postoperative seizures following drainage is comparable to that of seizures following excision.[7]

Multiple Aspiration. Trephination is performed over the suspected site, the abscess is located, and pus is aspirated. The abscess is repeatedly aspirated from day to day until the patient improves. Optimally, the abscess cavity may be followed by CAT scans. Lacking this, contrast media or air can be injected into the cavity for serial radiologic localization. Although this method has been used successfully, it requires a great deal of practice in tapping and in judging when to terminate the procedure. As with drainage the abscess may recur, or a daughter abscess may be missed. Infection may be spread into the overlying brain by multiple punctures of the abscess. Despite these drawbacks, aspiration may be curative or may tide an extremely sick individual over until excision can be undertaken. Antibiotic therapy should be maintained during active treatment and for several weeks thereafter.

Aspirated pus should be immediately sent to the laboratory for Gram stain and aerobic and anaerobic cultures. Great care must be taken to ensure that truly anaerobic cultures are taken. This is best accomplished if the neurosurgeon works conjointly with the infectious disease specialist. Special stains and cultures may be required for unusual organisms.

Sometimes, it is necessary to intervene surgically before infected brain (area of cerebritis) has been walled off. While the initial therapy of cerebritis consists of broad-spectrum antibiotics, if neurologic deterioration occurs because of increasing intracranial pressure, operation may be necessary. A generous brain decompression may be accomplished by resection of the necrotic and edematous focus, and this may reverse the patient's course. Steroids should be used to combat concomitant cerebral edema.

Postoperative Management. Because brain abscesses may recur whatever their form of therapy, all postoperative patients require diagnostic studies to assure that their abscess has been successfully treated. When available, CAT scans provide an ideal way to ascertain whether the surgically treated abscess itself is regressing and whether associated cerebral edema and hemispheral shift are resolving. After successful drainage, the abscess capsule is rarely enhanced on follow-up CAT scans.[22] When follow-up capsule enhancement persists on repeat CAT scans following initial surgical therapy, the abscess either has refilled or has spread. If CAT scanning is unavailable, postoperative cerebral arteriography or even pneumoencephalography is mandatory to make absolutely sure that the brain infection has been eradicated. Clinical observation alone is inadequate because an incompletely treated abscess may recur after hospital discharge.

Medical Treatment. Experience has indicated that operation is the appropriate treatment for brain abscess. Nevertheless, in 1971, Heineman et al [39] reported the successful antibiotic treatment of 6 patients with neurologic signs, and in some cases EEG findings suggestive of localized intracranial infection. Chow et al [40] reported the successful antibiotic treatment of a patient presumed to have multiple *Listeria monocytogenes* brain abscesses. Traditionalists who felt that pus must be drained or otherwise removed surgically viewed these reports with skepticism. Because no operative intervention occurred, there were no histologic specimens so these medically cured abscesses may have been areas of cerebritis which antibiotics might be expected to penetrate and cure. Furthermore, Black et al [34] had not had a good experience with antibiotics alone in the treatment of several surgically confirmed brain abscesses. Although antibiotics seemed to penetrate the abscess adequately, viable bacteria were subsequently cultured from them.

The development of CAT scanning made early direct visualization of the abscess possible. The acuteness of the infection and the extent of the intracranial mass could be quickly appreciated. The course of the abscess could be followed while antibiotics were given, presumably in preparation for operation. With close radiologic observation possible for the first time, reports began to appear on occasional abscesses or small groups of abscesses cured by antibiotics alone. I have found documented medical cures of 16 additional patients with brain abscesses (April, 1981). CAT scans were used to diagnose and follow the abscesses in 6 of the 7 reports. Radionuclide imaging was used once. It thus appears that in some instances brain abscesses may indeed by cured by antibiotics, without the aid of operation. While these reports appear encouraging, the results of Enzmann et al in dogs,[40a] which correlated CAT scans with histologic features, indicated that cerebritis may appear with a peripheral enhancing ring on CAT scans and thus may be confused with a true abscess. Thus some of the so-called medical cures of brain abscess may have been cures of cerebritis instead. This caveat notwithstanding, the growing number of clinical reports which are appearing strongly suggest that some brain abscesses may be cured by antibiotics alone. While this may be an impressive stride, by all measures the number of medical cures of brain abscesses is quite low. Furthermore, when medical therapy has been conscientiously tried it has only succeeded about 60 percent of the time.

Brain abscess acts as a rapidly expanding mass and operation on the lesion must be anticipated. In my judgement, medical management of a brain abscess should be undertaken by a neurosurgeon in conjunction with an internist knowledgeable in antibiotics and their potential for blood brain barrier and brain abscess penetration. Because medical therapy alone may fail and the patient may undergo neurologic decompensation quickly, I do not feel that antibiotics should be administered to an individual with a brain abscess without the close attendance of a neurosurgeon.

Rosenblum et al,[40b] with a series of 6 patients cured on antibiotics alone, suggest that medical management be undertaken for surgically high-risk patients if they are in good neurologic status despite their brain abscess. High-risk patients include those with congenital heart disease, multiple or deep-lying abscesses, as well as those with concurrent meningitis, ependymitis or hydrocephalus requiring a shunt. In undertaking the medical treatment of brain abscess penicillin and chloramphenicol are started and periodic CAT scans obtained. After 2 weeks of treatment, the patient is rescanned. Operation is performed if the abscess has enlarged, significant mass effect is present, or if any neurologic deterioration has occurred. If the clinical course is stable or improving, antibiotics are continued for 2 additional weeks. The patient is rescanned weekly or whenever new symptoms warrant. If the abscess has not decreased in size after 4 weeks an operation is performed. If the abscess does decrease in size with medical management, antibiotics are continued for 6 to 8 weeks and periodic CAT scans are done up to a year to ensure that the abscess does not recur. This therapy was successful in 6 of 10 cases initially tried on medical treatment alone by Rosenblum et al.[40b] Medical treatment is most successful with abscesses 3 cm or less in diameter. Steroids are avoided whenever possible because they retard abscess capsule formation.

Prognosis

Mortality. Tables 28-3 and 28-4 depict the mortality associated with brain abscess as determined by major series reported in the antibiotic era. Clearly, the operative mortality remains high despite sophisticated diagnostic means, neurosurgical availability, and a wide range of antibiotics. The major reasons for the continued high mortality for brain abscess are diagnostic failure and the poor neurologic condition of the patient at operation (Table 28-5). Poor neurologic condition usually results from brain stem compromise consequent to mass effect of the abscess. The larger mass effect, in turn, usually is a result of delayed diagnosis.

Tables 28-3 and 28-4 reveal that no particular form of initial therapy appears to enjoy a clear-cut lower mortality than others, particularly when one realizes that simpler surgical techniques as aspiration or drainage are apt to

TABLE 28-3. BRAIN ABSCESS MORTALITY AND FAVORED FORM OF OPERATIVE TREATMENT, 1946–1978

Author	Year	Total Surgical Cases	Deaths	% Mortality	Preferred Treatment
Le Beau [43]	1946	14	0	0	Excision
Pennybacker, Sellors [12]	1948	100	39	39	Excision
Jooma, Pennybacker, Tutton [44]	1951	150	41	27	Excision
Botterell, Drake [45]	1952	27	4	15	Excision
Tutton [46]	1953	59	12	20	Aspiration
Lewin [47]	1955	36	7	19	Aspiration
Loeser, Scheinberg [48]	1957	82	30	37	Excision
Gurdjian, Webster [49]	1957	16	4	25	Aspiration
Kerr, King, Meagher [50]	1958	47	14	30	Excision
Sperl, MacCarty, Wellman [51]	1959	60	10	17	Excision
Ballantine, Shealy [52]	1959	44	15	34	Excision
Martin, Brihaye, Martin [53]	1960	42	15	36	Excision
Liske, Weikers [54]	1964	93	46	50	—
Newlands [55]	1965	80 *	22	28	Aspiration
Krayenbühl [56]	1967	104	23	22	Excision
Eberhard [57]	1969	23 †	7	30	—
Garfield [30]	1969	142	47	33	Aspiration
Snyder, Farmer [58]	1971	10 †	5	50	—
Kapsalakis, Askitopoulou, Gregoriades [59]	1972	12	1	8	Aspiration
Carey, Chou, French [7]	1972	62	22	35	Drainage or excision
Gerszten, Dalton, Allison [60]	1973	36	14	40	—
Le Beau et al [61]	1973	99	32	32	Excision
Bhatia, Tandon, Banerji [6]	1973	55	17	31	Excision
Beller, Saher, Praiss [62]	1973	82	33	40	Aspiration, then excision
Morgan, Wood, Murphey [8]	1973	79	23	29	Aspiration/drainage or excision
Sampson, Clark [31]	1973	28	5	18	Excision
Martin [13]	1973	24 ‡	15	63	Aspiration
French, Chou [63]	1974	17	0	0	Excision
Fischbein, et al [9]	1974	23 §	7	30	—
Yoshikawa, Goodman [64]	1974	24	8	33	—
Brewer, MacCarty, Wellman [65]	1975	60	10	17	—
van Alphen, Dreissen [42]	1976	89	26	29	Drainage
Jefferson, Keogh [14]	1977	49	13	28	Aspiration
de Louvois, Gortvai, Hurley [17]	1977	44	9	20	—
Choudhury, Taylor, Whitaker [15]	1977	16	1	6	Excision
Joubert, Stephanov [11]	1977	23	4	17	Aspiration
Rosenblum et al [41]	1978	18	8	44	—
		20	0	0	Excision
TOTAL		1,989	589	29.6	

* All otogenic.
† All children < 15 years.
‡ All metastatic abscesses.
§ All in patients with congenital heart disease.

TABLE 28-4. CEREBELLAR ABSCESSES, MORTALITY AND FAVORED FORM OF OPERATIVE TREATMENT

Author	Year	Total Surgical Cases	Deaths	Percent Mortality	Preferred Treatment
Schreiber [66]	1941	9	1	11	Tap
Pennybacker [67]	1948	9 *	7	77	
Pennybacker [67]	1948	9 †	1	11	Excision
Shaw, Russell [68]	1975	41	13	32	Excision or aspiration
Morgan, Wood [69]	1975	13	3	23	Drainage or excision
TOTAL	1941–1978	81	25	31	

* Prepenicillin.
† Postpenicillin.

TABLE 28-5. PREOPERATIVE LEVEL OF CONSCIOUSNESS AND PERCENT MORTALITY IN SEVEN SERIES

		Clinical Status			
Author	No. of Patients	*Alert*	*Drowsy*	*Purposeful Response to Pain*	*Decerebrate or No Response to Pain (%)*
Kerr et al [50]	47	0	17	—	60
Newlands [55]	80	11	29	50	—
Garfield [30]	200	18	32	65	72
Carey et al [7]	86	21	21	44	89
Morgan et al [8]	79	9	27	40	70
Bhatia et al [6]	55	20	31	40	67
Van Alphen, Dreissen [42]	88	16	26	33	58

be used on more neurologically impaired patients (Table 28-5). Thus, it would appear that one should have a flexible approach to the treatment of brain abscess and be prepared to utilize all modalities as the individual case warrants. All forms of therapy should be designed to prevent increased intracranial pressure, brain stem compromise, and associated decompensation of the level of consciousness.

The introduction of computerized brain scans in the mid 1970s has lead to fewer deaths caused by brain abscesses. In seven series where CAT scans were used for diagnosis, only 16 of 112 patients (14 percent) died.

The ease of CAT scanning will certainly allow brain abscesses to be diagnosed and treated earlier when patients are in better neurologic condition. This fact in itself should greatly lessen mortality. Not only will the presence of the abscess be known but so will the acuteness of the process and the relative danger to the patient by the mass effect. This knowledge will allow the surgeon more freedom of action to (1) pursue a vigorous course of antibiotic therapy, (2) simply tap or drain the abscess, (3) consider formal excision in a neurologically intact individual, or to (4) tap and allow further encapsulation prior to later excision.

Unfortunately CAT scanning may not be available in underdeveloped countries where brain abscesses may be most prevalent. Many abscesses in these countries arise consequent to trauma and sinus/mastoid disease, however, and are relatively easily diagnosed. Clinical suspicion plus the relatively accurate and often available diagnostic modalities of EEG, angiography and radionuclide scanning should allow early diagnosis and decreased mortality.

Reports indicate that the mortality associated with metastic brain abscesses ranges from 55 to 78 percent, primarily because diagnosis has been hardest in this group. The efficacy of CAT scanning in reducing brain abscess mortality should be analyzed especially for these abscesses, but so far these data are not available for a significant number of cases.

Long-term Residua. Following successful treatment of brain abscess, 15 to 30 percent of individuals have paresis, while 10 to 20 percent have varying degrees of speech and language defects. Some postabscess disability may be expected in 30 to 50 percent of all patients, while 7 to 17 percent are totally disabled.[71] The quality of survival may be poorer in children,[71] but individuals who survive a cerebellar abscess may show surprisingly little disability.[69] Seizures occur in 15 to 55 percent of patients, but an even higher percentage may report seizures if they are followed for long periods of time.[71,72] Seizure development has been shown to be independent of the mode of surgical therapy and has its peak incidence four to five years after abscess occurrence and treatment. Because of this, anticonvulsants should be continued for five years after successful brain abscess therapy.

SUBDURAL ABSCESS (EMPYEMA)

Incidence and Pathogenesis

Subdural suppuration accounts for approximately 10 to 20 percent of all cases of intracranial abscess. Pus in the subdural space can be either loculated (subdural abscess) or diffuse (subdural empyema). In approximately 50 percent of cases, the subdural pus occurs as an empyema, spread widely over a hemisphere (Fig. 28-5). In the remaining half, the subdural abscess is a loculated, hemispherical convex mass (30 percent) in the interhemispheric fissure (10 percent) or in the posterior fossa (10 percent). Acute frontal sinusitis and chronic mastoid infections are the two most common antecedent causes.

The infecting bacteria may spread in a contiguous fashion from an infected sinus or bone to the adjacent dura and subdural space, or they may spread from the infected sinus to veins which lie within the subdural space. A septic thrombus forming in a cortical vein creates a nidus of infection that spreads in the subdural compartment, which has few boundaries.[73] Subdural empyema also may occur as a consequence of trauma, cavernous sinus thrombosis, partially treated meningitis, scalp infection, or infected cephalohematoma. In addition, a preexisting subdural hematoma may become infected as a result of concomitant sepsis or iatrogenically, as from needle aspirations.

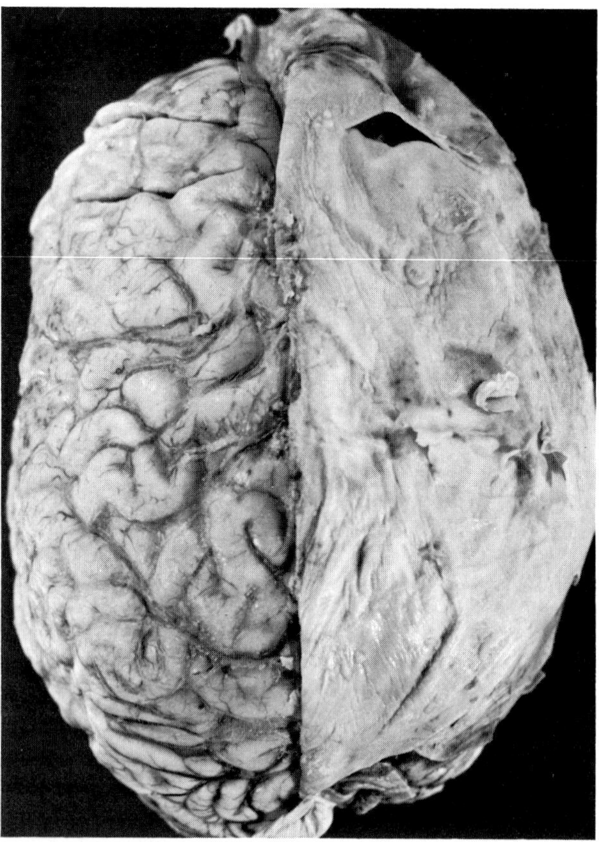

Fig. 28-5. Subdural empyema. This subdural empyema covered almost the entire left hemisphere. The thickened subdural membranes are adherent to the overlying dura and are reflected to the right. The leptomeninges covering the central portions of the left hemisphere are thickened. (Courtesy of Carlos Garcia, MD, State University Medical School, New Orleans, Louisiana.)

Etiology

Yoshikawa et al [74] have reviewed the bacteriology of subdural empyema, and the data showed that of 324 cases from the literature, 35 percent were caused by aerobic streptococci, 17 percent by staphylococci, 2 percent by pneumococci, and 12 percent by miscellaneous organisms. Interestingly, 12 percent of cases were caused by anaerobic organisms, while 27 percent of cultures were sterile. If the sterile cultures are assumed to be largely comprised of inadequately cultured anaerobic organisms, almost 40 percent of subdural infections are caused by anaerobes.

Clinical Manifestations

Local infection about the involved sinus, scalp, or skull may be evident early, but infection within the subdural space is heralded by intense generalized headache, fever, drowsiness, meningeal signs, and focal neurologic findings, such as jacksonian seizures, aphasia, or hemiparesis. Interhemispheric pus often produces a contralateral lower-monoparesis because it involves the medial portion of the motorstrip. Many clinicians fail to recognize subdural empyema as a complication of sinusitis and confuse subdural suppuration with aseptic meningitis or even viral encephalitis. Subdural infection is usually less fulminant than bacterial meningitis but more rapidly progressive than a brain abscess. In bacterial meningitis, focal signs are rare, and preceding sinus or mastoid infection need not be present. Clinically, the differentiation between subdural abscess and brain abscess may be quite difficult. Subdural abscess and brain abscess may be present concomitantly, but for some unknown reason this is uncommon.

Diagnosis

The cerebrospinal fluid usually contains only a few hundred cells per mm^3, the protein is elevated, glucose is near normal, and the fluid is sterile. Roentgenograms usually demonstrate sinus or mastoid infection. They may show a focus of osteomyelitis about the involved sinus or, possibly, of the skull itself if this is the underlying source of infection.

Plain CAT scans may show unilateral ventricular displacement, while enhanced scans usually demonstrate a dense curvilinear line separated from the inner surface of the skull, supposedly representing the cortical surface or inner membrane surrounding the subdural pus. Isodense subdural empyemas have been missed on CAT scanning, however, so this technique is not infallible. Angiography remains an excellent diagnostic tool to demonstrate the subdural or interhemispheric pus collection. If one is concerned about a frontal subdural abscess (consequent to frontal sinusitis), oblique arteriograms may be necessary to clearly demonstrate the frontal poles.

Treatment

Subdural empyema represents a neurosurgical emergency. Early drainage is essential because antibiotics may not eradicate the infection. The rapid accumulation of subdural pus can dangerously increase intracranial pressure. Once the diagnosis is suspected, large doses of broad-spectrum antibiotics (penicillin, methicillin, and chloramphenicol) should be started, and the patient should be prepared for operation. Some surgeons drain the pus via multiple burr holes placed over the area of infection, while others prefer limited craniectomies or even large craniotomy flaps to expose widely the subdural suppuration. Areas of subdural abscess are copiously irrigated with such antibiotic solutions as bacitracin (500 units per ml). Extreme care should be exercised to protect the arachnoid membrane to prevent subarachnoid spread of the infection. Some surgeons prefer to irrigate and drain the subdural space postoperatively.

When an interhemispheric subdural abscess is suspected, the head should be draped, allowing trephinations or craniectomies to be performed parasagitally from front to back, so that the entire interhemispheric region may be inspected, drained, and irrigated with antibiotic solution. Inspection of the area must be thorough, because any undetected, undrained pus pockets may lead to a continuance of the intracranial infection.

When osteomyelitis of the frontal sinus is present, the infected bone should be removed. The frontal sinus must be completely exenterated at the same time. When the skull and inner sinus wall appear intact, the infected sinus should be drained by an otolaryngologist. Mastoid infection is treated in the same manner. It is axiomatic that the underlying infective focus must be properly treated to prevent abscess recurrence. The subdural fluid should be Gram stained at the time of operation to aid in the choices of antibiotics. A specimen of pus should be sent for aerobic and anaerobic cultures and sensitivities so that more specific antibiotics may be given.

Prognosis

In the preantibiotic era, almost all patients died.[73,75] Even now, the overall mortality rate is between 25 and 30 percent (Table 28-6) because diagnosis is frequently delayed, and the course of the disease can be fulminating. I am hopeful that more widespread availability of computer scanning will increase the rate of diagnosis and contribute to a lowered death rate.

OSTEOMYELITIS OF THE SKULL

Osteomyelitis of the skull is frequently associated with an overlying subgaleal infection and an underlying epidural abscess. A subgaleal infection may spread directly or via vascular channels to contiguous structures and result in osteomyelitis of the skull, epidural or subdural infection, or brain abscess.

Osteomyelitis of the skull may result from direct spread of infection from sinus or mastoid suppuration, from open skull fractures from penetrating skull wounds, or via hematogenous spread from another infective focus. Osteomyelitis following open skull fracture is usually caused by inadequate initial treatment of the skin or underlying bone. In such cases, the edges of the fracture may contain minute foreign bodies, hair, or other contaminated debris. Closure of a scalp laceration without adequate debridement and irrigation may result in residual devitalized tissue or foreign bodies being left behind, which may cause local scalp infection and eventual osteomyelitis or intracranial infection.

Clinical Manifestations

When patients have osteomyelitis of the skull, pain, erythema, swelling, and tenderness are present about the

TABLE 28-6. MORTALITY ASSOCIATED WITH SUBDURAL EMPYEMA

Author	Year	Total Surgical Cases	Deaths	Percent Mortality
Schiller, Cairns, Russell [75]	1948	10 *	3	30
Botterell, Drake [45]	1952	10	0	0
Stern, Boldrey [76]	1952	16 *	7	44
Wood [77]	1952	11 *	4	36
Gurdjian, Webster [49]	1957	6	0	0
Hitchcock, Andreadis [78]	1964	26 *	7	27
Bhandari, Sarkari [79]	1970	37 *	12	34
Weinman, Samarasinghe [80]	1972	47 *	12	26
Le Beau et al [61]	1973	37	15	40
Anagnostopoulos, Gortvai [81]	1973	32	5	16
Farmer, Wise [82]	1973	14 *	4	29
Galbraith, Barr [83]	1974	14 *	2	14
van Alphen, Dreissen [42]	1976	16	4	25
Joubert, Stephanov [11]	1977	7	2	28
TOTAL	1948–1977	283	77	27

* Series devoted exclusively to subdural empyema.

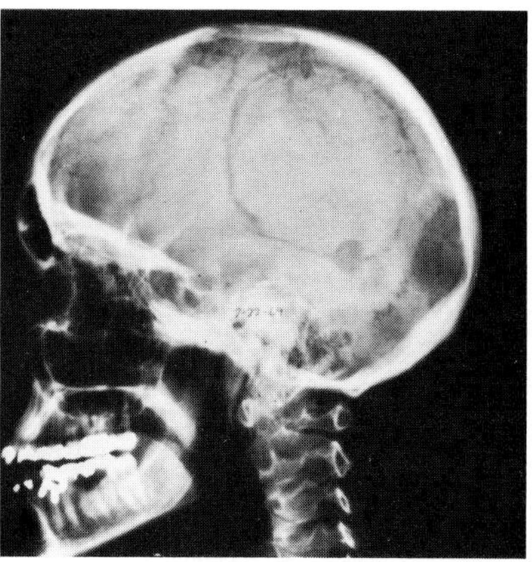
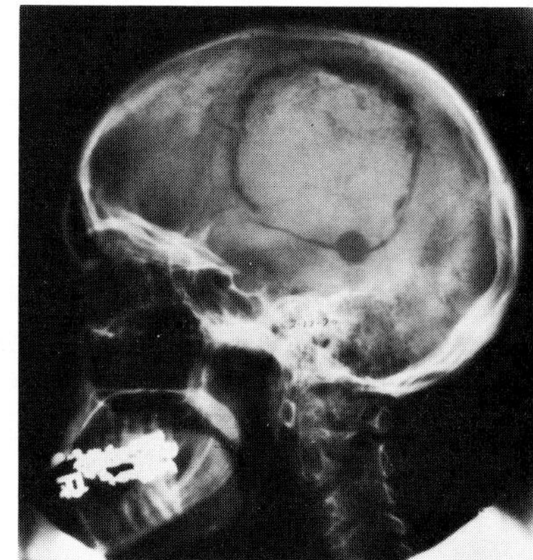
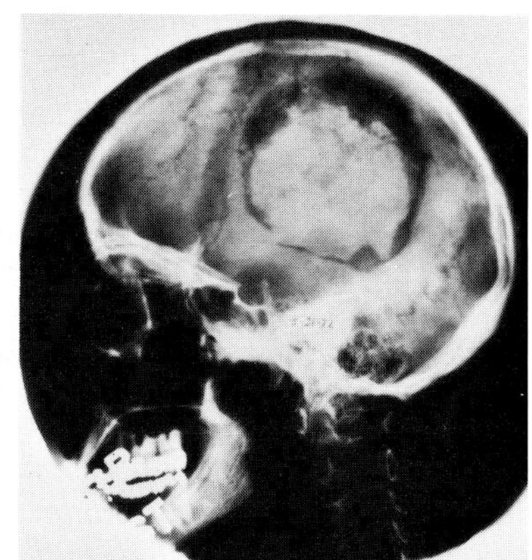

Fig. 28-6. **Osteomyelitis of the skull after craniotomy for glioma. Normal postoperative base line (left). Progressively enlarging areas of bone destruction involving margins of the bone flap (middle, right). (Courtesy of Lawrence H. A. Gold, MD, and Mathis P. Frick, MD, University of Minnesota.)**

area of infection. The patient is usually febrile. Focal neurologic signs, such as mental confusion, paresis, or convulsions, may supervene if the bone infection spreads to the epidural or subdural spaces or the brain itself.

Diagnosis

Roentgenograms of the skull can show clouding of an involved sinus, but the typical moth-eaten appearance of osteomyelitis usually takes several weeks to appear. In the interim, the involved bone may only appear radiolucent or trabeculated (Fig. 28-6). Radioactive bone scanning will, however, detect osteomyelitis before it is visible on skull roentgenogram.

Treatment

Treatment should begin with massive antibiotic therapy to cover a broad spectrum of organisms. Surgical therapy consists of removing the infected bone. Wide excision of necrotic bone is preferred, but the periosteum should be left intact so that new bone may regenerate. Infected sinuses should be exenterated, and the wound may be closed without drainage. When present, an epidural abscess should be drained, and the dura should be inspected carefully for evidence of penetration into the subdural space. Generally, the dura should not be opened if subdural spread has not occurred. If one feels compelled to inspect the subdural space when not completely sure that subdural spread has occurred, new, sterile surgical instruments should be used, and the dural incision should be made away from the area of epidural pus. After evacuation of an epidural abscess, drains may be left in the epidural space for a few days.

INTRACRANIAL TUBERCULOMAS

The incidence of intracranial tuberculomas varies according to the prevalance of tuberculosis in the community (Table 28-7).[84-90] Thirty-two to 50 percent of patients with intracranial tuberculomas are less than 10 years of age, while approximately 85 percent are younger than 25.[86,89] Tuberculomas may occur anywhere in the brain, but affected children have a high incidence of infratentorial lesions.

Pathology

Grossly, a mature tuberculoma presents as a well-defined avascular mass with multiple nodular extensions and a yellowish, gritty, caseating central core (Fig. 28-7A). In its immature form, it consists of multiple small tubercles with caseating or cystic centers surrounded by edematous brain. Over half become adherent to the dura. Microscopically, the central core of caseous necrosis is surrounded by tuberculous granulation tissue consisting of epithelioid cells, Langhans' giant cells, lymphocytes, polymorphonu-

TABLE 28-7. INCIDENCE OF INTRACRANIAL TUBERCULOSIS IN VARIOUS SURGICAL SERIES

Author	Country	Year	No. Intracranial Mass Lesions	No. Tuberculomas	Percent Tuberculomas
Vincent [84]	France	1938	1,248	34	2.5
Arsenjo [85]	Chile	1951	610	97	16
Arseni [86]	Rumania	1958	2,757	201	7.3
Katsura [87]	Japan	1959	3,094	80	2.6
Obrador [88]	Spain	1959	1,300	47	3.6
Dastur [89]	India	1963	373	114	30.5
Mathai [90]	India	1967	1,487	143	10
Dastur [89]	India	1972	201	32	15.6

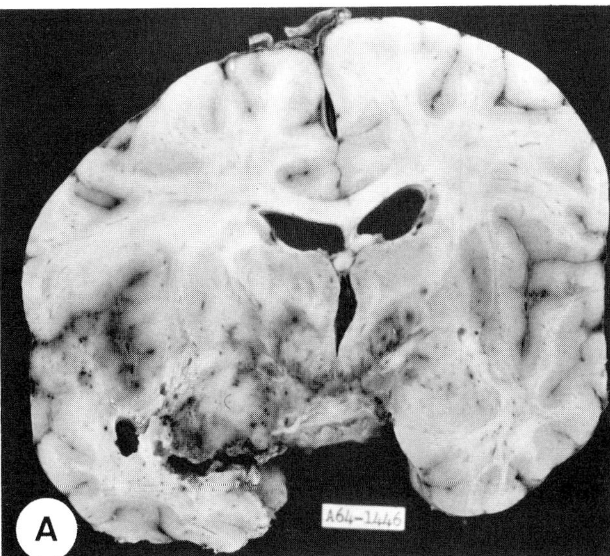

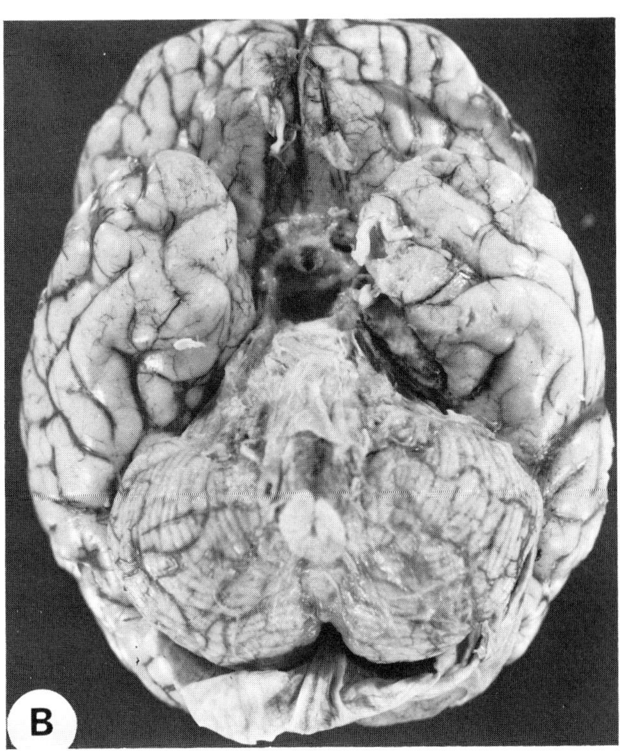

Fig. 28-7. **Tuberculosis. A. Hemorrhage and necrosis from widespread tubercular involvement of the brain. B. Basilar meningitis with widespread involvement of the cranial nerves. The basilar adhesions may also obstruct flow of cerebrospinal fluid and cause hydrocephalus and increased intracranial pressure. (Courtesy of Carlos Garcia, MD, State University Medical School, New Orleans, Louisiana.)**

clear cells, and plasma cells. Acid-fast bacilli may be seen in either layer. The surrounding brain shows degenerated nerve cells and fibers, swollen astrocytes, and oligodendroglia, as well as thrombosed vessels and multiple microinfarcts. Though rare, frank tuberculous abscess resembling a pyogenic abscess occasionally occurs.[91,92] Several cysic tuberculomas resembling a glioma have also been observed.[89] Tuberculomas of the brain are most often multiple.

Clinical Manifestations and Diagnosis

Patients with intracranial tuberculomas have evidence of the disease elsewhere or have had tuberculosis. Fever of a few weeks duration usually precedes the onset of neurologic findings. Tuberculomas in children often occur in the posterior fossa. Children, therefore, often give evidence of a posterior fossa mass—headaches, nausea, vomiting, papilledema, nystagmus, ataxia, and separated cranial sutures or an enlarging head. If the tuberculoma is supratentorial the neurologic findings will depend upon its location. Convulsions are common.

Definitive neuroradiologic diagnostic studies are indicated prior to operation because tuberculomas are often multiple, and the lesion causing increased intracranial pressure may not actually be the one that brings the patient in for medical treatment (eg, a small tuberculoma about the motor strip causing focal seizures in association with a large silent frontal tuberculoma causing intracranial hypertension). CAT scanning is the ideal diagnostic procedure, but it may be unavailable in developing nations where intracerebral tuberculomas are most common. Plain skull roentgenograms, electroencephalography, angiography, and ventriculography are still useful. Approximately 5 percent of intracranial tuberculomas calcify, but even if a calcified tuberculoma is seen, further contrast studies are indicated to identify all intracranial lesions. Angiographically, a tuberculoma presents as an avascular mass. Vessels in the vicinity may show a reduced caliber, and the midline shift may be small relative to the size of the tuberculoma. Tuberculomas near the surface may occasionally show a blush from meningeal or cortical vessels. Ventriculography may be used to identify space-occupying tuberculomas, particularly in the posterior fossa. This test is also used to evaluate hydrocephalus or the occurrence of tuberculomas following tuberculous meningitis.

Treatment

Specific antituberculosis drugs have made successful operations of intracranial tuberculomas possible. Total excision of the tuberculoma is preferred, but partial excision may be done when large tuberculomas impinge upon vital structures, such as the brain stem,[86,88,89] In such cases, a rim of tuberculoma may be left adjacent to the brain.

All surgeons give various combinations of streptomycin, para-aminosalicylic acid, and isoniazid before, during, and after operation (Chapter 18). Occasionally, medical therapy alone has brought about clinical amelioration, but clearly this course is not without inherent risks, especially in populations who may not understand their disease and who may not continue taking antituberculosis medicines. On the other hand, medical treatment alone may be best for tuberculomas of the brain stem or basal ganglia (Fig. 28-7B).

Prognosis

Prior to the use of streptomycin, the operative mortality was 10 percent, and subsequent mortality from tuberculous meningitis ranged from 40 to 75 percent.[86,88] Radical

TABLE 28-8. SURGICAL MORTALITY OF INTRACRANIAL TUBERCULOMAS

Author	Year	No. of Cases	Deaths	% Mortality
Arseni [86]	1958	124	17	14
Obrador [88]	1959	32	6	19
Mathai [90]	1967	143		16–27
Dastur [89]	1965	108	8	7
Dastur [89]	1972	224	23	10

operations resulted in an 85 percent mortality.[86] Now, surgical mortality ranges from 6 to 27 percent, and the mortality from postoperative tuberculous meningitis is 6 percent [7,88,89] (Table 28-8).

HERPES SIMPLEX ENCEPHALITIS

Etiology and Pathology

Two antigenically different strains of herpesviruses have been identified (Chapter 10). Type 1 herpesvirus is almost invariably associated with sporadic encephalitis. Type 2 causes neonatal encephalitis, which is frequently related to maternal genital infection. The latter strain also may cause a benign form of meningitis or radiculitis in adults.[93]

Herpes is probably the most frequent cause of sporadic viral infection with severe sequelae in the United States.[93-96] Pathologically, perivascular lymphocytic infiltration is seen, along with severe necrosis of the medial temporal lobes and orbital frontal lobes. Type A Cowdry eosinophilic inclusions are seen in both neurons and glia.[96,97] On electron microscopy, herpesvirus particles may be seen within affected cells.[93] Often, severe temporal lobe swelling accompanies the infection, and this swelling may be large enough to cause a significant intracranial mass lesion. Other areas of the brain are involved less often.[98]

Clinical Manifestations and Diagnosis

Clinically, the disease is manifest by headache, drowsiness, fever, seizures, and focal neurologic signs. Paradoxically, meningeal signs are not prominent. These findings may be seen with many types of encephalitis, but herpes infection is characterized by prominent psychologic symptoms early in the disease (global confusion, disorientation, clouding of consciousness, and hallucinations, particularly olfactory and gustatory) because of the predilection for the temporal lobe.[97] Early and accurate diagnosis of herpes is paramount because the disease has a high mortality, neurologic sequelae are severe, and treatment is available. Roentgenographic findings are normal, but radionuclide brain scan results may be positive because of the breakdown of the blood-brain barrier consequent to the infection. CAT scanning reveals low density in the involved areas. The EEG usually demonstrates high-voltage, sharp waves in the temporal area.[93] Fluorescent antibodies of the herpesvirus antigen and a passive hemagglutinating antibody may be demonstrated in the cerebrospinal fluid.[95] A brain biopsy (usually of the temporal lobe) is considered necessary for accurate diagnosis. When temporal lobe swelling becomes life threatening, temporal lobe resection may also be necessary.

Treatment

The mortality is quite high. Whitley et al [99] reported that 70 percent of untreated patients died. The mortality of herpes can be reduced to 28 percent by adenine arabinoside (Ara-A, Vidarabine).[99-101] Despite the availability of fairly adequate immunologic and cytologic means of diagnosis, Whitley feels that brain biopsy should be performed prior to the start of therapy.[99] If the biopsy culture is positive for the virus, a full 10-day course of treatment is given. If biopsy results are negative (encephalitis being caused by another virus), treatment with adenine arabinoside should be stopped in 5 days. Despite the favorable influence on mortality in several series, neurologic sequelae can be severe in survivors.

BACTERIAL ANEURYSMS

Subarachnoid hemorrhage can be caused by bacterial (mycotic) aneurysms [102,103] involving the intracranial blood vessels. These aneurysms usually occur with bacterial endocarditis, wherein a septic embolus from an infected heart valve lodges in an intracranial artery. This produces infection and necrosis in the arterial wall, which leads to vascular dilatation and possible rupture. Occasionally, a bacterial aneurysm will develop in association with meningitis. Bacterial aneurysms are usually found on distal branches of the middle or anterior cerebrospinal arteries. They can be multiple, and occasionally on serial arteriograms, additional aneurysms may be observed to develop.

The treatment of bacterial aneurysms has been both medical and surgical. According to Bingham's collected series,[103] 3 of 20 patients treated with antibiotics alone died, while 6 of 25 treated by antibiotics plus operation died. Many deaths in the latter group, however, were patients who were poor surgical risks, who had cardiac failure, or who succumbed to their underlying infection.

Bingham's conclusion was that serial arteriograms (every two to three weeks) were necessary. Antibiotic treatment alone may suffice for a mycotic aneurysm that is shown to disappear on serial angiograms. If, on repeated studies, a bacterial aneurysm has increased in size, an operation should be undertaken. If the aneurysm has not receded after antibiotic therapy, it should also be operated upon. Postoperative angiography always should be performed to make sure that no new lesions have developed.

CENTRAL NERVOUS SYSTEM CONDITIONS SIMULATING INFECTION [104,105]

Occasionally, acute demyelinating disease, brain tumors, or bleeding will incite a severe leptomeningeal inflammatory reaction. Extension of malignant conditions into the meninges can also incite such meningitic signs and symptoms as headache, fever, nausea, vomiting, and stiff neck. Several types of brain tumors (eg, dermoids or tumors abutting onto the ventricular or subarachnoid spaces) have presented as inflammatory central nervous system diseases.

When cases of purulent meningitis occur and bacteria cannot be identified, it becomes essential to look for other causes of cerebrospinal fluid pleocytosis—fungal, viral, amebic, neoplastic, or degenerative. The spinal fluid should be examined for fungi, amebas, malignant cells, blood, and fat. A CAT scan or arteriogram should be done to evaluate all suspected intracranial processes.

SPINAL INFECTIONS

PYOGENIC VERTEBRAL OSTEOMYELITIS

Pyogenic vertebral osteomyelitis most commonly follows pelvic or urinary infections,[106] as bacteria from the primary site metastasize to the vertebral column, either by arteries or via the veins of Batson's plexus. Vertebral osteomyelitis occasionally follows spinal surgery as well.[107] Osteomyelitis in adults has a predilection for the vertebral bodies because of the increased vascularity of these bones.[106] Generally, more than one vertebra is involved, and the body is affected more commonly than the posterior elements. The lumbar and thoracic areas are most frequently infected.[106,107] Pus from an infected vertebra may form a paravertebral abscess or, more importantly, an epidural collection that may compress neural structures. Collapse of a vertebral body may result in gibbus formation and impingement upon the spinal cord or cauda equina as well. Either epidural pus or bony collapse may lead to paralysis. In one series,[108] 3 of 28 patients with vertebral body infection subsequently developed paralysis. *S. aureus* has been the most common organism responsible for vertebral osteomyelitis,[106,107] but gram-negative organisms have also been implicated.[106,108] *Pseudomonas aeruginosa* has frequently been isolated from vertebral osteomyelitis among heroin addicts.[109]

Vertebral osteomyelitis in children usually has an abrupt onset of malaise, fever, back pain, and spine tenderness, and diagnosis in these cases is usually easy. In adults, however, the onset of symptoms is usually gradual, and up to three months may be required to make the diagnosis.[107] Little or no fever is present, and patients usually have no malaise. Back pain occurs about two thirds of the time. This is more likely if the mobile cervical and lumbar areas are afflicted rather than the fixed, thoracic spine. Usually, point tenderness to palpation is evident at the involved site. In adults, the leukocyte count is seldom raised, but the erythrocyte sedimentation rate is usually elevated. Some authors [107] have noted an association of vertebral osteomyelitis with diabetes, but others have not.[108]

Roentgenographic findings lag behind pathologic changes, signs, and symptoms by six to eight weeks.[106] These findings consist of rarefaction, loss of bony trabeculation close to the cartilaginous plate, and narrowing of the vertebral disc space (Fig. 28-8A). Bony collapse may also be present. Simultaneously, evidence of rapid bone regeneration occurs with the development of bone spurs and dense new bone. More than one vertebral body usually shows these changes.

Treatment of uncomplicated vertebral osteomyelitis consists of bed rest and immobilization, along with antibiotic therapy. Needle aspiration of the involved vertebra is mandatory to obtain material for culture and antibiotic sensitivities. Traction may prove a useful adjunct for cervical osteomyelitis to prevent bony collapse. Significant paravertebral abscesses may require drainage. Should the spinal cord be compressed by epidural pus or gibbus, decompression of the spinal cord will be necessary either by laminectomy or by an anterior or lateral approach.

PYOGENIC SPINAL EPIDURAL ABSCESS

Pyogenic spinal epidural abscess is a relatively rare but neurologically devastating disease, which is quite amenable to drainage. In two United States hospitals, the incidence was between 0.2 and 1.2 per 10,000 admissions from 1947 to 1974.[110] Acute or chronic forms have been described depending upon whether the clinical course evolves over a few days or several weeks.[111] Either may arise from hematogenous spread or from adjacent vertebral osteomyelitis (Fig. 28-8B).

Etiology and Pathogenesis

Skin infections are the most common antecedent distant source.[110-112] *S. aureus* has been the most common infecting organism, but streptococci and gram-negative bacteria from preexistent urinary tract infections may also be found fairly frequently.[110,111] Spinal trauma occurring just before the onset of symptoms has been reported in 10 to 40 percent of patients, but its significance is difficult to assess unless small, clinically insignificant traumatic hematomas subsequently become colonized with bacteria.[110,111,113]

Most epidural spinal abscesses involve the dorsal aspect of the spinal dura in the thoracic region. The dura is closely approximated to the vertebral bodies anteriorly, and the epidural fat, which is susceptible to bacterial invasion, lies dorsally.[110,111] Anterior epidural abscesses were found, however, in 7 of 39 cases reviewed by Baker et al.[110] In the acute hematogenous case, granulation tissue admixed with pus extends axially over an average of four spinal segments. Chronic epidural abscesses tend to have a more extensive axial spread than do acute lesions. The dura itself is resistant to bacterial penetration, and spread of infection to the subdural or subarachnoid spaces from the epidural focus is rare.

Intuitively, one would imagine that the space-occupying effect of the epidural pus compromises the spinal cord by pressure. Often, however, the neurologic involvement appears out of proportion to any observed pressure effects, and it has been proposed that the neurologic sequelae result from epidural arterial or venous thrombosis with resultant spinal cord infarction.[114]

Clinical Manifestations

Individuals with acute abscesses are febrile and septic, while those with chronic abscesses are afebrile and may appear relatively well. All spinal epidural abscesses evolve through four clinical stages: (1) focal spinal pain and tenderness, (2) root pain, (3) paresis, and (4) paralysis.[111,112] In the acute case, this sequence of events occurs over an average of seven days, while chronic cases may take several weeks or months. Once paresis ensues, however, total paralysis generally occurs within 24 hours.[112] *Because the ultimate quality of neurologic recovery varies inversely with the degree and duration of paresis or paralysis, spinal epidural abscess is a true neurosurgical emergency. Immediate operative decompression is mandatory.*

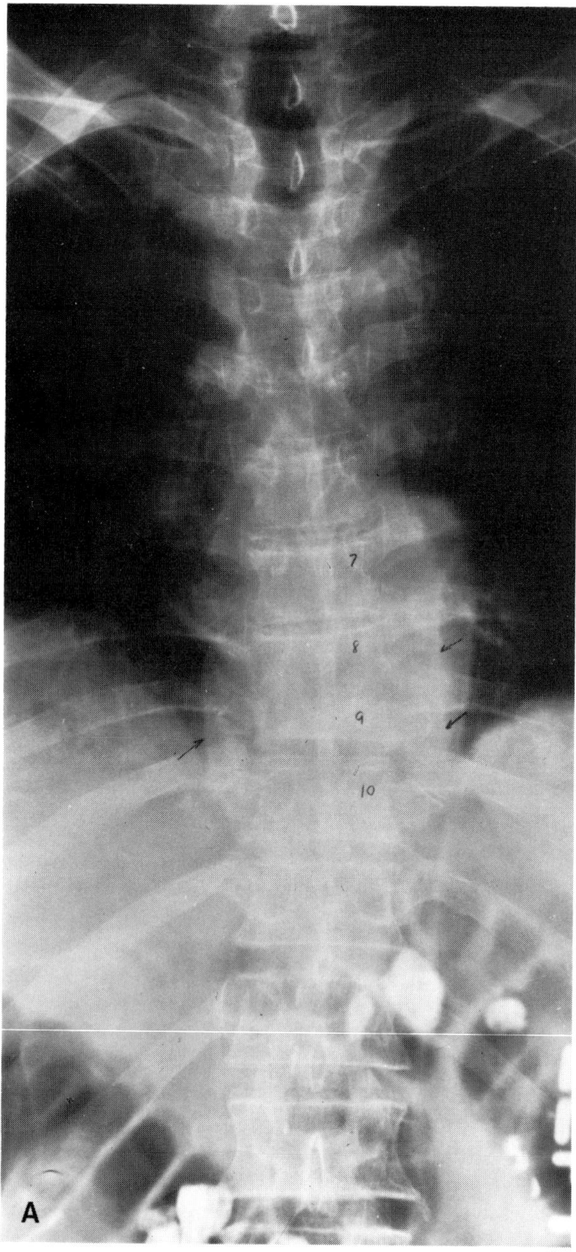

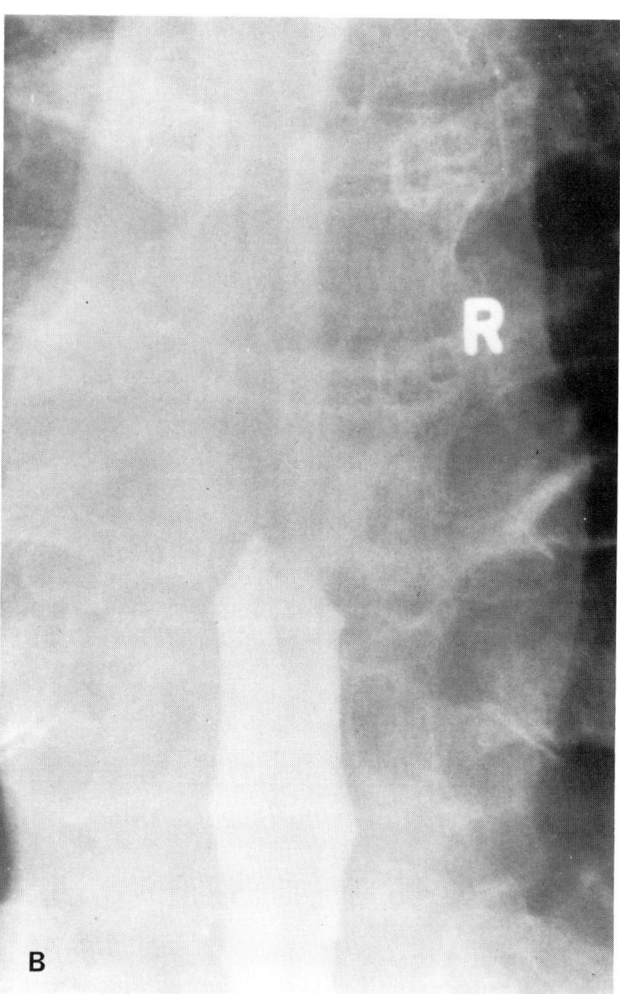

Fig. 28-8. **A. Pyogenic osteomyelitis of thoracic spine. Destruction of the inferior aspect of the body of T-8 and superior aspect of the body of T-9. The intervening disc space has been lost, and the two vertebrae are irregularly compressed together. Note paravertebral mass (arrows). B. Myelography shows complete extradural block at level T-8/T-9. (Courtesy of Lawrence H. A. Gold, MD, and Mathis P. Frick, MD, University of Minnesota.)**

If an individual has the classic clinical syndrome plus carious vertebral elements on plain roentgenograms, the diagnosis and approximate locus will be evident. In the acute metastatic case, however, no osteomyelitis will be evident, and while the diagnosis may be suspected, the exact area of involvement may be in question. In either case, but particularly in the acute case, myelography is indicated in order to delineate the rostral and caudal spread of epidural pus (Fig. 28-8B). Contrast medium may be put in above and below the lesion, the extent of the lesion may be outlined, and the most efficient operative approach may be planned. Care must be taken when advancing the spinal needle not to introduce bacteria from the epidural to the subarachnoid space.

The differential diagnosis of spinal epidural abscess includes meningitis, spinal subdural abscess, acute transverse myelopathy, herniated intervertebral disc, vascular lesions, and spinal canal or cord tumors.

Treatment

Antibiotics should be started as soon as the diagnosis is suspected while the patient is being prepared for operation. Intravenous penicillin, methicillin, and chloramphenicol should be given to completely cover the likely bacterial flora. At operation, a specimen of pus or granulation tissue should be obtained for a Gram stain and aerobic, anaerobic, and mycobacterial cultures and sensitivities. Once the specific organism is identified and its sensitivities determined, a specific antimicrobial agent may be selected for further therapy.

All free pus in the epidural space is drained by a generous laminectomy, and the epidural space is irrigated with saline containing antibiotics (eg, penicillin, methicillin, and chloramphenicol). Hulme and Dott[112] recommend excision of chronic granulation tissue to prevent subsequent dural stricture by scar tissue. In the series of Baker et al,[110] when chronic epidural abscesses were found, the laminectomy wound was closed primarily without difficulty. When acute pyogenic epidural abscess was found, the wound was either packed open for subsequent secondary closure or was loosely closed over soft irrigation catheters that could be used to irrigate the epidural space with antibiotic solution in the postoperative phase.[110]

Acute hematogenous abscesses are not usually associated with vertebral body destruction and spinal instability. If vertebral osteomyelitis coexists with body collapse and gibbus formation has occurred, or if spinal instability is present because of the infection, orthopedic measures are subsequently indicated to stabilize the spine.

Prognosis

Before the use of antibiotics, the mortality for epidural abscess ranged from about 30–90 percent.[111,112] Recent mortality approximates 18 percent. In general, the neurologic outcome depends upon the degree of cord function remaining prior to drainage. Those patients with no paresis or with weakness of less than 36 hours' duration make excellent neurologic recoveries. Those who have been paralyzed for longer than 48 hours make no neurologic recovery. Recently, Baker et al reported on the outcome with aggressive diagnosis and neurosurgery, of 32 patients who survived their epidural abscesses: 4 were permanently paralyzed, while 5 had paresis, and 23 were neurologically intact following drainage.

INTRAMEDULLARY PYOGENIC SPINAL CORD ABSCESS

The incidence of intramedullary spinal cord abscesses[112,115] approximates 1 per 40,000 autopsies. The peak incidence is in the first and third decades, and males are more commonly affected than females. The thoracic region of the spinal cord is most commonly infected. Among 55 reported cases,[115] 42 individuals had a single intramedullary abscess, and the remainder had multiple abscesses. A variety of culture results were obtained, including *Staphylococcus, Streptococcus,* actinomycosis, gram-negative organisms, *S. pneumoniae,* multiple organisms, sterile.

Antecedent infections in the respiratory tract, spine (including fractures), heart valves, genitourinary tract, soft tissues, and midline spinal skin defects, such as dermoid sinus, are present in 80 percent of patients. No apparent infective focus can be found in the rest. Bacteria can reach the spinal cord by (1) direct implantation secondary to trauma, (2) the hematogenous route, or (3) lymphatics from the retropharyngeal space, mediastinum, or abdominal cavity that course along spinal nerves and communicate with the subarachnoid space and Virchow-Robin spaces.

Acute intramedullary abscesses are typical of other central nervous system abscesses. They lack the widespread venous infarction seen with epidural abscesses, which may account for their often favorable prognosis.

Clinically, intramedullary abscesses can have acute, subacute, or chronic courses. The neurologic symptoms and signs vary according to abscess location. Acute cases have fever and transverse myelitis. Pain in the neck or back, urinary incontinence, dysesthesias, and monoparesis that progress to paraparesis or quadraparesis typically occur. Patients with chronic intramedullary abscesses have a stuttering course which simulates that of a spinal tumor. Examination of the cerebrospinal fluid is generally unrewarding, and the presence of white blood cells may suggest meningitis. Myelography demonstrates a spinal block and an intraspinal mass.

An intramedullary spinal abscess should be thoroughly incised and drained following an appropriate laminectomy. Occasionally, an intraspinal abscess will masquerade as arachnoiditis. Therefore when localized spinal arachnoiditis is discovered during a laminectomy, the surgeon must make sure that no cord abscess is present. Because of the high recurrence rate the patients should be followed closely for a long time. Twenty of the 55 patients had the abscesses drained. Five patients died, all before the advent of antibiotics. Six patients recovered neurologically, six were improved, but three remained unchanged.[115]

As with all abscesses, antibiotics (penicillin, methicillin, or chloramphenicol) should be started as soon as infection is recognized. The pus should be Gram-stained and cultured for aerobic, anaerobic, and acid-fast bacteria, as well as fungi, so that specific antimicrobial drugs can be given.

PARASPINAL TUBERCULOSIS

Tuberculous Spondylitis (Pott's Paraplegia)

Tuberculous destruction of the spine, with subsequent spinal cord compression, is a common finding in persons in developing nations. Mathai and Chandy[90] indicated that 42 percent of their spinal operations for nontraumatic paraplegias were for compression consequent to tuberculous spondylitis. In the United States, this disease is rare. Tuberculous spondylitis most frequently involves the lower thoracic and upper lumbar vertebrae. Usually more than one vertebra is affected, and the disease most commonly affects the vertebral body. Neurologic complications occur in 10 to 25 percent of patients, particularly if the thoracic spine is involved. Pott's paraplegia has been divided into early-onset cases, where the neurologic dysfunction starts within two years of the tuberculous spondylitis, and late-onset paraplegia which occurs after this time. Early cases occur when the disease is active, while late cases are associated with a recurrence or persistence of the infection despite apparent quiescence.

In general, the disease starts in the first decade of life, but the diagnosis is most frequently made during the patient's third decade, when neurologic complications are seen. No distinctive pattern of neurologic signs or symptoms exists with Pott's disease.[116] The primary neurologic manifestations are paraparesis or quadraparesis caused by upper motor neuron dysfunction. Pain and local spine tenderness occur in over 70 percent of patients. Radicular and referred pains also occur, as do sphincter disturbances and impotence. The actual cause of the cord compression may be epidural infection, bony compression, or both.

Radiographically, early decalcification is often seen about the disc or anteriorly with slight diminution of the disc space. Later, frank vertebral erosion and collapse are seen, and paravertebral or psoas abscesses may appear. Sclerotic changes also may be present because of concomitant bone regeneration and fusion of vertebral bodies. Scalloping of the anterior vertebral border may be seen from caseation occurring under the anterior spinal ligament (Fig. 28-9). Myelography can sometimes reveal a block at the infection site.

Spinal tuberculosis can be treated medically or surgically. Friedman[117] treated 64 patients with Pott's disease by prolonged administration of antituberculous drugs, bed rest, and braces. Spinal fusion was not done, and laminectomy was reserved for 8 patients with paresis from spinal cord involvement. Fifty patients were cured by this approach, but 10 others had relapses, and 4 others died. Hodgson and Stock,[118] on the other hand, have long been strong advocates of direct operative attack on tuberculous vertebrae. The diseased bone is approached anteriorly or laterally and curetted away. Granulation tissue around the dura is stripped away, and the vertebral bodies are stabilized by strut grafts. This approach has had beneficial effects on concomitant paralysis. In 1960, Hodgson and Stock reported 35 paralyzed patients, of which 26 made complete neurologic recoveries after operation. There were graft complications (slips, fractures, angulations) in 13 patients, and 4 others died. Several years later, Hodgson and his colleagues stated that 19 of 23 paretic children made complete neurologic recoveries following decompression and fusion, as did 17 of 20 who had been completely paralyzed.[119] Antituberculous drugs are given for at least 18 months after operation. It would appear that Hodgson's patients had much more serious bony and neurologic involvement than did Friedman's patients.

Tuli[120] reported on the results of aggressive medical and surgical therapy in 200 cases of spinal tuberculosis. Medical treatment for adults consisted of daily intramuscular injections of 1 gm of streptomycin for 3 months, sodium para-aminosalicylate 12 gm daily in divided doses for 18 months, and isoniazid 300 mg daily for 24 months. Rest on a hard bed or plaster jacket was enforced. Gradual mobilization of the patient in a spinal brace was begun after 6 to 9 months. Paravertebral abscesses were aspirated or drained. Decompression of the cord was eventually performed on the patients who failed to show progressive recovery of neurologic function on the medical treatment. Tuli's data indicate that 94 percent of patients who have spinal tuberculous without neural involvement make a satisfactory recovery without operation. Thirty-eight percent of those with neurologic involvement recovered without operation.

Spinal Tuberculosis

Tuberculosis may involve the dura, arachnoid, or spinal cord, in addition to the vertebral column.[89,90,121]

Spinal Cord

Intramedullary spinal tuberculomas are rare. Tuberculosis of the brain occurs 30 to 100 times as commonly as that of the spinal cord.[86,89,90] Dastur[89] reported that of six excised spinal tuberculomas, three made good neurologic recoveries.

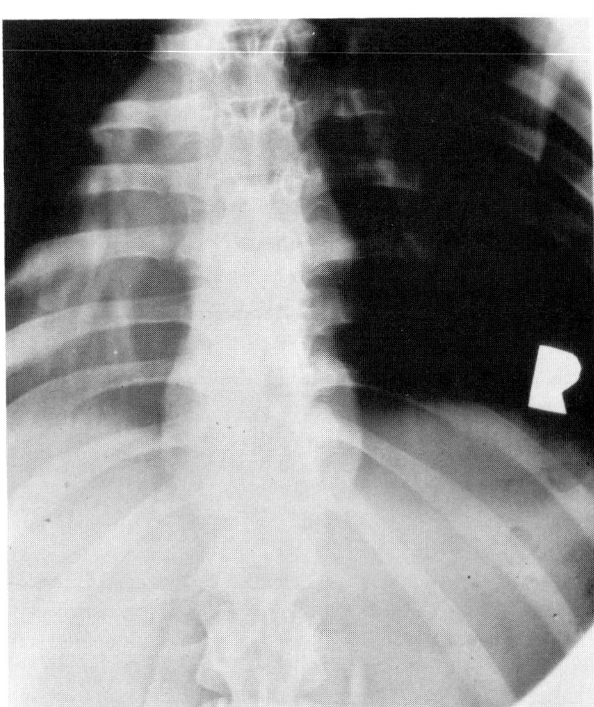

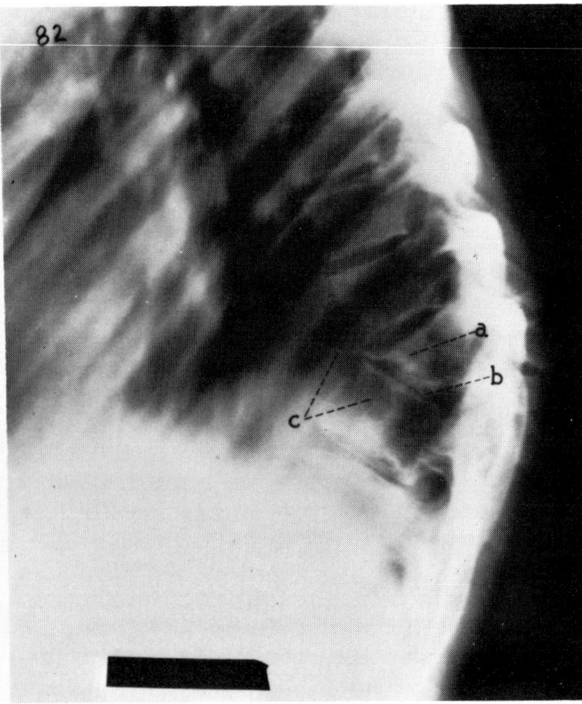

Fig. 28-9. **Tuberculosis of the spine with destructive (c) and sclerotic (a) changes of vertebral body. Note paravertebral soft tissue abscess and kyphosis. The vertebral interspace is maintained longer than in pyogenic infection (b). (Courtesy of Lawrence H. A. Gold, MD, and Mathis P. Frick, MD, University of Minnesota.)**

Tuberculomas Involving the Meninges

Tuberculous disease can transgress all anatomic planes from the bony vertebrae to the pia arachnoid, but often the disease is discrete and confined to one anatomic plane only.[121] Besides an intramedullary location, spinal tuberculomas can occur in the extradural or subdural spaces. Additionally, paraplegia can result from tuberculous arachnoiditis or from an associated vasculitis.

While Pott's paraplegia with its bony abnormalities may be fairly easily recognized, a tuberculoma of the spinal canal that is unaccompanied by bony changes is much more difficult to diagnose. In areas where tuberculosis is endemic, the onset of gradual spinal cord findings can reasonably be ascribed to a tubercular process. In more advanced countries, however, spinal cord tumor, epidural metastases, abscess, and multiple sclerosis are more likely diagnoses. When spinal cord findings occur in indigent individuals, immigrants, or those having recently had tuberculosis, an intraspinal tubercular lesion should be considered.

SPECIFIC BACTERIAL AND FUNGAL INFECTIONS OF THE CENTRAL NERVOUS SYSTEM

Fungal infections of the central nervous system occur sporadically among normal individuals. More commonly, however, they are found in the debilitated, the diabetic, or the immunocompromised person. Transplant recipients, therefore, are particularly susceptable.

ACTINOMYCOSIS

Actinomycoses are filamentous bacteria found in animals and in the oral cavity of man (Chapter 6). Spread to the central nervous system is usually hematogenous, but occasionally direct extension to the brain occurs from a nearby site, such as a sinus (Chapter 28). Only 1 to 3 percent of all actinomycotic infections involve the central nervous system.[122]

Signs and symptoms of an actinomycotic brain abscess depend upon location and may include focal neurologic findings as well as increased intracranial pressure. Meningitis is rare. Specific diagnosis can be made by the demonstration of basophilic or amphophilic sulfur granules on microscopic examination of tissue exudates. The organisms are not visible on hematoxylin and eosin sections but may be seen with a Gomori stain. These organisms grow best anaerobically. Penicillin, 2 to 20 million units per day for 6 to 18 months, is the best treatment.

NOCARDIOSIS

Nocardia is a strictly aerobic, gram-positive, filamentous bacterium that has an unusual propensity to spread from a primary pulmonary focus to the brain[123] (Chapter 7). Approximately 20 to 30 percent of patients with nocardial pulmonary infections subsequently develop a central nervous system infection. The mortality of central nervous system nocardiosis approaches 90 percent. Sulfonamides are the most useful drugs.

ASPERGILLOSIS

Aspergillosis[124] is caused by a fungus of the genus *Aspergillus* and can involve the meninges, cerebral parenchyma, or cerebral blood vessels (Chapter 9). Aspergillosis is particularly apt to be associated with drug addiction, diabetes, carcinomatosis, leukemia, transplantation, and steroids. About half the cases of generalized aspergillosis involve the central nervous system, where the lesion can be either acute (necrotizing and purulent) or chronic (granulomatous). Naturally, the clinical findings depend upon the sites and extent of the lesion. Although amphotericin B (perhaps in combination with 5-fluorocytosine) can be effective in some cases, the prognosis is usually guarded because of the underlying systemic disease.

NORTH AMERICAN BLASTOMYCOSIS

Blastomycosis is a fungal disease caused by *Blastomyces dermatitidis,* a soil saprophyte that is common in the central part of the United States[125] (Chapter 9). About 6 percent of the patients have chronic meningitis. Blastomycotic brain abscess alone is quite rare. Clinically, patients can have headache, coma, confusion, memory loss, aphasia, paresis, and increased intracranial pressure. It is difficult to make a diagnosis unless overt blastomycosis is present elsewhere. Skin testing is of limited value because blastomycosis antigen cross reacts with *Histoplasma* and *Coccidioides.* Amphotericin B is the most effective drug, but a blastomycotic abscess may require excision.

PHYCOMYCOSIS (MUCORMYCOSIS)

Cerebral mucormycosis[126] is an acute, rarely curable disease that affects the nasal sinuses, orbit, and brain (Chapter 9). This true fungus usually becomes pathogenic for man in association with predisposing conditions, such as diabetes, acidosis, altered immune mechanisms, and the use of antibiotics and corticosteroids. Cerebral mucormycosis following open brain injury alone also has been reported.[127] Patients with mucormycosis often have proptosis, orbital cellulitis, and total ophthalmoplegia. Central nervous system invasion (acute meningoencephalitis and purulent meningitis) occurs along arteries that traverse the lamina cribrosa. The fungus has a predilection for vascular invasion, particularly of arteries, which can lead to thrombosis and cerebral infarction, hemorrhage, or dissecting aneurysms. Treatment includes control of the underlying cause, local drainage or debridement of the involved tissue, and amphotericin B, both systemically and via local irrigations.

HISTOPLASMOSIS

Histoplasmosis[128] is caused by the dimorphic fungus *Histoplasma capsulatum* (Chapter 9), which rarely infects the central nervous system. When the central nervous system is infected, meningitis usually results, but occasionally parenchymal granulomas occur (Fig. 28-10). Amphotericin B is used for treatment.

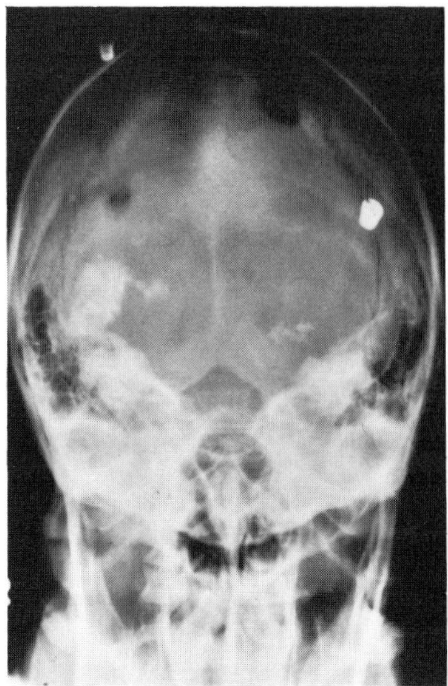
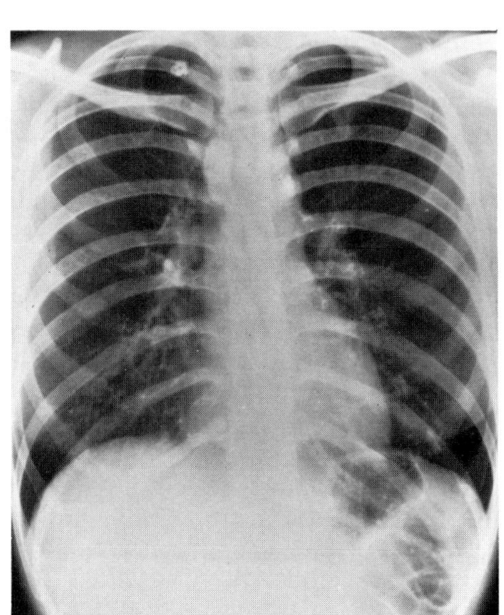

Fig. 28-10. **Calcified granulomas in cerebrum and cerebellum (left), as well as in lungs, hila, and spleen, due to histoplasmosis. (Courtesy of Lawrence H. A. Gold, MD, and Mathis P. Frick, MD, University of Minnesota.)**

CANDIDIASIS

Candidiasis[129] is usually a chronic infection caused by various species of the imperfect fungus, *Candida.* Central nervous system infection usually follows systemic disease in debilitated people with diabetes, malignancies, or immunologic problems or in those who have been treated with antibiotics, steroids, or other immunosuppressive drugs. The usual infection is meningitis, but parenchymal involvement also occurs. Amphotericin B, 5-fluorocytosine, and clotrimazole are effective drugs, but the ultimate prognosis is often poor because of the underlying disease.

COCCIDIOIDOMYCOSIS

Coccidioidomycosis[130] is caused by a fungus that exists in the mycelial form in hot desert soils and occurs as spherules in the human host (Chapter 9). Brain infection usually occurs as a meningitis, which leads to hydrocephalus and increased intracranial pressure. Amphotericin B is given either by repeated lumbar injections or through a shunt placed into one lateral ventricle of the brain. Because the ventricular shunts can become infected after repeated injections, some prefer to use the lumbar route of administration.

CRYPTOCOCCOSIS

Infection of the central nervous system by *Cryptococcus*[131] occurs usually in debilitated patients. The organism, *Cryptococcus neoformans,* reaches the brain or spinal cord by way of the blood and usually produces a meningitis, although space-occupying lesions that require excision have been reported. Currently, 60 percent of cryptococcosis patients who receive amphotericin B are cured (Chapters 9 and 47).

PARASITIC INFESTATIONS

CYSTICERCOSIS

Incidence

Human cysticercosis[132,133] is caused by the larval form of the pork tapeworm, *Taenia solium.* The disease is rare in developed countries but remains an important problem in such economically underdeveloped areas as Mexico, Central and South America, Africa, India, and Asia. In certain Central and South American countries, 1–4.5 cases of cysticercosis occur per 1,000 population, and 1 percent of the affected individuals subsequently develop neurocysticercosis. At the Mexico City General Hospital, cysticercosis was found in 2.4 percent of 1,770 autopsies, while neurocysticercosis was responsible for 30 percent of all space-occupying intracranial lesions. In the United States, Courville[134] found 22 cases of cysticercosis among 3,000 cerebral tumors (Chapter 11).

Pathogenesis and Pathology

People usually develop the disease by ingesting eggs of the parasite. The larvae of the parasite then pass through the gastric mucosa, enter capillaries, and spread throughout the body, and the brain is preferentially affected. Neurocysticercosis exists (1) as a space-occupying cyst or cysts within the brain parenchyma, (2) as a racemose lesion primarily involving the basal and chiasmatic cisterns, and (3) as a mixed cystic and racemose type. An intense inflammatory reaction is usually present. Some evidence suggests that intraparenchymal brain cysts form if spread to the central nervous system occurs via the cartoid artery, while the racemose form appears when cerebral spread has been via the vertebral artery.

Clinical Manifestations and Diagnosis

Clinical symptomatology depends upon the number of cysts, their size, multiplicity, location, and the toxic quality of the parasite. There are three basic clinical disorders: convulsions, intracranial hypertension, and psychiatric disturbances. If the basal leptomeningitis is severe and extends to involve the cord, amyotrophy and spastic paresis can also occur.

Spinal cysticercosis[135] occurs in only 2 to 5 percent of all cases of neurocysticercosis. Although spinal cysticercosis can occur by itself, it usually results from downward spread of intracranial disease.

Cerebrospinal fluid glucose is usually low, but protein and cell counts are elevated. A severe cerebrospinal fluid eosinophilia may be present. Cerebrospinal fluid complement-fixation tests against the cysticercosis parasite generally yield 70 percent positive results, but the assay can be difficult to perform and antigens cross-reacting with echinococcus may be a problem. Roentgenograms of the skull can reveal evidence of increased intracranial pressure or intracranial calcifications, while CAT scanning can be expected to reveal intraparenchymatous cysts. Pneumoencephalography may delineate intraventricular cysts.

Treatment

The best operative results (75 percent improvement, 24 percent mortality) have been obtained with extirpation of cysticerci which form a single, discrete, space-occupying lesion within the brain and produce focal signs. The poorest results (28 percent improvement, 67 percent mortality) have been seen in patients who developed basal leptomeningeal infection. [136] Cysts within the posterior fossa are the major problems. These may be extirpated or broken up via an initial posterior fossa exploration. Cysts elsewhere in the brain can then be approached directly. Others experienced with cysticercosis cerebri advocate leaving the basal cysts in situ. They prefer to deal with the problem of obstruction of cerebrospinal fluid by communicating the temporal horn with the cisterna ambiens or to simply shunt the cerebrospinal fluid. Further organism dissemination by this means is probably unlikely because cysticercosis cysts are rarely found in the lateral ventricles.

If operation fails, the prognosis is grim because there is no effective medical treatment for the disease. In most instances, death eventually occurs consequent to the parasitic brain infestation.

ECHINOCOCCOSIS [137]

Central Nervous System Echinococcosis

Incidence

Hydatid disease is caused by the larval stage of the tapeworm *Echinococcus granulosus* (Chapter 11). Only about 2 percent of those who develop echinococcal disease have central nervous system involvement.[138] Hydatid cysts account for about 3 percent of intracranial space-occupying lesions in Ankara, Turkey.[139] Children are affected 2.5 times more frequently than adults. Morquio from Uruguay stated that 50 percent of childhood tumors of the central nervous system turned out to be hydatid cysts.

Pathology

The disease exists in two forms. The discrete and encapsulated hydatid cysts act as space-occupying lesions in the brain. In the craniovertebral form, the parasite is unencapsulated, and it invades the bone and surrounding structures. Both forms can cause neurologic damage through compression and irritation of surrounding structures.

Because cerebral hydatid cysts are often single, surgical therapy is often successful. Most cysts start in the subcortical area and spread to the white matter. The cerebral hemispheres are more often infected than is the cerebellum.

Clinical Manifestations

In children, the peak incidence occurs between ages 5 and 10. Affected children usually have raised intracranial pressure, diminished visual acuity, mental changes, homonymous field cuts, and hemiparesis. The characteristic setting for the childhood disease is a child in good general condition who lives in a rural endemic area and has elevated intracranial pressure without focal findings.[140] In the adult, the clinical picture is less well defined. Increased intracranial pressure is usually evident, but the differentiation between echinococcal cyst and tumor may be difficult.

Roentgenograms of the skull in the child may show suture separation or thinning of the cranial vault, while isotopic scan reveals absence of uptake at the cyst site. Angiography may reveal significant vascular displacement. CAT scanning nicely delineates intracranial hydatid cysts.[139]

Treatment

Surgical therapy of encapsulated cerebral cysts is directed at removing the cyst without damaging its walls. This can be done by wide osteoplastic craniotomy, cortical incision, exposure of the cyst, and gentle irrigation between cyst wall and brain.

Echinococcosis of Bone

Vertebral hydatid disease occurs when the echinococcal embryo is carried to a vertebral body. In this environment, the parasite invades, infiltrates, and destroys bone. Thoracic involvement is most common. Spinal cord impingement can occur as the unencapsulated parasite invades the spinal canal or as collapsed bone presses upon the cord. Clinical progression of the disease is slow because the parasite enlarges slowly. The common signs and symptoms are pain, motor and sensory deficits, difficulty with bowel and bladder function, paravertebral swelling, and gibbus formation.

Laminectomy and evacuation of the extradural collection will decompress the spinal cord and nerve roots. Irrigating the wound with hypertonic saline for five minutes will destroy the residual organism. Occasionally, total vertebrectomy is necessary.

Cranial hydatid disease also represents an unencapsulated form of the parasite and can occur in either the cranial base or vault, with increased intracranial pressure, focal neurologic disturbances, skull deformity, and cranial nerve palsies. Involved bone of the vault may be widely resected, but this is not possible with a basal lesion.

SCHISTOSOMIASIS

Infestation by the trematode worm *Schistosoma* causes 200 million cases of schistosomiasis worldwide [141] (Chapter 11). Acute cerebral schistosomiasis can cause a fulminating encephalitis. Chronic cerebral schistosomiasis produces intracranial granulomas with obstruction to cerebrospinal fluid flow, elevated intracranial pressure, and localizing signs. Unfortunately, no specific features suggest the disease. Spinal schistosomiasis can present as an acute myelitis, with destruction and atrophy of the cord, a discrete, space-occupying, intrathecal granuloma, or a radicular process caused by microscopic granulomas on the cauda equina. The granulomatous form of the disease can produce chronic, progressive neurologic loss. In endemic areas spinal schistosomiasis should be considered when patients have spinal cord symptoms.

PARAGONIMIASIS

Paragonimiasis [142] is a parasitic disease caused by the ingestion of crustacea contaminated by *Paragonimus.* The disease is prevalent in the Far East, Southeast Asia, some parts of Africa, and South America. The lung is the primary site of infection and is thought to always precede central nervous system infestation. Most investigators feel that immature or mature worms enter the brain via foramina at the base of the skull as they follow vascular structures from the chest to the head. Entrance through the jugular foramen is highly suspect because most cerebral lesions are posterior, particularly in the occipital, parietal, and temporal lobes. Cerebral paragonimiasis may present as an acute meningoencephalitis, a well-encapsulated granuloma, or a chronic calcified lesion. Seizures, headache, visual disturbances and hemiparesis are the most common symptoms and signs. Roentgenograms of the skull may reveal posterior calcifications. There are no specific angiographic findings. Cerebrospinal fluid may be normal or abnormal. Occasionally, *Paragonimus* ova may be seen in the cerebrospinal fluid. Complement-fixation tests of cerebrospinal fluid against *Paragonimus* antigen are positive in 40 to 80 percent of cases of cerebral infestation. The parasite may also involve the spinal cord. The worms probably migrate into the spinal epidural space directly from the lungs because an extradural thoracic location is most common.

While medical therapy with bithionol [2,2′-thiobis(4,6-dichlorophenol)] affords primary treatment, surgery may be performed for intracranial mass lesions that elevate intracranial pressure. Twenty-four percent of space-occupying lesions within the brain were caused by *Paragonimus* in one endemic area. Small cysts may be entirely removed, while large cysts are evacuated, but the walls are left behind.

ENTAMOEBA HISTOLYTICA

Brain abscesses caused by *Entamoeba histolytica* [143-145] usually have a hematogenous origin from *E. histolytica* abscesses of the lung or liver, although at least five cases of direct spread of this organism from bowel to brain have been reported. *E. histolytica* brain abscess is usually solitary and unencapsulated. The abscess progresses rapidly and frequently ends fatally, but several instances have been recorded of survival following aspiration and antiamebic drug therapy (Chapter 11).

INFECTIONS AFTER NEUROSURGICAL OPERATION

GENERAL

Tables 28-9 [146-154] and 28-10 [147,149,151-159] indicate that an individual undergoing craniotomy runs a 3–6 percent risk of postoperative infection, while one having a laminectomy has approximately a 0.5–4 percent chance of infection. Virtually all authors indicate that *S. aureus* is the most frequent infecting organism.

Velghe [150] took postoperative wound swabs in approximately 1,000 operative cases, and about 25 percent of wound swabs grew bacteria. Despite this fact, only 10 percent of neurosurgical patients manifested clinical infection. The incidence of wound contamination rose sharply when procedures exceeded three hours. Room air conditioning lowered the wound contamination rate. Local application of antibiotics to the wound did not alter the incidence of infection.

Wright [151] made a detailed analysis of craniotomy wound infections and observed an increased likelihood of infection with increasing length of operation, use of postoperative drains, and wound reopening. Diabetes, malignancy, utilization of postoperative antibiotics, steroids, or hypothermia did not predispose to infection.

Where ultraviolet lights have been utilized, the neurosurgical infection rates are low.[147,149,160]

Balch [152] analyzed postoperative neurosurgical infections and determined that about half occurred in the subdural space and half were epidural. Twenty-eight patients in his series developed subdural infections consisting of ventriculitis, meningitis, brain abscesses, or subdural abscesses. Two died (7 percent), and four others (14 percent) sustained severe neurologic residua. Extradural infections included epidural abscess soft tissue infection, osteomyelitis, and septicemia. No patient with an extradural infection died, and only one sustained any neurologic sequelae.

In most instances, postoperative infection of the craniotomy bone flap with ensuing epidural abscess necessitates removal of the bone flap. Chou and Erickson [161] have salvaged 15 of 25 infected bone flaps by continuous irrigation of antibiotic solution through catheters placed over and under these bone flaps. The catheters are placed by means of a formal operative procedure. Saline-antibiotic solution is instilled through one catheter, while this irrigating solution drains out through another dependent catheter attached to a suction apparatus. One to two liters of antibiotic-irrigating solution are administered daily for approximately one week while systemic antibiotics are administered concomitantly. The antibiotics are chosen according to specific cultures and sensitivities.

TABLE 28-9. INFECTIONS FOLLOWING CRANIOTOMY

Surgeon	Year	Number of Craniotomies	Number of Infections	% Infection
Cushing, Eisenhardt [146]	1938	522	5	0.95
Woodhall, et al [147]	1949	1,228	13	1.05
Pool, Pava [148]	1957	122	7	5.70
Odum, et al [149]	1962	2,342	16	1.30
Wright [151]	1966	2,148	122	5.70
Balch [152]	1967	450	23	5.10
Green, et al [153]	1974	692	18	2.60
Savitz [154]	1974	214	9	4.20

TABLE 28-10. INFECTIONS FOLLOWING LAMINECTOMY

Surgeon	Year	Number of Laminectomies	Number of Infections	% Infection
Elsberg [155]	1925	100	2	2.0
Woodhall, et al [147]	1949	1,791	29	1.6
Gurdjian, et al [156]	1961	1,176	14	—
Odum, et al [149]	1962	3,774	21	0.6
Wright [151]	1966	2,085	85	4.1
Balch [152]	1967	271	9	—
Wright [157]	1970	579	2	0.3
Green et al [153]	1973	529	12	2.3
Savitz, et al [154]	1974	239	9	3.8
Horwitz, Curtin [158]	1975	495	16	3.2
Mayfield [159]	1976	1,408	14	1.0

While most authors have indicated that staphylococci are the most frequent organisms found in postoperative neurosurgical infections, Buckwold et al [160] found a preponderence of gram-negative organisms in a study of postoperative meningitis at McGill University. Nineteen gram-negative and four staphylococcal infections occurred after craniotomies, cerebrospinal fluid shunts, cerebrospinal fluid leaks, and skull fractures. Alarmingly, the outcome in these patients was unaffected by subsequent administration of antibiotics. Eleven of the 19 patients with gram-negative infections died, as did 1 of 4 with staphylococcal meningitis. All 23 of these patients had received prophylactic antibiotics at the time of their original neurosurgical operation, and the high number of gram-negative infections may have been influenced by prior antibiotic administration.

Several reports [162–164] indicate that the postoperative infection rate for subdural hematomas is in the range of 4 percent. Dohn [165] reported 3 instances of osteomyelitis in 201 anterior cervical fusions (1.5 percent), but this rate may be somewhat higher than usual. In spite of this complication, all infected interspaces fused in good position after drainage and immobilization.

Because of the nasal approach for transphenoidal pituitary surgery, a potential exists for the direct infection of the subarachnoid space with bacteria or the subsequent development of meningitis as a consequence of cerebrospinal fluid leakage. This complication occurs in 1 percent or less of transnasal hypophysectomies.[166–169]

INFECTIONS FOLLOWING CEREBROSPINAL FLUID SHUNTING PROCEDURES

The modern cerebrospinal fluid shunt for the control of hydrocephalus was developed in the early 1950s.[170] The so-called ventriculoatrial (VA) shunt consists of a flexible ventricular catheter that is connected to a subcutaneous pumping device affixed to the skull. The pump, in turn, is attached to a subcutaneous tube, which usually leads to the right atrium of the heart via the common facial or internal jugular vein. Cerebrospinal fluid pressure is controlled by a valve in the pumping device or in the cardiac catheter. Because of complications associated with this form of shunt, many other types of shunt were tried, and eventually the ventriculoperitoneal (VP) shunt, using flexible Silastic tubing [171] emerged. Intraventricular pressure is controlled as in the VA shunt, but spinal fluid is diverted to the peritoneal cavity for absorption. Some surgeons have reported fewer infections with VP shunts,[172,173] some with VA shunts,[174] while still others [175] have observed no difference in the infection rate between the two types.

Incidence

The incidence and mortality of shunt infections are listed in Table 28-11.[172,173,175-198] Infection has been and still remains the most serious complication of cerebrospinal fluid shunting procedures, whichever shunt is used. It has varied from 3–40 percent and has caused a 1.3–8 percent post-shunt mortality (Table 28-11). Because the probability of infection increases with duration of implantation, all data showing shunt infection rates are subject to upward revision during ensuing years.[186]

Clinical Manifestations

Early infections are usually caused by *S. aureus* or gram-negative bacteria.[184] They appear within a few days or weeks and exhibit obvious signs of wound sepsis or erythema along the course of the subcutaneous catheter. Delayed shunt infections (one third of cases) [185,186] occur more than one month after implantation and are usually not associated with obvious wound suppuration. In these infections, bacteremia, peritonitis, or meningitis develops with *Staphylococcus epidermidis* or other opportunists.[178,199-201] Chronic, low-grade shunt infections may be difficult to diagnose because symptoms are often minimal, apart from malaise, occasional nausea and vomiting, and unexplained fever of 100F to 102F. The blood leukocyte count may be elevated but has been shown to be less than 10,000 per mm^3 in 25 percent of patients with bacteremia from colonized shunts.[175] As the bacteremia becomes more advanced, anemia and splenomegaly may develop.[175,199,202,203] Blood cultures are usually positive in cases of infected VA shunts [175] but are usually negative in patients with infected VP shunts because these shunts are isolated from the bloodstream. Cerebrospinal fluid cultures are also positive in a high proportion of patients with chronic ventricular shunt infections, but as the infecting organism usually is not highly pathogenic, the cerebrospinal fluid cellular reaction may be minimal. *Because of the common occurrence of delayed bacterial colonization of ventriculoatrial and ventriculoperitoneal shunts, all shunted individuals with unexplained fever should have blood and cerebrospinal fluid cultures as an initial part of their fever work-up.* Since the infecting bacteria may be inside the shunt assembly and not in the bloodstream at the time of evaluation, a VA shunt should be pumped just prior to blood culture. The cerebrospinal fluid sample should be obtained percutaneously by needle from the shunt reservoir.

TABLE 28-11. CEREBROSPINAL SHUNT INFECTION AND MORTALITY FROM INFECTION

Author	Year	No. of Cases and Shunt *	Number of Infections	Infection † Rate %	Deaths Shunt-related Septicemia/ Meningitis	Infection-related Mortality %
Anderson [176]	1959	36 VA	8	22.7	7	19.4
Carrington [177]	1959	50 VA	3	6.0	3	6.0
Schimke, et al [178]	1961	54 VA	11	20.4	2	3.7
Bruce, et al [179]	1963	300 VA	17	5.7	4	1.3
Overton, Snodgrass [180]	1965	48 VA	7	14.6	4	8.3
Guthkelch [181]	1967	166 VA	—	—	4	2.0
Nulsen, Becker [182]	1967	VA	44	—	8	—
Forrest, Cooper [183]	1968	455 VA	49	11.0	13	2.9
Luthardt-Hemmer [184]	1967–1970	183 VA	18	10.0	3	1.6
McLaurin, Dodson [185]	1971	170 VA	20	11.8	0	—
Villani, et al [172]	1971	217 VA, VP	20	9.2	—	—
Shurtleff, et al [186]	1971	102 VA	18	15.7	—	—
Illingworth, et al [187]	1971	101 VA	9	8.9	2	1.9
Salmon [188]	1972	80	10	12.5	5	6.3
Little, et al [173]	1972	74 VA, VP	10	13.5	5	6.8
Morrice, Young [189]	1974	364 VA	67	19.3	8	2.2
Schoenbaum, et al [175]	1975	289 VA, VP	77	26.6	—	—
Mori, Raimondi [190]	1975	623 VA, VP	77	12.4	8	1.3
Ignelzi, Kirsch [191]	1975	300 VA, VP	18	6.0	—	—
Renier, et al [192]	1975	150	24	6.3	—	—
Sayers [193]	1976	730	—	—	26	3.6
Steinbok, Thompson [194]	1976	323 VA, VP	36	11.1	—	—
Venes [195]	1976	150 VA, VP	10	6.7	—	—
Raimondi, et al [196]	1977	161 VP	17	10.6	—	—
O'Brien, et al [197]	1978	VA, VP	—	—	—	—
Welch [198]	1979	404	13	3.2	—	—

* VA = ventriculoatrial; VP = ventriculoperitoneal

† The case infection rate is given. Because some patients have multiple procedures upon their shunts, the case infection rate will be somewhat higher than the operative procedure infection rate.

Mechanisms of Shunt Infection

Most investigators [175,178,195,199] regard the patient's skin as the most important bacterial reservoir for both early and late sepsis. Contact of the shunt catheter with skin may allow bacteria to adhere to the outside of the tubing or gain entrance to the shunt lumen. Some surgeons [175,182,186,194] have found an increased incidence of shunt infection in hydrocephalics with associated myelomeningoceles, while others [184,185] have not confirmed this association. In denying any correlation, these latter investigators note that myelomeningoceles are often colonized by gram-negative organisms, but these bacteria are relatively uncommon causes of shunt infection. Furthermore, patients with myelomeningocele comprise a large proportion of those requiring shunts but do not constitute a disproportionately large portion of the population whose shunts become infected.

Burke [204] has accumulated experimental evidence that airborne contamination may account for significant wound colonization during surgical procedures, and Velghe et al [150] have implicated airborne contamination for neurosurgical operations in general. Bayston and Lari [205] performed wound cultures upon 100 patients undergoing shunts and obtained 58 positive cultures. Thirty-two were probably skin contaminants, while 26 were felt to have been caused by airborne bacteria.[186]

Colonization of venous shunts by incidental bacteremias is another mechanism proposed to explain ventriculoatrial shunt infection. Not uncommonly, the distal shunt tubing of a ventriculoatrial shunt within the right atrium is heavily colonized with bacteria, while the proximal ventricular catheter is lightly colonized or sterile.[206] This bacterial distribution indicates an ascending infection from blood to brain along the shunt tube. This mechanism, however, would be unlikely to explain infection associated with VP shunts.[182,206]

Pathology of Shunt Infections

Colonized shunts are lined with a single layer of bacteria that appear to adhere to the tubing, possibly as a consequence of electrostatic attraction [179] or by a gummy substance secreted by the bacteria. Atrial or vena caval thrombi are frequently associated with the infected ventriculoatrial shunts,[176,186] and such thrombi may lead to septic pulmonary emboli. Endocarditis [178] is also associated with infected atrial catheters, and occasionally, frank tricuspid valvular vegetations may form.[182]

If bacteria ascend into the ventricular system, ventriculitis and meningitis occur. Ventriculitis can lead to stenosis of the aqueduct and change a communicating to a noncommunicating hydrocephalus. Infections of the peritoneal catheter may produce a frank peritonitis or a walled-off intraabdominal abscess. Unique infectious complications sometimes arise from shunts. Brook et al [207] for instance, reported two cases of meningitis consequent to enteric organisms where the peritoneal catheters had perforated the colon.

Prevention of Shunt Infections

Obviously, a thorough skin preparation, isolation of the skin by plastic drapes,[195] prevention of contact between shunt and skin during insertion,[195] meticulous surgical care, and brief operations [181,208] will minimize the chances of wound and shunt colonization. Nulsen and Becker [182] felt that placement of the atrial catheter into the inferior vena cava (below the T-6 vertebral level on operative roentgenograms) greatly increased the chance of infection and urged intracardiac placement above this level. McLaurin and Dodson,[185] however, could not confirm a correlation between catheter level and subsequent infection rate. Raimondi et al [196] indicated that a one-piece shunt has significantly lessened the need for shunt revisions and concomitant infection. Renier et al [192] perform their shunt operations with the patient in a surgical isolator to shield the operative field from airborne bacteria. Some series now report only a 3–6 percent infection rate (Table 28-11).

Prophylactic antibiotics have also been utilized in an attempt to prevent infection. While some [188,195] have reported encouraging results in uncontrolled trials with prophylactic antibiotics, others [175,185,190,191] have observed no beneficial results. Bayston [210] undertook a controlled study on the question of antibiotic prophylaxis on 132 patients. Twenty individuals received gentamicin, and 34 were given cloxacillin one hour preoperatively and at six hours after surgery. Seventy-eight patients got no antibiotics. Despite this prophylaxis, 50 to 60 percent of all wounds grew bacteria. Clinical wound infections occurred in no patient receiving gentamicin, in one receiving cloxacillin, and in only two controls. These data do not indicate that prophylactic gentamicin or cloxacillin affected the shunt infection rate.

Treatment of Established Shunt Infections

Elimination of bacteria that have colonized implanted foreign bodies is extremely difficult. Infected shunts, in particular, prove a challenge because bacteria may lie inside the hollow valve and tubes, shielded from host defense mechanisms. Systemically administered antibiotics will not diffuse through the shunt to reach bacteria within it, and systemic antibiotics in ordinary doses often do not transit the blood-brain barrier to establish bactericidal cerebrospinal fluid drug concentrations. Removal of the infected foreign body plus appropriate antibiotics has long been recognized as effective, but if an infected cerebrospinal fluid shunt is removed, means must be provided to handle the cerebrospinal fluid. Ventricular taps, external ventricular drainage, or cerebrospinal fluid drainage through the in-place ventricular catheter have been utilized following removal of all or part of an infected shunt or the atrial catheter. These techniques, however, are not without their own inherent risks: patients may deteriorate from increased intracranial pressure or may develop secondary infections of the central nervous system (Table 28-12).

Initially, surgeons were discouraged with attempts to sterilize infected shunts, and most recommended removal, antibiotics, and ventricular taps or venticular drainage for control of cerebrospinal fluid (Table 28-12). New shunts would be inserted after infection had cleared. It might be noted, however, that Schimke et al [178] in one of the earliest reports, obtained cures in 4 of 11 patients treated

TABLE 28-12. RECOMMENDED THERAPY OF SHUNT INFECTIONS

Author	Year	Recommended Treatment
Schimke, et al [178]	1961	Remove shunt, antibiotics
Callaghan, et al [202]	1961	Remove shunt, antibiotics
Bruce, et al [179]	1963	Remove shunt, antibiotics
Guthkelch [181]	1967	If no ventriculitis: antibiotics, remove shunt, immediate reinsertion If ventriculitis is present: remove shunt, sterilize CSF and prevent pressure by taps, replace shunt
Nulsen, Becker [182]	1967	Remove shunt, antibiotics
Nicholas, et al [211]	1970	Antibiotics, remove infected shunt, wait 20 minutes, insert new shunt
Luthardt [184]	1970	Remove infected auricular catheter, sterile, open drainage for ventricular catheter, antibiotics to sterilize patient, insert new valve in different location
Illingworth, et al [187]	1971	Try antibiotics, if fail, remove shunt
Salmon [188]	1972	Remove shunt, antibiotics (adults)
Morrice, Young [189]	1974	Antibiotics, remove shunt, immediate replacement If this becomes infected, remove and start external drainage, antibiotics to sterilize patient, insert new valve after patient sterilized
Shurtleff, et al [212]	1974	*S. epidermidis* only: initial treatment—intraventricular and systemic antibiotics, if fail, remove shunt
Schoenbaum, et al [175]	1975	Remove shunt, ventricular drainage if necessary, antibiotics to sterilize patient, replace shunt in new location
Mori, Raimondi [190]	1975	Remove shunt, external drainage, antibiotics to sterilize patient, replace shunt
Perrin, McLaurin [213] McLaurin, Dodson [185] McLaurin [214] McLaurin [215]	1967 1971 1973 1975	Initial treatment: systemic and intraventricular antibiotics for 2 weeks, if fails, give second course. If second course fails, remove shunt and replace immediately with new valve. If this fails, remove shunt, sterilize patient with antibiotics, replace shunt
Venes [195]	1976	Gram-positive infections: intraventricular and intravenous antibiotics for 7 days, shunt replacement within 24 hours of beginning intraventricular antibiotics, oral antibiotics for 1 additional week after parenteral antibiotics Gram-negative infections: ventricular drainage, antibiotics to sterilize patient, then replace shunt
Sells, et al [216]	1977	Gram-negative bacteria: remove shunt, antibiotics
Scarff, et al [217]	1978	External ventricular drainage plus intraventricular and systemic antibiotics
O'Brien, et al [197]	1979	Asymptomatic internal infections: IV antibiotics for 14 days Symptomatic gram-positive internal infections: remove shunt and replace a new one in the same site, 14 days of intraventricular and intravenous antibiotics Symptomatic gram-negative internal infections: shunt removed and appropriate intraventricular and intravenous antibiotics, external ventricular drainage if necessary.

with high doses of systemic antibiotics. Nevertheless, they too endorsed shunt removal as the best treatment.

Because of the risks associated with repeated ventricular taps or external drainage, some surgeons [211,213] began treating their patients with high doses of antibiotics, removing the infected shunt and immediately inserting a new one. They reasoned that with concomitant antibacterial coverage, bacteria would not colonize a new valve. Nicholas et al [211] stated that immediate reinsertion could be performed if the bacteremia was caused by *S. epidermidis* (but not if it was caused by more virulent organisms), if the ventricle was free from infection, and there was no local wound infection. They reported a 91 percent cure rate with this technique.

McLaurin [185,214] felt that antibiotics alone often failed to eradicate shunt infection because high cerebrospinal fluid concentrations were not obtained. He, therefore, began using intraventricular (via a Rickham reservoir) as well as systemic antibiotics and obtained several clinical cures. He currently [215] recommends staged treatment as follows:

1. An initial two-week course of intraventricular and systemic antibiotics (selected according to sensitivity determinations),
2. If infection recurs, institute a second course,
3. If the second course is unsuccessful, antibiotics are maintained, and the infected shunt is removed and immediately replaced by a new shunt. Intraventricular and systemic antibiotics are continued.
4. If this is unsuccessful, the new shunt is removed, and the patient is placed on cerebrospinal fluid drainage and sterilized with antibiotics. After cerebrospinal fluid and blood cultures are sterile, a new shunt is inserted in a new location.

Using antibiotics as the primary treatment, McLaurin reported cure in 10 of his 25 patients (1 death) with antibiotics alone. Salmon,[188] however, was less successful with this therapy in adults—5 of 10 patients so treated died. Shurtleff et al [212] reported 2 cures among 22 patients with *S. epidermidis* shunt infections treated by intraventricular and systemic antibiotics but no cures among 4 treated by systemic antibiotics alone. Despite the low overall cure rate, they concluded that a trial of systemic and intraventricular antibiotics was justified in *S. epidermidis* infections in order to preserve a functioning shunt. They observed, however, that intraventricular antibiotics could only be given if an implanted shunt reservoir was already available. If operation was necessary to insert such a device, complete shunt removal and replacement in a different site would be preferable. Sells et al [216] analyzed 20 cases of gram-negative shunt infection and concluded that immediate shunt removal should be undertaken in these cases because only 2 cases (both *Haemophilus influenzae*) were cured with antibiotics alone and because gram-negative infections are neurologically devastating.

Mori and Raimondi [190] and Scarff et al [217] have favored prolonged external ventricular drainage and antibiotics for shunt infections. This technique is not without its hazards. Mori and Raimondi reported 4 deaths among 26 patients so treated, while 4 others developed severe dehydration, electrolyte imbalance, hyponatremia, convulsions, or subdural hematoma. Reigel's group [217] reported successful treatment of 54 of 57 infections by external drainage without serious complications.

Shunt Infections and Glomerulonephritis

Chronic bacteremia from an infected shunt may be associated with immune-mediated glomerulonephritis.[218,219] Laboratory investigations have shown complement depletion and activation as well as bacterial antigen deposits along the glomerular basement membrane.

Shunts in Association with Operations for Brain Tumors

Ventriculoatrial shunts have been used in conjunction with craniotomy for brain tumor as a preliminary measure to reduce intracranial pressure and to allow more normal cerebral circulation and brain metabolism. The infection rate may be prohibitive if the shunt is left in place,[220,221] but the rate is negligible if the shunt is electively removed three to four days after tumor removal.

External Ventricular Drainage

External drainage [222-224] also has been used for the reduction of intracranial pressure secondary to the obstruction to cerebrospinal fluid flow. *S. epidermidis* ventriculitis is an occasional complication (10 to 30 percent).

Closed ventricular drainage [222] systems are safer than are drainage systems open to the air.[223,224] Nevertheless, open systems are commonly used for external drainage because of the ease by which ventricular pressure may be controlled. Use of double-bottle systems or of bottles with filtered air vents and bacitracin appear to help decrease associated infection. The use of large-bore ventriculostomy tubes (as No. 9 French infant feeding tube), which continue to drain and do not require manipulation, would also appear prudent. Most surgeons would probably feel safer instituting prophylactic antibiotics (eg, methicillin or cloxacillin), but the issue is not entirely clear because their use has not prevented infections secondary to the monitoring of intracranial pressure, which is also done using intraventricular catheters.

INFECTION IN SPINA BIFIDA AND MYELOMENINGOCELE

Children born with myelomeningocele can develop meningitis and ventriculitis, and these sequelae can cause further neurologic damage, leading to educationally subnormal individuals.[225]

Early closure of the myelomeningocele defect (within 24 to 48 hours) would logically eliminate bacterial colonization of the nervous system by skin organisms.[226] However, early closure only reduces this threat: Sharrard et al [227] demonstrated that 5 of 20 infants with myelomeningocele who underwent early closure subsequently developed meningitis, while 8 of 20 infants with late closures (>48 hours) developed central nervous system infection. The incidence of local wound infection is reduced by about 50 percent with early defect closure. The use of prophylactic antibiotics in patients with myelomeningocele encourages the development of gram-negative infections,[228] so that some surgeons who practice early closure do not use antibiotics until a specific infection develops.

INFECTION ASSOCIATED WITH INTRACRANIAL PRESSURE MONITORING

Systematic intracranial pressure monitoring has been used widely to measure and control intracranial pressure since its introduction by Lundberg in 1960. Subarachnoid screws or intraventricular catheters are employed most commonly, although epidural sensors have been tried. Although infection may be introduced into the epidural, subdural, subarachnoid, or ventricular spaces by these pressure-recording techniques, the risk is small provided that sterile techniques are used during insertion.

Sundbärg et al [229] summarized the monitor-associated infections in almost 1,000 intracranial pressure recordings performed between 1956 and 1972. Intraventricular catheters were inserted with strict asepsis, and cerebrospinal fluid samples were taken for culture immediately upon ventricular entry and thereafter at two- to three-day intervals. Recordings lasted an average of eight days, and the catheter tip was cultured after removal. No prophylactic antibiotics were given, but many patients received antibiotics for other reasons. In 997 recordings on 938 patients, 12 (1.3 percent) definite and 37 (3.9 percent) suspected cerebrospinal fluid infections occurred. No patients developed an epidural, subdural, or brain abscess. A definite infection was defined as one with positive clinical signs of meningitis, cerebrospinal fluid leukocytosis, and growth of bacteria in cerebrospinal fluid cultures. Suspected infections were characterized by cerebrospinal fluid leukocytosis and positive cerebrospinal fluid cultures but no overt clinical infection. All patients developing definite or suspected spinal fluid infection were successfully treated with antibiotics. In addition to this 5.2 percent infection rate, an additional 57 patients (6.1 percent) were felt to have contaminated cerebrospinal fluid cultures. Though bacteria grew from the cerebrospinal fluid specimens, the patients themselves had no cerebrospinal fluid leukocytosis nor signs of central nervous system infection. These patients were not treated with antibiotics. One hundred-six positive cultures were obtained in the following distribution; 50 percent *S. epidermidis*, 5.6 percent *S. aureus*, 5.6 percent *Pseudomonas*, 3.7 percent *E. coli*, and 11.3 percent various water saprophytes, such as *Sarcina*. Whereas no correlation occurred between duration of recording and cerebrospinal fluid infection, approximately 90 percent of those who developed definite and suspected infection had undergone ventriculography—only 53 percent of all patients underwent this diagnostic study.

Rosner and Becker [230] monitored 112 severely traumatized patients with subarachnoid screws and ventricular catheters. Many individuals had potentially infected vault and base fractures, which accounts for the fact that 24 had other minor or major infections. Only 3 major (2 meningitis, 1 subdural empyema) and 2 minor scalp infections and 1 death, the subdural empyema, occurred from monitoring alone (4.5 percent infection rate). No data on the value of prophylactic antibiotics are available from this series because the number of screw-related infections was so small.

Smith and Alksne [231] reported 3 infections solely caused by intracranial pressure monitoring among 65 patients, a 4.6 percent rate. Antibiotics were routinely given usually ampicillin or methicillin 500 mg every six hours. Initially, these authors used an air-vented bottle for cerebrospinal fluid removal, but they later switched to a closed drainage system. No infections occurred when the closed system was used. These authors felt that infection could be minimized by a snug dural opening around the ventricular catheter, a closed cerebrospinal fluid drainage system, and, possibly, antibiotic coverage.

One might expect a higher incidence of monitor-related intracranial infections in children because their thinner scalp and skull might allow an easier ingress of bacteria from the surrounding skin. Fortunately, this does not appear to be so. Mickell et al [232] observed only 1 case of frank ventriculitis among 42 monitored children (2.4 percent). Two other patients (4.8 percent) had asymptomatic contamination of their ventricular fluid.

PROPHYLACTIC ANTIBIOTICS IN NEUROSURGERY

Few studies on the effectiveness of prophylactic antibiotics in neurosurgery have been reported, but some of the more recent studies and their results are enumerated in Table 28-13. There are no randomized prospective studies on the worth of prophylactic antibiotics for general neurosurgical procedures, probably because so few infections occur in clean neurosurgical cases. Pavel et al [235] for instance, had to evaluate 1,600 patients in their prospective, double-blind study on the value of prophylactic cephaloradine for clean orthopedic cases. The studies, worthwhile though they are, are difficult to interpret because they are generally not randomized or are without adequate controls. These methodologic problems, as well as different patient populations and different mean length of operating time, may account for the different conclusions reached by Malis,[233] who thought that gentamicin, vancomycin, and streptomycin significantly reduced postoperative infection, and Llewellyn et al,[234] who reached the opposite conclusion. In a large and elaborate study, Pavel, et al [235] demonstrated that for clean orthopedic cases, prophylactic antibiotics had a mild but significant effect in reducing postoperative infections: those who received cephaloradine before and during operation had a 2.8 percent infection rate, while control patients had a 5 percent postoperative infection rate.

The studies of MacGee et al [236] and Ignelzi and VanderArk [237] (one retrospective, the other prospective) indicate that prophylactic antibiotics do not significantly reduce the threat of meningitis after traumatic cerebrospinal fluid fistula. In the former study, 1 of 41 patients who received antibiotics developed meningitis, as did 2 of 17 patients who did not. In the latter work, none of 50 patients not treated with prophylactic antibiotics developed intracranial infection, while 2 of 54 treated with antimicrobials developed either meningitis or a brain abscess. This study also demonstrated that prophylactic antibiotics encouraged gram-negative bacteria to develop in the nasopharynx, which might lead to meningitis that would be more difficult to treat should this condition develop.

TABLE 28-13. PROPHYLACTIC ANTIBIOTICS IN NEUROSURGERY

Surgeon	Year	Type of Study	No. of Cases	% Infection	Antibiotics	Conclusion
Wright [151]	1966	Retrospective	1,146	5.8	Postop penicillin and streptomycin, local bacitracin irrigation	Prophylactic antibiotics do not alter the postoperative infection rate
		Nonrandomized	1002	5.5	None	
Savitz, Malis, Meyers [154]	1974	Retrospective Nonrandomized	216	5.6	Postop ampicillin	No difference in antibiotic regimens
		No controls	237	2.5	Lincomycin at start of and during operation, none thereafter	
Horwitz, Curtin [158]	1975	Retrospective Nonrandomized	402	1.0	Pre-1965: multiple antibiotics, 1965–67: oxacillin	Prophylactic antibiotics reduce postoperative infections
			128	9.3	1968–75: no antibiotics	
Malis [233]	1976	Prospective Nonrandomized No controls	700	0.0	Gentamicin 80 mg IM and vancomycin 1.0 gm IV with anesthesia, 50 mg streptomycin to each liter of irrigating solution	This combination of antibiotics effectively reduces infection
Llewellyn, et al [234]	1978	Prospective Nonrandomized	174	1.0	Gentamicin 80 mg IM and vancomycin 1.0 gm IV with anesthesia, 50 mg streptomycin to each liter of irrigating solution	This combination of antibiotics does not affect the postoperative infection rate
			236	1.2	No antibiotics	

BIBLIOGRAPHY

Ojemann RG, Shillito J Jr (eds.): Clinical Neurosurgery, Vol 14. Baltimore, Williams and Wilkins, 1967.

Thompson RA, Green FR (eds): Advances in Neurology, Vol 6. New York, Raven, 1974.

Vinken PJ, Bruyn GW, Klawans H (eds.): Handbook of Clinical Neurology, Infections of the Nervous System, Part III, Vol 35. Amsterdam, North-Holland Publishing Company, 1978.

REFERENCES

1. Groff RA: Experimental production of abscess of the brain in cats. Arch Neurol Psychiatry 31:199, 1934.
2. Falconer MA, McFarlan AM, Russell DS: Experimental brain abscess in the rabbit. Br J Surg 30:245, 1943.
3. Hassler O, Forsgren A: Experimental abscesses in brain and subcutis. A microangiographic study in the rabbit. Acta Pathol Microbiol Scand 62:59, 1964.
4. Gregorius FK, Johnson BL Jr, Stern WE, Brown WJ: Pathogenesis of hematogenous bacterial meningitis in rabbits. J Neurosurg 45:561, 1976.
5. Molinari GF: Septic cerebral embolism. Stroke 3:117, 1972.

BRAIN ABSCESS

6. Bhatia R, Tandon PN, Banerji AK: Brain abscess—an analysis of 55 cases. Int Surg 58:565, 1973.
7. Carey ME, Chou SN, French LA: Experience with brain abscesses. J Neurosurg 36:1, 1972.
8. Morgan H, Wood MW, Murphey F: Experience with 88 consecutive cases of brain abscess. J Neurosurg 38:698, 1973.
9. Fischbein CA, Rosenthal A, Fischer EG, Nadas AS, Welch K: Risk factors of brain abscess in patients with congenital heart disease. Am J Cardiol 34:97, 1974.
10. Jennett B, Miller JD: Infection after depressed fracture of skull. Implications for management of nonmissile injuries. J Neurosurg 36:333, 1972.
11. Joubert MJ, Stephanov S: Computerized tomography and surgical treatment in intracranial suppuration: Report of 30 consecutive unselected cases of brain abscess and subdural empyema. J Neurosurg 47:73, 1977.
12. Pennybacker JB, Sellors TH: Treatment of thoracogenic brain abscess. Lancet 225:90, 1948.
13. Martin G: Non-otogenic cerebral abscess. J Neurol Neurosurg Psychiatry 36:607, 1973.
14. Jefferson AA, Keogh AJ: Intracranial abscess: A review of treated patients over 20 years. Q J Med 183:389, 1977.
15. Choudhury AR, Taylor JC, Whitaker R: Primary excision of brain abscess. Br Med J 2:1119, 1977.
16. Heineman HS, Braude AI: Anaerobic infections of the brain: Observations on eighteen consecutive cases of brain abscess. Am J Med 35:682, 1963.
17. de Louvois J, Gortvai P, Hurley R: Bacteriology of abscesses of the central nervous system: A multicentre prospective study. Br Med J 2:981, 1977.
18. Ingham HR, Selkon JB, Roxby CM: Bacteriological study

of otogenic cerebral abscesses: Chemotherapeutic role of metronidazole. Br Med J 2:991, 1977.
19. Ingham HR, Selkon JB, Roxby CM: The bacteriology and chemotherapy of otogenic cerebral abscesses. J Antimicrob Chemother 4:63, 1978.
20. Chernik NL, Armstrong D, Posner JB: Central nervous system infections in patients with cancer. Medicine 52:563, 1973.
21. Feigin RD, Shearer WT: Opportunistic infection in children. I. In the compromised host. II. In the compromised host. III. In the normal host. J Pediatr 87:507, 677, 852; 1975.
22. Claveria LE, du Boulay GH, Moseley IF: Intracranial infections: Investigations by computerized axial tomography. Neuroradiology 12:59, 1976.
23. Kaufman DM, Leeds NE: Computed tomography (CT) in the diagnosis of intracranial abscess. Brain abscess, subdural empyema, and epidural empyema. Neurology 27:1069, 1977.
24. Stevens EA, Norman D, Kramer RA, Messina AB, Newton TH: Computed tomographic brain scanning in intraparenchymal pyogenic abscess. Am J Roentgenol Radium Ther Nucl Med 130:111, 1978.
25. New PFJ, Davis KR, Ballantine HT Jr: Computed tomography in cerebral abscess. Radiology 121:641, 1976.
26. Steinhoff H, Lanksch W, Kazner E, Grumme T, Meese W, Lange S, Aulich A, Schindler E, Wende S: Computed tomography in the diagnosis and differential diagnosis of glioblastomas: A qualitative study of 295 cases. Neuroradiology 14:193, 1977.
27. Vignaendra V, Ghee LT, Chawala J: EEG in brain abscess: Its value in localization compared to other diagnostic tests. Electroencephalogr Clin Neurophysiol 38:611, 1975.
28. Suwanwela C, Poshyachinda V, Poshyachinda M: Brain scanning in the diagnosis of intracranial abscess. Acta Neurochir 25:165, 1971.
29. Tarcan Y, Fajman W, Marc J, Berg D: "Doughnut" sign in brain scanning. Am J Roentgenol Radium Ther Nucl Med 126:842, 1976.
30. Garfield J: Management of supratentorial intracranial abscess: A review of 200 cases. Br Med J 2:7, 1969.
31. Sampson DS, Clark K: A current review of brain abscess. Am J Med 54:201, 1973.
32. Katzman R, Pappius HM: The blood-brain barrier. In Katzman R, Pappius HM (eds): Brain Electrolytes and Fluid Metabolism. Baltimore, William & Wilkins, 1973, p 49.
33. Davson H: Discussion on the penetration of drugs into the cerebrospinal fluid. Proc R Soc Med 50:963, 1957.
34. Black P, Graybill JR, Charache P: Penetration of brain abscess by systemically administered antibiotics. J Neurosurg 38:705, 1973.
35. de Louvois J, Gortvai P, Hurley R: Antibiotic treatment of abscesses of the central nervous system. Br Med J 2:985, 1977.
36. de Louvois J: The bacteriology and chemotherapy of brain abscess. J Antimicrob Chemother 4:395, 1978.
37. Long WD, Meacham WF: Experimental method for producing brain abscesses in dogs with evaluation of the effect of dexamethasone and antibiotic therapy on the pathogenesis of intracerebral abscesses. Surg Forum 19:437, 1968.
38. Quartey GR, Johnston JA, Rozdilsky B: Decadron in the treatment of cerebral abscess: An experimental study. J Neurosurg 45:301, 1976.
39. Heineman HS, Braude Al, Osterholm JL: Intracranial suppurative disease: Early presumptive diagnosis and successful treatment without surgery. JAMA 218:1542, 1971.
40. Chow AW, Alexander E, Montgomeria JZ, Guze LB: Successful treatment of nonmeningitic listerial brain abscess without operation. West J Med 122:167, 1975.
40a. Enzmann DR, Britt RH, Yeager AS: Experimental brain abscess evolution: computed tomographic and neuropathologic correlation. Radiology 133:113, 1979.
40b. Rosenblum ML, Woff JT, Norman D: Nonoperative treatment of brain abscess in selected high-risk patients. J Neurosurg 52:217, 1980.
41. Rosenblum ML, Hoff JT, Norman D, Weinstein P, Pitts L: Decreased mortality from brain abscesses since advent of computerized tomography. J Neurosurg 49:658, 1978.
42. van Alphen HAM, Dreissen JJR: Brain abscess and subdural empyema: Factors influencing mortality and results of various surgical techniques. J Neurol Neurosurg Psychiatry 39:481, 1976.
43. Le Beau J: Radical surgery and penicillin in brain abscess. A method of treatment in one stage with special reference to the cure of three thoracogenic cases. J Neurosurg 3:359, 1946.
44. Jooma OV, Pennybacker JB, Tutton GK: Brain abscess: Aspiration drainage or excision? J Neurol Neurosurg Psychiatry 14:308, 1951.
45. Botterell EH, Drake CG: Localized encephalitis, brain abscess and subdural empyema (1945-1950). J Neurosurg 9:348, 1952.
46. Tutton GK: Cerebral abscess—the present position. Ann R Coll Surg Engl 13:281, 1953.
47. Lewin W: Recent developments in the management of brain abscess. Br Med J 1:631, 1955.
48. Loeser E Jr, Scheinberg L: Brain abscess: A review of ninety-nine cases. Neurology 7:601, 1957.
49. Gurdjian ES, Webster JE: Experiences in the surgical management of intracranial suppuration. Surg Gynecol Obstet 104:205, 1957.
50. Kerr FWL, King RB, Meagher JN: Brain abscess—a study of forty-seven consecutive cases. JAMA 168:868, 1958.
51. Sperl MP, MacCarty CS, Wellman WE: Observations on current therapy of abscess of the brain. Arch Neurol Psychiatry 81:439, 1959.
52. Ballantine HT, Shealy CN: The role of radical surgery in the treatment of abscess of the brain. Surg Gynecol Obstet 109:370, 1959.
53. Martin P, Brihaye J, Martin PH: A propos de 53 cas d'abcès encéphaliques. Neurochirurgie 6:299, 1960.
54. Liske E, Weikers NJ: Changing aspects of brain abscesses. Review of cases in Wisconsin 1940 though 1962. Neurology 14:294, 1964.
55. Newlands WJ: Otogenic brain abscess: A study of eighty cases. J Laryngol Otol 79:120, 1965.
56. Krayenbühl HA: Abscess of the brain. Clin Neurosurg 14:25, 1967.
57. Eberhard S: Diagnosis of brain abscess in infants and children. A retrospective study of twenty-six cases. North Carolina Med J 30:301, 363, 1969.
58. Snyder BD, Farmer TW: Brain abscess in children. South Med J 64:687, 1971.
59. Kapsalakis Z, Askitopoulou HC, Gregoriades A: Analysis of the treatment of twelve consecutive cases of brain abscess. J Neurosurg 37:182, 1972.
60. Gerszten E, Dalton HP, Allison MJ: Brain abscesses: A ten-year review. South Med J 66:593, 1973.
61. Le Beau J, Creissard P, Harispe L, Redondo A: Surgical treatment of brain abscess and subdural empyema. J Neurosurg 38:198, 1973.

62. Beller AJ, Saher A, Praiss I: Brain abscess: Review of 89 cases over a period of 30 years. J Neurol Neurosurg Psychiatry 36:757, 1973.
63. French LA, Chou SN: Treatment of brain abscesses. Adv Neurol 6:269, 1974.
64. Yoshikawa TT, Goodman SJ: Brain abscess. West J Med 121:207, 1974.
65. Brewer NS, MacCarty CS, Wellman WE: Brain abscess: A review of recent experience. Ann Intern Med 82:571, 1975.
66. Schreiber F: Cerebellar abscesses of otitic origin in nine children. Ann Surg 114:330, 1941.
67. Pennybacker J: Cerebellar abscess: Treatment by excision with the aid of antibiotics. J Neurol Neurosurg Psychiatry 11:1, 1948.
68. Shaw MDM, Russell JA: Cerebellar abscess: A review of 47 cases. J Neurol Neurosurg Psychiatry 38:429, 1975.
69. Morgan H, Wood MW: Cerebellar abscesses: A review of seventeen cases. Surg Neurol 3:93, 1975.
70. Shaw MDM, Russell JA: Value of computed tomography in the diagnosis of intracranial abscess. J Neurol Neurosurg Psychiatry 40:214, 1977.
71. Carey ME, Chou SN, French LA: Long-term neurological residua in patients surviving brain abscess with surgery. J Neurosurg 34:652, 1971.
72. Legg NJ, Gupta PC, Scott DF: Epilepsy following cerebral abscess: A clinical and EEG study of 70 patients. Brain 96:259, 1973.

SUBDURAL ABSCESS

73. Kubic CS, Adams RD: Subdural empyema. Brain 66:18, 1943.
74. Yoshikawa TT, Chow AW, Guze LB: Role of anaerobic bacteria in subdural empyema. Report of four cases and review of 327 cases from English literature. Am J Med 59:99, 1975.
75. Schiller F, Cairns H, Russell DS: The treatment of purulent pachymeningitis and subdural suppuration with special reference to penicillin. J Neurol Neurosurg Psychiatry 11:143, 1948.
76. Stern WE, Boldrey E: Subdural purulent collections. Surg Gynecol Obstet 95:623, 1952.
77. Wood PH: Diffuse subdural suppuration. J Laryngol Otol 66:496, 1952.
78. Hitchcock E, Andreadis A: Subdural empyema: A review of 29 cases. J Neurol Neurosurg Psychiatry 27:422, 1964.
79. Bhandari YS, Sarkari NBS: Subdural empyema, a review of 37 cases. J Neurosurg 32:35, 1970.
80. Weinman D, Samarasinghe HHR: Subdural empyema. Aust NZ J Surg 41:324, 1972.
81. Anagnostopoulos DI, Gortvai P: Intracranial subdural abscess. Br J Surg 60:50, 1973.
82. Farmer TW, Wise GR: Subdural empyema in infants, children and adults. Neurology 23:254, 1973.
83. Galbraith JG, Barr VW: Epidural abscess and subdural empyema. Adv Neurol 6:257, 1974.

INTRACRANIAL TUBERCULOSIS

84. Vincent C: Sur les tubercules cerebraux. Ann Med Chir 3:151, 1938.
85. Asenjo A, Valladares H, Fierro J: Tuberculomas of the brain, report on one hundred and fifty-nine cases. Arch Neurol Psychiatry 65:146, 1951.
86. Arseni C: Two hundred and one cases of intracranial tuberculoma treated surgically. J Neurol Neurosurg Psychiatry 21:308, 1958.
87. Katsura S, Suzuki J, Wada T: A statistical study of brain tumors in the neurosurgical clinics in Japan. J Neurosurg 16:570, 1959.
88. Obrador S: Intracranial tuberculomas: A review of 47 cases. Neurochirurgia 1:150, 1959.
89. Dastur HM: A tuberculoma review with some personal experiences: Part I—Brain. Part II—Spinal cord and its coverings. Neurol India 20:111, 131, 1972.
90. Mathai KV, Chandy J: Tuberculous infections of the nervous system: Clin Neurosurg 14:145, 1967.
91. Rab SM, Bhatti IH, Ghani A, Khan A: Tuberculous brain abscess: Case report. J Neurosurg 43:490, 1975.
92. Whitener DR: Tuberculous brain abscess: Report of a case and review of the literature. Arch Neurol 35:148, 1978.

HERPES SIMPLEX ENCEPHALITIS

93. Baringer JR: Human herpes simplex virus infections. Adv Neurol 6:41, 1974.
94. Johnson RT: Treatment of herpes simplex virus encephalitis. Arch Neurol 27:97, 1972.
95. Johnson KP, Rosenthal MS, Lerner PI: Herpes simplex encephalitis: The course in five virologically proven cases. Arch Neurol 27:103, 1972.
96. Boyle RS, Landry PJ: Herpes simplex encephalitis. Aust NZ J Med 7:408, 1977.
97. Drachman DA, Adams RD: Herpes simplex and acute inclusion body encephalitis. Arch Neurol 7:45, 1962.
98. Feldman RA, Shende MC: Herpes simplex virus encephalitis simulating a frontoparietal convexity neoplasm. Surg Neurol 3:329, 1975.
99. Whitley RJ, Soong SJ, Dolin R, Galasso GJ, Ch'ien LT, Alford CA: Adenine arabinoside therapy of biopsy-proven herpes simplex encephalitis (National Institute of Allergy and Infectious Diseases Collaborative Antiviral Study). N Engl J Med 297:289, 1977.
100. Taber LH, Greenberg SB, Perez FI, Couch RB: Herpes simplex encephalitis treated with Vidarabine (adenine arabinoside). Arch Neurol 34:608, 1977.
101. Maxwell GM, Thong YH, Manson JI, Robertson CF: Herpes simplex encephalitis: Treatment with adenine arabinoside and cytosine arabinoside. Med J Aust 24:181, 1978.

MYCOTIC ANEURYSMS

102. Ojemann RG, New PFJ, Fleming TC: Intracranial aneurysms associated with bacterial meningitis. Neurology 16:1222, 1966.
103. Bingham WF: Treatment of mycotic intracranial aneurysms. J Neurosurg 46:428, 1977.
104. Brown I, Peyton WT: Brain tumors simulating meningitis. J Neurosurg 8:459, 1951.
105. Soffer D: Brain tumors simulating purulent meningitis. Eur Neurol 14:192, 1976.

VERTEBRAL OSTEOMYELITIS

106. Waldvogel FA, Medoff G, Swartz MN: Osteomyelitis: A review of clinical features, therapeutic considerations and unusual aspects (third of three parts). N Engl J Med 282:316, 1970.
107. Stone DB, Bonfiglio M: Pyogenic vertebral osteomyelitis: A diagnostic pitfall for the internist. Arch Int Med 112:491, 1963.
108. Griffiths HED, Jones DM: Pyogenic infection of the spine:

A review of twenty-eight cases. J Bone Joint Surg 53B:383, 1971.

109. Jabbari B, Pierce JF: Spinal cord compression due to pseudomonas in a heroin addict: Case report. Neurology 27:1034, 1977.

EPIDURAL AND INTRAMEDULLARY SPINAL CORD ABSCESSES

110. Baker AS, Ojemann RG, Swartz MN, Richardson EP: Spinal epidural abscess. N Engl J Med 293:463, 1975.
111. Heusner AP: Nontuberculous spinal epidural infections. N Engl J Med 239:845, 1948.
112. Hulme A, Dott NM: Spinal epidural abscess. Br Med J 1:64, 1954.
113. Hancock DO: A study of 49 patients with acute spinal extradural abscess. Paraplegia 10:285, 1973.
114. Browder J, Meyers R: Pyogenic infections of the spinal epidural space: A consideration of the anatomic and physiologic pathology. Surgery 10:296, 1941.
115. Menezes AH, Graf CJ, Perrett GE: Spinal cord abscess: A review. Surg Neurol 8:461, 1977.

PARASPINAL TUBERCULOSIS

116. Ginsburg S, Gross E, Feiring E, Scheinberg L: The neurological complications of tuberculous spondylitis: Pott's paraplegia. Arch Neurol 16:265, 1967.
117. Friedman B: Chemotherapy of tuberculosis of the spine. J Bone Joint Surg 48A:451, 1966.
118. Hodgson AR, Stock FE: Anterior spine fusion for the treatment of tuberculosis of the spine: The operative finding and results of treatment in the first one hundred cases. J Bone Joint Surg 42A:295, 1960.
119. Bailey HL, Gabriel M, Hodgson AR, Shin JS: Tuberculosis of the spine in children: Operative findings and results in one hundred consecutive patients treated by removal of the lesion and anterior grafting. J Bone Joint Surg 54A:1633, 1972.
120. Tuli SM: Results of treatment of spinal tuberculosis by "middle-path" regimen. J Bone Joint Surg 57B:13, 1975.
121. Kocen RS, Parsons M: Neurological complications of tuberculosis: Some unusual complications. Q J Med 39:17, 1970.

UNUSUAL CENTRAL NERVOUS SYSTEM INFECTIONS

122. Causey WA: Actinomycosis. In Vinken PJ, Bruyn GW, Klawans H (eds): Handbook of Clinical Neurology, Infections of the Nervous System. Amsterdam, North Holland, 1978, Vol 35, Part III p 383.
123. Causey WA, Lee R: Nocardiosis. In Vinken PJ, Bruyn GW, Klawans H (eds): Handbook of Clinical Neurology, Infections of the Nervous System. Amsterdam, North Holland, 1978, Vol 35, Part III, p 517.
124. Saravia-Gomez J: Aspergillosis of the central nervous system. In Vinken PJ, Bruyn GW, Klawans H (eds): Handbook of Clinical Neurology, Infections of the Nervous System. Amsterdam, North Holland, 1978, Vol 35, Part III, p 395.
125. Leers WD: North American blastomycosis. In Vinken PJ, Bruyn GW, Klawans H (eds): Handbook of Clinical Neurology, Infections of the Nervous System. Amsterdam, North Holland, 1978, Vol 35, Part III, p 401.
126. Dhermy P: Phycomycosis (mucormycosis). In Vinken PJ, Bruyn GW, Klawans H (eds): Handbook of Clinical Neurology, Infections of the Nervous System. Amsterdam, North Holland, 1978, Vol 35, Part III, p 541.
127. Ignelzi RJ, VanderArk GD: Cerebral mucormycosis following open head trauma: Case report. J Neurosurg 42:593, 1975.
128. Lawrence RM, Goldstein E: Histoplasmosis. In Vinken PJ, Bruyn GW, Klawans H (eds): Handbook of Clinical Neurology, Infections of the Nervous System. Amsterdam, North Holland, 1978, Vol 35, Part III, p 503.
129. Tveten L: Candidiasis. In Vinken PJ, Bruyn GW, Klawans H (eds): Handbook of Clinical Neurology, Infections of the Nervous System. Amsterdam, North Holland, 1978, Vol 35, Part III, p 413.
130. Goldstein E, Lawrence R: Coccidioidomycosis of the central nervous system. In Vinken PJ, Bruyn GW, Klawans H (eds): Handbook of Clinical Neurology, Infections of the Nervous System. Amsterdam, North Holland, 1978, Vol 35, Part III, p 443.
131. Weenink HR, Bruyn G: Cryptococcosis of the nervous system. In Vinken PJ, Bruyn GW, Klawans H (eds): Handbook of Clinical Neurology, Infections of the Nervous System. Amsterdam, North Holland, 1978, Vol 35, Part III, p 459.
132. Trelles JO, Trelles L: Cysticercosis of the nervous system. In Vinken PJ, Bruyn GW, Klawans H (eds): Handbook of Clinical Neurology, Infections of the Nervous System. Amsterdam, North Holland, 1978, Vol 35, Part III, p 291.
133. Dixon HB, Lipscomb FM: Cysticercosis: An analysis and follow-up of 450 cases. Med Res Counc Spec Rep Ser (Lond) 299:1, 1961.
134. Courville CB: Intracranial tumors. Notes upon three thousand verified cases with some current observations pertaining to their mortality. Bull Los Angeles Neurol Soc 32[Suppl 2]:1, 1967.
135. Roy RN, Bhattacharya MB, Chatterjee BP, Pal NC: Spinal cysticercosis. Surg Neurol 6:129, 1976.
136. Stepien L: Cerebral cysticercosis in Poland: Clinical symptoms and operative results in 132 cases. J Neurosurg 19:505, 1962.
137. Arana-Iniguez R: Echinococcus. In Vinken PJ, Bruyn GW, Klawans H (eds): Handbook of Clinical Neurology, Infections of the Nervous System. Amsterdam, North Holland, 1978, Vol 35, Part III, p 175.
138. Kaya U, Özden B, Türker K, Tarcan B: Intracranial hydatid cysts: Study of 17 cases. J Neurosurg 42:580, 1975.
139. Özgen T, Erbengi A, Bertan V, Sağlam S, Gürcay Ö, Pirnar T: The use of computerized tomography in the diagnosis of cerebral hydatid cysts. J Neurosurg 50:339, 1979.
140. Anderson M, Bickerstaff ER, Hamilton JG: Cerebral hydatid disease in Britain. J Neurol Neurosurg Psychiatry 38:1104, 1975.
141. Bird AV: Schistosomiasis of the central nervous system. In Vinken PJ, Bruyn GW, Klawans H (eds): Handbook of Clinical Neurology, Infections of the Nervous System. Amsterdam, North Holland, 1978, Vol 35, Part III, p 231.
142. Oh SJ: Paragonimiasis in the central nervous system. In Vinken PJ, Bruyn GW, Klawans H (eds): Handbook of Clinical Neurology, Infections of the Nervous System. Amsterdam, North Holland, 1978, Vol 35, Part III p 243.
143. Mousa AH: Amebiasis in the tropics (a historical review). J Egypt Public Health Assoc 48:148, 1973.
144. Rananavare MM: Evolution of amoebic lesions. Indian J Pathol Bacteriol 12:101, 1969.
145. Reddy DR, Rao JJ, Krishna RV: Amoebic brain abscess. J Indian Med Assoc 63:61, 1974.

POSTOPERATIVE INFECTIONS

146. Cushing H, Eisenhardt L: Meningiomas: Their Classification, Regional Behavior, Life History and Surgical End Results. Springfield, Ill, Thomas, 1938.

147. Woodhall B, Neill RG, Dratz HM: Ultraviolet radiation as an adjunct in the control of post-operative neurosurgical infection. II. Clinical experience 1938–1948. Ann Surg 129:820, 1949.
148. Pool JL, Pava AA: Acoustic Nerve Tumors: Early Diagnosis and Treatment. Springfield, Ill, Thomas, 1957.
149. Odum GL, Hart D, Johnson Smith W, Brown I: A seventeen-year survey of the use of ultraviolet radiations. Presented at the 24th meeting of the American Academy of Neurological Surgery, New Orleans, Louisiana, November 1962.
150. Velghe L, Dereymaeker A, Voorde H Van de: Lécouvillon du champ opératoire en neurochirurgie. Analyse d'un millier de controles. Acta Neurochir (Wien) 11:686, 1964.
151. Wright RL: A survey of possible etiologic agents in post-operative craniotomy infections. J Neurosurg 25:125, 1966.
152. Balch RE: Wound infections complicating neurosurgical procedures. J Neurosurg 26:41, 1967.
153. Green JR, Kanshepolsky J, Turkian B: Incidence and significance of central nervous system infection in neurosurgical patients. Adv Neurol 6:223, 1974.
154. Savitz MH, Malis LI, Meyers BR: Prophylactic antibiotics in neurosurgery. Surg Neurol 2:95, 1974.
155. Elsberg CA: Tumors of the Spinal Cord and the Symptoms of Irritation and Compression of the Spinal Cord and Nerve Roots. Pathology, Symptomatology, Diagnosis, and Treatment. New York, Paul B Hoeber, 1925.
156. Gurdjian ES, Ostrowski AZ, Hardy WG, Lindner DW, Thomas LM: Results of operative treatment of protruded and ruptured lumbar discs. Based on 1,176 operative cases with 82% follow-up of 3 to 12 years. J Neurosurg 18:783, 1961.
157. Wright RL: Septic Complications of Neurosurgical Spinal Procedures. Springfield, Ill, Thomas, 1970.
158. Horwitz NH, Curtin JA: Prophylactic antibiotics and wound infections following laminectomy for lumbar disc herniation: A retrospective study. J Neurosurg 43:727, 1975.
159. Mayfield FH: Complications of laminectomy. Clin Neurosurg 23:435, 1976.
160. Buckwold FJ, Hand R, Hansebout RR: Hospital-acquired bacterial meningitis in neurosurgical patients. J Neurosurg 46:494, 1977.
161. Chou SN, Erickson DL: Craniotomy infections. Clin Neurosurg 23:357, 1976.
162. Svein HJ, Gelety JE: On the surgical management of encapsulated subdural hematoma. A comparison of the results of membranectomy and simple evacuation. J Neurosurg 21:172, 1964.
163. Vieth RG, Tindall GT, Odom GL: The use of tantalum dust as an adjunct in the post-operative management of subdural hematomas. J Neurosurg 24:514, 1966.
164. Raskind R, Glover MB, Weiss SR: Chronic subdural hematoma in the elderly: A challenge in diagnosis and treatment. J Am Geriatr Soc 20:330, 1972.
165. Dohn DF: Anterior interbody fusion for treatment of cervical disk conditions. JAMA 197:897, 1966.
166. Guiot G: Transsphenoidal approach in surgical treatment of pituitary adenomas: General principles and indications in non-functioning adenomas. In Kohler PO, Ross GT (eds): Diagnosis and Treatment of Pituitary Tumors. New York, American Elsevier, 1973, p 159.
167. Collins W: Hypophysectomy: Historical and personal perspective. Clin Neurosurg 21:68, 1974.
168. U HS, Wilson CB, Tyrrell JB: Transsphenoidal microhypophysectomy in acromegaly. J Neurosurg 47:840, 1977.
169. Tindall GT, McLanahan CS, Christy JH: Transsphenoidal microsurgery for pituitary tumors associated with hyperprolactinemia. J Neurosurg 48:849, 1978.
170. Nulson FE, Spitz EB: Treatment of hydrocephalus by direct shunt from ventricle to jugular vein. Surg Forum 2:399, 1951.
171. Ames RH: Ventriculo-peritoneal shunts in the management of hydrocephalus. J Neurosurg 27:525, 1967.
172. Villani R, Paoletti P, Gaini SM: Experience with ventriculo-peritoneal shunts. Dev Med Child Neurol 13[Suppl 25]:101, 1971.
173. Little JR, Rhoton AL Jr, Mellinger JF: Comparison of ventriculoperitoneal and ventricoloatrial shunts for hydrocephalus in children. Mayo Clin Proc 47:396, 1972.
174. Lajat Y, Lebatard-Sartre R, Guihard D, Ito I, Fresche F, Collet M, Descuns P: Étude comparative des complications observées dans les dérivations ventriculo-atriales et ventriculo-péritonéales (a propos de 106 cas). Neurochirurgie 21:147, 1975.
175. Schoenbaum SC, Gardner P, Shillito J: Infections of cerebrospinal fluid shunts: epidemiology, clinical manifestations, and therapy. Infect Dis 131:543, 1975.
176. Anderson FM: Ventriculo-auriculostomy in the treatment of hydrocephalus. J Neurosurg 16:551, 1959.
177. Carrington KW: Ventriculo-venous shunt using the Holter valve as a treatment of hydrocephalus. J Mich State Med Soc 58:373, 1959.
178. Schimke RT, Black PH, Mark VH, Swartz MN: Indolent *Staphylococcus albus* or *aureus* bacteremia after ventriculoatriostomy. Role of foreign body in its initiation and perpetuation. N Engl J Med 264:264, 1961.
179. Bruce AM, Lorber J, Shedden WIH, Zachary RB: Persistent bacteremia following ventriculo-caval shunt operations for hydrocephalus in infants. Dev Med Child Neurol 5:461, 1963.
180. Overton MC III, Snodgrass SR: Ventriculo-venous shunts for infantile hydrocephalus. A review of five years' experience with this method. J Neurosurg 23:517, 1965.
181. Guthkelch AN: The treatment of infantile hydrocephalus by the Holter valve. Br J Surg 54:665, 1967.
182. Nulsen FE, Becker DP: Control of hydrocephalus by valve-regulated shunt: Infections and their prevention. Clin Neurosurg 14:256, 1967.
183. Forrest DM, Cooper DGW: Complications of ventriculo-atrial shunts: A review of 455 cases. J Neurosurg 29:506, 1968.
184. Luthardt T: Bacterial infections in ventriculo-auricular shunt systems. Dev Med Child Neurol 12[Suppl 22]:105, 1970.
185. McLaurin RL, Dodson D: Infected ventriculo-atrial shunts: Some principles of treatment. Dev Med Child Neurol 13[Suppl 25]:71, 1971.
186. Shurtleff DB, Christia D, Foltz E: Ventriculo-auriculostomy-associated infection: a 12-year study. J Neurosurg 35:686, 1971.
187. Illingworth RD, Logue V, Symon L, Uemura K: The ventriculo-caval shunt in the treatment of adult hydrocephalus: Results and complications in 101 patients. J Neurosurg 35:681, 1971.
188. Salmon JH: Adult hydrocephalus, evaluation of shunt therapy in 80 patients. J Neurosurg 37:423, 1972.
189. Morrice JJ, Young DG: Bacterial colonization of Holter valves: A ten-year study. Dev Med Child Neurol 16[Suppl 32]:85, 1974.
190. Mori K, Raimondi AJ: An analysis of external ventricular drainage as a treatment for infected shunts. Childs Brain 1:243, 1975.
191. Ignelzi RJ, Kirsch W: Follow-up analysis of ventriculo-peritoneal and ventriculo-atrial shunts for hydrocephalus. J Neurosurg 42:679, 1975.
192. Renier D, Pierre-Kahn A, Hirsch JF: Neuro-chirurgie en asepsie stricte: Influence de l'isolateur d'óperation sur le taux

des infections après derivations par valve pour hydrocéphalie. Neurochirurgie 21:571, 1975.
193. Sayers MP: Shunt complications. Clin Neurosurg 23:393, 1976.
194. Steinbok P, Thompson GB: Complications of ventriculo-vascular shunts: Computer analysis of etiological factors. Surg Neurol 5:31, 1976.
195. Venes JL: Control of shunt infection: Report of 150 consecutive cases. J Neurosurg 45:311, 1976.
196. Raimondi AJ, Robinson JS, Kuwawura K: Complications of ventriculo-peritoneal shunting and a critical comparison of the three-piece and one-piece systems. Childs Brain 3:321, 1977.
197. O'Brien M, Parent A, Davis B: Management of ventricular shunt infections. Childs Brain 5:304, 1979.
198. Welch K: Residual shunt infection in a program aimed at its prevention. Presented at 23rd annual meeting of the Society for Research into Hydrocephalus and Spina Bifida, Newcastle Upon Tyne, June 1979.
199. Cohen SJ, Callaghan RP: A syndrome due to the bacterial colonization of Spitz-Holter valves. A review of five cases. Br Med J 2:677, 1961.
200. Everett ED, Eickhoff TC, Simon RH: Cerebrospinal fluid shunt infections with anaerobic diphtheroids (*Propionibacterium* species). J Neurosurg 44:580, 1976.
201. Raphael SS, Donaghue M: Letter: Infection due to *Bacillus cereus*. Can Med Assoc J 115:207, 1976.
202. Callaghan RP, Cohen SJ, Steward GT: Septicaemia due to colonization of Spitz-Holter valves by staphylococci. Five cases treated with methicillin. Br Med J 1:860, 1961.
203. Fokes EC Jr: Occult infections of ventriculo-atrial shunts. J Neurosurg 33:517, 1970.
204. Burke JF: Indentification of the sources of staphylococci contaminating the surgical wound during operation. Ann Surg 158:898, 1963.
205. Bayston R, Lari J: A study of the sources of infection in colonized shunts. Dev Med Child Neurol 16[Suppl 32]:16, 1974.
206. Holt RJ: Bacteriological studies on colonized ventriculo-atrial shunts. Dev Med Child Neurol 12[Suppl 22]:83, 1970.
207. Brook I, Johnson N, Overturf GD, Wilkins J: Mixed bacterial meningitis: A complication of ventriculo- and lumboperitoneal shunts: Report of two cases. J Neurosurg 47:961, 1977.
208. Tsingoglou S, Forrest DM: A technique for the insertion of Holter ventriculoatrial shunt for infantile hydrocephalus. Br J Surg 58:367, 1971.
209. Tsingoglou S, Forrest DM: Complications from Holter ventriculo-atrial shunts. Br J Surg 58:372, 1971.
210. Bayston R: Antibiotic prophylaxis in shunt surgery. Dev Med Child Neurol 17[Suppl 35]:99, 1975.
211. Nicholas JL, Kamal IM, Eckstein HB: Immediate shunt replacement in the treatment of bacterial colonization of Holter valves. Dev Med Child Neurol 12[Suppl 22]:110, 1970.
212. Shurtleff DB, Foltz EL, Weeks RD, Loeser J: Therapy of *Staphylcoccus epidermidis* infections associated with cerebrospinal fluid shunts. Pediatrics 53:55, 1974.
213. Perrin JC, McLaurin RL: Infected ventriculo-atrial shunts. A method of treatment. J Neurosurg 27:21, 1967.
214. McLaurin RL: Infected cerebrospinal fluid shunts. Surg Neurol 1:191, 1973.
215. McLaurin RL: Treatment of infected ventricular shunts. Childs Brain 1:306, 1975.
216. Sells CJ, Shurtleff DB, Loeser J: Gram-negative cerebrospinal fluid shunt-associated infections. Pediatrics 59:614, 1977.
217. Scarff TB, Nelson PB, Reigel DH: External drainage for ventricular infection following cerebrospinal fluid shunts. Childs Brain 4:129, 1978.
218. Dobrin RS, Day NK, Quie PG, Moore HL, Vernier RL, Michael AF, Fish AJ: The role of complement immunoglobulin and bacterial antigen in coagulase-negative staphylococcal shunt nephritis. Am J Med 59:660, 1975.
219. Moss SW, Gary NE, Eisinger RP: Nephritis associated with a diphtheroid-infected cerebrospinal fluid shunt. Am J Med 63:318, 1977.
220. Abraham J, Chandy J: Ventriculo-atrial shunt in the management of posterior-fossa tumours. J Neurosurg 20:252, 1963.
221. Naito H, Toya S, Shizawa H, Lizaka Y, Tsukumo D: High incidence of acute postoperative meningitis and septicemia in patients undergoing craniotomy with ventriculoatrial shunt. Surg Gynecol Obstet 137:810, 1973.
222. Poppen JL: Ventricular drainage as a valuable procedure in neurosurgery. Report of a satisfactory method. Arch Neurol Psychiatry 50:587, 1943.
223. Bering EA Jr: A simplified apparatus for constant ventricular drainage. J Neurosurg 8:450, 1951.
224. Wyler AR, Kelly W: Use of antibiotics with external ventriculostomies. J Neurosurg 37:185, 1972.
225. Hunt GM, Holmes AE: Factors relating to intelligence in treated cases of spina bifida cystica. Am J Dis Child 130:823, 1976.
226. Raine PA, Young DG: Bacterial colonization and infection in lesions of the central nervous system. Dev Med Child Neurol 17[Suppl 35]:111, 1975.
227. Sharrard WJW, Zachary RB, Lorber J, Bruce AM: A controlled trial of immediate and delayed closure of spina bifida cystica. Arch Dis Child 38:18, 1963.
228. Lorber J, Bruce AM: Prospective controlled studies in bacterial meningitis in spina bifida cystica. Dev Med Child Neurol 5:146, 1963.
229. Sundbärg G, Kjällquist A, Lundberg N, Ponten U: Complications due to prolonged ventricular fluid pressure recording in clinical practice. In Brock M, Dietz H (eds): Intracranial Pressure: Experimental and Clinical Aspects. New York, Springer-Verlag, 1972, p 348.
230. Rosner MJ, Becker DP: ICP monitoring: Complications and associated factors. Clin Neurosurg 23:494, 1976.
231. Smith RW, Alksne JF: Infections complicating the use of external ventriculostomy. J Neurosurg 44:567, 1976.
232. Mickell JJ, Reigel DH, Cook DR, Binda RE, Safar P: Intracranial pressure: Monitoring and normalization therapy in children. Pediatrics 59:606, 1977.
233. Malis LI: Control of neurosurgical infections by intra-operative antibiotics. Presented at the annual meeting of the American Association of Neurological Surgeons, San Francisco, Cal, April 1976.
234. Llewellyn RC, Jarrott DM, Meriwether RP: Intra-operative prophylactic antibiotic therapy: a prospective study of the effectiveness cost and complications. Presented at the annual meeting of the American Academy of Neurological Surgery, Munich, Germany, October 1978.
235. Pavel A, Smith R, Ballard A, Larsen IJ: Prophylactic antibiotics in clean orthopedic surgery. J Bone Joint Surg 56A:777, 1974.
236. MacGee EE, Cauthen JC, Brackett CE: Meningitis following acute traumatic cerebrospinal fluid fistula. J Neurosurg 33:312, 1970.
237. Ignelzi RJ, VanderArk GD: Analysis of the treatment of basilar skull fractures with and without antibiotics. J Neurosurg 43:721, 1975.

CHAPTER 29
Infections of the Breast

Gordon F. Schwartz

Infections of the breast are rarely life threatening, although they are annoying and uncomfortable. Any soft tissue infection may occur in the breast (Chapter 25), and the breast is a relatively common site of soft tissue infection in women seen by emergency room physicians. Serious infections are a product of the breast's unique function of lactation and its anatomic and physiologic development in response to this functional demand.

ANATOMY OF THE BREAST

An understanding of the specific anatomic considerations that may influence the development, containment, or dissemination of infectious processes is necessary as an initial measure.[1] Breast tissue extends from the infraclavicular margin superiorly, the midline medially, down to the sixth or seventh costal cartilage inferiorly, over the rectus sheath, laterally to the edge of the latissimus dorsi muscle. The breast also extends in a teardrop shape into the axilla, to a variable degree, as the axillary tail, at times all the way into the hairbearing area itself. Accessory breast tissue may occur in 2 to 3 percent of females, along the milk line between the axilla and groin. If there is parenchyma present in the accessory breast tissue, all the diseases that affect the breasts in their usual position are also possible in this ectopic tissue.

The arterial blood supply of the breast comes mainly from perforating branches 1 to 4 of the internal mammary artery. Additionally, several branches of the axillary artery nourish the breast, the major ones being (1) the highest thoracic artery, above the upper, medial border of the pectoralis minor muscle, (2) the pectoral branch of the thoracoacromial artery, which enters the deep surface of the breast, (3) the lateral thoracic artery to the lateral portion of the breast, and (4) the subscapular artery.

The venous drainage of the breast is more important, not only because of its role as an avenue of dissemination of both infection and cancer but also because the lymphatics generally parallel the course of the veins. These venous pathways are divided into several groups. The superficial subcutaneous veins lie below the superficial fascia and may be seen through the intact skin in many patients. These superficial veins usually converge (becoming confluent with veins of the central atrial breast) and drain into the internal mammary veins or into the lower neck veins. Within the parenchyma of the breast, there are three groups of veins: the internal mammary veins, the intercostal veins, and the axillary vein, which receives its tributaries in an irregular manner from the entire deep surface of the breast.

The breast lymphatics begin around the lobules, with collecting channels following mammary ducts centripetally to the areola and the rich subareolar lymphatic plexus. The retroareolar lymphatics and network of cutaneous lymphatics course to the axilla. The details of lymphatic drainage have been exhaustively reviewed elsewhere.[1] In addition to the five identifiable groups of axillary nodes, the internal mammary route of lymphatic drainage of the breast is also important. From the internal mammary nodes, the lymphatic drainage is to the thoracic duct on the left and the lymphatic duct on the right.

The breast itself is situated between two layers of fascia, the superficial and deep layers of the superficial fascia. The superficial layer of this fascia is within 2–3 mm of the skin and the deep layer of the superficial fascia, which itself lies superficial to the fascia and muscles of the chest wall. Behind this deeper layer of the fascia and the actual muscle fascia is a theoretical space, often called the retromammary bursa, composed of loose areolar tissue. It is this layer that allows the breast to move on the chest wall. Projections of the deep layer of fascia traverse the retromammary bursa and pierce the pectoralis fascia, forming the posterior suspensory ligaments of the breast. Small projections of glandular tissue may accompany these fascial projections right onto the surface of the pectoralis major muscle.

Throughout the breast parenchyma are Cooper's ligaments, toothlike projections of areolar tissue that reach superficially to the undersurface of the skin. Cooper's ligaments may be seen and palpated through incisions in the breast as fine white strands, invariably accompanied by small blood vessels that perforate the breast tissue. Involvement of the Cooper's ligaments by any process that invades or infiltrates them, whether inflammatory or neoplastic, may produce retraction within the breast because the ligaments are shortened by the infiltrative process.

These fascial projections may act as temporary barriers to the extension of inflammatory processes through the breast and tend to keep the process confined. As the architecture of the breast is maintained, the fluctuance that normally accompanies abscess formation can be masked so that infections may burrow into the parenchyma and be more extensive than the outward appearance of the breast may suggest.

MASTITIS AND BREAST ABSCESS

LACTATIONAL MASTITIS AND LACTATIONAL BREAST ABSCESS

The most common breast infection, that which accompanies pregnancy or nursing, is called lactational mastitis or abscess.[2–6] Although the threat to life is small, impressive symptoms, such as malaise and fever, may be produced. Abscess is more a local threat to the breast because, if it is not treated early, a large portion of the mammary parenchyma can be destroyed before the abscess spontaneously drains through the skin.

Etiology

The most common organism associated with lactational mastitis or abscess has been hemolytic, coagulase-positive *Staphylococcus aureus,* reported in from 65 percent to over 90 percent of collected cases.[4–9] *Staphylococcus epidermidis* and species of *Streptococcus* have also been found.[4] Lactational abscess has been associated with other aerobic and anaerobic organisms, such as *Bacteroides,* in the past few years.[7,9–12] Finegold has recently reviewed the anaerobes.[12] If the milk is cultured, the causative organism will sometimes be isolated. If the organism comes from the baby's nasopharynx, the milk from the contralateral breast may harbor the same organism without clinical evidence of infection.

Incidence and Epidemiology

The majority of lactational infections occur sporadically after childbirth, but they can also be encountered during pregnancy. Postpartum mastitis affects less than 2 percent of women after delivery, but sporadic epidemics affecting up to 10 percent of postpartum women have occurred.[6,9] At one time, it was thought that these represented two forms of infection, the epidemic variety being less acute with less constitutional symptoms than the sporadic ones, but this arbitrary division is no longer tenable.

For some mysterious reason, either real or because of the manner in which they are reported, about two thirds of these infections have been associated with first pregnancies. Perhaps the first-time pregnant breast is more susceptible to infection. It has been claimed, although not confirmed, that a woman who has experienced postpartum mastitis once is more likely to develop an infection after subsequent deliveries.

Pathogenesis and Pathology

By definition, these infections occur in the breasts of pregnant or lactating women and are seemingly related to lactational physiology. During the first trimester of pregnancy, the breasts are characterized by ductal sprouting and branching, induced by luteal and placental hormones. Near the end of the first trimester, there is hypertrophy of the lobular-alveolar units, as well as an actual increase in their number. In the second trimester, secretory activity is initiated, and colostrum appears within the alveoli. Enlargement of the breast continues, attributed to alveolar dilatation and the accumulation of colostrum, along with increased vascularity. Fat and connective tissue within the breast actually decrease during pregnancy. In the final trimester, the secretory cells of the alveoli continue their function as the breast fills with colostrum. The blood supply continues to increase, so that flow through the breast at the end of pregnancy may have doubled.

Under the influence of prolactin, after the postpartum withdrawal of placental lactogen and other sex steroids, lactation begins as milk is released into the mammary alveoli and collecting ducts. At the same time, in the first few days after delivery, venous and lymphatic stasis occurs, and the breast parenchyma itself becomes edematous. The composition of colostrum begins to change, so that mature milk is available about two weeks later. Breast edema, lymphatic stasis, colostrum and milk secretion, and partial ductal obstruction probably all play a role in the increased susceptibility of the postpartum breast to infection.

Why some women develop lactational infections is poorly understood. It is generally assumed that a cracked or fissured nipple, secondary to the continual irritation by the suckling infant, provides a portal of entry for pathogenic organisms from the infant's nasopharynx.[9] This assumes that the infant has been colonized by some carrier, and the organisms are then passed to the ducts or lymphatics of the nursing mother through the excoriated nipple. Many more mothers develop cracked nipples than develop infections of their breasts. It has also been suggested that milk stasis may be a contributing factor, because a missed feeding or weaning has been noted to precipitate infection in some women. There seems to be no single common denominator to explain the origin of most infections.

Another unsubstantiated explanation is the altered hormonal status of nursing women. Perhaps the hormonal milieu of the postpartum, nursing mother creates an environment that encourages the growth of organisms that might otherwise be unable to establish a foothold. Pregnancy seems to lower resistance to a variety of microbes.

Clinical Manifestations

The typical case of lactational mastitis begins in the second, third, or fourth week after delivery.[2,13] The range is as early as four or five days after childbirth to as late as one year later.[4] Tenderness is usually the first symptom, accompanied by erythema that is usually adjacent to the areolar margin.[13] Induration and edema may follow. A general malaise, as with any infectious process, may occur, although at this stage usually no systemic symptoms are present. Fever may occur as the infection continues.

Mastitis, inflammation without progression to actual abscess, is the most common lactational infection. Only about 5 percent of the infections will require surgical drainage if early detection and treatment are instituted. Even prior to the advent of antibiotics, mastitis did not always progress to abscess.

If lactational mastitis progresses without treatment, or if it is not detected until late in its course, a breast abscess can result. At this time, the erythema becomes more pronounced, tenderness and induration increase, and the breast becomes more edematous. Palpation of the breast reveals a mass, which is usually exquisitely painful and which may be fluctuant. Fever is almost always present, and the systemic signs may be impressive, including malaise, chills, and leukocytosis, as with any acute bacterial infection. Although bacteremia may occur, the organisms cannot usually be cultured from the blood.

Diagnosis

The usual surgical dictum of waiting for fluctuance to initiate drainage of an abscess does not apply here. Considerable tissue necrosis may occur within the breast without palpable evidence of fluctuance—mass and induration may be the only signs. Ancillary diagnostic studies, such as mammography, thermography, or ultrasonography, are usually not necessary because the diagnosis is evident clinically. Mammography is more unpleasant for the nursing patient or the patient with an already painful abscess because the squashing of the breast by the mammographic equipment is necessary to achieve an optimal image. Needless to say, mammography should not be used in the pregnant patient without especially good reason, such as the suspicion of carcinoma. Confirming the presence of mastitis or abscess does not seem to be sufficient reason for a pregnant woman to undergo this examination. Certainly, the same precautions do not pertain for the use of thermography or ultrasonography, but their value as diagnostic aids in this situation is, at best, superfluous. In other words, once the clinical diagnosis of breast abscess in the lactating patient is made, no further confirmatory studies are necessary, and treatment may be instituted forthwith.

Treatment

If treatment is begun promptly after the diagnosis of mastitis is made, further progression may be halted and the process resolved. Oral penicillin or a synthetic penicillin is the best treatment, with erythromycin as an alternative for the allergic patient.

If both mother and child are capable of continuing, nursing should not be stopped, particularly if milk stasis is a factor in the pathogenesis of infection, since it may have a beneficial effect.[2,4] If nursing must be discontinued, it is probably a good idea to express the milk from the breasts with a pump. Only a purulent exudate from the nipple or an actual abscess should stop nursing. In the past, diethylstilbestrol (DES) was advocated to help stop lactation [9] as part of the treatment for these infections, but this is no longer recommended.

If the infection is found early and treatment is begun, the erythema, tenderness, and induration diminish within three or four days. If the symptoms continue without improvement, an abscess must be suspected.

Rarely, a suspected breast abscess can be aspirated. If the abscess is small, aspiration with a No. 18 gauge needle and vigorous antibiotic therapy may avoid the need for open surgical drainage. If aspiration is attempted, several criteria should be fulfilled. The patient should be reexamined daily. If the purulence reaccumulates or if the inflammation does not improve quickly, open surgical drainage should be performed without delay. The aspirate should be submitted for immediate Gram stain, culture, and sensitivity studies so that the appropriate antibiotic, usually a synthetic penicillin, may be chosen.

When drainage of a breast abscess is necessary, it is best done under general anesthesia in the operating room. Invariably, such attempts in the physician's office, under local anesthesia, fail either because the light is poor, there is a lack of proper instruments and assistance, or the patient's discomfort does not allow the wound to be probed sufficiently.

Although many surgical textbooks describe radial incisions in the breast to drain abscesses (supposedly to avoid cutting across ducts), they are perpendicular to the natural skin lines and leave conspicuous scars, especially when these wounds are left open to heal secondarily (Fig. 29-1). Breast abscesses should be approached through incisions placed in the natural skin lines, parallel to the areolar

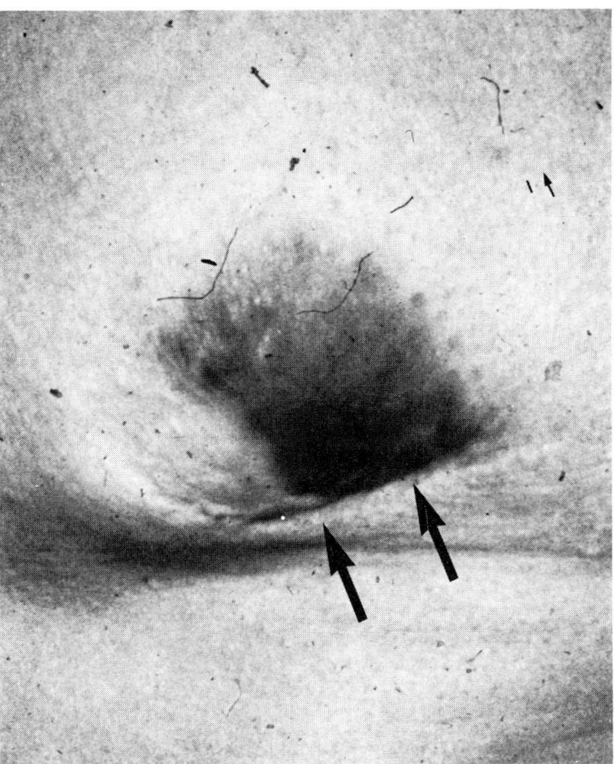

Fig. 29-1. **Conspicuous scar and deformity of breast following injudicious choice of incision and overzealous excision of inflamed tissues.**

margin, the same incisions used for breast biopsy.[13,14] These incisions heal with minimal scarring, even when they are left open (Fig. 29-2). Most breast abscesses occur adjacent to the areolar margin, and, therefore, a circumareolar incision can be used, which leads to the least conspicuous scar possible. Finger dissection within the breast may be required to fracture the loculations that have formed and to insure adequate drainage. Although some surgical atlases recommend the use of counter incisions to afford dependent drainage, these are seldom necessary and can leave conspicuous scars. If counter incisions are needed, they should be placed in the inframammary fold, so that the resultant scar will be hidden by the overhanging breast.

A sample of the wall of the abscess cavity must be histologically examined each time a breast abscess is drained. Carcinoma can mimic an abscess, although the coincidence of lactational abscess and carcinoma is rare. Carcinoma itself is unusual in young women and even more rare in the pregnant or lactating patient, but histologic examination of all tissues excised at operation is always indicated. A separate specimen should also be submitted to the microbiology laboratory for both aerobic and anaerobic cultures, as well as Gram stain, even if previous specimens have been sent.

Copious irrigation of the wound with saline solution helps debride the wound. Whether the addition of antibiotic to the irrigant is effective is questionable. Probably more important is a large volume of irrigant. A drain is necessary—a latex drain for small abscesses or a packing soaked in peroxide or Dakin solution for large ones. A single drain should remain in place a minimum of 48–72 hours. Antibiotics are usually continued for 7–10 days and may be switched from parenteral to oral form when the patient is better. The blood supply to the breast is relatively poor, and, therefore, the antibiotic should be continued until the cellulitis that accompanies the infection has nearly subsided.

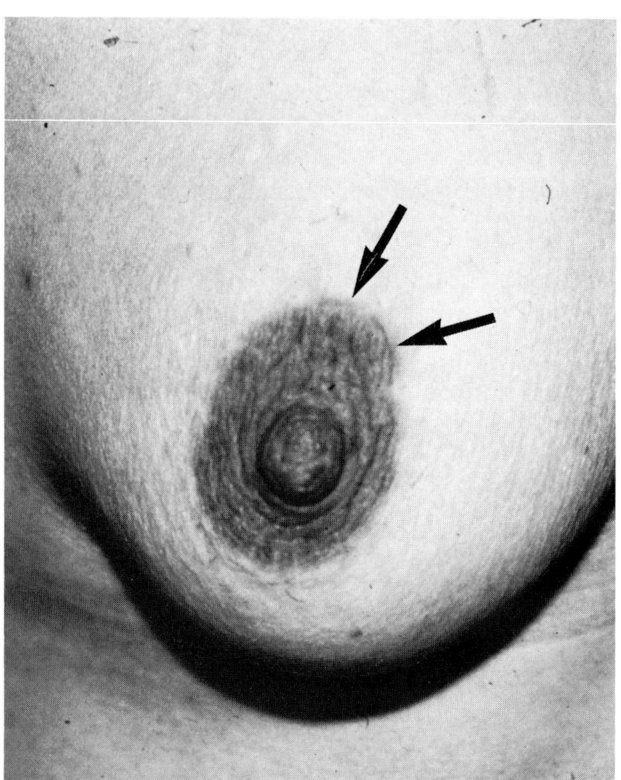

Fig. 29-2. **Arrows point to healed circumareolar incision used for drainage of abscess. Judicious choice of incision results in an almost invisible scar following healing.**

Prognosis

Despite the size of the cavity or the depth of the wound, if the drainage incision has been placed in the skin lines, both patient and physician are usually pleasantly surprised by the final appearance of the healed wound. If the amount of necrosis within the breast is minimal, there is usually no significant distortion of the breast nor large scar as a reminder of the event.

Prevention

Except for the obvious admonitions about personal hygiene, there is no feasible manner in which these infections can be completely avoided.

NONLACTATIONAL MASTITIS AND ABSCESS

The signs and symptoms, diagnosis, and treatment of breast infections in nonpregnant, nonlactating women are similar to those previously described. What is perhaps unusual about these infections is their mysterious origin. As with the lactational infections, these infections have a predilection for young women.[10,14] Almost all are found in premenopausal patients and seem to appear more commonly during patients' premenstrual phases of their cycle. A history of antecedent factors that may predispose to infection is obtained rarely, although embarrassment of the inquiring physician or the patient may cause omission of details about minor trauma to the nipples from "love bites."

After the inflammation or infection has begun, the same course of events and treatment pertain for the nonlactating breast as they did for the patient with a postpartum infection. The organisms are similar, and the treatment and outcome are no different.[10]

Differential Diagnosis

What is most important in the nonlactating female, however, is the differential diagnosis of those conditions of the breast that may mimic infection, which must be excluded when this problem presents itself.

The several diseases of the breast that must be differentiated from mastitis or abscess are mammary duct ectasia, Mondor's disease, and carcinoma. Although these conditions are not infectious in nature, they must all be discussed in enough detail to make this differentiation possible.

Mammary Duct Ectasia (Plasma Cell Mastitis, Comedomastitis). Mammary duct ectasia is a relative of cystic disease that is characterized by dilatation of the subareolar ducts with contiguous fibrosis and inflammation.[5,15] Unlike most breast infections, ectasia usually affects the breast of the menopausal or postmenopausal woman. As the collecting ducts beneath the nipple become dilated, they fill with cellular debris. A thick, blood-stained, toothpastelike nipple discharge may occur. If, instead, the process continues peripherally into the breast, the walls of the ducts become thickened, and the area is infiltrated by lymphocytes and plasma cells. If the intraductal material, a crystalline, lipid substance, ruptures through the duct wall, an intense inflammatory response ensues, with proliferation of giant cells, polymorphonuclear leukocytes, and lymphocytes. The center of the lesion may break down, even cavitate, becoming a sterile abscess filled with the same material. At this point, a mass is often palpable. Fibrosis within the breast produces retraction signs, so that the mass may be mistaken for carcinoma.

In a variable proportion of patients with mammary duct ectasia, the initial clinical signs may mimic exactly those of an infectious mastitis, with erythema, induration, tenderness, and axillary adenopathy. If it is incised, sterile pus is obtained. If treated with antibiotics, it resolves—as it does without treatment in 7–10 days. More likely, the ectatic lesion in the breast mimics cancer rather than infection, and biopsy is required to make the diagnosis.

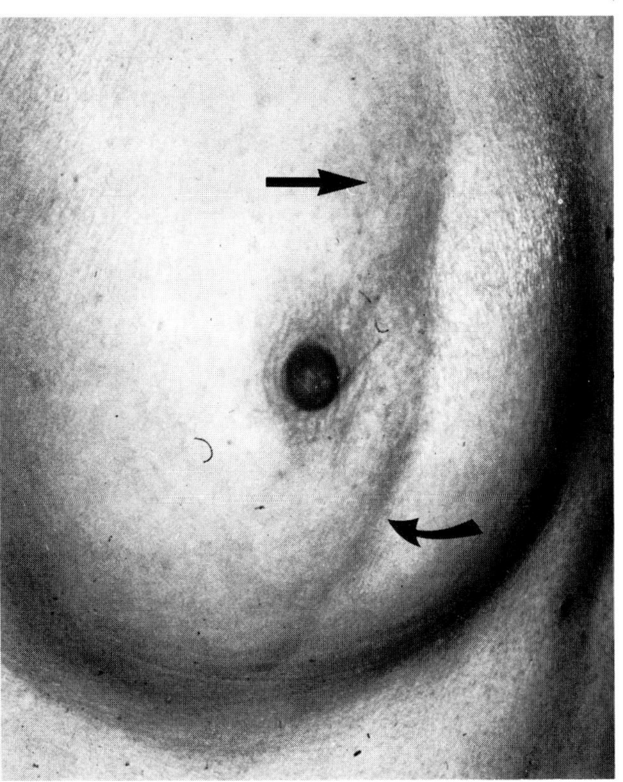

Fig. 29-3. **Mondor's disease. Upper arrow denotes area of erythema. Lower arrow points to cordlike thrombotic vein, with retraction.**

Mondor's Disease (Superficial Phlebitis of the Breast). Mondor's disease, an uncommon lesion that can mimic infection, is named after the French physician who first described it. Usually this phlebitic process involves the thoracoepigastric vessels in the lateral half of the breast, and the process may course down across the costal margin onto the abdominal wall (Fig. 29-3).[1] A history of trauma is often noted, and Mondor's disease may follow breast biopsy about three weeks after operation. Pain, tenderness, and erythema overlie a cordlike structure, which may demonstrate retraction along its course. Healing occurs spontaneously in two to four weeks, although it may take as long as six to eight weeks before the cord disappears. Neither biopsy nor treatment is necessary. About one fourth of the cases of Mondor's disease reported in the literature have been biopsied unnecessarily.

Carcinoma. Cancer associated with inflammation or infection of the breast is most unusual, and inflammatory cancer comprises less than 2 percent of all breast cancer. However, when the inflammatory type of breast carcinoma does occur, it may resemble an infection, and this diagnosis must be considered when an inflammatory lesion of the breast is encountered.[1]

Inflammatory carcinoma first appears as tenderness or discomfort. Although a mass may be present, it is often overlooked. The hallmark of this, the most virulent form of breast cancer, is the apparent inflammatory response of the breast with actual enlargement of the indurated, edematous breast. There is a characteristic pink flush to the skin, but this may be so faint that it is missed. The erythema is most often over the dependent portion of the breast, and the breast itself may be mottled in color. The reddened skin may feel warm to the touch, but there are few, if any, systemic manifestations of inflammation—fever, leukocytosis. The majority of these patients will have palpable, firm nodes in the axilla, and about one fourth of these patients will have foci of metastatic carcinoma elsewhere, such as bones, lungs, or liver.

Obviously, the important differential diagnosis is between inflammatory carcinoma and infection. Many patients with inflammatory cancer have been given antibiotics mistakenly. Infection or abscess is usually more well localized than is inflammatory cancer, which tends to affect the entire breast. Mammary duct ectasia must also be considered. Not only is ectasia a well-localized rather than a diffuse process, but also the inflammatory response to ectasia resolves spontaneously within a few days.

In addition to the generalized inflammatory response of this special form of cancer, the secondary infection that may accompany an ulcerated breast cancer may lead to a similar presentation (Fig. 29-4). Secondary infections evolve slowly and remain more localized. Redness and edema of the breast associated with ulceration are late signs of advanced localized disease. Medullary carcinoma, and even papillary carcinoma and comedocarcinoma, may undergo central necrosis, which may, in turn, be followed by erythema and edema of the overlying skin. Biopsy is the only way of making this diagnostic distinction. Carcinoma en cuirasse is a slow process in which the skin of the entire chest wall becomes fibrotic and thickened as

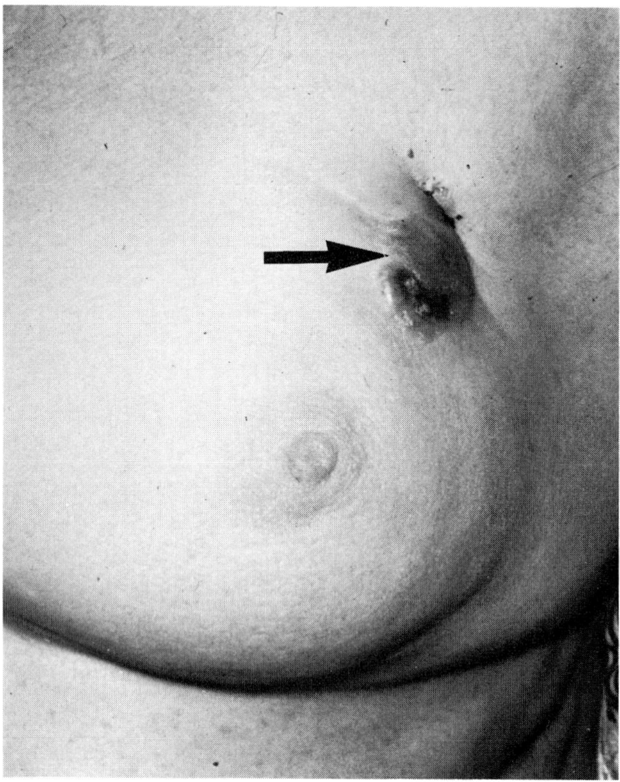

Fig. 29-4. **Carcinoma of the breast, with erythema and incipient ulceration. This is not inflammatory carcinoma.**

carcinoma advances. Although redness and apparent inflammation may accompany this process, it is usually easy to differentiate from acute inflammation, because carcinoma en cuirasse is so slow to evolve.

RECURRENT SUBAREOLAR ABSCESS

Recurrent subareolar abscess is a poorly understood and infrequently recognized chronic infection of the breast. It produces repeated episodes of inflammation and abscess and has sometimes led to total mastectomy in an attempt to control the infection. This is most unfortunate because if the diagnosis is made and the appropriate treatment undertaken, mastectomy should never be necessary.

It is possible that the majority of the breast abscesses that occur in the periareolar area, that are not associated with lactation, or for which a definite portal of entry cannot be established, may be related to this particular lesion. The lesion is not usually diagnosed until several attempts at cure by incision and drainage have been made.[15,16] In those abscesses that do not become recurrent, the initial attempt at drainage probably halts the continuing process.

Etiology

The most common infecting organisms have been *S. aureus, Proteus, Bacteroides,* and nonhemolytic *Streptococcus,* and the most recent reports have implicated anaerobic organisms in a greater proportion of these abscesses than heretofore appreciated.[7,10-12]

Pathogenesis and Pathology

In normal lactiferous ducts, there is an abrupt change from squamous to columnar epithelium 1–2 mm beneath the surface of the nipple. Hyperplasia of this squamous epithelium with accumulation of keratin within the lumen of the duct plugs the duct.[17] Dilatation and rupture of the proximal duct occur. Bacterial invasion then supervenes, and an abscess is formed, complicated by the keratinized material, which acts as an adjuvant foreign body.[5,18] Even if surgical drainage is performed, the suppurative process continues until the squamous epithelium is removed or destroyed. This process may produce a fistula at the edge of the areola, which, if probed, winds its way to the base of the nipple (Figs. 29-5 and 29-6).[16,17] True squamous metaplasia of the nipple ducts may occur, as manifested by transition from squamous to columnar, back to squamous epithelium deeper in the breast. It had been suggested that this condition must be accompanied by or is a result of inverted nipples,[19,20] but this does not seem to be substantiated, since about half of the patients with these recurring abscesses do not have inverted nipples.[10]

Diagnosis

If an abscess encountered in the breast seems to be associated with a sinus tract or fistulous opening adjacent to the areolar margin, Gram-stained smears and cultures should be done. If gram-negative bacilli are present, anaerobic cultures should be performed because *Bacteroides* is a common pathogen. Clindamycin, chloramphenicol, or metronidazole may be required. Most such infections are caused by staphylococci, and antibiotic therapy may not be necessary.

The acute abscess must be treated by incision and drainage, as for any breast abscess, but the involved duct(s) must be excised when the infection is quiescent, or the abscess will recur. It is sometimes difficult to convince the patient, after only the first or even the second abscess, that an operation is necessary when she is feeling well. After these patients have undergone repeated operations for drainage of their recurrent abscesses, however, ready agreement is obtained.

The sinus tract or fistula must be removed in its entirety.[15,17] This is done by including the opening within a small ellipse of skin at the areolar margin, then dissecting the duct or fistula from the retroareolar area toward the base of the nipple, removing that small area of nipple where the duct emerges, and coring it out (Fig. 29-7).[18] The nipple itself may be closed without drainage, although it is usually preferable to leave a soft sliver of rubber drain in the circumareolar incision for 24–48 hours. This procedure is minimal and done as the first attempt at eliminating the problem. In some patients, further recurrence may result from the involvement of additional ducts, and in these patients, a larger segment of nipple may have to be removed. If there is a second or third recurrence, the entire nipple and underlying major ducts may have to be removed (nipple only, not areola). This will cure the disease without resorting to mastectomy.

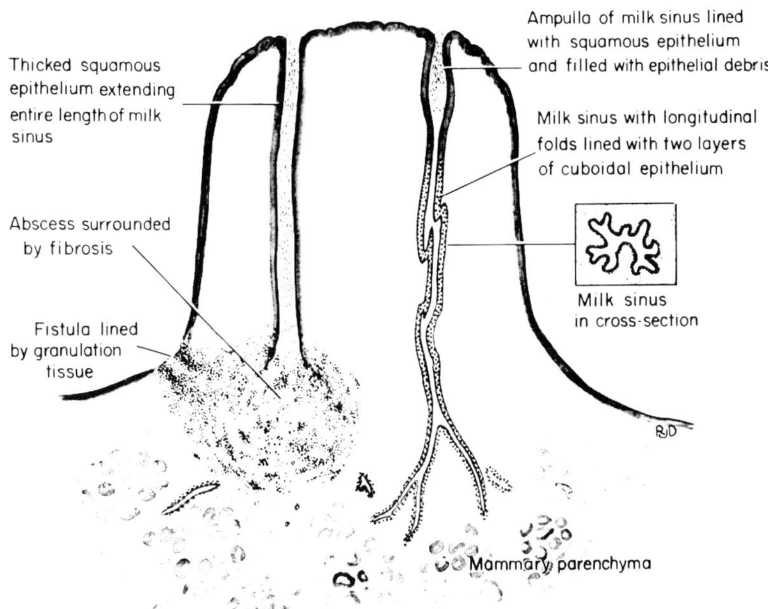

Fig. 29-5. **Recurring subareolar abscess shown diagrammatically. (From Haagensen CD: Diseases of the Breast, 2nd ed, 1971. Courtesy of WB Saunders Co.)**

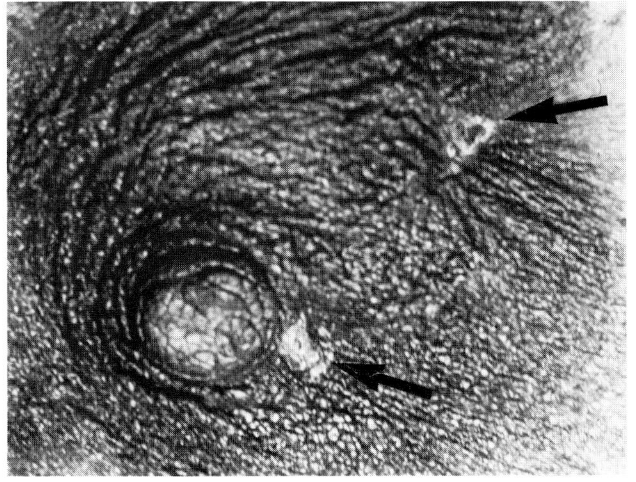

Fig. 29-6. **Recurring subareolar abscess. Arrows denote openings of sinus tracts beneath nipple-areolar complex.**

UNCOMMON INFECTIOUS DISEASES OF THE BREAST

MASTITIS OF THE AXILLARY TAIL

The normal extension of the breast into the axilla, known as the axillary tail or tail of Spence, is quite variable and forms a visible mass that enlarges in the premenstrual period or during lactation. If there is no communication between this axillary prolongation and the remainder of the lactating breast, it becomes enlarged, inflamed, and tender and may form a sterile abscess. If this occurs in the primipara, excision of the axillary breast tissue should be carried out after weaning. Excision may be performed under local anesthesia, and the resultant scar can be hidden inconspicuously in the hairbearing portion of the underarm.

NEONATAL MASTITIS

About one third of normal newborn infants develop conspicuous breast enlargement at three to four days after birth, which peaks by two or three weeks and is gone by one month of age. During the time of maximum swelling, a few drops of milky or clear discharge may escape from the baby's nipple (witch's milk). All this is normal.

The only complication of neonatal hypertrophy is infection, most probably the result of the repeated poking and prodding by parents who are overly concerned about the hypertrophy, especially in male infants. This may introduce organisms into the breast. When this type of infection occurs, it is signaled by erythema, swelling, induration, and pain and sometimes progresses to abscess.[21-23]

Simultaneous infection of the breast in mother and child is not rare, and the treatment is the same for both. The organisms implicated in neonatal infections are predominantly *S. aureus,* with reports of gram-negative organisms as well, eg, *Escherichia coli,* and even *Salmonella.*[21-23] In the case of *Salmonella* mastitis, the mastitis was a secondary complication of systemic infection.

If the mastitis in an infant is not cured by antibiotics and requires drainage, it becomes a more formidable undertaking, not because of the intrinsic danger of the infection to the child but because of the threat of the operative procedure to the breast itself, especially in a female child. The damage to the breast bud from the infection or from the required drainage may lead to asymmetry of growth or even failure of the breast to develop at puberty. For this reason, surgical drainage of a breast abscess in the neonate or in any prepubertal girl must be approached with caution.

PREPUBERTAL AND PUBERTAL MASTITIS

The prepubertal and pubertal breast, in both boys and girls, may be the site of an inflammatory reaction, manifested by erythema, tenderness, and even the development of a small mass. Such an occurrence is rare, and

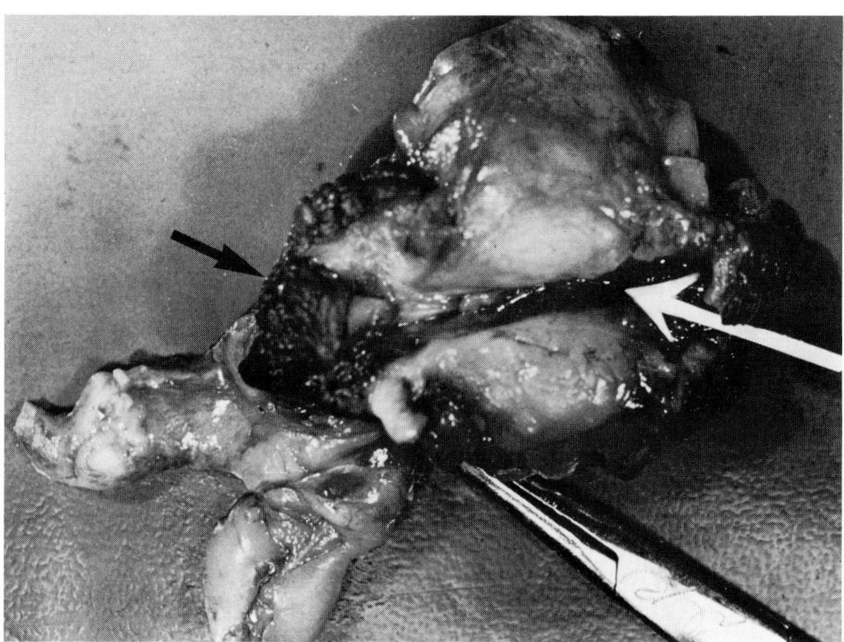

Fig. 29-7. **Recurring subareolar abscess, gross specimen following excision. White arrow points to squamous lined tract. Black arrow indicates small portion of excised areola with fistulous opening.**

even fewer go on to actual infection or abscess. The breast is a modified apocrine gland, so it is not unreasonable to imagine that it might also become active when the other apocrine glands become stimulated. Treatment for this condition is symptomatic, plus the prescription of an appropriate antistaphylococcal antibiotic.[24]

In a similar fashion, the adolescent female breast may be the target of an inflammatory mastitis. This is perhaps related to ductal obstruction because the ducts of the breast are being intensely stimulated by the hormones being produced at this time of life. Treatment is the same as for pubertal mastitis.

GRANULOMATOUS DISEASE OF THE BREAST

A newly described inflammatory lesion of the breast, which occurs in premenopausal women, has been called granulomatous mastitis.[25,26] A painless mass that resembles carcinoma on clinical examination leads to biopsy.[27] Rather than a central lesion, as with most other inflammatory conditions of the breast, this mass is usually peripheral in location and confined to the lobular elements of the breast. On histologic examination, small, sterile abscesses are found within typical granulomatous changes—but without ductal dilatation. The initial histologic impression often has been that of mammary duct ectasia, even tuberculous mastitis, but the lack of dilated ducts makes the diagnosis of ectasia untenable, and failure to demonstrate acid-fast organisms makes tuberculosis unlikely.

Two differing explanations for this lesion have been suggested. The first is akin to the pathogenesis of mammary duct ectasia, a granulomatous response to the contents of ruptured ducts.[26] Another theory is that this lesion resembles the histology of cat-scratch fever and, thus, may be a response to a similar agent, presumably viral in origin, or may even represent an unusual autoimmune phenomenon.[25]

Treatment is simple excision of the mass.

TUBERCULOSIS OF THE BREAST

Now an extremely rare lesion of the breast, in the days before specific antituberculous therapy, tuberculous mastitis occasionally accompanied generalized tuberculosis.[28] Even in its heyday, tuberculous mastitis accounted for only 2 percent of the breast diseases seen in specialized breast clinics. Most breast specialists today will never encounter a case. Tuberculosis of the breast was once divided arbitrarily into primary (breast only) and secondary (disseminated) forms. In the latter form, the breast was thought to be involved by retrograde lymphatic spread of organisms from the axillary nodes or as direct extension from pulmonary intrathoracic lymphatics. For the primary cases, a direct hematogenous source was postulated, with growth of the organisms directly in the breast itself. The most common finding was a painless mass in the breast progressing to retraction, ulceration, and abscess formation.[28] In its early stages, tuberculosis of the breast was confused with carcinoma.[29] The axillary nodes were enlarged in 50–75 percent of cases. Most patients seemed otherwise healthy and did not have the characteristic phthisic appearance. Nipple discharge was rarely present, and if it was cultured or smeared, the characteristic acid-fast organisms could be demonstrated in the discharge.

Treatment ranged from total mastectomy to antituberculous therapy only. The most reasonable suggestion for treatment would seem to be eradication of the tuberculous focus by local excision of the mass, accompanied by systemic antituberculous therapy.[29] There should be no need for total mastectomy unless the lesion is so immense that local excision and mastectomy would be synonymous.

Although this diagnosis is extremely rare, if a patient with known tuberculosis develops a breast mass, tuberculous mastitis must be considered. At one time, it was taught that breast cancer and tuberculosis were mutually exclusive diseases, and that the patient with tuberculosis was immune to the development of breast cancer. This is not true, and there are case reports of patients with cancer of one breast and tuberculosis of the other or the two diseases coexisting, not only in the same breast but within the same axillary nodes.

SILICONE MASTITIS

This general term has been coined to refer to all those forms of iatrogenic and self-induced infections related to the introduction of foreign bodies into the breast in an attempt to augment its size.[30] These reactions have occurred in response to the implantation or injection of a myriad of substances into the breast, some of which almost defy the imagination—beeswax, silicone wax, shellac, putty, epoxy resin, and even spun glass.

The characteristic histologic appearance is a nodal histiocytosis and a local inflammatory reaction to the injected or implanted material. Treatment for these infections must include removal of the offending foreign body. Unfortunately, in some patients who have undergone injection of these materials directly into the breast, total mastectomy has been the unpleasant result because the injected substance had permeated the entire breast.

Even the most carefully performed augmentation mammoplasty can be accompanied by infection of the wound or extrusion of the prosthesis through the skin. When either of these complications occurs, it is usually fruitless to attempt to salvage the situation. The prosthesis must be removed and the wound allowed to heal. At a later date, another attempt at augmentation may be undertaken.

MISCELLANEOUS INFECTIONS

The breast has been reported as the locus for many other unusual infectious diseases of bacterial, fungal, or protozoal origin. For example, syphilis of the breast has been described as both primary chancre and secondary gumma, although even large clinics may not have a case in their records.

In areas where the diseases are endemic, hydatid disease, filariasis, leprosy, blastomycosis, sporotrichosis, and actinomycosis of the breast have been reported.

There is a more complete discussion in Chapter 25.

POSTOPERATIVE WOUND INFECTIONS

Despite the relatively poor blood supply of the breast, operations on the breast are complicated infrequently by postoperative wound infections. Breast surgery is considered clean, and prophylactic antibiotics are not indicated unless preexisting infection is present. A possible exception to this dictum is augmentation mammoplasty, which requires the permanent implantation of a foreign body into the wound. Even with this procedure, the efficacy of preoperative and postoperative antibiotic prophylaxis has not been established unequivocally.

Breast biopsies are rarely uncomfortable after the first 24–48 hours, and a wound complication should be suspected if the pain continues, even if fever, erythema, and fluctuance are absent. Usually, there is some demonstrable serosanguineous or purulent drainage through the incision, and most often, all that is necessary is to open the wound and establish drainage, inserting a small gauze wick or peroxide-soaked packing into the wound to insure that the edges do not seal before effective drainage has been attained. It is customary to initiate a course of a synthetic penicillin at the time the wound is opened, while awaiting the reports of Gram-stained smear and culture. Most would respond to effective drainage alone, but the addition of the appropriate antibiotic may hasten resolution.

During major operative procedures on the breast, the thin skin flaps created during modified or radical mastectomy are relatively ischemic and, therefore, more vulnerable to infection. The likelihood of postoperative infection may be minimized by gentle handling, sharp dissection with scalpel, and wound closure using the finest (00000) sutures. Even during lengthy breast operations, the blood vessels and other structures that must be secured are small in caliber, even if numerous, and may be tied with the finest (00000) nonabsorbable sutures. Mastectomy flaps may be reapproximated quite satisfactorily with 00000 synthetic absorbable subcuticular sutures of Dexon or Vicryl and 00000 nylon sutures, even plastic tapes, for the skin. No heavier sutures are necessary in the breast!

When and if wound infection does occur, the same principles of treatment apply as pertain to other soft tissue infections. Indeed, most of the patients scheduled for these operations are otherwise healthy, and their natural defense mechanisms are intact.

The most common organism, even in hospital-acquired infections, is again *S. aureus*. Occasionally, an infection by a group A beta-hemolytic *Streptococcus* will occur after mastectomy. This particular infection is manifested by fever out of proportion to other symptoms, accompanied by leukocytosis and wound tenderness, along with considerable erythema in the wound and an exudate. The diagnosis may be made by Gram stain of the exudate, which reveals the characteristic gram-positive cocci in chains. Cultures of blood and wound should be followed by the use of high doses of penicillin—or erythromycin in the allergic patient.

Other wound infections, such as those caused by gram-negative organisms, anaerobic organisms, or clostridia, are extremely rare. The Gram-stained smear and culture should be able to rule these out at the time the infection is recognized and treatment is initiated.

BIBLIOGRAPHY

Haagensen, CD: Diseases of the Breast, 2nd ed. Philadelphia, Saunders, 1971.

REFERENCES

1. Haagensen CD: Diseases of the Breast, 2nd ed. Philadelphia, Saunders, 1971.
2. Devereux WP: Acute puerperal mastitis: Evaluation of its management. Am J Obstet Gynecol 108:78, 1970.
3. Gibberd GF: Sporadic and epidemic puerperal breast infections: A contrast in morbid anatomy and clinical signs. Am J Obstet Gynecol 65:1038, 1953.

4. Marshall BR, Hepper JK, Zirbel CC: Sporadic puerperal mastitis: An infection that need not interrupt lactation. JAMA 233:1377, 1975.
5. Sandison AT, Walker JC: Inflammatory mastitis, mammary duct ectasia, and mammillary fistula. Br J Surg 50:57, 1962.
6. Sherman AJ: Puerperal breast abscess: I. Report of an outbreak at Philadelphia General Hospital. Obstet Gynecol 7:268, 1956.
7. Monro JA, Markham NPL: Staphylococcal infection in mothers and infants. Maternal breast abscesses and antecedent neonatal sepsis. Lancet 2:186, 1958.
8. Sawyer CD, Walker PH: A bacteriologic and clinical study of breast abscess. Surg Gynecol Obstet 99:368, 1954.
9. Soltau DHK, Hatcher GW: Some observations on the aetiology of breast abscess in the puerperium. Br Med J 1:1603, 1960.
10. Ekland DA, Zeigler MG: Abscess in the nonlactating breast. Arch Surg 107:398, 1973.
11. Leach RD, Phillips I, Eykyn SJ, Corrin B: Anaerobic subareolar breast abscess. Lancet 1:35, 1979.
12. Finegold SM: Anerobic Bacteria in Human Disease. New York, Academic, 1977, p 467–470.
13. Newton M, Newton NR: Breast abscess: A result of lactation failure. Surg Gynecol Obstet 91:432, 1973.
14. Knight ICS, Nolan B: Breast abscess. Br Med J 1:1224, 1959.
15. Abramson DJ: Mammary duct ectasia, mammillary fistula, and subareolar sinuses. Ann Surg 169:217, 1969.
16. Zuska JJ, Crile G Jr, Ayres WW: Fistulas of lactiferous ducts. Am J Surg 81:312, 1951.
17. Patey DH, Thackray AC: Pathology and treatment of mammary duct fistula. Lancet 2:871, 1958.
18. Habif DV, Perzin KH, Lipton R, Lattes R: Subareolar abscess associated with squamous metaplasia of lactiferous ducts. Am J Surg 119:523, 1970.
19. Caswell HT, Burnett WE: Chronic recurrent breast abscess secondary to inversion of the nipple. Surg Gynecol Obstet 102:439, 1956.
20. Caswell HT, Maier WP: Chronic recurrent periareolar abscess secondary to inversion of the nipple. Surg Gynecol Obstet 128:597, 1969.
21. Burry VF, Beezley M: Infant mastitis due to gram-negative organisms. Am J Dis Child 124:736, 1972.
22. Schwarz MD, Rosen RA: Neonatal mastitis due to *Escherichia coli*. Clin Pediatr 13:86, 1974.
23. Stetler H, Martin E, Plotkin S, Katz M: Neonatal mastitis due to *Escherichia coli*. J Pediatr 76:611, 1970.
24. Mayer TC: Treatment of prepubertal mastitis. Lancet 2:721, 1975.
25. Cohen C: Granulomatous mastitis: A review of 5 cases. S Afr Med J 52:14, 1977.
26. Murthy MSH: Granulomatous mastitis and lipogranuloma of the breast. Am J Clin Pathol 60:432, 1973.
27. Kessler E, Wollock Y: Granulomatous mastitis: A lesion clinically simulating carcinoma. Am J Clin Pathol, 58:642, 1972.
28. Schaefer G: Tuberculosis of the breast. A review with the additional presentation of 10 cases. Am Rev Tuberc 72:810, 1955.
29. Cohen C: Tuberculous mastitis: A review of 34 cases. S Afr Med J 52:12, 1977.
30. Symmers WStC: Silicone mastitis in "topless" waitresses and some other varieties of foreign-body mastitis. Br Med J 3:19, 1968.

CHAPTER 30
Thoracic Surgical Infections

TIMOTHY TAKARO, GULSHAN K. SETHI,
STEWART M. SCOTT, AND THOMAS J. ENRIGHT

INFECTIONS of the chest can be divided into four regions: (1) the chest wall, (2) pleural spaces, (3) lungs and airways, and (4) the mediastinum. In each area, both primary and postoperative infections will be considered.

These divisions are somewhat artificial, of course, because infections in one area commonly involve neighboring areas. For example, pneumonias or lung abscesses are a major cause of pleural empyema. In turn, a loculated empyema may burrow through the chest, simulating an abscess of the chest wall (empyema necessitatis). Chronic mediastinal infections may result from primary lung infections, such as histoplasmosis or tuberculosis, while acute mediastinal infections that result from perforations of the esophagus or bronchopleural fistulas quickly cause infections of the pleural cavities.

The mouth and nasopharynx are normally host to many microorganisms and, being in continuity with the upper and lower airways of the lungs, provide natural and major portals of entry into this region. The result can be aspiration pneumonitis, lung abscess, or a communicable infectious disease transmitted by droplet from patient to patient, as in tuberculosis. Noncommunicable diseases may also result from inhaled or aspirated endogenous or exogenous agents, such as bacteria, viruses, fungi, protozoa, or gastric contents. Pathogenic organisms can also enter the thoracic contents through the bloodstream or lymphatics, via the fascial spaces from the neck, or from beneath the diaphragm.

Disturbances of normal physiologic pressure differentials may also cause serious consequences. For instance, if the normally negative intrapleural pressure is lost, the potential pleural space becomes an actual space, with partial or complete collapse of the lung and an invitation for intrapleural infection. Abnormal mediastinal masses, unusual enlargement or infection of mediastinal lymph nodes, and intense fibrous tissue inflammatory mediastinal reaction can produce a variety of clinical syndromes (superior vena caval syndrome, middle lobe syndrome), or abnormal fistulous communications between organs and adjoining spaces.

Pathogenetic factors will be discussed regionally. It is enough to point out the congenital anatomic disorders (tracheoesophageal fistulas, pulmonary sequestration, mediastinal cysts of almost any variety), acquired conditions, such as trauma, airway or esophageal obstruction, operative procedures, ischemia (pulmonary thromboembolic disease), or compromised host defense mechanisms *all* play important roles in surgical infections of the chest.

Fortunately, this region lends itself to examination by the traditional methods of physical examination, by roentgenographic methods including angiography, and by techniques involving radionuclides.

Aside from the brain, the human organism is most vulnerable in this region, housing, as it does, the organs of respiration and circulation. Thus, surgical infections of the chest can rapidly become critical.

INFECTIONS OF THE CHEST WALL

The thorax constitutes approximately 20 percent of the total body surface. Only those infections that are specific to the chest wall and that may require special considerations in management will be discussed here. Infections of the skin and subcutaneous tissue are discussed in Chapter 25.

ABSCESS OF THE CHEST WALL

Etiology and Pathogenesis

An abscess of the chest wall may arise as a primary infection or as a complication of septicemia. However, an abscess can result from an intrathoracic infection that penetrates the thoracic wall.[1-5] Thus, abscesses may be associated with osteomyelitis of the ribs or sternum or with costal chondritis of pyogenic, mycobacterial, or fungal origin. Actinomycosis, discussed in detail later, is the most common granulomatous infection of the chest wall and is characterized by chronically draining sinuses, the discharge typically containing sulfur granules.[2,3] Uncommon now, an undrained empyema may erode through the chest wall and present as a subcutaneous abscess. This so-called empyema necessitatis may drain spontaneously, forming an intermittently draining sinus.[4]

Subscapular and Subpectoral Abscesses. Subscapular and subpectoral abscesses are two specific, but uncommon, infections peculiar to the chest wall. A subscapular abscess may arise from an infected posterolateral thoracotomy incision and was formerly a common complication of Schede's thoracoplasty performed for the treatment of chronic empyema. A subpectoral abscess can occur from a suppurative lymphadenitis that involves the lymph nodes underlying the axillary portion of the pectoralis muscle following infection of the upper extremity or upper chest wall.[5]

Clinical Manifestations

Acute pyogenic abscesses of the chest wall may cause chills, fever, severe local pain, and tenderness. Leukocytosis is usually present. Empyema necessitatis caused by tuberculosis produces a cold abscess without signs of local inflammation.

Treatment

Pyogenic abscess of the chest wall requires surgical drainage, as with any soft tissue infection, combined with the use of antibiotics. The treatment of the underlying cause (actinomycotic infections, empyema necessitatis) is discussed in subsequent sections.

INFECTIONS OF THE COSTAL CARTILAGES: COSTAL CHONDRITIS

Pathogenesis

Costal cartilage, being composed of hyaline cartilage devoid of blood vessels, derives its nutrition by diffusion from the perichondrium. Because of this avascularity, costal cartilage, especially if it has been exposed, injured, or denuded of perichondrium, is especially vulnerable to infection. The cartilage then acts as a foreign body, with the development of chronic infection and draining sinuses. Healing often occurs only after the infected cartilage has been completely removed.

Incidence and Etiology

Costal chondritis now arises most often after operation and trauma, especially as a consequence of infected median sternotomy wounds. In former times, bloodborne infection or that arising from adjacent structures by way of the regional lymphatics occurred.[6-11] Consequently, all those pyogenic microbacterial and fungal organisms that infect the sternum are found.[6-11]

Clinical Manifestations

The clinical manifestations of costal chondritis vary with the offending organisms. With pyogenic infections, the area over the infected cartilage can develop signs of acute inflammation, including erythema, swelling, and tenderness, and there may be systemic signs of sepsis. Infections caused by mycobacteria, fungi, or bacteria of low virulence may produce minimal local, and often no, systemic symptoms. Only local tenderness followed by spontaneous drainage may occur. Infections of the costal arch on one side may extend to the opposite side either through the involvement of the xiphisternum or as a result of secondary osteomyelitis of the sternum. Thoracic roentgenograms are usually not helpful but occasionally show evidence of associated bony destruction. The diagnosis is usually confirmed at operation. Incision of pyogenic infections may release copious amounts of pus and liquefied cartilage. With *Candida* infections, the cartilage may be partly liquefied and replaced with pink, poorly vascularized loose granulation tissue.[8] Smears with Gram stain and acid-fast stain should suggest the appropriate diagnosis.

Treatment

Infections of costal cartilage are notoriously chronic but can be controlled by early and adequate therapy. Appropriate antibiotics should be administered, and complete excision of the involved cartilage should be performed promptly. Here, anatomic considerations become important. The first four and sometimes five costal cartilages are individually attached to the sternum and can be completely resected separately. The sixth and seventh costal cartilages and sometimes the fifth are joined not only to the sternum but to each other and to the eighth, ninth, and tenth costal cartilages as well, the lowermost four forming one side of the costal arch. Complete excision of this large cartilagenous plate is undesirable because it compromises chest wall stability. Therefore, as a first step, that portion of cartilage that is infected and 1–2 cm of adjacent normal cartilage may be excised subperichondrially and the denuded ends of the cartilage covered by preserved perichondrium. Other tissues, such as muscle, if available, may also be used to cover the cartilage.[12] If the infection persists, complete excision of the costal arch is necessary. The wound should be left open, in whole or in part, for topical irrigation with one of the antimicrobial solutions. Wray et al[10] found that 0.25 percent acetic acid irrigation was better than antibiotics, amphotericin B, or local packing with iodoform gauze, especially with chondritis caused by *Candida albicans*.

Prevention

Postoperative costochondritis can be prevented by proper precautions in draining intrathoracic or upper abdominal infections, as well as in closing the sternum. Wire sutures should not be placed through the costal cartilages. Chest tubes should be placed adjacent to ribs rather than cartilages. When an empyema or pulmonary abscess is drained, a portion of a rib rather than cartilage should be excised. If an infection lies beneath one of the upper four cartilages, the entire cartilage should be removed, and the denuded rib ends should be covered by perichondrium and muscles.

INFECTIONS OF THE STERNUM AND RIBS: MEDIAN STERNOTOMY WOUND INFECTIONS

Osteomyelitis of the sternum and ribs as a result of bloodborne infection is rare and does not differ significantly from osteomyelitis in any other part of the skeletal system (Chapter 42). Sternal osteomyelitis occurs most commonly after median sternotomy, an incision used for the majority of cardiac operations.[13] Postoperative infection is a dreaded complication because anterior mediastinitis with extension to the aortic and cardiac suture lines, prosthetic grafts, and intracardiac protheses can occur.

Incidence

The incidence of wound infections following median sternotomy has ranged from 0.5–6 percent.[14-18] In a review of 2,594 median sternotomy incisions, Culliford et al [15] reported 39 instances of postoperative sternal or costochondral infections (1.5 percent). This is consistent with the incidence observed by us and by others.[19]

Etiology

A wide spectrum of microbial organisms may be involved either singly or in combination. Staphylococci and gram-negative enteric bacilli alone or in combination with other organisms are the most commonly reported,[11,20,21] but a remarkable epidemic of sternal and secondary mediastinal infections due to *Mycobacterium fortuitum* contaminating bone wax has recently occurred.[22] Smears, Gram stains, KOH preparations, and acid-fast stains may all be indicated if proper therapy for the unusual organism is to be chosen.

Pathogenesis

As in all wound infections, sternal infections and associated mediastinitis apparently occur more frequently in association with chronic debilitation and malnutrition, the use of corticosteroids, and prolonged operative time. External cardiac massage and prolonged mechanical ventilation postoperatively predispose toward sternal instability and infection. Opinions differ regarding the significance of the technique of dividing or reapproximating the sternum, reoperation for bleeding, the low cardiac output syndrome, and other factors.[17,18] For example, Culliford et al [15] noted sternal wound infections in 1.1 percent of patients who underwent aortocoronary bypass graft procedures alone. However, dissection and mobilization of a single internal mammary artery resulted in doubling of the infection rate (2.3 percent), and use of both internal mammary arteries increased the infection rate eightfold (8.5 percent). The number and types of complications associated with the use of peristernal nylon bands make this technique unacceptable for closure of a median sternotomy.[17]

Clinical Manifestations and Diagnosis

The diagnosis of sternal wound infection and underlying anterior mediastinitis is not difficult if the patient has persistent, unexplained fever, drainage through the incision, and dehiscence of the sternum early in the postoperative period. When the infection is indolent, however, the diagnosis can be extremely difficult. Cellulitis that involves the incision or local tenderness over the sternum and costal cartilages, along with unexplained fever, should raise suspicion. Thoracic roentgenograms may show air under the sternum. Aspiration of the sternal wound as well as of the anterior mediastinal space may be necessary to prove the diagnosis. A radioactive gallium scan will occasionally help detect a mediastinal abscess. With sternal wound infections caused by mycobacteria, patients generally do not appear ill. There may be no or minimal elevation of temperature and only slight redness and moderate tenderness in the area of the incision. The watery drainage from the wound may not appear until several weeks after operation.[22]

Treatment

Systemic antibiotic administration is essential, especially if intracardiac prosthetic grafts or valves have been used. If the Gram stain of purulent material reveals gram-positive cocci, antistaphylococcal therapy should be started. Culture and sensitivity tests should be performed and antibiotics chosen accordingly.

The conventional method of wound infection treatment, such as opening of the wound and maintenance of wide-open drainage, may not be feasible because the heart, mediastinum, or pleural cavities may be exposed. Fortunately, it may not always be necessary. Selection of the appropriate method of therapy depends upon the time of appearance and duration of the wound infection and its possible association with an anterior mediastinitis. Superficial wound infections may be managed by debridement, local wound packing, and antibiotics. Major infections, with sternal instability, osteomyelitis of the sternum, or obvious mediastinal involvement, require a more aggressive approach.

For infections of limited extent and short duration, prompt reopening of the entire sternotomy, removal of sutures, and debridement of mediastinum, sternum, and subcutaneous tissues should be carried out.[15,16,23-25] Two chest tubes are placed under the sternum, one for irrigation and the other for drainage. (If the pleural cavity has been opened, an additional tube is inserted into the pleural cavity.) The sternal edges are reapproximated with multiple wire sutures, and the subcutaneous tissues are packed with gauze soaked with povidone-iodine. Continuous irrigation with antibiotic solution is initiated and continued for 10–14 days (Fig. 30-1). Neomycin–bacitracin solutions (2 gm neomycin, 100,000 units of bacitracin in 1 liter of normal saline, 50–100 ml per hour) have been suggested,[16] but the toxic effects of neomycin require caution.[26] Equally effective results should be obtainable by using solutions that contain other antibiotics selected on the basis of bacterial sensitivity. We, and others, use an irrigant of 0.5 percent povidone-iodine (Betadine solution), which is both bactericidal and fungicidal but also has some toxic effect on tissue.[27] Its short-term use until the wound surface is granulating is not dangerous.[28] If antibiotic irrigants are chosen, frequent cultures of the irrigant effluent should be taken to see if overgrowth with fungi or other organisms has occurred. If so, the addition of antifungal therapy is required.[29] Adequate dosages of appropriate systemic antibiotics should also be administered, and repeated blood cultures should be obtained to detect the occurrence of endocarditis.

Healing of the sternum in an afebrile patient is successful in more than 90 percent of patients.[15,16,23-25] If the infection continues or appears late (more than four to six weeks postoperatively) or the osteomyelitis is complicated by adjacent costal chondritis, a more radical procedure

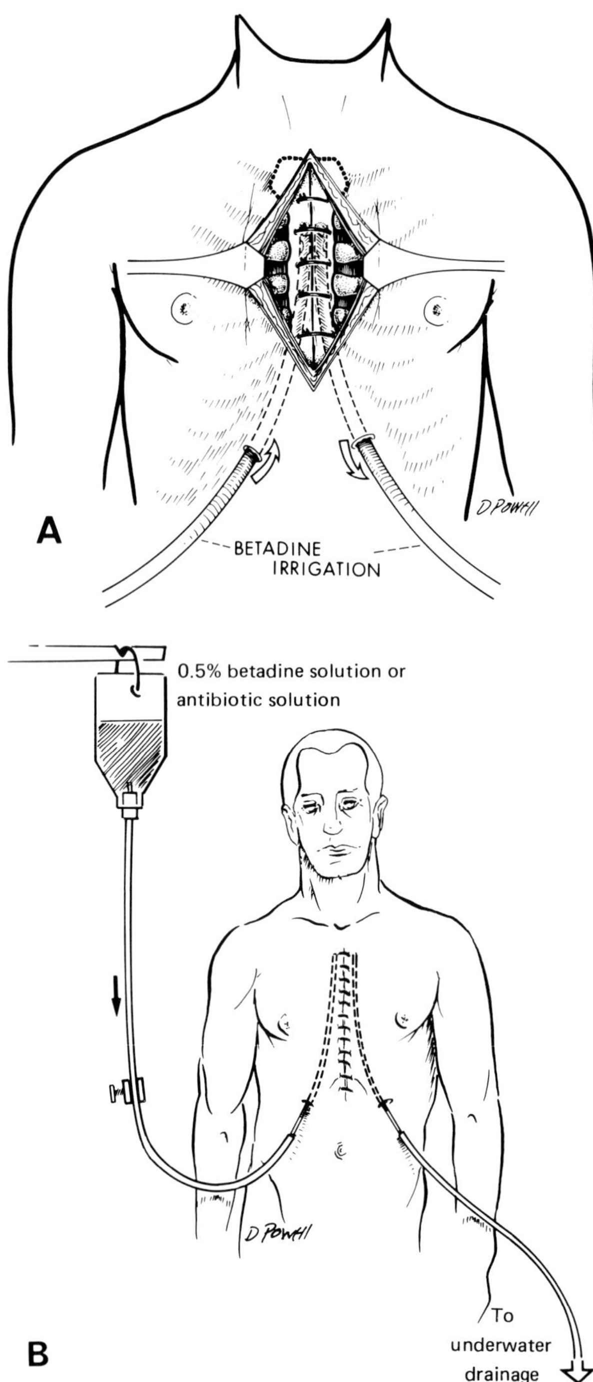

Fig. 30-1. A. Method of management of median sternotomy wound infection: The subcutaneous tissues, sternum, and mediastinal tissues are thoroughly debrided. The necrotic tissues are cultured and antibiotic sensitivities performed. The entire wound is irrigated with copious amounts of betadine or antibiotic solution. Two chest tubes are placed under the sternum, and the sternum is approximated with interrupted wires. Fascia, subcutaneous tissues, and skin are approximated. If the pleural cavity is entered, it is drained by a separate chest tube. B. Continuous irrigation with 0.5 percent povidone-iodine (50–100 ml per hour) or antibiotic solution is begun immediately after the operation and continued for seven to ten days. Care is taken to ensure that appropriate amounts of solution are retrieved by the drainage tube each hour.

is necessary to eradicate the infection. Resection of the entire sternum and adjacent costal cartilages with secondary wound healing may be required.[15] Local antibiotic irrigation and frequent dressing changes are necessary for a prolonged period. Removal of the sternum unfortunately eliminates the important anterior protective barrier for the heart and great vessels and leaves a serious cosmetic defect. To provide protection for the mediastinal contents and to accelerate healing, Lee et al.[30] recommended transposition of a pedicle of omentum to the anterior mediastinum, after total resection of the sternum. Robicsek et al.[22] successfully treated six patients using this method.

Prevention

A review of the predisposing factors suggests the measures to be taken to avoid median sternotomy wound infections.

First, adequate preoperative and intraoperative skin preparation must be used. Patients should receive 0.5 percent povidone-iodine whirlpool baths for 15 minutes, twice a day for two days prior to operation. Shaving is done approximately 18 hours before operation, and abrasion of the skin must be avoided. Many authorities think that shaving should be postponed until immediately prior to operation (Chapters 21 and 22). At operation, the skin is thoroughly scrubbed for 10 minutes with povidone-iodine soap and then the povidone-iodine scrub solution is applied over the skin. Disposable drapes in which the transparent plastic drape is already incorporated are used.

Wound infections can also be avoided by the prophylactic use of antibiotics.[31-33] The principles of their use are discussed extensively in Chapter 23. It is only necessary to reiterate here that the agent chosen should achieve therapeutic blood and tissue concentrations during the operation itself. Many cephalosporins (cephalothin) are excreted so rapidly that tissue levels are negligible unless the drug is administered every two hours.

Intraoperative preventive measures include avoidance of excessive tissue damage and prolonged operative time. Accurate midline incision and sternal divisions with the high-speed oscillating saw avoid injury to the cartilage and damage to the sternal periosteum. Minimal use of bone wax to control the bleeding from sternal marrow reduces the amount of foreign material left behind (a possible factor in one serious epidemic).[22] Both meticulous hemostasis and early detection and correlation of coagulation abnormalities are necessary to reduce postoperative bleeding. If reexploration of the mediastinum is necessary, the patient must be returned to the sterile operating room. It is important to place tubes in the mediastinum and pleural cavity to avoid cardiac tamponade and mediastinal hematoma. Complete closure of the pericardium is advocated by some,[14] including the use of pleural flaps or free grafts of fascia lata, with the hope that a closed pericardium might retard the extension of infection. Closure of pericardium is usually easily accomplished in patients who are undergoing operations for congenital heart disease and valvular disease. However, it may produce compression or kinking of bypass conduits in patients undergoing aortocoronary bypass grafting. We close the pericardium with interrupted nonabsorbable sutures in all patients except those undergoing aortocoronary bypass procedures. In these patients, the thymus tissue and mediastinal pleurae are approximated.

Interrupted wire sutures in adults and nonabsorbable sutures in infants and small children should be placed either through the bone or parasternally and not through the costal cartilages. Occasionally a figure-of-eight suture technique or other modification of the interrupted technique may be necessary for firm closure.[34] Basically, a stable closure of the sternum is essential—instability of the chest wall repair is an important predisposing factor to sternal dehiscence and secondary infection.[14]

Postoperatively, mechanical ventilation should be given through a nasotracheal tube to avoid the use of tracheostomy, at least until the tissue planes have become obliterated. All precautions should be taken to avoid pulmonary and systemic infections.

Prognosis

The prognosis for patients with sternal wound infections appears to be related to the time of appearance of the infection, the period of time until the institution of treatment, the adequacy of initial therapy, and perhaps the type of invading organism. The mortality in these patients has ranged from 10 to 26 percent.[15,19,24,25] It was 14 percent in our institution. Depending upon the difference in timing of initial treatment, Culliford et al [15] were able to distinguish three groups of patients. In those treated in the first postoperative month, the mortality rate was 7 percent, and an average of 25 days was required for resolution of the infection. If therapy was begun more than a month after the primary operation, the mortality rate was 20 percent, and an average of 73 days was required for resolution of the infection. An additional 10 percent of all patients who required multiple procedures died. An average of 141 days were required for resolution of infections in this group.

Patients with mycobacterial infections of the mediastinum tend to have a poorer prognosis. Only 3 out of 19 patients with this infection were cured with antibiotics and repeated wound debridement, while 5 patients died within four months after operation. Six patients required total resection of the sternum and an omental flap transposition. All of these patients survived. The late follow-up in the remaining 5 is not available.[22]

INFECTIONS INVOLVING IMPLANTED PROSTHESES

Pacemakers

Incidence

Various modifications in the designs and materials of implantable cardiac pacemakers have decreased the incidence of both primary wound infections of the pulse generator pocket and necrosis of the overlying skin. Siddons and Nowak [35] reviewed 7,205 pacemaker implantations. The results of their own experience with 1,543 implants are listed in Table 30-1. The incidence of skin necrosis is 3–10 times higher following reimplantations (changing the pulse generator) than in the initial procedure.[35-38]

TABLE 30-1. COMPLICATIONS AMONG 1,543 PACEMAKER IMPLANTATIONS

Group	Number of Complications	Total	% of 1,543 Implantations
Inflammatory		39	2.5
Wound infection			
Early	25		
Sinus	11		
Septicemia	3		
Skin necrosis		64	4.1
Over pacemaker	52		
Over wire	12		
Miscellaneous		15	1.0
Pain	5		
Wound dehiscence	5		
Pacemaker rotation	2		
Haematoma	2		
Muscle twitch	1		
TOTAL		118	7.6

From Siddons H, Nowak K: [35] Surgical complications of implanting pacemakers. *Brit J Surg 62:929, 935* 1975.

Treatment

The traditional treatment of the infected pacemaker has been to remove the pulse generator and electrode and replace it at a distant site or to insert a temporary pacemaker until the infection clears and then implant a new pacemaker. More recently, infected pacemaker sites have been treated with debridement, local and systemic antibiotics, and secondary closure of the wound.[39-42] A trial of this conservative method seems worthwhile because the electrode and pulse generator may not need to be replaced, and temporary transvenous pacing may also be avoided. In addition, potential sites for implantation are preserved for future use if needed. This treatment is illustrated in Figure 30-2.[40,41]

Occasionally, the pacemaker infection may lead to septicemia, bacterial endocarditis, and septic emboli to the lungs and to other parts of the body. Although, occasionally, such a patient may be managed successfully with antibiotics,[43] usually, the pacing unit must be removed to gain control of the infection.[44] Similarly, local wound revision for infection of a myocardial lead is usually ineffective because of residual infection at the myocardium. In such cases, complete removal of the epicardial lead is usually necessary.[45]

Prevention

The infections can be kept to a minimum by taking certain precautions:

1. The procedure should not be performed in a radiology suite—only in the operating room.[35]
2. The subcutaneous pocket should be larger than the pulse generator to avoid tension on the skin suture line.
3. The pocket should be created as far medially as possible because gravity causes the pulse generator to shift laterally, especially in bedridden patients. Lateral migra-

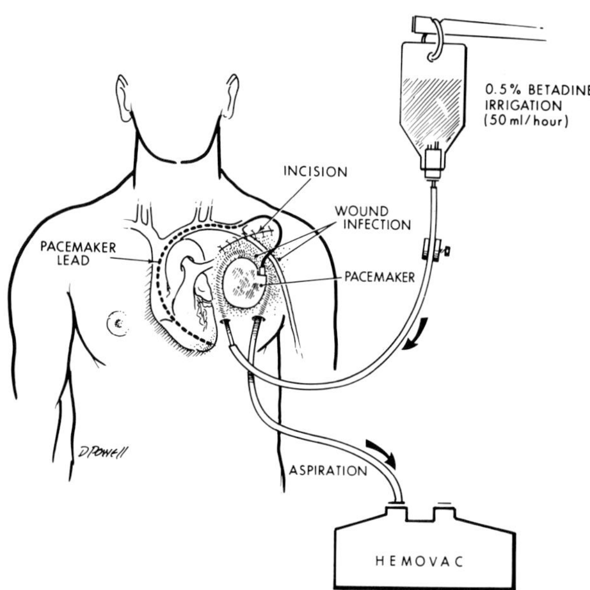

Fig. 30-2. **Method of management of infected pacemaker pocket. The wound is opened and thoroughly debrided. A hemovac catheter with multiple holes is inserted percutaneously for povidone-iodine or antibiotic solution irrigation. Another catheter is placed in the dependent portion of the pacemaker pocket and connected to a hemovac for aspiration of the irrigation solution. The wound is closed in two layers with 2:0 Dexon, and the skin is closed with 3:0 Dexon. Irrigation is continued at 50 ml per hour for five to seven days.**

tion is arrested in the anterior axillary line, where the pulse generator can produce considerable pressure and cause skin necrosis and infection.

4. The pacemaker unit should be placed under muscle in thin and elderly patients.

5. Hemostasis should be complete.

6. At the time of replacement of a pulse generator, the subcutaneous pocket should be enlarged in a medial direction.

7. Long-lived, lithium-powered or nuclear-powered pulse generators should be used to avoid multiple changes of the pulse generator.

In addition, Conklin et al,[46] with the lowest reported wound infection rate, stress the need for meticulous skin cleansing, prophylactic antibiotics, topical antibiotic irrigation, and closed suction drainage.

Vascular Prosthetic Grafts

Infections of vascular prosthetic grafts are discussed in detail in Chapter 33. Since vascular procedures involving the axillary artery are being performed with increasing frequency, axilloaxillary [47,48] and axillofemoral bypass in grafts are special cases that involve the thoracic wall. Infections of these grafts are common, unfortunately, because the patients who require them are old and debilitated and already have systemic infections in preexisting prosthetic grafts.[49] In a patient with a thin layer of subcutaneous tissue, the constant pressure and pulsations of the arterial prosthesis, especially over the costal arch, may cause necrosis and erosion of overlying skin and result in graft infection. Local signs of acute infection include warmth, erythema, swelling, local tenderness, and, ultimately, drainage of pus from the wound. Exposure of a graft in the wound is evidence enough for the presumptive diagnosis. Systemic signs, such as fever, night sweats, and tachycardia, may also occur.

The principles of treatment of all infected vascular protheses are discussed in Chapter 33. Only total graft excision results in resolution of infection, though appropriate parenteral antibiotics must be used. The arterial reconstruction should be performed via a noncontaminated route and delayed if possible.

Miscellaneous Infections of the Chest Wall

Two conditions that produce nonsuppurative inflammatory swelling of the chest wall should be noted. Both are usually self-limiting and may be confused with infections of the chest wall.

1. Mondor's syndrome is a superficial phlebitis of the thoracoepigastric vein and its branches. It is characterized by the presence of a subcutaneous cord, with variable inflammatory signs. This condition does not require specific therapy, and complete resolution can be expected within weeks or months [50] (Chapter 29).

2. Tietze's syndrome is a painful, nonsuppurative swelling of one or more costal cartilages, usually the second. Adults of either sex may be affected. The clinical picture may be suggestive of chondritis or cartilaginous tumor. The symptoms are usually self-limiting, but recurrences may occur. Appropriate specific treatment has not been defined.[51]

INFECTIONS OF THE PLEURAL CAVITIES (EMPYEMA)

Purulent collections in the pleural cavities are among the oldest conditions that surgeons have been called upon to treat, judging from the Hippocratic literature. "Pus in the chest" is no less important today to the thoracic surgeon, although the clinical circumstances that cause this condition are considerably different from ancient times. Since the availability of antibiotics, the incidence of empyemas has dropped sharply, and the causative organisms have changed.[52-54]

In this section, pleural empyemas will be discussed in general terms. It must be recognized, however, that there are important differences between empyemas of pyogenic origin and those caused by actinomycotic, fungal, or protozoan organisms and that empyemas of aerobic, anaerobic, and postoperative origin also differ.

Etiology and Pathogenesis

Pleural empyemas are not ordinarily primary infections. They usually occur in response to a primary infection elsewhere, most commonly pneumonia. This, however, may not be apparent when the empyema is fully developed. Probably the most common pathogenetic mechanism is rupture of a necrotic subpleural lung abscess or pneumonitis into the pleural cavity, although spread from lymphatic and hematogenous sources may also occur. The primary pneumonic process or abscess may, in turn, be the result of a variety of conditions, including bronchial obstruction (tumor, foreign body), bronchial infection (bronchiectasis), or emphysema (ruptured infected bleb). The mediastinum, subdiaphragmatic areas, chest wall, and dorsal spine can also be the sites of the primary infections that lead to an empyema (Fig. 30-3).

Such conditions as esophageal perforation, bronchopleural fistula, ruptured infected mediastinal lymph node, or subphrenic or intrahepatic abscess, including amebic abscess, have all been recognized as causes of empyema, as have external sources, such as trauma, needle aspiration, and thoracotomy tubes.[55] Infection of the pleural cavity (empyema) occurs if a hemothorax or a residual air space becomes infected following thoracotomy or if the pleural cavity is significantly contaminated during pulmonary resection or esophageal surgery (Fig. 30-3).

Posttraumatic empyema is a serious problem in wartime.[56] The incidence was 6 percent during the war in Vietnam.[57] Bacterial contamination of the pleural space can readily occur from penetrating injuries of the thorax, but infection is uncommon unless foreign material, such as clothing or organic matter, is retained in the pleural cavity. Air in the pleural space, especially in combination with hemothorax, doubles the likelihood of an empyema.[58]

Etiologic Agents. In the preantibiotic era, empyema was usually produced by pneumococci or streptococci. As effective antibiotics against these organisms became available, the incidence of empyema dropped significantly. In the late 1950s, however, pleuropulmonary infections caused by *Staphylococcus aureus*, resistant to all available antibiotics, increased for a time, especially in the young.[59,60] In the Johns Hopkins Hospital from 1955 to 1958, *Staphylococcus* caused 92 percent of empyemas in children under the age of 2 years.[59]

In addition most infections are mixed (Table 30-2). With the use of anaerobic culture techniques, anaerobes

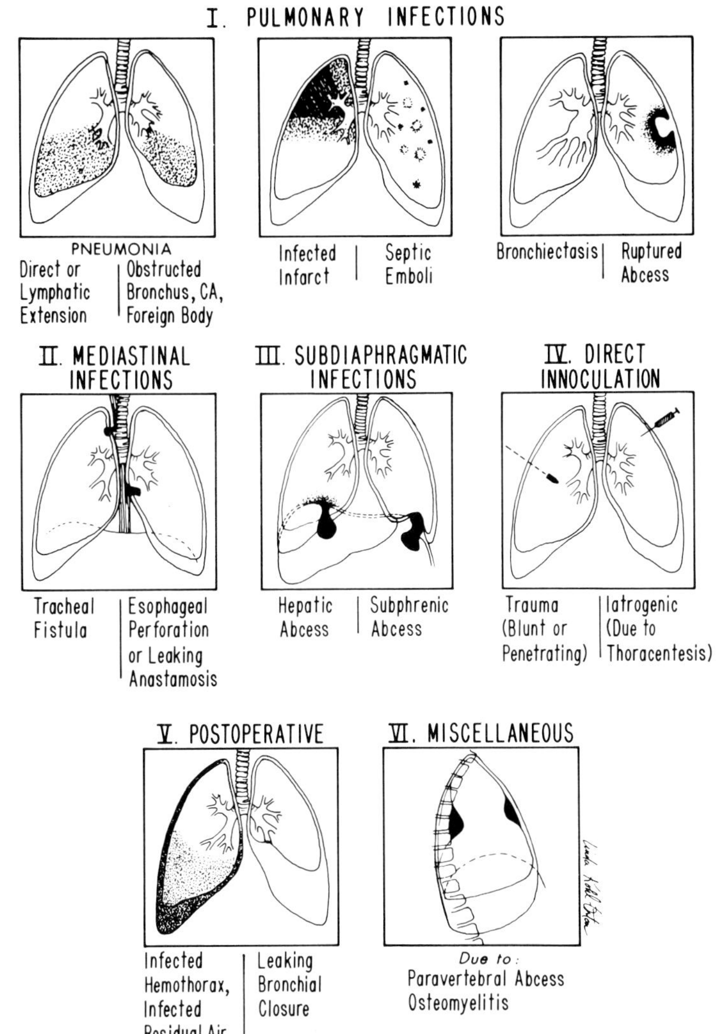

Fig. 30-3. **Etiology of thoracic empyema. (Redrawn after Snider GL, Saleh SS: Dis Chest 54:410, 1968; From Takaro T, et al: Curr Probl Surg 14:6, 1977.)**

and microaerophilic organisms have been identified with increasing frequency in empyema fluids.[61] Anaerobes are particularly common in empyemas arising from aspiration pneumonitis or in association with subdiaphragmatic infections. Table 30-2 lists the organisms identified from 83 patients with empyema in a laboratory with a strong interest in anaerobic bacteria. Tuberculous empyema is now rare. Amebic empyema and actinomycotic and nocardial empyemas also occur and are referred to in later sections.

Pathology. Empyemas may be encapsulated and localized to various regions of the pleural cavity, such as an interlobular location or a mediastinal or intrapulmonary region. They may also involve the entire pleural space. At first, during the exudative stage, the fluid is thin and has a low cell content, and the visceral pleura is still elastic, so that the lung can be reexpanded.[62] When increasing numbers of polymorphonuclear leukocytes and fibrin deposition begin to appear, the fibrinopurulent stage has been reached, and the visceral and parietal pleural surfaces begin to adhere. Finally, when the exudate has thickened so that more than 75 percent of an empyema fluid sediments on standing and fibroblasts have invaded the fibrinous layer over the pleural membranes, it is called an organizing empyema. Recognition of these distinctions in the natural course of pneumococcal and streptococcal empyemas by Graham and Bell in 1918 led to the use of closed drainage.[63] These three stages correspond only roughly with temporal conceptions of acute, subacute, and chronic empyema. Initially, all empyemas are acute, and chronicity develops if they are inadequately treated or if the primary condition is not controlled.

Empyema necessitatis (Fig. 30-4) is an encapsulated empyema that has burrowed through the chest wall into the subcutaneous tissues. It is still occasionally seen after pneumonectomy.[64] A bronchopleural fistula occasionally can be the result of a neglected empyema rupturing through a fresh or old bronchial closure or into the lung. The reverse is usually the case—the diseased lung or the bronchopleural fistula gives rise to the empyema.

TABLE 30-2. BACTERIOLOGY OF LUNG ABSCESS (45 CASES) AND EPYEMA (83 CASES)

Bacteriologic Results	Lung Abscess	Epyema
Only anaerobes recovered	26/45 (58%)	29/83 (35%)
Anaerobes and aerobes recovered concurrently	19/45 (42%)	34/83 (41%)
Anaerobic isolates		
Fusobacterium nucleatum	19 (3) *	16/3
F. necrophorum	1	
Bacteroides melaninogenicus	18 (1)	13
B. fragilis	9	13 (1)
B. oralis	5	8
B. corrodens	2	
Unidentified gram-negative bacilli	4	3
Peptostreptococcus	14 (4)	12
Peptococcus	14 (1)	14 (1)
Microaerophilic streptococcus	6 (3)	15 (5)
Veillonella	4	6
Eubacterium lentum	4	
Eubacterium sp.	3	5 (1)
Catalase-negative, non-spore-forming gram-positive bacilli	3	9
Propionibacterium sp	6	4
Clostridium sp	2 (1)	13 (1)
Aerobic and facultative isolates		
Staphylococcus aureus	6	17 (6)
Streptococcus faecalis	3	5
Streptococcus pneumoniae	2	5 (2)
Streptococcus pyogenes	1	4
Klebsiella pneumoniae	3	6 (1)
Escherichia coli	6	11
Proteus mirabilis	2	2
Haemophilus influenzae	1	1
Pseudomonas aeruginosa	3	10 (2)

Data from Wadsworth and Sepulveda Veterans Hospitals.

* Numbers in parentheses are numbers recovered in pure culture.

Reproduced, with permission, from Finegold.[436]

Clinical Manifestations

The symptoms and signs of the empyema may be continuous with those of the primary infection. Pleuritic pain and persistence of fever in spite of adequate chemotherapy, especially when the pneumonic process has largely subsided, suggest the diagnosis. The patient looks toxic and has chills and fever. The physical findings of empyema are typical of pleural effusion and include diminished movement of the affected hemithorax, impaired note on

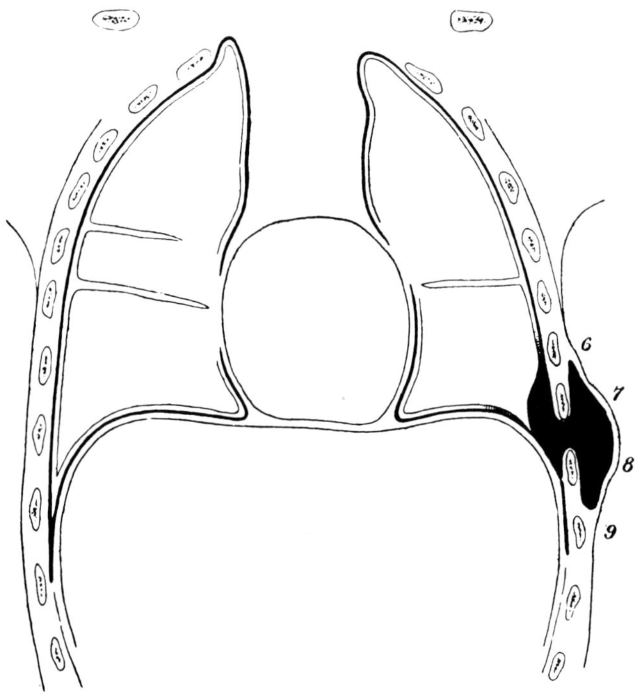

Fig. 30-4. **Diagram of empyema necessitatis showing its characteristic components: encapsulated pleural empyema, the narrow opening between the ribs through which the empyema has burrowed, and the externally presenting collection of pus in the subcutaneous tissues. (From Ashurst APC: Int Clin 4:173, 1916.)**

percussion, and reduced breath sounds and tactile and vocal resonance over the involved area. A large empyema may displace the mediastinum to the contralateral side and produce significant cardiopulmonary dysfunction on a mechanical basis alone.

Anemia, dyspnea, lassitude, debility, and clubbing of the fingers may develop in the chronic stages. The signs of empyema necessitatis have been described. If the pus takes another route and erodes into a bronchus, forming a bronchopleural fistula, sudden emptying of a large empyema into a bronchus may flood the bronchial tree and even drown the patient. Should this situation be suspected, the patient must be instructed to lie on the affected side to prevent leakage of empyema contents into the bronchus until the empyema can be definitely drained. Figures 30-5, and 30-6 are representative of the many appearances empyema may have.

In chronic empyema, movement of involved hemithorax can be severely restricted. If fibrothorax occurs, the trachea may be displaced toward the affected side, and the size of the involved hemithorax can decrease significantly. Amyloidosis may ultimately develop after a longstanding chronic empyema.

Diagnosis

In the preantibiotic era, thoracentesis, with the aspiration of purulent fluid from the pleural space, established the diagnosis unequivocally. Today, a patient may have clear pleural fluid, and organisms may not even be cultured from aspirates by conventional techniques. Yet, a pleural infection that is masked by antibiotics or caused by anaerobic organisms can be present. Even though the patient is usually febrile, the pleural infection may not become clinically evident until the antibiotics have been discontinued.

Aspirated material is sent to the laboratory for bacteriologic examination, including Gram stain, culture, and antibiotic sensitivity testing. The use of anaerobic culture techniques is essential. The possibility that the empyema may be the result of tuberculosis, actinomycosis, or fungal infections should be considered if response to therapy is slow, if the patient has chronic empyema or a draining sinus, or if the pus contains sulfur granules (the hallmark of an actinomycotic infection). In cases of amebic empyema, the characteristic anchovy sauce type of pus can be aspirated from the pleural cavity. This fluid and stools should be examined for *Entamoeba histolytica* and serologic procedures carried out (Chapter 11). A hepatic source must be sought and eliminated.[65]

Occasionally, bronchoscopy may be necessary in order to exclude the possibility of an intrabronchial tumor, an inhaled foreign body, or a bronchopleural fistula. The presence of a bronchial fistula can be confirmed by injecting 1 percent methylene blue into the empyema cavity and observing the expectorated material for blue dye.

Treatment

There are three major objectives in the treatment of an empyema. The first is control of the etiologic agent, usually by specific antimicrobial therapy. The second is evacuation of the contents of the empyema. The third, intimately related to the second, is restoration of normal lung function by reexpansion of the underlying lung.

Thoracentesis or needle aspiration of an empyema is nearly always the primary step. This single maneuver can establish the diagnosis, obtain material for identification of the etiologic agent, and at least in the exudative stage, evacuate the contents of the empyema space.

Tube Thoracotomy. Even in the exudative stage of an empyema, however, it is often wise to insert an intercostal tube for continuous closed drainage, especially when complete evacuation of the empyema space is unlikely to be achieved safely by needle aspiration alone. Thoractomy tube drainage is especially important if systemic toxicity has not been adequately controlled. This will ensure achieving the twin objectives of complete evacuation of the empyema space and reexpansion of the lung, provided the closed drainage procedure is carried out in the exudative or fibrinopurulent stages (Fig. 30-5).

The course of disease is followed by the clinical response of the patient and by frequent roentgenograms of the chest. Fluid should be cultured frequently, and the antibiotic treatment should be modified as indicated. After two to three weeks, the tube may be converted to open drainage if it seems necessary. Before conversion to open drainage, however, the fibrinopurulent stage of empyema must have been reached, so that the lung does not collapse. The size of a residual cavity can be assessed by injecting saline into the cavity. The tube can be removed safely when the volume of the cavity is less than 10 ml (Fig. 30-5).

Open Drainage. Open drainage should be instituted if there are multiple pus pockets, if the pus is very thick and contains fibrin flakes, if the empyema is first seen in the organizing stage, or if it appears to be inadequately drained. Langston[66] pointed out that overly long persistence in closed intercostal drainage for adults is a serious and common error.

Chronic empyema can result from inadequate or delayed earlier drainage procedures, some underlying primary condition such as a bronchopleural fistula, or esophagopleural fistula. A full investigation into the possible causes for the chronicity should always be made.

Because of prolonged infection, patients with chronic empyema often have anemia, depleted plasma proteins, and low blood volume. These should be corrected by blood transfusions as well as by a high-vitamin, high-protein diet. A positive nitrogen balance is essential for control of chronic infection and healing of fistulas or wounds. Appropriate and adequate antibiotic coverage is necessary before, during, and after operations.

The mainstay of management for chronic empyema should be adequate open drainage at the most dependent part of the cavity. Open drainage can be modified by creation of an Eloesser flap or one of its modifications.[67] This procedure is especially valuable in the treatment of postpneumonectomy empyema or for a large secondarily infected tuberculous empyema. It is also useful in the man-

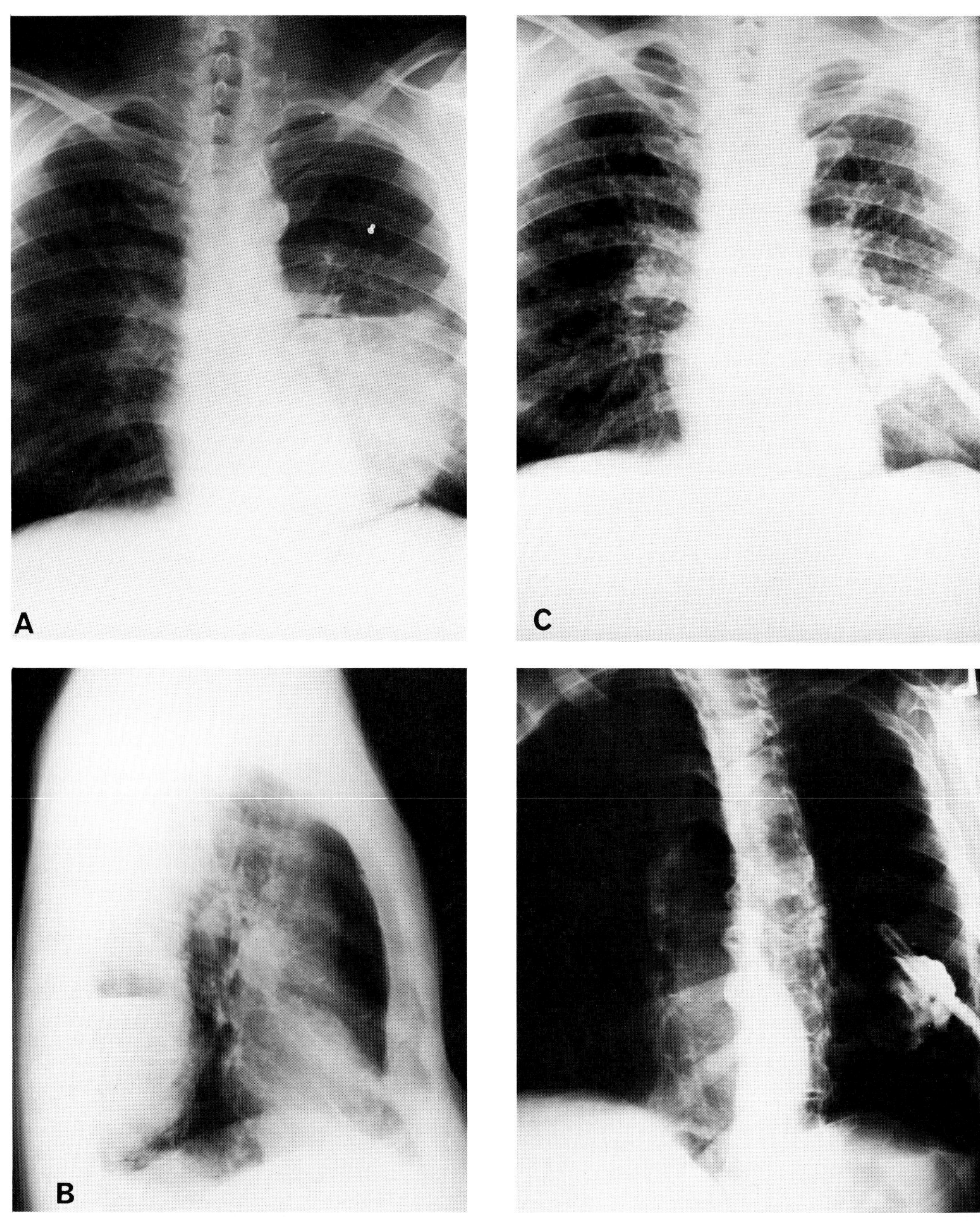

Fig. 30-5. Postpneumonic empyema for which rib resection and open drainage were carried out. *Streptococcus pneumoniae* was cultured from aspirate. A. Posteroanterior and B. lateral views showing posterior location of empyema cavity containing air-fluid level. C. and D. Sinograms five weeks after open drainage show residual space. A wide-bore tube was left in place until the space was completely obliterated six weeks later. (From Takaro T, et al: Curr Probl Surg 14(II):6, 1977.)

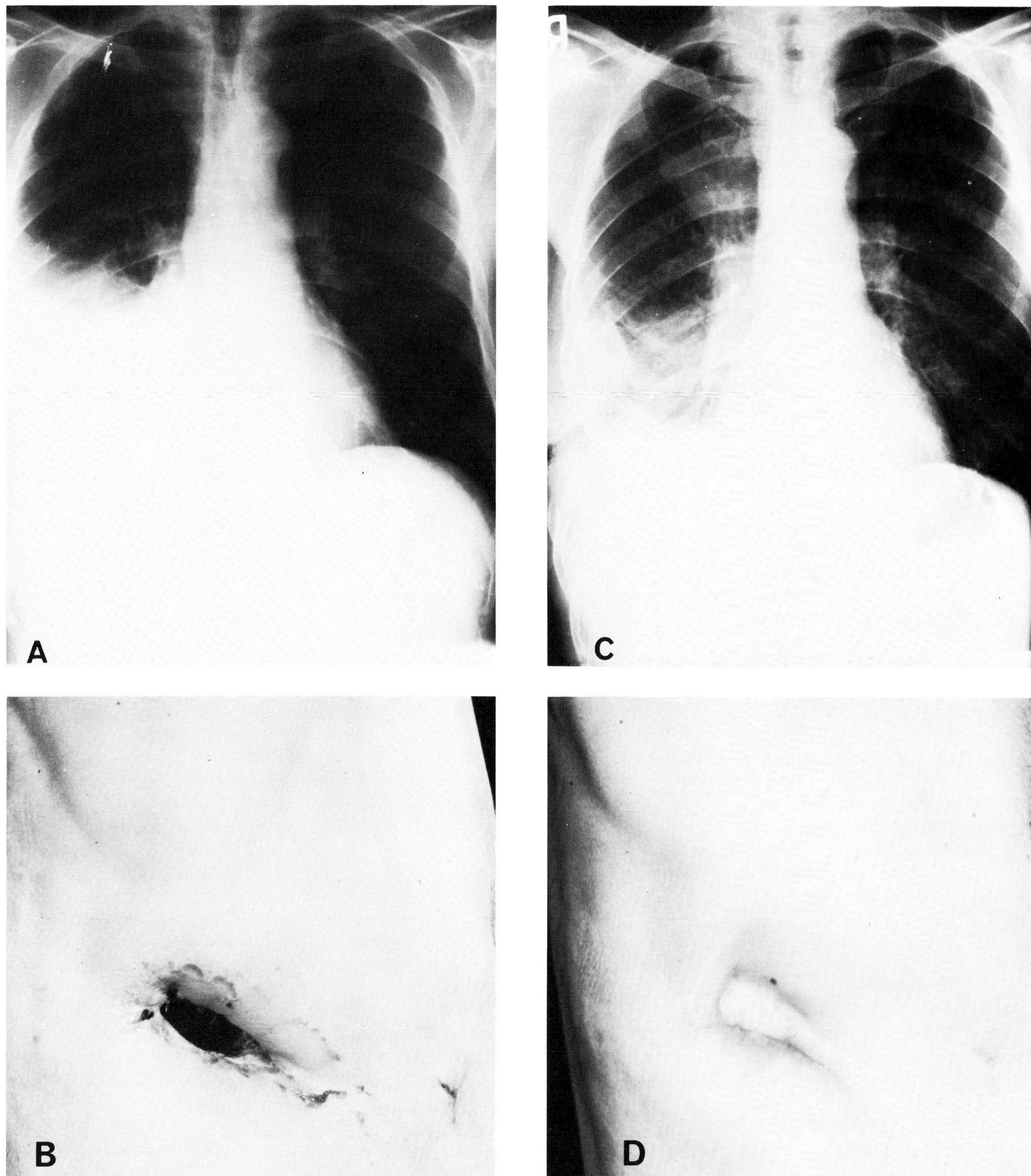

Fig. 30-6. Management of chronic empyema of three months' duration, using a modified Eloesser pedicled skin flap (see Fig. 30-7). Cultures of material from the empyema space grew a mixture of aerobic and anaerobic bacteria. A. Roentgenogram on admission. B. Appearance of chest wall three weeks after resection of segments of the eighth and ninth ribs and establishment of the flap. C. roentgenogram and D. chest wall four months after drainage procedure. (From Takaro T, et al: Curr Probl Surg 14(II):6, 1977.)

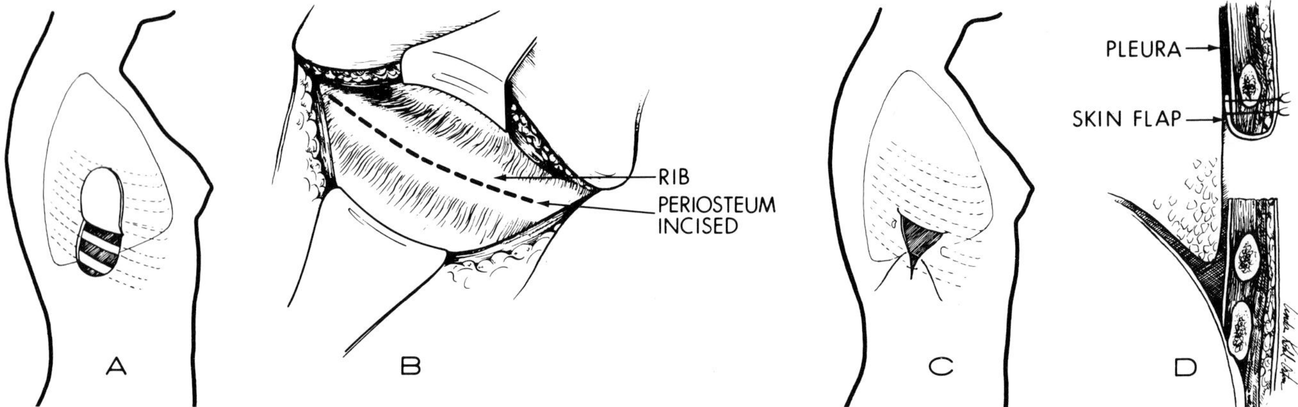

Fig. 30-7. **Eloesser flap drainage procedure. A. Full-thickness skin flap is elevated. We sometimes resect portions of two ribs rather than one. B. Preparation for subperiosteal resection of rib. C. Completed operation, showing skin flap inverted and sutured to parietal pleura at superior edge of thoracotomy wound. In most instances, fewer sutures than shown would be used inferiorly, to avoid diminishing the opening. D. Cross-section of thoracic wall, showing relationship of inverted skin flap to the parietal pleura. (Redrawn after Eloesser L: Ann Thorac Surg 8:355, 1969; From Takaro T, et al: Curr Probl Surg 14(II):6, 1977.)**

agement of empyema where the tube drainage would be uncomfortable, such as high in the axilla or in the paravertebral area. Its virtue is to maintain the drainage indefinitely, preventing premature closure (Figs. 30-6 and 30-7).

Sterilization of an empyema cavity, as described by Stafford and Clagett,[68] is especially useful for patients who develop empyema after pneumonectomy. A window is created by suturing the subcutaneous tissues to the pleura after rib resection. The empyema cavity is irrigated daily with half strength Dakin's solution for six to eight weeks. After the pleural cavity has diminished in size and become lined with clean, healthy granulation tissue, the sinus tract or window is excised, the cavity is irrigated with saline and filled with 0.25 percent neomycin solution, and the chest wall is closed in layers. The dangers of systemic neomycin administration must be recalled and literal application of this technique should be avoided.[26]

A modification of this method, which is more convenient for the patient and avoids a two-stage procedure, is advocated by Provan [69] and by Kärkölä et al.[70] Intrapleural antibiotic irrigation using two thoracostomy tubes—one near the apex of the space to instill the solutions, the other for drainage—has been successfully applied even when an open bronchopleural or esophagopleural fistula is present. The problem of bronchial aspiration is circumvented by careful positioning of the patient until the fistula is closed.

Decortication. Occasionally, in chronic empyema, the thick peel which forms over the visceral pleura may trap enough underlying lung to produce respiratory embarrassment. This peel may also prevent healing of the empyema, because with the rigid thickened lining, the cavity cannot close. Decortication to remove the thick pleural peel may improve function and encourage healing.[71,72]

In certain other circumstances also, decortication can be more efficient than open drainage. For example, in the management of an infected hemothorax, the intrinsically normal lung becomes imprisoned by its nonelastic, fibrin-purulent investment.[73,74] With few exceptions, however, decortication is not generally advocated as primary treatment for most types of empyema.[75]

Occasionally, a relatively small empyema cavity may be excised en masse (empyemectomy) without opening it, thus avoiding spillage of its contents into the uninvolved pleural space. This might be especially applicable in cases where the empyema pocket has never been subjected to open drainage or where the chronic encapsulation is either obviously infected or of unknown origin.[76]

Thoracoplasty. To obliterate a large (especially an apical) empyema cavity or close a coexistent bronchopleural or esophagopleural fistula, it is sometimes necessary to collapse the chest wall. The procedures available include the conventional thoracoplasty, the classic Schede's thoracoplasty, and modifications of them (Fig. 30-8). Andrews has used a thoracomediastinal plication operation.[77]

Additional special procedures may be necessary when an empyema is present along with a chronic bronchopleural or esophagopleural fistula. The empyema cavity is obliterated, if possible, by a pedicled muscle flap (fashioned from the serratus anterior, latissimus dorsi, pectoralis major, or subscapularis muscles, or from intercostal muscle bundles). The muscle flap is brought down (or in) to fill the empyema space and to seal the fistula.[78-81] Some tailoring of the chest wall may be necessary to permit these muscle flaps to reach their objectives (Fig. 30-9).

The management of postoperative empyemas following pulmonary resection has recently been reviewed by Kirsh et al,[82] and procedural details for the operations have been described.[83]

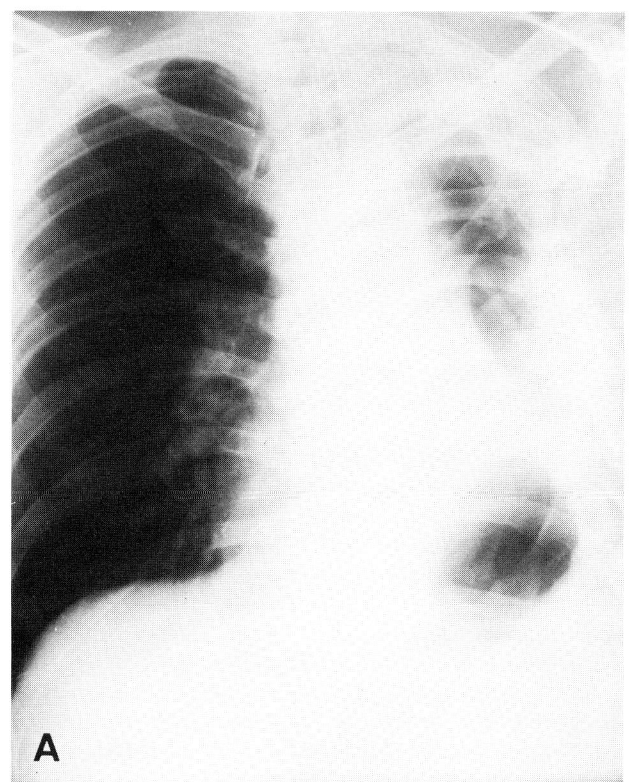

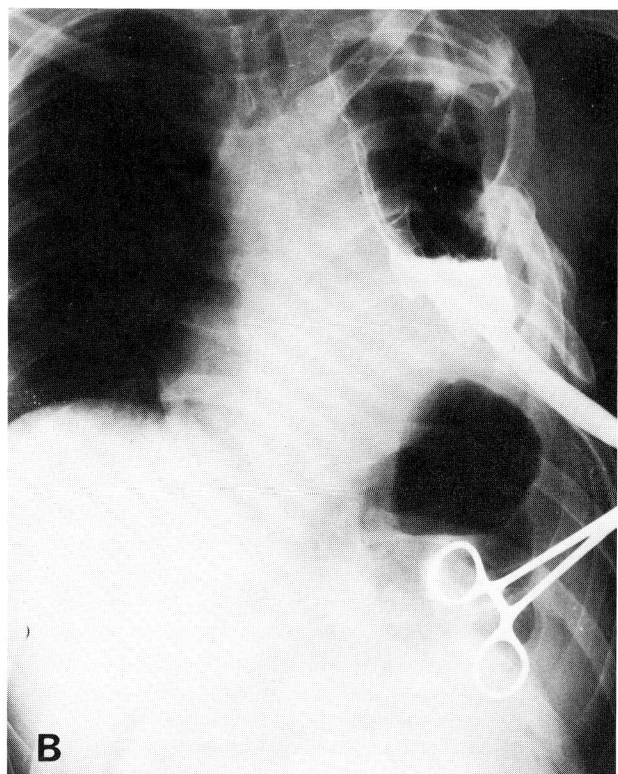

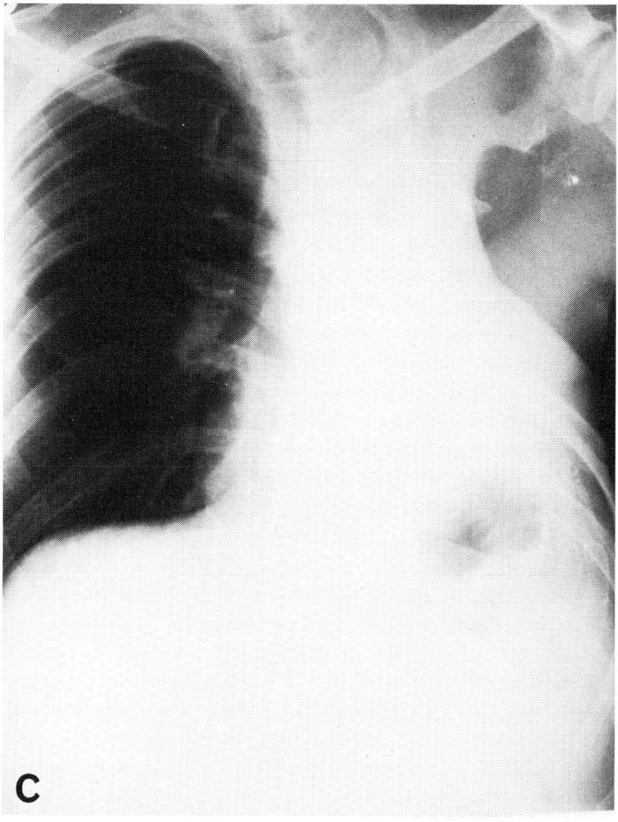

Fig. 30-8. Management of intractable, chronically draining empyema space, using a modified Schede's thoracoplasty, in young Vietnam veteran who had emergency pneumonectomy four years before admission. This was followed by empyema, with several previous unsuccessful attempts elsewhere to reduce or to sterilize the empyema space. Bronchoscopy and bronchography showed a healed left bronchial stump. Mixed flora (*Pseudomonas, Enterobacter* species, and enterococci) were cultured from purulent contents of the empyema space. The large space was completely unroofed of its calcific external wall after resection of portions of six ribs. The wound was packed and only partially closed, leaving a large opening for drainage and changes of dressing. Healing was uneventful and was essentially complete in approximately three months. A. Roentgenogram after previous rib resections and attempts to sterilize empyema space. B. Sinogram outlining extent of space. C. Appearance one year postoperatively. (From Takaro T, et al: Curr Probl Surg 14(II):6, 1977.)

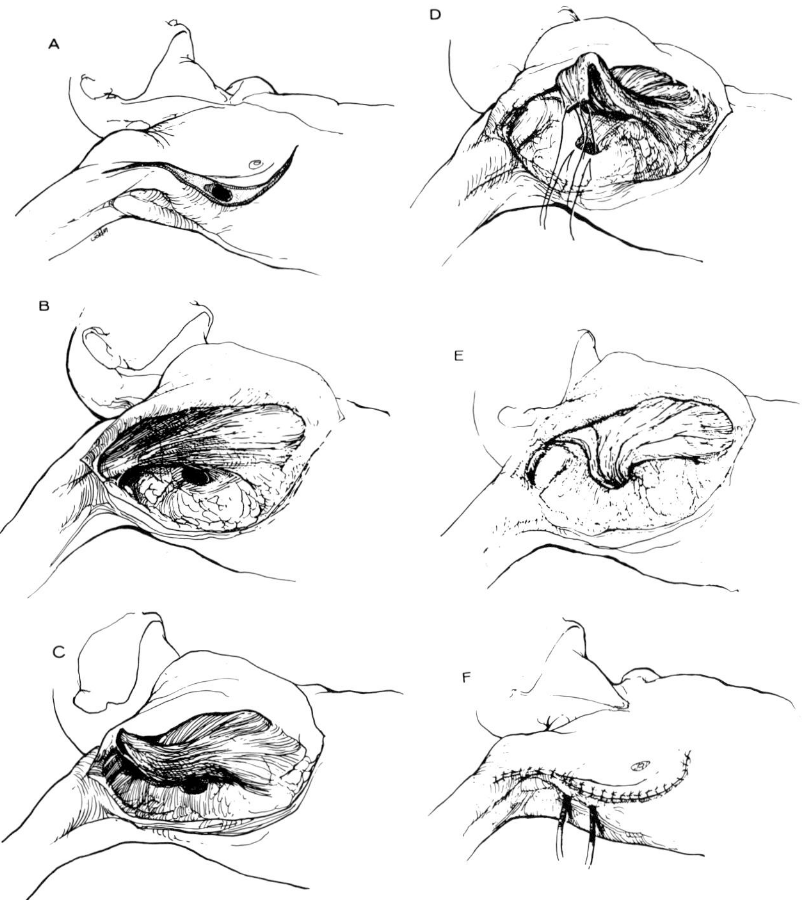

Fig. 30-9. **Steps in closure of a bronchopleural fistula using a pedicled muscle graft. A. Incision extends along border of pectoralis major muscle into axilla and includes fistulous tract. B. Pectoralis major muscle is dissected to its insertion on the humerus. C. The muscle is detached from its insertion and is unfolded to provide an adequate graft. D. It is then sutured into the space and stump with absorbable sutures. E. The muscle is shown sutured in place. F. The wound is closed, with subcutaneous drainage only. (From Barker WL, et al: J Thorac Cardiovasc Surg 62:393, 1971; in Takaro T, et al: Curr Probl Surg 14(II):6, 1977.)**

INFECTIONS OF THE LUNGS AND AIRWAYS

LUNG DEFENSE MECHANISMS AGAINST INFECTION

The defense mechanisms of the lung have been extensively reviewed by Newhouse et al.[84,85] The majority of potentially harmful particles and microbes in inhaled air is eliminated before reaching the alveoli. In fact, the normal lung is sterile from the first bronchial division to the terminal lung segments.

Inhaled particles can be deposited in the respiratory tract as a result of impaction, sedimentation, brownian motion,[86] turbulent diffusion,[87] and even electrostatic forces.[88] Whether or not the particle is retained depends on how it was inhaled (through the nose or the mouth), its size, shape, and density, and the air flow velocity and aerodynamic characteristics of the airway. For example, large particles are eliminated as the air passes the nasal vibrissae. Particles larger than 10 μm encounter the moist surface of the nasal septum and turbinates [89,90] and impact on the posterior wall of the pharynx, where the tonsils and adenoids are conveniently located. The few particles larger than 10–15 μm that remain will impact at the carina or within one or two bronchial divisions.[91,92]

Because of the rapid increase in the cross-sectional area of the bronchial tree beyond the tenth bronchial division, air flow rates fall rapidly. Beyond this division, particles of 0.2–5 μm in size sediment by gravity. The majority of bacteria thus sediment to the distal bronchial walls in these areas of stagnant air flow.

Particles of 0.1 μm and smaller are deposited mainly as the result of brownian motion because of their constant bombardment by gas molecules.[92] Particles between 0.5 and 0.1 μm are least affected by inertial, gravitational, and brownian forces, and only about 20 percent are retained in the lung.[93]

Despite these defenses, some large, irregular particles, such as asbestos fibers, are capable of reaching the lung periphery. This is possible because their aerodynamic characteristics prevent their retention in the upper airways. Similar factors may govern other particles.

Airway Reflexes

Basically, two airway reflexes exist, bronchoconstriction and cough. Stimuli of various types can produce vagally mediated reflex contraction of the airway smooth muscle and mucosal edema in both the upper and lower respiratory tract. Such stimuli, including mechanical irritation of the nose, trachea, or larynx, inhalation of irritant gases, some droplet aerosols, and chemically inert dusts can produce bronchoconstriction or trigger the cough reflex.[84,85] Bronchoconstriction is characterized by a concurrent reduction in airway caliber without decreasing the number of ventilated pulmonary units. The protection resides in the prevention of the deep penetration by mechanical or chemical irritants.

The cough reflex helps remove excess secretions and foreign bodies in the trachea or major bronchi. The reflex begins with a deep inspiration, after which expiration is initiated against a closed glottis with an elevation of intrapleural pressure to well over 100 mm of mercury. When the glottis is suddenly opened, the pressure within the trachea and major bronchi falls to a much lower level, resulting in a high transbronchial pressure and rapid reduction in bronchial caliber. Two effects then result: (1) secretions retained on the walls of the bronchus occupy a larger proportion of the cross-sectional area of the narrowed lumen and can temporarily occlude it, and (2) the flow rates throughout the bronchial tree are greatly augmented. The resulting high air flow velocity propels the mucous plug toward the mouth. Compression from the high intrathoracic pressures may also produce a milking action, which clears mucus into larger airways for subsequent expulsion. Cough is an effective means of expelling foreign bodies and secretions, but chronic bronchitis, emphysema, or cystic fibrosis can retard the cough mechanism, and an inefficient cough can cause retrograde movement of secretions to the lung periphery or aspiration from one lung into the other.[94]

Tracheobronchial Secretions and Mucociliary Transport

The respiratory airways from distal nasopharynx to terminal bronchioles are lined by mucus-covered, ciliated epithelium that removes deposited particles by means of mucociliary transport mechanisms. The larger particles that impact or sediment on the mucosa are swept upward by this mechanism, to be swallowed or spit out. The smaller particles that sediment in regions distal to the terminal bronchioles are not handled in this way.

Structure of Mucociliary Transport System

The mucociliary transport system has two components. The respiratory epithelium is lined by cells, each of which bear 200 cilia, whose sweep is coordinated by complex mechanisms. Airway secretions are produced by both mucosal goblet cells and submucosal mucus-secreting glands. The resulting mucous blanket consists of two layers: a 5 μm high-shear periciliary fluid that has the physical characteristics of a sol that bathes the cilia from the surface of the epithelial cell to their apex. Above this level is found a 2 μm lower-shear gel with greater viscoelasticity.

The gel layer is impermeable to water and may protect the subjacent epithelium and periciliary fluid from dehydration, ionic disequilibrium, and penetration of toxic substances. The gel layer also probably provides an important barrier to biologic agents because it contains secretory IgA and a number of nonspecific soluble factors that can act as defenses:

1. Alpha$_1$-antitrypsin can inhibit bacterial enzymes as well as collagenase, plasmin, thrombin, and proteases and elastase derived from lysosomes of neutrophils.[95-97] In addition, alpha$_1$-antitrypsin is probably identical to the chemotactic factor inactivator present in normal serum, and Ward and Talamo[97] have suggested that a deficiency in alpha$_1$-antitrypsin may permit neutrophils to damage the lung. In fact, emphysema is one consequence of congenital alpha$_1$-antitrypsin deficiency.

2. Lactoferrin, a potent bacteriostatic agent that binds free iron needed by proliferating bacteria, is apparently synthesized by glandular mucosal cells,[98,99] as well as by polymorphonuclear leukocytes.[100]

3. Lysozyme is abundant in bronchial mucus and can lyse bacterial cell walls.[101]

4. Complement is also present. Some components of the complement system are present at low levels in normal bronchial secretions, but the biologic activity may be important. In inflammation presumably most components of the complement system present in serum may have access to the bronchial and lung parenchyma.

Cilia and Mucociliary Transport

Cilia do not beat in synchrony but sequentially, in metachronal waves. The mucous blanket appears to provide a mechanical linkage between cilia, and a neuroidal pacemaker network has been hypothesized to explain the coordinated movement. The cilia beat at a frequency of between 1,000 and 1,500 cycles per minute. The tip of the cilium is in contact with the undersurface of the mucous gel only during the maximum velocity of the effector stroke.[102-104]

There is a progressive increase in the velocity of the mucous blanket toward the upper airways. Particles in the proximal bronchi are cleared with a half-time of about 30 minutes, whereas particles on the distal mucosa are removed with half-times up to several hours. All material deposited on the normal ciliated epithelium is removed in less than 24 hours.[105-107]

Ciliary movement is influenced by many physical and chemical stimuli. In the mammalian respiratory tract, cilia do not respond to neural stimuli. Autorhythmicity of cilia may be controlled by physiologic amines, such as serotonin, that might act as local pacemaker substances. Oxygen appears to be essential for ciliary motion. A number of agents appear to be toxic to cilia. High concentrations of carbon dioxide[108] and oxygen,[109] cigarette smoke,[110] pentobarbital, atropine, and alcohol[111] are toxic to cilia. Viruses damage mucociliary clearance,[112] and *Mycoplasma pneumoniae* infection can slow tracheobronchial clearance for as long as one year.[113]

PHAGOCYTIC DEFENSES (ALVEOLAR MACROPHAGES)

Although the major clearance mechanism of the lung consists of the mucociliary transport system, alveolar macrophages are responsible for the physical removal of inhaled particles. Alveolar macrophages can be specifically or nonspecifically activated during infections.[114] Activated macrophages have a higher lysosomal enzyme level,[114] are more phagocytic,[115] and possess more bactericidal activity[116,117] than do nonactivated cells. Once activated, macrophages display a nonantigen-specific capacity to ingest and kill apparently irrelevant organisms. It should be emphasized, however, that specific inactivation of bacteria by activated macrophages is nearly always quantitatively greater than nonspecific activation.[118] The primary bactericidal activity in the resting lung is dependent on this macrophage system.[119]

IMMUNOLOGIC DEFENSES

The lungs are not generally regarded as lymphoid organs, but submucosal lymphoid deposits respond to both systemic [120,121] and aerosolized antigens. Local mucosal presentation of antigen is a more efficient mode of obtaining local immunity.

It is now known that secretory IgA antibody acts as a primary defense mechanism at all mucosal surfaces (Chapter 13). IgA antibody present in nasal and upper respiratory tract secretions is better correlated with resistance to viral or bacterial infection than is serum antibody.[122-125]

IgA in bronchial mucus is in the secretory form, consisting of a dimer IgA together with two additional nonimmunoglobulin moieties, known as secretory component and J chain.[101,126] IgA-containing cells predominate at lymphoid sites in the lamina propria,[94,127] and relatively few cells containing IgM or IgG are normally found at these sites. Although normally only a few IgE-containing cells are found in these mucosal tissues, the relative number of such cells is greater in the respiratory tract and associated lymphoid tissue (such as tonsils and adenoids) than in peripheral lymphoid tissue.[128] In chronic respiratory tract disease, the number of cells that produce IgA and IgE tends to rise at a rate disproportionate to that in other classes.[129-131]

Intratracheal immunization is most effective in elicitation of IgE serum antibody.[132] Local attenuated viral vaccines given by nose drops or aerosol produce greater local IgA responses than when the vaccine is administered parenterally. Most evidence now supports the concept of immunologic memory within the local respiratory IgA system.[133-135]

Recent evidence indicates a predominantly IgG response in the lower respiratory tract to several antigens.[136,137] IgA-containing cells predominate in the upper and middle portions of the tract but are rarely, if ever, seen around bronchioles, even in infection.[138]

IgA appears, at first glance, to be an ineffectual antibody. It cannot fix complement [139] and can, therefore, not serve to lyse microorganisms. It cannot opsonize microbes for phagocytosis by neutrophils or macrophages.[140] More likely, IgA acts to neutralize toxins [141,142] or viruses [101] and to prevent bacterial colonization of mucosal surfaces, since bacteria sensitized with IgA appear unable to adhere to mucous membranes.[143,144] This property is shared with antibody classes,[145] but IgA resists proteolysis better than IgG or IgM.[101,126] IgA antibody can inhibit bacterial growth,[146] and Heremans and Crabbé [147] have referred to IgA in secretions as antiseptic paint [148] because it is adherent, through a noncovalent interaction with mucin,[149] to the apical surface of the columnar epithelium.

IgA-deficient patients do, on the average, suffer more often from respiratory tract infections, but some deficient patients are normal. Such people appear capable of replacing the IgA with IgM.

IgA may have an additional function—namely, to limit absorption of antigen. IgA-deficient patients have a higher incidence of autoimmune responses and atopy.

The reaginic or anaphylactic antibody, IgE, appears to be predominantly synthesized locally in mucous membranes.[128,150,151] No role in terms of antibacterial immunity has been demonstrated, but IgE antiviral antibody has been found.[152] The only role known for this class is the sensitization of mast cells or basophils for subsequent release of chemical mediators of inflammation and smooth muscle contraction after interaction with the appropriate antigen. Mast cells are found in the bronchial and bronchiolar lamina propia,[153] where they can be sensitized locally by locally produced IgE.

In addition to local humoral immunity, endobronchial instillation of antigen elicits a local cell-mediated immune response. These primary responses exceed the systemic response, and protection against subsequent respiratory challenge surpasses systemic protection.[154]

Both luminal lymphocytes [155] and bronchus-associated lymphoid tissue similar to Peyer's patches [156,157] have been described, although their interrelationships are unknown.[158]

The mucosal lymphoid aggregates are covered by a specialized follicle-associated epithelium, which, in Peyer's patches and the bursa of Fabricius,[159] appears to serve as a specialized sampler of the luminal environment. They may serve as a reservoir for IgA-producing cells similar to Peyer's patch cells.[160] In fact, a common immunologic mucosal system may exist, in which cells sensitized at one mucosal site will eventually provide protection for another.[158,161] Specific IgA antibody was found in large amounts in colostrum even though this class of antibody was absent in the serum. If this system is at work, one might expect that local immunization against respiratory pathogens might be achieved equally well with aerosolized or ingested antigens.

SPECIAL PROCEDURES IN THE DIAGNOSIS OF PULMONARY INFECTIONS

Special techniques are available to aid in the diagnosis of pulmonary infiltrates. These techniques are especially helpful in the diagnosis of pulmonary infiltrates in immunologically compromised hosts. Infiltrates in these patients—those treated with cancer chemotherapeutic agents, radiation therapy, and immunosuppressive drugs and patients with lymphoproliferative disorders and congenital immunodeficiency disorders—are frequently due to organisms that do not result in sputum production or are impossible or difficult to culture, such as *Pneumocystis carinii* and viruses. To diagnose these infections, tissue specimens are frequently required. Rapid diagnosis is required in these patients so that specific therapy can be instituted.

Sputum collection can be helpful when sputum production is copious. It is not helpful in the diagnosis of *P.*

carinii and viral infections. Because sputum is necessarily contaminated with oral bacteria, culture results are unreliable. Many laboratories will not even culture sputum for anaerobes, because contamination with oral bacteria makes interpretation impossible. Transtracheal needle aspiration avoids oral contamination, but in compromised patients with low platelet levels, the danger of bleeding is increased.

Bronchoscopy with the rigid bronchoscope has long been used for diagnosis and therapy to culture and wash out thickened bronchial secretions. This technique suffers from some of the same drawbacks as sputum collection, since the bronchoscope must be passed through the mouth and can become contaminated by oral bacteria. More recently, bronchoscopy with a flexible bronchoscope has largely replaced the rigid bronchoscope for diagnosis. The flexible bronchoscope can be directed into the subsegmental bronchi of the affected pulmonary segments to collect secretions from the specific location affected. Any obstruction—such as that due to tumor—can be visualized and biopsied. Lung can also be biopsied through the bronchoscope by penetrating the bronchus with the biopsy forceps to obtain lung tissue. *P. carinii* and viral infections can be diagnosed in this manner. Hanson et al [162] reported a 62 percent accuracy in the diagnosis of infectious lung disease in 37 patients with transbronchial biopsy through the flexible fiberoptic bronchoscope. Hemorrhage (>100 ml) occurred in 26 percent of the patients, and pneumothorax occurred in 19 percent. However, Anderson [163] reported only a 1 percent incidence of bleeding and a 12 percent incidence of pneumothorax. Low platelet levels in many of these patients increases the risk of hemorrhage that cannot be directly controlled. Recently, special sheathed catheters have been developed to try to circumvent contamination with oral bacteria. A sheathed catheter is passed through the flexible bronchoscope into the bronchus. A gelatin plug at the end is then punched out by the culture tip, and cultures are obtained. The sheathed catheters may provide more reliable culture results. One drawback to the use of flexible bronchoscopy is that these patients are frequently severely hypoxic, and the bronchoscope can occupy a substantial portion of the airway, especially in children. Supplementary oxygen cannot be given, as it can with the rigid bronchoscope.

The lack of reliability of cultures and risk of uncontrolled hemorrhage in many of these severely immunocompromised hosts has led to more direct sampling of lung tissue. In general, three methods are used: (1) percutaneous needle biopsy, (2) thoracoscopic biopsy, and (3) open lung biopsy.

Needle biopsy can be performed under fluoroscopic control to ensure that the diseased portion of the lung has been entered. This technique can be helpful for diffuse pulmonary infiltrates as well as for solid tumors.[164-166] There are several biopsy needles available, including the Vim-Silverman needle, aspiration biopsy with a thin (No. 18 to 20) needle, and trephine biopsy using a pneumatic drill. Trephine air drill biopsy was able to provide the diagnosis in up to 82 percent of immunocompromised patients with diffuse lung disease.[164] Hemorrhage occurred in 18 percent (3 of 17) of the patients. One patient required transfusion, and 60 percent (10 of 17) developed a pneumothorax; 8 of the 10 patients required a chest tube. This technique has the advantage of being performed under local anesthesia as long as the patient is cooperative. Aspiration of diffuse pulmonary infiltrates with a thin needle has not yielded reliable results.

Thorascopic biopsy allows direct visualization of the diseased lung and biopsy of the involved tissue. A thoracoscope is inserted through a small skin incision via a trocar. The lung and pleural surfaces can be viewed. A biopsy forceps is inserted through a separate stab wound, and several biopsies can be taken of the involved lung under direct vision. Any bleeding can be cauterized by touching the electrocautery to the biopsy forceps as it grasps the bleeding point. A chest tube is left in place to control the pneumothorax. This procedure can be performed with the patient awake, even in the pediatric age group.[167,168] Rogers et al [168] reported a 100 percent diagnostic accuracy in the diagnosis of pulmonary infiltrates in immunosuppressed patients. Chest tubes were left in place afterward, but 6 of 57 patients still developed pneumothorax.

Open lung biopsy for diffuse pulmonary infiltrates can be done safely through a small anterior thoracotomy. Leight and Michaelis [169] obtained diseased tissue in 100 percent of 42 consecutive open lung biopsies. A specific diagnosis was made in 30 patients (74 percent). Delayed pneumothorax occurred in 3 patients and wound dehiscence in 1 patient. In cooperative patients, open lung biopsy can be performed under local anesthesia.[170]

VIRAL INFECTIONS

Cytomegaloviral Infections

The viral infections are discussed in Chapter 10. Those of importance to immunosuppressed patients are discussed in Chapter 47. Aside from the occasional need to perform a lung biopsy or remedy a complication of the invasive diagnostic maneuvers discussed in the preceding section, only cytomegalovirus has major surgical significance. Cytomegaloviral pneumonias occur frequently after renal transplantation (70–96 percent of patients), bone marrow transplantation (40 percent of patients), cardiac transplantation (30 percent of patients), and, less commonly, after cardiac surgery involving extracorporeal circulation.[171-173] It may also predispose the patient to significant bacterial and fungal superinfection of the lungs. This is especially true in patients who are seronegative for the virus prior to operation and who develop cytomegaloviral infection postoperatively.

While there is a case on record of cytomegaloviral infection presenting as a solitary pulmonary nodule,[174] ordinarily the disease begins as a diffuse interstitial pneumonitis, suggestive of pulmonary edema, or as bilateral nodular infiltrates. Fever is an invariable concomitant finding, and leukopenia is common. Viremia carries a more grave prognosis, and seroconversion generally, but not always, is a sign that recovery is imminent. There is no treatment except generalized support and reduction in dosage of immunosuppressive drugs.[175] Trials with an attenuated vaccine are in progress, and interferon therapy is still experimental.

BACTERIAL INFECTIONS

Postoperative Lung Complications

While many postoperative complications that involve the lungs are associated with infection, the infection is often overshadowed by other clinical problems, such as mechanical airway obstruction, pleural space problems, respiratory insufficiency, or graft rejection. Nevertheless, postoperative lung complications will be discussed briefly, chiefly in relation to the element of lung infection.

Definition

Pulmonary complications associated with lung infection include retained secretions, localized pneumonitis, atelectasis, pneumonia, lung abscess, and the adult respiratory distress syndrome from sepsis or other causes. Any of these can be exacerbated by previous conditions, most notably chronic obstructive pulmonary disease, and by operations on any of the thoracic contents, the chest, or the abdominal wall.

Pathogenesis

Retention of pulmonary secretions, the most common complication, results from aspiration of saline or gastric juice into the airways or ineffective cough and hampered ventilation. If the atelectasis is unrelieved, infection will occur.

Aspiration pneumonia results from the inhalation of oronasopharyngeal secretions laden with microorganisms or gastric contents of high acidity, with the development of either a bacterial or a chemical pneumonia. It can also lead to lung abscess. Sepsis is the most commonly identified factor in the adult respiratory distress syndrome in the absence of preexisting pulmonary dysfunction. The pathogenesis of this complex state is unclear (Chapter 17), but circulating endotoxins from gram-negative organisms appear to be involved, as do such factors as recumbency, pulmonary or peritoneal infection, aspiration, fluid overload, fat or particulate microaggregate embolism, oxygen toxicity, and left ventricular failure.[176]

Clinical Manifestations

The symptoms and signs of retained secretions are easily recognized—pneumonitis and atelectasis may be heralded by low-grade fever, rales, or rhonchi, with roentgenographic evidence of patchy areas of pneumonitis. Aspiration pneumonia may be difficult to distinguish from atelectasis if it is localized to one lobe or lung. Under some circumstances, it may resemble pulmonary edema. The adult respiratory distress syndrome associated with sepsis usually begins with symptoms and signs of respiratory insufficiency, which may at first be mild. As it progresses, it is characterized by fever, hypotension, hyperventilation, oliguria, arterial hypoxemia, and hypocarbia. Blood cultures are usually positive. In the patient with full-blown adult respiratory distress syndrome, the symptoms and signs are more severe and less responsive to elevated inspired oxygen concentrations.

Treatment and Prevention

For retained secretions, a methodical progression of measures should be used. First, the patient should be encouraged to cough effectively and repeatedly with the aid of analgesics and physical support. If this is ineffective in eliminating secretions, transnasal aspiration of the trachea and main bronchi should be done, using a sterile catheter. Hypoxia can be avoided by hyperoxygenating the patient prior to suctioning and keeping the length of active suctioning brief.[177]

The next step should be a bedside bronchoscopy using the fiberoptic bronchoscope if secretions are thin. Otherwise, the rigid bronchoscope should be used.[178] If bronchoscopy is unsuccessful, endotracheal intubation and mechanical ventilation should follow. Tracheostomy allows ready and repeated access to the lower respiratory tract and should be resorted to if secretions cannot be managed through the endotracheal tube or if prolonged mechanical ventilation is anticipated.

For pneumonitis and atelectasis, essentially the same measures are used, but with increased vigor. Appropriate antibiotics should be administered as determined by culturing material aspirated from the lower respiratory tract for both aerobic and anaerobic organisms.[179]

Aspiration pneumonia will also require close monitoring of blood gases, elevated levels of inspired concentrations of humidified oxygen, and possibly, assisted ventilation.

Septic shock lung and adult respiratory distress syndrome almost always require careful and frequent monitoring of arterial blood gases and pH levels and continuous monitoring of hemodynamic parameters. These include systemic and pulmonary arterial and central venous pressures, electrocardiography, and cardiac and urinary output. In addition, knowledge of alveolar-arterial gradients, degree of pulmonary arteriovenous shunting, and measurements of lung mechanics may be required. Other principles of management include early recognition of the syndrome, search for and prompt evacuation of localized suppuration, antibiotic therapy appropriate for the organisms isolated, intravascular volume replacement, and mechanical ventilatory support. Ventilatory support may require the use of positive end-expiratory pressures. Attention to all other contributory factors, as discussed under pathogenesis, is also important.

By far the best course, for both patient and surgeon, is prevention. Careful assessment of the patient's respiratory reserve prior to operation and individualized preparation are vital, especially for patients with chronic obstructive lung disease. Smoking must be stopped, tracheobronchial secretions must be reduced or eliminated, and localized infection must be brought under control or eliminated.

Chest physiotherapy instituted prior to operation appears to be helpful, although proof of this is lacking. All measures to prevent aspiration of gastric contents during the induction of anesthesia, the course of the operation, and the postoperative period are essential.[180] Prompt postoperative institution of a coughing regimen and of transnasal endotracheal aspiration for retained secretions is mandatory.

The prevention and management of postoperative lung infections will probably occupy more time and cause more concern to the surgeon than any other condition described in this chapter.

Lung Abscess

Definition

Not all localized collections of "pus in the lung" qualify for our definition of lung abscess. A lung abscess is a localized area of suppuration in the lung followed by central necrosis of tissue and (usually) cavitation. A lung abscess, by this definition, excludes collections of pus in preexisting cavities or potential spaces. For the purposes of clarity, therefore, encysted and interlobar empyemas and infected pulmonary or bronchial cysts are not being considered in this section, although they can be construed by some as abscesses in the lung.

Historical Note

Putrid lung abscesses has been recognized for centuries, but treatment was always relatively ineffective. Incision and drainage, although described over a century and a half ago,[181] were rarely performed, even though the beneficial effects of providing prompt egress for collections of pus were understood. Usually, the diagnosis of lung abscess was delayed, and patients were in a debilitated and toxic state when submitted for surgical drainage, with understandably discouraging results. In 1942, however, a series of early, open drainage procedures was reported in 122 patients with putrid lung abscesses, with only a 3 percent mortality.[182] It was this unprecedented success that led to the need for greater precision in this diagnosis and topographic localization of lung abscesses on the chest wall based upon segmental bronchial anatomy. Lord Brock [183] provided the groundwork for the evolution of appropriate treatment, and the principles he emphasized remain valid. In the two-stage procedure of drainage, adherence of the visceral pleura to the parietal pleura was either identified as having already occurred or was deliberately provoked by packing the rib bed with gauze after segmental rib resection. In the second stage, drainage of the lung abscess was carried out through the prepared area, thereby avoiding contamination of the pleural space and resulting empyema. Later, resective procedures for chronic lung abscesses were introduced, almost completely displacing the two-stage procedure.

The most important advance in managing lung abscesses, however, was the introduction of antibiotics in the late 1940s. As a result, far fewer pneumonias developed into abscesses.[184] Even when an abscess developed, effective antibiotic treatment controlled most acute lung abscesses. Surgical treatment declined in popularity, and open drainage became rare.

In recent years, however, the microbes that cause lung abscesses have changed. This is due to the extensive use of the antibiotics as well as other agents, including antineoplastic drugs, corticosteroids, and immunosuppressive drugs. Opportunistic organisms have replaced primary pathogens as the cause of lung abscesses, so that, as the incidence of primary lung abscesses has decreased, the incidence of opportunistic lung abscesses has increased.[185-187]

Pathogenesis

Primary lung abscesses usually occur in patients with dental or oral infections during a period of decreased consciousness, which is usually accompanied by suppression of the normally protective cough reflexes, as in alcoholism, anesthesia, neurologic disorders, and submersion. Other causes of aspiration include drug ingestion or addiction, diabetic coma, and esophageal disorders. Infectious debris slips by gravity into the airway or is inhaled by the obtunded patient, preferentially into one of the three segmental bronchi most directly in line with the upper airways. Approximately three quarters of primary lung abscesses occur in three lung segments: the superior segments of the lower lobes of both lungs and the posterior segment of the right upper lobe (Fig. 30-10).[188,189] Such is not the case for opportunistic lung abscesses, which can occur in all segments with approximately equal frequency, although the right lung is more commonly involved than the left. The old adage that primary aspiration lung abscess almost never occurs in edentulous patients has been repeatedly shown to be incorrect.[190,191]

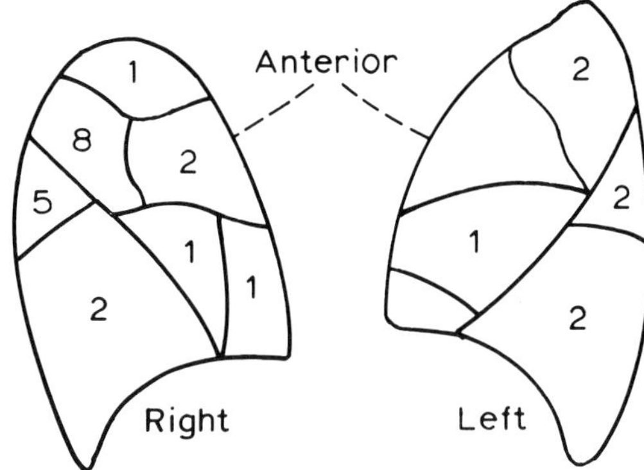

Fig. 30-10. **Localization of lung abscess by pulmonary segment (lateral view). (From Finegold SM: Anaerobic Bacteria in Human Disease, 1977. Courtesy of Academic Press.)**

The aspirated material causes bronchial occlusion and produces atelectasis of the lung tissue supplied by the blocked bronchus. This area may become infected by the organism carried down with the aspirate, producing a suppurative pneumonia. If the infection progresses, an area of focal necrosis and liquefaction can be produced.

The pathogenesis of opportunistic lung abscesses is not as readily understood. These abscesses occur in patients who are either very young or very old and who have serious, associated conditions ranging from prematurity to incurable malignancy. Intensive therapeutic efforts may have saved their lives but without the normal host defenses for successfully combating infections. In these patients, lung abscesses occur as a complication of a systemic disease. Prematurity, bronchopneumonia, congenital defects that require surgical treatment, the postoperative state itself, the presence of other infections, blood dyscrasias, and systemic diseases are all common predisposing conditions in early infancy. Systemic diseases, malignancies (especially of the lung and oropharynx), prolonged use of corticosteroids, immunosuppressive or radiation therapy, and, again, the postoperative period constitute the common conditions of the older age group in which opportunistic lung abscesses are seen.[187] Such conditions often cause multiple (rather than single) abscesses, the majority of which are acquired in the hospital.

Etiology

The most common organisms responsible for primary aspiration lung abscesses are anaerobic bacteria (Table 30-2). The fusobacteria, *Bacteroides* species, peptostreptococci, and peptococci are most commonly seen.[191] Aerobic bacteria (*Streptococcus pneumoniae, S. aureus,* beta-hemolytic streptococci, *Klebsiella* species, *Pseudomonas aeruginosa, E. coli*) are less commonly true etiologic agents but are often implicated because they are cultured from expectorated sputum by simple aerobic cultural techniques. Bartlett et al [192,193] have demonstrated the need for anaerobic cultural methods, preferably using percutaneous transtracheal aspiration, if accurate bacteriologic studies uncontaminated with nasopharyngeal flora are to be obtained. In common practice, the organisms often cannot be isolated because antibiotic therapy has already been started. Often, however, the technique for obtaining material for study is self-defeating because the bacteriostatic additives in injectable saline solutions that are used to obtain lung washings or the bacterial suppressive action of local anesthetic agents used at bronchoscopy or bronchography have inhibited bacterial growth.[193-197]

The types of bacteria isolated in opportunistic lung abscesses differ from those that cause aspiration disease. While *S. aureus* is still a common causative organism, alpha streptococci, *Neisseria catarrhalis,* pneumococci, *Pseudomonas, Proteus, E. coli,* and *Klebsiella* all appear. Occasionally, after prolonged antibiotic treatment, rather unusual bacteria and fungi are all that remain to be cultured from the sputum.

Clinical Manifestations

The typical onset of lung abscess is insidious, with cough and fever, sometimes in association with chest pain. Hemoptysis often signals the evacuation of the necrotic contents of the abscess cavity, following which purulent and sometimes foul-smelling sputum is produced. The color (green, brown, gray, or yellow) is usually not helpful, although the production of anchovy- or chocolate-colored sputum should suggest amebic abscess.[65,198] After the contents of the abscess are evacuated, clinical evidence of toxicity subsides.

The early physical signs of lung abscess are similar to those of localized pneumonia or consolidation. Later, the signs of cavitation may be elicited, as well as those of a pleural effusion, if empyema supervenes. Clubbing of the digits occurs only in patients with long-standing infection.[199]

Somtimes, severe toxemia, dyspnea, cyanosis, and septic shock overshadow symptoms and signs of staphylococcal pneumonia or lung abscess in infants or children, especially if rupture of the abscess and pyopneumothorax have occurred.

Thoracic Roentgenograms. Initially, an area of nonspecific, dense pneumonic consolidation may be seen. After evacuation of the necrotic center through a connecting bronchus, a typical air-fluid level is observed on films taken with the patient in the upright position or in the lateral decubitus position if the patient is too ill to sit up (Fig. 30-11). In time, the cavity may shrink and disappear, but occasionally a cavity will assume a cystlike appearance. Atelectasis, pneumothorax, pleural thickening, or effusion may confuse the typical picture. For example, complete or partial opacification of an entire hemithorax is occasionally seen in infants with staphylococcal pneumonias, because of their predilection to develop into infected, thin-walled pneumoceles associated with pleural effusion, empyema, or pyopneumothorax. Even such extensive roentgenographic changes can disappear rather dramatically after appropriate therapy.

Diagnosis

A significant infection in a dependent pulmonary segment in combination with known orogingival or dental disease, and a probable history of obtunded consciousness should suggest the possibility of a lung abscess. This diagnosis is strongly supported by the presence of purulent sputum and even more strongly if a fluid level can be identified in a characteristic lesion on the thoracic roentgenogram taken in the upright position. Any pneumonia can rapidly lead to a lung abscess in immunocompromised patients.

Differential Diagnosis. Many conditions can be mistaken for a lung abscess, especially from roentgenograms. These include lung tumors, tuberculosis, fungal infections of the lung, actinomycosis, bronchiectasis, pneumonia, aseptic necrosis of a tumor, and secondary infection of cysts or bullae.

Bacteriologic examination of the sputum for fungi and tubercle bacilli, sputum cytology, chest tomography, bronchoscopy, and bronchography may be needed in the differential diagnosis of atypical cases. The radiographic appearance of a carcinoma that has excavated can sometimes be confusing. The irregular lobulated contour containing an irregular central cavity with a thickened wall is helpful. A bronchogenic carcinoma should also be suspected if the lesion responds poorly to antibiotic therapy. An encysted subacute or chronic pleural or interlobar empyema may appear as a well-defined shadow which closely resembles an abscess. In a lateral roentgenogram, however, the empyema shadow is usually oval-shaped and interlobar or subpleural. Tuberculous or fungal cavities do not usually appear with a fluid level or in the clinical setting described. Bacteriologic and mycologic studies are obviously essential for differential diagnosis.

Cysts of the lung are spherical (often without a clear-cut outline) and thin-walled, with little or no inflammation surrounding them. Infected hydatid cysts are problems only in endemic areas—Utah, Canada, and Alaska.[200-202] It may be difficult to differentiate an abscess from a hydatid cyst after the latter has ruptured and become secondarily infected because then it has become a chronic lung abscess. A positive Casoni skin test (not completely reliable) or eosinophilia and the occurrence of urticaria are helpful in diagnosing echinococcosis.

Treatment

Medical. Prolonged antimicrobial therapy is the best treatment for primary aspiration lung abscess.[192,203,204] If all patients with primary lung abscesses were appropri-

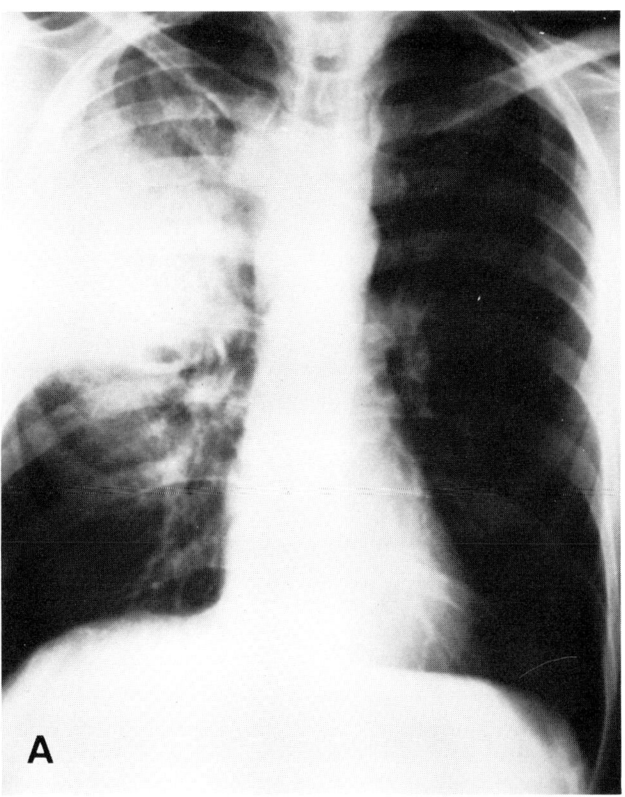

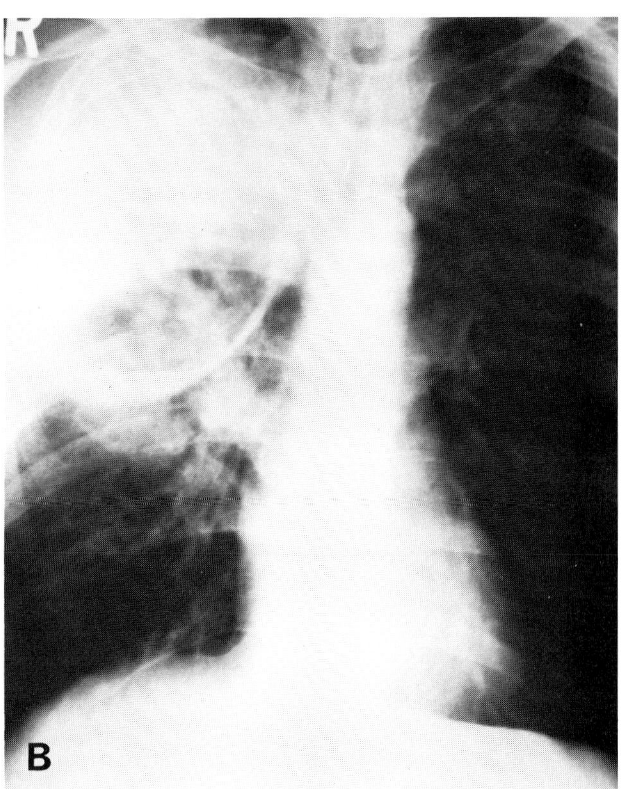

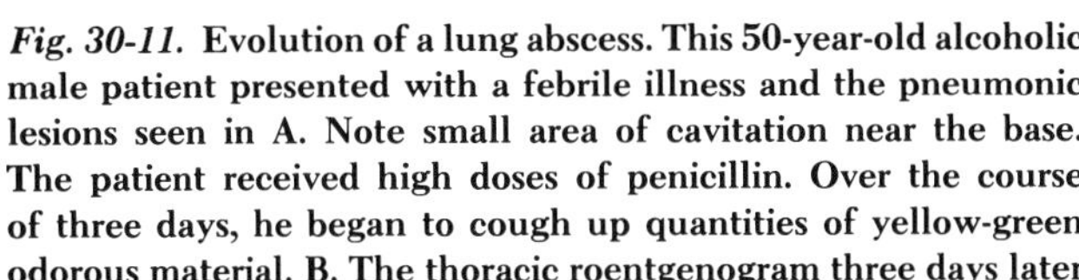

Fig. 30-11. **Evolution of a lung abscess. This 50-year-old alcoholic male patient presented with a febrile illness and the pneumonic lesions seen in A. Note small area of cavitation near the base. The patient received high doses of penicillin. Over the course of three days, he began to cough up quantities of yellow-green odorous material. B. The thoracic roentgenogram three days later shows a large cystic lesion with a fluid level. It is probable that a small lung abscess ruptured into and was loculated by the interlobar fissure, forming an interlobar empyema. With continued therapy, the process resolved, leaving only a thickened pleura and moderate reduction in lung volume.**

ately treated, there would be little place for operation in this disease.[192] Appropriate management involves percutaneous, transtracheal aspiration of secretions from the lungs prior to the institution of antimicrobial therapy. Unfortunately, most physicians are unfamiliar with the technique and are discomforted by the paroxysm of coughing induced. Therefore, few physicians use this method to obtain material for culture. The surgeon, more at home with invasive techniques, may be of help in allaying these anxieties.

At any rate, an effective regimen is penicillin G, 5–20 million units per day, either orally (the lower dose) or intravenously (the higher dose).[205] Other drugs, such as carbenicillin 6 gm intravenously every 6 hours [206] and clindamycin 600 mg intravenously every 6 hours,[207] have been equally effective. Four weeks of treatment have been recommended,[205] but the parenteral administration need not be this long. Parenteral therapy is continued until the patient's fever and toxicity have subsided and roentgenographic evidence of improvement is seen. After this, antibiotics are given orally, and treatment is continued until cavitation disappears and clinical cure is attained. Oral antibiotics may be required for 3–20 weeks, but with this treatment, operation for primary lung abscess has not been required over a 4.5-year period at two cooperating Veterans Administration Medical Centers.[191] Kanamycin may be the best drug for *Klebsiella* infection. Combinations of drugs may be needed in drug-resistant cases.

Bronchoscopy is often appropriate to look for foreign bodies, to rule out endobronchial tumor, and to aid in evacuating abscesses. If bronchoscopic manipulation to achieve transbronchial drainage of large abscesses is required, great care should be exercised to avoid spillage of pus into the opposite lung.[207] In fact, drowning has been reported in these circumstances. The recent refinement of transbronchoscopic drainage by catheterization of the appropriate bronchus by an arteriographic catheter (through a rigid bronchoscope, with or without fluoroscopic guidance) is more helpful than the flexible fiberoptic bronchoscope (Fig. 30-12).[208] Physical measures, including postural drainage [209] and percussion of the thorax, may be helpful, but proof of this is lacking.

Surgical Treatment. Operations are reserved for the complications of lung abscess. These include chronicity, serious hemoptysis, the development of bronchopleural fistula, and empyema. Operation should not often be required [191,210,211] but is occasionally useful in neglected or inadequately treated patients, in older males with suspected malignancy, and for giant abscesses where the risk of contralateral aspiration is great.[212]

Pulmonary resection (usually lobectomy) should be

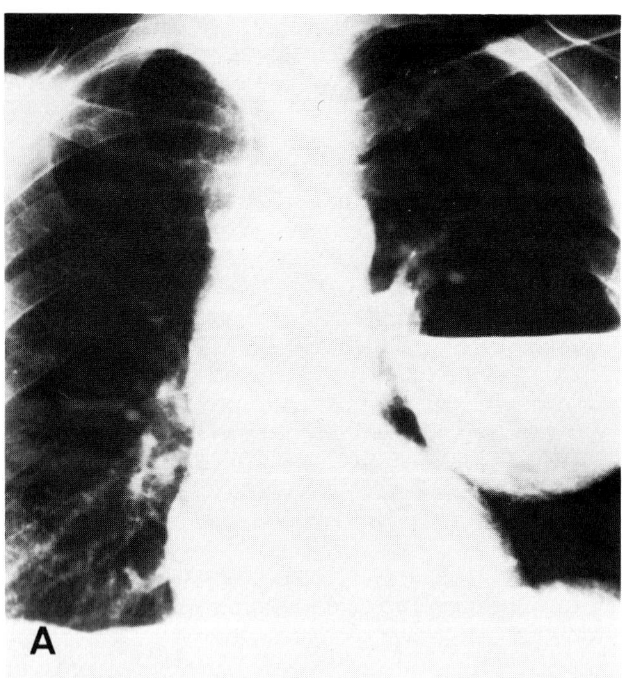

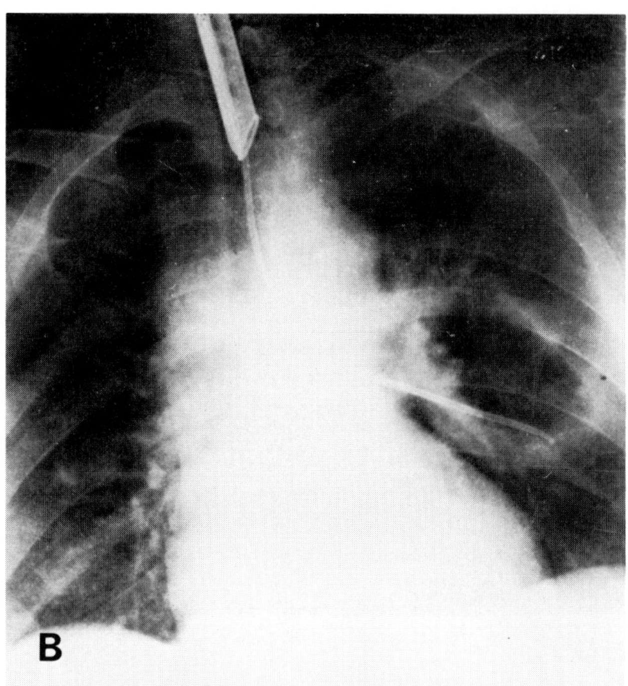

Fig. 30-12. **Transbronchial catheter drainage of a huge lung abscess in the superior segment of the left lower lobe, from which *K. pneumoniae* was cultured, in a 47-year-old alcoholic male. A. Thoracic roentgenogram before drainage. B. Immediately after drainage, showing catheter in the cavity. A Cordis right coronary angiographic catheter was used. The procedure was repeated three days later, again with evacuation of pus. The patient was ultimately discharged with a thin-walled, 2 cm cavity in the left lower lobe. (From Connors JP, et al: Ann Thorac Surg 19:254, 1975. Courtesy Little, Brown and Company.)**

used if a large (6 cm or more) or smaller, thick-walled, residual cavity remains after eight weeks of intensive antibiotic therapy, especially if there are continuing or recurring symptoms. Patients with sizable hemoptysis are at risk not so much because of the threat of exsanquination as because of the hazard of asphyxiation and may require emergency operation.[213,214] Radiologic features that can be seen in patients with severe hemoptysis include (1) alternate empyting and refilling of the abscess cavity in serial chest films (the emptying may correlate with an episode of hemoptysis, the refilling with periods of minimal or no hemoptysis), (2) an air-fluid level with differences in the radiolucency of the fluid phase and changes in location in the abscess cavity on changes in position, and (3) a persistent density with patchy radiolucencies. The persistent density may indicate an abscess cavity filled with blood clots.[213]

Special care is necessary when operating upon patients with lung abscesses because of the possibility of flooding the airways with blood or pus. Appropriate anesthestic and operative techniques must be used to prevent this material from entering the uninvolved portions of the lung. These techniques include the use of a tracheal divider (Carlens, Robertshaw) or placing the patient in the prone or supine position to prevent contralateral lung contamination and airway obstruction. The involved bronchus should be clamped as soon as possible after the chest is opened. A long, cuffed endotracheal tube passed into the main bronchus on the nonoperative side or blockage of a draining bronchus with a Fogarty-type catheter during bronchoscopy prior to intubation are less satisfactory methods but are sometimes necessary. Obviously, empyemas must be drained, and a pulmonary abscess that ruptures into the pleural cavity can be treated as an empyema. Closed-tubed thorascostomy drainage of a lung abscess is generally contraindicated because a large bronchopleural fistula may result. Nevertheless, giant abscesses and neglected abscesses can sometimes be rapidly cured with simultaneous closure of the abscess and the fistula by closed drainage. Aspiration will thereby be avoided. This is particularly useful in seriously ill patients who would not be expected to tolerate a formal thoracotomy. When patients with life-threatening hemoptysis cannot safely undergo major thoracic operations because of severe respiratory insufficiency, bilateral disease, inability to locate the site of bleeding, or because the patient refuses operation, nonsurgical treatment must be used. Several radiologists have reported successful control of pulmonary hemorrhage by embolizing the bronchial and nonbronchial arteries.[215,216]

Opportunistic Abscesses. Because of effective antibiotic therapy, the mortality rate in primary lung abscesses has declined from approximately 25 percent to less than 5 percent. Unfortunately, this is not true of opportunistic lung abscesses. Opportunistic lung abscesses require more aggressive diagnostic and therapeutic measures. Invasive diagnostic methods, such as percutaneous transtracheal aspiration and even direct needle aspiration of the lung, may be justified to determine the etiologic agent because specific therapy may be necessary.[217]

Occasionally, percutaneous transthoracic drainage can cause dramatic decompression of an abscess cavity, which can result in its obliteration and subsequent healing.[218,219] Newsom et al [219] successfully treated desperately ill patients by inserting a plastic intravenous catheter directly into the abscess cavity, aspirating the pus and instilling antibiotics. The mortality rate continues to be high, however (75–90 percent), in immunodepressed patients who have lung abscesses.[187]

Prevention

Lung abscesses can be prevented in some circumstances. Whenever possible, tonsillectomy, tooth extraction, and operations on paranasal sinuses should be performed under local rather than general anesthesia. If a foreign body is inhaled, it should be promptly removed by bronchoscopy. All acute lung infections should be promptly treated with appropriate antimicrobial drugs. Prevention of aspiration during the postanesthetic state, as well as during any state of altered consciousness, will prevent aspiration pneumonitis and abscess formation. Finally, maintenance of good oral hygiene would probably reduce the risk of putrid lung abscesses.

Hematogenous Lung Abscesses and Septic Pulmonary Infarcts

Hematogenous lung abscesses have not been considered here. They are usually associated with bacteremia, are almost always multiple, and do not usually require operative intervention. Vidal et al [220] have suggested surgical intervention for lung abscesses secondary to pulmonary infarction in patients who respond poorly to medical treatment. McMillan et al [221] reported that of 12 patients (many heroin addicts) with septic embolism and infected infarcts who required thoracotomy, only 1 died.

Bronchiectasis

To Laennec and his pupils belongs the credit for the earliest descriptions of bronchiectasis, although the term was not introduced until 1846 (by Hasse). Not much could be done about this "loathsome disease" for a century after its recognition, but in 1922 Sicard and Forestier introduced bronchography, which permitted visualization, localization, and assessment of its severity.[222] Treatment by drainage procedures similar to those used for empyema or lung abscess were predictably accompanied by disastrous results. Surgical treatment of bronchiectasis became firmly established only after Kent and Blades [223] pioneered lung resection using individual ligation of the lobar hilar structures. The frequency of the disease has happily declined since the introduction of effective antibiotics.

Pathogenesis

Acquired Bronchiectasis. Infection and bronchial obstruction are the two major factors contributing to the development of acquired bronchiectasis. The decline in the incidence of bronchiectasis in children is probably the result of the control of pertussis, measles, influenza, and bronchopneumonia by immunization and antibiotics.[224]

Causes of bronchial obstruction include aspiration of foreign bodies, retained mucopurulent secretions, bronchial tumors, and external bronchial compression by enlarged peribronchial lymph nodes associated with chronic lung infections (tuberculosis, histoplasmosis, and coccidioidomycosis).

The middle lobe syndrome refers to the particular susceptibility of this lobe to bronchiectasis. Two factors appear to be involved in its susceptibility: the acute angle at which the middle lobe bronchus arises from the bronchus intermedius, making it more susceptible to compression, and the poor collateral ventilation of the middle lobe, which leads to atelectasis and pneumonitis when the proximal bronchus becomes obstructed.[225]

Because bronchiectasis is frequently preceded by pneumonitis but not bronchial obstruction, the traction theory for the origin of bronchiectasis has evolved.[226] According to this hypothesis, after pneumonia, scarring and contracture of the tissue that surrounds the entrapped bronchi occur. Traction on the external circumference of the bronchi causes dilatation. The distal branches of the segmental bronchi, having the least cartilagenous support, then become dilated. The bronchial dilatation that follows the healing of a tuberculous infection or a chronic lung abscess can leave a residual bronchiectatic segmental or subsegmental bronchus.

Congenital Factors. The strongest evidence for a congenital link in the etiology of bronchiectasis is found in Kartagener's syndrome, a triad of conditions including situs inversus, pansinusitis, and bronchiectasis.[227] Whereas bronchiectasis at one time affected about 0.5 percent of the general population, it has been identified in 20 to 25 percent of patients with situs inversus and dextrocardia. A genetic abnormality, carried as an autosomal recessive, has been suggested, but such a relationship was not identified in the 1972 series from the Mayo Clinic.[227] Ultrastructural studies of a genetic disorder associated with the dynein arms of cilia [228] or with a lack of radial spokes [229] suggest abnormalities of mucociliary transport as a factor in the pathogenesis of some forms of bronchiectasis. Homozygous alpha$_1$-antitrypsin deficiency, a condition which is associated with pulmonary emphysema, is occasionally accompanied by bronchiectasis.[230]

Bronchiectasis is also seen in children with cystic fibrosis. These patients with tenacious bronchial secretions, abnormal bronchial mucosa, and impaired ciliary function ultimately die of complications of diffuse pulmonary disease.[231]

Pathology

Bronchiectasis is most frequently located in the basal segments of the lower lobes. While the superior segments are usually free of disease, the lingula may be involved in 60–80 percent of patients with left lower lobe bronchiectasis, and the right middle lobe may be bronchiectactic in 45–60 percent of patients with right lower lobe disease.[232]

The bronchi are dilated, and if secondary infection is present, they can be filled with mucopurulent secretions. The bronchial wall is partially destroyed and replaced with fibrous tissue. Both acute and chronic inflammatory changes may be present. The bronchial arteries are hypertrophied, and enlarged anastomoses between the bronchial and pulmonary arteries can be found. These anastomoses can cause significant arteriovenous shunting. Severe hemoptysis may be a consequence of this rich network of high pressure vessels.

Etiology

Infection is secondary to obstruction in bronchiectasis, and the infecting organisms are frequently mixed. When anaerobes are found, *Bacteroides, Fusobacterium,* and anaerobic streptococci are most frequently cultured.

Clinical Manifestations

Symptoms of cough, production of mucopurulent sputum, fever, and pleuritic pain occur intermittently when secondary infection supervenes. Much of the time, the patient may be asymptomatic. Recurrent episodes of bronchopneumonia are often accompanied by pleuritic pain and an increase in copious, foul-smelling sputum so severe that the social consequences exceed the threat to health. Patients with upper lobe bronchiectasis may be asymptomatic. Chronic or recurring hemoptysis, rather than productive cough, may be the primary symptom. Hemoptysis occurs in 41 percent of patients with localized disease and in 66 percent of patients with diffuse disease.[233] Bronchiectasis is the most common cause of hemoptysis in children.[234] Malnutrition and pulmonary insufficiency can develop when the disease is advanced. The classic physical findings of cyanosis, clubbing, and weight loss are rarely seen.

Percussion may reveal localized dullness. Moist, bubbling rales may be heard on ausculation over the affected areas, and coarse expiratory rhonchi are present during acute exacerbations.

Diagnosis

The diagnosis of bronchiectasis should be suspected in a patient with frequent respiratory infections, chronic productive cough, and hemoptysis. Because of the impact of antibiotics on the natural course of this disease, its symptoms are likely to be subtle.[235] Thoracic roentgenograms may demonstrate only nonspecific findings, such as atelectasis, fibrosis, and pleural thickening. In severe cases, dilated bronchi partially filled with purulent secretions may be identified by the presence of multiple air-fluid levels.

The only definitive method of diagnosing bronchiectasis is by bronchography. This is ordinarily performed only if operation is contemplated. It is also used occasionally to help exclude a tumor, foreign body, or a rare congenital abnormality. It is best performed after appropriate treatment of acute infection and after special efforts, such as postural drainage, have been made to evacuate secretions. The bronchi must be relatively free of secretions if a technically good bronchogram is to be obtained (Fig. 30-13).

Bronchoscopic examination may be performed at the same time as bronchography and may provide additional information, such as the specific segments that are the sources of purulent secretions and the visualization of bronchostenosis, foreign body, or neoplasm. Bacteriologic study of secretions obtained directly through the bronchoscope, uncontaminated with nasopharyngeal secretions (or local anesthetic agents), can give a more accurate diagnosis, so that more specific antibiotic therapy can be used. Finally, removal of thick purulent secretions is, in itself, therapeutic.

The differentiation between acute or chronic purulent bronchitis that causes cylindrical bronchiectasis, which may be reversible by vigorous antibiotic treatment, and true nonreversible bronchiectasis can be difficult to determine during bronchoscopy. Chronic bronchitis may be the cause of secondary infection in bronchiectasis.[236] The bronchographic appearance of cylindrical ectasia, with bronchi of uniform caliber crowded together and with rather diffuse involvement of both lungs, is more suggestive of chronic bronchitis or reversible bronchiectasis than of true surgical bronchiectasis.[237]

Treatment

Control of infection and relief of bronchial obstruction are the two most important measures in the treatment of bronchiectasis. The most common secondary infecting organisms are *Haemophilus influenzae,* a variety of streptococci, and *S. aureus,* as well as *K. pneumonia, E. coli,* fusiform bacilli, and Vincent's spirochetes.[238] When the patient's sputum is purulent, appropriate antibiotics should be given. Broad-spectrum antibiotics that have been effective are tetracycline, oxytetracycline, and ampicillin. Ampicillin combined with cloxacillin or benzylpenicillin is effective against *S. aureus* infections.[239] Vigorous antibiotic treatment and pulmonary toilet will reverse many of the bronchoscopic and bronchographic findings of chronic bronchitis and cylindrical bronchiectasis.

Coughing, endotracheal suction, and postural drainage are all effective in removing bronchial secretions. Postural drainage requires training and conscientious performance to be effective.[209] In addition to the use of postural drainage to remove bronchial secretions, the patient's cough can be enhanced with the use of bronchodilators and humidifiers. Isoproterenol, epinephrine, and phenylephrine are useful bronchodilators and can be used in nebulizers. Endotracheal aspiration of secretions is used when coughing and postural drainage are ineffective.

Should symptoms remain or recur after an adequate trial of medical therapy, an operation should be considered. These symptoms would include continuing episodes of pneumonitis, continuing production of 30–60 ml of purulent sputum daily, or frequent episodes of hemoptysis. The patient's general condition and pulmonary reserve, in particular, must be considered.

The best results can be anticipated in patients with limited or localized disease, especially in patients with unilateral disease restricted to the basal segments.[240] Eighty percent of patients with localized disease were relieved of all symptoms by operation. Only 36 percent with diffuse or multisegmental disease were rendered asymptomatic, although 50 percent were improved.[233] With bilateral disease, the side with the greater degree of involvement should be resected first. A maximum amount of pulmonary tissue should be conserved. Resection of the opposite lung will not always be necessary.[233]

Operative mortality for pulmonary resection for bronchiectasis is now less than 1 percent, and the incidence

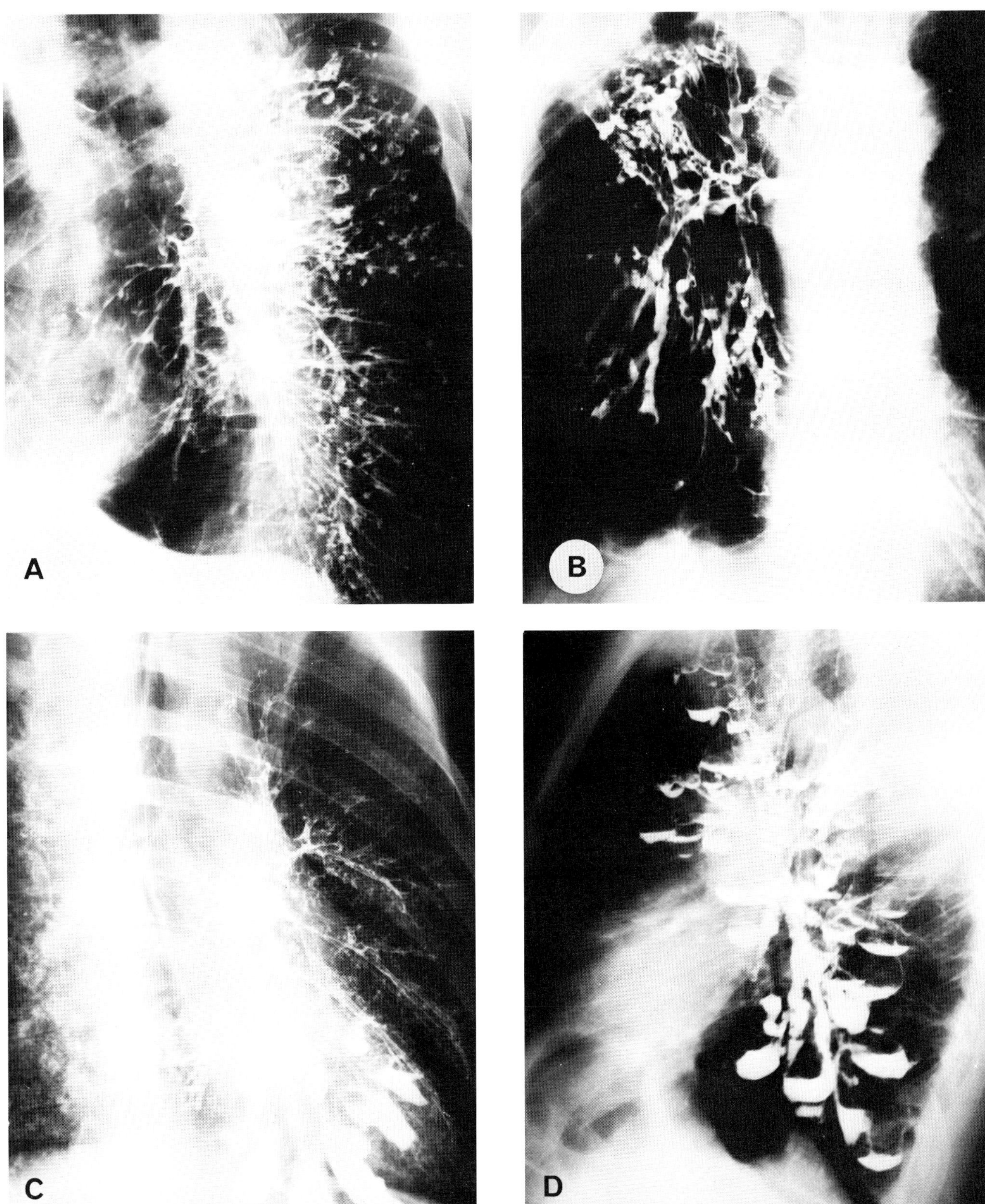

Fig. 30-13. Varieties of bronchiectasis revealed during bronchography. A. Bronchiolectasis, generalized involvement of very small bronchi, best seen in upper lung field. This is not a surgical condition. B. Marked distortion of bronchi following tuberculous infection, right upper lobe. This is also not usually a surgical condition per se. C. Localized postpneumonic saccular bronchiectasis, basal segments, left lower lobe. This patient was treated successfully by resection of the basal segments of the left lower lobe. D. Saccular bronchiectasis involving the entire left lung. The right lung was normal. This patient was treated successfully by left pneumonectomy. (From Takaro T, et al: Curr Probl Surg 14(II):6, 1977.)

of bronchopleural fistula and empyema has been between 3 and 5 percent.[241,242]

Prognosis

Bronchiectasis is no longer of considerable prominence in thoracic surgery. Prior to the advent of the antibiotic era, the average life expectancy of patients with bronchiectasis was less than 10 years.[222] Most patients now have a nearly normal life span.

PULMONARY TUBERCULOSIS

Definition and Etiology

Lung disease caused by mammalian tubercle bacilli (*Mycobacterium tuberculosis* and *Mycobacterium bovis*) is designated pulmonary tuberculosis. Nontuberculous mycobacterial lung infection is caused by mycobacteria other than mammalian tubercle bacilli (*Mycobacterium* Types I–IV).[243] The bacteriologic characteristics of these organisms are described more completely in Chapter 7.

Thoracic surgeons once called pulmonary tuberculosis the "King of Diseases," a title earned eight centuries ago. Surgeons formerly devised a number of ingenious operations to collapse the portions of the lungs occupied by cavities. These included artificial pneumothorax and pneumoperitoneum, extrapleural thoracoplasty, and plombage operations, to name a few. After antimicrobial agents became available, pulmonary resection became the operation of choice, and since the advent of effective antimicrobial therapy, operations for tuberculosis are rarely required today.[244]

Incidence

The decline in deaths from this disease (from 63 to just 2 per 100,000 in four decades) and the fall in active cases (from 77 to 16 per 100,000) was one of the more remarkable developments of this century.[245] Most of the decline in mortality occurred prior to the advent of antituberculous agents. Thus, the initial decline is attributable to improvements in public health. The more recent decline was associated with the discovery of effective chemotherapy. Nevertheless, the disease has not disappeared, and there are still 30,000 new cases in the United States per year.

Pathogenesis

The pathogenesis of this disease is discussed in Chapter 7. Typically, inhalation of tubercle bacilli leads to a peripheral, pulmonary, necrotizing pneumonitis and hilar lymph node involvement, which is sometimes very prominent, especially in children.[246] This comprises the primary Ghon complex, which nearly always heals. In a minority of cases, a caseous necrotic focus will excavate and empty its liquefied contents into a bronchus to produce cavitation and signal reinfection. There may then be either intrabronchial, lymphatic, or hematogenous spread of disease, or it may regress, fibrose, and calcify. A tuberculoma is formed when the contents of a caseating focus become inspissated. Bronchiectasis or atelectasis may result from partial or complete bronchial obstruction due to intrinsic disease (endobronchial disease with ulceration and scarring) or from extrinsic obstruction due to enlarged hilar lymph nodes. Rupture of a caseous subpleural focus into the pleural cavity may produce a tuberculous effusion or empyema. Tuberculosis of the larynx, mediastinal, supraclavicular, and cervical lymph nodes, pericardium, and chest wall may all occur. Extrathoracic hematogenous spread to any of the organs of the body, especially meninges, bones, joints, or peritoneal cavity, was common in earlier years.

Clinical Manifestations

The onset of pulmonary tuberculosis can be insidious, with vague complaints of anorexia, fatigue, weight loss, and low-grade fever. A more acute onset includes fever, cough, aching, sweating, and hemoptysis. Chest pain is usually caused by tuberculous pleurisy. Physical signs are not often helpful but should be sought in cases of pleural effusion, atelectasis, bronchiectasis, consolidation, or appreciable cavitation. Hoarseness may indicate laryngitis.

Thoracic roentgenograms can vary in appearance, depending on the extent and type of disease. Tuberculosis can mimic almost any other pulmonary disease roentgenographically. The lesions of surgical interest are the open cavity, the tuberculoma, bronchiectasis, and various combinations of atelectatic or destroyed lobes or lungs that can mimic bronchogenic carcinoma.

A number of roentgenographic patterns may be identified in patients with postprimary tuberculosis (Fig. 30-14).

1. Local exudative lesions represent alveolar consolidation of a patchy or confluent nature. The lymphatic drainage markings radiating toward the hilus are accentuated.

2. Local fibroproductive lesions are defined more sharply, although their size and shape may vary. Fibrosis and contracture are evidenced by a decrease in lung volume, and retraction of the hilus and trachea toward the lesion is common.

3. Cavitary lesions have moderately thick walls, but with healing these tend to become quite thin, the inner surface linings are smooth, and air-fluid levels are seen (Fig. 30-14). The cavities may disappear following adequate therapy, but some persist as open negative cavities. Tomography may be necessary to verify the persistence of some cavities after therapy.

The roentgenographic manifestations of pulmonary disease due to mycobacteria other than *M. tuberculosis* cannot be differentiated from those due to *M. tuberculosis.* Some features are more characteristic, however. There is a greater tendency for cavitation with multiple thin-walled cavities than with infection with the tubercle bacillus, and exudative lesions are uncommon, as are hematogenous dissemination and pleural effusion.

Diagnosis

The diagnosis of tuberculosis is solely dependent upon identification of the infecting organisms or the histologic

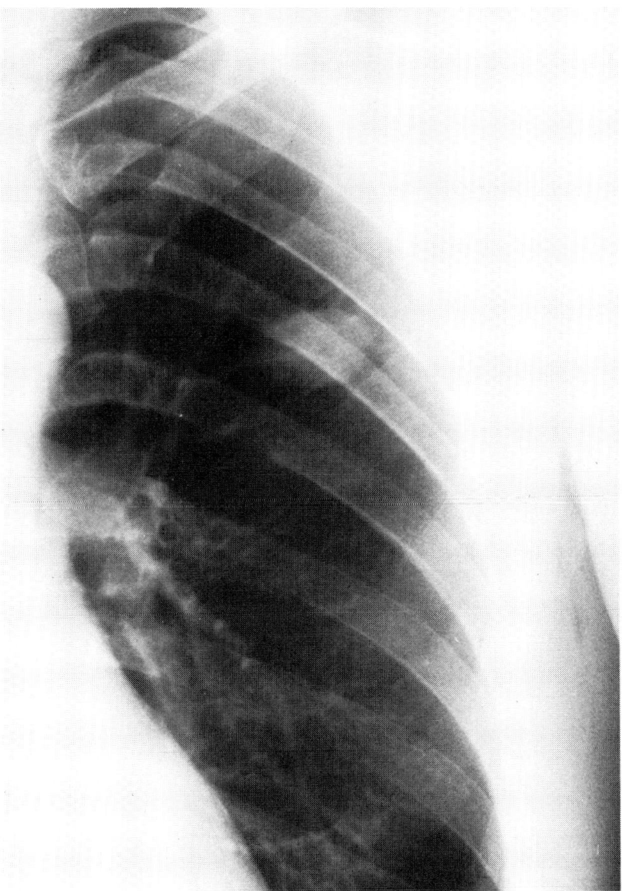

Fig. 30-14. **Thoracic roentgenogram of a 56-year-old male, a severe diabetic, who was found to have a new, noncalcified, solitary, pulmonary nodule. On suspicion of bronchogenic carcinoma, a left upper lobectomy was done. This lesion proved to be a tuberculoma.**

features and demonstration of the organism in the lung. A negative skin test result excludes the diagnosis unless miliary tuberculosis is present or an immunosuppressed patient is being examined. The principal differential diagnosis is cancer, but any chronic pulmonary infection can have a similar presentation.

Treatment

The contemporary treatment of tuberculosis by chemotherapeutic agents is summarized in an official statement of the American Thoracic Society.[247] The need for therapy and the duration of treatment depend upon the category of disease.

There are four universally recognized first-line drugs: isoniazid, ethambutol, streptomycin, and rifampin (Table 18-42), and all are associated with some degree of toxicity. There are also several second-line drugs, which are generally less effective and more toxic.

Certain principles in the use of drug therapy in pulmonary tuberculosis must be adhered to: (1) never use a single drug when there is clinical evidence of disease, (2) a failing regimen (ie, continued sputum positivity) indicates drug resistance, (3) never add only a single drug to a failing regimen, and (4) add two drugs to which sensitivity has been demonstrated.

Surgical treatment should be strongly considered under the following circumstances [248]:

1. The persistence of cavitary disease, bronchial disease, or granulomatous nodular disease, with sputum smears and cultures that remain positive for *M. tuberculosis* for three to six months when appropriate antimicrobial therapy with at least two drugs is being used.

2. The persistence of significant (>2 cm in diameter) nodular disease or a destroyed lobe or lung even without positive sputum cultures. The rationale here is that the antimicrobial agents penetrate dense fibrous tissue in insufficient concentration to adequately sterilize the lesion.

3. The presence of thick-walled cavities even when sputum cultures are negative (ie, open negative cavities in patients who cannot be relied upon to continue long-term antimicrobial therapy—18 months).

4. Lesions suspected of being bronchogenic carcinoma. Carcinomas can occur in an area previously damaged by tuberculous infection (scar carcinoma). A tuberculoma can usually be resected when carcinoma is suspected even without drug coverage (Fig. 30-14).[249]

5. Significant hemoptysis or hemorrhage if the source can be located and is resectable (bronchiectasis, broncholithiasis).

6. A lobe or lung trapped by a tuberculous empyema that is unexpandable even after decortication.

Operation is rarely required for childhood tuberculosis. Purulent tuberculous empyema is seldom encountered, but when it is, decortication may be necessary, with or without resection of a portion of the underlying diseased lung.

The complications of operations for tuberculosis include the usual problems that follow major thoracotomy and lung resection, especially persistent pleural air space, bronchopleural fistula, empyema, or spread of tuberculosis.[250] Patients should be treated prior to operation with a drug to which their bacilli are sensitive, since the complication rate is high if the organisms are resistant.[251,252] Ideally, at least one primary drug to which the organisms are sensitive should be used.[253] When an upper lobectomy plus resection of the superior segment of the lower lobe is required, a prior concomitant posterolateral thoracoplasty involving the upper three to five ribs can prevent the development of a significant space problem, empyema, or bronchopleural fistula.[254] If these complications develop, they should be managed like pleural empyemas. The problem of the long-term effects of thoracoplasty on cardiorespiratory function following pneumonectomy has been reviewed.[255]

The operative management of massive hemoptysis (200–300 ml in 24 hours) requires special attention. Success with this difficult problem requires locating the source of hemorrhage by bronchoscopy during active bleeding, the use of double-lumen endotracheal dividers, and judicious selection of patients.[244] Bronchial arterial embolization might be considered in inoperable candidates.[215,216]

In general, the long-term prognosis is excellent, 90–96 percent of patients who have had operations are free of disease at five years.[256] Even in developing countries, excellent results are noted.[257]

LUNG INFECTIONS BY ATYPICAL MYCOBACTERIA (TYPES I–IV)

Etiology

Infections with mycobacteria other than *M. tuberculosis* and *M. bovis* are now called "nontuberculous mycobacterial lung infections," rather than atypical tuberculosis.[243]

The microbiologic characteristics of these organisms are discussed in Chapter 7. The causative organisms in human disease are still largely confined to *Mycobacterium kansasii, Mycobacterium avium-intracellulare, Mycobacterium fortuitum-chelonei,* and *Mycobacterium scrofulaceum* (Table 7-2).

Pathogenesis

The pathogenesis of these diseases is obscure. The disease is not transmitted by droplet infection from person to person but appears instead to be acquired from natural sources in the environment. The majority of cases are reported in adult males with preexisting pulmonary lesions (pneumoconiosis, previous tuberculosis, chronic bronchitis, bronchiectasis, chronic obstructive lung disease, and chronic aspiration pneumonitis) or immunologic deficiency disease. Cases do occur, however, in men and women without apparent lung disease or immunologic deficiency states. Malignant disease is a recognized risk factor.

Clinical Manifestations and Diagnosis

Symptoms are insidious, often overshadowed by preexisting chronic lung disease, and include persistent and productive cough, weakness, dyspnea, and weight loss. Occasionally, hemoptysis and chest pain are present. Cervical lymphadenitis may be observed in children.

The diagnosis may be difficult to make, because symptomatically, roentgenographically, and histologically, nontuberculous lung infections caused by mycobacteria cannot reliably be distinguished from pulmonary tuberculosis. Skin tests may be helpful, but extensive cross-reactions may interfere with proper interpretation. Ultimately, the diagnosis depends upon microbiologic evidence—the characteristic appearance of *M. kansasii* on smears—and on cultures of material attained by sputum collection, transtracheal aspiration, or bronchoscopy. Other clinical syndromes include lymphadenitis, skin lesions, and infections of the bones and joint, as well as urologic infections. Cases of disseminated diseases have also been reported.

Treatment

A combined medical-surgical approach is favored.[258] For *M. kansasii* infection, isoniazid, ethambutol, and rifampin should be used for a minimum of 24 months. In most instances, this will result in cure.[259] For *M. avium-intracellulare* infection, which responds less readily to drug therapy, four drugs are recommended, one of which should be daily intramuscular streptomycin for at least two years. This expensive, uncomfortable, intensive treatment may also be toxic and can be modified by subsequent drug susceptibility studies and by the course of the disease (Table 18-43).

Operation is reserved for medical treatment failures and should be used without inordinate delay. If the residual disease is localized enough to be resectable after six to eight months of appropriate drug treatment, it should be excised. This will rarely be necessary with *M. kansasii* infection but will be required in an appreciable percentage of *M. avium-intracellulare* infections. Even with adjunctive surgical treatment, the relapse and late mortality rates can be high.[260] However, the overall late results in surgically treated patients are distinctly better than in those patients in whom operation is not carried out.[258,261,262]

MELIOIDOSIS

Incidence and Epidemiology

Melioidosis is a glanderslike infection of man and animals that occurs endemically in Southeast Asia. Natural immunity is probably attained in the indigenous population, but military personnel during the Vietnam war acquired the disease in skin abrasions, burns, and by ingestion or inhalation.[263]

Etiology

The organism responsible is *Pseudomonas pseudomallei,* a gram-negative bacillus that is ordinarily a saprophyte in damp tropical soils. While the organism grows readily on standard culture media, it probably is not often recognized.[264,265] A characteristic wrinkling of the colonies occurs at about 72 hours and can be hastened by culturing at room temperature.

Clinical Manifestations

This rare disease occurs in several forms: (1) asymptomatic cases identified only by positive serologic findings, (2) acute localized suppuration, (3) acute pulmonary infection (the most common form), (4) acute septicemia, a highly lethal form, (5) chronic suppuration, in which abscesses may be found in any organ, and (6) recrudescent infection, in which any of the preceding overt forms may occur months or years after exposure. The outcome is fatal in over 50 percent of these cases, even with vigorous and appropriate therapy.[266]

Clinically, the disease resembles either pulmonary tuberculosis or chronic fungal infection. Many of the cases seen at large military medical centers were initially diagnosed as pulmonary tuberculosis.[264] The full spectrum of roentgenographic findings—infiltration, cavitation, pleural effusion, and empyema—can be seen. Hemagglutination, direct agglutination, and complement-fixation tests are aids in diagnosis if a fourfold or greater rise in titer occurs in paired sera.[266]

Treatment

Antibiotics found to be effective in vitro, usually tetracycline, should be used for a minimum of 30 days.[266] Other antibiotics might have to be called upon singly or in a variety of combinations—novobiocin, chloramphenicol, trimethoprim, sulfadiazine, and kanamycin.

If pulmonary lesions remain after six months of antibiotic therapy, an operation is probably indicated. Ideally, sputum cultures should be negative at the time of operation, but this is not likely to be the case. Lobectomy, rather than segmental resection, is the best operation to avoid the development of bronchopleural fistula.[267,268] Good results can be expected.

INFECTIONS WITH THE ACTINOMYCETES
Actinomycotic and Nocardial Infections

Actinomyces and *Nocardia* morphologically resemble fungi because they form hyphae with true branching and are spore producing, but they are true bacteria. Their microbiologic and pathologic characteristics have been discussed in Chapters 6 and 7. This distinction is clinically important because these two diseases do not respond to the major antimycotic agent, amphotericin-B, but rather to antibacterial agents, such as penicillin and sulfonamides.

ACTINOMYCOSIS

Definition

Actinomycosis is a chronic infection caused by the anaerobic Actinomycetaceae, *Actinomyces israeli.* The disease is characterized by suppuration, with the formation of abscesses and sinuses, in association with dense scarring. Characteristic yellow-brown granules, sulfur granules, are sometimes seen in material draining from abscesses or sinuses. Such material must be cultured under anaerobic conditions.[269,270]

A. israeli is a normal inhabitant of the oral cavity. Therefore, the diagnosis can only be confirmed if the organism is recovered from closed tissue spaces, from draining sinuses or abscesses, or is shown to be invasive in histopathologic sections.

Clinical Syndromes

Three clinical forms of actinomycosis are recognized: cervicofacial (Chapter 27), thoracic, and abdominal (Chapters 6 and 34).

Thoracic actinomycosis can develop as an extension of the cervicofacial variety or even by extension from a subphrenic collection. Most commonly, it results from bronchopulmonary invasion from aspirated material. It appears first as a pneumonic suppurative process which may be associated with an abscess similar to suppurative pneumonia caused by other agents. Hemoptysis may occur. The infection may be so indolent that symptoms are few until pleural or chest wall involvement becomes apparent. Thus, while empyema and chronically draining chest wall sinuses are characteristic, they are usually late stages of an insidious pulmonary process in the form of a nonspecific-appearing pulmonary infiltration, consolidation, or hilar mass sometimes strongly suggestive of bronchogenic carcinoma (Fig. 30-15).[2,3,271]

Roentgenographic signs that are helpful clinical clues for actinomycosis are pleural fluid with chest wall involvement including ribs and periosteum, penetration of interlobar fissures, and vertebral destruction.[272,273] The infection rarely extends into the pericardium.[274,275]

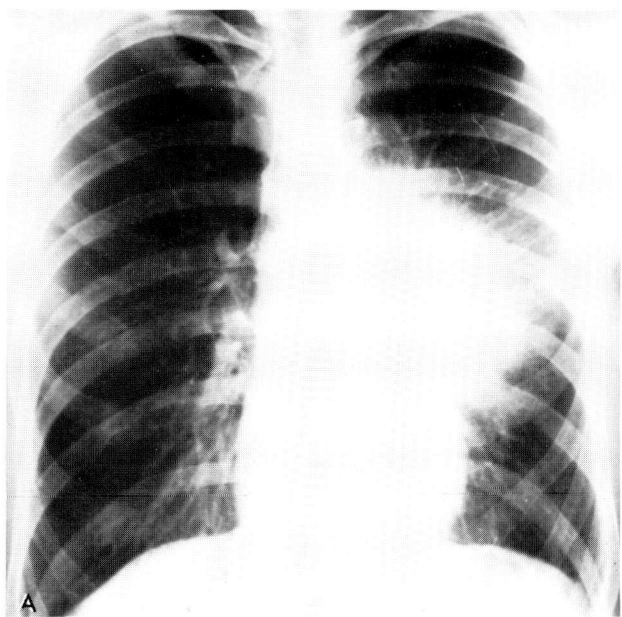

Fig. 30-15. **Thoracic roentgenogram of a patient with actinomycosis. A left pneumonectomy was performed because the lesion was suggestive of bronchogenic carcinoma. (From Takaro T: Lung infections and interstitial pneumonopathies. In Sabiston D, Spencer F (eds): Gibbon's Surgery of the Chest, 1976. Courtesy of W. B. Saunders Company.)**

Treatment

Penicillin should be used in high doses for a prolonged period—20 million units of penicillin daily for one to three months is recommended.[3] The prognosis after effective treatment is good.

Operations are sometimes indicated to remove a destroyed lobe, to drain an empyema, or to excise a sinus, but drug therapy is usually curative.[276] Suspicion of bronchogenic carcinoma is the most common indication for operation. Adequate and prolonged drug therapy to prevent reactivation of disease or development of empyema is important during and after thoracotomy.

The main problem with actinomycosis appears to be diagnosis rather than treatment. Fewer than 10 percent of these patients were correctly diagnosed in one series.[277]

NOCARDIOSIS

The microbiology and pathogenesis of nocardiosis are discussed in Chapter 7. Nocardiosis is a chronic infection usually caused by *Nocardia asteroides* (but also by several other species) and characterized by primary pulmonary involvement, with secondary hematogenous dissemination to other organs, especially the central nervous system.[278-280] The diagnosis is very difficult to make, but infection may be fatal unless adequate specific antimicrobial therapy is used.[269,270] In most recent reports, nocardiosis is seen as an opportunistic infection in patients with disordered immune systems associated with malignancy, organ transplantation, or immunosuppressive therapy.[279-281]

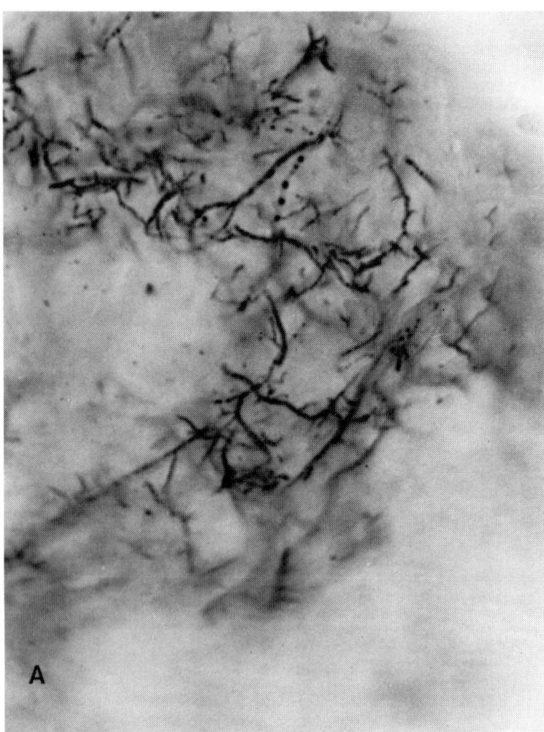

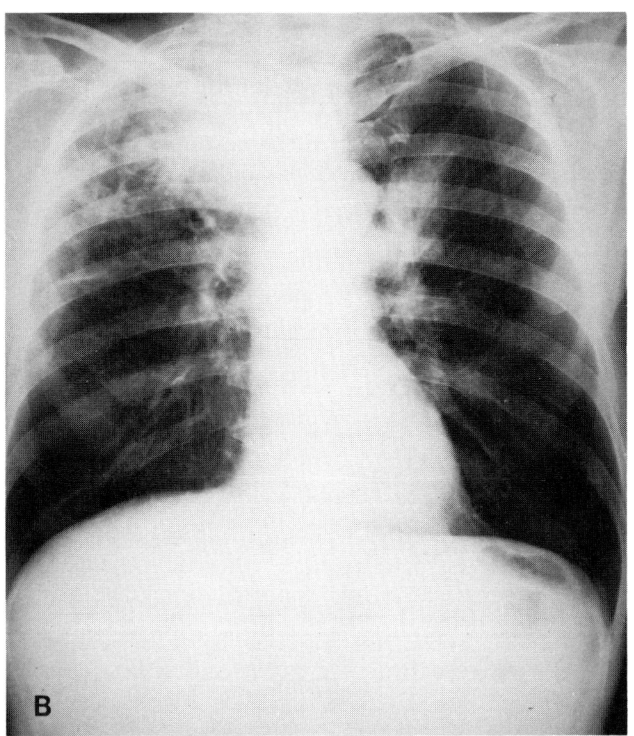

Fig. 30-16. **A. *N. asteroides.* These organisms have been mistaken for tubercle bacilli because of acid-fast staining characteristics. Gram. × 1,000. B. Roentgenogram of thorax shows pneumonic lesion of nocardiosis, right lung, and left parahilar infiltrate. *N. asteroides* was cultured from the sputum. The patient received a course of sulfadiazine and recovered. (From Takaro T: In Goldsmith EI (ed): Practice of Surgery, 1978. Courtesy of Harper and Row.)**

Pathogenesis and Pathology

Nocardia is aerobic and widely disseminated in soil, grains, grasses, and several species of animals.

The organism apparently enters via the respiratory tract and produces a necrotizing pneumonitis, progressing to abscess formation. Encapsulation is incomplete, so that spread to adjacent pulmonary tissue, pleura, and chest wall, as well as dissemination, is common. All organs may be involved, and brain abscesses are especially common. The histopathologic appearance is not diagnostic, although clumps of organisms may be seen and mistaken for *M. tuberculosis* (Fig. 30-16).

Clinical Manifestations

Classical nocardiosis, like actinomycosis, is characterized by fever, a necrotizing pneumonia productive of thick, purulent sputum, and chronic or subacute progression to involvement of the chest wall, with subcutaneous abscesses and draining sinuses. The exudate rarely will contain sulfur granules similar to those observed in actinomycosis. Most commonly, however, an immunosuppressed patient will have nonspecific flulike symptoms of cough, malaise, fever, weakness, night sweats, weight loss, and, occasionally, hemoptysis and pleuritic chest pain. On thoracic roentgenograms, a variety of presentations, including solitary nodules, nonspecific infiltrates, or cavitary disease, may be seen, and confusion with tuberculosis is common (Fig. 30-16).[282] Localized pneumonic or infiltrative lesions may suggest bronchogenic carcinoma. In the clearly opportunistic form of the disease, the progress to cavitation and dissemination can be accelerated.[278]

Diagnosis

Diagnosis is difficult and is frequently made at autopsy. A chronically ill or immunologically depressed patient with a subacute pulmonary infection (perhaps with evidence of nonspecific central nervous system involvement) is suggestive. The isolation of *Nocardia* from sputum, transtracheal aspiration, bronchoscopic washings, sinus drainage, or lung biopsy is diagnostic because the organism is not a respiratory tract saprophyte. The diagnosis can be missed in the laboratory if the technicians are not informed of the possibility of nocardiosis.

Nocardia grows so slowly that the cultures are frequently discarded. Antibiotics in fungal media suppress its growth. Overgrowth by oropharyngeal or sinus tract bacteria can obscure it, and histopathologic evidence is inconclusive because hematoxylin and eosin stain does not stain it. The Gram stain, methenamine silver stain, and acid-fast stain do. Serologic tests are useless. Because the differential diagnosis includes most of the fungi for which treatment is amphotericin B, empiric treatment is not attempted. Diagnosis of chronic pneumonias in compromised patients requires direct lung biopsy and culture of the specimen.[164,280,283-285] Identification is simple if the diagnosis of nocardiosis is considered.

Treatment

Sulfadiazine, 4–8 gm daily, or sulfisoxazole (Gantrisin) in divided doses totaling 12 gm daily, is recommended. A minimum of two to three months of therapy is usually necessary, but treatment may have to be prolonged up to six to eight months.[279] Recently, minocycline HCl and the combination of trimethoprim and sulfamethoxazole have been indicated as effective drug therapies.[279,286]

The drainage of abscesses may be necessary, but pulmonary resection is rarely indicated. Sulfonamide coverage of any operation is recommended even though resection has been done safely without drug coverage.

FUNGAL PNEUMONIA

The microbiologic characteristics of the fungi and the diagnostic problems that they present have been discussed in Chapters 9 and 47. This section will focus on the clinical problems of thoracic mycotic infections. Asymptomatic, self-limited forms of North American blastomycosis, histoplasmosis, coccidioidomycosis, and even cryptococcosis are common. Surgeons encounter these infections under two circumstances: the treatment of residual disease in immunosuppressed patients[287-290] and biopsy of the lung to achieve diagnosis.

North American blastomycosis, coccidioidomycosis, and histoplasmosis share a number of characteristics. All three are exogenous infections, endemic within sharply demarcated areas (Fig. 30-17), and share a pathologic and clinical resemblance to tuberculosis. Even serologic cross-reactions occur.

HISTOPLASMOSIS

Histoplasmosis is an acute or chronic infectious disease caused by the fungus *Histoplasma capsulatum* (Chapter 9). The endemic area is shown in Figure 30-17.

Pathology

The early lesion is pneumonitis with necrosis (rarely with cavitation), associated with an inflammatory response in the adjacent lymph nodes.[291] Both become calcified as in the familiar Ghon complex of primary pulmonary tuberculous. However, multiple dense infiltrations or calcifications are more characteristic of histoplasmosis. In the chronic progressive form, granulomatous infiltration, caseation, cavitation, and fibrosis occur, as well as lesions of centrilobular and bullous emphysema. Nodular histoplasmosis, often solitary but sometimes multiple, is characterized by concentric deposition of dense collagen, in the necrotic center of which can often be found (using Grocott's stain) the stained shells or capsules of nonviable yeast cells. In living tissue, these yeast cells are usually found packed in macrophages (Fig. 30-18). Recently, a progressive, multinodular form of the disease has been observed.[292]

Clinical Manifestations

The acute pulmonic form of histoplasmosis may be mild. The symptoms may be confused with those of an ordinary respiratory infection, or the disease may go undetected. Rarely, a more violent reaction is seen, with fever, prostration, weakness, and chest pains lasting for weeks to months. Diffuse nodular densities may be noted on the thoracic roentgenogram, which may subsequently either disappear completely or calcify (Fig. 30-19).

With chronic granulomatous histoplasmosis, again there may be no symptoms at all, the disease being discovered on a routine thoracic roentgenogram. Chronic cavitary histoplasmosis resembles chronic pulmonary tuberculosis both symptomatically and roentgenographically. Pulmonary fibrosis can occur after healing has taken place. Areas of emphysema are common and may give rise to pulmonary insufficiency and cor pulmonale.

Mediastinal involvement may take the form of either granuloma formation or fibrosis. These are discussed under infections involving the mediastinum.

Diagnosis

The details, with the interpretation of the skin test and serologic tests, are reviewed by many authors[293-296] (Chapter 9). Briefly, all the tests are of little clinical value in the individual patient, especially in endemic areas.

A definitive diagnosis depends upon the demonstration of *H. capsulatum* on sputum cultures or histologic evidence of organisms compatible with *H. capsulatum* in sputum or tissues. The organisms may be recovered occasionally from bone marrow and blood, from biopsy material (lymph nodes or lung lesions), or from resected lung tissue (Fig. 30-18). Needle or open lung biopsy is useful

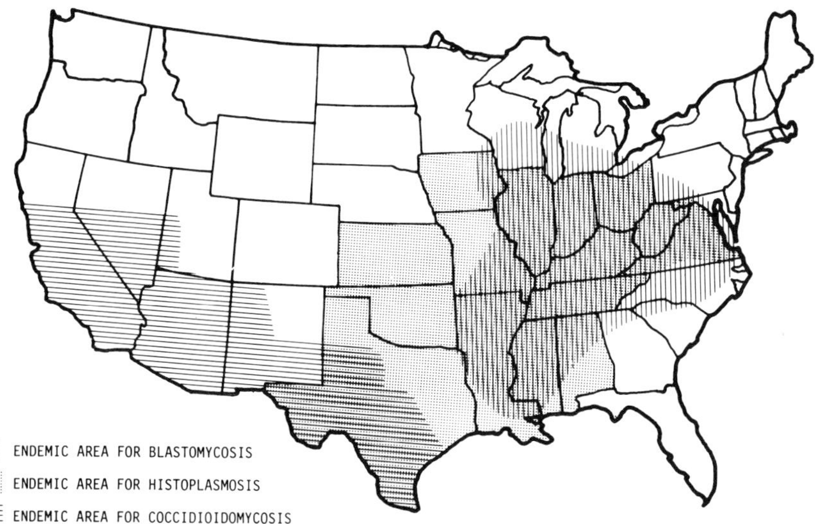

Fig. 30-17. **Map showing approximate areas in the United States recognized as endemic for North American blastomycosis, histoplasmosis, and coccidioidomycosis. (From Takaro T: In Goldsmith EI (ed): Practice of Surgery, 1978. Courtesy of Harper and Row.)**

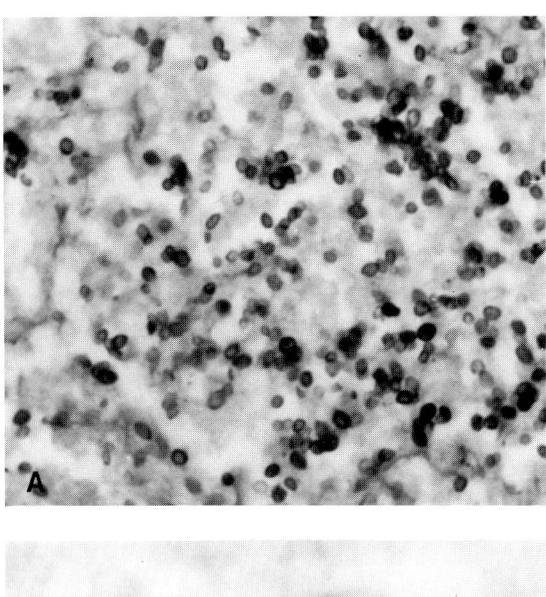

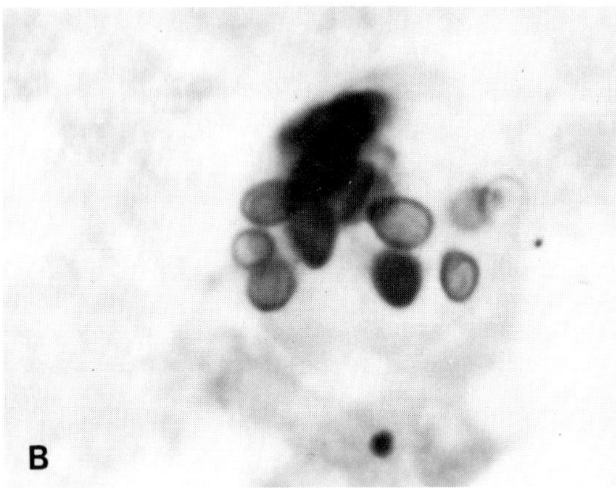

Fig. 30-18. Forms of *H. capsulatum* found in tissues. A. Nonviable capsules of *H. capsulatum* in necrotic center of a histoplasmoma. Gomori. × 1,000. B. Intracellular organisms. H & E. × 2,000. (A. from Takaro T: In Goldsmith EI (ed): Practice of Surgery, 1978. Courtesy of Harper and Row. B. From Takaro T: In Lewis' Practice of Surgery. New York, Hoeber, 1968.)

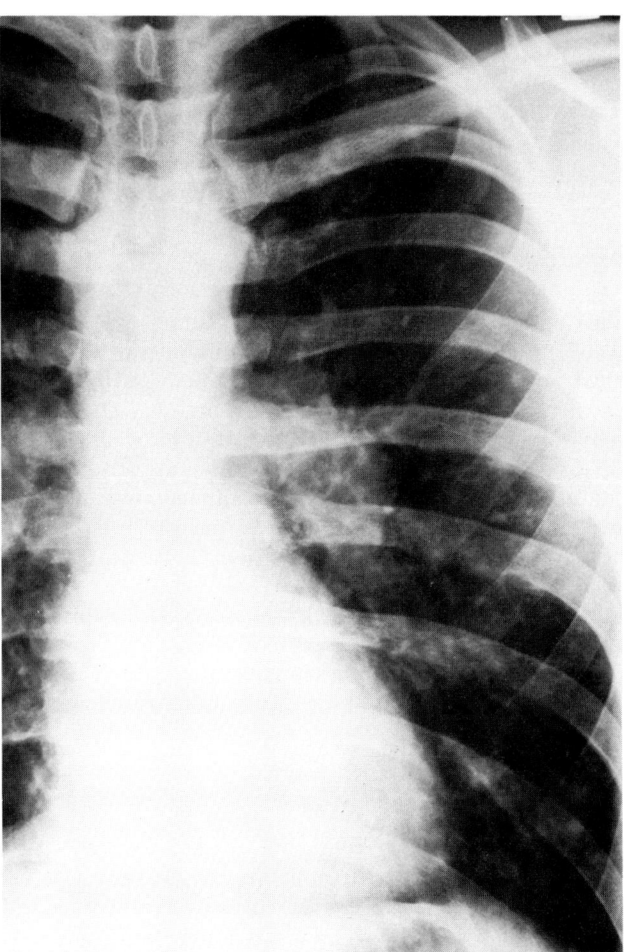

Fig. 30-19. Acute histoplasmosis. Thoracic roentgenogram of a 26-year-old male construction worker with a febrile illness of 10 days' duration, accompanied by malaise and weight loss. Note fine nodular infiltrates, especially on the left. Histoplasmin skin test was strongly positive. Mediastinal lymph node biopsy showed a gramuloma with central necrosis. In this area, on Gomori silver methenamine stains, innumerable small oval yeast cells were seen. The patient made an uneventful recovery without specific therapy, and the fine nodular infiltrates cleared.

in immunodepressed patients with subacute pulmonary disease.

Treatment

Acute pulmonary histoplasmosis may not require specific antifungal therapy unless symptoms are severe. In that case, amphotericin-B has been used successfully in relatively low dosage. For chronic histoplasmosis, amphotericin-B is the only effective drug.[270,293,297] At least 0.25 mg per kg body weight daily for a total dose of 2.5 gm of amphotericin-B is recommended.[297] The pharmacologic effects of antimycotic agents, their toxicity, and method of administration are outlined in detail by Bennett [298] and by Hermans [299] and in Chapters 9 and 18). Goodwin and his colleagues found that treated patients fared better than untreated in every category of disease except the early lesion without persistent cavitation.[300]

The surgical dilemma, ie, the proper management of the solitary pulmonary nodule, is not easily resolved. Steele [301] reported that 36 percent of 1,000 such lesions were malignant tumors and 53 percent were granulomas. Fungi, most commonly *H. capsulatum* or *Coccidioides immitis,* were isolated from the majority of these granulomas. Since malignancy was found in such a high percentage of cases and since the presence of calcium in a nodule is thought to be inadequate grounds for ruling out carcinoma unless the calcification is central, concentric, stippled, or dense, exploratory thoracotomy for the undiagnosed nodule will often be indicated, especially in adult males older than 40. On the other hand, if the diagnosis of a benign granuloma can be made by transbronchial brushing of the lesion, by the characteristic calcification, or by evidence of an unchanging lesion over a period of several years, neither thoracotomy nor drug therapy may be necessary (Fig. 30-20).[302,303]

The arguments for or against immediate open thora-

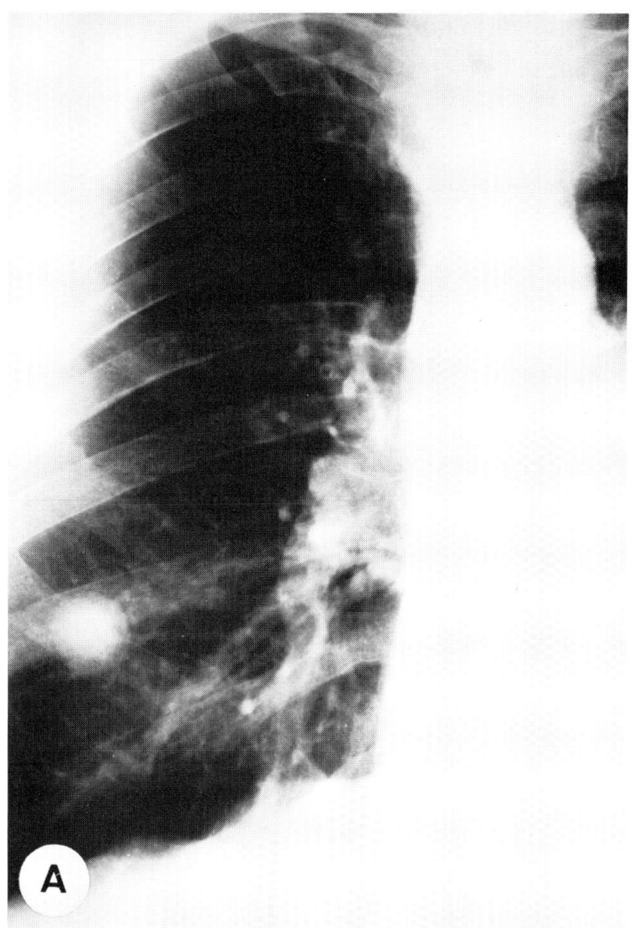

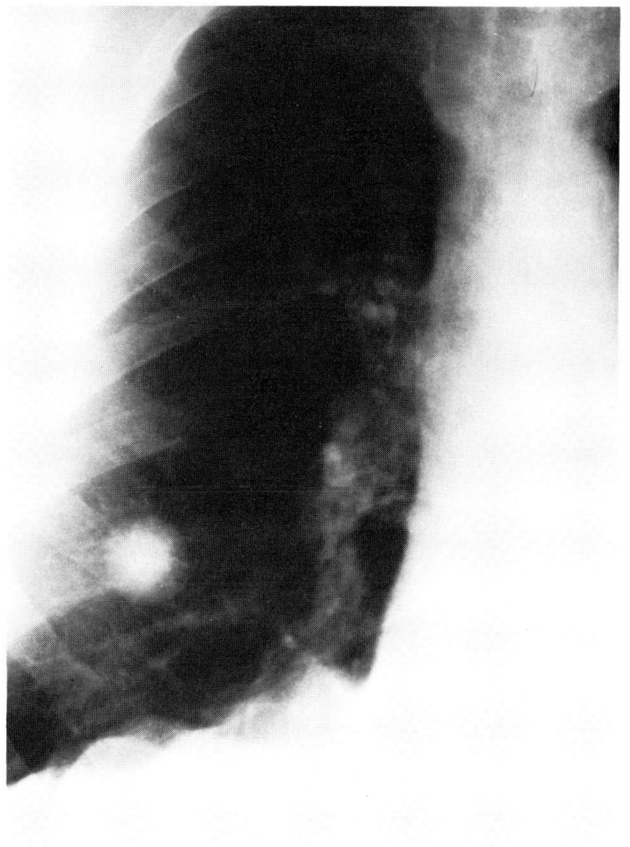

Fig. 30-20. **Probable histoplasma granuloma. A. The solitary nodule in the right lower lung field, first documented in 1968 in a 45-year-old male with severe chronic obstructive lung disease, can be seen to have a dense, laminated calcific center. B. Roentgenogram obtained 10 years later. There has been remarkably little change in the appearance of the nodule. No specific treatment is required.**

cotomy for a solitary pulmonary nodule in any individual patient are unending. According to two studies, 94 to 98 percent of all patients with carcinoma of the lung are 40 years of age or older.[304,305]

Cavitary histoplasmosis, proven by culturing the organism in the sputum or by transbronchial brush biopsy, should be treated primarily with amphotericin-B. Resection does not lower the relapse or death rate.[306] If resectional surgery is undertaken, a full course of amphotericin-B therapy should also be given.[307,308]

COCCIDIOIDOMYCOSIS

Coccidioidomycosis is a suppurative and granulomatous infectious disease whose etiologic agent, *Coccidioides immitis,* is usually inhaled from spore-laden dust. The microbiologic, pathogenetic features of this disease, as well as its generalized form, are reviewed in Chapter 9. The endemic area is shown in Figure 30-17.

Pathology

The gross lesions resemble those of pulmonary tuberculosis. The primary complex is composed of a parenchymal pneumonitis with regional lymph node involvement. This phase may not be detected clinically. Reinfection, which may be due to reactivation of the primary complex, results in caseous nodules, effusions, pneumonic areas, cavities, and calcified, fibrotic and ossified areas (Fig. 30-21). Dissemination can occur (Chapter 9).

The histologic lesions of coccidioidomycosis are those of granuloma formation with suppuration. With special stains, large (15 to 80 μm) spherules, packed with tiny endospores when mature, or the endospores themselves, can be seen (Fig. 30-22). Rarely, a mycetoma or fungus ball,[309,310] as seen in aspergillosis, is observed.

Clinical Manifestations

Most cases of primary infection are asymptomatic. However, about 25 percent of patients are symptomatic, especially Filipinos and blacks. Coccidioidomycosis begins with nonspecific respiratory tract symptoms or a flulike illness with malaise, headaches, and fever. There may be pleuritic pain and cough productive of mucoid or, rarely, bloody sputum. Erythema multiforme, erythema nodosum, or less specific morbilliform rashes are observed occasionally, especially in females. Mild arthritic manifestations that commonly pass under the name of desert rheumatism are also sometimes seen. The roentgenographic findings are nonspecific. In the acute stage, miliary lesions, pneumonic infiltrates, hilar adenopathy, or pleural and pericardial effusions can be observed. With chronic coccidioidomycosis, solitary nodules or coin lesions representing coccidioidal granulomas, chronic, thin-walled cavities sometimes with a fluid level, pneumothorax, fibrosis, or empyema can be seen.

Diagnosis

A positive culture of sputum (or other body fluid or tissue) is necessary for a definitive diagnosis. In acute coccidioidal pleural effusion, cultures of pleural biopsy specimens can be more rewarding than cultures of the fluid.[311] The details of skin tests and serologic tests are discussed in Chapter 9. Strongly suggestive evidence of coccidioidomycosis is provided by a recent conversion of the coccidioidin skin test to positive or by positive serology. While four serologic tests are available, early coccidioidal infection is usually detected only by the tube precipitin or the latex agglutination test. Rising serial complement-fixation tests mean severe disease or even dissemination, and a falling titer usually indicates regression or improvement.[294]

Treatment

Amphotericin-B is time-tested, but miconazole may prove to be useful. Treatment should be restricted to those patients with (1) severe acute pulmonary disease, (2) disseminated disease, (3) threatened dissemination, ie, a persistently high (>1:64) complement-fixation test titer, (4) cavitary disease with positive sputum cultures, (5) progressive chronic pulmonary lesions, (6) prophylaxis during pulmonary resection or excision or drainage of abscesses, sinus tracts, lymph nodes, or necrotic bone, and (7) prophylaxis in patients with active coccidioidomycosis, during corticosteroid therapy for whatever reason, during pregnancy, or in the diabetic patient.[312]

The indications for resective surgery for coccidioidomycosis include localized granulomatous lesions and cavitary disease (Fig. 30-23). While the majority of undiagnosed solitary pulmonary nodules occurring in patients in the endemic area prove to be coccidioidomas, 26 to 35 percent are found to be malignant.[313,314] Therefore, even in the endemic area, a coccidioidal granuloma must be resected if the diagnosis cannot be proven, especially if the patient is an adult 35 to 40 years of age or older with a history of cigarette smoking.[315]

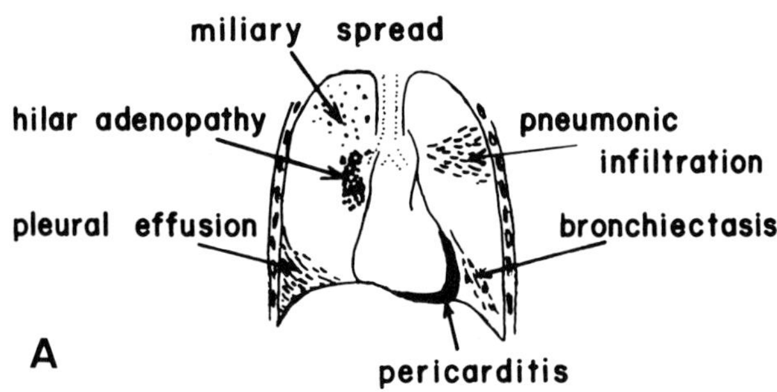

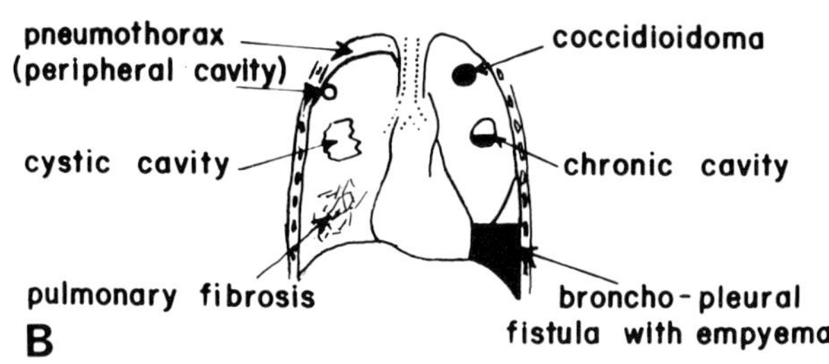

Fig. 30-21. **Varieties of pulmonary manifestations of coccidioidomycosis. A. Acute stage. B. Chronic stage. (From Paulson GA: In Ajello L (ed): Coccidioidomycosis, 1967. Courtesy of University of Arizona Press.)**

Known coccidioidal granulomas do not require resection. Localized resection in over 700 cases collected by Marks et al[316] was accompanied by a complication rate of approximately 10 percent, many of them minor air leaks or small bronchopleural fistulas.

For cavitary lesions, the indications for thoracotomy are clearer. They include persisting cavities 2 cm or

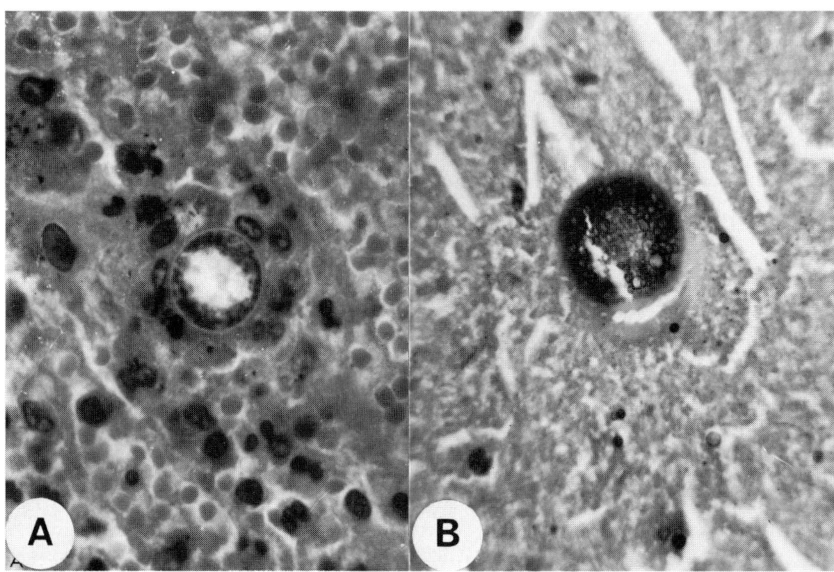

Fig. 30-22. **Spherules of *C. immitis* packed with endospores. A. In a giant cell. H. & E. × 372. B. In necrotic tissue. Gomori × 185. (From Takaro T: In Goldsmith EI (ed): Practice of Surgery, 1978. Courtesy of Harper and Row.)**

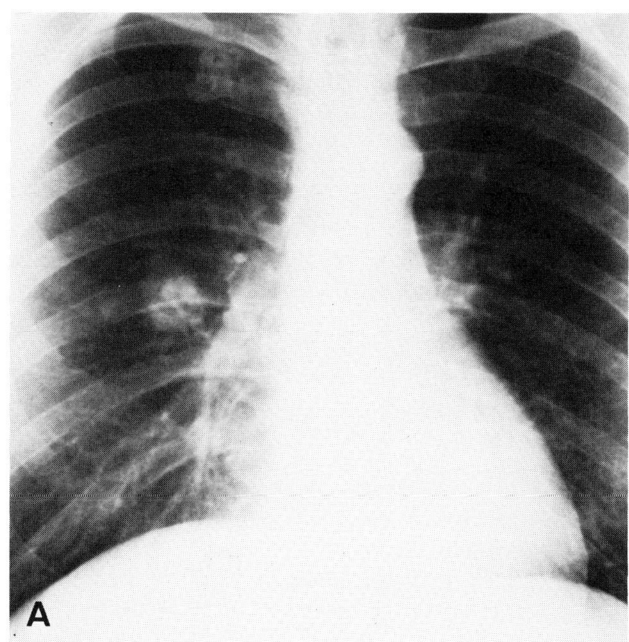

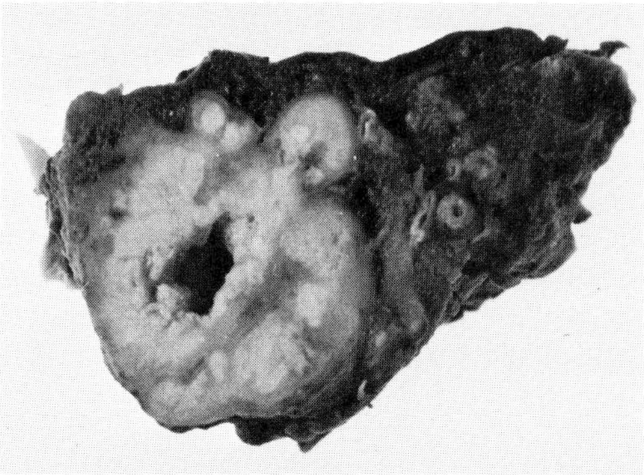

Fig. 30-23. Coccidioidal granuloma. A. Thoracic roentgenogram of a 45-year-old asymptomatic male chronic smoker from Texas who was refused a job as a foodhandler because of this dense, irregularly shaped nodule in the superior segment of the right lower lobe. All diagnostic studies proved negative or normal. B. Chronic granuloma containing central cavitation found in resected segment. A small satellite nodule was also resected. Fungal stains showed typical spherules packed with endospores. (From Takaro T: In Sabiston D, Spencer F (eds): Gibbon's Surgery of the Chest, 1976. Courtesy of W.B. Saunders Company.)

greater in diameter despite drug therapy, those that are enlarging, thick-walled, or ruptured, those associated with severe or recurrent hemoptysis, those occurring in diabetic or pregnant patients, and those coexisting with pulmonary tuberculosis.[316] Drug coverage with amphotericin-B is recommended by some, but it is not clear that the use of amphotericin-B has resulted in significantly fewer complications of bronchopleural fistula, empyema, and recurrent cavitation.[312,317-319]

Successful pericardiectomy for constrictive pericarditis due to coccidioidomycosis has been reported.[320]

NORTH AMERICAN BLASTOMYCOSIS

North American blastomycosis is a suppurative and granulomatous infectious disease caused by *Blastomyces dermatitidis,* which attacks primarily the lungs, skin, bone, and genitourinary tract.[269] The microbiologic, epidemiologic, and pathogenetic aspects of this fungus are discussed in Chapter 9. The endemic areas of the United States are shown in Figure 30-17.

Pathology

North American blastomycosis characteristically induces a granulomatous and pyogenic reaction, with microabscesses and giant cells and, occasionally, caseation, cavitation, and fibrosis. Special stains reveal the round, thick-walled yeast cell, measuring 5–20 μm in diameter with a single budding cell. Endogenous reinfection, as in pulmonary tuberculosis, has recently been documented.[321,322]

Clinical Manifestations

As in histoplasmosis and coccidioidomycosis, the acute pulmonary infection is usually mild or asymptomatic. If clinically evident, a bilateral basilar pneumonia is seen, which usually resolves spontaneously, though progression can occur (Chapter 9).

Chronic pulmonary blastomycosis is characterized by cough (usually productive only of mucoid sputum), chest pain, and occasional hemoptysis, though fever, malaise, weight loss, weakness, and other nonspecific symptoms may be the only complaints. Physical signs are not characteristic or particularly helpful.

Concomitant involvement of distant sites, especially bone, prostate, epididymis, and skin, is frequent. The skin is involved in two thirds of the cases as papules or papulopustules, which enlarge slowly, ulcerate, and exhibit elevated, cyanotic edges with peripheral microabscesses (Chapter 25). The organisms are found in the edges. The lesions may appear anywhere, both on exposed and unexposed portions of the skin, and are characterized by chronicity. Healing may occur, leaving a soft noncontracting scar.

Thoracic Roentgenographic Findings. Consolidation is characteristic of acute disease. Chronic blastomycosis [323] may present most commonly with fibronodular lesions with or without cavitation (reminiscent of pulmonary tuberculosis), but consolidation, mass lesions, diffuse patterns, pleural involvement, and hilar lymphadenopathy are also observed. Bronchogenic carcinoma is always in the differential diagnosis.

Diagnosis

A definitive diagnosis requires positive identification of the organism. This is made most commonly by culture of the sputum, aspirates, or biopsies of skin or bone.[318] The examination of bronchial washings or sputum by cytologic techniques (Papanicolaou) for *B. dermatitidis* has recently proven valuable.[324,325] Lung biopsy may be necessary to make the diagnosis, but, unfortunately, it is occasionally followed by dissemination of the disease. The major differential diagnostic problem in the endemic areas of blastomycosis is bronchogenic carcinoma.[326] A preoperative diagnosis is of importance in order to avoid an unnecessary radical resection. Serologic and intracutaneous diagnostic tests cannot be relied upon for a definitive diagnosis [294] (Chapter 9).

Treatment

Blastomycosis should be treated whenever the definitive diagnosis can be made. A presumptive diagnosis is not an adequate basis for therapy because the drugs used for treatment, 2-hydroxystilbamidine and amphotericin-B, are toxic.

Because of its wider margin of safety, 2-hydroxystilbamidine is considered the drug of first choice for noncavitary disease that is not extensive or has disseminated only to skin. For cavitary lesions, extensive disease, or systemic dissemination, amphotericin-B is preferred.[327] Ketoconazole may prove to be valuable (Chapter 18).

Surgery is indicated if bronchogenic carcinoma is suspected after efforts have been made, especially in endemic areas, to rule out North American blastomycosis. Drug treatment with amphotericin-B should follow operation if the diagnosis is made at operation. Cavitary lesions should be resected if they persist after adequate drug therapy (a total of at least 2 gm of amphotericin-B or 16 gm of 2-hydroxystilbamidine) because viable organisms usually persist in unresolved cavities even if they cannot be recovered in the sputum. Pulmonary blastomycosis is still a serious disease, with a five-year mortality rate of approximately 20 percent.

CRYPTOCOCCOSIS

Definition

Cryptococcosis is a subacute or chronic infection caused by *Cryptococcus neoformans* (formerly known as *Torula histolytica*) that primarily attacks the bronchopulmonary tree but also has a special predilection for the central nervous system.[269,270] Though meningitis is the most feared clinical manifestation, benign bronchopulmonary forms are more common. The number of patients with opportunistic infections with *C. neoformans* has increased.[328] The microbiologic, epidemiologic, and pathogenetic aspects of the fungus and its systemic diseases are discussed in Chapter 9.

Pathology

The respiratory tract is the portal of entry, and a primary complex (a pulmonary granuloma) with hilar node involvement, as in pulmonary tuberculosis, is characteristic.[329,330] However, there is little acute inflammatory response. The lesions are often solid, and the cut surface may be shiny, as in a mucoid carcinoma. Central necrosis, cavitation, and calcification are uncommon. The organisms can be easily identified in properly stained tissue. Pleural effusions and empyemas occur,[328,331] and dissemination to parts of the body other than the central nervous system is also described.[328]

Clinical Manifestations

Pulmonary symptoms are nonspecific, insidious, and frequently absent. Cough, bloody sputum, low-grade fever, weakness, and lethargy are sometimes seen. Spontaneous remission sometimes occurs. Since it is often an opportunistic infection, the manifestations of the primary disease may overshadow those of cryptococcosis, and the diagnosis may become apparent only if abnormalities on thoracic roentgenograms call attention to the lungs or symptoms referable to the central nervous system suggest meningitis. The roentgenographic features are not sufficiently characteristic to be of diagnostic help. Infiltrative, mass, nodular, and diffuse miliary lesions have all been described. Pleural effusion is unusual but is becoming recognized more frequently.[328,331-333] Cavities are rare.

Diagnosis

Cryptococcus may be isolated from sputum, bronchial washings, bronchial brushing, or percutaneous needle aspiration, as well as from cerebrospinal fluid, where it should always be sought (India ink preparation). Often the diagnosis is made from a resected lung specimen or at autopsy. No specific skin test for cryptococcosis is available, and serologic tests are not helpful.[328]

Treatment

Amphotericin-B and 5-fluorocytosine should be used in combination to treat all patients with proven disease.[334-339] In the unusual event that the diagnosis of pulmonary cryptococcosis has been firmly established prior to operation and pulmonary resection is being considered, drug therapy should be tried.[298,338]

If the diagnosis is made only after thoracotomy (the usual situation), fungal therapy may not be necessary,[340-342] but most recommend it to prevent subsequent meningitis.

ASPERGILLOSIS

The usually saprophytic *Aspergillus fumigatus* (or some other member of the species) can cause three distinctly different clinical syndromes: aspergillous bronchitis (an allergic disease), aspergilloma (fungous ball), or invasive, necrotizing aspergillous infection.[343] The organisms and all three types of disease are discussed in Chapter 9.

Pathology

In pathologic materials, the coarse, fragmented, septate, branching hyphae are found, either as short strands or ball-like clusters, which can be identified only by isolation in culture (Fig. 30-24).

Most of the surgically resected lesions of aspergillosis are aspergillomas.[344-351] A fungous ball is actually a matted sphere of hyphae, fibrin, and inflammatory cells, which appears grossly as a round or oval, friable, gray, red, brown, or yellow necrotic-looking mass. It is ordinarily found lying in an upper lobe cavity, the wall of which is often smooth and may be thick or thin, with relatively little evidence of inflammatory reaction. There usually is evidence, however, of previous chronic lung disease in this area, eg, tuberculosis, sarcoidosis, histoplasmosis, bronchiectasis, bronchogenic cyst, chronic lung abscess, or cavitating carcinoma, but sometimes there is no obvious evidence of preexisting pulmonary damage (Fig. 30-25). A true necro-

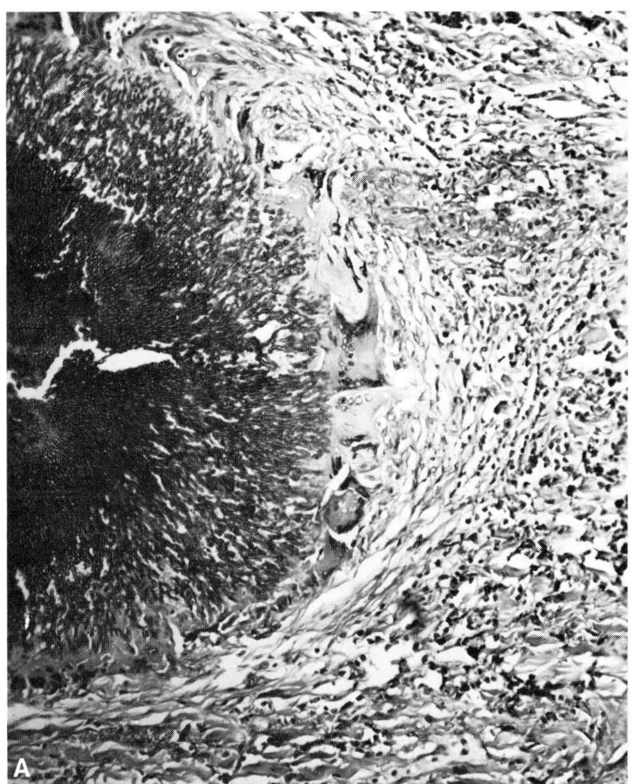

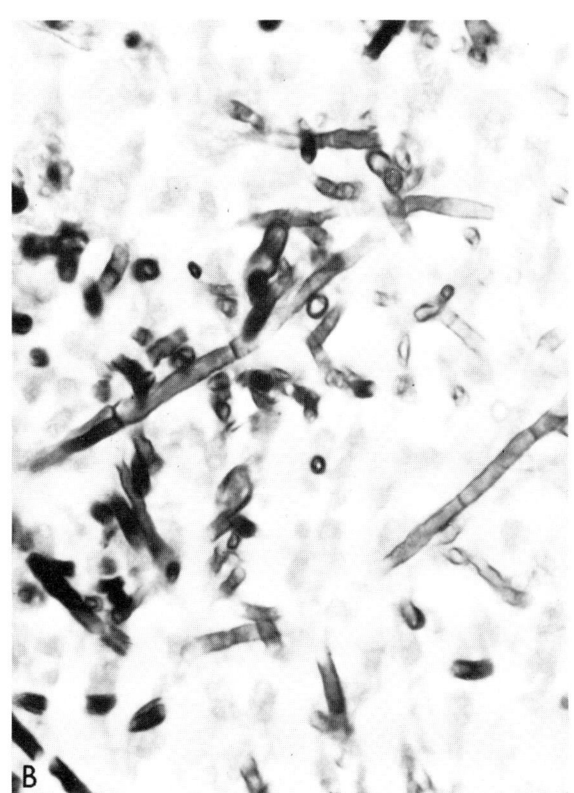

Fig. 30-24. A. fumigatus in tissues. A. Small colony of aspergilli found in a resected carcinomatous lesion of the lung. Note mycelia radiating outward from darker center of the colony. × 250. B. Close-up of coarse, septate, fragmented mycelia of *A. fumigatus.* Round bodies are mycelia seen end-on. Gomori. × 950. (From Takaro T: In Lewis' Practice of Surgery. New York, Hoeber, 1968.)

tizing pneumonia with abscess formation is found in immunologically compromised patients.

Clinical Manifestations

Aspergillomas occupying preexisting cavities usually produce no symptoms. Sometimes, cough with bloody or blood-streaked sputum is seen. An aspergilloma can be identified as a mass shifting within a cavity or cyst on changes in position of the patient. Thus, in a roentgenogram of the thorax exposed in the upright position, a crescentic radiolucency above a rounded radiopaque lesion is suggestive of aspergilloma (Fig. 30-25).

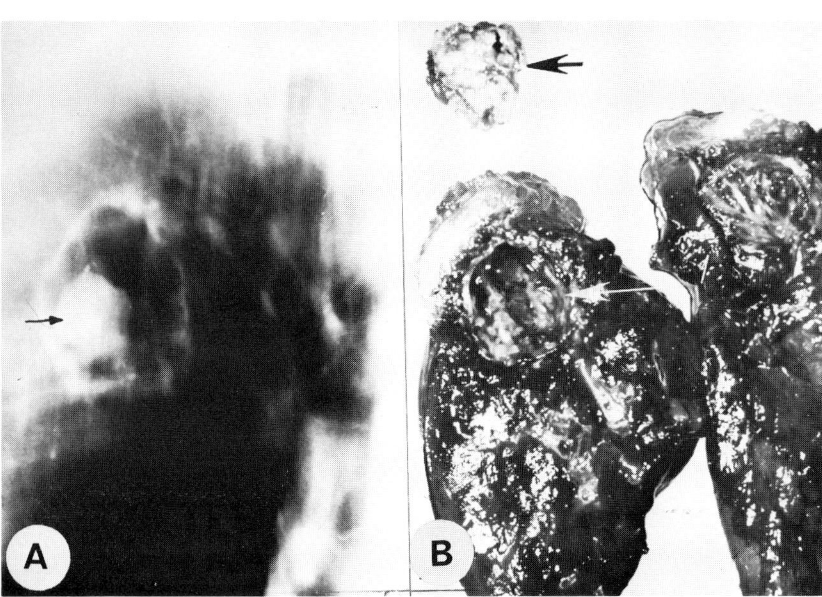

Fig. 30-25. Aspergillosis. A. Tomogram showing cavitary lesion, right upper lung field, containing a fungous ball or aspergilloma (arrow), lying free in a cavitary lesion. The ball characteristically will alter its location in the cavity as the patient changes position. B. Resected specimen of a right upper lobe, showing smooth-lined chronic cavity (white arrow) from which fungous ball (black arrow) was lifted out. (A. From Aslam: Chest 57:94, 1970. B. From Takaro T: In Goldsmith EI (ed): Practice of Surgery, 1978. Courtesy of Harper and Row.)

Invasive *Aspergillus* pneumonias present with chronic fever, cough, and sputum, which may progress to involve the pleura. Multiple abscesses can be seen within the lung and in other tissues, especially the brain.

Diagnosis

The finding of *Aspergillus* cells in the sputum alone does not justify the diagnosis of aspergillosis. If the clinical picture of aspergilloma is present and sputum cultures are positive for *Aspergillus,* the diagnosis is probable.

Transtracheal aspirates or direct lung aspirates by thin-walled 18-gauge needles may provide a definitive diagnosis and are especially useful in immunosuppressed patients.[351]

Treatment

Medical treatment of aspergilloma has been generally unsatisfactory,[352] but experience is limited. Amphotericin-B is the most satisfactory treatment and may be curative even in immunodeficient patients.[298,351,353] Diiodohydroxyquinoline and rifampin have been reported to be helpful in combination with amphotericin-B.[354,355] Persistent, long-term, high-dose therapy may be required. The indications for a resection of an aspergilloma are not clear. Severe hemoptysis is an obvious indication, but routine surgical excision probably is not indicated.[345,346,350,356,357] The reported complication rates are high.[348,349,358,359]

In difficult situations, where resection is indicated but cannot be carried out safely, cavernostomy or the endobronchial or endocavitary instillation of sodium iodide or amphotericin-B has occasionally been helpful.[345,353,360,361]

Aspergillous empyema, or pleural aspergillosis, has been treated by intrapleural amphotericin-B or nystatin and by pleural drainage, pleurectomy, thoracoplasty, and repair of bronchopleural fistulas.[362–364]

CANDIDIASIS

Although *Candida* species commonly affect mucous and cutaneous surfaces, deep or systemic infections of the lungs and other tissues also occur. *C. albicans* and other fungi of this species, *Candida guilliermondi, Candida stellatoidea, Candida parakrusei,* and *Candida tropicalis,* can all cause disease.[339,269] Microbiologic and pathogenic features are discussed in Chapter 9.

Clinical Manifestations and Diagnosis

Invasive candidiasis is an opportunistic infection rarely seen [365] except in the presence of intensive or prolonged antibiotic therapy, especially with multiple drugs or immunosuppressive or cytotoxic therapy.[290] Debility, senescence, prematurity, starvation, prolonged shock, multiple operations, multiple or mixed infections, bone marrow depression by lymphomas or antitumor drugs, radiation therapy, disseminated malignancies, and antibiotic or steroid therapy render the patient susceptible. Under these conditions, normal bacterial flora of patients may be suppressed, allowing an overgrowth of the often-present saprophytic species of *Candida.*

Invasion can take place through the skin, the bloodstream (via needles or catheters used for intravenous therapy), the lungs, or the gastrointestinal tract. *Candida* pneumonia, abscess, septicemia, and generalized infection may result, frequently with a fatal outcome.[366] Even tracheal obstruction associated with a *Candida* fungous ball has been reported.[367] *Candida* species in the sputum are of no diagnostic or prognostic importance, so that the diagnosis depends on finding *Candida* in bronchial or lung biopsies, the bloodstream, or evidence of *Candida* ophthalmitis. Candiduria frequently accompanies candidiasis but is not diagnostic. Biopsy proof of tissue invasion in immunosuppressed or otherwise compromised patients who have symptoms and signs of pneumonia or septicemia requires that drug therapy be given promptly.[339] On the other hand, Rosenbaum et al [368] suggest that some forms of *Candida* pneumonia are self-limited and require no treatment.

Treatment

The combination of amphotericin-B and 5-fluorocytosine is the most promising regimen available.

Prevention

Stone [369] has hypothesized that most systemic candidiasis arises from persorption of *Candida* from the gastrointestinal tract.[363] Prophylactic nystatin therapy by mouth has been shown to suppress gastrointestinal *Candida* and reduce the infection rate in debilitated patients who are taking antibiotics.[370,371]

SPOROTRICHOSIS

Sporotrichum schenckii, discussed in detail in Chapter 9, usually causes a cutaneous and lymphatic disease but rarely produces pulmonary disease.[372]

Clinical Manifestations

Pulmonary sporotrichosis is reported so rarely that it is hazardous to make generalizations. When recognized, however, the symptoms resemble pulmonary tuberculosis, and the course is slow. Localized cavitary disease has been reported in about 50 cases,[373,374] but a variety of clinical patterns, including hilar lymphadenopathy, pleural effusion, lobular consolidation, fibrosis, and multiple nodules, has been reported. Many patients with pulmonary disease work with plants and plant products. Such occupations put persons in contact with the plant and soil fungus.

Diagnosis

Although the organism is a saprophyte,[375,376] it is not a commensal of man. The diagnosis is based on its culture and identification from the resected specimens, sputum, or bronchial brushings. The preculture diagnosis is usually tuberculosis, sarcoidosis, or opportunistic fungus. Biopsy diagnosis may be difficult because the organism is sparse in tissue. The pathogenicity for animals can be established by inoculation. The serum agglutinins for *Sporotrichum* should be 1:50 or greater.

Treatment

Combined lung resection of localized cavitary disease, together with potassium iodide, amphotericin-B, or both, is probably the best treatment, although there are few patient data available.[375] A saturated solution of potassium iodide is given in a dosage of 9–12 gm per day. Amphotericin-B (Table 9-2) should be used as well for pulmonary disease.

MUCORMYCOSIS (PHYCOMYCOSIS)

Mucormycosis (phycomycosis, zygomycosis) is a rare fungal infection caused by genera belonging to the class zygomycetes, discussed in Chapter 9). Disease-causing organisms in this group include species of *Absidia, Rhizopus, Mucor, Mortierella,* and *Basidiobolus.*[269,377] Many of these organisms are saprophytes in nature, occurring as molds on manure and foods and producing spores that can be inhaled. Characteristically, direct blood vessel invasion, thrombosis, and infarction of invaded organs occur, with tissue destruction and cavitation in patients with compromised host defenses.

Clinical Manifestations

As noted in Chapter 9, mucormycosis is usually a rapidly fatal disease, occurring especially in acidotic diabetics, in patients with lymphomas or leukemias, or in persons receiving intensive or prolonged antimetabolite, antibiotic, or steroid therapy. Extensive necrosis of areas around the face (paranasal sinuses, orbit, mucous membranes) and the brain may be seen, in addition to cutaneous and subcutaneous infection. Pulmonary mucormycosis usually develops rapidly as a nonspecific bronchitis and pneumonia. Signs and symptoms of thrombosis and infarction manifested by severe chest pain, pleural friction rub, and bloody sputum appear. Massive fatal pulmonary hemorrhage has been reported.[378] Two fatal cases of necrotizing chest wall infections followed aortocoronary bypass surgery in which Elastoplast dressings were used.[379] Kidney transplant patients usually develop a necrotizing pneumonia with abscess formation.

Diagnosis

Biopsy is essential, since the diagnosis depends on the identification of wide (6–50 μm), nonseptate, branching hyphae in and around thrombosed vessels, especially well seen with hematoxylin and eosin. Culture permits identification of the particular species but does not alter therapy.

Treatment

Most patients die.[380,381] Drug therapy with amphotericin-B plus excision and drainage are necessary in debilitated, desperately ill patients.[305,382,383] Transthoracic drainage of a necrotic lobe was life saving in one patient (R.L. Simmons, personal communication). Control of diabetes is obviously essential, but control of the other predisposing conditions may be impossible.

PARACOCCIDIOIDOMYCOSIS (SOUTH AMERICAN BLASTOMYCOSIS)

This is a chronic granulomatous infection that involves the skin, mucous membranes, lymph nodes, and visceral organs (including the lungs), caused by *Paracoccidioides brasiliensis* (Chapter 9).[269,384,385]

Cavitary pulmonary disease occurs in about a third of the cases, and bilateral disseminated and polymorphic lung lesions seem to be the rule.[384-386] Surgery is indicated only for diagnostic biopsy. The disease is fatal unless treated. Amphotericin-B can be curative.

MONOSPOROSIS

Monosporium apiospermum (Allescheria boydii) is an inhabitant of soil which appears to act as a secondary invader of previously damaged lung tissue, such as a tuberculous cavity, a cyst, or a bronchial saccule. A fungous ball is sometimes formed. Amphotericin-B has not been effective. Localized resections have been performed in 10 cases, with 2 deaths.[387] Conservative management is recommended for asymptomatic patients without cavitary disease or bronchiectasis. Resection is advocated for good risk patients with localized cavitary disease or to help make a definitive diagnosis when bronchogenic carcinoma is suspected.

PROTOZOAN INFECTIONS

THORACIC AMEBIASIS

Thoracic complications of amebiasis are rare. They occur secondary to amebic hepatic abscess, usually on the right. The liver abscess (Chapter 36) may erode or rupture through the diaphragm without the formation of a subphrenic abscess. The second abscess, in the superadjacent, right lower, or middle lobe of the lung, or an empyema may lead to a hepaticobronchial fistula.[388]

In 90 percent of the cases, pathologic changes are confined to the right lower hemithorax.[65] Chest pain, fever, cough, and the expectoration of material variously described as resembling chocolate or anchovy sauce or catsup are characteristic. The liver is tender and enlarged. A history of dysentery or diarrhea may be suggestive (Chapters 11, 36, and 39).

Roentgenographic manifestations include moderate fixation, elevation, or localized bulge of the right diaphragm, pleural effusion, pneumonic consolidation, or abscess formation, usually in the right lower lung field.

Entamoeba histolytica organisms are reported in pus, sputum, or aspirated material only in about one quarter of the cases. In many patients, a presumptive diagnosis must be made, which is supported by the finding of *E. histolytica* in stools and by a positive serologic test for the organism.

Therapy should be directed toward cure of the liver abscess.[389,390] Aspiration and drug therapy are described in Chapter 36. Thoracic procedures are rarely indicated.

PNEUMOCYSTIS CARINII PNEUMONIA

This is an opportunistic infection in the form of a diffuse interstitial pneumonitis, which occurs largely in congenitally immunodeficient or pharmacologically immunosuppressed patients (Chapter 47). It first came to be recognized in epidemic form during World War II in people of central Europe whose nutritional status was presumably at a low level.[391]

Etiology

The protozoan *P. carinii* is so named for its discoverer, Carini. This organism occurs in thick-walled or thin-walled cystic forms, 5–12 μm in diameter. It has a double-walled outer membrane, and within are three to eight intracystic bodies. The organism stains with silver methenamine stains (Gomori).

Clinical Manifestations

Infection is quite rare. The disease almost invariably occurs in patients with impaired cellular immunity.[391,392]

The peculiar combination in patients at risk, often infants or children, of dyspnea, tachypnea, dry nonproductive cough, fever, flaring of the nasal alae, intercostal retraction, and sometimes cyanosis with minimal auscultatory signs and the roentgenographic findings of unilateral or bilateral diffuse (ground-glass) infiltrates should lead to a suspicion of *P. carinii* pneumonia. An air bronchogram silhouetted against a ground-glass infiltrate is a typical radiographic appearance. Marked hypoxemia and hypocapnia characterize this clinical picture. Less often, localized areas of pneumonitis or consolidation are seen.

Diagnosis

The diagnosis depends on the demonstration of the organisms in sputum (usually unreliable), bronchial brushings, or lung tissue. Because of the need for diagnostic open lung biopsy or thoracoscopic biopsy, the thoracic surgeon is often called.[167,168,393-395] The morbidity and mortality of open biopsy in desperately ill hypoxemic patients should not be underestimated. Other methods of biopsy, namely, percutaneous needle aspiration or transbronchoscopic lung biopsy, can also be followed by pneumothorax and hemorrhage and are less reliable.[396,397] Touch preparations of biopsy material stained with silver methenamine are used to identify the organisms. Since multiple coexistent infections may be present, bacterial and fungal cultures and histopathologic examinations should also be performed. Serologic techniques now being developed may eliminate the need for invasive diagnostic techniques.

Treatment

The need for precise diagnosis derives from the toxicity of the only treatment formerly available, pentamidine isethionate. Currently, trimethoprim-sulfamethoxazole appears to be an excellent alternative: if all attempts at diagnosis have failed, empirical therapy can be carried out. Because of severe hypoxemia, supplemental oxygen therapy is often necessary. The use of membrane oxygenator therapy has been reported.[393] With progression, lung compliance is seriously reduced, and the use of respirator support becomes essential.

Prognosis

Untreated, *P. carinii* pneumonia is often fatal. In patients treated early and adequately, approximately 65 to 75 percent may survive.

Prevention

Trimethoprim-sulfamethoxazole has been shown to be an effective prophylactic agent in high-risk patients, ie, children with acute leukemia. It may also be effective in transplant patients.

PULMONARY ECHINOCOCCOSIS: HYDATID DISEASE OF THE LUNG

Etiology

Pulmonary echinococcus disease is caused by the larval form of the small tapeworm *Echinococcus granulosus*, or rarely, *Echinococcus multilocularis* (Chapters 11 and 36).

Pathology

The cyst itself consists of a germinal layer and cyst fluid containing brood capsules and scoleces. A succession of acellular, white, hyaline layers are laid down outside the cyst, which is thus enclosed by a laminated cyst membrane. As the cyst enlarges, it usually reaches the pleural surface. Compression of the surrounding lung produces a thin fibrous layer of atelectatic lung around the hydatid, variously called capsule, adventitia, or pericyst.

The cyst may remain dormant for many years. However, it poses a hazard to the patient because rupture may occur at any time, which can result in the formation of daughter cysts or, uncommonly, in death due to asphyxiation or to a hypersensitivity reaction to the contents of the cyst. In any event, a ruptured cyst may become infected, forming a chronic lung abscess or a localized bronchiectactic area.

Clinical Manifestations and Diagnosis

Symptoms are minimal unless there is significant compression of an airway or a mediastinal structure (eg, esophagus, great veins) or unless the cyst ruptures. At such a time, there may be dramatic expectoration of cyst fluid, followed by an allergic rash and sometimes fever. If secondary infection occurs, the symptoms of lung abscess or bronchiectasis predominate.

The diagnosis is suspected most commonly by the characteristic roentgenographic appearance of round or oval radiopaque shadows of a very homogeneous waterlike density, with clear-cut borders and little or no evidence of reaction around them (Fig. 30-26), usually located in the mid or lower lung fields. When air enters the perivesicular space, a characteristic thin crescentic shadow is seen, which is quite unlike the semilunar shadow seen with aspergillomas. The most unusual and unique roentgenographic sign, the water lily sign, consists of a lenticular shadow rising from a fluid level in a cyst. This is seen after rupture of the cyst and partial evacuation of its contents, with the torn vesicular or germinal layer floating on the surface of the retained fluid.[398] The Casoni skin test for echinococcus disease is not completely reliable.

Treatment

The diagnosis of such a lesion in an area where pastoral as opposed to sylvatic echinococcosis is found, that is, where sheep and cattle are raised, is an indication for excision. Operations that conserve pulmonary parenchyma are advocated wherever possible. There are surprisingly vehement differences of opinion about the appropri-

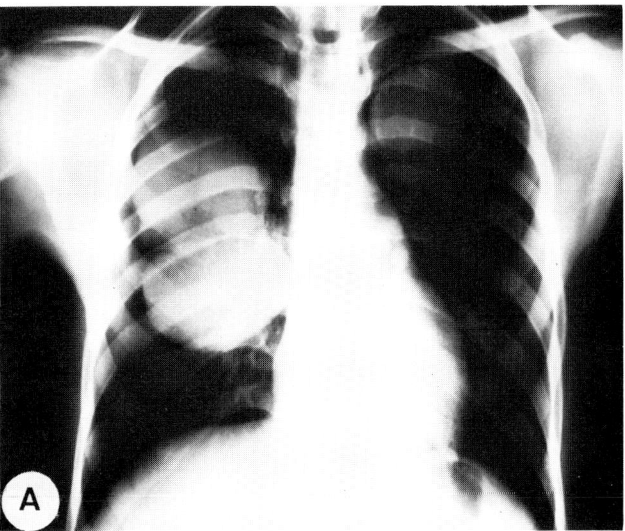

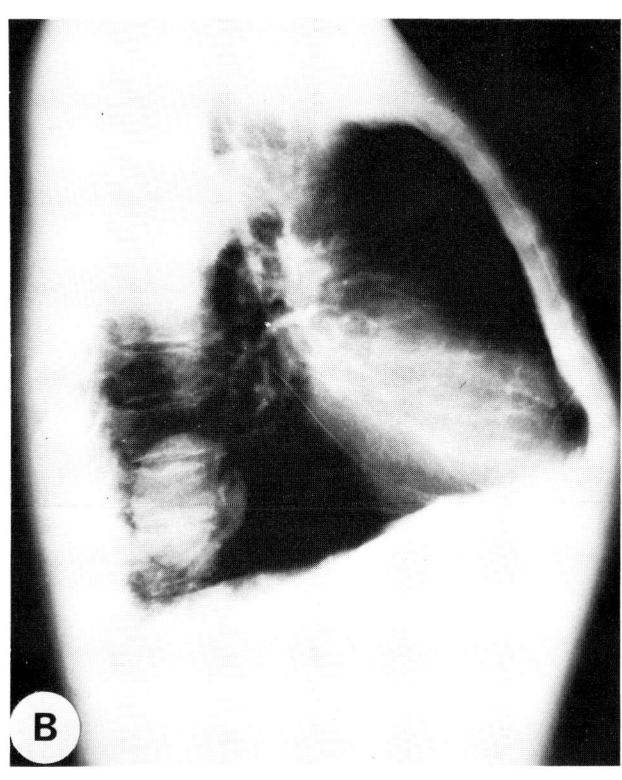

Fig. 30-26. **Thoracic roentgenograms showing echinococcus cysts. A. Multiple and bilateral cysts. In both roentgenograms, the characteristic appearance of large, rounded shadows of homogeneous density with clear-cut borders is well shown. B. Solitary cyst lying posteriorly behind the heart. (A. From Harris, et al: J Thorac Cardiovasc Surg 62:465, 1971. B. From Lichter I: Thorax 27:529, 1972.)**

ate procedure for cystectomy.[398] Peschiera,[398] who reports a large series of cases from Peru, is certain that the best method is partial aspiration of the cyst at open thoracotomy first, with instillation of formalin into the cyst. After that, the cyst is opened and removed together with the adventitial pericyst formed by the patient's own lung. On the other hand, others favor simple enucleation of the intact cyst, especially if it is not under tension (Fig. 30-27).[200,399,400] First, the nonadherent cleavage plane between cyst and pericyst is widely opened. Then, the anesthetist is requested to inflate the lung. This allows the fragile intact cyst to roll out or to be extruded into a waiting spoon, hand, or basin without the need to grasp or touch the cyst. Sometimes 10 ml of 10 percent sodium chloride solution is instilled into the cyst as a preliminary maneuver.[400] The remaining space in the lung parenchyma in both methods is obliterated after careful control of small and large bronchial fistulas with or without removal of the fibrous pericyst. If lung tissue has been destroyed by prolonged compression or infection, segmental resection or lobectomy may be necessary after removal of the cyst. Nonoperative treatment is recommended for the asymptomatic patient with the less common sylvatic or forest type of echinococcosis, which is observed in Alaska and Northern Canada where moose and caribou are hunted, as opposed to the more common and more serious pastoral disease in which operation is clearly indicated.[401]

Whatever operation is performed, it must be done carefully so that contents of the cyst are not spilled, which will lead to anaphylaxis and formation of daughter cysts. Recently, the instillation of a 10 percent povidone-iodine solution has been recommended to sterilize the cyst prior to attempts at excision.[401a]

INFECTIONS OF THE MEDIASTINUM

Infections of the mediastinum are uncommon but serious. They are often iatrogenic and pose many management problems.

The mediastinum extends from the thoracic inlet to the diaphragm and partitions the two pleural cavities. It is bounded anteriorly by the sternum and posteriorly by the thoracic vertebrae. Because of the many structures within this portion of the thoracic cavity, it is usually subdivided for easier description. The superior mediastinum lies above a plane that extends between the lower manubrium and the fourth thoracic vertebra. It contains the thymus gland, trachea, esophagus, and the aortic arch, and it is in direct continuity with the neck and its fascial planes. The inferior mediastinum is separated into anterior, middle, and posterior compartments. The anterior mediastinum contains only lymph nodes and connective tissue. The middle mediastinum contains, in addition to these, the trachea, mainstem bronchi, the heart and pericardium, and the ascending aorta. The posterior mediastinum contains the esophagus, vagus nerves, descending thoracic aorta, azygos veins, and the thoracic duct.

Infections of the mediastinum may result either from disease or from injury primarily affecting mediastinal structures or by extension of infection from adjacent regions, such as the neck, the pleural cavities, the lungs, or the abdominal cavity. Metastatic infections of the mediastinum by way of the bloodstream are rare.

Three fascial spaces in the neck—the pretracheal, the retrovisceral, and the perivascular—communicate with the mediastinum and thus provide ready avenues for the spread of infections into this vital area (Chapter 27). The pretracheal space is formed from the pretracheal fascia

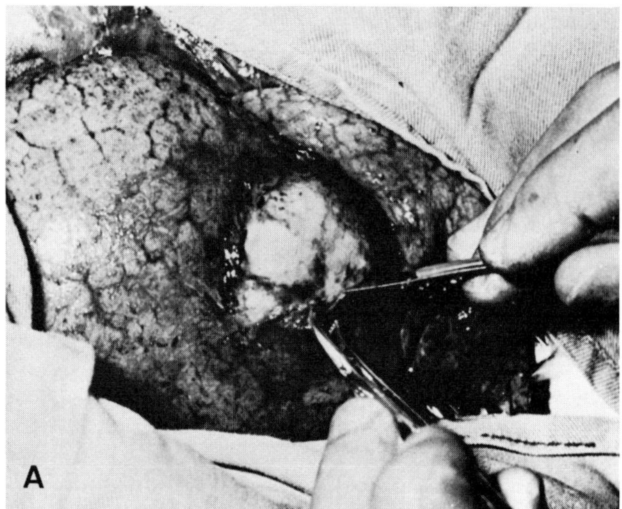

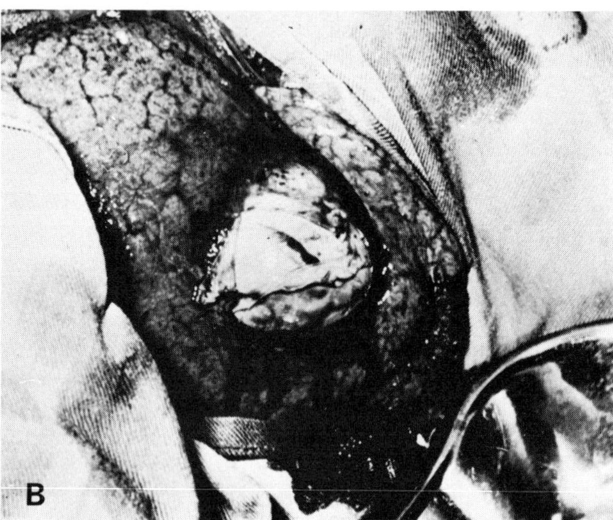

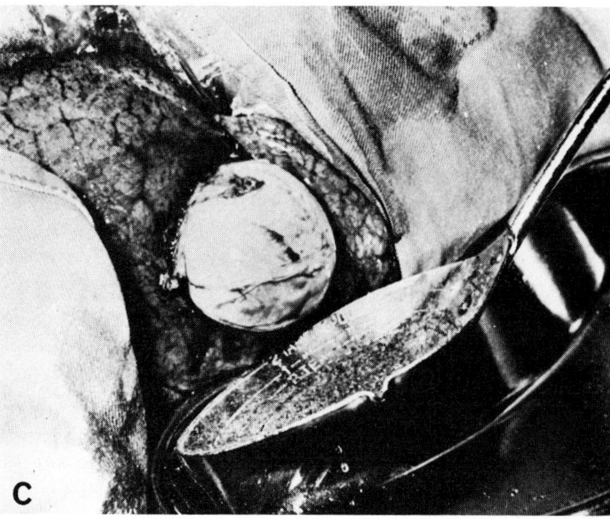

Fig. 30-27. Excision of Echinococcus cyst. A. Adventitia of subpleural cyst is carefully incised. B. Opening is widened promptly so cyst does not extrude through too small an opening and rupture. C. Anesthetist inflates lung, extruding cyst gradually into spoon or basin. Cyst must not be grasped or touched for fear of rupturing it. (From Lichter I: Thorax 27:529, 1972.)

and its fusion with the buccopharyngeal fascia and the carotid sheaths. It extends from the thyroid cartilage to the anterior mediastinum, where the pretracheal fascia blends into the pericardium. The retrovisceral space lies between the esophagus and the prevertebral fascia. It extends from the base of the skull to the posterior mediastinum. The perivascular space, containing carotid arteries, jugular vein, and vagus nerve, extends into the mediastinum along with these structures (Fig. 30-28).

Negative intrathoracic pressures may cause infection in these classic cervical fascial spaces to spread to the mediastinum, but the infectious process may not be contained or confined to these spaces.[402] Likewise, positive pressures relative to intrathoracic pressures may cause the fluid contents of a ruptured trachea, bronchus, or esophagus to be introduced into the mediastinum.

Retroperitoneal infections may extend into the mediastinum through the various openings in the diaphragm. However, this is rarely a cause of mediastinitis since the advent of antibiotic therapy.

ACUTE INFECTIONS OF THE SUPERIOR MEDIASTINUM

Pathogenesis

Acute mediastinitis involving the superior mediastinum is rarely a primary infection. It occurs most commonly by extension from the cervical region, including the oropharyngeal area, via the fascial planes or the lymphatics. Currently, esophageal perforation due to instrumentation is the most common cause,[403] but extensions of retropharyngeal abscess can also occur.[404] Surprisingly, mediastinitis due to tracheostomy, a common operative procedure invariably contaminated with microbes, is quite rare.

Retropharyngeal abscesses may extend into the retrovisceral space and from there into the mediastinum. A number of reports describe acute mediastinitis arising from retropharyngeal infections which are secondary to dental caries.[404-406] These may be severe or even fatal. When spread of infection from the root space of a tooth does occur, it is usually controllable with antibiotics. Rarely, it may extend from the mandible either into the pterygomandibular or infratemporal spaces or to the area above or below the mylohyoid muscle (Ludwig's angina). Once the retropharyngeal tissues become infected, an abscess may form, which can then spread along the retrovisceral, pretracheal, or perivascular spaces into the mediastinum (Fig. 30-28).[407] (See Chapter 27.)

Mediastinal infections due to esophageal perforation are always serious, and the mortality is high unless the perforation is recognized early and promptly treated. It is usually due to perforation of the cervical esophagus with a rigid esophagoscope, often because of pressure of the posterior esophageal wall against a cervical vertebral spur.[408]

Etiology

Infections caused by dental abscesses are usually mixed infections, because of the synergistic effects of anaerobic streptococci and *Bacteroides,* which together can cause a necrotizing inflammation.[405] Routine culture results may be reported as negative unless anaerobic organisms are

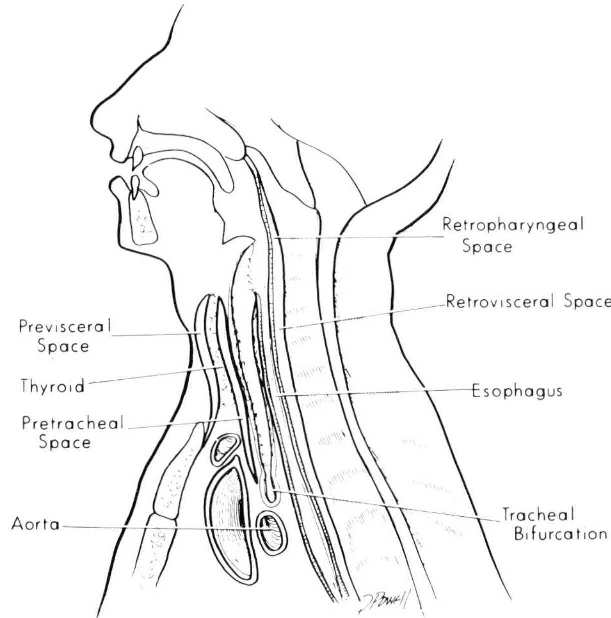

Fig. 30-28. **Three fascial planes along which infections may extend from the neck into the mediastinum are illustrated in this diagram. These are the previsceral space, the pretracheal space, and the retropharyngeal or retrovisceral space. Infections due to retropharyngeal abscesses or to perforations of the cervical esophagus usually extend along the retrovisceral space. (Adapted from Pearse HE Jr: Ann Surg 108:508, 1938.)**

suspected and anaerobic culture techniques are used.[409] However, gram-negative, pleomorphic rods on a smear may suggest *Bacteroides,* and since gas-forming organisms may be present, air in the retropharyngeal space may be seen on roentgenograms.[410]

Infections due to esophageal perforations contain oral flora, ie, mixed organisms, principally gram-positive aerobes and anaerobes at first. Later the flora resembles that recovered from retropharyngeal infections, as anaerobes proliferate.

Clinical Manifestations

Pain is the most prominent symptom of cervical esophageal rupture.[411] It occurs suddenly and is usually localized near the site of perforation. Occasionally, it is referred to the chest. Pain occurring with swallowing and cervical flexion are also common manifestations. There may be fever and localized cervical tenderness. Crepitation is usually present, and there may be radiographic evidence of cervical emphysema.[411] A lateral view of the cervical spine will show anterior displacement of the trachea and an air fluid level if a retrovisceral abscess has formed.[408] Contrast studies using a thin opaque material will usually demonstrate an esophageal leak.

Treatment

Retropharyngeal and Dental Origin. The treatment of mediastinitis caused by cervical and dental infections consists of surgical drainage and antibiotics. *S. aureus, Streptococcus,* and *Bacteroides,* the most common infecting organisms, are usually sensitive to clindamycin and chloramphenicol.

Cervical abscesses should be drained widely. A lateral incision along the posterior border of the sternocleidomastoid muscle can be extended to inspect and drain the pretracheal, perivascular, or retrovisceral spaces. Adequate drainage of the superior mediastinum can be obtained by this approach (Fig. 30-29). If the infection has spread to the inferior mediastinum, transthoracic drainage is necessary.

Esophageal Perforation due to Instrumentation. The treatment of cervical esophageal perforation is surgical drainage of the retrovisceral space, as described above. This procedure is prophylactic and will prevent abscess formation and the spread of infection to the mediastinum if the esophageal perforation is recognized early. If treatment is delayed, both cervical suppuration and superior mediastinitis may be adequately drained through the cervical approach. The wound should be cultured for both aerobic and anaerobic organisms, and appropriate antibiotics should be instituted. Penicillin G is usually found to be an excellent first choice antibiotic unless a preexisting infection with a penicillin-resistant organism was present, since most oral flora are sensitive. (See Chapter 28.)

ANTERIOR MEDIASTINITIS DUE TO STERNAL WOUND INFECTIONS

One of the most frequent causes of mediastinitis is infection following median sternotomy. The etiology and management of this condition have already been described in the section on chest wall infections.

Rarely, mediastinitis may develop in the postoperative period in the absence of sternal dehiscence or sternal wound infection. If the patient has only fever and leukocytosis, the diagnosis may be difficult to establish. If the chest roentgenogram shows a pleural effusion, increasing substernal opacification, or mediastinal widening, and the patient does not respond to antibiotic treatment, mediastinal exploration and drainage may be required, as described previously.

The presence of foreign material, such as Teflon pledgets, Dacron grafts, and epicardial pacemaker electrodes, poses a special problem. All foreign material should be removed when possible. Engleman et al[412] reported healing of mediastinitis following ventricular aneurysmectomy only after they removed the Teflon-felt used to buttress the ventricular suture line. Moseley et al,[413] however, reported success in sterilizing an infected Hancock prosthesis used to repair a truncus arteriosus. Only rarely does a chronic abscess develop from an acute infection unless a foreign body is present. The complications of mediastinitis may take a long time to become evident, as illustrated by one patient with postoperative sternal dehiscence, who developed a large mycotic aortic aneurysm at the site of aortic cannulation two years following aortocoronary arterial bypass surgery.[414]

INFECTIONS OF THE MIDDLE MEDIASTINUM

The pathogenesis and treatment of cardiac and pericardial infections are discussed in Chapters 31 and 32.

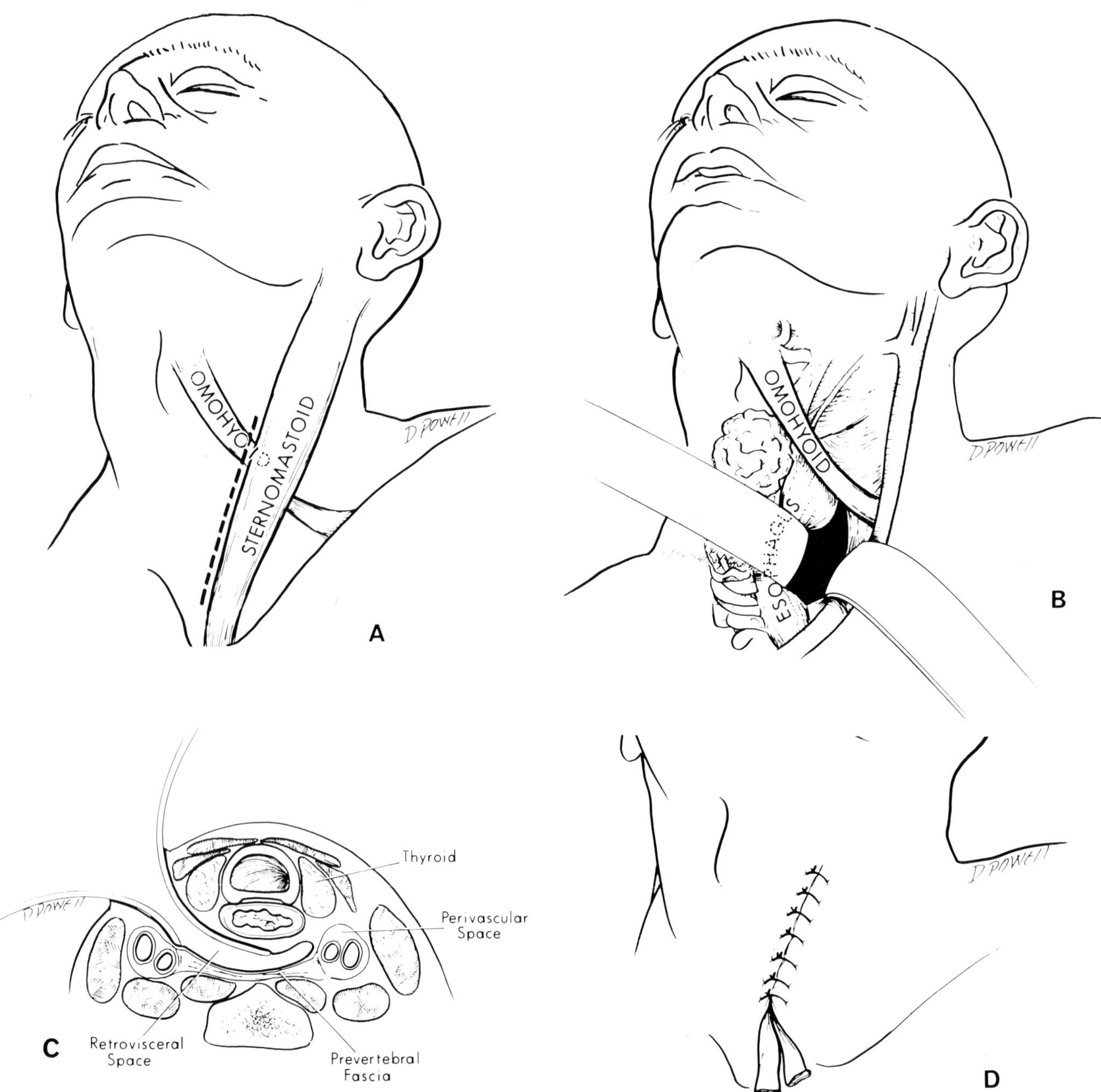

Fig. 30-29. **Cervical approach for draining the fascial planes of the neck and the upper mediastinum to the level of the fourth thoracic vertebra. A. Line of skin incision along anterior border of the sternomastoid muscle. B. Exposure of the retrovisceral space. C. Cross-sectional view of the approach to the retrovisceral space and the adjacent perivascular spaces. D. Rubber drains inserted into the dependent portion of the retrovisceral space. (Adapted from Payne WS, Larson RH: Surg Clin North Am 49:999, 1969.)**

Mediastinal Granulomas and Chronic Fibrosing Mediastinitis

These are probably different stages of the same disease.[415] They are most frequently located in the right paratracheal region and are due to *Histoplasma*, tuberculosis, or, more rarely, to sarcoidosis, nocardiosis, actinomycosis, or syphilis.[415-417] In the granulomatous phase, the large yellow and white masses of lymph nodes are often cystic and filled with caseous material. Microscopically, various stages of caseating granuloma are seen, and with Gomori methenamine silver nitrate stain, the yeastlike structures of *Histoplasma* are sometimes found. Cultures for *Histoplasma* and *Mycobacterium* are almost always negative.

Most patients are asymptomatic, but occasionally they may have symptoms caused by encroachment on important structures traversing the mediastinum, such as the superior vena cava, the esophagus, the trachea, or a bronchus.[418] Such encroachment may produce severe symptoms, depending on the structure which is compromised. They may include cough, hemoptysis, or the expectoration of broncholiths. Productive cough and wheezing may result if bronchiectasis develops. When the middle lobe alone is involved, the so-called middle lobe syndrome may be recognized on thoracic roentgenograms or on bronchography. The formation of an esophageal traction diverticulum may follow the development of an abscess in a mediastinal node, with erosion into the esophageal wall.[419] Fistula formation between the trachea and esophagus, with harrassing cough on taking fluids, may be another complication.[420]

Treatment

Fibrosis of the mediastinum can produce superior vena caval obstruction and, thus, the superior vena caval syndrome, signifies airway obstruction, or pulmonary hypertension primarily caused by pulmonary venous obstruction.[421-423] When the pericardium is involved, a granulomatous pericarditis can result. Constrictive pericarditis, however, is rare.[424]

Because of the seriousness of some of the complications of healed mediastinal granulomas and chronic mediastinitis—such as the middle lobe syndrome, the superior vena caval syndrome, broncholithiasis, esophagotracheal fistula, and pericarditis—appropriate corrective or extirpative surgical therapy may be required, depending on the severity of the symptom and the feasibility of relieving it surgically.[420,425-427] Some lesions may be difficult to manage by operation. Therefore, early resection of asymptomatic mediastinal granulomas to forestall such more intractable problems has been recommended and is probably appropriate.[418,428]

POSTERIOR MEDIASTINITIS

Posterior mediastinitis is largely caused by esophageal perforation. Other causes, such as paravertebral abscess, are much less common.

Esophageal Perforation (See also Chapter 38.)

Pathogenesis

After the cricopharyngeal area, the second most common site of instrumental perforation of the esophagus is the lower third of the esophagus where it narrows just above the diaphragm. Less commonly, the midesophagus, weakened by tumor or fresh caustic burn, can be perforated. Introduction of the flexible fiberoptic esophagoscope has greatly reduced the incidence of instrumental perforations.

Other causes of esophageal perforation include ingestion of foreign bodies, penetrating injuries, blunt trauma, caustic burns, and anastomotic leak after esophageal resection. Belsey and Hiebert[429] reported a 12 percent incidence in his series, and Payne and Larson[403] stated that 50 percent of the deaths that occur after esophageal surgery are the result of an anastomotic leak. Improved operative techniques (for example, the right-sided approach to esophageal resection and possibly automatic stapling devices) may help to reduce the incidence of this dreaded complication.

Perforation of the esophagus from either blunt or penetrating injury seldom occurs but is usually in association with multiple injuries that can obscure the diagnosis. The ingestion of foreign bodies is likewise an infrequent cause of esophageal perforation, but when it does occur, the foreign body must be removed by endoscopy or at operation.

Postemetic esophageal tear, Boerhaave's syndrome, still has a 20 percent mortality as a result of the severe necrotizing mediastinitis.[430]

Clinical Manifestations

Symptoms of esophageal perforation include substernal or epigastric pain, fever, dysphagia, and shortness of breath. Sometimes, the pleura is involved and there may be signs of pleural effusion or pneumothorax. Roentgenographic signs include widening of the mediastinum or emphysema, pleural effusion, and pneumothorax. A mediastinal air fluid level may be present.

Boerhaave's syndrome resembles an acute abdominal crisis (eg, perforated peptic ulcer), a spontaneous pneumothorax, or a myocardial infarction but not a ruptured esophagus. Subcutaneous and mediastinal emphysema are early signs of a ruptured esophagus, and the diagnosis can be confirmed by roentgenogram by having the patient swallow a thin aqueous contrast medium to demonstrate extravasation.

The diagnosis of an anastomotic leak is not always clear. There may be an insidious onset of symptoms, with low-grade fever and leukocytosis. If chest tubes are still in place, the instillation of methylene blue into the esophagus and its identification in drainage fluid confirms the presence of a leak between the esophagus and the pleural space. A swallow of thin radiopaque contrast medium also may demonstrate either an anastomic fistula or a paraesophageal abscess. Rarely will the disruption of an anastomosis be manifest as an acute catastrophic event with chest pain and hypotension. If this occurs, pleural drainage must be maintained, oral intake stopped, antibiotic coverage given, and appropriate fluid and volume replacement provided.

Pain is the most prominent symptom of an esophageal perforation caused by a foreign body. Fever and leukocytosis will also occur in time. If the foreign body is radiopaque, a roentgenogram may be diagnostic, or a rent in the esophagus may be found at the time esophagoscopy is performed for removal of the foreign body.

Treatment

There are two contrasting schools of thought regarding the management of acute perforations of the lower third of the esophagus, whether the result of instrumental perforation or postemetic rupture. One school advocates immediate operative intervention with direct suture repair of the esophagus. Although this approach was associated with a 23 percent mortality rate in 30 patients in Sawyers' series, there was only 1 death in the patients who had early suture closure and drainage.[431] On the other hand, of 17 patients treated conservatively in this study (including drainage procedures and nonreparative treatment), there were 10 deaths (59 percent). Against these data should be contrasted those of Lyons et al,[430] in which of 11 patients treated conservatively with drainage procedures, antibiotics, and decompressive procedures there was 1 death (9 percent), while of 18 patients treated by direct reparative surgery, 7 died (39 percent). The problem in reconciling these differing results probably stems from differences in the types of patients being reported and in the length of time between the perforation and its recognition.

Apparently, if the injury is recognized promptly (within 20 hours), oral intake is immediately stopped, and nasogastric and intrapleural drainage are initiated, together with the administration of antibiotics and steroids, many of these patients will do well even without direct reparative surgery. In any event, after 20 to 24 hours, direct suture repair often fails. Unfortunately, late recognition of perforation is associated with a higher mortality rate for *both* conservative and direct reparative modes of treatment. Prompt recognition and initiation of treatment are the key to success.

If a patient should survive beyond one month without surgery, an excisable fibrous tract may form, and then the fistula can be closed. The problem of esophagopleural fistula is discussed briefly in the section dealing with empyemas.

Postoperative esophagopleural fistula formations can usually be managed with intrapleural drains and without direct operative repair. If, however, reflux from the stomach or jejunum cannot be controlled or the breakdown of the anastomosis is so large that salivary flow is profuse, diversion of the refluxing intestine or of the proximal esophagus will be necessary.

Paravertebral Abscess

Although uncommon, a paravertebral abscess may develop from pyogenic osteomyelitis of the spine. The diagnosis of this condition is characteristically delayed by the patient's obscure symptoms, which are usually limited to back pain, muscle spasm, and fever. Roentgenograms of the chest may reveal vertebral destruction and a paravertebral abscess. A gallium scan has been reported to be helpful in identifying pyogenic osteomyelitis.[432] *S. aureus* is most frequently isolated. However, when there has been a history of antecedent urinary tract infection, gram-negative organisms are usually present. Identification of the organism is not always possible, and nonoperative treatment is generally successful.

Tuberculosis was another well-known cause of vertebral osteomyelitis and paravertebral abscess in earlier years. These abscesses developed from the upper thoracic vertebrae and either remained localized or extended inferiorly. When they extended along the psoas muscle, a cold abscess appeared in the abdominal wall or upper thigh. In addition to back pain, symptoms were those related to the presence of tuberculosis—fever, cough, and malaise. A chest x-ray often revealed a sharp convex shadow between the vertebrae and the esophagus. Posterior mediastinal abscesses were and still may be drained by excising short segments of one or more posterior ribs and entering the abscess extrapleurally (Fig. 30-30).[433]

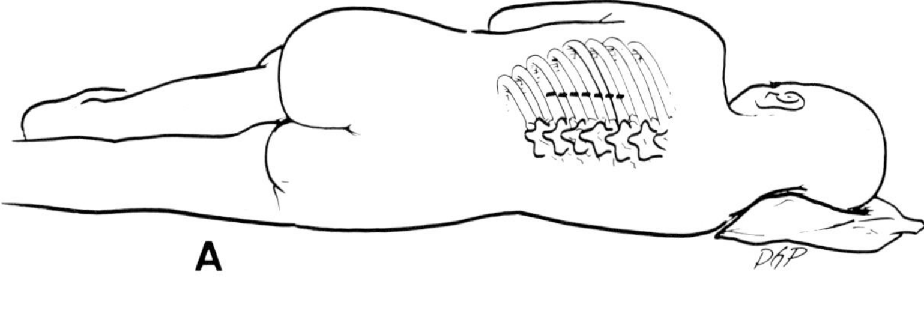

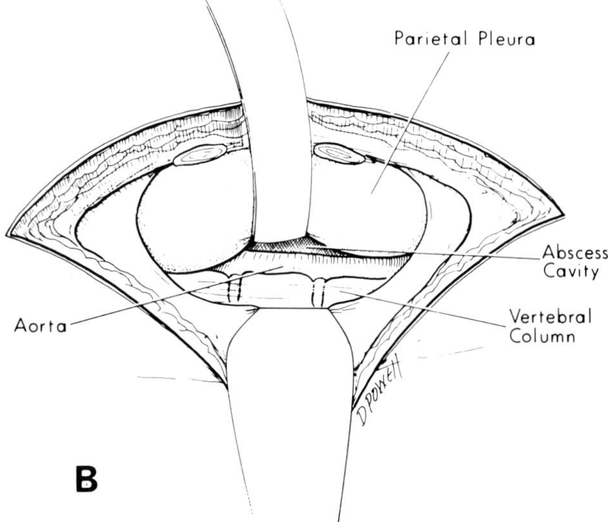

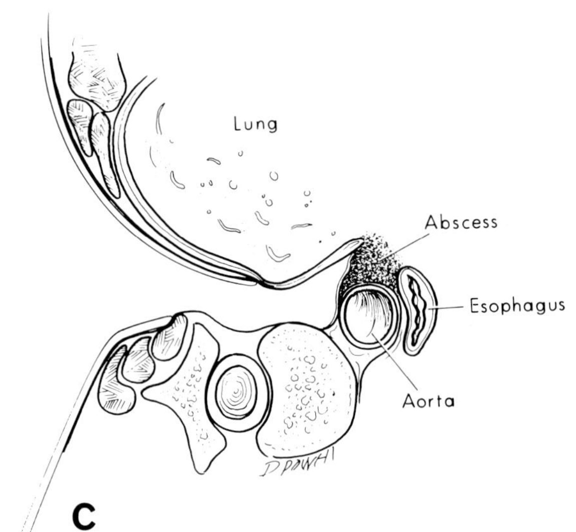

Fig. 30-30. **Drainage of posterior mediastinum. A. Skin incision lateral and parallel to vertebral bodies. B. Parietal pleura is retracted laterally to expose abscess cavity. C. Cross-section showing exposure of abscess cavity. (Adapted from Seybold WD, et al: Surg Clin North Am 30:1155, 1950).**

Echinococcus Mediastinal Cysts

Hydatid cysts due to *E. granulosus* occur anywhere in the human body, although the liver is the most common organ affected. Occasionally, the primary site of the disease will be the mediastinum, usually the posterior mediastinum where rib and vertebral body erosion sometimes occurs. They may cause compression of the spinal cord, superior vena cava, or branches of the aortic arch. When the anterior mediastinum is involved, hydatid cysts may cause tracheal compression or produce a Horner's syndrome.[428] Myocardial and pericardial disease are discussed in Chapters 31 and 32, respectively.

Anthrax

Anthrax is discussed in Chapter 7. Anthrax spores inhaled into the lungs may become phagocytosed and transported to mediastinal lymph nodes. Spores germinate there and cause a host reaction, which in turn results in an acute hemorrhagic mediastinitis. *Bacillus anthracis* is sensitive to both penicillin and streptomycin.

INFECTIONS OF THE ESOPHAGUS

Candida Esophagitis

Infections of the esophagus are extremely rare, and most are of no surgical significance. However, esophagitis due to *Candida* is not only the most common fungous infection of the esophagus, but it is the most frequent of all forms of esophagitis.[434] Esophageal candidiasis is seen in debilitated patients receiving cancer chemotherapy and antibiotics and in patients with diabetes mellitus and primary hypoparathyroidism.

C. albicans is the usual organism, although *C. krusei, C. tropicalis,* and *Torulopsis glabrata* are sometimes present. The disease may be acute or chronic. Symptoms include dysphagia and odynophagia, and esophagitis can occur without the presence of thrush in the mouth. The esophagus develops a green or white pseudomembrane. The mucosa under the membrane is red and necrotic. These areas may become scarred and strictured. An esophagogram often shows changes, especially in the lower two thirds of the esophagus. There may be spasm and lack of peristalsis, and the mucosa is irregular or sometimes ulcerated.

Orringer and Sloan recently reported three patients with esophageal stricture caused by monilial esophagitis and reviewed the literature.[435]

Candida esophagitis usually responds to nystatin taken as an oral suspension, 400,000 units every two hours while awake. The severely debilitated patient may require much greater concentrations of nystatin, and Kramer [434] recommends 2,400,000 units of dry nystatin suspended in 12 ml of distilled water and an equal volume of 1 percent methyl cellulose containing 0.5 percent chlorobutanol preservative. Miconazole, another potent antifungal drug, is also effective against *Candida*.[435] For systemic candidiasis, intravenous amphotericin B is most effective. Once a fibrous stricture develops, antifungal drugs are of little value. Chronic esophageal dilatation may be necessary and, occasionally, esophageal bypass surgery.

Herpes Esophagitis

Herpetic esophagitis is an occasional complication in the surgery of immunodepressed patients. It may or may not be associated with herpetic gingivostomatitis. In transplant patients, reactivation of the disease usually occurs in the first four posttransplant weeks and is characterized by dysphagia. Herpetic vesicles are seen on the pharynx and can be visualized by esophagoscopy. Superinfection with *Candida* can be prevented by nystatin. Most often the disease resolves spontaneously without stricture.

BIBLIOGRAPHY

Buechner HA: Management of Fungus Diseases of the Lung. Springfield, Ill, Thomas, 1971.

Cordell AR, Ellison RG: Complications of Intrathoracic Surgery. Boston, Little, Brown, 1979.

Sabiston DCJ: Textbook of Surgery. Philadelphia, Saunders, 1977.

Sabiston DC, Spencer FC (eds.): Surgery of the Chest. Philadelphia, Saunders, 1976.

Schwartz SI, Shires GT, Spencer FC, Storer EH (eds.): Principles of Surgery, 3rd ed. New York, McGraw-Hill, 1979.

REFERENCES

INFECTIONS OF THE CHEST WALL

1. Franz JL, Grover FL, Craven PR, Matthew EB, Trinkle JK: Pulmonary coccidioidomycosis presenting by direct extension through the chest wall. J Thorac Cardiovasc Surg 67:474, 1974.
2. Eastridge CE, Prather JR, Hughes FA Jr, Young JM, McCaughan JJ Jr: Actinomycosis: A 24-year experience. South Med J 65:839, 1972.
3. McQuarrie DG, Hall WH: Actinomycosis of the lung and chest wall. Surgery 64:905, 1968.
4. Marks MI, Eickhoff TC: Empyema necessitatis. Am Rev Respir Dis 101:759, 1970.
5. Bryant LR, Morgan C: Chest wall, pleura, lung and mediastinum. In Schwartz SI, Shires GT, Spencer FC, Storer, EH (eds): Principles of Surgery, 3rd ed. New York, McGraw-Hill, 1979, pp 635–738.
6. Pontius JG, Clagett OT, McDonald JR: Costal chondritis and perichondritis. Surgery 45:852, 1959.
7. Maier HC: Infections of the costal cartilages and sternum. Surg Gynecol Obstet 84:1038, 1947.
8. Williams CD, Cunningham JN, Falk EA, Isom OW, Chase RN Jr, Spencer FC: Chronic infection of the costal cartilages after thoracic surgical procedures. J Thorac Cardiovasc Surg 66:592, 1973.
9. Reckler JM, Flemma RJ, Pruitt BA Jr: Costal chondritis: An unusual complication in the burned patient. J Trauma 13:76, 1973.

STERNAL WOUND INFECTIONS

10. Wray TM, Bryant RE, Killen DA: Sternal osteomyelitis and costochondritis after median sternotomy. J Thorac Cardiovasc Surg 65:227, 1973.

11. Firor WB: Infection following open-heart surgery, with special reference to the role of prophylactic antibiotics. J Thorac Cardiovasc Surg 53:371, 1967.
12. Churchill ED: The technic of rib resection and osteomyelitis of the rib ends. JAMA 92:644, 1929.
13. Julian OC, Lopez-Belio M, Dye WS, Javid H, Grove WJ: The median sternal incision in intracardiac surgery with extracorporeal circulation: A general evaluation of its use in heart surgery. Surgery 42:753, 1957.
14. Stoney WS, Alford WC Jr, Burrus GR, Frist RA, Thomas CS Jr: Median sternotomy dehiscence. Ann Thorac Surg 26:421, 1978.
15. Culliford AT, Cunningham JN Jr, Zeff RH, Isom OW, Teiko P, Spencer FC: Sternal and costochondral infections following open-heart surgery. J Thorac Cardiovasc Surg 72:714, 1976.
16. Bryant LR, Spencer FC, Trinkle JK: Treatment of median sternotomy infection by mediastinal irrigation with an antibiotic solution. Ann Surg 169:914, 1969.
17. Sanfelippo PM, Danielson GK: Complications associated with median sternotomy. J Thorac Cardiovasc Surg 63:419, 1972.
18. Brown AH, Braimbridge MV, Panagopoulos P, Sabar EF: The complications of median sternotomy. J Thorac Cardiovasc Surg 58:189, 1969.
19. Nelson JC, Nelson RM: The incidence of hospital wound infection in thoracotomies. J Thorac Cardiovasc Surg 54:586, 1967.
20. Cerat GA, McHenry MC, Loop FD: Median sternotomy wound infection and anterior mediastinitis caused by *Bacteroides fragilis*. Chest 69:231, 1976.
21. Miller DR, Murphy K, Cesario T: Pseudomonas infection of the sternum and costal cartilages. J Thorac Cardiovasc Surg 76:723, 1978.
22. Robicsek F, Daugherty HK, Cook JW, Selle JG, Masters TN, O'Bar PR, Fernandez CR, Mauney CU, Calhoun DM: *Mycobacterium fortuitum* epidemics after open-heart surgery. J Thorac Cardiovasc Surg 75:91, 1978.
23. Cheanvechai C, Travisano F, Effler DB: Treatment of infected sternal wounds. Cleveland Clin Q 39:43, 1972.
24. Thurer RJ, Bognolo D, Vargas A, Isch JH, Kaiser GA: The management of mediastinal infection following cardiac surgery: An experience utilizing continuous irrigation with povidone-iodine. Cardiovasc Surg 68:962, 1974.
25. Jimenêz-Martínez M, Argüero-Sánchez R, Pérez-Alvarez JJ, Mina-Castañeda P: Anterior mediastinitis as a complication of median sternotomy incisions: Diagnostic and surgical considerations. Surgery 67:929, 1970.
26. Gruhl VR: Renal failure, deafness, and brain lesions following irrigation of the mediastinum with neomycin. Ann Thorac Surg 11:376, 1971.
27. Hau T, Ahrenholz DH, Simmons RL: Secondary bacterial peritonitis: The biologic basis of treatment. Curr Probl Surg 16:1, 1979.
28. Garnes AL, Davidson E, Taylor LE, Felix AJ, Thidhevsky BA, Prigot A: Clinical evaluation of povidone-iodine aerosol spray in surgical practice. Am J Surg 97:49, 1959.
29. Engelman RM, Williams CD, Gouge TH, Chase RM Jr, Folk EA, Boyd AD, Reed, GE: Mediastinitis following open-heart surgery. Arch Surg 107:772, 1973.
30. Lee AB Jr, Schimert G, Shatkin S: Total excision of the sternum and thoracic pedicle transposition of the greater omentum; useful strategems in managing severe mediastinal infection following open heart surgery. Surgery 80:433, 1976.
31. Burke JF: The effective period of preventive antibiotic action in experimental incisions and dermal lesions. Surgery 50:161, 1961.
32. Reed WA: Antibiotics and cardiac surgery. J Thorac Cardiovasc Surg 50:888, 1965.
33. Holswade GR, Dineen P, Redo SF, Goldsmith EI: Antibiotic therapy in open-heart operations. Arch Surg 89:970, 1964.
34. Robicsek F, Daugherty HK, Cook JW: The prevention and treatment of sternum separation following open-heart surgery. J Thorac Cardiovasc Surg 73:267, 1977.

PACEMAKER INFECTIONS

35. Siddons H, Nowak K: Surgical complications of implanting pacemakers. Br J Surg 62:929, 1975.
36. Kennelly BM, Piller LW: Management of infected transvenous permanent pacemakers. Br Heart J 36:1133, 1974.
37. Van Der Heide JNH, Bosma GJ, Kleine JW, Thalen HJT, Nieveen J, Bartstra M: Results with pacemaker implantations. In Thalen HJT (ed): Cardiac Pacing. Assen, The Netherlands, Van Gorcum, 1973, p 253.
38. Parsonnet V: Critical review: Power sources for implantable cardiac pacemakers. Chest 61:165, 1972.
39. Dargan EL, Norman JC: Conservative management of infected pacemaker pulse generator sites. Ann Thorac Surg 12:297, 1971.
40. Bonchek LI: New methods in the management of extruded and infected cardiac pacemakers. Ann Surg 176:686, 1972.
41. Furman RW, Hiller AJ, Playforth RH, Bryant LR, Trinkle JK: Infected permanent cardiac pacemaker: Management without removal. Ann Thorac Surg 14:54, 1972.
42. Golden GT, Lovett WL, Harrah JD, Wellons HA Jr, Nolan SP: The treatment of extruded and infected permanent cardiac pulse generators: Application of a technique of closed irrigation. Surgery 74:575, 1973.
43. Gordon AJ: Catheter pacing in complete heart block: Techniques and complications. JAMA 193:1091, 1965.
44. Sedaghat A: Permanent transvenous pacemaker infection with septicemia. NY State J Med 74:868, 1974.
45. Castberg T: Complications from the pacemaker pocket: Prophylaxis, treatment and results. Acta Med Scand [Suppl] 596:51, 1976.
46. Conklin EF, Giannelli S, Ayres SM, Mueller HS, Grace WJ: Prevention of pacemaker infections. NY State J Med 73:2675, 1973.
47. Sethi GK, Scott SM, Takaro T: Extrathoracic bypass for stenosis of innominate artery. J Thorac Cardiovasc Surg 69:212, 1975.
48. Sethi GK, Scott SM: Subclavian artery laceration due to migration of a Hagie pin. Surgery 80:644, 1976.
49. Wilson SE: Arterial infection. Curr Probl Surg 15:51, 1978.
50. Bircher J, Schirger A, Clagett OT, Harrison EG Jr: Mondor's disease: A vascular rarity. Proc Mayo Clinic 37:651, 1962.
51. Lewis FJ: Infections of the chest wall. In Shields TW (ed): General Thoracic Surgery. Philadelphia, Lea & Febiger, 1972, p 437.

EMPYEMA

52. Lindskog GE: Present-day management of pleural empyema in infants and adults. N Engl J Med 255:320, 1956.
53. LeRoux BT: Empyema thoracis. Br J Surg 52:89, 1965.
54. Snider GL, Saleh SS: Empyema of the thorax in adults: Review of 105 cases. Dis Chest 54:410, 1968.
55. Takaro T: The pleura and empyema. In Sabiston DC Jr (ed): Textbook of Surgery. Philadelphia, Saunders, 1977, p 2087.
56. Levitsky S, Annable CA, Thomas PA: The management of empyema after thoracic wounding. Observations on 25 Vietnam casualties. J Thorac Cardiovasc Surg 59:630, 1970.
57. Patterson LT, Schmitt HJ Jr, Armstrong RG: Intermediate care of war wounds of the chest. J Thorac Cardiovasc Surg 55:16, 1968.

58. Ogilvie AG: Final results in traumatic haemothorax: Report of 230 cases. Thorax 5:116, 1950.
59. Ravitch MM, Fein R: The changing picture of pneumonia and empyema in infants and children. A review of the experience at the Harriet Lane Home from 1934 through 1958. JAMA 175:1039, 1961.
60. Stiles QR, Lindesmith GG, Tucker BL, Meyer BW, Jones JC: Pleural empyema in children. Ann Thorac Surg 10:37, 1970.
61. Bartlett JG, Finegold SM: Anaerobic infections of the lung and pleural space. Am Rev Respir Dis 110:56, 1974.
62. American Thoracic Society: Management of nontuberculous empyema. Am Rev Respir Dis 85:935, 1962.
63. Recollections: Evarts A. Graham. Ann Thorac Surg 9:272, 1970.
64. Kerr WF: Late-onset postpneumonectomy empyema. Thorax 32:149, 1977.
65. Takaro T, Bond WM: Pleuropulmonary, pericardial, and cerebral complications of amebiasis: A twenty year survey. Surg Gynecol Obstet 107:209, 1958.
66. Langston HT: Empyema thoracis. Ann Thorac Surg 2:766, 1966.
67. Eloesser L: Recollections: Of an operation for tuberculous empyema. Ann Thorac Surg 8:355, 1969.
68. Stafford EG, Clagett OT: Postpneumonectomy empyema: Neomycin instillation and definitive closure. J Thorac Cardiovasc Surg 63:771, 1972.
69. Provan JL: The management of postpneumonectomy empyema. J Thorac Cardiovasc Surg 61:107, 1971.
70. Kärkölä P, Kairaluoma MI, Larmi TK: Postpneumonectomy empyema in pulmonary carcinoma patients: Treatment with antibiotic irrigation and closed-chest drainage. J Thorac Cardiovasc Surg 72:319, 1976.
71. Samson PC: Empyema thoracis: Essentials of present-day management. Ann Thorac Surg 11:210, 1971.
72. Bryant LR, Chicklo JM, Crutcher R, Danielson GK, Malette WG, Trinkle JK: Management of thoracic empyema. J Thorac Cardiovasc Surg 55:850, 1968.
73. Burford TH, Parker EF, Samson PC: Early pulmonary decortication in the treatment of posttraumatic empyema. Ann Surg 122:163, 1945.
74. Valle AR: Management of war wounds of the chest. J Thorac Surg 24:457, 1952.
75. Mayo P, McElvein RB: Early thoracotomy for pyogenic empyema. Ann Thorac Surg 2:649, 1966.
76. Maurer ER, Bellamah H, Mandez FL Jr: The forgotten problem of chronic empyema: Its successful surgical treatment. Arch Surg 81:275, 1960.
77. Andrews NC: The surgical treatment of chronic empyema. Dis Chest 47:533, 1965.
78. Barker WL, Faber LP, Ostermiller WE Jr, Langston HT: Management of persistent bronchopleural fistulas. J Thorac Cardiovasc Surg 62:393, 1971.
79. Virkkula L, Eerola S: Use of pectoralis skin pedicle flap for closure of large bronchial fistula connected with postpneumonectomy empyema. Scand J Thorac Cardiovasc Surg 9:144, 1975.
80. Hankins JR, Miller JE, McLaughlin JS: The use of chest wall muscle flaps to close bronchopleural fistulas; experience with 21 patients. Ann Thorac Surg 25:491, 1978.
81. Virkkula L: Treatment of bronchopleural fistula. Ann Thorac Surg 25:489, 1978.
82. Kirsh MM, Rotman H, Behrendt DM, Orringer MB, Sloan H: Complications of pulmonary resection. Ann Thorac Surg 20:215, 1975.
83. Takaro T, Scott SM, Bridgman AH, Sethi GK: Suppurative diseases of the lungs; pleurae and pericardium. Curr Probl Surg 14:1, 1977.

PULMONARY DEFENSE MECHANISMS

84. Newhouse M, Sanchis J, Bienenstock J: Lung defense mechanisms. New Engl J Med 295:990, 1976.
85. Newhouse M, Sanchis J, Bienenstock J: Lung defense mechanisms. New Engl J Med 295:1045, 1976.
86. Hatch TF, Gross P: Pulmonary Deposition and Retention of Inhaled Aerosols. New York, Academic, 1964, pp 31–43.
87. Owen PR: Turbulent flow and particle deposition in the trachea. In Wolstenholme GEW, Knight J (eds): Circulatory and Respiratory Mass Transport. Boston, Little, Brown, 1969, p 236.
88. Wehner AP: Negatively charged aerosols: effect on pulmonary clearance of inhaled $^{239}PuO_2$ in rats. Chest 60:468, 1971.
89. Proctor DF, Wagner HN: Mucociliary particle clearance in the human nose. In Davies CN (ed): Inhaled Particles and Vapours. II. London, Pergamon, 1967, p 25.
90. Proctor DF: Physiology of the upper airway. In Fenn WO, Rahn H (eds): Handbook of Physiology. *Respiration.* Baltimore, Williams & Wilkins, 1964, Vol 1, p 309.
91. Landahl HD: On the removal of air-borne droplets by the human respiratory tract. II. The nasal passages. Bull Math Biophysiol 12:161, 1950.
92. Morrow PE: Some physical and physiological factors controlling the fate of inhaled substances. I. Deposition. Health Phys 2:366, 1960.
93. Muir DCF, Davies CN: The deposition of 0.5μ diameter aerosols in the lungs of man. Ann Occup Hyg 10:161, 1967.
94. Newhouse MT, Sanchis J, Dolovich M, Rossman C, Wilson W: Mucociliary clearance in children with cystic fibrosis. In Mangos JA, Talamo RC (eds): Fundamental Problems of Cystic Fibrosis and Related Diseases. New York, Stratton, 1973, pp 319–344.
95. Talamo RC, Allen JD, Kahan MG, Austen KF: Hereditary $alpha_1$-antitrypsin deficiency. N Engl J Med 278:345, 1968.
96. Talamo RC: The α_1-antitrypsin in man. J Allergy Clin Immunol 48:240, 1971.
97. Ward PA, Talamo RC: Deficiency of the chemotactic factor inactivator in human sera with α_1-antitrypsin deficiency. J Clin Invest 52:516, 1973.
98. Tourville DR, Adler RH, Bienenstock J, Tomasi TB: The human secretory immunoglobulin system: immunohistological localization of γA secretory "piece," and lactoferrin in normal human tissues. J Exp Med 129:411, 1969.
99. Masson PL, Heremans JF, Schonne E, Crabbe PA: New data on lactoferrin, the iron-binding protein of secretions. Protides Biol Fluids Proc Collog Burgges 16:633, 1968.
100. Masson PL, Heremans JF, Schonne E: Lactoferrin, an iron-binding protein in neutrophilic leukocytes. J Exp Med 130:643, 1969.
101. Tomasi TB Jr, Bienenstock J: Secretory immunoglobulins. Adv Immunol 9:1, 1968.
102. Lucas AM, Douglas LC: Principles underlying ciliary activity in the respiratory tract: a comparison of nasal clearance in man, monkey and other mammals. Arch Otolaryngol 20:518, 1934.
103. Dalhamn T: Mucus flow and ciliary activity in the trachea of healthy rats and rats exposed to respiratory irritant gases (SO_2, H_3N, HCHO): A functional and morphologic (light microscopic and electron microscopic) study, with special reference to technique. Acta Physiol Scand [Suppl] 123:1, 1956.
104. Hilding AC: Experimental studies on some little understood aspects of the physiology of the respiratory tract and their clinical importance. Trans Am Acad Ophthalmol Otolaryngol 65:475, 1961.
105. Sanchis J, Dolovich M, Rossman C, Wilson W, Newhouse M: Pulmonary mucociliary clearance in cystic fibrosis. N Engl J Med 288:651, 1973.

106. Camner P, Helström PA, Philipson K: Carbon dust and mucociliary transport. Arch Environ Health 26:294, 1973.
107. Booker DV, Chamberlain AC, Rundo J, Muir DCF, Thomson ML: Elimination of 5μ particles from the human lung. Nature 215:30, 1967.
108. Marin MG, Morrow PE: Effect of changing inspired O_2 and CO_2 levels on tracheal mucociliary transport rate. J Appl Physiol 27:385, 1969.
109. Laurenzi GA, Yin S, Guarneri JJ: Adverse effect of oxygen on tracheal mucus flow. N Engl J Med 279:333, 1968.
110. Wanner A, Hirsch JA, Greeneltch DE, Swenson EW, Fore T: Tracheal mucous velocity in beagles after chronic exposure to cigarette smoke. Arch Environ Health 27:370, 1973.
111. Laurenzi GA, Guarneri JJ: Effects of bacteria and viruses on ciliated epithelium. A study of the mechanisms of pulmonary resistance to infection: the relationship of bacterial clearance to ciliary and alveolar macrophage function. Am Rev Respir Dis [Suppl 3] 93:134, 1966.
112. Hers JF: Disturbances of the ciliated epithelium due to influenza virus. Am Rev Respir Dis [Suppl 3] 93:162, 1966.
113. Jarstrand C, Camner P, Philipson K: *Mycoplasma pneumoniae* and tracheobronchial clearance. Am Rev Respir Dis 110:415, 1975.
114. Mackaness GB: The monocyte in cellular immunity. Semin Hematol 7:172, 1970.
115. Mackaness GB: The relationship of delayed hypersensitivity to acquired cellular resistance. Br Med Bull 23:52, 1967.
116. Blanden RV, Mims CA: Macrophage activation in mice infected with ectromelia or lymphocytic choriomeningitis viruses. Aust J Exp Biol Med Sci 51:393, 1973.
117. Collins FM, Boros DL, Warren KS: The effect of *Schistosoma mansoni* infection on the response of mice to *Salmonella enteritidis* and *Listeria monocytogenes.* J Infect Dis 125:249, 1972.
118. Collins FM: Vaccines and cell-mediated immunity. Bacteriol Rev 38:371, 1974.
119. Green GM, Kass EH: The role of the alveolar macrophage in the clearance of bacteria from the lung. J Exp Med 119:167, 1964.
120. Humphrey JH, Sulitzeanu BD: The use of (^{14}C) amino acids to study sites and rates of antibody synthesis in living hyperimmune rabbits. Biochem J 68:146, 1958.
121. Askonas BA, Humphrey JH: Formation of specific antibodies and gamma-globulin in vitro: a study of the synthetic ability of various tissues from rabbits immunized by different methods. Biochem J 68:252, 1958.
122. Perkins JC, Tucker DN, Knopf HLS, Wenzel RP, Kapikian AZ, Chanock RM: Comparison of protective effect of neutralizing antibody in serum and nasal secretions in experimental rhinovirus type 13 illness. Am J Epidemiol 90:519, 1969.
123. Perkins JC, Tucker DN, Knopf HLS, Wenzel RP, Hornick RB, Kapikian AZ, Chanock RM: Evidence for protective effect of an activated rhinovirus vaccine administered by nasal route. Am J Epidemiol 90:319, 1969.
124. Waldman RH, Mann JJ, Small PA Jr: Immunization against influenza. Prevention of illness in man by aerolized inactivated vaccine. JAMA 207:520, 1969.
125. Smith CB, Purcell RH, Bellanti JA, Chanock RM: Protective effect of antibody to parainfluenza type I virus. N Engl J Med 275:1145, 1966.
126. Tomasi TB, Grey HM: Structure and function of immunoglobulin A. Prog Allergy 16:81, 1972.
127. Brandtzaeg P, Fjellanger I, Gjeruldsen ST: Localization of immunoglobulins in human nasal mucosa. Immunochemistry 4:57, 1967.
128. Tada T, Ishizaka K: Distribution of γE-forming cells in lymphoid tissues of the human and monkey. J Immunol 104:377, 1970.
129. Martinez-Tello FJ, Braun DG, Blanc WA: Immunoglobulin production in bronchial mucosa and bronchial lymph nodes, particularly in cystic fibrosis of the pancreas. J Immunol 101:989, 1968.
130. Gerber MA, Paronetto F, Kochwa S: Immunohistochemical localization of IgE in asthmatic lungs. Am J Pathol 62:339, 1971.
131. Callerame ML, Condemi JJ, Ishizaka K, Johansson SGO, Vaughan JH: Immunoglobulins in bronchial tissues from patients with asthma, with special reference to immunoglobulin E. J Allergy Clin Immunol 47:187, 1971.
132. Van Hout CA, Johnson HG: Synthesis of rat IgE by aerosol immunization. J Immunol 108:834, 1972.
133. Rossen RD, Kasel JA, Couch RB: The secretory immune system: its relation to respiratory viral infection. Prog Med Virol 13:194, 1971.
134. Reynolds HY, Thompson RE: Pulmonary host defenses. I. Analysis of protein and lipids in bronchial secretions and antibody responses after vaccination with *Pseudomonas aeruginosa.* J Immunol 111:358, 1973.
135. Gerbrandy JLF, Van Dura EA: Anamnestic secretory antibody response in respiratory secretions of intranasally immunized mice. J Immunol 109:1, 46, 1972.
136. Kaltreider HB, Kyselka L, Salmon SE: Immunology of the lower respiratory tract. II. The plaque-forming response of canine lymphoid tissues to sheep erythrocytes after intrapulmonary or intravenous immunization. J Clin Invest 54:263, 1974.
137. Hand WL, Cantey JR: Antibacterial mechanisms of the lower respiratory tract. I. Immunoglobulin synthesis and secretion. J Clin Invest 53:354, 1974.
138. Kaltreider HB, Chan M: Immunoglobulin composition of fluid obtained from various levels of the canine respiratory tract. Abstract presented at the International Congress on Lung Diseases, Montreal, PQ, Canada, May 18–21, 1975.
139. Colten HR, Bienenstock J: Lack of C3 activation through classical or alternate pathways by human secretory IgA anti-blood group A antibody. In Mestecky J, Lawton AR (eds): The Immunoglobulin A System. Adv Exper Med Biol 45:305, 1974.
140. Eddie DS, Schulkind ML, Robbins JB: The isolation and biologic activities of purified secretory IgA and IgG anti-*Salmonella typhimurium* O antibodies from rabbit intestinal fluid and colostrum. J Immunol 106:181, 1971.
141. Curlin GT, Carpenter CCJ: Antitoxic immunity to cholera in isolated perfused canine ileal segments. J Infect Dis 121:S132, 1970.
142. Kaur J, McGhee J, Burrows W: Immunity to cholera: the occurrence and nature of antibody-active immunoglobulins in the lower ileum of the rabbit. J Immunol 108:387, 1972.
143. Williams RC, Gibbons RJ: Inhibition of bacterial adherence by secretory immunoglobulin A: A mechanism of antigen disposal. Science 177:697, 1972.
144. Freter R: Studies of the mechanism of action of intestinal antibody in experimental cholera. Texas Rep Biol Med 27:299, 1969.
145. Freter R: Mechanism of action of intestinal antibody in experimental cholera. II. Antibody-mediated antibacterial reaction at the mucosal surface. Infect Immunol 2:556, 1970.
146. Brandtzaeg P, Fjellanger I, Gjeruldsen ST: Adsorption of immunoglobulin A onto oral bacteria in vivo. J Bacteriol 96:242, 1968.
147. Heremans JF, Crabbé PA: Immunohistochemical studies on exocrine IgA. In Killander J (ed): Gamma Globulins: Structure and Control of Biosynthesis. Proceedings of the Third Nobel Symposium, Södergarn, Lidingö, June 12–17, 1967. Stockholm, Almqvist and Wiksell, 1967, p 129.

148. Burnet FM: The Colonal Selection Theory of Acquired Immunity. Nashville, Tenn, Vanderbilt Press, 1959, p 86.
149. Heremans JF: The Immune System and Infectious Diseases. Basel, S Karger (in press)
150. Ishizaka K, Ishizaka T, Tada T, Newcomb RW: Site of synthesis and function of gamma-E. In Dayton DH Jr, Small PA, Chanock RM, Kaufman HB, Tomasi TB Jr (eds): The Secretory Immunologic System. Bethesda, National Institute of Child Health and Human Development, 1971.
151. Deuschl H, Johansson SGO: Immunoglobulins in tracheobronchial secretion with special reference to IgE. Clin Exp Immunol 16:401, 1974.
152. Day RP, Bienenstock J, Rawls WE: Basophil-sensitizing antibody response to herpes simplex viruses in rabbits. J Immunol 117:73, 1976.
153. Brinkman GL, Brooks N, Bryant V: The ultrastructure of the lamina propria of the human bronchus. Am Rev Respir Dis 99:219, 1969.
154. Barclay WR, Busey WM, Dalgard DW, Good RC, Janicki BW, Kasik JE, Ribi E, Ulrich CE, Wolinsky E: Protection of monkeys against airborne tuberculosis by aerosol vaccination with bacillus Calmette-Guerin. Am Rev Respir Dis 107:351, 1973.
155. Daniele RP, Altose MD, Salisbury GB, Rowlands DT Jr: Characterization of lymphocyte subpopulations in normal human lungs. Chest 67[Suppl 2]:52S, 1975.
156. Bienenstock J, Johnston N, Perey DYE: Bronchial lymphoid tissue. I. Morphologic characteristics. Lab Invest 28:686, 1973.
157. Emery JL, Dinsdale F: The postnatal development of lymphoreticular aggregates and lymph nodes in infants' lungs. J Clin Pathol 26:539, 1973.
158. Bienenstock J, Johnston N, Perey DYE: Bronchial lymphoid tissue. II. Functional characteristics. Lab Invest 28:693, 1973.
159. Bockman DE, Cooper MD: Pinocytosis by epithelium associated with lymphoid follicles in the bursa of Fabricius, appendix and Peyer's patches: an electron microscopic study. Am J Anat 136:455, 1973.
160. Craig SW, Cebra JJ: Peyer's patches: An enriched source of precursors for IgA-producing immunocytes in the rabbit. J Exp Med 134:188, 1971.
161. Bienenstock J: The physiology of the local immune response and the GI tract. In Brent L, Holborow J (eds): Progress in Immunology II, Amsterdam, North Holland, 1974, Vol 4, pp 197–207.

DIAGNOSIS OF PULMONARY INFECTIONS

162. Hanson RR, Zavala DC, Rhodes ML, Keim LW, Smith JD: Transbronchial biopsy via flexible fiberoptic bronchoscope: Results in 164 patients. Am Rev Respir Dis 114:67, 1976.
163. Anderson HA, Transbronchoscopic lung biopsy for diffuse pulmonary disease: Results in 939 patients. Chest 73:734, 1978.
164. Cunningham JH, Zavala DC, Corry RJ, Keim LW: Trephine air drill, bronchial brush, and fiberoptic transbronchial lung biopsies in immunosuppressed patients. Am Rev Respir Dis 115:213, 1977.
165. Nordenström B, Sinnor WN: Needle biopsy of pulmonary lesions: Precautions and management of complications. Fortschr Röntgenstr 129:414, 1978.
166. Lalli AF, McCormack LJ, Zelch M, Reich NE, Belovich D: Aspiration biopsies of chest lesions. Radiology 127:35, 1978.
167. Rogers BM, Mozam F, Talbert JL: Thoracoscopy: Early diagnosis of interstitial pneumonitis in the immunosuppressed child. Chest 75:126, 1979.
168. Rogers BM, Mozam F, Talbert JL: Thoracoscopy in children. Ann Surg 189:176, 1978.
169. Leight GS Jr, Michaelis LL: Open lung biopsy for the diagnosis of acute, diffuse pulmonary infiltrates in the immunosuppressed patient. Chest 73:499, 1978.
170. Thompson DT: Lung biopsy with local anesthesia: Report on 100 cases with the use of a recently introduced technique. J Thorac Cardiovasc Surg 75:429, 1978.

VIRAL INFECTIONS OF THE LUNG

171. Nankervis GA, Kumar ML: Diseases produced by cytomegaloviruses. Med Clin North Am 62:1021, 1978.
172. Howard RJ, Balfour HH Jr, Simmons RL: The surgical significance of viruses. Curr Probl Surg 14:3, 1977.
173. Rand KH, Pollard RB, Merigan TC: Increased pulmonary superinfections in cardiac-transplant patients undergoing primary cytomegalovirus infection. N Engl J Med 298:951, 1978.
174. Ravin CE, Smith GW, Ahern MJ, McLoud T, Putman C, Milchgrad S: Cytomegaloviral infection presenting as a solitary pulmonary nodule. Chest 71:220, 1977.
175. Simmons RL, Matas AJ, Rattazzi LC, Balfour HH Jr, Howard JR, Najarian JS: Clinical characteristics of the lethal cytomegalovirus infection following renal transplantation. Surgery 82:537, 1977.
176. Anderson RW: Shock and circulatory collapse. In Sabiston DC, Spencer FC (eds): Surgery of the Chest. Philadelphia, Saunders, 1976, pp 107–145.
177. Padula RT: Postoperative management. In Sabiston DC, Spencer FC (eds): Surgery of the Chest. Philadelphia, Saunders, 1976, pp 174–194.
178. Wanner A, Landa JF, Nieman RE Jr, Vevaina J, Delgado I: Bedside bronchofiberscopy for atelectasis and lung abscess. JAMA 224:1281, 1973.

PNEUMONIA, LUNG ABSCESS, AND BRONCHIECTASIS

179. Bartlett JG, Gorbach SL: Treatment of aspiration pneumonia and primary lung abscess. Penicillin G vs Clindamycin. JAMA 234:935, 1975.
180. Cameron JL, Mitchell WH, Zuidema GD: Aspiration pneumonia. Clinical outcome following documented aspiration. Arch Surg 106:49, 1973.
181. Hochberg LA: Thoracic Surgery before the Twentieth Century. New York, Vantage Press, 1960.
182. Neuhof H, Touroff ASW: Acute putrid abscess of the lung; hyperacute variety. J Thorac Surg 12:98, 1942.
183. Brock RC: Lung Abscess. Oxford, Blackwell, 1952.
184. Abernathy RS: Antibiotic therapy of lung abscess: Effectiveness of penicillin. Dis Chest 53:592, 1968.
185. Perlman LV, Lerner E, D'Esopo N: Clinical classification and analysis of 97 cases of lung abscess. Am Rev Respir Dis 99:390, 1969.
186. Mark PH, Turner JAP: Lung abscess in childhood. Thorax 23:216, 1968.
187. Pappas G, Schröter G, Brettschneider L, Penn I, Starzl TE: Pulmonary surgery in immunosuppressed patients. J Thorac Cardiovasc Surg 59:882, 1970.
188. Bernhard WF, Malcolm JA, Wylie RH: Lung abscess: A study of 148 cases due to aspiration. Dis Chest 43:620, 1963.
189. Shafron RD, Tate CF Jr: Lung abscesses; A five-year evaluation. Dis Chest 53:12, 1968.
190. Anderson MN, McDonald KE: Prognostic factors and results of treatment in pyogenic pulmonary abscess. J Thorac Cardiovasc Surg 39:573, 1960.
191. Bartlett JG, Gorbach SL, Tally FP, Finegold SM: Bacteriology and treatment of primary lung abscess. Am Rev Respir Dis 109:510, 1974.

192. Bartlett JG, Rosenblatt JE, Finegold SM: Percutaneous transtracheal aspiration in the diagnosis of anaerobic pulmonary infection. Ann Intern Med 79:535, 1973.
193. Bartlett JG, Alexander J, Mayhew J, Sullivan-Sigler N, Gorbach SL: Should fiberoptic bronchoscopy aspirates be cultured? Am Rev Respir Dis 114:73, 1976.
194. Kleinfeld J, Ellis PP: Inhibition of microorganisms by topical anesthetics. Appl Microbiol 15:1296, 1967.
195. Conte BA, Laforet EG: The role of the topical anesthetic agent in modifying bacteriologic data obtained by bronchoscopy. N Engl J Med 267:957, 1962.
196. Davidson M, Tempest B, Palmer DL: Bacteriologic diagnosis of acute pneumonia: Comparison of sputum, transtracheal aspirates, and lung aspirates. JAMA 235:158, 1976.
197. Rein MF, Mandell GL: Bacterial killing by bacteriostatic saline solutions—potential for diagnostic error. N Engl J Med 289:794, 1973.
198. Sethi JP, Gupta ML, Kasliwal RM: Amebic pulmonary suppuration. Dis Chest 51:148, 1967.
199. Schweppe HI, Knowles JH, Kane L: Lung abscess: An analysis of the Massachusetts General Hospital cases from 1943 through 1956. N Engl J Med 265:1039, 1961.
200. Wolcott MW, Harris SH, Briggs JN, Dobell ARC, Brown RK: Hydatid disease of the lung. J Thorac Cardiovasc Surg 62:465, 1971.
201. Spruance SL, Klock LE, Chang F, Fukushima T, Anderson FL, Kagan IG: Endemic hydatid disease in Utah. A review. Rocky Mt Med J 71:17, 1974.
202. Wilson JF, Diddams AC, Rausch RL: Cystic hydatid disease in Alaska. A review of 101 autochthonous cases of *Echinococcus granulosus* infection. Am Rev Respir Dis 98:1, 1968.
203. Chidi CC, Mendelsohn HJ: Lung-abscess. A study of the results of treatment based on 90 consecutive cases. J Thorac Cardiovasc Surg 68:168, 1974.
204. Gopalakrishna KV, Lerner PI: Primary lung abscess: Analysis of 66 cases. Cleveland Clin Q 42:3, 1975.
205. Weiss W, Cherniack NS: Acute nonspecific lung abscess: A controlled study comparing orally and parenterally administered penicillin G. Chest 66:348, 1974.
206. Thadepalli H, Niden AH, Huang JT: Treatment of anaerobic pulmonary infections: Carbenicillin compared to clindamycin and gentamicin. Chest 69:743, 1976.
207. Groff DB, Marquis J: Transtracheal drainage of lung abscesses in children. J Pediatr Surg 12:303, 1977.
208. Connors JP, Roper CL, Ferguson TB: Transbronchial catheterization of pulmonary abscesses. Ann Thorac Surg 19:254, 1975.
209. Jaffe HJ, Katz S: Current ideas about bronchiectasis. Am Family Physician 7:69, 1973.
210. Barnett TB, Herring CL: Lung abscess. Initial and late results of medical therapy. Arch Intern Med 127:217, 1971.
211. Rubin PE, Block AJ: Nonspecific lung abscess. A perspective. Geriatrics 27:125, 1972.
212. Jensen HE, Amdrup E: Nonspecific abscess of the lung: 129 cases. I. Diagnosis and treatment. Acta Chir Scand 127:487, 1964.
213. Thoms NW, Wilson RF, Puro HE, Arbulu A: Life-threatening hemoptysis in primary lung abscess. Ann Thorac Surg 14:347, 1972.
214. Crocco JA, Rooney JJ, Fankushen DS, DiBenedetto RJ, Lyons HA: Massive hemoptysis. Arch Intern Med 121:495, 1968.
215. Remy J, Arnaud A, Fardou H, Giraud R, Voisin C: Treatment of hemoptysis by embolization of bronchial arteries. Radiology 122:33, 1977.
216. Harley JD, Killien FC, Peck AG: Massive hemoptysis controlled by transcatheter embolization of the bronchial arteries. Am J Roentgenol 128:302, 1977.
217. Monaldi V: Endocavitary aspiration in the treatment of lung abscess. Chest 29:193, 1956.
218. Morris JF, Okies JE: Enterococcal lung abscess: Medical and surgical therapy. Chest 65:688, 1974.
219. Newson SWB, Milstein BB, Stark JE: Local chemotherapy for pseudomonas lung abscess. Lancet 2:530, 1974.
220. Vidal E, LeVeen HH, Yarnoz M, Piccone VA Jr: Lung abscess secondary to pulmonary infarction. Ann Thorac Surg 11:577, 1971.
221. McMillan JC, Milstein SH, Samson PC: Clinical spectrum of septic pulmonary embolism and infarction. J Thorac Cardiovasc Surg 75:670, 1978.
222. Ochsner A: Bronchiectasis. A disappearing pulmonary lesion. NY State J Med 75:1683, 1975.
223. Kent EM, Blades B: Surgical anatomy of pulmonary lobes. J Thorac Surg 12:18, 1942.
224. Field CE: Bronchiectasis. Third report on a follow-up study of medical and surgical cases from childhood. Arch Dis Child 44:551, 1969.
225. Bradham RR, Sealy WC, Young WG Jr: Chronic middle lobe infection: Factors responsible for its development. Ann Thorac Surg 2:612, 1966.
226. Lindskog GE, Liebow AA, Glenn WWL: Thoracic and Cardiovascular Surgery with Related Pathology. New York, Appleton, 1962, p 176.
227. Miller RD, Divertie MB: Kartagener's syndrome. Chest 62:130, 1972.
228. Afzelius BA: A human syndrome caused by immotile cilia. Science 193:317, 1976.
229. Sturgess JM, Chao J, Wong J, Aspin N, Turner JAP: Cilia with defective radial spokes: A cause of human respiratory disease. N Engl J Med 300:53, 1979.
230. Longstreth GF, Weitzman SA, Browning RJ, Lieberman J: Bronchiectasis and homozygous alpha$_1$-antitrypsin deficiency. Chest 67:233, 1975.
231. Di Sant'Agnese PA, Talamo RD: Pathogenesis and physiopathology of cystic fibrosis of the pancreas: Fibrocystic disease of the pancreas (mucoviscidosis). N Engl J Med 277:1399, 1967.
232. Campbell GS: Bronchiectasis. In Sabiston DC Jr (ed): Textbook of Surgery. Philadelphia, Saunders, 1972, p 1823.
233. Sealy WC, Bradham RR, Young WG Jr: The surgical treatment of multisegmental and localized bronchiectasis. Surg Gynecol Obstet 123:80, 1966.
234. Mitchell RS: Bronchiectasis and bronchial complications of hilar lymph node infection. In Baum GL (ed): Textbook of Pulmonary Diseases. Boston, Little, Brown, 1974, p 395.
235. Ferguson TB, Burford TH: The changing pattern of pulmonary suppuration: Surgical implications. Dis Chest 53:396, 1968.
236. Rayl JE, Morada AO: Chronic bronchitis and bronchiectasis. In Gordon BL (ed): Clinical Cardiopulmonary Physiology, 3rd ed. New York, Grune & Stratton, 1969, p 523.
237. Blades B, Dugan D: Pseudobronchiectasis. J Thorac Surg 13:40, 1944.
238. Streete BG, Salyer JM: Bronchiectasis. An analysis of 240 cases treated by pulmonary resection. J Thorac Cardiovasc Surg 40:383, 1960.
239. Editorial: Bronchiectasis today. Br Med J 4:604, 1975.
240. Ripe E: Bronchiectasis. I. A follow-up study after surgical treatment. Scand J Respir Dis 52:96, 1971.
241. Borrie J, Lichter I: Surgical treatment of bronchiectasis: Ten year survey. Br Med J 2:908, 1965.
242. Sanderson JM, Kennedy MCS, Johnson MF, Manley DCE: Bronchiectasis: Results of surgical and conservative management. A review of 393 cases. Thorax 29:407, 1974.

TUBERCULOSIS

243. Wolinsky E: Nontuberculous mycobacteria and associated diseases. Am Rev Respir Dis 119:107, 1979.
244. McLaughlin JS, Hankins JR: Current aspects of surgery for pulmonary tuberculosis. Ann Thorac Surg 17:513, 1974.
245. Johnston RF, Wildrick KH: The impact of chemotherapy on the care of patients with tuberculosis. Am Rev Respir Dis 109:636, 1974.
246. Jenkins DE, Wolinsky E: Mycobacterial diseases of the lung and bronchial tree: Treatment of active pulmonary tuberculosis. In Baum GL (ed): Textbook of Pulmonary Diseases. Boston, Little, Brown, 1974, pp 323–366.
247. American Thoracic Society. Treatment of mycobacterial disease. Am Rev Respir Dis 115:185, 1977.
248. Young WG, Moore GF: The surgical treatment of pulmonary tuberculosis. In Sabiston DC, Spencer FC (eds): Surgery of the Chest. Philadelphia, Saunders, 1976, pp 567–590.
249. Prytz S, Hansen JL: Surgical treatment of "tuberculoma." A follow-up examination of patients with pulmonary tuberculosis resected on suspicion of tumour. Scand J Thorac Cardiovasc Surg 10:179, 1976.
250. Sethi GK, Takaro T: Management of complications following pulmonary resection for infections of mycobacterial, actinomycetic, and fungal origins. In Cordell AR, Ellison RG (eds): Complications of Intrathoracic Surgery, Boston, Little, Brown, 1979.
251. Anderson RP, Leand PM, Kieffer RF Jr: Changing attitudes in the surgical management of pulmonary tuberculosis. Ann Thorac Surg 3:43, 1967.
252. Teixeira J: The present status of thoracic surgery in tuberculosis. Dis Chest 53:19, 1968.
253. Rzepecki WM, Lodziak A: Pre- and postoperative treatment of chronic multiresistant cases of pulmonary tuberculosis with rifampicin. Chemotherapy 20:12, 1974.
254. Tamimi TM, Hankins JR, Miller JE, Sauer EP, McLaughlin JS: The value of thoracoplasty before extensive unilateral resection for pulmonary tuberculosis. Am Surg 42:71, 1976.
255. Huang CT, Lyons HA: Cardiorespiratory failure in patients with pneumonectomy for tuberculosis. Long-term effects of thoracoplasty. J Thorac Cardiovasc Surg 74:409, 1977.
256. Johnson G Jr, Peters RM: Pulmonary resection for tuberculosis: Life table analysis of results. Ann Thorac Surg 1:634, 1965.
257. Das PB, David JG: Role of surgery in the treatment of pulmonary tuberculosis. Can J Surg 18:512, 1975.

OPPORTUNISTIC INFECTIONS

258. Yeager H Jr, Raleigh JW: Pulmonary disease due to *Mycobacterium intracellulare.* Am Rev Respir Dis 108:547, 1973.
259. Harris GD, Johanson WG Jr, Nicholson DP: Response to chemotherapy of pulmonary infection due to *Mycobacterium kansasii.* Am Rev Respir Dis 112:31, 1975.
260. Rosenzweig DY: Course and long-term follow-up of 100 cases of pulmonary infection due to *M. avium-intracellulare* complex. Am Rev Respir Dis 113:55, 1976.
261. Elkadi A, Salas R, Almond CH: Surgical treatment of atypical pulmonary tuberculosis. J Thorac Cardiovasc Surg 72:435, 1976.
262. Oliver WA: Surgical management in atypical pulmonary tuberculosis (MAIS complex). Med J Aust 1:993, 1976.
263. Spencer H: Pathology of the Lung: Excluding Pulmonary Tuberculosis, 3rd ed. Oxford, Pergamon, 1977, Vol 1, pp 258–261.
264. Spotnitz M, Rudnitzky J, Rambaud JJ: Melioidosis pneumonitis. Analysis of nine cases of a benign form of melioidosis. JAMA 202:950, 1967.
265. Everett ED, Nelson RA: Pulmonary melioidosis. Observations in thirty-nine cases. Am Rev Respir Dis 112:331, 1975.
266. Sanford JP: Melioidosis and glanders. In Thorn GW, Adams RD, Braunwald E, Isselbacher KJ, Petersdorf RG (eds): Principles of Internal Medicine, 8th ed. New York, McGraw-Hill, 1977, pp 865–868.
267. Flemma RJ, DiVincenti FC, Dotin LN, Pruitt BA: Pulmonary melioidosis: a diagnostic dilemma and increasing threat. Ann Thorac Surg 7:491, 1969.
268. Zajtchuk R, Guiton CR, Sadler TR, Heydorn WH, Strevey TE: Surgical treatment of pulmonary melioidosis. J Thorac Cardiovasc Surg 66:838, 1973.
269. Steele JD (ed): The Treatment of Mycotic and Parasitic Diseases of the Chest. Springfield, Ill, Thomas, 1964.
270. Buechner HA: Management of Fungus Diseases of the Lungs. Springfield, Ill, Thomas, 1971.
271. Slade PR, Slesser BV, Southgate J: Thoracic actinomycosis. Thorax 28:73, 1973.
272. Flynn MW, Felson B: The roentgen manifestations of thoracic actinomycosis. Am J Roentgenol Radium Ther Nucl Med 110:707, 1970.
273. Balikian JP, Cheng TH, Costello P, Herman PG: Pulmonary actinomycosis. Radiology 128:613, 1978.
274. Datta JS, Raff MJ: Actinomycotic pleuropericarditis. Amer Rev Respir Dis 110:338, 1974.
275. Schlossberg D, Franco-Jove D, Woodward C, Shulman J: Pericarditis with effusion caused by *Actinomyces israelii.* Chest 69:680, 1976.
276. Foley TF, Dines DE, Dolan CT: Pulmonary actinomycosis. Report of 18 cases. Minn Med 54:593, 1971.
277. Weese WC, Smith IM: A study of 57 cases of actinomycosis over a 36-year period. A diagnostic "failure" with good prognosis after treatment. Arch Intern Med 135:1562, 1975.
278. Pinkerton JA, Lawler MR, Foster JH: Pulmonary nocardiosis. Am Surg 37:729, 1971.
279. Frazier AR, Rosenow EC III, Roberts GD: Nocardiosis. A review of 25 cases occurring during 24 months. Mayo Clin Proc 50:657, 1975.
280. Krick JA, Stinson EB, Remington JS: *Nocardia* infection in heart transplant patients. Ann Intern Med 82:18, 1975.
281. Beaman BL, Burnside J, Edwards B, Causey W: Nocardial infections in the United States, 1972–1974. J Infect Dis 134:286, 1976.
282. Balikian JP, Herman PG, Kopit S: Pulmonary nocardiosis. Radiology 126:569, 1978.
283. George RB, Jenkinson SG, Light RW: Fiberoptic bronchoscopy in the diagnosis of pulmonary fungal and noncardial infarctions. Chest 73:33, 1978.
284. Ellis JH Jr: Diagnosis of opportunistic infections using the flexible fiberoptic bronchoscope. Chest [Suppl] 73:713, 1978.
285. Sagel SS, Ferguson TB, Forrest JV, Roper CL, Weldon CS, Clark RE: Percutaneous transthoracic aspiration needle biopsy. Ann Thorac Surg 26:399, 1978.
286. Maderazo EG, Quintiliani R: Treatment of nocardial infection with trimethoprim and sulfamethoxazole. Am J Med 57:671, 1974.

FUNGAL INFECTIONS OF THE LUNG

287. Procknow JJ: Treatment of opportunistic fungus infections. Lab Invest 11:1217, 1962.
288. Mills SA, Seigler HF, Wolfe WG: The incidence and management of pulmonary mycosis in renal allograft patients. Ann Surg 182:617, 1975.
289. Schröter GPJ, Hoelscher M, Putnam CW, Porter KA, Starzl TE: Fungus infections after liver transplantation. Ann Surg 186:115, 1977.

290. Howard RJ, Simmons RL, Najarian JS: Fungal infections in renal transplant recipients. Ann Surg 188:598, 1978.
291. Chick EW, Dillon ML, Tahanasab A: Acute cavitary histoplasmosis. Chest 71:674, 1977.
292. Palayew MJ, Frank H: Benign progressive multinodular pulmonary histoplasmosis. A radiological and clinical entity. Radiology 111:311, 1974.
293. Goodwin RA Jr, DesPrez RM: State of the art: Histoplasmosis. Am Rev Respir Dis 117:929, 1978.
294. Chick EW, Baum GL, Furcolow ML, Huppert M, Kaufman L, Pappagianis D: The use of skin tests and serologic tests in histoplasmosis, coccidioidomycosis, and blastomycosis, 1973. Am Rev Respir Dis 108:156, 1973.
295. Sbarbaro JA: Skin test antigens: An evaluation whose time has come (editorial). Am Rev Respir Dis 118:1, 1978.
296. Lowell JR, Shuford EH: The value of the skin test and complement-fixation test in the diagnosis of chronic pulmonary histoplasmosis. Am Rev Respir Dis 114:1069, 1976.
297. Furcolow ML: Comparison of treated and untreated severe histoplasmosis: A communicable disease center cooperative mycoses study. JAMA 183:823, 1963.
298. Bennett JE: Chemotherapy of systemic mycoses. N Engl J Med 290:30, 320, 1974.
299. Hermans PE: Antifungal agents used for deep-seated mycotic infections. Mayo Clin Proc 52:687, 1977.
300. Goodwin RA Jr, Owens FT, Snell JD, Hubbard WW, Buchanan RD, Terry RT, Des Prez RM: Chronic pulmonary histoplasmosis. Medicine 55:413, 1976.
301. Steele JD: The Solitary Pulmonary Nodule. Springfield, III, Thomas, 1964.
302. Nathan H: Management of solitary pulmonary nodules. An organized approach based on growth rate and statistics. JAMA 227:1141, 1974.
303. Moser KM: Solitary pulmonary nodules. JAMA 227:1167, 1974.
304. Kyriakos M, Webber B: Cancer of the lung in young men. J Thorac Cardiovasc Surg 67:634, 1974.
305. Putnam JS: Lung carcinoma in young adults. JAMA 238:35, 1977.
306. Parker JD, Sarosi GA, Doto IL, Bailey RE, Tosh FE: Treatment of chronic pulmonary histoplasmosis. N Engl J Med 283:225, 1970.
307. Hughes FA Jr, Eastridge CE, Aslam PA: Surgical treatment of pulmonary histoplasmosis. In Ajello L, Chick EW, Furcolow ML (eds): Histoplasmosis. Springfield, Ill, Thomas, 1971, p 429.
308. Baum GL, Larkin JC Jr, Sutliff WD: Follow-up of patients with chronic pulmonary histoplasmosis treated with amphotericin-B. Chest 58:562, 1970.
309. Bayer AS, Yoshikawa TT, Galpin JE, Guze LB: Unusual syndromes of coccidioidomycosis: Diagnostic and therapeutic considerations. A report of 10 cases and review of the English literature. Medicine 55:131, 1976.
310. Thadepalli H, Salem FA, Mandall AK, Rambhatla K, Einstein HE: Pulmonary mycetoma due to *Coccidioides immitis.* Chest 71:429, 1977.
311. Lonky SA, Catanzaro A, Moser KM, Einstein H: Acute coccidioidal pleural effusion. Am Rev Respir Dis 114:681, 1976.
312. Baker EJ, Hawkins JA, Waskow EA: Surgery for coccidioidomycosis in 52 diabetic patients, with special reference to related immunologic factors. J Thorac Cardiovasc Surg 75:680, 1978.
313. Cohen SL, Gale AM, Liston HE: Report of a pilot study on noncalcified discrete pulmonary coin lesions in a coccidioidomycosis endemic area. Ariz Med 29:40, 1972.
314. Read TC: Coin lesion, pulmonary, in the Southwest (solitary pulmonary nodules). Ariz Med 29:775, 1972.
315. Paulsen GA: Pulmonary surgery in coccidioidal infections. In Ajello L (ed): Coccidioidomycosis. Tucson, Ariz, University of Arizona Press, 1967, p 69.
316. Marks TS, Spence WF, Baisch BF: Limited resection for pulmonary coccidioidomycosis. In Ajello L (ed): Coccidioidomycosis. Tucson, Ariz, University of Arizona Press, 1967, p 73.
317. Nelson AR: The surgical treatment of pulmonary coccidioidomycosis. Curr Probl Surg 11:1, 1974.
318. Melick DW, Grant AR: Surgery in primary pulmonary coccidioidomycosis and in the combined diseases of coccidioidomycosis and tuberculosis. Dis Chest [Suppl] 54:278, 1968.
319. Fosburg RG, Baisch BF, Trummer MJ: Limited pulmonary resection for coccidioidomycosis. Ann Thorac Surg 7:420, 1969.
320. Schwartz EL, Waldmann EB, Payne RM, Goldfarb D, Kinard SA: Coccidioidal pericarditis. Chest 70:670, 1976.
321. Landis FB, Varkey B: Late relapse of pulmonary blastomycosis after adequate treatment with amphotericin-B. Am Rev Respir Dis 113:77, 1976.
322. Laskey W, Sarosi GA: Endogenous reinfection in blastomycosis. Am Rev Respir Dis 115:266, 1977.
323. Cush R, Light RW, George RB: Clinical and roentgenographic manifestations of acute and chronic blastomycosis. Chest 69:345, 1976.
324. Sanders JS, Sarosi GA, Nollet DJ, Thompson JI: Exfoliative cytology in the rapid diagnosis of pulmonary blastomycosis. Chest 72:193, 1977.
325. Sutliff WD, Cruthirds TP: *Blastomyces dermatitidis* in cytologic preparations. Am Rev Respir Dis 108:149, 1973.
326. Poe RH, Vassallo CL, Plessinger VA, Witt RL: Pulmonary blastomycosis versus carcinoma—A challenging differential. Am J Med Sci 263:145, 1972.
327. Busey JF: Blastomycosis. III. A comparative study of 2-hydroxystilbamidine and amphotericin-B therapy. Am Rev Respir Dis 105:812, 1972.
328. Duperval R, Hermans PE, Brewer NS, Roberts GD: Cryptococcosis, with emphasis on the significance of isolation of *Cryptococcus neoformans* from the respiratory tract. Chest 72:13, 1977.
329. Salyer WR, Salyer DC, Baker RD: Primary complex of *Cryptococcus* and pulmonary lymph nodes. J Infect Dis 130:74, 1974.
330. Baker RD: The primary pulmonary lymph node complex of cryptococcosis. Am J Clin Pathol 65:83, 1976.
331. Salyer WR, Salyer DC: Pleural involvement in cryptococcosis. Chest 66:139, 1974.
332. Littman ML, Walter JE: Cryptococcosis: Current status. Am J Med 45:922, 1968.
333. Epstein R, Cole R, Hunt KK Jr: Pleural effusion secondary to pulmonary cryptococcosis. Chest 61:296, 1972.
334. Taylor ER: Pulmonary cryptococcosis: An analysis of 15 cases from the Columbia area. Ann Thorac Surg 10:309, 1970.
335. Hatcher CR Jr, Sehdeva J, Waters WC III, Schulze V, Logan WD, Symbas P, Abbott OA: Primary pulmonary cryptococcosis. J Thorac Cardiovasc Surg 61:39, 1971.
336. Lewis JL, Rabinovich S: The wide spectrum of cryptococcal infections. Am J Med 53:315, 1972.
337. Smith FS, Gibson P, Nicholls TT, Simpson JA: Pulmonary resection for localized lesions of cryptococcosis (torulosis): A review of eight cases. Thorax 31:121, 1976.
338. Utz JP, Garriques IL, Sande MA, Warner JF, Mandell GL, McGehee RF, Duma RJ, Thadomy S: Therapy of cryptococcosis with a combination of flucytosine and amphotericin-B. J Infect Dis 132:368, 1975.
339. Williams DM, Krick JA, Remington JS: Pulmonary infection in the compromised host. Am Rev Respir Dis 114:359, 593, 1976.
340. Soll EL, Bergeron RB: Pulmonary cryptococcosis—a case

diagnostically confirmed by transbronchial brush biopsy. Chest 59:454, 1971.
341. Hammerman KJ, Powell KE, Christianson CS, Huggin PM, Larsh HW, Vivas JR, Tosh FE: Pulmonary cryptococcosis: Clinical forms and treatment. Am Rev Respir Dis 108:1116, 1973.
342. Geraci JE, Donoghue FE, Ellis FH Jr, Whitten DM, Weed LA: Focal pulmonary cryptococcosis: Evaluation of necessity of amphotericin-B therapy. Mayo Clin Proc 40:552, 1965.
343. Campbell MJ, Clayton YM: Bronchopulmonary aspergillosis: A correlation of the clinical and laboratory findings in 272 patients investigated for bronchopulmonary aspergillosis. Am Rev Respir Dis 89:186, 1964.
344. Henderson RD, Deslaurier J, Ritcey EL, Delarue NC, Pearson FG: Surgery in pulmonary aspergillosis. J Thorac Cardiovasc Surg 70:1088, 1975.
345. Eastridge CE, Young JM, Cole F, Gourley R, Pate JW: Pulmonary aspergillosis. Ann Thorac Surg 13:397, 1972.
346. Karas A, Hankins JR, Attar S, Miller JE, McLaughlin JS: Pulmonary aspergillosis: An analysis of 41 patients. Ann Thorac Surg 22:1, 1976.
347. Sarosi GA, Silberfarb PM, Saliba NA, Huggin PM, Tosh FE: Aspergillomas occurring in blastomycotic cavities. Am Rev Respir Dis 104:581, 1971.
348. Bower GC, Ranga V, Coates EO Jr, Kvale PA: Pulmonary aspergilloma. A report of 25 patients. Am Rev Respir Dis 115:90, 1977.
349. Varkey B, Rose HD: Pulmonary aspergilloma. A rational approach to treatment. Am J Med 61:626, 1976.
350. Saab SB, Almond C: Surgical aspects of pulmonary aspergillosis. J Thorac Cardiovasc Surg 68:455, 1974.
351. Grow BG Jr, Griepp RB: In discussion of Henderson RD, Deslaurier J, Ritcey EL, Delaure NC, Pearson FG. Surgery in pulmonary aspergillosis. J Thorac Cardiovasc Surg 70:1093, 1975.
352. Hammerman KJ, Sarosi GA, Tosh FE: Amphotericin-B in the treatment of saprophytic forms of pulmonary aspergillosis. Am Rev Respir Dis 109:57, 1974.
353. Eastridge CE: Opportunistic infections due to aspergillosis. Ann Thorac Surg 22:102, 1976.
354. Ribner B, Keusch GT, Hanna BA, Perloff M: Combination amphotericin B-rifampin therapy for pulmonary aspergillosis in a leukemic patient. Chest 70:681, 1976.
355. Horsfield K, Nicholls A, Cumming G, Hume M, Prowse K: Treatment of pulmonary aspergillosis with di-iodohydroxyquinoline. Thorax 32:250, 1977.
356. Solit RW, McKeown JJ Jr, Smullens S, Fraimow W: The surgical implications of intracavitary mycetomas (fungus balls). J Thorac Cardiovasc Surg 62:411, 1971.
357. Strutz GM, Rossi NP, Ehrenhaft JL: Pulmonary aspergillosis. J Thorac Cardiovasc Surg 64:963, 1972.
358. Belcher JR, Plummer NS: Surgery in bronchopulmonary aspergillosis. Br J Dis Chest 54:335, 1960.
359. Faulkner SL, Vernon R, Brown PP, Fisher RD, Bender HW Jr: Hemoptysis and pulmonary aspergilloma: Operative versus nonoperative treatment. Ann Thorac Surg 25:389, 1978.
360. Eguchi S, Endo S, Sakashita I, Terashima M, Asano K, Yanagida H: Surgery in the treatment of pulmonary aspergillosis. Br J Dis Chest 65:111, 1971.
361. Ramirez-R J: Pulmonary aspergilloma: Endobronchial treatment. N Engl J Med 271:1281, 1964.
362. Krakowka P, Rowinska E, Halweg H: Infection of the pleura by *Aspergillus fumigatus*. Thorax 25:245, 1970.
363. Irani FA, Dolovich J, Newhouse MT: Bronchopulmonary and pleural aspergillosis. Am Rev Respir Dis 103:552, 1971.
364. Herring M, Pecora D: Pleural aspergillosis: A case report. Am Surg 42:300, 1976.
365. Louria DB, Stiff DP, Bennett B: Disseminated moniliasis in the adult. Medicine 41:307, 1962.
366. Rubin AHE, Alroy GG: *Candida albicans* abscess of lung. Thorax 32:373, 1977.
367. Spear RK, Walker PD, Lampton LM: Tracheal obstruction associated with a fungus ball. Chest 70:662, 1976.
368. Rosenbaum RB, Barber JV, Stevens DA: *Candida albicans* pneumonia. Diagnosis by pulmonary aspiration, recovery without treatment. Am Rev Respir Dis 109:373, 1974.
369. Stone HH: Candida sepsis. In Polk HC Jr, Stone HH (eds): Hospital-acquired Infections in Surgery. Baltimore, University Park Press, 1977, pp 51–58.
370. Carpentieri U, Haggard ME, Lockhart LH, Gustavson LP, Box QT, West EF: Clinical experience in prevention of candidiasis by nystatin in children with acute lymphocytic leukemia. J Pediatr 92:593, 1978.
371. Ezdinli EZ, O'Sullivan DD, Wasser LP, Kim U, Stutzman L: Oral amphotericin for candidiasis in patients with hematologic neoplasms. JAMA 242:258, 1979.
372. Baum GL, Donnerberg RL, Stewart D, Mulligan WS, Putnam LR: Pulmonary sporotrichosis. N Engl J Med 280:410, 1969.
373. Scott SM, Peasley ED, Crymes TP: Pulmonary sporotrichosis: A report of two cases with cavitation. N Engl J Med 265:453, 1961.
374. Jay SJ, Platt MR, Reynolds RC: Primary pulmonary sporotrichosis. Am Rev Respir Dis 115:1051, 1977.
375. Michelson E: Primary pulmonary sporotrichosis. Ann Thorac Surg 24:83, 1977.
376. Lowenstein M, Markowitz SM, Nottebart HC, Shadomy S: Existence of *Sporothrix schenckii* as a pulmonary saprophyte. Chest 73:419, 1978.
377. Utz JP, Buechner HA: Mucormycosis (phycomycosis). In Buechner HA (ed): Management of Fungous Diseases of the Lungs. Springfield, Ill, Thomas, 1971, p 175.
378. Murray HW: Pulmonary mucormycosis with massive fatal hemoptysis. Chest 68:65, 1975.
379. Gartenberg G, Bottone EJ, Keusch GT, Weitzman I: Hospital-acquired mucormycosis (*Rhizopus rhizopodiformis*) of skin and subcutaneous tissue. N Engl Med 299:1115, 1978.
380. Record NB Jr, Ginder DR: Pulmonary phycomycosis without obvious predisposing factors. JAMA 235:1256, 1976.
381. Murray HW: Pulmonary mucormycosis: One hundred years later. Chest 72:1, 1977.
382. Gale AM, Kleitsch WP: Solitary pulmonary nodule due to phycomycosis (mucormycosis). Chest 62:752, 1972.
383. Hauch TW: Pulmonary mucormycosis: Another cure. Chest 72:92, 1977.
384. Murray HW, Littman ML, Roberts RB: Disseminated paracoccidioidomycosis (South American blastomycosis) in the United States. Am J Med 56:209, 1974.
385. Bouza E, Winston DJ, Rhodes J, Hewitt WL: Paracoccidioidomycosis (South American blastomycosis) in the United States. Chest 72:100, 1977.
386. Restrepo A, Robledo M, Giraldo R, Hernández H, Sierra F, Gutierrez F, Londono F, Lopez R, Calle G: The gamut of paracoccidioidomycosis. Am J Med 61:33, 1976.
387. Jung JY, Salas R, Almond CH, Saab S, Reyna R: The role of surgery in the management of pulmonary monosporosis. A collective review. J Thorac Cardiovasc Surg 73:139, 1977.

PROTOZOAL AND HELMINTH INFECTIONS

388. Rodriguez C: Pulmonary and pleural amebiasis. In Shields TW (ed): General Thoracic Surgery. Philadelphia, Lea & Febiger, 1972, p 650.
389. Powell SJ, MacLeod I, Wilmot AJ, Elsdon-Dew R: Metronidazole in amoebic dysentery and amoebic liver abscess. Lancet 2:1329, 1966.

390. Metronidazole (Flagyl) for amebiasis. Med Lett Drugs Therapeut 14:39, 1972.
391. Burke BA, Good RA: *Pneumocystis carinii* infection. Medicine 52:23, 1973.
392. Charles MA, Schwartz MI: *Pneumocystis carinii* pneumonia. Postgrad Med J 53:86, 1973.
393. Geelhoed GW, Levin BJ, Adkins PC, Joseph WL: The diagnosis and management of *Pneumocystis carinii* pneumonia. Ann Thorac Surg 14:335, 1972.
394. Gentry LO, Ruskin J, Remington JS: *Pneumocystis carinii* pneumonia. Problems in diagnosis and therapy in 24 cases. Calif Med 116:6, 1972.
395. Michaelis LL, Leight GS, Pouell RD Jr, DeVita VT: *Pneumocystis* pneumonia: The importance of early open lung biopsy. Ann Surg 183:301, 1976.
396. Finely R, Kieff E, Thomsen S, Fennessy J, Beem M, Lerner S, Morello J: Bronchial brushing in the diagnosis of pulmonary disease in patients at risk for opportunistic infection. Am Rev Respir Dis 109:379, 1974.
297. Hodgkin JE, Andersen HA, Rosenow ED III: Diagnosis of *Pneumocystis carinii* pneumonia by transbronchoscopic lung biopsy. Chest 64:551, 1973.
398. Peschiera CA: Hydatid cysts of the lung. In Steele J (ed): The Treatment of Mycotic and Parasitic Diseases of the Chest. Springfield, Ill, Thomas, 1964, p 201.
399. Lichter I: Surgery of pulmonary hydatid cyst—the Barrett technique. Thorax 27:529, 1972.
400. Xanthakis D, Efthimiadis M, Papadakis G, Primikirios N, Chassapakis G, Roussaki A, Vernnis N, Krivaskis A, Aligizakis CJ: Hydatid disease of the chest. Report of 91 patients surgically treated. Thorax 27:517, 1972.
401. Pinch LW, Wilson JF: Nonsurgical management of cystic hydatid disease in Alaska. A review of 30 cases of *Echinococcus granulosus* infection treated without operation. Ann Surg 178:45, 1973.
401a. Hau T. personal communication.

MEDIASTINITIS

402. Pearse HE Jr: Mediastinitis following cervical suppuration. Ann Surg 108:588, 1938.
403. Payne WS, Larson RH: Acute mediastinitis. Surg Clin North Am 49:999, 1969.
404. Moncada R, Warpeha R, Pickleman J, Spak M, Cardoso M, Berkow A, White H: Mediastinitis from odontogenic and deep cervical infection. Anatomic pathways of propagation. Chest 73:497, 1978.
405. McCurdy JA Jr, MacInnis EL, Hays LL: Fatal mediastinitis after a dental infection. J Oral Surg 35:726, 1977.
406. Hendler BH, Quinn PD: Fatal mediastinitis secondary to odontogenic infection. J Oral Surg 36:308, 1978.
407. Enquist RW, Blanck RR, Butler RH: Nontraumatic mediastinitis. JAMA 236:1048, 1976.
408. Ellis FH: Disorders of the esophagus in the adult. In Sabiston DC Jr, Spencer FC (eds): Surgery of the Chest, 3rd ed. Philadelphia, Saunders, 1976, pp 678–726.
409. Sprinkle PM, Veltri RW, Kantor LM: Abscesses of the head and neck. Laryngoscope 84:1142, 1974.
410. Janecka IP, Rankow RM: Fatal mediastinitis following retropharyngeal abscess. Arch Otolaryngol 93:630, 1971.
411. Sandrasagra FA, English TAH, Milstein BB: The management and prognosis of oesophageal perforation. Br J Surg 65:629, 1978.
412. Engelman RM, Saxena A, Levitsky S: Delayed mediastinal infection after ventricular aneurysm resection. Ann Thorac Surg 25:470, 1978.
413. Moseley PW, Ochsner JL, Mills NL, Chapman J: Management of an infected Hancock prosthesis after repair of truncus arteriosus. J Thorac Cardiovasc Surg 73:306, 1977.
414. Crosby IK, Tegtmeyer C: Mycotic aneurysm of the ascending aorta following coronary revascularization. Ann Thorac Surg 25:474, 1979.
415. Schowengerdt CG, Suyemoto R, Main FB: Granulomatous and fibrous mediastinitis. A review and analysis of 180 cases. J Thorac Cardiovasc Surg 57:365, 1969.
416. Kunkel WM Jr, Clagett OT, McDonald JR: Mediastinal granulomas. J Thorac Surg 27:565, 1954.
417. Keefer CS: Acute and chronic mediastinitis: A study of sixty cases. Arch Intern Med 62:109, 1938.
418. Ferguson TB, Burford TH: Mediastinal granuloma. A 15-year experience. Ann Thorac Surg 1:125, 1965.
419. Jenkins DW, Fisk DE, Byrd RB: Mediastinal histoplasmosis with esophageal abscess. Two case reports. Gastroenterology 70:109, 1976.
420. Hutchin P, Lindskog GE: Acquired esophagobronchial fistula of infectious origin. J Thorac Cardiovasc Surg 48:1, 1964.
421. Hewlett TH, Steer A, Thomas DE: Progressive fibrosing mediastinitis. Ann Thorac Surg 2:345, 1966.
422. Fairbank JT, Tampas JP, Longstreth G: Superior vena caval obstruction in histoplasmosis. Am J Roentgenol Radium Ther Nucl Med 115:488, 1972.
423. Greenwood MF, Holland P: Tracheal obstruction secondary to histoplasma mediastinal granuloma. Chest 62:642, 1972.
424. Picardi JL, Kauffman CA, Schwarz J, Holmes JC, Fowler NO: Pericarditis caused by *Histoplasma capsulatum*. Am J Cardiol 37:82, 1976.
425. Pate JW, Hammon J: Superior vena cava syndrome due to histoplasmosis in children. Ann Surg 161:778, 1965.
426. Rosenbaum AE, Schweepe HI Jr, Rabin ER: Constrictive pericarditis, pneumopericardium, and aortic aneurysm due to *Histoplasma capsulatum*. N Engl J Med 270:935, 1964.
427. Cooley DA, Hallman GL: Superior vena caval syndrome treated by azygos vein-inferior vena caval anastomosis: Report of successful case. J Thorac Cardiovasc Surg 47:325, 1964.
428. Zajtchuk R, Strevey TE, Heydorn WH, Tresure RL: Mediastinal histoplasmosis: Surgical considerations. J Thorac Cardiovasc Surg 66:300, 1973.
429. Belsey R, Hiebert CA: An exclusive right thoracic approach for cancer of the middle third of the esophagus. Ann Thorac Surg 18:1, 1974.
430. Lyons WS, Seremetis MG, deGuzman VC, Peabody JW Jr: Ruptures and perforations of the esophagus: The case for conservative supportative management. Ann Thorac Surg 25:346, 1978.
431. Sawyers JL, Lane CE, Foster JH, Daniel RA: Esophageal perforation: An increasing challenge. Ann Thorac Surg 19:233, 1975.
432. Goldberg M, Balthazar E, Nichols R: Subacute pyogenic osteomyelitis of the thoracic spine diagnosed by gallium scan. Case report. Ill Med J 148:62, 1975.
433. Seybold WD, Johnson MA III, Leary WV: Perforation of the esophagus. An analysis of 50 cases and an account of experimental studies. Surg Clin North Am 30:1155, 1950.
434. Kramer P: Infections of the esophagus. In Bockus HL (ed): Gastroenterology. Philadelphia, Saunders, 1974, pp 329–338.
435. Orringer MB, Sloan H: Monilial esophagitis: An increasingly frequent cause of esophageal stenosis? Ann Thorac Surg 26:364, 1978.
436. Finegold SM: Anaerobic Bacteria in Human Disease. New York, Academic, 1977.

CHAPTER 31
Infections of the Heart

RAYMOND A. AMOURY

CARDIAC DEFENSES AGAINST INFECTION

SEVERAL anatomic and physiologic characteristics of the heart serve to prevent infection. The most important is the combined effect of the rapid flow of blood through the heart, which normally washes out any organism before it can proliferate, and the smooth endothelial surface, to which bacteria cannot adhere. When the endothelium is damaged by whatever cause, platelets and fibrin form a nonbacterial thrombotic vegetation to which bacteria can adhere. In addition, the slower turbulent flow that results impairs washout and permits proliferation in situ.

Similar protective factors are at work within the myocardium itself. The coronary arteries supply a capillary bed in extensive ultrastructural communication with the myofibrils of the heart. Myocardial contraction eliminates stasis from this rich vascular network. Any organism that enters the coronary circulation is rapidly washed out. The rich lymphatic supply of the myocardium has a similar function. Miller et al [1] found that dogs with impaired cardiac lymph drainage are more prone to develop acute endocarditis and myocarditis following intravenous injection of staphylococci than are dogs with normal lymphatics. For these reasons, myocardial infection is rarely seen even after myocardial infarction, unless endocarditis is also present.

Of minor importance is the action of the pulmonary vascular bed to filter microbes from the circulation before they reach the coronary vessels.

Certain other characteristics of the heart serve to localize or restrict infections when they occur. The pericardial sac is the best example (Chapter 32), but several other factors are at work as well. The thick, fibrous, and elastic subendocardial tissues appear to act as a natural barrier against the spread of endocardial infection to the myocardium.[2] The trabeculae carneae tend to entrap foreign bodies (eg, cardiac pacing wires), which tend to become infected.[3] The sinuses of Valsalva are obviously sites of turbulent blood flow and are well recognized sites of infection.[4]

INFECTIONS OF THE MYOCARDIUM

MYOCARDITIS AND MYOCARDIAL ABSCESS

Myocardial Infection in Patients With Coronary Artery Disease

Infection is a rare complication of coronary artery disease, even with advanced ischemia and myocardial necrosis. The same may be said for patients with hypertension, left ventricular hypertrophy, and secondary ischemia. In fact isolated abscesses of the myocardium seldom occur except in association with endocarditis. Gopalakrishna et al [2] reported a case of myocardial abscess which developed within a myocardial infarction. The infection was caused by group F streptococci, which had metastasized from a metatarsal osteomyelitis. They found 11 other cases in the English literature: *S. aureus* (4), *E. coli* (2), *Clostridium perfringens* (2), pneumococcus, beta-hemolytic *Streptococcus, Bacteroides.* A primary distant focus of infection was recognized as the source in six cases.

The mechanism of abscess formation within a myocardial infarction is uncertain, but it does not appear to be the result of septic embolization to a major coronary artery, because the artery is usually occluded by a bland thrombus. In addition, the artery walls show no evidence of arteritis. Bacteria probably penetrate the infarct via surrounding collaterals.[2]

Myocardial Infection in Patients with Septicemia

Interstitial myocarditis, myocardial abscess, and mural endocarditis limited to nonvalvular endothelium without valvular lesions or vegetations and with patent coronary arteries are extremely rare. Milstoc and Berger [3] have described a case caused by coagulase-negative *Staphylococcus.* The sequence of events is presumed to be septicemia, usually from an obvious site, with production of a focus of interstitial myocarditis and subsequent formation of an abscess. The abscess and surrounding interstitial exudative myocardial process then extends to and disrupts the endothelial surface, with deposition of a necrotic mass of fibrin, bacteria, and blood elements on the endocardial surface.

Myocardial Infection in Patients With Bacterial Endocarditis

Most myocardial abscesses appear in the upper interventricular septum of patients with aortic (or less often mitral) endocarditis.[4] The organisms are those that infect the valve. The diagnosis of myocardial abscess is seldom made during the patient's life but should be suspected when a patient with aortic or mitral endocarditis develops conduction disturbances resulting from septal involvement. Echocardiography can be used to support the diagnosis if septal thickening is found. The use of isotopic gallium 67 citrate imaging can be helpful when all other diagnostic maneuvers fail. Drainage and valvular replacement have been effective.[4]

Echinococcus Infection of the Myocardium

Echinococcus is an uncommon cause of infection of the heart and is treatable only by operation. The diagnosis should be considered in patients with cardiac symptoms who have been in an endemic area.[5]

Epidemiology, Incidence, and Pathogenesis

The epidemiology of echinococcosis is discussed in Chapter 11. Echinococcosis is endemic in sheep-raising countries. People are accidental hosts after ingesting ova on contaminated vegetables or after handling dogs that shed ova in their feces.

Less than 2 percent of the patients with echinococcosis have cardiac involvement because the larvae must first escape the hepatic and pulmonary filters to reach the coronary arteries. The left ventricular wall and the interventricular septum are most frequently infected, perhaps because of their more extensive blood supply.

Clinical Manifestations

Most patients with echinococcus disease of the heart are asymptomatic, and the diagnosis is first made on routine roentgen examination. When symptoms occur, they are generally caused by the enlarging cyst or its rupture. Arrhythmias can result from interference with the conduction system of the interventricular septum. In some cases, heart murmurs are caused by papillary muscle dysfunction that causes valvular insufficiency. A pulmonary systolic ejection murmur can result from the establishment of flow gradients between the right ventricular chamber and pulmonary artery, because of the projection of a cyst into the right ventricular outflow tract. Precordial pain appears to be related to episodes of partial cyst rupture into the pericardium causing pericarditis, which in turn causes either severe fibrosis (constrictive pericarditis) or pericardial effusion with tamponade. Rupture into a chamber is even more common, as there is no overlying pericardium to reinforce the cyst wall. Rupture into the left ventricle results in systemic emboli which, if not fatal, can produce metastatic lesions or infarcts. Acute and chronic cor pulmonale and metastatic pulmonary echinococcosis can follow rupture into the right ventricle.

Diagnosis

The most important historic point in the diagnosis is previous hydatid disease in other organs (liver or lung). The Casoni intradermal test and the less specific complement-fixation test results are corroborative when positive, but do not rule out the diagnosis when they are negative (Chapter 11). Eosinophilia is found in less than 25 percent of the patients and may indicate recent infection or rupture. Absence of eosinophilia may indicate death or degeneration of the cyst. Electrocardiographic abnormalities have been noted with hydatid cysts and help to distinguish them from ventricular aneurysms.

The roentgen findings are not diagnostic but vary with the stage of the disease. Plain films in various projections will help locate the cysts, and fluoroscopy can reveal an absence of paradoxical pulsation, but the most specific finding is the appearance of a calcification within a mass or in its periphery. Such peripheral calcification, if constrictive pericarditis is not present, indicates ecchinococcus disease of the heart.

Angiocardiography is the most informative of the radiologic studies, because it indicates the degree of penetration of a cyst into a cardiac chamber and differentiates a cyst from a ventricular aneurysm. Coronary arteriography shows displacement of vessels by a cyst and its lack of vascularization. The differential diagnosis includes mediastinal and cardiac tumors, pericardial cysts, and ventricular aneurysms.

Treatment

Excision is the only effective treatment for cardiac echinococcosis. If the cyst is accessible, it can be aspirated and any remaining viable scolices can be killed by the instillation of 2 percent formalin, ether, or preferably concentrated (30 percent) sodium chloride to prevent dissemination if the contents are spilled. The cyst can then be opened to remove its germinative lining.

When a cyst projects into a cardiac chamber with danger of rupture, a cardiopulmonary bypass is recommended for greater mobilization of the heart and adequate control should an intracavitary cyst rupture or a ventricle be perforated. In addition, bypass allows for resection of the heart wall if necessary, as in treating an aneurysm of the ventricle.

Myocardial Infections in the Immunologically Compromised Patient

Many factors can alter host resistance to make a patient abnormally susceptible to myocardial infections (Chapter 47). Candidal myocardial infections have been reported in patients treated with steroids, in leukemia patients treated with chemotherapeutic drugs, and in patients with burns. Most of these patients have small, diffuse abscesses that are not amenable to drainage (Fig. 31-1).

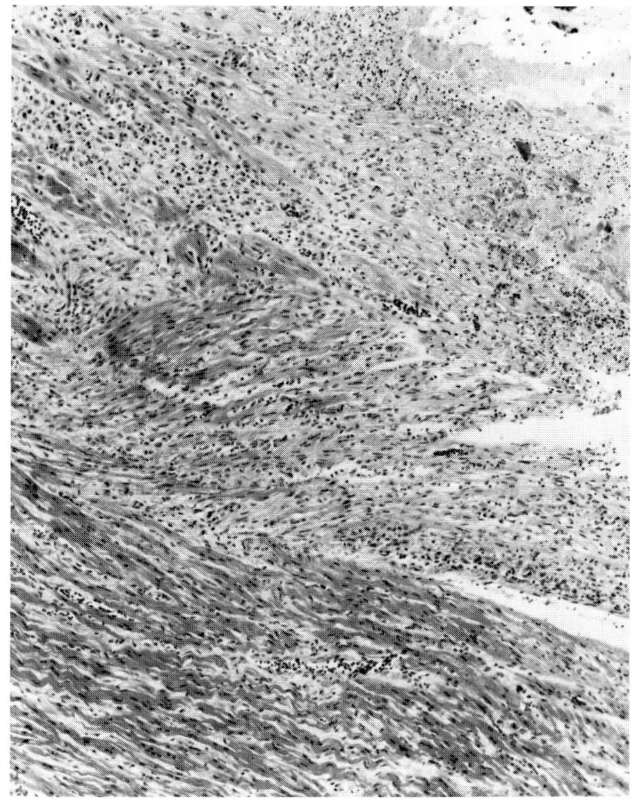

Fig. 31-1. Microabscesses in the myocardium of a severely burned child. Multifocal abscesses were present at postmortem examination. She died as a consequence of *S. aureus* (coagulase-positive) sepsis.

Myocardial Infections Caused by Trauma

Nonpenetrating chest trauma can cause cardiac contusion and occasionally valvular injury, such as aortic insufficiency. Infection of a traumatically damaged valve is rare. Penetrating wounds of the heart can cause both pericarditis and endocarditis. Enders et al [6] emphasize that both wound infection and intracardiac infection are less common than expected. *P. aeruginosa* and *S. aureus* [7] have been reported as etiologic agents. Projectiles embedded in the heart for a long time may also be sites for infection.[8]

INFECTIOUS ENDOCARDITIS

Infectious endocarditis is the most important infection of the heart. This subject has been reviewed in detail in monographs edited by Kaye,[9] Kaplan and Taranta,[10] and Rahimtoola.[11] This section will discuss only infections of the native endocardium. Subsequent sections will deal with prosthetic valve endocarditis.

Classification, Incidence, and Underlying Heart Disease

The established classification of endocarditis into acute and subacute forms has given way to a classification based on the identity of the causative microorganism, because both clinical features and treatment vary according to the organism.[9] The incidence of infectious endocarditis ranges between 0.3 to 3 per 1,000 hospital admissions. More than one-half of the patients are older than 50. Because endocarditis is found at areas of turbulence, such as at damaged or deformed valves and at sites of high pressure, a number of cardiac conditions predispose to these infections.[12]

Rheumatic Heart Disease. Nearly 50 percent of the patients with endocarditis have rheumatic heart disease, but the incidence is falling. The mitral valve is most frequently deformed by the rheumatic process and is the most common site for endocarditis. The aortic valve is next most commonly deformed, and in endocarditis it is infected alone or in combination (usually with the mitral valve) in over half the patients. Infection of the tricuspid valve occurs in less than 10 percent of patients with rheumatic heart disease and is usually accompanied by infection of the left heart valves.

Congenital Heart Disease. Approximately one-fifth of the patients with infective endocarditis initially have congenital heart lesions. Patent ductus arteriosus, ventricular septal defects, bicuspid aortic valve, coarctation of the aorta, pulmonic stenosis, and tetralogy of Fallot are the most commonly associated lesions.

No Apparent Heart Disease. Certain organisms can attack normal valves and cause endocarditis in patients without underlying heart disease. As many as 50 percent or more of the patients with endocarditis caused by *S. aureus, S. pneumoniae,* group A beta-hemolytic *Streptococcus,* and enterococcus may have no underlying heart disease. Opportunistic infections also occur on normal valves in patients with defects in host defense, in those receiving antibiotic therapy, and in drug addicts.

Degenerative Heart Disease. Degenerative or atherosclerotic lesions seldom predispose to infection, but the incidence appears to be increasing in the older population, especially in males with calcific aortic stenosis. Rare cases of endocarditis in patients with coronary artery disease have been reported.

Arteriovenous Fistulas. Peripheral arteriovenous fistulas have been created in animals to produce endocarditis, and this association has been found in humans with acquired arteriovenous fistulas. Patients with hemodialysis shunts in place can also develop endocarditis, and Quintiliani and Ganguli [12] reported a rare association of splenic arteriovenous fistula with bacterial endarteritis and endocarditis caused by coagulase-negative *Staphylococcus.* Coronary arteriovenous fistulas are rare lesions and are seldom complicated by bacterial endarteritis.

Other Predisposing Lesions. Subaortic stenosis was a major cause of endocarditis in the preantibiotic era, and acute endocarditis is occasionally seen in a patient with idiopathic hypertrophic subaortic stenosis. Mitral involvement can also occur. Mitral valve prolapse syndrome is

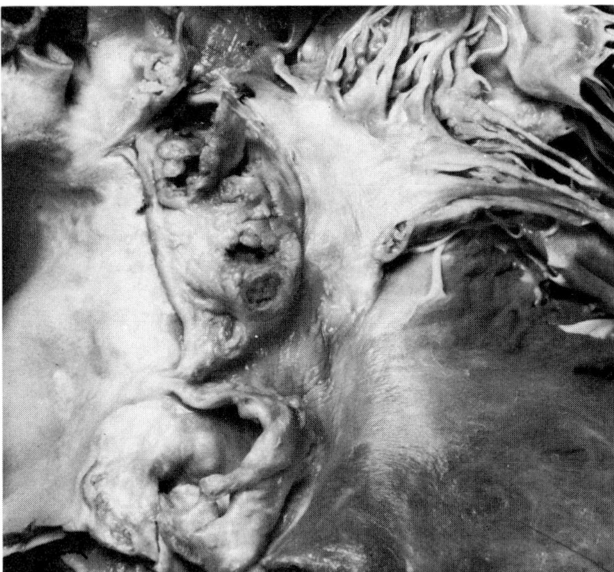

Fig. 31-2. Aortic valve showing background of rheumatic fibrosis and retraction of one cusp. Other two cusps show numerous perforations from bacterial endocarditis caused by beta-hemolytic *Streptococcus.* (From Dr. Jesse E. Edwards, Department of Pathology, United Hospitals, Inc., Miller Division, St. Paul, Minnesota.)

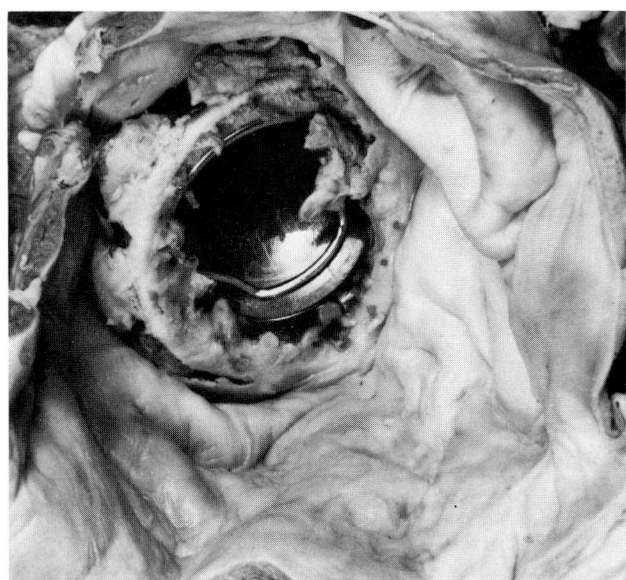

Fig. 31-3. Interior of left atrium and view of Bjork-Shiley prosthesis from above. Vegetations and dehiscence of prosthetic valve seat are the result of bacterial infection. (From Dr. Jesse E. Edwards, Department of Pathology, United Hospitals, Inc., Miller Division, St. Paul, Minnesota.)

a recently defined lesion which predisposes to infective endocarditis. Syphilitic aortitis is seldom found in patients with endocarditis, and does not appear to increase a patient's susceptibility.

Pathology of Infective Endocarditis

The pathology of infective endocarditis must include the pathologic alterations in the heart and in other organs.

Cardiac Pathology. Vegetations are classically found on the valves of patients with infective endocarditis. (Fig. 31-2). These lesions vary in number, size, color, and consistency, and tend to localize on the atrial surfaces of the atrioventricular valves and on the ventricular surfaces of the semilunar valves. Histologically, the vegetation consists of an amorphous mass of fibrin, leukocytes, and masses of red cell debris and bacteria. These may be suppurative, or show destruction of the underlying valve, or both. Granulation tissue is seen at the base of the lesion, with a nonspecific inflammatory response. The bacteria may be difficult to identify or may be seen at the surface or in the interior of the vegetation. If antibiotic therapy is successful, fibrosis, hyalinization, and calcification of the vegetation occurs with reendothelialization. Outpouchings, or aneurysms, of portions of a valve can develop in an area of valvulitis from scarring and altered hydrodynamics. Other destructive effects produced by vegetations are perforation, erosive aneurysms of the sinus of Valsalva, rupture of a papillary muscle or of chordae tendineae, and abscesses of the valve ring, at times with fistula formation and rupture of the interventricular septum.[13,14] (Fig. 31-3).

Myocarditis is an important complication of endocarditis and is recognized with increased frequency. Its pathogenesis is unclear, but ischemic damage secondary to coronary artery occlusion by emboli, damage as a result of microbial toxins, invasion of the myocardium by microorganisms, and the activity of immune complexes resulting in a vasculitis of arterioles and capillaries have all been suggested as causes. Myocardial abscesses containing bacteria have been found in about one-fifth of cases. Involvement of the pericardium is rare.[14]

Pathogenesis of the Cardiac Lesions. The characteristic lesion in infective endocarditis is an infected thrombus or vegetation on the endocardial surface, usually along the closing edges of the valve leaflets or cusps. There seem to be two mechanisms by which valves can become infected. The first is embolization of microorganisms to the valvular interstitium. This mechanism is unlikely because valves are vascularized only at their proximal parts, which are rarely colonized early in the disease. The more likely mechanism is infection of the endocardium by implantation of microorganisms on the endocardial surfaces of the valve.

The primary valvular lesion appears to be the result of platelet aggregation induced by contact with a foreign surface, ie, the endocardial surface previously damaged by disease or hemodynamic alteration. A nonbacterial thrombus composed largely of platelets becomes adherent to the site of endothelial damage.[14] Such sterile thrombi are found in rheumatic heart disease, as well as in patients with malignant and wasting disease and with connective tissue disorders, such as systemic lupus erythematosus. They serve as predisposing sites for bacterial endocarditis in rheumatic heart disease, but for obscure reasons are often harmless in the other conditions. Subsequent bacteremia can result in colonization of the platelet fibrin mass with the establishment of infection.

Nonbacterial and bacterial endocarditis share the same location and frequency of involvement. For example, in both acute rheumatic fever and bacterial endocarditis, the atrial surface of the mitral valve and the ventricular surface of the aortic valve are most frequently involved, followed by the aortic, tricuspid, and rarely the pulmonic valves.

Platelet aggregation can be induced by a variety of stimuli, in addition to thrombin, epinephrine, and adenosine diphosphate.[15] Clawson [15] has pointed out that some common bacterial pathogens such as staphylococci and streptococci may themselves act to stimulate platelet aggregation. This results in the incorporation of the bacteria into the aggregate. The location of large numbers of bacteria deep within the sanctuary of a platelet-fibrin mass provides a mechanical barrier to their elimination by phagocytes and probably to penetration by antibiotics and antibodies. Clawson has reviewed other interactions between platelets and bacteria.[15] Once the sterile thrombus is in place, bacteremia from any source can infect the damaged valve—a local infection in the skin, infected thrombi within the bloodstream, and direct inoculation of bacteria into the circulation. Most cases of clinical endocarditis, however, appear to arise from transient bacteremia, which occurs in normal individuals without a septic focus. Manipulation of contaminated mucosal surfaces can produce transient bacteremia. For example, people develop bacteremia after brushing their teeth or using an oral irrigation apparatus (Table 31-1). Tooth extraction causes a mixed bacteremia, with *S. viridans* and *B. melaninogenicus* as the predominant organisms in a majority of patients. The frequency of bacteremia from these sources is related to the degree of peridontal disease and the degree of trauma inflicted during the procedure, with infection being the more important factor. In addition, sigmoidoscopy and barium enema can both induce bacteremia, as does transurethral prostatic resection, cytoscopy, urethral dilatation and catheterization, abortion, delivery, and instrumentation of the female reproductive tract.[16] The properties of certain bacteria which enable them to adhere to endothelium are discussed in a subsequent section.

Valve dysfunction can result from either obstruction or destruction of the valve. As a result of continued deposition of platelets and fibrin, the vegetation can grow and obstruct the orifice. This is especially likely in fungal endocarditis but has also been reported with staphylococcal endocarditis of the mitral valve.[17] In other instances, especially in *S. aureus* endocarditis, destruction of tissue with resulting valvular insufficiency can result. In still other cases, healing with scar formation can produce valvular insufficiency or stenosis. Infection can also extend into the myocardium from the periphery of a valve, as into the mitral annulus or along the sinus of Valsalva into the aortic ring and produce burrowing abscesses. Septic emboli from infected, necrotic, calcified vegetations can produce infarcts in the lung, heart, brain, kidneys, spleen, liver, and extremities. Abscesses may develop when *S. aureus* endocarditis is the source of the emboli. Septic embolization to the vasa vasora or direct bacterial invasion of the arterial wall can predispose to the formation of mycotic aneurysms in the sinus of Valsalva and the aorta and its branches with the potential for rupture.

TABLE 31-1. INCIDENCE OF BACTEREMIA AFTER VARIOUS PROCEDURES

Procedure/Manipulation	Percentage of Positive Blood Cultures
DENTAL	
Dental extraction	18–85
Periodontal surgery	32–88
Chewing candy or paraffin	17–51
Tooth brushing	0–26
Oral irrigation device	27–50
UPPER AIRWAY	
Bronchoscopy (rigid scope)	15
Tonsillectomy	28–38
Nasotracheal suctioning/intubation	16
GASTROINTESTINAL	
Upper GI endoscopy	8–12
Sigmoidoscopy/colonoscopy	0–9.5
Barium enema	11
Percutaneous needle biopsy of liver	3–13
UROLOGIC	
Urethral dilatation	18–33
Urethral catheterization	8
Cystoscopy	0–17
Transurethral prostatic resection	12–46
OBSTETRIC/GYNECOLOGIC	
Normal vaginal delivery	0–11
Punch biopsy cervix	0
Removal/insertion of IUD	0

Scheld WM, Sande MA: Endocarditis and intravascular infections. In Mandell G, Douglas RG, Bennett JE: *Principles and Practice of Infectious Diseases* (Vol I). New York, Wiley, 1979, p 653.

Experimental Endocarditis. Some experimental models of endocarditis have shed light on the pathogenesis of the disease. For example, endocarditis occurs naturally in the opossum, in which the stress of captivity appears to produce the infection. As in man, the infection is caused by *S. viridans*, and the mitral and aortic valves are primarily involved. Bacterial inoculation consistently produces the disease in this species. Experimental endocarditis can be produced in many other animals: transarterial trauma to the aortic and mitral valves, high altitude, hypothermia, polycythemia, and the administration of vasoactive substances all predispose to valvulitis and vegetations.

Lillehei, Bobb, and Visscher [18] created arteriovenous (AV) fistulas in dogs as a method of producing endocardial changes and increasing the likelihood of valve deformities and endocarditis. The shunt must be large enough to increase cardiac output; the number and dimension of the fistulas required varied inversely with the age of the animal; younger animals required significantly more peripheral shunt flow to produce endocarditis. These investigators concluded that any condition that increased cardiac output could cause endocardial damage, leading to a nonbacterial thrombotic endocarditis that subsequently became infected.

Experimental endocarditis can be achieved in rabbits

or rats positioning a polyethylene catheter within the heart. The catheter induces vegetations, which can then be infected. If the catheter is removed long enough before microbial inoculation for the valve to reendothelialize, susceptibility to colonization is reduced.[19]

The level of metabolic activity of bacterial colonies in these vegetations was determined using tritiated L-alanine. The colonies in the periphery of the vegetation are the most active, while those in the interior were less active. Since some antibiotics depend on cell wall synthesis and cell division for their bactericidal action, the interior organisms may be difficult to eradicate. Hooke and Sande[20] prevented development of thrombotic vegetations by anticoagulation, but this did not prevent valvular colonization. The authors suggested that the fibrin vegetation actually retarded the disease by containing the bacteria. In the treated animals, the absence of vegetations allowed for more rapid eradication of infection, suggesting that rapid bacterial division on the outside of the vegetation makes them more susceptible to penicillin. These studies have definite correlates in clinical disease, especially in prosthetic valve infections.

A number of investigators have studied the possible role of cardiac lymphatic obstruction in the pathogenesis of cardiac disease, but the exact role in endocarditis is not yet clear. Symbas et al[21] studied the susceptibility to endocarditis in three groups of dogs. In six dogs no surgical procedure was done; in six dogs the cardiac lymphatics were interrupted; and in six animals two arteriovenous fistulas were created. Five million *S. aureus* organisms were injected intravenously three times at 3-day intervals. None of the control dogs developed endocarditis, and only one dog in the group with interrupted cardiac lymphatics developed chronic myocarditis without endocarditis. In the group with arteriovenous fistulas, three out of the six dogs developed endocarditis with gram-negative rods but not with the injected staphylococci.

Animal models of endocarditis are important in planning prophylactic and therapeutic antimicrobial regimens. For example, bacteriostatic drugs were of no value in experimental streptococcal endocarditis even when used on a sensitive organism for a prolonged period; bactericidal regimens were necessary. Multiple factors are involved in models using *S. viridans, S. aureus, S. fecalis, Pseudomonas, Candida,* and *Aspergillus.*[22] These studies indicate that effective prophylaxis is dependent on use of a microbicidal regimen that will achieve high blood levels for 6 or more hours after an episode of bacteremia.

Noncardiac Pathologic Features Associated With Infective Endocarditis.

Kidney. Diffuse glomerulonephritis may be a reaction to circulating antigen-antibody complexes. This concept is supported by electron microscopic studies showing dense, subepithelial deposits in the glomeruli of patients with endocarditis and nephritis, as well as deposits of immune globulins in glomerular basement membranes. Chronicity of infection may be important, as it is necessary for the organism or its antigens to stimulate antibody production and also to supply antigen for the formation of soluble complexes. The site of deposition in the glomeruli appears to depend on the size of the complex. In this way, small complexes formed under conditions of antigen excess are found in a subepithelial locus and are associated with diffuse proliferation. Large antigen-antibody complexes formed under conditions of antibody excess are deposited on the inside of the glomerular basement membrane and are accompanied by focal nephritis.

Skin. Petechiae and subungual splinter hemorrhages may be due to emboli or a hypersensitivity vasculitis. *Osler nodes* are the painful, erythematous elevations found in the digital pads, and these may be due to hypersensitivity vasculitis, probably immune complex deposition. Janeway nodes are painless hemorrhagic lesions that occur on the palms, soles, or tips of the digits. They are necrotic and contain polymorphonuclear leukocytes and bacteria.[14]

Spleen. Splenomegaly is frequently found. Microscopically, there is hyperplasia of lymphoid follicles and often considerable proliferation of reticuloendothelial cells. Splenic infarcts are noted in about one-third of patients coming to autopsy.

Central Nervous System and Eye. Mycotic aneurysms, embolic infarcts, and arteritis are all common. Additional findings include intracerebral and subarachnoid hemorrhage and encephalomalacia. Meningitis is uncommon. In the eye, petechial hemorrhages in the conjunctiva and retina are common, as are flame-shaped retinal hemorrhages.[14]

Immunologic Phenomena. A number of immunologic phenomena accompany endocarditis. Circulating antibodies against the pathogen appear. Hypergammaglobulinemia is associated with an increase in the plasma cells of the bone marrow. Approximately half the patients have positive serum tests for rheumatoid factor within 6 weeks. Complement levels may be low in patients in whom immune complex glomerulonephritis develops. Circulating cryoglobulins may appear and cause vascular occlusions in the digits of some patients. Hyperstimulation of the macrophage system is manifested by histiocytes in the peripheral blood. The role, if any, of each of these findings in the pathogenesis of the clinical manifestations is as yet not clear.[16]

Etiology of Infective Endocarditis

Common Infectious Agents. Although almost any bacteria are capable of producing bacterial endocarditis, streptococci and staphylococci account for 90 to 95 percent of cases in which an infecting organism can be identified (Table 31-2).

Streptococci. Streptococci are the causative microorganisms in 60 to 80 percent of blood culture–positive cases of infective endocarditis. The viridans streptococci account for more than one-half of cases of streptococcal endocarditis. Enterococci cause between 10 and 20 percent of the cases, but the relative incidence is increasing. Microaerophilic and anaerobic streptococci, nonhemolytic streptococci, group A beta-hemolytic streptococci, and streptococci of other groups account for the rest. Almost all cases of anaerobic endocarditis are due to streptococci.[23]

TABLE 31-2. ETIOLOGIC AGENTS OF INFECTIVE ENDOCARDITIS

Agent	Percent of Total Cases
The viridans streptococci	60–70
Staphylococcus aureus	10–20
S. faecalis (enterococcus)	5–15
S. epidermidis	5–10
Gram-negative rods	2–3
Fungi (*Candida, Aspergillus* species)	1–2
Miscellaneous bacteria	5
Blood culture negative	5–15

Sande MA, Strausbaugh LJ: Infective Endocarditis. In Hook EW, Mandell GL, Gwaltney JM Jr, Sande MA (eds): *Current Concepts of Infectious Diseases.* New York, Wiley, 1977, p 55.

The biology and taxonomy of the streptococci are discussed in Chapter 4. The dextran-forming strains were more often found in endocardial infection than the non-dextran-producing strains, although the role of dextran is not completely known. Dextran-like polysaccharides (eg, glucan) may be important in adherence of these bacteria to both teeth and endocardial tissue.

Striking differences to adherence of bacteria to endocardial tissue can be observed. Enterococci are most adherent, followed by staphylococci and viridans streptococci. *P. aeruginosa,* and *E. coli* were much less adherent. The ability to adhere to valvular endothelium may be an essential characteristic of the bacteria that cause human endocarditis.

Staphylococci. Staphylococci are the causative microorganisms in 10 to 30 percent of cases with positive blood cultures. The biology of the staphylococci is discussed in Chapter 4. Coagulase-positive staphylococci are isolated much more frequently than coagulase-negative staphylococci, especially in patients with the acute form of bacterial endocarditis. Coagulase-positive staphylococci can attack either normal or previously damaged heart valves and cause rapid destruction of valve substance with a fulminant and often fatal course. Death can occur within days from overwhelming bacteremia and within weeks from heart failure. Multifocal abscesses also occur from septic emboli and infarcts.

Coagulase-negative staphylococci account for only 1 to 3 percent of blood culture–positive endocarditis and are seen in patients with more subacute disease. These organisms usually attack heart valves with preexisting abnormalities or damage without causing rapid destruction.

The incidence of coagulase-positive staphylococcal endocarditis is increasing in drug addicts and patients with endocarditis following prosthetic valve replacement. In the latter group, coagulase-negative staphylococci are also a major cause of endocarditis.[24]

Uncommon Infectious Agents. Table 31-3 lists the less common and rare organisms associated with endocarditis. Almost all species of bacteria have been reported. Pneumococci have become uncommon causes of infective endocarditis (5 percent of cases) since effective therapy of pneumonia and otitis became available. Once established, pneumococci can attack normal or previously damaged valves and can cause rapid destruction. The gonococcus can attack and destroy either normal or previously damaged heart valves and was once a common cause of right heart endocarditis. It is now seldom seen.

Aside from the anaerobic streptococci, the most common anaerobes causing endocarditis are *Bacteroides* and *Actinomyces.*[23]

Mixed Infections. Two or more organisms are seldom involved simultaneously except in *Candida* infections, in which bacteria such as *S. aureus* may coexist with and probably precede the *Candida* infection. Prolonged antibiotic treatment of bacterial endocarditis can predispose to fungal superinfection.

Fungi. Fungal endocarditis is uncommon (Table 31-3), occurring principally in: (1) narcotics addicts, (2) patients receiving intravenous hyperalimentation, (3) patients receiving steroids, cytotoxic agents, and broad-spectrum antibiotics, and (4) patients with infected intracardiac prostheses.[24] *Candida, Aspergillus,* and *Histoplasma* species are the most common causes of fungal endocarditis, with *Candida* leading in overall frequency. *C. albicans* is the most common candidal organism isolated, but *C. tropicalis, C. krusei, C. parapsilosis,* and other candidal species have also been found.

Cell Wall-deficient Forms. These forms are usually isolated using hypertonic media when routine blood cultures are sterile. They are induced by antibiotics, and their presence does not necessarily implicate them in the pathologic process. Their persistence during therapy and subsequent reversion to the parent form may explain some relapses. The failure of penicillin as the sole therapy against enterococcal endocarditis is an illustration. In this situation, cell wall-deficient forms may be induced by penicillin. Successful therapy requires the addition of an aminoglyco-

TABLE 31-3. UNCOMMON AND RARE ORGANISMS IN ENDOCARDITIS

PYOGENIC COCCI	OTHER RARE CAUSES
Pneumococci	Meningococci
N. gonorrhoeae	*Coxiella burnetii*
GRAM-NEGATIVE BACILLAE	Diphtheroids
Salmonella	*Spirillum minus*
Streptobacillus moniliformis	*Listeria*
Serratia marcescens	Micrococci
Bacteroides	Propionibacterium
Hemophilus	FUNGI
Brucella	*Candida* } Most common
	Aspergillus } Most common
	Histoplasma } Most common
	Blastomyces
	Cryptococcus
	Mucor
	Torulopsis

side that is active against these bacterial forms. The frequency of cell wall-deficient bacteria in endocarditis is unknown.

Coxiella burnetii. The cause of Q fever has been found also to cause endocarditis in patients with underlying heart disease. Although the course of the disease is characteristic of infectious endocarditis, antibiotic therapy is unsuccessful, and valve replacement plus antimicrobial therapy is required. It is possible to isolate the organism by inoculating the patient's blood into guinea pigs; however, a rise in titer of complement-fixing antibody to *C. burnetii* is usually necessary to make the diagnosis (Chapter 7).

Virus Infections. These can cause valve lesions in animals, but there is no evidence that viral infections can cause a clinical syndrome resembling bacterial or fungal endocarditis.

Clinical Manifestations

Infective endocarditis is capable of multiple organ system involvement, and clinical manifestations can therefore show marked variability. Variations in the patient's course will also depend on the offending organism. Endocarditis caused by viridans-type streptococci will have an insidious onset, with nonspecific complaints such as fever and malaise, which may persist for weeks. Acute endocarditis caused by *S. aureus* will have a more fulminant course with high fever, congestive heart failure, and emboli as possible complications. In short, the clinical diagnosis is unreliable—only persistently negative blood cultures exclude the diagnosis.

Fever is virtually always found. It is usually remitting and seldom exceeds 39C unless the infection is staphylococcal, pneumococcal, or gonococcal in origin.

A cardiac murmur is present in almost all patients but may be absent in acute endocarditis and in drug addicts in whom tricuspid valve involvement may not be accompanied by a murmur. Changing murmurs—once thought to be characteristic of the disease—are not common. An aortic diastolic murmur is significant and can be seen in some patients with staphylococcal endocarditis.

Splenomegaly is a frequent finding. A number of cutaneous signs can be seen. Osler nodes and Janeway nodes have been discussed in preceding sections. Petechiae are found in 20 to 40 percent of patients and are thought to represent blood extravasated from superficial capillaries damaged by the vasculitis.

Neurologic complications occur in 20 to 40 percent of patients and represent a major symptom in one-half of them. Manifestations are varied and include major cerebral emboli and mycotic aneurysms. Cerebral emboli most frequently involve the middle cerebral artery and its branches and can cause hemiplegia, cortical sensory loss, aphasia, ataxia, and confusion. Mycotic aneurysms can result from septic emboli. These lesions occur at bifurcations of small arteries and are most often seen with *S. viridans* infections. Mycotic aneurysms are small and seldom cause space-occupying neurologic signs. Rupture is a grave threat, and subarachnoid, cortical, or intraventricular hemorrhage can be disastrous.

An acute brain syndrome ranging from mild personality changes to frank psychosis has been reported in patients even without focal neurologic findings. Cerebrospinal fluid analysis shows increased numbers of cells, increased protein, and a normal glucose concentration. *S. aureus* is usually the causative organism and can occasionally produce acute purulent meningitis. Meningoencephalitis should be considered when signs and symptoms of toxic encephalopathy and meningitis are found in the same patient. Small, multifocal brain abscesses can also result from an embolic shower in staphylococcal endocarditis. They are usually too scattered and minute for surgical treatment and respond to antibiotics in most cases.

The renal changes have been noted in preceding sections. Microscopic hematuria is found in approximately one-half of patients. Reversible renal failure is more typical of subacute or chronic endocarditis. Renal infarction is usually associated with staphylococcal endocarditis.

Laboratory Findings in Infective Endocarditis

Hematology. Normochromic and normocytic anemia is found in nearly all patients. The low reticulocyte count, low serum iron, and reduced percent saturation of iron-binding capacity are found in spite of adequate iron stores in the bone marrow. These findings are seen in many chronic infections and are attributed to decreased erythrocyte production in the marrow caused by slow release of iron from tissue macrophages.[16]

Except for patients with acute endocarditis, a normal white blood count and normal differential counts or a mild shift to the left are seen. Leukopenia and thrombocytopenia are found in a minority of patients.[25]

Large mononuclear cells of the monocyte-macrophage lineage have been found in the marrow and in capillary blood; the ear lobe is a good source. Ingested organisms can sometimes be seen in these phagocytic cells, but more often they contain vacuoles and cellular debris.[25]

Powers and Mandell [26] have described a technique for the preparation of a concentrated monolayer of neutrophils and monocytes using a drop of venous blood. There is good correlation between the finding of bacteria within leukocytes, a clinical diagnosis of endocarditis, and the presence of positive blood cultures. A positive result may be considered as a strong indication to start therapy.

Erythrocyte sedimentation rates are consistently elevated. Although the test is nonspecific, a normal value is presumptive evidence against the diagnosis unless the patient is in congestive heart failure.

Urine. Microscopic hematuria, proteinuria, red blood cell casts, and white blood cell casts may all be found. Proteinuria is seen more commonly than hematuria.[25]

Teichoic Acid Antibodies. The presence of precipitating antibodies to teichoic acid may be useful in the diagnosis of serious staphylococcal infections (Chapter 4). Positive reactions are found in over three-fourths of patients with staphylococcal endocarditis,[25] and the technique may be of value in patients with negative blood cultures.

Diagnosis

Blood Cultures. The most important examination in establishing a diagnosis of infective endocarditis is a positive blood culture. Since the bacteremia of endocarditis is usually continuous, timing of venipuncture is not critical. Two or three separate sets of blood cultures should be collected within a 24-hour period. Skin preparation and collection of separate sets are most important, as some organisms found in the skin can cause endocarditis. In similar fashion, too large a volume of blood contaminated during a single venipuncture can result in a false-positive diagnosis. An adequate volume in adults is approximately 20 ml drawn at each venipuncture and inoculated in equal parts into two 100-ml vacuum blood culture bottles. One bottle should be used for anaerobic culture and the other vented transiently to allow for recovery of both anaerobic and aerobic organisms. Werner et al [27] report that the first blood culture was positive in 96 percent of the cases of streptococcal endocarditis, and one of the first two blood cultures was positive in 98 percent of the cases. In endocarditis caused by microorganisms other than streptococci, the first blood culture was positive in all cases. The incidence of positive results was slightly reduced when the patient had received an antimicrobial agent within 2 weeks.

Echocardiography. Localization of the valvular site may be helpful in planning surgical therapy. Obtaining quantitative cultures of blood proximal and distal to a valve is dangerous, because vegetations can be dislodged. The best current procedure is echocardiography. Vegetations are best seen on aortic and mitral valves, but even there they must be large.[28] Thomson et al [28] reviewed the ultrasound characteristics of vegetations on the aortic, mitral, and tricuspid valves in a total of 17 patients. Echocardiography correctly identified the abnormality in 11 valves. They found 8 valves with false-negative results and indicated that a negative echocardiogram does not exclude infective endocarditis. The echocardiographic criteria for diagnosis of infective endocarditis are noted in Table 31-4. Riba et al [29] demonstrated in rabbits that Indium 111 labeled platelets resulted in cardiac imaging sensitive enough to detect endocardial lesions. The clinical utility of this test has not been proved.

TABLE 31-4. ECHOCARDIOGRAPHIC CRITERIA FOR DIAGNOSIS OF INFECTIVE ENDOCARDITIS

AORTIC VALVE
Shaggy nonuniform thickening in systole and/or diastole with unrestricted leaflet motion
Shaggy echoes moving longitudinally across the aortic valve
MITRAL VALVE
Thick shaggy echoes from either leaflet, with unrestricted leaflet motion either attached to or moving behind the leaflets
Systolic flutter of the prolapsing segments of the mitral valve
TRICUSPID VALVE
Shaggy thickening of the anterior leaflet with a mass of echoes behind the anterior leaflet

From Thomson KR, Nanda, NC, Gramiak R: The reliability of echocardiography in the diagnosis of infective endocarditis. *Radiology* 125:473, 1977.

Treatment

Medical Management. The therapy of infective endocarditis has been extensively reviewed.[30] In theory, bactericidal therapy is best determined on the basis of in vitro sensitivity studies and is administered parenterally for the most consistent results. The duration of therapy is determined by the organism. Serum bactericidal activity should be monitored. Treatment with the selected agent should not be shortened or interrupted without good reason such as a documented hypersensitivity reaction.

Streptococcal Endocarditis. Hook and Guerrant [30] have advocated determining the minimal inhibitory concentration of penicillin for an isolate and base their therapy on whether or not a strain of streptococci is inhibited at an arbitrary level of 0.1 μg per ml of penicillin. Streptococci (usually *S. viridans*) are best treated with penicillin alone or in combination with streptomycin. Almost all patients respond, but bacteriologic cure is not achieved in all and relapses have occurred. Penicillin (1.2 million units intramuscularly every 6 hours, or 20 million units a day by constant infusion) should be given for 4 weeks, plus streptomycin (0.5 intramuscularly every 12 hours) for 2 weeks.

In patients with hypersensitivity to penicillin, cephalothin or cefazolin should be substituted in doses of 2 gm every 4 hours or 1 to 2 gm every 6 hours respectively. For organisms resistant to cephalosporins as well as penicillin, vancomycin (0.5 gm every 6 hours for 4 weeks with streptomycin for the first 2 weeks) should be used intravenously.

Streptococci resistant to 0.1 μg per ml of penicillin G are usually enterococci. In view of the in vitro synergism between streptomycin and penicillin against most enterococci, both drugs are used for 6 weeks. The dose schedule for streptomycin for adults is 1 gm every 12 hours intramuscularly for 2 weeks, then 0.5 gm every 12 hours for an additional 4 weeks. Penicillin G is given by constant intravenous infusion 20 million units daily for 6 weeks. Ampicillin (6 to 12 gm per day) may be substituted for penicillin, and gentamicin (3 to 5 mg per kg per day divided into three doses) may be substituted for streptomycin.

In patients in whom disturbances of vestibular function occur, streptomycin may need to be stopped after 4 weeks. Aminoglycoside levels should be measured periodically, since the pharmokinetics of these drugs is variable and doses may need readjustment frequently even in the absence of obvious renal functional impairment. Cephalosporins have no place in the treatment of enterococcal endocarditis, because enterococci are generally resistant.

Staphylococcal Endocarditis. Only penicillinase-resistant penicillins are reliable and must be used for 4 to 6 weeks. Methicillin, nafcillin, oxacillin, or the cephalosporins such as cephalothin can be used at doses of 2 gm every 4 hours intravenously. Some physicians add gentamicin or tobramycin to these regimens.

Pneumococcal, Gonococcal, and Meningococcal Endocarditis. Endocarditis due to these organisms will usually respond to high doses of penicillin (20 million units per day) given continuously by the intravenous route for 4 weeks.

Endocarditis Caused by Gram-Negative Organisms. Therapy should be based on the results of in vitro sensitivity tests. A cephalosporin with or without an aminoglycoside is frequently selected. Penicillin G or ampicillin (for *E. coli, Proteus mirabilis,* or *Salmonella*); cephalosporins (for *E. coli, P. mirabilis,* or *Klebsiella* species); and carbenicillin (for *Enterobacter* species, *Proteus* species other than *P. mirabilis,* or *Pseudomonas aeruginosa*) are common choices.[30]

Endocarditis Caused by Anaerobes. Anaerobic organisms are uncommon causes of endocarditis. Penicillin is the treatment of choice for most anaerobes, but *B. fragilis* strains are highly resistant to penicillin. Most strains of *B. fragilis* are sensitive in vitro to clindamycin and chloramphenicol, but the prognosis is grave. Both are bacteriostatic rather than bactericidal. Metronidazole may prove more effective.

Fungal Endocarditis. Fungal endocarditis remains a challenging problem as the drug of choice, amphotericin B, is highly toxic. Combination with flucytosine may be more effective. In general, however, surgical intervention in addition to antifungal therapy is necessary for cure in most cases (see subsequent section).

Endocarditis with Negative Culture. The management of the uncommon patients with typical findings of endocarditis and negative blood cultures is empirical. Most clinicians treat such patients as they would those with enterococcal endocarditis unless the course is fulminant, in which case they are treated as if they had staphylococcal endocarditis. Agents that may be implicated include fungi, anaerobes, diphtheroids, cell wall-defective bacteria, and *C. burnetii.*

Most patients with infective endocarditis will be cured of their disease by appropriate antibiotic therapy and have a 5-year survival rate of 50 to 85 percent.[31] The mortality in viridans-type streptococcal endocarditis is about 10 to 15 percent and is due to damage that had occurred by the time therapy was initiated. Some patients will require surgical intervention to control the infection or the hemodynamic consequences of infection.

Surgical Management of Infective Endocarditis. In 1964, Yeh et al[32] first demonstrated the feasibility of valve replacement with a prosthesis in six patients with endocarditis of the aortic valve who had been successfully treated with antibiotics before operation. The following year, Wallace et al[33] accomplished valve replacement successfully in a patient with active infection. Since that time, an increasing number of cases of surgically treated endocarditis have been reported,[34-36] and infective endocarditis has become a well-recognized indication for cardiac surgery when congestive failure persists or worsens in spite of aggressive medical management.

Indications for Operations. In their detailed review of 293 cases of left-sided endocarditis, Jung, Saab, and Almond[35] found the mean age of the surgical patient to be 30 to 40 years, with males predominating approximately 3:1. A history of a preexisting congenital or acquired heart disease can be elicited in 60 percent of patients, and where identified, streptococci (mostly of the viridans type) were the commonest infecting organisms, followed by staphylococci and pneumococci. The most common indication for surgical intervention was congestive heart failure with hemodynamic deterioration caused by destruction of heart valves and their supporting structures.[35] It was the only indication in 84 percent of the patients and was combined with embolization or resistant organisms in 12 percent. Resistant infection with repeated septic embolization or drug toxicity constituted the indication in the remaining 4 percent. Despite the fact that the mitral valve is the most common valve infection, the aortic valve was replaced in 71 percent, the mitral valve in 19 percent, and both valves in 10 percent of the patients.[35] This experience reflects the devastating consequences of aortic insufficiency as compared with mitral insufficiency.

The valves demonstrated the usual vegetations, disruption of leaflets and supporting structures, perforations, and tears of valve cusps. Abscesses of the annulus, which sometimes extended into the interventricular septum or myocardium, mycotic aneurysm of the sinuses of Valsalva, or fistulous connections between cardiac chambers or into the pulmonary artery were also found.

Operative Correction. The operative procedure consists of valve replacement in the great majority of patients. In some of the earlier cases, aortic and mitral cusp replacement and valvuloplasty were generally unsuccessful.

Results of Surgical Treatment. Patients with "active" disease are at high risk. The early mortality was 30 percent and the late mortality 7 percent. For inactive patients whose indications were hemodynamic or embolic, the early and late mortality figures were 12 percent and 11 percent respectively. The early mortality rates were comparable (approximately 20 percent) in patients undergoing aortic, mitral, or aortic and mitral replacement. The most significant factor affecting mortality rate was the degree of cardiac decompensation present at the time of operation. Procedures carried out because of severe congestive heart failure carried a mortality of 34 percent, in contrast to elective operations where the mortality rate was 15 percent.

One of the potential dangers of valve replacement in endocarditis is infection of the prosthetic valve. Only 12 of 293 patients with infective endocarditis developed infection of the prosthesis, and only 5 of 162 operated on during the active phase developed infection by the original organism. One patient developed infection by a different organism. Of six additional patients who developed infection of the prosthesis, three were in the inactive stage and the stage was not specified in three other patients.[35] All the patients with infected prostheses died. It appears that the procedure is safer than delaying operation in patients with uncontrolled heart failure. Bacteria have usually been eliminated from the circulation and the infected valve within days of starting effective antibiotic treatment unless the organisms are drug-resistant or inaccessible, as in a bulky vegetation or nidus of calcification. In the case of organisms that are inaccessible, operative excision and debridement may actually be essential to eliminate the infection. Jung, Saab, and Almond [35] feel that this explains why the variable duration of antibiotic therapy preoperatively had no bearing on the mortality rate or rate of recurrence of infection on the implanted prosthesis. If one can assume that patients reported in most surgical series would succumb to their disease without operative intervention, a combined early (22 percent) and late (9 percent) mortality rate of 31 percent, though high, is better than a 100 percent mortality. It is probable that the results could be improved if operation were undertaken before irreversible congestive heart failure occurs and before such anatomic complications as aortic root abscesses, sinus of Valsalva aneurysms, and fistulas occur. The emphasis on earlier operation is clearly seen in the series of Boyd et al.[36] In their 45 patients with primary endocarditis, survival was improved when operation was carried out promptly in those with both controlled and uncontrolled infection.

Valve replacement is almost always necessary for fungal and *Pseudomonas* endocarditis, which rarely respond to chemotherapy alone. If the tricuspid valve is infected (see subsequent section on drug addiction), excision of the valve without immediate replacement is in order.

Prophylaxis

Patients with suspected congenital or acquired valvular heart disease should be given antibiotics immediately before dental manipulation, obstetric delivery, urethral catheterization, or other forms of mucosal manipulation (Table 31-1). A practical regimen is a single dose of 1.2 million units of aqueous procaine penicillin administered with 1 gm streptomycin within 30 minutes of dental surgery. A loading dose of a 2 gm penicillin V followed by 0.5 gm of the drug at 6-hour intervals for 48 hours is probably equally effective. Patients who are allergic to penicillin should receive 2 gm cefazolin plus 1 gm streptomycin intramuscularly, or 1 gm vancomycin intravenously. The best regimen for preventing enterococcal endocarditis is ampicillin plus gentamicin. No firm dosage schedules have been established, but 2 gm ampicillin followed by 0.5 gm every 6 hours plus 3 to 5 mg per kg gentamicin in three divided doses for a total of 48 hours given simultaneously should be adequate. The prophylactic doses of penicillin used to prevent group A streptococcal infection and recurrent rheumatic fever will not prevent bacterial endocarditis.[9,10]

Infective Endocarditis in Drug Addicts

Infective endocarditis in drug addicts is an entity of increasing concern. Bacteremia obviously arises by injection of unsterile material, use of unclean needles, syringes, and other paraphernalia. Most often, endogenous skin or oral bacteria are inoculated. In addition to direct intravenous inoculation, bacteria may enter the circulation from foci of phlebitis or through regional lymphatic absorption from areas of bacterial cellulitis.

Preexisting heart disease is present in only about 20 percent of narcotic addicts presenting with their initial episode of endocarditis, in sharp contrast to the 60 percent of nonaddicts with endocarditis. The mechanism of endocarditis beginning on normal structures is uncertain. Repeated intravenous injections of foreign material may traumatize the endocardial surfaces, causing roughened areas that serve as sites for aggregation of platelets and development of platelet thrombi. Highly contaminated systemic venous flow could explain the frequency of right heart endocarditis in drug abusers. The tricuspid valve was infected in 55 percent of 270 cases, the aortic in 35 percent, the mitral valve in 30 percent, and the pulmonary valve in only 2 percent of these patients.[37]

Etiology

The microbiology of infective endocarditis in drug addicts is different from that in nonaddicts. *S. aureus* is the most common pathogen (45 to 56 percent). Aerobic gram-negative bacilli account for approximately 15 percent; fungi (usually *Candida*), 11 percent; streptococci other than enterococci, 10 percent; and enterococci, 8 percent. Enterococcal endocarditis may occur more frequently in some series.[37] *Pseudomonas* is identified in one-third of the gram-negative bacillary infections and often involves the tricuspid valve. Borow, Alpert, and Pennington [38] caution that transient *Pseudomonas* bacteremia in an addict may mimic right-sided endocarditis and may actually require a much shorter course of therapy. It may be that virulent organisms (eg, staphylococci) are necessary to initiate endocardial infection in addicts without preexisting heart disease, but once valvular damage has occurred, the addict becomes susceptible to infection with organisms of lesser virulence.

Clinical Manifestations

The patients are generally young adult males with symptoms of acute onset and short duration. Fever is present in 90 percent, with pleuritic chest pain, increased sputum production, or hemoptysis occurring in about 30 percent. Exertional dyspnea, orthopnea, and paroxysmal nocturnal dyspnea occurs in 15 percent and are manifestations of heart failure. The other manifestations and complications of endocarditis are those noted previously in nonaddicts. Pulmonary complications often dominate the clinical picture due to emboli from the right heart.

Three specific syndromes have been identified: [37]

1. Staphylococcal endocarditis. Valve destruction occurs early, and septic pulmonary emboli with pulmonary infiltrates are common. Although right-sided involvement predominates, either or both sides of the heart may be involved. The mortality increases with aortic or mitral valve involvement over that from isolated tricuspid valve involvement because of the hemodynamic derangements of valvular insufficiency of the left side of the heart.

2. Gram-negative bacillary endocarditis. The most

commonly involved organisms are of the *Klebsiella-Enterobacter* group, *E. coli* and *Pseudomonas. Serratia marcesens* and *Herellea vaginicola* have also been found. Infection of both sides of the heart can result from gram-negative bacteria, although left-sided endocarditis predominates and is associated with a mortality of approximately 90 percent. This is due in part to the relative resistance of these bacteria to antibiotics—*Pseudomonas* being especially difficult to treat.

3. Candida endocarditis. These very serious infections are often superimposed on a previous episode of bacterial endocarditis. A mixed fungal and bacterial infection was present in four of the five addicts with *Candida* endocarditis reported by Harris et al.[39] The clinical course is less acute, and the left side of the heart is most often involved. Large vegetations occur in fungal endocarditis, and those in the left heart may embolize to other organs and to large peripheral arteries (eg, the aortic or femoral bifurcation). The prognosis in fungal endocarditis is dismal.[37]

Treatment

The treatment is the same in addicts as in nonaddicts, with the exception of the addict with (bacterial or fungal) tricuspid endocarditis caused by resistant organisms. In these circumstances, the best results are achieved when the tricuspid valve has been excised without replacement. Four of the five patients so treated by Arbulu et al[40] were alive and free of infection and hemodynamic problems from 7 to 17 months after operation. On the basis of their experience, the authors recommended 6 weeks of intensive antibiotic treatment followed by total excision of the tricuspid valve where medical therapy has failed.

Prognosis

Reinfection of addicts with successfully treated endocarditis is a common problem. Some[10] have suggested remedies such as antibiotic prophylaxis and personal hygiene. Obviously, the surgeon will require professional social and psychologic assistance in the rehabilitation of these patients.

PACEMAKER ENDOCARDITIS

The advent of permanent cardiac pacemakers has revolutionized the management of patients with cardiac arrhythmias. As with any procedure involving the implantation of foreign bodies, pacemaker infection is a threat that may involve the pacing system at any point outside the heart or within the endocardium. The infections of the subcutaneous pacemaker pocket are discussed in Chapter 30. This section focuses on infections within the heart.

Incidence

Intravascular infection is an uncommon complication. Schwartz and Pervez[41] reported the first case of acute bacterial endocarditis in a patient with a permanent transvenous pacemaker. In 1972, Imparato and Kim[42] reviewed the complications found in 200 patients with permanent cardiac pacemakers. Six patients (5 percent) developed skin erosions by the hardware, and all but one developed secondary infection of the pacemaker pockets and catheter tracts. In none of the five could the electrodes be extracted at the time of removal of the pacemakers from their infected pockets (trapped endocardial electrode). In three cases, the trapped electrodes were severed distal to the infected pacemaker pockets and left within their venous tracts. This resulted in the delayed appearance of septicemia in one, persistent septicemia in another, and migration of the electrode in the third. The rate can be reduced. Conklin et al[43] reported an infection rate on all pacemaker procedures of 0.13 percent (1 of 726), but these results are unusual. Grogler et al[44] reported a 3.2 percent incidence of infection of generator pocket infections in 1,376 pacemaker operations and a 1.9 percent incidence of infected electrode channels. In most cases, infection could be directly related to operation, but a few appeared months to years after implantation.

Pathogenesis and Bacteriology of Pacemaker Endocarditis

Endocardial electrodes can become infected by one of two major mechanisms. In the more frequent type, the infected pacemaker generator site acts as a foreign body which allows a direct extension of organisms along pacemaker wires with or without systemic bacteremia. Cultures most often reveal *S. aureus* followed by *S. epidermidis* and *Klebsiella.* Other organisms that have been rarely encountered include *E. coli, Candida, Serratia, Flavobacterium,* and other Enterobacteriaceae. The less frequent type is caused by metastatic implantation of bacteria from a distant site. As expected, any microorganism can be involved.[45]

Treatment

High doses of antibiotic drugs should be used in all cases of prosthetic endocarditis. The surgical treatment of the infected pacemaker generator and external wires has been discussed in Chapter 30. The standard treatment is removal of all infected foreign bodies including extrathoracic electrode segments, drainage, and antibiotics; sterile electrode tracts seldom need to be disturbed. The in situ management of the infected pulse generator has been reported by Dargan and Norman[46] and is described in Chapter 30.

When infection has spread from the pulse generator or external wires into the heart or has involved the endocardial electrode by metastatic spread from a distant focus, all foreign material must be removed. Removal of the electrode is usually accomplished by graded traction on the electrode. The wire is tensed until the tugging caused by ventricular motion is felt. The wire is then taped to the chest and the procedure repeated as slack is developed in the wire and the electrode wire removed completely.[42] Obviously, a new pacemaker system must be in place before removal is attempted.

The most difficult problem is the trapped electrode. Retention is due to ensheathment of the larger tip of the electrode by fibrous tissue, which prevents its easy withdrawal through the fibrous ring just proximal to it. Trapped electrodes have sometimes required thoracotomy, cardiopulmonary bypass, and cardiotomy for removal.[46]

Prophylaxis of Pacemaker Infections

Hartstein et al [47] retrospectively analyzed 298 pacemaker procedures. There was no significant difference in infection rate between the group given prophylactic antibiotics and the group given no or inadequate prophylactic antibiotics. Prospective studies have not been completed. Hartstein et al [47] concluded that drains should be avoided in battery pack plus pacing wire procedures. Conklin et al [43] noted that the one infection in their series resulted from repeated efforts to aspirate a pouch hematoma. They recommend that a pouch hematoma be treated by prompt operation, evacuation of the hematoma, and primary closure of the pouch.

Although late intracardiac infections are unusual, chemoprophylaxis with antibiotics (see preceding section on prophylaxis of endocarditis) should be carried out in patients with intravascular pacemakers whenever bacteria-inducing procedures are contemplated (Table 31-1).

INFECTIONS FOLLOWING HEART SURGERY

Chest wall wound infections have been discussed in Chapter 30. The following sections will discuss intracardiac infections following heart surgery.

ENDOCARDITIS IN THE ABSENCE OF AN INTRACARDIAC PROSTHESIS

Incidence and Consequences

There is limited information regarding the incidence of endocarditis after cardiac surgery in the absence of an intracardiac prosthesis. An incidence of 2 percent was once estimated. Geraci et al [48] reported on the experience of the Mayo Clinic from 1946 through 1962 with bacterial endocarditis and endarteritis following approximately 4,300 cardiac or large vessel operations, excluding coarctation of the aorta and lesions distal to this site. There were 24 patients (0.5 percent) with bacterial or fungal endocarditis, 12 of whom had undergone intracardiac operations. Four had congenital aortic stenosis, four had mitral stenosis, and four had atrial septal defects (with associated pulmonic stenosis and patent ductus arteriosus in one patient each). Seven patients died. The patients of Geraci et al [48] and Looser et al [49] are described in Table 31-5.

Pathogenesis

Experience is so limited that the pathogenetic factors are not clear. Cardiopulmonary bypass probably plays an important role in many cases of postoperative endocarditis (see subsequent section), as must preexisting infection, suture material, and extracardiac foreign bodies. Damaged valves and suture lines are most often affected. Late infections have involved teflon-reinforced, ventricular suture lines.[49] The role of sepsis and additional factors such as operative contamination and intravascular catheters in postoperative endocarditis is better documented in patients with prosthetic valve endocarditis and will be discussed in that section.

Etiology

S. aureus is responsible for more than half of the cases, with *S. epidermidis*, *S. pyogenes* (group A), *P. aeruginosa*, and other gram-negative rods responsible for the rest.[48,49] Fungi are rare etiologic agents: *C. albicans*,[49] *Mucor*, and *Histoplasma* [48] have been cultured from suture lines and damaged valves.

Pathology

The pathologic changes of postoperative endocarditis in the absence of an intracardiac prosthesis are similar to those previously described for endocarditis when the valves are affected. Most of the nonvalvular infections involve cardiotomy and aortotomy suture lines. The highest incidence of fatal infections have followed operations for aortic stenosis—aortic suture line separation, mycotic aneurysm formation, and aortic valve cusp infection have all been noted. Mitral (and sometimes aortic) vegetations were a dominant feature in heart infections following mitral commissurotomy, and myocardial abscess and atrial thrombi were also seen.[48,49]

Clinical Manifestations

The clinical diagnosis of postoperative endocarditis in the absence of an intracardiac prosthesis can be elusive. Embolic signs and splenomegaly were each noted in four instances.[48] The appearance of new or changing murmurs is not as striking as in patients with infected intracardiac prostheses. Persistent early or late unexplained fever is often the only sign. When combined with positive blood cultures, intracardiac infection should be suspected. Conventional roentgenograms and lung scans can be useful in detecting pulmonary emboli and infarcts, and ultrasound studies can at times document intracardiac vegetations as well as pericarditis with effusion. Angiocardiography is useful in suture line disruption and where an exact assessment of a residual defect is important before reoperation.[48]

Treatment

Medical Therapy. The patient should be started on a bactericidal antibiotic regimen, giving adequate doses for a sufficiently long period and regulating the course of treatment by determination of bactericidal levels of antibiotics in the patient's serum. Most of Geraci's et al [48] patients cured with antibiotic therapy alone had undergone repair of an atrial septal defect with silk suture or commissurotomy for valve stenosis. The diagnosis of bacterial endocarditis in patients successfully treated can never be proved, but three patients with similar signs clearly received inadequate courses of antibiotic therapy and died of their infection, as did four patients treated aggressively with antibiotic therapy.

In some patients, infection cannot be eradicated but can be suppressed by indefinite antibiotic administration. This approach can be better appreciated in patients with infected prostheses.

Surgical Treatment. In hemodynamically stable patients, surgical treatment should be considered only after

TABLE 31-5. PERTINENT DATA ON 14 PATIENTS WITH POSTOPERATIVE ENDOCARDITIS IN THE ABSENCE OF AN INTRACARDIAC PROSTHESIS

Ref.	Sex/ Age	Cardiac Lesion	Intracardiac Foreign Body	Pathogen	Postmortem/ Cultures Results	Pathology and Comment
Geraci et al [48]	M 14	Congenital aortic stenosis	Silk sutures, Ivalon sponge around aorta	*P. aeruginosa*	*P. aeruginosa* from Ivalon sponge, aortic & mitral vegetations	Mycotic aneurysm of ascending aorta. Infection around aorta at suture line and sponge
	F 13	Atrial septal defect (ASD), patent ductus arteriosus	Silk sutures	*P. aeruginosa*	—	Survived. Dangling, vegetation; encrusted silk suture in left atrium. Vegetation grew *P. aeruginosa*
	M 53	Mitral stenosis	Commissurotomy, silk sutures in left atrium	*H. capsulatum* (autopsy)	*H. capsulatum* cultured from mitral valve	Vegetation on mitral valve, organisms compatible with *H. capsulatum* histologically
	M 47	Mitral stenosis	Commissurotomy, silk sutures in left atrium	Unidentified gram-negative bacilli	—	Survived
	F 9	Subvalvular aortic stenosis	Aortotomy closed with silk sutures	*S. aureus*	Same phage type Staph. cultured from spleen & vena caval blood	Vegetations on aortic valve with perforation of right & posterior cusps. Mycotic aneurysm at aortotomy site. Organisms present in aortic valve vegetations
	M 57	Congenital aortic stenosis	Silk sutures in aorta	*S. aureus*	*S. aureus* from aortic valve, lung, & heart blood	Separation of aortic sutures, with false aneurysm of aorta & active infection. Extension acute subendocardial & myocardial infarcts
	M 35	Mitral stenosis	Commissurotomy, silk sutures in left atrium	*S. epidermidis*	Vegetation on mitral valve & heart blood, negative for *S. epidermidis*	Vegetations & bacteria on mitral & aortic valves. One aortic cusp perforated. Thrombus of left atrium. *S. aureus* cultured from mitral valve, felt to be a contaminant
	F 9	Congenital aortic stenosis	Silk sutures at aortotomy site	*S. aureus*	No necropsy	Reoperation 16 days postop., infection limited to aortotomy site, with purulent material & infected sutures & tissue. Died after reoperation. No necropsy

	F 45	Mitral & tricuspid stenosis	Commissurotomy, silk sutures in left atrium	*S. aureus* only at postmortem; three ante mortem cultures negative	*S. aureus* from kidney, cerebrospinal fluid & cerebellum. Mitral valve negative	Microabscesses in myocardium. Vegetation on mitral & aortic valves. Thrombus in left atrium extending into left ventricle; gram-positive cocci noted in valve vegetations
	F 26	Atrial septal defect & pulmonic stenosis	Silk sutures used to close foramen ovale & pulmonary artery	*S. aureus*	—	Survived. This patient could have had bacteremia only without endocardial or suture infection
	F 56	Atrial septal defect	Silk suture used to close ASD	Beta-hemolytic streptococcus	—	Survived
	F 36	Atrial septal defect	Silk suture used to close ASD	*S. aureus*	—	Survived
Looser et al [49]	M 49	Ventricular aneurysm	Teflon-felt reinforced ventricular suture line	*S. aureus* & *Peptostreptococcus*		Died 5 weeks after resection of large pseudoaneurysm of the left ventricle using cardiopulmonary bypass. The pseudoaneurysm was in continuity with the Teflon-felt reinforced suture line of the original repair, done more than 1 year previously. Infection of the suture line probably followed a left lower lobe pneumonia & septicemia. There was no evidence of recurrent infection at time of death
	M 63	Coronary artery disease & ventricular aneurysm	Teflon-felt reinforced ventricular suture line	*C. albicans*		Died 6 months after excision of ventriculocutaneous fistula, and infected Teflon-felt reinforced suture line of the original repair, done more than 4 years previously. A draining sinus appeared in the chest wall 2 years after operation, & over the next 2 years several attempts were made to debride the tract. Success was finally achieved using cardiopulmonary bypass but the patient succumbed from intractable congestive heart failure. No evidence of recurrent infection was found at autopsy

an adequate trial of effective bactericidal antibiotic therapy for 4 or more weeks. Those in whom relapse occurs after therapy or where bacteremia is not controlled are candidates for reoperation. In this way, the surgeon can ascertain whether the foreign body suture or prosthetic material has become infected, and if it can be removed. In 1961, Kelsch and Thomson [50] reported cure of a patient with postoperative endocarditis by removing the infected silk sutures used to close a ventricular septal defect. Hemodynamic instability requires urgent operations as in native endocarditis.

Prevention

Technical. The principles of bacterial control in the operating room, in the patient's preparation, and during operation are the same as in patients in whom prostheses are inserted (this will be touched on in a subsequent section discussing technical aspects of prophylaxis of infection during implantation of a prosthesis).

Antibiotic Prophylaxis. Prophylactic antibiotics are usually employed in patients undergoing open heart surgery, but for shorter times than in patients who require valve replacement. Endocarditis developed in spite of prophylactic antibiotics used in the Mayo Clinic series.[48] This may be related to the dosages and in some cases to drugs used for prophylaxis. With current methods of prophylaxis, the rate of postoperative endocardial infection is low in the absence of an intracardiac prosthesis. Most trials reflecting the beneficial effects of antibiotic prophylaxis have been performed during the implantation of intracardiac prostheses.

PROSTHETIC VALVE ENDOCARDITIS

In the 1960s, postoperative endocarditis became more frequent—especially in patients with acquired heart disease and in those in whom intracardiac prostheses were used. In 1966, Amoury, Bowman, and Malm [51] reported an early experience with 13 instances of postoperative endocarditis following a total of 568 open heart operations. In this group, 357 patients required intracardiac prostheses, with 223 intracardiac patches and 134 patients receiving 154 valve prostheses. Clinical details are noted in Table 31-6. Endocarditis was most common after aortic valve replacement, less common after intracardiac patch prosthesis, and least common when no prosthesis was used. Other studies in the 1960s confirmed these findings.[52] Although the incidence has been further reduced, prosthetic valve endocarditis (PVE) is still a major complication, with serious consequences.

Epidemiology and Incidence

In order to more accurately assess the incidence of PVE, it is necessary to define the diagnostic criteria. Wilson [53] considers PVE to be present if two of three criteria are fulfilled: (1) at least two positive blood cultures contain the same microbial species, (2) surgical or autopsy specimens show evidence of bacterial endocarditis, and (3) at least two of the following clinical signs are found—fever, appearance of a new regurgitant murmur, newly developed splenomegaly, and signs of peripheral emboli.

The disease can be further divided into early and late groups. Early PVE, appearing within 2 months of operation, and later PVE. Wilson found PVE in 45 of 4,586 patients (0.98 percent) given 4,706 prosthetic valves. Early PVE occurred in 16 (0.35 percent) and late PVE in 29 (0.63 percent). In patients with early PVE, the mean time from operation to onset of symptoms was 17 days (range 1 to 45 days). In the late group, the mean delay was 26 months (range 72 days to 10 years). The aortic valve was involved more frequently than the mitral. All age groups were equally susceptible. A wound infection was the portal of entry in five of the 16 early cases (31 percent), but no obvious portal was present in the rest. In the late group, five of the patients with endocarditis caused by *S. viridans* had either antecedent trauma, surgical procedures, or dental work. Two of three patients with late onset PVE due to group D streptococci had prior or concomitant urinary tract infection with the same organism. None of the remaining 22 patients with late onset PVE had an obvious portal of entry.

Both early and late onset PVE may follow contamination of prostheses in the perioperative period, and considerable attention has been focused on this period in a patient's course. Ankeney and Parker [54] studied 383 open heart operations during which 1,555 intraoperative blood cultures were secured. *S. epidermidis* grew out in 7.5 percent of these samples and diphtheroids in 9.8 percent. The greatest number of positive cultures were in specimens taken from the recently assembled and primed pump and from the suction line during bypass, when the pump and blood are most exposed to the operating room air.

In similar studies of 400 patients, Yeh et al [52] obtained positive cultures from the primed oxygenator preoperatively in 37: *Staphylococcus* (7), *Streptococcus* (2), diphtheroids (7), *Alcaligenes* (20), *Paracolobactrum* (1). Nineteen had positive blood cultures from the pump equipment following bypass: *Staphylococcus* (2), diphtheroids (6), *Alcaligenes* (5), and *Proteus, Mima, Bacillus, Aerobacter, Pseudomonas,* and unidentified gram-negative rod (1 each). Only two developed bacterial endocarditis due to the same organism (diphtheroid and *P. maltophilia*) found in the pump equipment. Of these 400 patients,[52] 32 had positive blood cultures at some time following cardiopulmonary bypass, and 18 of these were considered to have PVE. Thus, most infections arise postoperatively rather than intraoperatively. Contamination most often arises from arterial and venous cannulations, cannulation of the heart, tracheostomy, endotracheal intubation, and bladder catheterization.

Etiology (Bacteriology)

A variety of organisms have been reported in patients with PVE (Tables 31-7 to 31-9). Both gram-positive and gram-negative organisms are found. Staphylococci and streptococci are the most frequently encountered gram-positive organisms in almost all series, but almost any pathogen or saporophyte can be encountered. Tables 31-8 and 31-9 cite case reports of the rarely encountered bacte-

TABLE 31-6. TYPES AND SITES OF UNITS AND OCCURRENCE OF ENDOCARDITIS

	Number of patients	Type	Number of units	Endocarditis	Comment
Intracardiac patch	223	Teflon	223	1	
Mitral replacement	61	Ball	61	1	
Double valve replacement	18	Ball	35	2	1 mitral, 1 aortic
		Teflon cloth	1		
Aortic replacement	55	Ball	43 *	5	
		Teflon cloth	6	2	
		Hinged, graphite unicusp	3	0	

* Two reoperations.

From Amoury RA, Bowman FO Jr, Malm JR: Endocarditis associated with intracardiac prostheses. *J Thorac Cardiovasc Surg* 51:36, 1966.

TABLE 31-7. BACTERIAL ETIOLOGY OF PROSTHETIC VALVE ENDOCARDITIS

	Early Cases		Late Cases	
Bacteria	***No.***	***Percent***	***No.***	***Percent***
Streptococci (except enterococci)	9	6.0	41	26.6
Enterococci	6	4.0	14	9.1
S. aureus	30	20.0	22	14.3
S. epidermidis or *Micrococcus* spp	41	27.1	36	23.4
S. pneumoniae	2	1.3	—	—
Diphtheroids	12	8.0	6	3.9
Enterobacteriaceae	19	12.5	12	7.8
Pseudomonas spp	5	3.3	2	1.3
Haemophilus spp	—	—	3	1.9
Vibrio fetus	—	—	1	0.6
Other gram-negative rods	6	4.0	1	0.6
Candida or *Torulopsis* spp	14	9.3	4	2.6
Aspergillus	4	2.6	5	3.3
Culture-negative	3	2.0	7	4.6
	151	100.0	154	100.0

Data compiled from experience at Massachussetts General Hospital and from 12 published series.

From Karchmer AW, Swartz MN: Infective endocarditis in patients with prosthetic heart valves. In Kaplan EL, Taranta AV (eds): Infective Endocarditis. Dallas, American Heart Association, Inc., 1977, p. 58.

ria that cause PVE.[55-82] Mixed infections are uncommon—most involve *Staphylococcus* and another bacterium or a fungus. The special characteristics of fungal infections will be described in a subsequent section.

Pathology of Prosthetic Valve Endocarditis

The pathologic findings seen in endocarditis following valve replacement have been extensively documented.[83] Thrombotic vegetations on prostheses of various types, separation sutures anchoring prostheses, pseudoaneurysm and mycotic aneurysms of the ascending aorta, microabscesses in the myocardium, and abscess of the aortic valve ring are frequently noted (Fig. 31-3). There are no pathologic alterations distinctive for a given organism.[51] Thrombi are typically located at the junction of the struts and the metallic rings of the prosthesis, with extension up the struts. Ring abscesses are almost always present and most often involve the entire valve annulus and spread to adjacent structures in more than half the cases. For example, aortic ring abscesses frequently burrow through the ascending aorta into the periaortic space, through the atrial septum into the right atrium, into the left atrium, through the ventricular septum into the right ventricle, or into the anterobasal left ventricular wall. The ring abscess of infected mitral protheses can burrow through the atrial wall into the pericardial space. These features are apparently the result of the rolling motion of the rigid frame of the valve prostheses. The more severe changes around the aortic valve may be due to the greater turbulence across the aortic prosthesis than the mitral.[83]

TABLE 31-8. PROSTHETIC VALVE ENDOCARDITIS: UNCOMMON BACTERIA

Author/Ref.	Micro-organism	Valve(s) Involved	Early or Late Onset	Clinical Features	Blood Culture Results	Other	Indications for Reoperation/ Comment	Outcome
Clark, Patton [55]	*Neisseria perflava*	Dacron graft for aneurysm of ascending aorta & Cutter aortic prosthesis	Early—4 weeks	Chills, fever, digital & upper abdominal pain, splenomegaly, normal prosthetic heart sounds, systolic ejection murmur	Negative at 4 weeks postop; positive at 5–6 weeks postop		Not reoperated. First report of PVE due to this organism	Died—leak in suture line of aortic graft. No evidence of infection at autopsy (preceding antibiotics)
Levin et al [56]	*N. meningitidis*	Starr-Edwards mitral prosthesis	Late—6½ months	Lethargic, confused, purpuric rash, meningitis, changing murmurs	Positive	Cerebrospinal fluid	Not reoperated. First report PVE due to this organism	Died—calcified granulations beneath the mitral valve annulus containing gram-negative diplococci
Jephcott, Hardisty [57]	*N. meningitidis*	Bjork-Shiley aortic prosthesis replacing an initial prosthesis	Late—3 months	Fever, headache chills, pyoarthrosis, appearance of a diastolic murmur	Positive	Joint fluid	Not reoperated. Probable but not certainly case of PVE	Survived—antibiotic therapy
Goldsweig, Matsen, Castaneda [58]	*Haemophilus aphrophilus*	Starr-Edwards mitral prosthesis	Late—4 months	Chills, fever, anorexia,	Positive at 4 months		Not reoperated. 28 cases of PVE due to *H. aphrophilus* reviewed; 7 died	Survived—antibiotic therapy
Stauffer, Goldman [59]	*Actinobacillus actinomycetemcomitans*	Starr-Edwards aortic prosthesis	Late—5 years	Fever, chills, weight loss, splenomegaly, anemia, hematuria, changing murmurs	Positive		Not reoperated. May originate in oral lesions	Survived—antibiotic therapy
Juffe et al [60]	*Actinobacillus*	Aortic ball valve	Late—3 years	Fever, anemia, splenomegaly, aortic diastolic murmur	Positive		Not reoperated	Survived—antibiotic therapy. Died 2⅓ years later of PVE due to *S. viridans*

Buchanan [61]	*Mima polymorpha (Acinetobacter)*	Artificial mitral & aortic	Late—2½ years	Fever, headache, paresthesias, other evidence of emboli. Roth spots, petechiae, multiple neurologic findings, no changing murmurs	Positive		Not reoperated. First reported case of PVE due to this organism	Survived—antibiotic therapy
Fischer [62] Yeh [63]	*Pseudomonas maltophilia*	Starr-Edwards mitral prosthesis	Early—3 weeks	Fever, petechiae, apical systolic murmur which disappeared	Positive		Not reoperated	Survived—antimicrobial therapy (trimethoprim methoxazole-sulfate)
Vlachakis, Gazez, Hairston [64]	*Nocardia asteroides*	Beall mitral prosthesis	Late—3¾ months	Fever, congestive failure, cutaneous abscesses	Negative	Multiple skin abscesses grew *N. asteroides*	Not reoperated	Died—*Nocardia* abscesses in myocardium, thyroid, adrenals, kidneys, spleen
O'Meara et al [65]	*Brucella melitensis*	Starr-Edwards mitral prosthesis	Late—10.5 months	Fever, congestive heart failure	Positive	Elevated agglutinins & complement-fixation titers to *Brucella* antigens. *B. melitensis* (type 3) cultured from vegetations on prosthesis	Mitral valve obstruction. First report of de novo PVE due to this organism. A previous case of brucellosis endocarditis with subsequent PVE reported by Ehrenhaft [66]	Survived—mitral valve replacement & antimicrobial therapy (cotrimoxazole)
Weinstein et al [67]	*Listeria monocytogenes*	Starr-Edwards aortic prosthesis	Late—2¼ years	Fever, chills, arrhythmias, changing murmurs	Positive		Congestive heart failure. First report of PVE due to this organism	Died—during replacement with another valve. Coronary embolism from a vegetation with an extensive early myocardial infarct
Saravolatz et al [68]	*L. monocytogenes*	Xenograft (porcine) mitral prosthesis	Late—7¼ months	Splenomegaly, systolic ejection murmur	Positive		Not reoperated. Review of 13 cases	Survived—antibiotic therapy

(Continued)

TABLE 31-8. ***(Continued)***

Author/Ref.	Micro-organism	Valve(s) Involved	Early or Late Onset	Clinical Features	Blood Culture Results	Other	Indications for Reoperation/ Comment	Outcome
Jackson, Saunders [69]	Diphtheroids	All types	Early and late	4 of 7 cases	Usually positive		Literature reviewed—commonly reported in larger series and many other reported cases	4 of 7 survived on sodium fusidate and erythromycin. Others report cure after valve replacement
Juffe et al [60]	*Corynenbacterium diptheriae*	Bjork-Shiley mitral prosthesis	Early—2 months	Fever, anemia, splenomegaly, no unusual murmurs	Positive		Not reoperated	Survived—antibiotic therapy
Block, Levy, Fritz [70]	*Bacillus cereus*	Bjork-Shiley mitral prosthesis	Early—17 days	Anemia, jaundice, splenomegaly, splinter hemorrhages, diminished pulses in leg & hemiplegia, prosthetic sounds clear, diastolic murmur present	Positive at 2–3 weeks		Not reoperated. First report of PVE due to this organism. Natural valve endocarditis reviewed by Tuazon et al [71]	Died—24 days
Geraci et al [72]	*Cardiobacterium hominis*	Bjork-Shiley aortic prosthesis, saphenous vein bypass	Late—2 years. First valve replacement (leak) 13 months, second valve replacement (PVE & leak)	Followed dental work. Fever, cough, orthopnea, dyspnea, widened pulse pressure, aortic diastolic murmur	Positive. Slow, growing gram-negative bacilli	Valve cultures negative	Aortic insufficiency & congestive heart failure	Survived—third valve replacement & antibiotic therapy
Spernoga et al [73]	*C. hominis*	Xenograft (porcine) mitral prosthesis	Late—16 months	Splenomegaly. Patient appeared well, unchanging apical systolic murmur	Positive at 17 months		Not reoperated. Reviews 12 cases of natural and prosthetic endocarditis-organism causes no other disease than endocarditis	Survived—antibiotic therapy

Several important clinical events can be clearly related to the pathologic findings. The appearance of an aortic diastolic murmur probably coincides with the formation of a discrete paravalvular leak and aortic insufficiency. An alternate explanation could be the interposition of a tail of thrombus onto the rim of the cage, thereby preventing complete seating of the ball during ventricular diastole.[83] The appearance of abnormal rhythms and defects in impulse propagation are probably the result of extension of the infection into the interventricular septum. Complete first-degree heart block frequently means that an abscess involves the AV node or bundle of His. Left bundle branch block does not correlate with infection of the conduction system. In such patients, idiopathic atrophy and fibrosis of the proximal portion of the left bundle is found. The principal causes of death are congestive heart failure (85 percent), central nervous system embolus, and generalized infection.

Aortic valves are more commonly infected than mitral. In patients with two prosthetic valves, only the "downstream" valve becomes infected, ie, the aortic valve becomes infected in patients with mitral and aortic prostheses, and the mitral valve becomes infected in patients with tricuspid and mitral prostheses. Infected aortic prostheses tend to become detached more often than mitral, and infected mitral prostheses tend to become obstructed by vegetations more often than aortic.

Pathogenesis

From the foregoing, the pathogenesis of PVE can be deduced and the major factors summarized. Transient bouts of bacteremia from contaminated intravascular catheters or examinations (dental, rectal, gynecologic) serve as microbial sources (Table 31-1). The bacteria lodge in areas of turbulence, stasis, and microthromboses. Such disturbances are seen wherever significant pressure gradients exist across a defect or valve. High-velocity flow through a narrow orifice produces diminished lateral pressure locally and determines the sites of endocardial bacterial lesions. The use of metal frame prostheses within the heart introduces a well-defined area of rigidity, producing local turbulence and often a small gradient.

The cloth fixation ring and sutures provide an inert foreign body anchored in the turbulent stream. Barney et al[84] found that 100 percent of dogs inoculated intravenously with a predetermined dose of *S. mitis* developed endocarditis if a prosthesis was inserted or if an aortic valve had been damaged. No infection occurred in a similarly exposed control group and in a group with right ventriculotomies.

The changes in systemic host defense caused by pump oxygenators should also be noted, although their contribution to PVE is probably minor. The bactericidal activity in the serum of patients following open heart surgery using standard nonmembrane oxygenators is depressed, and transient defects in the phagocytic functions of leukocytes concurrently appear. Jacob and his colleagues[85] have shown that exposure of blood to cellophane membranes activates the complement cascade in the fluid phase. Circulating leukocytes become aggregated and embolize to capillary beds, especially in the lung. There, activation of the oxidative and enzymatic digestive processes may take place. This scenario, for which there is convincing experimental and clinical evidence, would account for both the humoral and transient cellular antimicrobial defects after cardiopulmonary bypass.

The further effects of cardiopulmonary bypass on platelets may have an indirect bearing on infection by predisposing to abnormal hematomas and sternal instability. Blood collections are easily infected.

The extracardiac effects of extracorporeal circulation may be important here. Intestinal necrosis is a rare but grave complication following open heart surgery, as is necrotizing enterocolitis.[86] These clear-cut episodes of loss of intestinal viability testify to the possibility that transient compromise of the gastrointestinal barrier may occur during bypass, which may permit endogenous intestinal organisms to seed the bloodstream.

Experimental Studies in the Pathogenesis of PVE.

The Role of Preexisting Thrombosis. The experimental production of infective endocarditis has been discussed in a previous section. The same basic designs have been applied to PVE, and these methods have been reviewed by Archer.[87] In small animals, the most consistent model of endocarditis has resulted from passage of a polyethylene catheter into either side of the heart. This abrades the ventricular endocardium and produces the sterile vegetations characteristic of nonbacterial thrombotic endocarditis. Such lesions can be consistently colonized with inoculated bacteria. These thrombi resemble the thrombi often found on the struts of prosthetic valves.

Archer[87] studied colonization of catheter-induced vegetations by inoculated *S. aureus, S. fecalis,* and *P. aeruginosa.* He showed that gram-negative bacteria adhere to or multiply in endocardial vegetations at a slower rate than gram-positive bacteria and that most bacteria adhere passively to nonbacterial thrombotic endocarditis lesions without prior interaction with other blood elements. The latter observations stand in contrast to other studies, which suggest that bacteria agglutinate platelets during the production of vegetations. It is likely that turbulent flow around natural valves or prostheses, plus the inherent characteristics of individual organisms, are the most important factors determining the deposition of microorganisms on natural and prosthetic valves. Archer[87] also made the important observation that tightly interwoven fibrin acts as a barrier to the effective migration of phagocytes. He found that although fibrin is loose at the surface of a vegetation, it is packed tightly in the region just below the surface and contains colonies of bacteria in areas that are devoid of phagocytes. Bacterial agglutination of platelets is necessary for bacteria to localize on vegetations. Bacterial infection of a sterile platelet-fibrin thrombus may occur after organisms are caught on the surface of a platelet-fibrin lattice and are buried by accretion of platelets and fibrin from the circulation. Multiplication occurs in the depths of this lattice unimpeded by phagocytes.

The Role of Bacteremia. A somewhat different view, which assigns bacteria a primary role in thrombus formation, should be noted. Jones et al[88] related the frequency of massive thrombus accumulation on prosthetic heart valves in dogs to the common occurrence of bacteremia in these animals. If the dogs could be rendered free of

TABLE 31-9. PROSTHETIC VALVE ENDOCARDITIS: MYCOBACTERIA, RICKETTSIAE

Author/Ref.	Micro-organisms	Valve(s) Involved	Early or Late Onset	Clinical Features	Blood Culture Results	Other	Indication for Reoperation/ Comment	Outcome
Norenberg et al [74]	*Mycobacterium fortuitum* (group IV)	Starr-Edwards aortic prosthesis	Late—2½ months	Chills, fever, weight loss, changing murmurs	Negative	Cultures of valve ring positive	Perivalvular leak. An epidemic of sternal wound infections reported by Robicsek et al [75]	Died 17 days after valve replacement
Altmann et al [76]	*M. chelonei* (group IV)	Bjork-Shiley aortic prosthesis (natural) replaced valve destroyed by endocarditis gram-positive	Late—3–4½ months	Fever, weakness, pulsating lesion at right cardiac border (no mention of murmur)	Positive	Cultures of vegetations positive	Not reoperated. First report of PVE due to this organism	Died—vegetation on valve, aortotomy with aneurysmal dilatation of aorta & aorto-atrial fistula
Repath [77]	*M. chelonei*	Starr-Edwards mitral & aortic prostheses	Late—3¾ months	Fever, chills, cough, cardiomegaly, petechiae, delirium, soft systolic murmur, LSB, audible valve sounds	Positive	Cultures of vegetations positive	Not reoperated. Organism commonly found in porcine xenograft valves Tyras et al [78]	Died
Lohr [79]	*M. gordonae* (group II)	Braunwald-Cutter aortic prosthesis	Late—13 months	Dental without antibiotic prophylaxis, fever, dyspnea, unchanging systolic murmur	Negative	Cultures of spinal fluid & bone marrow negative, liver biopsy noncaseating granulomas, *M. gordonae* cultured from vegetation	Valve dehiscence & annular abscess. Only report of PVE due to this organism	Survived valve replacement and antituberculous chemotherapy

O'Rourke, Shanahan, Harkness [80]	Acid-fast, not identifiable	Xenograft (porcine)	Probably early	Fever, splenomegaly, anemia, appearance of a loud precordial murmur	Negative (venous & arterial)	Bone marrow culture negative. Histologic-acid-fast organisms in excised vegetations & aortic wall. Bacteria never cultured	Aorta-RV fistula, valve dehiscence	Survived xenograft replacement with a mechanical prosthesis
Kristinsson, Bentall [81]	*Rickettsia burnetii (Coxiella burnetii)*	Fascia lata aortic prosthesis	Late—4 months	Breathlessness night sweats, clubbing	*S. albus* X 2 approx- 4 months. No response to 6 week antibiotic therapy	Complement-fixation titer to *R. burnetii* elevated. Microcolonies suggestive of *R. burnetii* seen in destroyed valve. Organism isolated on guinea pig inoculation		Survived—tissue valve replaced with Starr-Edwards prosthesis
Morgans, Cartwright [82]	*R. burnetii (C. burnettii)*	Starr-Edwards aortic prosthesis	Late—1 year	Hyperdynamic heart, Osler's nodes, clubbing	Negative	Complement-fixation titer to *R. burnetii* elevated. Guinea pig inoculations of blood showed elevation of complement-fixing antibodies. Aortic prosthesis showed a large vegetation with *Rickettsiae* demonstrated on special stains		Died 2 weeks after starting tetracycline therapy

bacteremic episodes by means of an elemental diet, preoperative gut decontamination, and systemic antibiotics, the valves remained free of thrombus.

The Role of Cloth Covering to the Prosthesis. Prostheses with the base and struts entirely covered with thin, porous fabric have been designed to minimize thromboembolism, though totally cloth-covered valves remain susceptible to infection with large inocula of *S. aureus.*

Clinical Manifestations

The diagnosis of PVE is more difficult to establish in patients who have undergone open heart operations than in unoperated patients. Although the same symptoms and signs are found (Table 31-10), they require cautious interpretation, as they can all occur in the absence of bacteremia following cardiopulmonary bypass. In general, patients with early PVE have shaking chills and splenomegaly. Changing murmurs usually appear at the same time as the first positive blood culture, both in the early and late cases, but in some changing murmurs are not noted until more than 1 month after the first positive blood culture. Embolic accidents can occur at any time.

Although the single consistent finding in all patients is still fever, a febrile response occurs commonly in patients following bypass in the absence of infection. For example, in infants, overheating by the environment is a common artifact. More detailed investigation must be instituted for daily unexplained temperature elevations of above 38.4C which persist postoperatively beyond 10 to 14 days. Evaluation should be particularly thorough in patients who demonstrate the triad of fever, splenomegaly, and a change in heart sounds.

The most significant change in heart sounds is usually the appearance of an aortic diastolic murmur. Dysfunction of a prosthetic mitral valve is indicated by the progression of a systolic murmur, and thrombosis of a mitral prosthesis can be heralded by the disappearance of the characteristic clicking sound. Cheng et al [89] state that this change should arouse immediate suspicion of massive thrombosis of the prosthesis. They reported a patient with an infected mitral prosthesis where the infection provided a nidus for progressive, fatal thrombosis.

Laboratory Examination in Diagnosis of PVE

Hematologic Findings. Anemia is uncommon, and leukocytosis is mild. Differential counts generally show predominance of neutrophils, and atypical lymphocytes are rarely noted. Erythrocyte sedimentation rates are consistently elevated. Leukocytosis in the diagnosis of infection after cardiac valve surgery has been previously emphasized,[51] but only a third of the patients with PVE have leukocytosis.

Urinary Findings. Microscopic hematuria and variable degrees of proteinuria are present in the majority of the patients. The degree of hematuria is not impressive, nor is the associated microscopic pyuria. Urine cultures are usually sterile.[51]

TABLE 31-10. CLINICAL FINDINGS IN PATIENTS WITH PROSTHETIC VALVE ENDOCARDITIS

Finding	Patients (%)	
	Early Group	*Late Group*
Fever	93	96
Chills	62	72
New regurgitant murmur	62	38
Shock	31	0
Leukocytosis (>12,000/mm³)	37	31
Congestive heart failure	25	31
Splenomegaly	19	20
Peripheral emboli *	6	27

* Includes Osler nodes.

From Wilson WR: Prosthetic valve endocarditis: incidence, anatomic location, cause, morbidity, and mortality. In Duma RJ (ed): *Infections of Prosthetic Heart Valves and Vascular Grafts.* Baltimore, University Park Press, 1977, p 5.

Nitroblue-Tetrazolium (NBT) Test. Freeman et al [90] monitored 74 consecutive patients undergoing open heart surgery for evidence of infection using the nitroblue tetrazolium (NBT) test as one method of surveillance. They felt that bacterial infection can be ruled out if the test is negative.

Roentgenographic and Other Special Diagnostic Examinations in PVE.

Roentgenographic Examinations. Stinson et al [91] reviewed some of the radiologic signs in endocarditis following prosthetic valve replacement. They noted that loosening of a prosthesis may occur with or without infection, but that extensive disruption of a suture line with gross valve movement is more likely caused by a destructive infectious process. The authors described the double exposure appearance of a disrupted prosthesis on prolonged exposure roentgenograms and distinguished between the gross angulation of a loose mitral prosthesis and the slight angulation that occurs with normal mitral valve action. In contrast, an aortic prosthesis normally moves very little during the cardiac cycle, and minor degrees of tilt on prolonged exposure may be significant. Gross angulation usually signifies detachment of most of the suture line. Fluoroscopy characteristically shows a rapid tilt or "flip" as the base of partially detached prosthesis changes its axis during systole.

Cinefluoroscopy allows more deliberate examination, and if there is still doubt, appropriate contrast studies are done using a cine or multiple frame technique. Kittredge and McCord [92] felt the degree of partial detachment and resultant insufficiency of a valve should be evaluated by intracardiac or aortic root injection of contrast material. Regurgitation in large amounts throughout systole usually results from a leak around the valve ring; however, the differential diagnosis would have to include a malfunctioning valve with the poppet lodged in the open position. Contrast material is especially important in evaluating the opening and closing function of a valve when the poppet is nonopaque.

The diagnostic features of malfunction of mitral valve prostheses has been outlined by Stross, Willis, and Kahn.[93] The authors studied two patients with disk prostheses in whom valve clicks were heard over the precordium in both cases. Routine films of the chest were diagnostic of valve malfunction with incomplete closure of the mitral disc evident in both cases. The authors note valve opening or closure occurs in approximately 1/30 of a second. Because the usual x-ray is 1/20 of a second, the valve is usually shown in the opened or closed position. Cine studies or rapid frame exposures will usually clarify valve motion and angulation. As in aortic valve dysfunction, cardiac catheterization and cineangiography should be done promptly when noninvasive studies are inconclusive.

The clinical and roentgenographic examinations are not only useful in a diagnostic sense, but they can also have therapeutic implications, eg, by dictating the removal of an unstable valve before the hemodynamic alterations are too advanced.

Echocardiography. The use of echocardiography in the diagnosis of infective endocarditis on natural valves is well established.[28] The use of echocardiography for the detection of valve vegetations in the diagnosis of PVE has increased of late.

Isotope Scanning. The experimental imaging of infective endocarditis with Indium 111 labeled blood cellular components has been noted. Riba et al [29] demonstrated in rabbits that Indium 111 labeled platelets (but not leukocytes) resulted in cardiac imaging that was sensitive enough to detect endocarditis. Isotope angiocardiography has been used clinically in detecting a malfunctioning tricuspid valve prosthesis by Malcolm, Ahuja, and Chamberlain.[94] They used technicium-99 pertechnetate and isotopically outlined a large right atrium with a striking hold-up of isotope in the great veins and right atrium. Isotope scanning may be a useful noninvasive adjunct in diagnosis of PVE where infection has caused valve dysfunction. The technique would be more valuable in right-sided prostheses, where imaging and activity-time curves for intravenously administered isotope are maximal before forward flow and dilution.

Diagnosis

The definitive diagnosis is established only by a positive venous blood culture. This is the most critical examination performed in both the diagnostic evaluation and subsequent assessment of patients developing intracardiac infections postoperatively. If the patient is receiving antibiotics, therapy is discontinued for 2 days. Venous samples from different sites are taken daily for 3 consecutive days and each specimen inoculated into one or more flasks. The venipuncture site must be well prepared, and sterile gloves must be worn. The cultures should then be incubated in aerobic and anaerobic media for 3 weeks. Penicillinase is added to the media as indicated. If the cultures remain sterile, bacterial endocarditis is highly unlikely. When indicated, the specimens should also be studied for fungi which, like the bacteria, usually show growth within 10 days. Antibiotic therapy can be resumed while awaiting the results.

Single isolated positive cultures should not be disregarded as contaminants. If the culture results are equivocal, a series of cultures should be repeated before either embarking on a prolonged course of therapy or discarding the diagnosis. The diagnosis of endocarditis is more certain if a large proportion of separately drawn blood cultures and inoculated flasks show growth of the same organism.

In a few cases, it may be difficult to identify the site of infection in a patient with sustained bacteremia when there is no clinical or roentgen evidence of valve dysfunction. Bach et al [95] localized infection in an aortic bypass graft which extended from the thoracic to the abdominal aorta using intra-arterial catheters and quantitative bacterial counts on blood samples taken upstream and downstream from the graft. The same principle can be applied to those rare patients with intracardiac prostheses and bacteremia in whom there is no definite evidence of endocarditis and no other obvious extracardiac source for bacteremia.

Treatment

The management of patients with PVE can be divided into three areas: (1) general care, (2) antimicrobial therapy, and (3) surgical considerations.[96]

General Care. Special attention should be directed to the organ systems most commonly affected in PVE. The major complications of PVE have been noted in the preceding sections and include congestive heart failure, arrhythmias, myocardial infarction secondary to coronary artery emboli, and myocardial abscess. Standard parameters that merit serial studies include repeated physical examinations, electrocardiograms, and roentgenograms of the chest. Other tests that may be useful in specific cases include fluoroscopy, echocardiography, and cardiac catheterization for hemodynamic studies and at times for quantitative cultures to assist in localization of a focus of infection.

Careful repeated evaluation of renal function is also indicated to adjust antibiotic dosage. Diminished renal function significantly alters the pharmacokinetics of most antibiotics, and antibiotic dosages should be reviewed daily in any patient who is uremic. Acute tubular impairment in PVE can be due to aminoglycoside toxicity, and prerenal azotemia can be due to cardiac failure as well as the glomerulonephritis seen as part of the vasculitis of PVE. The central nervous system, the skin, and the reticuloendothelial system should also be evaluated and followed.

Antimicrobial Therapy. After a microbiologic diagnosis is established by means of blood cultures, therapy can be initiated. If the illness is more acute, therapy can be started following the collection of three blood cultures several hours apart. Initial therapy, when possible, should include two drugs with synergistic bactericidal activity against the suspected or identified pathogen (Table 31-7).

The principles outlined in the sections on infective endocarditis also apply to the patient with PVE. Samples of organisms isolated from the blood cultures should be saved until treatment has been completed, so that susceptibility tests using a viable isolate can be done. Serum bactericidal activity and direct measurement of the agent in blood should be done to study the adequacy of drug dosage. Serum levels should be assessed at standardized times after administration. Synergism assays of the bactericidal activity of cell wall active agents such as penicillin and aminoglycosides can be carried out. As noted, this is especially important in patients with changing renal function.

Prolonged parenteral therapy with appropriate doses of antibacterial drugs is the most dependable approach. Oral antibiotics have not gained wide recognition for the treatment of patients with PVE. In their review, Gardner et al [96] note that the average duration of parenteral therapy was 5 weeks. Patients infected with staphylococci or gram-negative bacilli were usually treated longer, whereas patients infected with *S. viridans* or non-group D streptococci often received shorter treatment courses.

Surgical Considerations. The management of most patients with PVE hinges on antimicrobial therapy. Reoperation and replacement of the prosthesis must be carried out for patients with congestive heart failure, valve dysfunction, multiple septic emboli, or when medical therapy fails.[97,98] Utilizing these common criteria, however,[99] the overall mortality for patients with PVE averages 56 percent.

In view of these poor results, Gardner, Saffle, and Schoenbaum [96] reexamined the concept of prompt valve replacement versus medical treatment alone. The obvious goal is to excise the diseased prosthesis before the infection spreads into critical structures (septic emboli, interventricular septum, myocardial abscesses, etc.) or produces congestive heart failure. Arguments against prompt valve replacement include the risks of persistent or recurrent infection that could necessitate a second reoperation. One of the consequences of recommending early operations is that valve replacement will be done in some patients who could have been cured with antibiotics alone. In rebuttal, Gardner et al [96] argue that the operative mortality in cardiac surgery is correlated chiefly with a degree of congestive heart failure at the time of operation and that a policy of prompt valve replacement would probably lower the operative mortality to that seen in elective valve replacement (less than 10 percent).

Prognosis

Gardner et al [96] reviewed three large series, which included a total of 134 patients (Table 31-11). The mortality in the three series ranged from 51 to 60 percent (average 56 percent). Patients with an early onset of PVE had a high mortality (78 percent) and were infected chiefly by staphylococci, gram-negative bacilli, or *Candida*. Patients with late onset PVE had a lower mortality (38 percent) and were more commonly infected with streptococci.

Twenty-two percent of patients were treated by valve replacement. The indications for surgery were: (1) significant valvular leak and congestive heart failure (64 percent), (2) persistent or recurrent bacteremia (35 percent), and (3) peripheral emboli (22 percent). Several of the patients had more than one indication for operation. The overall mortality was 63 of 103 cases (61 percent) for patients treated with antibiotics alone and 39 percent (12 of 32 cases) for patients treated by valve replacement plus antibiotics (Table 31-12). Gardner et al [96] emphasize that patients who died shortly after diagnosis were frequently too ill to be benefited by any therapy, and that this group unfairly prejudiced the treatment results. Consequently, they analyzed a subgroup of patients who survived at least 1 week after the diagnosis of PVE. Table 31-13 clearly shows that surgical intervention was more advantageous when the unsalvageable patients were excluded from the analysis.

Gardner et al [96] concluded that the results of therapy with antimicrobial drugs alone approaches the success rate of valve replacement only for patients with late onset infection caused by highly sensitive organisms such as *S. viridans* who do not have valve dysfunction, congestive heart failure, multiple septic emboli, or refractory infection (Table 31-14). They suggest that the more liberal indications for surgery would yield a greater salvage.

Prevention of PVE. Intraoperative Prophylactic Antibiotics. The principles and practice of antibiotic prophylaxis is reviewed in Chapter 23. The use of prophylactic antibiotics following open heart surgery is now considered a major factor in the prevention of postoperative endocarditis.[51] The value of prophylactic antibiotics was questioned before it became clear that preoperative and intraoperative bactericidal serum levels must be maintained and that the antibiotic choice should be made from

TABLE 31-11. MORTALITY BY CAUSATIVE ORGANISM IN PROSTHETIC VALVE ENDOCARDITIS

Organism	Early Onset, No. Deaths/No. Cases	Late Onset, No. Deaths/No. Cases	Total No. Deaths/No. Cases	Mortality (%)
Staphylococcus epidermidis	7/13	3/7	10/20	(50)
S. aureus	13/15	8/10	21/25	(84)
Viridans streptococci	2/2	4/18	6/20	(30)
Group D streptococci	3/4	3/12	6/16	(37)
Other streptococci		3/9	3/9	(33)
Gram-negative bacilli	13/15	3/12	16/27	(59)
Candida spp	7/8	2/2	9/10	(90)
Other	2/3	2/4	4/7	(57)
Total (% mortality)	47/60 (78)	28/74 (38)	75/134	(56)

From Gardner P, Saffle JR, Schoenbaum SC: Management of prosthetic valve endocarditis. In Duma RJ (ed): *Infections of Prosthetic Heart Valves and Vascular Grafts.* Baltimore, University Park Press, 1977, p 132.

TABLE 31-12. RESULTS OF TREATMENT BY VALVE REPLACEMENT VERSUS ANTIBIOTICS ALONE FOR PVE PATIENTS (NO. DEATHS/NO. CASES)

	Early Onset *		Late Onset †		Total	
Series	*Medical*	*Valve Replacement*	*Medical*	*Valve Replacement*	*Medical*	*Valve Replacement*
Mayo Clinic	13/15	1/1	9/21	2/8	22/36	3/9
University of Oregon	19/22	1/1	6/17	3/8	25/39	4/9
Massachusetts General Hospital	10/15	3/6	6/13	2/7	16/28	5/13
Total (% mortality)	42/52 (81)	5/8 (63)	21/51 (41) ‡	7/23 (30) ‡	63/103 (61) ‡	12/31 (39) ‡

Based on 134 cases in 131 patients.
* Within 60 days of prosthetic valve insertion.
† More than 60 days from prosthetic valve insertion.
‡ $P < 0.05$

From Gardner P, Saffle JR, Schoenbaum SC: Management of prosthetic valve endocarditis. In Duma RJ (ed): *Infections of Prosthetic Heart Valves and Vascular Grafts.* Baltimore, University Park Press, 1977, p 133

TABLE 31-13. RESULTS OF TREATMENT BY VALVE REPLACEMENT VERSUS ANTIBIOTIC ALONE FOR PVE PATIENTS WHO SURVIVED AT LEAST ONE WEEK AFTER DIAGNOSIS (NO. DEATHS/NO. CASES)

	Early Onset *		Late Onset †		Total	
Sources	*Medical*	*Valve Replacement*	*Medical*	*Valve Replacement*	*Medical*	*Valve Replacement*
Mayo Clinic	11/13		11/21	1/7	22/34	1/7
University of Oregon Hospital	18/21	1/1	5/16	0/5	23/37	1/6
Massachusetts General Hospital	7/11	2/4	4/11	1/5	11/22	3/9
Total (% mortality)	36/45 (80)	3/5 (60)	20/48 (42) ‡	2/17 (12) ‡	56/93 (60) ‡	5/22 (23) ‡

Based on 115 cases in 112 patients.
* Within 60 days of prosthetic valve insertion.
† More than 60 days from prosthetic valve insertion.
‡ $P < 0.05$

From Gardner P, Saffle JR, Schoenbaum SC: Management of prosthetic valve endocarditis. In Duma RJ (ed): *Infections of Prosthetic Heart Valves and Vascular Grafts.* Baltimore, University Park Press, 1977, p 135.

TABLE 31-14. PVE: MORTALITY BY ORGANISM ACCORDING TO METHOD OF THERAPY (NO. DEATHS/NO. CASES)

	Early Onset		Late Onset		Total	
	Medical	*Valve Replacement*	*Medical*	*Valve Replacement*	*Medical*	*Valve Replacement*
Staphylococcus epidermidis	5/10	2/3	2/3	1/4	7/13	3/7
S. aureus	12/14	1/1	6/7	2/3	18/21	3/4
Viridans streptococci	2/2		3/15	1/3	5/17	1/3
Group D streptococci	3/3	0/1	2/8	1/4	5/11	1/5
Other streptococci			2/6	1/3	2/6	1/3
Gram-negative bacilli	12/14	1/1	3/9	0/3	15/23	1/4
Candida	6/7	1/1	1/1	1/1	7/8	2/2
Others	2/2	0/1	2/2	0/2	4/4	0/3
Total (% mortality)	42/52 (81)	5/8 (63)	21/51 (41)	7/23 (30)	63/103 (61)	12/31 (39)

Based on 134 cases in 131 patients.

From Gardner P, Saffle JR, Schoenbaum, SC: Management of prosthetic valve endocarditis. In Duma RJ (ed): *Infections of Prosthetic Heart Valves and Vascular Grafts.* Baltimore, University Park Press, 1977, p. 136.

those that kill the organisms most likely to cause the infection.

Using these principles, almost all investigators have reduced the incidence of positive blood cultures during surgery [54,100] and the incidence of PVE.[48,51,54,100]

The drug regimens vary somewhat according to institution, but a typical regimen for antibiotic coverage includes the use of penicillin, methicillin or oxacillin, and streptomycin or kanamycin starting on the day before operation and continuing for 1 week postoperatively.[101] This type of regimen is in contrast to the heavy and sustained parenteral coverage noted before.

Long-Term Antibiotic Prophylaxis. A patient with a prosthetic intracardiac device has a chance of contracting endocarditis when undergoing dental or other procedures long after complete recovery has taken place (Table 31-1). Bacteremia can even result from gingival ulcers caused by ill-fitting dentures, and late endocarditis may result from this mechanism. A vigorous prophylactic antibiotic program should be begun in patients with prosthetic cardiac valves who are about to undergo dental or other procedures. The prophylactic program must be more intensive than the prophylactic penicillin regimen recommended for patients with rheumatic heart disease who are candidates for surgical procedures. It includes the use of broad-spectrum antibiotics for 2 days before a dental procedure to reduce the number of organisms in the mouth. On the day before, the day of, and for 3 to 5 days following the procedure, parenteral procaine penicillin (600,000 units every 6 hours) and streptomycin (0.5 gm every 12 hours) are given. Methicillin (5 gm) is given intravenously during the day of operation and oxacillin (4 gm) orally for 3 to 5 days following the procedure.

In penicillin-sensitive patients, a cephalosporin is commonly substituted, although erythromycin or lincomycin could be used. Cephalothin is so rapidly excreted that repeated doses need to be given at 2-hour intervals. Cephazolin would seem to be a better choice for intraoperative prophylaxis.

Fungal Prosthetic Valve Endocarditis

Although intracardiac fungus infection is uncommon following open heart surgery, the diagnosis should be considered in those patients suspected of having endocarditis in whom routine blood cultures are sterile. Characteristically, *Aspergillus* and *Candida* vegetations are found impairing the function of the prosthetic valve and widespread septic emboli are present.[102] McLeod and Remington [102] collected more than 300 cases of fungal endocarditis from the literature. More than half occurred on prosthetic valves. Many of the case reports contained only partial information, and their analysis was based only on those cases in which a specific factor was mentioned. Their tabulated information is most useful, and the percentages stated in their tables refer solely to the percentage of patients in whom a specific parameter was defined.

Etiology

Table 31-15 lists the valves involved by various fungi in 170 cases of endocarditis that occurred after cardiac surgery.[102] Obviously, *Aspergillis* and *Candida* species predominate. Table 31-16 [103-112] lists the clinical characteristics of the more unusual fungal prosthetic valve infections.

Incidence

Fungal PVE is uncommon—its incidence relative to bacterial PVE is shown in Table 31-7. McLeod and Remington [102] found no apparent preferential predisposition of any specific type of valve for fungi and no predilection of any specific fungus for a particular valve.

TABLE 31-15. VALVES INVOLVED BY VARIOUS FUNGI IN 170 CASES OF FUNGAL ENDOCARDITIS OCCURRING AFTER CARDIAC SURGERY

	Total	No Implant	Prosthesis *	Homograft	Heterograft	Fascia lata	Other Cardiac Surgery
Aspergillus	43	4	28(30)	3	0	5	3
Candida albicans	65	11	34(36)	16	1	0	3
Candida (non-*albicans*)	32	10	15(26)	4	0	0	3
Candida (species not specified)	15	0	9	4	1	0	1
Coprinus species	1	0	1	0	0	0	0
Cryptococcus neoformans	1	0	1	0	0	0	0
Curvularia geniculata	1	0	0	1	0	0	0
Histoplasma capsulatum	2	2	0	0	0	0	0
Paecilomyces varioti	2	0	1	1	0	0	0
Penicillium spp	3	0	3	0	0	0	0
Phialophora	2	0	1	0	1	0	0
Phycomyces	1	0	1	0	0	0	0
Saccharomyces cerevisiae	2	0	2	0	0	0	0
Torulopsis glabrata	1	0	0(1)	0	0	0	0
Total	171	27	112	29	3	5	10

* Figures in parentheses include cases in which infection recurred on prosthesis after fungal infection on a different valve.

From McLeod R, Remington JS: Postoperative fungal endocarditis. In Duma RJ (ed): *Infections of Prosthetic Heart Valves and Vascular Grafts.* Baltimore, University Park Press, 1977, p 171.

Pathogenesis

Fungi are everywhere in ventilating systems near and in the operating room and recovery rooms. Operating room equipment and anesthesia equipment are both contaminated—as are occasional homograft valves, porcine heterograft valves, and suture material. Fungi may also be introduced into the circulation by trauma to the trachea or colonization of the lower airways during intubation and mechanical ventilation. Other wound infections and intravenous catheters and solutions are well-known sources.

The turbulence and jet effect, which produce endocardial surface trauma and thereby predispose to platelet deposition and adherence of organisms, has been stressed by Robboy and Kaiser.[113] They found four lethal cases in which the fungi had implanted on patches of neoendocardium consisting of platelets, fibrin, and fibroblasts that developed as ingrowth of host endocardium onto the sewing cloth rather than on the cloth or the metallic parts of the valve.

Concomitant bacterial and fungal infections have been reported in a number of cases. In fact, antibiotics had been administered before the development of fungal endocarditis in 68 percent of McLeod and Remington's cases.[102] Intravenous catheters had been used in 43 percent. The same bacteria that occur as common causes of bacterial endocarditis also occur in conjunction with fungal endocarditis. These are organisms that have a greater ability to adhere to heart valves in vitro, and the adherence properties of bacteria may well be related to fungal implantation on a valve. In addition, staphylococci grow better in vitro in the presence of *C. albicans* than in pure culture.[102]

Role of Antibiotics in Predisposing to Fungal Infection. The role of antibiotics in predisposing to fungal infection has received considerable attention (Chapters 9 and 47). Antibiotics may predispose to fungal infection by eliminating intestinal bacteria that normally compete for nutrients and produce antifungal agents, thereby allowing fungal overgrowth which in turn leads to fungemia. In addition, antibiotics are thought to interfere directly with cellular fungicidal mechanisms. Cooper et al [114] found that antibiotics were necessary in dog models to produce *C. guilliermondi* endocarditis.

Pathology

One of the most characteristic features of fungal endocarditis are the large, bulky vegetations (2–8 cm in largest diameter). Fungal vegetations can produce aortic insufficiency by valvular destruction, interference with valve closure by a vegetation, and destruction of paravalvular tissue and secondary paravalvular leaks. Fungal vegetation in a prosthetic valve may also prevent proper seating of the ball in the metallic ring and thereby lead to regurgitation. In addition, stenosis of a valve orifice may be caused by vegetations interfering with flow across the valve.

The vegetations histologically reveal debris, fibrin, and large colonies of organisms with either yeast or hyphal forms or both. Organisms are present both on the surface and within the vegetation. In addition, histiocytes, lymphocytes, and neutrophils are seen within vegetations and at their periphery. Patches of neoendocardium, which appear to have developed as ingrowths of host endocardium onto the sewing ring of artificial valves, have been involved with foci of infection.

Nonvalvular cardiac involvement in fungal endocarditis includes myocardial abscesses, fistulas, coronary emboli and infarction, aneurysms of the atrioventricular valve ring, and destruction and perforation of the interventricular septum and papillary muscles. In addition, myocarditis and pericarditis have also been seen.

Hepatic involvement most frequently consists of chronic passive congestion or small hepatic abscesses. Enlarged spleens are commonly found and show congestion and at times splenic infarcts and abscesses. Renal abnormalities are present in the majority of patients, with infarction, abscesses, and fungal pyelonephritis. Focal glomerulitis as seen in bacterial endocarditis has also been noted.

Emboli can occur to almost any site within the body, most commonly the kidney, the central nervous system, the lower extremities, and the spleen. Cerebral emboli have been associated with mycotic aneurysms. *Aspergillus* is an especially virulent embolic agent in that it invades and causes necrosis of walls of small to medium sized arteries and veins.

Clinical Manifestations

McLeod and Remington [102] noted that an antemortem diagnosis of fungal endocarditis had been made in only one-half of the reported cases.

Special attention should be paid to intravenous drug abusers, patients who have received antibiotics, those in whom intravenous catheters have been used for any length of time, and patients with infected catheter sites. Fungal endocarditis should also be suspected in patients with disseminated fungal disease. These historical features can be deceptive in that they may antedate an obvious illness by months and at times even years. Fungal endocarditis should also be suspected in patients who have persistent fever even after therapy for proven bacterial endocarditis, and those in whom endocarditis is suspected, but where blood culture results are repeatedly negative. The most common clinical features are the same as those seen in bacterial PVE, except that embolic phenomena are more prevalent.[102] Seventy-two percent of the patients with fungal PVE had emboli, in contrast to 27 percent of those with bacterial endocarditis.[115]

Laboratory Findings

The laboratory and electrocardiographic findings in fungal endocarditis are the same as in all endocarditis. The roentgen findings may be useful. Lesions in the lungs secondary to septic pulmonary emboli include consolidations, streaks in the parenchyma, pleural effusions, or at times nodular densities. Areas of increased lucency secondary to pulmonary ischemia may at times be seen. McLeod and Remington [102] note that the inflammatory response is deficient in leukopenic patients, and pulmonary findings may be much less impressive even during an active fungal infection. Arteriograms may demonstrate bulky emboli in the lungs. Abnormal echoes may be produced by the large vegetations, which modify the motions of prosthetic devices.

TABLE 31-16. PROSTHETIC VALVE ENDOCARDITIS—UNCOMMON FUNGAL INFECTIONS

Author/Ref.	Micro-organisms	Valve(s) Involved	Early or Late Onset	Clinical Features	Blood Culture Results	Other	Indication for Reoperation/Comment	Outcome
Uys et al [103]	*Paecilomyces varioti*	Ivalon mitral baffle	Late—12½ months	Fever, clubbing, cerebral embolus, infarction	Positive	Microcerebral vessel and brain infarct containing fungal elements	Not reoperated. First reported case of PVE due to this organism	Died—received short course of antifungal therapy
Silver, Tuffnell, Bigelow [104]	*P. varioti*	Aortic valve allograft	Late—8–12 months	Fever, emboli, systolic and diastolic murmurs	Negative	Valve vegetations	Aortic insufficiency	Died 3 weeks after allograft replacement with a mechanical prosthesis
McClellan et al [105]	*P. varioti*	Starr-Edwards aortic prosthesis	Late—7½ months	Fever, anorexia, weight loss, clubbing, petechiae, prosthetic opening sound louder than closing sound, systolic ejection murmur	Negative	Embolectomy specimen; thrombus on replaced aortic prosthesis	Emboli First report of PVE of a mechanical prosthesis due to this organism	Died—mediastinal hemorrhage following aortic valve replacement
Weaver, Batsakis, Nishiyama [106]	*Histoplasma capsulatum*	Teflon aortic prosthesis	Late—10 months	Fever, probable emboli	Negative	Microorganisms seen, *H. capsulatum* cultured from vegetations on aortic valve prosthesis	Not reoperated. First report of PVE due to this organism. Review of 16 cases of natural valve *Histoplasma* endocarditis. Diagnosis difficult because cultures usually negative	Died—disseminated noncaseating granulomas
Alexander et al [107]	*H. capsulatum*	Bjork-Shiley aortic prosthesis	Late—3–6 months	Fever, weight loss, hemiparesis, aphasia (3–4 months), fever, cough, neurologic deterioration (6 months). Prosthetic valve sounds unremarkable. No diastolic murmur heard	Negative at 3–4 months	CSF culture negative, *H. capsulatum* cultured from meninges and valvular vegetations	Replacement of initial tissue valve with Bjork-Shiley valve not reoperated	Died—aortic prosthesis infected but there was no impediment to function

Kaufman [108]	*Curvularia geniculata*	Aortic valve homograft	Late—7¾ months	Fever, splinter hemorrhages, multiple neurologic signs, peripheral emboli, murmurs noted, no mention of change	Negative	Organisms cultured from vegetations on homograft valve	Emboli. First report of PVE due to this organism	Died 6 days following homograft valve replacement with a mechanical prosthesis
Khicha et al [109]	*Mucor* species	Beall mitral prosthesis	Early	Pulmonary edema, hypotension	Negative	Characteristic mucor forms in thrombotic vegetation	Not reoperated	Died 26 days postop
Upshaw [110]	*Penicillium chrysogenum*	Starr-Edwards aortic prosthesis	Early—45 days postop	Probable emboli to central nervous system, legs, increased intensity of systolic ejection murmur	Not stated	Fungal thromboemboli to iliac arteries	No cardiac reoperation. First report of PVE due to this organism	Died 74 days after embolectomy
Hall [111]	*Penicillium* species	Starr-Edwards aortic and mitral prostheses	Early—less than 1 month	Fever, headache anorexia, petechiae, prosthetic heart sounds heard, no murmurs	Sterile negative	Innumerable hyphae in prostheses vegetations. Cultures grew *Penicillium* spp	No reoperation. Ceiling ventilator above pump oxygenator assembly colonized	Died—less than 1 month
Hall [111]	*Penicillium* species	Starr-Edwards aortic prosthesis	Early—2 weeks	Fever, systemic emboli, petechiae, cerebrovascular accident, no change in heart sounds	Sterile	Numerous septate hyphae in prosthesis vegetations. Culture grew *Penicillium* spp	No cardiac reoperation	Died—2 weeks
Roberts, Allen, Maybee [112]	*Petriellidium boydii (Allescheria boydii)*	Xenograft (porcine) mitral prosthesis	Late—2½ months	Fever, hepatomegaly, petechiae	Positive	Thrombus on valve contained hyphae & thick-walled *Candida*	Not reoperated. Organism common in mycetoma	Died

Serologic Studies. Serologic studies in the diagnosis of fungal disease are discussed in Chapter 9. McLeod and Remington [102] note that among the more promising methods in detecting candidiasis are those which detect precipitating antibodies, mannan (a surface polysaccharide of *Candida*), antigenemia, and gas-liquid chromatography. None are diagnostic, since false-positive reactions are too common.

Cultures. All thromboemboli should be cultured for fungi. Histologic examination of tissue can also be very helpful in identifying fungal elements and is independent of cultures that may be sterile. Bone marrow cultures may also be useful.

McLeod and Remington [102] tabulated the results of blood cultures in fungal endocarditis (Table 31-17). Blood cultures were frequently positive in *Candida* endocarditis (64 to 93 percent), but they were seldom positive in endocarditis due to *Aspergillus.* Several reasons have been proposed for the negative blood cultures: (1) differences in growth characteristics of certain fungi; (2) low numbers of organisms due to the fact that fungi grow in mycelial masses rather than as separate organisms—it may be necessary to culture larger volumes of blood than usually necessary for bacterial endocarditis; (3) fungi may be trapped in capillary beds, and arterial cultures may be more useful than venous blood cultures in some cases; (4) the possible emergence of L-forms in patients with fungal endocarditis has also been postulated; in patients with negative cultures, hypertonic media should be used to pick up possible L-form transformation; [102] (5) fungi may not cloud the culture medium as bacteria do, so that the cultures are erroneously discarded.

Blood cultures should be examined by a Gram stain even when the culture media appears to be negative. Therefore, variations in media may be helpful in achieving growth of some of the fungi.[102]

Treatment and Prognosis

The results of therapy are dismal—only 16 percent of patients with *Candida* infections and 5 percent of those with *Aspergillus* survive.[108]

Patients with fungal PVE seldom survived when given amphotericin (22 percent) alone, while 11 of 22 who received both amphotericin and operation survived. In brief, drugs alone are not adequate therapy for fungal prosthetic valve endocarditis. Replacement of the valve is necessary in the vast majority of cases. Delay is rarely justified. Preoperative amphotericin B does not improve the outcome, but intravenous doses of the drug should be started on the day of operation, to be continued for long periods. Local irrigations of the endocardium with a 1 percent solution of amphotericin B may be helpful.[102]

The drugs useful for fungal PVE are those useful for fungal infections in general—amphotericin B, 5-fluorocytosine, and miconazole (Chapter 18). The combinations of amphotericin B and flucytosine are additive or synergistic. Synergy of a combination of amphotericin B and rifampin have been noted against *C. albicans* and combinations have been fungicidal against *Histoplasma.* Rifampin and low-dose amphotericin B have been used successfully in inhibiting growth of *Saccharomyces.*

PVE-Involving Tissue Valves

The use of tissue valves has increased in the past decade because the incidence of thromboembolism is reduced when compared to mechanical prostheses. Various tissue substitutes have been employed and the experiences with prosthetic valve endocarditis documented.[116]

Aortic Homograft Valves

In 1962, Ross [117] carried out the first clinical placement of an aortic valve homograft in the subcoronary position. In an earlier series, the homografts were sterilized and

TABLE 31-17. DATA ON BLOOD CULTURES, SEROLOGY, AND SURVIVAL IN PATIENTS WITH ENDOCARDITIS CAUSED BY DIFFERENT FUNGI

Fungus	Total Cases Reported	% with Positive Blood Cultures	% with Positive Serology	% Surviving
Aspergillus	43	13 (4/30)		5
Candida albicans	65	81 (47/58)	100 (9/9)	18
Candida (Non-*albicans)*	32	93 (26/28)	100 (4/4)	14
Candida (species not specified)	15	64 (7/11)	100 (2/2)	13
Coprinius spp	1	0 (0/1)		0
Cryptococcus neoformans	1	100 (1/1)	0 (0/0)	0
Curvularia geniculata	1	0 (0/1)		0
Histoplasma capsulatum	2	0 (0/2)	0 (0/0)	0
Paecilomyces varioti	2	50 (1/2)		0
Penicillium spp	3	0 (0/2)		0
Phialophora	2	50 (1/2)		0
Phycomyces	1	0 (0/0)		0
Saccharomyces cerevisiae	2	100 (2/2)		50
Torulopsis glabrata	1	0 (0/0)		0

Figures outside parentheses: percentage of patients with the parameter. Numerators of figures inside parentheses: patients with the parameter. Denominators of figures inside parentheses: those patients in whom it was possible to define this parameter from the data presented.

From McLeod R, Remington JS: Postoperative fungal endocarditis. In Duma RJ (ed): *Infections of Prosthetic Heart Valves and Vascular Grafts.* Baltimore, University Park Press, 1977, p 163.

preserved in 4 percent formaldehyde solution buffered to a pH of 5.6. Acute bacterial endocarditis *(S. aureus)* was one of the most important postoperative complications and accounted for one of five deaths. Gonzalez-Lavin et al [118] reported on 259 patients who had undergone aortic valve replacement with preserved homograft valves. Most valves showed fragmentation of collagen fibers, resulting in diminution in tensile strength. For this reason, Malm et al [119] adopted sterilization by activated gamma irradiation and preservation of valves in the frozen state.

Although the incidence of endocarditis was not increased by the use of preserved aortic homografts, graft failure requiring reoperation was too common. Sometimes, endocarditis appeared to precede valve failure. Sterilization of homograft valves by either irradiation or beta-propiolactone solution produced acellularity with a loss of fibrillar structure, separation of collagen fibers, and disruption of elastic fibers. The changes were accentuated in most cusps removed for dysfunction. The most pronounced changes were found in cusps that had been affected by a previous episode of bacterial endocarditis. These valves had thickening, fibrosis, and areas of calcification. These findings encouraged the search for other tissue valve prostheses.

Fascia Lata Grafts

The use of strut supported autologous fascia lata grafts was first reported by Ross et al.[120] The grafts apparently maintained viability, but functional deterioration in the tricuspid and mitral positions and a high incidence of endocarditis has led to the abandonment of this technique.

Homologous Dura Mater Valves

In a continuing exploration of material for tissue valves, Zerbini [121] reported on 533 patients in whom homologous dura mater grafts were used for cardiac valve replacement. In these patients, the dura was harvested from cadavers within 12 hours of death and sterilized and preserved in 98 percent glycerol solution for 12 days. There were only two instances of prosthetic valve endocarditis, both due to *Aspergillus fumigatus.*

Porcine Aortic Xenograft (Hancock) Valves

In view of the shortcomings already noted in tissue valves, the use of xenografts has gained in popularity. Porcine aortic xenografts have been studied extensively and closely resembles its human counterpart. In 1975, Buch et al [122] reported on 120 patients who underwent mitral valve replacement with a Hancock "stabilized glutaraldehyde process: porcine aortic xenograft." Enterococcocal endocarditis developed in only one patient, 20 months after surgery and responded to ampicillin and probenicid therapy. Further experience has suggested that the Hancock porcine xenograft is: (1) as susceptible to infection as are rigid prostheses, (2) relatively resistant to early postoperative bacteremia, (3) easier to sterilize than rigid prostheses, and (4) more durable than other tissue valves in the face of PVE.[116]

The Hancock porcine valve continues to gain acceptance in many centers, but some later failures may be due to low-grade infection. A fastidious atypical mycobacteria which can be cultured only after prolonged incubation in special media has been found in eight of 24 Hancock values (Table 31-9). Whether this organism is the *M. avium–M. intracellulare* complex, which commonly infects pigs, or some other atypical mycobacterium is unknown. Currently, glutaraldehyde stabilization of the collagen matrix of the valve is an effective sterilizing agent as well. Valves are not released to users until a quarantine period has passed and control cultures have been proved to be sterile. An extensive study was undertaken comparing heterograft tissue valves and mechanical valves by Rossiter et al [116] in 1978.

Norenberg et al [74] found half the cases of bacterial PVE were caused by opportunistic bacteria, and 13 to 20 percent were caused by fungi. Unusual organisms have been especially noted in tissue valves (Tables 31-8, 31-9, 31-15, and 31-16).

POSTOPERATIVE SYNDROMES

Three identifiable postoperative syndromes have been described in patients after cardiac surgery, with and without the use of extracorporeal circulation: the postpericardiotomy, postperfusion, and postcardiotomy syndromes.[123]

POSTPERICARDIOTOMY SYNDROME

The postpericardiotomy syndrome is delayed in onset and follows trauma, myocardial infarction, or a variety of cardiac surgical procedures. Fever and chest pain are the predominant symptoms, with evidence of pericarditis confirmed by physical examination, electrocardiogram, roentgen examination, or echocardiography. The incidence can be as high as 30 percent. Heart-reactive antibodies have been found in many patients, particularly in association with serologic evidence of infection with coxsackie B1-B6 or cytomegalovirus. Engle et al [124,125] suggest that a recent viral illness or reactivation of a latent illness may trigger the immunologic response that constitutes the postpericardiotomy syndromes.

The syndrome is usually mild and self-limited, although pericardial tamponade has been reported. Rest, fluid restriction, and diuretics are commonly recommended. Systemic steroids are effective in patients with severe or prolonged symptoms.

POSTPERFUSION SYNDROME

The postperfusion syndrome consists of fever, an atypical lymphocytosis, and splenomegaly appearing most commonly 2 to 6 weeks after an episode of extracorporeal circulation. Pericarditis and pleurisy are not dominant findings. Rising titers of antibodies to cytomegalovirus during the course of the syndrome, and isolation of the virus from body fluids has implicated this virus as the causative agent. Identification of the parainfluenza virus in tissue cultures from patients with a similar disorder suggested that multiple viruses or virus strains may be producing different clinical varieties of the syndrome in various parts of the world. Since the cytomegalovirus resides in the leukocyte fractions of fresh blood, primary CMV infections could be acquired. Other evidence suggests that latent CMV may become reactivated by alterations in host defense induced by extracorporeal circulation (Chapter 10).[124,125] This syndrome is benign and usually mildly symptomatic. The importance of correct diagnosis lies in differentiating more serious causes of fever, such as bacterial endocarditis and hepatitis.

POSTCARDIOTOMY SYNDROME

The postcardiotomy syndrome exhibits features of both postpericardiotomy and the postperfusion syndromes. Kirsh et al[123] characterized it by the onset of prolonged fever, tachycardia, and mucosal lesions within a few days after operation. Recurrent fever, pleuropericardial friction rub, hepatomegaly, and splenomegaly develop three to six weeks later. The course is benign, and only supportive treatment is necessary.

Fever After Heart Surgery

Undiagnosed febrile illnesses are common after open heart surgery and may or may not conform to the clinical syndromes discussed. Freeman et al[90] identified a group of febrile but clinically well patients with strongly positive NBT tests with no identifiable bacterial cause. These patients recovered completely in a few days, and the NBT test became negative. There was a fourfold or greater rise in complement-fixing antibody titer to cytomegalovirus in three (4 percent), and to *M. pneumoniae* in 14 (19 percent) of 74 patients. There was no serologic evidence of infection with influenza A and B, mumps, the psittacosis-lymphogranuloma venereum group of agents *(Chlamydia)* or *Coxiella burnetii.* Caul and co-workers[126] found complement-fixing antibodies to cytomegalovirus in 21 of 55 cardiac surgical patients. There was no correlation between cytomegalovirus infection and age, sex, blood group, or season. All the patients received fresh blood, but none of those receiving less than 5 pints became infected. The authors speculated, as have others, on whether some of these infections are due to fresh blood used in extracorporeal circuits.

Burch and Colcolough[127] have suggested that some viruses, especially the coxsackie B group, are capable of infecting the heart and remaining dormant for long periods of time to be activated when conditions are suitable. They found a number of instances in which viral antigen was detected within the myocardium and valves of experimental animals many months after the initial infection. They felt that some instances of chronic valvular and myocardial disease, thought previously to be rheumatic in origin, might have been due to viruses. In addition, these findings make it conceivable that the postperfusion and perhaps the postpericardiotomy and postcardiotomy syndromes may result from activation of a dormant cardiac virus following the trauma of operation, transfused blood, and extracorporeal circulation.

Hornick[128] emphasizes that in addition to bacterial contamination of parenteral solutions, other agents may also be transfused with debilitating effects (ie, cytomegalovirus, hepatitis viruses, and EB viruses). These agents can both induce infection and depress host defenses so that superinfection can occur.

Infection with *M. pneumoniae* after open heart surgery has been studied by Freeman et al[90] who screened 119 heart surgery patients using the nitroblue tetrazolium (NBT) test and routine serologic examination for evidence of viral infection. A group of patients emerged in whom the NBT test was strongly positive but in whom no evidence of bacterial infection could be found by conventional methods. Twenty-five of the 119 heart surgery patients (21 percent) showed serologic evidence of infection with *M. pneumoniae.* There were no details about the clinical manifestations of the infections, except that no patient exhibited the radiologic features of primary atypical pneumonia.

Obviously, not all febrile illnesses are infective in origin. The role of transfused blood per se, and altered host immunologic reactivity has been investigated by Roses et al.[129] They studied the etiology of postoperative fevers in 97 patients after cardiac surgical procedures. Of this group, 26 had unexplained fevers, while only 6 of all the patients had a postpericardiotomy syndrome. The pathogenetic mechanisms have included exacerbation of rheumatic fever, an inflammatory response to blood in the pericardial cavity, autoimmune responses to traumatized cardiac tissue, and reaction of the patient to leukocytes in transfused blood. Atypical lymphocytes occurred almost twice as frequently in patients with prolonged fevers after the first postoperative week, in whom no specific etiology could be defined, compared with subjects who were afebrile after the first postoperative week. This group also received more units of transfused blood during operation. There was no correlation, however, between such cellular activation and the appearance of lymphocytotoxic antibodies against a standard reference panel of lymphocytes obtained from 30 normal donors of different HLA phenotypes. This suggested that the atypical lymphocytes reflected a cellular rather than a serologic immune response to massive blood transfusions.

BIBLIOGRAPHY

Brewer LA (ed): Prosthetic Heart Valves. Springfield, Ill, Charles C Thomas, 1969.

Duma RJ (ed): Infections of Prosthetic Heart Valves and Vascular Grafts. Baltimore, University Park Press, 1977.

Kaplan EL, Taranta AV (eds): Infective Endocarditis. Dallas, American Heart Association, 1977.

Kaye D (ed): Infective Endocarditis. Baltimore, University Park Press, 1976.

Rahimtoola SH (ed): Infective Endocarditis. New York, Grune and Stratton, 1978.

REFERENCES

MYOCARDIAL INFECTIONS

1. Miller AJ, Pick R, Kline IK, Katz LN: The susceptibility of dogs with chronic impairment of cardiac lymph flow to staphylococcal valvular endocarditis. Circulation 30:417, 1964.
2. Gopalakrishna KV, Kwon KH, Shah A: Metastatic myocardial

abscess due to group F streptococci. Am J Med Sci 274:329, 1977.
3. Milstoc M, Berger AR: True bacterial mural endocarditis. Chest 59:103, 1971.
4. Mildvan D, Goldberg E, Berger M, Altchek MR, Lukban SB: Diagnosis and successful management of septal myocardial abscess: a complication of bacterial endocarditis. Am J Med Sci 274:311, 1977.
5. Tellez G, Nojek C, Juffe A, Rufilanchas J, O'Connor F, Figuera D: Cardiac echinococcosis: report of three cases and review of the literature. Ann Thorac Surg 21:425, 1976.
6. Enders GC, Graeber GM, Poirier RA: Wounds traversing two or more cardiac chambers. Case presentation of two survivors and review of the literature. J Thorac Cardiovasc Surg 76:83, 1978.
7. Pate JW, Richardson RL: Penetrating wounds of cardiac valves. JAMA 207:309, 1969.
8. Symbas PN, DiOrio DA, Tyras DH, Ware RE, Hatcher CR Jr: Penetrating cardiac wounds: significant residual and delayed sequelae. J Thorac Cardiovasc Surg 66:526, 1973.

INFECTIOUS ENDOCARDITIS

9. Kaye D (ed): Infective Endocarditis. Baltimore, University Park Press, 1976.
10. Kaplan EL, Taranta AV (eds): Infective Endocarditis. Dallas, American Heart Association, 1977.
11. Rahimtoola SH (ed): Infective Endocarditis. New York, Grune and Stratton, 1978.
12. Quintiliani R, Ganguli P: Splenic arteriovenous fistula with bacterial endoarteritis and endocarditis. JAMA 214:727, 1970.
13. Roberts WC: Characteristics and consequences of infective endocarditis (active or healed or both). In Rahimtoola SH (ed): Infective Endocarditis. New York, Grune and Stratton, 1978.
14. Krause JR, Levison SP: Pathology of infective endocarditis. In Kaye D (ed): Infective Endocarditis. Baltimore, University Park Press, 1976, p 55.
15. Clawson CC: Role of platelets in the pathogenesis of endocarditis. In Kaplan EL, Taranta AV (eds): Infective Endocarditis. Dallas, American Heart Association, 1977, p 24.
16. Levison ME: Pathogenesis of infective endocarditis. In Kaye D (ed): Infective Endocarditis. Baltimore, University Park Press, 1976, p 29.
17. Reeve R, Reeve JS, Matula G, Lawson W: Mitral obstruction by vegetations of staphylococcal endocarditis. JAMA 228:75, 1974.
18. Lillehei CW, Bobb JR, Visscher MB: The occurrence of endocarditis with valvular deformities in dogs with arteriovenous fistulas. Ann Surg 132:577, 1950.
19. Sande MA: Experimental endocarditis. In Kaye D (ed): Infective Endocarditis. Baltimore, University Park Press, 1976, p 11.
20. Hook EW, Sande MA: Role of the vegetation in experimental streptococcus viridans endocarditis. Infect Immun 10:1433, 1974.
21. Symbas PN, Cooper T, Gantner GE Jr, Willman VL: Lymphatic drainage of the heart: effects of experimental interruption of lymphatic vessels. Surg Forum 14:254, 1963.
22. Sande MA: Antibiotic therapy of experimental endocarditis. In Kaplan EL, Taranta AV (eds): Infective Endocarditis. Dallas, American Heart Association, 1977, p 33.
23. Finegold SM: Cardiovascular infections. In Finegold SM (ed): Anaerobic Bacteria in Human Disease. New York, Academic, 1977, p 182.
24. Amoury RA: Infection following cardiopulmonary bypass. In Norman JC (ed): Cardiac Surgery. New York, Appleton-Century-Crofts, 1972, Chapter 29.
25. Mandell GL: The laboratory in diagnosis and management. In Kaye D (ed): Infective Endocarditis. Baltimore, University Park Press, 1976, p 155.
26. Powers DL, Mandell GL: Intraleukocytic bacteria in endocarditis patients. JAMA 227:312, 1974.
27. Werner AS, Cobbs CG, Kaye D, Hook EW: Studies on the bacteremia of bacterial endocarditis. JAMA 202:199, 1967.
28. Thomson KR, Nanda NC, Gramiak R: The reliability of echocardiography in the diagnosis of infective endocarditis. Radiology 125:473, 1977.
29. Riba AL, Thakur ML, Gottschalk A, Andriole VT, Zaret BL: Imaging experimental infective endocarditis with Indium-111 labeled blood cellular components. Circulation 59:336, 1979.
30. Hook EW, Guerrant RL: Therapy of infective endocarditis. In Kaye D (ed): Infective Endocarditis. Baltimore, University Park Press, 1976, p 167.
31. Lerner PI, Weinstein L: Infective endocarditis in the antibiotic era. N Engl J Med 274:199, 259, 323, 388, 1966.
32. Yeh TJ, Hall DP, Ellison RG: Surgical treatment of aortic valve perforation due to bacterial endocarditis. A report of six cases. Am Surg 30:766, 1964.
33. Wallace AG, Young WG Jr, Osterhout S: Treatment of acute bacterial endocarditis by valve excision and replacement. Circulation 31:450, 1965.
34. Manhas DR, Hessel EA II, Winterschied LC, Dillard DH, Merendino KA: Open heart surgery in infective endocarditis. Circulation 41:841, 1979.
35. Jung JY, Saab SB, Almond CH: The case for early surgical treatment of left-sided primary infective endocarditis. J Thorac Cardiovasc Surg 70:509, 1975.
36. Boyd AD, Spencer FC, Isom OW, Cunningham JN, Reed GE, Acinapura AJ, Tice DA: Infective endocarditis. An analysis of 54 surgically treated patients. J Thorac Cardiovasc Surg 73:23, 1977.
37. Cannon NJ, Cobbs CG: Infective endocarditis in drug addicts. In Kaye D (ed): Infective Endocarditis. Baltimore, University Park Press, 1976, p 111.
38. Borow KM, Alpert JS, Pennington J: Transient *Pseudomonas* bacteremia in a heroin addict. JAMA 240:560, 1978.
39. Harris PD, Yeoh CB, Breault J, Meltzer J, Katz S: Fungal endocarditis secondary to drug addiction. J Thorac Cardiovasc Surg 63:980, 1972.
40. Arbulu A, Thomas NW, Wilson RF: Valvulectomy without prosthetic replacement. J Thorac Cardiovasc Surg 64:103, 1972.
41. Schwartz IS, Pervez N: Bacterial endocarditis associated with a permanent transvenous cardiac pacemaker. JAMA 218:736, 1971.
42. Imparato AM, Kim GE: Electrode complications in patients with permanent cardiac pacemakers. Ten years experience. Arch Surg 105:705, 1972.
43. Conklin EF, Giannelli S Jr, Nealon TF Jr; Four hundred consecutive patients with permanent transvenous pacemakers. J Thorac Cardiovasc Surg 69:1, 1975.
44. Grogler FM, Frank G, Greven G, Dragojevic D, Oelert H, Leitz K, Dalichav H, Brinke U, Lohlein D, Rogge D, Hetzer R, Hennersdorf G, Borst HG: Complications of permanent transvenous cardiac pacing. J Thorac Cardiovasc Surg 69:895, 1975.
45. Charez CM, Conn JH: Septicemia secondary to impacted infected pacemaker wire. J Thorac Cardiovasc Surg 73:796, 1977.
46. Dargan EL, Norman JC: Conservative management of infected pacemaker pulse generator sites. Ann Thorac Surg 12:297, 1971.

47. Hartstein AI, Jackson J, Gilbert DN: Prophylactic antibiotics and the insertion of permanent transvenous cardiac pacemakers. J Thorac Cardiovasc Surg 75:219, 1978.

POSTOPERATIVE ENDOCARDITIS

48. Geraci JE, Dale AJD, McGoon DC: Bacterial endocarditis and endoarteritis following cardiac operations. Wis Med J 62:302, 1963.
49. Looser KG, Allmendinger PD, Takata H, Ellison LH, Low HBC: Infection of cardiac suture line after ventricular aneurysmectomy. J Thorac Cardovasc Surg 72:280, 1976.
50. Kelsch JV, Thomson NB Jr: Bacterial endocarditis complicating repair of a ventricular septal defect. Report of a case cured after removal of silk sutures. N Engl J Med 265:1245, 1961.

PROSTHETIC VALVE ENDOCARDITIS

51. Amoury RA, Bowman FO, Malm JR: Endocarditis associated with intracardiac prostheses. Diagnoses, management, and prophylaxis. J Thorac Cardiovasc Surg 51:36, 1966.
52. Yeh TJ, Anabtawi IN, Cornett VE, White A, Stern WH, Ellison RG: Bacterial endocarditis following open-heart surgery. Ann Thorac Surg 3:29, 1967.
53. Wilson WR: Prosthetic valve endocarditis: incidence, anatomic location, cause, morbidity, and mortality. In Duma RJ (ed): Infections of Prosthetic Heart Valves and Vascular Grafts. Baltimore, University Park Press, 1977, p 3.
54. Ankeney JL, Parker RF: Staphylococcal endocarditis following open heart surgery related to positive intraoperative blood cultures. In Brewer LA (ed): Prosthetic Heart Valves. Springfield, Thomas, 1969, p 719.
55. Clark H, Patton RD: Postcardiotomy endocarditis due to *Neisseria perflava* on a prosthetic aortic valve. Ann Intern Med 68:386, 1968.
56. Levin S, Balagtas R, Susmano A, Edwards L, Dainauskas J: Meningococcus endocarditis at the site of Starr-Edwards mitral prosthesis. Arch Intern Med 129:963, 1972.
57. Jephcott AE, Hardesty CA: Meningococcal septicemia in a patient with a prosthetic valve. A successfully treated case. Br J Clin Pract 30:180, 185, 1976.
58. Goldsweig HG, Matsen JM, Castaneda AR: *Hemophilus aphrophilus* endocarditis in a patient with a mitral valve prosthesis: case report and review of the literature. J Thorac Cardiovasc Surg 63:408, 1972.
59. Stauffer JD, Goldman MJ: Bacterial endocarditis due to *Actinobacillus actinomycetemcomitans* in a patient with a prosthetic aortic valve. Calif Med 117:59, 1972.
60. Juffe A, Miranda AL, Rufilanchas JJ, Maronas JM, Figuero D: Prosthetic valve endocarditis by opportunistic pathogens. Arch Surg 112:151, 1977.
61. Buchanan TM: *Mima polymorpha* endocarditis: a patient with two artificial heart valves. South Med J 65:693, 702, 1972.
62. Fischer JJ: *Pseudomonas maltophilia* endocarditis after replacement of the mitral valve: a case study. J Infect Dis 128:S771, 1973.
63. Dismukes WE, Karchmer AW: The diagnosis of infected prothetic heart valves: Bacteremia versus endocarditis. In Duma RJ (ed): Infections of Prosthetic Heart Valves and Vascular Grafts. Baltimore, University Park Press, 1977, p 61.
64. Vlachakis ND, Gazez PC, Hairston P: Nocardial endocarditis following mitral valve replacement. Chest 63:276, 1973.
65. O'Meara D, Eykyn S, Jenkins BS, Braimbridge MV, Phillips I: *Brucella melitensis* endocarditis: successful treatment of an infected prosthetic mitral valve. Thorax 29:377, 1974.
66. Ehrenhaft JL: Discussion of Kaiser GC, Willman VL, Thurmann M, Hanlon CR: Valve replacement in cases of aortic insufficiency due to active endocarditis. J Thorac Cardiovasc Surg 54:491, 1967.
67. Weinstein GS, Nichols NJ, Rogers MR, Franzone AJ, Stertzer SH, Wallsh E: Endocarditis of aortic valvular prosthesis due to *Listeria monocytogenes.* Chest 69:807, 1976.
68. Saravolatz LD, Burch KH, Madhavan T, Quinn EL: Listerial prosthetic valve endocarditis: successful medical therapy. JAMA 240:2186, 1978.
69. Jackson G, Saunders K: Prosthetic valve diphtheroids endocarditis treated with sodium fusidate and erythromycin. Br Heart J 35:931, 1973.
70. Block CS, Levy NL, Fritz VU: *Bacillus cereus* endocarditis: a case report. SA Med J 53:556, 1978.
71. Tuazon CU, Murray HW, Levy C, Solny MN, Curtin JA, Shaegren JN: Serious infections from *Bacillus* sp. JAMA 241:1137, 1979.
72. Geraci JE, Greipp PR, Wilkowske CJ, Wilson WR, Washington JA II: *Cardiobacterium hominis* endocarditis, four cases with clincal and laboratory observations. Mayo Clin Proc 53:49, 1978.
73. Spernoga JF, Laskowski L, Marr JJ, Burmeister RW: Cardiobacterium hominis endocarditis. South Med J 72:85, 1979.
74. Norenberg RG, Sethi GK, Scott SM, Takaro T: Opportunistic endocarditis following open heart surgery. Ann Thorac Surg 19:592, 1975.
75. Robicsek F, Daugherty HK, Cook JW, Selle JG, Masters TN, O'Bar PR, Fernandez CR, Mauney CU, Calhoun DM: *Mycobacterium fortuitum* epidemics after open-heart surgery. J Thorac Cardiovasc Surg 75:91, 1978.
76. Altmann G, Horowitz A, Kaplinsky N: Prosthetic valve endocarditis due to *Mycobacterium chelonei.* J Clin Microbiol 1:531, 1975.
77. Repath F, Seabury JH, Sanders CV, Dumer J: Prosthetic valve endocarditis due to *Mycobacterium chelonei.* South Med J 69:1244, 1976.
78. Tyras DH, Kaiser GC, Barner HB, Laskowski LS, Marr JJ: Atypical mycobacteria and the xenograft valve. J Thorac Cardiovasc Surg 75:331, 1978.
79. Lohr DC, Goeken JA, Doty DB, Donta ST: *Mycobacterium gordonae* infection of a prosthetic aortic valve. JAMA 239:1528, 1978.
80. O'Rourke MF, Shanahan MX, Harkness JL: Endocarditis with an acid-fast organism after porcine heart-valve replacement. Lancet 2:686, 1978.
81. Kristinsson A, Bentall HH: Medical and surgical treatment of Q-fever endocarditis. Lancet 2:693, 1967.
82. Morgans CM, Cartwright RY: Case of Q-fever endocarditis at site of aortic valve prosthesis. Br Heart J 31:520, 1969.
83. Arnett EN, Roberts WC: Clinicopathology of prosthetic valve endocarditis. In Duma RJ (ed): Infections of Prosthetic Heart Valves and Vascular Grafts. Baltimore, University Park Press, 1977, p 17.
84. Barney JD, Williams GR, Cayler GG, Bracken EC: Influence of intracardiac prosthetic materials on susceptibility to bacterial endocarditis. Circulation 26:684, 1962.
85. Jacob HS, Craddock PR, Hammerschmidt DE, Moldow CF: Complement-induced granulocyte aggregation: an unsuspected mechanism of disease. N Engl J Med, 302:789, 1980.
86. Amoury RA: Necrotizing enterocolitis. In Holder TM, Ashcraft KW (eds): Pediatric Surgery. Philadelphia, Saunders, 1981, Chapter 29.
87. Archer GL: Experimental endocarditis. In Duma RJ (ed): Infections of Prosthetic Heart Valves and Vascular Grafts. Baltimore, University Park Press, 1977 p 43.
88. Jones RD, Akao M, Cross FS: Bacteremia and thrombus accu-

mulation on prosthetic heart valves in the dog. J Surg Res 9:293, 1969.

89. Cheng, TO, Kinhal V, Tice DA: Fatal thrombosis of the Starr-Edwards mitral valve prosthesis associated with bacterial endocarditis. Diagnostic significance of a disappearing prosthetic click. Chest 57:151, 1970.
90. Freeman R, King B, Hambling MH: Infective complications of open-heart surgery and the monitoring of infections by the NBI test. Thorax 28:617, 1973.
91. Stinson EB, Castellino RA, Shumway NE: Radiologic signs in endocarditis following prosthetic valve replacement. J Thorac Cardiovasc Surg 56:554, 1968.
92. Kittredge RD, McCord CW: Roentgenographic diagnosis of complications in heart valve replacements. Am J Roentgenol 107:392, 1969.
93. Stross JK, Willis PW III, Kahn DR: Diagnostic features of malfunction of disk mitral valve prostheses. JAMA 217:305, 1971.
94. Malcolm AD, Ahuja SP, Chamberlain MJ: Malfunction of tricuspid valve prosthesis shown by isotope angiocardiography. J Thorac Cardiovasc Surg 71:134, 1976.
95. Bach MC, Lewin EB, Sheaff ET, Schwartz L, DeBakey ME: Localization of endovascular infection by selective catheterization with serial cultures. J Thorac Cardiovasc Surg 69:377, 1975.
96. Gardner P, Saffle JR, Schoenbaum SC: Management of prosthetic valve endocarditis. In Duma RJ (ed): Infections of Prosthtetic Heart Valves and Vascular Grafts. Baltimore, University Park Press, 1977, p 123.
97. Killen DA, Collins HA, Koenig MG, Goodman JS: Prosthetic cardiac valves and bacterial endocarditis. Ann Thorac Surg 9:238, 1970.
98. Schrire V, Beck W, Hewitson RB, Barnard CN: Immediate and long-term results of aortic valve replacement with University of Cape Town aortic valve prosthesis. Br Heart J 32:255, 1970.
99. Wilson WR, Jaumin PM, Danielson GK, Giuliani ER, Washington JA III, Geraci JE: Prosthetic valve endocarditis. Ann Intern Med 82:751, 1975.
100. McGoon DC, Pluth JR: Postoperative care of the open-heart patient. General considerations. In Burford TH, Ferguson TB (eds): Cardiovascular Surgery and Current Practice, Vol 1. St. Louis, Mosby, 1969, p 33.
101. Braunwald NS: Artificial heart valves. Prosthetic devices. In Burford TH, Ferguson TB (eds): Cardiovascular Surgery, Current Practice, Vol 1. St. Louis, Mosby, 1969, p 116.
102. McLeod R, Remington JS: Postoperative fungal endocarditis. In Duma RJ (ed): Infections of Prosthetic Heart Valves and Vascular Grafts. Baltimore, University Park Press, 1977, p 163.
103. Uys CJ, Don PA, Schrire V, Barnard CN: Endocarditis following cardiac surgery due to the fungus *Paecilomyces.* S Afr Med J 37:1276, 1963.
104. Silver MD, Tuffnell PG, Bigelow WG: Endocarditis caused by *Paecilomyces varioti* affecting an aortic valve allograft. J Thorac Cardiovasc Surg 61:278, 1971.
105. McClellan JR, Hamilton JD, Alexander JA, Wolfe WG, Reed JB: *Paecilomyces varioti* endocarditis on a prosthetic aortic valve. J Thorac Cardiovasc Surg 71:472, 1976.
106. Weaver DK, Batsakis JG, Nishiyama OH: *Histoplasma* endocarditis. Arch Surg 96:158, 1968.
107. Alexander WJ, Mowry RW, Cobbs CG, Dismukes WE: Prosthetic valve endocarditis caused by *Histoplasma capsulatum.* JAMA 242:1399, 1979.
108. Kaufman SN: *Curvularia* endocarditis following cardiac surgery. Am J Clin Pathol 56:466, 1971.
109. Khicha GJ, Berroya RB, Escano SB Jr, Lee CS: Mucormycosis in a mitral prosthesis. J Thorac Cardiovasc Surg 63:903, 1972.
110. Upshaw CB Jr: *Penicillium* endocarditis of aortic valve prosthesis. J Thorac Cardiovasc Surg 68:428, 1974.
111. Hall WJ III: *Penicillium* endocarditis following open heart surgery and prosthetic valve insertion. Am Heart J 87:501, 1974.
112. Roberts FJ, Allen P, Maybee TK: *Petriellidium boydii (Allescheria boydii)* endocarditis associated with porcine valve replacement. Can Med Assoc J 117:1251, 1977.
113. Robboy SJ, Kaiser J: Pathogenesis of fungal infection of heart valve prostheses. Human Pathol 6:711, 1975.
114. Cooper T, Morrow A, Roberts W, Herman L: Postoperative endocarditis due to *Candida:* clinical observations in the experimental production of the lesion. Surgery 50:341, 1961.
115. Utley J, Mills J, Hutchinson J, Edmunds L, Sanderson R, Roe B: Valve replacement for bacterial and fungal endocarditis: A comparative study. Circulation 48 (Suppl. 3):42, 1973.
116. Rossiter SJ, Stinson EB, Oyer PE, Miller DC, Schapira JN, Martin RP, Shumway NE: Prosthetic valve endocarditis: comparison of heterograft tissue valves and mechanical valves. J Thorac Cardiovasc Surg 76:795, 1978.
117. Ross DN: Homograft replacement of the aortic valve. Lancet 2:487, 1962.
118. Gonzalez-Lavin L, Al-Janabi N, Ross DN: Long-term results after aortic valve replacement with preserved aortic homografts. Ann Thorac Surg 13:594, 1972.
119. Malm JR, Bowman FO Jr, Harris PD, Kowalik ATW: An evaluation of aortic valve homografts sterilized by electron beam energy. J Thorac Cardiovasc Surg 54:471, 1967.
120. Ross D, Gonzalez-Lavin L, Dalichau H: A two-year experience with supported autologous fascia lata for heart valve replacement. Ann Thorac Surg 13:97, 1972.
121. Zerbini EJ: Results of replacement of cardiac valves by homologous dura mater valves. Chest 67:706, 1975.
122. Buch WS, Pipkin RD, Hancock WD, Fogarty TJ: Mitral valve replacement with a Hancock stabilized glutaraldehyde valve. Arch Surg 110:1408, 1975.

POSTCARDIOTOMY SYNDROMES

123. Kirsh, MM, McIntosh A, Kahn DR, Sloan H: Postpericardiotomy syndrome. Ann Thorac Surg 9:158, 1970.
124. Engle MA, Klein AA, Hepner S, Ehlers KH: The postpericardiotomy syndromes. Cardiovasc Clin North Am 1976, p 211.
125. Engle MA, Ehlers KH, O'Loughlin JE Jr, Linday LA, Fried R: The postpericardiotomy syndrome: Iatrogenic illness with immunologic and virologic components. In Engle MA (ed): Pediatric Cardiovascular Disease. Philadelphia, FA Davis Company, 1981, p 381.
126. Caul WO, Clarke SKR, Mott, MG, Perham TGM, Wilson RSE: Cytomegalovirus infections after open-heart surgery. Lancet 1:777, 1971.
127. Burch GE, Colcolough HL: Postcardiotomy and postinfarction syndromes—a theory. Am Heart J 80:290, 1970.
128. Hornick RB: Source of contamination in open-heart surgery. In Duma RJ (ed): Infections of Prosthetic Heart Valves and Vascular Grafts. Baltimore, University Park Press, 1977, p 81.
129. Roses DF, Rose MR, Rappaport FT: Febrile responses associated with cardiac surgery: Relationships to the postcardiotomy syndrome and to altered host immunologic reactivity. J Thoracic Surg 67:251, 1974.

CHAPTER 32
Pericardial Infections

VALLEE L. WILLMANN

PERICARDIAL INFECTIONS

ANATOMY

THE pericardium is a serous-lined, tough, fibrous enclosure of the heart normally present in most vertebrates. There are no known serious defects in cardiac function attendent upon its absence,[1] although there are several circumstances in which its presence is disadvantageous. Most of these are associated with or are the result of inflammation.

Two serous layers of the pericardium enclose a space normally filled with a small amount of serous exudate, containing macrophages, desquamated mesothelial cells, small lymphocytes, and eosinophils. The inner layer, the epicardium or visceral pericardium, is a monocellular layer of cuboidal cells overlying the epicardial fat and myocardium.[2] Myocardial lymphatics, nerves, and superficial vessels lying in the epicardial fat are covered by this single layer of cells. This same cellular layer reflects from the heart to cover the inner side of the tough layer of fibrous tissue, and with this tissue forms the parietal pericardium. The parietal pericardium attaches to the heart at its base close to the origin of the great vessels and dorsal to the heart at the confluence of the pulmonary veins, pulmonary arteries, and vena cavae. The nonserosal surface of the pericardium opposes the diaphragm, sternum, thymus, and pleura. Dorsally, it is separated from the trachea, bronchi, and esophagus by tissues of the posterior and superior mediastinum.

The fibrous pericardium is made up of a superficial, middle, and deep layer of collagenous fibers with interspersed elastic fibers, scattered fibroblasts, macrophages, mast cells, fat cells, nerves, lymphatics, and blood vessels. The nature of the collagen and elastic relationship makes the structure essentially unyielding to acute tension, yet subject to stretching with chronic stress. The loss of this elasticity as a result of infection and inflammation contributes to conditions of the pericardium that impair cardiac function. Constrictive pericarditis is the flagrant example of this, although a stiffened pericardium might contribute to cardiac dysfunction in other conditions in which the heart enlarges.

Although laced with blood vessels, the pericardium is not really a vascular structure, and except for the areas of attachment at the aorta, diaphragm, and pulmonary veins, the blood vessels rarely require control when severed. The arterial supply is by branches of the internal mammary and musculophrenic arteries. Many current cardiac procedures surely interrupt most of these branches. The effect of this deprivation is not grossly observable; it is unknown what effect it has on resistance to infection or alteration in the inflammatory response. Nerve fibers enter the pericardium from the vagus, the left recurrent laryngeal, and the esophageal plexus.

Lymphatics are present in both the epicardium and the parietal pericardium. They are sparse and drain into the nodes at the base of the heart, where there is communication with the lymphatics from the lungs, esophagus, and mediastinum.[3]

The pericardium is close to several organs which predispose it to infection. It is broadly attached to the diaphragm at the dome and extends down to the aortic and esophageal hiatuses. Lymphatics of the diaphragm, along with esophageal and hepatic lymphatics, have common pathyways in this area.

Posteriorly, where the pericardium reflects from the pulmonary veins and left atrium, it lies adjacent to the posterior mediastinum, which contains the esophagus and the major bronchi. The major lymphatic drainage of these systems communicates with lymphatics from the pericardium.

PHYSIOLOGY

The pericardium functions as a mechanical support to the heart and as a mechanism for chemical and fluid exchange. The capacity of the pericardial space is ordinarily limited to less than 100 ml of fluid.[4] Overdistention impairs the capability of the heart to expand in diastole and limits stroke volume. When this occurs acutely, the full-fledged syndrome of cardiac tamponade occurs. In this condition, there are high-filling pressures (high venous pressure), low blood pressure and narrow pulse pressure, distant heart sounds, increased peripheral vascular resistance.[5] The accompanying bradycardia is unexplained, as one would anticipate baroreceptor-induced acceleration. There is some evidence that it is a vagal efferent phenomenon.

When the restriction to filling occurs more slowly as a result of fibrotic or calcific changes, constrictive pericarditis develops. Many of the same hemodynamic alterations as in tamponade appear, except for the cardiac rate alterations. Hepatomegaly and ascites develop as a result of longstanding venous back pressure.

The character as well as the amount of the pericardial fluid is related to lymphatic drainage, osmosis, and capillary permeability. These are all interrelated and affected by inflammation. Although the fluid transfer mechanisms of the pericardium are not well understood, in normal circumstances they are bidirectional.[6] Pericardial fluid reflects changes in serum electrolyte content and serum injected into the pericardium is removed by the lymphatics.[7,8] With inflammation of the pericardium, the increased amount of fluid might represent impaired resorption or increased exudation. There is no proof of the common belief that the latter is the principal mechanism.

PATHOGENESIS AND PATHOLOGY

Acute inflammation of the pericardium, induced by infectious agents, can result from direct extension from contiguous areas, through lymphatic spread, by bloodborne agents, trauma, operation, or from infections of the heart.[9-14] Pericarditis is most commonly associated with infection in neighboring structures, particularly the lungs, but also the esophagus, mediastinum, pleura, heart, and liver.[12,14,15] Pneumonia and empyema have been the chief causes of acute purulent pericarditis.[16,17] Abscess of the liver, pyogenic, amebic, ecchinococcal, or subdiaphragmatic abscess may penetrate the diaphragm to involve the pericardium[11,15] (Chapter 36). Tuberculous pericarditis is generally associated with caseating tuberculous mediastinal lymphadenitis.[18] Esophagitis and mediastinitis, secondary to esophageal ulceration or penetration, can result in pericarditis by direct extension.[12,14] Lymphatic permeation can account for infection when there is adjacent but noncontiguous infection.

The pericardium, like most serous membranes, responds to infection and inflammation by interstitial swelling and by production of an exudate. The nature of the exudate varies with the infecting organism and the severity of the process. In the early stages, the effusion is generally serous, becoming more fibrinous as the process ages. The development of frank pus can alter this process and can even be associated with hemorrhage. Whatever the character of the fluid, cardiac function is impaired. In the presence of effusion, this can progress to life-threatening cardiac tamponade. Even simple inflammation and fibrinous adhesions between the two serosal layers undoubtedly have some adverse effect on the overall cardiac compliance. In the presence of distention to the point of increased pressure, it is difficult to escape the notion that blood flow to and lymphatic drainage from the pericardium itself are impaired, thus further inhibiting the control of the infection.

In viral pericarditis, the myocardium is usually infected as well (myopericarditis).[19] Acute benign interstitial inflammatory response is usually seen, and recovery is complete. Occasionally, myocardial cellular necrosis will occur with scarring and calcification. Calcification within the pericardium always suggests a restrictive lesion. Some cases of myocarditis primarily affect the subendocardial myocardium (eg, mumps) and after healing produce endocardial fibroelastosis.[20]

In pyogenic pericarditis, the pericardium is usually thickened and contains 500–2,000 ml of purulent exudate or granulation tissue under varying degrees of tension. The pericardial sac may be filled with cheesy material, or a fibrinous granulomatous pericarditis can be present without fluid accumulation.

Infections following operations, particularly in association with wound infections, are increasing in frequency.[9,21] It remains unclear whether or not the frequently occur-

TABLE 32-1. ASSOCIATED CONDITIONS IN 200 AUTOPSY REPORTS OF PURULENT PERICARDITIS

	Before 1944	After 1944
Underlying condition or disease	21 (14%)	43 (78%)
Thoracic surgery	4	12
Chronic renal failure	7	9
Carcinoma	5	8
Myocardial infarction	0	2
Diabetes, myeloproliferative disorders	4	6
Sickle cell	1	2
Miscellaneous	0	4
Primary infectious disease	124 (86%)	12 (22%)
Pneumonia	72	3
Meningitis	4	4
Osteomyelitis	9	0
Skin and otitis media	11	0
Subacute bacterial endocarditis	11	3
Endometritis	4	0
Miscellaneous	13	2

Klacsmann PG, Bulkley BH, Hutchins GM: The changed spectrum of purulent pericarditis: an 86 year autopsy experience in 200 patients. *Am J Med* 63:666, 1977.

TABLE 32-2. SOURCE OF INFECTING ORGANISM IN 200 AUTOPSY REPORTS OF PURULENT PERICARDITIS

	Before 1944		After 1944	
Source	***No.***	**%**	***No.***	**%**
Direct pulmonary extension	93	64	11	20
Hematogenous spread	28	19	16	29
Myocardial abscess/endocarditis	18	12	12	22
Perforating injury chest wall (surgery, trauma)	5	4	13	24
Subdiaphragmatic suppurative lesion	1	1	3	5

Klacsmann PG, Bulkley BH, Hutchins GM: The changed spectrum of purulent pericarditis: an 86 year autopsy experience in 200 patients. *Am J Med* 63:666, 1977.

ring postoperative pericardial inflammations, resulting in the postpericardiotomy syndrome, is infective. The evidence for a noninfective, autoimmune etiology is considerable,[22,23] although viral associations have been reported.[24]

Purulent pericarditis has been described since the time of Galen.[25] Before the introduction of antibiotics, the disease was seen principally in conjunction with pneumonia in children. The course was frequently fulminant and carried a grave prognosis. During the past 30 years, there has been a change in the etiologic agents and in clinical manifestations [13,16,17] for two reasons: pneumococcal pneumonia now responds to treatment, and the immunocompromised patient survives sufficiently to develop this complication of the underlying disease.

Table 32-1 lists the conditions associated with 200 fatal cases of purulent pericarditis. Before 1944, direct extension from pulmonary infections was considered the mechanism in nearly two-thirds of the instances. Since that time, hematogenous spread, extention from myocardial infections,[10,26] and postoperative (traumatic) infections have become relatively more common (Table 32-2).

ETIOLOGY

Pericarditis and pericardial effusions can be infectious or noninfectious. Some noninfectious causes are listed in Table 32-3. Table 32-4 lists all the major infectious causes of myopericarditis. The most common causes of viral myopericarditis are the enteroviruses (coxsackieviruses and echoviruses) (Chapter 10). These viruses are rarely isolated from pericardial fluid, and the diagnosis requires serologic confirmation. In contrast, in cases of bacterial or fungal pyogenic pericarditis, isolation from the fluid is almost uni-

TABLE 32-3. SOME NONINFECTIOUS CAUSES OF PERICARDITIS AND MYOPERICARDITIS

Myocardial infarction
Pericardiotomy
Uremia
Neoplasia
Collagen-vascular disease (including drug-induced)
Familial Mediterranean fever
Acute rheumatic fever
Radiation therapy

Adapted from Lerner MA: Myocarditis and pericarditis. In Mandell GL, Douglas RG Jr, Bennett JE (eds): *Principles and Practice of Infectious Diseases,* Vol 1. New York, Wiley, 1979, p 711.

TABLE 32-4. INFECTIOUS CAUSES OF MYOPERICARDITIS

Viruses
- Adenoviruses
- Cytomegalovirus
- Coxsackieviruses A and B *
- Epstein-Barr virus
- Echoviruses *
- Hepatitis A virus
- Polioviruses
- Herpes simplex viruses, type 1 and type 2
- Influenza viruses A and B
- Lymphocytic choriomeningitis virus
- Mumps virus
- Rubella virus
- Vaccinia virus
- Varicella-zoster virus

Bacteria
- *Corynebacterium diphtheriae*
- *Neisseria gonorrhoeae*
- *N. meningitidis*
- *Pasteurella (Francisella) tularensis*
- *Pseudomonas pseudomallei*
- *Staphylococcus aureus* *
- *Streptococcus pneumoniae* *
- *S. pyogenes*
- *Treponema pallidum*
- Aerobic gram-negative bacilli *
- Anaeroblic bacteria including *Bacteroides* and pepto-streptococci

Mycobacteria
- *Mycobacteria chelonei*
- *Mycobacteria tuberculosis* *

Fungi and Actinomycetes
- *Actinomyces israelii*
- *Aspergillus* spp *
- *Blastomyces dermatitidis*
- *Candida* spp *
- *Coccidioides immitis*
- *Cryptococcus neoformans*
- *Histoplasma capsulatum* *
- *H. mucorales*
- *Nocardia asteroides*

Parasites
- *Echinococcus granulosus* *
- *Entamoeba histolytica* *
- *Plasmodium* spp
- *Schistosoma* spp
- *Toxoplasma gondii* *
- *Trichinella spiralis* *
- *Trypanosoma cruzi*

Rickettsia
- *Rickettsia burnetii*
- *R. mooseri*
- *R. rickettsii*

Other
- *Chlamydia psittaci*
- *Mycoplasma pneumoniae* *

* These infectious agents are probably most frequently found in the United States.

Adapted from Lerner MA: Myocarditis and pericarditis. In Mandell GL, Douglas RG Jr, Bennett JE (eds): *Principles and Practice of Infectious Diseases,* Vol 1. New York, Wiley, 1979, p 711.

TABLE 32-5. ORGANISMS ISOLATED FROM 200 AUTOPSIED CASES OF PURULENT PERICARDITIS

	Before 1944		After 1944	
Organisms	***No.***	***%***	***No.***	***%***
Gram-positive				
Pneumococcus	62	51	6	9
Staphylococcus	23	19	15	22
Streptococcus	12	10	9	13
Gram-negative				
Proteus, Escherichia coli, Pseudomonas, Klebsiella	3	2	22	32
Salmonella/Shigella	1	1	3	4
Neisseria meningitidis	3	2	2	3

Klacsmann PG, Bulkley BH, Hutchins GM: The changed spectrum of purulent pericarditis: an 86 year autopsy experience in 200 patients. *Am J Med* 63:666, 1977.

versal. The agent can be isolated in about half the cases with tuberculous pericarditis. Bacterial pericarditis was once caused by the pyogenic gram-positive cocci which caused the adjacent bacterial pneumonias (Table 32-5). Now hematogenous spread to the pericardium from distant infections with gram-negative organisms are most often seen. Tuberculous pericarditis is now rare.[27] Cases of pericarditis due to *Actinomyces*[28] *H. influenza,* and *Mycoplasma*[29] have been reported in addition to those listed in Table 32-5.

Fungal pericarditis is still rare. Histoplasmosis may cause both benign pericarditis or chronic constrictive pericarditis in previously healthy people. *Candida* and *Aspergillus* species cause pericarditis in immunocompromised patients and have together become the second most common cause of purulent pericarditis in some series.[17] American trypanosomiasis (Chagas' disease), trichinosis, toxoplasmosis, amebiasis, and echinococcosis can all produce myopericarditis.[30]

CLINICAL MANIFESTATIONS

General Symptoms and Signs

Pain, generally taken as the principal symptom of acute pericarditis, varies considerably with etiologic agents and can be entirely absent in up to half the cases.[31] Pain can be of varying quality and intensity. The diversity of its location and areas of referral can lead to considerable confusion. The pain can be precordial, substernal, nuchal, dorsal, epigastric, generalized abdominal, right chest, to either arm, or even pleuritic. This spectrum cannot be attributed to the distribution of fibers entering the pericardium. More likely it relates to the probability of confluent inflammation of surrounding structures. The pain of a thoracic incision obviously confuses the pain that might arise from pericarditis occurring in the postoperative period. Pain is clearly a function of the etiologic mechanisms. The slow course of tuberculous pericarditis probably accounts for its usual silence, whereas purulent pericarditis is more likely to be acutely uncomfortable. Of great importance is the understanding that the pain of pericarditis can mimic that of many other entities.

The other signs of inflammation also vary in relation to the causative agents and the host capacity to respond. It is typical that nonspecific pericarditis and that associated with the postpericardiotomy syndrome have low-grade temperature elevations and lymphocytosis. Purulent pericarditis, on the other hand, would be expected to elicit high temperatures and granulocytosis. Often, however, a patient nutritionally depleted by long-standing heart disease, carcinoma, or uremia, or immunosuppressed during treatment of collagen disease or transplant rejection, will fail to show such a response even with flagrant infection.

Viral Myopericarditis

Coxsackie and echoviral infections are discussed in Chapter 10. There are many serologic subtypes. Pericarditis usually appears as part of a general, mild, undifferentiated febrile illness with upper respiratory symptoms, exanthems, lymphadenitis, pleurodynia, orchitis, gastroenteritis. Less often, pericarditis occurs as part of a life-threatening meningoencephalitis, hepatitis, pneumonia, or hemolytic-uremic syndrome.

A postvaccinial myopericarditis has been observed 10 to 14 days after primary smallpox vaccination.

Viral pericarditis is usually a milder disease than bacterial pericarditis. Patients with coxsackie virus B pericarditis usually first have dyspnea, pain in the chest, malaise, and fever. Symptoms of preceding upper respiratory infection, myalgia, arthralgia, or gastroenteritis are unusual.[32] The common clinical findings in coxsackievirus B pericarditis are listed in Table 32-6.

Pyogenic Pericarditis

Patients with pyogenic pericarditis are toxic and acutely ill with anorexia, fever, chills, and chest pain, raised jugular venous pulsations, adynamic pericardium with impalpable apical pulses, and muffled heart sounds. Hepatomegaly, parodoxical pulses, and cardiac tamponade are striking features of pyogenic pericarditis. Pleural effusions, ascites, and pitting edema are also more common in purulent pericarditis and are unusual signs in viral pericarditis.

Pericardial friction rubs are best heard to the left of the midsternal border with the patient sitting, leaning forward, and holding his or her breath. The rubs are accentuated during inspiration or expiration and may be heard in one or several of the phases of the cardiac cycle. The rubs may even be palpable (Table 32-6).

Laboratory Features

A leukocytosis, enlarged cardiac silhouette, and abnormal electrocardiogram findings are common in both pyogenic and coxsackie virus B pericarditis. Arrythmias are rare with pyogenic and common with coxsackie virus B pericarditis, and pericardiocentesis always yields the organism with bacterial pericarditis and rarely with viral pericarditis (Table 32-6).

The cardiac silhouette, when there is effusion, would be expected to enlarge and to broaden at the diaphragm

TABLE 32-6. CLINICAL FINDINGS IN PYOGENIC PERICARDITIS AND COXSACKIEVIRUS B MYOPERICARDITIS

	Pyogenic * (percent)	Coxsackievirus B * (percent)
Symptoms/signs		
Acutely ill (toxic, fever, dyspnea)	100 * †	58
Raised jugular venous pulse	100	21
Enlarged cardiac dullness	100	74
Adynamic pericarditis	100	11
Muffled heart sounds	94	11
Hepatomegaly	94	21
Paradoxical pulse	88	11
Cardiac tamponade	88	0
Pleural effusion	56	5
Pericardial friction rub	38	26
Ascites	31	0
Pitting edema	25	5
Apical systolic murmur	10	68
Laboratory features		
Polymorphonuclear leukocytosis	100	74
Enlarged cardiac silhouette	100	74
Abnormal EKG (low voltage; ↓ST, ↑ST segments)	100	100
Arrhythmia	Rare	Common
Pericardiocentesis with isolation of bacterium or virus from fluid	100	Rare
Pericardial fluid	Exudate	Usually exudate

* Estimates of occurrence of symptoms/signs are made from data reported in Klacsman, Bulkley, and Hutchins [13] and in Sainani, Dekate, and Rao.[32]

From Lerner AM: Myocarditis and pericarditis. In Mandell GL, Douglas RC Jr, Bennett JE (eds): Principles and Practice of Infectious Disease, Vol 1. New York, Wiley, 1979, p 711.

in the erect position. This, however, by experience rarely proves helpful. The electrocardiogram can be of assistance in diagnosis if the S-T segment changes, characteristics of an injury-current appear, or if T wave abnormalities develop secondary to myocarditis. Decreasing amplitude can also suggest the development of effusion.[33,34] Unfortunately, these findings are neither always present or pathognomonic and frequently the electrocardiogram is of only suggestive value.

Echocardiography is currently the most useful noninvasive measurement providing evidence of effusion, ventricular motion, and pericardial thickening.[35,36] A negative result does not exclude a significant effusion, and cardiac tamponade can even be missed. Angiocardiography is sometimes definitive in that it outlines discrepancies between chambers and external borders; its limitation is its need for instrumentation.

Infections after Cardiac Surgery

Along with the increased frequency in operative procedures on the heart and thorax, there has occurred an increased incidence of postoperative pericarditis.[21] The nonspecific pericarditis resulting in pain, tachycardia, lymphocytosis, and mild temperature elevation, generally categorized as postcardiotomy pericarditis, is diagnosed on the basis of the clinical picture and in the absence of an identified infective organism. That some instances so classified are truly infective and suppressed by antibiotic and supportive therapy is highly probable. In some circumstances, the acute purulence does develop and presents a diagnostic difficulty even greater than when there has been no recent operation in the region. A pericardial rub, temperature elevation, pain, S-T segment changes, and altered cardiac silhouette are all frequently altered postoperatively and are for the most part lost as diagnostic aids. The echocardiogram remains useful, but even it is less definitive, considering the frequency of some trapped pericardial blood or fluid.

The diagnosis is still missed in half the cases.[5,17] There are certainly others missed that contribute to morbidity and mortality. A consciousness of the potential existence of purulent pericarditis existing in the postoperative patient is the principal advantage one has in working toward the diagnosis and treatment. The echocardiogram and computerized tomography are the most useful tools short of exploration. Negative exploration results will certainly be a part of the cost of more frequent diagnosis.

Even with diagnoses and appropriate therapy, the mortality rate remains high. Early recognition and adequate drainage offer the best opportunity for success.

DIAGNOSIS OF PERICARDITIS

Aspiration and analysis of pericardial fluid may be helpful in reaching specific diagnoses, but pericardiocentesis has the risk of hemopericardium and cardiac tamponade.[39] It is best performed in the operating room with electrocardiographic monitoring. A pericardiogram at the time of pericardiocentesis may suggest that simple aspiration or operative drainage and debridement is required. A pericardial biopsy can be useful for diagnosis of chronic pericarditis. Smear, Gram stain, acid-fast stain, and potassium hydroxide preparations for fungi yield tremendous amounts of information. Tubercle bacilli can be isolated in only 40 percent of tuberculous cases. Methenamine silver stains should also be done. If the smears and culture results are negative, serial viral serologic tests should be performed for enteroviruses. The high prevalence of neutralizing antibody within the population precludes the diagnosis on the basis of a single elevated neutralizing antibody titer in the absence of a fourfold or greater increase in titer. Finding of IgM antibodies is a reliable indicator of recent infection, but heterotypic reactions may also occur. The serologic interpretations are complicated and have been reviewed by Lerner.[19]

TREATMENT

The treatment of pericarditis is directed toward the relief of pain, the correction of the circulatory abnormalities caused by cardiac compression, and the treatment of the etiologic agent or process.

The management of pain is frequently accomplished by analgesic agents in low dosage. In chronic infections, this may be unsatisfactory, and one looks to the control of pain by treating the disease. Where there is not a specific etiology, the pain is often relieved by the use of corticosteroids. Keep in mind, however, especially in the postoperative patient, that if there is a bacterial agent associated with the process, corticosteroids might reduce the inflammation and pain but subject the patient to greater risk of sepsis.

In viral pericarditis, digitalis, diuretics, and antiarrhythmic agents are useful for symptomatic relief. Repeated pericardiocentesis and even pericardiectomy may be required for resistant or persistent cases. Steroids and anticoagulants should be avoided for the first 2 weeks. After that, local or systemic steroids may be indicated.[37] The instillation of nonabsorbable steroids through an indwelling catheter for 24 to 48 hours is useful for uremic pericarditis, but it has not been evaluated for viral pericarditis and is definitely contraindicated in bacterial or fungal pericarditis.

Patients with viral pericarditis and associated endocarditis should be treated according to the protocol associated with myocardial infarction. One to 3 months' rest may be required in these patients. If steroids are used during the chronic phase, approximately 20 mg of prednisone four times a day is useful.

In pyogenic pericarditis, a Gram stain of the pericardial aspirate should be used as a guide to antibiotic choice. The gram-positive cocci are likely to be penicillin-resistant; penicillinase-resistant penicillin or cephalosporin is indicated. For gram-negative bacilli or mixed organisms, a cephalosporin plus an aminoglycoside should be used. Fungal pericarditis requires amphotericin B. Tuberculous pericarditis requires not only antituberculous drugs (Chapter 18) but also corticosteroids, which appear to suppress inflammation within the pericardium and enhance reabsorption of the effusion and retard pericardial constriction.[38] In pyogenic pericarditis, drainage of the pericardium is important both in diagnosis and in temporary relief of any compression on the heart. It has also been advocated as a means of definitive therapy,[16] but has not proven reliable in pyogenic pericarditis. This method of drainage has value only in unusual circumstances where even a minor operation might have major adverse consequences.

Operative drainage is usually necessary for pyogenic pericarditis. Although the earliest operative approach to the pericardium was directly from the front, it became popular at one time to drain the pericardium into a pleural space and then treat the pleural space according to the nature of the pericardial fluid. Infective material was drained by a thoracostomy tube; noninfective fluid was left for absorption by the pleura. The choice of operation for drainage of acute purulent pericardial effusions remains controversial. Avoidance of median-sternotomy incision would seem advisable, as the spreading of infection to the anterior mediastinum and sternum could have serious consequences. Those who argue for thoracotomy with wide drainage into the pleural spaces cite the advantage of wide resection of the pericardium and the lessening of the possibility of later constriction by a fibrotic pericardium.[40-44] The soiling of the pleural space is probably not consequential. Exposure by thoracotomy also ensures better exploration of the pericardium and drainage of all areas, should the process be compartmentalized. The disadvantage of this approach, of course, is the need for general anesthesia and the extensiveness of the procedure with its connotation for pulmonary dysfunction.

The increasingly prevalent use of pericardial drainage by the subxyphoid route has, in the minds of many, essentially eliminated the consideration of transpleural drainage in infective pericarditis.[17,45-47] Subxyphoid drainage can be established under local or general anesthesia. The pericardium is exposed at the base of the heart, separating the rectus abdominus muscles and reflecting the diaphragm inferiorly. In most instances, it is useful to resect the xyphoid, although adequate exposure can usually be obtained by dissecting along either of its sides. With limited dissection, the pericardium can be exposed and a defect made adequate for insertion of a finger and exploration of most of the pericardial space and insertion of irrigation and drainage catheters. With more extensive dissection, a large amount of the base and anterior wall of the pericardium can be exposed and resected. In all cases, it is to be emphasized that more than a window be created. This approach allows for dependent drainage and avoids extensive tissue space or pleural contamination.

When pericardial sepsis is suspected, we perform pericardiotomy in combination with systemic antibiotic therapy (usually oxacillin). We then modify the antibiotic therapy to conform to the results of Gram stain culture and in vitro antibiotic sensitivity studies. In the presence of relatively small amounts of thick, purulent material, we place irrigating catheters in the pericardium along with soft drainage catheters. Both are advanced and removed as drainage decreases.

The subxyphoid approach can, of course, be unsuitable when there is loculation of the effusion, high and anterior, particularly on the right between the right atrium and the superior vena cava.

CHRONIC CONSTRICTIVE PERICARDITIS

The cause of chronic constrictive pericarditis is usually unknown, although it may be the end-stage of an undiagnosed viral pericarditis. Whereas tuberculosis was formerly thought to be the most frequent cause, it rarely has any infectious etiology. Sometimes traumatic hemopericardium can evolve to a constrictive pericarditis. The pericardial cavity is found to be obliterated and may be calcified. Diastolic filling is severely restricted, resulting in decreased stroke volume, tachycardia, decreased cardiac output, and increased right ventricular diastolic pressure. Central venous pressures reach levels of 25–30 cm of water. Hepatic enlargement, ascites, peripheral edema, and venous distention occur so that the diagnosis is easily confused with cirrhosis. Unlike other patients with congestive heart failure, the heart is normal size without murmurs or abnormal sounds, although atrial fibrillation may be present as well as pleural effusion. The pulse pressure is normally decreased to a variable degree, and paradoxic pulse (obliteration of the pulse during deep inspiration) is found in some patients. The venous pressure is elevated, the heart is of normal size on chest roentgenogram, and calcification is present in half the cases. Cardiac catheterization is confirmatory. Pericardiectomy gives good short-term results, and since the disease is not now thought to be of infective etiology, no unusual antimicrobial therapy is required.

BIBLIOGRAPHY

Klacsmann PG, Bulkley BH, Hutchins GM: The changed spectrum of purulent pericarditis. An 86-year autopsy experience in 200 patients. Am J Med 63:666, 1977.

Lerner AM: Myocarditis and pericarditis. In Mandell GL, Douglas RG Jr, Bennett JE (eds): Principles and Practice of Infectious Diseases. New York: Wiley, 1979, p 711–724.

REFERENCES

1. Moore TC, Shumacker HB Jr: Congenital and experimentally produced pericardial defects. Angiology 4:1, 1953.
2. Holt JP: The normal pericardium. Am J Cardiol 26:455, 1970.
3. Drinker CK, Field ME: Lymphatics, lymph and tissue fluid. Baltimore, Williams and Wilkins, 1933.
4. Fineberg MH: Functional capacity of the normal pericardium. An experimental study. Am Heart J 11:748, 1936.
5. Dellenback RJ, Chien S, Usami S, Potter RT, Gregersen MI: Hemodynamic effects of pericardial tamponade. Proc Soc Exp Biol Med 123:623, 1966.
6. Drinker CK, Field ME: Absorption from the pericardial cavity. J Exp Med 53:143, 1931.
7. Burch GE, Ray CT: Rates of transfer of Rb^{86}, K^{36}, Ma^{24}, Na^{20}, Cl^{36}, and Cl^{35} across the pericardium in normal dogs. Am J Med 25:115, 1958.
8. Stewart HJ, Crane NF, Deitrick JE: Absorption from the pericardial cavity in man. Am Heart J 16:198, 1938.
9. Bulkley BH, Humphries JO, Hutchins GM: Clinical Pathologic Conference: purulent pericarditis with asymmetric cardiac tamponade: a cause of death months after coronary bypass surgery. Am Heart J 93:776, 1977.
10. Canning B, Mulcahy R, Towers R: Abscess formation in an acute cardiac infarct. Br Med J 1:164, 1969.
11. Devin J, Merdinger WF: Pericardioperitoneal communication—an additional etiologic factor in purulent pericarditis. Dis Chest 56:454, 1969.
12. Hankins JR, McLaughlin JS: Pericarditis with effusion complicating esophageal perforation. J Thorac Cardiovasc Surg 73:225, 1977.
13. Klacsmann PG, Bulkley BH, Hutchins GM: The changed spectrum of purulent pericarditis: an 86-year autopsy experience in 200 patients. Am J Med 63:666, 1977.
14. Symbas PN, Logan WD, Hatcher CR Jr, Abbott OA: Factors in the successful recognition and management of esophageal perforation. South Med J 59:1090, 1966.
15. Ochsner A, DeBakey M: Subphrenic abscess. Collective review and analysis of 3,608 collected and personal cases. Int Abstr Surg 66:426, 1938.
16. Boyle JD, Pearce ML, Guze LB: Purulent pericarditis: review of literature and report of eleven cases. Medicine 40:119, 1961.
17. Rubin RH, Moellering RC Jr: Clinical, microbiologic and therapeutic aspects of purulent pericarditis. Am J Med 59:68, 1975.
18. Barrett AM, Cole L: A case of tuberculous pericarditis. Br Heart J 6:185, 1944.
19. Lerner AM: Myocarditis and pericarditis. In Mandell GL, Douglas RG Jr, Bennett JE (eds): Principles and Practice of Infectious Diseases. New York, Wiley, 1979, p 711.
20. St Geme JW Jr, Noren GR, Adams P Jr: Proposed embryopathic relation between mumps virus and primary endocardial fibroelastosis. N Engl J Med 275:339, 1966.
21. Bulkley BH, Klacsmann PG, Hutchins GM: A clinicopathological study of postthoracotomy purulent pericarditis. A continuing problem of diagnosis and therapy. J Thorac Cardiovasc Surg 73:408, 1977.
22. Engle MA, McCabe JC, Ebert PA, Zabriskie J: The postpericardiotomy syndrome and antiheart antibodies. Circulation 49:401, 1974.
23. Kahn DR, Ertel PY, Murphy WH, Kirsh MM, Vathayanon S, Stern AM, Sloan H: Pathogenesis of the postcardiotomy syndrome. J Thorac Cardiovasc Surg 54:682, 1967.
24. Burch GE, Colcolough HL: Postcardiotomy and postinfarction syndromes. A theory. Am Heart J 80:290, 1970.
25. Siegel RE: Galen on surgery of the pericardium. An early record of therapy based on anatomic and experimental studies. Am J Cardiol 26:524, 1970.
26. Katz A: Abscess of the myocardium complicating infarction. Report of two cases. Can Med Assoc J 91:1225, 1964.
27. Ortbals DW, Avioliv LV: Tuberculous pericarditis. Arch Intern Med 139:231, 1979.
28. Dutton WP, Inclan AP: Cardiac actinomycosis. Dis Chest 54:65, 1968.
29. Lewes D, Rainford DJ, Lance WF: Symptomless myocarditis and myalgia in viral and *Mycoplasma pneumoniae* infections. Br Heart J 36:924, 1974.
30. Turner JA: Parasitic causes of pericarditis. West J Med 122:307, 1975.
31. Herrmann CR, Marchand EJ, Greer GH, Hejtmancik M: Pericarditis. Clinical and laboratory data of 130 cases. Am Heart J 43:641, 1952.

32. Sainani GS, Dekate MP, Rao CP: Heart disease caused by coxsackie virus B infection. Br Heart J 37:819, 1975.
33. Soffer A: Electrocardiographic abnormalities in acute, convalescent, and recurrent stages of idiopathic pericarditis. Am Heart J 60:729, 1960.
34. Surawicz B, Lasseter KC: Electrocardiogram in pericarditis. Am J Cardiol 26:471, 1970.
35. Horowitz MS, Schultz CS, Stinson EB, Harrison DC, Popp RL: Sensitivity and specificity of echocardiographic diagnosis of pericardial effusion. Circulation 50:239, 1974.
36. Teicholy LE: Echocardiographic evaluation of pericardial effusion. In Grannac R, Wang RC (eds): Cardiac Ultrasound. St. Louis, Mosby, 1975, p 106.
37. Buselmeier TJ, Davin TD, Simmons RL, Najarian JS, Kjellstrand CM: Treatment of intractable uremic pericardial effusion. JAMA 240:1358, 1978.
38. Rooney JJ, Crocco JA, Lyons HA: Tuberculous pericarditis. Ann Intern Med 72:73, 1970.
39. Krikorian JG, Hancock EW: Pericardiocentesis. Am J Med 65:808, 1978.
40. Caird R, Conway N, McMillan I: Purulent pericarditis followed by early constriction in young children. Br Heart J 35:201, 1973.
41. Cosgrove DM, Echeverria P, Sade RM: The management of *Hemophilus influenzae,* type B, pericarditis. Ann Thorac Surg 21:281, 1976.
42. Sethi GK, Nelson RM, Jenson CB: Surgical management of acute septic pericarditis. Chest 63:732, 1973.
43. Symbas PN, Ware RE, DiOrio DA, Hatcher CR Jr: Purulent pericarditis: a review of diagnostic and surgical principles. South Med J 67:46, 1974.
44. Wychulis AR, Connolly DC, McGoon DC: Surgical treatment of pericarditis. J Thorac Cardiovasc Surg 62:608, 1971.
45. Cameron EWJ: Surgical management of staphylococcal pericarditis. Thorax 30:678, 1975.
46. Dai ND, Pate JW: Purulent pericarditis in South Vietnam: report of 16 cases. South Med J 67:1306, 1974.
47. Garvin PJ, Danis RK, Lewis JE, Willmann VL: Purulent pericarditis in children. Surgery 84:471, 1978.

CHAPTER 33
Vascular Infection

WESLEY S. MOORE AND JAMES M. MALONE

ARTERIAL INFECTION

ARTERIAL infections usually are not diagnosed preoperatively. In spite of modern antibiotic and surgical treatment, these lesions are still associated with a high morbidity and mortality because they rupture prior to surgical intervention, or there is recurrent infection after repair. The most complete classification of spontaneous arterial infections, which stresses both the arterial pathology and the infectious etiology, is the system suggested by Wilson et al (Table 33-1).[1]

Incidence of Arterial Infection

The incidence of arterial infection, in normal or atherosclerotic arteries, caused by endocardial infection has decreased with the advent of antibiotic therapy. In 1923, Stengel and Wolferth [2] reported that bacterial endocarditis was the source of 86 percent of arterial infections. Pneumonia and osteomyelitis were the next most common causes of arterial infection.[1,3] Aortic infections were much more common than visceral or peripheral arterial infections in most early series.[1,4] Ninety-five percent of arterial infections with aneurysm formation were etiologically related to endocarditis as recently as 1949.[1] In 1951, penicillin treatment of bacterial endocarditis lowered the rate of arterial infection caused by septic emboli from 80 percent to 47 percent.[5] Because bacterial endocarditis and mycotic aneurysms are not reportable diseases, the exact incidence is unknown. Wilson et al [1] estimate the incidence of bacterial endocarditis at 1 in 1,000 to 6,000 hospital admissions but suggest that the actual incidence may be much higher. Pelletier and Petersdorf [3] recently reported that 18 percent of 125 patients with bacterial endocarditis had mycotic aneurysms and that 13 percent died of aneurysm rupture.

Infected atherosclerotic aneurysms are being reported with increasing frequency. An autopsy series by Sommerville et al [6] of 20,201 cadavers suggests an incidence of over 3 percent (6 of 170) with infected atherosclerotic abdominal aortic aneurysms. Essentially all types of soft tissue and organ infections have been associated with infected atherosclerotic aneurysms, but the primary source of infection is unknown in one third to one half of the cases. The true incidence of infected atherosclerotic aneurysms may be higher, but most vascular surgeons do not culture abdominal aortic aneurysms at the time of operation.

The invasion of preexisting arterial lesions during noncardiac bacteremia is probably more common than is suspected, and many early bacterial arterial lesions are probably sterilized by high-dose intravenous antibiotic therapy. This type of lesion is best termed "microbial arteritis." [1] Preexisting arterial lesions include congenital cardiovascular abnormalities, atherosclerotic vascular disease, hypertensive vascular disease, and prior traumatic vascular insult. The differentiating feature between microbial arteritis and mycotic aneurysms is that the source of arterial infection in microbial arteritis is noncardiac.

We recently reported a surprisingly high incidence of bacteremia with clinical diagnostic tests or invasive procedures that involve mucous membrane trauma.[7] The incidence of bacteremia ranged from 8 percent for hemodialysis to 60 to 90 percent for dental extractions. Bacteremias have been documented in healthy individuals without mucous membrane trauma, but the incidence is probably less than 1 percent. In healthy patients with mucous membrane trauma, bacteremia is usually of no consequence. However, patients with vascular lesions, either intrinsic (eg, rheumatic heart disease, atherosclerotic vascular disease) or extrinsic (eg, vascular surgery, vascular trauma) are at increased risk for arterial or valvular infection (5 to 15 percent).[7] The exact incidence of microbial arteritis, however, is unknown. The potential for arterial infection to occur must be considered in any patient with congenital or acquired cardiovascular disease, or prior cardiovascular surgery, who has sustained a clinically significant episode of either bacteremia or septicemia.

False aneurysms differ from true arterial aneurysms in that the wall of the false aneurysm is made of compressed periarterial tissue and clot rather than of adventitia, media, and intima. The use of invasive diagnostic tests and vascular operations and the larger number of traumatic injuries have increased the incidence of infected arterial false aneurysms in recent years. The poor prognosis associated with any untreated infected aneurysm demands that any patient with bacteremia or septicemia and a history of vascular surgery or vascular trauma must be evaluated closely.[1,4,8]

Although the reported incidence of secondary or contiguous arterial infections caused by periarterial infections (including periarterial abscess, lymphangitis with lymph

TABLE 33-1. DIFFERENTIAL FEATURES OF SPONTANEOUS ARTERIAL INFECTIONS

	Mycotic Aneurysm	Infected Aneurysm	Microbial Arteritis	Traumatic Infected Pseudoaneurysm
Etiology	Endocarditis	Bacteremia	Bacteremia	Trauma, narcotic addiction
Sex	F > M	M	M	M or F
Age	30–50	Over 50	Over 50	Under 30
Incidence	Rare	Unusual	Common	Common
Number	Multiple	Single	Single	Multiple
Site	Visceral, intracranial, aorta, and peripheral arteries	Distal aorta	Aortoiliac, superficial femoral arteries; congenital or traumatic vascular defects	Femoral, carotid, or sites of injection
Bacteriology	Gram-positive cocci	*Staphylococcus, Escherichia coli*	*Salmonella* species	Polymicrobial flora
Mortality	Moderate (25%)	High (90%)	High (75%)	Low (10%)

From Wilson SE, Van Wagenen P, Passaro E Jr: Arterial infection. *Curr Probl Surg* 15:1, 1978.

node involvement, osteomyelitis, phlebitis, and infected pseudocysts) is low,[9] most commonly occurring after vascular surgery, these types of periarterial infections must be suspected in patients with a history of arterial trauma or surgery who have evidence of a systemic infection. Host immunocompetence is an important etiologic factor with this type of arterial infection. Kyriakides et al [10] and Walsh et al [11] have noted an increased incidence of arterial infections caused by periarterial infections in immunosuppressed renal transplant patients. Contiguous arterial infections in nonimmunosuppressed hosts have also been documented after gastrointestinal procedures. Kerr and Tilney [12] noted an external iliac arterial infection that resulted from a pelvic abscess after a routine colonic resection. Although any artery theoretically can be infected through extension of a perivascular infection, infections of the thoracic and abdominal aortas are most common.[1] While the incidence of contiguous arterial infection is unknown, this diagnosis must be considered when there is an abscess or inflammatory process adjacent to an artery.

The invasion of preexisting arterial lesions during endocardially induced bacteremia, the creation of iatrogenic arterial injuries that subsequently become infected, and secondary septic pulmonary parenchymal abscess and pulmonary arterial mycotic aneurysms are almost entirely diseases of the twentieth century, which result most often from iatrogenic, diagnostic, or operative intervention or intravenous drug abuse. Intravenous drug addiction is the leading cause of septic emboli in the arterial tree.[1] Septic emboli to the pulmonary artery or lung parenchyma may also result from septic thrombophlebitis of the arm, pelvis, or leg. Most often, septic thrombophlebitis also is associated with either iatrogenic procedures or intravascular drug abuse. The subject of venous infection will be covered in more detail in a later section of this chapter. Griffith et al [13] have reported that the incidence of infected arterial emboli is approximately 2 to 3 percent of all arterial emboli. The diagnosis of septic arterial emboli or secondary pulmonary or parenchymal infection should be suggested in patients with a recent history of intravenous drug abuse or iatrogenic arterial manipulation.

The last type of arterial infection to be considered results from arterial erosion into the gastrointestinal tract. This infection is often not diagnosed prior to death and is almost always fatal unless it is treated before it becomes an arterial infection. The abdominal and thoracic aorta is most commonly involved, and a typical example is an aortoenteric fistula with erosion into the duodenum caused by an untreated expanding abdominal aneurysm. The incidence of these lesions is extremely low. The significance of the lesion is that expanding major arterial aneurysms, in proximity to the gastrointestinal tract, have a substantial risk for erosion with rapid hemorrhage and subsequent death.

Location

While spontaneous infections have the potential to occur in any artery larger than the digital vessels, large arterial degenerative changes predispose the thoracic and abdominal aorta and its major branches to arterial infection (Fig. 33-1).[1,2,4] An obvious exception to this rule is the high incidence of peripheral arterial infections without aortic involvement associated with arterial trauma, operations, invasive diagnostic tests, and intravenous drug abuse (Fig. 33-2).[14] Overall, however, the occurrence of arterial infections usually involves the aorta, the visceral arteries, and the peripheral arteries in decreasing frequency. The distal extremity vessels and intracranial vessels are not as commonly involved, with the exception of intracranial fungal infections secondary to fungal endocarditis.[1,14] Arterial infections caused by bacterial endocarditis usually involve visceral, peripheral, or intracranial vessels primarily. Arterial infections that result from noncardiac-related bacterial invasion usually involve the aorta and its major branches or the extremity vessels. This variability of location associated with infectious etiology is probably related to the pathogenesis of the infection.

Pathogenesis

The etiology of arterial infections depends upon the size of the artery. In small arteries, which are predisposed to degenerative changes, bacteria or septic emboli probably

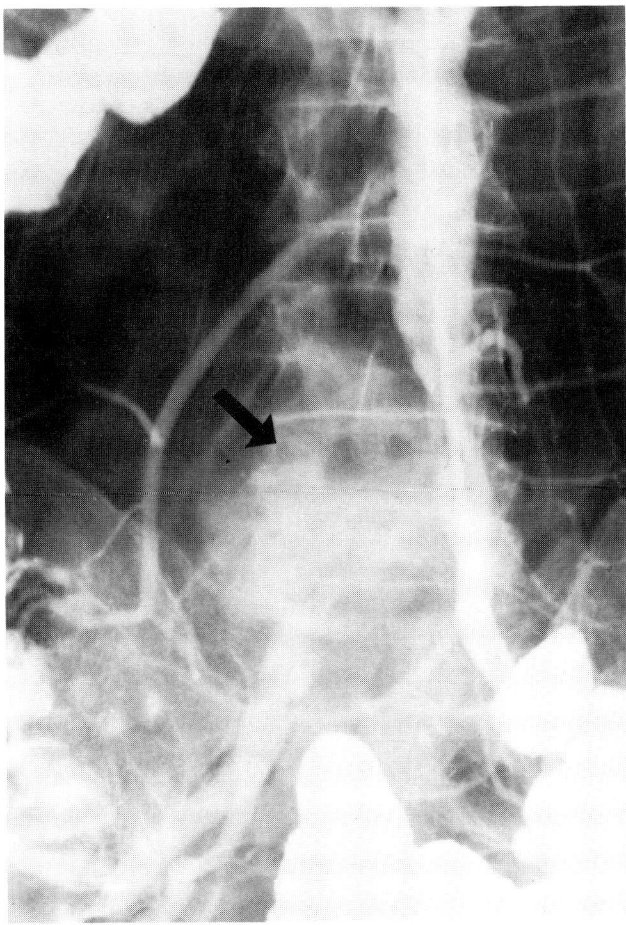

Fig. 33-1. *Salmonella* arteritis of the aortoiliac bifurcation resulting in rupture and pseudoaneurysm formation (arrow). (From Wilson SE, Van Wagenen P, Passaro E Jr: Curr Probl Surg 15:1, 1978.)

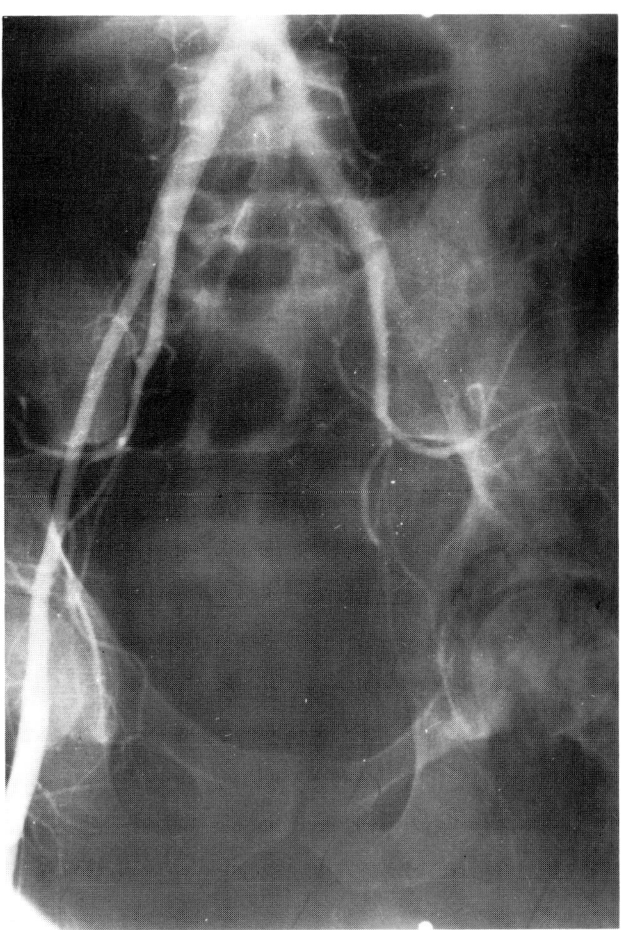

Fig. 33-2. Arteriogram in heroin addict with mycotic aneurysm of common femoral artery that caused thrombosis of vessel. Abundant gas production in soft tissue of thigh resulted from anaerobic peptostreptococcal infection. (From Anderson CB, Butcher HR, Ballinger WF: Arch Surg 109:712, 1974.)

lodge in the vessel wall and lead to locally invasive intimal infections. This will result in secondary transmural arteritis and subsequent aneurysm formation from arterial wall degeneration. In large arteries, however, bacteremia or emboli may lodge in areas of intimal or medial disease on the luminal side of the artery, or they may lodge in the vasa vasorum, with secondary ischemic degeneration of the media. This medial degeneration will be followed by aneurysmal degeneration of the arterial wall. Arterial bifurcations, congenital cardiovascular abnormalities, areas of localized cardiovascular trauma, and primary noninfected arterial aneurysms all predispose to arterial infection.

In the embolic type of arterial infection, there is usually an identifiable source of infection, such as bacterial endocarditis.[1,2,15] Arterial infection may also occur as a direct result of inoculation at the time of vascular trauma or operation. Examples of this latter etiology include intravenous drug abuse,[14] brachial arterial infection after coronary catheterization, osteomyelitis, and infection after vascular surgery.[1,7] Finally, arterial infection may occur as a direct extension (contiguous arterial infection) from a perivascular infection, such as thoracic tuberculous aortitis adjacent to tuberculous mediastinal lymph nodes, arterial infection from contiguous periarterial abscesses,[9] or erosion into the superior mesenteric artery or aorta by a pancreatic pseudocyst.[1,12] As noted earlier, host immunocompetence and host debilitation are important in the pathogenesis of arterial infections.[10,11]

Systemic diseases that are associated with medial degeneration or obliterative endarteritis of the vasa vasorum, such as Marfan's syndrome and Behcet's disease,[16] have been associated with an increased incidence of arterial aneurysm formation and subsequent infection. Arteries with primary disease caused by noninfective inflammatory processes are at increased risk of infections that can result from bacteremia or emboli. These lesions, therefore, can be loosely grouped in the category of predisposing lesions. Discussion of the arteritides and subsequent secondary arterial infection has been purposely excluded from this discussion. Rosenberg et al[17] provide an excellent review of noninfective arterial inflammatory diseases.

Microbiology

The bacteriology of spontaneous arterial infections is essentially that of bacterial endocarditis. Historically, hemolytic streptococci, *Streptococcus pneumoniae,* and

Haemophilus were the most common organisms. More recently, an increasing incidence of *Salmonella* species and staphylococci have been reported. Other organisms include enterococci, gonococci, diphtheroids, *Serratia, Escherichia coli, Yersinia, Pseudomonas, Klebsiella, Proteus, Citrobacter,* and anaerobic organisms, including *Clostridium, Peptostreptococci,* and *Bacteroides.* Mycobacterial infections have been reported throughout the entire history of spontaneous arterial infections. Arterial infections caused by endocardial emboli tend to be of primarily gram-positive cocci, while infections in preexisting arterial lesions caused by nonendocardial bacteremia are more commonly the result of *Salmonella* and a variety of gram-negative rods. Arterial infections that result from perivascular spread are most commonly associated with *Salmonella,* staphylococci, mycobacteria, and fungi. The bacteriology of arterial infection is reviewed in detail by Wilson et al.[1]

The morbidity and mortality of arterial infections are related to the infecting bacteria. Gram-negative infections result in a much higher morbidity and mortality than do gram-positive infections.[1,4]

Of special note are arterial infections caused by *Salmonella* species (Fig. 33-1). Three types of arterial lesions have been noted with *Salmonella:* (1) focal arteritis with aneurysm formation and rupture, (2) diffuse suppurative arteritis with aneurysm and rupture, and (3) secondary infection complicating degenerative arterial lesions. Unlike other bacterial arterial infections which require 6 to 12 weeks of antibiotic therapy, *Salmonella* infections require at least six months of oral therapy after acute intravenous therapy is concluded.[1]

Almost all reports of fungal arterial infections have been associated with fungal endocarditis [18] or iatrogenic cardiovascular trauma. These would include intravenous drug abuse, arterial surgery, and invasive diagnostic procedures.[14] Fortunately, fungal endocarditis or arteritis is a rare disease and is most commonly seen in debilitated or immunosuppressed patients.[18] The most commonly reported fungal organisms include *Candida, Histoplasma, Rhodotorula, Aspergillus,* and *Blastomyces.* Prognosis for either fungal endocarditis or fungal mycotic aneurysms, even with excision and intensive antifungal treatment, is often poor.

Viral arterial infections have not been documented in humans. However, herpesvirus and measles virus have caused arterial lesions that are similar to immunologic connective tissue disorders demonstrated in animals.[19]

Manifestations

The signs and symptoms of arterial infections depend on the infectious etiology and the location of the arterial infection. The relationship between bacterial endocarditis and infection in normal or atherosclerotic arteries or arteries with other predisposing lesions is dependent upon the timing, duration, and success of treatment of the endocardial disease. Patients are usually in the second to fourth decades. The signs and symptoms of mycotic aneurysms will be those of bacterial endocarditis and include fever, weight loss, cardiac murmur, signs of peripheral embolization (petechiae, rose spots, splinter hemorrhages), neurologic symptoms caused by central nervous system emboli, or organic failure.

Unlike arterial infections related to bacterial endocarditis, noncardiac-induced arterial infections are characterized by their lack of specific clinical symptoms. The usual clinical features are those of any systemic infection. Signs of vascular insufficiency in the setting of systemic infection should alert one to the possibility of arterial infection or infected arterial emboli. Sommerville et al [6] emphasized the difficulty of distinguishing patients with infected abdominal aortic aneurysms from those with noninfected aneurysms.

Depending on the location of the arterial infection, history and physical examination may be of value. The presence of a pulsatile mass in a patient with signs of a systemic infection is diagnostic of infected arterial aneurysm. Symptoms suggestive of systemic illness after previous arterial trauma, including vascular surgery, cardiac catherization, intravenous drug abuse, or bacterial endocarditis, should alert one to the possibility of arterial infections. The clinical presentation of a contiguous arterial infection is not different from other types of arterial infection caused by noncardiac infections, except for the presence of a previous abscess.

Laboratory tests are relatively unhelpful and usually demonstrate only evidence of a systemic infection. The most helpful laboratory result is a positive blood culture, which will occur more frequently if arterial samples are taken downstream from the site of an arterial infection, rather than by routine venipuncture.[1]

Routine roentgenograms may reveal vascular calcifications, which suggest aneurysm formation or bone erosion due to contiguous osteomyelitis, but the primary diagnostic procedure, after physical examination and blood cultures, is arteriography. Arteriograms can often be used to differentiate between arterial embolization and primary arterial disruption or thrombosis caused by localized infection. Most importantly, however, the precise location of the lesion is revealed, allowing adequate preoperative evaluation.

Ultrasonography is of limited value in the diagnosis of either infected or noninfected arterial aneurysms. Computer assisted tomographic (CAT) body scanning, however, is sometimes helpful and offers the advantage of being a noninvasive test. CAT scans appear to be of most value for aortic, extremity, and central nervous system lesions and are of unknown value for the diagnosis of visceral arterial lesions.

There are several reports that suggest that radionuclear scans are valuable in both diagnosis and localization of mycotic and infected aneurysms.[46,47] In addition, radiologic or radionuclear evidence of an infection adjacent to a major vessel in a patient with signs of a systemic infection suggests an arterial infection.

The sudden onset of bacteremia, localized pain, localized murmur or bruit, or pulsatile mass in the area of a suspected abscess indicates an arterial infection.[4,22] It is difficult to diagnose abdominal, thoracic, and intracranial arterial infections without arteriography or CAT scans. Most particularly, we cannot overemphasize the difficulty in diagnosing visceral arterial aneurysms without using arteriography. Typically, physical examination and routine laboratory evaluations in a patient with an infected visceral arterial aneurysm will reveal fever, abdominal pain, and signs of systemic illness. Although some visceral aneurysms, such as those involving the proper hepatic artery, may be associated with specific symptom complexes (signs of cholecystitis, hepatitis, or hematobilia), they are not, by themselves, diagnostic in any individual patient. The high morbidity and mortality of untreated infected visceral arterial aneurysms can only be reduced through a high degree of suspicion and angiography.

Treatment and Results

The management of arterial infections is a combination of antibiotic therapy and operation. However, successful treatment is also related to their location.

Large doses of culture-specific antibiotics are commenced preoperatively and continue through the operation and at least six to eight weeks postoperatively or longer, depending upon the aneurysm and the organism.[1,4] Adequate serum antibiotic levels must be checked and maintained during all phases of therapy. Bactericidal, rather than bacteriostatic, drugs should be used. Without operative treatment, infected arterial lesions may continue to enlarge and either rupture or remain a reservoir for continued bacteremic infection in spite of antibiotic therapy. Sterilization of a preexisting endocarditis is especially important to minimize the risk of contaminating newly implanted vascular prostheses.

Surgical treatment should include excision of the infected artery and surrounding tissue, exclusion from the arterial circulation if excision is not possible, and vascular reconstruction through uninfected tissues if simple ligation or excision is not adequate. Simple ligation and excision are the best treatment if the arterial infection involves a noncritical artery or as immediate treatment if the arterial infection involves a critical artery but the collateral flow is acceptable. Reconstruction should be performed as needed but as late as possible (preferably three to six months) after the primary operation. In many cases, immediate arterial reconstruction is required. The principles of arterial reconstruction in infected fields will be discussed in a later portion of this chapter. However, there are two basic rules: (1) prosthetic grafts must be routed outside any potentially infected area to avoid recurrent graft infection, and (2) arterial continuity through an infected area can only be assured with fresh autogenous tissue grafts.[1,7]

Successful management of aortic or other large retroperitoneal arterial vascular infections will be possible only with total excision of the involved arterial segment and surrounding tissue. We prefer to use a monofilament suture for oversewing the proximal and distal portions of the remaining artery. If possible, we use a two-layer closure, using a continuous suture reinforced with interrupted sutures. The area should be retroperitonealized, if possible, and drained, using retroperitoneal flank drains. Copious amounts of intraoperative local antibiotic irrigation should be used. A closed-system antibiotic irrigation during the postoperative period, much like the closed systems used for open fractures, can be employed.

Successful management of visceral arterial infections is difficult because the vessels are often end organ in nature, with poor collateral supply. In addition, extensive dissection may injure the surrounding structures. Techniques used for management of infected visceral arterial aneurysms include endoaneurysmorrhaphy, ligation and excision, and excision with primary grafting. All the various vascular techniques attempt to minimize dissection because the aneurysm is usually densely adherent to surrounding structures, a result of the inflammatory process. Because it is not usually possible to route a visceral graft through an uninfected area, it is best to use fresh autogenous arteries or veins for reconstruction of infected visceral arterial lesions. It must be emphasized that drainage of infected vascular lesions must be thorough and that any revascularization procedures must be performed through clean tissue planes, if possible.

Infected peripheral arterial lesions are usually the easiest lesions to diagnose and treat because of the ease of both examination and operative access, the amount of potential collateralization, and the presence of noninfected tissue compartments that can be used for extraanatomic vascular reconstruction.

Regardless of the location of the vessel, the presence of a perivascular abscess or infection is an absolute indication for surgical drainage.

Several types of arterial lesions, especially atherosclerotic abdominal aneurysms, are often not recognized as being infected prior to operation. All atherosclerotic abdominal aneurysms or questionable and unusual arterial lesions should have their wall or intraluminal contents cultured and Gram stained. If an infection is suspected, based upon operative findings or Gram stain, excision of the lesion and management as previously described are mandatory. If the cultures return to positive during the postoperative period, antibiotic therapy should be continued for six to eight weeks with culture-specific antibiotics.

Excised specimens also should always be cultured, not only because blood cultures will not always be positive but also because cardiovascular infections may be polymicrobial, and adequate adjunctive antibiotic therapy depends upon identification of specific organisms. The increased appearance of antibiotic-resistant organisms in arterial infections emphasizes the need for accurate culture information.

The relatively poor long-term results in management of arterial lesions in critical arteries strongly suggest that both postoperative arteriography and long-term follow-up with noninvasive tests, such as CAT scan, are mandatory. In addition, strong consideration should be given for extended oral antibiotic coverage (6 to 12 months) after the completion of acute surgical antibiotic therapy.

Fungal organisms, *Candida* species in particular, tend to preferentially embolize to both intracranial and extremity vessels. The tendency for these fungal lesions to embolize is related to the poor adherence of fungal vegetation to the vascular surfaces. Surgeons should be aggressive in exploring arteries suspected of being occluded by fungal emboli, especially those suspected of being infected with *Candida* because embolectomy can be performed safely, even in the most debilitated patient.[22]

INFECTIONS IN VEINS

Unlike arteries, veins are rarely infected unless a foreign body lies in the venous system. The most notable exception to such a general statement is the occurrence of pyelophlebitis with appendicitis, necrotic bowel, abdominal abscesses, and other types of abdominal sepsis.[23] The intrinsic venous resistance to bacteremia-induced infection is probably related to the lack of degenerative changes in the venous system which predispose veins to bacterial seeding and subsequent infection. The low incidence of venous infection in postphlebitic limbs or in venous segments that have sustained trauma suggests that venous injury alone is not a predisposing lesion. The best hypotheses to explain the low incidence of spontaneous venous infection (without the introduction of extrinsic organisms into the venous system) include (1) the lack of predisposing lesions in the venous system, (2) differences in flow and pulsatility compared to the arterial system, and (3) differences in morphology of the veins, such as the lack of a vasa vasorum, as seen in large and medium-sized arteries. We can neither explain adequately with specific facts nor understand objectively the pathophysiology associated with the relatively low incidence of venous infections in the absence of direct inoculation.

The subsequent sections on venous infection will emphasize postinfusion phlebitis and suppurative phlebitis. Nonsuppurative venous inflammatory diseases have been reviewed by Abruzzo.[24]

UMBILICAL ARTERIAL AND VENOUS CATHETERS

The increased use of both umbilical arterial and venous catheters in neonatal units has brought with it a host of complications, including vascular thrombosis, organ infarction, and visceral ischemia.[25] Balagtas et al [26] reviewed the infectious risks of umbilical venous catheterization in 86 newborn infants. They reported that 52 percent of all umbilical venous catheters were colonized with bacteria within 48 hours of insertion (primarily with staphylococci and coliform organisms). Most importantly, they found that the incidence of catheter colonization was not related to the duration of catheterization.[26] A prospective study by Anagnostakis et al [25] of 65 newborn infants with umbilical venous catheters revealed that 53 percent of the umbilical cord stumps were contaminated prior to catheter placement, even though the stump was cleaned before catheterization, and that 62 percent of the umbilical venous catheters were colonized at the time of removal. In addition to the high rate of catheter bacterial colonization, both studies documented an 8 to 10 percent incidence of catheter-related bacteremia and sepsis.[25,26] Balagtas et al [26] showed that, although prophylactic antibiotics (penicillin and kanamycin) did not decrease the overall incidence of catheter colonization, the antibiotics significantly decreased the incidence of bacteremia.[26] Most studies (except Balagtas et al [26]) suggest that prophylactic antibiotics did not significantly change the risk of sepsis, the incidence of positive umbilical catheter blood cultures, or the incidence of catheter bacterial colonization.[25] This is consistent with studies of other intravascular catheters.[27-29] Everyone agrees that umbilical arterial and venous catheters should be removed as rapidly as possible.[25]

PERIPHERAL CATHETER-RELATED PHLEBITIS

The reported incidence of postinfusion or suppurative phlebitis ranges from 0.2 to 15 percent.[27] This variation is related to (1) the type of catheter used, because steel scalp venous needles are associated with a lower incidence of infection than are plastic catheters,[27] (2) techniques of venipuncture and catheter care and maintenance,[28,29] and (3) the high incidence of inflammatory but nonsuppurative phlebitis seen with all types of venous catheters.

Intravenous catheter tips often show positive cultures without the occurrence of local suppurative phlebitis. The incidence of culture-positive intravenous catheter tips in some studies is as high as 47 percent, although the incidence of suppurative phlebitis can range from 5 to 16 percent. This apparent discrepancy suggests that there are errors in culture technique (which can introduce nonpathogenic bacteria onto the catheter) or differences in the parameters of the clinical diagnosis of suppurative phlebitis versus nonsuppurative postinfusion phlebitis. This also suggests that there are two etiologies—irritation and infection—important to the pathogenesis of true suppurative phlebitis. The histopathologic changes noted in postinfusion phlebitis strongly support irritation as one of the important etiologic factors. Early phlebitis demonstrates endothelial swelling and increased numbers of polymorphonucleocytes in the media of the vein. As the degree of the phlebitis becomes more severe, endothelial cell loss increases, and increased numbers of polymorphonucleocytes are noted in the media. In additon, there is pyknosis of many medial muscle cells. Finally, in the most severe form, phlebitic veins demonstrate wall necrosis. These changes are noted with and without bacteria, and it is, therefore, difficult to suggest that the changes are due only to localized infection or irritation. There is little question, however, that infection is involved in the pathophysiology of suppurative phlebitis (pus in vein lumen). The most common organisms are skin organisms, *Staphylococcus aureus* and streptococci, although almost all major groups of gram-positive and gram-negative organisms have been reported, as well as yeasts and fungi.[28]

Cannula-related sepsis is a risk with intravenous therapy, and the risk is higher with plastic indwelling catheters than with steel scalp venous needles (Chapter 24). Although there are no comparable double-blind studies, the incidence of cannula-related sepsis for scalp venous needles and for plastic catheters would appear to be less than 0.5 percent and over 5 percent, respectively. Postinfusion phlebitis or catheter-related infections, excluding true suppurative phlebitis, usually respond to treatment after the catheter is removed. True suppurative phlebitis, however, is lethal unless the involved venous segment is excised.[24,26,27,30] Suppurative phlebitis is seen most commonly with leg intravenous catheters [27] and with prolonged intravenous cannulation with plastic catheters (longer than 48 hours).[24,26,27] In addition, there is an increased risk of suppurative phlebitis in burn patients,[27] debilitated or immunosuppressed patients, and in patients with cancer.[27]

The clinical signs of inflammation or an unexplained fever in a patient with no obvious source of infection all suggest intravenous catheter-related infection. The local signs of inflammation and infection are often absent, however, in patients with cancer, burns, immunoincompetence, or severe debilitation. If suppurative phlebitis is suspected, exploratory venotomy is indicated.

INFECTIONS WITH CENTRAL VENOUS CATHETERS

All of our previous statements regarding infections related to peripheral intravenous cannulation also apply to central venous catheters. However, a few specific points deserve emphasis. The technique of insertion and intravenous catheter care are extremely critical to both catheter patency and catheter-related infections, especially in immunologically compromised patients. Properly inserted and maintained central venous catheters can be used for total parenteral nutrition for extended times without the occurrence of catheter-related sepsis. These same lines cannot be used, however, for administration of medication, for central venous pressure measurements, or for routine intravenous administration, without a high risk of catheter-related sepsis after 48 to 72 hours (Chapter 24).

The risk of central venous catheter-related infection varies with the infection status of the patient. In a review of 130 consecutive percutaneous subclavian catheters, Mogensen et al [28] noted no catheter-related infections in 64 noninfected patients and both a 10 percent (9 of 66) incidence of catheter-related sepsis and a 25 percent (17 of 66) incidence of positive catheter cultures in patients with previous septic foci. In the 17 patients with positive catheter cultures, 14 had positive cultures of catheter contents, and 9 had positive blood cultures drawn from other venipuncture sources. In addition, in the group with previous septic foci, the incidence of catheter-related sepsis varied directly with the duration of catheter placement.[28]

In addition to improper catheter insertion, improper catheter maintenance, or errors in the use of a hyperalimentation line, an often overlooked and not unusual source of sepsis is the contamination of the intravenous solution itself.

DEEP VENOUS THROMBOSIS AND INFECTION

In the absence of iatrogenic or penetrating traumatic injury, the incidence of suppurative phlebitis with deep venous thrombosis is exceedingly low. In fact, the occurrence of suppurative phlebitis with routine deep venous thrombosis is rare. Iatrogenic septic deep venous thrombosis occurs most commonly after intravenous drug abuse, pelvic or urologic surgery, peripheral arterial, or venous surgery. Traumatic septic deep venous thrombosis is most often related to intravenous drug abuse and, much less commonly, to severe crushing injuries of the lower extremities. There has always been a suspicion that primary or routine deep venous thrombosis was caused by infection, especially with L-forms (wall-deficient bacteria). Nicolaides et al [31] reviewed 420 surgery patients screened by I-125 fibrinogen for deep venous thrombosis. They found a statistically significant increase of deep venous thrombosis with postoperative infection and with the perioperative use of antibiotics in the absence of postoperative infection. While there is little question that the incidence of deep venous thrombosis is increased with operation, it is difficult, at best, to suggest that the Nicolaides study conclusively proves an infectious cause of deep venous thrombosis. The bulk of data suggests that deep venous thrombosis is related to local vascular trauma, local hypercoagulation, stasis, and possibly hypofibrinolysis of the venous endothelium. There are no conclusive data to suggest a primary infection in most cases of deep venous thrombosis.

INFECTION IN IRRADIATED ARTERIES AND VEINS

Radiation probably induces vascular damage by obliterating small nutrient wall vessels, such as the vasa vasorum, that supply the media of small, medium, and large arteries. Obliteration of these nutrient vessels causes tissue (media) hypoxemia and subsequent wall degeneration. Radiation treatment can cause both arterial aneurysm formation and arterial stenosis and occlusion. The type of arterial injury caused by a specific form of radiation therapy is unpredictable. The predilection of irradiation to disproportionately injure small nutrient vessels probably accounts for the lesser incidence of recognized radiation-associated venous injury because there are few nutrient vessels in most veins. As discussed in our sections on arterial and venous infection, any histopathologic changes caused by radiation would predispose the artery or vein to an increased risk of infection (both cardiac and noncardiac bacteremia and septicemia). The relative resistance of the venous system to infection from bacteremia accounts for the low incidence of irradiation-related venous infections. Svanberg et al [32] demonstrated decreased endothelial fibrinolytic activator activity in irradiated vessels, compared to nonradiated control vessels, and a decreased rate of endothelial fibrinolytic activity in irradiated vessels with passage of time after radiation therapy. Intravascular thrombus must be considered as not only adequate nutrient media for bacterial and fungal organisms but also a predisposing lesion for arterial and venous infection with respect to a bacteremic challenge, especially in a debilitated, immunosuppressed, or cancer patient (Fig. 33-3). The relationship between the vascular changes, the venous and arterial endothelial fibrinolytic activity, and the subsequent vascular thrombosis and infection is unknown. There is no question that the loss of endothelial fibrinolytic activator activity denotes biochemical, if not histologic, injury and that decreased endothelial fibrinolysis is associated with an increased incidence of local vascular thrombus formation or vessel thrombosis. It is attractive to hypothesize that radiation-induced changes in endothelial fibrinolytic activity may be associated with either an increased incidence

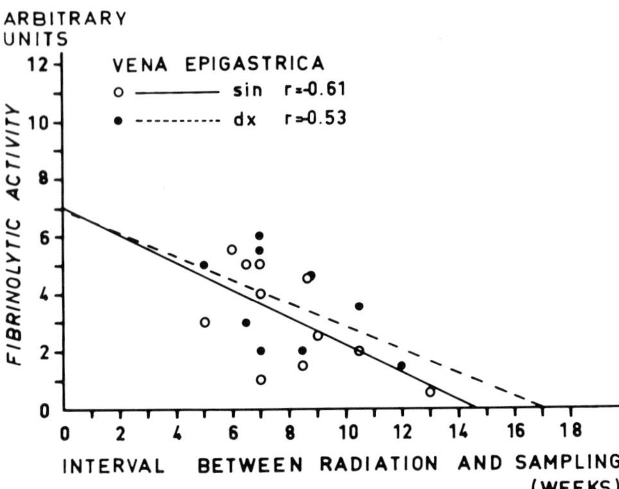

Fig. 33-3. **Comparison between fibrinolytic activity in superficial veins and interval between radiation and sampling. (From Svanberg L, Åstedt B, Kullander S: Acta Obstet Gynecol Scand 55:49, 1976.)**

of arterial and venous infection or a decreased resistance of irradiated arteries and veins to infection from bacteremic challenge.

It is recognized that irradiated tissues have severely decreased resistance to infection, and it is reasonably safe to predict that there should be an increased incidence of contiguous arterial infection in those patients who have had local irradiation over the artery in question. However, there is only the common clinical observation that carotid arterial rupture after combined excision and radiation therapy for head and neck cancer is much more frequent than that following either treatment alone.

INFECTION IN VASCULAR GRAFTS

Infection that involves a vascular graft is a rare but disastrous complication. Morbidity and mortality from graft infection have been extremely high because of the critical location of the graft as well as the necessity to remove the graft material, particularly in the instance of a prosthetic graft, after infection has been established. The incidence, natural history, and management are influenced by the type of material used for grafting, the location of the graft, and the functional distribution of the arterial blood supply for which the graft was intended.

Historic Perspective

The first reported clinical series of infected prosthetic grafts appeared in the late 1950s. Schramel and Creech [33] collected six cases of infected prostheses. Of four grafts located in the femoral or femoropopliteal regions, three were treated by excision, resulting in two major amputations—one hip disarticulation and one high above-knee amputation. Two grafts were in the aortic or iliofemoral region, and both were treated by excision. One patient had above-knee amputation, and the other died from continued sepsis.

Harrison [34] used dogs to compare the effect of infection on aortic homografts with experimental infection in Teflon prostheses. Two groups were employed: in the first group, grafts were implanted in an infected wound, and in the second group, the grafts were placed in a contaminated wound. In the first group, 5 of 11 dogs died from disruption of an infected homograft, and 5 of 10 dogs experienced complications of infection in a Teflon prosthesis, but only 2 disrupted. In the second group of implants, in contaminated wounds, 6 of 9 dogs developed infection in a homograft, and 5 of the 6 dogs died from disruption. Seven out of 11 Teflon grafts became infected, and there were 3 deaths from disruption. The authors concluded that the only difference between the behavior of Teflon and homografts in the presence of infection or contamination was the incidence and mode of death. The Teflon graft harbored sepsis, while the homograft promptly disrupted, leading to exsanguination.

Humphries et al [35] reported a clinical series of 11 infected homografts collected in 525 arterial reconstructive procedures, an incidence of 2 percent. All of these 11 homografts ruptured from lysis of the grafts, presumably the result of the proteolytic effect of the infection.

Prompted by a clinical experience of having an aortic homograft lyse and exsanguinate following resection and replacement of a mycotic aortic aneurysm, Foster et al [36] carried out a similar study to compare the effect of infection on Teflon grafts and homografts. They observed that all the homografts that became infected disrupted and exsanguinated, while the plastic prostheses remained intact. They cautioned, however, that the plastic prostheses appeared to continue to harbor infection.

Following these initial clinical and experimental reports, many case reports were published that confirmed the serious nature of infection that complicates vascular grafts. This led the way toward an in-depth search for the etiology, methods of management, and prevention of graft infection.

Incidence

The incidence of graft infection is difficult to quantitate for several reasons. First, the actual number of graft infections is few, and, second, graft infections do not necessarily appear in the immediate postoperative course. They may be delayed for several months to several years before they become clinically manifest. There are a number of factors that appear to affect the reported incidence of graft infection in the various series. These factors include the type of graft (autogenous vs prosthetic) and the type of fabric employed in the construction of the prosthetic material. Live autogenous grafts appear to be far more resistant to infection and, therefore, have a lower incidence of infection in contrast to a foreign body implant.[37-39] In addition, the type of fabric used for the prosthetic graft will have a major effect upon the healing properties of the graft. Late infections are considerably fewer in grafts that have a more complete healing response than in those that are more inert to tissue ingrowth.[40] The location of the graft appears to have a major effect on the likelihood of subsequent infection. Infection is also influenced by the appropriate use of antibiotic prophylaxis.[41,42] In analyzing various series, it is important to evaluate the number of operations per year, the number of grafts at risk in a given time interval, and the relative proportion of types of operative procedures and locations when comparing the incidence of graft infection from one series to another.

The overall incidence of graft infection ranges from 1.34 to 6 percent.[43,44] The larger, current series gives the best idea of the problem. In 1972, Szilagyi et al,[45] in a detailed review, evaluated their experience between the years 1952 and 1971, which included 3,347 arterial reconstructive procedures. Of the 2,145 prosthetic grafts, 40 became infected, an incidence of 1.9 percent. Of the 445 vein grafts, 2 (0.4 percent) became infected. There was 1 (0.2 percent) arterial infection in 492 endarterectomies, and 265 reconstructions were performed with arterial allografts, in which there was 1 (0.4 percent) infection. These authors also analyzed the incidence of infection by the site of insertion and noted that the incidence of infection in aortoiliac grafts was 0.7 percent, in aortofemoral grafts, 1.6 percent, in femorofemoral grafts, 0.9 percent, and in femoropopliteal grafts, 3.0 percent.[45] In 1974, Goldstone and Moore [41] reviewed 566 prosthetic graft implantations performed between 1959 and 1973. Fourteen infections were reported, for an overall incidence of 2.5 percent. These data were broken down into two time intervals, corresponding to a change in the regimen used for antibiotic prophylaxis. Between 1959 and 1965, antibiotics were used in an inconsistent fashion, usually beginning antibiotic treatment in the postoperative period. Nine of the 222 grafts inserted during this interval became infected, for an overall infection rate of 4 percent. Between 1966 and 1973, modern methods of antibiotic prophylaxis, which included preoperative, intraoperative, and postoperative administration of antibiotic medication, were instituted. There were 344 grafts placed during this second period, of which 5 became infected, for an overall incidence of 1.5 percent. An analysis of the incidence of graft infection as a function of location is shown in Table 33-2, which also compares the incidence of graft infection in the two periods analyzed.

Pathogenesis

There are many causes of graft infection. Some have been proven either by clinical observation or by experimental means, and others represent hypothetical ways in which a prosthesis can become contaminated.[40,46-48]

Traumatic Wounds. Arterial trauma from war or civilian injuries represents an obvious source of bacterial contamination that can subsequently compromise a vascular repair by producing a combination of wound and graft sepsis. Since every traumatic wound is contaminated, the arterial repair should be performed with autogenous tissues. If this is done properly, the chance of successful repair will be remarkably improved. In those instances in which prosthetic grafts have been implanted directly in contaminated or infected wounds, the incidence of subsequent infectious complications is extremely high, and, as such, contaminated wounds represent a major cause of vascular graft sepsis.

TABLE 33-2. INCIDENCE OF GRAFT INFECTION AS A FUNCTION OF GRAFT LOCATION AND ERA OF IMPLANTATION

	Infection Rate		
Anatomic Location	*1959–65* %	*1966–73* %	*1959–73* %
Aortoiliac	1.3	1.2	1.2
Aortofemoral	5.7	1.2	3.0
Axillofemoral	8.0	3.1	5.3
Femorofemoral			7.7
Femoropopliteal			2.3

Modified from Goldstone J, Moore WS: Infection in vascular prostheses. *Am J Surg* 128:225, 1974.

Improper Sterilization of Graft or Surgical Instruments. This mechanism probably represents an infrequent source of contamination of a vascular graft.

Break in Sterile Technique. Strict aseptic technique must be followed throughout the procedure.

Skin Contact. Since the skin cannot be sterilized, large exposed areas of skin will continue to harbor organisms on the surface. A prosthetic graft, if allowed to come in contact with the skin, can pick up skin organisms. Skin contact with a graft may occur most commonly in relatively superficial grafting sites, such as the femoral, popliteal, and axillary arteries. This may account for the relatively higher incidence of graft infection when prostheses are implanted in these locations. In addition to the skin surface as a source of organisms, the cut edges of skin represent another source of skin contact and transfer of organisms.

Infected Lymph Glands or Lymphatics. Lymph glands or lymphatics may be a source of organisms, particularly when there is infection present in the extremity, such as a toe or web space. Incisions to expose arteries that must pass through lymph glands or lymphatic channels will liberate contaminated lymph and may represent a major source of contamination of prostheses placed in those anatomic areas. Femoral incisions represent the most obvious source for this mode of contamination.

Intestinal Transudate. It is common practice to place the loops of small bowel in a sack when preparing the exposure of the abdominal aorta. There have been reports that the liquid that collects in the plastic bag is contaminated with bacteria. Return of this liquid to the abdominal cavity may bathe the prosthesis and increase the likelihood of graft infection. Other reports, however, have failed to confirm bacterial contamination in this fluid, which may reflect a beneficial effect of prophylactic antibiotics.

Infected Arterial or Aneurysm Content. On occasion, an abdominal or peripheral aneurysm may be infected prior to repair. The prosthetic graft will inevitably be contaminated. There is also evidence that bacteria are always present in the laminated thrombus lining an abdominal aortic aneurysm. If this is true, this would be another source of contamination of the prosthetic graft.

Combined Operations. The performance of another operation at the time of vascular repair may also be a source of bacterial contamination of the arterial graft. This is particularly true with appendectomy, cholecystectomy, and colectomy. A clean vascular surgical procedure should never be intentionally combined with a contaminated or clean contaminated operation.

Transient Bacteremia. External contamination of the prosthetic graft is most common, but internal contamination during transient bacteremia also occurs. Bacteria in the arterial blood may deposit on the luminal surface of the graft and ultimately lead to a prosthetic infection. Sources of transient bacteremia in the perioperative period include Foley catheters, endotracheal tubes, such secondary infection as pneumonia or urinary tract infection, and, in general, any vigorous mucous membrane manipulation. Transient bacteremia may also be a cause of late graft infection in those instances where the lining of the graft is incomplete. We strongly recommend the use of vigorous antibiotic therapy as prophylaxis in those patients undergoing mucous membrane manipulation (dental surgery, cystoscopy, proctoscopy) with vascular prostheses in place.

Etiology

It is possible for any organism to infect a graft, and there is a wide spectrum of organisms reported to have infected prostheses. These include such unlikely organisms as *Mycobacterium tuberculosis* and *Histoplasma capsulatum*. Most infections are due to *S. aureus* and fewer to gram-negative organisms.[43] Table 33-3 lists the organisms found in prosthetic graft infections in several recent series.[41,44,45,48] Multiple organisms are frequently found.

Each of the groups [41,44,45,48] also analyzed the type and frequency of infection as a function of the interval between operation and clinical presentation and of the location of the clinical infection. They noted that the median time interval between graft implantation and the appearance of infection was 3.5 months. Table 33-4 identifies the infecting organism and frequency of those infections that occurred earlier and later than 3.5 months, as a function of location.

Exposure of the graft to skin bacteria in a superficial subcutaneous site like the groin is the most important factor in graft infection. The low-virulence skin organism, *Staphylococcus epidermidis*, is most often found late after grafting, and it is conceivable that a dormant period intervenes between contamination and clinical infection. The increased risk of graft infection when the graft extends below the inguinal ligament should encourage a greater degree of care when extending prosthetic reconstruction in that area. Finally, the association between the frequency of the *Staphylococcus* as the infecting organism should direct one to antibiotic prophylaxis that includes *Staphylococcus* in its bactericidal spectrum.[41]

Clinical Manifestations

Infection in a vascular graft may have a wide spectrum of clinical manifestations. The clinical appearance of a graft infection is dependent upon three major factors: the duration between implantation and appearance of sepsis, the type of graft material involved in the infectious process, and the location of the vascular conduit.

Acute Graft Infection. Acute vascular graft infections usually occur as a consequence of a postoperative wound infection. Therefore, acute graft infections are most often limited to those reconstructive procedures that come in close proximity to the skin (femoral, popliteal, axillary, and carotid-subclavian anastomoses). The initial manifestations of sepsis include the characteristics of a wound infection:

TABLE 33-3. SPECTRUM OF ORGANISMS INFECTING VASCULAR GRAFTS

	Percent of Patients with Cultured Organisms			
Organism	*Conn et al*[44]	*Szilagyi et al*[45]	*Liekweg and Greenfield*[48]	*Goldstone and Moore*[41]
Aerobacter	10.25	—	—	—
Bacteroides	—	2.5	0.6	—
Corynebacterium	—	2.5	0.6	—
Escherichia coli	10.25	22.5	13.4	15.0
Enterococcus	10.25	—	1.8	—
Enterobacter	2.5	—	—	—
Klebsiella	7.5	—	5.4	
Proteus	13.0	7.5	4.8	
Providencia	—	—	—	4.0
Pseudomonas	13.0	2.5	6.1	7.0
Salmonella	—	—	1.2	—
Serratia marcescens	10.25	—	—	—
Staphylococcus, coagulase negative	—	15.0	—	—
Staphylococcus albus	2.5	—	3.6	26.0
Staphylococcus aureus	18.0	32.5	50.0	41.0
Streptococcus	2.5	5.0	8.5	—
Unknown	—	10.0	16.0	7.0
TOTAL INFECTIONS	39	40	188	27

TABLE 33-4. SPECTRUM AND LOCATION OF INFECTIONS WITHIN OR AFTER 3.5 MONTHS OF OPERATION

Organism	Within 3.5 Months		After 3.5 Months	
	Groin	*Elsewhere*	*Groin*	*Elsewhere*
Entamoeba coli	0	2	1	1
Providencia	—	—	0	1
Pseudomonas	1	1	—	—
Staphylococcus albus	—	—	7	0
Staphylococcus aureus	9	0	1	1
Unknown	—	—	2	0

From Goldstone J, Moore WS: Infection in vascular prostheses. *Am J Surg* 128:225, 1974.

fever, leukocytosis, redness, induration, and abscess formation. The specific manifestations of acute sepsis in the vascular conduit depend upon the type of material used for the vascular graft. The details of infection in various graft materials will be discussed later.

Late Graft Infection. The most common manifestation of graft infection usually occurs months to years after a vascular reconstructive procedure. In this setting, the signs of sepsis can be quite subtle. The patient may be afebrile, the white blood count is often normal, and the actual manifestations of sepsis will depend upon the type of graft material and the location of implantation. One consistent laboratory finding, both clinically and experimentally, has been an elevated erythrocyte sedimentation rate.

Manifestations of Sepsis as a Function of the Graft Material

Plastic Prostheses. Once infecting organisms contaminate a plastic prosthesis, they continue to be harbored in the graft fabric, since the prosthetic graft represents a multifibered foreign body. It is impossible to clear contaminating organisms from the plastic prosthesis by systemic antibiotic therapy. Sepsis in a plastic prosthesis can manifest itself in several ways, including anastomotic breakdown with formation of a false aneurysm, graft thrombosis, a purulent draining sinus, wound breakdown with exteriorization of the prosthesis, systemic sepsis, and septic emboli.

Table 33-5 lists the mode of onset and clinical manifestations of graft infections in an older [43] and more recent [41] series. The clinical manifestations can be divided into two general patterns. In the first, the diagnosis is readily evident. There is persistent purulent wound drainage, wound abscess, or exteriorization of the graft. In the second the diagnosis is subtle—persistent low-grade fever, systemic sepsis, septic embolization, graft thrombosis, ureteral obstruction, an abdominal mass, a false aneurysm, and gastrointestinal hemorrhage.

Liekweg and Greenfield [48] analyzed the mode of presentation of 164 cases from the literature as a function of anatomic location (Table 33-6).

Preserved Homografts. Freeze-dried preserved homografts were introduced by Gross et al in 1949 [49] and represented a major breakthrough in the availability of materials for grafting of large vessels. Sepsis complicating the use of this material, however, is particularly disastrous. Since the material is nonviable, sepsis results in rapid proteolytic digestion of the graft material, which promptly leads to disruption and massive hemorrhage. Early experimental studies by Foster et al [36] confirmed this observation and indicated that plastic prostheses, while continuing to harbor infection as a foreign body, at least remain intact, thus preventing disruption and hemorrhage from the body of the graft. The various manifestations of sepsis in preserved homografts are again dependent upon the location of the homografts, but, ultimately, hemorrhage is the final common pathway. Freeze-dried preserved arterial homografts are not in clinical use at the present time. However, a new material has been introduced to the market and is currently being employed for vascular reconstruction and dialysis access. This is the tanned, externally supported

TABLE 33-5. PRESENTING CLINICAL MANIFESTATIONS OF GRAFT SEPSIS

Complications	Number	
	Fry and Lindenauer [43]	*Goldstone and Moore* [41]
Graft occlusion	4	8
Localized infection and draining sinus	3	14
False aneurysm	1	13
Local hemorrhage	1	7
Systemic sepsis or shock	2	5
Persistent pelvic abscess	1	—
Septic emboli	—	2
TOTAL	12	49

TABLE 33-6. CLINICAL MANIFESTATION OF GRAFT SEPSIS AS A FUNCTION OF LOCATION

Mode	Aortoiliac %	Aortofemoral %	Iliofemoral %	Femoropopliteal %
Wound purulence	10.4	43.6	42.8	74.5
Sepsis	24.1	18.2	7.1	0.0
False Aneurysm	10.4	9.1	14.2	9.1
Hemorrhage	20.8	7.2	7.1	7.2
Sinus tract	6.9	9.1	21.4	7.2
Upper gastrointestinal bleeding	27.5	18.2	0.0	0.0
Graft occlusion	0.0	9.1	7.1	1.8

Modified from Liekweg WG Jr, Greenfield LJ: Vascular prosthetic infections: Collected experience and results of treatment. *Surgery* 81:335, 1977.

umbilical vein, harvested from umbilical cords. This material is not viable and possesses the identical characteristics of freeze-dried preserved homografts when their clinical use is complicated by sepsis.

Bovine Heterografts. Carotid arteries, obtained from cows and processed by digestion and tanning to yield a collagen tube, are in common use today. These materials are primarily used for dialysis access procedures. When sepsis complicates a bovine heterograft, the sequence of events is identical to that of the freeze-dried preserved homograft, namely, disruption and hemorrhage.

Fresh Autogenous Grafts. Fresh autogenous artery and vein have been used for a variety of vascular grafting operations. Specifically, the autogenous saphenous vein has been used for femoropopliteal replacement, patch angioplasty, coronary bypass, and extrathoracic cerebrovascular bypass procedures. Fresh autogenous arteries (eg, hypogastric, external iliac, reconstituted thrombectomized superficial femoral) have been used as renal arterial replacements or as replacements in septic fields as a vascular replacement material. These conduits tend to be quite resistant to the immediate complications of sepsis, provided there is prompt treatment of the surrounding septic processes, including drainage, irrigation, and antibiotic therapy. However, if the surrounding sepsis is profound and is not treated in time, infection will lead to proteolytic disruption of the autogenous vascular material, with breakdown and hemorrhage.

Sepsis as a Function of Graft Location. Sepsis as a function of graft location will produce not only the evidence of the systemic problem but also features that are unique to the organ being supplied or organs adjacent to the infected graft. For example, infection in an abdominal graft can produce a fistula into adjacent duodenum, small bowel, or large intestine. Thus, the first presenting manifestation of graft sepsis will be massive upper or lower gastrointestinal bleeding. It is well to remember this fact when any patient with a history of vascular replacement in the abdomen presents with gastrointestinal bleeding. Under such circumstances, gastrointestinal bleeding *is* graft sepsis until proven otherwise.[50]

As long as the sepsis is confined to the shaft of the graft, it may remain relatively quiet for some time. If the shaft is superficial to skin surface, the septic process may ultimately become visible as an abscess or a draining sinus. Once the septic process extends to the anastomosis between the plastic prosthesis and host artery, the sepsis ultimately destroys the host tissue at the union and leads to the formation of a septic false aneurysm. If the anastomosis is relatively close to the skin surface, the presence of a false aneurysm will easily be appreciated upon physical examination. If the anastomosis is within the abdomen or chest cavity, the false aneurysm may not be obvious until it produces a mass effect, obstructs an adjacent organ, such as a ureter, or produces exsanguinating hemorrhage. The specific manifestations as a function of the type of reconstructive procedure as documented by Liekweg and Greenfield[48] are summarized in Table 33-6.

Natural History, Morbidity, and Mortality. Uncontrolled infection involving a tissue graft (fresh autograft, preserved homograft, and heterograft) results in proteolytic digestion of the graft, disruption, and exsanguinating hemorrhage. The natural history of a prosthetic graft infection often takes a slower and more insidious course. The foreign material continues to harbor infecting organisms, but the rate at which infection spreads along the course of the prosthesis to involve the anastomoses is quite variable. If the organism is of low virulence, such as *S. epidermidis,* the infection may remain quiescent for years. If the infecting exudate has egress, as through an exposed graft or a draining sinus, the progression of the infection to the anastomotic areas may be quite delayed. On the other hand, if the infecting organisms are virulent or if the infection remains confined to a closed space, the infection will progress rapidly along the course of the graft to ultimately involve the anastomosis. Once the anastomosis is involved, anastomotic disruption occurs, resulting in exsanguinating hemorrhage.

The morbidity and mortality associated with graft infection are great even when a management program is appropriately instituted. Bouhoutsos et al[46] reported their experience with 14 infected grafts, 7 aortofemoral or iliofemoral and 7 femoropopliteal grafts. Three patients died, in the aortofemoral series, in spite of treatment (mortality,

TABLE 33-7. MORBIDITY AND MORTALITY OF INFECTED GRAFTS AS A FUNCTION OF LOCATION

Anatomic Location	Szilagyl et al [45] Mortality (%)	Szilagyl et al [45] Amputation (%)	Liekweg et al [51] Mortality (%)	Liekweg et al [51] Amputation (%)
Aortoiliac	40.0	0.0	58.6	34.5
Aortofemoral	52.6	10.5	43.5	13.0
Femoropopliteal	0.0	50.0	9.9	32.7
TOTAL GRAFTS	34		153	

29 percent). Two major lower extremity amputations were required in the femoropopliteal group (amputation rate of 28.6 percent). Fry and Lindenauer,[43] reporting their experience with 12 infected grafts, had 9 deaths (mortality rate of 75 percent) in spite of a vigorous attempt at surgical management. Conn et al,[44] in their series of 22 graft infections, had a 40.9 percent mortality rate and a 27 percent lower extremity amputation rate. Goldstone and Moore,[41] reporting on 27 patients with graft infection, had 10 deaths (a mortality rate of 37 percent), and another 6 patients underwent major lower extremity amputation (an amputation rate of 22 percent). Szilagyi et al [45] and Liekweg et al [51] have looked at mortality and amputation as a function of the graft location (Table 33-7).[45]

When a graft infection presents primarily with bleeding into the gastrointestinal tract, the prognosis is grave in spite of aggressive management. Elliot et al [50] report a mortality rate of 73.7 percent despite aggressive management in 19 patients with aortic or paraprosthetic enteric fistulas.

Diagnosis

History. Anyone with a vascular graft in place, particularly a plastic prosthesis, is a candidate for infection, regardless of length of time between implantation and subsequent presentation of the clinical problem. In evaluating a patient with suspected graft infection, the following points are of value:

1. The surgeon's operative report from the original implantation should be carefully reviewed to elicit any potential intraoperative problems that may have predisposed to graft infection. These would include an inadvertent enterotomy, grafting in the presence of a coexistent septic problem (eg, infected, gangrenous extremity, intraabdominal sepsis, or trauma), or combined operations, such as simultaneous appendectomy, cholecystectomy, or colectomy.

2. A history of postoperative wound complications may suggest continued wound sepsis.

3. A history of repeated re-do operations. Recurrent false aneurysms or graft thrombosis may have been signs of a subtle graft infection that was not obvious at the time of initial repair.[50a] Also, each time a graft is reexposed, the possible de novo introduction of sepsis must be considered.

4. A history of infection or potential bacteremic exposure. An acute urinary tract infection, pulmonary infection, or mucous membrane manipulation or instrumentation, such as dental extraction or endoscopy, may have provided an opportunity for introduction of bacteria into the bloodstream.

5. Any patient with a history of intraabdominal vascular grafting who has gastrointestinal bleeding must be considered a candidate for graft infection and paraprosthetic-enteric fistula until proven otherwise.

Physical Examination. In performing a physical examination on a patient with suspected graft sepsis, the examiner must keep in mind the specific manifestations that the more overt presentations of graft sepsis may demonstrate. These include absence of pulsation associated with a graft limb thrombosis, a palpable pulsatile mass that accompanies a false aneurysm at one of the anastomotic sites of the graft, a draining sinus through one of the incision sites at the extremity of the graft, abscess formation along the course of the graft or in the area of a healed incision, wound breakdown with obviously exposed graft, fever, wound erythema, and petechiae over the skin in the distribution of blood flow from a prosthetic graft, indicating the possible presence of septic emboli.

Laboratory Studies. Routine laboratory studies should be performed, enabling one to identify evidence for nonspecific inflammation or infection. These include a white cell and differential blood count, erythrocyte sedimentation rate, and several blood cultures. It should be noted that some of the less virulent forms of graft infection may be present with a totally normal white blood cell count, as well as a normal differential. The erythrocyte sedimentation rate has been uniquely accurate in identifying possible sepsis. The sedimentation rate is invariably elevated if sepsis is present. Finally, blood cultures may be helpful, if positive. However, many patients with graft sepsis will have sterile blood at the time cultures are obtained.

Special Studies. Special diagnostic studies are often helpful in establishing the presence of graft sepsis.

Arteriography. An arteriogram is helpful. The arteriogram may reveal irregularity in the area of an anastomosis, a frank false aneurysm, or graft thrombosis, all of which may be indirect evidence of sepsis. In instances of gastrointestinal bleeding, the arteriogram sometimes reveals the arterioenteric fistula.

Sinogram. If the patient has a draining sinus, the insertion of a small catheter with the careful injection of contrast material is often helpful in making the diagnosis of prosthetic infection. If the sinogram demonstrates a tract around the graft, as evidenced by the appearance of corrugations corresponding to the prosthesis, the diagnosis of graft sepsis is confirmed.

Aspiration. A careful attempt at needle aspiration of the perigraft space under sterile conditions can be helpful if there is a fluid collection around the graft. The fluid obtained is cultured, and a positive culture confirms graft sepsis.

CAT Scan or Ultrasonography. CAT scanning or diagnostic ultrasound scanning is often helpful in identifying a false aneurysm, a retroperitoneal hematoma, or a fluid collection around a prosthetic graft. These findings would provide good evidence for possible graft sepsis.

Treatment

The management of infection in a vascular graft will depend upon the type of material involved (autograft, homograft, heterograft, or plastic prosthesis), the location, the physiologic distribution of blood flow through the prosthesis, and the extent to which the graft is involved in the septic process.

General Principles. If the vascular graft is constructed of fresh, viable materials, such as an autograft or homograft artery or vein, it may be possible to manage the infection by conservative means. Open wound drainage, debridement, and intensive antibiotic therapy while the patient is kept under careful observation are quite appropriate. On the other hand, if the graft consists of preserved tissue, such as a freeze-dried homograft or a preserved heterograft, sepsis cannot be controlled by conservative measures, and radical therapy including the removal of the graft must be instituted. The same is true of a plastic prosthesis, which can never be sterilized and will always harbor infection once it is established. Therefore, the entire infected graft must be removed to eradicate the septic problem. The general principles for management of an infected plastic prosthesis or a preserved tissue graft would observe the following sequence:

1. Remove the entire graft. Only by removing the entire graft will total control of the septic process be assured, since any portion of the foreign body left behind may continue to harbor infection.

2. Close arteriotomy sites with monofilament suture. Once the graft has been removed, the anastomotic sites must be oversewn. In the instance of an end-to-side anastomosis, closing the arteriotomy simply without compromising apparent flow through the artery is ideal. On the other hand, if a considerable circumference of the artery has been effaced or destroyed by the septic process, it may be necessary to close the arteriotomy site with a patch in order to maintain flow through the parent or recipient vessel. Obviously, prosthetic materials cannot be used for this purpose; the ideal material would be fresh autogenous vein. It should be recognized that there is some risk in this maneuver because there may be septic destruction of the patch or parent artery if the septic process is not adequately controlled. The use of monofilament suture is essential, since monofilament suture functions better in a contaminated wound than does multifilament suture, which behaves in much the same way as any multifibered foreign body. Monofilament sutures that have been used include stainless steel and polypropylene.

3. Debridement, irrigation, and drainage. Once the graft has been removed, any septic tissue or exudate must be carefully debrided, the wound generously irrigated with an antibiotic, such as kanamycin, and drainage provided. Closed suction drainage is sufficient in the retroperitoneum, but in superficial wounds (ie., the groin), the wound must be left open to close secondarily.

4. Long-term systemic antibiotics. The principle cause of management failure in the surgical treatment of graft sepsis is persistent sepsis in the periarterial tissues or continued sepsis in the arterial wall proper. Massive doses of antibiotics to which the organisms are sensitive will help to eradicate this major cause of management failure. Treatment with intravenous therapy during the two weeks following graft excision is followed by three months of oral antibiotics.

5. Extraanatomic revascularization. If the patient has an organ or an extremity that was totally dependent upon blood flow through the removed graft, blood flow must be reestablished or the organ or extremity sacrificed. In the case of a peripheral vascular graft, it is our practice to remove the infected graft first and then evaluate the circulation to the extremity. Many times it is not possible to predict whether an extremity is dependent upon the graft or whether there will be adequate collateral blood flow to maintain viability. The only reliable way to establish dependence of the extremity upon blood flow through the prosthetic graft is to evaluate the extremity following graft removal. If collateral circulation is adequate to maintain viability, we do not recommend immediate revascularization because it increases the possible contamination of the newly placed graft. On the other hand, if the extremity is clearly nonviable following graft removal, every attempt should be made to provide for some form of extraanatomic revascularization.

Specific Problems

Aortoenteric Fistula. After appropriate blood replacement, a rapid exploration should be carried out. The fistula site is usually obvious because the bowel is adherent to the phlegmon. If the fistula is between the proximal anastomosis and the duodenum, proximal control of the aorta is best obtained immediately below the diaphragm. The iliac arteries distal to the iliac anastomoses are then mobilized and controlled. Careful dissection can now be carried out between the graft and the duodenum. Once the duodenum is disconnected, the graft is excised from the distal anastomoses, and debridement is carried out, the arteriotomy sites are closed with monofilament suture, providing an adequate cuff of both proximal and distal artery. The posterior aspect of the duodenum is closed transversely. It is desirable to interpose tissue between the aortic closure and the duodenal closure, and this is best accomplished by developing an omental pedicle to place over the aortic stump. Prior to clamping the aorta, it is advisable to administer heparin (5,000 units intravenously). Following closure of the arteriotomies, the proximal and distal clamps are removed. The perigraft tissues are carefully debrided and generously irrigated with kanamycin solution. Closed suction drains are placed, and the abdomen is closed. The drapes are then removed, and the extremities are carefully evaluated for evidence of capillary blood flow to the toes. If the extremities are obviously ischemic, the patient is reprepped and redraped, and an axillary–bifemoral bypass is performed. High-dose systemic antibiotic therapy is administered in the postoperative period and should be continued for up to three months. Antibiotic therapy is based on the assumption that polymicrobial intestinal flora are present.

Aortoiliac Graft Sepsis. The management of infection of an aortofemoral bypass graft depends upon the extent to which the graft is involved in the infectious process. It is possible for the infection to be confined to the distal end of one femoral limb, leaving the proximal graft and opposite femoral limb sterile. It is also possible for the entire prosthesis to be infected, which necessitates the complete removal of the bifurcation graft. The initial surgical maneuver is to establish the extent of the septic process. If the patient has localized sepsis at one groin, the approach we recommend is a suprainguinal, retroperitoneal exposure of the proximal limb of that graft. If that portion of the graft demonstrates a good fibrous tissue reaction around the prosthesis, and no evidence of perigraft exudate is present, the graft limb is divided near the bifurcation, a segment of graft is removed, and the proximal and distal portions of the excised segment are oversewn. The objective of this maneuver is to disconnect the proximal sterile portion of the graft from the distal infected portion and to allow an interposition of viable soft tissue between the divided segments of the graft. At a second procedure, the femoral incision is reopened, the infected limb of the graft is disconnected from the femoral artery, and the femoral arteriotomy is oversewn. The distal portion of the graft is then pulled out from the retroperitoneal tunnel, thus leaving the proximal graft and opposite graft limb functioning with flow to the opposite extremity. Usually, if there is good blood flow to the opposite extremity, ligation of one side of the bifurcation graft will not endanger the viability of the extremity on that side. There is usually good cross-pelvic collateral flow through the ipsilateral leg from the contralaterally grafted iliofemoral arterial system. The femoral wound on the infected side is usually packed open, and a Penrose drain is carefully placed up the retroperitoneal tunnel to ensure good drainage of the contaminated tunnel site. This wound is allowed to close secondarily. Once again, topical antibiotic irrigation is carried out, as well as long-term administration of systemic antibiotics.

If both graft limbs are involved, or if the body of the graft is involved, total graft removal through a transabdominal and transfemoral approach is required. Following graft removal, if the extremities appear nonviable, an extraanatomic bypass is necessary. If the superficial femoral arteries are open, an axillary bypass skirting wide of the contaminated femoral wound can be carried down and anastomosed to the midsuperficial femoral artery. If the superficial femoral arteries are occluded, an axillary-to-popliteal bypass can be performed.

When sepsis is confined to one femoral site, an alternative mode of grafting is possible. A new graft limb is anastomosed to the proximal aortic graft and brought through the obturator foramen to the superficial femoral artery. This is a more extensive operative method of circumventing the contaminated femoral site and is, therefore, less desirable.

Femoropopliteal Graft Sepsis. Sepsis of a femoropopliteal bypass graft can occur acutely with an autogenous reconstruction as part of a wound infection, or it can occur late in association with prosthetic graft bypass. In the instance of autogenous tissues, open drainage and irrigation will usually clear the sepsis and allow wound closure. When a prosthetic graft is involved, the entire graft must be removed. If the viability of the extremity is compromised, reconstruction is best carried out with an autogenous saphenous vein, but if one is not available, a superficial femoral endarterectomy can be performed.

Sepsis in a Dialysis Access Arteriovenous Fistula. An emerging problem in graft sepsis has to do with an increasing number of patients with chronic renal failure in whom subcutaneous dialysis access is utilized. The dialysis access grafts may consist of a bovine heterograft, an externally supported umbilical vein graft, or an expanded polytetrafluorethylene graft. Since the dialysis access grafts are always superficial and usually confined to an easily accessible area of the extremity, more conservative means of managing graft sepsis are possible. Considerable success has been reported with local excision of the segment of septic graft, with replacement of a new segment of graft around the open septic area. This is in contrast to the usual approach of total graft excision and replacement in a new uninfected zone. The local excision and bypass have the advantage of preserving the proximal and distal anastomotic portions of the access graft.

New Concepts in the Management of Graft Sepsis

Fresh Tissue Graft Replacement. In 1961, Moore et al [37] experimentally demonstrated that fresh autogenous veins could be placed in infected fields and would function as a vascular conduit and the local infection could still be eradicated. In a clinical study, Wylie [38] demonstrated that autogenous arterial grafts could be placed in an infected field and function while the systemic sepsis was clearing. This is an exciting concept, but the availability of autogenous arteries is somewhat limited, and the portion of autogenous artery removed must be replaced with a plastic graft to maintain arterial continuity. Theoretically, this is a disadvantage, since the arterial graft replacing the donor site of the autogenous artery may become secondarily infected. Moore et al [39] demonstrated in an experimental study that fresh allograft arteries could be implanted in infected fields, would permit infection to be cleared, and would function as a viable conduit. The fresh allograft did as well as the fresh autograft control. Studies are currently under way to find means of harvesting and preserving fresh allograft artery so that it can be used as a reserve conduit for the management of graft sepsis.

Local Antibiotic Irrigation. There are occasional reports documenting the success of topical irrigation of an exposed graft with antibiotic solution, which permits the development of granulation tissue and closure of the septic wound site. The only cases that were successful, however, were those in which only a segment of the shaft of the graft was exposed. In no instance was this method successful if an anastomotic site was exposed.[52,52a]

Local Excision, Drainage, Suppressive Antibiotic Therapy. On occasion, when the total excision of an infected graft is impossible, due either to the critical location or to systemic illness, another approach has been used with some success. Local excision of the obviously infected portion of the graft, particularly that involving a distal femoral anastomosis, is carried out. The wound is generously irrigated with antibiotic solution. The proximal septic process can frequently be controlled by the permanent systemic administration of antibiotics. Thus, the high-risk patient is permitted to live out his or her abbreviated remaining lifespan.

Prevention of Graft Sepsis

Obviously, the best method of managing graft sepsis is prevention. Recognition of the causative factors in prosthetic sepsis is helpful in designing a program to reduce the incidence and thus help prevent this dreaded complication.

Antibiotic Prophylaxis. Experimental reports and a recent, controlled, clinical trial have demonstrated that the perioperative use of prophylactic antibiotics is effective in reducing the incidence of graft infection.[41,42,53,53a] Antibiotic prophylaxis should ensure bacterocidal tissue levels during the entire operation (Chapter 23). Since the most common organism associated with graft sepsis is *Staphylococcus,* prophylactic antibiotics should be selected with this organism in mind. Our drugs of choice are cephalosporins, which are bactericidal not only for *Staphylococcus* but also for the several gram-negative organisms that have been identified as causes of graft sepsis. During the course of operation, another dose of prophylactic antibiotic is administered, and postoperative antibiotic prophylaxis is continued until all of the lines, such as Foley catheter, nasogastric tube, arterial and venous cannulas, are out of the patient.

Prevention of Intraoperative Graft Contamination. The skin is a potential source of organisms that may contaminate a graft. Every attempt should be made to avoid bringing the graft in contact with the skin. This is best accomplished by the use of plastic adhesive drapes that will cover the large exposed area of skin often present during vascular surgical procedures. Plastic drapes are far superior to cloth drapes, since cloth drapes become moistened and permit the migration of contaminated fluids through the cloth surface. One other source of skin contamination not often recognized is the cut edge of skin. This is particularly important in superficial grafting sites, such as femoral or popliteal wounds. Bringing a graft into contact with the cut edge of skin is as bad as allowing direct surface skin contact with the prosthesis. Skin edge contact can be avoided by appropriate draping and by keeping this potential source of contamination in mind when handling a graft in a superficial site.

Another source of intraoperative contamination is the contaminated lymphatic, particularly in femoral incisions. In making a femoral incision, it is important to avoid incising directly through lymph nodes, particularly in patients who have gangrenous changes of the extremities, since there may well be bacterial contamination of lymphatic channels or the lymph nodes themselves.

Particular care should be paid to the closure of superficial grafting sites, since wound sepsis, if it occurs, offers a major risk for extension and graft contamination. We advocate closing wounds in several layers and using subcuticular rather than transcutaneous sutures, particularly in incisions over the femoral artery.

Another way to help maintain the sterility of the operative field and the graft during placement is to practice generous irrigation of the graft and wound with antibiotic solutions, such as kanamycin. Experimental data have demonstrated that topical wound irrigation will significantly reduce the risk of graft sepsis.[53a,54]

Late Antibiotic Prophylaxis. Prosthetic vascular grafts will inevitably have incomplete healing of their linings, and these raw spots are always susceptible to implantation from circulating bacteria.[40] Patients should be instructed to inform their other physicians of the presence of the vascular graft and the need for using prophylactic antibiotic therapy when undergoing such procedures as dental extraction, mucous membrane manipulation, or endoscopy. Patients with prosthetic grafts should also be more concerned about superficial infection and the prompt treatment of systemic infection by antibiotic therapy.

BIBLIOGRAPHY

Duma RJ (ed): Infection of Prosthetic Heart Valves and Vascular Grafts. Baltimore, University Park Press, 1977.

Wilson SE, Van Wagenen P, Passaro E Jr: Arterial infection. Curr Probl Surg 15(9): 1, 1978.

REFERENCES

1. Wilson SE, Van Wagenen P, Passaro E Jr: Arterial infection. Curr Probl Surg 15(9):1, 1978.
2. Stengel A, Wolferth CC: Mycotic (bacterial) aneurysms of intravascular origin. Arch Intern Med 31:527, 1923.
3. Pelletier LL Jr, Petersdorf R: Infective endocarditis. In Harrison T (ed): Harrison's Principles of Internal Medicine, 8th ed. New York, McGraw-Hill, 1977, Vol 1, p 797.
4. Jarrett F, Darling RC, Mundth ED, Austen WG: The management of infected arterial aneurysms. J Cardiovasc Surg 18:361, 1977.
5. Cates, J, Christie R: Subacute bacterial endocarditis: A review of 442 patients treated in 14 centers appointed by the Penicillin Trials Committee of the Medical Research Council. Q J Med 20:93, 1951.
6. Sommerville RL, Allen EV, Edwards JE: Bland and infected arteriosclerotic abdominal aortic aneurysms—a clinicopathologic study. Medicine 38:207, 1959.
7. Moore WS, Malone JM: The use of prophylactic antibiotics in vascular surgery. J Surg Pract 6:24, 1977.
8. Sullivan JJ Jr, Mangiardi JL: Surgical management of mycotic aneurysms. Ann Surg 148:119, 1958.
9. Shapiro SL: Carotid artery erosion secondary to pharyngeal infection. Eye Ear Nose Throat Mon 52:513, 1974.

10. Kyriakides GK, Simmons RL, Najarian JS: Mycotic aneurysms in transplant patients. Arch Surg 111:472, 1976.
11. Walsh TJ, Zachary JB, Hutchins GM, Sterioff S: Mycotic aneurysm with recurrent sepsis complicating post-transplant nephrectomy. Johns Hopkins Med J 141:85, 1977.
12. Kerr AI, Tilney NL: Mycotic aneurysm from unrecognized colonic sepsis. J R Coll Surg Edinb 22:271, 1977.
13. Griffith G, Maull K, Sachatello C: Septic pulmonary embolization. Surg Gynecol Obstet 144:105, 1977.
14. Yellin AE: Ruptured mycotic aneurysm: a complication of parenteral drug abuse. Arch Surg 112:981, 1977.
15. Bennett DE, Cherry JK: Bacterial infection of the aortic aneurysms: A clinicopathologic study. Am J Surg 113:321, 1967.
16. Jenkins A, MacPherson A, Nolan B, Housley E: Peripheral aneurysms in Behcet's disease. Br J Surg 63:199, 1976.
17. Rosenberg TF, Medsger TA Jr, DeCicco FA, Fireman P: Allergic granulomatous angiitis (Churg-Strauss syndrome). J Allergy Clin Immunol 55:56, 1975.
18. Collins GS Jr, Rich NM, Hobson RW, Andersen CA, Green D: Multiple mycotic aneurysms due to candida endocarditis. Ann Surg 186:136, 1977.
19. Smith KO, Gehle WD, Sanford BA: Evidence for chronic viral infections in human arteries. Proc Soc Exp Biol Med 147:357, 1974.
20. Michal JA III, Coleman RE: Localization of gallium^{67} citrate in a mycotic aneurysm. Am J Roentgenol 129:1111, 1977.
21. Sukerkar AN, Dulay CC, Anandappa E, Asokan S: Mycotic aneurysm of the hepatic artery. Case diagnosed with radionuclide imaging and ultrasound. Radiology 124:444, 1977.
22. Gladstone JL, Friedman SA, Cerruti MM, Jomain SL: Treatment of candida endocarditis and arteritis. J Thorac Cardiovasc Surg 71:835, 1976.
23. Liebman PR, Patten MT, Manny J, Benfield JR, Hechtman HB: Hepatic-portal venous gas in adults: Etiology, pathophysiology, and clinical significance. Ann Surg 187:281, 1978.
24. Abruzzo JL: The spectrum of systemic vasculitis. J Med Soc NJ 74:227, 1977.
25. Anagnostakis D, Kamba A, Petrochilou V, Arseni A, Matsaniotis N: Risk of infection associated with umbilical vein catheterization: A prospective study in 75 newborn infants. J Pediatr 86:759, 1975.
26. Balagtas RC, Bell CE, Edwards LD, Levin S: Risk of local and systemic infections associated with umbilical vein catheterization: A prospective study in 86 newborn patients. Pediatrics 48:359, 1971.
27. Maki DG, Drinka PJ, Davis TE: Suppurative phlebitis of an arm vein from a "scalp-vein needle." N Engl J Med 292:1116, 1975.
28. Mogensen JV, Frederiksen W, Jensen JK: Subclavian vein catheterization and infection. A bacteriological study of 130 catheter insertions. Scand J Infect Dis 4:31, 1972.
29. Rubio T, Riley HD Jr: Serious systemic infection associated with the use of indwelling intravenous catheters. South Med J 66:633, 1973.
30. Stein JM, Pruitt BA Jr: Suppurative thrombophlebitis: A lethal iatrogenic disease. N Engl J Med 282:1452, 1970.
31. Nicolaides AN, Kakkar VV, Field ES, Yates-Bell AJ, Taylor S, Clarke MB: Prostatectomy and deep-vein thrombosis. Br J Surg 59:487, 1972.
32. Svanberg L, Åstedt B, Kullander S: On radiation-decreased fibrinolytic activity of vessel walls. Acta Obstet Gynecol Scand 55:49, 1976.
33. Schramel RJ, Creech O Jr: Effects of infection and exposure on synthetic arterial prostheses. Arch Surg 78:271, 1959.
34. Harrison JH: Influence of infection on homografts and synthetic (Teflon) grafts. A comparative study in experimental animals. Arch Surg 76:67, 1958.
35. Humphries AW, Hawk WA, DeWolfe VG, LeFevre FA: Clinicopathologic observations on the fate of arterial freeze-dried homografts. Surgery 45:59, 1959.
36. Foster JH, Berzins T, Scott HW Jr: An experimental study of arterial replacement in the presence of bacterial infection. Surg Gynecol Obstet 108:141, 1959.
37. Moore WS, Blaisdell FW, Gardner M, Hall AD: Effect of infection on autogenous vein arterial substitutes. Surg Forum 13:235, 1962.
38. Wylie EJ: Vascular replacement with arterial autografts. Surgery 57:14, 1965.
39. Moore WS, Swanson RJ, Campagna G, Bean B: The use of fresh tissue arterial substitutes in infected fields. J Surg Res 18:229, 1975.
40. Roon A, Malone JM, Moore WS, Bean B, Campagna G: Bacteremic infectibility: A function of vascular graft material and design. J Surg Res 22:489, 1977.
41. Goldstone J, Moore WS: Infection in vascular prostheses: Clinical manifestations and surgical management. Am J Surg 128:225, 1974.
42. Kaiser AB, Clayson KR, Mulherin JL Jr, Roach AC, Allen TR, Edwards WH, Dale WA: Antibiotic prophylaxis in vascular surgery. Ann Surg 188:283, 1978.
43. Fry WJ, Lindenauer SM: Infection complicating the use of plastic arterial implants. Arch Surg 94:600, 1967.
44. Conn JH, Hardy JD, Chavez CM, Fain WR: Infected arterial grafts: Experience in 22 cases with emphasis on unusual bacteria and technics. Ann Surg 171:704, 1970.
45. Szilagyi DE, Smith RF, Elliott JP, Vrandecic MP: Infection in arterial reconstruction with synthetic grafts. Ann Surg 176:321, 1972.
46. Bouhoutsos J, Chavatzas D, Martin P, Morris T: Infected synthetic arterial grafts. Br J Surg 61:108, 1974.
47. Fry WJ: Vascular prosthesis infections. Surg Clin North Am 52:1419, 1972.
48. Liekweg WG Jr, Greenfield LJ: Vascular prosthetic infections: Collected experience and results of treatment. Surgery 81:335, 1977.
49. Gross RE, Bill AH Jr, Peirce EC: Methods for preservation and transplantation of arterial grafts: Observations on arterial grafts in dogs. Report of transplantation of preserved arterial grafts in 9 human cases. Surg Gynecol Obstet 88:689, 1949.
50. Elliott JP Jr, Smith RF, Szilagyi DE: Proceedings: Aortoenteric and paraprosthetic-enteric fistulas. Problems of diagnosis and management. Arch Surg 108:479, 1974.
50a. Satiani B: False aneurysms following arterial reconstruction. Surg Gynecol Obstet 152:357, 1981.
51. Liekweg WG Jr, Levinson SA, Greenfield LJ: Infection of vascular grafts: Incidence, anatomic location, etiologic agents, morbidity, and mortality. In Duma RJ (ed): Infections of Prosthetic Heart Valves and Vascular Grafts. Baltimore, University Park Press, 1977, p 239.
52. Golden GT, Lovett WL, Harrah JD, Wellons HA Jr, Nolan SP: The treatment of extruded and infected permanent cardiac pulse generators: Application of a technique of closed irrigation. Surgery 74:575, 1973.
52a. Popovsky J, Singer S: Infected prosthetic grafts. Arch Surg 115:203, 1980.
53. Parsa F, Gordon HE, Wilson SE: Intraoperative antibiotics in the prevention of experimental Dacron graft infection. Vasc Surg 10:64, 1976.
53a. Pitt HA, Postier RG, MacGowan WAL, Frank LW, Surmak AJ, Sitzman JV, Bouchier-Hayes D: Prophylactic antibiotics in vascular surgery. Topical, systemic, or both? Ann Surg 192:356, 1980.
54. Lord JW Jr, Rossi G, Daliana M: Intraoperative antibiotic wound lavage: An attempt to eliminate postoperative infection in arterial and clean general surgical procedures. Ann Surg 185:634, 1977.

CHAPTER 34
Peritonitis and Other Intra-abdominal Infections

DAVID H. AHRENHOLZ AND RICHARD L. SIMMONS

PATHOBIOLOGY OF PERITONITIS

PERITONEAL fluid, like pleural, synovial, and cerebrospinal fluid, is normally sterile. When it becomes infected, it is a catastrophic event. In this chapter, the anatomy and physiology of the peritoneal cavity, the pathophysiology of peritonitis, and the local and systemic sequelae of such infections will be reviewed.

ANATOMY AND PHYSIOLOGY OF THE PERITONEAL CAVITY

The peritoneal cavity represents the largest preformed extravascular space in the body, with a huge surface area. Normally, however, the cavity contains less than 50 ml of clear fluid, and the viscera are in contact along their serosal surfaces. Normal peritoneal fluid is clear yellow, with a specific gravity less than 1.016 and less than 3 gm per dl of protein, predominantly albumin. Fibrinogen is not present, and the fluid will not clot. Peritoneal fluid has a minimal antibacterial activity, mostly complement-mediated.[1] Solute concentrations are nearly identical to those in the plasma. The normal fluid contains less than 3,000 cells per mm^3, with 50 percent macrophages, 40 percent lymphocytes, a few eosinophils, mast cells, and a rare mesothelial cell.

In adults the area of peritoneal surface approximates that of the total cutaneous surface (1.7 m^2). Most of this membrane behaves as a passive, semipermeable barrier to the diffusion of water and low-molecular-weight solutes, making peritoneal dialysis an effective treatment for chronic renal failure.

Fluid Exchange

Studies of dialysis patients have shown that the functional exchange surface of the peritoneal cavity is approximately 1 m^2. The efficiency of fluid exchange is increased by agents that increase local splanchnic blood flow or vascular permeability. During peritoneal dialysis, hyperosmolar solutions can induce a net flow of 300–500 ml of water per hour into the peritoneal space.[2] The inflammatory process in peritonitis has a similar effect, so that hypovolemic shock rapidly kills the untreated patient. Chemical irritants, such as pancreatic enzymes, bile, and gastric acid, can potentiate this exudation. It has been proposed that acute generalized peritonitis has the same hemodynamic effect as a 50 percent or greater body surface burn and requires a correspondingly massive fluid infusion, at least during the first 24 hours.

Particulate and Microbial Absorption

Although the entire peritoneal surface participates in fluid and low-molecular-weight solute exchange, particulate matter can be absorbed only via the diaphragmatic lymphatics because of specialized features of the diaphragmatic mesothelium and the lymphatics in this area. In most areas of the peritoneal cavity, the mesothelial cells form a carpet of closely packed, flattened cells covered with numerous microvilli and with indistinct boundaries (Fig. 34-1B).[3] On the inferior surface of the diaphragm, however, special lymphatic collecting vessels (lacunae) are present just under the mesothelial basement membrane (Figs. 34-1 and 2). These stomata serve as channels for the lymphatic drainage of the peritoneal cavity. Passive stretching of the diaphragm results in a rapid influx of fluid through the stomata into the lacunae. Contraction of the diaphragm then empties the lymphatics into efferent ducts, with the aid of the simultaneous drop in intrathoracic pressure during inhalation. Reverse flow during exhalation is prevented by one-way valves in the thoracic lymphatics. In most animals, the chief route of drainage of the diaphragmatic lymphatics is via the right thoracic duct. The exact drainage route for the human diaphragmatic lymphatics is uncertain, but the anterior mediastinal lymphatics of patients who are dying of peritonitis contain bacteria, even though the remainder of the thoracic cavity is sterile.

The size of the stomata (8–12 mm) determines the maximum size of particles that are readily absorbed from

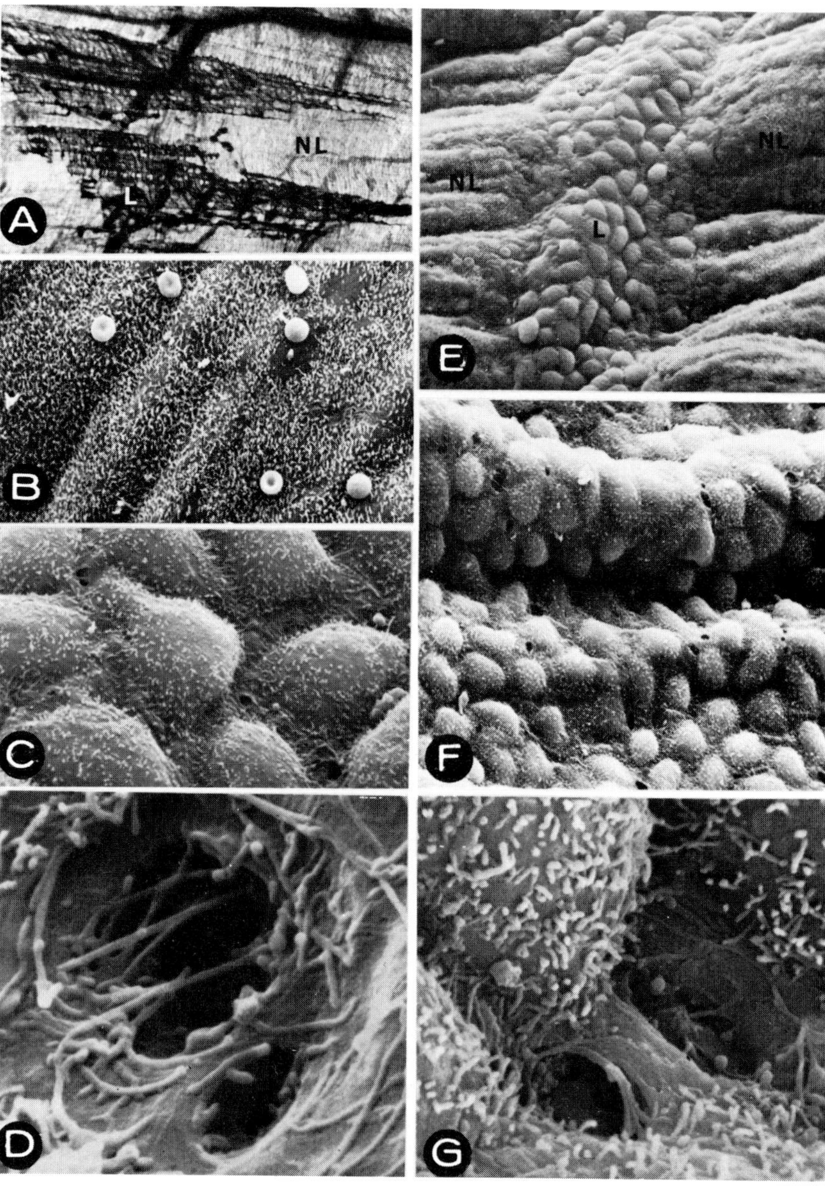

Fig. 34-1. The topography of the peritoneal surface by light and scanning electron microscopy (SEM). *A.* Low-power photomicrograph of the peritoneal surface of the diaphragm showing the lacunar areas labeled with India ink. Lacunar areas (L) are sharply delineated from nonlacunar areas (NL). ×8. *B.* Higher power of a nonlacunar area. The mesothelial cells lining the surface are flat, and they have many microvilli. Boundaries between individual cells are not seen. ×713. *C.* Mesothelial cells of a lacunar area. Each cell is distinctly outlined. Many interdigitating processes and a few small stomata between them are seen at the border of each cell. ×1800. *D.* High-power micrograph of a complex stoma. The upper portion of the stoma overlies a deep pit and is encircled at its rim by several cell processes. The lower portion of the stoma is smaller, and the surface of another cell can be seen beneath its opening. ×12,300. *E.* Peritoneal surface of the diaphragm observed with the SEM. The mesothelial cells over nonlacunar areas are flattened, and individual cells cannot be distinguished. The mesothelial cells overlying a lacunar area protrude toward the lumen of the peritoneal cavity and have distinct boundaries. A muscular contraction, probably due to the action of the fixative, caused folding of the surface of the diaphragm. ×360. *F.* Higher power of a lacunar area. The mesothelial cells lie on ridges over the lacuna. The nucleus of each individual cell is represented by a round swelling in the center of each cell. Numerous stomata can be seen between adjacent cells. ×680. *G.* A stoma between two adjacent mesothelial cells is shown. Processes extend between the cells and bridge the opening of the stoma. Underneath the opening is seen the surface of another cell. ×6,888. (From Tsilibary EC, Wissig SL: Am J Anat 149:127, 1977.)

the peritoneal cavity. Only a few polystyrene beads 20 μm in diameter can be absorbed, but 10 μm-sized beads pass through easily.[4] There is no evidence that particles can be absorbed from nondiaphragmatic peritoneal surfaces, except the omentum.

Bacteria, which average 0.5–2 μm in diameter, are cleared rapidly from the peritoneal cavity. Organisms are recoverable from the right thoracic duct lymph of dogs within 6 minutes and from the blood within 12 minutes after injection.[5] In 1900, Fowler[6] used the semi-upright position in nine patients with peritonitis to prevent the rapid absorption of "toxins" from the peritoneal cavity. In 1944, Steinberg[5] showed that absorption of bacteria from the peritoneal cavity was delayed by the upright position and accelerated by the head-down position.

Other factors have been found that indirectly affect the peritoneal clearance of particulate material. In dogs, omentectomy has no effect on clearance of peritoneal graphite particles, but laparotomy with manipulation of the viscera leading to ileus causes a delayed clearance time.[7] Phrenic neurectomy, with resultant diaphragmatic paralysis, initially delays absorption on the denervated side: the absorption is later accelerated as the muscles atrophy. Florey[8] found that increased intraperitoneal pressure accelerates the clearance of material from the peritoneal cavity. Depression of spontaneous respiration by general anesthetic agents decreases the clearance in proportion to the depression of the respiratory rate. Conversely, high concentrations of CO_2 within inspired air accelerate particle clearance. The effects of positive pressure ventilation have not been investigated, but we hypothesize that positive intrathoracic pressure decreases efferent lymph flow and may thereby decrease clearance of bacteria from the peritoneal cavity.

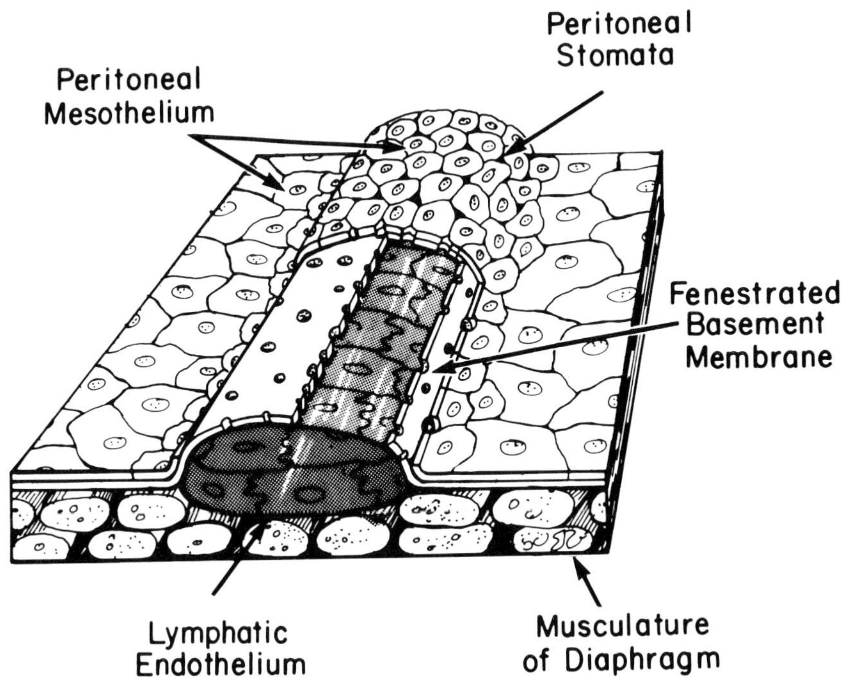

Fig. 34-2. Schematic view of lymphatic lacunae on the peritoneal surface of the diaphragm. The mesothelial cells are flattened and polygonal everywhere but over the lymphatics, where they are smaller, with stomata between the cells. These stomata correspond to fenestrations of the underlying basement membrane. The lymphatic endothelium lines the lymphatic lacuna and probably communicates with the peritoneal cavity through the stomata. (Modified from Allen L: Anat Rec 67:89, 1936.)

The Intraperitoneal Circulation

The removal of fluid via the diaphragmatic lymphatics creates a relative negative pressure in the upper abdomen and leads to a cephalad flow of peritoneal fluid. This upward circulation of peritoneal fluid is resisted by gravity (Fig. 34-3). Autio[9] found that contrast material injected into the ileocecal region after routine appendectomy or cholecystectomy rapidly accumulated in the pelvis and, to a lesser degree, in the right paracolic and subhepatic areas. Lesser amounts accumulated along the left paracolic gutter to the left subphrenic space. When contrast medium was injected into the right infrahepatic space near the duodenum, the dye spread to the right suprahepatic space, the left infrahepatic space, the right paracolic gutter, and the pelvis. Such studies defined the routes of spread of contaminated material from a ruptured viscus and coincide with the pattern of abscess location after peritonitis in man (Fig. 34-3B).

Placing a patient in Fowler's position tends to pool peritoneal fluid in the pelvis and other dependent areas and to retard fluid and bacterial absorption, probably facilitating formation of both pelvic and subdiaphragmatic abscesses. Prior to the development of antibiotics and adequate surgical therapy, Fowler's position might have delayed the onset of septicemia and occasionally facilitated patient survival. Currently, however, if patients are promptly treated by operative removal of grossly infected material, any method that impairs the clearance of residual bacteria from the peritoneal cavity could actually increase the incidence of recurrent intra-abdominal infection. Since the flat or even the head-down position experimentally accelerates the removal of bacteria from the peritoneal cavity, it is theoretically preferable to Fowler's position after continued peritoneal contamination has ceased.

RESPONSE OF THE PERITONEUM TO INJURY AND INFECTION

Mesothelium is so easily damaged that it sloughs even after exposure to air or saline (Fig. 34-4A).[10] Regeneration, however, is rapid. Round cells of uncertain origin cover the denuded surface within four hours, and healing is complete within a week.[10] Whether the round cells arise from the local proliferation of submesothelial cells (macrophages of fibroblasts) that differentiate into mesothelium or whether mesothelial cells from opposing peritoneal surfaces seed the denuded site is unclear.

The ready susceptibility of the mesothelium to injury may be important in the formation of fibrinous adhesions, which, in turn, act to prevent the dissemination of infection (Fig. 34-5). When the serosa is injured, peritoneal mast cells release histamine and other permeability factors, such as nucleosides and polypeptides, which increase vascular permeability. A protein-rich, fibrinogen-laden plasma then exudes into the peritoneal cavity. The injured cells also release thromboplastin, which converts fibrinogen to fibrin, which adheres to adjacent tissue surfaces. A plasminogen activator present in the mesothelial and submesothelial cell membranes normally activates fibrinolytic enzymes, and fibrin adhesions are lysed. Peritoneal injury depresses this activity and bacterial peritonitis completely abolishes it. Fibrinous adhesions, therefore, persist in areas of mesothelial injury until fibroblasts lay down collagen to form fibrous adhesions. Whole blood also potentiates adhesion formation because it also produces fibrin deposits. In untreated peritonitis, adhesion formation may be lifesaving by sealing a perforated viscus or by loculating bacteria away from the subdiaphragmatic areas of bacterial absorption.

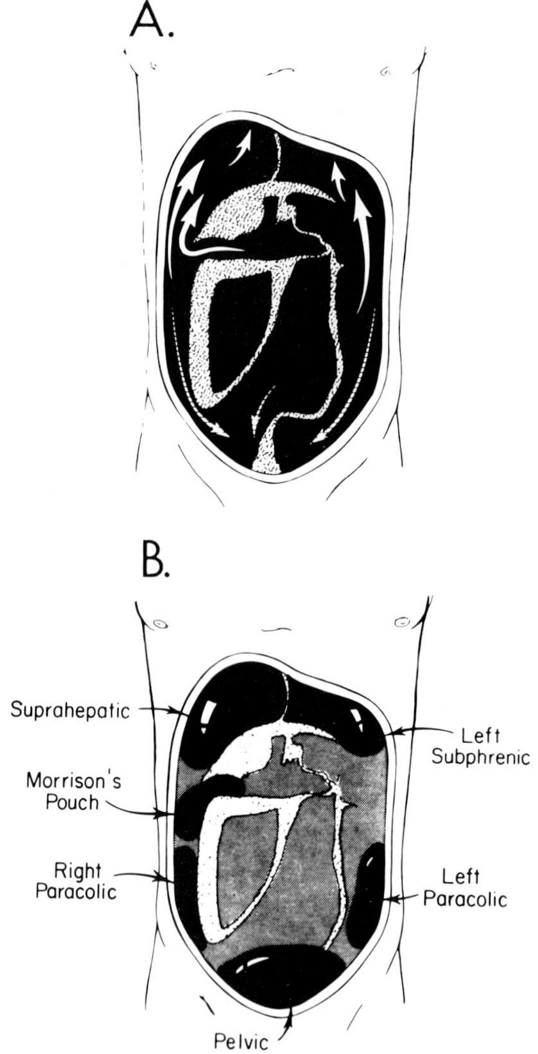

Fig. 34-3. ***A.*** **Circulation of fluid in the peritoneal cavity. Solid arrows indicate the flow generated by diaphragmatic movement and absorption of material from the diaphragmatic lymphatics. Dashed arrows demonstrate the effect of gravity in the upright position. (Modified from Autio V: Acta Chir Scand 123 [Suppl 321]:5, 1964.)** ***B.*** **The sites of abscess formation in the peritoneal cavity. The labeled sites are most commonly involved. (Modified from Altemeier WA, Culbertson WR, Fuller W, Shook C: Ann Surg 125:70, 1973.)**

HOST DEFENSES AGAINST PERITONEAL INFECTION

When a pure suspension of bacteria is injected into the peritoneal cavity of an experimental animal, the bacteria begin to disappear immediately—even before the influx of phagocytic cells.[11] Bacteria can be found within the diaphragmatic lymphatics of dogs within 6 minutes and the blood stream in 12 minutes.[5] These results suggest that the first defense of the peritoneal cavity against bacterial contamination is physical removal of the bacteria, which are carried cephalad by the intraperitoneal circulation and absorbed into the diaphragmatic lymphatics (Figs. 34-2 and 34-6).

The peritoneal cavity has a single response to noxious stimuli (Fig. 34-6). This acute inflammatory response includes degranulation of peritoneal mast cells with release of vasoactive substances and outpouring of fluid rich in complement and serum opsonins that bind to the bacteria. The opsonized bacteria are either passed into the regional lymph nodes or are engulfed in situ by the phagocytic cells, which take several hours to migrate to the area in quantity. In addition, fibrin deposits isolate the perforated viscus from the free peritoneal cavity and retard bacterial absorption which might lead to endotoxin shock.[12] These fibrin deposits persist because, as noted earlier, the inflammatory process depresses peritoneal fibrinolysis (Fig. 34–6).

Because of its great mobility, the omentum contributes to the defense of the peritoneal cavity by adhering to a perforated viscus and walling it off. In experimental studies, the omentum can contribute a collateral vascular supply to an ischemic viscus. If a segment of bowel is devascularized and wrapped in omentum, collaterals form to maintain bowel viability. The omentum also participates directly in bacterial absorption, isolation of foreign matter, and influx of phagocytic cells into the peritoneal cavity. Tracer studies indicate that uptake of particulate matter by the omentum is rapid, but systemic absorption is slow.

The rapid cellular influx of neutrophils (within four hours) followed later by macrophages, is probably the most important defense of the abdominal cavity against major contamination. Specific mediators that trigger this phagocytic cell response include C3a and C5a released during complement activation, products of bacterial growth, and other products of inflammation (Chapter 13). The vasodilatation characteristic of acute inflammation also speeds the influx of neutrophils into the free peritoneal cavity. Phagocytic cell function in the acute inflammatory response is discussed in Chapter 13 (Fig. 34-6).

ADVERSE EFFECTS OF THE HOST RESPONSE TO PERITONEAL CONTAMINATION

The defenses of the peritoneal cavity (Fig. 34-6) unfortunately can have deleterious as well as favorable effects for the host. For example, the rapid absorption of bacteria via the diaphragmatic lymphatics reduces their number within the peritoneal cavity at the expense of inducing septicemia. Similarly, the same factors that increase peritoneal vascular permeability so that bacteria can be opsonized and phagocytosed also produce hypovolemic shock.

The fluid influx may have other adverse effects. The long distance from the nearest capillary, the poor solubility of oxygen, and bacterial oxygen consumption lead to a lowered redox potential, which favors the growth of anaerobic bacteria.[13] Oxygen is also required for efficient bacterial killing by neutrophils.

Normally, fluid from the peritoneal cavity is removed by the lymphatics of the diaphragm, taking with it suspended bacteria, although small molecules readily equilibrate across the peritoneal surface. However, large volumes of fluid exceed the lymphatic absorptive capacity,

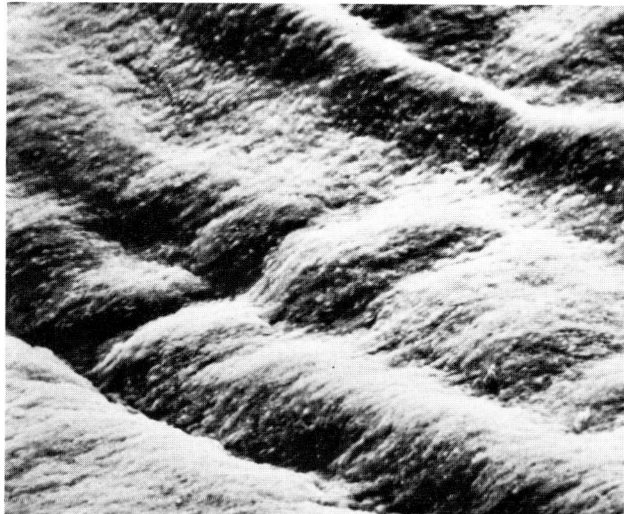

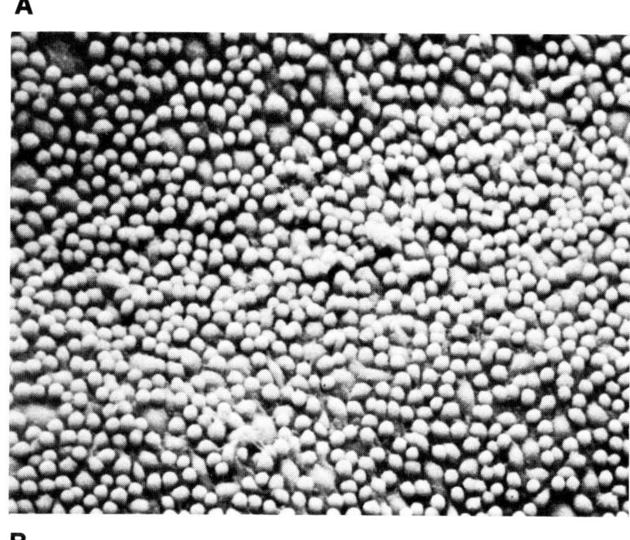

Fig. 34-4. A. Scanning electron microscopic views of parietal peritoneum immediately after removal of the mesothelium by application and stripping of a dry gelatin film. *B.* Four hours later, the surface is covered with closely spaced round cells, a few of which have already begun to flatten out. (From Watters WB, Buck RC: Lab Invest 26:604, 1972.)

allowing bacteria to remain and proliferate. Inflammatory fluids become rapidly depleted of bacterial opsonins, and surviving bacteria suspended in nonopsonic fluids cannot be phagocytosed. In addition, fibrin deposits on the diaphragm may physically occlude the stomata and decrease fluid absorption or clot within lymphatics.

Fibrin deposits normally localize infection and prevent generalized peritonitis by entrapping bacteria and reducing mortality. However, contaminated clots always produce abscesses in experimental animals.[12] Fibrin deposits allow bacterial growth, protected from neutrophils. As an abscess forms, localized bacteria are isolated from opsonins and antibiotics by the abscess wall. Many bactericidal antibiotics are effective only on rapidly growing bacteria, and organisms that grow slowly are unaffected. Bacteriostatic agents have little effect on inactive bacteria within an abscess.

Although neutrophils usually function to kill bacteria, neutrophilic enzymes are capable of digesting normal tissue. Extracellular release of neutrophilic enzymes normally occurs to a limited extent during phagocytosis but is markedly exaggerated during attempted phagocytosis of large particles, such as particulate intestinal contents. Neutrophils moving along fibrin strands that have trapped activated complement components also prematurely release their enzymes. Preliminary data indicate that a small degree of extracellular bacterial killing takes place within contaminated fibrin clots as a result of this release.[14]

Neutrophils themselves are sufficient for abscess formation.[15] If sites of experimental bacterial inoculation are sterilized by antibiotics after the tissues have been infiltrated by large numbers of neutrophils, an abscess can develop. It is not the bacteria alone but the neutrophil and its intracellular contents that ultimately lead to the development of an abscess.[15]

Abscess cavities tend to persist once they have developed. A large number of enzymes are present that are capable of digesting surrounding tissue. Oxygen-dependent bacterial killing systems of neutrophils are depressed by the lowered local oxygen tension. The abscess contents are usually hypertonic, allowing survival of bacteria even in the presence of antibiotics, such as penicillin, that kill bacteria by disrupting cell wall formation. The bacteria lack cell walls but persist as L-forms in the hypertonic

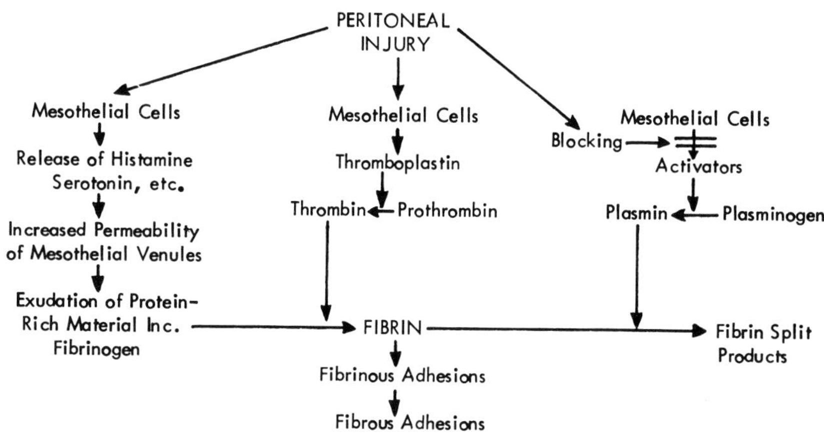

Fig. 34-5. Diagram of the events postulated to lead to adhesion formation. (From Hau T, Payne WD, Simmons RL: Surg Gynecol Obstet 148:415, 1979.)

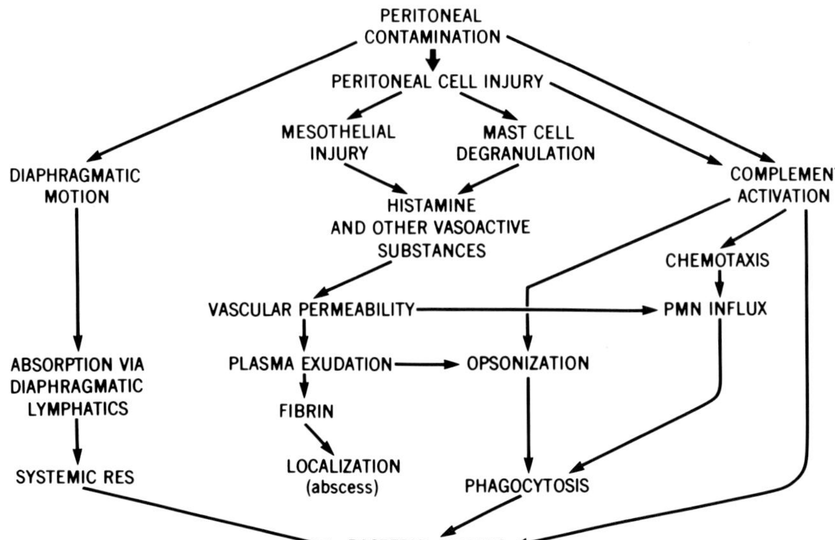

Fig. 34-6. Diagram of the peritoneal response to contamination. Diaphragmatic motion is the principal means of systemic absorption of peritoneal contents. There is an influx of phagocytic cells that kill the bacteria in situ. Fibrin deposits tend to wall off the process but interfere with clearance and phagocytosis, often resulting in an abscess. (From Hau T, Ahrenholz DH, Simmons RL: Curr Probl Surg 16:1, 1979.)

environment. Antibiotics poorly penetrate mature abscess walls because of the fibrotic wall or thrombosis of local blood vessels. It is not surprising that mechanical evacuation is usually required for the resolution of infections that reach the abscess stage.

PERITONITIS

Peritoneal infection can be the result of obvious contamination of the peritoneal cavity by external trauma or visceral disruption. This is called "secondary peritonitis." In contrast, primary peritonitis is caused by microbial contamination from a cryptic source. Because of its relative clinical importance, especially to the surgeon, secondary peritonitis will be discussed first.

SECONDARY BACTERIAL PERITONITIS

Etiology

Secondary bacterial peritonitis is defined as peritoneal infection caused by contamination from a perforated hollow viscus. Because the normal gastrointestinal tract contains in excess of 10^{12} bacterial organisms at any given time and is the most common source of peritonitis, the microflora of the gastrointestinal tract must be briefly reviewed (Chapters 3, 27, 38, and 39).

Bacteriology of Secondary Peritonitis

When the continuity of the gastrointestinal tract is breached, bacteria are released from the lumen. There is a definite relationship between the level of perforation of the intestine and the bacteria subsequently isolated from the peritoneal cavity. Experimental perforations of the empty stomach of dogs results in only a 7 percent mortality, and bacteria can rarely be cultured from the peritoneum.[16] When the stomach contains fluid, the mortality is 87 percent, and many types of organisms, including staphylococci and the aerobic and anaerobic streptococci, can be cultured. Duodenal perforation in dogs results in an 81 percent mortality, with gram-positive organisms predominating. Gram-negative organisms can be cultured from less than half the animals. Similar results have been found clinically. Stone et al [17] found that no bacteria could be cultured after traumatic duodenal perforation in the human. Culture results were positive after some gastric perforations, 50 percent of the time for aerobic bacteria and 20 percent of the time for anaerobic bacteria. If the small bowel was perforated, 30 percent of patients had aerobes cultured and 10 percent anaerobes cultured. If the colon or rectum was perforated, both anaerobic and aerobic bacteria were always isolated. Aerobic bacteria were found almost exclusively, however, if local suppuration lead to perforation. In gangrenous processes, aerobic bacteria were cultured from 90 percent and anaerobic bacteria from 60 percent of the patients. Inflammatory diseases apparently eliminate certain species. One remarkable fact has repeatedly been noted—the number of bacterial species isolated from a given case of clinical or experimental peritonitis is inversely proportional to the duration of the infection in the absence of continued soilage of the peritoneal cavity.[18] Obviously, the peritoneal cavity more effectively eliminates some organisms than others. Those that survive are, by definition, the virulent organisms.

Peritonitis is still a polymicrobial infection (Table 34-1). Stone et al [17] found a mean of 1.8 aerobic species and 2.4 anaerobic species per patient. Lorber and Swenson [20] recovered 1.3 aerobic and 2.6 anaerobic isolates per patient. Although the host defenses are able to eliminate most of the several hundred bacterial species that are released by a colonic perforation, a number of species survive.

About 30 percent of all patients with peritonitis have blood cultures that most often contain *Bacteroides fragilis* or *Escherichia coli* (Table 34-1). Fry et al [21] have suggested that *B. fragilis* septicemia in a postoperative patient is an indication for urgent exploration for residual intraabdominal sepsis. *E. coli* septicemia does not correlate with

TABLE 34-1. BACTERIOLOGY OF SECONDARY PERITONITIS IN THREE STUDIES

	Gorbach et al 1974 [19]		Lorber and Swenson 1975 [20]		Stone et al 1975 [17]		Total	
	No.	*%*	*No.*	*%*	*No.*	*%*	*No.*	*%*
Aerobic Bacteria								
E. coli	28	61	43	43	164	67	235	60
Streptococci	3	11	28	37	11	28	108	28
Enterococci	2	4	9	9	55	23	66	17
Staphylococci	16	34	—	—	13	6	29	7
Enterobacter/Klebsiella	17	37	6	6	78	32	101	26
Proteus	10	22	8	8	69	28	87	22
Pseudomonas	8	17	2	2	20	8	30	8
Candida	4	9	—	—	2	1	6	2
Anaerobic Bacteria								
Bacteroides	36	84	45	59	136	85	288	72
B. fragilis	28	26	71	36	54	34	153	38
Eubacteria	11	65	8	4	75	47	94	24
Clostridia	31	72	7	4	29	18	67	17
Peptostreptococci	11	26	22	11	22	14	55	14
Peptococci	3	7	21	10	18	11	42	11
Propionibacteria	2	5	—	—	34	21	36	9
Fusobacteria	6	14	15	8	13	8	34	8

From Hau T, Ahrenholz DH, Simmons RL: Secondary bacterial peritonitis: The biologic basis of treatment. *Curr Prob Surg* 16:1, 1979.

recurrent peritonitis but may represent other sites of infection, such as the urinary tract or lungs.

Pathogenesis of Secondary Peritonitis

The Role of Adjuvant Substances

Large numbers of bacteria in pure culture injected into the peritoneal cavity of animals are rapidly removed by normal host defense mechanisms. Death results only when the dose exceeds that which induces septicemic shock.[5] If sublethal doses of bacteria are administered, the animal may develop bacteremia but will survive without residual intra-abdominal infection. In bacterial peritonitis secondary to trauma, with the escape of intestinal content, the mixed organisms are always accompanied by other substances that facilitate the establishment of local infection. These include necrotic tissue, feces, barium sulfate, gastric secretions, bile salts, and hemoglobin.[22-26]

Hemoglobin. Of all the adjuvant substances, hemoglobin has been the most extensively studied. In an attempt to understand the toxicity of fluid trapped in the lumen of ischemic loops of intestine, Yull et al [25] found that intraperitoneal hemoglobin increased the lethality of intraperitoneal *E. coli* inocula. The phenomenon has been extensively reproduced. Hemoglobin appears to act locally, rather than systemically, to increase the number of bacteria in the peritoneal cavity. Our initial in vitro studies demonstrated that commercial crystalline hemoglobin preparations which contain stroma interfered with chemotaxis, phagocytosis, and bacterial killing by human neutrophils.[14] Our most recent evidence indicates that compounds which contain heme-iron act directly on some bacteria to facilitate their proliferation.[26]

Intraperitoneal Fluid and Fibrin. Intraperitoneal fluid and fibrin, two important components of the peritoneal inflammatory response, also appear to play adjuvant roles. Saline infused intraperitoneally with nonlethal numbers of *E. coli* renders the combination lethal in direct proportion to the volume of saline infused. The adjuvant effect is apparently related to interference with two host defenses against bacteria—the need for opsonic proteins, which are apparently diluted by the saline, and the need for surfaces on which phagocytes can trap and ingest unopsonized bacteria. Large volumes of fluid within the peritoneal cavity suspend the bacteria, isolating them from neutrophils on the peritoneal surface and permitting bacterial proliferation to lethal numbers.

Although fibrin is considered to be an intraperitoneal defense that functions to isolate infection and seal visceral perforations, it may have deleterious effects as well.[27] We first showed that heparin could decrease mortality in dogs with necrotic bowel.[28] Ahrenholz and Simmons [12] have shown that fibrin clots that are full of bacteria will protect against a lethal peritonitis, but only for a few days. Thereafter, abscesses appear around the fibrin clot. Abscesses can be produced in rats with as few as 10^2 *E. coli* implanted within a pure fibrin clot. Phagocytes are delayed in reaching fibrin-entrapped bacteria. Hemoglobin increases the mortality of *E. coli* even when fibrin is present.[14]

Although the mechanisms for action of all intraperitoneal adjuvants are not known, meticulous hemostasis, copious lavage to remove all types of adjuvant substances from the peritoneal cavity, and aspiration of all excess irrigant may reduce the incidence of recurrent intra-abdominal infection after an operation. Even fibrin and fluid exudates may be harmful in combination with residual, otherwise easily tolerated numbers of bacteria.

Bacterial Synergism

The previous discussion illustrates that many types of substances allow bacteria to survive and proliferate within the peritoneal cavity. There is also evidence that some bacterial species interact with the host in ways that favor their survival in the peritoneal cavity.[29] Since secondary peritonitis is usually a polymicrobial infection, some understanding of these interactions is necessary.

Solid feces can contain 10^{10} to 10^{11} bacteria per gm, with more than 500 bacterial species. After intestinal perforation, many species are rapidly eliminated by the combination of host defenses and the lack of suitable environment outside the bowel lumen. This clinical observation is not simply a reflection of the inability of clinical microbiology laboratories to isolate all the species in feces. Onderdonk et al [18] implanted gelatin capsules containing barium sulfate and rat feces into the peritoneal cavities of rats. At least 27 species of organisms were isolated from the initial inoculum, but few (including those most abundant in the original isolates) could be isolated after intraperitoneal implantation. A two-stage disease was found: in the acute stage all animals developed free peritonitis and *E. coli* bacteremia. Peritoneal cultures yielded *E. coli* (10^6 per ml), enterococci (10^5 per ml), and *B. fragilis* (10^6 per ml). If the animals survived, intraabdominal abscesses were found, yielding *B. fragilis* (10^9 per ml), *E. coli* (10^8 per ml), and enterococci (10^6 per ml). Thus, a dramatic reduction in the number of bacterial species is found as peritonitis progresses to the localized abscess stage. Furthermore, anaerobic species predominate in abscesses of fecal origin.

Onderdonk et al [30] extended their studies in rats by mixing sterile feces with known quantities of bacteria within gelatin capsules. Pure cultures of *B. fragilis, Fusobacterium varium, E. coli,* or *Streptococcus faecalis* could not induce intra-abdominal abscesses. Neither could combinations of the two aerobes nor the two anaerobes. When an anaerobic organism was combined with an aerobe, however, intraperitoneal abscesses were consistently produced.

A number of mechanisms for bacterial synergism have been proposed: (1) the production of a growth factor or nutrient by one bacterium that allows survival and growth of another, (2) a bacterial secretion that protects against host defense mechanisms, and (3) the production of a suitable environment for growth of a pathogenic organism (Chapter 8).

Experimentally, antibiotic therapy directed against one synergistic partner early in an infection appears to abort abscess formation.[31] It appears, however, that after an abscess is established, the elimination of one organism will not reverse the infection. This may be because an abscess is a self-sustaining inflammatory process or because, within the abscess, the bacterial growth is retarded, making it resistant to many types of antimicrobial killing.

Clinical Manifestations

Textbook descriptions of secondary bacterial peritonitis tend to equate it with the acute abdomen. In fact, the manifestations are variable depending upon the specific disease, its location in relation to the other viscera and serosal surfaces, and host factors, such as immunosuppression or recent operations.

Visceral perforation is a frequent cause of secondary bacterial peritonitis. The resulting rapid contamination of the peritoneal cavity often produces the classic acute abdomen. Pain is of recent onset and may be sudden or appear over several hours. Whereas the pain at onset could be localized, generalized pain develops rapidly. Movement, coughing, or jarring the bed aggravates the symptoms. In diffuse peritonitis, tenderness is found over the entire abdomen, and rebound tenderness is diffuse and severe. At first, the patient lies still, with shallow respirations and voluntary muscular guarding of the abdomen. As the parietal peritoneum becomes inflamed, rigidity ensues due to reflex muscular spasm. Anorexia, nausea, and vomiting are present from the onset, but the patient is thirsty, and urine output is low. Ileus results in abdominal distention and hyperresonance, and bowel sounds are usually diminished or absent.

Fever and tachycardia are almost always present, except in patients being treated with steroids. The patient is initially alert and irritable but, without treatment, gradually becomes obtunded. The patient normally dies of dehydration and hypovolemic shock, not sepsis. If a patient is being carefully monitored, the development of a hyperdynamic shock, drop in arteriovenous oxygen extraction, hyperglycemia, and acidosis may be detected before any other symptoms appear. Hypotension is more common in the elderly and young, who frequently have less obvious symptoms as well. Septic shock is usually a late event except in cases of ruptured abscess.

Peritonitis developing from a prior site of visceral inflammation, such as appendicitis, diverticulitis, or tuboovarian abscess, usually has a less dramatic presentation unless an abscess suddenly ruptures to contaminate the entire peritoneal surface. These patients usually first note a dull aching pain in the abdomen. This referred pain is due to irritation of the pain fibers of the visceral peritoneum, which have little power of localization. Rectal or vaginal exam may reveal tenderness or fluctuance of a pelvic abscess. The parietal peritoneum of the anterior abdominal wall is affected, and the distribution of pain fibers here permits the perception of localized pain. If the abscess remains deep in the pelvis or under the diaphragm, abdominal tenderness may be difficult to elicit.

Similarly, postoperative patients with peritonitis have unreliable signs of developing intraperitoneal infection. Incisional pain, postoperative analgesics, or respiratory complications may mask the intraperitoneal irritation. Fever and ileus are such common, nonspecific signs in postoperative patients that their significance tends to be ignored.

Even when sepsis becomes obvious, other sources of infection must be ruled out.

Patients who are immunodepressed for any reason also have diminished abdominal signs. Patients receiving steroids have few conclusive findings, and patients with malignancy, uremia, diabetes, or other chronic illness may also present difficult diagnostic challenges.

Laboratory Studies

In diffuse peritonitis, peripheral leukocytosis usually exceeds 15,000 white blood cells per ml^3, with polymorphonuclear predominance and a moderate shift to the left. Normal or even depressed counts may be encountered. Patients being treated with steroids may also have a depressed leukocyte response.

Dehydration is reflected by a rise in hematocrit and blood urea nitrogen values. The sedimentation rate may be increased, especially with subacute infection. Microscopic hematuria and pyuria occur with infection adjacent to the urinary tract. As the patient becomes more ill, acidosis and hypernatremia may occur. Amylase levels are usually normal or mildly elevated except in perforated ulcer disease or bowel strangulation. Blood cultures drawn at this time are frequently positive, usually for only one organism, but a polymicrobial infection is almost invariably present in the peritoneal cavity.

Radiologic examination is also useful. A roentgenogram of the chest will frequently reveal free air below the diaphragms if a viscus is ruptured and help rule out pulmonary infection. Supine, decubitus, and upright abdominal films will demonstrate evidence of mechanical intestinal obstruction, volvulus, intussusception, or vascular occlusion. More commonly, mild distention of the small and large intestine with air fluid levels and bowel loops separated by intraperitoneal fluid are found. The properitoneal fat lines and psoas shadow may be obliterated if a retroperitoneal infection is present. Gas within the biliary tree or gallbladder suggests fistulous communication or emphysematous cholecystitis. Gas within the portal vein or liver is diagnostic of pyelophlebitis. Extraluminal gas with a fluid level or gas bubbles in an abscess or hematoma suggest areas of anaerobic bacterial metabolism.

In diffuse generalized peritonitis, needle aspiration of the peritoneal cavity or peritoneal lavage are diagnostic if gross pus, feces, or blood is obtained. The presence of bacteria on Gram stain of centrifuge sediment is also diagnostic. In cases of intraperitoneal infection where loculation is efficient, peritoneal lavage may provide no evidence of intraperitoneal infection, except for a few leukocytes, which are found in many other conditions. Any fluid obtained should be cultured and examined microscopically for red and white cell counts.

Diagnosis

The diagnosis is usually based on clinical and radiographic signs in patients who have sepsis and minimal abdominal findings, secondary to corticosteroid use or other immunosuppression. Exploratory laparotomy may be empirically necessary to make the diagnosis. Patients with mesenteric infarction or other gangrenous processes also have minimal findings other than a profound unexplained acidosis, and operation is necessary to make the diagnosis. The problem of diagnosis in the postoperative patient will be considered in detail in the sections dealing with abscesses.

Treatment of Secondary Bacterial Peritonitis

General Preoperative and Postoperative Treatment. Every patient with an intraperitoneal infection is at least potentially critically ill and requires adequate monitoring of vital functions in the preoperative and postoperative periods (Chapter 16). Repeated and systematic clinical evaluations yield the greatest amount of information and are critical in the management of these patients. Determinations, such as blood pressure, pulse, central venous pressure, urine output, and specific gravity, and such laboratory values as hematocrit, peripheral leukocyte count and differential, serum electrolytes, serum creatinine, and assessment of pulmonary function with arterial blood gases have become routine evaluations. Arterial cannulation offers some advantages in providing direct access to the blood pressure and serves as a convenient source of blood for serial determinations of blood gases and other laboratory values. We believe that a Swan-Ganz catheter should be used routinely in elderly patients and others who have evidence of compromised cardiorespiratory function. Since early hypovolemia is characteristic of all patients with peritonitis, pulmonary artery wedge pressure determinations can be used to estimate the volume of crystalloid required for rapid adequate rehydration of the patient.

The controversy over use of colloid versus crystalloid in resuscitation of the hypovolemic patient continues. Adequate resuscitation with crystalloid requires a larger volume than with colloid, but systemic sepsis causes an increased permeability of the pulmonary vasculature, and studies with labeled serum albumin have shown that large quantities of albumin can enter the alveoli and result in hypoxemia. Recent studies indicate that colloid has no advantages over crystalloid solutions, and the latter should be used.[32] We reserve the use of whole blood for patients found to be anemic on admission.

Hourly urine outputs should be measured to assure adequate renal function. A controversy exists whether diuretics actually prevent renal failure when they are used after adequate fluid resuscitation has failed to restore urine output.

Hypoxemia is often found in these septic patients. Increased permeability of the pulmonary vasculature may result in transudation of fluid into the alveoli, decreasing oxygen exchange. Reflex abdominal rigidity and diaphragmatic spasm may contribute to hypoventilation. Hypoxemia is treated by increasing the inspired oxygen to 40 percent based on blood gas determinations. Intubation and respiratory assistance with a volume control respirator are indicated if the patient still remains hypoxemic (Chapter 17). If the intraperitoneal infection is controlled, the respiratory assistance is usually required only for a limited period of time.

Some patients are first seen in septic or hypovolemic

shock. The clinical approach to this problem is outlined in Chapter 16. In addition to rapid fluid resuscitation and the administration of antibiotics, we give such patients pharmacologic doses of corticosteroids, even though this therapy remains controversial. Schumer [33] demonstrated beneficial effects of methylprednisolone or dexamethasone on survival after septic shock in a double-blind trial. Nevertheless, his remarkable findings have not been confirmed in other clinical studies. Inotropic and vasoactive agents may also be required if adequate hemodynamic indices are not obtained after fluid resuscitation. We favor dopamine or dobutamine at levels that do not cause vasoconstriction of the visceral microcirculation, with associated local tissue acidosis. These agents are useful for pharmacologic cardiac support (Chapter 16).

Ileus is characteristically present in acute peritonitis. Swallowed air and the intestinal contents distend the bowel, and diaphragmatic motion is impeded. Preoperative intubation with either a nasogastric tube or a long intestinal tube may rapidly decompress the bowel, relieving pressure on the diaphragm and increasing pulmonary ventilation. Abdominal closure at the end of an operation is easier with the bowel decompressed. Many clinicians believe that decompression facilitates early return of intestinal mobility, with decreases in morbidity, postoperative starvation, and adhesion formation, but objective evidence is not available.

We routinely withhold sedatives and analgesics in patients until the diagnosis of the intraperitoneal process has been made. Thereafter, however, analgesics and sedatives are given as needed.

Metabolic and Nutritional Therapy. The nutritional requirements of these septic patients are enormous, and the metabolic effects of sepsis have been discussed in detail in Chapters 15 and 16. Enteral alimentation is usually impossible, so that total parental nutrition, using the guidelines discussed in Chapters 15 and 16, should be instituted.[34]

Antibiotic Therapy. Antibiotic therapy should always be initiated as soon as the clinical diagnosis of peritonitis is made. Careful aerobic, anaerobic, and fungal cultures should be taken at operation, and sensitivity studies obtained. Almost all antibiotics reach therapeutic levels in normal intraperitoneal fluid. The aminoglycosides, ampicillin, and cephalosporins reach intraperitoneal levels equivalent to serum levels. The level of clindamycin in intraperitoneal fluid is approximately one-half that of the serum concentration.[35]

Upper gastrointestinal perforations usually release predominantly gram-positive organisms that are sensitive to the penicillins or cephalosporins, and lesser quantities of gram-negative organisms are released. With peritonitis due to perforations of the distal gastrointestinal tract, antibiotics should be chosen to eradicate three classes of bacteria—the coliforms (Enterobacteriaceae), enterococci (group D *Streptococcus*), and the anaerobic organisms (especially *Bacteroides* species) (Table 34-1). Of the available bactericidal agents, we prefer the combination of an aminoglycoside, ampicillin, and clindamycin. Although there are several reports citing the effectiveness of single-drug therapy in peritonitis,[36] we believe that triple-drug treatment eliminates the maximum number of bacteria in the preoperative periods before antibiotic sensitivity tests are available. Single-drug therapy appears especially effective in trauma patients with acute peritoneal contamination before infection is established or local host defenses are impaired.

The aminoglycosides (gentamycin, tobramycin, amikacin, and others) are bactericidal to most facultative gram-negative organisms and are indicated in peritonitis caused by these bacteria. Activity against *Pseudomonas* is variable, although tobramycin is quite effective. Plasmid-mediated resistance to aminoglycosides is common among gram-negative organisms, and it is often necessary to change the therapeutic drug in recurrent infections. Aminoglycosides are excreted in the urine, and patients with impaired renal function require reduced dosages to prevent toxicity. Peak blood levels of at least 6 μg per ml of gentamycin or tobramycin are necessary. Peak blood levels should not exceed 12 μg per ml, and trough levels should remain below 2 μg per ml. Because the volume of distribution and rate of excretion are so variable from patient to patient, individualized dosage regimens should be determined for each patient based upon peak and trough blood levels of antibiotic after intravenous administration to minimize complications. Dosage schedules based upon body weight and serum creatinine are so unreliable as to be dangerous. Aminoglycosides are effective agents in clinical peritonitis due to coliforms and readily penetrate infected peritoneal fluid.[35]

Most anaerobic bacteria are resistant to aminoglycosides, especially the anaerobic gram-negative rods, such as the *Bacteroides* species. In fact, experimental *B. fragilis* infections are potentiated by aminoglycosides. Clindamycin is a bactericidal antibiotic effective against essentially all strains of *Bacteroides*, including those resistant to penicillin and tetracycline, although clindamycin-resistant strains do occur.

Not all clinicians agree that clindamycin is indicated in peritonitis. Stone et al [17] found that an operation so alters the redox potential of the peritoneal cavity that anaerobic bacteria cannot be recovered after 20 minutes. These results have been difficult to confirm. The use of an aminoglycoside plus operation resulted in cures of more than 90 percent of the patients with diffuse peritonitis or intraabdominal abscesses. However, anaerobes were still isolated from a majority of intraperitoneal abscesses that occurred after antibiotic therapy.

Trauma patients usually do well even after single antibiotic therapy for peritoneal contamination. A prospective study of trauma patients treated with either cephalothin or clindamycin revealed no difference in abscess formation or wound infection rates between the two groups.[17] In contrast, Thadepalli et al [37] compared cephalothin and kanamycin versus clindamycin and kanamycin in 100 patients with penetrating abdominal trauma. The aerobic infection rate was identical, but anaerobic infections developed in 11 of 52 patients treated with cephalothin and kanamycin versus 1 of 48 patients treated with clindamycin and kanamycin.

The special role of anaerobes in the pathogenesis of intraperitoneal abscesses was studied by Nichols et al.[31] They injected human feces intraperitoneally into rats. The lowest abscess formation rates were found with tobramycin–clindamycin treated animals, whereas antibiotic combinations not directed toward the eradication of both coliform and anaerobes were not as effective overall. The data provide the best experimental evidence of the importance of antibiotic therapy directed against both aerobes and anaerobes in peritonitis.

The major objection to the use of clindamycin is the risk of diarrhea and pseudomembraneous colitis—a risk with all broad-spectrum antibiotics, not only clindamycin.[38] This colitis is usually due to overgrowth of an enterotoxin-producing *Clostridium* (probably *Clostridium difficile*), and the incidence of pseudomembranous colitis is higher with oral than with parenteral therapy. Furthermore, the risk can be reduced if the drug is discontinued at the first sign of diarrhea (Chapter 39).

Several recent treatment failures of mixed bacterial infections with an aminoglycoside and clindamycin have been the result of enterococcal sepsis. Although it has been suggested that the enterococcus is not a pathogenic organism,[39] it is a frequent isolate from clinical peritonitis, and Onderdonk et al [30] have found it to be an important synergistic partner with anaerobes in experimental peritonitis. The enterococcus is usually sensitive to ampicillin, and we routinely have administered this antibiotic to our patients who have peritonitis.

The aim of antibiotic therapy is to reduce the systemic and local infectious complications of peritonitis. For this reason, the best current results should be obtained by triple-antibiotic therapy designed to eliminate the three groups of commonly isolated bacteria—enterococci, coliforms, and anaerobes.

Despite our preference for this combination, single- or double-antibiotic therapy combined with early operative management will result in a high success rate in many cases of uncomplicated peritonitis. For example, carbenicillin and ticarcillin are semisynthetic penicillins effective against many coliforms, *Pseudomonas*, and most anaerobes. Each may be a useful alternative to clindamycin [39a] in combination with an aminoglycoside. Carbenicillin inactivation of aminoglycosides occurs in vitro but is clinically significant only in patients with renal failure.

Chloramphenicol is a potent drug effective against a wide spectrum of bacteria, including enterococci and *Bacteroides*. It does not require adjustments in dosage for patients with renal failure and has been widely used in azotemic patients. However, chloramphenicol is a bacteriostatic rather than bactericidal agent. Further, there is evidence that in vitro a variety of anaerobic organisms can inactivate chloramphenicol, even though they are sensitive to the drug by the usual antibiotic sensitivity testing procedures. There are reports of clinical failures of chloramphenicol in anaerobic infections.[40] Many patients develop neutropenia during chloramphenicol administration. Therapy should be discontinued immediately to minimize the risk of aplastic anemia, a rare but lethal complication.

The combination of an aminoglycoside with penicillin or cephalosporin has been popular because of their wide gram-positive and gram-negative spectrum and synergism against some organisms. Penicillin in high dosages, although effective against virtually all of the anaerobes, is ineffective against *B. fragilis*, a defect shared by the cephalosporins. In addition, the cephalosporins may potentiate aminoglycoside renal toxicity.

The newer cephalosporins, especially cefamandole, cefotaxime, moxalactam, and ecfoxitin, have extended gram-negative and anaerobic efficacy. Studies are underway to determine the usefulness of these drugs in both experimental and clinical peritonitis.[41] Cefoxitin appears to be the most effective against *B. fragilis*, and has been shown to be as effective as clindamycin in the treatment of anaerobic surgical infections.[41a]

Metronidazole is a potent antianaerobic agent that has been used in Europe and Canada to treat *Bacteroides* infections. It appears to be as effective as clindamycin against intraperitoneal anaerobes.

The preceding discussion refers to the choice of presumptive antibiotic therapy. Much confusion surrounds the indications for change of antibiotic therapy as culture and antibiotic sensitivity results return from the laboratory. Unfortunately, clinical microbiology laboratories cannot identify all of the components in mixed fecal flora and may fail to report some of the organisms present. Furthermore, if antibiotics were started prior to operation, cultures may fail to identify all the pathogens. For these reasons, clinically effective therapy should not be prematurely discontinued on the basis of laboratory reports that suggest that some drugs may not be necessary. On the other hand a change of antibiotics will be necessary if a confirmed isolate is resistant to the drug therapy already being used.

There are no precise criteria for duration of postoperative antibiotic therapy. A period of 10 days to two weeks is usually adequate if clinical improvement continues. Breakthrough bacteremia during adminstration of appropriate antibiotics is presumptive evidence of residual or recurrent infection, although other nosocomial infection must be ruled out.[21]

Operative Therapy. The goal of operative therapy of peritonitis is to control the source of contamination, reduce or eliminate the bacterial inoculum, and prevent the recurrence of sepsis. A variety of operative therapies have been advocated, but it must be stressed that no prospective randomized study of the operative approaches to peritonitis has been published.

Nonoperative therapy is the treatment of choice for primary peritonitis, which will be dealt with in a subsequent section. In the days when anesthesia was unsafe, operation was delayed or avoided in patients with secondary bacterial peritonitis. The principles of fluid and electrolyte resuscitation were not understood, and antibiotics were not available. Nonoperative therapy was popularized by Ochsner, who proposed a regimen of (1) nothing by mouth, (2) gastric lavage with warm water, (3) hydration by proctoclysis, (4) head high, pelvic low position, (5) morphine, and (6) heat applied to the abdomen.

Today, aggressive operative management of secondary peritonitis is the treatment of choice, even though a rare patient will survive nonoperative therapy because of the normal defenses of the peritoneal cavity and the availability of potent antibiotics.[42]

Operative therapy attempts to eliminate continuing bacterial contamination by closing, excluding, or resecting the perforated viscus and evacuating obvious loculated fluid. Management of the intraperitoneal residua of the perforation is controversial, however. In the more traditional approach, peritonitis is treated by making the incision as small as possible to adequately visualize and close the visceral perforation. The peritoneal cavity is not explored to evacuate other loculations or to remove fibrinous exudate. Irrigation of the cavity is avoided for fear of spreading infection. Drains are placed into abscess cavities to permit escape of exudate or to provide an exit route for potential fistulas from insecurely closed viscera, the damaged pancreas, or the retroperitoneal area. This approach is successful for the majority of patients with peritonitis.

It is especially successful if preexisting inflammation due to visceral disease has facilitated localization of the infection to one part of the peritoneal cavity. The most unfavorable features of this therapy are that synchronous abscesses at other sites will go undetected and that the bacteria left behind will cause abscesses.

An alternative approach has emerged that is especially useful in the treatment of diffuse peritonitis or in patients with impaired host defenses. Hudspeth[43] has presented a remarkable series of 92 patients with advanced generalized peritonitis treated by radical peritoneal debridement. His technique utilizes a vertical midline incision from xiphoid to pubis, so that the abdomen can be completely explored and all loculations and abscess cavities identified and eliminated. The bowel is decompressed by a long intestinal tube, and all fibrin and necrotic material is debrided. All spaces and potential spaces within the peritoneal cavity are opened and cleaned. The abdomen is then irrigated with saline until clear. Drains are not placed unless hysterectomy is part of the procedure. In his series, there were no deaths and no recurrent intra-abdominal infections. Confirmatory clinical studies using this operative approach have not yet been published and one randomized prospective study has shown no advantage of the radical over the conservative approach.[43a]

Several objections have been raised to this procedure. Experimentally, drying the mesothelium or exposing it to saline for prolonged periods causes desquamation of the cells. Damage to these cells, however, has never been demonstrated to interfere with translymphatic clearance of bacteria or intraperitoneal killing by phagocytes.

Traditionally, surgeons have dreaded the spread of localized bacterial infection. Bacterial contamination of the previously uninflamed peritoneal cavity is, however, rapidly disseminated throughout by the intraperitoneal circulation. As the inflammatory process develops, bacteria in many areas are eliminated, and in the other areas, the bacteria are contained as abscesses develop. Surgeons have feared that opening these areas and irrigating them with fluid would result in recurrent infection elsewhere. However, the risk of leaving an undrained abscess that almost certainly will require reoperation outweighs the risk of disseminating bacteria as long as irrigation is used to minimize the bacterial inoculum.

The most serious objection to radical peritoneal debridement is that it causes bleeding from damaged peritoneal surfaces. Thereby two of the most potent adjuvants to infection, hemoglobin and fibrin, are infused.

The conservative and radical approaches cannot be successfully combined. If pus escapes into the peritoneal cavity during an attempt at localized drainage, the cavity becomes highly contaminated and almost certainly will develop new areas of infection if not properly evacuated by irrigation. Conversely, if incomplete debridement of the peritoneal cavity takes place, residual necrotic debris may develop into pockets of infection. Therefore, we believe that radical peritoneal debridement, by minimizing the bacterial inoculum left behind, is probably the best treatment. Despite our preference, some chronic abscess cavities may be so fibrotic or vascular that debridement carries a prohibitive risk of bleeding. In these cases, only lavage and drainage are possible. The details of peritoneal lavage are discussed in a subsequent section.

Bacteriologic Specimen Collection at Operation. Immediately upon opening the peritoneal cavity, any free fluid is aspirated with a syringe and injected without air bubbles into a suitable anaerobic transport container (Chapter 12). This is sent for immediate Gram stain and culture for aerobic and anaerobic organisms. We have not found the Gram stain to be particularly helpful in determining antibiotic therapy for our patients. In our series of proven bacterial peritonitis, 12.5 percent were false-negative. If the results had been taken literally, antibiotics would have been discontinued in patients with bacterial peritonitis. A direct smear, however, is only able to detect bacteria at concentrations greater than 10^5 per ml. In the presence of neutrophils and other debris, even greater numbers of bacteria probably must be present for detection. Gram stains performed at operation are useful in warning the surgeon that a specific organism (eg, pneumococcus, *Clostridium*) is present, but clinical evidence is a more reliable indicator of infection than is the Gram stain alone.

The belief that *E. coli* produces a foul-smelling process has long been laid to rest. The free fatty acids and their esters, which are responsible for the penetrating foul odor often found in peritonitis, are the result of anaerobic bacteria. These pungent by-products of bacterial growth are so characteristic that anaerobic bacteria are routinely identified in the clinical laboratory by gas chromatographic analysis of the volatile fatty acids.

Peritoneal Irrigation and Local Application of Antibiotics. Local irrigation and antibiotic therapy can take several forms. These include intraoperative crystalloid lavage, intraoperative antibiotic lavage, postoperative instillation of antibiotics, postoperative crystalloid lavage, and postoperative antibiotic lavage. The use of intraoperative lavage does not necessarily commit one to radical peritoneal debridement although the objectives of each may be the same.

Intraoperative Saline Irrigation. Many surgeons fear that peritoneal irrigation spreads bacteria throughout the peritoneal cavity, but peritoneal lavage unquestionably reduces the number of bacteria present,[44] as well as reducing the concentration of adjuvant substances.[45] Unfortunately the mortality and infectious complications of experimental peritonitis are not much reduced by saline irrigation.[45] Crystalloid irrigation alone is only curative if carried out using large volumes within hours of peritoneal contamination. After this time, fibrin deposits probably have trapped bacteria locally,[12] and irrigation alone will not be effective in removing them. Intraoperative lavage is a useful part of operative therapy even if it is not curative because it reduces the bacterial inoculum. However, residual saline dilutes bacterial opsonins and suspends the bacteria in a fluid medium, decreasing phagocytosis and permitting bacterial proliferation.[45a] If the abdomen is irrigated with saline, *all* residual fluid should be aspirated prior to abdominal closure. It is not clear whether this precaution was carried out in the published experimental studies.

Intraoperative Antibiotic Irrigation. In contrast to the controversy that surrounds the use of saline irrigation, both experimental and clinical studies have shown that intraoperative irrigation with antibiotic solution is definitely beneficial to the host. Those investigators who found no improvement in survival with saline irrigation found that adding antibiotics to the intraoperative irrigation fluid significantly reduced the mortality.[44] In 1967, Noon et al [46] randomized 404 carefully stratified patients to treatment with normal saline irrigation or saline irrigation with 1 gm of kanamycin and 50,000 units of bacitracin. Although there was no difference in mortality, the infectious complication rate was 12 percent in the antibiotic-treated group vs 24 percent with the saline-treated group. All patients received comparable systemic antibiotics. Nevertheless, Rambo,[47] using cephalothin, and Sherman et al,[48] using kanamycin, were unable to show an advantage of intraoperative antibiotic irrigation over saline irrigation in patients with peritonitis who received systemic antibiotics.

Locally instilled antibiotics have concentrations 10^2 to 10^4 times higher than serum levels achieved by parenteral administration. Gerding et al [35] found that systemic administration of antibiotics produces intraperitoneal levels comparable to serum levels in patients with generalized peritonitis. Antibiotics rapidly penetrate into uninfected peritoneal fluid, but penetration into infected spaces resembling abscesses is markedly reduced.

Because of the clinical and experimental evidence showing the efficacy of intraoperative antibiotic irrigation, we currently use cephalothin irrigation (1 gm per liter) in addition to the systemic antibiotics described previously. At a concentration of 1,000 μg per ml, the agent is effective against even the gram-negative and anaerobic bacteria. McMullan and Barnett [49] have used concentrations as high as 100,000 μg per ml. Aminoglycosides are also effective as local irrigants, but they are nephrotoxic and ototoxic and potentiate the effect of muscle relaxant drugs used during anesthesia (Chapter 18). Postoperative respiratory depression has been reported.

Postoperative Intraperitoneal Antibiotic Instillation. Several investigators have shown the beneficial effect of continuous intraperitoneal antibiotic instillation in dogs with experimental peritonitis.[49-52]

DiVincenti and Cohn [51] treated 101 patients with perforated appendicitis. All patients received systemic antibiotics, usually penicillin and streptomycin. The patients were randomly allocated to receive intraperitoneal kanamycin once at the time of operation or daily via intraperitoneal catheter for three days. There was a significant decrease in wound and intraperitoneal infections with the more prolonged local kanamycin treatment. Fowler [52] found that 48 hours of postoperative treatment with intraperitoneal cephaloridine produced a significant reduction in intraperitoneal abscesses in children with perforated appendicitis. McMullan and Barnett [49] have used up to 12 gm of cephalothin per 24 hours, intraperitoneally, without adverse effects even at concentrations of 1 gm per 10 ml saline.

Continuous Postoperative Peritoneal Lavage. Continuous postoperative peritoneal lavage with crystalloid has also been used to treat peritonitis.

Kiene and Troeger [53] treated 90 peritonitis patients conventionally, with a mortality of 52 percent. Those patients receiving postoperative peritoneal lavage with antibiotics had a mortality of 36 percent. Hunt et al [54] studied patients with gynecologic peritonitis and reduced their mortality from 47 percent (historical controls) to 24 percent when peritoneal lavage with 15 μg per ml of gentamycin was begun. The only randomized clinical trial has been reported by Bhushan et al [55] from Agra, India. Sixty patients with diffuse peritonitis were randomly divided into intraoperative and postoperative peritoneal lavage with saline solution, with or without kanamycin and penicillin. The control group had a mortality of 60 percent, whereas the antibiotic treatment group had a mortality of 20 percent.

The indications for continuous postoperative peritoneal lavage are not yet well defined. Such aggressive therapy is only rarely indicated. However, in those patients with massive peritoneal contamination or markedly depressed host defenses, such as tumor chemotherapy or immunosuppressive drug treatment, continuous peritoneal dialysis may be worthwhile. Postoperative antibiotic lavage delivers antibiotics locally and washes away bacteria and their toxic products. It is standard therapy for peritonitis associated with chronic peritoneal dialysis. Antibiotics used in postoperative peritoneal lavage fluid are added in concentrations equal to the desired serum concentration of the drug. In this way, serum levels of antibiotics, which are rapidly exchanged across the peritoneal surface, are maintained continuously without reaching the toxic range. There may be some advantage to this continuous administration of antibiotic, since continuous, high serum

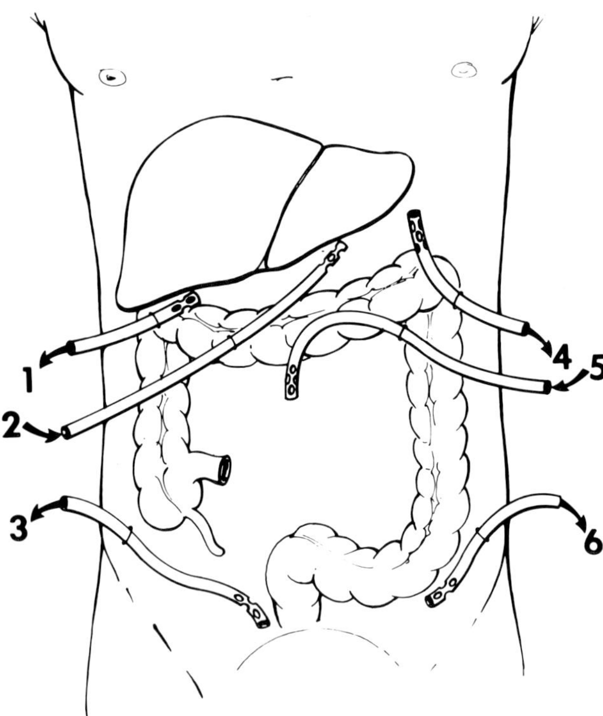

Fig. 34-7. **One possible arrangement of postoperative peritoneal irrigation catheters. Numbers 2 and 5 are used for inflow and the others for outflow of fluid. Number 1 can be placed above the dome of the liver. Number 2 can be placed in the lesser sac. Number 5 can be placed beneath the transverse mesocolon. (Modified from Parneix M, Mayeux CI, Laporte F: Chirurgie 98:779, 1972.)**

levels are maintained without the risk of toxicity.

Figure 34-7 shows one method of instituting postoperative peritoneal dialysis. Two inflow catheters and four outflow catheters are used. Several liters of dialysis solution are infused into the peritoneal cavity and allowed to rest there for 20 to 30 minutes. The fluid is then removed by suction through the outflow catheters, and fresh, warm solution is reinfused. The alternative technique of continuous suction encourages development of adhesion-lined tracts between the inflow and outflow catheters, which prevent adequate lavage. During dialysis, disturbances in electrolytes are corrected, and protein losses, which may be massive, must be replaced. Lavage is carried out until bacteria and feculent debris have disappeared from the fluid. After four or five days, loculations usually occur even with vigorous dialysis, although small doses of heparin (3,000 to 5,000 units every 8 to 12 hours) may delay this.

Many patients with severe peritonitis develop renal failure. Continuous peritoneal lavage has some advantages, since hemodialysis in septic patients is frequently associated with hemodynamic instability and a high incidence of death. Complement activation results in trapping of leukocytes in the lungs during hemodialysis, which may add to the respiratory dysfunction in patients with sepsis.

Peritoneal Irrigation with Antiseptic Agents. A variety of studies have appeared recently documenting the effects of intraperitoneal antiseptic agents in peritonitis. Such agents are attractive because they have an almost universal bactericidal spectrum, with rapid killing of bacteria. In addition, they are cheap and readily available. Notoxylin [56] and taurolin,[57] which release formaldehyde locally, have been used in the United Kingdom. Povidone iodine (PVP-I) has been used clinically in both Europe and the United States.[58] Sindelar and Mason [58] lowered the abscess rate in contaminated abdominal operations from 10.2 percent with intraoperative saline lavage to 1.3 percent by using a liter of 1:10 dilution of PVP-I. Other studies have indicated topical PVP-I yields fewer wound infections than saline lavage [59] but more wound infections than topical antibiotics.[60] Concentrated PVP-I solutions can actually increase wound infection rates.[61] Despite clinical enthusiasm for intraperitoneal povidone iodine, results from our laboratory [62] show that this agent is a potent inactivator of such neutrophil functions as chemotaxis and phagocytosis even at dilutions of 1:10. Under experimental conditions, the antiseptic can increase the mortality of experimental peritonitis, presumably by damaging host defenses.[62] In Europe, a different preparation of povidone iodine is available, and even postoperative povidone iodine lavage has been used.[63] This alternate formulation may be more suitable for intraperitoneal use. Antiseptic agents that have the potential for inducing damage to mammalian as well as microbial cells would seem, on theoretical grounds, to have little advantage over the local use of high concentrations of antibiotics that are not toxic to tissues. Antiseptics have a short duration of action in vivo,[62] whereas local antibiotics remain effective for prolonged periods. Systemic absorption of povidone iodine may produce iodine toxicity,[63] but antibiotics achieve therapeutic serum levels after intraperitoneal use. We prefer antibiotics.

Drains. It is impossible to drain the free peritoneal cavity in peritonitis. An exception may be in patients with severe ascites in whom a drain results in a continuous ascitic fistula. The inflammation initiated by the presence of a foreign body drain, however, is sufficient to rapidly isolate the drain tract from the rest of the peritoneal cavity. In addition to being ineffective, drains act as foreign bodies, potentiating intraperitoneal infection. Drains also allow external bacteria to enter the peritoneal cavity. Haller et al [64] found that children with penrose drains placed during operations for free peritonitis secondary to ruptured appendicitis averaged 3.7 more hospital days than undrained children. Drains designed to remove bacteria and fluid are never effective in free peritonitis unless peritoneal lavage is also used. Drains are effective only if their purpose is to evacuate abscesses, establish controlled fistulas, or offer a preferential pathway for the escape of visceral secretions after extensive damage to pancreas or biliary tree.

Abdominal Closure. When a vertical midline incision has been used, the fascia is closed in a single layer with interrupted monofilament sutures, such as proline, nylon, or wire. A major technical consideration is taking generous bites of tissue on each side to prevent dehiscence should a localized subfascial infection develop. Retention sutures tied over multiple red rubber catheters lateral to the wound are useful in the elderly, the severely malnourished, or the recipients of steroids or other catabolic drugs. If these retention sutures are too tight, one or more sections of the catheters can later be removed from beneath a given retention suture.

There are many reports of the presumed benefits of leaving the peritoneal cavity open in patients with extensive peritonitis—especially when enteric fistulas are expected. Sometimes the defect is temporarily closed by porous Marlex mesh, and sometimes the defect is merely packed open. If a prosthesis is used it usually must be removed after firm granulations have formed but before it has become totally incorporated into the abdominal wall. Leaving it in place is often followed by chronic infected sinuses.

Steinberg[65] treated 14 patients with suspected peritonitis. He used a paramedian incision and closed the wound with only a large gauze pack placed over the viscera and loose 000 wire through the fascia. External dressings were held in place with an abdominal binder. After two to three days, the dressings were soaked in 2 percent lidocaine and removed. The wires were pulled up and tied, allowing the wound to heal secondarily. Steinberg believes that this technique allows complete drainage of the peritoneum and reduces the incidence of recurrent sepsis. One patient died, and one had a subhepatic abcess.

Delayed Primary Closure of the Subcutaneous Tissue and Skin. Patients with extensive peritonitis will develop wound infection if the skin and subcutaneous tissue are closed primarily. Instead, sterile gauze should be packed in the wound, which should be kept covered by an occlusive dressing for four days. The gauze is then removed, and clean wounds are closed with tape. If there is a question of infection, a quantitative bacterial count can be done. Wounds with fewer than 10^5 bacteria per gm of tissue can safely be closed. Primary closure over suction catheters that are irrigated with antibiotic solution is an alternative technique.[66]

Prognosis

The ultimate outcome of an episode of secondary peritonitis is determined by many factors, some of which are controlled directly by the surgeon.[67] These include the delay in operative therapy, adequacy of debridement, lavage, and closure, correct choice and administration of antibiotics, and nutritional and hemodynamic support. The patient with peritonitis has already sustained a major traumatic episode and will not tolerate even the smallest of technical errors.

Other factors are beyond the physician's control. These include the patient's delay in seeking therapy, the source of sepsis, the patient's age, previous nutritional status, and concomitant disease states, including immunosuppressive diseases or medications. Figure 34-8 correlates the patient's age and source of sepsis with mortality. Mortality is consistently higher in the young and the elderly, and increases with more distal gastrointestinal sources of contamination.[67] The highest incidence of death is found in patients with peritonitis after operation. Often this is due to delay in diagnosis and treatment because the symptoms have been masked by postoperative analgesics or by the surgeon's failure to admit the possibility of failure. In addition, most patients have received antibiotics at least some time during their hospital course and, therefore, have selected out a resistant bacterial flora. The massively traumatized patient also probably has a decreased host resistance for many reasons, including operative factors that decrease the local resistance of the peritoneum to bacterial insult.

Burke et al[68] in 1963 analyzed the causes of death in patients with peritonitis and found that early deaths were the result of fluid and electrolyte imbalances. With better control of these problems, early deaths are rare. But in the 1960s and 1970s, a syndrome of distant or multiple organ system failure was noted in patients with sepsis

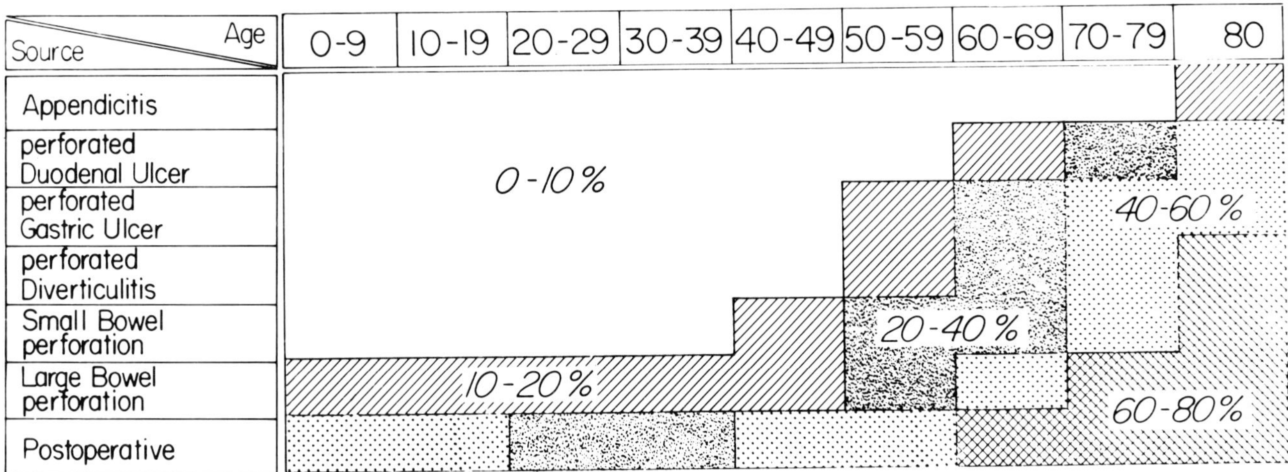

Fig. 34-8. **Estimated mortality of peritonitis according to age of patients and level of gastrointestinal tract perforation. Note the markedly higher mortality of postoperative peritonitis in all age groups. (From Hau T, Ahrenholz DH, Simmons RL: Curr Probl Surg 16:1, 1979.)**

or massive trauma [68] (Chapter 17). Organ systems are characteristically affected in a distinct chronologic order.[67] Acute hypovolemia may result in cardiovascular system dysfunction, and in severe cases, acute renal failure can result from systemic hypotension. More often, however, after the hemodynamic problems are corrected, a progressive respiratory decompensation is noted. The patients may require intubation and respiratory support on a volume-cycled respirator. With persistent sepsis, an insidious renal failure can occur, usually along with an ileus, which may be either a local or a systemic effect of sepsis. This associated renal failure has an extremely high mortality (over 85 percent) in postoperative patients, and those who survive long enough can develop liver failure.[67] Stress ulceration with massive upper gastrointestinal bleeding is also a major problem. Gastric hyperacidity refractory to cimetadine has been proposed as a valid indicator of occult sepsis.[69]

Recently, Saba et al [70] have proposed that distant organ failure is a toxic effect of the by-products of sepsis, which normally are opsonized and removed by a plasma protein (fibronectin) for phagocytosis by the fixed reticuloendothelial systems (Chapter 17). In infected patients, these opsonins can become depleted. Preliminary data suggest that replacement therapy with cryoprecipitate may temporarily reverse the organ failure until aggressive surgical control of the source of infection is obtained.

Fry et al [21] have presented data that *Bacteroides* septicemia is a sensitive indicator of recurrent intraabdominal infection in postoperative patients. They do not, however, routinely use antibiotics effective against anaerobes, and this may bias their data somewhat.

PRIMARY PERITONITIS

Not all bacterial peritonitis arises from a perforated viscus or from external trauma that contaminates the peritoneal cavity. Patients with impaired host defenses can develop a primary intraperitoneal infection without an obvious source of sepsis. In 1581, Fernel described a 7-year-old girl who developed painless diarrhea and died. At autopsy, the abdomen was distended with putrid purulent peritoneal fluid. This probably represents the first description of primary bacterial peritonitis.

At least five subgroups of primary peritonitis can be identified: (1) in apparently normal infants and young children, (2) associated with the nephrotic syndrome (characteristically in children), (3) in cirrhosis (alcoholic or postnecrotic), usually associated with ascites, (4) in immunocompromised hosts, eg, lupus erythematosus, and (5) in Fitz-Hugh-Curtis syndrome due to gonococci.

Incidence

Normal Infants and Children. Primary peritonitis is declining in frequency. It once accounted for 10 percent of all abdominal emergencies in children, with 75 percent of the cases occurring in children less than 5 years old.[71] McDougal et al [72] found that primary peritonitis accounted for 2.1 percent of all pediatric abdominal emergencies, 17.6 percent of diffuse peritonitis in infants, and 13.4 percent of diffuse peritonitis in children. Primary peritonitis follows a bimodal age distribution.[71] In infants, it occurs within the first two months of life, and females predominate. In childhood, the peak incidence is from 5 to 9 years of age (mean 8.5), and a more equal distribution of males and females is seen.

Cirrhosis. The incidence of this illness appears to be increasing. Spontaneous bacterial peritonitis in cirrhotic patients was largely unrecognized until 1958, when Caroli and Platteborse [73] reported a series of 20 cirrhotic patients with *E. coli* or pneumococcal peritonitis. In 1975, Correia and Conn [74] reported an additional 25 cases among approximately 400 cirrhotic patients—an overall incidence of about 6 percent. Among the patients with ascites, the incidence was 18 percent. Recurrent infections occurred in 12 percent, not significantly different from the group overall.

Systemic Lupus Erythematosus. Primary peritonitis is rare in patients with systemic lupus erythematosus, although 10 to 35 percent of these patients will manifest abdominal pain as a part of their symptomatology.[75] A small percentage of these patients will have an acute abdomen, the medical peritonitis of lupus.

Nephrotic Syndrome. Wilfert and Katz [76] found 7 cases of intraperitoneal bacterial infections during the hospital admission of 280 nephrotic children between 1963 and 1967. Speck et al [77] found 39 episodes of primary peritonitis in 22 children, with a 2:1 predominance of males. The mean age was 3.5 years, and one-half the children developed peritonitis in the first year after the diagnosis of nephrotic syndrome.

Fitz-Hugh-Curtis Syndrome. Gonococcal perihepatitis in women was described in the 1930s—one man has been reported.[78] The diagnosis is rarely made clinically. Instead, perihepatic adhesions are found incidently during operation or at autopsy.

Etiology

In the early part of the century, the pneumococcus was the dominant cause of primary peritonitis. Several factors were contributory:

1. The pneumococcus commonly colonizes the genital tract of baby girls, and retrograde ascent of the fallopian tubes may result in intraperitoneal contamination.
2. Pneumococcal bacteremia is characteristic of pneumococcal respiratory infections, so that hematogenous seeding of the peritoneal cavity is possible.
3. The pneumococcus is an encapsulated organism, and once it reaches the peritoneal cavity, it cannot be phagocytosed without a specific opsonizing antibody.

In more recent years, the incidence of pneumococcal peritonitis has decreased in parallel with the general decrease in pneumococcal infections of all types. The widespread use of antibiotics, not only in children but even in animal feed, may have led to a generalized suppression of human pneumococcal colonization. Pneumococcal vaccination of susceptible children may further reduce the incidence.

Table 34-2 illustrates that the coliform organisms now are more commonly isolated from cases of primary peritonitis. Even such uncommon organisms as the meningococcus, *Haemophilus influenzae*, enterococcus, and the anaerobic bacteria are sometimes found.[79] Unlike the situation in secondary peritonitis, anaerobes are rarely isolated, probably because of the relatively high oxygen tension within the normal peritoneal cavity. In patients with ascites, however, the large volumes of fluid and poor solubility of oxygen may account for this finding, although Sheckman et al [79] found that the Po_2 of normal ascitic fluid was 43 ± 3.1 mm Hg, equal to mixed venous blood.

Half the children with postnecrotic cirrhosis have gram-positive and half gram-negative infections, although the latter are increasing.[77]

Fitz-Hugh-Curtis syndrome results from gonococcal perihepatitis after pelvic inflammatory disease in females. This organism is venereally transmitted and has an affinity for urogenital epithelium. The resulting ascending infection reaches the peritoneal cavity. *Chlamydiae* can also cause this syndrome in females with or without gonococci.

Pathogenesis

Mechanisms of Bacterial Contamination. There are at least four mechanisms by which bacteria reach the peritoneal cavity. The most likely route in male children with pneumococcal peritonitis is hematogenous. Hematogenous spread is the most likely source of infection in cases associated with a noncontiguous infection or an intravascular infection, such as an infected plastic catheter.

The female genital tract is a frequent route of infection, especially in Fitz-Hugh-Curtis syndrome. The single reported case of gonococcal perihepatitis in a male was presumably the result of hematogenous spread.[78] In female children, the vaginal tract secretions are alkaline, and most pathogens are inhibited by the acidic secretions that develop after puberty. In cases of gonococcal peritonitis and pneumococcal primary peritonitis in children, the organism can be cultured from the vagina.[80] Whether this represents ascending or descending disease is unclear. Beale and Hackett [81] also documented reflux of urine into the uterus of a child; this may aid the spread of bacteria to the peritoneal cavity. Prior or concurrent urinary tract infections are frequent in female children who develop primary peritonitis.[72]

A third source is the contiguous spread of infection. Frequently a simultaneous infection of the lungs, pancreas, or urinary tract will be found in adults. Of course, an episode of sepsis may lead to hematogenous spread, but it is difficult to disprove the contiguous spread of infection across the visceral peritoneum. Primary peritonitis is often associated with lower lobe pneumonia in adults.[82]

A fourth possibility is transmural migration of endogenous intestinal bacteria. Many patients, especially adults with cirrhosis, will develop primary peritonitis with enteric organisms. Bacteria probably cross the bowel wall during local ischemia or systemic shock states.

Patients dying of primary pneumococcal peritonitis can have microscopic evidence of enteritis. Patients dying of septicemia secondary to perforated appendix or peptic ulcer do not have microscopic enteritis. Bacterial enteritis may lead to peritoneal contamination in primary peritonitis.

The documented association with hepatic malfunction suggests that diminished clearance of enteric bacteria by the liver may contribute to the pathogenesis of primary peritonitis. Under normal conditions, the portal venous blood is sterile, but bacteria can be released into this system by enteric infections or local anatomic lesions, such as those found in regional enteritis. These are usually trapped by the sinusoidal phagocytes of the liver. In cirrhosis, however, much of the portal flow is shunted around the liver sinusoids to the systemic circulation via collaterals. The abnormal hepatic circulation also permits contamination of the portal lymph, which becomes ascitic fluid in cirrhotic patients.

The cirrhotic patient is susceptible to unusual opportunistic infections of many types, even *Vibrio fetus* and *Pasteurella multocida*.[83] Patients with these infections have low serum protein levels,[84] but the pattern is not the same as in nephrotic children who lack gamma globulins. Alcoholics have a neutrophil dysfunction caused by ethanol or serum inhibitors. Simberkoff et al [84] found that cirrhotic patients had a small but significant depression of serum bactericidal and opsonic activity against *Serratia marcescens* but not against *E. coli*. More impressive, however, was a profoundly decreased bactericidal and opsonic activity of ascitic fluid against both organisms, along with decreased IgG, IgM, and complement levels in this fluid.

TABLE 34-2. PATHOGENS ISOLATED FROM PERITONEAL CULTURES IN PATIENTS WITH CIRRHOSIS AND PRIMARY PERITONITIS

	No.
Number of episodes	54
Single organism	50
Total organisms observed	62
Organisms	
E. coli	20
Klebsiella	7
Pneumococcus	8
Streptococcus	11
Bacteroides	3
Pseudomonas aeruginosa	2
Aeromonas hydrophila	1
Enterobacter aerogenes	1
Citrobacter	1
Proteus morganii	1
Unidentified gram-positive rod	1
Staphylococcus aureus	1
Pasteurella multocida	1
Anaerobic diphtheroids	1
Candida albicans	1
Peptococcus	1
Unidentified gram-negative rod	1
Enteric	41
Nonenteric	21

From Correia JP, Conn HO: Spontaneous bacterial peritonitis in cirrhosis: Endemic or epidemic? *Med Clin North Am* 59:963, 1975.

Cirrhotic patients are also prone to spontaneous infections of other fluid collections, such as pleural effusions.

In either cirrhosis or nephrosis, the presence of ascites is probably the principal host factor in the pathogenesis of primary peritonitis. Bacteria entering the fluid are in a relatively protected environment.

Spontaneous peritonitis may also occur in patients who receive systemic steroids for systemic lupus erythematosus,[75] other collagen vascular disease, or in patients who receive immunosuppression after transplantation or chemotherapy for neoplasia.[85] It is rare in normal adults.

Systemic lupus erythematosus is characterized by an entire spectrum of peritoneal inflammatory syndromes.[86] Ten to 37 percent of patients will have abdominal pain at one time or another. Fewer will develop an acute abdomen—lupus peritonitis—due to aseptic peritonitis, vasculitis, or pancreatitis. Fewer still will develop bacterial peritonitis secondary to intestinal infarction. Lupus patients may also develop primary peritonitis, usually with encapsulated bacteria.[75] Most of these patients have been treated with steroids.

In patients receiving chemotherapy for malignancy, however, a specific primary peritonitis syndrome has been described. The ileocecal syndrome usually occurs in patients with leukemia or lymphoma.[85] The bacterial peritonitis arises in the area of the ileocecal valve and may be due to a transmural migration of enteric bacteria, as a result of either tumor necrosis or microscopic mucosal ulceration. Operation is of little benefit in these patients. High-dose antibiotics, which cover the spectrum of bowel organisms, are given if cecitis is found on barium exam. Occurrence of the syndrome during relapse of the malignancy is uniformly fatal. Perforation of the bowel is also lethal, regardless of surgical intervention. In contrast, the acute appendicitis that also occurs in these patients responds to immediate surgery.

Predisposing Factors. A number of procedures increase the incidence of primary peritonitis, especially in patients with cirrhosis and ascites. A recent paracentesis, upper gastrointestinal endoscopy, portacaval anastomosis, arterial or umbilical vein catheterization, barium enema, or sigmoidoscopy appear to increase the risk of primary peritonitis.[87] Flood's syndrome is primary peritonitis associated with an ulcerated umbilical hernia and ascitic fistula.[88] Any patient with an ascitic fluid leak has a high risk of peritonitis.

In nephrotic children, peritonitis appears during an active stage of the renal disease, with increased urinary loss of protein, hypoproteinemia, and probably subclinical ascites. Peritonitis may precede the diagnosis of nephrotic syndrome, and any child with primary peritonitis should be evaluated for renal disease.

In adults, foreign bodies, such as IUDs in the genital tract, may predispose to primary peritonitis.

Clinical Manifestations

Unlike secondary bacterial peritonitis, which often begins with an acute or even catastrophic picture, primary peritonitis usually develops over a period of days to weeks. McDougal et al [72] found that infants and neonates often develop poor feeding, a decreased temperature, and decreased platelet count over a period of one to two days and ultimately become distended with infected ascites. Older children will have a rapid onset of abdominal pain, nausea, vomiting, diarrhea, fever, and a diffusely tender abdomen, with guarding, rigidity, and rebound and local tenderness. Acute appendicitis is frequently the preoperative diagnosis. Diarrhea is more common in the younger age group. A brisk leukocytosis is characteristic, and the abdominal roentgenograms show no mass or free air.[82]

Abdominal pain is a variable symptom in cirrhotic patients. At least one half have fever and one third have increasing hepatic encephalopathy.[89] Abdominal tenderness, decreased bowel sounds, hyperthermia, and hypotension occur less commonly. Rapid accumulation of ascites highly suggests intraperitoneal infection in cirrhotics.[74]

Gonococcal perihepatitis begins as a sudden pain in the right upper quadrant, which radiates to the shoulder. A hepatic rub may be heard during respiration. Fever, tenderness, guarding, and rebound may be present. Genital infection may or may not be evident.

Diagnosis

Primary peritonitis is most easily diagnosed by analysis of ascitic fluid obtained by paracentesis with or without peritoneal lavage. An ascitic fluid leukocyte count >300 per mm^3 with more than 30 percent neutrophils is diagnostic of intraperitoneal infection, although after aggressive diuresis, some cirrhotics will have cell counts of 300 to 500 per mm^3 without infection. A specimen is centrifuged, and a Gram stain is made of the sediment. The finding of only gram-positive organisms is highly suggestive of primary peritonitis, but the presence of a surgically correctable lesion cannot be excluded, especially if gram-negative bacilli are seen on smear. Mixed gram-positive and gram-negative organisms are characteristic of a perforated viscus. The fluid is cultured to insure rapid identification of the responsible organisms. Blood cultures in symptomatic patients often yield the same organism that is found intraperitoneally. Recovery of more than a single organism is highly suggestive of a perforated viscus.

The direct Gram stain in cirrhotic ascites has a high false-negative rate.[89] Kline et al [90] have prospectively performed paracentesis on 50 cirrhotic patients admitted for management of their cirrhosis. Three patients were found to have bacteria in the ascitic fluid and subsequently developed evidence of primary peritonitis. The authors suggest that prospective taps are useful because of the high morbidity and mortality associated with this disease.

Primary peritonitis in children is often associated with urinary tract infections or pneumonia.[82] Cultures of the urine and sputum may aid in rapid identification of the causative organisms in such cases. Although the organisms may reach the peritoneal cavity via the genital tract in females, vaginal cultures have not proved helpful in the modern era.

Reichert and Valle [91] have used laparoscopy to confirm the diagnosis of gonorrheal perihepatitis. This may give a higher yield than paracentesis in selected patients.

Treatment

Any patient in whom a surgically correctable lesion cannot be excluded should undergo exploratory laparotomy. This is especially true when gram-negative organisms are seen on the smear of the sediment from a peritoneal tap. Golden and Shaw [82] recommend surgery in children even if pneumococci are recovered in pure culture.

Two patient subgroups have an increased risk of complications from exploratory laparotomy. Patients with nephrotic syndrome have increased morbidity from depressed wound healing. Therefore, Fowler [71] withholds operation in patients with abdominal pain and proteinuria if only gram-positive organisms are obtained on peritoneal tap. If gram-negative organisms are obtained, laparatomy and appendectomy are carried out. Appendectomy adds little morbidity or mortality to the operation and is done in children to rule out a source of subsequent diagnostic confusion.[82] No drains are left in the patients. Any child with gram-positive primary peritonitis should be evaluated for occult renal disease. Five of ten patients in one series had nephrotic syndrome that was not suspected until peritonitis developed.

Cirrhotic patients with rapid hepatic decompensation also do poorly after laparotomy.[74] If clinical data indicate primary peritonitis, peritoneal dialysis with antibiotic-containing fluids may be indicated. This permits rapid removal of large numbers of bacteria but necessitates massive parenteral protein replacement therapy. Disseminated intravascular coagulation is frequently a lethal complication of this infection.

Relative contraindications to peritoneal tap include previous abdominal operation or possible meconium peritonitis in neonates. These patients often have bowel adherent to the anterior abdominal wall, which may be punctured by the procedure. Major complications including bowel perforation have been reported following diagnostic paracentesis in 7 of 242 procedures.[87]

Antibiotic therapy for *Streptococcus pneumoniae* or *Streptococcus pyogenes* is parenteral penicillin G. All other patients, including all those with gram-negative infections, should be treated initially with an aminoglycoside and ampicillin unless anaerobes are suspected. The antibiotic therapy is then adjusted on the basis of culture and sensitivity results as they are received.

Prognosis

In the early part of this century, the mortality of primary peritonitis in children approached 100 percent, even though many of these children were operated upon.[80] Intraperitoneal pneumococcal infection is a lethal disease in the absence of specific therapy. With the advent, first, of specific pneumococcal vaccines and, ultimately, of antibiotics, the mortality of primary peritonitis in childhood has fallen to between 5 and 10 percent.[72] In neonates, the mortality may still be 40 to 50 percent.[72]

Approximately half of cirrhotic patients expire from sepsis after primary peritonitis.[74] Nevertheless, the overall mortality is much higher (approaching 95 percent) because the majority of patients die of complications of their cirrhosis. The prognosis in those patients with hepatic encephalopathy, hypothermia, hypotension, azotemia, or concurrent infection is poor.

UNUSUAL FORMS OF INFECTIVE PERITONITIS

GRANULOMATOUS PERITONITIS

Granulomatous peritonitis is an infection or sterile inflammation characterized by an intense peritoneal reaction, with formation of local granulomas. Ultimately, dense adhesions form, with subsequent risk of bowel obstruction. The infectious causes are considered first.

Tuberculous Peritonitis

Incidence

Public health measures have diminished the incidence of tuberculosis, and the development of effective chemotherapeutic agents has closed most of the large sanitoria where patients with tuberculosis were once confined. Lougheed et al,[92] in 1963, found tuberculous peritonitis in 40 of 3,750 patients treated for tuberculosis over an 8-year period. Other large series have reported an incidence of 0.004 to 0.7 percent of all cases of tuberculosis.[93] The incidence is especially low in countries that monitor dairy herds for tuberculosis. Characteristically, this is a disease of younger people, with approximately 50 percent of the cases occurring between the ages of 20 and 40, with a 2:1 predominance of females.[93] Blacks have an increased susceptibility to all forms of tuberculosis, including tuberculous peritonitis.

Etiology

The microbiologic characteristics of *Mycobacterium tuberculosis* have been discussed in Chapter 7. Mycobacterium types I, II, III, and IV are rare causes of abdominal tuberculosis.

Pathogenesis and Pathology

Patients with a documented exposure to active tuberculosis, evidence of previous pulmonary tuberculosis, or poor nutrition are at high risk. Patients susceptible to other forms of primary peritonitis may also develop tuberculous peritonitis.

In the last century, primary infection of mesenteric lymph nodes often occurred after ingestion of the organism in contaminated milk. Patients with achlorhydria or malabsorption syndromes were particularly susceptible. Infection after partial gastrectomy is well known, and Yu [94] reported seven cases after jejunoileal bypass for obesity.

Dineen et al [93] propose five possible sources of infection: (1) reactivation of latent peritoneal tuberculosis, (2) a primary extraperitoneal focus, usually in the lung, (3) an infected mesenteric lymph node, (4) contamination from tuberculous enteritis, or (5) tuberculous salpingitis in the female. Most cases are associated with a primary pulmonary focus, which may be occult. The peritoneum is usually infected by hematogenous spread.[92]

Clinical Manifestations

The disease develops over weeks to months, with increased abdominal girth and dull cramping or aching pain aggravated by movement. Abdominal pain is found in 93 percent of patients, and most patients have fever, night sweats, weight loss, and ascites leading to abdominal enlargement. Acute fever and rigors suggest acute bacterial infection. Abdominal tenderness and a doughy abdominal mass are frequent but inconstant signs. Leukocytosis is mild or absent. Positive PPD skin test results are usually found.

Diagnosis

The diagnosis of tuberculous peritonitis should be suspected in patients with insidious onset of abdominal pain, fever, and tenderness but with a normal white blood cell count.[95] A positive history of exposure to tuberculosis, a positive PPD test, or roentgenographic findings that are consistent with tuberculosis are helpful. A sputum examination positive for acid-fast bacilli provides presumptive evidence for the diagnosis. A paracentesis rarely yields visible organisms, but if a liter of ascites is cultured, the organism will be recovered in 80 percent of cases.[95] Singh et al [95] recommend needle biopsy of the peritoneum and recovered caseating granulomas in 64 percent of their cases. Blind peritoneal needle biopsy is contraindicated in the absence of ascitic fluid. A high protein content (> 2.5 gm per dl) and low glucose level (<30 mg per dl) of peritoneal fluid are characteristic.[93] A peritoneal lymphocytosis of 70 percent or greater is also usual.

The roentgenographic findings of tuberculous peritonitis are rather nonspecific. Abdominal films show mild ileus, ascites, elevation of the diaphragm, and loss of the psoas outline. Barium enema studies usually show a rapid transit time, with fixation of the small intestine and a slightly widened space between the intestinal loops. Occasionally, spasm of the cecum characteristic of tuberculous enteritis can be demonstrated.

Laparotomy is frequently required for definitive diagnosis, but laparoscopy may permit suitable biopsies under direct vision. Tubercles are scattered throughout the peritoneal cavity, especially the omentum. Laparoscopy is contraindicated in the absence of ascites.

Treatment

Triple antituberculosis drug therapy alone is curative if the diagnosis can be made without operation (Chapter 18). The need for ancillary operation is controversial. Some surgeons recommend laparotomy to evacuate ascites, excise caseating lesions, and lyse adhesions.[92] In Dineen's series, 36 patients underwent abdominal operations without mortality, and in 20 the diagnosis was made only at operation.[93] Adhesions may be decreased by early operation and evacuation of caseous material; [92] steroids have also been advocated. Chemotherapy is maintained for 18 months after operation.[95]

Prognosis

Prior to the advent of chemotherapy, the mortality of this disease was 49 percent. Now it is less than 7 percent in most series.[95]

Abdominal Actinomycosis

Actinomycosis is a chronic, progressive, suppurative disease characterized by formation of multiple abscesses, draining sinuses, fibrous adhesions, and abundant granulation tissue. The appearance of sulfur granules in the lesions, sinus walls, or discharges of involved tissues is characteristic. Prior to the discovery of antibiotics, the abdominal form of actinomycosis generally presented as a disease process of many years' duration that was ultimately fatal.[96]

Etiology

The *Actinomyces* organisms are gram-positive, non-spore-forming microaerophilic or obligate anaerobes (Chapter 6). *Actinomyces israelii* is usually responsible for the disease in humans.

Incidence

Actinomycosis is encountered worldwide but is unusual in the United States. Young adult males are most often affected. Putman et al [97] reported only 122 cases of abdominal actinomycoses during a 35-year period.

Pathogenesis

Actinomyces organisms are normal inhabitants of the oral cavity and tonsillar crypts. They are swallowed and reach the distal bowel. Abdominal actinomycosis is most commonly discovered after appendectomy or drainage of a periappendiceal abscess. The colon, stomach, liver, gallbladder, pancreas, small bowel, anorectal region, pelvis, abdominal wall, and other sites can also be involved.[96] Usually, a single organ is infected, and disseminated intra-abdominal actinomycosis is uncommon. Pelvic actinomycosis can follow introduction of intrauterine contraceptive devices.

A. israelii probably cannot invade the intact mucous membrane, but disruption of gastrointestinal mucosa by disease or trauma allows the organisms to pentrate into adjacent tissue. The organism becomes aggregated into sulfur granules, and the resulting suppurative granulomatous reaction produces abscesses, draining sinuses, and fistulas.

Other pathogenic bacteria are virtually always associated with actinomycotic abscess, and a synergistic interaction between *Actinomyces* and other microorganisms has been postulated. Coliforms and anaerobic, gram-negative bacilli are commonly found in abdominal actinomycosis, while *Actinobacillus actinomycetemcomitans* and *Eikenella corrodens* are found more commonly in those with thoracic and pulmonary lesions. The latter is a normal inhabitant of the oropharynx. All are susceptible to penicillin.

Clinical Manifestations

Abdominal actinomycosis is one of the great imitators in clinical practice. Granules are not always present, and other organisms capable of producing chronic infections can form loose aggregates or even granules. Actinomycosis generally presents as a chronic, localized, inflammatory process associated with fever and leukocytosis, but the diagnosis is often not suspected in the absence of a draining sinus. There is usually a latent interval of days to weeks between the onset of symptoms and presentation with a persistent, draining sinus.

In the early stages, abdominal actinomycosis may be indistinguishable from other processes. Acute appendicitis with or without perforation, inflammatory bowel disease, carcinoma, or acute cholecystitis can all be simulated. The majority of patients have had an episode of acute abdominal inflammation, which, in retrospect, represented actinomycosis. The diagnosis is not recognized until a enterocutaneous fistula develops. Nonspecific constitutional disturbances may be particularly severe. Pyrexia, anemia, elevated erythrocyte sedimentation rate, leukocytosis, weight loss, nausea, vomiting, and pain are among the more frequent findings.

Bacteriologic cultures of a sinus reveal secondary infection with other enteric or saprophytic microbes. Only curettings from the depth of the tract will recover the organism. Sulfur granules, when seen, are diagnostic.

Diagnosis

The diagnosis is confirmed by histologic identification of the actinomycotic granule or culture of the organism.

Nocardia asteroides and *Nocardia brasiliensis,* gram-positive, acid-fast, branching, higher bacteria, produce a chronic infection similar to actinomycosis. The organisms may form loose aggregates of organisms or even granules. However, fibrosis is rare, and liquefaction is evident in most cases. This differentiation is extremely important because penicillin cures most patients with actinomycosis, but treatment of nocardiosis with penicillin is inadequate and usually lethal. Actinomycosis must also be distinguished from all other causes of granulomatous peritonitis and intraperitoneal infections.

Prognosis

Before the advent of antibiotics, the prognosis of patients with abdominal actinomycosis was grave, with a mean survival of seven months after diagnosis. Now, cure rates of 88–96 percent are reported with antibiotics, and deaths are rare.[97]

Treatment

Before antibiotics, surgical treatment included incision, evacuation, and scraping of abscesses, followed by repeated irrigations with an antiseptic solution, such as iodine or hydrogen peroxide. In the antibiotic era, incision and drainage, with curettage of abscess cavities or sinus tract, remain essential in many instances of abdominal actinomycosis. Penicillin is the antibiotic of choice. Erythromycin and rifampin are most active in vitro, followed by penicillin G, cephaloridine, minocycline, and clindamycin. Aminoglycoside activity is negligible. Combination antibiotic therapy is desirable in many instances because of the frequency of associated bacteria with abdominal actinomycosis. Antibiotics alone are generally curative even in advanced disease, but operation may be required to resolve draining fistulas. Massive doses of penicillin are required for weeks in the majority of patients to effect a cure, but months of antibiotic treatment may be required in the more refractory instances.[96]

Amebic Peritonitis

Amebic peritonitis is unusual in the United States, although numerous cases have been reported in men returning from Vietnam. The asymptomatic carrier state in the United States may reach 5 percent,[98] and amebic dysentery may be misdiagnosed as ulcerative or granulomatous colitis. Progression to toxic megacolon is common. Three or four percent of patients with amebic dysentery are first seen by their doctors with perforation of the colon or small bowel and profound shock. The mortality of mixed amebic and fecal peritonitis is 75–100 percent but can be lowered by early operation. Chronic cases, with formation of pericecal ameboma, have been reported.[99] Patients treated by simple appendectomy often develop fecal fistulas, which fail to heal until appropriate antiamebic therapy is begun.

Amebic peritonitis occurs in 6–9 percent of patients with hepatic abscess,[100] and rupture may be preceded by increasing right upper quadrant pain. These patients present with abdominal distention and fever and may deteriorate quite rapidly, but a rigid abdomen is not always present.

Abscesses of the left lobe or the inferior surface of the liver can rupture into the peritoneal cavity, even though most amebic abscesses of the liver are situated on the superior hepatic surface and tend to perforate into the pleural space (Chapter 36).

In the United States, most of these patients are male, have emigrated from or have recently traveled to Latin America, or have served in Vietnam. The organisms may be overlooked in Gram-stained specimens of peritoneal exudates and are best seen in fixed specimens stained with iron-hematoxylin. Shaggy perforations of the cecum or ruptured liver abscesses discovered at laparotomy suggest the diagnosis, and the microbiology laboratory should be notified. Serologic test results, so valuable for the diagnosis of hepatic abscess, are almost always negative in acute peritonitis secondary to amebic bowel perforation (Chapter 11).

In the United States, the diagnosis is usually made at laparotomy because the disease is rare and is not considered preoperatively. The trophozoites are best seen on biopsy of the liver abscess or cecal wall. For cecal perforation, resection with exteriorization of the bowel ends is indicated because suture closure or primary anastomosis usually fails.[99] Drains usually result in formation of sinus tracts. Combinations of antibiotics are given because of the polymicrobial bacterial contamination. Drug therapy with a systemic amebicide is necessary—the current drug of choice is metronidazole for at least 10 days; a parenteral form is now available. Eradication of the amebic reservoir (Chapters 11 and 36) requires both intestinal and extraintestinal amebicidal drugs.

Candida Peritonitis

Candida can cause both suppurative and granulomatous infections (Chapter 9). *Candida* peritonitis is frequently associated with a mixed bacterial peritonitis because *Candida* colonization of the gastrointestinal tract is common. Cohen et al [102] found that greater than 50 percent of patients cultured carried *Candida* as part of their stable flora somewhere in the gastrointestinal tract. Colonization rates increased proximally to distally with 59 percent of patients carrying *Candida* in the colon. Numerous factors increase the rate of *Candida* colonization, including antibiotic therapy, prolonged hospitalization, local radiation therapy, ostomy sites, and antacid therapy.

Patients who develop any type of *Candida* infection are usually immunodepressed. Malignancy, corticosteroid therapy, antineoplastic therapy, radiation therapy, malnutrition, uremia, severe burns, and concomitant infection are important factors.

The incidence of *Candida* peritonitis may be increasing with the greater use of cimetidine to manage peptic ulcer disease. The decreased acid production may allow *Candida* overgrowth and mycotic perforation rather than peptic perforation as seen in the past. Operations on the achlorhydric stomach may permit peritoneal contamination with gastric *Candida*. In addition, aminoglycosides appear to inhibit the candicidal ability of human neutrophils, so these antibiotics may potentiate candidal infections.

Candida enteritis in debilitated or immunosuppressed patients can result in bowel invasion by pseudohyphal forms and bowel perforation with secondary peritonitis. This disease is rare, and most causes of *Candida* peritonitis result when *Candida* cells reach the peritoneal cavity either by perforation of the gastrointestinal tract or via paracentesis or peritoneal dialysis catheter. When the gastrointestinal tract is the source, *Candida* are always found with bacterial microorganisms. Dialysis peritonitis is usually a monomicrobial infection.

Candida peritonitis associated with gastrointestinal tract perforation has a high mortality for two reasons: (1) the compromised host mounts an inadequate response to the infection,[103] and (2) most physicians ignore the *Candida* when treating peritonitis with antibiotics. Disseminated *Candida* sepsis sometimes results.[103a]

If *Candida* is found as part of the polymicrobial flora secondary peritonitis, systemic antifungal agents should be administered until the patient is well. Long-term therapy, so necessary for adequate treatment of disseminated *Candida* infections, can be avoided in these patients if they respond to combined operative and antimicrobial therapy within a week or two. A total dose of 0.5 to 1.0 gram of amphotericin B will usually suffice.

Dialysis peritonitis usually responds to peritoneal amphotericin B lavage [104] unless the patient develops abdominal pain, ileus, distention, and fever when systemic therapy is indicated.

Probably the best treatment for this disease is prevention. Oral nystatin or clotrimazole effectively decrease candidal colonization of the gastrointestinal tract in patients at risk. We use oral nystatin as chemoprophylaxis in patients receiving systemic antibiotics for severe surgical infections, as well as in immunosuppressed patients.

Other Granulomatous Infections

Almost any disseminated fungal disease (Chapter 9) or parasite (Chapter 11) can reach the peritoneal cavity to produce a granulomatous intra-abdominal infection. *Pityrosporum, Nocardia,* and *Strongyloides* have been occasional causes of intraperitoneal infection by invasion of the bowel wall and perforation or, more rarely, by hematogenous dissemination.

PERITONITIS ASSOCIATED WITH INTRAPERITONEAL PROSTHESES

PERITONEAL DIALYSIS

Since most forms of peritoneal dialysis require an indwelling Silastic catheter that passes from the peritoneal cavity to the skin, these patients with renal failure are at increased risk for peritonitis.

Incidence

With general improvements in cuffed catheter design (eg, the Tenckhoff catheter), the incidence of peritonitis for each peritoneal dialysis has fallen to 0.3 to 0.7 percent.[105,106] Since these patients are usually dialyzed three times per week, the risk is approximately 75 percent per year of dialysis. If patients undergo chronic dialysis in intensive care units, the risk is 3.6 percent per dialysis, possibly because the dialyses are done by relatively inexperienced nurses who care for other seriously ill (and sometimes septic) patients, thereby increasing the risk of contamination.[107]

Vaamonde et al [108] found that the risk of peritonitis in acute renal failure is 6.3 percent per dialysis. In contrast to patients who are on chronic peritoneal dialysis, these patients are seriously ill, and the temporary catheters usually lack a Dacron cuff so that the risk of contamination from the catheter track is increased.

Etiology

The organisms causing peritonitis in chronic dialysis patients are usually skin organisms—staphylococci, diphtheroids, coliforms, or *Candida* (Table 34-3). The organisms isolated during acute peritoneal dialysis are those found in the intensive care unit (ie, *Pseudomonas, Serratia*),[107] those isolated from other sites in the patient, or enteric organisms.[108] In 15 to 35 percent of clinical episodes, no bacteria can be isolated. Presumably, the clinical findings are due to pyrogen contamination of the dialysis fluid.[106]

Pathogenesis

Large numbers of bacteria can normally be cleared by peritoneal defense mechanisms without establishing overt peritonitis. Foreign bodies of all kinds, however, increase the risk of infection, although the risk is lower with the cuffed Silastic catheters than others. In addition, fluid deprived of opsonins potentiates intraperitoneal infection, allowing a small bacterial inoculum to proliferate, partially protected from local defense mechanisms.[45a] The tract associated with percutaneously placed dialysis catheters may become secondarily infected, leading to direct contamination of the peritoneal fluid from the skin.

Clinical Manifestations and Diagnosis

The diagnosis of intraperitoneal infection is first suspected when the dialysate fluid becomes cloudy. Quantitative bac-

TABLE 34-3. ORGANISMS CAUSING PERITONEAL INFECTIONS IN PATIENTS RECEIVING PROLONGED PERITONEAL DIALYSIS

Organism	Number of Infections: *First Episode*	*Subsequent Episodes*	*Total*
Staphylococcus albus	14 (58%)	12 (36%)	25 (46%)
Staphylococcus aureus	6 (25%)	4 (12%)	10 (17%)
Acinetobacter anitratum	0	5	5
Escherichia coli	1	2	3
Proteus mirabilis	1	2	3
Streptococcus faecalis	1	2	3
Pseudomonas aeruginosa	0	2	2
Others *	1	4	5
TOTAL	24	33	57

* One each of *Streptococcus pyogenes, Streptococcus viridans, Bacillus cereus, Enterobacter aerogenes,* and *Candida albicans.*

From Cohen SL, Percival A: Prolonged peritoneal dialysis in patients awaiting renal transplantation. *Br Med J* 1:409, 1968.

terial counts of dialysis fluid have not been used but might prove to be a sensitive test for intraperitoneal infection. The outflow dialysis fluid should always be cultured and often is contaminated, but this is not a reliable indicator of infection. Brewer et al [107] found that 11 of 568 routine cultures of fluid were positive in the absence of clinical infection. In Vaamonde's series, there were 39 positive cultures not associated with infection.[108]

The usual peritoneal signs of tenderness, guarding, and rebound pain are variable, probably because the dialysate dilutes or removes the local products of inflammation even though infection persists. Abdominal pain is frequent, even in the absence of infection. Brewer et al [107] discovered the dialysis catheter was in contact with the diaphragm in several patients who developed signs of an acute abdomen. Repositioning the catheter resolved the symptoms. Even temperature measurements are not reliable. Many uremic patients remain afebrile or become hypothermic in response to infection, especially if cold dialysate is used.[108] Patients develop chills and fever after infusion of endotoxin-contaminated dialysate or, in a small group of patients, hypertonic dialysate.[108]

A reliable finding in peritonitis in these patients is a rapid increase in the protein loss into the peritoneal dialysate. Peritoneal dialysis patients have a chronic protein loss secondary to dialysis but seldom become hypoalbuminemic if they eat a well-balanced, high-calorie, high-protein diet. When peritonitis supervenes, however, protein losses may be multiplied 10-fold and dietary intake falls, so that a severe catabolic state results. These patients frequently require hyperalimentation and protein supplementation during their episode of peritonitis.

Factors that increase the risk of peritoneal infection include severe debility or multiple trauma, the use of open rather than closed dialysis systems, the use of noncuffed catheters, dialysis done by inexperienced personnel who care for acutely ill patients, prolonged dialysis, and leakage of fluid around the catheter.

Cultures and Gram stains of the dialysate are obtained once the diagnosis of intraperitoneal infection is suspected. Centrifugation of the fluid will increase the yields of the Gram stain.

Treatment

Black et al [109] have proposed a specific treatment protocol. Continuous dialysis is instituted to prevent fluid loculation and loss of exchange surface secondary to adhesion formation. Parenteral and intraperitoneal antibiotics are given and dosages are adjusted on the basis of serum and peritoneal fluid antibiotic levels (Table 34-4). Dialysis is carried out until culture results are negative for three days and the patient is asymptomatic. Then intermittent dialysis is done for an additional one to three days, and oral antibiotics are administered for another one to three weeks. Patients are instructed in a high-protein diet to make up for protein losses during dialysis.

The catheter itself rarely requires removal unless there is infection of the subcutaneous tunnel. The catheter should be replaced if the patient develops recurrent infection with the same organism, however. In these cases, the peritoneal cavity is explored to rule out occult intraperitoneal or subcutaneous abscess. In patients who develop peritonitis while awaiting imminent transplantation, the catheter should be removed and systemic antibiotics administered. Hemodialysis is instituted. Peritoneal dialysis can safely be performed up to the time of transplantation, however, if the dialysate remains sterile.

If the bowel is perforated by the dialysis catheter during percutaneous placement, most authors advocate immediate laparotomy, with repair of the perforation and placement of another catheter so that immediate lavage can be started. These patients are treated by Black's protocol [109] and do well. Some authors recommend that if perforation occurs, another catheter should be placed percutaneously and the patients should not undergo laparotomy unless the symptoms increase during treatment for peritonitis.[110] We do not recommend this procedure.

Inadequately treated generalized peritonitis in patients with indwelling peritoneal dialysis catheters usually results in adhesion formation and rapid fall in the dialysis

TABLE 34-4. Doses of Antibiotics

Drug *	Systemic Dose	Intraperitoneal Dose
Oxacillin	50–100 mg/kg/day	10 mg/l
Ampicillin	50–100 mg/kg/day	20–25 mg/l
Penicillin G	100,000–150,000 units/kg/day	1,000–1,500 units/l
Carbenicillin	50–100 mg/kg/day	200 mg/l
Cephalothin	40–80 mg/kg/day	10–25 mg/l
Gentamicin	1–2 mg/kg/every third day	5 mg/l
Kanamycin	7.5 mg/kg/every third day	10–15 mg/l
Lincomycin	10–15 mg/kg/day	5–10 mg/l
Clindamycin	5–15 mg/kg/day	5–10 mg/l
Amphotericin B†	0.5–1.0 mg/kg/day or every other day	3 mg/l

* Tetracycline, chloramphenicol, and erythromycin should not be used.

† Therapy should be instituted with small doses (1–5 mg/day), with subsequent increments depending on clinical condition. Pretreatment with aspirin and hydrocortisone reduces febrile reactions.

From Black HR, Finkelstein FO, Lee RV: The treatment of peritonitis in patients with chronic indwelling catheters. *Trans Am Soc Artif Intern Organs* 20:115, 1974.

capability of the peritoneal cavity. These patients most often require hemodialysis, but recovery of peritoneal clearance over weeks or months following peritonitis can occur.

PERITONITIS ASSOCIATED WITH PERITONEOVENOUS SHUNT

Recently, peritoneovenous shunts have been implanted for the palliation of intractable ascites.[111] These patients have a high risk of primary infection of the ascitic fluid. The removal of the ascites from the peritoneal cavity may decrease the incidence of peritonitis in these patients, but it is too early to demonstrate this from the published data.

The incidence of infection associated with shunts is unknown, but preliminary reports indicate that the shunts should be removed to allow eradication of the infection. The shunt apparently acts as a foreign body, which potentiates the infection.

INFECTIONS ASSOCIATED WITH VENTRICULOPERITONEAL SHUNTS

The diagnosis and treatment of infected ventriculoperitoneal shunts is discussed in detail in Chapter 28. Ventriculoperitoneal shunts drain cerebrospinal fluid from the obstructed ventricles to the peritoneal cavity. A shunt infection rate of 20 percent has been reported.[112] The patients usually present with septicemia, headache, neck stiffness, and evidence of increased intracranial pressure.

Acute abdominal infection is rare with ventriculoperitoneal shunts,[112] but primary shunt infection can lead to seeding of the peritoneal cavity. Usually, central nervous system symptoms are minimal compared to the abdominal findings. The children usually have a history of several days of anorexia, fever, abdominal pain, nausea, and vomiting. A leukocytosis is characteristic. All patients with a shunt and abdominal pain should have a percutaneous puncture of the shunt. Analysis of the fluid usually shows decreased glucose, and recovery of organisms is diagnostic. *Staphylococcus aureus* and *S. epidermidis* are the most common pathogens. Gram-positive organisms suggest primary shunt infection, but gram-negative organisms may indicate an ascending infection from primary or secondary peritonitis.

The recommended treatment is high-dose intravenous and intraventricular antibiotics for two weeks, followed by shunt replacement and an additional two weeks of antibiotics.

DISEASES MIMICKING BACTERIAL PERITONITIS

Other, noninfectious diseases can present with acute abdominal pain and may mimic peritonitis. Periodic peritonitis (Mediterranean fever, periodic polyserositis), porphyria, and hyperlipemic crisis can all mimic an acute abdominal catastrophe, but laparotomy fails to demonstrate pathologic findings.

INTRA-ABDOMINAL ABSCESS

Intra-abdominal abscesses are purulent collections of fluid separated by a more or less well defined wall from surrounding tissue. These abscesses usually contain necrotic debris and bacteria, although truly sterile abscesses can be produced. An abscess, by definition, is the result of a subacute or chronic inflammation because the accumulation of neutrophils and formation of a fibrinous or fibrous capsule requires time. Thus, free peritonitis, which is characteristically an acute inflammation, may lead to abscess formation during the resolution phase as infected fluid becomes loculated into anatomic recesses. Perhaps two thirds of abscesses, however, occur adjacent to an inflamed viscus without the intervening stage of free peritonitis.

ANATOMY OF ABSCESS FORMATION

Intraperitoneal Spaces

The posterior peritoneal reflections and mesenteric attachments of the intra-abdominal viscera divide the intraperitoneal space into anatomic areas where abscesses can form (Figs. 34-3, 34-9 and 34-10).[113] The transverse mesocolon divides the peritoneal cavity posteriorly into an upper and lower space. The greater omentum lies immediately adjacent to the anterior abdominal wall and functionally completes the division. The lower peritoneal space is, in turn, divided into right upper and left lower portions by the diagonal origin of the small bowel mesentery.

The intraperitoneal circulation described previously follows the pattern shown in Figure 34-9.[114,115] The most dependent recess is the pelvis, where the pouch of Douglas lies between the rectum and the body of the uterus, and the perirectal and perivesical fossas lie lateral to the rectum and bladder. The peritoneal circulation favors unilateral spread of exudate because the phrenocolic ligament, which spans the diaphragm, spleen, and splenic flexure of the colon, interrupts the flow into the left subphrenic space during respiration (Fig. 34-9).[114] Left subphrenic abscesses are, therefore, commonly associated with retrogastric (lesser sac) lesions. Bilateral subphrenic abscesses are uncommon, since the right and left subhepatic spaces are separated by the falciform ligament. The left subhepatic space is divided by the gastrohepatic omentum into an anterior space and a lesser sac (Figs. 34-9 and 34-10). Abscesses can form in any of these areas.

The lesser sac communicates with the general peritoneal cavity via the foramen of Winslow between the free border of the gastrohepatic omentum and the posterior parietal peritoneum. The opening is small, so visceral performations elsewhere in the peritoneal cavity rarely produce suppuration of the lesser sac. Primary lesser sac abscesses can spread downward via the foramen of Winslow, across the hepatic flexure of the colon, into the right gutter, and then upward into the subphrenic space. The movement of water-soluble contrast material selectively injected into various intraperitoneal spaces is depicted in Figure 34-9.[114] In general, the distance a material spreads depends upon its volume, viscosity, and specific gravity. The mobility of the small bowel tends to limit the accumulation of fluid in the central portion of the peritoneal cavity under normal circumstances. However, truly massive abscesses (horseshoe abscesses) may extend down one gutter to the pelvis and up the opposite side.[116] Pelvic abscesses occur below the brim of the true pelvis.

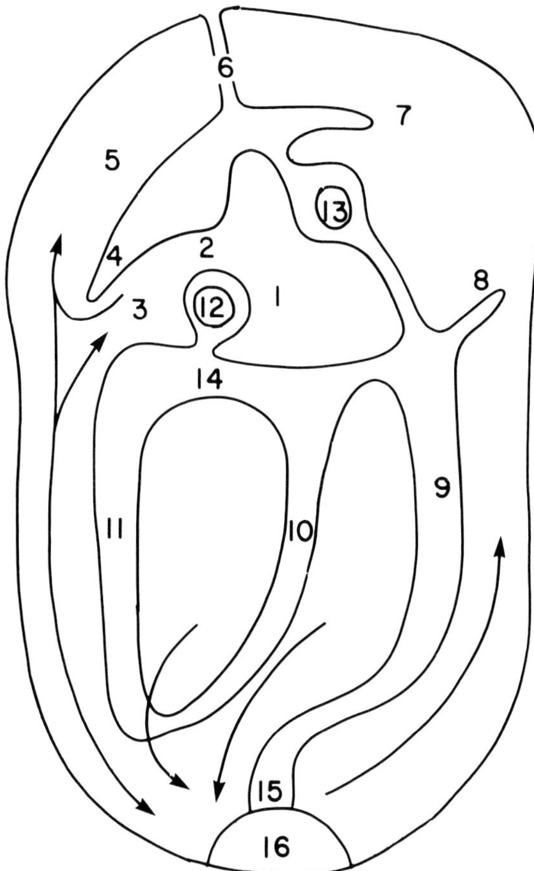

Fig. 34-9. **Schematic diagram of the posterior peritoneal reflections and recesses of the peritoneal cavity. *1.* Lesser sac. *2.* Foramen of Winslow. *3.* Morison's pouch. *4.* Right triangular ligament. *5.* Right subphrenic space. *6.* Falciform ligament. *7.* Left subphrenic space. *8.* Phrenicocolic ligament. *9.* Bare area of the descending colon. *10.* Root of the small bowel mesentery. *11.* Bare area of ascending colon. *12.* Duodenum. *13.* Esophagus. *14.* Root of the transverse mesocolon. *15.* Bare area of rectum. *16.* Bladder. (From Levison ME: In Mandell GL, Douglas RG Jr, Bernett JE (eds): Principles and Practice of Infectious Diseases, 1979, Vol 1, p. 609. Courtesy of John Wiley & Sons.)**

Retroperitoneal Spaces

There is a potential space between the peritoneum and the transversalis fascia [115,116] that extends from the diaphragm superiorly to the brim of the true pelvis inferiorly and to the lateral borders of the quadratus lumborum muscles. The retroperitoneal space extends across the midline, but most infections are unilateral.

The renal fascia surrounding the kidneys and enclosing the great vessels separates the retroperitoneal space into anterior and posterior compartments (Fig. 34-10). The anterior retroperitoneal space is bordered by the posterior peritoneum and the anterior portion of the renal fascia (Fig. 34-11).[117] The posterior peritoneal space is subdivided into superior and inferior divisions by the posterior leaf of the renal fascia. The renal compartment of the posterior retroperitoneal space is closed superiorly and open inferiorly, favoring the downward spread of infection.

The retrofascial space is posterior to the transversalis fascia and encloses the dorsal spine and muscles. It is not strictly a part of the retroperitoneal space but is included in most studies because its position is truly retroperitoneal.

The anterior retroperitoneal space contains the esophagus, duodenum, pancreas, bile duct, portal and splenic veins, appendix, ascending and descending colon, and rectosigmoid. The posterior (perinephric) space contains the kidneys, ureters, gonadal vessels, aorta, inferior cava, and lymph nodes. The retrofascial (ileopsoas) space encloses the twelfth rib, spine, and paraspinous muscles.

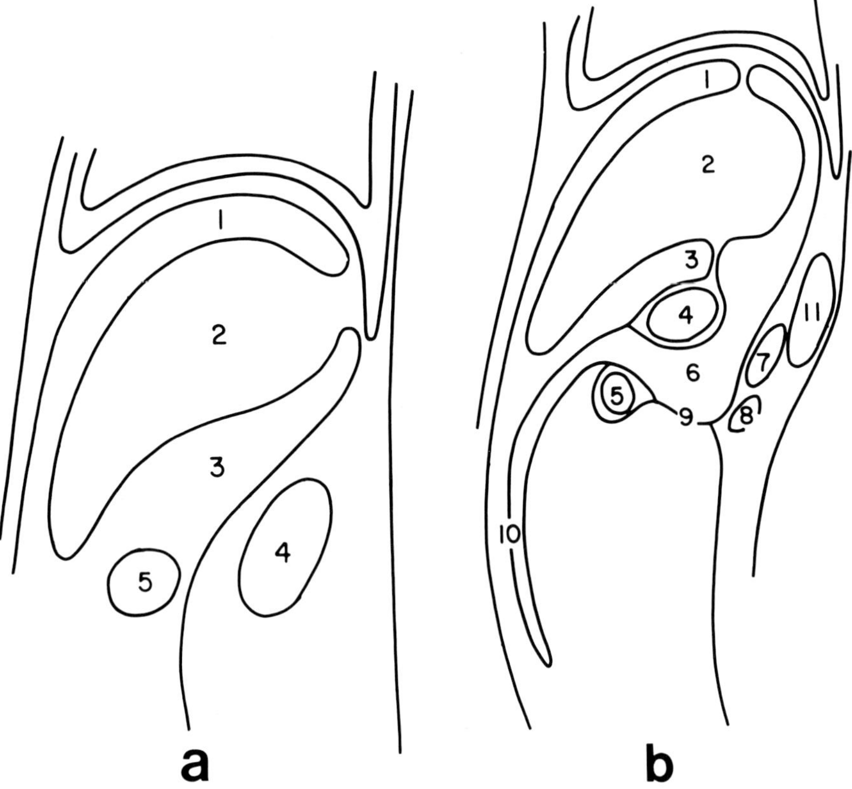

Fig. 34-10. Schema of a sagittal section of the peritoneal cavity. *A.* Right upper quadrant. *1.* Subphrenic space. *2.* Liver. *3.* Subhepatic space. *4.* Right kidney. *5.* Transverse colon. *B.* Left upper quadrant. *1.* Subphrenic space. *2.* Liver, left lobe. *3.* Subhepatic space. *4.* Stomach. *5.* Transverse colon. *6.* Lesser sac. *7.* Pancreas. *8.* Duodenum. *9.* Transverse mesocolon. *10.* Omentum. *11.* Left kidney. (From Levison ME: In Mandell GL, Douglas RG Jr, Bernett, JE (eds): Principles and Practice of Infectious Diseases, 1979, Vol 1, p. 609. Courtesy of John Wiley & Sons.)

Incidence of Intra-abdominal Abscesses

The literature dealing with intraperitoneal abscesses is severely limited in scope. Most papers describe abscesses restricted to a single anatomic area, such as subphrenic abscesses, or arising from a specific disease process, such as diverticulitis or appendicitis. Only one paper takes a comprehensive view of all abscesses below the diaphragm and above the inguinal ligament.[113]

The incidence of some types of intraperitoneal abscesses is definitely changing. A marked decrease in appen-

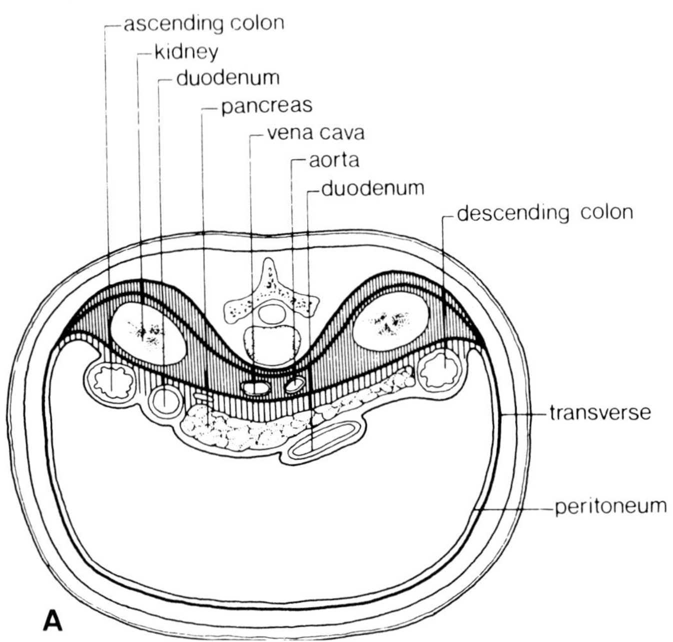

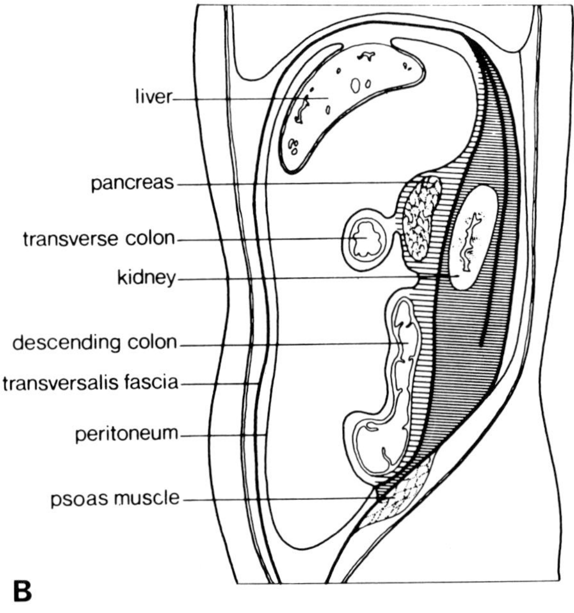

Fig. 34-11. Details of the retroperitoneal space. *A.* Cross section. *B.* Sagittal section. Note the anterior compartment and the perinephric-perivascular posterior compartment. The retroperitoneal muscles are not strictly considered part of the retroperitoneum. (From Goris RJA, Lubbers EJC, Oostveen HW, van den Dries ACP: In de Boer HHM (ed): Intraabdominal Sepsis, 1979, p. 47. Courtesy of Bunge Scientific Publishers.)

diceal abscesses parallels the general decreasing incidence of appendicitis and the increasing quality of medical care.[118] A perforated appendix was formerly the most common cause of subphrenic abscess and is now third or fourth.[119] However, the incidence of abscesses secondary to colonic diverticulitis is increasing as the age of the population increases. Subphrenic abscesses are relatively uncommon infections whose incidence has remained rather constant. As the incidence of spontaneous disease falls, the relative incidence secondary to operation and trauma has risen.[120]

Table 34-5 lists the location and type of intraabdominal abscess found by Altemeier et al[113] over an 11-year period. Thirty-six percent occurred within the peritoneal cavity, 38 percent in the retroperitoneal spaces, and 26 percent were visceral. Table 34-6 shows the many primary diseases that caused these intra-abdominal abscesses. Table 34-7 shows the abscess locations associated with the primary disease. Most abscesses derive from perforations of nearby viscera. Distant spread by the intraperitoneal circulation occurs less often.

Subphrenic Abscesses. The distribution of subphrenic abscesses is changing.[119] These abscesses are increasingly a disease of the elderly (Fig. 34-12), with a peak incidence in the sixth and seventh decades.[121,122] Currently, only about 15 percent of all subphrenic abscesses develop without previous abdominal operation or trauma, most occurring after gastric or duodenal peptic perforation, appendiceal perforation, or acute cholecystitis.[121] Procedures upon the pancreas, spleen, stomach, and duodenum have the highest absolute incidence of postoperative (iatrogenic) subphrenic abscess (Table 34-8).[121]

Formerly, more than 80 percent of subphrenic abscesses occurred on the right side, but most abscesses are now occurring after operation, and left-sided lesions outnumber right-sided abscesses in some series.[115,119] Incidental splenectomy during operation on the gastrointestinal tract has an especially high incidence of left subphrenic abscess formation. Splenectomy during elective gastric resection for ulcer disease has a 3.4 to 6 percent incidence of abscess formation, which increases to 16 percent after operations for gastric carcinoma.[123,124] Splenectomy during colon resections has a 5 percent abscess rate.[125] Splenectomy for blunt trauma has a 1.5 percent abscess rate vs 5 percent for penetrating trauma.[123] Subphrenic abscesses occurring after gastric resection in the absence of splenectomy usually occur on the right side.[126]

Many subphrenic abscesses are associated with synchronous abscesses elsewhere in the abdomen, and 6 to 19 percent are bilateral (Table 34-9).[127]

Abscesses after Appendicitis. Certain diseases predispose to characteristic intra-abdominal abscesses. In the past, appendicitis has been the major cause of intra-abdominal abscess formation, including subphrenic and pelvic abscesses. Bradley and Isaacs,[118] however, reviewed 2,621 patients with acute appendicitis seen between 1962 and 1976 and found only 68 cases (2.6 percent) of appendiceal abscess. This compares to a 21 percent incidence between 1931 and 1939[128] and a 3 percent incidence from 1937

TABLE 34-5. LOCATION AND TYPE OF INTRA-ABDOMINAL ABSCESS

Location and Type	Number of Cases	Percent
Intraperitoneal		
Right lower quadrant	86	16
Left lower quadrant	28	5
Pelvic	27	5
Subphrenic	27	5
Morison's pouch or subhepatic	10	2
Interloop	8	1
Giant horseshoe	6	1
Lesser sac	2	0.3
SUBTOTAL	194	36
Retroperitoneal		
Anterior retroperitoneal	92	17
Posterior retroperitoneal	79	15
Retrofascial	32	6
SUBTOTAL	203	38
Visceral		
Hepatic	69	13
Pancreatic	34	6
Tubo-ovarian	26	5
Gallbladder and biliary tract	13	2
Kidney	1	0.2
SUBTOTAL	143	26
TOTAL	540	100

From Altemeier WA, Culbertson WR, Fullen WD, Shook CD: Intra-abdominal abscesses *Am J Surg* 125:70, 1973.

TABLE 34-6. SOURCES OF INFECTION IN INTRA-ABDOMINAL ABSCESS

Primary Disease	Number of Cases	Percent
Appendicitis	97	19
Pancreatitis or pancreatic tumor	60	12
Lesions of genitourinary tract (male	59	12
and female)	32	6
Lesions of biliary tract	41	8
Diverticulitis	37	7
Actinomycosis	19	4
Septicemia	20	4
Osteomyelitis of spine or twelfth rib	18	4
Perforating tumors	17	3
Trauma	17	3
Peptic ulcer	8	2
Leaking anastomotic suture line	7	2
Amebiasis	5	1
Regional enteritis	3	0.6
Miscellaneous	19	4
Unknown	42	9
TOTAL	501	

From Altemeier WA, Culbertson WR, Fullen WD, Shook CD: Intra-abdominal abscesses. *Am J Surg* 125:70, 1973.

TABLE 34-7. RELATIONSHIP OF LOCATIONS TO PRIMARY DISEASES

Primary Disease	Location of Abscess	Number
Appendicitis	Right lower quadrant	76
	Pelvic	16
	Anterior retroperitoneal	19
	Subphrenic	8
	Interloop	3
Diverticulitis of Colon	Left lower quadrant	20
	Pelvic	9
	Right lower quadrant	5
	Anterior retroperitoneal	2
	Interloop	2
	Subphrenic	1
	Subhepatic	1
Pancreatitis and pancreatic tumor	Retroperitoneal	19
	Lesser sac	16
	Intraperitoneal	4
Peptic ulcer	Left lower quadrant	5
	Right upper quadrant	2
	Subphrenic	5
	Subhepatic	2
	Pelvic	1
	Interloop	1

From Altemeier WA, Culbertson WR, Fullen WD, Shook CD: Intra-abdominal abscesses. *Am J Surg* 125:70, 1973.

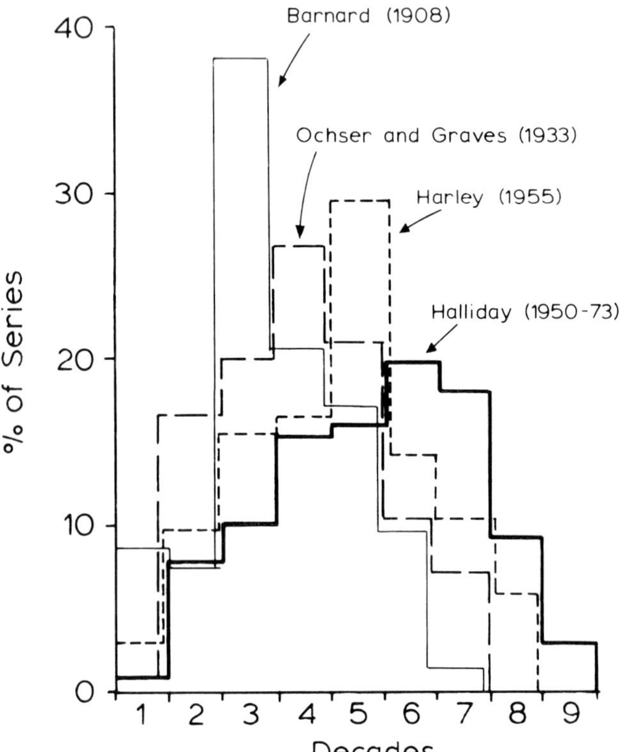

Fig. 34-12. **Comparison of the age distributions of subphrenic abscesses in various series. (Adapted from Halliday P, Halliday JH: Br J Surg 63:352, 1976.)**

through 1959.[129] In the 1930s, 1 percent of patients with appendicitis developed a subphrenic abscess. Abscesses still occur in the very young or elderly. The abscess is typically located in the right lower quadrant, pelvis, or pelvic retroperitoneum (Table 34-7).

Abscesses after Diverticulitis. Diverticulitis is the second most common cause of intraperitoneal abscess. By definition, the disease is an acute inflammation of an obstructed colonic diverticulum that arises where blood vessels penetrate the bowel wall (Chapter 39). In some series, almost half of the patients surgically treated for diverticulitis had abscess formation or free perforation with peritonitis, but usually only about 7 percent perforate.[130] The inflamed diverticulum may drain spontaneously into the colon, resolving the inflammation. Most gross abscesses are found in the left lower quadrant or pelvis (Table 34-7).

Abscesses Associated with Inflammatory Bowel Disease. Of patients with Crohn's disease, 12 to 28 percent develop an abscess.[131] Such abscesses are of three types: (1) Enteroparietal abscesses having at least one wall of the abscess in contact with the abdominal wall, (2) interloop abscesses completely surrounded by adjacent intestinal segments, and (3) intramesenteric abscesses due to perforations into the leaves of the mesentery. The latter abscesses can dissect into the true retroperitoneal space.[132] Abscess are uncommon with ulcerative colitis but can develop months to years after proctocolectomy for this disease.

Abscesses Associated with Colonic Carcinoma. Approximately 6 percent of colonic or rectal carcinomas are complicated by perforation.[133] Generalized peritonitis can result, with cecal perforation due to distal obstruction, but with cecal carcinomas, extraperitoneal perforation into the paracolonic tissues or the anterior abdominal wall is more common. Perforations of rectal and colonic tumors lead to paracolonic abscesses in the pelvis or retroperitoneum.

Pelvic Abscesses. Pelvic abscesses result most commonly from pelvic inflammatory disease or obstetric complications, but ruptured appendicitis, rectosigmoid diverticulitis, or sigmoid colon perforations are also sources. Generalized peritonitis rarely causes pelvic abscesses even if the patient is maintained in Fowler's position. In the past, pelvic abscesses had a better prognosis than did subphrenic abscesses and could be drained through the rectum or vagina.[134] Low anterior anastomoses or abdominoperineal resections are common causes of pelvic abscesses postoperatively.

Retroperitoneal Abscesses. Retroperitoneal infections arise from complications of trauma, infections, or malignancy of adjacent retroperitoneal or intraperitoneal organs, osteomyelitis of the vertebral column or lower ribs, suppurative lymphadenitis, or bacteremia.[117] In the past, pyelonephritis was the most common cause of retroperitoneal infections (Table 34-10). Now, infected pancreatic pseudocysts, posterior duodenal perforations, and intramesenteric abscesses are more frequent causes.

TABLE 34-8. INCIDENCE OF POSTOPERATIVE SUBPHRENIC ABSCESS

System	No. Operations	Percent
Stomach, duodenum	3,000	1.4
Biliary tract	3,700	0.3
Intestine	1,900	0.9
Pancreas, spleen	1,350	1.5
Appendix	1,800	0.2

From Sherman NJ, Davis JR, Jesseph JE: Subphrenic abscess. A continuing hazard. *Am J Surg* 117:117, 1969.

Etiology

The bacteria that cause intraperitoneal abscesses are the same ones that cause secondary bacterial peritonitis—a mixture of aerobic and anaerobic enteric organisms (Tables 34-1 and 34-11). Exceptions are pneumococcal abscesses after primary pneumococcal peritonitis[71] or gonococcal pelvic abscesses after pelvic inflammatory disease, although mixed anaerobic organisms are now isolated more frequently from the latter than they were previously.[135] In the past, retroperitoneal abscesses were frequently tuberculous (Table 34-10) but are now usually mixed infections.[117]

Pathogenesis of Intra-abdominal Abscess Formation

The precise conditions that precede abscess formation are not known. Under normal conditions, the tissue lymphatics efficiently remove bacteria and other small particulate matter. The slow but constant flow of extracellular fluid washes bacteria into the efferent lymphatics and lymph nodes, where they are phagocytosed by the fixed macrophages.

A similar flow of extracellular fluid occurs within the peritoneal cavity. For this reason, it is extremely difficult to establish intraperitoneal abscesses by injecting bacteria alone. In animal experiments, the bacterial counts begin to fall immediately after intraperitoneal innoculation.[11] Bacteria can be recovered from the lymphatic duct within 6 minutes and from the bloodstream within 12 minutes.[5] This physical removal of bacteria from the peritoneal cavity is the most important early defense mechanism of the peritoneal cavity.

TABLE 34-9. INCIDENCE OF MULTIPLE SYNCHRONOUS SUBPHRENIC ABSCESSES REPORTED IN THE LITERATURE

Author	Multiple	Bilateral
Harley, 1949	12	6
Wetterfors, 1959	42	19
Yonehiro, 1961	35	—
Ozeran, 1967	15	—
Johnson, 1968	—	17
Miller and Talman, 1969	—	10
Sherman et al, 1969	15	8
Halasz, 1970	26	11

From Halasz NA: Subphrenic abscess. Myths and facts. *JAMA* 214:724, 1970.

Local inflammation, however, disrupts the usual bacterial clearance mechanisms. First, there is a transudation of protein-rich fluid. Fibrin deposits bind adjacent viscera to the inflamed organ and tend to seal any perforation. Subsequently, fibrin deposits wall off this area of the peritoneal cavity, slowing lymphatic uptake of bacteria that might otherwise produce a lethal bacteremia. The isolated bacteria have a slowed growth rate because of a decreased nutrient flow (Fig. 34-6).

Although these acute inflammatory mechanisms are initially protective, they establish the groundwork for abscess formation. The fibrinous capsule around the abscess probably impedes the influx of phagocytic cells, complement, antibodies, and other opsonins that are capable of immobilizing and killing the bacteria. Antibiotic penetration is also impaired. The contents of the abscess become relatively anaerobic, allowing the proliferation of virulent anaerobic bacteria that ordinarily are unable to grow within tissues.

Neutrophils are necessary for abscess formation. Miles et al[15] demonstrated that local injection of bacteria resulted in an influx of neutrophils within four hours. If the bacteria were killed with antibiotics before four hours, no abscesses resulted. If antibiotics were administered after four hours when the neutrophils already were present, however, abscesses resulted even if the bacteria all died. Neutrophils are end-stage cells that do not return to the systemic circulation after entering the tissues. When they degranulate during phagocytosis and bacterial digestion or when they die, they release their component of digestive enzymes, which lyse not only living bacteria but host tissue as well. These enzymes are normally neutralized by plasma inhibitors, such as alpha-1 antitrypsin. In abscesses, the neutrophil enzyme levels apparently exceed the neutralizing ability of the alpha-1 and alpha-2 globulins present.

In addition, the contents of abscesses are hypertonic, resulting in an influx of fluid and a gradual expansion of the abscess cavity, which tends to dissect along planes of least resistance. Digestion of host tissue produces a rich growth medium for the bacteria. Most bactericidal antibiotics block bacterial cell wall formation, causing spontaneous bacterial lysis at normal serum osmotic pressure. Within hypertonic abscess cavities, however, these bacteria may survive and reproduce as L-forms.

An abscess appears to form when a residual bacterial inoculum is trapped in situ relatively protected from recruited phagocytic cells. Fibrin is central to this mechanism, because fibrin binds bacteria and neutrophils.[12]

The fibrinolytic apparatus within normal clots and within the peritoneal mesothelium would be expected to oppose abscess formation. However, peritoneal fibrinolysis is profoundly inhibited by peritonitis, and the products of lysed red cells are known to block neutrophil function.[11]

Other inflammatory changes in the peritoneal cavity may be detrimental. The diaphragmatic lymphatics absorb peritoneal fluid at a relatively fixed rate. If bacteria are suspended in large volumes of intraperitoneal fluid, fewer organisms will be absorbed per unit time. In addition, phagocytosis is depressed in a fluid depleted of opsonins. Products of inflammation recruit neutrophils, but these same factors may interfere with cell function. Neutrophils

TABLE 34-10. RETROPERITONEAL ABSCESSES: SOURCE AND ANATOMIC LOCATION OF INFECTION

Organ	Lesion	No.
ANTERIOR RETROPERITONEAL SPACE		
Appendix	Appendicitis	15
Colon	Actinomycosis	13
	Carcinoma	6
	Amebiasis	1
	Foreign body	1
	Diverticulitis	3
	Trauma	2
Duodenum	Trauma	3
	Peptic ulcer	2
Stomach	Carcinoma	1
	Trauma	1
	Penetrating ulcer	1
Bile ducts	Sarcoma	1
	Trauma	2
Ileum	Radiation ileitis	1
	Regional ileitis	2
Pancreas	Carcinoma	2
	Pancreatitis	8
	Trauma	2
Kidney	Tuberculosis	1
Metastatic		3
Miscellaneous		4
Unknown		9
	TOTAL	84
POSTERIOR RETROPERITONEAL OR PERINEPHRIC SPACE		
Kidney	Pyelonephritis	44
	Tuberculosis	5
	Carbuncle	2
	Carcinoma	1
	Trauma	4
Colon	Actinomycosis	1
Metastatic		1
Miscellaneous		4
Unknown		14
	TOTAL	76
RETROFASCIAL SPACE		
Spine	Tuberculosis	15
Metastatic		7
Twelfth rib	Actinomycosis	2
Miscellaneous		2
Unknown		3
	TOTAL	29

From Altemeier WA, Alexander JW: Retroperitoneal abscess. *Arch Surg* 83:512, 1961.

exposed to high concentrations of chemotactic factors lose their sensitivity to chemotactic attraction. Thus, the neutrophils may have a decreased ability to locate and phagocytose bacteria in the presence of the same factors that attract them to the site of infection.

After the abscess becomes established, few mechanisms for its absorption are known. The intrinsic fibrinolytic system of the peritoneal surface is totally inhibited in the presence of inflammation and infection. The fibrin deposits persist and ultimately are replaced by the ingrowth of fibroblasts, resulting in dense adhesion formation. The neutrophil digestive enzymes can be neutralized by serum protease inhibitors, but penetration of these globulins through the abscess capsule appears poor. The bacteria themselves can be killed by antibodies, complement, opsonins, and phagocytic cells or even antibiotics, but penetration is inhibited by the relatively avascular abscess wall. In animal models, abscesses may be well tolerated and resolve gradually with dense adhesion formation. It is not surprising, however, that spontaneous or surgical drainage results in more rapid resolution.

TABLE 34-11. BACTERIOLOGY OF SUBPHRENIC ABSCESS IN 24 PATIENTS

Organism	No. (%)
Aerobic flora	
E. coli	23 (96)
Streptococcus (enterococcus)	16 (67)
Proteus	9 (38)
Klebsiella	5 (21)
Pseudomonas	2 (8)
Staphylococcus	2 (8)
Anaerobic flora	
B. fragilis	20 (83)
Anaerobic cocci	12 (50)
Clostridium	12 (50)
Fusobacterium	9 (38)
Eubacterium	2 (8)

Modified from Wang SMS, Wilson SE: Subphrenic abscess. The new epidemiology. *Arch Surg* 112:934, 1977.

Clinical Manifestations

Whereas diffuse generalized peritonitis usually produces such intense abdominal pain that the diagnosis is obvious, intra-abdominal abscesses have fewer and less impressive symptoms. Enteroparietal abscesses are the easiest to diagnose. There are pain, tenderness, and a palpable abdominal mass. Interloop, intramesenteric, and subphrenic abscesses give much less pain because the visceral peritoneum is innervated by splanchnic rather than somatic pain fibers, and no mass can be palpated. Retroperitoneal abscesses may only produce lumbar or ileopsoas muscle spasm. Pelvic abscesses can be palpated but usually give few symptoms, and so the appropriate examination is not performed.

The clinical diagnostic dilemma is compounded by the fact that over 90 percent of subphrenic abscesses now occur after an abdominal operation, and one third of all intra-abdominal abscesses result after an episode of generalized peritonitis—usually treated by a surgeon. In the postoperative patient, the abdominal symptoms are much less obvious, being masked by incision pain, postoperative analgesics, and the reluctance of the surgeon to admit even temporary defeat. Physical examination is notoriously unreliable in this period—all patients are distended and tender.[126] Only if serial detailed examinations are carried out by the same examiner can any but the most easily palpable abdominal abscesses be diagnosed. More importantly, if a physical examination reveals nothing, all thoughts of the diagnosis tend to be dispelled, and other suggestive historical or laboratory findings are discarded.

The most important diagnostic information in a patient who has not been operated upon is a history suggestive of visceral inflammation (urinary tract infection, purulent vaginal discharge, gastroenteritis, partial intestinal obstruction, fever, abdominal pain) that improved spontaneously or after empiric antibody therapy. When the symptoms recur, an intra-abdominal abscess is likely. Physical examination usually yields only vague tenderness, with or without rebound.

In postoperative patients, a history of difficulty with operative dissection or lysis of adhesions, an anastomosis under tension, or any operation on the esophagus, duodenum, pancreas, or colon suggests the presence of abscesses. The immediate postoperative period is often free of complications other than prolonged ileus, although basilar atelectasis or a fever that responded to empirical antibiotic treatment is common. The patient who requires reinsertion of a nasogastric tube to relieve recurrent ileus or partial intestinal obstruction should be suspect. Special diagnostic techniques are almost always required for a precise preoperative diagnosis. Even with such assistance, however, the diagnosis will frequently require empiric reoperation.

Subphrenic Abscess. Most recent reports have focused on subphrenic abscesses for reasons first detailed by Whipple in 1926. These abscesses occur after the most severe intraperitoneal infections, they appear late in the illness, they are insidious in onset and course, they are difficult to diagnose, the drainage is difficult and frequently inadequate, and the disease has a high mortality. Bonfils-Roberts et al[136] found that abdominal pain was present in over 90 percent of patients. All patients manifested fever and tachycardia, and two-thirds had abdominal guarding or distention. Other suggestive findings included hiccoughs, tachypnea, cough, or jaundice.[121] In the preantibiotic era, the large abscesses ultimately produced characteristic patterns of abdominal tenderness, especially over the twelfth rib or costal margin.[137] With the use of antibiotics, however, the clinical presentation of subphrenic abscesses has changed considerably.[138] Patients currently demonstrate a decreased incidence of abdominal tenderness, an attenuated pattern of fever, and less leukocytosis than previously, probably because the abscesses are smaller. The earliest findings are generally a persistent ileus or signs suggesting partial intestinal obstruction after a period of improving function. Nonspecific thoracic manifestations include pleural effusion, elevation of the diaphragm, and decreased basilar breath sounds.[138,139]

Pelvic Abscess. Women usually have evidence of a genital tract infection for days to weeks before the abscess develops. In those who develop a tubo-ovarian abscess, pelvic inflammatory disease is manifested by diffuse low abdominal pain, high fever, leukocytosis, and occasionally ileus. On pelvic examination, the uterine corpus is exquisitely tender, and lateral masses may be palpated. Postdelivery or postoperative pelvic infections cause fever and a purulent vaginal discharge. Abdominal pain is a variable finding, but the patient appears toxic. This usually represents a pelvic or uterine cellulitis, which may progress to a true pelvic abscess (Chapter 44).

Five presentations of pelvic abscesses in the female have been noted: (1) unilateral or bilateral parametrial abscesses that bulge into the vagina or inguinal area, (2) cul de sac collections palpable in the posterior fornix, (3) tubo-ovarian abscesses fixed high on the pelvic wall, (4) tubo-ovarian or ovarian abscesses that present as an abdominal mass, and (5) rupture of an abscess with peritonitis.

Development of a pelvic abscess of gastrointestinal tract origin may be quite insidious, with low-grade fever, mild abdominal discomfort, and diarrhea or constipation, progressing to anorexia, nausea, and abdominal distention. A leaking colonic anastomosis may cause only postoperative fever, persistent low-grade leukocytosis, and prolonged ileus. There may be a sudden fever spike, hypotension, and bacteremia, compelling an aggressive search for the abscess. A mass is often palpable on rectal examination. Abdominal findings are consistently minimal because the abscess is so distant from the anterior abdominal wall.

Retroperitoneal Abscess. Abdominal or flank pain and fever are present in over 90 percent of patients with retroperitoneal infections. Other symptoms include nausea, vomiting, anorexia, chills, and lumbar or psoas muscle spasm. About half the patients have a flank mass and tenderness with or without overlying edema. An unexplained limp may be the earliest sign of retroperitoneal abscess. The patients frequently lie in bed with the psoas muscle relaxed by flexing and abducting the thigh. Extension of the thigh increases the pain. This may progress to a tightly flexed hip and ipsilateral rectus muscle spasm. Sigmoid carcinoma perforation can present with pelvic, thigh, perirectal, or gluteal abscesses. Rarely, the first manifestation will be subcutaneous emphysema. Splenic flexure carcinoma may produce left perinephric abscesses.

Laboratory Investigations

The diagnosis of intra-abdominal abscess is first made clinically and is only supported by laboratory and radiographic findings and confirmed at operation or autopsy. Sherman et al[121] noted that "once the suspicion of a subphrenic abscess is raised, confirmation . . . is most challenging and often frustrating. The first and most essential step is to entertain this suspicion and then retain it, in spite of negative investigations, until the outcome is certain."

Other than leukocytosis and a late finding of elevations of liver function tests and decreasing respiratory or renal function, laboratory tests add little to confirm the diagnosis. The exception is a finding of gonorrhea in the female, which suggests gonococcal pelvic inflammatory disease or gonococcal abscess. Hyperglycemia or hypertriglyceridemia in a patient receiving parenteral nutrition is suggestive of an occult septic focus. Tachycardia, increased cardiac output, with a decreased arteriovenous oxygen difference are other observations that suggest sepsis in a well-monitored patient (Chapter 16).

Conventional Radiographic Studies

Subphrenic Abscess. Conventional chest radiographic examinations are most helpful in patients with subphrenic abscess (Table 34-12). The use of antibiotics, unfortunately, has made the chest radiograph less diagnostic (Fig. 34-13).[122]

Over half of the patients in one series had evidence of intra-abdominal extraluminal air indicative of an intraperitoneal abscess (Table 34-12),[126] but intraperitoneal air may persist for days to weeks after abdominal operations, especially in thin patients, so that it is an unreliable sign by itself.

DeCosse et al [126] noted that subhepatic abscesses have fewer thoracic manifestations of sepsis than do true subphrenic abscesses. In their series, all patients with a subdiaphragmatic abscess had a pleural effusion or pulmonary infiltrate, but patients with subhepatic abscess had minimal thoracic signs. Elevation of the diaphragm during fluoroscopy was evident in 75 percent of patients with subdiaphragmatic abscess but in only 30 percent of those with subhepatic abscess.

Approximately one half of the patients will have abdominal roentgenographic evidence of ileus, and 14 to 40 percent will exhibit an extraluminal air fluid level indicative of an abscess (Table 34-12). Other findings may include extraluminal compression of the stomach or duodenum or increased distance between the gastric bubble and the diaphragm. Gastric or colonic contrast studies may be helpful, especially in delineating left-sided abscesses. [121]

Pelvic Abscess. Although plain abdominal films rarely show any but the most massive pelvic abscesses, cystograms often show bladder compression or spasm, and barium enema examinations can show colonic spasm.

TABLE 34-12. RADIOGRAPHIC FINDINGS IN SUBPHRENIC ABSCESS

	Sherman et al [121]	DeCosse et al [126]
	Percent	*Percent*
Chest roentgenogram		
Effusion	43	72
Elevated diaphragm	33	60
Atelectasis	18	
Pneumonitis	6	[70]
Fluoroscopy		
Decreased motion	51	[55]
No motion	31	
Normal	18	45
Abdominal roentgenogram		
Air/fluid level	61	
Mass	19	
Normal	20	

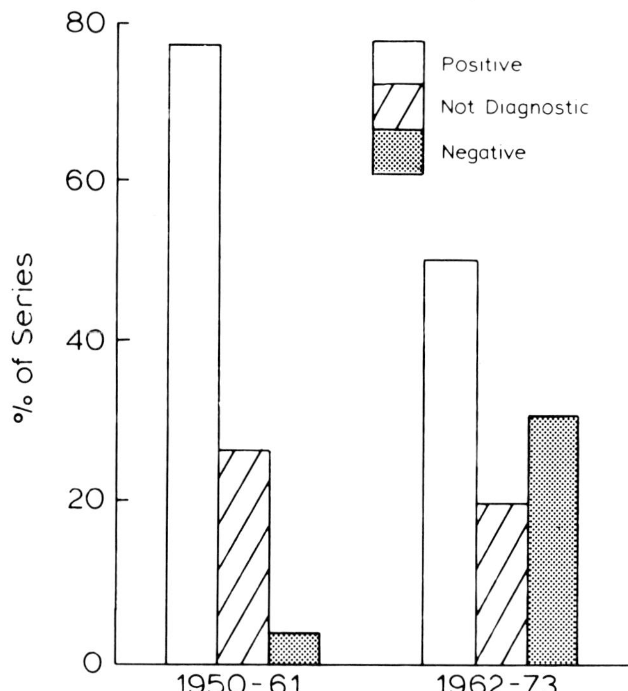

Fig. 34-13. **Changes in the value of radiologic examination in suphrenic abscess. (Adapted from Halliday P, Halliday JH: Br J Surg 63:352, 1976.)**

Retroperitoneal Abscess. Retroperitoneal abscesses often have radiographic evidence of a soft tissue mass. Barium enemas and intravenous pyelograms frequently show displacement of the colon or ureters.

Sinugrams. Many postoperative abscesses are already partially drained by drainage tubes placed into abdominal recesses at operation. Persistent infection commonly rests within these inadequately evacuated pockets. Contrast studies of the drainage tracts or spontaneous fistulas will often reveal residual abscess cavities which act as the septic source, or which communicate with viscera. A water-soluble contrast medium should be used.

Other Diagnostic Methods

Although intra-abdominal abscess must be diagnosed clinically, few surgeons operate without exhausting the current repertory of diagnostic tests to localize the abscess. In addition to conventional roentgenographic studies, these tests include fluoroscopy, simultaneous liver and lung scanning, ultrasound, gallium-67 scanning, CAT scanning, and indium-111 autologous leukocyte scans (Table 34-13).[139a] The surgeon hopes that correctly localizing the abscess will guarantee its presence. An extraserous drainage, rather than a complete exploration, can then be undertaken. Unfortunately, the time required for localization may seriously delay therapy.

Of all these diagnostic techniques, fluoroscopy is the

TABLE 34-13. DIAGNOSTIC EXAMINATIONS IN SUBPHRENIC ABSCESS

Procedure	No. (%) of Patients Examined	No. (%) Abnormal	No. (%) Normal
Anteroposterior chest roentgenogram	44 (100)	41 (93)	3 (6.8)
Plain abdominal x-ray film	34 (77)	21 (61.7)	13 (38)
Hepatic Tc-99m sulfur colloid scan	21 (48)	12 (57)	9 (42.8)
Ultrasound	22 (50)	13 (59)	9 (41)
Fluoroscopy of diaphragm	11 (25)	6 (54.4)	5 (45.5)
Gallium-67 citrate scan	11 (25)	7 (64)	4 (36)
Liver–lung scan	11 (25)	5 (45.5)	6 (54.5)

From Deck KB, Berne TV: Selective management of subphrenic abscesses. *Arch Surg* 114:1165, 1979.

oldest. Limitation of diaphragmatic motion or paradoxical motion is found in 25–70 percent of patients with subphrenic abscess.[126] Simultaneous liver and lung scanning with technetium-99 may demonstrate a purulent collection between liver and lung, but the test is not specific or sensitive because only relatively large right subphrenic abscesses are visualized. The majority of these patients will have a right pleural effusion, which also separates the lung and liver. No other abscesses can be visualized with this technique.

Grey-scale ultrasonography has several potential advantages compared to other methods of evaluation.[140] It is cheap and noninvasive and does not expose the patient to further irradiation. The test can be completed and interpreted within an hour. The disadvantages of the system are that it requires an intact abdominal wall overlying the abscess, it cannot penetrate air or bone so that deep structures often cannot be evaluated, and it requires considerable operator skill in performance and interpretation. In experienced hands, the accuracy can be remarkable. Taylor et al [141] presented 220 patients in whom an abscess was suspected: 36 of 40 abscesses within the abdominal cavity were correctly diagnosed, and all but 1 of 113 were correctly excluded. Thirty-two of 33 pelvic abscesses were diagnosed and correctly excluded in 33 out of 34. The overall accuracy in their hands was 96.8 percent. Unfortunately, other centers have not been able to duplicate their remarkable results.[139a] Ultrasonography has also been used to define retroperitoneal abscesses.

Computerized axial tomography (CAT) of the abdominal cavity has become available within the last few years. Its advantages include higher resolution, little need for operator skill in interpretation, and an ability to see deep to bone and gas-filled structures without the need for an intact abdominal wall. Its greatest disadvantages are the extreme cost in setting up a facility and the radiation absorbed. Daffner et al [142] reported five patients in whom intra-abdominal abscess was diagnosed by CAT scan. He listed as criteria required for diagnosis: (1) a low-density mass, (2) extraluminal gas, (3) the presence of a mass distinct from bowel, which did not enhance following the administration of intravenous or oral contrast material, and (4) extraluminal gas.

Gallium-67 scanning has had an enthusiastic trial in the diagnosis of intraperitoneal inflammatory processes.[143] Numerous problems exist. It is a very nonspecific test and readily images neoplasms as well as abscesses. The material is excreted in the gastrointestinal tract, and a vigorous bowel prep is necessary (but impossible in patients with ileus) in order to evaluate the abdominal cavity. Because of the short half-life of the isotope, there is considerable cost in generating and rapidly transporting the dose necessary for the test. In addition, 24 to 72 hours are required for uptake before scanning. The biggest disadvantage, however, is the lack of specific labeling of inflammatory foci. Experimental abscess:blood ratios of only 8:1 are found.[144]

The clinical reports have been variable. Caffee et al [143] presented 50 patients undergoing scan with presumed intra-abdominal abscess. There were 12 true-positive, 7 false-positive, 2 false-negative, and 30 true-negative scans, an overall accuracy of 84 percent.

In an attempt to increase the accuracy rate over that of gallium-67 scanning, indium-111 has been used as an in vitro label for autologous neutrophils, which are then infused intravenously.[144] The leukocytes subsequently migrate to sites of inflammation. Several advantages have been found. The neutrophils can be separated in vitro and specifically labeled, giving amazingly high abscess: blood ratios (as high as 81:1 in experimental models).[144] A correspondingly lower total dose of radiation can be used. The test is quite specific for sites of inflammation and relatively insensitive to neoplasms. A few disadvantages remain—it still is relatively expensive and involves a moderate radiation dose to the patient. Twenty-four hours are required for the neutrophils to localize at the inflammatory site. Fully functional neutrophils are necessary, and neutrophil dysfunction is common in the severely septic patient [145] or the patient being treated with steroids. In the neutropenic patient, heterologous neutrophils must be labeled in vitro and then injected.

Relatively few reports of this new technique are available. Segal et al [146] reported a correct diagnosis of abscess in three patients and exclusion of abscess in an additional five patients initially tested. Ascher et al [147] reported 66 scans performed in 43 surgical patients, with an overall accuracy rate of 85 percent.

These complex studies are primarily useful in localizing rather than in diagnosing intra-abdominal abscesses. Those patients with a single abscess have the highest incidence of positive findings. In contrast, those patients with multiple abscesses are the sickest and tend to have the fewest positive results. Bacteremia with more than one bacterial organism, especially *Bacteroides* bacteremia, is virtually diagnostic of intra-abdominal sepsis.[21] Such patients require operation to diagnose as well as to evacuate abscesses. Thus, the appearance of signs of respiratory, renal, or hepatic organ failure should prompt operation rather than a host of diagnostic studies. The use of more subtle indications for reoperation requires much experience and clinical judgment. It is especially important, therefore, to rule out extra-abdominal sources of infection, ie, infected intravascular catheters or infections of the urinary or respiratory tracts, before a diagnostic and therapeutic laparotomy is carried out.

Treatment

Operative Therapy. The therapy of most intra-abdominal abscesses has become stereotyped by surgical tradition. There is no question that pockets of liquid pus, solidly walled-off from the intra-abdominal contents, can be incised, aspirated, packed, and drained. Accessible pelvic abscesses can be drained transrectally or transvaginally after needle aspiration.[134] Periappendiceal abscesses are drained readily through a right lower quadrant incision,[148] and extraparietal drainage of most retroperitoneal abscesses is easily accomplished.

To assume, however, that all or even the majority of abscesses can be drained via extraserous routes is a serious mistake. Extraserous drainage is useful only if synchronous abscesses elsewhere can be convincingly excluded. Furthermore, in the preantibiotic era, intra-abdominal abscesses were most often the residue of heavy peritoneal contamination or the result of spontaneous disease, localized by intact host defenses. Currently, however, most abscesses are the sequelae of surgical therapy, and most represent continued communication with contaminated visceral contents. For these reasons, the approach to therapy must be individualized.

The history of surgical therapy for subphrenic abscess has been reviewed by Halliday.[137] Initially, subphrenic abscesses were drained through the chest, and, later, suturing of the diaphragm to the intercostal muscle was introduced to avoid spillage into the pleural cavity. However, because of the high morbidity and mortality associated with this procedure, intercostal incision without rib resection was introduced. Later, a two-stage procedure was introduced, in which the pleural cavity was packed for several days to allow adhesions to form between the pleural surfaces of the chest wall and the diaphragm. The pleura was then incised, and the abscess was drained. In 1922, Nather and Oschner[149] introduced posterior extraserous drainage of the subphrenic space through the bed of the resected twelfth rib. With this procedure, they were able to lower the operative mortality from 32 to 11.7 percent, a remarkable accomplishment in the preantibiotic era.[150]

The extraserous approach became the accepted procedure prior to the antibiotic era for several reasons: (1) the abscesses were large and relatively easy to locate, (2) spillage of large volumes of purulent material into the peritoneal cavity would cause septicemia and hypovolemic shock, and (3) with large abscesses, loculations were usually not a problem, and the cavities were evacuated readily.[137]

The alternative to transthoracic or extraserous drainage[151] is laparotomy. In the 1960s, however, high complication and mortality rates with this approach were reported.[121] Halasz, in 1970,[127] reemphasized the rationale for this procedure: multiple abscesses are so common (Table 34–9) that total exploration is necessary. Halasz had only a 12 percent mortality and 6 percent reoperation rate, and 5 of 17 patients had multiple abscesses at the first operation.

The transperitoneal approach allows visualization of all potential spaces, aspiration of all loculated purulent material, debridement of some if not all fibrin deposits, precise placement of drains, and lavage of the freshly contaminated peritoneal cavity with antibiotics. The available data indicating the increasing mortality from transserous drainage probably do not reflect the advances in surgical therapy of the 1970s and are biased by patient selection. Whenever doubt exists about the precise cause of intra-abdominal infection, the transperitoneal approach should be taken.

Many patients can still be managed by extraserous drainage. Deck and Berne[152] have been successful in selecting such patients, who are characterized by having clearcut localizing findings without serious signs of systemic sepsis. By definition, these patients have the best prognosis. For example, abscesses contiguous with the abdominal wall can be drained by local incision over the abscess, making extensive intraperitoneal explorations unnecessary. In general, interval appendectomy for periappendiceal abscess is acceptable, but primary resection of this or other sources of contamination is preferred (eg, diverticulitis). This removes the septic focus primarily and allows much more rapid resolution of the infectious process. Primary anastomosis is carried out only if gross peritoneal soiling is not present. Similarly, pelvic abscesses can be frequently drained through the vagina or rectum after needle aspiration of the abscess.

Clearly, definitive guidelines for modes of treatment for each of the clinical varieties of infection are difficult to make. Large unilocular abscesses that are statistically single (eg, left subphrenic abscess after left colectomy and splenectomy, right subphrenic abscess after Billroth II gastric resection and a difficult duodenal stump, pelvic abscess after low anterior resection of the left colon) can be drained by extraserous approach and needle localization. Rapid resolution of clinical infection will be evidence that the approach was correct. If the abscess is difficult to localize or arises from an obscure source, however, every abdominal recess should be explored transperitoneally. The failure to clearly discriminate the therapeutic efficacy of various approaches to clearly defined subcategories of disease must be corrected.

Antibiotic Therapy. The choice of antibiotic is usually determined by the culture and sensitivity reports obtained on fluid aspirated at operation. Based on the polymicrobial nature of such abscesses (Table 34-11), the choice of empiric antibiotics should be those recommended in the treatment of peritonitis. Experimental evidence and clinical trials suggest that certain antibiotics are especially efficacious in treating abscesses. These include cefoxitin, carbenicillin, clindamycin, and cefamandole.

Prognosis

Intra-abdominal abscesses which do not communicate with contaminating viscera sometimes follow a relatively indolent course in the antibiotic era. Case reports have appeared detailing patients with cryptic subphrenic abscesses for months to years. The majority of intra-abdominal abscesses are, however, associated with considerable morbidity and mortality. Altemeier et al [113] tabulated the average hospital stay in days for patients with various types of intra-abdominal abscesses (Table 34-14).[113] The average ranged from 21 to 47 days, with isolated patients staying 120 to 210 days. Many of the shorter stays were terminated by the rapid deterioration and death of the patient. Retroperitoneal abscesses had a mean stay of 57 to 80 days.

The mortality of intra-abdominal abscesses remains high. For example, appendiceal abscesses, biliary tract abscesses, and genitourinary tract abscesses had a 2, 4, and 10 percent mortality, respectively.[113] In the older literature,[119] subphrenic abscesses treated with drainage alone had a mortality of 25 to 60 percent (median 35 percent).[119,121,138] Antibiotic therapy has probably reduced the number of subphrenic infections that require drainage but a number of authors noted that the mortality rates for surgical therapy had not decreased over the 30-year period through the early 1960s. Older patients do less well (Fig. 34-14).[120,122] Sherman et al [121] found that patients whose abscesses were drained between two to four weeks after development of the abscess had a lower mortality than those drained at any other time (Table 34-15), but no one recommends delay in operative therapy for well defined abscesses.

TABLE 34-14. MORBIDITY OF INTRA-ABDOMINAL ABSCESSES

	Hospital Stay in Days		
Type of Abscess	*Longest*	*Shortest*	*Average*
Intraperitoneal			
Right lower quadrant	210	7	24
Pelvic	65	2	24
Left lower quadrant	120	1	31
Morison's pouch	120	20	47
Suphrenic	90	1	41
Lesser sac	37	37	37
·Interloop	42	3	21
Horseshoe	58	10	37
Retroperitoneal			
Anterior retroperitoneal	45	19	57
Posterior retroperitoneal	126	35	80
Retrofascial	104	38	67
Visceral			
Liver	84	31	53
Pancreas	126	21	74
Tubo-ovarian	29	9	19
Gallbladder and biliary tract	54	16	37
Kidney	35	—	35

From Altemeier WA, Culbertson WR, Fullen WD, Shook CD: Intra-abdominal abscesses. *Am J Surg* 125:70, 1973.

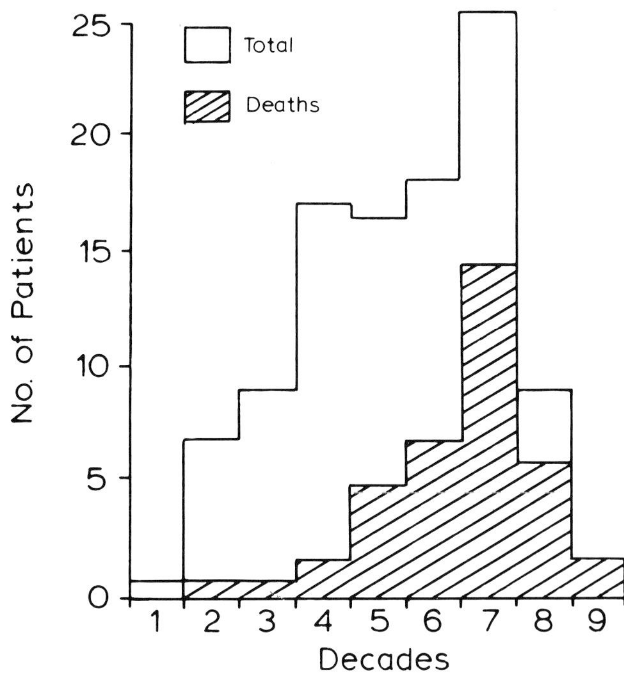

Fig. 34-14. **Mortality of subphrenic abscess by decades of age. (Adapted from Halliday P, Loewenthal J: Aust NZ J Surg 33:260, 1964.)**

The data regarding the mortality for extraserous versus transperitoneal drainage are somewhat confusing and contradictory. Sherman et al,[121] Halliday and Halliday,[122] and DeCosse et al [126] found an increased mortality with transperitoneal drainage vs. extraserous drainage (Table 34-16). Wang and Wilson [119] found that half of all deaths were caused by uncontrolled sepsis, and 20 percent of their patients had more than one abscess at the time of first drainage. This corresponds to the finding of Halasz [127] that 12 to 42 percent of patients have more than one abscess (Table 34-9). In his series, extraserous drainage had a 22 percent mortality vs 8 percent for transperitoneal drainage. Patterson [115] found that the posterior approach to left-sided subphrenic abscesses was unsatisfactory when compared to the anterior approach, and Sherman et al 1969 [121] found that 48 percent of deaths in their series were due to inadequate drainage. Deck and Berne [152] found that 7 percent of the extraserously drained patients developed distant abscesses (Table 34-16). In the transperitoneal group, 1 of 16 patients developed a recurrent abscess and another a heterotopic abscess. These numbers are too small to be statistically significant. DeCosse et al [126] found that none of the patients drained through the right twelfth rib was adequately drained and advocated the lateral approach, which was uniformly effective in their hands (Table 34-16). Most surgeons have agreed that the

TABLE 34-15. MORTALITY AND TIME OF DRAINAGE

Interval from Surgery to Drainage (weeks)	Percent with Drainage	Mortality Percent
0–2	37	28 %
2–4	32	17 %
4–8	20	33 %
8 or more	10	25 %

From Sherman NJ, Davis JR, Jesseph JE: Suphrenic abscess: A continuing hazard. *Am J Surg* 117:117, 1969.

transthoracic route is contraindicated and that rib resection is not necessary.

INTRA-ABDOMINAL FISTULA

Many authors do not distinguish between intra-abdominal infections that are fed by continuous contamination (ie, abscess due to a fistula) and those that result from a discrete episode of contamination. Similarly, all fistulas are not necessarily infections, but most acquired enteral fistulas involve a primary or secondary intraperitoneal infectious component that is important either in pathogenesis or prognosis.

Fistulas that traverse a portion of the normal peritoneal space can arise by several mechanisms: (1) a congenital communication, (2) penetrating trauma, including operation, (3) inflammatory adherence with degeneration of the common wall, (4) perforation of the gastrointestinal tract with abscess formation that subsequently perforates adjacent structures, (5) an abscess outside the gastrointestinal tract that perforates into the intestine. Table 34-17 represents an alternative classification scheme. A recent monograph by Webster and Carey [153] reviews all aspects of the problem.

Acquired fistulas may be either spontaneous or iatrogenic. Spontaneous fistulas can be traumatic but are usually the result of intrinsic bowel disease (cancer, peptic ulcer, inflammatory bowel disease, diverticulitis). Most enterocutaneous fistulas result from iatrogenic causes because the surgical wound allows ready egress to the surface. A technical error (eg, inadequate closure of the duodenal stump or unrecognized injury to the bowel) or local intrinsic disease (eg, Crohn's disease or irradiated bowel) may result in the formation of fistulas. Distal obstruction and consequent increased intraluminal pressure may cause leakage of an otherwise technically adequate anastomosis. Para-anastomotic infection can cause the breakdown of virtually any anastomosis in the early postoperative period. Rare infectious causes of nonoperative fistula include tuberculosis, syphilis, and typhoid. Table 34-18 is a classification scheme of the common causes of enterocutaneous fistulas.

Incidence and Pathogenesis

The incidence of various fistulas is closely related to the factors that control local infection and healing at that site. Most enterocutaneous fistulas follow some type of operative procedure.[153]

After Esophageal Surgery. The well-developed defense mechanisms of the peritoneal cavity make intraperitoneal sites rather resistant to anastomotic breakdown. The esophagus is prone to anastomotic dehiscence because of its extraperitoneal location, the absence of a well-developed seromuscular layer to hold sutures, and tension across the anastomosis. Presternal esophagogastrostomies have a higher incidence of fistula formation compared to retrosternal anastomoses. End-to-side esophagogastrostomy and esophagojejunostomy have lower leakage rates than end-to-end anastomosis, probably because tension is less frequent with the end-to-side anastomosis. Colon interposition for total esophageal replacement is frequently followed by leaks in the neck.[154]

After Gastric Surgery. Gastrostomy sites frequently (6 to 10 percent) become persistent fistulas after removal of the gastrostomy tube.[153] Anastomotic leakage is common acutely after gastric bypass for obesity because swallowed air can readily distend the partially devascularized proximal gastric pouch and rupture a suture line if the nasogas-

TABLE 34-16. METHODS OF INITIAL SUBPHRENIC DRAINAGE IN 44 PATIENTS

Operative Approach	No. (%) of Patients	Abscesses, No. (%)	
		Recurrent	*Heterotopic*
Extraserous	28 (63)	4 (14)	2 (7)
Anterior	20 (45)	1 (3.5)	1 (3.5)
Anterolateral	5 (11.3)	1 (3.5)	1 (3.5)
Posterior	3 (6.8)	2 (7)	0 (0)
Celiotomy	16 (36)	1 (6)	1 (6)
Transperitoneal	14 (32)	1 (6)	1 (6)
Guided extraserous	2 (4.5)	0 (0)	0 (0)

From Deck KB, Berne TV: Selective management of subphrenic abscesses. *Arch Surg* 114:1165, 1979.

tric tube fails to function. Gastrojejunostomy with or without antrectomy has a low anastomotic leak rate.[155]

The blown-out duodenal stump is a feared complication after gastrectomy and Billroth II reconstruction, since one half of the deaths after gastrectomy are caused by this complication.[156] Suture line failures account for the majority of these fistulas, and the operative report usually notes that stump closure was difficult. The incidence of leak is decreasing, however. Soeters et al [155] report that only 0.6 percent of 280 gastrectomy patients (1960–1975) develop fistulas.

Duodenal Fistula. The lateral duodenal fistula arising with the duodenum in continuity (ie, after blunt trauma or unrecognized operative duodenal perforation) has traditionally been considered a more serious complication.[157] Rarely, perforation of a duodenal diverticulum may be the cause. These fistulas have a serious prognosis because all the gastric and duodenal contents exit into the fistula site, whereas only biliary and pancreatic secretions are lost to the skin surface from the end fistula after a Billroth-II reconstruction.

Small Bowel Fistula. Fistulas from the small bowel are typically iatrogenic, but the incidence is increased by intrinsic bowel disease, such as Crohn's disease or irradiation injury. Early suture closure of traumatic small bowel perforation rarely results in a fistula. Few patients with intestinal obstruction spontaneously develop fistulas, although small bowel diverticuli may perforate.

The more proximal small intestinal fistulas typically have a high output, but spontaneous closure will frequently occur if adequate nutrition is maintained. Failure to close under these circumstances is commonly the result of distal obstruction, intrinsic bowel disease, foreign body, or total disruption of the anastomosis.[153] The construction of excretory reservoirs (the Kock pouch-continent ileal reservoir and ileal conduit for urinary tract diversion) is associated with a high rate of leakage.

TABLE 34-17. CLASSIFICATION OF ENTERIC FISTULAS

- I. Congenital
- II. Acquired
  - A. Nonoperative
    - Inflammatory bowel disease
    - Infection
      - Intrinsic
      - Extrinsic
    - Trauma
      - Blunt
      - Penetrating
      - Foreign body
      - Irradiation
    - Neoplastic
      - Benign
      - Malignant
  - B. Operative
    - Intentional
    - Unintentional
      - Technical error
      - Residual intrinsic disease
      - Distal obstruction
      - Compromised host
      - Local sepsis with anastomotic failure

From Webster MW Jr, Carey LC: Fistulae of the intestinal tract. *Curr Probl Surg* 13:5, 1976.

TABLE 34-18. COMMON CAUSES OF ENTEROCUTANEOUS FISTULAS

Orocutaneous	Trauma
Pharyngocutaneous	Carcinoma
Esophagocutaneous	Postoperative
Gastrocutaneous	Trauma
Gastrojejunocutaneous	Gastric ulcer
	Stomal ulcer
	Radiation therapy
	Postoperative
	Anastomotic failure
	Gastrostomy
Duodenocutaneous	Trauma
	Postoperative
	Duodenotomy
	Duodenal stump leak
Enterocutaneous or colocutaneous (fecal fistula)	Congenital vitelline duct
	Crohn's disease
	Ulcerative colitis
	Diverticulitis
	Tuberculosis
	Foreign body (intraperitoneal)
	Trauma (intraextraluminal)
	Extrauterine pregnancy
	Carcinoma of colon
	Amebiasis
	Strangulated hernia
	Postoperative
	Intestinal injury
	Anastomotic failure
Appendicocutaneous	Perforated appendicitis
Appendicoumbilical	Appendiceal trauma
Enteroperineal or coloperineal	Following pelvic exenteration

From Webster MW Jr, Carey LC: Fistulae of the intestinal tract. *Curr Probl Surg* 13:5, 1976.

After Colonic Surgery. Colonic anastomotic leaks are decreasing in frequency. The incidence of fecal fistula is around 12 percent in controlled randomized prospective studies using mechanical bowel preparation without parenteral or oral antibiotics. When oral antibiotic bowel preparation is added (neomycin, erythromycin), the rate falls dramatically [158,159] (Chapter 23).

Intraperitoneal anastomoses have a lower fistula rate than do extraperitoneal anastomoses. In fact, a rate as high as 50 percent has been reported in low anterior anastomosis studied routinely with radiocontrast enemas in the early postoperative period.[160] Clinical leakage rates after such anastomoses are much lower (10 to 30 percent). For this reason, routine proximal protective colostomy is no longer recommended. The use of the automatic circumferential stapling device for the creation of low anterior anastomoses has further reduced the fistula rate (1.1 percent).[161]

After Operation for Crohn's Disease or Radiation Enteritis. These conditions particularly predispose to fistula formation as a complication of the disease or as a consequence of operative therapy. Cases of pseudo-Crohn's disease have also been reported in which a persistent fistula associated with a retained foreign body was not recognized during the initial evaluation. The histologic picture is similar to classic Crohn's disease.

In patients who received intra-abdominal irradiation with radiation injury to the bowel, spontaneous fistula developed in less than 1 percent, but 16 of 51 (31 percent) patients undergoing laparotomy after radiation bowel injury developed an enterocutaneous fistula.[162]

General Aspects of the Pathogenesis of Acquired Fistulas

Fistula formation after enterotomy is sometimes the result of inadequate operative technique: an incomplete closure of the enterotomy, sutures that impair local blood supply, excessive tension across an anastomosis that pulls apart repaired bowel, or placement of a foreign body (eg, a drain) near a fresh anastomosis so that healing is impaired. After extraluminal bacterial contamination, paraenteric abscesses form and penetrate into adjacent structures, out through incisions, or along drainage tracts.

Other factors can increase the incidence of fistulas:

1. Intestinal bacterial counts may be increased by preexisting disease, such as gastric achlorhydria or small bowel obstruction, resulting in a colonic flora within the proximal small bowel. Subsequent enterotomy spills a larger or more virulent local bacterial inoculum.

2. Adhesions may prevent removal of spilled bacteria from the peritoneal cavity by the diaphragmatic lymphatics, allowing local proliferation with abscess formation.

3. Preexistant fibrosis can decrease the influx of phagocytic cells normally capable of eliminating a small bacterial inoculum.

4. Unresolved obstruction distal to an entrectomy may cause increased intraluminal pressure with blowout of weakened areas.

Local bacterial infection of the enterotomy site is critically important to the breakdown of otherwise technically adequate intestinal anastomoses. Cohn and Rives [159] have demonstrated convincingly that even ischemic anastomoses are protected from dehiscence if antibiotics are infused upstream from the anastomosis. Preoperative administration of oral antibiotics has reduced the anastomotic leak or fistula rate dramatically after elective colonic surgery.[158] Furthermore, limbs of bowel with no function seldom develop fistulas. Thus, in the relative absence of both intraluminal contents containing bacteria and intraluminal pressure, small holes rapidly seal themselves unless foreign bodies isolate the anastomosis from normal peritoneal defenses.

Abscesses induce fistulas, but the mechanisms are poorly defined. Several processes appear to be at work:

1. The contents of abscesses are hyperosmolar as a result of the release of lysosomal enzymes and tissue digestion. The cavity expands as fluid accumulates.

2. Phagocytic cells release their enzymes, including elastase and collagenase which break down the newly formed collagen. Collagenase inhibitor therapy reduces the rate of fistula formation and speeds healing of anastomoses.[163]

3. Many bacteria secrete extracellular enzymes, including collagenase. If the bacterial inoculum can be reduced by antibiotics, the whole process can be aborted.

An impaired local blood supply, ie, atherosclerosis, radiation fibrosis, or hypovolemic shock, also markedly increases the risk of fistulas. Hermreck and Crawford [164] found that anastomotic leak occurred in 80 percent of patients who developed a period of shock after esophageal surgery vs an 8 percent leak rate in patients not experiencing shock.

Any factor that adversely affects wound healing (chronic steroid administration, malnutrition, vitamin deficiency, diabetes mellitus) can increase the incidence of fistula formation. Intrinsic bowel disease that affects the wall of the bowel, such as Crohn's disease, enteric tuberculosis, actinomycosis, amebiasis, typhoid, syphilis, or carcinoma, predisposes to fistula formation.[165] Biliary stones within the gallbladder, common duct, or intestine can erode into the bowel. Similarly, drains within abscess cavities or along fistula tracts can induce fistulas between adjacent organs.

Host defenses function to wall off the contamination when a leak develops. For practical purposes, enteric bacteria are always present and induce diffuse or local peritonitis. When the intestinal breakdown is so sudden that no preexisting peritoneal inflammation has taken place, the entire peritoneal cavity will become contaminated. This is characteristic of perforated gastric and duodenal ulcers, of traumatic and operative enterotomies, and of occasional cases of perforated diverticulitis. If inflammation has been present for several days, as in penetrating carcinoma or Crohn's disease, a localized leak is more likely. The fistula may not be discovered until the abscess is evacuated and the cavity continues to drain gastrointestinal contents.

A drain placed prophylactically at operation creates a fibrinous and later fibrous tract. This provides rapid removal of extravasated intestinal contents if there is leakage of gastrointestinal contents. The preformed fistula tract is narrow, isolated from free peritoneal cavity, and in direct connection with the skin. These are the characteristics of the ideal fistula, which will heal rapidly.[153] However, drains may impair healing of enterotomy sites or erode into normal bowel. Prophylactic drainage may, therefore, become a self-fulfilling prophecy for fistula formation.

In the absence of a preformed tract, enterocutaneous fistulas usually emerge at incision sites. The dissection pathway is unhealed and susceptible to breakdown from pressure and enteric, pancreatic, or neutrophilic enzyme digestion. Enteric leaks that do not become fistulas in this way develop into abscesses, which either remain localized or dissect along tissue planes to emerge at unexpected sites, eg, the pleural space, pericardium, bronchus, biliary tract, bladder, vagina. Because fistulous tracts usually drain via a nonmucosa-lined tract, they have a tendency to close spontaneously (albeit slowly) if adequate patient nutrition is maintained. Factors that preclude spontaneous tract closure include distal obstruction to the normal flow of enteric contents, a high enzyme content of the draining material, a foreign body remaining within the tract, total disruption of bowel continuity, or growth of mucosa along the tract.[153]

Cancer, irradiation, and negative nitrogen balance reduce the probability of spontaneous closure. An insidious problem is pooling of the gastrointestinal tract contents in a large stagnant abscess cavity at the base of the fistula inadequately drained by a long, narrow fistula tract. This pooling fosters abscess formation, and these patients usually remain septic. Conversely, patients with well-formed fistula tracts may feel healthy, especially if it is a low-output fistula. Fistulograms are necessary to define the extent of the fistula tract and its associated abscesses in most instances.

Etiology

With the exception of congenital communications, fistulas arise from the same pathologic causes as peritonitis and intra-abdominal abscesses—traumatic, operative, inflammatory, or neoplastic visceral disruption. Consequently, the same mixed aerobic and anaerobic flora are associated with intra-abdominal fistulas (Tables 34-1 and 34-11). With antibiotic treatment, resistant organisms appear, such as *Pseudomonas, Serratia* and *Candida* species. In addition, any intrinsic intestinal parasites that elicit necrosis or granulomatous host reactions can lead to fistula formation. Table 34-19 lists some of these rare infectious causes that will require the special treatment described in Chapters 7, 11, 38, and 39.

TABLE 34-19. RARE PRIMARY INFECTIOUS ETIOLOGIES OF INTRA-ABDOMINAL FISTULAS

	Rare Primary Infectious Etiology
Enterocutaneous	Tuberculosis Amebiasis Actinomycosis
Enteroenteric	Tuberculosis Typhoid Syphilis
Enterorespiratory	Tuberculosis Histoplasmosis Actinomycosis Nonspecific adenitis Syphilis Aortic aneurysm Gumma
Biliary respiratory and biliary pericardial	Amebiasis Echinococcosis
Nephroenteric or ureteroenteric	Tuberculosis Echinococcosis Bilharziasis
Enteropericardial	Tuberculous adenitis

From Webster MW Jr, Carey LC: Fistulae of the intestinal tract. *Curr Probl Surg* 13:5, 1976.

Clinical Manifestations

Table 34-20 lists the clinical problems created by gastrointestinal fistulas. The septic problems will be stressed first, since these may be life-threatening, and the other problems frequently persist even after the infectious element is controlled.

Acute acquired fistulas due to operative or accidental trauma present with the general symptoms and signs of a cryptic intra-abdominal abscess. Fever, leukocytosis, prolonged ileus, and poorly localized abdominal pain are characteristic.[166] Signs consistent with partial intestinal obstruction are common. Steadily increasing drainage from a drain site may be found, but more often a wound infection is opened only to subsequently drain enteric contents. Occasionally, patients will rapidly improve after drainage is established, but, more often, the patient continues to look and feel ill. This correlates with the degree of pooling within the abscess cavity. The most proximal small bowel fistulas are usually the most symptomatic because of the corrosive nature of pancreatic-duodenal contents. Activated pancreatic exocrine secretions can digest both the external skin and peritoneal surfaces. Acute internal fistulas will resemble abscesses unless, by chance, they decompress themselves into adjacent organs.[165] If enteroenteric or biliary enteric fistulas result, the diagnosis may be delayed until symptoms of malabsorption appear. Spontaneous drainage of intra-abdominal contents into bronchial tree, renal pelvis, or bladder may occasionally be life threatening.

Diagnosis

The noninvasive methods previously described for the diagnosis of intra-abdominal abscesses can all be useful.[139a,153] The diagnosis of enterocutaneous fistulas is usually readily apparent when enteric contents appear at the skin surface. Sinograms and enteric contrast studies usually are successful in outlining the tract, diagnosing abscesses that lie along it, and establishing their origin.

The oral administration of methylene blue or powdered charcoal may document a fistula in doubtful cases, whereas the water-soluble contrast materials available sometimes fail to detail an anatomic defect. Chemical analysis of the drainage fluid is sometimes valuable in determining its source (eg, amylase, bilirubin, creatinine).

Treatment

The therapeutic goals are dictated by the problems that threaten the patient. The initial treatment of acute enterocutaneous fistulas has been outlined by Fischer [166] and can be adapted to all acute fistulas:

1. Correct the fluid and electrolyte imbalances. These

TABLE 34-20. COMPLICATIONS OF ENTEROCUTANEOUS FISTULA

Nutritional	Septic
Dehydration	Peritonitis
Electrolyte shifts	Abscess
Malnutrition	Septicemia
Vitamin deficiencies	Distant organ failure
Trace element deficiencies	Local
Catheter related	Bleeding
Sepsis	Skin excoriation
Thrombosis	Persistent fistula
Pneumothorax	Wound infection
	Wound dehiscence
	Psychologic depression

are especially troublesome in upper intestinal fistulas from which fluid losses can be enormous.

2. Control infection by early adequate drainage of the tract and of any abscess cavities. Reber et al[167] found that 81 percent of 186 fistula patients were septic on admission.

3. Provide adequate nutrition. Total parenteral nutrition has revolutionized the therapy of enteric fistulas.[166-169] Adequate calories must be administered with sufficient amino acids, free fatty acids, vitamins, and trace elements. Enteral alimentation, either proximal to a colonic fistula or distal to an esophageal or gastric fistula, may be possible and preferable to parenteral alimentation.

4. Radiographic evaluations, including sinograms and contrast studies, should be performed to precisely identify the enteric origin, the presence of preexisting disease (lymphoma, carcinoma, Crohn's), an associated inadequately drained abscess, and the likelihood of spontaneous closure. Because complete distal obstruction or anastomotic dehiscence virtually precludes spontaneous closure, early surgical intervention must be undertaken in selected patients. The contrast studies must be repeated at intervals to document healing and identify those patients requiring surgical correction.

5. Control skin excoriation, especially in patients with proximal gastrointestinal tract fistulas. Skin problems may be especially troublesome while awaiting spontaneous closure. Karaya gum, Stomadhesive, and fitted acrylic appliances all offer improved care in this area.

6. Reduce the volume of secretions entering the fistula from the bowel and avoid pooling within the tract.

7. Definitive operation is indicated for fistulas that fail to close spontaneously after four to six weeks of total parenteral nutrition and in patients with spontaneous fistulas due to malignancy or Crohn's disease.[167,170]

Early Management of Enteric Fistulas. The therapeutic goal of early management is to convert the fistula from the state of a partially drained abscess cavity into a narrow linear tract as rapidly as possible. As soon as an enteric fistula is recognized, oral intake is stopped. The majority of fistulas occur in the postoperative patient when ileus is still present. Therefore, nasogastric or long-tube intestinal decompression is usually indicated as soon as the intestinal leak is suspected in order to prevent further distention of anastomoses and to minimize the output of enteric contents.

Rapid control of sepsis is life saving in these patients.[171] All acute fistulas represent inadequately drained intraperitoneal infections until proved otherwise. Pooled secretions within the abdominal cavity must be continuously and efficiently evacuated along with loculated intraperitoneal abscesses. Antibiotic therapy must be directed toward the polymicrobial enteric flora. Proximal small bowel fistulas typically have low numbers of bacteria per milliliter of fluid, but because of their large fluid volume and high content of digestive enzymes, pooling of the secretions can yield virtual autodigestion of peritoneal surfaces. Distal fistulas have a less caustic output but so many pathogenic bacteria that abscesses are inevitable if adequate drainage is not immediately established.

Antibiotic usage in these patients is controversial. Soeters et al[155] advise that antibiotics should be reserved for septicemia and cholangitis or used for intraperitoneal infection only in conjunction with surgical drainage. This point of view probably reflects a broad experience with chronic spontaneous fistulas without major infectious components. However, if one regards all *early* acute fistulas as an external manifestation of ongoing sepsis within a relatively limited portion of the peritoneal cavity, antibiotics become necessary until the septic component can be controlled. Athanassiades et al[171] found severe intraperitoneal infection in 35 of 70 fistula patients. In 21 patients, clinical signs of sepsis preceded the appearance of the fistula, but in 14 patients it appeared after the fistula presented. With time and adequate drainage, the body walls off this septic focus and a fibrous tract relatively resistant to bacterial invasion is formed. Only at that time do antibiotics become unnecessary.

The choice of antibiotics depends upon the organisms cultured. Presumptive therapy should include those antibiotics discussed in the section on therapy for peritonitis, since mixed aerobic and anaerobic infections will be found in most cases of enteric fistula. Adjustment of antibiotics will be necessary depending on the clinical course and the changing flora. Fistulas caused by the unusual organisms listed in Table 34-19 require additional treatment with the appropriate antimicrobial agents described in Chapters 11 and 18.

Ideally, the patient with enterocutaneous fistula should be positioned so that gravity can continuously assist the drainage of enteric contents. A circle bed or a Stryker frame is useful for this purpose. Unfortunately, the awkward positions that result are uncomfortable. An alternative choice, which has the additional advantage of protecting the skin from the digestive enzymes, is suction drainage of the cavity. Sump tubes offer the most efficient fluid removal. Hard plastic tubes that are capable of eroding into the bowel or slipping into the bowel should be avoided. On the other hand, pliable drainage tubes (eg, Jackson-Pratt drains) are relatively difficult to position unless they are placed during operation. One option is a large-diameter, soft latex tube with a smaller intraluminal sump tube introduced into the fistula at bedside and placed to low continuous suction. Persistence of a well-drained fistula in the absence of distal obstruction or malignancy, however, may be due to the drain itself. When the tract is long and fibrous, most drains can be removed, allowing spontaneous closure of the fistula.

Radiographic studies are then carried out under fluoroscopic control, using water-soluble contrast media introduced via the drain catheter to evaluate the relationship of the catheter tip to the fistula and determine the cavity size. The surgeon should be present during these examinations. Discovery of complete anastomotic dehiscence, retained foreign body, or complete distal obstruction mandate early operation because continued high output and uncontrolled sepsis are more frequent in these settings. On the other hand, chronic, well-walled-off, short, straight fistulous tracts require a far less aggressive approach.

All patients require long-term nutritional support to facilitate spontaneous closure of enteric fistulas. Unless enteral tube feeding is possible, early institution of total parenteral nutrition via central venous catheter is indicated.[155,166,168] Because of the high output of many enterocutaneous fistulas, 4,000 to 5,000 calories per day may be required.[166] High caloric intake correlates with a higher spontaneous closure rate and a lower mortality (Table 34-21). Most patients with enterocutaneous fistulas will require total parenteral nutrition for a minimum of several weeks, so careful attention should be paid to free fatty acid, vitamin, and trace element requirements.[169] Some authors feel that high-dose vitamin C administration augments wound healing.[166] Zinc deficiency is an occasional finding in patients with enterocutaneous fistulas.[166] Symptoms respond dramatically to addition of zinc to the hyperalimentation solution. Several patients have developed hypocalcemia with tetany due to unsuspected magnesium deficiency. The hypocalcemia is totally refractory until adequate magnesium levels are obtained. Severe hypophosphatemia also can occur. Central venous catheter care is also important in these patients. Ryan et al[172] noted a 20 percent incidence of sepsis when the catheters received poor local care vs 3 percent with excellent care (Chapter 24).

It is sometimes possible to collect the drainage from duodenal or high jejunal fistulas for reinfusion into a distal limb of small bowel.[156] Although this is applicable only in selected patients, a reduced complication rate for fluid, electrolyte, and protein losses justifies its use when possible.

The proximal, high-output fistulas have been especially difficult management problems because of the resulting skin excoriation. Reber et al[167] found a significant decrease in output of proximal fistulas if gastric acid secretion was suppressed by cimetadine.

Many different devices have been described to aid in the collection of fluid from enterocutaneous fistulas and reduce pooling on the skin surface. These include configurations to hold a sump tube in position on the fistula surface.[173] Several investigators propose that acidification of the output prevents activation of the proteolytic pancreatic enzymes responsible for digestion of the abdominal wall.[173] Lactic acid solution (0.45 percent) has been dripped into the wound and aspirated continuously in an attempt to flush away the highly caustic material.[173] Similarly, adherent ion exchange resin pads with an acidic pH have been applied around fistula tracts in an attempt to prevent activation of these enzymes. Stomadhesive pads are useful in protecting the skin and allowing healing of the excoriated areas. Custom silicone castings of the abdominal wall defect have been used in management of enterocutaneous fistulas that were so irregular that conventional stoma appliances could not be used. Silicone castings of the abdominal wall are made after occluding the fistula with a disposable syringe. After the casting hardens, the syringe is removed and karaya paste is applied to the undersurface of the casting. A conventional stoma appliance is applied to the surface of the casting. Such castings allow patients to be ambulatory, and, in one series, five of the six patients so treated were discontinued from total parenteral nutrition and treated as outpatients.[169] Although none had spontaneous closure of the fistula, their direct hospital costs were reduced and adequate nutrition was maintained during this period.

Operative Management of Specific Fistulas

Drainage of Abscesses. A common problem in many fistulas is a concurrent, localized intraperitoneal infection or associated abscess. Management includes elimination

TABLE 34-21. CLOSURE RATE AND MORTALITY IN DIFFERENT SERIES WITH AND WITHOUT TOTAL PARENTERAL NUTRITION (TPN)

	Year	Spontaneous Closure %	Operative Closure %	Total Closure Rate %	Average Closure Time (Days)	Mortality %
No TPN						
Chapman et al	1964	—	—	89 *	—	
		—	—	37 †	—	55
Halversan et al	1969	29	27	56	59	40
Lorenzo and Beal	1969	—	—	61	—	30
TPN						
Sheldon et al	1971	—	—	78	—	16
Ali and Leffall	1972	25	45	70	—	30
Roback and Nicoloff	1972	—	—	—	—	31
MacFadyen et al	1973	70	22	92	35	8
Kessler	1974	—	—	100	24	0
Himal et al	1974	56	36	92	—	8
Aquirre et al	1974	29	50	79	—	21
Freund et al	1975	60	13	73	40	27

* More than 1,600–2,000 cal per day.
† Less than 1,000 cal per day.
From Freund H, Anner C, Saltz NJ: Management of gastrointestinal fistulas with total parenteral nutrition. *Int Surg* 61:273, 1976.

of the contaminating source by intestinal resection, exclusion, or exteriorization. Then the abscess cavity can be treated as described previously. The source cannot be eliminated in all cases, especially in patients with high gastrointestinal fistulas or preexisting disease. Only efficient drainage can be offered to some patients.

Specific Management Problems in Enteric Fistulas. Specific levels of fistulization cause different problems that require brief consideration. Webster and Carey [153] provide further discussion and an extensive bibliography.

ESOPHAGEAL FISTULAS. After total esophagectomy, fistulization at the proximal suture line of the interposed bowel in the neck is a rather common occurrence.[154] Generalized necrosis of the bowel must be ruled out, since this is a surgical emergency. Saliva is relatively nontoxic if adequately drained, so drainage and maintenance of nutrition usually result in a spontaneous closure of these fistulas unless there is intestinal discontinuity.

Esophagogastrostomy and esophagojejunostomy leakage within the chest represent somewhat more formidable problems. After a Roux-en-Y anastomosis, there is no pancreatic or biliary flow through the anastomosis, and only saliva passes into the mediastinum. Leakage is usually manifested by a pleural effusion and systemic toxicity. Penicillin plus an aminoglycoside should be used for early antibiotic therapy, since the hospitalized patient most often has altered oral flora. Placement of a chest tube transpleurally to lie near the site of leakage will be adequate therapy only if the pleural cavity is drained and the reexpanded lung contacts the site of leak, allowing it to seal. If prompt control is not gained, however, thoracotomy with suture closure of the leak, decortication of the pleura, drainage of pleural loculations, and reexpansion of the lung will all be required to seal the fistula. Diverting cervical esophagostomy may be necessary.[164]

A more complicated situation is produced if the esophagus has been anastomosed to the side of a jejunal loop or a partially obstructed stomach. In these cases, an enteropleural or gastropleural fistula is created, which will continue to contaminate the pleura with feculent flora. Consistent patient survival will only be achieved by taking down the anastomosis and diverting salivary flow.[164]

Esophageal perforation can result from esophagoscopy or bouginage. If the perforation is recognized early, successful primary suture can be undertaken. In contrast, postemetic rupture has a poor prognosis because the rupture usually forces a large quantity of contaminated gastric contents into the mediastinum. Early primary suture repair is indicated but usually fails if extensive mediastinitis is present. Buttressing the closure with the stomach fundus may reinforce the repair. The mediastinum must be drained into the pleura, and a drainage tube can be left near the suture line in the event that it fails. Esophageal diversion and drainage rather than operative closure have been advocated for late cases because of the high failure rate.[174] Operation is lifesaving in severely toxic patients, however.

Postoperatively, the patient must be maintained on parenteral feeding. The saliva must be aspirated via a tube placed just above the leak. Constant aspiration of the stomach via a gastrostomy may be required to prevent regurgitation of gastric contents. If the fistula volume remains large, cervical esophagogastrostomy or bowel interposition procedure is necessary. This has been advocated as a primary procedure in cases of severe mediastinitis with esophageal necrosis.

GASTROCUTANEOUS FISTULAS. Gastrocutaneous fistulas most commonly result after removal of a temporary gastrostomy.[153] Most other gastrocutaneous fistulas appear when an inflammatory or neoplastic process binds the gastric wall to the anterior abdominal wall or after gastric surgery, especially if distal obstruction is present. A short tract without associated extensive abscess formation usually occurs. Excision of the mucosa-lined tract is curative in the absence of obstruction.

Gastrojejunocutaneous fistulas may follow an anastomotic disruption or as a late complication of perforated anastomotic ulcer.[165] An associated abscess is common. Drainage of the abscess and closure of the inflamed bowel wall lead to recurrence. A preferred treatment is drainage of the fistula, proximal gastric decompression, and elimination of gastric obstruction. The fistulas will usually close. If operative intervention is necessary, resection of the stomach and reconstruction of the gastrojejunostomy will be required. Abscesses associated with gastrojejunocutaneous fistulas can penetrate into adherent colon to produce a gastrojejunocolonic fistula. Treatment thereafter will require simultaneous transverse colostomy and excision of the colonic fistula at the time of the abscess drainage. When associated with Zollinger-Ellison syndrome, total gastrectomy is indicated.

DUODENOCUTANEOUS FISTULAS. There are two types of duodenocutaneous fistulas: (1) an end duodenal fistula, which usually results from a blown duodenal stump closure following gastrectomy and gastrojejunostomy (Billroth II reconstruction), and (2) a lateral duodenal fistula, which follows the inadvertent or planned duodenotomy. The lateral fistulas are more lethal because of the severe loss of food, fluid, and electrolytes and digestion of the skin by pancreatic or duodenal contents.[159]

Prevention may be the best therapy, since placement of an end or lateral duodenostomy tube routinely for difficult duodenal stump closure nearly eliminates this complication.[156] Anderson et al [157] noted that placement of a periduodenal drain at operation reduces the mortality if a leak later occurs.

A subhepatic abscess is an almost constant feature of such fistulas. After control of the infection, the fistulas have been classified as high output (> 500 ml per day) or low output. Lateral duodenal fistulas have a higher mortality and may persist chronically.[157] Control of the fistula may be obtained by sump drainage and proximal gastric decompression.[157] A few authors advocate prophylactic placement of a drainage tube through the duodenal stump, securing it with a chromic catgut suture. Subsequent aspiration of the duodenum minimizes peritoneal soilage and skin excoriation and allows the formation of a thin, direct drainage tract. The aspirate can be reinfused distally into a feeding jejunostomy tube via a closed system.[156] This distal tube can also be used for supplemental enteral feeding.

Welch and Edmond [175] have advocated early surgical closure with an omental patch to reinforce the suture line. Nassos and Braasch [176] suggested control of sepsis and malnutrition, followed by delayed surgical closure. Recent evidence suggests that, with aggressive nutritional support and control of sepsis, many of these fistulas will close spontaneously.[177]

With the lateral fistula even control of secretions and local infection may be difficult. Diverticulization of the duodenum requires closure of the duodenal perforation, accompanied by antrectomy, vagotomy, duodenostomy, and Billroth II gastrojejunostomy, with conversion of the lateral duodenal fistula to an end duodenal fistula. This is indicated only with associated pancreatic trauma—even then pancreatectomy or duodenectomy may be required.

GASTROCOLIC, GASTROJEJUNOCOLIC, OR DUODENOCOLIC FISTULAS. The infectious problems with these types of fistulas are different. Fecal contamination of the stomach and duodenum leads to bacterial overgrowth in the upper intestine. Upper abdominal pain, weight loss, vomiting, and severe watery diarrhea are common. Barium enema will usually determine the diagnosis.[153] After control of any associated intra-abdominal abscesses, resection of the adjacent loops of bowel will usually cure the fistula if the primary problem (duodenal ulcer, carcinoma of colon) is also adequately treated. In debilitating illnesses, a prior proximal diverting colostomy may be helpful.[140]

JEJUNAL AND ILEAL FISTULAS. Operation to relieve intestinal obstruction secondary to extensive adhesions is the usual cause.[155,171] Such patients must be evaluated early for unrelieved distal obstruction. If obstruction remains, early reoperation to relieve the problem or divert the fecal stream is necessary. In the absence of obstruction, hyperalimentation is indicated in cases of radiation bowel injury unless there is evidence of localized injury.[162]

Anastomotic leaks due to residual Crohn's disease will, on occasion, heal with conservative management, but perforation due to recurrent anastomotic malignant disease rarely does. Massive fluid and electrolyte losses in high-output syndromes and skin excoriation are the principal problems encountered in these patients.

Leaking intraperitoneal ileocolonic anastomoses often spontaneously close on a minimal residue diet once sepsis is controlled. An exception is ileocolonic anastomotic failure because of intrinsic colonic disease, such as residual Crohn's disease. In these cases, resection with primary ileostomy is preferred therapy.

CECAL OR APPENDICEAL FISTULAS. Cecal fistula after drainage of a ruptured appendix is seldom a major problem if the infection is adequately controlled. The fistula behaves much like a cecostomy and usually closes spontaneously.

COLONIC FISTULAS. When no intrinsic disease is present, diverting proximal colostomy has been advocated for colonic fistulas, especially if sepsis persists. An alternative is direct attack on the leaking site. Experience with perforated diverticulitis indicates that patients with primary resection of a perforated colon have fewer septic complications.[130] In those cases, resection and primary anastomosis are possible if the surgeon feels that the septic problem has been surgically controlled. For complete anastomotic dehiscence or generalized peritonitis after diverticular perforation, a Hartman's procedure and end-on colostomy will allow more rapid control of life-threatening sepsis (Chapter 39).

ENTEROENTERIC FISTULAS. In contrast to all the enterocutaneous fistulas, enteroenteric fistulas rarely cause gross intraperitoneal soiling. They usually represent spontaneous internal drainage of a localized abscess or perforation of a local inflammatory process. As a result, the patients have fewer septic episodes and frequently will appear as chronically ill rather than acutely ill. Enteroenteric fistulas, however, seldom close spontaneously and usually require segmental resection of the diseased bowel. On occasion, additional procedures are indicated, such as total gastrectomy in patients who present with marginal ulcer causing a gastrojejunocolonic fistula secondary to unsuspected Zollinger-Ellison syndrome. Many of the patients require intensive nutritional therapy because of chronic malnutrition but seldom present with fluid and electrolyte problems, skin excoriation, or sepsis. In this respect, they represent much less complex clinical management problems. Webster and Carey [153] review this subject in detail.

Special Problems. Internal fistulas to the respiratory tract or pleura will require tube or open thoracostomy drainage of the empyema to evacuate enteral or biliary secretions so that they cannot contaminate the bronchial tree. Associated pneumonia and lung abscesses will require the approaches described in Chapter 30. In the case of esophagopleural fistulas, however, it is important to recognize that failure to achieve rapid and complete pleural drainage with tube thoracostomy may be the result of pleural adhesions or restrictive fibrosis of the lung. In either case, open thoracotomy is necessary with proper placement of drainage tubes and decortication of the pleural surface to permit full expansion of the lung and obliteration of the abscess cavity. Prompt recognition of this problem is required to permit healing.

The special problems of fistulas to the pericardium are those of acute pericarditis, namely, tamponade and adequate drainage of a purulent pericarditis (Chapter 32).

Prognosis

Table 34-21 lists the tabulated mortality and closure rates in several series of enterocutaneous fistulas collected by Freund et al.[169] Two more recent series by Reber et al [167] and Soeters et al [155] reported 433 patients with an overall mortality of 20 percent. Fluid and electrolyte problems previously were a major cause of death. Soeters et al [155] found this complication in 49 percent of their patients, but it was not responsible for any deaths.

Numerous studies have documented that prognosis is directly related to how rapidly infection is controlled. Athanassiades et al [171] reported twice the number of fistula-related deaths in septic vs nonseptic fistula patients. Soeters et al [155] found that if sepsis were controlled, the mortality was 0 vs 81 percent for uncontrolled sepsis. Reber et al [167] reported that if sepsis were controlled within one month, mortality was 8 percent and the spontaneous closure rate was 48 percent. If sepsis were not controlled within one month, the mortality was 85 percent and the closure rate was 6 percent.

Many patients are malnourished as a result of their enterocutaneous fistulas. Chapman et al [177] reported 100 percent mortality for the combination of a high-output fistula plus malnutrition. The mortality was 14 percent in patients receiving more than 3,000 calories per day and 55 percent for those receiving less. Soeters et al,[155] however, have emphasized that adequate nutrition is of little benefit unless the sepsis is first controlled.

Other factors that affect mortality of enterocutaneous fistulas are listed in Table 34-22.[167] The prognosis is poor for older patients and patients with Crohn's disease, cancer, or previous bowel irradiation. Prior bowel irradiation is frequently complicated by abdominal carcinomatosis and intractable intestinal obstruction.[162]

Table 34-23 [167] relates the spontaneous enterocutaneous fistula closure rate and mortality with the site of enteric origin. The small bowel fistulas closed spontaneously far less often than did esophageal, gastric, or colocutaneous fistulas. The gastric, biliary, and jejunal fistulas had higher mortality than esophageal, ileal, or colocutaneous fistulas.

Although the prognosis is somewhat better since the advent of total parenteral nutrition, high-output fistulas are still associated with a higher mortality (8 to 65 percent, with an average of approximately 30 percent).

Other factors affecting the rate of spontaneous fistula closure are listed in Table 34-22. No one has approached the excellent results reported by MacFayden et al,[178] an 82 percent spontaneous enterocutaneous fistula closure rate and a 6.5 percent mortality rate with total parenteral nutrition.

When adequate calories were administered by either hyperalimentation or tube feeding, Reber et al [167] found no statistically significant difference in mortality (7 percent enteral vs 14 percent parenteral) or closure rate (22 percent enteral vs 37 percent parenteral). But tube-fed patients are a selected group with a significant length of small bowel in continuity. Patients with watering-pot abdomen or midsmall bowel fistulas are probably excluded. Reber concluded that parenteral nutrition had not altered mortality but had greatly simplified the management of these patients, who could be provided with adequate caloric and nitrogen requirements within 2 days rather than the 7 to 10 days required with tube feeding.[167]

TABLE 34-22. FACTORS AFFECTING SPONTANEOUS FISTULA CLOSURE

Factor	Closure Rate (%)
Local sepsis	Virually zero
Complete anastomotic dehiscence	Virtually zero
Retained foreign body	Virtually zero
Epithelialization of tract	Virtually zero
Distal obstruction	Virtually zero
Crohn's disease of small bowel	8
Irradiation of small bowel	14
Tract less than 2 cm	17
Cancer	26
Closure rate with none of these adverse factors	32

From Reber H, Roberts C, Way LW, Dunphy JE: Management of external gastrointestinal fistulas. *Ann Surg* 188:460, 1978.

Soeters et al [155] also investigated the role of hyperalimentation and the mortality for fistulas. In their series, hyperalimentation did not lower the mortality, but there were twice as many septic patients in the hyperalimented group as in the control group. In the esophageal, gastric, and duodenal fistula group, the mortality fell from 62 percent for historical controls to 40 percent in the nonhyperalimented group and 23.5 percent in the hyperalimented group, suggesting an improvement with hyperalimentation.

The spontaneous closure rate has not obviously improved with hyperalimentation. The closure rate still remains 20 to 35 percent in collected series.

Monod-Broca [170] showed that more than 80 percent of all enterocutaneous fistulas that underwent spontaneous closure did so within 40 days. Similarly, Reber et al [167] reported that greater than 90 percent of all fistulas that

TABLE 34-23. RELATION OF ORIGIN OF FISTULA TO MORTALITY AND SPONTANEOUS CLOSURE RATE OF ENTEROCUTANEOUS FISTULAS

Origin of Fistula	Number of Patients	Percent of all Fistulas	Fistula-related Deaths (%)	Spontaneous Closure (%)
Esophagus	11	6	0 (0)	9 (82)
Stomach	14	8	4 (29)	6 (43)
Duodenum (end)	8	4	2 (25)	4 (50)
Duodenum (side)	11	6	0 (0)	3 (27)
Jejunum	48	26	13 (27)	10 (21)
Ileum	72	39	8 (10)	14 (19)
Pancreas	9	5	1 (11)	6 (67)
Bile ducts	19	5	2 (20)	6 (60)
Cecum/appendix	8	5	0 (0)	4 (44)
Colon	40	22	5 (13)	12 (30)
Rectum	10	5	1 (10)	3 (30)

Adapted from Reber H, Roberts C, Way LW, Dunphy JE: Management of external gastrointestinal fistulas. *Ann Surg* 188:460, 1978.

ultimately closed did so within one month. For this reason, both authors recommend operative closure at one month if continuing improvement is not evident. This is supported by Monod-Broca's data that the highest success and lowest mortality for operative closure occurs if the procedure is carried out *more* than 15 days after fistula formation.

In general, resection with primary anastomosis is the therapy of choice if sepsis is not present. There are two important exceptions, however. One is the patient whose bowel cannot be resected because of extensive adhesions. In these patients, exclusion or bypass procedures are preferable. Similarly in patients with irradiated bowel, the rate of leakage is so high after resection and primary anastomosis that several authors have advocated exclusion procedures as the therapy of choice. Operative closure is least likely to succeed in patients with irradiated bowel, Crohn's disease, and residual malignant tumor.[167]

Enterocutaneous fistulas remain a feared complication for the general surgeon because of their extreme morbidity and frequently iatrogenic etiology. We have stressed the enteric fistula in this chapter on intra-abdominal sepsis. Early control of sepsis and careful attention to fluid and electrolyte problems will decrease the early mortality of this disease. Late prognosis will continue to be limited in the majority of cases by the initiating disease process.

These fistulas represent one end of the spectrum of intraperitoneal sepsis where a perforated viscus continues to pour contaminated material into and through the peritoneal cavity. Control of peritoneal infection requires removal of the bacteria and agents that potentiate their virulence, administration of appropriate antimicrobial chemotherapeutic agents, prevention of ongoing or recurrent contamination, nutritional and hemodynamic support, and careful observance of the indications of recurrent sepsis. These general principles are applicable to all types of intraperitoneal bacterial infections.

BIBLIOGRAPHY

Hau T, Ahrenholz DH, Simmons RL: Secondary bacterial peritonitis: The biological basis of treatment. Curr Probl Surg 16(10):1, 1979.

Steinberg B: Infections of the Peritoneum. New York: Hoeber, 1944.

Webster MW Jr, Carey LC: Fistulae of the intestinal tract. Curr Probl Surg 13:5, 1976.

REFERENCES

PATHOBIOLOGY OF PERITONITIS

1. Bercovici B, Michel J, Miller J, Sacks TG: Antimicrobial activity of human peritoneal fluid. Surg Gynecol Obstet 141:885, 1975.
2. Henderson LW, Nolph KD: Altered permeability of the peritoneal membrane after using hypertonic peritoneal dialysis fluid. J Clin Invest 48:992, 1969.
3. Tsilibary EC, Wissig SL: Absorption from the peritoneal cavity: SEM study of the mesothelium covering the peritoneal surface of the muscular portion of the diaphragm. Am J Anat 149:127, 1977.
4. Allen L, Weatherford T: Role of fenestrated basement membrane in lymphatic absorption from the peritoneal cavity. Am J Physiol 197:551, 1959.
5. Steinberg, B: Infections of the Peritoneum. New York, Hoeber, 1944.
6. Fowler GR: Diffuse septic peritonitis, with special reference to a new method of treatment, namely, the elevated head and trunk posture, to facilitate drainage into the pelvis. With a report of nine consecutive cases of recovery. Med Rec 57:617, 1900.
7. Higgins GM, Beaver MG, Lemon WS: Phrenic neurectomy and peritoneal absorption. Am J Anat 45:137, 1930.
8. Florey H: Reactions of, and absorption by, lymphatics, with special reference to those of the diaphragm. Br J Exp Pathol 8:479, 1927.
9. Autio V: The spread of intraperitoneal infection. Studies with roentgen contrast medium. Acta Chir Scand 123 [Suppl 321]:5, 1964.
10. Watters WB, Buck RC: Scanning electron microscopy of mesothelial regeneration in the rat. Lab Invest 26:604, 1972.
11. Hau T, Hoffman R, Simmons RL: Mechanisms of the adjuvant effect of hemoglobin in experimental peritonitis. I. In vivo inhibition of peritoneal leukocytosis. Surgery 83:223, 1978.
12. Ahrenholz DH, Simmons RL: Fibrin in peritonitis: I. Beneficial and adverse effects in experimental *E. coli* peritonitis. Surgery 88:41, 1980.
13. Renvall S, Niinikoski J: Intraperitoneal oxygen and carbon dioxide tensions in experimental adhesion disease and peritonitis. Am J Surg 130:286, 1975
14. Ahrenholz DH: Unpublished data.
15. Miles AA, Miles EM, Burke J: The value and the duration of defense reactions of the skin to the primary lodgement of bacteria. Br J Exp Pathol 38:79, 1957.

PATHOGENESIS OF SECONDARY BACTERIAL PERITONITIS

16. Bergh GS, Bowers, WF, Wangensteen OH: Perforation of the gastrointestinal tract: An experimental study of factors influencing the development of peritonitis. Surgery 2:196, 1937.
17. Stone HH, Kolb LD, Geheber CE: Incidence and significance of intraperitoneal anaerobic bacteria. Ann Surg 181:705, 1975.
18. Onderdonk AB, Weinstein WM, Sullivan NM, Bartlett JG, Gorbach SL: Experimental intra-abdominal abscesses in rats: Quantitative bacteriology of infected animals. Infect Immun 10:1256, 1974.
19. Gorbach SL, Thadepalli H, Norsen J: Anaerobic microorganisms in intra-abdominal infections. In Balows A., DeHann RH, Dowell VR, Guze LB (eds): Anaerobic Bacteria: Role in Disease. Springfield, Ill, Thomas, 1974, p 339.
20. Lorber B, Swenson RM: The bacteriology of intra-abdominal infections. Surg Clin North Am 55:1349, 1975.
21. Fry DE, Garrison RN, Polk HC Jr: Clinical implications in *Bacteroides* bacteremia. Surg Gynecol Obstet 149:189, 1979.
22. Sharbaugh RJ, Rambo WM: A new model for producing experimental fecal peritonitis. Surg Gynecol Obstet 133:843, 1971.
23. Sisel RJ, Donovan AJ, Yellin AE: Experimental fecal peritonitis. Influence of barium sulfate or water-soluble radiographic contrast material on survival. Arch Surg 104:765, 1972.
24. Schneierson SS, Amsterdam D, Perlman E: Enhancement

of intraperitoneal staphylococcal virulence for mice with different bile salts. Nature 190:829, 1961.
25. Yull AB, Abrams JS, Davis JH: The peritoneal fluid in strangulation obstruction. The role of the red blood cell and *E. coli* bacteria in producing toxicity. J Surg Res 2:223, 1962.
26. Lee JT Jr, Ahrenholz DH, Nelson RD, Simmons RL: Mechanisms of the adjuvant effect of hemoglobin in experimental peritonitis. V. The significance of the coordinated iron component. Surgery 86:41, 1979.
27. Rodeheaver G, Wheeler CB, Rye DG, Vensko J, Edlich RF: Side-effects of topical proteolytic enzyme treatment. Surg Gynccol Obstet 148:562, 1979.
28. Hau T, Simmons RL: Heparin in the treatment of experimental peritonitis. Ann Surg 187:294, 1978.
29. Mackowiak PA: Microbial synergism in human infections (2 parts). N Engl J Med 298:21, 87, 1978.
30. Onderdonk A, Bartlett J, Louie T, Sullivan-Seiger N, Gorbach S: Microbial synergy in experimental intra-abdominal abscess. Infect Immun 13:22, 1976.
31. Nichols RL, Smith JW, Fossedal EN, Condon RE: Efficacy of parenteral antibiotics in the treatment of experimentally induced intra-abdominal sepsis. Rev Infect Dis 1:302, 1979.

TREATMENT OF SECONDARY BACTERIAL PERITONITIS

32. Lucas CE, Weaver D, Higgins RF, Ledgerwood AM, Johnson SD, Bouwman DL: Effects of albumin versus non-albumin resuscitation on plasma volume and renal excretory function. J Trauma 18:564, 1978.
33. Schumer W: Steroids in the treatment of clinical septic shock. Ann Surg 184:333, 1976.
34. Dudrick SJ, Rhoades JE: Metabolism in surgical patients: protein, carbohydrate and fat utilization by oral and parenteral routes. In Sabiston D (ed): Davis-Christopher Textbook of Surgery. Philadelphia, Saunders, 1977, p 150.
35. Gerding DN, Hall WH, Schierl EA: Antibiotic concentrations in ascitic fluid of patients with ascites and bacterial peritonitis. Ann Intern Med 86:708, 1977.
36. Stone HH, Morris ES, Kolb LD, Geheber CE: Management of peritonitis: cefamandole vs gentamicin. Contemp Surg 15:21, 1979.
37. Thadepalli H, Gorbach SL, Broido PW, Norsen J, Nyhus L: Abdominal trauma, anaerobes, and antibiotics. Surg Gynecol Obstet 137:270, 1973.
38. Dowell VR Jr: Antibiotic-associated colitis. Hosp Pract 14:75, 1979.
39. Horvitz RA, Von Graevenitz A: A clinical study of the role of enterococci as sole agents of wound and tissue infection. Yale J Biol Med 50:391, 1977.
39a. Harding GKM, Buckwold FJ, Ronald AR, Marrie TJ, Brunton S, Koss JC, Gurwith MJ, Albritton WL: Prospective, randomized comparative study of clindamycin, chloramphenicol and ticarcillin, each in combination with gentamicin, in therapy for intra-abdominal and female genital tract sepsis. J Infect Dis 142:384, 1980.
40. Thadepalli H, Gorbach SL, Bartlett JG: Apparent failure of chloramphenicol in the treatment of anaerobic infections. Curr Ther Res 22:421, 1977.
41. Louie TJ, Onderdonk AB, Gorbach SL, Bartlett JG: Therapy for experimental intra-abdominal sepsis: comparison of four cephalosporins with clindamycin plus gentamicin. J Infect Dis 135[Suppl]:S18, 1977.
41a. Tally FP, McGowan K, Kellum JM, Gorbach SL, O'Donnell TF: A randomized comparison of cefoxitin with or without amikacin and clindamycin plus amikacin in surgical sepsis. Ann Surg 193:318, 1981.
42. Donovan AJ, Vinson TL, Maulsby GO, Gewin JR: Selective treatment of duodenal ulcer with perforation. Ann Surg 189:627, 1979.
43. Hudspeth AS: Radical surgical debridement in the treatment of advanced generalized bacterial peritonitis. Arch Surg 110:1233, 1975.
43a. Polk HC, Fry DE: Radical peritoneal debridement for established peritonitis: The results of a prospective randomized clinical trial. Ann Surg 192:350, 1980.
44. Schumer W, Lee DK, Jones B: Peritoneal lavage in postoperative therapy of late peritoneal sepsis. Preliminary report. Surgery 55:841, 1964.
45. Rosato EF, Oram-Smith JC, Mullis WF, Rosato FE: Peritoneal lavage treatment in experimental peritonitis. Ann Surg 175:384, 1972.
45a. Ahrenholz DH: Effect of intraperitoneal fluid on mortality of *Escherichia coli* peritonitis. Surg Forum 30:272, 1979.
46. Noon GP, Beall AC Jr, Jordan GL Jr, Riggs S, DeBakey ME: Clinical evaluation of peritoneal irrigation with antibiotic solution. Surgery 62:73, 1967.
47. Rambo WM: Irrigation of the peritoneal cavity with cephalothin. Am J Surg 123:192, 1972.
48. Sherman JO, Luck SR, Borger JA: Irrigation of the peritoneal cavity for appendicitis in children: a double-blind study. J Pediatr Surg 11:371, 1976.
49. McMullan MH, Barnett WO: The clinical use of intraperitoneal cephalothin. Surgery 67:432, 1970.
50. Smith EB: Adjuvant therapy of generalized peritonitis with intraperitoneally administered cephalothin. Surg Gynecol Obstet 136:441, 1973.
51. DeVincenti FC, Cohn I Jr: Prolonged administration of intraperitoneal kanamycin in the treatment of peritonitis. Am Surg 37:177, 1971.
52. Fowler R: A controlled trial of intraperitoneal cephaloridine administration in peritonitis, J Pediatr Surg 10:43, 1975.
53. Kiene VS, Troeger H: Intraperitoneale Antibiotikaspuldrainage bei diffuser Peritonitis (2. Mitteilung), Zentralbl Chir 99:833, 1974.
54. Hunt JA, Rivlin ME, Clarebout HJ: Antibiotic peritoneal lavage in severe peritonitis. A preliminary assessment. S Afr Med J 49:233, 1975.
55. Bushan C, Mital VK, Elhence IP: Continuous postoperative peritoneal lavage in diffuse peritonitis using balanced saline antibiotic solution. Int Surg 60:526, 1975.
56. Pickard RG: Treatment of peritonitis with pre- and postoperative irrigation of the peritoneal cavity with noxythiolin solution. Br J Surg 59:642, 1972.
57. Browne MK, MacKenzie M, Doyle PJ: A controlled trial of taurolin in established bacterial peritonitis. Surg Gynecol Obstet 146:721, 1978.
58. Sindelar WF, Mason GR: Intraperitoneal irrigation with povidone-iodine solution for the prevention of intra-abdominal abscesses in the bacterially contaminated abdomen. Surg Gynecol Obstet 148:409, 1979.
59. Gilmore OJA, Sanderson PJ: Prophylactic interparietal povidone-iodine in abdominal surgery. Br J Surg 62:792, 1975.
60. Pollock AV, Evans M: Povidone-iodine for the control of surgical wound infection: a controlled clinical trial against topical cephaloridine. Br J Surg 62:292, 1975.
61. Viljanto J: Disinfection of surgical wounds without inhibition of normal wound healing. Arch Surg 115:253, 1980.
62. Ahrenholz DH, Simmons RL: Povidone-iodine in peritonitis. I. Adverse effects of local instillation in experimental *E. coli* peritonitis. J Surg Res 26:458, 1979.

63. Guignier M, Brambilla C, Brabant A, Debru J-L, Hernandez J-L, Pircher C, Muller J-M: Les lavages péritonéaux a la polyvinylpyrrolidone iodée. A propos de 11 cas. Nouv Presse Med 23:1559, 1974.
64. Haller JA Jr, Shaker IJ, Donahoo JS, Schnaufer J, White JJ: Peritoneal drainage versus non-drainage for generalized peritonitis from ruptured appendicitis in children: A prospective study. Ann Surg 177:595, 1973.
65. Steinberg D: On leaving the peritoneal cavity open in acute generalized suppurative peritonitis. Am J Surg 137:216, 1979.
66. McIlrath DC, van Heerden JA, Edis AJ, Dozois RR: Closure of abdominal incisions with subcutaneous catheters. Surgery 80:411, 1976.
67. Hau T, Ahrenholz DH, Simmons RL: Secondary bacterial peritonitis: The biologic basis of treatment. Curr Probl Surg 16:1, 1979.
68. Burke JF, Pontoppidan H, Welch CE: High output respiratory failure: an important cause of death ascribed to peritonitis or ileus. Ann Surg 158:581, 1963.
69. Martin LF, Max MH, Polk HC: Failure of gastric pH control in the critically ill: A valid sign of occult sepsis. Surgery 88:59, 1980.
70. Saba TM: Reticuloendothelial defense: Its relevance to cardiopulmonary function in septic surgical, trauma, and burn patients. Contemp Surg 14:64, 1979.

PRIMARY PERITONITIS

71. Fowler R: Primary peritonitis; changing aspects 1956–1970. Aust Paediatr J 7:73, 1971.
72. McDougal WS, Izant RJ Jr, Zollinger RM Jr: Primary peritonitis in infancy and childhood. Ann Surg 181:310, 1975.
73. Caroli J, Platteborse R: Septicemie porto-cave: cirrhoses du foie et septicemie a colibacille. Sem Hop Paris 34:472, 1958.
74. Correia JP, Conn HO: Spontaneous bacterial peritonitis in cirrhosis: endemic or epidemic? Med Clin North Am 59:963, 1975.
75. Lipsky PE, Hardin JA, Schour L, Plotz PH: Spontaneous peritonitis and systemic lupus erythematosus. Importance of accurate diagnosis of gram-positive bacterial infections. JAMA 232:929, 1975.
76. Wilfert CM, Katz SL: Etiology of bacterial sepsis in nephrotic children 1963–1967. Pediatrics 42:840, 1968.
77. Speck WT, Dresdale SS, McMillan RW: Primary peritonitis and the nephrotic syndrome. Am J Surg 127:267, 1974.
78. Kimball MW, Knee S: Gonococcal perihepatitis in a male. N Engl J Med 282:1080, 1970.
79. Scheckman P, Onderdonk AB, Bartlett JG: Anaerobes in spontaneous peritonitis. Lancet 2:1223, 1977.
80. Donovan EJ: Surgical aspects of primary pneumococcic peritonitis. Am J Dis Child 48:1170, 1938.
81. Beale G, Hackett AH: A case of uterine reflux of urine in a girl and its suggested role in primary peritonitis. NZ Med J 69:158, 1969.
82. Golden GT, Shaw A: Primary peritonitis. Surg Gynecol Obstet 135:513, 1972.
83. Gerding DN, Khan MY, Ewing JW, Hall WH: *Pasteurella multocida* peritonitis in hepatic cirrhosis with ascites. Gastroenterology 70:413, 1976.
84. Simberkoff MS, Moldover NH, Weiss G: Bactericidal and opsonic activity of cirrhotic ascites and nonascitic peritoneal fluid. J Lab Clin Med 91:831, 1978.
85. Sherman NJ, Woolley MM: The ileocecal syndrome in acute childhood leukemia. Arch Surg 107:39, 1973.
86. Pollak VE, Grove WJ, Kark RM, Muehrcke RC, Pirani CL, Steck IE: Systemic lupus erythematosus simulating acute surgical condition of the abdomen. N Engl J Med 259:258, 1958.
87. Mallory A, Schaefer JW: Complications of diagnostic paracentesis in patients with liver disease. JAMA 239:628, 1978.
88. Flood FB: Spontaneous perforation of the umbilicus in Laennec's cirrhosis with massive ascites. N Engl J Med 264:72, 1961.
89. Conn HO, Fessel JM: Spontaneous bacterial peritonitis in cirrhosis: variations on a theme. Medicine 50:161, 1971.
90. Kline MM, McCallum RW, Guth PH: The clinical value of ascitic fluid culture and leukocyte count studies in alcoholic cirrhosis. Gastroenterology 70:408, 1976.
91. Reichert JA, Valle RF: Fitz-Hugh-Curtis syndrome. A laparoscopic approach. JAMA 236:266, 1976.

GRANULOMATOUS PERITONITIS

92. Lougheed JC, Saporta J, Holmes J: Treatment and current status of tuberculous peritonitis. Am Surg 29:850, 1963.
93. Dineen P, Homan WP, Grafe WR: Tuberculous peritonitis: 43 years' experience in diagnosis and treatment. Ann Surg 184:717, 1976.
94. Yu VL: Onset of tuberculosis after intestinal bypass surgery for obesity. Guidelines for evaluation, drug prophylaxis, and treatment. Arch Surg 112:1235, 1977.
95. Singh MM, Bhargava AN, Jain KP: Tuberculous peritonitis. An evaluation of pathogenetic mechanisms, diagnostic procedures and therapeutic measures. N Engl J Med 281:1091, 1969.
96. Berardi RS: Abdominal actinomycosis. Surg Gynecol Obstet 149:257, 1979.
97. Putman HC Jr, Dockerty MB, Waugh JM: Abdominal actinomycosis; analysis of 122 cases. Surgery 28:781, 1950.
98. Brooke MM: Epidemiology of amebiasis in the US. JAMA 188:519, 1964.
99. Judy KL: Amebiasis presenting as an acute abdomen. Am J Surg 127:275, 1974.
100. DeBakey ME, Ochsner A: Hepatic amebiasis; 20 year experience and analysis of 263 cases. Int Abstr Surg 92:209, 1951.
101. Monga NK, Sood S, Kaushik SP, Sachdeva HC, Sood KC, Datta DV: Amebic peritonitis. Am J Gastroenterol 66:366, 1976.
102. Cohen R, Roth FJ, Delgado E, Ahearn DG, Kalser MH: Fungal flora of the normal human small and large intestine. N Engl J Med 280:638, 1969.
103. Hurwich BJ: Monilial peritonitis. Report of a case and review of the literature. Arch Intern Med 117:405, 1966.
103a. Solomkin JS, Flohr AB, Quie PG, Simmons RL: The role of *Candida* in intraperitoneal infections. Surgery 88:524, 1980.
104. Bortolussi RA, MacDonald MRA, Bannatyne RM, Arbus GS: Treatment of candida peritonitis by peritoneal lavage with amphotericin B. J Pediatr 87:987, 1975.

PERITONITIS AND INTRAPERITONEAL PROSTHESES

105. Tenckhoff H, Blagg CR, Curtis KF, Hickman RO: Chronic peritoneal dialysis. Proc Eur Dial Transplant Assoc 10:363, 1973.
106. Oreopoulos DG: Chronic peritoneal dialysis. Clin Nephrol 9:165, 1978.
107. Brewer, TE, Caldwell FT, Patterson RM, Flanigan WJ: Indwelling peritoneal (Tenckhoff) dialysis catheter. Experience with 24 patients. JAMA 219:1011, 1972.

108. Vaamonde CA, Michael UF, Metzger RA, Carroll KE Jr: Complications of acute peritoneal dialysis. J Chronic Dis 28:637, 1975.
109. Black HR, Finkelstein FO, Lee RV: The treatment of peritonitis in patients with chronic indwelling catheters. Trans Am Soc Artif Intern Organs 20:115, 1974.
110. Rubin J, Oreopoulos DG, Lio TT, Mathews R, De Veber GA: Management of peritonitis and bowel perforation during chronic peritoneal dialysis. Nephron 16:220, 1976.
111. LeVeen HH, Wapnick S, Diaz C, Grosberg S, Kinney M: Ascites: its correction by peritoneovenous shunting. Curr Probl Surg 16:3, 1979.
112. Hubschmann OR, Countee RW: Acute abdomen in children with infected ventriculoperitoneal shunts. Arch Surg 115:305, 1980.

PATHOGENESIS OF INTRA-ABDOMINAL ABSCESSES

113. Altemeier WA, Culbertson WR, Fullen WD, Shook CD: Intra-abdominal abscesses. Am J Surg 125:70, 1973.
114. Mitchell GAG: The spread of acute intraperitoneal effusions. Br J Surg 28:291, 1941.
115. Patterson HC: Left subphrenic abscesses. Am Surg 43:430, 1977.
116. Altemeier WA, Culbertson WR, Fidler JP: Giant horseshoe intra-abdominal abscess. Ann Surg 181:716, 1975.
117. Goris RJA, Lubbers, EJC, Oostveen HW, van den Dries ACP: Retroperitoneal infection. In de Boer HHM (ed): Intra-abdominal Sepsis. Utrecht, Bunge Scientific Publishers, 1979, p 47.
118. Bradley EL, Isaacs J: Appendiceal abscess revisited. Arch Surg 113:130, 1978.
119. Wang SMS, Wilson SE: Subphrenic abscess. The new epidemiology. Arch Surg 112:934, 1977.
120. Halliday P, Loewenthal J: Subphrenic abscess. Aust NZ J Surg 33:260, 1964.
121. Sherman NJ, Davis JR, Jesseph JE: Subphrenic abscess. A continuing hazard. Am J Surg 117:117, 1969.
122. Halliday P, Halliday JH: Subphrenic abscess: a study of 241 patients at the Royal Prince Edward Hospital, 1950–73. Br J Surg 63:352, 1976.
123. Naylor R, Coln D, Shires GT: Morbidity and mortality from injuries to the spleen. J Trauma 14:773, 1974.
124. Klaue P, Eckert P, Kern E: Incidental splenectomy: early and late postoperative complications. Am J Surg 138:296, 1979.
125. Cioffiro W, Schein CJ, Gliedman ML: Splenic injury during abdominal surgery. Arch Surg 111:167, 1976.
126. DeCosse JJ, Poulin TL, Fox PS, Condon RE: Subphrenic abscess. Surg Gynecol Obstet 138:841, 1974.
127. Halasz NA: Subphrenic abscess. Myths and facts. JAMA 214:724, 1970.
128. Stafford ES, Sprong DH Jr: The mortality from acute appendicitis in the Johns Hopkins Hospital. JAMA 115:1242, 1940.
129. Barnes BA, Behringer GE, Wheelock FC, Wilkins EW: Treatment of appendicitis at the Massachusetts General Hospital (1937–1959). JAMA 180:122, 1962.
130. Berne CJ, Pattison AC: Diverticulitis of the colon. California West Med 52:225, 1940.
131. Nagler SM, Poticha SM: Intra-abdominal abscess in regional enteritis. Am J Surg 137:350, 1979.
132. Greenstein AJ, Dreiling DA, Aufses AH Jr: Crohn's disease of the colon. V. Retroperitoneal lumbocrural abscess in Crohn's disease involving the colon. Am J Gastroenterol 64:306, 1975.
133. Welch JP: Unusual abscesses in perforating colorectal cancer. Am J Surg 131:270, 1976.
134. Rubenstein PR, Mishell DR Jr, Ledger WJ: Colpotomy drainage of pelvic abscess. Obstet Gynecol 48:142, 1976.
135. Meislin HW: *Bacteroides* in pelvis abscesses. N Engl J Med 297:788, 1977.

DIAGNOSIS AND TREATMENT OF INTRA-ABDOMINAL ABSCESSES

136. Bonfils-Roberts EA, Barone JE, Nealon TF Jr: Treatment of subphrenic abscess. Surg Clin North Am 55:1361, 1975.
137. Halliday P: The surgical management of subphrenic abscess: a historical study. Aust NZ J Surg 45:235, 1975.
138. Carter R, Brewer LA III: Subphrenic abscess: a thoracoabdominal clinical complex. Am J Surg 108:165, 1964.
139. Boyd DP: The intrathoracic complications of subphrenic abscess. J Thorac Cardiovasc Surg 38:771, 1959.
139a. Ascher NL, Forstrom L, Simmons RL: Radiolabeled autologus leukocyte scanning in abscess detection. World J Surg 4:395, 1980.
140. Doust BD, Quiroz F, Stewart JM: Ultrasonic distinction of abscesses from other intra-abdominal fluid collections. Radiology 125:213, 1977.
141. Taylor KJW, Wasson JFM, Graaff CD, Rosenfield AT, Andriole VT: Accuracy of grey-scale ultrasound diagnosis of abdominal and pelvic abscesses in 220 patients. Lancet 1:83, 1978.
142. Daffner RH, Halber MD, Morgan CL, Trought WS, Thompson WM, Rice RP: Computed tomography in the diagnosis of intra-abdominal abscesses. Ann Surg 189:29, 1979.
143. Caffee HH, Watts G, Mena I: Gallium-67 citrate scanning in the diagnosis of intra-abdominal abscess. Am J Surg 133:665, 1977.
144. Thakur ML, Coleman RE, Welch MJ: Indium-111 labeled leukocytes for localization of abscesses: Preparation, analysis, tissue distribution and comparison with gallium-67 citrate in dogs. J Lab Med 89:217, 1977.
145. Christou NV, Meakins JL: Neutrophil function in anergic surgical patients: neutrophil adherence and chemotaxis. Ann Surg 190:557, 1979.
146. Segal AW, Thakur ML, Arnot RN, Lavender JP: Indium-111 labelled leukocytes for localisation of abscesses. Lancet 2:1056, 1976.
147. Ascher NL, Ahrenholz DH, Simmons RL, Weiblen B, Gomez L, Forstrom LA, Frick MP, Henke C, McCullough J: Indium-111 autologous tagged leukocytes in the diagnosis of intraperitoneal sepsis. Arch Surg 114:386, 1979.
148. Foran B, Berne TV, Rosoff L: Management of the appendiceal mass. Arch Surg 113:1144, 1978.
149. Nather C, Ochsner EWA: Retroperitoneal operation for subphrenic abscess with the report of two cases. Surg Gynecol Obstet 37:665, 1923.
150. Ochsner A: Reappraisal. The value of extraserous drainage in subphrenic abscesses. Surgery 43:319, 1958.
151. Halliday P, Grant AF, Nicks GR, Leckie BD, Loewenthal J: Combined transpleural exploration and extraserous drainage of subphrenic abscess. Br J Surg 61:453, 1974.
152. Deck KB, Berne TV: Selective management of subphrenic abscesses. Arch Surg 114:1165, 1979.

INTRA-ABDOMINAL FISTULAS

153. Webster MW Jr, Carey LC: Fistulae of the intestinal tract. Curr Probl Surg 13:5, 1976.

154. Yamato T, Hamanaka Y, Hirata S, Sakai K: Esophagoplasty with an autogenous tubed gastric flap. Am J Surg 137:597, 1979.
155. Soeters PB, Ebeid AM, Fischer JE: Review of 404 patients with gastrointestinal fistulas. Impact of parenteral nutrition. Ann Surg 190:189, 1979.
156. Welch CE, Rodkey GV: A method of management of the duodenal stump after gastrectomy. Surg Gynecol Obstet 98:376, 1954.
157. Anderson GW, Goss JC, Lawrence GH: External duodenal fistula. Am Surg 43:666, 1977.
158. Condon RE, Bartlett JG, Nichols RL, Schulte WJ, Gorbach SL, Ochi S: Preoperative prophylactic cephalothin fails to control septic complications of colorectal operations: results of controlled clinical trial. A veterans administration cooperative study. Am J Surg 137:68, 1979.
159. Cohn I Jr, Rives JD: Antibiotic protection of colon anastomoses. Ann Surg 141:707, 1955.
160. Sharefkin J, Joffe N, Silen W, Fromm D: Anastomotic dehiscence after low anterior resection of the rectum. Am J Surg 135:519, 1978.
161. Chassin JL, Rifkind KM, Sussman B, Kassel B, Fingaret A, Drager S, Chassin PS: The stapled gastrointestinal tract anastomosis: incidence of postoperative complications compared with the sutured anastomosis. Ann Surg 188:689, 1978.
162. Mortensen E, Nilsson T, Vesterhauge S: Treatment of intestinal injuries following irradiation. Dis Colon Rectum 17:638, 1974.
163. Amlicke JA, Ponka JL: Gastrocolic and gastrojejunocolic fistulas. A report of sixteen cases. Am J Surg 107:744, 1964.
164. Hermreck AS, Crawford DG: The esophageal anastomotic leak. Am J Surg 132:794, 1976.
165. Miller HI, Dorn BC: Postoperative gastrointestinal fistulas. Am J Surg 116:382, 1968.
166. Fischer JE: The management of high-output intestinal fistulas. Adv Surg 9:139, 1975.
167. Reber H, Roberts C, Way LW, Dunphy JE: Management of external gastrointestinal fistulas. Ann Surg 188:460, 1978.
168. Thomas RJS, Rosalion A: The use of parenteral nutrition in the management of external gastrointestinal tract fistulae. Aust NZ J Surg 48:535, 1978.
169. Freund H, Anner C, Saltz NJ: Management of gastrointestinal fistulas with total parenteral nutrition. Int Surg 61:273, 1976.
170. Monod-Broca P: Treatment of intestinal fistulas. Br J Surg 64:685, 1977.
171. Athanassiades S, Notis P, Tountas C: Fistulas of the gastrointestinal tract. Experience with eighty-one cases. Am J Surg 130:26, 1975.
172. Ryan JA Jr, Abel RM, Abbott WM, Hopkin C, Chesney T, Colley R, Phillips K, Fischer J: Catheter complication in total parenteral nutrition. N Engl J Med 290:757, 1974.
173. Hollender LF, Otteni F: Treatment of postoperative external fistulas of the small intestine. Surg Annu 7:295, 1975.
174. Patton AS, Lawson DW, Shannon JM, Risley TS, Bixby FE: Reevaluation of the Boerhaave syndrome. A review of fourteen cases. Am J Surg 137:560, 1979.
175. Welch CE, Edmunds LH: Gastrointestinal fistulae. Surg Clin North Am 42:1311, 1962.
176. Nassos TP, Braasch JW: External small bowel fistulas: Current treatments and results. Surg Clin North Am 51:687, 1971.
177. Chapman R, Foran R, Dunphy JE: Management of intestinal fistulas. Am J Surg 108:157, 1964.
178. MacFadyen BV Jr, Dudrick SJ, Ruberg RL: Management of gastrointestinal fistulas with parenteral hyperalimentation. Surgery 74:100, 1973.

CHAPTER 35
Biliary Tract Infections

RONALD LEE NICHOLS

ANATOMIC AND PHYSIOLOGIC ASPECTS OF BILIARY TRACT INFECTIONS

ANATOMY OF BILIARY TREE

ALTHOUGH there are many anatomic variations in the human biliary tract, the blood supply to the gallbladder is usually a single cystic artery, which arises from the right hepatic artery and passes to the gallbladder above and behind the cystic duct. The venous drainage of the gallbladder is primarily by small veins, which enter the liver directly. A cystic vein can sometimes be identified as it passes parallel to the cystic artery into the portal vein or its right branch. The lymphatic vessels of the entire extrahepatic biliary tree drain into the cystic nodes at the neck of the gallbladder and to the node of the epiploic foramen. The lymph flows through these nodes to more proximal hepatic nodes and then to the celiac group. Retrograde lymphatic drainage to the hilum of the liver occurs but is rare.

The arterial supply of the common bile duct consists of a number of small vessels arising from the right hepatic, cystic, hepatic, supraduodenal, gastroduodenal, and pancreaticoduodenal arteries. Each of these vessels supplies one segment of the choledochus. The venous return is to the portal vein via an epicholedochal venous plexus.

The interrelationships of vascular and lymphatic supply are important in the spread of infection within the biliary tree but are of little clinical interest.

INTERACTION BETWEEN BILE AND BILIARY TRACT MICROORGANISMS

The normal adult secretes 250–1,000 ml of bile each day. The main constituents of bile include electrolytes, bile salts, proteins, cholesterol, fats, and bile pigments. Many enteric microorganisms, especially the coliform bacilli, grow luxuriantly in bile. The data of Lou et al [1] suggest that bile may exert an inhibitory effect on some gastrointestinal anaerobes. Maki [2] has presented evidence that suggests that calcium bilirubinate stones are the result of infection of the bile with *E. coli.* He suggests that the beta-glucuronidase of bacterial origin hydrolyzes bilirubin glucuronide (the usual water soluble form of bilirubin in the bile) into free bilirubin and glucuronic acid. Calcium in the bile combines with the carboxyl radical of the liberated bilirubin to form calcium bilirubinate. As a result of electrostatic effects, these particles then coagulate to form stones, which can contain varying amounts of cholesterol. In other experiments, however, gallstones have been formed, without infection, by the production of biliary stasis or by altering the composition of the diet. Undoubtedly, all three factors, bacteria, stasis and diet, contribute to the development of calculi in humans.

INFLUENCE OF GASTRIC BACTERIAL INHIBITORY MECHANISMS ON THE MICROORGANISMS INHABITING THE BILIARY TRACT

The presence of a gastric microflora increases the likelihood of increased concentrations of microorganisms within the duodenum and perhaps the biliary tract. Bacterial counts seldom exceed 10^3 per ml in the empty stomach of healthy people because both gastric acid and gastric motility successfully control the intragastric proliferation of swallowed or reflux bacteria. Arnold and Brody [3] noted as early as 1926 that bacterial overgrowth in the stomach occurred routinely in patients who had either decreased gastric acid output (the elderly or patients with pernicious anemia) or altered gastric motility (following peptic ulcer surgery).[3,4]

The organisms that inhabit the stomach in these altered states enter from the oropharynx by way of saliva or by reflux of intestinal contents through the pylorus (Chapters 3, 27). Primary bacterial contribution is made by saliva, with total aerobes and anaerobes numbering 10^8 to 10^9 bacteria per ml of saliva. The commonly isolated aerobes include streptococci, *Haemophilus,* and staphylococci, while the predominant anaerobes include *Fusobacterium,* peptostreptococci, and *Bacteroides oralis* and *B. melaninogenicus.* When present, the proximal small bowel contents account for small numbers of bacteria, and are usually isolated in concentrations of 10^2 to 10^4 per ml of intestinal contents. Colonic anaerobes, such as *B. fragilis,* are rarely isolated from proximal intestinal contents.

The microflora of the duodenum, which ultimately become the microflora of the biliary tree, are sparse when gastric acid and motility are normal. After a meal, however, during which bacteria are protected by swallowed food, or in the presence of gastric hemorrhage during which the gastric acid is neutralized, duodenal bacteria counts will rise.[4]

ORIGIN OF MICROORGANISMS WITHIN THE BILIARY TRACT

The biliary tract of healthy individuals does not usually harbor bacteria.[5] Two recent studies, using modern bacteriologic techniques, found that the gallbladder bile of all normal persons was sterile.[6,7]

Three routes of biliary contamination potentially exist. Most evidence suggests the spread ascends from the duodenum. This hypothesis is supported by the fact that the number of intestinal organisms is higher in gallbladder bile than in the wall of the gallbladder.[8] It is further supported by the commonly reported finding that cholangitis is rare when tumors obstruct the distal biliary tree.[8a] In contrast, cholangitis is a common complication of choledocholithiasis or retrograde transduodenal instrumentation. There is some evidence, however, that bile can be contaminated by means of portal venous bacteremia or by translymphatic routes. The types of bacteria isolated from the biliary tract tend to negate the possibility that organisms arrive in the gallbladder from the general circulation during septicemia. However, the cholecystitis of typhoid or cholera probably does occur as a consequence of a transient arterial or portal-venous bacteremia which takes place during the primary intestinal disease.[9]

PHYSIOLOGIC FACTORS

The principal mechanism by which the biliary tree is kept relatively free of bacterial colonization from any of these routes is the large volume of bile produced, which must drain through a tract of small capacity. Bacteria cannot multiply rapidly enough in the unobstructed biliary tree to achieve a significant concentration. In addition, eating stimulates gallbladder contraction via humoral mechanisms. The normal biliary tree is thus flushed many times each day. Only when the free flow of bile is impaired by mechanical or functional disorders does the biliary tree become readily infected.

ANTIBIOTIC EXCRETION IN BILE

Historically, antibiotics chosen for use in biliary sepsis were those that achieved high bioactive concentrations in bile. Recently, Keighley et al [10] have stressed the importance of using antibiotics which attain adequate serum levels in biliary sepsis.

In the absence of biliary obstruction, the bioactive concentrations of penicillin, rifampin, and most tetracyclines are much higher in bile than in serum.[11] In contrast, biliary levels of carbenicillin, chloramphenicol, gentamicin, and streptomycin are generally lower than those in serum. Most studies of the cephalosporins have shown higher biliary levels with cefazolin or cephaloridine than with cephalothin.[11-13] Cefoxitin, a second-generation cephalosporin, has shown high levels in bile [14] (Table 18-25).

When the common duct is obstructed, biliary concentrations of most antibiotics, except the tetracyclines,[15] are dramatically reduced. In patients with obstruction of the cystic duct, levels of appropriate antibiotics will be high in common duct bile but low in gallbladder bile. Thus, patency of both the common and cystic ducts appears to be necessary to allow adequate penetration of the antibiotics into choledochal and cholecystic bile.

A recent study has demonstrated the failure of using preoperative radiographic studies of gallbladder function to predict which patients would attain high concentrations of antibiotic within gallbladder bile.[13]

REGIONAL INFECTIONS

ACUTE CHOLECYSTITIS

This condition occurs when there is blockage to the outflow of bile from the gallbladder into the common duct. This blockage is usually the result of gallstones. Rarely, carcinoma of the bile duct or gallbladder can cause acute cholecystitis. Bacterial contamination and infection occur secondarily in most cases.

Pathology and Pathogenesis

As the result of the blockage, the ability to empty the concentrated bile from the gallbladder is retarded and the gallbladder becomes tense, swollen, erythematous, and edematous. As the inflammation spreads to the serosa of the gallbladder, it involves the adjacent structures, ie, gastrohepatic omentum, common bile duct, and the porta hepatis. If the obstruction is not relieved, spontaneously or by medical or surgical management, the progressive tension of the gallbladder wall (which results from continued secretions) will cause vascular compromise and eventual gangrene. Gangrene will most frequently occur in the fundus of the gallbladder, where the blood supply is poorest. Perforation of the gangrenous area with bile peritonitis routinely occurs at this stage, unless operative intervention precedes it.

Most cases of acute cholecystitis do not progress further than the early chemical inflammatory phase. Resolution will follow the relief of obstruction. Bacterial infection plays a small role in early cholecystitis; however, as the period of stasis increases, so does the concentration of bacteria within the lumen of the gallbladder.

Rarely, acute cholecystitis occurs when no calculi are present. Acalculous cholecystitis can be produced by obstruction of the cystic duct by anomalies of vascular supply, internal valves of the cystic duct, pancreatic or bile duct tumors, or acute pancreatitis. Other predisposing conditions that lead to biliary stasis or mucosal injury include sepsis, hypotension, multiple transfusions, prolonged fasting, ventilatory support, and intravenous hyperalimentation.[16,16a]

Clinical Features

The most prominent local symptom of acute cholecystitis is biliary colic. The pain normally begins after a large evening meal with a gradual onset in the right upper quadrant of the abdomen, often radiating around the right costal margin to the angle of the scapula. The pain is constant and severe and is intensified by respiration and movement. Anorexia and nausea are regularly associated with the pain.

Vomiting is usually not reported in early cholecystitis. Pyrexia of varying degrees occurs as the inflammation progresses.

Physical findings include tenderness and muscular guarding, usually limited to the area below the right costal margin. As the disease progresses, the inflamed gallbladder and adjacent tissues may be palpated as a right upper quadrant tender mass. The development of muscular rigidity associated with absent bowel sounds and rebound tenderness signals the rupture of the gallbladder and the development of bile peritonitis.

Diagnosis

The diagnosis is clear in patients with proved gallbladder disease who report typical symptoms and signs. There is usually a slight elevation of the white blood cell count (10,000–15,000 WBC per mm³). Tests of liver function are normal early in the disease but are mildly elevated if the inflammation continues. Plain radiograms of the abdomen may show a mild and nonspecific ileus pattern. Calculi are seen in the right upper quadrant approximately 10 percent of the time. Oral cholecystograms are not indicated. The most helpful study is the echogram, which reveals stones and a distended gallbladder in a majority of patients. Intravenous cholangiography is expensive and exposes the patient to high doses of radiation and unfortunately has poor resolution. This technique has been replaced in most centers by a radionucleotide hepatobiliary scan, which shows the patent biliary tree without filling of the gallbladder.[16b]

Microbiology

Csendes et al[6] and Lou et al[1] reported that nearly 50 percent of patients with acute cholecystitis had positive gallbladder bile findings. There was no significant differences when gallbladder bile cultures were compared to gallbladder wall cultures. The organisms isolated were the aerobic enterics, most commonly *E. coli, S. fecalis* (enterococcus), and *Klebsiella*. Anaerobic bacteria were rare and no fungi were isolated[1] (Table 35-1).

TABLE 35-1. BACTERIOLOGY OF THE HUMAN BILIARY TRACT

Organism	Number of Patients *	Colony Counts
Klebsiella pneumoniae	6	1.2×10^5 to 1.33×10^7/ml
Enterococcus	4	1×10^4 to 5.64×10^6/ml
Escherichia coli	2	Nonquantitated
Proteus species	2	1.45×10^6; nonquantitated
Moraxella lwoffi	2	1.5×10^3 to 1×10^4/ml
Enterobacter hafniae	1	2.5×10^5/ml
Staphylococcus aureus	1	<100/ml
Salmonella typhi	1	7×10^5/ml
Clostridium perfringens	1	Nonquantitated

Total patients = 74.
* Four patients had more than one isolate.

Lou MS, Mandal AK, Alexander JL, Thadepalli H: Bacteriology of the human biliary tract and the duodenum. *Arch Surg* 112:965, 1977.

Treatment

Many, if not most, cases of acute cholecystitis spontaneously resolve, and the disease continues into the chronic phase. In cases that do not resolve spontaneously, the relative merits of early or late operative intervention are unclear. The advocates of early intervention (within 1 to 2 days of onset of symptoms) argue that: (1) the procedure is safe and entails the same morbidity as late operations, (2) resection is easier before the development of fibrosis and scar formation, (3) there is a substantial reduction in hospitalization time, allowing the patient a more rapid recovery and return to work, (4) delay of operation may mask a silent perforation or empyema of the gallbladder, which may be difficult to diagnose in older patients, and (5) a second attack or perforation can occur during the waiting period.

On the other hand, the proponents of delay in operation (4 to 8 weeks following the onset of symptoms) state that: (1) the patient would then be in optimal condition, fully hydrated and in normal electrolyte balance, (2) the additional time allows the diagnosis to be established beyond doubt, (3) the acute infection has completely subsided, thus making resection easier, and (4) the incidence of postoperative complications during an elective procedure at a later time is considerably reduced.

In recent years, the pendulum seems to be shifting toward early operative intervention.[17] In practice, however, basic surgical principles are observed by advocates of either school, and the patient's condition, rather than the surgeon's philosophy, usually dictates the necessary management.

The management of acute cholecystitis can be divided into three stages (Table 35-2). Some patients can move rapidly from one state to another, so that considerable clinical judgment is necessary.

The preferred operation for acute cholecystitis is cholecystectomy. An emergency cholecystostomy may be lifesaving in cases of serious deterioration in the clinical course, advanced age, or signs suggesting imminent perforation of the gallbladder. This operation can be performed under minimal general or even local anesthesia.

The use of antibiotics is recommended in all patients who require operative intervention for acute cholecystitis. The incidence of bacteria cultured from the bile and gallbladder wall, in the presence of obstructing stones, suggests that infection occurs in the majority of patients. Antibiotic therapy can be discontinued within 2 to 3 days of an uncomplicated cholecystectomy. In patients with extensive local infection, perforation, or gangrene, antibiotic treatment should be continued for at least 6 to 10 days.

The antibiotics should be effective against the aerobic, enteric, gram-negative rods. Initial therapy should be started preoperatively and can be altered if indicated, when intraoperative Gram stain of bile and subsequent culture results are available. Finding gram-positive rods on intraoperative stains should be an indication for the addition of penicillin therapy. The antibiotic agents currently recommended can be found in Table 35-3. When cephalosporin antibiotics are used, better results can be expected with the newer second-generation agents, which

TABLE 35-2. MANAGEMENT OF ACUTE CHOLECYSTITIS

Indications	Therapy
Stage I: Initial therapy and general support measures	
Biliary colic, with persistence of pain, requiring hospitalization	Nothing by mouth; insert Levine tube, if vomiting and distension are present; IV fluids and electrolytes; analgesics; antispasmodics
Stage II: Control of infection	
Fever Leukocytosis Ileus Tenderness or a mass in right upper quadrant	As in stage I, and parenteral antibiotics
Stage III: Relief of obstruction (decision should be made rapidly)	
Progression of sepsis; persistent or rising fever, shaking chills, hypotension, rising WBC Increasing signs in right upper quadrant; rigidity, rebound tenderness, or an enlarging mass. In some cases, a smooth mass may become irregular in shape; with surrounding peritoneal signs in the region Progressively abnormal liver function results The presence of diabetes or advanced age increases the risk of perforation, empyema and other complications	Surgical removal of the gallbladder; cholecystostomy (when indicated); parenteral antibiotics (before, during, and after operation)

in general offer a more predictable control of the aerobic enterics.[17] Combinations of antibiotics are theoretically necessary, however, if the entire spectrum of bacteria commonly found are to be eradicated.

Prognosis

Most patients do well after cholecystostomy for acute cholecystitis. Obviously, the longer the delay in treatment in the absence of resolution, the greater the probability will be for the septic complications. MacLean et al [18] found that operations for acute cholecystitis doubled the incidence of postoperative sepsis when compared to operations performed for chronic calculous cholecystitis. Similar findings were reported by Stone et al.[19]

Flinn et al [20] found that five of eight patients with acute cholecystitis had bacteria cultured from their bile, while 12 of 16 patients with acute cholecystitis showed acute inflammatory changes within the portal triads on liver biopsies done during the operation. They felt that finding polymorphonuclear leukocytes within the liver in patients with acute cholecystitis was significant and should be an indication for early cholecystectomy to prevent potential hepatocellular damage.

HYDROPS OF THE GALLBLADDER

Hydrops of the gallbladder is characteristically heralded by some degree of right upper quadrant biliary colic and development of a right upper quadrant, nontender, smooth mass. Occasionally, the developing mass is completely painless. The progressive enlargement of the gallbladder is due to obstruction of the cystic duct, usually

TABLE 35-3. ANTIBIOTIC SENSITIVITIES OF COMMONLY ISOLATED BILIARY BACTERIA

	Penicillin	Ampicillin	Cephalosporins	Aminoglycosides	Carbenicillin	Clindamycin
AEROBES						
Escherichia coli	−	+	++	++	+	−
Klebsiella spp	−	+	++	++	−	−
Enterobacter spp	−	+	++ †	++	+	−
Enterococcus	−	++ *	+	++ *	+	−
ANAEROBES						
Clostridium	++	+	+	−	+	+
Bacteroides fragilis	−	−	+ ‡	−	+	++

++ = Drug of choice. + = Other agents clinically useful.
− = Ineffective drugs or agents less useful because of irregular clinical responses.
* = Therapy of enterococcal *(S. faecalis)* infections requires both a penicillin and an aminoglycoside.
† = Cefamandole only has effective coverage.
‡ = Cefoxitin has most effective coverage.

by a calculus. The gallbladder continues to distend because of the accumulation of mucus which is being secreted by the mucosal lining cells. If bacteria are present within the gallbladder bile, empyema will develop.

Cholecystectomy is the best treatment for hydrops of the gallbladder. Antibiotics are used only if the bile-mucus mixture within the gallbladder shows the presence of bacteria on Gram stain at the time of operation. Because this entity is relatively rare, no good bacteriologic studies are available.

EMPYEMA OF THE GALLBLADDER

Prolonged obstruction of the cystic duct by a stone may lead to a large collection of pus within the gallbladder, a condition referred to as empyema. Increased intracystic pressure, along with infection and disintegrating leukocytes, causes necrosis of the gallbladder wall. The major complications of empyema are perforation and generalized peritonitis.

Clinical Features

Initially, the disease resembles acute cholecystitis. Within 48 hours, however, the abdominal findings escalate in severity. Right-sided abdominal tenderness is severe and is associated with tachycardia and a fever of 103 to 105F. The physical examination reveals a distinct, exquisitely tender mass in the right upper abdomen. Signs of generalized peritonitis indicate perforation of the diseased gallbladder—rebound tenderness, absent bowel sound, and abdominal rigidity. While these signs are classically found after perforation of the gallbladder, older patients may have a more cryptic course with a paucity of abdominal signs. Persistent systemic toxicity, in combination with medically treated cholecystitis, should raise the suspicion of empyema.

Diagnosis

The diagnosis is made on typical historical and clinical findings. The laboratory findings are similar to those of acute cholecystitis except that the white blood cell count may become elevated, often above 20,000 per mm^3.

Treatment

The treatment for empyema of the gallbladder is early operative intervention. Preoperative stabilization should include appropriate fluid therapy and parenteral antibiotics. This resuscitation should be done rapidly, however, to accomplish removal of the gallbladder before rupture and generalized peritonitis occur. Cholecystectomy is preferable to tube drainage in these cases because the gallbladder wall is frequently gangrenous and necrotic. A temporizing cholecystostomy may be necessary in critically ill patients who could not survive a prolonged procedure under general anesthesia.

EMPHYSEMATOUS CHOLECYSTITIS (PNEUMOCHOLECYSTITIS)

Emphysematous cholecystitis, although relatively rare, is a severe variant of acute cholecystitis. It is diagnosed by a roentgenogram of the abdomen, which should reveal air in the gallbladder lumen, blebs in the wall, and collections of gas in the pericholecystic tissue or the biliary radicles. The differential diagnoses of these radiologic findings include communication with the gastrointestinal tract, lipoma of the gallbladder, and incompetence of the sphincter of Oddi, which produces gas in the common duct as well as in the gallbladder and biliary tree.

Several clinical and laboratory findings help to distinguish acute cholecystitis from the emphysematous variety (Table 35-4). The gas is produced by both facultative and anaerobic microorganisms, and there is a higher incidence of positive bile cultures in the emphysematous variety. Coliforms, especially *E. coli* and *Klebsiella*, are frequently found, as well as clostridia, which are isolated in approximately 50 percent of the cases.[1,7] *C. perfringens* is the most common bacterial species isolated. The emphysematous form occurs more often in males, and is seen with unusual frequency in diabetics. Its tendency to produce gangrene and perforation is an index of its severity.

It is important to diagnose emphysematous cholecystitis early because of the lethal complications. For this reason, radiograms of the abdomen are required in all patients with acute cholecystitis. If gas is recognized in the gallbladder, the surrounding tissue, or the biliary radicles, there is a clear indication for early operative intervention. Antibiotic therapy, begun preoperatively, is aimed at both anaerobic clostridia and the facultative coliforms. When culture results are available, the unnecessary antibiotic agent can be discontinued.

ACUTE CHOLANGITIS

Cholangitis is defined as infection within the bile ducts. The milder form of acute cholangitis is associated with partial obstruction and an inflammatory reaction within the biliary tree—so-called ascending cholangitis. A further extension of the infection, suppurative cholangitis, is associated with frank pus under pressure in the bile ducts, a diagnosis that can only be established at operation. Such purulent collections are associated with a bacterial hepatitis, septicemia, and a higher mortality.[21]

Incidence

Stone disease of the biliary system is the most common hepatobiliary diagnosis in the United States, and the majority of patients with cholangitis have stones. But it is a rare complication; suppurative cholangitis accounts for less than 2 of every 1,000 hospital admissions [22] and only 17

TABLE 35-4. FEATURES DIFFERENTIATING ACUTE AND EMPHYSEMATOUS CHOLECYSTITIS

	Acute Cholecystitis	Emphysematous Cholecystitis
Male-female	1:2.5	2.5:1
Without stones	10%	30%
Gangrene of gallbladder at time of operation	2%	75%
Perforation of gallbladder at time of operation	4%	20%
Mortality	4%	15%
Clostridia in bile	<10%	>50%

of 955 patients with biliary disease in series seen by gastroenterologists.[23] In surgical series, however, almost 10 percent of patients with a prior diagnosis of biliary disease ultimately developed suppurative cholangitis and one-third of all patients undergoing a common duct operation had it.[24] In the United States, half the patients developing this disease are older than 70, and it is rare in patients under the age of 50. However, a subgroup of persons of Chinese extraction seem to be more susceptible to the disease at a younger age. In the Chinese population, it is characteristically found in the 30- to 40-year-old age group and is associated with soft choledochal stones (see subsequent section on cholangiohepatitis).

Pathogenesis

The normal pressure within the biliary tract is less than 10 cm H_2O, increasing to 30 cm H_2O with contraction of the gallbladder (compared to the 37.5 cm H_2O maximal secretory pressure of bile production by the liver). The sphincter of Oddi is normally competent to pressures up to 16 cm H_2O; pressures seldom exceed this level unless obstruction is present. When the gallbladder contracts, the flow of bile will open the sphincter and wash out contaminating material, including bacteria from the ductal system. However, in obstructive states, whether secondary to mechanical or functional obstruction, the pressure may be sufficient to reflux stones, bacteria, or other detritis into the liver itself.

Biliary stasis is the sine qua non of cholangitis, and the most frequent cause of obstruction in calculous biliary disease. Once the stones enter the common duct, they can become impacted in the papilla or reflux up and down, causing an intermittent ball-valve obstruction, disrupting normal ampullary competence, and permitting reflux of duodenal contents into the biliary tree. Biliary obstruction can also result from papillitis, tumors, pancreatitis, parasites, or choledochal cysts, but obstructing lesions which totally prevent reflux (like cancer) are seldom causes of cholangitis unless instrumentation has been used.

Choledocholithiasis not only permits duodenal-biliary reflux, it is associated with alterations of the intestinal bacterial flora itself. Interruptions to bile flow impairs fat absorption. Because fat is poorly absorbed, much greater amounts reach the distal small bowel and colon, where bacteria rapidly multiply in the extra food source, producing gas and organic acids. This results in a decreased transit time for food as peristalsis is stimulated. Not only is there an increase in the number of bacteria growing in the distal gastrointestinal tract (and presumably ascending to the jejunum) but with the absence of bile in the duodenum, bacteria mixed in food exiting the stomach rapidly proliferate.[25] The increased numbers of bacteria found in the duodenum are probably a major contributing factor to the development of cholangitis.

When bacteria contaminate the obstructed biliary tree, few host defenses exist to clear them. Bile contains normal levels of immunoglobulins, but neutrophils are almost completely immobilized by high bile salt concentrations.

Continued untreated cholangitis in the presence of complete obstruction may cause a build-up of pressure within the biliary tree. Bile secretion ceases above 36–38 cm H_2O pressure, but much lower pressures result in release of bacteria from the bile canaliculi. Huang et al[27] introduced *E. coli* into the partially obstructed common ducts of dogs after cannulating the thoracic duct and hepatic veins. At 20 cm H_2O pressure, bacteria appeared in thoracic duct lymph. At 25 cm of H_2O bacteria appeared in the blood. With increasing pressures, there was an exponential increase in the bacteria recovered from both lymph and blood cultures.

It is not surprising, therefore, that cholangiography in the presence of bacteria results in septicemia, whether it is done by the endoscopic retrograde choleangiopancreatography, T tube, or transhepatic route. Perhaps manometric monitoring of pressures during cholangiography should be done to prevent intrahepatic disruption of bile canaliculi.[26]

Clinical Manifestations

Cholangitis occurs in several characteristic clinical settings: (1) an older patient with long-standing symptomatic cholelithiasis; (2) a common duct stone retained from a recent cholecystectomy—the original operation is generally less than 1 year prior to the onset of new symptoms; (3) a common duct stone, formed as a primary concretion within the hepatic or common duct—such patients have undergone cholecystectomy 5 to 10 years or even longer before recurrence; (4) benign strictures following biliary tract or intestinal surgery; (5) biliary-intestinal reconstructive procedures; and (6) abnormal connections or fistulae between the biliary tract and the intestine.

The classic symptoms of acute cholangitis make up Charcot triad—fever, abdominal pain, and jaundice. Other common clinical and laboratory findings are listed in Tables 35-5 and 35-6.

Fever occurs in 95 percent of patients with cholangitis, although it may be observed in only two-thirds of patients at the time of hospital admission. Fever is sudden in onset and paroxysmal, often associated with shaking chills.

Abdominal pain and deep tenderness in the right upper quadrant occur in the majority of patients during the course of cholangitis. The pain may be constant or colicky, often radiating to the back or right shoulder. It may persist for several days even after the fever has subsided.

Jaundice can be noted clinically in two-thirds of the patients and by measurement of serum bilirubin in over 90 percent. It is generally of mild degree, although infrequently it may be pruritic. In general, jaundice progresses to a peak over 3 to 5 days and then gradually returns to a baseline level. Shock and central nervous system depression are diagnostic features of suppurative cholangitis, which carry a grim prognosis.[24]

Attacks of cholangitis, consisting of a constellation of signs and symptoms, occur intermittently and persist for several years if appropriate treatment cannot be instituted. Some patients, however, develop severe infection with suppuration and septic shock and may not survive the first acute episode.

Diagnosis

The diagnosis of cholangitis is based on the typical triad of symptoms, with a history of prior biliary operation or

TABLE 35-5. CLINICAL FINDINGS IN ACUTE CHOLANGITIS

Signs and Symptoms	Percent Present
History of fever	95
Fever on admission	65
RUQ tenderness	80
Abdominal pain	80
Jaundice	80
Nausea and vomiting	50
Peritoneal irritation	45
Shock	5

TABLE 35-6. LABORATORY FINDINGS IN ACUTE CHOLANGITIS

Laboratory Studies	Percent Abnormal
Bilirubin	90
Alkaline phosphatase	90
Transaminase	90
Positive blood cultures	40
WBC (>10,000 mm^3)	62
Amylase (serum)	35
Roentgenogram (flat plate)	15

partial obstruction caused by choledocholithiasis. Physical findings are localized to the right upper quadrant and may be minimal, consisting only of deep tenderness. These findings should be contrasted with the severe local findings which are seen with acute infections of the gallbladder.

Laboratory data and x-ray studies support the diagnosis (Tables 35-5 and 35-6) (Fig. 35-1A). A definitive diagnosis is easiest by a percutaneous transhepatic cholangiogram (Fig. 35-1B). If the bilirubin level is only modestly elevated, an intravenous cholangiogram can be performed, but this is far less useful. Transduodenal retrograde cholangiography also provides the diagnosis in most cases. An additional advantage of this approach is that a transduodenal sphincterotomy can be performed in high risk patients. If a liver biopsy is performed, the portal areas will show inflammatory changes, infiltration with leukocytes, fibrosis, and proliferation of bile ducts.

One or more liver function tests are almost invariably abnormal during an attack of acute cholangitis (Tables 35-5 and 35-6). On the other hand, the white blood cell count is unpredictable, normal in some cases and inordinately high in others, often in the range of a leukemoid reaction. It is important to obtain blood cultures before initiating antibiotics because the yield of positive results is over 40 percent.

Progressive elevation of the serum alkaline phosphatase to moderate levels when the serum bilirubin level is normal suggests the blockage of one of the main hepatic ducts. This complication usually occurs postoperatively when a stone has been pushed into a hepatic duct during exploration of the common duct.

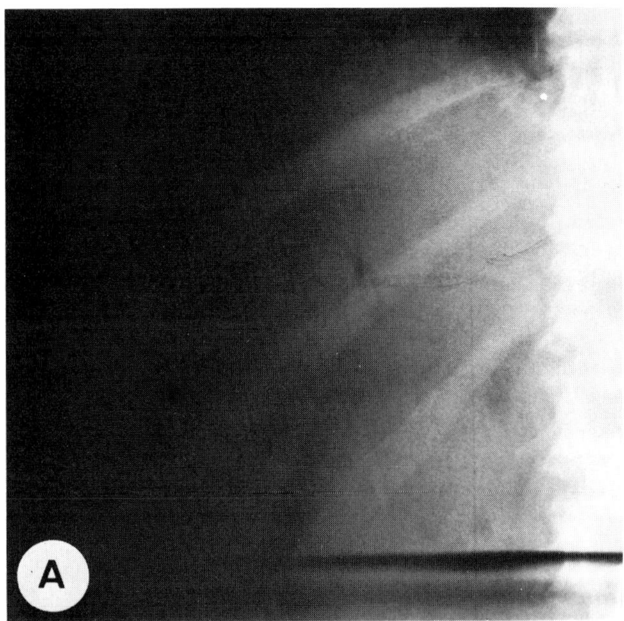

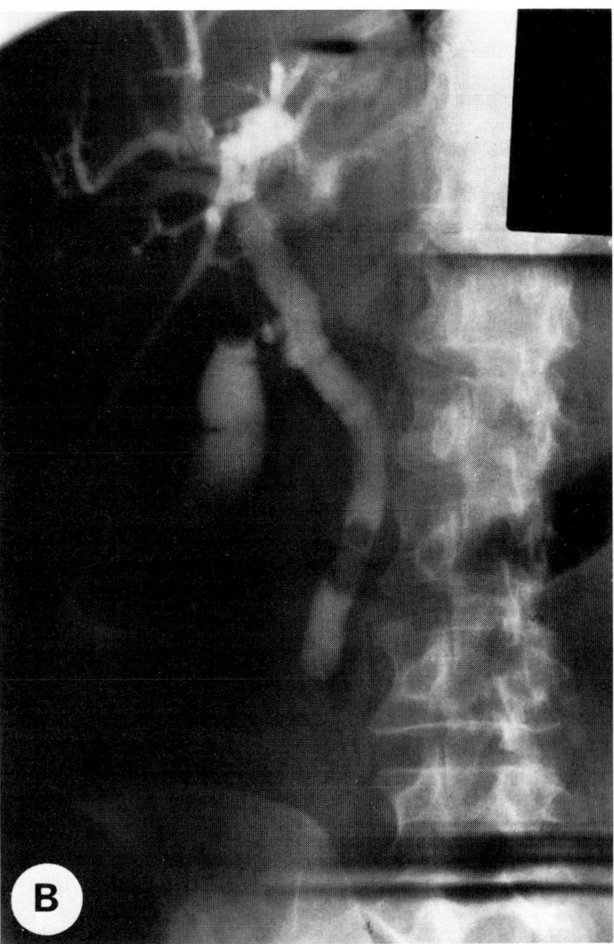

Fig. 35-1. A. Air in biliary tree of a jaundiced febrile woman with suppurative cholangitis. The air was not apparent on admission but developed over 12 hours. B. A percutaneous transhepatic cholangiogram was performed showing a dilated common duct, stones floating in the common duct and gallbladder. Two small stones are impacted at the ampulla. (Courtesy of Dr. R.L Simmons.)

Microbiology

The isolation of bacteria from common duct bile in cholangitis is greater than 85 percent.[7,8,20,28] During acute suppurative cholangitis, many species will be isolated from a single patient. The most frequently isolated bacteria are the enteric coliforms, just as in infections of the gallbladder. Unlike acute cholecystitis, anaerobic bacteria are frequently present in cholangitis.[28,29] *B. fragilis* and clostridia are isolated most frequently (Table 35-7).

Treatment

The treatment of cholangitis depends on the severity of symptoms and the underlying cause. All patients should undergo initial medical therapy, which includes: (1) initiation of parenteral antibiotics similar to those advised for acute cholecystitis—the major exception is that a drug with activity against *B. fragilis* (such as clindamycin) is also used; (2) intubation and aspiration of the upper intestine; (3) intravenous fluid and electrolytes; and (4) relief of pain.

Medical management is a delaying tactic to improve the patient's condition in preparation for primary operative treatment, which includes exploration of the common duct and removal of stones or repair, reconstruction, or bypass of strictures. Decompression of the biliary tree with a percutaneous transhepatic catheter may be useful while preparing the patient.[29a]

If the patient has not responded promptly (less than 24 hours) to initial medical management, an emergency operation is required. This is especially true in patients with bacteremia or who show signs of hemodynamic instability or cerebral malfunction.

Decompression of the common duct with a T tube is the essential procedure and may be all the patient can tolerate. Cholecystectomy or cholecystostomy are never sufficient in themselves. Under optimal conditions, the common duct should be explored, and the stones should be extirpated. The gallbladder is then removed and a T tube is placed in the common duct, thus obviating the necessity for a second operation. The liver should be examined for evidence of gross abscesses, which should be drained. Several surgeons recommend a biliary fenestration procedure (choledochoduodenostomy) at the time of biliary decompression, with the hope that the incidence of recurrence will be reduced. A common error in the surgical treatment of patients with suppurative cholangitis is to drain only the gallbladder, which does not properly drain the common duct, the primary site of the suppurative infection.

Complications of acute cholangitis include unrelenting sepsis and septic shock, liver abscess, and recurrent, relapsing cholangitis. The mortality rate is approximately 15 percent, and the usual cause of death is uncontrolled sepsis. Prompt operation when medical management fails will reduce the mortality.[23] Recognition that micro- and macroscopic liver abscesses may exist when patients fail to respond to appropriate decompression of the biliary tree should prompt reexploration for small liver abscesses and drainage. Long-term antibiotic therapy may be necessary.

TABLE 35-7. BACTERIA ISOLATED FROM BILIARY TRACT CULTURES

	Percent of 701 Isolates	Percent of 157 Isolates
Aerobic organisms *		
Escherichia coli	24	
Streptococcus, group D	19	
Klebsiella	17	
Pseudomonas aeruginosa	8	
Streptococcus, viridans group	7	
Enterobacter cloacae	3	
Proteus mirabilis	3	
Staphylococcus epidermidis	3	
Proteus morganii	3	
Citrobacter freundii	2	
Corynebacterium spp	2	
Pseudomonas spp	1	
Enterobacter aerogenes	1	
Staphylococcus aureus	1	
Citrobacter diversus	1	
Lactobacillus	1	
Anaerobic organisms †		
Anaerobic gram-negative bacilli		50
Bacteroides		45
B. fragilis		38
Fusobacterium		5
Clostridium		39
C. perfringens		32
Nonsporing gram-positive bacilli		8
Anaerobic cocci		3

* Total of 284 cultures obtained from 251 patients, including 98 mixed infections and 153 with aerobes only isolated.
† Total of 119 cultures obtained from 100 patients, including 98 mixed infections and 2 with anaerobes only isolated.

Adapted from England DM, Rosenblatt JE: Anaerobes in human biliary tracts. *J Clin Microbiol* 6:494, 1977.

Cholangiohepatitis

Cholangiohepatitis (recurrent pyogenic cholangitis) is found almost exclusively among the Chinese.[30-32] In Hong Kong, it is the most common biliary disease and is the third most common abdominal emergency after appendicitis and perforated ulcer. Young adults are most commonly afflicted. Stock and Fung [32] have summarized the pathogenetic mechanisms (Fig. 35-2) in the development of biliary obstruction. The intestinal bacteria are the etiologic agents for the acute attack (See Fig. 11-27).

The gallbladder is usually distended but not inflamed. The common bile duct is also usually grossly distended and contains pigment stones, the nuclei of which may contain the parasites. Intrahepatic bile ducts are both dilated and constricted. Inflammatory changes are present in the periductal tissue, and abscesses are common. The clinical manifestations and treatment resemble in almost all respects those of suppurative cholangitis. However, the prognosis is guarded and recurrence is frequent.

SALMONELLA INFECTIONS OF THE BILIARY TRACT

Acute Cholecystitis

Although rare, large numbers of typhoid bacilli can accumulate within the gallbladder during a systemic attack

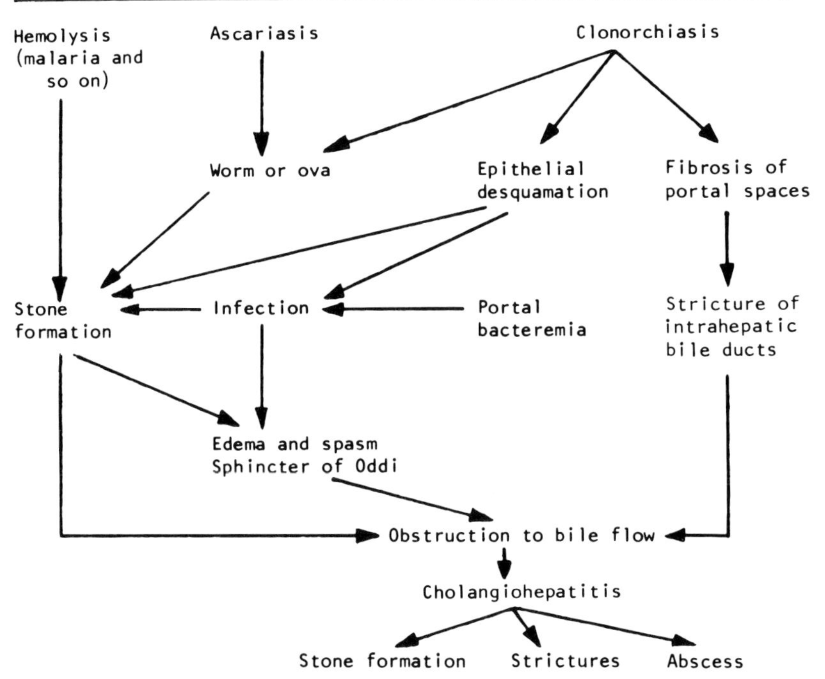

Fig 35-2. Schema of etiologic factors implicated in cholangiohepatitis. (After Stock FE, Fung JHY: Oriental cholangiohepatitis. In Smith R, Sherlock S: Surgery of the Gall Bladder and Bile Ducts, London, Butterworths, 1964.)

of typhoid fever. The organ can become inflamed, and classic acute cholecystitis is produced. The majority of patients with acute typhoidal cholecystitis can be managed medically with nasogastric suction and continuation of antibiotics (chloramphenicol). A small number of patients, however, will have intense inflammatory response in the gallbladder that requires cholecystectomy.

Surgical Management of Typhoid Carriers

A chronic carrier is defined as a person with positive stool cultures for at least 1 year following an episode of typhoid fever or, in some cases, positive stool culture results without a documented history of disease. The carrier state rarely disappears after persisting for 1 year. Chronic carriers are more common in older age groups, in women (a 3:1 ratio of women to men), and in people with gallstones. The organism is usually harbored in the gallbladder, often forming part of the gallstones and persists in symbiotic relationship with the host, causing neither local inflammation nor systemic symptoms. The bile contains enormous numbers of bacilli, up to 10^9 per ml, which are discharged in the feces in varying concentrations. The organisms are viable and fully infective so that the carrier may be a source of new infections.

The organism can be eradicated in some patients with prolonged antibiotic therapy. A regimen that works in approximately two-thirds of the patients is ampicillin, 6 gm per day in four divided doses for 4 weeks. Relapses of the carrier state are generally associated with stones and gallbladder disease. In individuals with gallstones or chronic cholecystitis, cholecystectomy cures the carrier state in 85 percent of the patients. This procedure, however, is only recommended for individuals whose profession—food handlers and health care providers—is not compatible with typhoid carrier state.

BILE PERITONITIS

The chemical inflammation that occurs when bile escapes from the interrupted biliary tract after trauma or disease causes varying degrees of clinical symptomatology (Chapter 34), eg, when associated with infection, gangrenous acute cholecystitis, or empyema, a highly virulent peritonitis is produced. Sterile bile by itself can be benign within the peritoneal cavity, although bacterial infection ultimately occurs if the biliary fistula is not controlled.

INFECTIONS FOLLOWING BILIARY SURGERY FOR CHRONIC CALCULUS CHOLECYSTITIS

In a collaborative study reported in 1964 by the National Research Council,[33] the infection rate after elective biliary tract surgery varied from 6.9 to 17.1 percent. The low figure was the average for simple cholecystectomy, while the higher infection rate was observed after choledochostomy. A recent large, one-hospital study, reported by Cruse,[34] showed that the infection rate for cholecystectomy alone or with cholecystectomy and cholangiography was around 2 percent, while the rate for choledochostomy was 7.9 percent. When elective appendectomy is added to cholecystectomy, divergent results are reported. Wolloch et al [35] found no significant increase in postoperative infection rates after biliary tract operations when routine appendectomy was added to the procedure, but Cruse [34] reported an increase from 2 percent to 4.8 percent.

Bacteriology of Bile in Patients Undergoing Cholecystectomy for Chronic Calculus Cholecystitis

As discussed previously, the healthy biliary tract rarely harbors significant concentrations of bacteria. In the presence of chronic calculus cholecystitis, bacteria have been isolated in 15 to 30 percent of cases.[36] Csendes et al [6] found bacteria in 30 percent of gallbladder bile cultures in a group of patients with chronic calculus cholecystitis, while results of gallbladder wall cultures in the same group of patients were not significantly different. Other reports showed significantly higher positive bile culture rates in a group of patients with juxtapapillary duodenal diverticula who were undergoing cholecystectomy for chronic calculus cholecystitis.[37] These findings were interpreted as supporting the ascending route in biliary tract infection.

The bacteria isolated from bile in all disease states of the biliary tract are primarily gram-negative enteric coliforms. *E. coli,* alone or mixed with another organism, is present in 50 percent of positive cultures. Other coliforms, ie, *Klebsiella, Enterobacter,* and *Proteus,* are less commonly isolated.

Anaerobic microorganisms are isolated in fewer than 20 percent of the cases. In most studies, *C. perfringens* is the most commonly isolated anaerobe, however, a recent investigation has shown *B. fragilis* to be most prevalent.[38] A polymicrobial infection, including both aerobes and anaerobes, is often found in liver abscess and in long-standing common duct obstruction caused by choledocholithiasis.

Quantitative bile cultures have shown concentrations of bacteria in most biliary disease states to be less than 10^5 viable organisms per ml of bile. In patients with choledocholithiasis, however, bacterial cholangitis is usually present, and the bile may harbor bacteria in the range of 10^5 to 10^9 microorganisms per ml.[36]

Clinical Risk Factors for Development of Postoperative Infection after Biliary Surgery

Positive bile cultures collected at the time of biliary operations are associated with a higher postoperative infection rate.[33] Delikaris et al [39] reported a 33 percent postoperative infection rate in patients undergoing a biliary tract operation who were found to have positive bile culture. Several studies [40-43] have elicited those clinical factors which favor bactobilia and a corresponding increased risk of postoperative sepsis (Table 35-8). Prophylactic antibiotics are indicated when one or more of these risk factors are present.

Immediate Gram-Staining of Bile in Patients Undergoing Biliary Surgery

Some patients who undergo elective cholecystectomy in the absence of risk factors (Table 35-8) will nevertheless have bactobilia. For this reason, a bile sample taken at the time of operation, usually from the gallbladder, should be sent to the microbiology laboratory for Gram staining and culture and sensitivity.[44,45] The overall accuracy rate of the Gram stains when compared to subsequent bile cultures is greater than 75 percent and allows the surgeon to start appropriate antibiotics during the operation in those patients who were not previously given them. It also allows for additions or changes in antibiotics when organisms are found that were not anticipated, such as gram-positive rods on immediate staining, which would call for antibiotic coverage of *Clostridium.* Numerous case reports of catastrophic clostridial infections following biliary surgery have been reported.[46-48]

TABLE 35-8. CLINICAL RISK FACTORS FAVORING THE PRESENCE OF BACTOBILIA IN BILIARY TRACT DISEASE

Previous biliary tract operation
Age over 70
Operation done as emergency
Jaundice present
Chills or fever within 1 week of operation
Empyema or pneumocholecystitis
Stone in common duct
Operation done within 1 month of an acute attack of cholecystitis

Antibiotic Recommendations in Surgery for Chronic Calculus Cholecystitis

Well-controlled studies have shown the benefits of prophylactic antibiotics, before or during surgery, in patients who had clinical risk factors or a positive intraoperative Gram stain showing the presence of bacteria in bile.[40,41,46-51] Authoritative committees have reported that antibiotic prophylaxis in chronic calculus cholecystitis appears to be justified.[52,53] The initial antibiotic agent chosen should be effective against the usual infecting organisms, the aerobic, gram-negative coliforms. The aminoglycosides or the second generation cephalosporins appear to be the best choice. If a gram-positive rod is seen on Gram stain, penicillin should be added to the regimen. The prophylactic antibiotics should only be continued for 24 to 72 hours after operation. As stated previously, equal benefit can be expected from antibiotic agents that give either high serum or bile levels. The prolonged use, however, of prophylactic antibiotics in all patients who undergo cholecystectomy for chronic calculus cholecystitis should be avoided.

BIBLIOGRAPHY

Andrew DJ, Johnson SE: Acute suppurative cholangitis, a medical and surgical emergency: A review of ten years experience emphasizing early recognition. Amer J Gastroenterol 54: 141, 1970.

Keighley MRB, Drysdale RB, Quoraishi AH, Burdon DW, Alexander-Williams J: Antibiotics in biliary disease: The relative importance of antibiotic concentrations in the bile and serum. Gut 17:495, 1976.

REFERENCES

1. Lou MA, Mandal AK, Alexander JL, Thadepalli H: Bacteriology of the human biliary tract and the duodenum. Arch Surg 112:965, 1977.
2. Maki T: Pathogenesis of calcium bilirubinate gallstone: role of *E. coli,* beta-glucuronidase and coagulation by inorganic ions, polyelectrolytes and agitation. Ann Surg 164:90, 1966.
3. Arnold L, Brody L: Bacterial flora and hydrogen ion concentration of the duodenum. J Infect Dis 38:249, 1926.
4. Nichols RL, Smith JW: Intragastric microbial colonization in common disease states of the stomach and duodenum. Ann Surg 182:557, 1975.

5. Scott AJ: Progress report. Bacteria and disease of the biliary tract. Gut 12:487, 1971.
6. Csendes A, Fernandez M, Uribe P: Bacteriology of the gallbladder bile in normal subjects. Am J Surg 129(6):629–31, 1975.
7. Nielsen ML, Justesen T: Anaerobic and aerobic bacteriological studies in biliary tract disease. Scand J Gastroenterol 11:437, 1976.
8. Edlund YA, Mollstedt BO, Ouchterlony O: Bacteriological investigation of the biliary system and liver in biliary tract disease correlated to clinical data and microstructure of the gallbladder and liver. Acta Chir Scand 116:461, 1959.
8a. O'Connor MJ, Schwartz ML, McQuarrie DG, Sumner HW: Cholangitis due to malignant obstruction of biliary flow. Ann Surg 193:341, 1981.
9. Tynes BS, Utz JP: Factors influencing the cure of salmonella carriers. Ann Intern Med 57:871, 1962.
10. Keighley MRB, Drysdale RB, Quoraishi AH, Burdon DW, Alexander-Williams J: Antibiotics in biliary disease: the relative importance of antibiotic concentrations in the bile and serum. Gut 17:495, 1976.
11. Brown RB, Martyak SN, Barza M, Curtis L, Weinstein L: Penetration of clindamycin phosphate into the abnormal human biliary tract. Ann Intern Med 84:168, 1976.
12. Ram MD, Watanatittan S: Biliary excretion and concentration of cefazolin. Am J Gastroenterol 66:540, 1976.
13. Trachtenberg L, Fagelman KM, Polk HC: The biliary tract kinetics of some cephalosporin antibiotics. Surgery 84:342, 1978.
14. Geddes AM, Schnurr LP, Ball AP, McGhie D, Brookes GR, Wise R, Andrews J: Cefoxitin: a hospital study. Br Med J 1:1126, 1977.
15. Zaslow J, Rosenthal A: The excretion and concentration of terramycin in the abnormal biliary tract. Ann Surg 139:478, 1954.
16. Howard RJ, Delaney JP: Acute acalculous cholecystitis. Minn Med 55:549, 1972.
16a. Peterson SR, Sheldon GF: Acute acalculous cholecystitis: A complication of hyperalimentation. Am J Surg 138:814, 1979.
16b. Szlabick RE, Catto JA, Fink-Bennett D, Ventura V: Hepatobiliary scanning in the diagnosis of acute cholecystitis. Arch Surg 115:540, 1980.
17. Järvinen HJ, Hästbacka J: Early cholecystectomy for acute cholecystitis. Ann Surg 191:501, 1980.
18. MacLean LD, Goldstein M, MacDonald JE, Demers R: Results of cholecystectomy in 1000 consecutive patients. Can J Surg 18:459, 1975.
19. Stone AM, Tucci VJ, Isenberg HD, Wise L: Wound infection: acute versus chronic cholecystitis. Am J Surg 133:285, 1977.
20. Flinn WR, Olson DF, Oyasu R, Beal JM: Biliary disease. Ann Surg 185:593, 1977.
21. Welch JP, Donaldson GA: The urgency of diagnosis and surgical treatment of acute suppurative cholangitis. Am J Surg 131:527, 1976.
22. Haupert AP, Carey LC, Evans WE, Ellison EH: Acute suppurative cholangitis: experience with 15 consecutive cases. Arch Surg 94:460, 1966.
23. Andrew DJ, Johnson SE: Acute suppurative cholangitis, a medical and surgical emergency: a review of ten years experience emphasizing early recognition. Am J Gastroenterol 54:141, 1970.
24. Saik RP, Greenburg AG, Farris JM, Peskin GW: Spectrum of cholangitis. Am J Surg 130:143, 1975.
25. Anderson RE, Priestley JT: Observations on the bacteriology of choledocal bile. Ann Surg 133:436, 1951.
26. Dellinger EP, Kirshenbaum G, Weinstein M, Steer M: Determinants of adverse reaction following postoperative T-tube cholangiogram. Ann Surg 191:397, 1980.
27. Huang T, Bass JA, Williams RD: The significance of biliary pressure in cholangitis. Arch Surg 98:629, 1969.
28. Shimada K, Inamatsu T, Yamashiro M: Anaerobic bacteria in biliary disease in elderly patients. J Infect Dis 135:850, 1977.
29. England DM, Rosenblatt JE: Anaerobes in human biliary tracts. J Clin Microbiol 6:494, 1977.
29a. Denning DA, Ellison EC, Carey LC: Preoperative percutaneous transhepatic biliary decompression lowers operative morbidity in patients with obstructive jaundice. Am J Surg 141:61, 1981.
30. Stock FE, Fung JHY: Oriental cholangiohepatitis. Arch Surg 84:409, 1962.
31. Mage S, Morel AS: Surgical experience with cholangiohepatitis (Hong Kong disease) in Canton Chinese. Ann Surg 162:187, 1965.
32. Stock FE, Fung JHY: Oriental cholangiohepatitis. In Smith R, Sherlock S (eds): Surgery of the Gall Bladder and Bile Ducts. London, Butterworth, 1964.
33. National Academy of Sciences-National Research Council, Division of Medical Sciences, Ad Hoc Committee of the Committee on Trauma: Postoperative wound infections: the influence of ultraviolet irradiation of the operating room and of various other factors. Ann Surg 160(suppl 2): 1, 1964.
34. Cruse PJE: Incidence of wound infection on the surgical service. Surg Clin North Am 55:1269, 1975.
35. Wolloch Y, Feigenberg Z, Zer M, Dintsman M: The influence of biliary infection on the postoperative course after biliary tract surgery. Am J Gastroenterol 67:456, 1977.
36. Nichols RL: Use of antibiotics in stomach, duodenal and biliary tract surgery. J Surg Prac 6:20, 1977.
37. Löveit T, Osnes M, Aune S: Bacteriological studies of common duct bile in patients with gallstone disease and juxta-papillary duodenal diverticula. Scand J Gastroenterol 13:93, 1978.
38. Gorbach SL, Bartlett JG: Anaerobic infections (Part 1). N Engl J Med 290:1177, 1974.
39. Delikaris PG, Michail PO, Klonis GD, Haritopoulos NC, Golematis BC, Dreiling DA: Biliary bacteriology based on intraoperative bile cultures. Am J Gastroenterol 68:51, 1977.
40. Chetlin SH, Elliot D: Preoperative antibiotics in biliary surgery. Arch Surg 107:319, 1973.
41. Keighley MRB: Prevention of wound sepsis in gastrointestinal surgery. Br J Surg 64:315, 1977.
42. Keighley MRB, Flinn R, Alexander-Williams J: Multivariate analysis of clinical and operative findings associated with biliary sepsis. Br J Surg 63:528, 1976.
43. Prytek LJ, Bartus SA: An evaluation of antibiotics in biliary tract surgery. Surg Gynecol Obstet 125:101, 1967.
44. Keighley MRB, McLeish AR, Bishop HM, Burdon DW, Path MRC, Quoraishi AH, Oates GD, Dorricott NJ, Alexander-Williams J: Identification of the presence and type of biliary microflora by immediate Gram stains. Surgery 81:469, 1977.
45. McLeish AR, Keighley MRB, Bishop HM, Burdon DW, Alexander-Williams J: Selecting patients requiring antibiotics in biliary surgery by immediate Gram stains of bile at operation. Surgery 81:473, 1977.
46. Aukee S, Alhava EM, Koskela E, Lahtinen J, Salmela J: Clostridium septicemia following biliary surgery in a gastrectomized patient. Scand J Gastroenterol 10:109, 1975.
47. Clancy MT, O'Brian S: Fatal *Clostridium welchii* septicemia following acute cholecystitis. Br J Surg 62:518, 1975.
48. Hitchcock CR, Haglin JJ, Arnar O: Treatment of clostridial infections with hyperbaric oxygen. Surgery 62:759, 1967.
49. Gunn AA: Antibiotics in biliary surgery. Br J Surg 63:627, 1976.
50. Keighley MRB, Baddeley RM, Burdon DW, Edwards JAC,

Quoraishi AH, Oates GD, Watts GT, Alexander-Williams J: A controlled trial of parenteral prophylactic gentamicin therapy in biliary surgery. Br J Surg 62:275, 1975.
51. Stone HH, Hooper CA, Kolb LD, Geheber CE, Dawkins EJ: Antibiotic prophylaxis in gastric, biliary and colonic surgery. Ann Surg 184:443, 1976.
52. Veterans Administration Ad Hoc Interdisciplinary Advisory Committee on Antimicrobial Drug Usage: 1. Prophylaxis in Surgery. JAMA 237:1003, 1977.
53. Antimicrobial prophylaxis: prevention of wound infection and sepsis after surgery. Med Lett Drugs Ther 19:37, 1977.

CHAPTER 36
Infections of the Liver and Spleen

Toni Hau

The structure and function of the liver and spleen can be altered during many systemic infections, and some infections can involve these organs diffusely (Table 36-1). Many cases of hepatitis lead to cirrhosis with associated portal hypertension, intestinal varices, hemorrhage, hypersplenism, and ascites, all of which may be surgical problems, the treatment of which lie outside the scope of this book. In addition, patients with cirrhosis are prone to develop systemic sepsis and primary peritonitis (discussed in Chapter 34), and infections of the biliary tract can lead to liver infection (dealt with in Chapter 35). This chapter will be limited to discussions of infections and infestations of the liver and spleen whose treatment or diagnosis frequently requires surgical consultation.

The liver and spleen are the major reservoirs of the fixed macrophage population in the body. As blood passes through both organs, it is in intimate and prolonged contact with sinusoidal macrophages, one of whose functions is to clear the filtered blood of microorganisms. The liver filters the portal blood so that pathogenic or opportunistic microbes that escape the gut are usually trapped by the Küpffer cells. Both the liver and the spleen clear the arterial blood of circulating organisms.[1]

LIVER

Despite continuous exposure to microbial organisms and their toxins, the liver of humans, unlike that of dogs and other experimental animals,[2-5] is normally sterile,[2,6-10] as is normal portal blood.[2,6] When portal bacterial showers occur,[11] however, the liver is able to eliminate bacteria from the blood stream. Berg et al [12] showed that animals with normal contaminated liver parenchyma have sterile bile. Beeson et al [1] demonstrated that patients with subacute bacterial endocarditis had a lower concentration of organisms in the hepatic vein blood than in the peripheral blood. In spite of the filtering function of the liver, bacterial infections are rare and usually occur in the form of abscesses. In most instances, the morphologic changes observed during septicemia are caused by toxic damage to the hepatocytes. Only a few cases of true bacterial hepatitis, mostly streptococcal, have been reported,[13-15] and it appears to be rare today.[13] Histologically, one can see the invasion of parenchyma by streptococci and scattered focal areas of hepatocellular necrosis. In contrast to toxic damage of the liver by viruses, which is centrilobular, these lesions are either periportal or intrazonal. The liver is involved in numerous other infections; only a few bacterial, mycotic, and protozoal infections assume surgical significance (Table 36-1). Abscesses can develop in granulomas caused by brucellosis, actinomycosis, and candidiasis, which require surgical drainage. Tuberculosis of the liver can develop as large caseating granulomas, which might require resection of the liver.[16] All other diseases that cause diffuse parenchymal damage or miliary abscesses and granulomas are not amenable to surgical therapy.

BACTERIAL ABSCESS OF THE LIVER

Incidence

Abscess of the liver has always been a rare finding. Two autopsy series conducted before 1900 reported incidences of liver abscesses between 0.4 and 1.75 percent.[17,18] Even in 1932, Collins found only 111 cases in 18,300 autopsies (0.606 percent).[19] At the same time, the incidence based on hospital admissions ranged from 0.04 percent to 0.007 percent.[20,21] Pyogenic liver abscesses occur even less frequently since the advent of antibiotic therapy. Knowles and Rinaldo [22] reported nine cases from the Henry Ford Hospital over the 10 years before 1960 (0.005 percent of all hospital admissions), and Ribaudo and Ochsner [23] found one liver abscess in every 1,628 patients in 1973. Furthermore, the peak incidence of the liver abscesses has shifted from the third and fourth decade to the seventh and eighth decades of life, a reflection of the previous importance of appendicitis as the main cause of liver abscesses.[24] The current autopsy incidence is not available.

Besides the decline in the incidence of pyogenic liver abscesses, a change in the relative frequency of bacterial and amebic abscesses has been observed. Whereas Ochsner et al [25] noted that 35 percent of all liver abscesses were amebic in 1938, they now constitute approximately 10 percent.[26,27]

TABLE 36-1. INFECTIOUS DISEASE WITH HEPATIC INVOLVEMENT

A. Bacterial infections
  1. Gram-positive cocci
    a. *Pneumococcus*
    b. *Staphylococcus* *
    c. *Streptococcus* *
  2. Gram-negative cocci
    a. *Gonococcus* (Fitz-Hugh-Curtis syndrome)
  3. Gram-negative enteric bacteria
    a. *E. coli* *
    b. *Salmonella*
    c. *Shigella*
    d. Other enteric bacteria *
  4. Other gram-negative bacilli
    a. *Brucellosis* *
    b. *Tuberculosis* *
    c. Granuloma inguinale
    d. Tularemia
  5. Spirochaetales
    a. Leptospirosis
    b. Borreliosis
    c. Syphilis
  6. Anaerobic bacteria
    a. *Clostridium* *
    b. *Bacteroides* *
    c. Other anaerobic bacteria *
  7. Rickettsial infections
    a. Q fever
  8. *Chlamydiae*
    a. Psittacosis

B. Mycotic infections
  1. Actinomycosis *
  2. Blastomycosis
  3. Candidiasis *
  4. Coccidioidomycosis
  5. Cryptococcosis
  6. Histoplasmosis
  7. Aspergillosis
  8. Mucormycosis

C. Protozoan infections
  1. Malaria
  2. Toxoplasmosis
  3. Amebiasis *

D. Viral infections
  1. Adenovirus
  2. Coxsackie virus
  3. Cytomegalovirus
  4. Echovirus
  5. Hepatitis virus A, B, non-A, non-B
  6. Herpes simplex virus
  7. Epstein-Barr virus
  8. "Marburg" virus
  9. Reovirus
  10. Rubella
  11. Varicella zoster

* Diseases of surgical significance.
Modified by Klatskin G: Hepatitis associated with systemic infections. In Schiff L (ed): *Diseases of the Liver,* 4th ed. Philadelphia, Lippincott, 1975.

Etiology

Virtually every bacterium known to medical microbiology has been mentioned as a causative agent of hepatic abscesses; however, reliable data are hard to come by. Ochsner et al [25] isolated *E. coli* in 30.4 percent, streptococci in 26.6 percent, and staphylococci in 26.0 percent of all cases of hepatic abscess; the cultures were sterile in 37.9 percent. In the older literature, sterile cultures were found in up to 60 percent of all cases.[28] Even in more recent reviews, the number of sterile abscesses still exceeds 10 percent.[29] Aside from 47 cases observed by Sabbaj et al,[30] only 165 cases of anaerobic liver abscesses have been reported. This low number is probably the result of inadequate anaerobic culture techniques. In a systematic search, Sabbaj found that anaerobic bacteria were present in 45 percent of all liver abscesses; the most commonly encountered organisms were anaerobic and microaerophilic streptococci, *B. fragilis,* and *Fusobacterium.* Of the 47 cases of Sabbaj et al,[30] 19 grew only aerobes, 15 grew only anaerobes, and 6 showed mixed anaerobic and aerobic cultures. In seven instances, either the cultures were sterile or the results were not available. In view of experimental data in which chronic liver abscesses could be reliably reproduced in mice only by the intraperitoneal injection of *Fusobacterium necrophorum,*[31] and the observations of Onderdonk et al [32] that the presence of anaerobic bacteria is necessary to produce intraperitoneal abscesses, it is likely that anaerobic bacteria are involved in a large percentage of hepatic abscesses. Unfortunately, there is little information about the relationship between the pathogenesis of liver abscess and its bacteriology. It seems, however, that anaerobic bacteria are prominent in abscesses secondary to hepatic tumors, and that the bacteriology of abscesses originating from lesions within the portal circulation closely resembles that of intraperitoneal infections, ie, *E. coli,* enterococci, and *Bacteroides.* A summary of the bacteriology of liver abscesses in Table 36-2 excludes the data of Sabbaj et al. Table 36-3 lists the anaerobes in 310 patients with liver abscesses collected by Finegold.[33] Rarely, some bacteria that normally elicit granulomatous reactions will cause hepatic abscess as a complication of systemic infection. Brucellosis is commonly complicated by hepatomegaly, splenomegaly, and microscopic hepatic granulomas. Although *B. abortis* is the common human pathogen, abscesses of the liver and spleen have been seen in *B. suis* infections.[34] In these cases, prolonged septic courses with calcific deposits in the liver or spleen were relieved by drainage.

Most tuberculous lesions of the liver are miliary granulomas. Abscesslike masses (tuberculomas) sometimes form and spread along the walls of the intrahepatic bile ducts (tuberculous cholangitis). Diagnosis may be difficult because both caseation and acid-fast organisms can be absent. Tuberculomas are often, but not always, accompanied by an abdominal focus. Drainage was sometimes curative in the prechemotherapeutic era.[35]

Miliary abscesses have been found in cases of disseminated granuloma inguinale.[36] Hepatic clostridial infections cause gas abscesses, but most of the jaundice in disseminated infections is hemolytic.

Pathogenesis

Table 36-4 lists the pathogenetic factors that are probably involved in the formation of liver abscesses. Primary hepatic causes include trauma, tumor, and ischemia. Direct extension of infections of neighboring organs to the liver has been described, but is rather rare. In Ochsner's series, trauma was responsible for approximately 10 percent of hepatic abscesses.[25] The same paper reports, however, that of the 575 cases collected from the world's literature, only 3 percent were caused by trauma. In a recent survey, trauma caused 5 percent of the liver abscesses.[29] According to Robertson et al,[37] 16 percent of all hepatic abscesses observed over a 25-year period originated from secondary infection of neoplastic lesions. Trump et al[38] have stated that of 1,262 liver abscesses described in the literature since 1934, only 32 patients had a lesion associated with either primary or metastatic tumor. Jochimsen et al[39] reported several cases of liver abscess that developed after the hepatic artery was ligated for the treatment of neoplasms (hepatic metastases).

Although abscesses that are associated with tumors may not be reported in surgical series, the association of infection with metastatic liver disease is probably underreported. Whether infection superimposed on hepatic metastasis is a common undiagnosed problem is speculative.

Because of the liver's dual blood supply, hematogenous spread of infections to the liver can occur via the portal vein or the hepatic artery, although the portal system is the more common pathway. Appendicitis was once the leading cause of hepatic abscesses. Ochsner et al [25] reported that 34 percent of all liver abscesses were caused by appendicitis; conversely, 0.38 percent of all cases of appendicitis developed a hepatic abscess. Today, 20 percent of all liver abscesses are secondary to an infection in the drainage area of the portal vein (Table 36-4).

Hepatic abscesses that originate from the arterial circulation of the liver constitute 13 to 15 percent of all liver abscesses, a number that has remained rather constant through the years.[25,29] Every infection associated with bacteremia can be the source of this kind of liver abscess.

The most common cause of pyogenic liver abscess today is ascending cholangitis that is secondary to biliary obstruction or manipulation. According to Ochsner,[25] infections of the biliary system were responsible for only 14 percent of all hepatic abscesses; this percentage has since increased to over 30 percent.

Even after thorough clinical and pathologic investigation, 20 percent of hepatic abscesses will remain, the source of which cannot be determined (cryptogenic abscesses). Perhaps they develop secondary to bacterial invasion from an unrecognized source within the portal system,[40] or even after dental manipulation. Focal areas of ischemia within the hepatic parenchyma may provide a local site of impaired defense so that bowel bacteria cannot be cleared.[41]

Patients with compromised host defenses have an increased risk of developing pyogenic liver abscesses. Diabetes mellitus was present in 15 percent of the patients of Altemeier et al,[42] and liver abscesses have been found in children with leukemia, chronic granulomatous disease, and other immune deficiency disorders.[43,44]

TABLE 36-2. BACTERIOLOGY OF HEPATIC ABSCESSES

Organisms	Number (%)	Number (%)
GRAM-POSITIVE AEROBES		
Staphylococci		34 (18.5)
S. aureus	27 (14.7)	
S. epidermidis	7 (3.8)	
Streptococci		36 (19.6)
Hemolytic strep	3 (1.6)	
Nonhemolytic strep	13 (7.1)	
Enterococci	20 (10.9)	
Others		4 (2.2)
GRAM-NEGATIVE AEROBES		
E. coli		82 (44.6)
Klebsiella/Enterobacter		61 (33.2)
Proteus		21 (11.4)
Pseudomonas		12 (6.5)
Others		16 (8.7)
ANAEROBES		
Bacteroides		16 (8.7)
Peptostreptococcus		11 (6.0)
Clostridium		7 (3.8)
Others		5 (2.7)

305 isolates from 184 patients.[24,26,29,68,70]

TABLE 36-3. ANAEROBIC ORGANISMS IN PYOGENIC LIVER ABSCESS (310 PATIENTS)

Organisms	Number of Isolates
Anaerobic streptococci	58
Microaerophilic streptococci	38
Anaerobic gram-positive cocci	7
Anaerobic gram-negative cocci	1
Bacteroides spp.	39
B. fragilis	33
B. oralis	2
B. serpens	3
B. melaninogenicus	7
Bacteroidaceae	6
Fusobacterium spp.	34
F. girans	3
F. necrophorum	47
Unidentified anaerobic gram-negative rods	16
Clostridium	38
Actinomyces	32
Eubacterium spp.	2
Lactobacillus spp.	1
Bifidobacterium	1
Propionibacterium	2
Bacterium halosepticum	1
Unidentified anaerobic gram-positive rods	5
"Anaerobe"	4
Total	379 strains

From Finegold SM: Anaerobic bacteria in human disease. New York, Harcourt, 1977, p 276.

TABLE 36-4. PATHOGENESIS OF PYOGENIC HEPATIC ABSCESSES

PRIMARY HEPATIC	Trauma Tumor Ischemia Hepatic parasites Foreign bodies
BY DIRECT EXTENSION	Penetrating peptic ulcers Penetrating carcinomas of the UGI tract Cholecystitis Pancreatitis Perihepatic abscess
VIA THE PORTAL CIRCULATION	Inflammatory disease of the small and large bowel Carcinoma of the GI tract with abscess formation Appendicitis Diverticulitis Pancreatitis Splenic infections Peritonitis and intraperitoneal abscesses Omphalitis
VIA THE ARTERIAL CIRCULATION	All infections associated with bacteremia
VIA THE BILIARY SYSTEM	Ascending cholangitis secondary to Stones Strictures Tumor
CRYPTOGENIC	

Pathology

The pathogenesis of liver absceses is reflected in the gross anatomic picture. If the cause of the abscess is a primary pathologic process of the liver, the abscess is single and corresponds to the primary lesion. Similar observations can be made if the abscess has been created as a direct extension of a perihepatic infection. If the primary lesion is located within the portal circulation, the abscesses are large, single or multiple, and in most cases confined to the right lobe of the liver; the left lobe alone is rarely affected. Kinney and Ferrebee,[45] in a study based on experiments of Sérégé in 1901,[46] showed that there is a separate flow of blood from the superior mesenteric vein to the right lobe of the liver, and from the splenic vein to the left lobe of the liver. This explains the preferential location of portal hepatic abscesses in the right lobe, which drains the intestines. Hepatic abscesses in both lobes will occur only when the portal vein is filled with a septic thrombus.

Bacteria originating from the systemic circulation reach the liver through the hepatic artery, and usually form many small abscesses—a frequent autopsy finding in debilitated and immunosuppressed hosts. If the hepatic abscesses originated from the biliary system, they are equally distributed over both lobes of the liver, are multiple, and the dilated biliary ducts are filled with pus. Approximately 65 percent of all hepatic abscesses occur in the right lobe, the left lobe less than 5 percent of the cases, and the remainder involve both lobes. The abscesses are multiple 40 percent of the time.[25,47]

Clinical Manifestations

The symptoms and signs associated with hepatic abscess are either systemic or local. The systemic symptoms are those of sepsis: fever, chills and profuse sweating. The fever is classically of the septic (picket fence) type, but continuous and intermittent fevers occur. Malaise and anorexia occur early, along with weight loss, weakness, nausea, vomiting, and lethargy. The most prominent local symptom, dull, constant, right upper quadrant pain, was present in over 90 percent of the cases reported by Ochsner et al [25]; it appears less frequently in more recent reports.[24,41] Often, the patient complains of pain that radiates into the right shoulder.[48]

The salient physical finding in two-thirds of these patients is a large, tender liver. Other findings include localized guarding and thoracic signs of pleural effusion or lower lobe infiltration. Jaundice occurs less commonly; Ochsner described it in only 8.3 percent of his patients. This holds true only for those hepatic abscesses that were not caused by an obstruction of the biliary tree.[25] Ascites is rare and is seen only as a terminal event.

Complications of Hepatic Abscess. Complications from hepatic abscess result from perforation of the abscess into neighboring structures. Pleural pulmonary complications, with a 15 percent occurrence in Ochsner's series,[25] result most often from direct extension of the hepatic abscess through the diaphragm into the parenchyma of the lung or the pleural space. Metastatic abscesses are rare. Even less frequently, a hepatic abscess will rupture into the peritoneal cavity and cause peritonitis or subhepatic abscess. In the preantibiotic era, this complication was observed in 7.2 and 2.5 percent of hepatic abscesses, respectively.[25] Perforations may also occur into the pericardium,[49] the hepatic vein,[50] the thoracic duct,[51] and the abdominal wall.[52] All these complications appear in less than 10 percent of the most recent series.[24,47,53] Block et

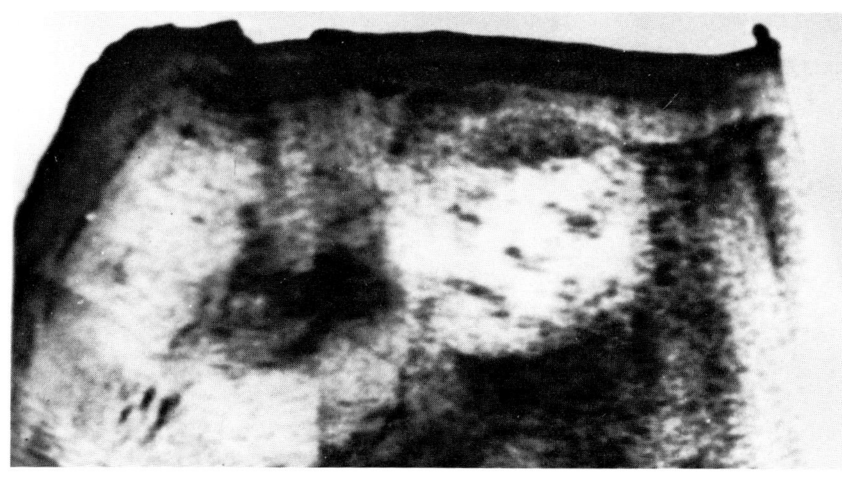

Fig. 36-1. Echogram of the liver revealing a large fluid-filled intrahepatic space, which was found to be a hepatic abscess at operation. (Courtesy of Dr. S. B. Feinberg, Department of Radiology, University of Minnesota, Minneapolis, Minnesota.)

al [26] state that eight of 26 patients with hepatic abscesses had other nonhepatic abscesses which required drainage.

Laboratory Evaluation. The laboratory findings in patients with a pyogenic abscess of the liver reflect systemic infection as well as impairment of the hepatic function. Leukocytosis is common, and occasionally microcytic anemia is present. Hepatic dysfunction is manifested by a moderate elevation of bilirubin, alkaline phosphatase, serum glutamic-oxaloacetic transaminase (SGOT), an increased retention of sodium sulfobromophthalein (BSP), decreased serum albumin, and prolonged prothrombin time. The abnormalities in the liver function are usually mild and do not correlate with the clinical picture of severe illness with hepatomegaly, or of systemic sepsis. Although it was once stated that blood cultures are sterile in most cases of hepatic abscesses,[21] Satiani and Davidson [47] recently found positive blood culture results in 58 percent of their patients.

Radiologic Evaluation. The most reliable methods to diagnose a hepatic abscess are radiologic. Certain abnormalities observed by roentgenograms of the chest and plain film of the abdomen may suggest the presence of a hepatic abscess. The roentgenogram may show an elevation of the right diaphragm, a right pleural effusion, atalectatic changes in the right lower lobe, or obliteration of the costophrenic angle. Fluoroscopy reveals that the motion of the diaphragm is limited. The plain film of the abdomen may also show signs of hepatic enlargement. Accumulation of gas within the liver indicates the presence of a hepatic abscess. Gas within the unoperated biliary tree suggests septic cholangitis; gas within the portal vein suggests gangrene of the bowel with extension of the infection to the liver. A right lateral view is especially helpful in locating the accumulation of gas and deciding if it is within, or outside, the liver parenchyma.[54] Large abscesses will also show displacement of the stomach or the duodenum, which can be better demonstrated by radiologic examination of the upper gastrointestinal tract. One of the most accurate methods to demonstrate and localize a hepatic abscess is a liver scan with technetium 99 sulfur colloid. A filling defect can be demonstrated in over 80 percent of the patients with hepatic abscess.[24,47] Sometimes an increased uptake of the isotope around the liver abscess can be observed as a result of the surrounding hyperemia.[55] The limitation of this method is that the nature of the filling defect cannot be determined, although the combination of the typically described clinical findings with the positive liver scan makes the presence of a liver abscess very likely.[56] Ultrasonography may be helpful, although the resolution of this method is no higher than that of hepatic scanning and masses smaller than 2–3 cm remain undetected.[57] Ultrasonography may give some hints about the nature of the hepatic defect because it can differentiate between a solid and a cystic process (Fig. 36-1).[58]

Other aids to the diagnosis and location of intrahepatic abscesses are scans with indium-111 labeled leukocytes and gallium-67. Both isotopes become concentrated around an infection and thus produce an increased uptake over the hepatic abscess. Intrahepatic abscess can be diagnosed with great accuracy if these images are superimposed on the technetium-99 scans (Fig. 36-2). Preliminary experimental and clinical evidence suggests that the indium-111 scan is superior to the gallium scan because the abscess-blood ratios of indium are higher than those of gallium.[59-61] Both techniques may be misleading if used alone, however, because both isotopes are normally concentrated in the liver.

Other radiologic methods used in the diagnosis of hepatic abscesses include intravenous radionuclear hepatography with technetium-99-sulfur colloid. According to Yeh et al,[62] the absence of uptake of the isotope in an area indicated the presence of abscesses. Tumors will show either a good or a poor uptake of isotope.[62] Morin et al [63] described total body opacification with urographin, which showed hypervascularities surrounding a filling defect in the liver. Hepatic abscesses, like other hepatic lesions, can be revealed by computerized tomography (Fig. 36-3). Robertson et al [37] diagnosed an intrahepatic abscess by T-tube cholangiogram, and Ascione et al [64] described two patients in whom an intrahepatic abscess was diagnosed by retrograde cholangiography and opacification of the abscess cavity by contrast material. Arteriography has also been used. An avascular area is surrounded by a halo, which is best seen during the capillary venous phase of the angiogram. This halo effect can be explained by the compression

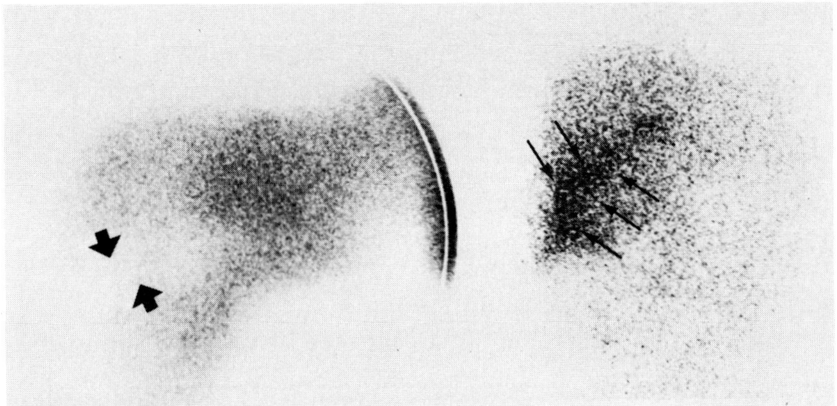

Fig. 36-2. Demonstration of a liver abscess by gallium-67 scan (right) and corresponding defect on technetium-99 liver scan (left). (Frick MP, Knight LC, Feinberg SB, Loken MK: Computer tomography, radionucleide imaging and ultrasound in hepatic mass lesions. *Comp Tomogr* 3:49, 1979.)

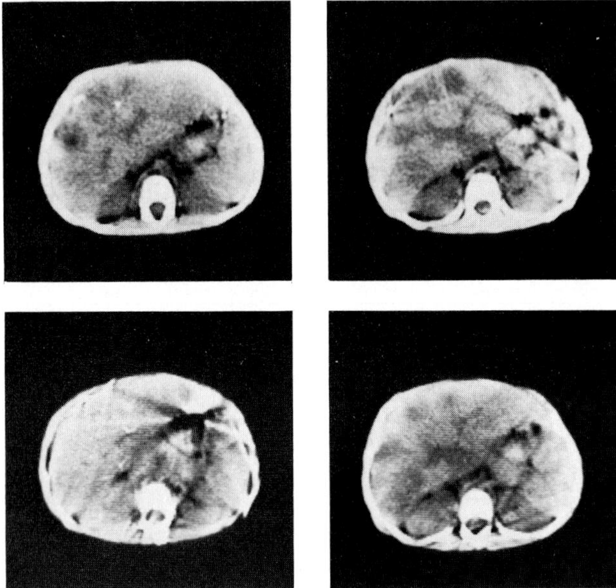

Fig. 36-3. Computerized tomography demonstrating the same defect as in Fig. 36-2. (Frick MP, Knight LC, Feinberg SB, Loken MK: Computer tomography, radionucleide imaging and ultrasound in hepatic mass lesions. *Comp Tomogr* 3:49, 1979.)

of the hepatic parenchyma by the abscess cavity, as well as by the hyperemia.[65,66]

Diagnosis

A combination of systemic sepsis with hepatomegaly, and hepatic tenderness without jaundice, is the characteristic clinical syndrome of hepatic abscesses. The diagnosis can seldom be made on clinical grounds alone. In two series, only 9 of 24 and 26 of 42 abscesses were diagnosed ante mortem.[37,56] Lee and Block [41] pointed out that the use of liver scans decreased the incidence of autopsy diagnosis from 26 percent to 8 percent, but Rubin et al [24] noted that none of 35 patients with liver abscesses was diagnosed clinically. Although the symptoms seem to be less acute than in the past,[67] they should at least arouse suspicion and lead to the institution of the proper diagnostic procedures. Liver scan in combination with an indium-111 or gallium-67 scan and ultrasonography, together with the clinical picture, should establish the presence of a hepatic abscess and make the routine use of more invasive diagnostic procedures unnecessary. An intensive search for the primary source of infection should be conducted, because it has significant prognostic and therapeutic implications. The differentiation from amebic abscesses will be discussed later.

Treatment

The treatment of pyogenic abscesses requires both antibiotic therapy and operative drainage, but no controlled studies have been carried out. The antibiotic treatment is usually started when a hepatic abscess is suspected, because systemic sepsis is obvious in most patients. If this is not the case, antibiotic treatment should be started before operation. The choice of antibiotics can be deduced from the microbiology of hepatic abscesses. As stated earlier, there are three groups of bacteria, which may be present singly or in combination: (1) pyogenic gram-positive cocci (staphylococci and streptococci), (2) enterobacteria (*E. coli*, *Klebsiella*, *Enterobacter*, *Proteus*, and others), and (3) anaerobic bacteria (*B. fragilis* and clostridia). Antibiotic treatment is usually started without knowledge of the causative organism or its sensitivity. No *one* antibiotic covers the entire spectrum of possible bacteria, however, so a combination of antibiotics, ie, a cephalosporin, an aminoglycoside, and clindamycin, is recommended. The cephalosporins and aminoglycosides cover the entire spectrum of pyogenic bacteria and nearly all enterobacteria, and clindamycin the anaerobic flora. If a newer cephalosporin (ie, cefotaxime or cefoxitin), which exhibits activity against anaerobic bacteria, is used, the need for a third antibiotic directed against anaerobic bacteria may be obviated. The treatment, of course, should be modified as soon as reliable cultures and sensitivity determinations are available. Because false-negative results of anaerobic cultures are frequent, a combination of antibiotics should be continued as long as is clinically indicated. Multiple abscesses may require long-term antibiotic suppression even if drainage is thought to have been accomplished.[24] Although Ranson et al [68] suggested that antibiotics should be infused into the portal system via the reopened umbilical vein to achieve a higher concentration of the antibiotic in the liver parenchyma, this is rarely done. If the hepatic abscess is of biliary origin, an antibiotic that achieves high concentrations in bile and has a broad spectrum covering all organisms commonly encountered in biliary sepsis, ie, cefamandole, should be used.

Antibiotic treatment alone is insufficient in the treatment of hepatic abscesses, because bactericidal concentrations of antibiotics may be difficult to achieve within the walled-off abscess cavity. Surgical drainage is therefore mandatory. Without drainage, the mortality of the disease approaches 100 percent. Several recent reports, which indicate the success of treating hepatic abscesses by repeated needle aspiration and instillation of antibiotics,[66,69] need to be confirmed. Similarly, long-term percutaneous catheterization for drainage of the abscess cavity may be a useful alternative.

Two operative approaches can be used to drain the liver abscess. Extraserous drainage was once considered mandatory to avoid contamination of the peritoneal cavity.[25] This method is effective only if a solitary abscess is located near the dome of the liver, because the incision permits only a limited exploration of the liver. Smaller abscesses can easily be overlooked, and the limited exposure will not permit any intra-abdominal septic source to be diagnosed. For these reasons, and because of the safety of the transperitoneal approach with appropriate antibiotic coverage and thorough peritoneal toilet, most authors prefer the transperitoneal approach.[42,47,70,71]

Extraperitoneal drainage of an anterior hepatic abscess can be done using a short right subcostal incision. After division of the rectus muscle, the dissection can be carried cephalad between the abdominal wall and the parietal peritoneum until the fluctuant abscess is reached. After needle aspiration confirms its location, the abscess is entered and evacuated. Soft suction drains are left within the cavity and led out through the abdominal wall (Fig. 36-4).

If the abscess is located in the posterior aspect of the dome of the liver, the transpleural approach through the bed of the tenth or eleventh rib can be used.[68] After the pleural space has been entered, a chest tube is inserted in the fifth intercostal space. The dome of the liver is palpated, and after the area of the abscess has been identified, the diaphragmatic pleura is mobilized and sutured to the parietal pleura above the level of the thoracotomy. The diaphragm is then incised, the abscess unroofed, and soft rubber suction drains left in the cavity (Fig. 36-5). Both these methods depend upon the preexistence of adhesions between the parietal and visceral peritoneum to prevent contamination of the peritoneal cavity.

Transperitoneal drainage of the hepatic abscess can usually be accomplished through a subcostal incision. A midline incision can be used if further exploration of the abdominal cavity is necessary to determine the source of sepsis. If the primary source of infection is not known, a thorough exploration should be carried out to exclude all possible sites. The liver is then palpated, and suspicious

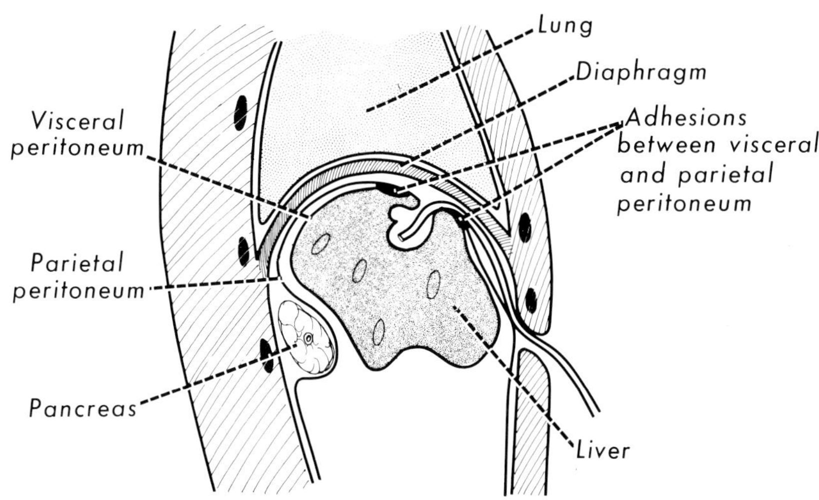

Fig. 36-4. **Extraserous drainage of a hepatic abscess located anteriorly close to the dome of the liver through a right subcostal incision.**

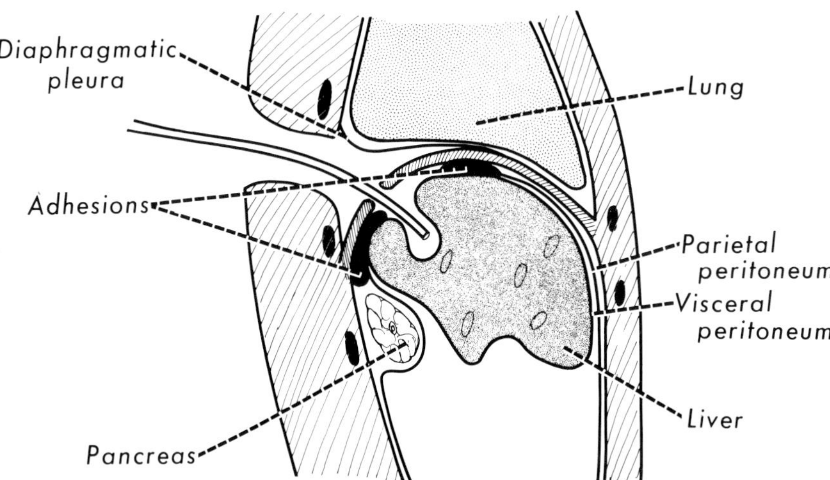

Fig. 36-5. **Transthoracic extraserous drainage of a posterior hepatic abscess close to the dome of the liver.**

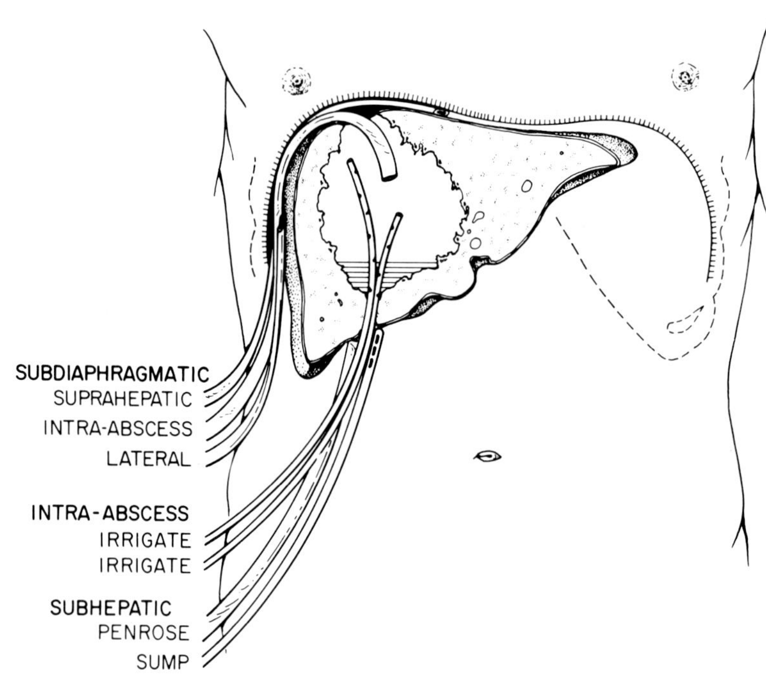

Fig. 36-6. **Transperitoneal drainage of a hepatic abscess. (Goldsmith HS, Chen WF: Management of a pyogenic abscess of the liver. *Surg Clin North Am* 53:711, 1973.)**

areas are aspirated with a needle. After the abscess has been located, its cavity is entered and the entire contents evacuated and irrigated till clear. Loculations should be broken up to create *one* large cavity. During this procedure, the peritoneal cavity should be protected by a heavy layer of antibiotic-soaked gauze pads. Traditionally, dependent drainage with soft rubber drains is established by appropriate placement of drainage incisions. Soft silastic suction drains will function better without reliance on a dependent position. In addition, the shutter action of the abdominal muscles will not interfere with a suction drain, as it does with Penrose drains brought out through a stab wound. In some cases, marsupialization of an anterior abscess can be used. If the drain tract traverses a long distance across the peritoneal cavity, peritoneal contamination will occur for the several days prior to the development of a fibrous tract. For this reason, additional drains should be placed in the parahepatic space to permit exit tracts for contaminated spillage. Some drainage catheters can be set up for irrigation of the cavity with an antibiotic solution in the postoperative period. Evacuation of all necrotic tissue during the operation should make this procedure unnecessary (Fig. 36-6).

It is possible to compromise between the transperitoneal and extraserous approaches. For example, after laparotomy and location of the abscess in the liver, a separate retroperitoneal tract can be developed for the actual drainage.[42]

Some patients with suppurative cholangitis will have concurrent or subsequent hepatic abscesses. In addition to drainage of the common duct and evacuation of the hepatic abscesses, they will need irrigation of the common duct to provide through-and-through drainage of hepatic abscess and common duct. This technique can help locate the smaller, less easily detected abscesses within the hepatic parenchyma. Also, hepatic resection for multiple liver abscesses confined to one lobe is possible.[72] Whatever the technique, postoperative management requires prolonged antibiotic treatment and nutritional support. If sepsis continues, or recurs, reexploration may be necessary to rule out the reaccumulation of pus within the liver, the appearance of additional abscesses, or the development of the perihepatic abscess. Our clinical experience with the serial use of indium-111-labeled leukocytes indicates that it might be a good diagnostic guide for the reaccumulation of pus in the abdominal cavity.

The postoperative complication rate is still approximately 30 percent. Santiani and Davidson[47] reported a 42 percent, and Rubin et al[24] a 28 percent rate of reabscesses in the liver, abscess formation within the peritoneal cavity, metastatic abscesses, and wound infections. The reaccumulation of pus, whether within the peritoneal cavity or the cavity of the hepatic abscess, requires reevacuation and drainage. Empyemas must also be drained. Metastatic abscesses in the lung, however, usually respond to antibiotic treatment. Hepatobronchial fistulas result in a spontaneous drainage of the abscess; once it is drained, antibiotic treatment usually leads to closure of the fistula.

Prognosis

In 1938, Ochsner et al[25] reported a mortality of 79.6 percent in a collected series of 432 liver abscesses. This figure did not change significantly, even after introduction of antibiotics, until the introduction of the liver scan in the middle 1960s. In the early 1970s, Brodine and Schwartz[29] reported a mortality of 68.3 percent in 532 cases. Pitt and Zuidema[70] reported a mortality of 65 percent in 80 cases. Altemeier et al[42] and Lee and Block[41] found the mortality in the prescan era to be between 70 and 85 percent; in the postscan era it dropped below 30 percent.

Block et al [26] reported eight consecutive cases without fatality. The improvement in prognosis is mainly the result of earlier and more accurate diagnosis. According to Lee and Block,[41] during the period from 1955 to 1965 the disease was diagnosed antemortem only 20 percent of the time and with an 80 percent mortality. Since 1965, the disease was diagnosed in 78 percent of the patients, resulting in a drop of mortality to 28 percent.[41]

The mortality in the prescan as well as in the postscan era was influenced by: (1) the number of abscesses, (2) the causative bacteria, (3) the mode of treatment, (4) the presence of complications, and (5) the age of the patient. Before the mid-1960s, the differences in prognosis are much more pronounced. Ochsner et al [25] described a mortality from solitary liver abscess of 37.5 percent, and for multiple abscesses of over 90 percent. There is still a mortality of over 70 percent when multiple abscesses are present.[29,70]

The reports of the influence of various etiologic agents on mortality are controversial. Pitt and Zuidema [70] describe a mortality of 78 percent for abscesses with pure aerobic organisms, 50 percent for patients with mixed bacteria, and 24 percent for patients with only anaerobic organisms. In contrast, Santiani and Davidson [47] observed a higher mortality with mixed aerobes and anaerobes (50 percent) than with purely aerobic organisms (20 percent).

Patients with hepatic abscesses secondary to biliary disease had the worst prognosis (90 percent mortality), followed by abscesses that originated in the portal circulation (70 percent mortality). When the abscess was secondary to trauma, primary liver processes, arterial bacteremia, or cryptogenic processes, the mortality was 30 percent.[70]

Mortality is proportional to age. Pitt and Zuidema [70] observed that the mortality of patients below the age of 70 was 57 percent and above the age of 70 was 81 percent. The presence of complications tripled the deaths in the preantibiotic era; more recent data on primary complications of pyogenic abscesses are not available. The mortality of an undrained hepatic abscess in the preantibiotic, as well as the postantibiotic, era is 100 percent. Today, the mortality for liver abscesses is approximately 30 percent. If the abscess is diagnosed early and the proper treatment is instituted, this can be reduced to less than 10 percent.

AMEBIC ABSCESS OF THE LIVER

Incidence

Contrary to general opinion, infestation with amebas is relatively common even in temperate zones. Hepatic involvement, though relatively uncommon, is serious. Ochsner and DeBakey [73] found clinical evidence of hepatic involvement in 5 percent of 9,696 patients with amebiasis. Of 5,211 amebiasis patients who died, however, 36 percent had liver involvement. Contrary to this low incidence, Adams [74] recently found an incidence of hepatic involvement in 41 percent of over 5,000 cases treated in South Africa between 1955 and 1974. Males are more commonly affected by hepatic amebiasis than females—in some series the ratio is 10 to 1. Though there is no race preference, the native population of endemic regions seems to be less frequently afflicted with hepatic amebiasis than others.

Etiology

Systemic amebiasis is discussed in Chapter 11.

Pathogenesis and Pathology

The ameba can theoretically reach the liver via three routes: (1) the portal system, (2) the lymphatic system, and (3) direct extension. The latter two routes, if used at all, are of little practical significance. It is generally agreed that amebas enter the liver from within the colon via the portal blood. Although it has not been possible to develop an animal model of hepatic amebiasis by creating intestinal amebiasis, Maegraith and Harinasut [75] created hepatic amebiasis in animals by direct injection of amebas into the portal system. On the basis of clinical and experimental observations, intrahepatic portal thrombosis and infarction are key features in the development of the typical lesions.[76,77] These lesions usually start in the portal triad and extend peripherally toward the capsule. In the early stages, an area of necrotic tissue, which may contain leukocytes, connective tissue cells, and occasional amebas, is surrounded by hyperemia. Later, a more or less well-defined capsule develops in which, unlike the necrotic center, amebas can be found. The contents of the abscess is a viscid, light to dark brown material, which has been classically described as anchovy paste.

The coexistence or preexistence of amebic hepatitis has been disputed. Regenerative changes, Küpffer cell hyperplasia, increased hyperfuchsin pigment, portal and sinusoidal infiltration, and occasional areas of focal necrosis have been described on light microscopy,[78] and injury to the mitochondria and to endoplasmic reticulum have been seen on electron microscopy.[27] Adams and McLeod [79] and Turrill and Burnham,[80] however, feel that there is no histologic evidence of amebic hepatitis. Aside from the typical abscesses, liver biopsies taken from patients with hepatic amebiasis fail to reveal any typical changes [81] even in patients who die of amebiasis.[82]

The right lobe of the liver is involved in a single abscess in over 90 percent of the cases. Multiple abscesses are found in only 10 percent. Amebic abscesses are usually bacteriologically sterile. Secondary bacterial infection has been observed in earlier reports in approximately 20 percent,[83,84] but more recently an incidence of less than 5 percent has been reported.[80,85]

Clinical Manifestations

The symptoms of liver abscesses are similar regardless of etiology. The main symptom is pain, located over the right hypochondrium, the chest, or the epigastrium, which radiates occasionally into the right shoulder and is accompanied by cough, fever, weakness, and weight loss. Over 80 percent of the patients have an enlarged, tender liver and tenderness below the right costal margin. An abnormal finding over the right lung base or localized intercostal tenderness can be found in 47 and 38 percent, respectively.[79]

Only one- to two-thirds of the patients have either clinical signs of intestinal amebiasis at the time of diagnosis or a history that suggests it.[73,79] If the diarrhea antedates the diagnosis of hepatic amebiasis, the symptom-free interval is less than 2 months in over two-thirds of the patients.[86]

The disease can occur in a chronic or acute form. Ochsner and DeBakey [73] stated that two-thirds of all the cases had a rather chronic course, but more recent reports indicate that over two-thirds of all patients have an acute form, with symptoms lasting approximately 2 weeks before hospital admission.[79,85] In some patients, a rectosigmoidoscopic examination will reveal signs of amebic colitis, manifested by mucosal edema, granularity, hyperemia, and increased friability.[86]

Radiologic Evaluation. Roentgenograms will reveal an elevated right diaphragm, the motion of which is decreased on fluoroscopy, pleural effusion or infiltrate at the base of the right lung, and occasionally a bulge in the right diaphragm. According to DeBakey and Ochsner,[83] positive radiologic signs on plain films are present in 80 percent of the patients. If the abscess is situated in the left lobe of the liver, there are usually no findings on roentgenograms of the chest, but an upper gastrointestinal series will show signs of external compression on the stomach.[87] A liver scan will nearly always locate the abscess. It has been generally assumed that the results of gallium-67 scans of amebic abscesses will be normal because of the lack of granulocytes in the abscess,[88] but Geslien et al [89] have found increased uptake in the periphery of amebic abscesses in two patients. Imaging of amebic abscesses with radioactive-labeled nitroimidazoles is still experimental.[90] Occasionally, ultrasound, angiography, splenoportography, and laparoscopy have been useful for diagnosis.

Complications. The most common complication of an amebic hepatic abscess involves direct extensions into the thorax. Hematogenous and lymphatic spread are rare. Ochsner and DeBakey [21] described a 15.7 percent incidence equally divided between pulmonary consolidation or abscess, bronchopleural fistula, or empyema. More recent reports give an incidence of 4 to 7 percent,[79,85] half of these presenting as bronchopleural fistula, and the rest as empyema or consolidation-pulmonary abscess.[79] Before the actual rupture of the liver abscess into the chest, signs of pleural irritation like effusion or atalectasis can be detected either clinically or by roentgenogram. After rupture, the patients complain of pain located over the right lower thorax that radiates toward the shoulder, a cough (sometimes with hemoptysis, or expectoration of large amounts of amebic pus, if a bronchopleural fistula is present), and dyspnea. Physical signs are similar to those of pleural effusion or consolidation, usually with an elevated diaphragm.

Rupture of the amebic abscess into the peritoneal cavity may occur in as many as 7 to 11 percent of cases.[73,85] In endemic areas, the incidence may be lower; Adams and McLeod [79] report an incidence of only 1.8 percent in over 2,000 cases of hepatic amebiasis. The rupture can result in either a perihepatic abscess or in diffuse peritonitis.

Rupture of an amebic abscess into the pericardium has been observed in less than 2 percent of all cases of hepatic amebiasis.[79] The abscess is often located in the left lobe of the liver. The rupture into the pericardial sac can occur suddenly or gradually, and is often preceded by a pericardial effusion or a pericardial friction rub. Three modes of presentation have been observed:[74,79]

1. About one-third of the patients have typical signs of a hepatic abscess followed by chest pain on the left side and midsternum and signs of pericarditis.

2. Two-thirds of the patients initially have pericardial effusion and congestive heart failure, without any suspicious liver findings—the correct diagnosis is seldom suspected in these patients.

3. Rarely, a patient presents in shock with signs of cardiac tamponade.[74,79]

The diagnosis of amebic pericarditis is based on clinical, electrocardiographic, and radiologic evidence of pericarditis, positive serology, and an elevated diaphragm on the left side. In addition, a defect in the left lobe of the liver can be seen on hepatic scan (Chapter 32).

Secondary bacterial infection, which has been previously quoted to be present in 10 to 20 percent of amebic abscesses,[83,84] is rarely encountered today.[79,85] If organisms other than amebas are found, open drainage of the abscess is mandatory. Other rare complications of hepatic amebiasis are the rupture of the abscess into the adjacent gastrointestinal tract, hematobilia and thoracobilia, and metastatic brain abscesses.[73,79,91]

Laboratory Evaluation. Patients with hepatic amebiasis usually have a moderate leukocytosis (white blood cell count of 16,000 per mm^3 with increased band forms), eosinophilia, and a mild microcytic anemia. The patients have liver dysfunction, as indicated by moderately elevated bilirubin and liver enzyme levels, decreased albumin, and prolonged prothrombin time. The results of the bromosulphophthalein retention are variable. Severe liver dysfunction and jaundice, although rare, can be the initial problem.[92] DasGupta [93] found that the IgG levels in intestinal amebiasis are significantly higher than in the extraintestinal form. The IgE levels were elevated equally in both forms of the disease, and the IgA and IgM levels do not show any changes. The C3 levels are elevated in invasive amebiasis.[94]

Amebas cannot regularly be found in the stools of patients with hepatic amebiasis, but Ochsner and DeBakey [73] recovered either trophoids or cysts in 36.4 percent. More recent reports show between 7 and 26 percent recovery of amebas from stools.[79,80,86,95] Healy [96] stressed that in more chronic cases the stool should be examined repeatedly for parasites. The direct wet mount is done to demonstrate trophoids as well as cysts. Polyvinyl alcohol preparations increase the yield in detecting the trophoids, and formalin preparations facilitate the detection of the cystic form [96] (Chapter 11).

Serologic tests are important in the diagnosis of hepatic amebiasis.[95-99] A summary of the accuracy of serologic tests is presented in Table 36-5.

Other diagnostic measures include the percutaneous aspiration of the abscess, which yields typical "anchovy paste" abscess fluid in over 80 percent of the cases. The aspirate is lacking in granulocytes and is usually sterile. Bacteria are cultured in only 4 percent, and amebas are rarely found.[79,80,86]

TABLE 36-5. SEROLOGIC TESTS FOR AMEBIASIS

	Percent Positive Reaction		
	CF	*IHA*	*GDP*
No amebiasis	0–6	0.6–18	0–18
Noninvasive intestinal amebiasis	11–90	0–90	1–85
Invasive intestinal amebiasis	67–90	33–100	81–95
Hepatic amebiasis	83–100	47–100	80–100

CF = Complement-fixation test.
IHA = Indirect hemagglutination test.
GDP = Gel-diffusion-precipitin test.

Modified from Juniper K Jr, Worrell CL, Minshew MC, Roth LS, Lypert H, Lloyd RE: Serologic diagnosis of amebiasis. *Am J Trop Med Hyg* 21:156, 1972.

Diagnosis

Neither the physical findings nor the roentgenographic examination offer a definite differentiation from bacterial abscesses either in the liver or under the diaphragm. The clinical symptoms of hepatic amebiasis are usually mild, and toxicity is rarely present. The history of diarrhea is unreliable. Because the treatment of bacterial and amebic abscesses differs considerably, it is important to make the differentiation. After the clinical and radiologic findings, a reliable diagnosis of the suspected hepatic amebiasis can be made by serologic testing. The most frequently used test is the gel-diffusion precipitin test with an accuracy of nearly 100 percent (Table 36-5). If this test is not available or the suspicion of amebiasis persists even after a negative result, diagnostic aspiration should be performed in the operating room. If aspiration yields the typical anchovy paste, open drainage should not be done unless bacterial superinfection is present.

The absence of amebas in the stool or in the aspirated abscess material does not exclude the presence of amebiasis. In endemic areas, the amebicidal drugs should be tried—the diagnosis of amebiasis can then be confirmed by the response of the patient to this treatment.[100]

Treatment

There is general agreement that amebicidal drugs, with or without a needle aspiration of the abscess, is the best treatment for hepatic amebiasis. Only a few authors recommend drainage of the amebic abscess.[101,102] Ochsner and DeBakey [73] had shown in 1943 that the open drainage of an amebic abscess leads to secondary bacterial infection of the cavity, and Turrill and Burnham [80] confirmed this earlier observation. Furthermore, the advocates of open drainage report a high mortality and morbidity rate.[102]

The essential treatment is both a systemic amebicide (metronidazole, emetine, dehydroemetine, chloroquine) and a luminal amebicide (diiodohydroxyquinoline, diloxanide furoate, tetracycline). Emetine is the classic drug to treat invasive amebiasis.[103] Although emetine has produced excellent results,[104] it is toxic to skeletal and cardiac muscle. Dehydroemetine is similarly cardiotoxic.[82,105]

Although chloroquine alone is not as effective as either emetine or dehydroemetine, combining it with either of the two resulted in 100 percent cure in 800 patients.[106]

The best drug is metronidazole, with a nearly 100 percent cure in hepatic amebiasis. Powell et al [107] subjected 100 patients to different dosage schedules of metronidazole, and all patients were cured. Side effects such as nausea, vomiting, drowsiness, headaches, skin rashes, and pruritus, as well as moderate leukopenia, can occur but are minimal and transient. Up to 10 gm of the drug have been ingested without serious harm by suicidal patients.[108] The recommended dosage schedule is 300 mg three times daily for 5 days. One treatment failure has been reported.[109] Other nitroimidazoles, for example, tinidazole, are also highly effective in the treatment of hepatic amebiasis.[110,111] Other drug schedules are noted in Table 36-6.

The effectiveness of metronidazole on intestinal amebiasis is not as constant as on hepatic amebiasis. Approximately 15 to 20 percent of the patients continue to pass cysts and must be treated with a luminal amebicide, such as diiodohydroxyquin (Table 36-6).

Although hepatic amebiasis can be cured by the oral administration of metronidazole alone,[95,112] some authors feel that the hepatic abscess should still be aspirated. Powell et al [107] had no treatment failures when they combined metronidazole with aspiration. We feel that the initial therapy for hepatic amebiasis is metronidazole alone. Indications for percutaneous aspiration are: failure to respond to medical management within five days, large left lobe abscesses (greater propensity for intrapericardial rupture), and suspected bacterial superinfection. The only indication for surgical drainage of amebic liver abscess is proven bacterial superinfection.[113]

The aspiration should be done at the point of maximal tenderness with a medium-gauge needle under local anesthesia. The needle rarely needs to be advanced more than 8 cm. A complete evacuation of the abscess can then be done with a larger needle. The most common sites are the right lower intercostal spaces and the right hypochondrium. The procedure must be repeated when more than 250 ml of pus are aspirated the first time.

The thoracic complications of amebiasis are generally treated conservatively. The hepatic abscess should be aspirated, and the patient should receive amebicidal drugs. An empyema should also be aspirated. Surgical intervention is rarely necessary for a persistent empyema or a pul-

TABLE 36-6. SUMMARY OF TREATMENT OF AMEBIASIS

Drug	Primary Clinical Usage	Daily Adult Dosage Employed	Duration of Therapy in Days
SYSTEMIC AMEBICIDES			
Nitroimidazole			
Metronidazole (Flagyl)	Symptomless carriers to moderate clinical nondysenteric amebiasis,	400–800 mg 3 times daily	5
	Amebic dysentery	800 mg 3 times daily	5
		or	
		2.4–4 gm every day	3
	Hepatic abscess and other forms of extraintestinal amebiasis	400 mg 3 times daily	5
		or	
		2.0–2.4 gm every day	2–3
Tinidazole (Fasigyn)	Mild clinical to dysenteric amebiasis	2 gm every day*	2–5
	Liver abscess	1.2 gm every day*	7
		or	
		400–800 mg 3 times daily*	1
LUMINAL AMEBICIDES			
Alkaloids			
Emetine hydrocholoride	Amebic dysentery; amebic liver abscess; and other forms of extraintestinal amebiasis	65 mg (1 gr) every day† intramuscularly	Up to 4–10‡
Dehydroemetine	Same as emetine	1–1.5 mg per kg intramuscularly or deep subcutaneous injection	Up to 5–10§
Halogenated hydroxyquinolines			
Diiodohydroxyquin (Diodoquin)	Symptomless carriers and *mild* clinical nondysenteric intestinal amebiasis	650 mg 3 times daily	20
Anilines			
Diloxanide furoate (Furanimide)	Symptomless carriers and mild and chronic nondysenteric intestinal amebiasis	500 mg 3 times daily	10
Aminoquinolines			
4-aminoquinoline Chloroquine diphosphate (Aralen, Nivaquine, Avloclor)	Amebic liver abscess	500 mg twice daily followed by 500 mg every day	2 and 12 or 19
Antibiotics			
Oxytetracycline (Terramycin)	Amebic dysentery; mild to moderate nondysenteric intestinal amebiasis	250–500 mg 4 times daily	Up to 10
Tetracycline (Achromycin, Tetracyn)	Same as oxytetracycline	250–500 mg 4 times daily	Up to 10

* Preliminary dosages; subject to change.
† Daily dosage of emetine hydrochloride is 1 mg per kg; total daily dose not to exceed 65 mg (1 grain).
‡ Maximum duration of therapy with emetine hydrochloride is 10 days; total dose for this period not to exceed 10 mg per kg (650 mg or 10 grains). For amebic liver abscess, 10 days; for amebic dysentery, 4 to 6 days as needed to control the dysentery.
§ Dehydroemetine, up to 5 days for amebic dysentery; 10 days for liver abscess.

From Hunter G, Swartzwelder J, Clyde D: *Tropical Medicine,* 5th ed. Philadelphia, Saunders, 1976.

monary abscess that does not respond to conservative therapy. Bronchopleural fistulas always heal under medical treatment.

Laparotomy for drainage purposes, as well as establishment of the diagnosis, is always indicated in suspected rupture of an intraperitoneal abscess, and is supplemented by treatment with amebicidal drugs. The treatment of amebic pericarditis consists of antiamebic drugs plus pericardial aspiration.

Prognosis

No one with uncomplicated hepatic amebic abscesses should die. Ochsner and DeBakey [73] reported no deaths, and Adams and McLeod [79] reported a mortality rate of 0.7 percent in 1,959 uncomplicated cases. The presence of complications, however, changes this favorable picture dramatically. Pulmonary complications carry a mortality of 6.2 percent.[81] Amebic peritonitis secondary to hepatic abscess rupture has a mortality of 18.4 percent, which is more favorable than amebic peritonitis secondary to the intestinal perforations, which uniformly involves bacterial superinfection.[79] The most serious complication is the rupture of the abscess into the pericardium, which has a mortality of 30 to 100 percent.[79,114] Secondary infection converts the amebic abscess to a pyogenic abscess of the liver, with the typical mortality of around 20 percent. Taking all possible complications into account, approximately 2 percent of all patients with hepatic amebiasis will die.

HYDATID CYST OF THE LIVER

Incidence

Echinococcal disease is rare in the United States. Katz and Pan [115] collected only 556 cases; of those the infestation of only 24 had occurred near the United States. In other countries, however, especially in the Mediterranean, infestation with *Echinococcus* is common. The largest endemic area in North America is Alaska, where an estimated 22 percent of all dogs are infested.[116] In northwestern Canada, approximately 40 percent of the indigenous human population is infested.[117]

Etiology

The details of echinococcal disease are given in Chapter 11. In brief, people can be infested with larvae of two species of *Echinococcus: E. granulosus* and *E. multilocularis.* The tapeworm is only a few millimeters in length and usually has four segments. It lives in the small bowel of canines, mainly dogs, wolves, and foxes. The terminal segment contains eggs, which are discharged into the intestinal contents of the host. The eggs reach the intermediate host via fecal contamination of food, fingers, or water. The capsule of the ova is dissolved in the stomach and the larvae hatch from the ova in the small intestine, penetrate through the intestinal mucosa, and are carried with the portal circulation to the liver where they develop the cyst. The intermediate hosts for *E. granulosus* are sheep, cattle, hogs, and man. The intermediate hosts for *E. multilocularis* are small silvan rodents. Since small wild canines feed on these animals, this variety of *Echinococcus* is found mainly in foxes.

Pathology

Infestation with *E. granulosus,* which accounts for over 80 percent of all human infestations, results in a large single cyst. The cyst wall has two layers, an outer layer of adventitia which represents the host's reaction to the parasite, and an inner layer, the laminated membrane, which contains the growing organism. The cyst fluid is clear and colorless and is often under considerable pressure. Cysts tend to grow slowly, so a person might be infested as a child and be asymptomatic until adulthood. Infestation with *E. multilocularis* results in the development of multiple small cysts replacing large segments of liver parenchyma. The liver is involved in three-fourths of the cases, and in half of the cases the liver is the only organ affected. Other organs frequently involved are the lung (10 percent), spleen (3 percent), and kidney (4 percent), as well as musculature, bone, bladder, pleura, breast, brain, and other structures. As is usually the case in enteric-derived liver disease, the cyst is located in the right lobe in 75 percent of the cases [118] and can reach gigantic size.[119]

Clinical Manifestations and Diagnosis

Most cysts are rather asymptomatic until they become large enough to create fullness and a mass in the abdomen.[120] Roentgenogram will reveal typical calcifications in the cyst wall, and the liver scan shows a filling defect (Fig. 36-7). Angiographic studies by Rizk et al [121] demonstrated a small rim of increased density surrounding the cyst during the capillary phase. Because the relationship of the biliary system to the cyst is important for the planning of the surgical management,[122] preoperative retrograde cholangiography should be considered.[123]

Laboratory test results are usually normal, except for moderate eosinophilia. Immunologic tests can confirm the diagnosis. The Casoni test consists of an intradermal injection of hydatid cyst fluid and the development of a large weal surrounding the site of injection is a positive reaction. This test is positive in over 80 percent of the cases and will always be positive even if the cyst has been removed or is inactive. The complement-fixation test is somewhat more specific but less sensitive, and is positive in only 50 to 60 percent of the cases. The diagnosis is established by the demonstration of parasitic elements in the cyst fluid—hooklets, scolices, and fragments of the membrane. These elements can also be found in the stool when the cyst has ruptured into the biliary tree, or into the bowel, or in the sputum if a rupture into the bronchial system has taken place.

Complications. The most common complication of cysts in the liver is the rupture into the biliary tree. Papadimitriou and Mandrekas [124] described this complication in 6.2 percent of 227 cases, and other authors report even higher incidence.[125,126] According to Bourgeon and Pietri,[127] a rupture of the cyst into the biliary tree occurs in two phases. In the first phase, minute communications between the cyst and the biliary duct are created by abruptly increased pressure within the cyst during trauma, deep inspiration, or cough. Because the pressure in the echinococcal cyst is higher than in the bile ducts, the contents of the cyst leak into the biliary system. The second phase—the rupture of the cyst into the biliary tree—is caused

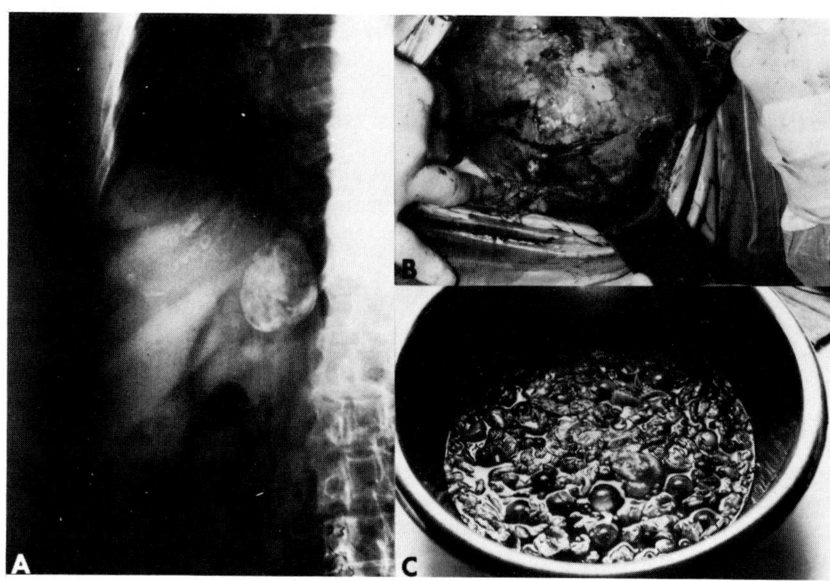

Fig. 36-7. **Hydatid cyst of the liver. A. Calcified cyst on plain film of the abdomen. B. Gross pathology seen during en-bloc excision. C. Daughter cysts after en-bloc excision of hydatid. (Courtesy of Dr. Basil Golematis, Athens, Greece.)**

by weakening of the wall of the bile ducts, through areas of recurrent cholangitis caused by the parasite.[127] The classic symptoms of this complication include biliary colic and jaundice, as fragments of the parasite are passed through the biliary tree into the bowel. Other signs and symptoms include a spiking fever, enlargement of the liver, allergic reaction manifested by a rash, and a high eosinophil count. Rarely, an anaphylactic reaction can occur. If a communication between the hydatid cyst and the biliary tree is suspected, a retrograde cholangiogram can help find the exact location and size of the fistula.[123] The treatment is directed at elimination of the parasitic cyst and internal drainage of the biliary fistula.

The next most common complication (2 percent) is rupture of the cyst through the diaphragm into the pleural space or the bronchial tree. Cysts in the dome of the right lobe of the liver are relatively common,[42,128,129] and the hepatopleural or hepatobronchial fistulas occur slowly with no dramatic symptoms in some of these. Fistulas between cysts and the bronchus result in productive cough, sometimes with bile-stained sputum. Parasites can be found in the sputum. The sudden rupture of the hydatid cyst into the pleural cavity, although uncommon, is accompanied by severe right-sided chest pain which radiates into the shoulder. A roentgenogram of the chest will show a pleural effusion on the right, or a consolidation of the right base as well as an elevated and immobile diaphragm.

Rupture of the hydatid cyst into the peritoneal cavity is rather rare. Barros [122] describes only one instance of spontaneous intraperitoneal rupture in 124 cases of hydatid cyst of the liver, and Papadimitriou and Mandrekas [124] describe an incidence of 3.5 percent. Rupture of the cyst and spillage of its contents into the peritoneal cavity, however, is not so rare during operation. Schiller [130] reported 30 cases of spillage of hydatid cyst contents into the abdominal cavity, an incidence of 13.5 percent. In nine of these cases, signs of anaphylaxis were present; two of the patients died of anaphylactic shock, and four others died of septic complications.

The last complication is that of superinfection of the cyst which, according to Papadimitriou and Mandrekas,[124] occurs in 7.8 percent of these patients. In those cases, the parasites are frequently destroyed by the bacterial infection, which should be treated like a pyogenic hepatic abscess.

Treatment

Although successful treatment of hydatid disease with mebendazole (400–600 mg three times daily for 21–30 days) has been reported,[130a,130b] the generally accepted treatment for echinococcal cysts is surgical. Operation should be undertaken as soon as the cyst is diagnosed, because the mortality increases significantly when complications develop. The aim of operation is to remove the entire parasitic cyst. During operation, any spillage of the cyst fluid might infect the entire peritoneal cavity. The operative field is therefore walled off with packs, and the cyst fluid is evacuated by aspiration. A solution designed to kill the parasite is then instilled into the cyst. Two percent formalin has been used in the past, although fatalities with this treatment have been reported.[122] The preferred solution now is absolute alcohol [122,131] or 30 percent saline,[132,133] or povidone-iodine.[120] The adventitia of the cyst is then incised, and the laminated membrane is removed. The laminated membrane containing the parasites must be removed meticulously to prevent relapses. If a fibrous capsule is present, this should be resected to reduce the size of the cyst.[132] A small cyst can usually be closed primarily; however, several methods have been proposed to deal with the resulting space of a large cyst. Harris [133] and Ekrami [132] recommend filling the entire cyst with water and closing the capsule tightly with a continuous suture. Barros[122] and Papadimitriou and Mandrekas [124] recommend filling the empty space with omentum. Marsupialization to the outside and drainage have been used, although this technique frequently resulted in persistent biliary fistulas. Papadimitriou and Mandrekas [124] reported bile leaks in 25 percent of marsupialized cases and 61 percent after drainage. With omentoplasty this complication occurred in only 2.5 percent. While resecting the laminated membrane, it is important to detect small bile leaks, which must be oversewn. The communication of a large bile duct with the cyst requires internal drainage of the cyst with a Roux-en-Y cyst-jejunostomy to prevent postoperative leaking of bile.[122] If many cysts are present, especially in the case of infestation with *E. multilocularis*, resection of the diseased part of the liver, usually a right hepatectomy, is required. Dintsman et al [134] reported a successful hepatectomy for echinococcal disease in 10 patients.

Yacoubian [129] and Barros [122] recommend a transthoracic approach for removal of cysts that extend into the thorax, whereas Reventos et al [128] prefer an abdominal approach. If a fistula into the pleural cavity has developed, the pleura has to be cleaned and drained, the diaphragm has to be closed, and the cyst treated as previously described. In case of rupture into the bronchial tree, a segmental resection of the lung may be required.

In treating peritoneal spillage, either spontaneous or operative, thorough cleansing of the peritoneal cavity is mandatory to diminish the number of parasites seeded in the abdomen. Secondary cysts have formed in 50 percent of the patients who were evaluated for prolonged periods after intraperitoneal seeding.[130]

Prognosis

The mortality for removal of an echinococcal cyst is approximately 3.5 percent.[124] When the thorax is involved, or intraperitoneal seeding occurs, however, this number increases to 20 percent.[130] Complications of cyst removal include external bile fistulas, which are observed in 2.5 to 3.8 percent, contamination of the peritoneal cavity, intraperitoneal abscesses, and wound infection.[130c] The multilocular hydatid disease caused by *E. multilocularis* is a slowly progressive disease and resection can be palliative but is rarely curative.[130d]

INFECTIOUS COMPLICATIONS OF LIVER TRAUMA AND HEPATECTOMY

Infectious complications after liver resection or liver trauma are common. Three recent series report an incidence of septic complications from 15 to 19 percent of patients with liver trauma.[135-137] Although approximately half of the infectious complications in each group were superficial wound infections, severe intraperitoneal infections appear in 5 to 10 percent of cases.[135,137,138] Intra-abdominal sepsis in approximately two-thirds of the cases was perihepatic abscess formation. Diffuse peritonitis and intrahepatic abscesses, as well as abscesses remote from the liver, were less common. The likelihood of postoperative infections is, of course, increased with the degree of hepatic injury. Fischer et al [138] noted intraperitoneal sepsis in only 1 percent of the patients with nonbursting liver injuries and 19.6 percent in patients with bursting injuries.

These septic complications contribute significantly to the mortality of liver injuries. Lim et al [139] describe a series of 681 patients with trauma of the liver, 71 of whom died soon after initial treatment (most commonly of hemorrhage), and 29 patients who died late in the course of their hospitalization (41 percent of septic complications).

An important pathogenetic factor for the development of those infections is thought to be the presence of blood, bile, and necrotic tissue in the right upper quadrant, all of which are known to be potent adjuvants in the development of intraperitoneal infections.[140-142] The risk of infection is, of course, increased if there is continuous hemorrhage or a bile leak. Complications similar to these after liver trauma have been observed after elective hepatic resections, although their frequency is somewhat less.[143]

Some guiding principles have emerged with regard to the prophylaxis of these complications. The preoperative administration of antibiotics is effective in reducing the incidence of infectious complications. Stone and Hester [144] have shown that the preoperative administration of a cephalosporin lowers the incidence of infectious complication after laparotomy for trauma, including injuries of the liver. In addition, all are agreed: (1) that nonbleeding lacerations should not be sutured, (2) that all devitalized tissue should be removed,[139,145] and (3) that hemostatic agents such as Gelfoam and Surgicell should not be left in the wound, because they seem to increase the risk of a postoperative infection.[136] A major controversy in infection prophylaxis centers around the question of drainage. Merendino et al [146] once advocated T tube drainage of the biliary tree in the treatment of intrahepatic injuries to decompress the biliary system and thereby avoid the development of a biliary fistula. In a randomized trial, however, Lucas and Walt [147] have shown that biliary drainage did not lower the incidence of complications but was instead detrimental.

The recommendation to drain all liver wounds goes back to Madding et al [148] in 1946 and is still advocated by many.[135,136,139,149] The purpose of these drains is to evacuate blood, bile, and serum which inevitably escape the cut or damaged surface of the liver. The theoretical disadvantages are the facts that foreign bodies are adjuvants for infection and that exteriorized drains permit the ingress of microbes. Fischer et al [138] reported a series of 303 patients, only 1.6 percent of whom were drained after liver injury treated in the usual way. Intraperitoneal infections developed in only 11 of the 127 patients (4.8 percent) who survived and were not drained. The authors state that most of these intraperitoneal infections would not have been prevented by drainage of the perihepatic space because the infections developed distant from the liver. Of the 27 surviving patients who were drained, two developed intraperitoneal sepsis. Although the incidence of infection is lower than other series, no randomization was carried out and one can reach no definitive conclusion. Similarly, one cannot comment on the efficacy, in the prevention of biliary fistula or infection, of suturing omentum to the cut surface of the liver—although it is aesthetically pleasing.

INFECTIONS OF THE SPLEEN

Many infections can involve the spleen and represent systemic infections which involve the reticuloendothelial system, and few are of special interest to the surgeon. Some of these infections will, on rare occasions, produce sufficient hypersplenism to indicate splenectomy, and others, most notably infectious mononucleosis, will cause such splenic hypertrophy that rupture—either spontaneous or after mild trauma—will occur, requiring operative control.

SPLENIC ABSCESS

Incidence and Pathogenesis

Splenic abscesses are rare today. Between 1964 and 1978, Chulay and Lankerani [150] found only ten cases in 94,460 hospital admissions (0.01 percent), and the incidence in 2,840 autopsy reports was 0.22 percent. Eighty percent of splenic abscesses occur in conjunction with systemic infection [151]—otitis, mastoiditis, peritonsillar abscess, suppurative parotitis, cutaneous infection, pulmonary abscesses, appendicitis, diverticulitis, cholecystitis, and osteomyelitis. Prior to the antibiotic era, splenic suppuration was found in 10 percent of all cases with bacterial endocarditis,[152] and the incidence of splenic abscesses was tripled in patients with typhoid fever compared to the normal population.[153] Lately, the entity has been described in patients addicted to self-administered intravenous drugs.[154]

The work of Caldarera [155] shed some light on the pathogenesis of splenic abscesses. Splenic abscesses could not be produced with an injection of *S. aureus* in experimental animals unless a branch of the splenic artery had been previously ligated or the spleen itself traumatized. Thus, it is not surprising that splenic abscesses are more frequent in patients with hemolytic disorders whose spleens undergo repeated infarction. Three-quarters of patients with splenic abscesses in Nigeria suffer from sickle cell disease.[156] The incidence is also increased in thalassemia,[157] malaria,[158] and leukemia.[159]

Fifteen percent of splenic abscesses follow splenic trauma.[160] With the advent of splenic embolization in the treatment of hypersplenism, cases of development of splenic abscess have been described after this procedure.[161]

Etiology

Table 36-7 lists the organisms most often found in splenic abscesses. As expected, staphylococci, streptococci, salmonellae, and other gram-negative bacteria predominate. Recently, a change in flora has been noted with an increase in the enteric and anaerobic bacteria as well as sterile cultures. *Salmonella* species have nearly disappeared, and the incidence of streptococci has declined. In drug addicts, splenic abscesses are nearly exclusively caused by *S. aureus*.[154]

Clinical Manifestations

Fever is present in nearly all patients, along with other symptoms of systemic sepsis—chills, malaise, nausea, and vomiting. In two-thirds of the patients, abdominal pain is present, which is often sharp in nature and radiates into the left shoulder and the left thorax; however, localization to the splenic area is only present in one-half the patients. One-third of the patients have a palpable spleen, and often an abdominal mass can be felt in the epigastrium or left upper quadrant. Laboratory test results reveal a leukocytosis with a shift to the left, and plain roentgenograms show a mass in the left upper quadrant, extraluminal gas, and elevated left diaphragm with pleural effusion (Fig. 36-8). A liver-spleen scan, in combination with a gallium-67 or indium-111 scan, are probably the most reliable methods to locate the splenic abscess.[159,162,163]

TABLE 36-7. BACTERIOLOGY OF SPLENIC ABSCESSES (PERCENT)

Staphylococci	21
Streptococci	16
Salmonellae	15
E. coli	8
Other gram-negative bacilli	17
Anaerobic organisms	5
Others	1
Sterile cultures	24

From Chulay JD, Lankerani MR: Splenic abscess: report of 10 cases and review of the literature. *Am J Med* 61:513, 1976.

Treatment and Prognosis

The generally accepted treatment for splenic abscesses is splenectomy, sometimes accompanied by distal pancreatectomy if the abscess is closely adherent to the tail of the pancreas.[150,154] The prognosis of the splenic abscess is basically that of the underlying disease. If the serious underlying disease is not present, all patients can be cured.[150] If, however, the diagnosis is not made in time and the splenectomy is delayed, rupture into the peritoneal cavity can occur and nearly always causes death.[164] In ten cases described by Chulay and Lankerani,[150] delay in diagnosis and appropriate therapy was responsible for the death of three of ten patients.

RUPTURE OF THE SPLEEN IN INFECTIOUS DISEASE

Rupture of the spleen in association with infectious diseases has long been recognized. The most common cause is infectious mononucleosis. However, only 14 percent of the reported cases fit rigid criteria of spontaneous rupture, and most are caused by trauma to an enlarged friable spleen.[165] Other infectious diseases that can cause a spontaneous rupture of the spleen are malaria,[53,166] endocarditis,[167,168] viral hepatitis,[169] and actinomycosis.[170,171] Rupture of the spleen is usually preceded by the development of upper abdominal pain. At the time of actual rupture, an acute abdomen, with shock, develops. Sokolowski and Kent [172] described certain rotengenologic features that might assist the diagnosis—these include distention of the stomach with a serrated margin of the greater curvature, downward displacement of the gastric cardia, and displacement of the stomach to the right from extrinsic pressure. There is also a downward displacement of the splenic flexure of the colon and elevation and decreased mobility of the left diaphragm.[172] If a splenic rupture is diagnosed immediately, there should be no deaths caused by the rupture itself. The long-time prognosis is the same as it is for the underlying disease.

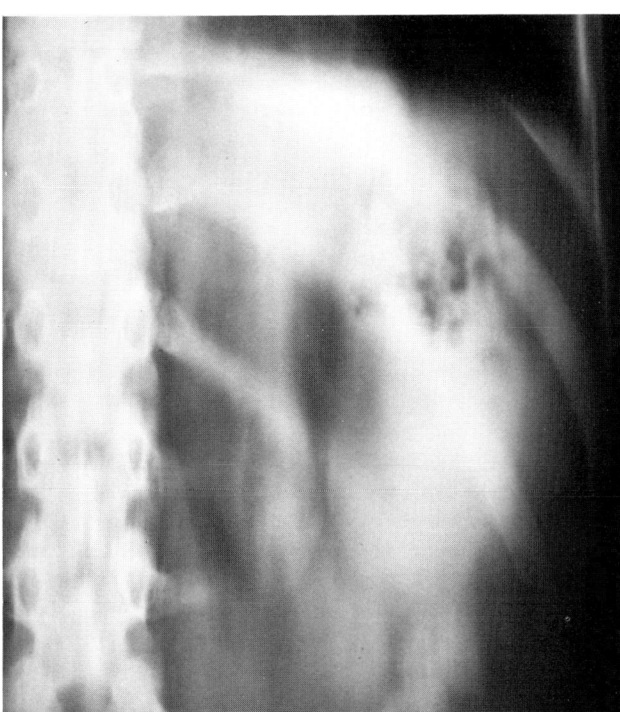

Fig. 36-8. **Gas formation in the spleen after splenic embolization on tomograms of the RUQ. The patient had a splenic abscess due to *Klebsiella.* (Courtesy of Dr. D. Spigos, Department of Radiology, University of Illinois Medical Center, Chicago, Illinois.)**

INFECTIOUS COMPLICATIONS AFTER SPLENECTOMY

The risk of infection after splenectomy is twofold. First, local infections can develop in the postoperative period, and second, splenectomized patients seem to succumb more often to fulminant sepsis with encapsulated bacteria.

LOCAL INFECTIONS

Local infectious complications occur in approximately 16 percent of all patients who undergo splenectomy. One-third of those are subphrenic abscesses, the remainder are subcutaneous wound infections.[173] Patients who undergo splenectomy for trauma or for hypersplenism associated with leukemia and other generalized disease have the highest incidence of suppurative infections.[173,174] Septic complications after splenectomy are especially common when the splenectomy is associated with peritoneal contamination by intestinal contents. Incidental splenectomy during intra-abdominal procedure increases the incidence of an intra-abdominal abscess from 0 to 10.5 percent.[175]

The pathogenesis of subphrenic abscesses after splenectomy is similar to that of the development of perihepatic abscesses after liver trauma and liver resection. Necrotic tissue, blood, and sometimes pancreatic juice from the contused pancreas accumulate in the left upper quadrant and function as adjuvants for a bacterial infection. Good hemostasis, operative evacuation of all fluid, and avoidance of pancreatic trauma will minimize the chances of development of septic complications after splenectomy.

The proper use of drains remains controversial. Several authors feel that the drainage of the subphrenic space after splenectomy significantly increases the incidence of the development of postoperative septic complications. Although all available studies are retrospective, clinical observation together with experimental evidence would lead one to avoid drainage of the splenic bed after splenectomy. In a retrospective study, Cohn [151] found intra-abdominal septic complications in 40 percent of the patients in whom drainage of the splenic bed had been carried out; the incidence of septic complications was only 4 percent without drainage. Olsen and Beaudoin [176] observed ten subphrenic abscesses and ten infections of the drainage tract in 228 patients who underwent splenectomy with drainage. In 87 patients who did not undergo splenic drainage, only one subphrenic abscess was found.[176] Experimental evidence suggests that bacteria can migrate from the skin surface along the drain tract into the abdominal cavity.[101,177] Nora et al [177] obtained positive cultures in 34 percent of intra-abdominal drains inserted in a previously sterile area. If drains are to be used, closed suction with soft silastic drains should be employed for as short a period as possible—preferably 24 hours. Drains are unnecessary in almost all cases. Soft latex (Penrose) drains were used in all the above studies.

OVERWHELMING SEPSIS AFTER SPLENECTOMY

Incidence

Recent attention has been directed toward the relatively high incidence of fulminant infections after splenectomy, long suspected after splenectomy in childhood. Evidence also supports an increased incidence even in otherwise healthy adults.

Singer [178] first reviewed 2,795 splenectomy patients and found an incidence of lethal, overwhelming sepsis in 2.5 percent. Similar results have been obtained by Eraklis and Filler,[179] who found an incidence of lethal overwhelming infections in 2.4 percent of patients who underwent splenectomy in childhood. The incidence of postsplenectomy sepsis was found to depend in part on the underlying disease. The highest incidence is observed in patients with thalassemia and reticuloendothelial disease. Splenectomy secondary to trauma or incidental during operative procedures carries a rather low risk of the development of lethal postsplenectomy fulminant sepsis, 0.53 and 0.86 percent respectively,[178] but both are substantially higher than similar healthy persons with spleen intact. Indeed, Gopal and Bisno [180] have recently collected 26 patients without underlying disease who developed fulminant pneumococcal sepsis after splenectomy for trauma, or incidentally during operation. Fifteen of these patients were adults, and none of them was under 7 years of age when the splenectomy was performed. More WW II veterans who had been splenectomized for trauma died from pneumonia and ischemic heart disease than did members of a nonsplenectomized control group.[178a]

Etiology

Approximately half of all cases of overwhelming postsplenectomy infections are caused by pneumococci; mortality is 50 percent. *N. meningitidis, E. coli, H. influenzae,* and *S. aureus* are found in decreasing frequency.

Pathology

At autopsy, the observations are typical of septicemia but also include adrenal hemorrhage in high proportion of cases (Waterhouse-Friderichsen syndrome).

Pathogenesis

Several lines of evidence suggest that splenectomized patients have compromised humoral defenses—both immunoglobulin and complement deficiencies have been reported.[181] Numerous defects in immunoglobulins have been reported after splenectomy. Antibody responses to intravenously administered particulate antigens and bacteriophage are reduced. Asplenic individuals have an inability to switch from IgM to IgG antibody.[182] The average serum IgM level in splenectomized patients is significantly depressed.[183] Proof that the IgM depression was the result of the splenectomy and not the underlying disease is best seen in patients with traumatic rupture of the spleen. The IgM level in the splenectomized group was 94 ± 48 mg per 100 ml compared to 159 ± 74 in age-matched controls.[183]

IgG and IgA immunoglobulins are frequently elevated in normal and splenectomized patients, and no reliable data on IgD or IgE levels has been gathered.

The IgM deficiency in splenectomized patients does not completely explain the failure to eradicate circulating bacteria. Host defense in most bacteria requires opsonization either by antibody (usually IgG) or by complement. Opsonized bacteria can be cleared by the spleen, and less effectively by the liver. However, in the absence of opsonins, pneumococci are nearly exclusively cleared by the spleen.[183a] Pneumococci obviously are best opsonized by specific antibody but can be opsonized by complement by the alternative complement pathway. In this regard, properdin activity, an alternate complement pathway factor, is reduced in asplenic man,[181] but this depression is not universal. Several investigators have been unable to show diminished serum opsonic activity after vaccination with a pneumococcal vaccine.[181] Finally, the spleen produces tuftsin, a polypeptide which promotes phagocytosis, and serum levels of this substance are significantly decreased after splenectomy.[183b]

Splenectomy also influences the numbers of lymphocytes. Circulating T lymphocytes are somewhat reduced following splenectomy; the lymphocyte mitogen proliferative response is initially decreased, but then returns to normal.[183c] Polymorphonuclear leukocyte functions and C3 levels are not changed in asplenic patients.

In short, although there are numerous defects of the immune response after splenectomy, none of them totally explain the failure to appropriately eliminate circulating encapsulated organisms. It is probable that the filtering effect of the spleen itself is important in eliminating these organisms and that the liver is far less efficient than the spleen in this regard.

Clinical Manifestations

Overwhelming postsplenectomy infection is characterized by the sudden onset of nausea, vomiting, and confusion, which leads to coma, and often proceeds to death, within hours. The case fatality rate ranges from 50 to 75 percent.[181] There is frequently evidence of disseminated intravascular coagulation, severe hypoglycemia, electrolyte imbalance, and shock.

Prevention

Penicillin prophylaxis has effectively reduced the incidence of pneumococcal sepsis after splenectomy. Penicillin should be continually administered for life. Unfortunately, compliance with daily penicillin ingestion is expected to decrease with time, so that it is important to educate the patient to the risks after splenectomy.

Pneumococcal vaccination can now be carried out: The present commercially available vaccine contains the capsular polysaccharides of 14 pneumococcal serotypes. These 14 types account for over 80 percent of the serious pneumococcal infections encountered in people. Since the polysaccharides are highly purified, few side effects of vaccination are seen. The antibody response of splenectomized patients is apparently normal when each antigen is used alone. Giebink [184] has noted that antibody responses of patients splenectomized for trauma respond to fewer of the antigens in the polyvalent vaccines. In addition, the titer of pneumococcal antibody decreases over time and reverts to prevaccination levels in less than 6 months. Whether boosters can be used is unknown. In addition, several patients who were previously vaccinated have died with overwhelming pneumococcal sepsis after splenectomy. Even though pneumococcal vaccination cannot be relied upon, it should be used in all patients, in addition to daily penicillin prophylaxis. The risk of death from overwhelming postsplenectomy infection is enough of a threat to maintain patient compliance.

The principal precaution for the surgeon is not to remove spleens from patients in whom hemostasis can be obtained by other methods. The conservative surgical management of splenic trauma has become common in the past 5 years.[185] The suspicion of bleeding from a ruptured spleen is no longer sufficient cause for laparotomy and splenectomy, and careful observation can be used as the first policy—particularly in pediatric patients. Stable vital signs, abdominal findings, and hematocrit are indications to continue clinical surveillance. Even if laparotomy is undertaken, remodeling, mattress suturing, and the repair of rents and holes in the spleen, which have heretofore been considered impossible, are now accepted procedures.[186] Newer hemostatics are on the market; splenic suture with omental tamponade or ligation of the main splenic artery are other techniques to be tried.

Experimental attempts to produce splenosis, the growth of splenic tissue in the peritoneal cavity after trauma, may be possible. Such heterotopic autotransplantation of splenic tissue at the time of original injury may ultimately be a useful clinical technique for managing the badly damaged spleen.

BIBLIOGRAPHY

Adams EB, McLeod IN: Invasive amebiasis. Am J Surg 111:424, 1966.

Golematis B: Hydatid disease: history, etiology, epidemiology, epizootiology, locations and prevention. Surg Ann 10:359, 1978.

Leonard AS, Giebink GS, Baesl TJ, Krivit W: The overwhelming post-splenectomy sepsis problem. World J Surg 4(4):423–426, 1980.

Kapoor OP: Amoebic Liver Abscess. Bombay, India, S.S. Publishers, 1979.

Klatskin G: Hepatitis associated with systemic infections. In Schiff L (ed): Diseases of the Liver, 4th ed. Philadelphia, Lippincott, 1975.

McDonald AP, Howard RJ: Pyogenic liver abscess. World J Surg 4(4):369–375, 1980.

REFERENCES

1. Beeson PB, Brannon ES, Warren JV: Observations on the sites of removal of bacteria from the blood in patients with bacterial endocarditis. J Exp Med 81:9, 1945.
2. Orloff MJ, Peskin GW, Ellis HL: A bacteriologic study of human portal blood: implications regarding hepatic ischemia in man. Ann Surg 148:738, 1958.
3. Schweinburg FB, Sylvester EM: Bacteriology of the healthy experimental animal. Proc Soc Exp Biol Med 82:527, 1953.
4. Wolbach SB, Saiki T: A new anaerobic spore-bearing bacterium commonly present in the livers of healthy dogs, and believed to be responsible for many changes attributed to aseptic autolysis of liver tissue. J Med Res 21:267, 1909.
5. Markowitz J, Rappaport AM: The hepatic artery. Physiol Rev 31:188, 1951.
6. Coblentz A, Kelly KH, Fitzpatrik J, Biermen HR: Microbiologic studies of the portal and hepatic venous blood in man. Am J Med Sci 228:298, 1954.
7. Perry JF, Herman B, Odenbrett PJ, Kremen AJ: Bacteriologic studies of the human liver. Surgery 37:533, 1955.
8. Romieu C, Brunschwig A: Bacteriologic study of the human liver. Surgery 30:621, 1951.
9. Sborov VH, Morse WC, Giges B, Jahnke EJ: Bacteriology of the human liver. J Clin Invest 31:986, 1952.
10. Lewis FJ, Wangensteen OH: Penicillin in the treatment of peritonitis due to liver autolysis in dogs. Proc Soc Exp Biol Med 73:533, 1950.
11. Klatskin G: Hepatitis associated with systemic infections. In Schiff L (ed): Diseases of the Liver, 4th ed. Philadelphia, Lippincott, 1975.
12. Berg BN, Zau ZD, Jobling JW: Bactericidal function of the liver. Proc Soc Exp Biol Med 24:433, 1926.
13. Weinstein L: Bacterial hepatitis: a case report on an unrecognized cause of fever of unknown origin. N Engl J Med 299:1052, 1978.
14. Helly K: Über die septische Leberfleckung. Verh dtsch path Ges 13:312, 1909.
15. McMahon HE, Mallory FB: Streptococcus hepatitis. Am J Pathol 7:299, 1931.
16. Gracey L: Tuberculous abscess of the liver. Br J Surg 52:442, 1965.
17. Baerensprung C: Der Leberabscess nach Kopfverletzungen. Arch klin Chir 18:586, 1975.
18. Kobler G: Zur Aetiologie der Leberabscesse. Arch path Anat 163:134, 1901.
19. Collins AN: Abscess of the liver. Minn Med 15:756, 1932.
20. Norris GW, Farley DC: Abscess of the liver. Med Clin North Am 10:17, 1926.
21. Ochsner A, DeBakey M: Pleuropulmonary complications of amebiasis. An analysis of 153 collected and 15 personal cases. J Thorac Surg 5:225, 1936.
22. Knowles R, Rinaldo JA: Pyogenic hepatic abscess secondary to sigmoid diverticulitis. Gastroenterology 38:262, 1960.
23. Ribaudo JM, Ochsner A: Intrahepatic abscess: amebic and pyogenic. Am J Surg 125:570, 1973.
24. Rubin RH, Swartz MN, Malt R: Hepatic abscess: changes in clinical, bacteriological and therapeutic aspects. Am J Med 57:601, 1974.
25. Ochsner A, DeBakey M, Murray S: Pyogenic abscess of the liver. II. An analysis of forty-seven cases with review of the literature. Am J Surg 40:292, 1938.
26. Block MA, Schuman BM, Eyler WR, Truant JP, DuSault IA: Surgery of liver abscess. Arch Surg 88:602, 1964.
27. Tandon BN, Tandon HD, Puri BK: An electronmicroscopic study of liver in hepatomegaly presumably caused by amebiasis. Exp Mol Pathol 22:118, 1975.
28. Elsberg CA: Solitary abscess of the liver. Ann Surg 44:209, 1906.
29. Brodine WN, Schwartz SL: Pyogenic hepatic abscess. NY State J Med 73:1657, 1973.
30. Sabbaj J, Sutter VL, Finegold SM: Anaerobic pyogenic liver abscess. Ann Intern Med 77:629, 1972.
31. Abe PM, Lennard ES, Holland JW: *Fusobacterium necrophorum* infection in mice as a model for the study of liver abscess formation and induction of immunity. Infect Immun 13:1473, 1976.
32. Onderdonk A, Bartlett J, Louis T, Sullivan-Seigler N, Gorbach SL: Microbial synergism in experimental intraabdominal abscess. Infect Immun 13:22, 1976.
33. Finegold SM: Anaerobic Bacteria in Human Disease. New York, Harcourt, 1977, p 276.
34. Spink WW: Host-parasite relationship in human brucellosis with prolonged illness due to suppuration of the liver and spleen. Am J Med Sci 247:129, 1964.
35. Herrell WE, Simpson WC: Recurrent hyperpyrexia due to solitary tuberculoma of the liver. JAMA 111:517, 1938.
36. Lyford J III, Johnson RW, Blackman S, Scott RB: Pathologic findings in a fatal case of disseminated granuloma inguinale with miliary bone and joint involvement. Bull Johns Hopkins Hosp 79:349, 1946.
37. Robertson RD, Foster JH, Peterson CG: Pyogenic liver abscess studies by cholangiography: case report and 25 year review. Am Surg 32:521, 1966.
38. Trump DL, Fahnenstock HM, Cloutier CT, Dickman MD: Anaerobic abscess and intrahepatic metastases: A case report and review of the literature. Cancer 41:682, 1978.
39. Jochimsen PR, Zinke WL, Shirazi SS, Pearlman NW: Iatrogenic liver abscess. Arch Surg 113:141, 1978.
40. Butler TJ, McCarthy CF: Pyogenic liver abscess. Gut 10:389, 1969.
41. Lee JF, Block GE: The changing clinical pattern of hepatic abscesses. Arch Surg 104:465, 1972.
42. Altemeier WA, Schowengerdt CG, Whiteley DH: Abscess of the liver: surgical considerations. Arch Surg 101:258, 1970.
43. Dehner LP, Kissane JM: Pyogenic hepatic abscess in infancy and childhood. J Pediatr 74:763, 1969.
44. Nebesar RA, Tefft M, Colodny AH: Angiography of liver abscess in granulomatous disease of childhood. Am J Roentgenol Radium Ther Nucl Med 108:628, 1970.
45. Kinney TD, Ferrebee JW: Hepatic abscess: factors determining its localization. Arch Pathol 45:41, 1948.
46. Sérégé H: Contribution à l'étude de la circulation du sang forte dans le foie et des localisation lobaires hépatiques. J méd Bord 31:208, 217, 291, 312, 1901.

47. Satiani B, Davidson ED: Hepatic abscess: improvement in mortality with early diagnosis and treatment. Am J Surg 135:647, 1978.
48. Young AE: The clinical presentation of pyogenic liver abscess. Br J Surg 63:216, 1976.
49. Zodikoff R: Multiple liver abscesses with rupture into the pericardium. Am Heart J 33:375, 1947.
50. Webber RJ, Coe JI: Rupture of pyogenic hepatic abscess into hepatic vein. Surgery 27:907, 1950.
51. Nieweg GA: Abscess of the liver and right psoas muscle secondary to gangrenous appendix. US Vet Bureau Med Bull 5:58, 1929.
52. Huard P, Meyer-May J: Début péritonéal aigu de certains abcés du lobe hépatique droit non-extériorisés. Press Med 44:654, 1936.
53. Bearn JG: Spontaneous rupture of the malarial spleen: a case and some anatomical and pathological considerations. Trans R Soc Trop Med Hyg 55:242, 1961.
54. Sanders RC: Radiological and radioisotopic diagnosis of perihepatic abscess. Crit Rev Clin Radiol Nucl Med 5:165, 1974.
55. DeNardo GL, Stadalnik RC, DeNardo SJ, Raventos A: Hepatic scintiangiographic patterns. Radiology 111:135, 1974.
56. Pyrtek LJ, Bartus SA: Hepatic pyemia. N Engl J Med 272:551, 1965.
57. Lawson TL: Hepatic abscess: ultrasound as an aid to diagnosis. Dig Dis 22:33, 1977.
58. Friday RO, Barriga P, Crummy AB: Detection and localization of intra-abdominal abscess by diagnostic ultrasound. Arch Surg 110:335, 1975.
59. Adatepe MH, Welch M, Evens RG, Potchen EJ: Clinical application of the broad spectrum scanning agent—indium-113m. Am J Roentgenol Radiother Nucl Med 112:701, 1971.
60. Thakur ML, Coleman RE, Welch MJ: Indium-111-labeled leukocytes for the localization of abscesses: preparation, analysis, tissue distribution, and comparison with gallium-67 citrate in dogs. J Lab Clin Med 89:217, 1977.
61. Thakur ML, Lavender JP, Arnot RN, Silvester DJ: Indium-111-labeled autologous leukocytes in man. J Nucl Med 18:1014, 1977.
62. Yeh S-H, Shih WJ, Liang JC: Intravenous radionuclide hepatography in the differential diagnosis of intrahepatic mass lesions. J Nucl Med 14:565, 1974.
63. Morin ME, Bauer DA, Marsan RE: Hepatic abscess: diagnosis in the adult by total body opacification. JAMA 236:1607, 1976.
64. Ascione A, Elias E, Scott J, Sherlock S: Endoscopic retrograde cholangiography (ERC) in nonamebic liver abscesses. Dig Dis 23:39, 1978.
65. Madayag MA, Lefleur RS, Braunstein P, Beranbaum E, Bosniak M: Radiology of hepatic abscess. NY State J Med 75:1417, 1975.
66. Novy SB, Wallace S, Goldman AM, Ben-Menachem Y: Pyogenic liver abscess: angiographic diagnosis and treatment by closed aspiration. Am J Roentgenol 121:388, 1974.
67. Palmer ED: The changing manifestations of pyogenic liver abscess. JAMA 231:192, 1975.
68. Ranson JHC, Madayag MA, Localio SA, Spencer FC: New diagnostic and therapeutic techniques in the management of pyogenic liver abscesses. Ann Surg 181:508, 1975.
69. McFadzean JS, Chang KPS, Wong CC: Solitary pyogenic abscess of the liver treated by closed aspiration and antibiotics. Br J Surg 41:141, 1953.
70. Pitt HA, Zuidema GD: Factors influencing mortality in the treatment of pyogenic hepatic abscesses. Surg Gynecol Obstet 140:228, 1975.
71. Goldsmith HS, Chen W-F: Management of a pyogenic abscess of the liver. Surg Clin North Am 53:711, 1973.
72. Hicken NF, McAllister AJ: Resection of entire left lobe of liver: intrahepatic abscesses, stones and foreign bodies. Am J Surg 105:278, 1963.
73. Ochsner A, DeBakey M: Amebic hepatitis and hepatic abscess: an analysis of 181 cases with review of the literature. Surgery 13:460–612, 1943.
74. Adams EB: Amoebic pericarditis. Med S Afr 17:1013, 1974.
75. Maegraith GB, Harinasut AC: Experimental amoebic infection of the liver in guinea pigs: infection via the mesenteric vein and via the portal vein. Ann Trop Med 48:421, 1954.
76. Palmer RB: Changes in the liver in amebic dysentery with special reference to the origin of amebic abscesses. Arch Pathol 25:327, 1938.
77. Ratcliffe HL, Geiman QM: Spontaneous and experimental amebic infections in reptiles. Arch Pathol 25:160, 1938.
78. Ravi VV, Tandon HD, Tandon BN: Morphological changes in the liver in hepatic amoebiasis. Indian J Med Res 62:1832, 1974.
79. Adams EB, McLeod IN: Invasive amebiasis. II. Amebic liver abscess and its complications. Medicine 56:325, 1977.
80. Turrill FL, Burnham JR: Hepatic amebiasis. Am J Surg 111:424, 1966.
81. Powell SJ, Wilmot AJ, Elsdon-Dew R: Hepatic amoebiasis. Trans R Soc Trop Med Hyg 53:190, 1959.
82. Wilmot AJ: Amoebiasis. In Woodruff AW (ed): Medicine in the Tropics. Edinburgh and London, Churchill Livingstone, 1974.
83. DeBakey ME, Ochsner A: Hepatic amebiasis: a 20 year experience and analysis of 263 cases. Surg Gynecol Obstet 92:209, 1951.
84. Manson-Bahr P: Secondary bacterial infections of amebic abscess of the liver. Trop Dis Bull 45:519, 1948.
85. Crane PS, Lee YT, Seel DJ: Experience in the treatment of two hundred patients with amebic abscess of the liver in Korea. Am J Surg 123:332, 1972.
86. Chavez FJZC, Cruz, I, Gomes C, Domingues W, DaSilva EM, Veloso FT: Hepatic amebiasis, analysis of 56 cases. Am J Gastroenterol 68:134, 1977.
87. Alkan WJ, Kalmi B, Kalderon M: The clinical syndrome of amebic abscess of the left lobe of the liver. Ann Int Med 55:800, 1961.
88. Grove RB, Madewell JE, Rapp GS, Pinsky SM, Johnson MC: Practical application of ^{67}Ga-citrate to the evaluation of liver pathology. J Nucl Med 14:402, 1973.
89. Geslien GE, Thrall JH, Johnson MC: Gallium scanning in acute hepatic amebic abscess. J Nucl Med 15:561, 1974.
90. Tubis M, Krishnamurthy GT, Endow JS, Stein RA, Suwanik R, Bland WH: Labeled metronidazoles as potential new agents for amebic abscess imaging. Nucl Med 14:163, 1975.
91. Amir-Jahed AK, Sadrieh M, Fappour A, Azar H, Namdaran F: Thoracolbilia: a surgical complication of hepatic echinococcosis and amebiasis. Ann Thorac Surg 14:198, 1972.
92. Ramachandran S, Pakianathan V, Aiyathurai JEJ: Severe obstructive jaundice due to amoebic liver abscess. Med J Austr 104:925, 1976.
93. DasGupta A: Immunoglobulin in health and disease. III. Immunoglobulin in the sera of patients with amoebiasis. Clin Exp Immunol 86:163, 1974.
94. Ravi VV, Mithal S, Malaviya AN, Tandon BN: Immunologic studies in amebic liver abscess. Indian J Med Res 63:1732, 1975.
95. Shabot JM, Patterson M: Amebic liver abscess: 1966–1976. Dig Dis 23:110, 1078.
96. Healy GR: The laboratory diagnosis of amebiasis. Am J Gastroenterol 42:191, 1964.
97. Powell SJ, Maddison SE, Wilmot AJ, Elsdon-Dew R: Amoebic gel-diffusion-precipitation test. Clinical evaluation in amoebic liver abscess. Lancet 2:602, 1965.

98. Milgram EA, Healy GR, Kagan IG: Studies on the use of the indirect hemagglutination test in the diagnosis of amebiasis. Gastroenterology 50:645, 1966.
99. Juniper K Jr, Worrell CL, Minshew MC, Roth LS, Lypert H, Lloyd RE: Serologic diagnosis of amebiasis. Am J Trop Med Hyg 21:156, 1972.
100. Cerise EJ, Pierce WA, Diamond DL: Abdominal drains: their role as source of infection following splenectomy. Ann Surg 171:764, 1970.
101. Balasegaram M: New concepts in hepatic amebiasis. Ann Surg 175:528, 1972.
102. Nuguid TP: Surgical drainage of amoebic abscess of the liver. Drug 15:53, 1978.
103. Rogers L: The rapid cure of amoebic dysentery and hepatitis by hypodermic injection of soluble salts of emetine. Br Med J 1:1424, 1912.
104. Wilmot AJ, Powell SJ, Adams EB: The comparative value of emetine and chloroquine in amebic liver abscess. Am J Trop Med Hyg 7:197, 1958.
105. Powell SJ: The cardiotoxicity of systemic amebicides. Am J Trop Med Hyg 16:447, 1967.
106. Wilmot AJ, Powell SJ, McLeod IN, Elsdon-Dew R: The treatment of amoebic liver abscess with dehydroemetine. Proc 3rd Int Congr Chemother. Stuttgart, Georg Thieme, 1964.
107. Powell SJ, Wilmot AJ, Elsdon-Dew R: Further trials of metronidazole in amoebic dysentery and amoebic liver abscess. Ann Trop Med Parasitol 61:511, 1967.
108. Lewis BV, Kenna AP: Attempted suicide with Flagyl. J Obstet Gynaecol Br Commenw 72:806, 1965.
109. Henn RM, Collin DB: Amebic abscess of the liver: treatment failure with metronidazole. JAMA 224:1394, 1973.
110. Powell SJ, Elsdon-Dew R: Some new nitroimidazole derivatives. Clinical trial in amebic liver abscess. Am J Trop Med Hyg 21:518, 1972.
111. Scragg JN, Proctor EM: Tinidazole in treatment of amebic liver abscess in children. Arch Dis Child 52:408, 1977.
112. Cohen HG, Reynolds TB: Comparison of metronidazole and chloroquine for the treatment of amebic liver abscess: a controlled trial. Gastroenterology 69:35, 1975.
113. Abuabara S, Barrett J, Hau T, Jonasson O: Amebic liver abscess. Arch Surg, 1981, in press.
114. DeBakey M, Jordan GL: Surgery of the liver. In Schiff L (ed): Diseases of the Liver, 4th ed. Philadelphia, Lippincott, 1975.
115. Katz AM, Pan L-T: Echinococcus disease in the United States. Am J Med 25:759, 1958.
116. Rausch RL: Recent studies on hydatid disease in Alaska. Parassitologia 2:391, 1960.
117. Cameron TM: Incidence and diagnosis of hydatid disease in Canada: *Echinococcus granulosus* var. *Canadiensis.* Parassitologia 2:381, 1960.
118. Romero-Torres R, Campbell JR: An interpretive review of the surgical treatment of hydatid disease. Surg Gynecol Obstet 121:851, 1965.
119. Dungal N: *Echinococcus* in Iceland. Am J Med Sci 212:124, 1946.
120. Golematis B: Hydatid disease: history, etiology, epidemiology, epizootiology, locations, and prevention. In Nyhus LM (ed): Surg Ann 10:359, 1978.
121. Rizk GK, Tayyarah KH, Ghabdur-Mnaymneh L: The angiographic changes in hydatid cyst of the liver and spleen. Diag Radiol 99:303, 1971.
122. Barros JL: Hydatid cyst of the liver. Am J Surg 135:597, 1978.
123. Cottone M, Amuso M, Cotton PB: Endoscopic retrograde cholangiography in hepatic hydatid disease. Br J Surg 65:107, 1978.
124. Papadimitriou J, Mandrekas A: The surgical treatment of hydatid disease of the liver. Br J Surg 57:431, 1970.
125. Kattan YB: Intrabiliary rupture of hydatid cyst of the liver. Br J Surg 62:885, 1975.
126. Al-Hashimi HM: Intrabiliary rupture of hydatid cyst of the liver. Br J Surg 58:228, 1971.
127. Bourgeon R, Pietri H: L'ouverture de kystes hydatiques du foie dans les voies biliaires. Sixième congrès international de l'hydatidose, Athènes 16:193, 1956.
128. Reventos J, Nogueras FM, Rius X, Lorenzo T: Hydatid disease of the liver with thoracic involvement. Surg Gynecol Obstet 143:570, 1976.
129. Yacoubian HD: Thoracic problems associated with hydatid cyst of the dome of the liver. Surgery 79:544, 1976.
130. Schiller CF: Complications of *Echinococcus* cyst rupture. JAMA 195:220, 1966.
130a. Bekathi A, Schaaps J-P, Capron M, Dessaint J-P, Santoro F, Capron A: The treatment of hepatic hydatid disease with mebendazole: Preliminary results in four cases. Brit Med J 2:1047, 1977.
130b. Beard TC, Richard MD, Goodman HT: Medical treatment for hydatids. Med J Aust 1:366, 1978.
130c. Sayek I, Yalin R, Sanac Y: Surgical treatment of hydatid disease of the liver. Arch Surg 115:847, 1980.
130d. Mosimann F: Is alveolar hydatid disease of the liver incurable? Ann Surg 192:118, 1980.
131. Hankins JR: Management of complicated hepatic hydatid cysts. Ann Surg 158:1020, 1963.
132. Ekrami Y: Surgical treatment of hydatid disease of the liver. Arch Surg 111:1350, 1976.
133. Harris JD: Rupture of hydatid cysts of the liver into the biliary tracts. Br J Surg 52:210, 1965.
134. Dintsman M, Chaimoff C, Woloch Y, Lubin E, Tikva P: Surgical treatment of hydatid cyst of the liver. Arch Surg 103:76, 1971.
135. Crosthwait RW, Allen JE, Murga F, Beall A, DeBakey ME: The surgical management of 640 consecutive liver injuries in civilian practice. Surg Gynecol Obstet 114:640, 1962.
136. McClelland RN, Shires T: Management of liver trauma in 259 consecutive patients. Ann Surg 161:248, 1965.
137. Stone HH, Ansley JD: Management of liver trauma in children. J Pediatr Surg 12:3, 1977.
138. Fischer RP, O'Farrell KO, Perry JF: The value of peritoneal drains in the treatment of liver injuries. J Trauma 18:393, 1978.
139. Lim RC, Lau G, Steele M: Prevention of complications after liver trauma. Am J Surg 132:156, 1976.
140. Altemeier WA: The pathogenicity of bacteria in appendiceal peritonitis: an experimental study. Surgery 11:374, 1942.
141. Hau T, Hoffman R, Simmons RL: Mechanisms of the adjuvant effect of hemoglobin in experimental peritonitis. I. In vivo inhibition of peritoneal leukocytosis. Surgery 83:233, 1978.
142. Schneierson SS, Amsterdam D, Perlman E: Enhancement of intraperitoneal staphylococcal virulence for mice with different bile salts. Nature 190:829, 1961.
143. Pinkerton JA, Sawyers JL, Foster JH: A study of the postoperative course after hepatic lobectomy. Ann Surg 173:800, 1971.
144. Stone HH, Tester TR Jr: Incisional and peritoneal infections after emergency celiotomy. Ann Surg 117:669, 1973.
145. Mays ET: The hazards of suturing certain wounds of the liver. Surg Gynecol Obstet 143:201, 1976.
146. Merendino KA, Dillard DH, Gammock EE: The concept of surgical biliary decompression in the management of liver trauma. Surg Gynecol Obstet 117:285, 1963.
147. Lucas CE, Walt AJ: Analysis of randomized biliary drainage in hepatic trauma in 189 patients. J Trauma 12:925, 1972.

148. Madding GF, Lawrence KG, Kennedy PA: War wound of the liver. Texas State J Med 42:267, 1946.
149. Trunkey DD, Shires GT, McClelland R: Management of liver trauma in 811 consecutive patients. Ann Surg 179:722, 1974.
150. Chulay JD, Lankerani MR: Splenic abscess: report of 10 cases and review of the literature. Am J Med 61:513, 1976.
151. Cohn LH: Local infections after splenectomy. Arch Surg 90:230, 1965.
152. Blumer G: Subacute bacterial endocarditis. Medicine 2:105, 1923.
153. Billings AE: Abscess of the spleen. Ann Surg 88:416, 1928.
154. Fry DE, Richardson JD, Flint LM: Occult splenic abscess: an unrecognized complication of heroin abuse. Surgery 84:650, 1978.
155. Caldarera E: Acute abscess of the spleen. Surg Gynecol Obstet 67(supp):265, 1938.
156. Anand SW, Davey WW: Surgery of the spleen in Nigeria. Br J Surg 52:335, 1965.
157. Bouvry M, Nordlinger B: Absès de la rate à salmonelles chez un thalassémique. Nouv Press Méd 3:206, 1974.
158. Anderson ARS: Splenic abscess in malarial fever. Lancet 2:1159, 1906.
159. Coopersmith A, Ritchey AK, Zinkham WH: Fever of unknown origin and the value of gallium-67 and technetium-99^m for defining abnormality of the spleen: a case report. Johns Hopkins Med J 137:51, 1975.
160. Elting AW: Abscess of the spleen. Ann Surg 62:182, 1915.
161. Spigos DG, Jonasson O, Felix E, Capek V: Transcatheter therapeutic embolization of hypersplenism. Invest Radiol 12:418, 1977.
162. Silva J Jr, Harvey WC: Detections of infections with gallium-67 and scinigraphic imaging. J Infect Dis 130:125, 1974.
163. Zook EG, Bolovar JC, Epstein LI: Value of scintiscans in the diagnosis of splenic abscess. Surg Gynecol Obstet 131:1125, 1978.
164. Asopa HS, Echence IP: Ruptured abscess of spleen. Indian J Med Sci 19:618, 1965.
165. Rutkow IM: Rupture of the spleen in infectious mononucleosis. Arch Surg 113:718, 1978.
166. Davis R: Spontaneous rupture of the pathological spleen in malaria. S Afr Med J 47:1801, 1973.
167. Cope Z, Maingot R: Abdominal Operations, 4th ed. New York, Appleton, 1961.
168. Gonin A, Berthou JD, Roques JC, Dufoix V: Rupture spontanée de la rate: manifestation révélatrice d'une endocardite infectieuse. Nouv Press Méd 2:1306, 1973.
169. Wood LJ: Pathologic aspects of acute epidemic hepatitis. Arch Pathol 41:345, 1946.
170. Franke D: Spontanruptur der gesunden Milz. Mschr Unfallheilk 68:465, 1965.
171. Sperling RL, Heredia R, Gillesby WJ, Chomet B: Rupture of the spleen secondary to actinomycosis. Arch Surg 94:344, 1967.
172. Sokolowski JW, Kent DC: Spontaneous rupture of the spleen in infectious mononucleosis: value of roentgenography. NY State J Med 68:1172, 1968.
173. Hodam RP: The risk of splenectomy: a review of 310 cases. Am J Surg 119:709, 1970.
174. Fabri PJ, Metz EN, Nick WV, Zollinger RM: A quarter of century with splenectomy. Arch Surg 108:569, 1974.
175. Kassum D, Thomas EJ: Morbidity and mortality of incidental splenectomy. Can J Surg 20:209, 1977.
176. Olson WR, Beaudoin DE: Wound drainage after splenectomy: indications and complications. Am J Surg 117:615, 1969.
177. Nora PF, Vanecuo RM, Bransfield JJ: Prophylactic abdominal drains. Arch Surg 105:173, 1972.
178. Singer DB: Postsplenectomy sepsis. In Rosenberg AS, Bolande RP (eds): Perspective in Pediatric Pathology, Vol I. Chicago, Year Book Medical Publishers, 1973.
178a. Robinette CD, Fraumeni JF: Splenectomy and subsequent mortality in the veterans of the 1939–45 war. Lancet 2:127, 1977.
179. Eraklis AJ, Filler RM: Splenectomy in childhood: a review of 1413 cases. J Pediatr Surg 7:382, 1972.
180. Gopal V, Bisno AL: Fulminant pneumococcal infections in "normal" asplenic hosts. Arch Intern Med 137:1526, 1977.
181. Krivit W, Giebink GS, Leonard A: Overwhelming post-splenectomy infection. Surg Clin North Am 59:2:223, 1979.
182. Sullivan JL, Ochs HD, Schiffman G, Hammerschlag MR, Miser J, Vichinsky A, Nedwood RJ: Immune response after splenectomy. Lancet 1:178, 1978.
183. Krivit W: Overwhelming post-splenectomy infection. Am J Hematol 2:193, 1977.
183a. Schulkind ML, Ellis EF, Smith RT: Effect of antibody upon clearance of I^{125}-labelled pneumococci by the spleen and liver. Pediat Res 1:178, 1967.
183b. Constantopoulus A, Najjar VA, Wish JB, Necheles TH, Stolbach LL: Defective phagocytosis due to tuftsin deficiency in splenectomized subjects. Am J Dis Child 125:663, 1973.
183c. Amsbaugh DF, Prescott B, Baker PJ: Effect of splenectomy on the expression of regulatory T cell activity. J Immunol 121:1483, 1978.
184. Giebink: Personal communication.
185. Morgenstern L: The avoidable complications of splenectomy. Surg Gynecol Obstet 145:525, 1977.
186. Sherman NJ, Asch MD: Conservative surgery for splenic injuries. Pediatrics 61:267, 1978.

CHAPTER 37
Infections of the Pancreas

ROBERT L. GOODALE, JR. AND THOMAS D. DRESSEL

PANCREATIC INFECTIONS

INFECTIONS of the normal pancreas are unusual except under two circumstances—hematogenous spread of systemic viral or bacterial infection, and infection associated with pancreatitis. A discussion of pancreatic infections must therefore consider pancreatitis as a concomitant event.[1]

NATURAL PANCREATIC DEFENSE MECHANISMS AGAINST INFECTION

The pancreas lies sheltered in its retroperitoneal location, protected against external injury posteriorly by the vertebral column and back muscles and anteriorly by the umbrella of the rib cage. Blunt trauma is more likely to damage liver, spleen, and other more superficial gas- and fluid-filled intra-abdominal organs. In addition, the pancreas lies adjacent to the portion of the gastrointestinal tract that normally contains the fewest organisms—stomach, duodenum, and biliary tree. Two sphincters at the ampulla of Vater act to prevent reflux of duodenal contents into the pancreatic duct.

The pancreatic sphincters maintain duct pressures at a low level, around 25 mmHg, which is usually sufficient to prevent reflux of duodenal contents. Intraductal pressures in biliary tree and pancreatic ducts normally exceed resting intraduodenal pressures by a mean of 10 mmHg in the pancreatic duct and 8 mmHg in the common duct.[2] Only during retching, straining, or duodenal obstruction do duodenal pressures exceed pancreatic duct pressure. In 42 percent of people, there is an alternate route for exocrine secretions via the duct of Santorini, should pressures in the main duct increase suddenly to harmful levels.[3] Because intraductal volume is small and the secretory volume exceeds 1 liter per day, the flow rate of secretions is high. Consequently, there is little time for bacteria to divide before being flushed into the duodenum.

When duodenal or biliary reflux into the pancreatic duct occurs, the pancreatic ductal epithelium serves as a barrier to organ damage. The ductal epithelium maintains a barrier to absorption of certain ions,[4] to conjugated bile acids, and probably many other substances. This barrier can be broken by aspirin and alcohol[4] but not by lipase and amylase, the only enzymes secreted in active form by the pancreas. All the proteolytic enzymes in the pancreatic ducts are secreted in inactive (zymogen) form. Bile itself does *not* activate trypsinogen,[5] as formerly believed. Normal bile and pancreatic juice actually contain trypsin inhibitors, further protecting the ductal epithelium.[6]

The lymphatics rapidly clear the secretory enzymes, which spill into the interstitial spaces during times of pressure build-up. After secretion is stimulated, lymphatic flow exceeds ductal flow.[7] The normal pancreas has a loose areolar capsule and can easily swell without altering intracapsular pressure or vascular perfusion.

Because duodenal reflux is the major potential source of contaminating organisms, normal gastric acidity is obviously an important factor in the maintenance of pancreatic sterility. In patients with gastric achlorhydria, however, 10^4 to 10^8 coliforms per ml can be found in the upper intestine.[8,9]

If intestinal contents reflux into the pancreas, bile acids play some bacteriostatic role. Unconjugated bile acids are bacteriostatic for the anaerobes[10] *Bacteroides* and *Lactobacillus* and bactericidal for *Clostridium perfringens.* Bile acids increase the rate of enterokinase activation of trypsinogen to trypsin, thereby increasing the concentrations of proteolytic enzymes, which are inhibitors to bacterial growth (eg, *Vibrio cholerae*)[11] and can detoxify *C. perfringens* exotoxin.[8,12] Lipase and lysolecithin, which are sometimes present in pancreatic secretions, are bactericidal for a variety of microorganisms.

PATHOGENESIS OF PANCREATIC INFECTION

Pancreatitis is the most common predisposing factor in pancreatic infection, and its pathogenesis is worth considering in detail (Fig. 37-1). In addition, pancreatitis may on occasion be the result of an infective agent acting in combination with another pathogenic factor. Pancreatic duct obstruction, caused by stones, strictures, tumors,

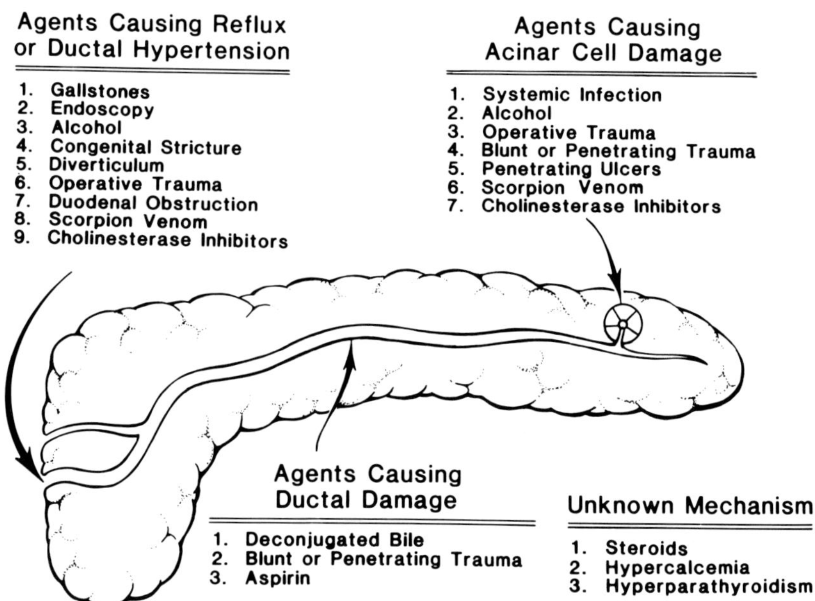

Fig. 37-1. **Known causes of pancreatitis.**

postoperative edema, parasites, or congenital or acquired anatomic abnormalities,[13-17] have all been described as important factors in the pathogenesis of pancreatitis. Direct operative or accidental trauma will also cause enzymatic extravasation and activation, setting the stage for infection.

GALLSTONE PANCREATITIS

The understanding of the pathogenesis of pancreatitis began with Opie's autopsy finding, in 1901,[18] of a 3-mm stone impacted in the ampulla of a patient who died with hemorrhagic pancreatitis. There was a common channel draining both the bile and pancreatic ducts. He postulated that regurgitation of bile caused the pancreatitis. Although an obstructing calculus in a common channel can only be found in a few patients, the migration of calculi through the ampulla is still thought to be an important cause of pancreatitis. In acute pancreatitis, gallstones are present in 36 to 68 percent of patients, depending on sex, socioeconomic, and racial factors.[19] The natural course of the disease is for attacks to recur in 30 percent of patients unless biliary surgery is done.

The mechanism by which biliary tract disease can cause pancreatitis is incompletely understood, but an infection is suspected. Bile within the normal or even the obstructed biliary tract is almost always sterile. In contrast, about 25 percent of patients with diseases of the gallbladder and almost 90 percent of patients with common duct stones have positive bile culture results. The aerobic bacteria are predominately *E. coli, Klebsiella, Proteus,* and enterococci. Anaerobes (especially *Bacteroides*) are present in 40 percent, either in pure (12 percent) or mixed culture (25 percent). Clostridia are occasionally found (Chapter 36).[20-22]

Patients with bactibilia frequently grow the same organisms from the liver, regional lymph nodes, and the duodenal lumen.[22] In fact, a colonic type of microflora within the duodenal lumen is a clue to choledocholithiasis. In patients undergoing biliary tract surgery,[9] 35 percent of those with predominantly colonic organisms (10^3 per ml) in duodenal aspirates had choledocholithiasis, stenosis, or dilation of the common duct. Of these, 90 percent grew intestinal bacteria from the biliary tree. In contrast, only 8 percent with normal duodenal microflora had choledocholithiasis, and only 9 percent with the common pharyngeal organisms (10^5 per ml aerobic streptococci, enterococci, *Neisseria,* yeasts, *Haemophilus,* pneumococci) had choledocholithiasis or extrahepatic pathology. With advancing age, there was a parallel increase in the incidence of choledocholithiasis, achlorhydria, and a colonic duodenal flora.[23] Since most evidence supports the idea that reflux through the partially or intermittently obstructed ampulla leads to bactibilia, it is likely that bacterial colonization of the pancreatic duct derives from a similar mechanism.

In one study, 31 percent of patients with chronic pancreatitis had organisms in pancreatic juice.[24] Two-thirds of patients with pancreatitis also showed infected bile. Fifty percent of patients with acute relapsing pancreatitis had a moderate infection. The most frequently cultured species were *E. coli,* enterococci, and *Enterobacter.* Interestingly, although fever was associated with infected pancreatic juice in less than 50 percent of the patients with pancreatitis, ductal abnormalities were present in all infected ducts.

Colonization of the pancreatic duct and biliary tree almost certainly arises by reflux of duodenal contents through an ampulla rendered incompetent by passage of a stone or iatrogenic manipulation. Sometimes, reflux results from pressures generated within the duodenal lumen from vomiting or obstruction. This can occur at duodenal pressures of 40 mmHg. Colonization does not by itself induce pancreatitis. Colonization plus mechanical or functional obstruction (stones within the common channel or an inflamed ampullary complex) will, however, cause stasis and permit bacterial proliferation. A number of untoward events may then ensue. *Clostridium, E. coli, Bacteroides,* and *Streptococcus* contain beta-glucuronidase and are capable of deconjugating bile.[25] Deconjugated chenodeoxycholic and deoxycholic acids are four to eight times more injurious to the pancreatic ducts than are the conjugated acids. The mechanism of injury is destruction of the mucopolysaccharide blanket protecting the ductal epithelium.[26]

Another pathogenic mechanism set in motion by gallstone pancreatitis is proenzyme activation. This occurs prematurely within the pancreas. Trypsinogen activation may be initiated by enterokinase refluxing from duodenal contents, by bacterial toxins or by plasminogen activators. With ductal hypertension resulting from obstruction, trypsin attacks at the acinar level, often leaving the ductal epithelium intact. Then activation of trypsinogen occurs autocatalytically along with activation of prophospholipase, elastase, chymotrypsinogen, and kallikreinogen. Lipase and colipase liberation [27] are responsible for the fat necrosis and hemorrhage within the pancreas. Kallikrein causes edema of the pancreas. Toxins of *E. coli* that are present in bile or duodenal contents will sensitize the pancreatic blood vessels of animals and cause microvascular thrombosis.[27-30] Arthus sensitization reaction and local Shwartzman reactions can be induced to demonstrate the role of severe local anoxia in acute pancreatitis. The clinical finding of diffuse hyaline capillary thrombosis, extensive necrosis of arterioles, venules and larger vessels in acute pancreatitis is similar to the dermal-Shwartzman reaction.

Not all evidence supports the role of bacteria in the pathogenesis of human pancreatitis. For example, the protective effect of systemic antibiotics in the treatment of experimental acute hemorrhagic pancreatitis can be shown in animals,[31,32] and infected bile causes a more severe pancreatitis when injected into the pancreatic duct of dogs than sterile bile.[28-30] But Nance and Cain [33] demonstrated typical hemorrhagic pancreatitis in Pfeffer loop preparations in germ-free dogs, and no clinical studies have ever demonstrated the effectiveness of antibiotics in the treatment of pancreatitis.

PANCREATITIS FOLLOWING ENDOSCOPY

The endoscopist may transmit bacterial pathogens to the normal and compromised pancreas. Tseng et al [34] report sepsis rates as high as 9 percent after endoscopic retrograde cholangiopancreatography (ERCP) for pseudocyst. The reported organisms are *Pseudomonas, Salmonella,* and *Bacteroides.*[34] It is easy to see how the injection of these pathogens into the pancreatic duct under pressure during ERCP might predispose to pancreatitis or pancreatic infections. The most likely routes of contamination were the biopsy and suction channels of the endoscope, which are irrigated with wash solutions and surfactants exposed to air-borne contaminants.[35]

ACUTE ALCOHOLIC PANCREATITIS

The mechanism by which alcohol ingestion causes pancreatitis is uncertain. It is postulated that pancreatic hypersecretion is induced by increased gastrin and secretin release, and that alcohol-induced duodenitis causes ampullary spasm.[36] The combination of hypersecretion and outflow obstruction causes regurgitation of proteolytic proenzymes into the pancreatic interstitial space. Activation of proenzymes, possibly by duodenal regurgitation secondary to retching, results in pancreatic autodigestion.

Another theory involves lipoprotein metabolism. Serum triglycerides rise after the drinking of alcohol and perhaps as a result of the inhibition of lipoprotein lipase.[37,38] When high levels of circulating triglycerides are exposed to pancreatic lipase in the pancreatic capillaries, intrapancreatic free fatty acids are formed and cause local capillary damage. Thus, the pancreatitis of chronic alcoholism, and that associated with hyperlipoproteinemia, Frederickson type I and V, may share a common mechanism.[15,39] Chronic alcoholism causes precipitation of protein plugs in the pancreatic duct.[36,40] Not only is an abnormal protein present,[41,42] but a state of hypersecretion or increased vagal tone has been described.[36,40] Recent studies suggest that protein-deficient states induced by ethionine may increase cholinergic tone within the pancreas which, if sustained, has been shown to be detrimental to the pancreas.[41] Furosemide, which occasionally causes acute pancreatitis, is also associated with hyperlipidemia.[44]

POSTOPERATIVE PANCREATITIS

Millbourn [50] has listed five etiologic factors in the pathogenesis of postoperative pancreatitis: (1) mechanical injury to the pancreatic tissue by traction or pressure, (2) vascular injury, (3) stagnation of duodenal contents with possible reflux into the pancreatic duct, (4) spasm of ampullary muscles, and (5) injury to pancreatic ducts.

The incidence ranges from 6.8 percent to 16 percent. Common bile duct exploration is the most common preceding operation,[51] but operations on the stomach, spleen, and aorta are common, and 22 percent had operations remote from the pancreas.[52]

POSTTRAUMATIC PANCREATITIS

The incidence of pancreatitis following major abdominal trauma ranges from 0.9 to 8 percent [53] and may be acute, subacute, or chronic. The failure to recognize pancreatic damage and provide for the controlled escape of activated pancreatic enzymes is the critical surgical error.[54] Amylase elevations can occur but do not correlate with severity of the injury. Many patients have an associated retroperitoneal organ or major vessel injury,[55] and 20 percent have combined pancreaticoduodenal injuries.

Overlooking a pancreatic injury almost always leads to a major complication, especially if contamination with enteric organisms occurs.[55] This can be an abscess, fistula, pseudocyst, or hemorrhage, and each one carries a heavy mortality. The problem, then, is recognition and control. An elevated serum amylase level is quite useful in detecting injuries to the pancreas secondary to blunt trauma [55] but is not useful in penetrating trauma, or pancreatic or lesser sac abscesses.

TABLE 37-1. CAUSES OF PANCREATITIS UNDERLYING PANCREATIC ABSCESSES

Author	# Patients with Abscess	Alcoholic (percent)	Gallstones (percent)	Postoperative (percent)	Trauma (percent)	Miscellaneous (percent)	Unknown Etiology (percent)
Holden [73]	28	72	18	—	—	—	10
Miller [65]*	63	23	27	48	4	15	11
Altemeier [61]	32	22	56	—	3	—	18
Grace [67]	20	40	—	55	—	—	5
Camer [67]	113	10	29	41	0.8	5	13
Kune [72]	19	21	26	21	—	15	15
Bolooki [71]	74	54	10	15	14	2	5

* Multiple etiologic factors in some patients.

OTHER CAUSES OF PANCREATITIS

Parathyroid Disease

Cope with one of the first to cite the relationship between pancreatitis and hyperparathyroidism.[45] Pancreas calcification occurs because of insolubility of increased calcium ions in pancreatic juice.[45,46]

Steroids

The association between corticosteroids and pancreatitis was established first by Stump and later by Carone and Liebow.[47] Acinar ectasia represents obstruction from a low flow state and accumulation of viscid secretions within acini.

Renal Transplantation

Pancreatitis is a recognized complication of renal transplantation,[48] with a reported incidence varying from 2 to 6 percent.[49] Steroids and hyperparathyroidism may play pathogenetic roles.

TABLE 37-2. THE 11 EARLY OBJECTIVE SIGNS USED TO CLASSIFY THE SEVERITY OF PANCREATITIS

At admission or diagnosis
- Age over 55 years
- White blood cell count over 16,000/mm^3
- Blood glucose over 200 mg/100 ml
- Serum lactic dehydrogenase over 350 IU/1
- Serum glutamic oxaloacetic transaminase over 250 Sigma-Frankel units/100 ml

During initial 48 hours
- Hematocrit fall greater than 10 percentage points
- Blood urea nitrogen rise more than 5 mg/100 ml
- Serum calcium level below 8 mg/100 ml
- Arterial Po_2 below 60 mmHg
- Base deficit greater than 4 mEq/liter
- Estimated fluid sequestration more than 6,000 ml

From Ranson JHC: Acute pancreatitis. *Curr Probl Surg* 16:1, 1979.

ROLE OF PANCREATIC DAMAGE IN THE PATHOGENESIS OF PANCREATIC ABSCESS

Whatever the etiology, acute pancreatitis is associated with tissue necrosis, lesser sac transudation of fluid, interstitial edema, lymphatic and venous congestion.[56-59] The general loss of normal circulatory dynamics compromises the cellular and humoral antibacterial defense mechanisms, thus setting the stage for invasive infection. The origin and route of bacterial contamination can arise in a variety of ways: spread along lymphatics from the liver, gallbladder, or colon; hematogenous seeding; regurgitation of infected bile or duodenal contents, and direct transmural penetration of the transverse colon. Invasive infection of necrotic pancreatic tissue and protein-rich edema fluid results in further pancreatic necrosis. Larger areas of the gland are soon involved, with increasing collections of fluid in the lesser sac. The infected pancreas is devascularized, mushy in character, and brown-black in color. Continuation of this necrotizing inflammatory process can eventually include the entire gland. Thus, the posterior wall of the lesser sac becomes a necrotic mass.

Abscesses of varying size and distribution may evolve and communicate with fistulous tracts to skin or gut. Microscopically, the necrotizing process extends along intralobular spaces. Even without ductal rupture, toxins permeate interstitial spaces through clefts between acinar cells, and vascular destruction is important for the progression of the lesion.

PANCREATIC ABSCESS

Incidence

Pancreatic abscess is an unusual complication in patients with acute pancreatitis (incidence from 1.5 to 4.5 percent).[60-64] Table 37-1 summarizes the various causes of pancreatitis that lead to abscess formation: alcohol, gallstones, and postoperative pancreatitis lead all reported causes of postoperative pancreatitis which resulted in pancreatic abscess. Biliary tract surgery comprised the majority (36 to 100 percent) of the postoperative abscesses.[64-68]

Thus biliary tract disease predisposes to pancreatic abscess, both as a primary cause of pancreatitis and as a condition which necessitates operative manipulation of the duodenum, ampulla, or head of the pancreas. In some studies, abscesses were more common with gallstone pancreatitis than with alcoholic pancreatitis.[68] The preponderance of patients with biliary tract disease may be a result of a combination of preexisting bactibilia and a greater enzyme content of the pancreas in this group of patients than in patients with more fibrotic, enzyme depressed, chronic pancreatitis, or alcoholic pancreatitis. Frey et al [68] suggest that patients with alcoholism and hemorrhagic pancreatitis

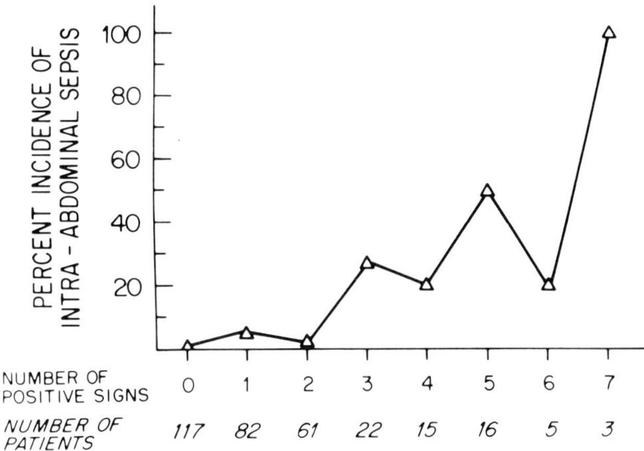

Fig. 37-2. **The incidence of peripancreatic sepsis related to the number of positive prognostic signs recorded during the initial 48 hours of treatment of pancreatitis. Patients who died without sepsis are not included. (From Ranson JHC: Acute pancreatitis. Curr Probl Surg 16:1, 1979.)**

may not survive the fluid loss phase of pancreatitis long enough to have a secondary infection. Ranson[69,70] analyzed objective parameters which correlated with the severity of pancreatitis. Table 37-2 summarizes these 11 parameters, which are established at the time of admission and during the first 48 hours of hospitalization. Sixty-two percent of patients with three or more early positive findings became seriously ill or died.[69] Figure 37-2 shows the positive correlation between the number of positive findings and the incidence of pancreatic abscess formation. Thus, the incidence of septic complications is related to the severity of the underlying episode of acute pancreatitis.[69,70]

Etiology

The organisms recovered from pancreatic abscesses are usually coliforms. Polymicrobial cultures were obtained in 107 of 253 abscesses reported by the seven groups in Table 37-1. Table 37-3 lists the organisms isolated by Holden et al.[73] They are typical of those found by all other investigators, and they are the characteristic organisms of biliary tract, hepatic, and most other mixed intra-abdominal infections. Whether anaerobes will be isolated more often in the future as anaerobic microbiologic techniques improve is not known.

TABLE 37-3. BACTERIA ISOLATED FROM PANCREATIC ABSCESSES IN 28 PATIENTS

Organism	Number of Isolates
Escherichia coli	12
Klebsiella	7
Bacteroides	4
Candida	3
Pseudomonas	3
Staphylococcus	3
Citrobacter	2
Streptococcus	2
Proteus	1
Salmonella	1
No growth	2

Modified from Holden JL, Berne TV, Rosoff L: Pancreatic abscess following acute pancreatitis. *Arch Surg* 111:858, 1976.

Holden et al[73] found all the bacteria isolated would have been sensitive to a combination of penicillin, gentamicin, and chloramphenicol. Eighty percent of 62 isolates reported by Bolooki et al[71] were sensitive to chloramphenicol. Owens and Hamit[74] reported all bacteria, except *Klebsiella*, isolated from 11 abscesses were sensitive to ampicillin. Although antibiotic therapy alone is inadequate treatment for pancreatic abscesses, antibiotics are a useful adjuvant to surgical drainage.

Clinical Manifestations

In a small series, 90 percent of abscesses followed the first, rather than subsequent, attacks of pancreatitis. Thirty percent of pancreatic abscesses develop within the first 48 hours following the onset of acute pancreatitis, but 70 percent occur following a more prolonged lull in the acute process.[73] The clinical course almost always begins with an attack of severe acute pancreatitis, usually associated with hypovolemic shock.[72] The patients survive the acute illness but then fail to make a satisfactory recovery. They have continued fever and leukocytosis for 10 to 14 days, at which point sudden deterioration may occur as a result of sepsis.[71] In other instances, the patient recovers completely only to develop nausea, vomiting, abdominal pain, tenderness, and mass. This latter presentation is usually misinterpreted as recurrent pancreatitis or a pseudocyst.

Ranson has compared the timing of the onset of septic

TABLE 37-4. TIMING OF PERIPANCREATIC SEPSIS IN PATIENTS WITH ACUTE PANCREATITIS

	Group 1	Group 2	Group 3
Early management of pancreatitis	Nonoperative	Late operation	Early operation
Number of patients	18	2	15
Onset of sepsis (days)			
Range	8–46	2–3	2–34
Median	16	—	6

Group 1 was managed nonoperatively prior to sepsis. Group 2 developed sepsis following laparotomy for possible sepsis. Group 3 had undergone early (day 0–7) laparotomy for pancreatitis without sepsis.

From Ranson JHC: Acute pancreatitis. *Curr Probl Surg* 16:1, 1979.

TABLE 37-5. SYMPTOMS, SIGNS, AND LABORATORY FINDINGS IN 113 PATIENTS WITH PANCREATIC ABSCESS

	Type of Pancreatitis		
Data	***Acute (37)***	***Chronic (29)***	***Postoperative (47)***
Epigastric pain	24	22	14
Flank and back pain	4	7	3
Generalized pain	1	1	4
Fever (101F)	27	21	40
Anorexia	11	9	10
Nausea and vomiting	8	6	7
Distention	3	5	21
Jaundice	6	3	16
Weight loss	20	14	10
Diabetes	2	6	3
Tenderness	10	8	19
Abdominal mass	12	16	9
External fistula	0	4	9
Anemia (hemoglobin < 11.0)	12	11	20
Leukocytosis (10,000/mm³)	26	13	32
Serum amylase elevation	15	4	12
Hypocalcemia (< 8.8 mg/100 ml)	5	2	5

From Camer SJ, Tan EGC, Warren KW, Braasch JW: Pancreatic abscess: a critical analysis of 113 cases. *Am J Surg* 129:426, 1975.

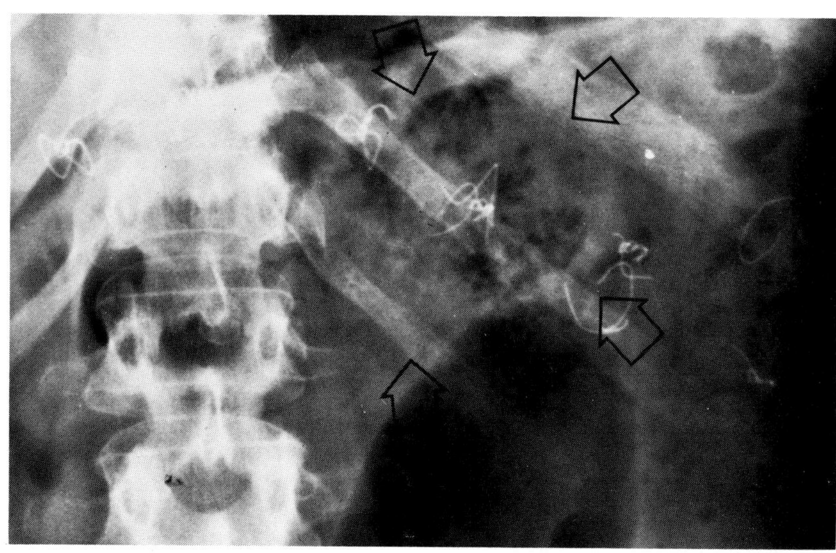

Fig. 37-3. **Typical roentgenographic appearance of a gas-filled pancreatic abscess cavity. This "soap bubble" sign may be confused with stool in the colon.**

complications of pancreatitis in three groups of patients (Table 37-4). In nonoperated patients, sepsis usually developed 2 to 3 weeks after the onset of pancreatitis. In patients undergoing laparotomy either early or late in the course of acute pancreatitis, sepsis tended to occur early (1 week) following laparotomy.

The presenting signs and symptoms vary, but abdominal pain, tenderness, nausea and vomiting, fever, and physical findings or roentgenographic evidence of retrogastric mass are commonly noted. Table 37-5 lists the symptoms, signs, and lab findings in 113 patients reported by Camer et al.[66] Table 37-6 lists the clinical and laboratory features of patients with pancreatic sepsis as reported by Ranson. Fever, leukocytosis (>10,000), epigastric pain, and an abdominal mass have been discussed by almost all investigators, but the mass is found in less than half of the combined series.

Serum amylase is not a reliable indicator of abscess formation. The serum amylase is normal in 33 to 73 percent of pancreatic abscess.[61,65,66] Abdominal roentgenograms are helpful in making the diagnosis by showing signs of subphrenic inflammation manifested by basilar atelectasis, diaphragmatic elevation, or pleural effusion. Displacement of the gastric air bubble has been noted; obliteration of the psoas shadow, or gas within the abscess itself are commonly observed. The latter finding, the so-called soap bubble sign (Fig. 37-3), is considered pathognomonic of a retroperitoneal abscess. Miller [65] reported routine roentgenograms helpful in making the diagnosis of pancreatic abscess in 87 percent of the cases. Recently, ultrasound,

TABLE 37-6. CLINICAL AND LABORATORY FEATURES OF PATIENTS AT THE TIME SEPSIS WAS DIAGNOSED (PERCENT OF PATIENTS) *

	Group 1	Group 2	Group 3
CLINICAL			
Early management of pancreatitis	Nonoperative	Late operation	Early operation
Number of patients	18	2	15
Fever			
> 101F	100	100	93
> 102F	89	100	73
> 103F	61	50	47
Abdominal distention	94	100	0
Abdominal mass	71	0	0
Hypotension (blood pressure < 90 mmHg)	39	0	60
Pneumonia or effusion	89	0	80
Respirator support	39	0	47
Renal failure (blood urea nitrogen > 40 mg/100 ml)	39	0	33
Coma	28	0	40
LABORATORY			
Elevated serum amylase (> 200 SU/100 ml)	28	50	29
White blood cell count			
> 10,000/mm³	78	100	79
> 15,000/mm³	72	50	50
> 20,000/mm³	33	50	29
Platelet count			
> 400,000/mm³	9	—	27
< 175,000/mm³	55	—	36
Prothrombin time prolonged (> 2 sec)	44	—	36
Serum bilirubin			
> 1.5 mg/100 ml	67	50	36
> 4.0 mg/100 ml	11	0	14
Serum glutamic oxaloacetic transaminase			
> 40 SFU/100 ml	50	50	62
> 150 SFU/100 ml	6	0	0
Serum lactic dehydrogenase			
> 225 IU/liter	81	50	91
> 400 IU/liter	25	0	64
Elevated alkaline phosphatase	39	100	23
Serum albumin			
< 3.5 gm/100 ml	75	0	64
< 2.0 gm/100 ml	13	0	29

From Ranson JHC: Acute pancreatitis. *Curr Probl Surg* 16:1, 1979.
* Table 37-4 defines groups.

computerized axial tomography, and gallium scans have been used to make the diagnosis of intra-abdominal fluid collections and abscesses (Fig. 37-4). Frey et al[1] state the echography is the most helpful tool if the abscess is well walled off.

The diagnosis of biliary calculi can be made by abdominal echography or by percutaneous transhepatic cholangiography (Chapter 35). Transduodenal retrograde endoscopic cholangiopancreatography is generally contraindicated during the acute process, unless emergency endoscopic sphincterotomy is contemplated.

The serum DNase-1 level may be a specific test for pancreatic necrosis. The activity of DNase-1 is higher in the pancreas than in other organs.[75] Patients with acute hemorrhagic pancreatitis showed elevations more than five times the normal DNase activity in the blood. DNase activity does not seem to be as elevated in other pancreatic disorders. A recent report indicates that the elevations of pancreatic isoenzyme of RNase may similarily indicate acute pancreatic necrosis.[76] Serum RNase levels were elevated in 11 of 13 patients who required surgical debridement of necrotic pancreatic tissue or drainage of abscess.

A

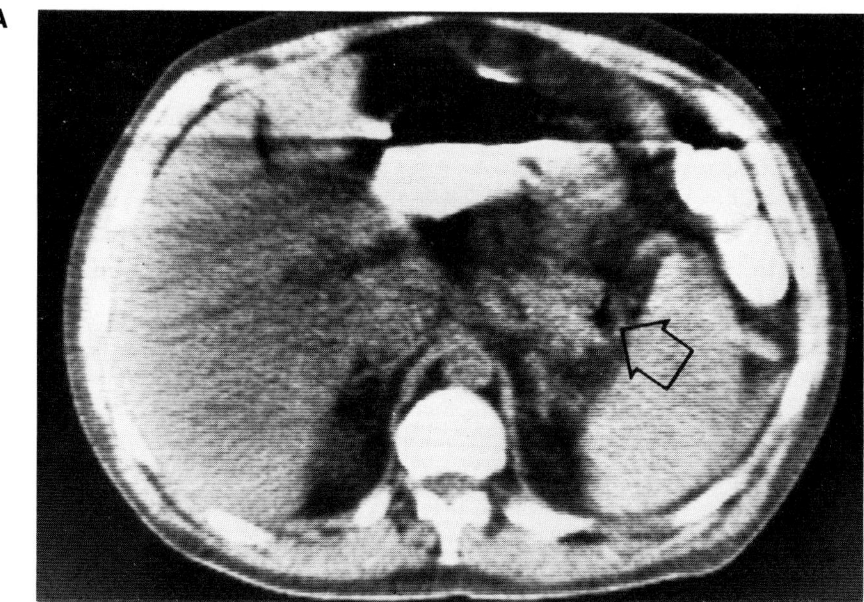

B

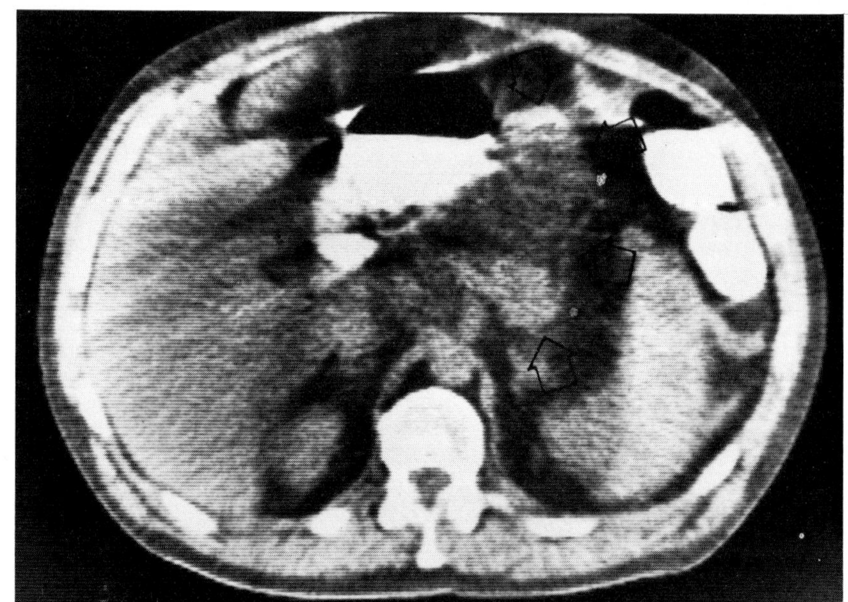

Fig. 37-4. **Computerized axial tomogram of a pancreatic abscess: *A.* showing gas in the tail of the pancreas, and *B.* extension of the abscess into the lesser sac with displacement of the contrast filled stomach.**

The value of the test may be in early detection of pancreatic necrosis and in those needing early debridement or drainage.

Methemoglobinemia or methemalbumin in peritoneal fluid was considered [77] to be highly specific finding in hemorrhagic or necrotic pancreatitis, but the specificity has been questioned.[78] In summary, diagnosis of the pancreatic abscess must be suspected in a patient, following acute pancreatitis or biliary tract surgery, who fails to make satisfactory progress and who also has an inordinate amount of abdominal pain, distension and tenderness, an abdominal mass and persistent fever greater than 101C.

Treatment

Table 37-7 compares the mortality of patients with surgically drained or undrained pancreatic abscesses. Unless correctly diagnosed and promptly treated, pancreatic abscess is almost uniformly fatal. A few spontaneous cures occur when an abscess ruptures into the gastrointestinal tract, usually at the splenic flexure of the colon.[79] This is a rare occurrence, however, since only 47 cases of internal fistula were reported before 1976. It thus appears that adequate surgical drainage is of paramount importance.

TABLE 37-7. MORTALITY IN PANCREATIC ABSCESS

Author	Patients	Overall (percent)	Drained (percent)	Undrained (percent)
Holden [73]	28	40	50	—
Miller [65]	63	53.9	37	100
Altemeier [61]	32	44	14	100
Camer [66]	113	22	17.7	100
Bolooki [71]	74	57	47	100

TABLE 37-8. THE INFLUENCE OF MANAGEMENT OF ACUTE PANCREATITIS ON THE INCIDENCE OF PERIPANCREATIC SEPSIS AND DEATH FROM SEPSIS

	Early Operation		Mean NPO Days		Dead without Sepsis		Sepsis			Death with Sepsis		
	No.	*%*	*< 3 Signs*	*≥ 3 Signs*	*No.*	*%*	*No.*	*%*	*Mean + Signs*	*No.*	*%*	*Mean + Signs*
First 100 patients	21	21	7	12	7	7.0	16	16	2.8	8	8.0	3.8
Second 230 patients *	13	5.7	8	16	2	0.9	5.2	5.2	4.8	8	3.5	5.0

* In the more recent 230 patients, early operation was avoided when possible and nasogastric suction was maintained until all evidence had subsided.
NPO = nil per os.

From Ranson JHC: Acute pancreatitis. *Curr Probl Surg* 16:1, 1979.

Most authors use adjuvant antimicrobial agents, but it is uniformly emphasized that adequate surgical debridement with external drainage is the only appropriate therapy for pancreatic abscess. Frequent reoperations for residual loculations may be required.[67] All authors strongly advise use of soft sump or closed suction drainage rather than stiff drains, to avoid pressure against bowel and major vessels. External drains are brought out through separate stab wounds. Operative placement of the catheters within the lesser sac is advocated because a large phlegmon of the pancreas has sealed off the lesser sac in a large proportion of patients (Fig. 37-5). In the eight patients so treated, there were two deaths. Many authorities [60,80-82] also advocate operative placement of soft rubber sump drains in the peripancreatic bed through the foramen of Winslow to remove the products of pancreatitis, feeling that the quantity and composition of the exudate from the pancreatic inflammation are responsible for the progression of the process. Most authors believe that this type of drainage operation on patients with uncomplicated acute edematous pancreatitis has not increased the mortality rate. However, Ranson has shown reduced mortality in acute pancreatitis by avoiding early surgical intervention and utilizing a prolonged period without oral feedings (Table 37-8). In patients with suspected abscess, formal exploration of the entire peripancreatic retroperitoneum is undertaken, and prolonged wide sump drainage is instituted.

Frey et al [1] point out that necrotic pancreatic tissue may not pass through drain tracts easily so that marsupialization is required.[71] Consequently, early reoperation must be considered if systemic toxicity persists or recurs after drainage of a pancreatic abscess.

The timing of more extensive operations and the necessity for debridement or sequestrectomy for necrotizing hemorrhagic pancreatitis is a controversial issue. Although the reported incidence of septic complications in hemorrhagic pancreatitis is from 47 to 60 percent,[64,83,84] and while all agree that the mortality is high (71 to 82 percent),[85,86] in unoperated patients, people do not agree on how or even when to proceed with resection surgery. Condon and Henry,[87] in a study of hemorrhagic pancreatitis in dogs, were not able to show an increased incidence

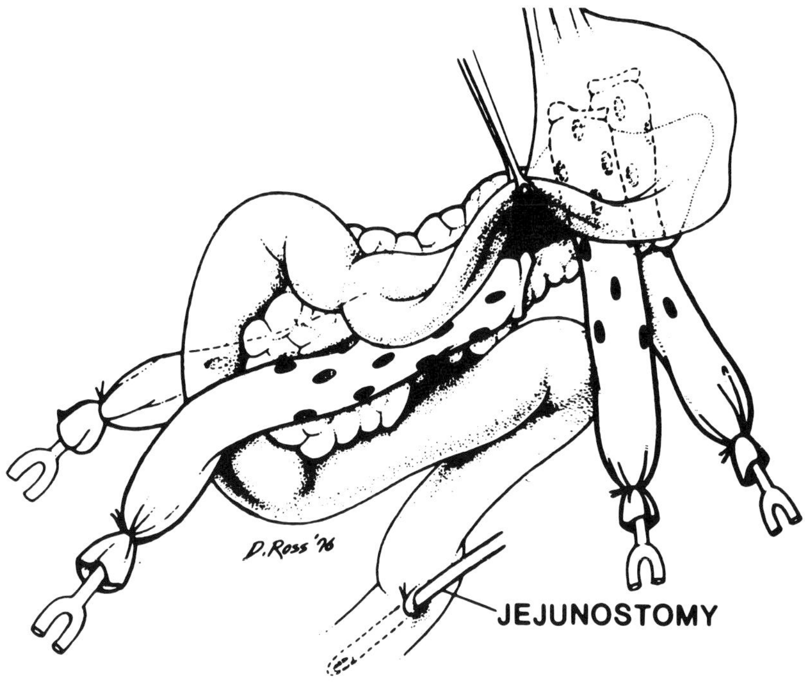

Fig. 37-5. Diagrammatic representation of the technique of wide sump drainage of the peripancreatic retroperitoneum recommended for patients with pancreatic abscesses. (From Ranson JHC: Acute pancreatitis. Curr Probl Surg 16:1, 1979.)

of survival after early subtotal pancreatectomy when compared to the results in controls who had fluid resuscitation.

On the other hand, White and Heimbach [83] reported only a 20 percent mortality in patients after early extensive sequestrectomy in hemorrhagic pancreatitis after failure of the initial operation, which was cholecystostomy with T tube drainage of the common bile duct. These results compare favorably with those obtained with peritoneal dialysis. It would appear that in centers where surgeons have developed the skill and interest in sequestrectomy [88,89] and resection, this method does work—the 30 to 40 percent mortality, however, is still high.

Nasogastric suction or gastrostomy are commonly used, and feeding jejunostomy may be useful because long periods of starvation are inevitable. Antibiotics should be started when abscess or necrosis is suspected against aerobic and anaerobic organisms.[62,71] Penicillin and chloramphenicol or cephalothin and lincomycin are recommended by Warshaw.[64] Steedman et al [62] recommend penicillin in combination with tetracycline, chloramphenicol, or kanamycin. We recommend coverage of the gram-negative enteric flora, with an aminoglycoside (gentamicin, tobramycin, or amikacin) in combination with clindamycin (to eliminate *Bacteroides*) and ampicillin (for enterococci). Modification of this regimen can be made as cultures and sensitivities dictate.

Complications of Pancreatic Abscesses

Table 37-9 reveals the spectrum of complications in 113 infected patients reported by Camer et al.[66] Frequently, complications include pulmonary problems, renal and hepatic failure, massive gastrointestinal hemorrhage, intra-abdominal hemorrhage, and fistula. Infectious complications comprise one-third of all complications.[66] The most common complication of pancreatic abscesses is recurrence of another abscess in the pancreas or retroperitoneum.[61] A second abscess develops in 8.5 to 20 percent of cases.[61,66,67] If not drained, recurrent abscesses may erode into major vessels and lead to lethal hemorrhage.

TABLE 37-9. POSTOPERATIVE COMPLICATIONS OF 113 PATIENTS WITH PANCREATIC ABSCESS

Complication	Patients	Deaths
Peritonitis	2	2
Septic shock	3	3
Septicemia	14	3
Renal failure	12	7
Pleural effusion	29	3
Atelectasis	6	1
Pulmonary embolus	4	2
Bronchopneumonia	6	3
Wound abscess	17	9
Wound dehiscence	3	1
Gastrointestinal hemorrhage	7	6
Intra-abdominal hemorrhage	6	5
Hepatic failure	3	3
Diabetes	14	2
Gastric retention	19	3
Ileus	19	5
Fistula	31	9
Pancreatic	12	
Biliary	4	
Duodenal	6	
Colonic	9	

From Cramer SJ, Tan EGC, Warren KW, Braasch JW: Pancreatic abscess: a critical analysis of 113 cases. Am J Surg 129:426, 1975.

Prevention of Pancreatic Abscess

There are a number of complications of pancreatitis which can result in pancreatitis or peripancreatic infection. Proper management may help prevent infection.

Pseudocysts. Pseudocyst formation (fluid collection in the lesser sac) is a relatively common result of pancreatic necrosis and autodigestion, especially alcoholic pancreatitis.[90,91] A few pseudocysts are secondary to carcinoma,[90] and most contain blood, pancreatic secretions, and tissue debris without an epithelial lining, and most are sterile. About two-thirds of pseudocysts communicate with the ductal system, although poorly. A few communicate with the peritoneal cavity and cause pancreatic ascites. As they enlarge, they may impinge on the lesser peritoneal sac, greater omentum, spleen, left kidney, colon, stomach, common bile duct, duodenum, and mediastinum. Pseudocysts can cause obstruction of the stomach, biliary tract, small bowel, or colon and often erode into the biliary tract or intestine.

Massive hemorrhage and abscess formation are the most feared complications. Septic complications occur in 14 to 40 percent of patients with pseudocysts.[92,93]

Gray scale ultrasonography has a diagnostic accuracy of 75 to 100 percent.[91,93] Computerized tomography and gallium citrate scans can be helpful as well. Retrograde pancreatography has a diagnostic accuracy of approximately 85 percent, but infection of a pseudocyst is an occasional but serious complication. Prophylactic antibiotics should be used during this procedure, and prompt operative drainage of the pseudocyst should follow localization to prevent infection of the cyst.

Treatment is aimed not only at control of symptoms but also at the prevention of complications. In a recent study of 93 patients having a combined clinical and ultrasonic diagnosis of pseudocyst,[92] urgent laparotomy and drainage was done in only 12 percent. Fifty-eight percent received repeated examinations. Twenty percent of these had spontaneous resolution, almost all within 6 weeks. There were no deaths in the 30 percent of patients who underwent elective surgery. Twenty-two patients who were followed expectantly had complications. The interval between the formation of a pseudocyst and development of complications averaged 13.5 weeks. Eleven ruptured into the intestine or peritoneal cavity, seven formed abscess, and four patients developed biliary duct obstruction. Therefore, observation of a pseudocyst for over 7 weeks exposed the patient to an unwarranted risk in which the mortality exceeded that of elective surgery.

Grace [95] followed a similar series of 54 patients with pseudocyst. Forty-eight percent subsequently required one or more hospitalizations for chronic pancreatitis, hemorrhage occurred in 13 percent, and the pseudocyst recurred in 3.8 percent within 3 years. The mortality was

11 percent, mostly as a result of hemorrhage and sepsis. To prevent these complications, cysts greater than 5 cm diameter which do not resolve in 6 weeks should be drained. External drainage (ie, marsupialization) is indicated if the wall of the cyst is thin or if free perforation of the cyst has occurred. Externally drained pseudocysts frequently drain for 9 months to 1 year and present a debilitating problem for the patient,[96] ie, necessity for dressings, skin excoriation, and a 31 percent incidence of complications.[95] There has been some promising experience with percutaneous catheter drainage. Surgeons favor internal drainage of pseudocyst if possible, either by cystogastrostomy or Roux-en-Y cystojejunostomy. Each has its advocates, and there is no intrinsic advantage of one technique over the other.

Anatomic location and adherence or lack of adherence of the pseudocyst will determine which viscus can most conveniently be used to establish drainage internally. Hence, if the pseudocyst wall is firmly attached to the posterior wall of the stomach, cystogastrostomy suffices. If not adherent, then a Roux-en-Y cystojejunostomy should be done. The objectives in either case are that the fistulous opening must be widely patent to permit adequate drainage, and that the cystic cavity not be debrided vigorously or irrigated because of the risk of hemorrhage.

Large bore rubber tubes should not be placed into the cavity for fear of vessel erosion. When pseudocyst hemorrhage occurs, it is not the anastomotic suture line that bleeds but the exposed vessels deep within the cavity that cause the disastrous exsanguinating complications. In multiple pseudocysts, localized to the body and tail of the pancreas, it may be preferable to perform a distal pancreatectomy instead of drainage.

Splenic vein thrombosis can occur as an extension of an inflammatory mass or pseudocyst into the splenic hilus. Sudden enlargement of the spleen, splenic infarction, hematoma, or rupture can all appear. The symptoms are marked by acute intense pain in the left flank and a mass. Abdominal echogram is quite accurate, and arteriography yields a definitive diagnosis.[78,97] Splenic vein thrombosis often causes bleeding from esophageal varices. It is best treated by splenectomy; for pseudocyst or abscess in the tail of the pancreas, a combined distal pancreatectomy and splenectomy is recommended.

Distant fat necrosis can occur in the retroperitoneal mesentery, and also at quite a distance, and can involve pleural, pericardial, and subcutaneous tissues. Fat necrosis in the subcutaneous tissue of the lower extremity indicates an especially serious prognosis. In the retroperitoneum and mesentery, fat necrosis can cause thrombosis of mesenteric vessels, and intestinal infarction or obstruction.[98]

Distal common bile duct obstruction is due to inflammation at the head of the pancreas and causes a smoothly tapering area of stricturing, either at the ampulla or for some length of duct proximal to the ampulla. The diagnosis is established by diffuse enlargement at the head of the pancreas by ultrasonography or CAT scan. Transhepatic cholangiography will rule out choledocholithiasis and yields the definitive diagnosis. ERCP is best avoided during the acute phase for risk of exacerbation of the pancreatitis and cholangitis. Surgical treatment is usually deferred unless there is an infection, because obstruction is temporary and relents in a few weeks.

Respiratory complications include pleural effusion, atelectasis, and pulmonary edema. The pleural effusion is probably the result of lymphatic spread of pancreatic enzymes or exudate through the lymphatic spaces in the diaphragm. A pseudocyst can also rupture into the pleural space, as can an abscess. The fluid has a high amylase content. Interstitial pulmonary edema may be the result of an increase in alveolarcapillary membrane permeability. Liberation of free fatty acids which damage the membrane, or phospholipase A which hydrolyzes lecithin (a normal component of surfactant), lowers the level of surfactant and disrupts alveolar stability. This condition is heralded by a drop in arterial pO_2 and may require assisted ventilation with positive pressure oxygen therapy and tracheostomy.

Coagulation defects, thought to be due to release of proteolytic enzymes such as trypsin in the blood, can lead to disseminated intravascular coagulation and microthrombi.[99,100,101] This is detected by increased fibrin split products, decreases in fibrinogen levels, and increases in prothrombin time.

Treatment of Pancreatitis. Pancreatic abscesses may be prevented by the prompt control of pancreatitis. Unfortunately, however, no specific therapy for pancreatitis exists. Nasogastric decompression and intravenous fluids remain the mainstays of therapy. Leven and Wangensteen [102] showed that feeding of animals with mild pancreatitis results in exacerbation of their diseases. Levant et al [103] questioned the therapeutic value of nasogastric suction, and recent controlled randomized studies in patients with mild acute alcoholic pancreatitis showed no therapeutic gain. Nasogastric decompression to treat ileus, vomiting, and pain, however, will probably never be abandoned.

Aprotinin (Trasylol) was first advanced by Fry (cited by Kirsch et al [104]) in 1933 for treatment of pancreatitis. Reports on its efficacy have been debated, and most prospective randomized studies have not demonstrated a beneficial effect.[104] Trasylol does not prevent amylase elevation or pain after endoscopic retrograde pancreatography,[105] and we have found no inhibiting effect of Trasylol on in vitro enzyme activation.[106]

Insulin infusion has been tried in acute pancreatitis because hormone-sensitive lipase in fat cells may be inhibited by glucose and insulin.[107] Patients given insulin infusions became free of pain in a shorter period of time than controls, but there was no difference between the two groups after 24 hours.[108]

Jejunal feeding of elemental diet in dogs results in enzyme-poor pancreatic secretion. When compared to feedings of blenderized diet, however, the total enzyme outputs are the same.[109] Unfortunately, the data show that the exocrine pancreas will respond to jejunal feedings, so that the merits of bypassing the duodenum with this treatment are of dubious value.

Although experimental studies have indicated therapeutic effect of antibiotics, no evidence has been presented that antibiotics reduce the severity of acute hemorrhagic pancreatitis or lower the incidence of pancreatic abscess.[57,110,111]

Peritoneal dialysis was first used for pancreatitis in 1937, but was discontinued because of an increase in mortality. In 1965, Wall[112] described encouraging results and this treatment has been popularized by Gliedman et al.[113] The benefit from peritoneal dialysis can be attributed as much to removal of enzymes and bacteria from the peritoneal cavity as to the correction of the fluid and electrolyte disturbances. Schmiedin and Sebening[114] obtained positive peritoneal fluid cultures in 53 percent of patients with acute pancreatitis. Ranson et al[70] randomly assigned 10 patients with three or more early signs of severe pancreatitis to peritoneal dialysis or continued conventional care. All five who received dialysis recovered in less than 9 days, whereas two of the other five patients died. Death occurred in 15 percent of dialyzed patients early in Ranson's experience, but in only 3.5 percent of a more recent series. Ranson believed improvement was a result of early identification of severe disease, avoidance of laparotomy, prolongation of nasogastric suction until all inflammation was resolved, early treatment of pulmonary complications, and peritoneal dialysis for severe disease. Some surgeons believe that peritoneal lavage tubes should be placed into the lesser sac to be effective, and that exploration does not exacerbate acute hemorrhagic pancreatitis, although this runs counter to the older views. Rosato et al[115] used dogs to support the hypothesis that the removal of toxic products from the peritoneal cavity by lavage improved survival (24-hour survival was 86 percent versus 33 percent in controls). They advocate utilizing peritoneal lavage as management of severe pancreatitis rather than excision or debridement, reserving surgical treatment for cases when the diagnosis is in doubt or in those patients who fail to improve after lavage. Gliedman[113] believes lavage has not lowered the incidence of necrotic complications and superinfection.

Surgical Treatment for Acute Gallstone Pancreatitis. The final solution to gallstone pancreatitis and its septic complications is elimination of the choledocholithiasis—the controversies revolve around the proper timing of the operation. In one retrospective study, when surgery was delayed, recurrence of pancreatitis forced an emergency readmission in 40 percent of patients, and the average hospital stay was 50 percent longer than for those who had prompt operation.[116] Of 23 patients with prompt operation, only two postoperative complications occurred, and no one died. Most writers argue in favor of an early cholecystectomy in gallstone pancreatitis.[117-119] None of these studies prove the benefit of early operation.

For acute gallstone pancreatitis, the operative techniques are governed by the severity of the process and condition of the patient. The surgeon still tries to decompress the biliary tree and establish free drainage by removal of obstructing stones, whether in the gallbladder or common duct. It may be safer and more expeditious to evacuate stones and decompress the common duct via a cholecystostomy rather than risk the dissection involved in a cholecystectomy in an unstable patient. It may be more efficacious to establish biliary drainage from the common duct with a T tube or a choledochoduodenostomy and leave a stone downstream in a distal common duct than to persist in attempts to remove impacted ampullary stones by repeated traumatic passage of stone forceps, or to forcefully dilate the sphincter of Oddi and thereby exacerbate the pancreatitis.

Endoscopic sphincterotomy has been extensively studied in Japan[120] and Germany[121] and now in this country,[23] with a mortality rate less than 1 percent and a success rate of 80 percent. It is possible to remove small stones 5–15 mm in diameter by endoscopic sphincterotomy. Whether this method will be effective in the treatment of acute gallstone pancreatitis is unknown. Similarly, little is known of the potential efficacy of decompression of the biliary tree via percutaneous transhepatic biliary catheterization.[122]

Prevention of Endoscopic Complications. Most endoscopists now use antibiotics, such as gentamicin, either in the contrast media used in ERCP or systemic antibiotics. Glutaraldehyde and povidone-iodine solutions are effective and permit disinfectant action on the outside of the endoscopes with a contact time of 10 to 30 minutes. More important, the irrigating solutions used in the flushing channels of the scopes should be changed daily and the containers sterilized. We recently reported two near-fatal cases of pancreatitis caused by *Pseudomonas* which contaminated the irrigating solution.

Patients with acute pancreatitis should not undergo ERCP. Acute edematous pancreatitis can be converted to necrotic pancreatitis by the retrograde injection of unsterile contrast into the pancreatic ducts. Pancreatic pseudocysts 5 cm or more in diameter, or which drain poorly into the duct, can safely be injected by ERCP provided that the operation is performed within 24 hours. Additionally, antibiotic coverage with aminoglycoside is needed in all cases of pseudocysts.[94]

POSTOPERATIVE PANCREATIC INFECTIONS

PREVENTION OF POSTOPERATIVE INFECTIONS

Infections of the pancreas or of the peripancreatic tissues occur after operations on the pancreas itself or other organs. In the latter instances, the infection is usually the consequence of postoperative pancreatitis.

Pancreatic Resection

The operation with the highest incidence of pancreatic complications is the partial or near total resection of the pancreas for cancer or chronic pancreatitis (Table 37-10). The complication of fistula and abscess has caused some surgeons to abandon partial pancreatectomy for cancer in favor of total pancreatectomy. In chronic pancreatitis, the pancreas is firm and less likely to fistulize after pancreatic-enteric anastomosis.[38] Abscess formation following partial pancreatectomy has not been prevented by the routine placement of sump or suction drains in the area

TABLE 37-10. INCIDENCE OF COMPLICATIONS AFTER PANCREATIC AND PERIPANCREATIC OPERATIONS

Operation	Author	Number of Patients	Fistula (percent)	Pseudocyst (percent)	Pancreatitis (percent)	Intra-abdominal Abscess (percent)	Wound Infection (percent)
Drainage or resection for trauma	Northrup [54]	523	19	12	—	5	7.8
	Jones [123]	267	4	1	—	20	—
	Karl [124]	25	20	—	16	24	16
Pseudocyst drainage	Shatney [125]	119	4.2	—	7	11.7	8.4
Pancreatic jejunostomy for chronic pancreatitis	Cox [126]	86	3.4	—	—	2	3
Resection for chronic pancreatitis							
Pancreaticoduodenectomy	Braasch [127]	55	1.8	—	—	16	—
Pancreaticoduodenectomy	Frey [68]	19	13	—	—	15	6
40–80% pancreatectomy	Frey [68]	53	16.9	—	—	28.3	2
80–95% pancreatectomy	Frey [68]	77	7.7	—	—	22	11.6
Resection for cancer (pancreaticoduodenectomy)	Braasch [127]	223	8.5	—	2.7	21.5	—
Splenectomy	Brenning [128]	167	—	—	—	4.7	—
	Danforth [129]	185	0.5	—	0.5	4.3	8.1
	Kassum [109]	76	—	—	2.6	10.5	17.1
Common bile duct exploration	Keighley [132]	116	—	—	4.3	2.5	25
	Heimbach [130]	885	—	—	1.9	—	—
	Bardenheier [51]	180	—	—	12.2	—	—
Sphincteroplasty	Schmitt [139]	167	—	—	0.5	—	—
Partial gastrectomy (overall)	Millbourn [50]	147	—	—	10	—	—
	Saidi [137]	3,018	—	—	0.08	—	—
Billroth II reconstruction	Wallensten [138]	1,769	—	—	0.6	—	—
Billroth I reconstruction	Wallensten [138]	605	—	—	0	—	—

of the pancreatic stump anastomosis. Drains should be avoided in the area of pancreatic intestinal anastomosis and should be used prophylactically only to direct a pancreatic fistula to the outside.

Biliary Tract Surgery

Biliary tract surgery with common duct exploration results in a high incidence of pancreatic complications (Table 37-10). Twenty-one percent of Bardenheier's patients with biliary tract operations developed pancreatitis.[51] In White's recent series,[131] 40 percent of postoperative pancreatitis cases were the result of previous common duct explorations. Pancreatitis is undoubtedly caused by traumatic manipulation of the ampullary region with metal dilators and probes. After choledochotomy, Keighley [132] reported a 4 percent incidence of postoperative pancreatitis. A long-limbed T tube placed through the sphincter of Oddi has also been incriminated.[133]

A side-to-side choledochoduodenostomy is sometimes preferable to traumatic disimpaction of common duct stones at the ampulla and may lower the incidence of postoperative pancreatitis.[134,135]

Splenectomy

Splenectomy occasionally (0.5 percent) [136] results in postoperative pancreatitis (Table 37-10). Injuries to the pancreas occur when pancreatic tissue is inadvertently crushed at the splenic hilus during clamping and suture ligature of the vascular pedicle. A more frequent complication of incidental (10.5 percent) [109] or planned splenectomy is the subphrenic abscess. When faced with a large and difficult spleen, the surgeon should remember that vascular control can be first secured by suture ligation of the splenic artery within the lesser sac before he attempts to remove the spleen. The spleen can usually be saved after inadvertent operative trauma—an ideal way to avoid the immediate and late complications. In any case, drainage of the splenectomy bed has no support as a measure to reduce incidence of subphrenic abscess (Chapter 36).

Gastrectomy

The incidence of pancreatitis after gastrectomy may be as high as 10 percent (Table 37-10). Saidi and Donaldson [137] emphasized the dangers of damage to the blood supply of the pancreas in suture ligation of the gastroduodenal or superior pancreaticoduodenal artery in cases of a penetrating duodenal ulcer. We prefer to undermine the adjacent mucosa surrounding the ulcer bed and cover the ulcer defect with normal mucosa, if it cannot be resected.

When confronted with a penetrating bleeding duodenal ulcer at the head of the pancreas, it is safer to locate and ligate the gastroduodenal arteries a few centimeters from the ulcer. The afferent-limb syndrome, or any condition that causes duodenal ileus or obstruction of the duodenal loop after a gastrojejunostomy, is more often associated with pancreatitis than is the Billroth I procedure. Reflux of infected duodenal contents into the ductal systems of the pancreas is the incriminating factor.[138]

Other technical maneuvers that will avoid trauma to

the pancreas during gastrectomy have been described. For example, it is unnecessary to excise the base of a penetrating ulcer at gastrectomy if the duodenal stump can be closed proximal or distal to the ulcer.

No attempt should be made to excise, cauterize, currette, or scrape the ulcer bed. Any openings in the ducts of Wirsung or Santorini which are seen at the surface of the ulcer should be closed carefully with nonabsorbable sutures, but it is not safe to ligate the duct of Santorini. If the anatomy is confusing, insert a rubber tube via a choledochotomy to ensure that the distal common duct is not injured by dissection.[131] The duodenum can also be dissected with the stump open so that the papilla can be visualized. If the duodenal stump is insecure, a decompressing duodenostomy tube or reinforcement with a patch of jejunum can be employed. A controlled duodenal stump fistula is preferable to a ligated pancreatic or biliary duct. The incidence of pancreatitis after gastrectomy is low (0.8 percent), but mortality is distressingly high (29 percent).[137]

In 1,700 Billroth II operations, there were 12 deaths caused by acute postoperative pancreatitis, whereas in 600 Billroth I resections, there were no deaths caused by pancreatitis. Wallensteen [138] attributed this difference in incidence to blind loop stagnation occurring in Billroth II anastomosis.

Sphincterotomy

Sphincterotomy results in pancreatitis only 0.5 to 1.0 percent of the time. At first this seems surprising. According to French authors, acute pancreatitis is more common after laborious or difficult sphincterotomy or sphincteroplasty, necessitating the use of metallic sounds or forceful passages. In certain institutions, the introduction of metallic sounds or dilators is not permitted during sphincterotomy, and the procedure is done over a soft rubber catheter.[139]

PREVENTION OF INFECTION FOLLOWING PANCREATIC TRAUMA

Abdominal exploration should not be done for elevated serum amylase alone. During exploration after trauma, a retroperitoneal hematoma found in the area of the pancreas should always be opened to permit inspection of the pancreas. This may also require mobilization of the duodenum. Small lacerations of the pancreas without ductal disruption can be carefully oversewn with nonabsorbable sutures, and closed suction drainage can be used. If one is not sure a duct has been transected, intravenous secretin may be given, 1 unit per killigram (bolus) and a clear gush of fluid indicates a transected duct. Transections of the main duct may be safely treated in the body by distal pancreatectomy. Pancreaticoduodenectomy is performed only when the head of the gland is completely shattered, and when the duodenum is disrupted. Debridement of the pancreas and resection of badly contused tissue may be necessary to avert subsequent necrosis and abscess. External drainage (preferably filtered sump drains) should be employed following operation for trauma. This may result in external fistula formation but, as pointed out by Northrup and Simmons,[54] a fistula is a desirable alternative to a pseudocyst or abscess becasue most external fistulas will close in a month.

MISCELLANEOUS INFECTIONS OF THE PANCREAS (VIRAL AND HELMINTHIC)

Mumps virus commonly causes mild self-limited pancreatitis. Rarely, chronic pancreatitis can result,[140] and has been reported in about 12 cases worldwide. Although amylase levels are elevated in 95 percent of mumps cases, the isoenzyme is of parotid rather than pancreatic origin.[141]

An unknown percentage of patients with acute pancreatitis have serologic evidence of infection with *Mycoplasma pneumoniae.* According to Hayflick et al,[142] 33 percent of patients with acute pancreatitis had some evidence of *Mycoplasma.* Of 27 consecutive patients with acute pancreatitis studied by Freeman and McMain,[143] nine had evidence of *Mycoplasma* infection by a fourfold or greater rise in antibody titers to *Mycoplasma.* Three patients without changes in *Mycoplasma* titers were shown to have antibody titer rises in Coxsackie virus group B, type II and type III. Whether the rise in antibodies is specific enough to prove infection or whether there was some nonspecific production of antibody is unknown. Other workers have also reported *M. pneumoniae* titer rises in association with acute pancreatitis.[144] Lysolecithin and lipase lyse *Mycoplasma* and should prevent colonization of the pancreatic duct with *Mycoplasma.* The pathogenicity of these organisms needs verification by further studies.

Enterovirus infections have been described in acute pancreatitis. Arnesjö et al [145] studied 91 patients with acute pancreatitis and found evidence of enteroviral infection in 18 (19.8 percent). Seventeen had enterovirus isolated from the feces or urine, and a significant rise in antibody titer was demonstrated in seven of them. The Coxsackie viruses, B-2, B-5, and echoviruses, 6, 11, 20, and 30, were the etiologic agents. When a history of gallstone disease or alcohol has been excluded, the authors conclude that about 9 percent of patients had an enteroviral infection.

Ascariasis is the most frequent helminthic infection in people, and the adult parasites usually live in the jejunum and ileum, producing few symptoms. The most frequent extraintestinal habitat of ascaris is the biliary tract, and this can cause biliary pain and obstructive jaundice. Pancreatitis and severe cholangitis also have been reported.[146] The ascaris has a powerful trypsin and lipase inhibitor, which protects it from the action of pancreatic juice.

Fifty cases of ascaris blocking the duct of Wirsung have been reported.[90] Retrograde endoscopic studies outline the parasite clearly and are now a valuable method in the diagnosis of this disease.[147]

The systemic effects of the sting of the Trinidad scorpion can cause fatal pancreatitis, especially in children. The symptoms resemble that of an acute cholinergic crisis,[148] and the treatment has been nonspecific supportive care. In our own laboratory,[149] Dressel has demonstrated that acute pancreatitis results from intoxication with the anticholinesterase type of insecticides which cause cholinergic crisis. The mechanism appears to be inhibition of a cholinesterase that is synthesized within the acinar cells.

BIBLIOGRAPHY

Frey CF, Lindenauer SM, Miller TA: Pancreatic abscess. Surg Gynecol Obstet 149:722, 1979.

Gambill EE (ed): Pancreatitis. St. Louis, Mosby, 1973.

Howard JM, Jordan GL Jr: Surgical Diseases of the Pancreas. Philadelphia, Lippincott, 1960.

Ranson JHC: Acute pancreatitis. Curr Probl Surg 16:1, 1979.

Ranson JHC, Spencer FC: Prevention, diagnosis, and treatment of pancreatic abscess. Surgery 82:99, 1977.

Wolfson P: Surgical management of inflammatory disorders of the pancreas. Surg Gynecol Obstet 151:689, 1980.

REFERENCES

1. Frey CF, Lindenauer SM, Miller TA: Pancreatic abscess. Surg Gynecol Obstet 149:722, 1979.
2. Rösch W, Koch H, Demling L: Manometric studies during ERCP and endoscopic papillotomy. Endoscopy 8:30, 1976.
3. Mairose UB, Wurbs D, Classen M: Santorini's duct—an insignificant variant from normal or an important overflow valve? Endoscopy 10:24, 1978.
4. Mosely JG, Fox JN, Reber HA: Aspirin secretion by the pancreas: effect on the pancreatic duct mucosal barrier. Surgery 86:17, 1979.
5. Elmslie R: The effect of bile on the activation of trypsinogen and the activity of trypsin in pancreatic juice. Br J Surg 52:465, 1965.
6. Allan BJ, White TT: Bile pancreatic cancer, and the activation of pancreatic juice. Biochem Biophys Res Comm 79:485, 1977.
7. Bainbridge FA: The lymph-flow from the pancreas. J Physiol 32:1, 1905.
8. Gorbach SL, Tabaqchali S: Bacteria, bile and the small bowel. Gut 10:963, 1969.
9. Engström J, Hellström K: The duodenal microflora in relation to various symptoms and manifestations in patients with extrahepatic biliary disease. Acta Med Scand 193:267, 1973.
10. Percy-Robb IW, Collee JG: Bile acids: a pH dependent antibacterial system in the gut? Br Med J 3:813, 1972.
11. Felsenfeld O, Gyr K: Action of some pancreatic enzymes on *Vibrio cholerae.* Med Microbiol Immunol (Berl) 163(1):53, 1977.
12. Hadorn B, Hess J, Troesch V, Verhaage W, Götze H, Bender SW: Role of bile acids in the activation of trypsinogen by enterokinase: disturbance of trypsinogen activation in patients with intrahepatic biliary atresia. Gastroenterology 66:548, 1974.
13. Osnes M, Myren J, Lötveit T, Swensen T: Juxtapapillary duodenal diverticula and abnormalities by endoscopic retrograde cholangio-pancreatography (ERCP). Scand J Gastroenterol 12:347, 1977.
14. Gregg JA: Pancreas divisum: its association with pancreatitis. Am J Surg 134:539, 1977.
15. Rösch W, Koch H, Schaffner O, Demling NL: The clinical significance of the pancreas divisum. Gastrointest Endosc 22:206, 1976.
16. Malik SA, Van Kley H, Knight WA Jr: Inherited defect in hereditary pancreatitis. Am J Dig Dis 22:999, 1977.
17. Robechek PJ: Hereditary chronic relapsing pancreatitis: a clue to pancreatitis in general? Am J Surg 11:819, 1967.
18. Opie EL: The etiology of acute hemorrhagic pancreatitis. Bull Johns Hopkins Hosp 12:182, 1901.
19. Howard JM, Jordan GL Jr: Surgical Diseases of the Pancreas. Philadelphia, Lippincott, 1960.
20. Nielsen ML, Asnaes S, Justesen T: Susceptibility of the liver and biliary tract to anaerobic infection in extrahepatic biliary tract obstruction. III. Possible synergistic effect between anaerobic and aerobic bacteria. An experimental study in rabbits. Scand J Gastroenterol 11:263, 1976.
21. England DM, Rosenblatt JE: Anaerobes in human biliary tracts. J Clin Microbiol 6:494, 1977.
22. Keighley MRB: Micro-organisms in the bile: a preventable cause of sepsis after biliary surgery. Ann R Coll Surg Engl 59:328, 1977.
23. Vennes JA, Silvis SE: Endoscopic sphincterotomy with electrocoagulation. Gastrointest Endosc 22:236, 1976.
24. Gregg JA: Detection of bacterial infection of the pancreatic ducts in patients with pancreatitis and pancreatic cancer during endoscopic cannulation of the pancreatic duct. Gastroenterology 73:1005, 1977.
25. Konok GP, Thompson AG: Pancreatic ductal mucosa as a protective barrier in the pathogenesis of pancreatitis. Am J Surg 117:18, 1969.
26. Hansson K: Experimental and clinical studies in aetiologic role of bile reflux in acute pancreatitis. Acta Chir Scand 375:1, 1967.
27. Lee PC, Nakashima Y, Appert HE, Howard JM: Lipase and colipase in canine pancreatic juice as etiologic factors in fat necrosis. Surg Gynecol Obstet 148:39, 1979.
28. Thal A: Studies of pancreatitis. II. Acute pancreatic necrosis produced experimentally by the arthus sensitization reaction. Surgery 37:911, 1955.
29. Thal A, Brackney E: Acute hemorrhagic pancreatic necrosis produced by local Schwartzman reaction: experimental study on pancreatitis. JAMA 155:569, 1954.
30. Thal A, Molestina JE: Studies on pancreatitis. III. Fulminating hemorrhagic pancreatic necrosis produced by means of staphylococcal toxin. Arch Pathol 60:212, 1955.
31. Byrne JJ, Joison J: Bacterial regurgitation in experimental pancreatitis. Am J Surg 107:317, 1964.
32. Lewis FJ, Wangensteen OH: Antibiotics in the treatment of experimental acute hemorrhagic pancreatitis in dogs. Soc Exp Biol Med Proc 74:453, 1950.
33. Nance FC, Cain JL: Studies of hemorrhagic pancreatitis in germ-free dogs. Gastroenterology 55:368, 1968.
34. Tseng A, Sales DJ, Simonowitz DA, Enker WE: Pancreas abscess: a fatal complication of endoscopic cholangiopancreatography (ERCP). Endoscopy 9:250, 1977.
35. Helgerson R: Unpublished data.
36. Sarles H: Alcohol and the pancreas. Ann NY Acad Sci 252:171, 1975.
37. Breckenridge WC, Little JA, Steiner G, Chow A, Poapst M: Hypertriglyceridemia associated with deficiency of apolipoprotein C-11. N Engl J Med 298(23):1265, 1978.
38. Jones DP, Losowsky MS, Davidson CS, Lieber CS: Low plasma lipoprotein lipase activity as a factor in the pathogenesis of alcoholic hyperlipemia. J Clin Invest 42:945, 1963.
39. Gennes JL, Turpin G, Truffert J: Les pancréatites des hyperlipidémies idiopathiques. Etude d'une série personnelle de 40 cas. Ann Med Interne (Paris) 125:333, 1974.
40. Sarles H, Sahel J: Pathology of chronic calcifying pancreatitis. Am J Gastroenterol 66:117, 1976.
41. Dressel, Goodale: Unpublished observations.

42. Cameron JL, Zuidema GD, Margolis S: A pathogenesis for alcoholic pancreatitis. Surgery 77:754, 1975.
43. Estevenon JP, Figarella C, Sarles H: Lactoferrin in the duodenal juice of patients with chronic calcifying pancreatitis. Scand J Gastroenterol 10:327, 1975.
44. Call T, Malarkey WB, Thomas FB: Acute pancreatitis secondary to furosemide with associated hyperlipidemia. Am J Dig Dis 22:835, 1977.
45. Cope O, Culver PJ, Mixter CG, Nardi GL: Pancreatitis, a diagnostic clue to hyperparathyroidism. Ann Surg 145:857, 1957.
46. Jackson CE: Hereditary hyperparathyroidism associated with recurrent pancreatitis. Ann Intern Med 49:829, 1958.
47. Carone FA, Liebow AA: Acute pancreatic lesions in patients treated with ACTH and adrenal corticoids. N Engl J Med 257:690, 1957.
48. Corrodi P, Knablauch M, Binswanger U, Schölzel E, Largiader F: Pancreatitis after renal transplantation. Gut 16:285, 1975.
49. Robinson DO, Alp MH, Grant AK, Lawrence JR: Pancreatitis and renal disease. Scand J Gastroenterol 12:17, 1977.
50. Millbourn E: On acute pancreatic affections following gastric resection for ulcer or cancer and the possibilities of avoiding them. Acta Chir Scand 98:1, 1949.
51. Bardenheier JA, Kaminski DL, Willmam VL: Pancreatitis after biliary tract surgery. Am J Surg 116:773, 1968.
52. White TT, Slavotinek AH: Results of surgical treatment of chronic pancreatitis. Report of 142 cases. Ann Surg 189:217, 1979.
53. Baggenstoss AH: Pathology of pancreatitis. In Gambill EE (ed): Pancreatitis. St. Louis, Mosby, 1973, p 183.
54. Northrup WF III, Simmons RL: Pancreatic trauma: a review. Surgery 71:27, 1972.
55. Shires T: Management of pancreatic injuries. In Najarian JS, Delaney JP (eds): Critical Surgical Care. New York, Symposia Specialists, 1977, p 109.
56. Bockman DE: Route of flow and micropathology resulting from retrograde intrabiliary injection of India ink and ferritin in experimental animals. Gastroenterology 67:324, 1974.
57. Howard JM, Smith AK, Peters JJ: Acute pancreatitis: pathways of enzymes into the blood stream. Surgery 26:161, 1949.
58. Nabseth DC, Goodale RL, Reif AE: Studies on the effect of intragastric cooling on acute experimental pancreatitis. Surgery 47:542, 1960.
59. Sim DN, Duprez A, Anderson MC: Alterations of the lymphatic circulation during acute experimental pancreatitis. Surgery 60:1175, 1966.
60. Evans FC: Pancreatic abscess. Am J Surg 117:537, 1969.
61. Altemeier WA, Alexander JW: Pancreatic abscess: a study of 32 cases. Arch Surg 87:80, 1963.
62. Steedman RA, Doering R, Carter R: Surgical aspects of pancreatic abscess. Surg Gynecol Obstet 125:757, 1967.
63. Lutwick LI: Pancreatic abscess with *Haemophilus influenza* and *Eikenella corrodens*. JAMA 236:2091, 1976.
64. Warshaw AL: Current concepts: pancreatic abscesses. N Engl J Med 287:1234, 1972.
65. Miller TA, Lindenauer SM, Frey CF, Stanley JC: Pancreatic abscess. Arch Surg 108:545, 1974.
66. Camer SJ, Tan EGC, Warren KW, Braasch JW: Pancreatic abscess: critical analysis 113 cases. Am J Surg 129:426, 1975.
67. Grace SG, State D: Septic complications of pancreatitis. Br J Surg 63:229, 1976.
68. Frey CF, Child CG III, Fry W: Pancreatectomy for chronic pancreatitis. Ann Surg 184:403, 1976.
69. Ranson JHC: Acute pancreatitis. Curr Probl Surg 16:1, 1979.
70. Ranson JHC, Rifkind DM, Turner JW: Prognostic signs and nonoperative peritoneal lavage in acute pancreatitis. Surg Gynecol Obstet 143:209, 1976.
71. Bolooki H, Jaffe B, Gliedman ML: Pancreatic abscesses and lesser omental sac collections. Surg Gynecol Obstet 126:1301, 1968.
72. Kune GA: Abscesses of the pancreas. Aust NZ J Surg 38:125, 1968.
73. Holden JL, Berne TV, Rosoff L: Pancreatic abscess following acute pancreatitis. Arch Surg 111:858, 1976.
74. Owens BJ III, Hamit HF: Pancreatic abscess and pseudocyst. Arch Surg 112:42, 1977.
75. Kowlessar OD, McEvoy RK: Desoxyribonuclease I activity in pancreatic disease. J Clin Invest 35:1325, 1956.
76. Warshaw AL, Lee KH: Serum ribonuclease elevations and pancreatic necrosis in acute pancreatitis. Surgery 86:227, 1979.
77. Winstone NE: Methaemalbumin in acute pancreatitis. Br J Surg 52:804, 1965.
78. Banks PA: Acute pancreatitis. Gastroenterology 61:382, 1971.
79. Henderson JM, MacDonald JAE: Fistula formation complicating pancreatic abscess. Br J Surg 63:233, 1976.
80. Ranson JHC, Spencer FC: Prevention, diagnosis, and treatment of pancreatic abscess. Surgery 82:99, 1977.
81. Paloyan D, Simonowitz D, Bates RJ: Guidelines in management of patients with pancreatic abscess. Am J Gastroenterol 69:97, 1978.
82. Waterman NG, Walsky R, Kasdan M, Abrams BL: The treatment of acute hemorrhagic pancreatitis by sump drainage. Surg Gynecol Obstet 126:963, 1968.
83. White TT, Heimbach DM: Sequestrectomy and hyperalimentation in the treatment of hemorrhagic pancreatitis. Am J Surg 132:270, 1976.
84. Leger L, Chiche B, Moullé P, Louvel A: Pancreatic necrosis and acute pancreatitis. Int Surg 63:41, 1978.
85. Foster PD, Ziffren SE: Severe acute pancreatitis. Arch Surg 85:252, 1962.
86. Jacobs ML, Daggett WM, Civetta JM, Yasu MA, Lawson DW, Warshaw AL, Nardi GL, Bartlett MK: Acute pancreatitis: analysis of factors influencing survival. Ann Surg 185:43, 1977.
87. Condon RE, Henry LG: Ablative surgery for necrotizing pancreatitis. Am J Surg 131:125, 1976.
88. Alexandre JH, Chambon H, de Hochepied F: La pancréatectomie totale dans la pancréatite aiguë nécrosante et hémorragique. J Chir (Paris) 110:405, 1975.
89. Norton L, Eiseman B: Near total pancreatectomy for hemorrhagic pancreatitis. Am J Surg 127:191, 1974.
90. Gambill EE, Baggenstoss AH, Priestley JH: Chronic relapsing pancreatitis. Fate of fifty-six patients first encountered in the years 1939 to 1943, inclusive. Gastroenterology 39:404, 1960.
91. Bradley EL, Gonzalez AC, Clements JL: Acute pancreatic pseudocysts: incidence and implications. Ann Surg 184:734, 1976.
92. Bradley EL, Clements JL, Gonzalez AC: The natural history of pancreatic pseudocyst: a unified concept of management. Am J Surg 137:135, 1979.
93. Ravelo HR, Aldrete JS: Analysis of 45 patients with pseudocysts of the pancreas treated surgically. Surg Gynecol Obstet 148:735, 1979.
94. Sugawa C, Walt AJ: Endoscopic retrograde pancreatography in the surgery of pancreatic pseudocysts. Surgery 86:639, 1979.
95. Grace RR, Jordan PH Jr: Unresolved problems of pancreatic pseudocysts. Ann Surg 184:16, 1976.
96. Parshall WA, Remine WH: Internal drainage of pseudocysts

of pancreas. Arch Surg 91:480, 1965.
97. Moreaux J, Bismuth H: Les complications splénique des pancréatities chroniques: a propos de cinco observations. Presse Med 77:1467, 1969.
98. Collins JJ, Peterson LM, Wilson RE: Small intestinal infarction as a complication of pancreatitis. Ann Surg 167:433, 1968.
99. Anderson MC, Schiller WR: Microcirculatory dynamics in the normal and inflamed pancreas. Am J Surg 115:118, 1968.
100. Kwaan HC, Anderson MC, Gramatica L: A study of pancreatic enzymes as a factor in the pathogenesis of disseminated intravascular coagulation during acute pancreatitis. Surgery 69:663, 1971.
101. Ranson JHC, Lackner H, Berman IR, Schinella R: The relationship of coagulation factors to clinical complications of acute pancreatitis. Surgery 81:502, 1977.
102. Leven NL, Wangensteen OH: Effect of gastrostomy feedings on occurrence of experimental acute pancreatic necrosis after ampullary obstruction. Soc Exp Biol Med Proc 27:965, 1930.
103. Levant JA, Secrist DM, Resin H, Sturdevant RAL, Guth PH: Nosogastric suction in the treatment of alcoholic pancreatitis: a controlled study. JAMA 229:51, 1974.
104. Kirsch A, Werner U, Weckner W: Etude prospective des résultats comparés du traitement des pancréatites aiguës avec ou sans inhibiteurs de protéinases. Lyon Chir 71:306, 1975.
105. Brust R, Thomson ABR, Wensel RH, Sherbaniuk RW, Costopoulos L: Pancreatic injury following ERCP: failure of prophylactic benefit of Trasylol. Gastrointest Endosc 24:77, 1977.
106. Goodale RL, Condie RM, Dressel TD, Taylor TN, Gajl-Peczalska K: A study of secretory proteins, cytology and tumor site in pancreatic cancer. Ann Surg 189:340, 1979.
107. Carlson LA: Inhibition of the mobilization of free fatty acids from adipose tissue. Physiological aspects on the mechanisms for the inhibition of mobilization of FFA from adipose tissue. Ann NY Acad Sci 131:119, 1965.
108. Svensson JO: Role of intravenously infused insulin in the treatment of acute pancreatitis: a double-blind study. Scand J Gastroenterol 10:487, 1975.
109. Kassum D, Thomas EJ: Morbidity and mortality of incidental splenectomy. Can J Surg 20:209, 1977.
110. Finch WT, Sawyers JL, Schenker S: A prospective study to determine the efficacy of antibiotics in acute pancreatitis. Ann Surg 183:667, 1976.
111. Kodesch R, DuPont HL: Infectious complications of acute pancreatitis. Surg Gynecol Obstet 136:763, 1973.
112. Wall AJ: Peritoneal dialysis in the treatment of severe acute pancreatitis. Med J Aust 2:281, 1965.
113. Gliedman ML, Bolooki H, Rosen RG: Acute pancreatitis. Curr Probl Surg VII:1, 1970.
114. Schmieden V, Sebening W: Chirugie die pankreas. Arch Klin Chir 148:319, 1927.
115. Rosato EF, Mullis WF, Rosato FE: Peritoneal lavage therapy in hemorrhagic pancreatitis. Surgery 74:106, 1973.
116. Paloyan D, Simonowitz D, Skinner DB: The timing of biliary tract operations in patients with pancreatitis associated with gallstones. Surg Gynecol Obstet 141:737, 1975.
117. Kelly TR: Gallstone pancreatitis. Arch Surg 109:294, 1974.
118. Dixon JA, Hillam JD: Surgical treatment of biliary tract disease associated with acute pancreatitis. Am J Surg 120:371, 1970.
119. Glenn F, Frey C: Re-evaluation of the treatment of pancreatitis associated with biliary tract disease. Ann Surg 160:723, 1964.
120. Kawai K, Akasaka Y, Murakami K, Tada M, Kohli Y, Nakajima M: Endoscopic sphincterotomy of the ampulla of Vater. Gastrointest Endosc 20:148, 1974.
121. Classen M, Demling L: Endoskopische sphinkterotomie der papilla vateri und steinextraktion aus dem ductus choledochus. Dtsch Med Wochenschr 99:469, 1974.
122. Ring EJ, Oleaga JA, Freiman DB, Husted JW, Lunderquist A: Therapeutic applications of catheter cholangiography. Radiology 128:333, 1978.
123. Jones R: Management of pancreatic trauma. Ann Surg 187:555, 1978.
124. Karl HW, Chandler JG: Mortality and morbidity of pancreatic surgery. Am J Surg 134:549, 1977.
125. Shatney CH, Lillehei RC: Surgical treatment of pancreatic pseudocysts. Analysis of 119 cases. Ann Surg 189:386, 1979.
126. Cox WD, Gillespie WJ: Longitudinal pancreaticojejunostomy in alcoholic pancreatitis. Arch Surg 94:469, 1967.
127. Braasch JW, Grey BN: Considerations that lower pancreatoduodenectomy mortality. Am J Surg 133:480, 1977.
128. Brenning G, Johansson H: Splenectomy: a surgical panorama. Uppsala J Med Sci 81:28, 1976.
129. Danforth DN, Thorbjarnson B: Incidental splenectomy: a review of the literature and the New York Hospital experience. Ann Surg 183:124, 1976.
130. Heimbach DM, White TT: Immediate and long term effects of instrumental dilation of the sphincter of Oddi. Surg Gynecol Obstet 148:79, 1978.
131. White TT, Heimbach DM: Sequestrectomy and hyperalimentation in the treatment of hemorrhagic pancreatitis. Am J Surg 132:270, 1976.
132. Keighley MRB, Burdon DW, Baddeley RM, Dorricott NJ, Oates GD, Watts GT, Alexander-Williams J: Complications of supraduodenal choledochotomy: a comparison of three methods of management. Br J Surg 63:754, 1976.
133. Smith SW, Barker WF, Kaplan L: Acute pancreatitis following transampullary biliary drainage. Surgery 30:695, 1951.
134. Burgess JN, Kidd HA: Choledochoduodenostomy in treatment of chronic pancreatitis and choledocholithiasis. Br Med J 2:607, 1967.
135. Capper WM: External choledochoduodenostomy, an evaluation of 125 cases. Br J Surg 49:292, 1961.
136. Danforth DN Jr, Throbjarnarson B: Incidental splenectomy: a review of the literature and the New York Hospital experience. Ann Surg 183:124, 1976.
137. Saidi F, Donaldson GA: Acute pancreatitis following distal gastrectomy for benign ulcer. Am J Surg 105:87, 1963.
138. Wallensten S: Acute pancreatitis and hyperdiastasuria after partial gastrectomy. Acta Chir Scand 115:182, 1958.
139. Schmitt JC, Mathieu P, Seror J: Notre expérience de la sphinctérotomie d'indication biliare. A propos de 167 observations. Ann Chir 30:447, 1976.
140. Wood CB, Bradbrook RA, Blumgart LH: Chronic pancreatitis in childhood associated with mumps virus infection. Br J Clin Pract 28:67, 1974.
141. Levitt M: Personal communication.
142. Hayflick L, Weyer EM, Kraus M, Sussel K, LaMirende AG (eds): Biology of the mycoplasma. Ann NY Acad Sci 143:1, 1967.
143. Freeman R, McMahon MJ: Acute pancreatitis and serological evidence of infection with microplasma pneumoniae. Gut 19:367, 1978.
144. Mardh PA, Ursing B: The occurrence of acute pancreatitis in *Mycoplasma pneumoniae* infection. Scand J Infect Dis 6:167, 1974.
145. Arnesjö B, Edén T, Ihse I, Nordenfelt E, Ursing B: Enterovirus infections in acute pancreatitis: a possible etiological connection. Scand J Gastroenterol 11:645, 1976.
146. Ramirez-Degollado J, Peniche-Bojorquez J, Olvera-Perez O:

Endoscopic cholangiographic diagnosis of ascaris in the common bile duct. Gastrointest Endosc 24:86, 1977.

147. Dobrilla G, Valentini M, Filippini M: A case of common bile duct ascariasis diagnosed by duodenoscopy. Endoscopy 8:211, 1976.

148. Bartholomew C, McGeeney KF: Experimental studies on the etiology of acute scorpion pancreatitis. Br J Surg 63:807, 1976.

149. Dressel TD, Goodale RL, Arneson MA, Borner BA: Pancreatitis as a complication of anticholinesterase insecticide intoxication. Ann Surg 189:199, 1979.

CHAPTER 38
Infections of the Upper Gastrointestinal Tract

M. David Tilson

Whereas a human being consists of approximately 10^{13} cells, he harbors an indigenous flora of 10^{14} microbes.[1] These organisms reside largely in the gastrointestinal tract, where they divide on the average of once each day, a rate much lower than the maximum possible. If maximal growth were permitted, the microflora would overwhelm the body in less than a day.[2]

The number and importance of the gastrointestinal microflora were underestimated until recently. The development and increasing use of anaerobic bacteriologic techniques, however, have led to a rapid growth of knowledge in this field. Anaerobic techniques permit the culture of microorganisms in an oxygen-free, high carbon dioxide atmosphere, so that it is now estimated 95 percent of the bacterial species in the gastrointestinal tract can be cultured. Indeed, culture techniques have jumped ahead of taxonomy, and a greater number of species can now be identified and cultured than can be classified. Estimates of the number of species from the gastrointestinal tract of a single person ranges between 200 and 500.[1]

Of significance to the general public health and underscoring the importance of continuing investigation of the intestinal microflora is the fact that gastrointestinal infection causes 200 million work days lost per year in the United States at a cost of 20 billion dollars.[3] In consideration of the problem of gastrointestinal infection worldwide, it has been estimated that there is enough diarrhea in a single day to equal the effluent over Victoria Falls in a minute.[4]

This chapter will deal with the microbiology of the stomach and small intestine, the mechanisms by which the flora is regulated, the consequences of breakdown of specific host defense mechanisms, and the disease entities and syndromes resulting from microbial overgrowth or infection of these organs.

MICROBIAL ECOLOGY OF THE UPPER GASTROINTESTINAL TRACT

ANATOMIC CONSIDERATIONS

Gross Features

The anatomic features of the stomach and small bowel most relevant to a discussion of surgical microbiology are the sphincters. Little importance has been attached to the lower esophageal sphincter as a mechanism of microbiologic significance, but the pylorus, ileocecal valve, and sphincter of Oddi play important roles. Of these three, the ileocecal valve is probably the most significant. The ileocecal valve is a physiologically important sphincter, and to some extent it isolates the small bowel from the fecal flora of the colon. Insofar as it also retards the passage of intestinal contents into the colon, the distal ileum becomes the only area of the small bowel with any significant stasis. Thus, according to some authorities, the ileum is the only locus within the upper gastrointestinal tract with any appreciable colonization by a nontransient or indigenous flora.[1] In this regard, the distal ileum is that segment most often directly involved in infectious processes.

The pylorus is a sphincter of obvious physiologic importance, which also plays a role in the regulation of the microflora by prolonging the exposure of the gastric contents to the bactericidal effects of gastric acid. When this sphincter is bypassed by gastroenterostomy, in conjunction with vagotomy to reduce gastric acid secretion, some investigators have found significant changes in the proximal flora while others have not. Subtotal gastrectomy almost always results in some degree of bacterial overgrowth, but it has been difficult to determine how much is due to loss of the sphincter and how much to reduced gastric acid.

The sphincter of Oddi probably serves to prevent colonization of the biliary tract and pancreas. Under conditions of bacterial overgrowth in the proximal small intestine (10^9 organisms per ml jejunal contents), clinical infection of the normal biliary tract is rare.

Microscopic and Fine Structure

The villous configuration of the small intestinal mucosa provides a surface of interstices and niches where bacteria may grow without being washed along with the lumen contents. Similarly, the glycolcalyx of the microvillous membrane is a mucous layer on the surface of the epithelial cells harboring a portion of the total flora. These organisms are not easily dislodged from this layer even by repeated washings. Culture of biopsy specimens from the surface epithelium yields a similar spectrum of organisms to that isolated from the lumen. Since peristalsis and pH are not effective in regulating the flora in immediate association with the epithelial cells, control of the microflora at this level of fine structure may be accomplished primarily by local immune mechanisms and the secretory immunoglobulins. These matters will be discussed in greater detail, along with the mechanisms for microbial attachment to the epithelium.

HOST DEFENSES

Physiologic Defenses

The primary mechanisms by which the gastrointestinal flora are controlled are the secretion of acid by the stomach and intestinal peristalsis. For example, if the transit time through the lumen were less than the doubling time of bacteria, it would not be possible to have any microbial residents except for those species that can attach to the intestinal wall. In addition, since a high concentration of hydrogen ion is bactericidal to most swallowed organisms, the acid environment of the stomach provides an environment that is relatively free of microorganisms. The lymphoid system and metabolic conditions prevailing in the lumen are only involved in the fine ecologic tuning of the intestinal microflora.

The natural defenses are so efficient that it has been difficult to simulate infectious diseases of the gastrointestinal tract using laboratory models. Since most pathogens are acid-sensitive, it is usually necessary to bypass the stomach by direct inoculation of the organism under study into the small intestine. Opiates have also been administered to animals to reduce peristalsis to initiate infection, and other manipulations have been used to reduce gastric acid.

Gastric Acid

The importance of the secretion of gastric acid in protecting the gastrointestinal tract from bacteria was postulated more than 50 years ago. Patients with normal secretion of gastric acid rarely have any appreciable number of microbes in the empty stomach. Swallowed food protects swallowed organisms, however, and hypochlorhydric stomachs are always colonized, as are those effectively treated with antacids or cimetidine.[5] In infants with chronic diarrhea, high bacterial counts and a high pH coexist in the stomach.[6]

The gastric juice has been examined repeatedly for evidence of other bactericidal mechanisms in addition to gastric acid. Bactericidal substances have been reported in the stomachs of suckling rabbits, but the evidence is limited. Some investigators have found that breast-fed babies have a higher gastric pH than bottle-fed babies, but the bacterial count remains low in the breast-fed infant. This finding has been taken to suggest that there are also bactericidal factors in breast milk that are as yet unidentified.[6] Other investigators have claimed that the breast-fed baby has a lower gastric pH, a higher redox potential, and an increase in the anaerobic lactobacterial flora. This state of affairs is possibly consistent with an increased resistance to pathogens, but again the evidence is inconclusive.

Intestinal Peristalsis

Beyond the pylorus, the most important factor in microbial control is peristalsis. Almost all predispositions toward clinically significant bacterial overgrowth in the small intestine are related to interference of one sort or another with peristalsis. A vast increase in intestinal microorganisms occurs in intestinal obstruction in animals and in man. Furthermore, after operations for the relief of intestinal obstruction, the intraluminal bacterial counts remain high until peristalsis returns. Then, the counts fall precipitously.[7] As important as peristalsis is, however, it probably cannot remove organisms with an efficient mechanism for epithelial attachment, so that other mechanisms of control probably come into play against certain pathogens.

Other Physiologic Factors

In addition to peristalsis and pH, the general physiologic and metabolic conditions in the gastrointestinal tract obviously dictate the kind of flora that can survive. Most bacteria thrive at 37C; thus, temperature is not a selective regulatory factor. The oxygen tension is so low all the way along the gastrointestinal tract that anaerobic species have a decisive advantage. For any species to survive in the stomach, it must tolerate a low pH. For a species to survive in the small intestine, it must accommodate to an alkaline environment. The nutritional requirements of indigenous flora are not comprehensively worked out, but it is obvious that for a species to thrive it must be able to satisfy its nutritional requirements from partially digested food, from secretions and desquamated cells, or from the metabolic products of other bacteria. Similarly, the distribution of bile acids and their state of conjugation are relevant to the species of bacteria that may survive. Bile acids are absent from the stomach, conjugated in the small intestine, and unconjugated in the colon.

Although the relationship of diet to the microflora, and in particular the possible changes in bile salt levels induced by diet, have been widely studied, so far there is little evidence to confirm early claims that the diet can alter the microflora. Indeed, some have reported that humans and other species of animals can tolerate drastic alterations in the diet without significant changes in the flora.[1] It is obvious that bacteria need never be vegetarians, since approximately 100 gm of epithelial cells slough into the lumen each day.

Dietary factors may be related to resistance to particular pathogens. An interesting example of this phenomenon has come from New Guinea, where enteritis necroticans caused by *C. perfringens* type C is endemic. The organism is 100 percent lethal in guinea pigs when inoculated into the stomachs along with raw sweet potatoes. However, when inoculated alone or with baked sweet potato, the animals are not infected. The raw sweet potato has a trypsin inhibitor that is believed to prevent the inactivation of the B toxin of the microorganism, so that the consumption of raw sweet potato in New Guinea may be related to the prevalence of the disease.[8]

There may be other bactericidal mechanisms on the mucosal surface that are not necessarily immunologic. For example, there is evidence for bacterial killing outside the epithelial cell that depends on an intact blood supply. The significance of this process requires further study.

The Gut Lymphoid System

In addition to discrete lymphoid follicles within the submucosa, there are large numbers of immunologically competent cells among the epithelial cells and in the lamina propria. It is estimated that these cells comprise about one-fourth of the mass of the entire gastrointestinal tract, a mass equivalent to the spleen.

The immunologic cells on the surface of the mucosa are scattered abundantly among the absorptive cells (intraepithelial lymphocytes). The intraepithelial lymphocytes appear to be T cells, since the population is drastically reduced in thymectomized animals and lymphocytes appear in the gut during embryonic life several weeks following the appearance of lymphocytes in the thymus gland.

The immunologic cells of the lamina propria are either lymphocytes or plasma cells. The plasma cells are part of the B cell system and are absent in congenital agammaglobulinemia. Plasma cells make secretory immunoglobulins (IgA), which may be an important line of defense against the contents of the lumen at the mucosal surface (Chapter 13).

Both intraepithelial lymphocytes and plasma cells reach the lamina propria by migrating as lymphocytes through the capillaries. The lymphocytes arriving at the epithelial layer migrate from the lamina propria and are eventually shed along with the epithelial cells at the villus tip. This loss of lymphocytes is estimated to amount to 0.05 percent of the total body lymphocyte population each day. There is also evidence from some species that small lymphocytes of T cell derivation may reenter the circulation after a sojourn in the gut.

Secretory Immunoglobulins

While the predominant immunoglobulin is IgG, the predominant immunoglobulin of secretions is IgA. In this respect, the secretions of the gut are no different from those of the bronchial epithelium or the salivary glands. The ratio of gut plasma cells making IgA to IgM to IgG is approximately 10:2:1.

Immunoglobulin A is predominantly a dimer of two 7s molecules made by plasma cells in the lamina propria. The complete secretory molecule has an additional component manufactured and attached by the epithelial cells. The complete secretory IgA molecule is believed to be delivered to the lumen by reverse pinocytosis. The secretory component added by the epithelial cell is probably responsible for the molecule's extraordinary stability in a proteolytic environment.

Secretory IgA binds to viruses and bacteria, and a primary function of the molecule may be to prevent bacterial adherence to the mucosa. An additional function of great potential importance may be to prevent the absorption of certain ingested macromolecules or products of bacterial metabolism. While the surface epithelium does pose a barrier against the absorption of potentially toxic complexes, absorption of some macromolecules can occur. Indeed, there is detectable absorption of endotoxins administered directly into the small intestine. Thus, a function of the secretory immunoglobulins may be to combine with certain of these antigens to reduce absorption. In overall function the barrier is efficient, since few complex molecules from food or bacteria are actually absorbed intact.

Another feature of the secretory immunoglobulin defense is that higher levels of immunity are accomplished after local than systemic introduction of antigens. Local immunity is illustrated by studies in patients with double-barreled colostomies. An attentuated poliovirus was used to immunize one limb of the colostomy. Subsequently, significant immunization was proven in the test limb of the colostomy by comparison to the control unimmunized limb.[9]

Not all bacterial inhabitants of the intestine appear to induce antibodies. Some bacterial inhabitants that were once believed to induce antibodies detectable in serum or secretions turned out on further investigation to be incapable of inducing antibodies on their own. The antibodies appear to be directed against bacteria that share antigens with the surface mucus or mucosa. This factor may select species with antigenic similarities to the host surface. On the other hand, some bacteria clearly evoke immune responses. For example, *Vibrio cholerae* induces antibodies that interfere with its attachment.

Paneth Cells

Paneth cells may also be a part of the gastrointestinal host defense system. These cells sit in the deepest reaches of the small intestinal crypts, and recent studies reveal evidence for active phagocytosis and degradation of microorganisms opsonized by IgA within these cells.[10] In addition, immunofluorescence studies show that lysozyme granules are present in Paneth cells and that these granules appear to be discharged into the lumen after stimulation with intravenous pilocarpine. Lysozyme can degrade the cell wall polymer of most bacteria, and in the intestinal lumen the bactericidal properties of lysozyme may be enhanced by secretory immunoglobulins.

Microbial Adherence as a Genetic Basis for Resistance

Microbial invasion of intact epithelial surfaces seems to require the presence on the surface of the bacteria of specific receptors for epithelial cells or vice versa. This property may represent an important virulence factor for certain bacteria. Consequently, the absence of certain epithelial receptors may render some animals genetically resistant to infection. Thus, in a strain of piglets with receptors for the virulence antigen of a species of *E. coli*, 95 percent of animals die after inoculation. On the other hand, if the piglet strain does not have receptors for the attachment antigen, 95 percent of inoculated animals survive. Similar phenomena related to the attachment of indigenous organisms may be important in the selection of the nonpathogenic local flora, whose function is to compete with potentially pathogenic species.

MICROBIAL FLORA OF THE UPPER GASTROINTESTINAL TRACT

INDIGENOUS FLORA

Until about the mid-1960s, when methods for culturing strict anaerobes came into wider use, coliforms were thought to be the chief inhabitants of the intestines. Now it is known that anaerobic species outnumber aerobic and facultative bacteria by a factor of a thousand. Although the organisms inhabiting the lumen are not necessarily identical to the organisms populating the epithelium or mucosal surface, most evidence suggests that the flora are similar. With present methods of culture techniques, well over half and perhaps as many as 90 percent of enteric organisms can be cultured.[1]

A continuing theme in the study of the intestinal flora relates to the questions of why particular organisms emerge as the predominant flora. Of even greater importance is the question of why certain organisms emerge as the pathogens. In addition to selective metabolic factors that have been discussed, adhesiveness factors have been identified for several species. These factors do not appear to be the same for all organisms. For example, *V. cholerae* adheres to intestinal epithelium by means of a calcium-dependent active metabolic adhesive process. *E. coli* has a filamentous surface protein that appears to be essential for virulence, and some strains of *Salmonella* show chemotaxis toward the mucosa.

The indigenous flora of the gastrointestinal tract are discussed in Chapter 3. Some features deserve emphasis here.

The Stomach

The microbes found in the human stomach probably depend on the methods used, the geographic locale, and even the time at which the gastric contents are sampled. Although the normal empty stomach is frequently sterile, more than 10^3 organisms per ml of many species including lactobacilli, aerobic streptococci, bifidobacteria, clostridia, and coliforms have been found. Indeed, such a variety of organisms has been recovered that some authorities believe all isolated species to be transients. On the other hand, some acid-tolerant species are isolated with such regularity (eg, aerobic streptococci, lactobacilli, and *Candida*) even from the fasting stomach that others believe them to be a part of the indigenous flora.[3]

Duodenum and Proximal Jejunum

The proximal small intestine has been described "as a microbial vacuum in the midst of plenty," [3] but several studies have identified a variety of organisms in concentration of greater than 10^3 per ml. Streptococci and lactobacilli usually predominate. Coliforms and obligate anaerobes like clostridia and *Bacteroides* are uncommon, but these species are isolated more frequently with sampling farther down the small bowel. The number of microorganisms recovered from the proximal small intestine depends on the time at which the contents of the duodenum and jejunum are sampled. For example, Dickman et al [11] found mean counts of $10^{1.8}$ per ml in man during the fasting state. After a meal, the number of organisms increased to 10^4 per ml. This flora qualitatively resembles the oral and gastric flora, but in decreasing numbers, suggesting that large numbers of organisms are killed by passage through the stomach.

Most studies of the small bowel microflora have demonstrated increasing bacterial counts with distance down the small bowel from the pylorus. Counts of anaerobes of 10^4–10^5 in the jejunum increase to 10^7–10^8 in the ileum, with gram-positive and gram-negative organisms in approximately equal numbers. Anaerobic species are isolated from only about half of normal control patients, and in these individuals the quantitative counts are lower. Anaerobic counts of approximately 10^2–10^5 in the jejunum rise to 10^5–10^7 in the ileum. Thus, the gradient from proximal to distal is also preserved for the anaerobic species.

Although segmented microorganisms that attach to epithelial cells have been described in animals with the bacterium inserted into an invagination of the cell membrane, such species have not yet been reported in man. Even in animals, these microorganisms have not yet been successfully cultured, so it will not be surprising if additional species are discovered that are not classified at the present time.

Lower Jejunum and Ileum

The distal small intestine has a microflora that represents a transition zone to the colon. Lactobacilli and streptococci are less common than proximally, although they are not rare. Clostridia, coliforms, and *Bacteroides* are more commonly identified in concentrations greater than 10^3. The total quantitative counts usually run between 10^6 and 10^8, with aerobes and anaerobes in approximately equal numbers. The predominant aerobes are *E. coli* and enterococci, and the predominant anaerobes are *Bacteroides* and bifidobacteria. On reaching the colon, the quantitative counts rise to approximately 10^{11} organisms per ml, and the microflora constitutes approximately 70 percent of the dry weight of colonic content. Although many have reported that the flora of the colon lumen is overwhelmingly anaerobic by ratios of 1000:1 or greater, others have reported that the ratio is approximately 1:1 in quantitative cultures taken from mucosal biopsy samples.[12]

As previously noted, the indigenous flora contributes to its own stability through nutritional competition; species not well adapted to the intraluminal environment starve.

In addition, toxic products of bacterial metabolism also select the species that predominate. Short-chain fatty acids produced by the metabolism of some bacteria are highly toxic to invaders at the low oxidation-reduction potentials maintained by the anaerobic microbial community.

ROLE OF THE INDIGENOUS FLORA IN NORMAL PHYSIOLOGY

Although much work in germ-free animals has focused on the responses of animals to shock or strangulating intestinal obstruction, the role of the indigenous flora in normal physiology has not been extensively studied. It is clear, however, that the intestinal microflora are essential for normal morphology, metabolism, and immunology of the small bowel.

Many of the "normal" characteristics of the small bowel do not develop without an intestinal flora. In germ-free animals, the mucosa is thin and the villi are slender, fingerlike, and sometimes short. The crypts are shallow, and the lamina propria is poorly developed with few plasma cells present. In addition, there is an overall decrease in cell turnover, as established by decreased crypt labeling with tritiated thymidine. The migration rate of cells is also slow, so that the lifespan of an epithelial cell is about 4 days instead of the normal 2 days.[13] After colonization, crypt hyperplasia takes place. Such animals develop taller ileal villi than conventional animals, persisting as long as 8 weeks in a conventional environment. There is some speculation that the relatively anaerobic environment maintained by the microflora in the lumen causes villous tip hypoxia, without which crypt hypoplasia occurs.

In some animals, intestinal microorganisms clearly carry on metabolic and digestive activities from which the host derives nutritional benefit. For example, fibrous food is delayed in the stomach of ruminants for microbial digestion, from which the host is the ultimate beneficiary. Similarly, rats derive vitamin B6 from their indigenous flora. These observations suggest that in some species bacterial metabolism does provide essential nutrients, but it has been difficult to prove that the microflora play any nutritional role in the normal human.

Since plasma cells are not seen in significant numbers until a few weeks after birth, the appearance of plasma cells may be related to the colonization of the intestine with indigenous microbes. Germ-free animals have decreased numbers of lymphocytes within the epithelium and the lamina propria, with a concurrent decreased production of immunoglobulin A.

The competition between the normal resident flora within the gastrointestinal tract and potential invasive pathogens has not been well studied. However, there is considerable evidence that it exists. One of the most striking demonstrations of this putative effect is the administration of antibiotics to human volunteers prior to an oral challenge with *Salmonella typhi*. Under these circumstances, the inoculum required to reduce typhoid fever was markedly reduced.[14] The presumed mechanism was the suppression of the normal inhibitory activities of the indigenous microflora. Similarly, conversion of asymptomatic chronic carriers to active cases of typhoid, clinical exacerbation of resolving *Salmonella* gastroenteritis, and precipitation of *Salmonella* bacteremia have all been described as consequences of antibiotic therapy.

As previously noted, the resident strains compete with each other and with pathogens for their own essential nutrients. They also maintain a pH and redox potential that puts alien invading organisms at a disadvantage. For example, the germ-free animal has an oxidation-reduction potential of approximately −50 millivolts, which decreases to −230 millivolts when the animal is colonized by a normal flora. The resident strains also produce short-chain organic acids that are bactericidal to foreigners and inhibit the growth of pathogens like *Salmonella*.

In summary, the indigenous flora carries out activities that are essential for the normal morphology of the intestine and its normal immunologic function, and the resident strains may also make contributions to host metabolism.

HOST PATHOGENETIC FACTORS

Intestinal Obstruction

Any disorder that interferes with intestinal motility can result in bacterial overgrowth within the intestine. For example, in scleroderma the peristaltic waves that ordinarily help to clear bacteria from the proximal small bowel may be diminished, and bacterial overgrowth may occur as a result of functional obstruction with a patent lumen. Syndromes associated with chronic bacterial overgrowth may ensue. In acute intestinal obstruction, intraluminal bacterial overgrowth also occurs and can be a major source of morbidity and mortality after operative relief. In fact, most deaths after surgery for intestinal obstruction result from sepsis.

Studies of the microbial flora in intestinal obstruction are difficult, because the intraluminal contents cannot be safely obtained and the laboratory resources for quantitative bacteriology are frequently not available during emergencies. Some recent studies have negotiated these obstacles. In one, the aerobic bacterial counts in obstructed jejunum were on the order of 10^8 per ml.[15] Anaerobes were isolated from 17 of 26 obstructed patients and averaged over 10^2 per ml in obstructed jejunum and over 10^4 per ml in obstructed ileum. In another study, total bacterial counts in obstructed small intestine were between 10^9 and 10^{11} per ml. The aerobic bacteria numbered between 5 and 6×10^9 per ml. More than 90 percent of patients had quantitative anaerobic cultures in the range of 5×10^5 per ml with a range of 10^5–10^7 per ml, while only about 50 percent of unobstructed patients cultured any anaerobic organisms at all.[16] There is a great increase in the frequency of isolation of *Bacteroides* species in obstructed small bowel.

The duration of intestinal obstruction also correlates with the quantitative bacterial counts. In intestinal obstructions of more than 12 hours duration, jejunal aerobic counts rise to 10^{10} per ml and higher. During the recovery phase after intestinal obstruction, the flora returns to normal after peristalsis resumes, and quantitative counts are back to normal after a few days.[16]

In large bowel obstruction, there is also an increase

in the number of bacteria in the small intestine. Larger numbers of organisms are isolated at both jejunal and ileal levels, and there is a loss of the normal gradient of bacterial counts. Indeed, 10^{10}–10^{11} organisms per ml may be cultured from the entire length of the small intestine. In one study, anaerobes were recovered from all of ten specimens, and *Bacteroides* were isolated from all specimens except one.[16]

Reduced Gastric Acid

Hypochlorhydria and achlorhydria, regardless of the etiology, are associated with bacterial overgrowth in the stomach and sometimes the small intestine. Overgrowth may occur in the course of chronic diseases such as pernicious anemia with reduced gastric acid secretion. Overgrowth also occurs in patients with gastric ulcer, either benign or malignant. Patients with carcinoma of the stomach are frequently achlorhydric, and those with benign gastric ulcer are often relatively hypochlorhydric. Septic complications are far more common after gastric operations for these conditions than for duodenal ulcers.

Massive bacterial overgrowth may also occur in the stomach when there is gastric hemorrhage. The blood buffers the gastric acid and provides a broth suited to the exuberant growth of microorganisms. Wound infection and other septic complications after emergency gastric surgery for hemorrhage are correspondingly more common.

Changes in Local and Systemic Immune Status

Gastrointestinal infection with some microorganisms, such as *Candida*, are virtually unknown except in patients with cancer, diabetes, or immunosuppression. Advanced malnutrition in cancer patients appears to predispose toward serious infection with *Candida*. In experimental animals, T cell-deficient mice have been found to be more susceptible to *Salmonella* enteritis.

Changes in local immune status also appear to predispose toward infections with certain organisms. Infection with *Giardia* is rare except in patients with congenital or acquired deficiencies in immunoglobulin A. IgA deficiency may be selective or caused by a global immunoglobulin deficiency.

It has been speculated that deficiencies in local antibody production may also result in a breakdown of the mucosal barrier function to macromolecules and result in the absorption of noxious materials that may be related to hepatic or systemic disease.

Intestinal Ischemia

The mortality of gangrenous small bowel remains high regardless of etiology. The major causes of intestinal gangrene—strangulating obstructions and mesenteric vascular accidents—have remained essentially the same, but little progress has been apparent in reducing the septic complications of these conditions. The importance of the microflora in intestinal gangrene is easily demonstrable in experimental models. Ischemic injury to bowel has been compared in germ-free versus monocontaminated species. Of the contaminating species studied, *C. perfringens* type A has been found to be extraordinarily toxic and lethal. This organism is capable of virtually dissolving an intestinal segment in animals.[17]

The concept of an intestinal factor in irreversible shock goes back to the 1950s. Fine[18] postulated a role for enteric organisms in contributing to the irreversibility of hemorrhagic shock, and he showed that denervation of the intestine protected an animal from longer periods of hypotension. Since the arterioles in the intestine undergo spasm during hypotension to redistribute the cardiac output to other organs, the gut becomes progressively ischemic and vulnerable to bacterial invasion and absorption of endotoxins that leak through the epithelial barrier. Denervation allows the arterioles to vasodilate and autoregulate blood flow, resulting in protection of the mucosa.

Genetic Susceptibility

Almost nothing is known in man about a genetic basis for the resistance to invasion of the small bowel by microorganisms. Recent work in piglets has suggested that receptors to certain antigens associated with bacteria enable pathogenic microorganisms to attach to the mucosa. The K-88 antigen of the surface of *E. coli* is a virulence determinant in piglets, since the adhesive properties of the antigen enable the bacteria to attach to the cell surface. Ninety-six percent of animals genetically lacking the K-88 receptor survive inoculation with the organism, while 95 percent of animals with the appropriate receptor die following inoculation.[19] Nothing is known in man about this possible mechanism of resistance to enteric infection.

Underlying Diseases and Metabolic Disorders

Enteric bacterial overgrowth is recognized in a number of systemic diseases. However, most of these associations are explained by the effect of the systemic disease on one of the mechanisms of host defense that has been previously discussed. For example, the bacterial overgrowth associated with diabetes may be related to a motility disturbance related to diabetic neuropathy. Gastric emptying may also be reduced in gastroparesis diabeticorum of diabetes mellitus. Similarly, scleroderma may predispose to bacterial overgrowth from a disturbance in motility. High coliform counts in the proximal bowel are seen in pernicious anemia, and this disturbance is probably due to gastric achlorhydria.

Anatomic Disorders

Several anatomic disorders predispose to bacterial overgrowth in the small intestine. Originally, the pathophysiology of blind loop syndrome was developed experimentally in animals with true antiperistaltic blind loops. Accordingly, the term blind loop syndrome carried over easily to patients with actual surgical blind loops. These may develop from poorly planned anastomoses, which leave segments of bowel that do not empty properly by peristalsis. Bacterial overgrowth is usually the conspicuous and presenting problem in patients with diverticulae of the small intestine. Other anatomic disorders such as strictures and fistulas that interfere with the peristaltic cleansing of the bowel predispose to bacterial overgrowth.

Extension from Other Infected Regions

The only ductal system from which bacterial overgrowth spreads to the small bowel is the pancreaticobiliary tree. Bacterial overgrowth has been reported in the small bowel in connection with common duct disease and obstruction of the biliary tract.[20] Once bacterial overgrowth is established in the small intestine, contamination spreads the length of the gastrointestinal tract. Accordingly, bacterial overgrowth originating in the small bowel, for example in a case of jejunal diverticulosis, tends to traverse the pylorus and to contaminate the stomach.

Relationship to Prior Operative Procedures

Infectious complications from operative procedures span a variety of problems that may be broken down into two groups. On the one hand, there are the wound infections and anastomotic leaks that may occur after surgery on the stomach and small bowel; on the other hand, there are the operative procedures that predispose to bacterial overgrowth in the lumen as chronic complications. The former are discussed in other chapters, while the latter predispose to blind loop syndrome. Another matter that merits comment here is the problem of bacteremia arising from the small bowel in association with diagnostic procedures. Bacteremias occur after peroral jejunal biopsy or upper gastrointestinal endoscopy; however, these bacteremias rarely induce significant infection elsewhere. Most endocarditis is caused by cocci, which form rigid chains in the bloodstream. However, most enteric organisms are motile rods that do not float in clumps and adhere to the cardiac valves. It may be advisable, though, in patients with rheumatic heart disease or intravascular prosthesis, to provide prophylactic antibiotic coverage against enterococci before instrumentation of the proximal gastrointestinal tract.

Surgical procedures that predispose to bacterial overgrowth as a late complication interfere either with peristaltic emptying or gastric acidity. Anatomic blind loops from side-to-side anastomoses have been mentioned. Perhaps the most common clinical form of this problem is a side-to-side ileotransverse colostomy to bypass Crohn disease, with the distal ileum terminating in a stricture or inflammatory mass. Although the defunctionalized small intestine after jejunoileal bypass for obesity should empty isoperistaltically, there is recent evidence that bypass enteropathy may be related to bacterial overgrowth in the excluded segment.

Hypochlorhydria has also been discussed as a predisposition for bacterial overgrowth, regardless of etiology. Bacterial overgrowth has been noted after a variety of gastric procedures for either benign or malignant disease. Manifestations of bacterial overgrowth may occur either as contaminated small bowel syndrome or as a predisposition toward infection with specific organisms such as *Salmonella*. A fecal flora in the small bowel with bacterial counts up to 10^8 per ml, predominantly enterobacteria and bifidobacteria,[21,22] has been reported after both Billroth I and Billroth II reconstruction of the stomach. Vitamin B12 malabsorption after gastrectomy is probably as likely to occur from bacterial overgrowth as it is from loss of intrinsic factor. Significant changes have also been reported after vagotomy and drainage. While some have shown major changes after gastroenterostomy,[23] others have claimed that the changes are small. A recent study has included the more contemporary acid lowering procedures in dogs with a variety of gastric operations.[24] A marked and persistent increase in the flora occurred after subtotal gastrectomy or total vagotomy with antrectomy; the bacterial overgrowth was prominent in the stomach as well as in the jejunum. Only after highly selective vagotomy was there no bacterial overgrowth. All animals were said to have the same degree of acid reduction at 30 and 90 days postoperatively, but acid secretion returned in the animals with highly selective vagotomy at 1 year.

INFECTIONS OF THE ESOPHAGUS

The esophagus serves as a conduit through which food passes from the hypopharynx to the stomach. Food and saliva contaminated by mouth organisms pass through the esophagus many times a day. The microbes found in the esophagus, then, are those organisms that have been carried down from the mouth.

The esophagus is almost entirely free of infectious problems. The main infection seen is mediastinitis as a result of esophageal perforation or rupture (Chapter 30).

Primary infections tend to occur only in compromised hosts. The only two infections seen in this population are *Candida* esophagitis and herpesvirus esophagitis, but the latter condition is rare and is only diagnosed at autopsy. Even rarer today are diseases such as tuberculosis, syphilis, scarlet fever, and diphtheria of the esophagus.

PERFORATIONS OF THE ESOPHAGUS

Perforations of the esophagus are discussed in Chapter 34.[25,26] The major cause of perforations is instrumentation. In one series of 199 perforations, 137 (70 percent) were due to instrumentation.[26] Endoscopy has a perforation rate of 0.2 to 0.5 percent; the rate is less with the flexible endoscope than with rigid instruments. Dilatations are accompanied by a perforation rate of 1.0 to 1.5 percent. Other causes of perforation were postemetic (spontaneous) (12 percent), paraesophageal surgery (10 percent), penetrating trauma (5 percent), foreign body (3 percent), and blunt trauma (2 percent). The site of perforation is cervical esophagus (39 percent), upper thoracic esophagus (12 percent), lower thoracic esophagus (40 percent), and abdominal esophagus (10 percent).

Infection Caused by Perforation

Perforations of the esophagus allow food and saliva contaminated by oral microorganisms to contaminate the neck, mediastinum, or abdomen. Perforations of the esophagus allow microbes to enter the perivertebral space. Because this space extends from the base of the skull to the diaphragm, infection of the entire space can occur. Perforations of the anterolateral wall of the esophagus or pyriform sinus allow the infection to extend anteriorly into the pretracheal space. The infection can extend from the pretracheal space into the thorax. If the esophagus is perforated immediately above the diaphragm, the pleural space can be entered, resulting in empyema, since the pleura, especially the left one, is immediately adjacent to the esophagus. Perforation of the abdominal esophagus results in peritonitis. Discussion of infectious problems of these different spaces can be found in Chapters 27 (cervical space infections), 30 (mediastinitis and empyema), and 34 (peritonitis). Of course, leaking anastomoses in these same regions can give rise to similar space infections as perforations.

Because these infections are due to mixed anaerobic and aerobic organisms, they can be rapidly necrotizing, leading to gangrene of the esophagus or eroding into the pleura, lung, and even major blood vessels. Infected lacerations of the esophageal mucosa can even result in direct extension of the inflammation without actual perforation.

With slower developing perforations, such as those that occur with esophageal carcinomas, fistulas into the trachea, bronchus, and pleural spaces can develop.

Treatment

A thorough discussion of the treatment of esophageal perforations can be found elsewhere.[25-27] In general, the treatment depends on the size and rapidity of perforation. With large perforations, there is immediate and continuous pouring of food, saliva, and bacteria into the mediastinum or abdomen. With postemetic perforations (Boerhaave syndrome), there is forceful ejection and flooding of the esophagus with food, bacteria, and irritating gastric juices. On the other hand, with some instrumental or foreign body perforations, the hole in the esophagus may be small and the leak is not continuous. In most esophageal perforations, there is no fibrosis to stop the free dissection of the inflammatory process, but with some perforations the esophageal penetration occurs slowly so that fibrosis and sealing off occurs, which prevents free spread of the infection. Perforation of tumors by instruments, however, is usually into the open mediastinum. Strictures occurring after lye ingestion can be accompanied by surrounding fibrosis, which may limit the spread of any infection as a result of perforation after dilatation.

Most esophageal perforations should be repaired operatively and the surrounding area drained.[25-27] Perforations of the lower and abdominal esophagus should all be operated on. A trial of nonoperative treatment can be done in selected circumstances *provided the patient is followed closely:* (1) when the perforation occurs high in the neck when there is no continuing leak of air or fluid; (2) when the perforation in the cervical region is due to a sharp foreign body such as a pin or fishbone, if the object has been removed; (3) when the patient is not seen until several days after the perforation, has no fever, leukocytoses, or radiographic evidence of spreading infection, and has minimal symptoms; (4) when a suspected diagnosis of perforation cannot be proved and the symptoms are minimal; and (5) perforation resulting from chronic lye stricture.[25] If symptoms persist, a fever continues or develops, or the white blood count remains elevated, however, prompt operation should be carried out, to direct the salivary and refluxing gastric fluids, and to drain the mediastinium and pleura.[27]

Candida Esophagitis

Incidence

Candida (monilial) esophagitis usually occurs in patients with compromised host defenses. It is found in patients with malignant neoplasms—especially the lymphoproliferative disorders—who have received radiation therapy or chemotherapy, in persons treated with antibiotics, and in some patients with chronic disorders such as diabetes mellitus and aplastic anemia. Only rarely is it found in otherwise healthy persons who have received antibiotics.

Candida can occur as a part of the normal flora of the mouth and gastrointestinal tract. *Candida* overgrowth is prevented by competing bacteria. When this bacterial population is reduced by antibiotic therapy or the balance is altered by malignant neoplasms or chronic diseases, excessive growth of *Candida* can occur.

Pathology

Candida esophagitis is characterized by a pseudomembrane which contains yeasts, hyphae, and necrotic debris. The esophageal mucosa is ulcerated, inflamed, and bleeds easily. Microscopically, the esophageal wall is inflamed.

Clinical Features

The esophageal inflammation gives rise to spasm of the esophageal musculature. This spasm results in dysphagia and retrosternal pain on swallowing. Gastrointestinal bleeding can accompany esophageal ulceration and necrosis in patients receiving cancer chemotherapy.[27a] These patients may also have oral candidiasis (thrush), but oral candidiasis is usually completely painless. Pain and dysphagia suggest esophageal involvement. Any patient receiving antibiotics, steroids, or chemotherapeutic agents who complains of dysphagia should be suspected of having *Candida* esophagitis.

Diagnosis

A barium study of the esophagus will show the typical pseudomembrane with ulcerations and pseudopolypoid changes comparable to that seen in the colon in patients with ulcerative colitis. Esophagoscopy shows a yellow to white pseudomembrane, ulcers, and marked inflammation. A biopsy of the pseudomembrane will show typical mycelia mixed with necrotic debris and bacteria.

Treatment

Nystatin, 400,000–600,000 units four times a day, should be administered promptly after diagnostic studies have been obtained and should be continued for 10 days. Improvement is usually prompt, and the dysphagia lessens in 24 to 48 hours. The roentgenographic appearance returns to normal in about 7 days. Systemic amphotericin B is recommended for severely ill patients.[27b]

INFECTIONS OF THE STOMACH

Spontaneous infections of the normal stomach are almost unknown because its acid environment is virtually sterile.

Almost all infections arise in achlorhydric stomachs or by extension from contiguous extragastric sources.

Suppurative Gastritis

This condition is so rare that an incidence of 2.5 cases per year in the world has been suggested. Obviously, many cases go unreported. The most severe form, emphysematous gastritis, was once considered to be uniformly fatal. Survival is said to have increased from 16 percent in 1938 to 67 percent in 1970.[28]

Etiology

Numerous organisms have been cultured, but 70 percent of patients have alpha-hemolytic streptococci in the stomach. Suppurative gastritis due to *S. pneumoniae* has been associated with pneumonia and endocarditis. Other organisms include *Staphylococcus, E. coli,* and, more rarely, *Proteus vulgaris* and *C. perfringens.*[29] *C. perfringens* is most commonly associated with emphysematous gastritis.

Pathogenesis and Pathology

The predisposing factors include chronic gastritis, hypoacidity, infections elsewhere in the body, and the debilitated, immunosuppressed state. Emphysematous gastritis is most often associated with gastric cancer, corrosive gastritis, and preceding gastric operation. The pathologic findings include a congested edematous gastric wall occasionally with gangrene and frequently containing pockets of pus. Submucosal blebs of gas may be present under the mucosa in emphysematous gastritis.

Clinical Manifestations

Patients usually present with the sudden onset of abdominal pain, nausea, vomiting, and the physical findings of an acute abdomen. Purulent emesis, though rare, is pathognomonic, and in emphysematous gastritis an entire coat of the stomach may be vomited. Fever, chills, prostration, and bacteremia are frequent, and peritonitis rapidly ensues. The roentgenographic findings in the usual case of suppurative gastritis are nonspecific. In emphysematous gastritis, however, bubbles can be seen in the thickened stomach wall. Submucosal gas blebs and intramucosal penetration of contrast medium along mural sinus tracts can be seen on upper gastrointestinal series. The differential diagnosis includes pneumatosis cystoides intestinalis and traumatic emphysema of the stomach.

Treatment

The usual treatment has been gastric resection and antibiotics. Near total gastrectomy is required for emphysematous gastritis. There are a few survivors who have recovered with antimicrobial treatment alone, but most have required gastric resection. One would expect that agents effective against gram-positive cocci or clostridia would be most efficacious. In the absence of careful bacterial studies, however, one must assume that a mixed oral and colonic flora will be found. Therefore, a combination of an aminoglycoside, clindamycin, and massive doses of penicillin seem rational. Many other agents have also been used with success.

Prognosis

Death is common, but increasing numbers of survivors are seen. In the rare survivor without gastric resection, cicatricial constriction of the stomach may result.

Gastric Diverticulitis

Gastric diverticulitis is a rare complication of a rare condition. A gastric diverticulum is found in only 0.0043 percent of hospital admissions, is most often asymptomatic, is rarely subject to obstruction, and occurs at a site where bacterial contamination is minimal. The complications of hemorrhage and perforation are likely not related to previous obstruction.[30]

Gastric Mycosis

Gastric fungus balls have been reported after gastric operation.[31] Only one of these patients had a vagotomy. They were not taking antibiotics, steroids, or immunosuppressive agents, and had no systemic diseases to account for the proliferation of *Candida* in their stomachs. All were achlorhydric, except one had narrowing of the surgical anastamosis. The fungus ball is not really an infection, but is rather a bezoar.

Granulomas of the Stomach

A variety of infectious and noninfectious granulomas of the stomach can occur. Noninfectious granulomatous diseases of the stomach include sarcoidosis, Crohn disease, eosinophilic granuloma, and isolated nonspecific granulomas. Infectious granulomas of the stomach can be due to tuberculosis, syphilis, histoplasmosis, and eosinophilic granulomas associated with nematode larvae.[32-36]

Tuberculosis

Gastric tuberculosis occurs in less than 0.6 percent of patients who die of tuberculosis and is rarely, if ever, seen in patients without severe primary or systemic tuberculosis.[32] Like all gastric granulomas, the symptoms are nonspecific and include epigastric pain, vomiting, weight loss, weakness, hematemesis, and gastric outlet obstruction. As with all gastric infections, hypochlorhydria or achlorhydria is common. X-ray studies reveal gastric ulceration, tumor, stenosis of the pylorus and antrum, constricting lesions, concurrent duodenal involvement, and a picture resembling linitis plastica. Gastric cytology can be confusing.

In tuberculosis of the stomach, fistula formation and ulceration of the antrum may be confused with Crohn disease. The diagnosis depends on demonstration of either acid-fast bacillae or caseating granulomas in the stomach by endoscopic or open biopsy. Organisms are rarely cultured from gastric washings in gastric tuberculosis.

Antibiotic therapy is effective for gastric tuberculosis, and surgery should be used only for the complications of stricture, fistulae, stenosis, and ulcers. Gastric tuberculosis can give rise to carcinoma.

Syphilis

Tertiary syphilis rarely affects the stomach, and the diagnosis is dependent on biopsy evidence of granulomatous gastritis, a diagnosis of untreated tertiary syphilis, a roentgen defect in the stomach, gastric symptoms, and biopsy evidence of a fibrosing obliterative panvasculitis. The most diagnostic roentgen findings include the so-called hourglass stomach and large shallow ulcerations. Differentiation from extensive involvement of stomach with cancer may be difficult. Penicillin is the treatment, but the response may be slow so that the suspicion of cancer may grow. If healing is progressing well and the definitive diagnosis of cancer cannot be made, operation should be delayed.[33] Secondary syphilis may be accompanied by syphilitic gastritis—the mucosa is hyperemic, edematous, and friable.

Histoplasmosis

The stomach is rarely involved in disseminated histoplasmosis, though occasionally patients treated with amphotericin B may present with apparent carcinomas of the fundus and cardia of the stomach, which reveal noncaseating granulomas. Special stains will demonstrate the organism (Chapter 9). Although the disease can be cured with amphotericin B, fibrosis and stricture may result in persistent gastric lesions and obstruction.[34]

Differential Diagnosis of Granulomas of Unknown Etiology

Granulomatous disease of the stomach of unknown etiology must always be considered to represent sarcoidosis or Crohn's disease. In the absence of other evidence of these diseases, the diagnosis of isolated sarcoid or isolated Crohn's is doubtful. Such patients are frequently considered to have isolated granulomatous gastritis until other systemic involvement appears. Since no case of isolated granulomatous gastritis which evolved into Crohn's disease or sarcoidosis has been described, isolated eosinophilic gastric granulomatosis must be considered an entity.

In Japan the eating of raw fish permits the larvae of *Anisakis* species (a nematode) to penetrate the human gastric mucosa and establish a symptomatic ulcerating eosinophilic granulomatous reaction. Resection is necessary for the diagnosis, which can be made during histopathologic examination (Chapter 11).[33]

INFECTIVE COMPLICATIONS AFTER GASTRIC SURGERY

The infections that follow gastric surgery are similar to wound infections following all clean-contaminated operations (Chapter 20). The more common intraperitoneal infections of subphrenic, subhepatic, and intra-abdominal abscess also follow gastric surgery (Chapter 34). The incidence is rather low following elective surgery for duodenal ulcer. Gardner et al [35] reported an overall wound infection rate of only 3.3 percent for elective gastric surgery. However, the incidence increases markedly for emergency surgery, especially that performed for massive bleeding or perforation. Snyder and Stellar [36] reported a wound infection rate of 10 percent in a large series of patients with duodenal ulcers on whom emergency surgery was performed. Rapid overgrowth of oral bacteria within the gastric blood clots and hemorrhagic shock probably accounted for the increased rate of sepsis in patients undergoing emergency surgery for hemorrhage. A similar increased rate is seen after surgery for chronic pyloric obstruction, which appears to permit bacterial growth secondary to gastric stasis. In patients with gastric ulcer, gastric cancer, or recovering from operations on achlorhydric or hypochlorhydric stomachs, septic complications can be extremely common because these stomachs are not sterile and may be obstructed or contain necrotic tissue.

In order to minimize infectious complications, the hypochlorhydric or obstructed stomach should be lavaged with either antibiotics or povidone-iodine before operation. In emergencies, gastric lavage with povidone-iodine (1:10 dilution) can be carried out just prior to operation.

In patients with gastric carcinoma, a full-fledged colonic bowel prep should be carried out if there is any possibility that a portion of the transverse colon will be resected. Systemic perioperative antibiotic prophylaxis should be used in patients with achlorhydria, gastric carcinoma, or obstruction (Chapter 23).

Subphrenic and Intra-abdominal Abscess after Gastric Surgery

Sherman and associates [37] reported that suphrenic abscess followed 1.4 percent of 3,000 gastric operations. This figure is consistent with other series. Most such abscesses appear because of leakage at the suture lines, especially duodenal stump dehiscence.

Late and Persistent Postgastrectomy Infections

Pulmonary tuberculosis and *Salmonella* enteritis seem to occur with increased frequency after gastric resection.[38] The increased susceptibility of the latter may be due to the lack of the protective effect of gastric acidity. Prophylactic isoniazid has even been recommended for patients undergoing gastrectomy.[38]

Gastric overgrowth syndromes are also common after Billroth II operations with anemia, steatorrhea, diarrhea, and malabsorption syndromes, even though the most common reason for anemia is iron deficiency associated with decreased iron intake, increased gastrointestinal blood loss, and malabsorption of dietary or organic iron in the achlorhydric patient whose duodenum has been bypassed. However, one must not assume that postgastrectomy malabsorption is due to bacterial overgrowth, because the usual postgastrectomy malabsorption can be related to mild pancreatic insufficiency or to a deficient gastric reservoir.

INFECTIONS OF THE UPPER SMALL INTESTINE

Jejunal Diverticulitis

Incidence

Diverticulosis of the jejunum is generally an asymptomatic condition, but it may produce a variety of confusing syndromes, which are surgically correctable. In a group of 62 patients with jejunal diverticulosis seen by Altemeier et al,[39] symptomatic complications occurred in 16, but only two developed inflammation with one perforation and death. Symptomatic diverticula are rarely seen before age 60.

Pathogenesis and Pathology

Acquired jejunal diverticula appear as thin-walled, round, elliptical, or multilobulated sacs continuous with the walls of the intestine and extending between the leaves of the mesentery. The opening into each diverticulum is large, varying from a few millimeters to 3 cm in diameter. The large ostium and the fluid contents of the duodenum and jejunum make conditions unfavorable for inspissation and prolonged retention of material within the lumen. The wall of the diverticulum consists largely of fibromucosal tissue, however, and consequently lacks the muscular motor power to empty its contents effectively.

The most frequent involvement is in the proximal jejunum, and the larger diverticula are found near the duodenal-jejunal flexure just proximal or distal to the ligament of Treitz. The multiple diverticula are usually in continuity, although skip areas may occur, and the entire length of the small intestine may occasionally be involved. If partly distended with air and fluid, the sacs are easily seen, but when empty they may be overlooked or their true extent not appreciated. Concomitant duodenal diverticula are present in about 20 percent of patients and ileal diverticula in 10 percent.

Manifestations

Most patients have no symptoms, but six clinical syndromes have been discussed by Altemeier et al: [39] (1) acute inflammation, (2) hemorrhage, (3) intestinal malabsorption, (4) chronic "dyskinesia," (5) acute high intestinal obstruction, and (6) spontaneous pneumoperitoneum (one patient). The malabsorption syndrome appears to be identical with the bowel overgrowth syndromes discussed elsewhere in this chapter. Neither the acute nor the chronic obstructive symptoms are related to infection. The rare cases of jejunal diverticulitis occurred in elderly patients with acute pain and tenderness progressing to peritonitis. Whether obstruction to the diverticulum orifice, vascular compromise, or bowel infection was important is unknown.

Treatment

Chronic symptoms are best treated symptomatically or with resection if severe or if a blind loop syndrome appears. Emergency operation, resection, and treatment of the peritonitis is necessary for acute diverticulitis or hemorrhage. The role of antibiotics here in the treatment is unknown though probably useful for the treatment of the acute peritonitis.

Antibiotic-Associated Gastrointestinal Problems

A wide spectrum of gastrointestinal toxicity results from the use of antimicrobial agents. These have recently been reviewed by Joiner and Gorbach [40] and are listed in Table 38-1. Many of these are mild and transient and are important only because they lead to discontinuation of the antimicrobial agents or can be confused with other complications. Life-threatening complications, however, can ensue from pseudomembranous colitis and enterocolitis, and clinical presentation may vary from mild diarrhea to a condition resembling ulcerative colitis with life-threatening illness.

INFECTIOUS ENTEROPATHIES

BACTERIAL DIARRHEAS

It has become customary to distinguish the "dysenteric" or inflammatory syndromes from the "choleric" or secretory syndromes. The inflammatory syndromes are characterized by abdominal cramps with blood and pus in the stool, while the secretory syndromes are characterized by profuse watery diarrhea.[41] The secretory syndromes are caused by organisms that elaborate an exotoxin (enterotoxin, pharmacotoxin) that stimulates intestinal secretion without actual invasion of the mucosa. The classic example, cholera toxin, is heat labile, water soluble, and antigenic. It probably binds to a site on the mucosal side of the cell and stimulates secretion.

The inflammatory syndromes, on the other hand, are caused by organisms that invade and destroy the mucosa by means of cytotoxins. Although some species of *Salmonella* work their damage on the gut by invasion alone without enterotoxin production, most organisms that cause dysentery (eg, most species of *Shigella*) produce both cytotoxins and enterotoxins and the illness produced is both inflammatory and secretory.

These toxins should not be confused with bacterial endotoxins, which are lipopolysaccharide components of the bacterial cell wall. Intestinal endotoxins have nothing to do with invasion or intestinal secretion, but endotoxin may be absorbed from the gut during invasion by bacteria and contribute to systemic illness. Endotoxemia from the small bowel most commonly occurs when ischemic or gangrenous bowel is invaded by anaerobic species.

Since this book is devoted to infectious diseases of primary relevance to surgeons, this interesting group of diseases will be summarized without elaborate detail (Tables 38-2 and 38-3). The reader may find more comprehensive discussions of these diseases in other sources.[41,42] The only bacterial enteropathy with important, though rare, operative indications are those due to *Salmonella typhi* and *Clostridium*.

Cholera

The organisms of the genus *Vibrio* are discussed in detail in Chapter 7. In cholera and its related diseases, the vibrios colonize the lumen but do not penetrate the wall of the bowel. The mucosa is not shed, its gross and microscopic appearance is normal, the permeability of the bowel is intact, and the epithelium does not leak large molecular species. The signs, symptoms, and metabolic derangements of cholera all result from the massive secretion of fluid and electrolytes into the lumen of the gut.

TABLE 38-1. GASTROINTESTINAL SIDE EFFECTS OF ANTIMICROBIAL AGENTS

NAUSEA, VOMITING—GASTROINTESTINAL UPSET	
Antibacterial	Aminoglycosides (with oral administration)
	Cephalosporins
	Chloramphenicol
	Macrolides (clindamycin, erythromycin, linconomycin)
	Penicillin
	Sulphonamides
	Tetracyclines
	Urinary tract antiseptics: Methenamine
	Nalidixic acid
	Nitrofurantoin
Antituberculous	Isoniazid
	Rifampicin
Antifungal	Amphotericin B
	5-fluorocytosine
Antiparasitic	Chloroquine
	Dehydroemetine, emetine
	Diiodohydroxyquin
	Diloxanide furoate
	Metronidazole
	Quinacrine
DIARRHEA: SPECIFIC ETIOLOGIES	
Malabsorption syndrome: (Binding of bile salts,	Neomycin
direct mucosal damage)	Paromomycin
Overgrowth syndrome	Ampicillin, amoxicillin
(staphylococci, fungi)	Chloramphenicol
	Tetracycline
Pseudomembranous colitis	Ampicillin
	Cephalosporins
	Chloramphenicol
	Clindamycin, lincomycin
	Cotrimoxazole
	Tetracycline
Ulcerative colitis,	Ampicillin
proctitis	Chloramphenicol
	Tetracycline
HEPATIC TOXICITY	
Antibacterial	Carbenicillin
	Erythromycin estolate
	Oxacillin
	Tetracycline
Antituberculous	Isoniazid
	Rifampicin
Antifungal	Amphotericin B
	5-Fluorocytosine
Antiparasitic	Quinacrine
MISCELLANEOUS	
Abdominal pain	Mebendazole (Vermox)
	Rifampicin
Antabuse-like reaction	Metronidazole
Esophageal ulceration	Tetracycline
Glossitis, stomatitis	Chloramphenicol
	Metronidazole
	Penicillin
	Tetracycline
Metallic or unpleasant taste	Metronidazole
	Tetracycline
	Vancomycin
Tooth discoloration	Tetracycline

Reproduced with permission from Joiner KA, Gorbach SL: *Clin Gastroenterol* 8:3, 1979.

TABLE 38-2. DISTRIBUTION AND PREVALENCE OF BACTERIAL DIARRHEAS

		In North America		In Developing Countries	
Causative Organism	**General Distribution**	***Age Group Principally Affected***	***Transmission Patterns***	***Age Group Principally Affected***	***Transmission Patterns***
Shigella	Global	Children	Custodial institutions	0–6 years	Direct contact
E. coli	Global	Newborn	Hospital nursery	0–6 years ?Adults	Direct contact ?Direct contact
V. cholerae	Asia and contiguous areas	—	—	0–10 years All ages	Epidemic Water; ?food (epidemic)
V. parahemolyticus	Japan; ?elsewhere	Adults	Raw shellfish	?	?Raw seafood
Salmonella	Global	All	Prepared foods; poultry; egg products	All	Food-borne; direct contact
C. perfringens	?Global	Adults	Cooked meat	Children; nonimmune adults	Pork feasts ("pigbel")
Staphylococci	Industrialized nations	All	Prepared foods	—	(Rare)

Reproduced with permission from Grady GF, Keusch GT: *N Engl J Med* 285:831, 1971.

TABLE 38-3. CLINICAL CORRELATIONS OF ENTEROPATHOGENICITY

Organism	Diarrhea/ Dysentery	Abdominal Pain	Vomiting	Incubation Period (hr)	Mucosal Penetration	Enterotoxin	Extraintestinal Manifestations
Shigella	+/+	+	±	24–72	+	+*	Seizures: meningismus
E. coli	+/0	±	0	24–72	0	+	Minimal
	0/+	+	0	24–72	+	0(?)	Variable
V. cholerae	+/0	0	±	24–72	0	+	Hypokalemic nephropathy
Salmonella	+/±	±	±	12–36	+	0(?)	Fever: bacteremia
C. perfringens	+/0	++	±	8–15	0	+†	Minimal
	+/+‡	++	+	18–48	±	0(?)	Shock
Staphylococci	+/0†	±	++	4–8	0	+†	Minimal
	+/+§	+	±	Indeterminate	±	+(?)	Shock

* ? only *S. dysenteriae* 1.
† Preformed toxin ingestion.
‡ Necrotizing jejunitis (enteritis necroticans) may be clinically similar to dysentery.
§ May occur when enterocolitis is produced by proliferating enterotoxin-producing organisms.

Reproduced with permission from Grady GF, Keusch GT: *N Engl J Med* 285:831, 1971.

The onset of cholera is an abrupt, painless, watery diarrhea, which can rapidly result in hypovolemic shock, since several liters of fluid may be lost in a few hours. If the losses are not replaced, death will occur. With prompt replacement therapy, however, the mortality is almost zero.

Cholera organisms produce an enterotoxin with a molecular weight of 84,000 daltons. The greatest effect of the enterotoxin is in the jejunum, and aspiration of the lumenal contents largely controls the diarrhea. The ileum is moderately sensitive to the enterotoxin, and the colon is little affected. Evidence from bidirectional fluxes of sodium with in vivo perfusion studies and with in vitro chamber methods suggests that sodium absorption is relatively unaffected. However, the massive diarrheal stool losses continue even when a patient receives nothing by mouth. All evidence suggests the activation of a secretory pump for chloride. Intermediate steps in the activation of the chloride pump are increased adenylcyclase and increased cyclic AMP. The empiric use of Coca-Cola syrup by mouth to treat the diarrhea derives its rationale from the evidence that sodium transport in the jejunum is strongly stimulated by lumen glucose, regardless of the state of activation of the secretory mechanism. Indeed, oral glucose and electrolyte are so effective in improving jejunal water absorption that fluid balance can often be maintained in adults by the oral route without additional intravenous support. As noted previously, cholera toxin is

TABLE 38-4. POSTOPERATIVE COMPLICATIONS OF TYPHOID PERFORATIONS OF THE BOWEL

	No Bypass (49)	Bypass (29)
None	8	7
Major wound infection or dehiscence	12	2
Fecal fistula	7	2
Chest infection	16	8
Septicemia	4	5
Intra-abdominal abscess	5	0
Encephalopathy	5	1
Minor wound infection	5	10
Miscellaneous	12	9

Reproduced with permission from Eggleston FC, Santoshi B, Singh CM: *Ann Surg* 190:31, 1979.

antigenic, and up to 10 gm of IgA can be found each day in the stool of patients in the convalescent phase.

Enteropathogenic *E. Coli*

Enteropathogenic ("toxinogenic") *E. coli* usually produces choleric or secretory symptoms (traveler's diarrhea) without morphologic damage, although some strains may cause inflammatory diarrhea. The episode is usually self-limiting in adults, lasting less than 24 hours. A heat-labile enterotoxin, which shares the mechanism of cholera toxin for activating the secretory chloride pump, is responsible for the illness. Severe cases should receive antibiotics (eg, trimethoprim-sulfamethoxazole).[42a]

Outbreaks of diarrhea due to *E. coli* in the United States usually occur in hospital nurseries, and about a dozen enteropathogenic serotypes have been identified. Typing of strains of *E. coli* may also be done by phages that can lyse the bacteria, but typing by the antigens O, K, and H has become more widely practiced. Invasive infections with *E. coli* occur less often and produce a dysenteric syndrome similar to shigellosis. Organisms producing this syndrome have a special K antigen.

Endotoxins are normally detectable in portal blood and are removed by the liver. The O antigens of *E. coli* contribute endotoxin activity, and absorption of these antigens may overwhelm the hepatic defense and contribute to the fever and cardiovascular collapse of severe enteropathogenic *E. coli* diarrhea. Secretory IgA has not yet been proved to be an effective defense against *E. coli* diarrhea, although circulating antibodies achieved by parenteral immunization show some protection.

Staphylococci

Two intestinal disturbances are caused by staphylococci. One is relatively mild food poisoning due to ingestion of an enterotoxin preformed in contaminated food by toxinogenic *S. aureus*. The other is an invasive, sometimes fatal enterocolitis that is usually described in hospitalized patients on bowel preps.

Food poisoning (staphylococcal gastroenteritis) is a syndrome of nausea, vomiting, cramps, and diarrhea with an onset within a few hours of ingestion of the contaminated food and a duration of 8 to 72 hours. As with other enterotoxins, the diarrhea is secretory, without morphologic gastrointestinal lesions. Interestingly, the diarrhea may be reproduced by intravenous administration of the toxin, so direct contact with the mucosal surface does not appear essential. Gram staining and culture of the suspected food or serologic assay for enterotoxin may establish the etiology. The offending dish usually looks fit to eat, since enough enterotoxin to produce a violent gastroenteritis may be in food of perfectly normal appearance. Cultured pathogenic organisms are usually coagulase-positive, since coagulase-negative strains rarely produce an enterotoxin. The guilty strain may sometimes be traced to the fingers of a foodhandler. Foods that were previously sterilized by cooking appear to support the growth of staphylococci better than uncooked foods, and custards or pastries at room temperature are often found to be the source. The best prevention is refrigeration of all perishable foods.

Staphylococcal enterocolitis is a much more serious condition, first described widely in surgical patients on antibiotic bowel preps, although cases were reported prior to the antibiotic era. It is an invasive infection of the bowel wall with ulceration and necrosis of the mucosa. It begins within a few days (or sometimes weeks) of the antibiotic and is characterized by sudden diarrhea with mucus and blood. Not long ago, a Gram stain of the stool positive for abundant staphylococci was considered to be virtually diagnostic. Presently, however, it seems likely that many of these patients may have always been suffering from the effect of a *Clostridium difficile* enterotoxin and that the *Staphylococcus* in stool may not have been etiologic. Whatever the cause, the treatment is Vancomycin. This topic is discussed more thoroughly in Chapter 39.

Shigella

Shigella is a gram-negative aerobe for which man is the apparent reservoir, and infection is primarily an inflammatory process (although the organisms may also produce a neurotoxin or an enterotoxin similar to *Cholera* toxin). Occasionally, an illness may be of such severity that it will mimic ulcerative colitis. The usual illness is an acute colitis characterized by fever and diarrhea with mucus and blood, although the organisms may also invade the small bowel mucosa. Sigmoidoscopy demonstrates diffuse involvement with shallow ulcerations. The usual course is about 3 days, and less than 1 percent of cases are fatal in the United States. The illness may be extremely toxic in children, producing a mental obtundation and seizures that mimic meningitis. Outbreaks of *Shigella* diarrhea usually occur in custodial institutions, and sanitation appears to be the key to prevention.

Nontyphoidal Salmonellosis

In addition to the organism *S. typhi* that causes typhoid fever, which will be discussed separately, the gram-negative aerobic *Salmonella* include over 1,000 nontyphoidal serotypes based on typing of somatic and flagellar antigens. The gastroenteritis of nontyphoidal salmonellosis is usually mild, with a mortality of less than a fraction of a percent. It is characterized by fever, abdominal pain, and diarrhea for 3 to 5 days, although the duration is quite variable.

It is an inflammatory diarrhea with inflammation of the lamina propria and swollen lymph follicles. The diagnosis is established by stool culture.

Salmonella outbreaks in the United States are due to contaminated food or drink and are often traceable to food handlers of poultry or egg products. Cholecystectomy cures the carrier state in about 85 percent of patients. Another source appears to be pet Easter chicks and baby turtles.

Salmonella organisms may also be associated with septicemias indistinguishable clinically from typhoid fever and focal infections, including arterial false aneurysms and osteomyelitis. There is evidence from experimental animals that a deficiency of T-dependent intramucosal lymphocytes increases susceptibility to infection with *Salmonella.*

Typhoid Fever

Typhoid fever is an acute febrile disease caused by *S. typhi,* although other *Salmonella* organisms can produce an identical clinical picture with fever, headache, apathy, prostration, cough, splenomegaly, rash, leukopenia, and diarrhea. Several important surgical complications occur.

Etiology

The etiology, epidemiology, and clinical features of this illness are discussed in some detail in Chapter 5. Typhoid fever is spread by food or drink contaminated by human excreta from a patient or an asymptomatic carrier. It is principally seen in areas of the world with poor standards of sanitation, but several hundred cases are reported in the United States yearly. The carrier state is more frequent in females.

Pathogenesis and Pathology

Enteric *S. typhi* pass from the intestinal lumen to the regional lymphoid tissue, where they are phagocytized but not killed. The pathologic hallmark is the proliferation of large mononuclear cells involving the lymphoid tissue of the gastrointestinal tract, particularly the terminal ileum. The bacteria multiply intracellularly, seed the blood, and infect the biliary tract. The organisms are then poured back into the gut, and appear in stool during the second week of the illness.

Typhoid perforations usually occur in the last 12 inches of the terminal ileum. The perforations are usually 5–10 mm in diameter and oriented in the long axis of the gut on its antimesenteric border. The edges of the perforations are edematous, but the margin is usually not so friable that it will not hold sutures. When typhoid perforations of the ileum occur, the abdomen is usually distended with 3–4 liters of purulent material or feces.

Clinical Manifestations

Typhoid fever has an incubation period of 1 to 2 weeks and a course of 3 to 4 weeks. Fever and headache are the first signs. The rash of typhoid is described as rose-colored spots on the upper abdomen. Splenomegaly and leukopenia are typical. Diarrhea is not a prominent symptom early in the course of the disease—in fact, constipation is a common complaint, though mild diarrhea occurs. During the second week of fever, diarrhea is more common and may be bloody, but vomiting and abdominal pain are more typical. Tenderness with guarding in the right lower quadrant and increasing distention suggest impending or perforated disease.

Severe hemorrhage occurs in about 2 percent of patients and perforation in 1 percent. Perforation is the most serious complication and is frequently preceded by minor or major episodes of bleeding. Pain, tenderness, and rigidity precede signs of generalized peritonitis.

In areas where typhoid is endemic, the diagnosis is rarely problematic. The author has not seen a case of typhoid perforation in the northeastern United States, but at a hospital in Haiti where the disease is endemic, patients presenting with a clinical syndrome resembling appendicitis were presumed to have typhoid until proved otherwise. The diagnosis may be established by blood culture during the first week or stool culture during the second or third weeks. A fourfold or greater increase in agglutinin titer against the O antigen should confirm the diagnosis.

Treatment

There seems to be little doubt that abdominal exploration should be performed for perforations with peritonitis. Some patients in underdeveloped countries are seen so late that they are moribund. Multiple perforations should be sutured in two layers, including areas of apparent incipient perforation. Even for multiple perforations, small bowel resection is inadvisable, since resection seems to increase the mortality rate. Patients treated with end-to-side ileotransverse colostomy in addition to closure of the perforations have fewer complications (Table 38-4).

If perforations are seen late, particularly with peritonitis for more than 48 hours, some authorities recommend drainage of the peritoneal cavity through a flank incision. This may be accomplished with local anesthesia, and it has even been carried out as a bedside procedure with local anesthesia, with some survivors. This appears to be a stopgap procedure, however, and cannot be recommended for routine therapy.

Typhoid fever should be treated with chloramphenicol. Early treatment may reduce the incidence of ileal perforation, but perforation and hemorrhage can still occur despite treatment. Ampicillin, amoxacillin, and trimethoprim-sulfamethoxazole are appropriate second choices for resistant strains. Peritonitis due to the perforation must be considered polymicrobial and not due to *S. typhi* alone.[41] The choice of antibiotics must take this polymicrobial contamination into account. As noted in Chapter 34, the use of chloramphenicol alone in this circumstance risks failure.

Prognosis

The two most important factors affecting outcome are duration of illness or perforation and fluid replacement. In one large series, the patients who lived had been ill for 6 days prior to admission, while those who died had been ill for 11 days. Similarly, duration of the interval between perforation and operation is a highly significant factor. Those who were operated on within 24 hours of perforation had a 14 percent mortality, while those who had been perforated for more than 72 hours had an 80 percent mortality.[43] In another study, those who had been perforated for less than 48 hours had a 14 percent mortality, while those who had been perforated for more than 72 hours had a 100 percent mortality. Finally, those patients who received less than 2 liters of intravenous fluids had a much higher mortality than those who received over 4 liters of fluid replacement.[44]

It is noteworthy that the mortality for typhoid perforation is still approximately 33 percent, which is said not to be appreciably lower than the mortality in the presurgical era when nonoperative management was the rule.[45] Also, the antibiotic era has not made much impact on mortality from perforation, although the overall mortality for typhoid fever is lower. About half of the patients who die with perforation succumb to myocarditis and toxemia. Nevertheless, in most series nonoperative management is associated with 100 percent mortality.

Clostridia

Species of clostridia are associated with three noteworthy problems: food poisoning, intestinal gangrene, and antibiotic-associated diarrhea.

Food Poisoning

C. perfringens, usually found in meat products but also in other foods, is a major cause of food-borne diarrhea, overshadowing its importance as a cause of dramatic infections like gas gangrene. It causes a secretory syndrome of cramps and diarrhea, with an onset of 10 to 24 hours and a duration of 24 hours or less (Table 38-3). The enterotoxin is produced by the type A organism that forms heat-resistant spores, which may not be killed by cooking. These spores may germinate and grow at room temperature. Since the organisms are anaerobic, it is important that anaerobic cultures be performed on suspected foods in search of enterotoxin-producing organisms.[46]

Pseudomembranous Enterocolitis

C. difficile has recently been implicated as the leading cause of pseudomembranous enterocolitis.[47] It is likely that many previously reported cases of antibiotic-associated colitis, often attributed to staphylococci, were actually due to overgrowth of this organism. The clue came from a study suggesting that 9 of 10 patients with pseudomembranous colitis had a bacterial toxin in the feces, which was neutralized by a clostridial antitoxin. These matters will be discussed in more detail in Chapter 39.

Necrotizing Enteritis

Certain clostridial species are associated with "enteritis necroticans," a rapidly progressive form of gas gangrene of the bowel with diarrhea and shock.[48]

C. perfringens and *C. septicum* can invade the intestinal wall in the absence of vascular compromise or obstruction. The best studied example is necrotizing enteritis (pigbel), found in New Guinea in association with traditional pig feasting where large amounts of contaminated pork are consumed. *C. perfringens* type C (beta toxin) appears to be the cause. Since this organism is frequently isolated from resected bowel, beta antitoxin levels are high, and mortality is reduced by beta antitoxin. Darmbrand is a form of necrotizing enteritis in Germany which appears after excessive consumption of rich food associated with type C (formerly thought to be type F) *C. perfringens.* Numerous other case reports have documented the association of *C. perfringens* infections of various serotypes. Finegold has summarized the literature through 1976.[46]

The need for overeating may be related to the need for partial intestinal obstruction or stasis to permit the organisms time to proliferate within the intestine. In the other cases scattered throughout the literature, other causes of gangrene of the bowel such as strangulation, volvulus, intussusception, and mesenteric arterial or venous occlusion have been excluded. It is possible that transient ischemic disease may also permit invasion by clostridia. Unfortunately, the extensive invasion of the bowel wall with gangrene and the tendency for clostridial overgrowth in the postmortem period does not permit clarification of the pathogenesis. It is possible that similar pathophysiologic events take place in toxic megacolon or necrotizing enterocolitis of the newborn (Chapter 39). Nausea, vomiting, and crampy abdominal pain rapidly progress to steady pain with distention and peritonitis leading to shock. In general, the clinical picture resembles enteric vascular occlusion with intestinal gangrene, except that the onset is less sudden than that due to vascular compromise. Since food poisoning and intestinal obstruction lie within the differential diagnosis, the diagnosis may be difficult.

When necrotizing enteritis is present, resection of the involved bowel segment is required in combination with antibiotics designed to eliminate intestinal organisms from the peritoneal cavity. A Gram stain of the peritoneal contents should show a predominance of clostridia. If the etiologic agent is recognized, high doses of penicillin are required. Even in the absence of the diagnosis, the combination of an aminoglycoside, clindamycin, and ampicillin is recommended for the treatment of polymicrobial peritonitis.

Yersinia and Campylobacter

Yersinia has recently been recognized as a pathogen of increasing importance. This organism can also cause a severe enterocolitis with necrosis of the intestinal epithelium. *Yersinia* has also been isolated from cases of acute appendicitis (Chapters 39, 40).

Campylobacter jejuni causes a broad spectrum of diarrheal illnesses from the mild to the bloody. The illnesses may mimic or exacerbate inflammatory bowel disease.[46a]

Bacteroides

Bacteroides species are ubiquitous intestinal anaerobes often isolated in cases of bacterial overgrowth associated with blind loop syndromes. *Bacteroides* is of particular importance in the steatorrhea of bacterial overgrowth, because it is one of the few bacteria with the enzyme to cleave the glycine or taurine conjugates of the bile salts (see subsequent sections).

UNCOMMON INFECTIOUS AGENTS

While the common bacterial infectious agents affecting the stomach and small bowel rarely produce complications that require surgery, some of the less common infectious and parasitic agents may lead to perforation and obstruction. The helminthic parasites and other unusual intestinal infections are discussed briefly (Chapter 11).

Roundworms (Nematodes)

Ascariasis is common worldwide and is seen with some frequency in the southern United States. It is the largest roundworm of man, and the adults live in the small intestine. The eggs laid in the small bowel must reach the soil to develop into an infective stage. After ingestion, the eggs hatch and the larvae begin a migration from the gut via the circulation to the lungs. Then they migrate via the airways and pharynx back to the gut, where they establish residence. Surgical complications arise when a bolus of worms obstructs the ileocecal valve. The mass of worms may also initiate a volvulus or intussusception. If the administration of an antihelminthic like piperazine through a long intestinal tube does not relieve the obstruction, laparotomy is required. The mass of worms can usually be milked down into the colon without the necessity for an enterotomy.[49]

Strongyloidiasis is also seen in the southern United States. It has the most complex reproductive cycle of the nematodes and can sometimes cause massive intestinal infestation with bloody diarrhea. Steroid drugs should be avoided in patients with strongyloidiasis, since systemic dissemination has been reported.

Four additional nematodes account for most of the other human infestations. Hookworms (*Ancylostoma* and *Necator*) inhabit the small bowel after the larvae enter the skin on contact with contaminated soil. Gastrointestinal complaints are unusual, and patients usually present with anemia. Pinworms and whipworms more commonly inhabit the colon, especially in children. Pinworms (enterobiasis) migrate at night and cause perianal pruritis. They are treated effectively by several antihelminthics.

Tapeworms

The tapeworms *Taenia saginata* and *Diphyllobothrium latum* may grow to extraordinary size in the gut, sometimes reaching 10 meters in length. They cause few symptoms other than anemia. The most dangerous tapeworm for man is *T. solium* (the pork tapeworm), since man may harbor a larval stage that migrates and encysts (eg cystercercosis).

Protozoans

The protozoan infections deserve comment. Amebiasis is primarily a colonic infestation and is discussed in Chapters 11, 36, and 39. Giardiasis, on the other hand, is ingested as cysts, and the trophozoites inhabit the duodenum and jejunum attached to the mucosa by sucking disks. Infestation is usually asymptomatic, but in patients with immunodeficiencies (hypo- or agammaglobulinemia), *Giardia* may cause diarrhea. Radiographic studies are nonspecific, and duodenal biopsy may resemble sprue. The most rewarding diagnostic step is to search duodenal aspirates for the cysts. There is evidence that *Giardia* can be invasive. In a series of 31 patients with trophozoites in stool, 12 had invasion of the lamina propria in jejunal biopsy specimens.

Other Agents

Complications of *Candida* overgrowth usually occur either in diabetes mellitus or in terminally ill patients with carcinoma. *Candida* has been reported to be responsible for multiple jejunal perforations.[50] When perforation occurs, yeasts have been seen deep in the intestinal mucosa and also cultured from the perforation site and the peritoneal fluid, supporting the possibility that the primary infection was an invasive process.

Tuberculosis of the small bowel is usually ulcerative and associated with pulmonary disease. Perforation is rare because of the fibrous adhesions to the bowel and the thick bases of the tuberculous ulcers. From a hospital with over 240 cases of abdominal tuberculosis, only three perforations were reported.[51] Tuberculosis of the bowel may also obstruct with strictures and adhesions.

BACTERIAL OVERGROWTH SYNDROMES

Blind Loop Syndrome

The syndrome of bacterial overgrowth in the small intestine that results in anemia, steatorrhea, and malabsorption is usually known as blind loop syndrome. Because several causes of blind loop syndrome do not involve an anatomic blind loop, the British prefer the term stagnant loop syndrome. Since any cause of bacterial overgrowth within the small intestine may produce the syndrome, the terms "blind loop" and "contaminated small bowel" may be used interchangeably.

Etiology and Pathogenesis

The two factors that keep the proximal small bowel relatively clear of fecal organisms are gastric acid and peristalsis. Thus, disturbances of either of these functions may result in bacterial overgrowth. Defects in gastric acid production and effective peristalsis arise from certain congenital or acquired anatomic defects (small intestinal diverticula, strictures, and fistulas), surgical procedures (gastrectomy, vagotomy and pyloroplasty, afferent loops, and other upper gastrointestinal operations), or disorders of small bowel function and motility (scleroderma, diabetic autonomic neuropathy, radiation enteritis). Achlorhydria from any cause leads to increased bacterial levels in the jejunum. Most of the abnormalities cause neither symptoms nor malabsorption, since the bacterial overgrowth is composed of coliforms, streptococci, and lactobacilli. Symptoms appear when stasis of small bowel contents is accompanied by overgrowth with anaerobes, especially *Bacteroides*, *Veillonella*, clostridia, and anaerobic cocci.

Jejunal diverticulosis is one of the more common predisposing factors in the elderly; it is likely to take many years for the symptoms to develop in some patients. An interesting cause of blind loop syndrome is the gastrojejunocolic fistula as a complication of gastrectomy. The diarrhea that results from this fistula is not due to direct passage of ingested nutrients to the colon but rather to the contamination of the small intestine with colonic organisms that work their pathophysiologic effects by mechanisms to be described.

Although bacterial overgrowth within the small intestinal lumen is the common pathogenetic factor, each of the components of the syndrome, anemia, steatorrhea, and malabsorption, is explained by different mechanisms.

Anemia. The first case of this syndrome was described in the nineteenth century in a patient with an intestinal stricture and anemia. Similar cases were described with macrocytic, hyperchromic anemia, glossitis, and neurologic symptoms. Although the illness mimics pernicious anemia, these patients produce both acid and intrinsic factor. Either antibiotics or parenteral vitamin B_{12} can correct the anemia, and it appears that some intestinal microorganisms compete directly with the host for vitamin B_{12}.

Binding of vitamin B_{12} to intrinsic factor normally protects the vitamin somewhat from bacterial uptake, but some bacteria can ingest the whole complex. The megaloblastic anemia is not related to malabsorption of folic acid, since serum folate may actually be increased above normal because of bacterial synthesis of folic acid.

Steatorrhea. Steatorrhea as a result of the blind loop syndrome is principally due to malabsorbed dietary fat. In addition, bacteria may synthesize hydroxylated fatty acids, which are poorly absorbed. Free fatty acids have a cathartic effect on the colon, which may further aggravate the diarrhea by mechanisms similar to the action of ricinoleic acid in castor oil.

The major cause of fat malabsorption is a short-circuiting of the enterohepatic circulation of bile salts.[52] Bile salts are steroids synthesized by the liver from cholesterol, conjugated there with either glycine or taurine, and excreted as conjugates into the bile. Bile salts are then absorbed through active transport sites in the ileum and reutilized. The enterohepatic circulation thus seems to temporarily provide the bile salts to the proximal small intestine to solubilize dietary fat and recover the bile salts from the ileum after fat absorption is complete. To solubilize fat for absorption, there must be a critical micellar concentration of at least 2–3 millimoles per liter of conjugated bile salts in the lumen. Under normal circumstances, the lumen concentration is 5–10 millimoles per liter.

Conjugation of the bile salts enables these molecules to perform two functions essential for normal fat absorption. First, conjugation enables the bile salts to form micelles efficiently and to solubilize dietary fat. Second, conjugation seems to protect the bile salts against premature passive reabsorption by the jejunum. If the bile salts become deconjugated in the jejunum, a jejunohepatic circulation occurs rather than the normal ileohepatic circulation, and the bile salts are not retained within the intestinal lumen to solubilize and to facilitate absorption of dietary fat.

Bacteroides, clostridia, and a few other strict anaerobes have enzymes, such as taurocholate amidase, which can cleave the glycine or taurine conjugate from the bile salt. Most coliforms do not have the enzyme to perform this cleavage. Indeed, *E. coli* may proliferate widely in the proximal small intestine, competing with the host for vitamin B_{12} and causing anemia but not producing steatorrhea. Thus, while most microorganisms can compete with the host for essential nutrients, only particular species with the appropriate amidases can conjugate the bile salts and disrupt the enterohepatic circulation. In patients in whom quantitative cultures of jejunal contents have identified organisms with the enzymatic machinery to split the bile salts, the same fluid has shown an increase in free bile acids and a decrease in conjugated bile salts. Indeed, the degree of deconjugation can be correlated with the degree of steatorrhea. This pathophysiology is the basis of the breath analyzer test for bile salt deconjugation. Isotopically tagged bile salts are administered orally, and the patient with bacterial deconjugation will rapidly exhale the isotope in his breath. In addition to hydrolyzing the bile salts, some bacteria can also dehydroxylate bile salts, leading to a further decrease in the ability of the bile acids to form micelles.

Other hypotheses to explain the pathogenesis of steatorrhea have been proposed over the years:

1. Some have suggested that unconjugated bile salts interfere with lipolysis by pancreatic lipase, but this claim has not been widely accepted.

2. In vitro studies have suggested that conjugated bile salts are essential for intracellular reesterification of lipids, but it is possible that the tissue was damaged in the in vitro preparation.

3. A direct toxic effect of unconjugated bile acids on the epithelium has been proposed and gained some support from demonstrations of metabolic and morphologic abnormalities in intestinal mucosa exposed to unconjugated bile salts in vivo.[53]

Most evidence still seems to favor decreased micelle formation by normal conjugated bile salts as the primary pathophysiologic mechanism. For example, unconjugated deoxycholic acid has been administered both orally and as a continuous intraduodenal infusion, without any evidence of producing steatorrhea or mucosal damage. In addition, patients may experience symptomatic relief on a regimen that includes feeding conjugated bile salts, even though the amounts of unconjugated bile salts in the jejunum increase. Finally, the presence of free bile acid has been demonstrated in patients who do not have steatorrhea, unless the level of unconjugated bile acid is also below the critical micellar concentration.

Panmalabsorption. Although the bile salt story seems to be a sufficient explanation for the steatorrhea of blind loop syndrome, other features of the illness are presently not well explained. Some patients with bacterial overgrowth have hypoproteinemia, edema, alopecia, depigmented hair, low essential amino acids in serum, and low-voltage electrocardiograms. These changes reflecting panmalabsorption of carbohydrate and protein are not easily explained by the micelle theory. Furthermore, the steatorrhea induced by cholestyramine is relatively mild.

Some laboratories have also found steatorrhea and bacterial overgrowth in the jejunum of patients after gastrectomy with no evidence of free bile acids in the lumen. Thus, there has been an impetus to search for other possible explanations.

Goldstein[54] has developed the concept of bacterial competition for essential nutrients to explain some of these problems. He has calculated that a liter of intestinal fluid in bacterial overgrowth syndromes may contain approximately 10 gm of bacteria. At known rates of bacterial multiplication, the nutritional requirements for this mass of organisms can easily run over 100 gm of sugar per day. Thus, the nutritional requirements of the mass of bacteria alone may pose a significant competitive burden for the host.

Low serum essential amino acids have also been noted in some blind loop patients, but protein-losing enteropathy is rare. It is possible that the bacteria also compete with the host for amino acids. A classic example of this possibility is the bacterial metabolism of tryptophan, which is so constant a pathophysiologic feature in blind loop syndrome that it is useful as a diagnostic test. Bacterial deamination of tryptophan leads to increased ammonia production and urea synthesis, which have been demonstrated in man. It also leads to the increased urinary excretion of a variety of indicans and 5-hydroxyindoleacetic acid. Indicans are indoles formed by coliforms which split the side chain of tryptophan. 5-hydroxyindoleacetic acid arises from hepatic monoamine oxidase activity on tryptamine. Thus, indole and tryptamine are the intermediaries formed by the bacteria in the eventual excretion of indicans and 5-hydroxyindoleacetic acid possessed by liver enzymes.

Carbohydrate malabsorption is also well established in experimental blind loop syndrome. Decreased urinary excretion of D-xylose may also be a result of bacterial competition for sugars. Although xylose is not metabolized by man, a number of bacterial species that include a variety of aerobic organisms do metabolize xylose. Thus, it is not established whether xylose malabsorption in blind loop syndrome is due to uptake and competition by the bacteria or to a possible toxic factor as previously outlined.

Deficiencies of fat-soluble vitamins are common in the steatorrheas, but vitamin K deficiency almost never occurs in blind loop syndrome. Vitamin K is synthesized by intestinal microorganisms, so in this one instance the bacterial mass contributes a molecule that is useful to the host.

Pathology

The mucosa is normal by light microscopy in syndromes of bacterial overgrowth except for infiltrates in the submucosa and lamina propria. The significance of these infiltrates is not clear, but they probably represent a development of the gut lymphoid system in defense against the bacterial flora. Increased concentration of Paneth cells have been noted in bypassed intestine, and this may also reflect a defense mechanism against the bacteria.

Clinical Manifestations

Anemia and steatorrhea are the hallmarks of blind loop syndrome, but symptoms of abdominal discomfort and cramps (depending on the underlying cause of bacterial overgrowth) may precede the development of the typical metabolic findings for years. In addition to the typical megaloblastic anemia, some patients with chronic hemorrhage also have iron deficiency. Weight loss and neurologic manifestations of vitamin B_{12} deficiency may occur, along with hypoproteinemia and edema. Watery diarrhea may result from the cathartic effects of bacterial synthesis of hydroxy-fatty acids.

Laboratory Findings

The steatorrhea should be documented and quantified by stool collection for fat analysis. A routine hematologic work-up should be done, including red cell indices and vitamin B_{12} levels, which may show evidence of vitamin B_{12} deficiency. A three-stage Shilling test will usually be abnormal in the first two steps, when vitamin B_{12} is given alone and then with intrinsic factor. However, in the third stage, when vitamin B_{12} is given after a course of oral antibiotics as described below, normal absorption of vitamin B_{12} should be restored.

Jejunal biopsy should be performed to rule out other causes of malabsorption, such as sprue. The small bowel should also be intubated for quantitative bacteriologic studies. If the combined anaerobic and aerobic count is greater than 10^7 per ml, the bacterial overgrowth syndrome should be suspected. The quantitative cultures should be repeated after a 5-to-7-day course of tetracycline along with follow-up stool fat determination and the three stages of the Shilling test. If these studies show improvement in vitamin B_{12} absorption and reduced stool fat excretion along with a reduction in bacterial count, the diagnosis may be considered confirmed. Additional niceties such as serum-free bile acids and jejunal levels of free and conjugated bile acids are interesting but not essential for the diagnosis.

The breath analyzer test for bile salt deconjugation has already been reviewed. Recent studies indicate that when a critical level of bacterial overgrowth is defined as greater than 10^3 anaerobes per ml or greater than 5×10^4 aerobes per ml in the jejunum, the test as presently performed has a sensitivity of 70 percent and a specificity of 90 percent.[55] There has also been an effort to find a stable isotope for a breath test that would be safe for infants and pregnant women. ^{13}C-labeled glycoholate appears to be suitable.

Diagnosis

Clues to bacterial overgrowth in blind loops and certain other conditions of special interest to surgeons are often present in the history of the patient. Previous gastric or small bowel surgery or a history of an intestinal disorder like Crohn disease with a tendency to stricture should arouse suspicion of bacterial overgrowth when noted in patients with steatorrhea or megaloblastic anemia. A history of Raynaud phenomenon or dysphagia may suggest scleroderma.

An upper gastrointestinal series with small bowel follow-through is usually definitive in establishing any predisposing malfunction that can be surgically corrected. Suspicion of the diagnosis should be sustained by the laboratory studies outlined above.

Treatment

Operative therapy is advisable for those patients with lesions that are correctable without massive resection of the intestine (e.g., solitary jejunal diverticulum, mechanical obstruction, gastrojejunocolic fistula). Patients with multiple jejunal diverticula or motility disorders should be treated medically.

If medical management is selected, tetracyline, 250 mg daily, is a satisfactory initial antibiotic, with further modifications based on jejunal culture results. Alternate regimens have been discussed by Joiner and Gorbach.[40]

Bypass Enteropathy

Incidence

Within a few years of the introduction and popularization of jejunoileal bypass for morbid obesity, the complication of bypass enteropathy was recognized.[56] Estimates of the incidence of this complication vary considerably. On the low side is an estimate of approximately 3 percent based on one patient with the complication in 31 procedures, while estimates on the high side approach 60 percent with 15 patients out of 26.[57,58] This variation no doubt relates to different criteria for diagnosis and the recognition of patients in some series with more subtle rather than fulminant signs of enteropathy.

Etiology and Pathogenesis

The available evidence strongly suggests that this complication is related to overgrowth in the bypassed intestine.[40] Although peristaltic activity in bypassed small bowel has not been studied in detail, it seems likely that the bypassed intestine develops a motility disturbance that predisposes toward bacterial overgrowth in the segment. There may be acquired deficiencies in the gut immune system within the bypassed bowel segment, but studies in experimental animals have actually shown Paneth cell hyperplasia, which may reflect a reaction by the gut immune system to the overgrowth of bacteria. Evidence for bacterial overgrowth in the bypassed loop in association with the enteropathic syndrome was found in three patients who had not been on systemic antibiotics. Aspirations of the secretions in the bypass revealed a flora with 10^6–10^7 aerobes per ml and 10^7–10^9 anaerobes per ml. This evidence of bacterial overgrowth, along with the observation that some patients improve on antibiotic therapy, strongly suggests that bacteria do play some pathogenetic role. On the other hand, an increase in flora may not be specific for the patients with signs of the disease. For example, Corrodi et al [59] have reported a "colonic" flora in the bypassed loops of patients who are asymptomatic.

Bacterial overgrowth in the small bowel has also been considered a possible cause of liver failure after jejunoileal bypass. Germ-free dogs with jejunoileal bypass do not develop liver failure, but antibiotics given to conventional dogs do not appear to protect them well.[60]

Pathology

In patients requiring revision of the jejunoileal bypass, the bowel has been found to be dilated in almost all cases. In addition, inflammation is apparent on the serosal surface, either of the whole bypassed loop or on the ileum adjacent to the colon anastomosis. Occasionally, the whole colon shows similar evidence of serosal inflammation. There may be evidence of pneumatosis cystoidis intestinalis.

On microscopic examination, the mucosa shows evidence of nonspecific inflammatory changes with blunted villi and infiltrates of lymphocytes and plasma cells in the lamina propria.

Clinical Manifestations

Virtually all patients have diarrhea and abdominal distension with air fluid levels apparent on radiographic examination. The severity and duration of symptoms are inconstant, however. Symptoms may begin early in the postoperative course, or they may be delayed for several years. Once bypass enteropathy has developed, the subsequent course is variable. Exacerbations and remissions are common even without antibiotic therapy, although remission is often induced by antibiotics.

Signs and symptoms of an acute abdomen may develop in as many as 25 percent of all patients with enteropathy. These patients have abdominal pain, tenderness, nausea, fever, and leukocytosis.

The clinical course may also be complicated by systemic symptoms—skin lesions resembling erythema nodosum, arthralgias and arthritis, and recurrent fevers. Hyperoxaluria and kidney stones do not seem to be more common in patients with enteropathy than in patients without intestinal complications. The systemic symptoms are relieved in some patients by courses of antibiotic therapy or by dismantling the bypass.

Diagnosis

In patients with the typical clinical findings of diarrhea and distension, the diagnosis should be suspected. Abdominal films showing distended bowel with air fluid levels are essential for the diagnosis. Liver biopsy may be performed if there is any evidence of liver failure, and a significant percentage of patients with bypass enteropathy have shown steatosis and fibrosis. Although steatosis is often seen in patients with jejunoileal bypass who do not have enteropathy, fibrosis is unusual without some degree of enteropathy, except in alcoholics.

Treatment

The place of antibiotics in the initial management of these patients seems well established. In a double blind antibiotic crossover study, five jejunoileal bypass patients with colonic pseudo-obstruction had only 9 of 34 pain-free days on placebo, while they had 31 out of 33 pain-free days on metronidazole. Metronidalzole also resulted in a precipitous decrease from 10^9–10^1 in the anaerobic counts per ml from the vicinity of the bypassed loop. Kanamycin was relatively ineffective and did not decrease the abdominal girth or bacterial cell counts in the patients studied.[61]

Operation is required under two circumstances: (1) if the symptoms cannot be controlled with antibiotics, an elective dismantling of the bypass should be performed; (2) emergency exploration should be carried out in the less common patient with an acute abdomen. If serosal inflammation is not intense, restoration of continuity may suffice. However, if there is severe inflammation of a portion of the bypassed bowel, it is safest to resect that portion of the bowel along with colon that appears severely involved.

Prognosis

Since the severity and duration are quite variable, and since exacerbations are common followed by remissions, it is difficult to be dogmatic about the prognosis in this condition. In patients with severe enteropathy with a poor response to antibiotics, dismantling of the bypass is advisable. The late sequelae of bypass enteropathy with long-term antibiotic control are as yet unknown.

Prevention

If the primary disturbance in the pathogenesis of the condition is a disorder of motility in the bypassed intestine, prevention of this complication may be difficult to achieve. Presently, experimental work has been directed toward the use of a modified Koch valve to prevent reflux of colon contents into the small intestine. Time will tell whether this maneuver will effectively prevent bypass enteropathy. The present trend toward abandonment of jejunoileal bypass in favor of other methods for control of morbid obesity may make the complication obsolete.[61a]

Ileostomy and Continent Ileostomy

The pathophysiology of bacterial overgrowth in ileostomy reservoirs is identical to that described for blind loop syndrome. Because the continent ileostomy is a relatively recent surgical innovation, it deserves separate discussion.

The flora of a conventional ileostomy is unique, occupying an intermediate portion of the spectrum between normal ileal flora and the flora of a transverse colostomy. Anaerobic flora are less prevalent than in transverse colostomy effluent, and counts are approximately 10^5 lower than typical feces. On the other hand, the counts are approximately 10^2 higher than the counts in normal contents of the ileum.[62] Since the purpose of the continent ileostomy is to induce stasis, the microbial ecology would be expected to come to resemble the colonic flora. Bacterial counts are 10^3 higher than effluents of conventional ileostomies.

Two recent studies have investigated the possible consequences of this increase in flora with respect to the pathophysiology of blind loop syndrome. Schjonsby and co-workers [63] compared steatorrhea in patients with continent ileostomy versus conventional ileostomy. Abnormal fat excretion was found in 57 percent of the reservoir patients versus 14 percent of the conventional patients. Similarly, abnormal vitamin B_{12} absorption was found in 71 percent of the reservoir patients versus 29 percent of the conventional patients. The reservoir patients had increased total anaerobic counts and also counts of *Bacteroides;* 29 percent had abnormal breath tests for bile salt deconjugation. Oral lincomycin increased vitamin B_{12} absorption, reduced fecal fat excretion, and reduced microbial counts of *Bacteroides* in four patients. Similarly, four of seven continent ileostomy patients evaluated by Halvorsen and coworkers [64] for blind loop syndrome had malabsorption of fat and vitamin B_{12}. Others have reported enteritis as a complication of continent ileostomy with an incidence of over 50 percent.[65] Thus, evaluation for blind loop syndrome should routinely be recommended for patients with ileostomy reservoirs, and attention should be given to possible vitamin B_{12} depletion in the remote postoperative period.

WOUND INFECTION AFTER SMALL BOWEL OPERATIONS

Bowel preps for small bowel operations have been studied, with results the author believes are inconclusive. In one series of 155 jejunoileal bypasses for morbid obesity,[67] positive jejunal and ileal cultures were obtained in 62 and 87 percent of cases respectively. The jejunal flora was predominantly streptococci, lactobacilli, and staphylococci, while the ileal flora contained these organisms with other coliforms and anaerobes. A mechanical preparation alone did not appreciably alter the incidence of positive cultures to 57 and 56 percent respectively. There was a statistically significant reduction in the percentage of patients with positive ileal cultures. The wound infection rate with mechanical preparation alone was 43 percent, in comparison to the infection rate of 11 percent in patients with mechanical and antibiotic preparations. However, a wound infection rate was zero in patients who had no preparation at all, and it renders the results of the entire study problematic.

It is known that the oral administration of doxycycline (200 mg 4 hours before operation) results in tissue levels in the ileum that are approximately twice the serum level.[68] Whether oral doxycycline decreases the incidence of wound infections, however, is unknown. Studies of the wound infection rates after parenteral antibiotics in small bowel surgery are not available.

Since asymptomatic bacteremias do occur during small intestinal operations, it seems advisable to cover patients with prosthetic vascular grafts or other unincorporated implants with prophylactic systemic antibiotics before operation.

BIBLIOGRAPHY

Corrodi P, Wideman PA, Sutter VL, Drenick EJ, Passaro E, Finegold SM: Bacterial flora of the small bowel before and after bypass procedure for morbid obesity. J Infect Dis 137:1, 1978.

Joiner KA, Gorbach SL: Indications for antimicrobial therapy of gastrointestinal disorders. In Weinstein L, Fields BN (eds): Seminars in Infectious Disease 3:153, 1980.

Savage DC: Microbial ecology of the gastrointestinal tract. Annu Rev Microbiol 31:107, 1977.

Shackleford RT: Perforations and ruptures of the esophagus. In Surgery of the Alimentary Tract, 2nd ed. Philadelphia, Saunders, 1978.

Sleisenger MH and Fordtran JS (eds): Gastrointestinal Disease: Pathology, Diagnosis and Management. Philadelphia, Saunders, 1977.

Walker WA, Isselbacher KJ: Intestinal antibodies. New Eng J Med 297:767, 1977.

REFERENCES

MICROBIAL ECOLOGY

1. Savage DC: Microbial ecology of the gastrointestinal tract. Ann Rev, Microbiol 31:107, 1977.
2. Gibbons RJ, Kapsimalis B: Estimates of the overall growth of intestinal microflora in hamsters, guinea pigs, and mice. J Bacteriol 93:510, 1967.
3. Luckey TD: Bicentennial overview of intestinal microecology. Am J Clin Nutr 30:1753, 1977.
4. Brandborg LL: Other infectious inflammatory and micellaneous diseases. In MH Sleisenger and JS Fordtran (eds): Gastrointestinal Disease. Philadelphia, Saunders, 1973, p 909.
5. Ruddell WSJ, Axon ATR, Findlay JM, Bartholomew BA, Hill MJ: Effect of cimetidine on the gastric bacterial flora. Lancet 1:672, 1980.
6. Maffei HVL, Nobrega FJ: Gastric pH and microflora of normal and diarrhoeic infants. Gut 16:719, 1975.
7. Sykes PA, Boulter KH, Schofield PF: Alterations in small bowel microflora in acute intestinal obstruction. J Med Microbiol 9:13, 1976.
8. Lawrence G, Walker PD: Pathogenesis of enteritis necroticans in Papua, New Guinea. Lancet 1:125, 1976.
9. Ogra PL, Karson DT: Distribution of poliovirus antibody in serum, nasopharynx and alimentary tract following segmental immunization of the lower alimentary tract with polio-vaccine. J Immunol 102:1423, 1969.
10. Rodning CB, Wilson SD, Erlandson SL: Immunoglobulins within human small intestinal Paneth cells. Lancet 1:984, 1976.
11. Dickman MD, Chapelka AR, Schaedler RW: The microbial ecology of the upper small bowel. Am J Gastroenterol 65:57, 1976.
12. Peach SL, Drasar BS, Hawley PR, Hill MJ, Marks CG: Mucosal flora of the human colon. Gut 16:824, 1975.
13. Rolls BA, Turvey A, Coates MF: The influence of the gut microflora and of dietary fibre on epithelial migration in the chick intestine. Br J Nutr 39:91, 1978.
14. Hornick RB, Greisman SE, Woodward TE, Dupont HL, Snyder MJ, Dawkins AT: Typhoid fever: Pathogenesis and immunologic control. N Engl J Med 283:686, 1970.
15. Sykes P: Small bowel microflora in intestinal obstruction and Crohn's disease. Proc R Soc Med 69:325, 1976.
16. Sykes PA, Boulter KH, Schofield PF: The microflora of the obstructed bowel. Br J Surg 63:721, 1976.
17. Yale CE, Balish E: The importance of clostridia in experimental intestinal strangulation. Gastroenterol 71:793, 1976.
18. Fine J: The intestinal circulation in shock. Gastroenterology 52:454, 1967.
19. Rutter JM, Burrows MR, Sellwood R, Gibbons RA: A genetic basis for resistance to enteric disease caused by *E. coli.* Nature 257:135, 1975.
20. Scott AJ, Khan GA: Partial biliary obstruction with cholangitis producing a blind loop snydrome. Gut 9:187, 1968.
21. Dellipiani AW, Girwood RH: Bacterial changes in the small intestine in malabsorptive states and in pernicious anaemia. Clin Sci 26:359, 1964.
22. Gorbach SL, Tabaquali S: Bacteria, bile and the small bowel. Gut 10:963, 1969.
23. Mortimer DC, Reed PI, Vidinli M, Finlay JM: The role of the upper gastrointestinal flora in malabsorption syndrome. Can Med Assoc J 90:559, 1964.
24. Greenlee HB, Gelbart SM, DeOrio AJ, Francescatti DS, Paez J, Reinhardt GF: The influence of gastric surgery on the intestinal flora. Am J Clin Nutr 30:1826, 1977.

ESOPHAGUS

25. Schackelford RT: Perforations and ruptures of the esophagus. In Surgery of the Alimentary Tract, 2nd ed. Philadelphia, Saunders 1978, pp 51–87.
26. Wichern WA Jr: Perforation of the esophagus. Am J Surg 19:534, 1970.
27. Skinner DB, Little AG, DeMeester TR: Management of esophageal perforation. Am J Surg 139:760, 1980.

27a. Jones JM: Necrotizing *Candida* esophagitis: failure of symptoms and roentgenographic findings to reflect severity. JAMA 244:2190, 1980

27b. Odds FC: *Candida* and Candidosis. Baltimore, University Park Press, 1979.

STOMACH

28. Stephenson SE Jr, Yasrebi H, Rhatigan R, Woodward ER: Acute phlegmasia of the stomach. Am Surg 36:225, 1970.
29. Nevin NC, Eakins D, Clarke SD, Carson DJL: Acute phlegmonous gastritis. Br J Surg 56:268, 1969.
30. Locolio SA, Stahl W: Diverticular disease of the alimentary tract: the esophagus, stomach, and duodenum and small intestine. Curr Probl Surg 51:3, 1968.
31. Konok G, Haddad H, Strom B: Postoperative gastric mycosis. Surg Gynec Obstet 150:337, 1980.
32. Chazan BI, Aitchison JD: Gastric tuberculosis. Br Med J 2:1288, 1960.
33. Raffin S: Granulomatous infectious disease of the stomach. In Sleisenger MH, Fordtran JS (eds): Gastrointestinal Disease: Pathophysiology, Diagnosis, Management. Philadelphia, Saunders, 1973, p 573.
34. Nudelman, HL, Rakatansky, H: Gastric histoplasmosis: a case report. JAMA 195:44, 1966.
35. Gardner B, Butler ED, Goldman L: Early complications of gastrectomy with particular reference to delayed gastric emptying. Arch Surg 89:475, 1964.
36. Snyder EN Jr, Stellar CA: Results from emergency surgery for massively bleeding duodenal ulcer. Am J Surg 116:170, 1968.
37. Sherman JN, Davis JR, Jesseph JE: Subphrenic abscess: a continuing hazard. Am J Surg 117:117, 1969.
38. Brummer DL: Prophylaxis of tuberculosis after gastrectomy (editorial). Am J Dig Dis 14:753, 1969.

SMALL INTESTINE

39. Altemeier WA, Bryant LR, Wulsin JH: The surgical significance of jejunal diverticulosis. Arch Surg 86:732, 1963.
40. Joiner KA, Gorbach SL: Antimicrobial therapy of digestive diseases. Clin Gastroenterol 8:3, 1979.
41. Grady GF, Keusch GT: Pathogenesis of bacterial diarrheas. N Engl J Med 285:831–841, 891–900, 1971.
42. Sleisenger MH, Fordtran JS (eds): Gastrointestinal Disease: Pathophysiology, Diagnosis, Management. Philadelphia, Saunders, 1973.

42a. Thorén A, Wolde-Mariam T, Stintzing G, Wadström T, Habte D: Antibiotics in the treatment of gastroenteritis caused by enteropathogenic *Escherichia coli.* J Infect Dis 141:27, 1980.

43. Archampong EQ: Typhoid ileal perforations: why such mortalities? Br J Surg 63:317, 1976.
44. Singh J, Singh B: Enteric perforation in typhoid fever: a study of 15 cases. Aust NZ J Surg 45:279, 1975.
45. Eggleston FC, Santoshi B, Singh CM: Typhoid perforation of the bowel. Experience in 78 cases. Ann Surg 190:31, 1979.
46. Finegold SM: Anaerobic Bacteria in Human Disease. New York, Academic, 1977.

46a. Newman A, Lambert JR: Campylobacter jejuni causing flare-up in inflammatory bowel disease. Lancet 2:919, 1980.
47. Larsen HE, Price AB, Honour P, Borriello SP: *Clostridium difficile* and the aetiology of pseudomembranous colitis. Lancet 1:1063, 1978.
48. Hitchcock CR, Bubrick MP: Gas gangrene infections of the small intestine, colon and rectum. Dis Colon Rectum 19:112, 1976.
49. Asao OG, Solanke TF: Surgical aspects of ascariasis. J Natl Med Assn 69:149, 1977.
50. Schlossberg D, Devig PM, Travers H, Kovalcik PJ, Mullen JT: Bowel perforation with candidiasis. JAMA 238:2520, 1977.
51. Asraf SM, Mital RN, Prakash A: Tuberculous bowel perforations, Am J Proctol 26:47, 1975.

BACTERIAL OVERGROWTH SYNDROMES

52. Rosenberg IH: Influence of intestinal bacteria on bile acid metabolism and fat absorption: contributions from studies of blind-loop syndrome. Am J Nutr 22:284, 1969.
53. Gracey M, Burke V, Oshin A, Barker J, Glasgow EF: Bacteria, bile salts, and intestinal monosaccharide malabsorption. Gut 12:683, 1971.
54. Goldstein F: Mechanisms of malabsorption and malnutrition in the blind loop syndrome. Gastroenterology 61:780, 1971.
55. Lauterburg BH, Newcomer AD, Hofmann AF: Clinical value of the bile acid breath test. Mayo Clin Proc 53:227, 1978.
56. Drenick EJ, Ament M, Finegold SM, Corrodi P, Passaro E: Bypass enteropathy: intestinal and systemic manifestation following small-bowel bypass. JAMA 236:269, 1976.
57. Francis WW, Eunnuccilli E: Acute fulminating transmural ileocolitis after small bowel bypass for morbid obesity. Am J Surg 135:524, 1978.
58. Drenick EJ, Ament M, Finegold SM, Passaro E: Bypass enteropathy: an inflammatory process in the excluded segment with systemic complications. Am J Clin Nutr 30:76, 1977.
59. Corrodi P, Wideman PA, Sutter VL, Drenick EJ, Passaro E Jr, Finegold SM: Bacterial flora of the small bowel before and after bypass procedure for morbid obesity. J Infect Dis 137:1, 1978.
60. Nelson JL, Rees R, Bonneval MM, Bornside GH, Cohn I: Jejunoileal bypass, liver morphology and intestinal microflora in conventional and germ-free dogs. Surg Forum 27:73, 1976.
61. Barry RE, Chow AW, Billesdon J, Benfield JR, Gorbach SL: Colonic pseudo-obstruction complicating jejuno-ileal bypass: the role of intestinal flora. Gut 16:825, 1975.
61a. Brolin RE, Mendelow H, Ravitch MM: The manifestations of bypass enteritis following jejunoileal bypass. Surg Gynec Obstet 151:209, 1980.
62. Brandberg A, Kock NH, Philipson B: Bacterial flora in intraabdominal ileostomy reservoir. Gastroenterology 63:413, 1972.
63. Schjonsby H, Halvorsen JF, Hofstad T, Hordenak N: Stagnant loop syndrome in patients with continent ileostomy (intra-abdominal ileal reservoir). Gut 18:795, 1977.
64. Halvorsen JF, Heimann P, Hoel R: The continent reservoir ileostomy: review of a collective series of 36 patients from 3 surgical departments. Surgery 83:252, 1978.
65. King SA: Enteritis and the continent ileostomy. Conn Med 41:477, 1977.
66. Nichols RL, Smith JW: Intragastric microbial colonization in common disease states of the stomach and duodenum. Ann Surg 182:557, 1975.
67. Parker TH, O'Leary JP: Effect of preparation of the small bowel on microflora and postoperative wound infections. Surg Gynecol Obstet 146:379, 1978.
68. Hojer H, Wetherfors J: Concentration of doxycycline in bowel tissue and postoperative infections. Scand J Infect Dis (Suppl) 9:100, 1976.

CHAPTER 39
Infections of the Colon

Frank E. Jones and Robert E. Condon

PATHOGENETIC FEATURES OF INFECTIONS ARISING IN THE COLON

ANATOMIC FEATURES

At some point in its course, the colon is situated near every intra-abdominal organ. Loss of bowel wall integrity can, therefore, lead to any of the intra-abdominal infections discussed in Chapter 34. Disease of the cecum or the sigmoid colon may remain localized in the right or left lower quadrant, or extend into the pelvis. Disease of the ascending or descending colon can be confined to the paracolic gutters. Hepatic or splenic flexure disease can cause subphrenic or subhepatic abscesses.

Only the transverse colon and sigmoid colon are supported by a mesentery. Disease may extend directly into the mesentery, remain confined there, or burst free. The result may be an abscess of the lesser sac originating from the transverse colon, or a pelvic or midabdominal (interloop) abscess originating from the sigmoid colon.

The posterior surfaces of the ascending and descending colon are retroperitoneal. Perforation can cause a retroperitoneal abscess with subsequent extension to perineum, thigh, groin, abdominal wall, or chest (posterior mediastinum, pericardium, pleural cavities). Infection arising within the retroperitoneal rectosigmoid or rectum can spread cephalad into the main retroperitoneal spaces, remain localized in the pelvis in the presacral, pararectal, rectovesical, and prevesical spaces, or extend through the levator diaphragm into the ischirorectal space and the perineum.

PHYSIOLOGIC FEATURES

The large bowel conducts the ileal effluent to the rectum, where it is stored until defecation is convenient. Propulsive activity differs in the right and left colon. On the right side, much of the motor activity consists of short runs of circular muscle contractions, involving only a portion of the bowel circumference; bidirectional flow results. Periodically, the cecum contracts, the ascending colon shortens, and a sequential wave of circular muscle contractions strip the luminal content into the transverse colon. Periodic contractions do not occur in the left colon. Rather, mass contraction of both circular and longitudinal muscle occurs from the left transverse to the proximal sigmoid colon. As a result, the left colon forms a semirigid tube through which the fecal mass is moved by contractions of the right colon. Mass contraction activity occurs most consistently after meals.

There is also some evidence for antiperistaltic activity in the left colon. Barium sulfate instilled into the rectum can be found in the ascending and transverse colon within several hours.

Segmental contractions also occur throughout the colon, particularly between meals. These localized, almost occlusive contractions temporarily separate the colon into a series of small compartments, producing a kneading action on the fecal bolus.

Considerable absorption of water, sodium, and chloride occurs during fecal passage through the large bowel. Whereas 1,500 ml of ileal content, containing about 185 mEq of sodium, enters the cecum each day, the daily fecal volume of 200–400 ml contains only 2–5 mEq of sodium. General peritoneal contamination is therefore more common after cecal than sigmoid perforation.

FECAL FLORA

The microbial ecology of the alimentary tract is discussed in Chapter 3. The gut is sterile at birth, but rapidly becomes populated by both aerobic and anaerobic organisms. Although *E. coli* and *Klebsiella* species appear quickly in infant feces, aerobic lactobacilli predominate while milk or formula is the primary food. Anaerobes are present in infant feces within 1 week of birth. *Bacteroides* species predominate in formula-fed babies, while *Bifidobacterium* species are more frequent in breast-fed infants.

The fecal flora remains remarkably stable and is only slightly affected by environmental or dietary changes. Up to 40 percent of stool bulk is composed of bacteria—10^{10}–10^{11} organisms per gram of stool. These numbers are close to the theoretical maximum number (10^{12} per ml) of bacteria that can be packed into such a volume.

The fecal flora is a mixture of aerobic and anaerobic bacteria (Fig. 39-1). The principal aerobic pathogen is *E.*

coli (10^7–10^9 per gram of feces). Other aerobic coliforms (*Klebsiella, Proteus, Enterobacter*) and the enterococcus are present in lower concentrations. Anaerobes are 100 to 1,000 times more numerous in stool than aerobic coliforms.[1] Oxidation-reduction potentials of less than 150 millivolts in the colon provide conditions promoting their growth.

The predominant anaerobic pathogen is *B. fragilis* (10^9–10^{11} organisms per gram) (Fig. 39-1). Of the several subspecies of *B. fragilis*, encapsulated *B. fragilis ssp. fragilis* is recovered most frequently from infections originating from the colon, even though its fecal concentration is low. Other species of *Bacteroides* as well as anaerobic streptococci, peptococci, and peptostreptococci are regularly present in stool (10^6–10^9 organisms per gram). *Clostridium* are also present (10^4–10^6 organisms per gram stool). *Bifidobacterium* and *Fusobacterium* are inconsistent findings, and their concentrations are low.

Staphylococci and fungi also inhabit the colon in small numbers, their concentration being inversely related to the concentration of *E. coli.* Antimicrobial agents, which act selectively against *E. coli,* will permit staphylococcal and fungal overgrowth. *Salmonella typhi* and *V. cholerae* cannot easily colonize the colonic contents unless the inoculum is very high or malnutrition is present.

PERFORATION OF LARGE BOWEL

GENERAL ASPECTS

Epidemiology and Incidence

The causes of large bowel perforation are listed in Table 39-1. In the United States, most perforations are due to carcinoma, diverticulitis, and violent trauma; in less developed areas, parasitic disease is important. Matolo et al [2] found that 30 percent of 102 patients with abdominal visceral perforation, seen during 1972–74, had problems originating in the large bowel. Altemeier et al [3] reported that 20 percent of 501 patients with intra-abdominal abscess had primary large bowel disease. Others [4] have found that 8 to 25 percent of cases of *Bacteroides* infection originated from colorectal disease.

Etiology and Pathogenesis

It is the bacterial component of feces that causes problems after perforation. Sterilized feces injected into the peritoneal cavity of experimental animals have no major adverse consequences. However, feces containing live bacteria produce peritonitis.[5]

Normal fecal organisms are isolated most frequently from patients with abdominal sepsis (Chapter 34).[1,6] *E. coli* is recovered in 9 of 10 cases of infection due to colon perforation and *Klebsiella, Enterobacter, Proteus,* and enterococci are frequent aerobic isolates. *Pseudomonas,* staphylococci, and *Candida* are found infrequently. The most common anaerobic organism is *B. fragilis,* isolated in 80 to 95 percent of patients with colorectal perforation. Also found are other *Bacteroides* species, *Clostridium, Fusobacterium,* peptococci, peptostreptococci, and *Eubacterium.* The number of anaerobic species recovered varies with the skill of the laboratory. The importance of synergistic infections caused by multiple organisms has been stressed by many authors [1,6,7] (Chapters 34, 8). While most enteric aerobes are relatively noninvasive pathogens, anaerobic organisms may be quite tissue-invasive when necrotic tissue, decreased tissue oxidation-reduction potentials, and iron derived from hemoglobin or myoglobin are present. The chief contribution of aerobic organisms in mixed infections may be the utilization of available tissue oxygen.

In addition to the presence of fecal contamination, the volume and consistency of spilled colon contents influence the clinical course after perforation of the large bowel. A right colon perforation is more likely to cause widespread contamination because it contains liquid feces and undergoes frequent contractions. In contrast, the contents of the left colon are solid and its motor activity infrequent.

In prolonged preliminary inflammation (eg, diverticulitis), the omentum and surrounding viscera may seal a leak almost immediately, resulting in a well-localized process. But in perforating trauma, peritoneal defenses are unlikely to be mobilized, and spillage may be extensive.

The site of perforation is another important factor influencing the outcome. If perforation occurs in the intraperitoneal colon, peritoneal contamination may be greater

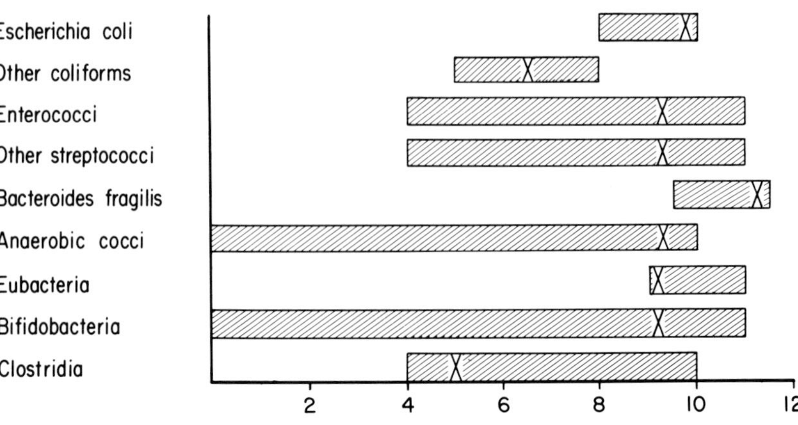

Fig. 39-1. **Concentrations of fecal bacteria. (X = Median; bars = Range.)**

TABLE 39-1. CAUSES OF PERFORATION

- Trauma
  - Penetrating injury
  - Blunt injury
  - Iatrogenic
    - Operative injury
    - Drain erosion
    - Enema
    - Endoscopic and diagnostic
    - Thermometer
  - Colostomy irrigation
  - Ingested foreign body
  - Pneumatic rupture
  - Rectal foreign body
- Diverticular disease
  - Sigmoid diverticula
  - Cecal diverticula
- Inflammatory bowel disease
  - Ulcerative colitis
  - Granulomatous colitis
- Carcinoma of large bowel
- Large bowel obstruction
  - Extrinsic tumor
  - Fecal impaction
  - Volvulus
  - Strangulated hernia
  - Intussusception
  - Pseudoobstruction of colon
- Ischemic colitis
  - Necrotizing colitis
  - Colitis of obstruction
- Ischemic colitis (cont)
  - Colitis of vascular surgery
  - Radiation colitis
  - Stercoral ulcer and perforation
  - Spontaneous ulcer and perforation
- Bacterial infections
  - Shigellosis
  - Salmonellosis, including typhoid
  - Yersiniosis
- Antibiotic-associated colitis
- Tuberculosis
- Actinomycosis
- Cytomegalovirus disease
- Amebiasis
- Schistosomiasis
- Diseases of infancy and childhood
  - Neonatal necrotizing enterocolitis
  - Idiopathic perforation
  - Obstructive lesions
    - Hirschprung disease
    - Atresia of colon or anus
    - Meconium ileus
    - Meconium plug syndrome
    - Neonatal small left colon syndrome
  - Trauma
  - Strangulation of colon
    - Intussusception
    - Hernia
    - Volvulus

but may be balanced by the ability of peritoneal defense mechanisms to localize the infection. On the other hand, retroperitoneal injury results in less initial contamination, but the probability of sealing the perforation is also less. Infection is likely to spread along tissue planes with greater freedom. However, the abscess is more likely to discharge via a sinus to the body surface in close proximity to the original leak, resulting in a milder systemic insult.

Finally, the degree of trauma associated with the perforation is important. A stab wound produces a clean injury associated with little surrounding tissue damage. In contrast, a shotgun blast or shrapnel causes massive injury of surrounding tissue, which promotes infection and interferes with healing.

Clinical Features

Leaking large bowel contents most often cause local peritonitis (Chapter 34). Abdominal pain is constant, aching, and aggravated by sudden change in position or by coughing or retching. Initially, the pain is localized; however, as the process expands the pain spreads, first across the lower abdomen and then upward over the entire abdomen. If the diaphragm is involved, unilateral or bilateral shoulder pain may develop. If the process is confined to the pelvis, little or no anterior abdominal pain may be present. Small amounts of blood in the stool are commonly found on rectal examination.

Peritonitis results in disordered secretory and absorptive function of the bowel. Initially, the bowel segments adjacent to the perforation become inflamed, leading to diarrhea. Later, as ileus develops, obstipation results.

Fever, most often low grade (39C), but sometimes spiking (41C) with shaking chills, is present in nearly all patients. With septicemia, the temperature may be subnormal. Usually, malaise and anorexia are present even if pain is absent. If generalized ileus results, nausea and vomiting may occur.

The clinical presentation combines the findings of hypovolemia and sepsis. At first, pain may induce tachycardia and mild hypertension. With peritonitis, diarrhea, ileus, and vomiting, and extracellular fluid volume becomes depleted, the heart rate increases, blood pressure declines, and shock eventually ensues. The patient is thirsty, lethargic, and weak, and becomes disoriented. Skin turgor may be decreased, and urine output is low. The patient may be flushed owing to septicemia or pale owing to poor capillary filling if hypovolemia predominates. Blood loss may contribute to pallor.

Inspection of the abdomen may show limited motion of respiration due to local guarding. If generalized peritonitis is present, the abdominal component of respiration may be entirely absent. Distension eventually occurs.

Palpation demonstrates localized or generalized guarding. If guarding is not severe, a mass may be palpated. Bowel sounds are hypoactive. The abdomen is distended, tympanitic to percussion, and normal dullness over the liver may be absent. Tenderness can be elicited by abdominal percussion and may be localized to the area of involvement, referred from the local area to elsewhere in the abdominal wall, or be generalized.

Rectal and pelvic examination may demonstrate exquisite tenderness in the presence of pelvic sepsis or generalized peritonitis. Gross or occult blood may be present in the stool. With a pelvic abscess, a fluctuant mass may bulge into the anterior rectum. With a retroperitoneal abscess, abdominal symptoms and signs may be totally absent.

Stone et al [6] note that septicemia caused by anaerobic organisms is often characterized by jaundice and disorientation, as well as high spiking fever. Occasionally, perforation of the colon and rectum is detected first as a perianal or perineal abscess, sometimes even as gangrene of the scrotum and perineum or as a psoas abscess. Motion at the hip joint may be limited because of muscle spasm or joint involvement. Thus, a patient presenting with buttock, perineal, groin, or thigh pain, associated with erythematous or dusky skin, perhaps with bullae or tissue emphysema, may have an occult colon perforation.

More bizarre clinical presentations of colon perforation such as mediastinitis, empyema, or pneumopericardium have been recorded. Polk and Shields [8] have described patients in whom remote systemic organ failure was the only clinical evidence of sepsis that originated in the large bowel.

Laboratory Findings

In most cases, the leukocyte count is elevated between 10,000 and 20,000 cells per mm^3. *Bacteroides* septicemia may elicit leukocyte counts as high as 50,000. The differential count usually shows increased numbers of immature neutrophils.

A normal urinalysis indicates that the urinary tract is not the source of the problem. However, an infection contiguous to any portion of the urinary system may induce a mild pyuria or hematuria. A fistula between the colon and the urinary tract directly contaminates the urine.

Abdominal roentgenograms should be taken in the recumbent, upright, and left and right lateral decubitus positions. Free air may be noted under the diaphragm on upright films (Fig. 39-2A) or in the flank on the lateral decubitus films (Fig. 39-2B). Loss of a flank preperitoneal fat stripe or a psoas shadow indicates local inflammation in these areas. The kidney outline may be obscured as a result of a perinephric infection. Inflammation in perirenal and pararenal tissues may impair the movement of the kidneys when the patient moves from a recumbent to an erect position. The presence of free intraperitoneal fluid may be suggested.

Examination of the bowel gas pattern can indicate ileus, obstruction, or volvulus. "Thumbprinting" suggests ischemic or inflamed colon. Displaced loops of bowel indicate an extrinsic mass, and extraluminal gas bubbles point to an abscess.

In most clinical situations, contrast studies are unnecessary. Intravenous pyelography may help document the location of the ureters, and in doubtful cases, water-soluble contrast studies of the colon can confirm the leak. Barium contrast studies should be avoided.

Endoscopy may be considered if the patient is stable and the diagnosis is unclear. The perforation itself, another lesion, or ischemic mucosa may be noted.

In cases of multiple trauma, and in obtunded patients or children, the diagnosis may be more difficult. Peritoneal lavage with a liter of crystalloid solution may yield helpful information; finding bacteria, vegetable fibers, or other fecal matter, or a white blood cell concentration greater than 500 per mm^3 of lavage fluid may help establish a diagnosis of perforation.

In patients with an obscure clinical picture, compatible with but not diagnostic of intra-abdominal or retroperitoneal sepsis, three recent techniques of detecting and localizing septic processes have been proposed (Chapter 34)—ultrasonography, radioisotopic scanning, and computerized tomography. Norton et al [9] found the overall accuracy of these techniques was 57, 54, and 67 percent respectively. In addition, agreement between tests was achieved in 57 percent of patients who had two examinations, but in only 22 percent of patients who had all three tests. No test was superior to the other. Thus, while there is a place for each examination, the information derived in individual patients must be interpreted in light of the total clinical picture.

Diagnosis

In order to provide optimum antimicrobial therapy, it is desirable, but probably impossible, to identify each organism involved in these infections. Chapter 34 lists those bacteria commonly found in feculent peritonitis, and the rationale for empiric choice of antibiotics. A Gram stain of the infected material is sometimes helpful in the tentative identification of organisms morphologically identifiable as anaerobes. Even when anaerobes cannot be cultured, anaerobes must be assumed as present in all fresh perforations. Stone et al [6] have documented that the ability to isolate anaerobic organisms from intra-abdominal pus decreases the longer the peritoneal cavity is exposed to air. The procedures best for anaerobic culture are described in Chapter 12.

Treatment and Prognosis

Treatment of a suspected large bowel perforation should be vigorous. The blood volume should be replenished with intravenous crystalloid solution or blood. A gastric tube should be placed to empty the stomach contents and reduce the risk of aspiration of vomitus.

Because human stool contains *Clostridium tetani* in 10 to 25 percent of patients,[1] tetanus prophylaxis should be administered (Chapter 44). Intravenous antibiotics should be administered immediately. Since fecal organisms are most likely to be present, a combination of an aminoglycoside and clindamycin is best. Alternative choices of antibiotics in secondary bacterial peritonitis are discussed in Chapter 34.

After the patient is prepared, surgical control of the perforation is obtained. The basic tasks to be accomplished at operation are closure or exteriorization of the perforation and removal of necrotic tissue and pus.

The site of leakage must be controlled. On occasion, this may be accomplished by simple suture closure if: (1)

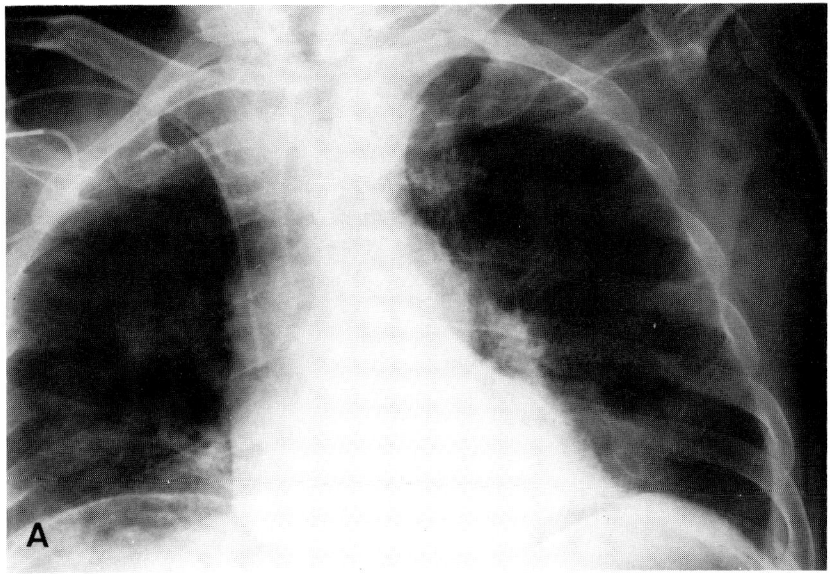

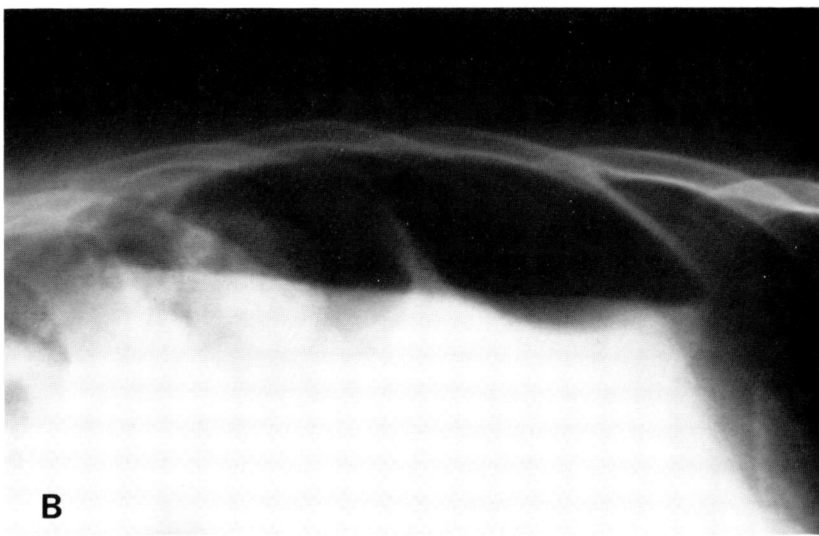

Fig. 39-2. **A. Colon perforation. Free air is seen under the diaphragm on an upright chest film. B. Colon perforation. Free air is seen under the right rib cage on a left lateral decubitus abdominal film.**

there is no fecal contamination, (2) the colon wound is small, and (3) the colon wall is otherwise structurally normal. More frequently, the involved bowel should be exteriorized or resected. Exteriorization or resection are preferred to closure and proximal colostomy in most situations. The circumstances in which drainage alone of a large bowel perforation suffices are few.

The rationale of thorough peritoneal toilet in the treatment of peritonitis is discussed in Chapter 34. As much necrotic tissue as possible should be debrided. Collections of pus must be aspirated completely. Abscess cavities are drained externally, using liberal numbers of soft Penrose drains and sump drains. The drains should be brought out through separate stab incisions placed so that the drainage track is as short, direct, and dependent as possible. The peritoneal cavity should be irrigated copiously with 10 to 20 liters of saline or other crystalloid solution to remove all fibrinous debris and to dilute the concentration of residual bacteria. A final irrigation is performed using a solution containing diluted kanamycin and bacitracin. In our hands, the use of indwelling inflow and outflow catheters for postoperative irrigation has often been unsatisfactory because of mechanical obstruction of one or more of the catheters.

The incision is closed using a running suture of monofilament nylon, prolene, or wire. The skin is not closed; the exposed subcutaneous tissues are covered with a single layer of fine mesh gauze under bulky dressings. The entire dressing is changed postoperatively as often as it is needed. The removal of the mesh serves to debride the wound. If the wound is clean and contains no necrotic tissue, delayed closure is accomplished by loose approximation of the wound edges after the fifth postoperative day.

Although the risk of death following perforation of the colon and rectum is still high, the mortality rate of patients with untreated intra-abdominal sepsis approaches 100 percent.[3] Thus, expeditious and thorough surgical therapy, combined with aggressive postoperative care and essential organ support, are essential to save as many patients as possible.

PERFORATION OF THE COLON IN INFANCY

Large bowel perforations account for about 18 percent of all gastrointestinal perforations in children. Cruze and Snyder [10] identified the apparent cause of colon perforation in 16 infants and children. Colitis (probably necrotizing enterocolitis) was the cause in five; Hirschprung disease, atresia of the anus or colon, and idiopathic perforation were present in three patients each. One patient had meconium ileus, and one had a perforation following closure of a colostomy.

Neonatal Necrotizing Enterocolitis

This disease causes one-fourth of all pediatric gastrointestinal perforations. Although the problem became increasingly apparent during the 1970s,[11,12] the need for operation has decreased of late as understanding of the pathogenesis of the disease has increased.

Pathology and Pathogenesis

Variable amounts of gut are affected in neonatal necrotizing enterocolitis. The ileocecal area and ascending colon are involved most often; the entire gut from stomach to rectum is affected in 5 to 15 percent of cases. Skip areas of necrotic and normal bowel are often found. The gut proximal to areas of involvement and the involved bowel are both dilated, the bowel wall being thin and friable. The affected bowel may demonstrate a spectrum of necrosis from areas of apparent subserosal ecchymosis to obvious full-thickness gangrene. Multiple perforations surrounded by deposits of fibrin and exudate are frequent and perforations may be sealed by adherent surrounding loops of bowel. The mucosa is edematous, hemorrhagic, or ulcerated. Frequently, pockets of gas are noted under the mucosa and, less frequently, subserosally. Gas bubbles may be detected in mesenteric veins.

Microscopic examination shows hemorrhagic, edematous, and ulcerated mucosa, which may progress to full-thickness necrosis of the bowel wall. Bacteria may be seen in the bowel wall. Ganglion cells are present between muscle layers. Intramural blood vessels are engorged, but thrombosis is rare except in autopsy specimens.

Certain predisposing factors appear to be critical to the pathogenesis of this condition. The Apgar score is often below seven, and most of these infants (68 to 80 percent) are premature or have low birth weights. Respiratory distress syndrome or apneic episodes occur in 50 to 60 percent, an umbilical artery catheter has been used in 25 to 60 percent, and exchange transfusion has been necessary in another 15 to 45 percent. Congenital heart disease and patent ductus arteriosus are present in 20 to 45 percent.

The common factor seems to be bowel ischemia. Thromboembolic phenomena may be involved, but vasospasm in response to hypoxia and stress seems to be more important. Barlow and Santulli [13] have been able to reproduce a similar condition in newborn rats subjected to hypoxia or to cold stress. After the mucosal barrier is injured, gut bacteria can invade and cause further damage.

Whether infection is ever a primary cause of neonatal necrotizing enterocolitis is debated. Clustering of cases of enterocolitis suggesting an infectious epidemic have been reported.[14,15] Book et al [14] were unable to identify any specific responsible organisms, but using infection control procedures, they reduced their incidence of necrotizing enterocolitis from 3.6 to 0.7 percent. On the other hand, Howard et al [15] were able to isolate *Clostridium butyricum* from the blood of nine of their ten patients. In contrast, Bell et al [16] found no unusual organisms in patients with enterocolitis, even though *E. coli* and *K. pneumoniae* were more prevalent in the feces of enterocolitis patients than control patients.

Many patients with necrotizing enterocolitis have been fed formula or glucose solution rather than breast milk, with its apparent protective effect due to its content of IgA and leukocytes.[13] Formula and glucose solutions are, in addition, hyperosmolar and may further injure ischemic mucosa.

Clinical Manifestations

Although the syndrome usually starts during the first 10 days of life, necrotizing enterocolitis can be delayed for 3 or 4 weeks. Initial changes may be subtle—lethargy, acrocyanosis, increased gastric retention between feedings, and vomiting or regurgitation of bile-stained gastric contents. Abdominal distention is almost always present, initially soft and nontender, but later tender with erythema and induration of the abdominal wall. The presence of an inflammatory mass in the scrotum or pneumoscrotum indicates bowel perforation.[11] In a thin neonate, intramural intestinal air blebs may be detectable by abdominal palpation, a sensation akin to that of feeling Rice Krispies.

Affected infants have usually passed meconium, and the anus is patent. Diarrhea sometimes appears, and one-fourth pass stools of mucus and visible blood. Hypothermia or thermal instability is frequent. As dehydration progresses, tachycardia and hypotension become apparent. Petechiae and oropharyngeal bleeding appear late in the course.

Diagnosis

Laboratory examination at first reveals only a mild anemia, leukocytosis or leukopenia, and thrombocytopenia (50,000–75,000). In later stages of the illness, diffuse intravascular coagulation, hypoxia, and acidosis will be evident. Stool analysis may reveal the presence of occult blood and of reducing substances (carbohydrate). These tests may be used to screen infants at risk for enterocolitis, but a positive result in the absence of other clinical signs does not establish a diagnosis.

All pediatric patients with findings suggestive of sepsis should have cultures of sputum, urine, feces, cerebrospinal fluid, and blood made before institution of antibiotic treatment. Positive blood culture findings are obtained from 20 to 70 percent of patients with necrotizing enterocolitis. In the majority of cases, *E. coli, Klebsiella, Enterobacter,* and *Proteus* are recovered. Positive anaerobic blood culture results are rare, although Howard et al [15] describe a group of patients from whom *C. butyricum* was isolated.

Repeated plain abdominal roentgenograms in the recumbent, upright, or lateral decubitus positions at 4- to

8-hour intervals are most useful for diagnosing and following necrotizing enterocolitis. The early picture is one of generalized ileus, with dilation of the stomach and small and large bowel. As the disease progresses, there is evidence of thickened bowel walls. Intramural collections of gas—pneumatosis cystoides intestinalis—are noted in 75 to 80 percent of patients. In addition, gas may be noted in the mesenteric and portal venous systems. Intra-abdominal fluid is found in later stages of the disease. Free intraperitoneal gas indicates bowel perforation. Fixed loops of bowel may indicate areas of sealed perforation. Early in the disease, one should resist the temptation to perform a contrast enema, because the risk of perforation is great while the diagnostic aid is small.

Treatment

The appropriate role of medical and surgical treatment of neonatal necrotizing enterocolitis has evolved rapidly. When operation was routine, the mortality rate was high.[11,17] Early enterocolitis can most often be cured by nonoperative treatment. Oral feedings should be stopped, gastric suction instituted, and intravenous antibiotics begun. On the basis of the organisms usually cultured, an aminoglycoside and a penicillin (usually ampicillin) are chosen as initial therapy. On the basis of the work of Cohn et al,[18] which indicates that topical antibiotics can help to heal ischemic bowel, Bell et al [17] also administer aminoglycosides by gastric tube.

Intravenous fluids and electrolytes help maintain vital signs, urine output, and normal electrolyte balance. Blood is replaced as necessary. Fresh whole blood or fresh frozen plasma is given if coagulation abnormalities develop. It may be necessary to transfuse platelets. Maintenance of nutrition with intravenous alimentation is essential. Nonoperative therapy is continued as long as improvement is noted.

The indication for operation in acute necrotizing enterocolitis is development of gangrene of the bowel, with or without actual perforation. The clinical task is to detect this state without performing unnecessary operations. Kosloske et al [19] recently reviewed 61 infants with this disease. A total of 10 proposed clinical, roentgenographic, and laboratory criteria for operation were considered. Each operative criterion was correlated with the documented presence or absence of intestinal gangrene. Indications for operation verified by this study were: (1) pneumoperitoneum, (2) paracentesis findings positive for gangrenous intestine, (3) erythema of the abdominal wall, (4) a fixed abdominal mass, and (5) a persistently dilated loop of intestine on serial abdominal radiographs. The first two signs occurred frequently; the latter three were rare. Operative indications that proved to be invalid in this study were: (1) clinical deterioration, (2) persistent abdominal tenderness, (3) profuse lower gastrointestinal hemorrhage, (4) the roentgenographic finding of a gasless abdomen with ascites, and (5) severe thrombocytopenia.

Surgical management involves resection of perforated and gangrenous segments of bowel. If any doubt exists as to whether bowel may survive, it is better to perform a second-look operation after 24 hours than to excise too much bowel and cause malabsorption problems. All free ends of bowel should be brought out as enterostomies instead of performing primary anastomoses.

Prognosis

Neonatal necrotizing enterocolitis used to be uniformly fatal. With earlier diagnosis and aggressive treatment, survival rates with nonoperative therapy now range from 29 to 100 percent (median 69 percent).[12,17] Kosloske et al [19] found the mortality of patients with perforation to be 64 percent—double that (30 percent) of patients who underwent operation for intestinal gangrene without perforation. Survival rates in the more severely ill surgical patients in other series range from 31 to 90 percent (median 54 percent).[12,17] The mortality rate is determined in part by the underlying condition that originally predisposed to necrotizing enterocolitis. Late complications include malabsorption when large lengths of bowel must be excised and obstruction resulting from stricture as the ischemic bowel heals. Obstruction usually necessitates operation, although Tonkin et al [20] document strictures that have resolved spontaneously.

Idiopathic Perforation of the Colon in Infants and Children

Although affected patients do not present the usual picture of necrotizing enterocolitis, ischemia of the gut may also account for these lesions.

Idiopathic perforation of the colon can be difficult to detect. The predominant sign is abdominal distension. Obstipation, bilious vomiting, and unstable vital signs usually develop but may be absent. The diagnosis is made by the presence of free air within the peritoneal cavity in the absence of any obstructive or traumatic lesion. The treatment is the same as any secondary bacterial peritonitis (Chapters 9 and 34), plus exteriorization or resection of the diseased bowel.

Obstructive Lesions Leading to Colonic Perforation in Infants and Children

Hirschprung disease,[21,22] atresia of the colon or anus, meconium ileus, meconium plug syndrome, and neonatal small left colon syndrome will result in perforation of the colon if left unattended. Patients with Hirschprung disease frequently develop an enterocolitis proximal to the obstructed segment. This condition is distinct from necrotizing enterocolitis in that necrosis of the bowel wall with perforation is unusual, even though septicemia can occur; the mucosa demonstrates only a nonspecific colitis.[23]

Hirschprung Disease

The clinical picture of Hirschprung disease may vary, but in all instances problems with defecation begin in the first few days of life. There may be no spontaneous passage of meconium, or only small amounts may be passed. Vigorous rectal examination or enemas may result in passage of a large quantity of normal meconium and stool. Typically, abdominal distension develops over weeks or months and peristaltic waves are sometimes visible on the abdominal wall. Feeding is less vigorous, bilious vomiting may occur, and food may be retained only intermittently. The infant is unusually listless and fails to gain weight. Cecal perforation or acute appendicitis in the newborn are commonly caused by Hirschprung disease.[22]

The enterocolitis of Hirschprung disease occurs in about one-fourth of patients and is responsible for most of the deaths.[22,23] Explosive diarrhea is associated with abdominal distension, fever, and prostration.

Some individuals with untreated Hirschprung disease survive infancy. These patients have problems with chronic constipation, abdominal distension, and flatulence, but encopresis does not occur. Both development and weight gain lag. Although mild, intermittent episodes of diarrhea are more prevalent; enterocolitis continues to be a risk.

Hirschprung disease is suspected when a dilated colon filled with feces is seen proximal to the involved narrow segment on barium enema. Usually, there is a rather definite demarcation between segments. To be certain of the diagnosis, a rectal biopsy demonstrating lack of intermuscular ganglion cells is required.

Often the obstruction of Hirschprung disease can be initially managed by enemas, but once the diagnosis has been proved by rectal biopsy, a colostomy proximal to the affected segment should be established. When the child has grown sufficiently, and the proximal bowel has returned to normal size, the abnormal bowel is resected and a coloanal or colorectal anastomosis is made in the manner of Swenson, Duhamel, or Soave. Usually, the enterocolitis can be managed for several days with frequent saline enemas. Careful observation by a physician or parent is necessary to prevent dehydration in severe cases.

Patients with Hirschprung disease rarely survive to adulthood without operation. Death occurs in 2 to 4 percent of patients who undergo elective resection.[22,24] Patients with enterocolitis, especially infants, have a much worse prognosis, because of the complications of dehydration, perforation, and septicemia. The mortality rate in enterocolitis is 30 to 55 percent.[22,23] The significance of enterocolitis in Hirschprung disease is indicated by the mortality rate of diverting colostomy performed in infants before or after the onset of enterocolitis—4 percent versus 33 percent, respectively. The incidence of postoperative enterocolitis is 5 to 25 percent[24] and is more likely to occur if it was present preoperatively. Sieber and Soave[22] report that the Swenson procedure results in the highest rate of postoperative enterocolitis.

Other Obstructive Colonic Lesions

These lesions, the meconium plug syndrome, atresia, and the small left colon syndrome, are unusual causes of perforation proximal to the obstruction, and rarely are associated with enterocolitis of the obstructed bowel. The diagnosis is usually apparent on barium enema.

The meconium plug syndrome and the small left colon syndrome do not require operative treatment unless perforation has taken place. Irrigation of the colon with Gastrografin usually suffices to clear obstructing meconium from the bowel. As the child matures and as the distal colon is used, the bowel attains normal caliber. Atresia and meconium ileus require operative correction of the obstruction.

Trauma

Children often swallow foreign objects, which may perforate the colon. Iatrogenic perforation with a thermometer or an enema also occurs. Patients with trauma to the colon usually present clinical features similar to those of adults. When the history of the accident is vague, the possibility of parental child abuse must be considered.

Strangulation of the Colon

This occurs most frequently as a result of an obstructing lesion, such as malrotation of the bowel or incarcerated hernia. In infants, hernia must be sought not only in the inguinal and umbilical regions, but also in unusual sites such as the diaphragm, perineum, and lumbar areas.

Treatment

The treatment of trauma and strangulation follows the usual principles—remove necrotic bowel, close or remove perforated bowel segments, relieve obstruction by resection, diversion, or bypass. The decision whether or not to perform primary anastomosis or primary closure of the bowel depends on a number of factors, including viability of the bowel, degree of peritonitis and fecal contamination, and the size of the structures to be anastomosed.

TRAUMATIC PERFORATION OF COLON AND RECTUM

Pathogenesis

Trauma to the colon and rectum usually leads to uncontrolled peritoneal contamination which, if left untreated for long, will produce a true infectious peritonitis.[25,26,27] Most (92 percent) injuries of colon and rectum are the result of *penetrating trauma.* Gunshot wounds predominate, 3 to 1. The transverse colon is involved most frequently (36 percent), followed by the left colon (32 percent), the right colon (24 percent), and the rectum (8 percent). Isolated large bowel injuries are present only about 20 percent of the time. Rectal injuries are frequently accompanied by injuries to the pelvic skeleton and genitourinary system. The severity of the resulting infection and the prognosis are usually determined by the gravity of the injuries to organs other than the colon.

The velocity and mass of the penetrating projectile determine the amount of energy delivered to the tissues (Chapter 22). Stab wounds usually cause little injury beyond the wound track. Multiple fragments obviously cause more damage than a single missile. The amount of foreign matter (bone, dirt, clothing) carried into the wound is an important infection-potentiating factor, and some missile materials, such as phosphorous, are injurious in themselves. The time between injury and definitive treatment is also important. The longer uncontrolled infection or impaired vascularity are present, the more severe the necrosis. After a perforating agent passes through feces, it becomes contaminated so that invasive infection may develop anywhere along the subsequent path of injury.[28]

Most (50 to 70 percent) blunt injuries are the result of vehicular trauma.[25,27] There are four mechanisms of *blunt injury* to intra-abdominal colon:

1. Rapid deceleration avulses bowel segments which are fixed at the ends to the retroperitoneum, eg, the transverse or sigmoid colon. Intramural hematoma, mesenteric tear producing bowel ischemia, or laceration of the bowel wall can all result.

2. Acute increases in intraluminal pressure can cause blow-out lesions.

3. Linear trauma is caused by direct impact.

4. Injury may result from general compression of the abdomen, as in crush trauma and explosions. Compression often produces primarily retroperitoneal injury, because the increased pressure is distributed evenly to all sides of intraperitoneal structures but unevenly to only part of the surface of the retroperitoneal portions of the bowel.

Rectal injuries associated with blunt trauma usually accompany fractures of the pelvis. The rectum may be lacerated by bone fragments. Avulsion injuries of the rectum occur most often at the level of attachment of the levator sling to the rectum. Avulsion of the rectum from the sphincter apparatus may occur.

Iatrogenic trauma is frequent, but is reported infrequently. Injuries at operation are usually recognized quickly, so that fecal spillage is minimal or absent. Erosion of the colon by an adjacent stiff drain usually appears as a fecal fistula. Injuries during enemas or colostomy irrigations are caused by the enema tip itself or excessive hydrostatic pressure. Injection of an irritating enema solution, such as hypertonic phosphate, may result in widespread necrosis of tissue. The most common cause of rectal injury in infants is perforation by a thermometer. If the perforation is limited to perirectal tissues, only a perirectal or ischiorectal abscess may develop.

Most iatrogenic injuries occur during diagnostic procedures. The rate of perforation after barium enema is about 0.02 percent.[29] Although the resting pressure developed by a barium enema with the reservoir 4 feet above the table is only 8–38 mmHg, spasms of the colon during the procedure can produce pressures of over 170 mmHg, which are sufficient to rupture a normal colon.[30] The risk of perforation is increased when a barium enema is performed through a colostomy stoma. Sterile barium sulfate injected into the peritoneal cavity induces a benign, self-limited, acute inflammatory reaction, granuloma formation, and adhesions.[5] In contrast, the experimental injection of feces together with barium uniformly produces death. Water-soluble contrast medium mixed with feces also is more lethal than feces alone in laboratory animals, but can be treated more successfully than barium peritonitis. Injection of barium and feces into the paracolic soft tissues leads to soft tissue infections. Intramesenteric perforation may occur, usually in patients with diverticular disease. Barium injected into the portal venous system [31] usually results in pylephlebitis and death.

Perforation during passage of the rigid proctoscope usually affects the anterior surface of the sigmoid colon near the sacral promontory where the sigmoid angulation is most acute. Most perforations, however, occur as a consequence of biopsy.

The rate of perforation during diagnostic fiberoptic colonoscopy is less than 1 percent. During colonoscopic polypectomy, the perforation rate is less than 1.6 percent.[32] Most perforations are caused by inexperienced endoscopists. Air insufflation carries the danger of overinflation, especially of the normal cecum and transverse colon. Particular care must be taken to avoid insufflation directly into the mouth of a diverticulum. In addition, perforation may occur through diseased segments of bowel or through seromuscular tears induced during the procedure.

Perforation may also occur because of mechanical trauma; the tip of the instrument may be forced through the colon wall, especially during the blind "slide-by" maneuver. As perforation is about to occur, one ceases to see the mucosa sliding by the tip of the scope and sees instead a red-out. If further pressure is applied, one sees a white-out, followed by perforation. Perforation may occur when trying to pass through a stricture or beyond a tumor. Application of pressure to advance the colonoscope can create great tension on the mesentery of a looped portion of colon, particularly the sigmoid colon. Seromuscular tears of the sigmoid colon are frequently seen when laparotomy is performed soon after colonscopy. Further pressure from the instrument or from insufflated air results in perforation. When such "bowing" of the bowel occurs, the forces that tend to cause trauma can be reduced by straightening maneuvers or by performing an alpha maneuver. But such maneuvers themselves may cause injury, particularly when the sigmoid colon is bound down by adhesions.

The unprepared colon contains inflammable gases in nearly half of patients, and there is a theoretical danger of an explosion occurring during electrocoagulation. Although most endoscopists no longer insufflate with carbon dioxide, episodes of explosion have not often been recorded.

Occasional perforations of the rectum may occur during cystoscopy and culdoscopy, often causing minimal damage. Small perforations of the colon may occur during paracentesis of the abdominal cavity.

Another potential infectious complication of diagnostic procedures is *septicemia.* Blood cultures taken during rectal examination have failed to document bacteremia, but bacteremia has been documented during, and for up to 30 minutes after, proctoscopy, barium enema, and colonoscopy. Transient bacteremia can be expected to cause no problem in healthy patients; however, a patient with leukemia died of anaerobic septicemia following a barium enema.[33] Antibiotic prophylaxis is mandatory in immunodepressed patients and in those subject to development of endocarditis.

Perforation of colon during *colostomy dilation* or *irrigation* is rare.[34] The most common mechanism is forcing an irrigation catheter through the wall of a redundant loop of colon. Such loops are frequently associated with paracolostomy hernia. Perforation may be intraperitoneal or into the abdominal wall. This type of perforation may be avoided by using a cone irrigation device rather than a catheter.

Colon perforation by an *ingested foreign body* occurs in children, denture wearers, and the mentally incompetent. More than 90 percent of all foreign objects and 80 percent of ingested sharp foreign bodies pass per rectum, without incident, usually within a week. After an object has passed out of the stomach, perforation is most likely to occur in the large bowel, especially the cecum and sigmoid colon. Perforation may be acute, resulting in peritonitis and abscess formation, or chronic resulting in an abscess adjacent to the site of the perforation while the perforation itself is found to have healed.

Pneumatic rupture of the large bowel [35] is usually the result of a prank in which the nozzle of a compressed air hose is placed near the anus.[30] The average bursting pressure of the colon in adults was found to be 184, 191, 131, and 94 mmHg for the rectum, sigmoid colon, transverse colon, and cecum respectively.[30]

Another type of trauma to the perineum and large bowel is *impalement injury,* usually a fall onto a rigid rod or stake. If the object is long enough, multiple injuries to the bowel and other organs may occur. A similar injury results from insertion of foreign bodies into the rectum for erotic purposes [36] or following a sexual assault with a foreign object. Perforation may occur through the extraperitoneal rectum or through the sigmoid colon.

Clinical Manifestations

The clinical presentation in the traumatic varieties of perforation are similar to the typical picture of nontraumatic large bowel perforation described previously.

When the colon has been injured by a penetrating injury, abdominal pain usually develops within an hour or two. The symptoms of colon injury may be overshadowed by those owing to other concomitant injuries. Entrance and exit wounds are examined to estimate the track of the missile or weapon. Omentum, bowel, or stool may be present in the wound. Marked abdominal distension suggests intraperitoneal free blood or occasionally air. Usually, the abdomen is quiet on auscultation and tender to palpation; signs of peritonitis are present. Blood may be present in the rectum. On occasion, no findings are present initially, and repeated examinations are necessary to detect signs of colon injury as early as possible.

Following *blunt trauma,* examination yields similar findings; ecchymoses may suggest the mechanism of injury. A fracture of the pelvis should make one suspect rectal injury. A quiet tender abdomen suggests significant injury, as does blood in the rectum.

Iatrogenic injuries of large bowel frequently produce immediate abdominal pain and progressive signs of peritonitis temporally related to the procedure (e.g., perforation by biopsy at proctosigmoidoscopy may not be apparent for hours or days). When the injury results from an enema or colostomy irrigation, the patient often reports that there was little or no return of the solution. Blood may be found on a catheter or thermometer. Perforation during endoscopy may be immediately apparent when the examiner sees omentum or small intestine, or free air may be seen in the peritoneal cavity on postcolonoscopy abdominal roentgenogram. Barium may be seen either leaking into the peritoneal cavity or in an extraluminal location in the evacuation films.

Diagnosis

Laboratory findings following traumatic perforation of the large bowel are similar to those for nontraumatic perforation. Roentgenograms of the chest, abdomen, and pelvis are essential in cases of penetrating and blunt trauma. These studies are most useful for helping to determine the path taken by bullets and other missiles. Pelvic fractures are detected or confirmed. Contrast studies of the large bowel are contraindicated when perforation is suspected. All patients with indwelling rectal foreign bodies should have biplanar roentgenograms taken of the pelvis to determine the orientation of the object.

Proctoscopy is indicated any time blood is detected on rectal examination. Proctoscopy should also be considered in any patient in whom a missile has traversed the pelvis or who has a pelvic fracture. In addition, proctoscopy is indicated in those with rectal injury or rectal foreign body—both before and after extraction.

When the patient is unable to communicate with the physician, as in cases of head trauma or young children, or when physical examination is otherwise inconclusive, peritoneal lavage may be useful to detect evidence of intra-abdominal injury. The finding of blood (100,000 RBC per mm^3), leukocytes (500 per mm^3), or feces in the lavage aspirate may indicate perforation of the colon. A Gram stain of the lavage return can offer definitive proof of bacterial contamination in doubtful cases.

Treatment

The general approach to intraperitoneal colonic perforation has been discussed in preceding sections of this chapter. Improved survival rates are achieved when intervention occurs within 6 hours of injury. Antibiotics, preferably an aminoglycoside and clindamycin, are administered intravenously, tetanus prophylaxis is given, and blood volume is restored. Appropriate arrangements for monitoring are made (CVP, Foley catheter, etc.).

The importance of separating injured colon segments from adjacent bone injuries at operation to prevent development of osteomyelitis has been stressed by Christy.[37] Devitalized bone fragments should be debrided whenever feasible. Most discussion concerning treatment of colon and rectal trauma centers on the method of control and repair of the traumatized bowel. Traditional treatment has taken four forms: (1) primary repair of the injury with protection of the repair with a proximal diverting colostomy or ileostomy, (2) exteriorization of the injury as a colostomy, (3) resection of the injured bowel with anastomosis protected by a proximal diverting enterostomy or colostomy, and (4) resection with an end-colostomy and mucus fistula or oversewing of the distal remnant. Subsequent stoma closure is always necessary with traditional management.

A primary repair, or resection with immediate primary anastomosis without a proximal diverting stoma, avoids a temporary colostomy and, if successful, shortens convalescence. Primary closure, with or without resection, has been found to be as safe as traditional methods, if *all* the following conditions prevail: (1) minimal injury to colon adjacent to the perforation, (2) repair conducted less than 6 hours after injury, (3) stable patient without preceding shock or severe hemorrhage, (4) good basic health prior to injury, (5) injury to no more than one other organ in addition to the large bowel, and (6) minimal or no fecal spillage or peritonitis.[38] Unfortunately, the necessary conditions are not often fulfilled. In addition, if a urinary tract injury coexists, primary anastomosis is inherently dangerous even if all other conditions for the direct approach are fulfilled.

A compromise procedure is proposed in which the injury is exteriorized, but primary closure is performed in order to obviate the need for colostomy. The segment is then "interiorized" after 7 to 10 days if the repair remains intact.

Primary repair and careful observation of rectal lacerations is feasible when there is no gross fecal leakage, significant hematoma, or necrosis of surrounding tissue. Otherwise, diverting sigmoid colostomy and primary repair or resection of the damaged segment is recommended. Whether or not diverting colostomy is carried out, washout of all fecal matter from the rectum and dependent drainage of traumatized perirectal tissues through the perineum will reduce the incidence and severity of subsequent pelvic infections.

Prognosis

The median mortality rate for a collected series of nearly 4,000 patients was 7.5 percent,[39-47] and the median incidence of infectious complications was 28 percent. Traditional management, including treatment by exteriorized primary repair, was employed in 55 percent of patients, with a median mortality rate of 10.5 percent and a median infectious morbidity rate of 32.5 percent. Primary repair was performed in 45 percent of patients. The median mortality rate was 6 percent, and the median morbidity rate was 24 percent.

Stone and Fabian [38] have reported a prospective, randomized study of traditional versus primary closure therapy in patients whose wounds fulfilled the six criteria listed in the previous section. The mortality rate (1 percent) was the same in each group. The infectious morbidity rates were greater in the group treated with colostomy (wound sepsis—57 percent, peritoneal sepsis—29 percent, anastomotic failure—10 percent) than in the group treated with primary closure without colostomy (48 percent, 15 percent, and 1 percent, respectively). However, significantly greater complication rates occurred only in patients having intraperitoneal drains.

Right colon injuries could be analyzed specifically in four series.[45-47] This subgroup was composed of 384 patients, 41 percent of whom were treated by traditional measures and 59 percent by primary repair. The overall mortality rate (4 percent) in patients with right colon trauma was better than for all colon trauma patients, and there was no difference in the mortality rates of patients treated traditionally (4 percent) or by primary repair (3 percent). However, the infectious morbidity rate in those treated traditionally (25 percent) was better than that for those treated by primary repair (40 percent).

Exteriorized primary repair was successful in avoiding colostomy in 66 percent of 153 patients. It is important to change the sterile moist dressings frequently to prevent serositis. The morbidity rate was only modestly better with primary repairs, and the mortality rate was essentially the same as for traditional treatment. The results of primary repair must be interpreted in light of the fact that primary repair was usually performed in patients with injuries much less severe than those of patients treated by traditional measures. Although primary repair of colon injuries may succeed under favorable circumstances, the available data indicate that traditional measures are indicated in most large bowel injuries. The use of methods of "instant bowel prep" may improve results of primary repair in carefully selected cases (see subsequent section on bowel preparation).

DIVERTICULAR DISEASE OF THE COLON

Incidence

The true incidence of diverticulosis of the colon in the general population is unknown, because estimates derived from either necropsy or barium enema studies are of necessity biased. Most studies cite an incidence of 6 to 8 percent.[48,49]

Diverticulosis is principally a disease of the elderly who reside in Western industrial nations. Patients less than 40 years of age make up less than 3 percent of the patients,[50] and patients older than 70 years of age have an incidence of about 25 percent. Most recent series document a higher incidence of diverticular disease in females—an observation that cannot be explained by the greater longevity of women.

Pathogenesis

The pathologic anatomy of diverticular disease has been reviewed by Morson.[51] Typical diverticula are pulsion-type outpouchings of mucosa protruding through the colon circular muscle at sites of apparent weakness, located adjacent to the mesenteric side of each of the antimesenteric taeniae, at the point where the blood vessels penetrate the wall. In addition, smaller vessels penetrate the bowel wall on either side of the mesenteric taenia. Thus, typically, there are two rows of diverticula on each side of the colon. The mucosa of the diverticulum is covered superficially by a thin layer of longitudinal muscle and peritoneum. Frequently, the diverticula are also invested with the fat of epiploic appendages. Marcus and Watt [52] describe a row of diverticula often found on the antimesenteric, intertaenial aspect of the colon in addition to the more usual locations.

Another structural characteristic of diverticular disease is thickness of the bowel wall, primarily due to prominence of the circular muscle layer but also due to thickening and apparent shortening of the taeniae. These muscular changes result in a apparent increase in the number and height of haustra and a narrowed lumen.

The sigmoid colon is affected in 95 percent of diseased patients and is the sole site of disease in 50 to 75 percent. The descending colon is next most frequently involved, with the transverse and right colon involved in less than 15 percent of patients.[53]

The uncomplicated presence of diverticula is thought to be the result of increased intraluminal colonic pressures. Diseased colonic segments manifest a high rate of muscle contraction and increased pressure responses to administration of prostigmine and morphine.[54] Arfwidsson [55] also noted a high resting intraluminal pressure.

The high pressures are apparently the result of strong segmental contractions of circular muscle. Cineradiographic studies in patients with diverticulosis have shown the formation of small segments of bowel with complete occlusion of the lumen at both ends of the segments. These little "bladders" are subjected to high pressures, and the diverticula in these segments become distended with the rise in pressure. The muscle alterations are thought to be caused by a deficiency of fiber in the diet, and the loss of bulk allows narrowing to occur. If bulk is present, exaggerated segmentation is prevented, narrowing inhibited, and development pressures noted in diverticulosis patients are avoided. Laboratory animals fed diets low in bulk develop diverticula.[56]

Solitary diverticula of the cecum seem to have a different pathogenesis. These diverticula are outpouchings from the cecum, within 2 cm of the ileocecal valve, containing all the coats of the bowel. They probably represent congenital lesions, although a pulsion mechanism has been postulated.

Diverticulitis represents, at the least, an inflammatory response in the vicinity of a diverticulum.[51] Stool and mucus collect in a diverticulum and cause an inflammatory response in the mucosa. Perforation can then occur, leading to a greater or lesser infection, which may include a phlegmon, abscess, or free perforation. Obstruction may be the result of scar formation, which thickens, narrows, and stiffens the bowel wall. Bleeding is said to be a consequence of the anatomic relationship of the colonic arteries to the diverticula whereby ulceration of a diverticulum can lead to hemorrhage. Recent clinical experience, however, demonstrates that many episodes of apparent diverticular bleeding are actually hemorrhages from arteriovenous malformations, often located in the right colon.

The so-called giant sigmoid diverticulum develops as the result of a localized perforation, which subsequently develops a ball valve so that a cyst lined by granulation and fibrous tissue develops.

Clinical Manifestations

Diverticulosis. Traditionally, diverticulosis was deemed an asymptomatic condition. That this is not the case is suggested by Morson's finding that 35 percent of colon specimens removed for "persistent diverticulitis" showed no evidence of inflammation. Abnormal bowel musculature was the predominant finding.

The pain is nonspecific—ranging from an uncomfortable sensation of fullness to intermittent cramps, usually felt in the lower abdomen.[48,49] Constipation is three to four times more frequent than diarrhea. Flatulence and bleeding are not characteristic of diverticulosis. The symptoms cannot be correlated with the number of diverticula or their location.[49] Patients with involvement of the entire colon are more likely to have symptoms, however, and symptoms increase as the size of the diverticula increases.

There are no specific physical findings. There may be tenderness in the left lower abdomen, and the left or sigmoid colon may be palpable as a firm, sausage-like structure, but often no mass is discernible.

Diverticulitis. The most frequent complaint is pain, which may be intermittent and cramping in nature but is more commonly steady, deep, and aching. Pain is usually located in the left lower quadrant but may be hypogastric or present on the right. Aching in the low back is common. Often, there is a history of altered bowel function, usually constipation. As in diverticulosis, diarrhea or intermittent constipation and diarrhea occur. Changes in bowel function are often the result of acute incomplete obstruction due to inflammation.

Nausea and vomiting may be due to obstruction but are usually the result of the inflammatory process. Weight loss occurs in about one of four patients. The reported incidence of chills and fever is variable—perhaps because the diagnosis of diverticulitis is difficult to make on clinical grounds alone. Blood in the stool is common, but bleeding is rarely profuse (less than 5 percent). Symptoms of suprapubic pain, dysuria, and frequency may indicate inflammation in the region of the urinary tract, or it may indicate the presence of a colovesical fistula. Pneumaturia and fecaluria are seen when a fistula is present.

When complications of diverticulitis develop, pain often intensifies and spreads as the abscess enlarges. If perforation occurs, the diffuse pain of generalized peritonitis ensues.

Colovesical fistula is suggested by dysuria and urinary frequency. If pneumaturia is present, it is described as a hissing or popping sound noted at the end of urination. Particles of feces may be seen in the urine. Symptoms of urinary sepsis may predominate.

Other fistulas may be recognized by passage of stool per vagina or through an abdominal cutaneous fistula site. The development of diarrhea suggests the presence of a fistula in the small bowel.

Diverticulitis in a cecal diverticulum usually produces symptoms similar to those of acute appendicitis. There is less nausea and vomiting than with appendicitis; otherwise, the two conditions cannot be differentiated until operation is performed. Giant sigmoid diverticula rarely produce distinctive symptoms. Sometimes, the patient becomes aware of an intra-abdominal mass.

Physical findings, in patients with diverticulitis or its complications, are like those of a localized or generalized intra-abdominal inflammation. Local tenderness, with guarding and localized rebound, is most frequent. If ileus or obstruction is present, distension will be noted. Frequently, an abdominal mass, most often in the left lower quadrant or pelvis, is noted on abdominal, pelvic, or rectal examination. Blood may be found on the examining finger after rectal examination.

Diagnosis

There are no blood tests specific for diverticular disease. The leukocyte count is usually elevated in diverticulitis. If there has been bleeding, anemia may be present. Urinalysis may be abnormal when there is impending or actual vesicosigmoid fistula. If only bladder irritation exists, pyuria alone might be noted. With fistulization, bacteria will be detected in the urine on Gram stain or culture. If the fistula is large enough, fecal matter will be noted on gross or microscopic examination.

Endoscopy of the rectum and colon is performed primarily to rule out other disease, especially carcinoma, and to determine the length of healthy rectum available for an anastomosis. Sigmoidoscopy is of limited value in making a diagnosis, because the involved segments are usually not visible with this instrument. Wychulis et al [57] list the following endoscopic observations in patients with diverticular disease: acute angulation at the lower level of the sigmoid, pronounced fixation of the colon, narrowing of the bowel lumen, edema and inflammation of the mucosa, sacculation of the bowel, blood and purulent material in the lumen, extrarectal mass. Rarely, diverticular ostia may be visualized. Ritchie [58] emphasizes the relationship of mucosal puckering with diverticulosis. Wychulis et al [57] noted one or more sigmoidoscopic findings in two-thirds of their patients, but Ochsner and Bargen [48] found abnormalities in only one-fifth. Care must be used in performing proctoscopy on patients with acute diverticulitis. Friable bowel may be injured, and confined areas of sepsis may be disrupted. Colonoscopy offers theoretical advantages, but in the presence of bowel angulation, fixation, and narrowing, it is difficult to perform. Only one-half of examinations are successful.

The diagnosis of colon carcinoma in patients with suspected diverticulitis requires visualization of abnormal mucosa. Morton and Goldman [59] were able to see only 38 percent of carcinomas in their series of patients with diverticular disease. Samuel and Dean [58a] were able to diagnose only 4 of 14 carcinomas in 19 patients in whom colonoscopy was successful.

Roentgen examinations are the most productive means of diagnosing diverticular disease. Plain films may demonstrate thickened bowel wall, displaced small bowel, and abnormal collections of air. Barium enema examination demonstrates goblet-like outpouchings from the bowel lumen, sometimes displaced by fecal matter within the diverticula. The lesions may also be obscured by the overlying column of barium. The use of air contrast overcomes this problem, but is a dangerous maneuver in patients with acute disease. The postevacuation film demonstrates residual barium-filled diverticula in most instances. Findings that have been suggested to indicate diverticulitis or abscess include spasticity and hyperactivity of the bowel, prominent sacculations, transverse folds, a "sawtooth" appearance of the bowel mucosa, stenosis of the bowel, and extraluminal barium in abscess cavities or fistulas (Figs. 39-3 and 39-4). Muscle abnormalities account for most of these findings, whether or not diverticulitis is present. The sawtooth deformity usually corresponds to the presence of diverticula in the antimesenteric intertaenial area.[52] Persistent narrowing suggests scarring in the bowel wall or extrinsic compression by abscess, but most abscesses manifest no roentgenographic changes. In addition, Parks [60] could demonstrate no significant correlation between roentgenologic appearance and clinical symptoms and signs of acute diverticulitis.

In the presence of narrowing, obstruction, or a mass lesion, one must rule out neoplasm. The following points are identified [59] as being indicative of diverticular disease: (1) long segments of bowel involvement, (2) gradual tapering of the ends of the segment, (3) preservation of the mucosal pattern, (4) the presence of diverticula and other signs of diverticular disease, (5) changing appearance of

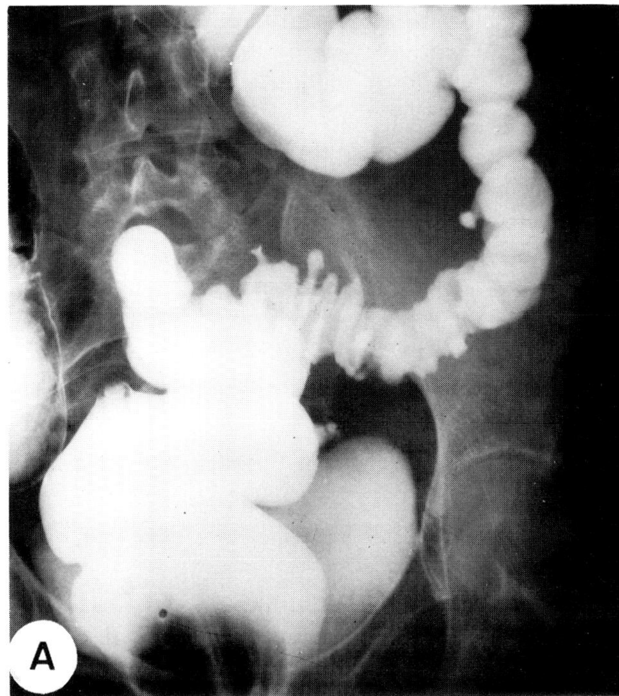

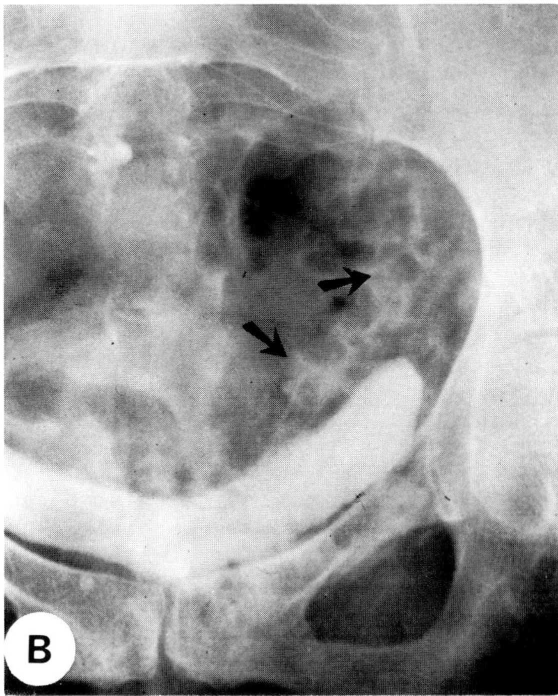

Fig. 39-3. **A. Diverticulitis. Barium enema demonstrates diverticula, prominent sacculations, and narrowing in the sigmoid colon. The presence of contrast in the bladder proves a colovesical fistula; the patient has received no urinary contrast media. B. Colovesical fistula. Cystogram demonstrates contrast leaking into the sigmoid colon (arrows) of a patient with diverticulitis—a rare finding.**

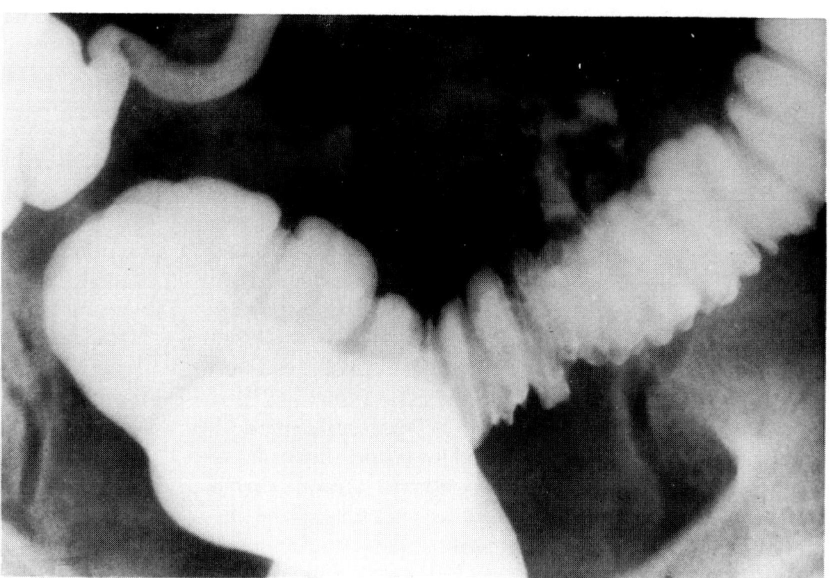

Fig. 39-4. **Diverticulitis. Barium enema demonstrates extraluminal contrast in a confined paracolic abscess.**

the lesion in the same examination or in different examinations, and (6) obstruction without demonstrable tumor. Carcinoma may coexist with diverticular disease.

The diagnosis of colon fistula is discussed in another section of this chapter. Sigmoidoscopy and colonoscopy almost never allow the fistula to be seen. Barium enema examination confirms the presence of diverticular disease and sometimes demonstrates the tract. A small bowel series will demonstrate a coloenteric fistula. Colovesical fistula are usually not seen during cystoscopy, cystography, or intravenous pyelography. An air fluid level or external bladder compression may be the only sign.[61]

Giant sigmoid diverticulum frequently becomes apparent initially on plain film of the abdomen or barium enema.[62]

Treatment

Nonoperative treatment of patients with diverticular disease is summarized by Eastwood[63] and Friedman and Janowitz.[64] Adding bulk to the diet appears to stop the progression and relieves the symptoms of diverticulosis. Although carrots, apples, brussels sprouts, and oranges offer such bulk, emphasis has been placed on bran because it is inexpensive and intake can be quantitated. Alternative but relatively expensive forms of bulk are psyllium colloids (Metamucil) and karaya gum. The estimated bulk requirements are 15 gm of bran and 200 gm of appropriate fruits and vegetables per day. The goal is to provide enough fecal bulk to prevent excess segmentation and to allow at least one effortless bowel movement per day.

Painter et al[65] offered dietary management with bran to 70 patients. Although 8 patients could not tolerate the diet, 62 experienced relief of their chronic symptoms. Three of the 62 were admitted during bran treatment to the hospital with acute left lower quadrant pain—one with acute suppurative diverticulitis. All but 7 patients were able to give up chronic use of other laxatives.

Most attacks of acute suppurative diverticulitis can be managed without operation. The patient should be hospitalized, given nothing by mouth, and maintained with intravenous fluids. If obstruction (partial and decompressible) or minimal signs of peritonitis exist, the gastrointestinal tract should be decompressed with a nasogastric tube. Antibiotics (an aminoglycoside and clindamycin) should be administered. As long as response is prompt, this treatment suffices for the specific episode. Painter and Truelove[54] have cautioned against the use of morphine or opiates other than meperidine for analgesia, because these drugs increase the pressure within the involved segment.

Surgical treatment is indicated for repeated attacks of diverticulitis or for the complications of obstruction, perforation, bleeding, and fistula formation. Another indication for resection is inability to rule out the presence of a neoplasm. In order to avoid the increased risks of an operation under urgent conditions, patients with persistent and recurrent symptoms of diverticulitis should be considered for elective resection of the diseased bowel segment. Chronic obstruction (34 percent), abscess (19 percent), acute obstruction (13 percent), perforation (12 percent), fistula (12 percent), and hemorrhage are the most common indications for operation.

Operative Treatment of Complications. The prime task in surgical treatment is to resect the diseased segment of colon, because colostomy has proved to be an unsatisfactory therapy for distal infection. Over 30 years ago, Smithwick[66] documented that colostomy fails to control infection. Mortality remained high (8 to 9 percent). Even if temporary control was achieved, exacerbation followed colostomy closure. Drainage of abscesses is equally unsatisfactory, as simple drainage resulted in persistent fecal fistula in 41 to 95 percent of patients,[66] and creation of a proximal colostomy did not result in permanent closure of either cutaneous or colovesical fistulas. Smithwick[66] concluded that a three-stage operative protocol was needed: (1) colostomy and drainage, (2) resection with anastomosis, and (3) closure of colostomy at 3- to 6-month intervals. The mortality was low (4 to 5 percent), and three-fourths of the patients were cured.

The three-stage treatment protocol is still useful in selected cases. The intervals between colostomy and closure can be shortened, and most surgeons now resect the diseased bowel at the initial operation.[67,68] The mortality rate ranges from 0 to 4 percent, and fecal fistulas and anastomotic leaks develop in less than 5 percent of patients.

In 1961, Madden and Tan [69] reported a 33 percent mortality rate in patients who had diverticular perforation with abscess or peritonitis treated by staged resection. They then successfully treated six patients with resection and primary anastomosis. Subsequently, Madden [70] promoted primary resection with anastomosis in patients with complicated diverticulitis.[70] Primary anastomosis, however, in the presence of peritonitis, abscess, or even partial obstruction, or in an extraperitoneal location, is still associated with a high rate of leak and other serious morbidity.[71] In the recent decade, there has been a trend away from primary anastomosis in the presence of acute sepsis or obstruction. The conditions necessary for a successful anastomosis include two healthy ends of bowel, with a good blood supply, which can be joined without tension. There should be no fecal matter remaining in the bowel. Tissues surrounding the anastomosis must be free of sepsis. Thickened bowel, inflamed bowel, or dilated obstructed bowel that does not return to a normal appearance upon decompression cannot be expected to heal.

Most studies have shown that patients do better when diseased bowel is excised at the first operation. A preliminary first-stage proximal colostomy will not be effective when there has been a prior resection, when there is a persistent distal column of feces, and when there is an enterocolic fistula which bypasses the colostomy. Sepsis will continue from an abscess that is not well drained, or if a leak from the perforation persists. Most authors recommend either exteriorization of the perforated segment, resection with double barrel colostomy, or Hartman resection if urgent or emergency operation is required.[72] One can expect a mortality rate of less than 10 percent with such an approach. Complicated diverticular disease is sometimes encountered in a patient who is operated on, following adequate bowel preparation, for pelvic mass, possible carcinoma, or fistula. In such patients, resection of the diseased bowel and adjacent disease or fistula with primary anastomosis of the bowel can sometimes be performed safely if conditions are ideal. Several authors stress the increased risk of anastomotic leak when extraperitoneal bowel is mobilized to make the anastomosis. Therefore, they suggest complementary colostomy for low anterior anastomosis in the presence of active disease.[70]

Elective Operation. Elective one-stage colectomy can be performed with a mortality rate of less than 3 percent.[73] Colcock [74] summarizes the current indications for elective resection: (1) two or more attacks of acute diverticulitis while on good medical management—the diagnosis of acute diverticulitis should be supported by the presence of acute pain, localized peritoneal signs, palpable mass during the attack, fever, leukocytosis, and roentgen signs of acute diverticulitis, (2) one or more attacks of diverticulitis associated with radiologic evidence of perforation, (3) attacks associated with persistent evidence of obstruction, (4) attacks associated with symptoms of urinary tract irritation, (5) repeated episodes of lower gastrointestinal hemorrhage (in the absence of arteriographic evidence of arteriovenous malformation), (6) inability to rule out the presence of neoplasm, and (7) attacks of diverticulitis in patients less than 50 years of age.

Resection of the diseased segment is successful in preventing the recurrence of symptomatic disease in nearly all patients. In order to achieve the best results, it is necessary to resect all bowel with thickened and hypertrophied muscle, but it is not necessary to remove all diverticula. It is especially important that the distal resection margin be free of both diverticula and hypertrophied muscle.

When the importance of colonic muscular hypertrophy was recognized, longitudinal myotomy of the antimesenteric intertaenial circular muscle was introduced for the treatment of patients with chronic symptoms,[75] but without inflammatory complications. The mortality rates with this procedure have ranged from 0 to 5 percent,[75,76] and successful relief of symptoms has been achieved in 85 to 90 percent. When the procedure is used in patients with complications of diverticulitis, however, septic complications occur more frequently. Smith [76] demonstrated that the procedure reduces the high intracolonic pressure seen in diverticular disease. However, 3 to 5 years following myotomy, high pressure has returned. A diet including bran tends to retard return of the high-pressure state.

Others have felt that shortening of the taeniae is more important as a factor contributing to diverticular disease and have performed multiple transverse myotomies in the antimesenteric taeniae. No circular muscle is incised, so that the risk of mucosal perforation is reduced. This procedure, too, has successfully relieved symptoms and led to reduction of intracolonic pressure. The two procedures have been combined by Kettlewell and Moloney.[77] Myotomy has not been adopted by surgeons in America, and further experience will be necessary to judge the merit of this technique.

Giant Sigmoid Diverticulum. A one- or two-stage elective resection of the cyst and associated segment of colon with primary anastomosis in the majority of cases is usually successful.[62]

Cecal Diverticulum. The diagnosis of cecal diverticulum must be considered in all periappendiceal inflammations. Digital invagination of the cecum may permit palpation of the diverticular os. If an inflamed cecal diverticulum with only minimal surrounding inflammation is detected, excision of the involved tissue is adequate treatment if care is taken to avoid both tension on the repair and obstruction of the ileocecal valve. More generalized cecitis with no apparent diverticulum may be left alone or drained. More advanced inflammation may require ileocecal resection. Perforation with abscess formation requires drainage of the abscess and exteriorization or two-stage resection of the cecum. If neoplasm cannot be ruled out, a formal right hemicolectomy should be performed. Primary anastomosis is safe if abscess or peritonitis is not present.

Prognosis

Diverticulosis is a progressive disease. Increase in the number, size, and distribution of diverticula occurred in 30 percent of patients followed an average of 5 years and 60 percent of patients followed 10 to 30 years.

About 25 percent of patients with diverticulosis will have at least one attack of diverticulitis (range 15 to 82 percent).[49] Factors that affect the incidence of diverticulitis are: (1) the number of diverticula, (2) the extent of involved colon, (3) the duration of follow-up, (4) progression of diverticulosis during follow-up, and (5) the criteria used to diagnose diverticulitis.[49]

Once a person has a single attack of diverticulitis, the incidence of recurrent disease ranges from 11 to 75 percent (median 30 percent).[53] Three or more episodes of diverticulitis are noted in 6 to 24 percent.[53]

When diverticulitis recurred, recurrence took place within 1 year in 46 to 83 percent.[53] Symptoms were noted in the interval between attacks in 73 to 92 percent.

Death due to diverticular disease in patients treated nonoperatively occurs in 2 to 6 percent.[53] Of patients who had diverticulitis, operation was eventually required in 11 to 55 percent (median 25 percent).[53,66]

Complications requiring surgical therapy were much more likely to occur in patients who had multiple attacks of diverticulitis. On the other hand, of patients requiring operation, 12 to 48 percent (median 37 percent) had never had symptoms before the acute attack that led to operation.[66,78]

Younger patients with diverticulitis have more complications.[50,53] Eusebio and Eisenberg [50] describe the course of diverticulitis in patients less than 40 years of age. Fifty-eight percent required surgical treatment; 76 percent of the operations were performed for an acute emergency, and in those treated medically, 53 percent continued to have symptoms when followed up to 4 years.

Colon resection is effective in preventing recurrent symptoms of diverticulitis. Long-term follow-up in numerous series shows that 69 to 100 percent (median 89 percent) of patients are asymptomatic following resection of the diseased colon.[50,66,78]

INFLAMMATORY BOWEL DISEASE

Most patients with inflammatory bowel disease (ulcerative colitis and granulomatous colitis) can be treated without operation. However, infectious etiologies have not been excluded, and significant morbidity and mortality in these diseases result from infectious complications.

Epidemiology

The epidemiologic features of granulomatous and ulcerative colitis are similar. Most cases appear in young adults, although ulcerative colitis is somewhat more likely to appear in children. Both sexes are equally affected. Caucasians are affected more often than members of other races, and these diseases are detected more frequently in industrialized countries.

The incidence of ulcerative colitis has remained stable recently, but there has been an increase in the incidence of granulomatous colitis (regional enteritis).[79] The proportion of patients with ulcerative colitis ranges from 32 to 87 percent, granulomatous colitis from 12 to 58 percent, and unclassified colitis from 1 to 11 percent. The reported relative incidence varies according to whether the histopathology has been analyzed using modern criteria, and whether the subsequent course of the disease has been taken into account. Tompkins et al [80] report that the proportion of their patients with ulcerative colitis decreased from 85 to 39 percent upon histologic review.

Etiology and Pathogenesis

The pathogenesis of inflammatory bowel disease has recently been reviewed.[81] Although theories abound, no specific causative factor has been proved. A number of conditions associated with the onset of ulcerative colitis [82] include pregnancy, severe purgation, a recent surgical procedure, emotional trauma, epidemic diarrhea, and infectious disease in general. Most recent work has attempted to identify infectious and immune factors.[83]

Current hypotheses include damage to the colon resulting from an abnormal immune response to a microbe—either an infectious agent or a part of the normal flora—and allergic responses to exogenous or endogenous antigens (autoimmune reaction).

Proof of an infectious etiology has long been sought. There is no difference in the fecal flora of patients with ulcerative colitis, granulomatous colitis, or a normal bowel. However, microbiologic techniques, especially those necessary to detect fastidious anaerobes, chlamydia, and rare opportunistic agents, continue to be improved and may yet detect a responsible organism. Monteiro et al [83] describe an antibody reacting with fecal anaerobic bacteria in the colonic mucosa of patients with ulcerative colitis.

Evidence supporting a viral agent in inflammatory bowel disease has been discussed by Brooke [81] and Kirsner.[79] Simonowitz et al [84] produced histologic changes similar to Crohn disease in rabbit colon by injecting a homogenate of bowel wall from Crohn disease patients. Hardin and Werder [85] produced a viral cytopathic effect in tissue culture of human amniotic membrane cells by adding sera from ulcerative colitis patients. Antibody to cytomegalovirus has been isolated from the sera of 65 percent of ulcerative colitis patients. In addition, a cytopathic effect similar to that of cytomegalovirus was detected in tissue cultures of the mucosa of three of six patients with ulcerative colitis and one of four with Crohn disease. Sidi et al [86] discussed 12 ulcerative colitis patients in whom cytomegalovirus inclusions were found in the granulation tissue of mucosal ulcers and in mucosal endothelial cells. Such findings constitute only circumstantial evidence and do not confirm an etiologic relationship between viruses and inflammatory disease of the bowel.

Pathology

Ulcerative colitis nearly always (90 to 96 percent) involves the rectum. The disease extends proximally without skip areas. The rectum alone is involved in 4 to 15 percent, the rectosigmoid and left colon in 6 to 10 percent, and the entire colon in 31 to 43 percent.[87] These figures are based on barium enema examinations, so that the extent of disease is probably underestimated.

Ulcerative colitis is a disease primarily of the mucosa. Grossly, there is edema, diffuse granularity, and friability. Extensive mucosal involvement results in denuding and pseudopolyp formation. Discrete ulcers are unusual. Fibrous thickening of the entire bowel wall is not seen, and strictures are uncommon in the absence of neoplasm. Enlargement of mesenteric lymph nodes is unusual.

Histologic examination confirms that ulcerative colitis is confined to the mucosa and the superficial submucosa. At first, abscesses are confined to the crypts; later, they also involve the lamina propria. There is a reduction in numbers of goblet cells in the mucosa, and premalignant changes may be seen. Lymphoid aggregates are sometimes found in the mucosa, but granulomas are not. Lymphedema of the submucosa is absent. Fissures are absent. Fibrosis is noted only in the mucosa and submucosa. In the absence of toxic megacolon, the muscular and serosal layers are not at all involved.

Granulomatous colitis, on the other hand, is more likely to be distributed segmentally with intervening normal bowel. The rectum is spared in 22 to 81 percent. The small bowel is involved in 27 to 58 percent, and the colon is involved in 35 to 90 percent of all patients with Crohn disease.[88]

Granulomatous colitis is a disease of all the bowel wall layers. Early discrete ulcers later coalesce to form serpiginous longitudinal ulcers with intervening normal mucosa. The development of transverse fissures produces the cobblestone effect of the mucosa. Pseudopolyps may be found. The bowel wall is thickened by fibrosis affecting all layers, and serositis is usually present. The mesentery is edematous with large, succulent lymph nodes. Spontaneous fistula is more likely to occur in this disease.

Microscopically, a subacute inflammatory response with thickening and fibrosis involves all layers of the bowel wall. Noncaseating granulomas and deep fistulas are common.

Toxic dilation of the colon is a potential serious complication of all inflammatory colon disease and leads to many infectious complications. The colon becomes dilated, and the wall thins. Serositis is severe, subserosal vessels are engorged, and a fibrinous exudate develops. Mucosal ulceration is severe. Histologically, there is transmural inflammation. Muscle cells are separated by exudate, and hyaline degeneration of muscle may be present. Often, inflammation of the ganglia of the intramuscular neural plexus is seen.[89]

Clinical Manifestations

Both ulcerative colitis and granulomatous colitis can have the same symptoms, signs, and complications. The cardinal symptoms are abdominal pain, diarrhea, and hematochezia. Infectious complications that occur in both diseases are perianal sepsis, bowel perforation, fistula, and toxic megacolon. In the following discussion, differences between the two conditions are stressed.

Typically, ulcerative colitis is characterized by acute exacerbations with intermittent periods of improvement or remission (relapsing-remitting type). Each attack may be mild or severe. Most exacerbations last less than 3 months, but some may remit after a year. Generally, if the disease has been active for 6 months, it remains so (chronic continuous type). Instead of undergoing some degree of healing, the colon progressively deteriorates, and the extent of involvement usually increases. There is an especially increased risk of developing large bowel cancer in the chronic-continuous form of the disease. Any acute attack may be characterized by a rapid, relentless progression of symptoms (the acute fulminating type). Acute fulminating attacks occur in 3 to 21 percent of patients.[90] Most deaths and complications occur in this form of the disease, largely the result of bleeding, perforation, or toxic megacolon.

Granulomatous colitis usually develops more slowly and is more relentlessly progressive. Acute fulminant attacks are rare, though symptoms wax and wane. There may be long periods of remission. Infectious complications may develop at any stage. Manifestations of associated small bowel disease may mask those of the colitis.

The most common symptom in both diseases is diarrhea. In ulcerative colitis, diarrhea occurs early, often with great frequency, and is associated with urgency. Hematochezia occurs almost universally and, in fulminating attacks, may be exsanguinating. Diarrhea in granulomatous colitis is of lesser frequency and urgency, and serious hemorrhage is rare. Hematochezia is seldom the first symptom of granulomatous colitis (5 percent).

Intermittent cramping abdominal pain, in the absence of complications, is usually periumbilical or hypogastric. In ulcerative colitis, cramps tend to occur prior to defecation and are accompanied by tenesmus, whereas in granulomatous colitis, cramps are more continuous and have no regular relationship to defecation.

Physical signs are not diagnostic in either condition unless complications are present. Fever and toxicity are noted in severe or fulminant acute attacks. There may be tenderness overlying the colon. Occasionally, an abdominal mass may be palpated in granulomatous colitis. Rectal examination may reveal blood or pus on the examining finger.

There are many noninfectious complications of inflammatory bowel disease (colon carcinoma, growth retardation, arthritis). Malnutrition is a serious accompaniment of acute attacks and can predispose to infectious complications.

The most frequent infectious complication of inflammatory bowel disease is perianal sepsis in the form of anal fissure, perianal abscess and fistula, or rectovaginal fistula (Chapter 41). Perianal sepsis is more common in patients with granulomatous colitis (25 to 81 percent),[91] and it is the first symptom in 27 percent of patients, especially those with colonic rather than small intestinal involvement.[92] The incidence of perianal sepsis in ulcerative colitis (6 to 23 percent) is not increased by steroid therapy.

Colon perforation and fistula occur infrequently in ulcerative colitis. Although the signs and symptoms of perforation may be masked in patients treated with steroids,[91,93] these drugs have not resulted in an increase in the incidence of perforation (1 to 12 percent). Most perforations occur during fulminant acute attacks, especially if toxic dilation of the colon develops. One-half to two-thirds of acute perforations are free; the rest are sealed or confined with abscess formation.[94] In older series, perforations and abscesses progressed so that external fistulas were seen in 1 to 2 percent of patients. Such fistulas are rare today.

Free perforation is unusual in granulomatous colitis (2 to 6 percent),[91] because most perforations occur slowly, resulting in abscess or a fistula formation. The reported incidence of internal and external fistula in patients with granulomatous colitis ranges from 3 to 59 percent (median 21 percent).[95] Even when perforation or fistula occurs, they more often originate in the small bowel rather than the colon.

Toxic dilation is a common complication of acute fulminating attacks of colitis (2 to 14 percent of patients hospitalized with ulcerative colitis),[91,93,94,96] but occurs in only 1 percent of patients with granulomatous colitis. Typically, patients show signs of toxicity (fever and tachycardia) and peritonitis (abdominal distension and tenderness). But Sirinek et al [96] stress that these signs may be absent, particularly if the patient is very ill; the diagnosis may be missed unless abdominal roentgenograms are made of all patients with an acute attack of colitis. If perforation occurs (24 percent), the mortality is high.

Diagnosis

The diagnosis of inflammatory bowel disease and the differentiation between ulcerative colitis and granulomatous colitis are determined by the clinical picture, endoscopic examination, and histologic appearance. Proctoscopy is abnormal in about 95 percent of patients with ulcerative colitis,[91] but reveals changes in only 5 to 25 percent of patients with granulomatous colitis. Colonoscopy increases the diagnostic yield to about 87 percent,[97] and the addition of biopsy results increases the yield to nearly 100 percent.

In ulcerative colitis, the endoscopic findings are edematous mucosa with petechiae, pits, pinpoint ulcerations, friability, and on occasion pseudopolyps. In granulomatous colitis, edematous, friable mucosa with aphthous ulcers and mucosal nodules may be seen. Biopsy of perianal lesions may confirm the presence of granulomatous disease. A key distinguishing feature is that ulcerative colitis is a general, diffuse process, whereas granulomatous colitis is characterized by discontinuous involvement with relatively normal mucosa between.

Roentgenographic examinations are more important than endoscopy in the diagnosis of infectious complications. Plain films of the abdomen should be taken in acute attacks to detect unsuspected toxic dilation of the colon (Fig. 39-5). In addition, there may be evidence of perforation or intra-abdominal sepsis. Barium enema should not be used during acute exacerbations for fear of precipitating toxic megacolon. In the early stages of ulcerative colitis (Fig. 39-6), the bowel may be irritable, haustra are thickened and irregular in width, and mucosal margins may be fuzzy or stippled due to tiny ulcers and exudate or may take on a shaggy appearance as ulcers become larger. Postevacuation films may show coarse longitudinal folds instead of the normal transverse folds. As the disease becomes more chronic, there is often progression to continuous involvement from distal to proximal, the mucosa is granular, haustra disappear, the lumen becomes narrowed and the bowel shortened. Pseudopolyps may become apparent. The presence of a stricture raises the possibility of carcinoma. Typically, there is no involvement of terminal ileum.

The barium enema findings of granulomatous colitis

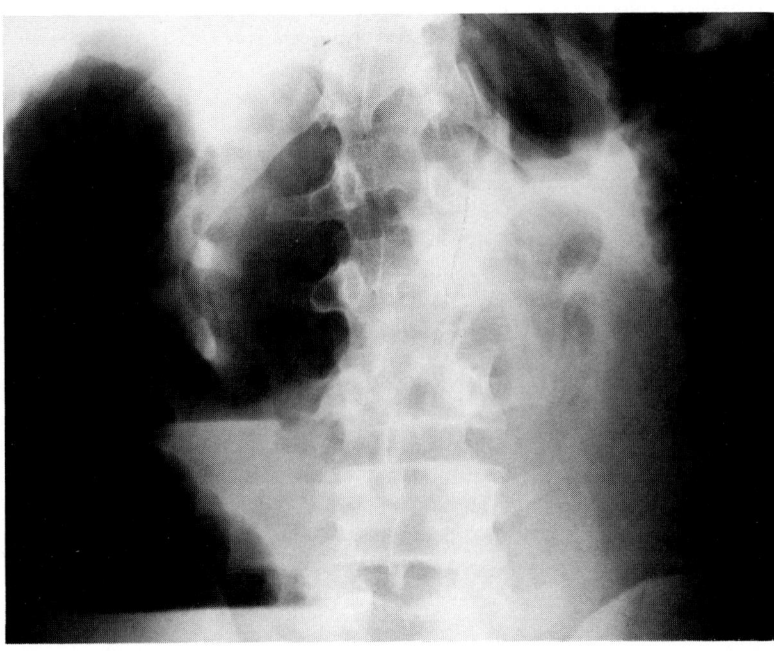

Fig. 39-5. Ulcerative colitis. Plain abdominal film demonstrates toxic dilation of the colon.

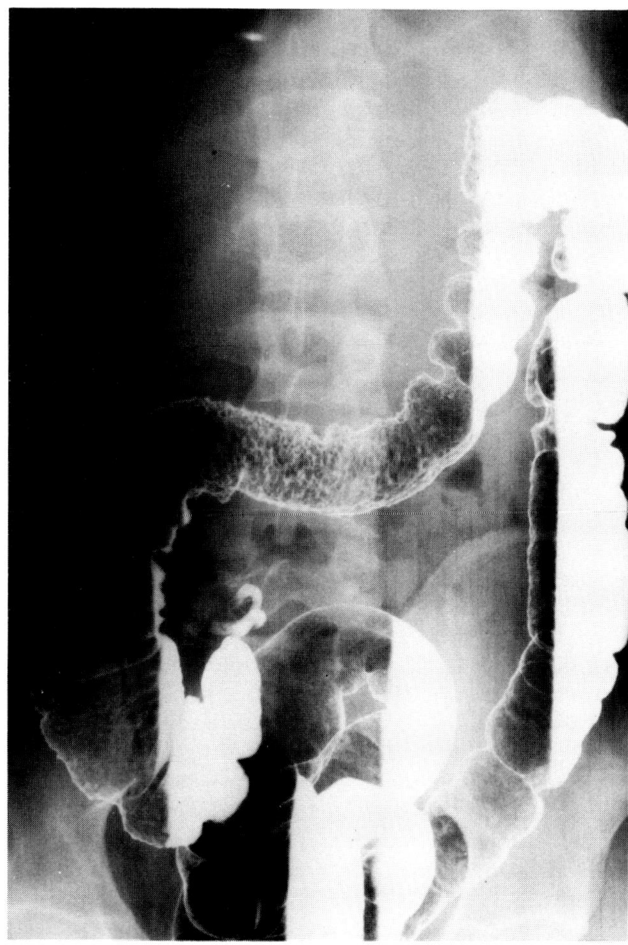

Fig. 39-6. **Ulcerative colitis. Air contrast barium enema (lateral decubitus position) demonstrates a shaggy mucosal pattern with ulcerated margins. Haustra are sparse in number and thickened. Shortening of the right colon has occurred.**

(Fig. 39-7) include an abnormal haustral pattern and ulcerations that eventually progress to typical longitudinal ulcers with transverse fissures. These produce a cobblestone pattern, and pseudopolyps are also seen. Involvement is often eccentric, and skip areas are apparent. As the disease progresses, strictures and internal fistulas are seen frequently. The terminal ileum is often involved.[97]

Treatment

In most instances, acute attacks of inflammatory bowel disease are treated without operation. Nutritional and fluid deficits should be replaced. It is desirable to reduce the fecal volume by an elemental diet, intravenous hyperalimentation, and a nasogastric tube.

Antidiarrheal agents (Lomotil, loperamide, codeine phosphate) may help control the diarrhea of mild disease, but should never be used during a severe attack, because they can precipitate toxic megacolon.

The most useful drugs for inflammatory bowel disease are corticosteroids and sulfasalazine.[98,99] Steroids do not increase the complication rate; neither do they prevent relapse of either ulcerative colitis or granulomatous colitis.[100] Steroids may be administered either orally or intravenously; ulcerative proctitis may be treated by steroid suppositories or retention enemas.

Sulfasalazine is a less effective antiinflammatory agent. It does not prevent relapse of Crohn disease,[100] but does reduce the early relapse rate in ulcerative colitis. Its antimicrobial effect is incidental. It must be broken down by gut flora, mainly in the colon, to its metabolites, sulfapyridine and 5-amino-salicylic acid (5-ASA). Antibiotics have no effect on either disease.

Treatment of Complications. Indications for surgical treatment in ulcerative colitis include fulminating acute disease that is unresponsive to nonoperative treatment, perforation, fistula (rare), hemorrhage, occurrence of systemic complications, growth failure in children, and persistent rectal disease. The risk of carcinoma in patients with chronic persistent disease also warrants operation. Although severe hemorrhage and cancer occur rarely in

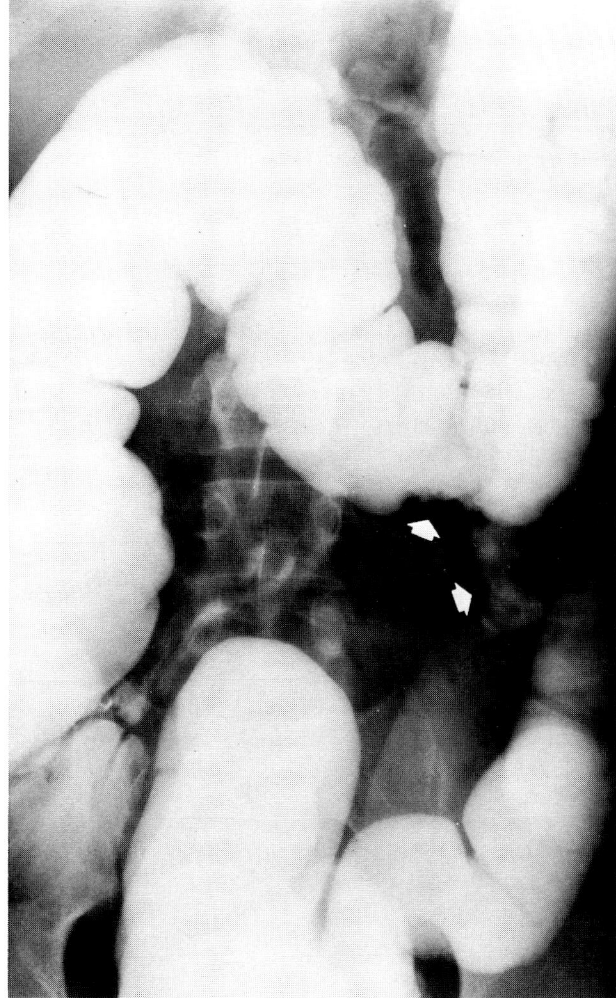

Fig. 39-7. **Granulomatous colitis. Barium enema demonstrates segmental involvement of transverse and descending colon; intervening colon is normal. Descending colon segment (arrow) is narrowed with ulcers and fissures apparent. Transverse colon involvement (arrow) is eccentric.**

granulomatous colitis, the indications for surgical treatment are otherwise the same as in ulcerative colitis.

The surgical treatment of ulcerative colitis requires, as a minimum, removal of the entire abdominal colon. Before 1960, ileostomy alone yielded an immediate postoperative mortality rate of about 25 percent, an eventual mortality rate of 46 to 84 percent (largely within the first postoperative year), and persistent disease requiring eventual colectomy in 41 to 45 percent.[101] Good results occurred in only 20 percent of surviving patients.[101] If the ileostomy was subsequently closed, only 13 percent had a good result, and 50 percent required a new ileostomy.

The overall mortality rate of total abdominal colectomy with or without proctectomy is 3 to 14 percent (median 8 percent),[93,94] being higher after emergency colectomy (14 to 54 percent; median 23 percent).[94] Infectious morbidity (incisional and intra-abdominal sepsis) of emergency procedures is 36 to 57 percent.[93]

No single operation is best for the treatment of granulomatous colitis. The disease is segmental, and cure cannot be assured by excising the involved segment of bowel. The basic choices in treatment of granulomatous colitis are diversion of the fecal stream from the diseased segment by proximal stoma or bypass, excision of the segment with subsequent anastomosis, colectomy and ileoproctostomy, or total coloproctectomy and ileostomy. In general, such operations are associated with a mortality rate of about 5 percent,[102] a wound infection rate of 18 percent, and an intra-abdominal sepsis rate of 3 percent. Five percent of anastomoses leak. The recurrence rate ranges from 16 to 94 percent (median 31 percent) and is less common when gross disease is restricted to the colon.

When infectious complications (abscess, perforation) are present, diversion (proximal stoma or bypass) is safer than resection (mortality range 0 to 24 percent).[103] Morbidity, including anastomotic leak, ranges from 4 to 10 percent.[103] Recurrence, however, is almost inevitable (94 percent).[102,104] Because of the frequent need for reoperation, Homan and Dineen [103] recommend that diversionary procedures be performed only when an important normal structure (such as a ureter) would be endangered or entry into an otherwise confined abscess would be needed to resect diseased bowel.

Resection of only grossly involved bowel segment with primary anastomosis is appealing because functioning colon is conserved and the need for ileostomy is avoided. Once again, the operative mortality rate is low (0 to 2 percent) and morbidity is acceptable (6 percent).[103] Following such resections, recurrence ranges from 39 to 85 percent (median 75 percent),[103,104,105] and the reoperation rate ranges from 11 to 59 percent (median 22 percent).[104,105]

Total colectomy with ileostomy succeeds in removing almost all diseased bowel with low operative mortality (0 to 8 percent),[88,104] and an acceptable recurrence (7 to 43 percent),[88,105] and reoperation rate (2 to 20 percent).[104] In an effort to achieve the benefits of total colectomy and avoid ileostomy, many surgeons perform total colectomy and ileoproctostomy. The following situations are accepted contraindications to this procedure: (1) emergency operations, (2) active disease in the rectum, (3) stricture and fibrosis of the anorectum due to chronic anorectal and perianal sepsis. Although it has been claimed that in ulcerative colitis rectal disease often resolves following total abdominal colectomy, subsequent ileorectal anastomosis is almost never possible in any ulcerative colitis patient whose rectum is retained. In patients with granulomatous colitis, the retained rectum frequently develops active disease (50 to 73 percent),[88] and proctectomy is required in 24 to 50 percent (median 30 percent).[88]

If ileoproctostomy is performed, the incidence of anastomotic leak (2 to 25 percent)[88,106] can be reduced by a proximal diverting ileostomy. The patient must be warned that the recurrence rate in the rectum is high,[106] and conversion to ileostomy may be necessary.[88,106]

Acute Toxic Megacolon. In no case is timing more important than in the management of acute toxic dilation of the colon. The mortality rate with nonoperative treatment is 27 percent, with surgical treatment, 20 percent. If perforation of the colon is allowed to occur (24 percent), the mortality rate is 41 percent; without perforation, the mortality rate is only 9 percent.

Turnbull et al [89] recognized the problem of intraoperative perforation. Many perforations found at operations had sealed, but in the process of performing total colectomy, were frequently opened again with subsequent fecal spillage. Turnbull proposed a temporizing procedure—ileostomy, transverse colostomy, and sigmoid colostomy—to avoid extensive dissection. This procedure resulted in a lower mortality rate (2 percent). However, 10 percent of the patients did not improve, and 31 percent reactivated their colitis (19 percent with recrudescence of toxic megacolon) before elective colectomy could be performed.

Fry and Atkinson [107] noted that when patients were operated on within four days of the onset of toxic dilation, no perforations occurred, and total colectomy was performed with no deaths. This experience has been confirmed by others.[96,108]

Therefore, operative treatment of acute fulminating disease, including toxic dilation of the colon, is indicated when nonoperative measures have failed to produce improvement within 48 to 72 hours. Total abdominal colectomy is the procedure of choice. Proctectomy is indicated in emergent cases only when severe rectal hemorrhage complicates the acute process.[108]

INFECTIOUS COMPLICATIONS OF CARCINOMA OF THE LARGE BOWEL

The acute mortality of large bowel cancer is due largely to infectious complications. In addition to the direct complications from the tumor and its surgical treatment, infections of other body systems (eg, the urinary and respiratory tracts) are common, there may be impaired immune resistance due to poor nutrition, and adjuvant treatment may impair body resistance. Two infectious complications of large bowel cancer are of pressing concern to the surgeon: (1) the acute perforation of a tumor, which necessitates emergency operation, and (2) the occurrence of certain opportunistic infections which suggest the diagnosis.

ACUTE CARCINOMATOUS PERFORATION

Epidemiology and Pathogenesis

Perforation most often occurs as a consequence of direct penetration by the tumor (3 to 8 percent).[109,110] The combination of obstruction and proximal perforation occurs in only about 1 percent of patients with large bowel cancer. Both obstruction and perforation occur more frequently in elderly females.

Most invasive perforations (about two-thirds) occur in the left colon; those in the right colon are more frequently the result of neglected obstruction. Perforation of nonobstructed colon is more likely to result in abscess or fistula formation, whereas peritonitis results from obstruction-perforation. The frequency of fistula formation ranges from 15 to 28 percent.[109] In contradistinction to fistulas resulting from diverticular disease, the structures most likely to be involved by the fistula are adjacent loops of small bowel and colon; stomach and duodenum are involved in 5 to 10 percent, bladder and female reproductive organs in about 20 percent, and colocutaneous fistulas in less than 10 percent.

Clinical Manifestations

The acute picture of perforated large bowel cancer, with or without obstruction, does not differ from perforation as discussed previously. Most patients have abdominal pains, local or general peritoneal signs, fever, and a palpable abdominal or rectal mass. Welch [111] stresses that abscesses may be found in unusual locations. A patient with a fistula, on the other hand, rarely presents an acute emergency.

It is desirable to be aware preoperatively that carcinoma is present. A prior history of change in bowel habits, weight loss, and gross rectal bleeding suggests the presence of cancer. Generally, the duration of symptoms prior to perforation is less than 5 months, often less than 2 months. Perforating tumors seem to be more aggressive, at least locally, than nonperforating tumors. A mass may be palpable on abdominal or rectal examination. Hepatomegaly is sometimes found.[109,110] Observations that suggest carcinoma include anemia or a stool positive for occult blood. Proctoscopy demonstrates the tumor in 44 to 67 percent; contrast enema (water soluble) shows the lesion in 95 percent of patients.

Treatment and Prognosis

The treatment of perforation of large bowel cancer has two goals: control of the acute sepsis and cure of the tumor. Although it is true that cancer cure rates for such patients are lower than those for unperforated large bowel cancer, cure is possible. Peloquin [110] found no difference in the proportion of patients with either positive nodes or distant metastases in his patients with perforation compared with all large bowel cancer patients. Peritoneal seeding following perforation is unusual.

Proximal diversion or bypass of a tumor perforation is a simple but inadequate procedure. The shortcomings of this approach are that the leaking bowel and an obstructed column of stool remain in situ, and that definitive treatment for the tumor is substantially delayed. Primary resection both removes the leaking bowel segment and provides definitive treatment for the cancer. Drawbacks of this approach are the added stress of the procedure and the risk that the tumor may be unresectable. If the tumor is adherent to adjacent structures, it may be impossible to tell whether these structures are involved by tumor or not. Thus, an attempt at curative resection often demands removal of adjacent organs and tissues, maneuvers that may be unwise in the infected patient. Resection, at least for palliation, is feasible in about 80 percent of patients.[109] Tumor must be assumed to be present in the walls of abscesses and along the fistula tract.

Our approach to patients with malignant perforation of the colon stresses aggressive resuscitation. Patients with small, localized abscesses, fistulas, or incomplete obstruction can be treated with fluids, electrolytes, intestinal decompression, parenteral nutrients, and antibiotics; a planned primary operation is then possible.

For most patients, however, an emergency operation is needed to treat the infection. At operation, the technical feasibility of curative resection, including necessity to resect adjacent tissues and organs, and the presence of distant metastasis are ascertained. We prefer to resect both perforated and obstructing tumors with proximal perforation and to turn out the bowel ends. We do not do primary anastomoses in the presence of peritonitis or obstruction. Although a Hartman resection of a rectal tumor might be necessary, emergency abdominoperineal resection is not performed. After the intra-abdominal infection is eradicated, staging of the lesion must be completed to rule out second primaries and to interdict further operative procedures in patients whose life expectancy is limited.

Large series report overall mortality rates for cancer patients with perforation from 30 [109] to 44 percent. Perforation with diffuse peritonitis is roughly twice as lethal as perforation with abscess; likewise the mortality rate of patients with obstruction-perforation is about twice that of penetration.[109] Patients with fistula have mortality rates from 5 to 11 percent.[109]

For primary resection, the mortality rate is 8 to 25 percent (median 19 percent).[109,112] Primary resection has half the mortality of diversionary procedures for perforated tumors. When the perforation occurs proximal to an obstructing tumor, however, Welch and Donaldson [113] report that preliminary decompression of the perforated bowel followed by staged resection yields a mortality half that of primary resection.

Anastomotic leak rates of 33 and 40 percent are noted in patients with perforated cancer treated by resection and primary anastomosis, even in the right colon. Three of five patients with an anastomotic leak in these series died. However, others report no leaks.[112]

Prognosis

A crude calculation indicates that the 5-year survival of patients with perforating carcinoma is less than half (8 to 25 percent) of that for all colon cancer patients (32 to 50 percent).[109,110,113] These results primarily reflect the immediate mortality of patients with perforated tumors. In patients with perforating tumors who survive the acute emergency, the survival ranges from 36 to 50 percent—

only slightly less than all colon cancer patients.[109,110] In contrast, patients with both obstruction and perforation remain at a disadvantage. Survival following curative operations ranges from 11 to 25 percent.[113]

OPPORTUNISTIC INFECTIONS IN COLON CANCER

Patients with early large bowel cancer are not overly susceptible to systemic opportunistic infections (Chapter 47). Instead, tumor ulceration allows fecal bacteria access to the bloodstream so that systemic infections caused by *Bacteroides* and *Clostridium* (especially *C. septicum*) occur more frequently in patients with colon cancer.

In addition, colon cancer fosters gut colonization by certain uncommon organisms. *Streptococcus bovis* is recovered from the feces of 56 percent of patients with large bowel cancer versus 10 percent of control patients.[114] Infection with *S. bovis*, a nonenterococcal, group D organism, is unique in that it often causes endocarditis, as well as septicemia.[114]

S. bovis can only be differentiated from enterococcus by special microbiologic techniques. One may suspect *S. bovis* if enterococcus, unusually susceptible to penicillin, cephalosporins, and clindamycin, is isolated. Usually, only one drug is necessary to treat septicemia with this organism, rather than the combinations of drugs usually used for enterococcus.

The special importance of these infections is that their presence may be the only early indication of large bowel cancer. Any patient with such infections without an obvious source should undergo evaluation for colon cancer.

INFECTIOUS MANIFESTATIONS OF LARGE BOWEL OBSTRUCTION

Obstruction of the large bowel can be complicated by perforation, strangulation, and colitis proximal to the point of obstruction. The infections that ensue account for much of the morbidity and mortality associated with large bowel obstruction. The conditions that cause most bowel obstructions are discussed elsewhere in this chapter and will not be treated in any detail here. Ischemia contributes importantly to the colitis of obstruction; this entity is discussed with ischemic and nonspecific colitis. Because they are not included elsewhere, volvulus, hernia, intussusception in adults, and pseudo-obstruction are discussed here.

Epidemiology and Pathogenesis

Large bowel obstruction occurs primarily in the elderly, with nearly equal distribution between sexes.[115-117] Perforation occurs in 8 to 9 percent [116,117] and, of these, 22 to 50 percent occur at the site of obstruction.

The degree of colon distension depends on the duration and completeness of the obstruction and the competence of the ileocecal valve. If the ileocecal valve is competent, decompression into proximal bowel cannot occur (closed-loop obstruction). Michel et al [118] estimate that the ileocecal valve is competent in about 50 percent of patients. With the development of the closed loop, intestinal content and gas (mostly swallowed air) flow into the colon, thereby increasing intraluminal pressure. Increased amounts of fluid are secreted, and absorption is inhibited.

Distension of the bowel may result in perforation in two ways. The first is mechanical rupture by increased pressure. The cecum is usually the segment that perforates proximal to an obstruction because it has a thinner wall and distends to a greater diameter at a given pressure in accordance with La Place's law (tension = pressure $\times$ diameter $\times$ π). The second mechanism of perforation is development of ischemic injury as intraluminal pressure increases. A role for fecal bacteria, promoting the process in obstructed ischemic colon that leads to perforation, is assumed but has not been documented.

Strangulation of the colon is usually a result of volvulus or an unusual incarcerated hernia. As the bowel wall loses viability, bacteria and their toxins gain access to the peritoneal cavity, even in the absence of actual perforation.

The more common lesions that account for large bowel obstruction are listed in Table 39-2. Large bowel obstruction is seldom caused by adhesions. Obstruction due to extrinsic cancer usually results from gynecologic tumors, although neoplasms of prostate, genitourinary tract, and presacral tumors may also cause obstruction. Massive fecal impaction may occur in patients with motility disorders, but occurs more frequently in elderly, senile, and institutionalized patients. Massive fecal impaction may occur in drug (opiate) abusers and in patients taking large quantities of narcotic analgesics. Aluminum and calcium containing antacids may produce fecal impaction.

Most cases of intussusception occur in young children; less than 10 percent are colonic in origin. Intussusception in adults originates in the ileocecal segment in 46 percent, the sigmoid in 18 percent, and the intervening colon in 36 percent.[119] The intussusceptum is usually a benign tumor.

Pseudo-obstruction of the colon occurs in adults of all ages. Although no organic obstructing lesion is present, the danger of colon perforation is as great as if one were present, and cecal perforation occurs in about one-fourth of reported cases. Causes include pregnancy, intra-abdominal inflammation, sepsis, cardiac failure, retroperitoneal disease, pelvic surgery, trauma, and cesarean section; 23 percent of cases are idiopathic.

TABLE 39-2. CAUSES OF LARGE BOWEL OBSTRUCTION

Lesion	Range (%)	Median (%)
Large bowel cancer	34–64	53
Volvulus	7–28	13
Congenital	9–16	13
Diverticulitis	3–12	7
Extrinsic cancer	2–13	3
Ileus	3–5	4
Hernia	0–3	2
Adhesions	1–4	3
Fecal impaction	1–6	4
Intussusception	—	1

Compiled from references 115–117, 120.

Clinical Manifestations

Patients with large bowel obstruction usually give a history of cramping hypogastric abdominal pain, associated with obstipation and abdominal distension.[118] There may have been preexisting diarrhea or constipation. Nausea and vomiting occur but are frequently absent, even in patients with advanced obstruction. If perforation or strangulation occurs, pain becomes localized and more constant as peritonitis develops. Typically, large bowel obstruction develops over days or even weeks.

Abdominal distension, active bowel sounds, tympany, tenderness, and peritoneal signs may be present, even in the absence of peritonitis, owing to stretching of the peritoneum. There are no typical signs of gangrenous bowel, although tenderness (86 percent), decreased bowel sounds (46 percent), rebound tenderness (45 percent), and fever (43 percent) are supposed to be classic.[117,120]

In cases of volvulus, there is sometimes a history of prior episodes of abdominal pain, distension, and constipation. The diagnosis of incarcerated hernia is usually obvious. When a diaphragmatic hernia is present, peristaltic sounds or a succussion splash may be heard in the chest. Intussusception in adults may have no distinctive findings, although a mass may be palpable. Pseudo-obstruction is associated with abdominal distension and obstipation, but pain is minimal or absent. Pain and signs of peritonitis develop only when perforation is imminent or has occurred.

Diagnosis

Radiologic studies are essential.[117] Plain films demonstrate distended colon and possibly a cutoff at the site of obstruction. Frequently, small bowel distension causes confusion as to the site of obstruction. Cecal distension greater than 9 cm diameter suggests impending perforation. All stable patients with bowel obstruction but no evidence of perforation or strangulation should have a contrast enema, which will demonstrate the lesion. Although frequently omitted,[117] proctoscopy is indicated in most obstructed patients. The obstructing lesion may be visualized, and diagnosis may be confirmed by biopsy.

Sigmoid volvulus is suggested by a greatly distended sigmoid colon bent upon itself, a loop extending as far as the diaphragm, and a pattern of mucosal spiraling or a bird's beak cut-off on contrast enema. Classic signs of cecal volvulus are: (1) a distended cecum located in the left upper quadrant, midabdomen, or right upper quadrant, (2) a large extragastric air-fluid level in the left upper quadrant, (3) an ileocecal valve seen on the right side of the cecum, (4) mucosal folds and "beaking," (5) small bowel in the right lower quadrant in place of the cecum, and (6) small bowel distension.

Intussusception mainly produces findings of small bowel obstruction, whereas contrast enema will outline an intussuscepted bowel.[119] Absence of an obstructing lesion on contrast enema indicates pseudo-obstruction.

Treatment

Nonoperative treatment is directed toward the prevention of perforation by nasogastric decompression and fluid resuscitation. Complete large bowel obstruction and perforation or strangulation are indications for immediate operation. Distension of the cecum to greater than 12 cm in diameter necessitates operation if the cecum does not decompress promptly.

The two alternative surgical approaches to large bowel obstruction are initial proximal decompression of the obstructed segment and primary resection of the obstructing lesion. Proximal decompression with left transverse colostomy or cecostomy [115-118,120] relieves the obstruction with minimal trauma. The danger of performing rapid decompression alone is that a gangrenous bowel or perforation can be missed. Furthermore, a second major procedure is necessary for definitive treatment. Payne and McAlpine [121] suggest making a stoma as close as possible to the obstruction so that the colostomy closure can be performed coincident with removal of the lesion.

We agree with those who prefer to resect the obstructing lesion at the first operation. We do not feel, however, that primary anastomosis in obstructed colon is ever indicated. Perforated segments should be exteriorized or resected; proximal cecal perforations may be managed with a cecostomy if the cecum is otherwise viable. Proximal decompression is performed if the lesion is unresectable or if a combined anterior-posterior resection is necessary for removal.

Uncomplicated fecal impaction is managed by manual disimpaction and saline or Gastrografin enemas.

Contrast enemas and endoscopy are successful in reducing sigmoid volvulus in 50 to 85 percent of patients.[122] Even so, the risk of recurrence makes elective resection of the involved loop of sigmoid colon desirable. Emergency resection is required if nonoperative reduction fails or strangulation occurs. Primary anastomosis must be avoided.

Cecal volvulus requires emergency reduction with cecopexy or cecostomy. There is an increased incidence of postoperative sepsis when cecostomy is added. If gangrenous bowel is present, right colectomy is indicated. If the patient is moribund, exteriorization may suffice. Volvulus of the transverse colon requires emergency resection.

If possible, incarcerated inguinal hernias should be reduced by gentle manipulation aided by mild sedation. If reduction is unsuccessful or if strangulation is believed present, operation should be performed promptly to reduce the hernia, repair the defect, and resect the strangulated bowel.

Because of the high incidence of malignancy, attempts to reduce adult colonic intussusception by any means are not indicated. The involved bowel should be resected. Only when rectosigmoid intussusception is present should manual reduction be performed, to avoid the need for anterior-posterior resection.

When signs of perforation are absent, pseudo-obstruction of the colon is treated with nasogastric decompression and intravenous fluids. If the cecal diameter exceeds 12 cm, or if distension persists for more than 48 hours, immediate decompression of the colon is necessary. Success has been reported with colonoscopic decompression, otherwise, cecostomy is indicated. If perforation has occurred, cecostomy must be performed.

Prognosis

The mortality rate for patients with large bowel obstruction in general ranges from 6 to 37 percent (median 32 percent).[115-117,120] This rate reflects the advanced age of the patients and associated illnesses, in addition to the cause of the obstruction and complications. Perforation and peritonitis increase the mortality considerably—almost 50 percent for perforated sigmoid or cecal volvulus and pseudo-obstruction.

ISCHEMIC DISEASES OF THE COLON

Ischemic colitis frequently passes unrecognized because it is actually a spectrum of conditions ranging from acute single ulcers of the colon to gangrenous necrotizing colitis. Ischemia alone does not account for the entire clinical picture; although unproved, the fecal flora may account for additional tissue necrosis, as well as toxemia and septicemia. In this discussion, the following disorders are considered: ischemic colitis, necrotizing colitis, colitis complicating large bowel obstruction, ischemic colitis complicating vascular surgery, radiation colitis, stercoral ulcer and perforation, spontaneous ulcer or perforation of the colon.

Epidemiology and Pathogenesis

Most ischemic diseases of the colon occur in the elderly with atherosclerotic disease and carcinoma of the colon. Institutionalized patients, many of them elderly, with poor bowel habits, younger patients with radiation damage to the colon following treatment for gynecologic cancer, and those with autoimmune disorders are also susceptible.

An obvious cause of ischemia of the colon is spontaneous, traumatic, or operative occlusion of the visceral arteries.

Decreased perfusion due to heart disease, shock, or sepsis and drugs used to treat such disorders (digitalis, vasopressors) may also divert blood from the splanchnic circulation. Enterocolitis, apparently ischemic in nature, is described in a child with pheochromocytoma. The effects of distension and increased intraluminal pressure on blood flow were discussed in the section on colon obstruction.

Proliferative intimal changes in the small arterioles and moderate medial hypertrophy have been seen in ischemic colitis. Thrombosis of small submucosal vessels is associated with thrombotic disorders such as the hemolytic-uremic syndrome. Use of estrogen compounds is described in patients with ischemic colitis, and discrete colonic ulcers have been noted following use of oral contraceptives.[123] Autoimmune disease may induce a vasculitis of the small vessels to the colon.[124] Although early radiation injury of the bowel involves mucosal cells, the late changes include a vasculitis, characterized by subendothelial proliferation and medial thickening.

Whereas ischemia may produce initial mucosal injury in the colon, the indigenous bacteria certainly exacerbate the situation. This concept is supported by the ability of local antibiotic instillation to protect ischemic bowel anastomoses.[18]

Although any fecal organism might be expected to increase the damage to ischemic bowel wall, the anaerobic environment particularly encourages growth of anaerobic organisms such as clostridia. Stasis of stool behind a colon obstruction promotes increased concentrations of anaerobic organisms. Invasion of the colon by clostridia has been implicated in necrotizing enterocolitis of infancy and antibiotic associated colitis. Likewise, clostridia have been identified in patients reported to have ischemic colitis [125] and necrotizing colitis. Infectious influences may play an important role in the development of ischemic colitis,[126] necrotizing colitis, and cecal perforation in leukemia patients who are receiving chemotherapy. Similar influences may account for some of the same problems seen in renal transplant patients. LeVeen et al [127] feel that the occurrence of some acute ulcerative lesions in patients with uremia may be the result of the action of urease-producing gut bacteria resulting in large local concentrations of ammonia.

Early changes of colon ischemia are mucosal and submucosal edema and hemorrhage. Mucosal necrosis follows, and with more severe involvement, transmural infarction develops with acute inflammatory changes and bacterial penetration. During the healing phase, mucosal ulcers with granulating bases are present.[128] The surrounding mucosa regenerates over the ulcer. When only the mucosa and submucosa are involved, complete healing is expected. When the muscularis propria is invaded and replaced with scar tissue, stricture results. The other forms of ischemic colon disease produce a similar histologic picture.

Clinical Manifestations

The clinical features of classical ischemic colitis have been extensively reviewed.[128] Usually, the patient presents with lower abdominal pain, vomiting, and diarrhea. Minimal to moderate amounts of blood are passed per rectum. Frequently, the patient gives no past history of significant bowel disease or other illness, but many patients are already hospitalized for shock, heart disease, sepsis, or other predisposing illnesses. Typical physical findings include a normal blood pressure, no more than a mild fever, and minimal, if any, abdominal tenderness. Peristaltic sounds are active to hyperactive.

One group of patients with ischemic colitis had transient disease, which rapidly healed and caused no further trouble (45 percent).[128] A second group recovered within a week but presented 1 to 12 months later with a large bowel obstruction due to a segmental ischemic stricture (13 percent). The third group developed transmural gangrenous colitis (19 percent),[128] with severe abdominal pain, generalized abdominal distension, and peritoneal signs. Occasionally, patients presented with milder disease and progressed to transmural involvement over the next 1 to 4 days. Boley et al [128] observed a fourth group of patients (19 percent) whose symptoms continued over the next 1 to 4 months and who later developed perforation, stricture, or a protein-losing enteropathy. The clinical features of necrotizing colitis are similar to those of a gangrenous or transmural ischemic colitis, and most surgeons now consider these entities identical.[129,130]

Patients with the colitis associated with bowel obstruction usually present with the findings of carcinomatous large bowel obstruction. The presence of local abdominal tenderness, diarrhea, and toxicity may suggest colitis, but the diagnosis cannot be made. Obstructive colitis may not be suspected until an anastomotic leak occurs following resection of a colon tumor.[131]

The findings of colon ischemia complicating aortic surgery are similar to those of typical colonic ischemia. Unfortunately, postoperative pain obscures the clinical picture. The diagnosis is first considered when diarrhea, often developing into bloody diarrhea, appears within the first postoperative week.[132] Although this complication is said to occur in 1 to 2 percent of patients undergoing aortic surgery, Ernst et al [132] report that 6 percent of their patients, examined routinely in the postoperative period, have endoscopic evidence of colon ischemia. Preoperative antibiotic and mechanical bowel preparation decrease the incidence of this complication.

Radiation enteritis complicates abdominopelvic radiation therapy in 5 percent of patients. Most damage is done to the rectum and small bowel; colon, especially sigmoid, damage accompanies 17 percent of bowel injuries. Sigmoid injury most frequently follows pelvic operation and irradiation for carcinoma of the cervix. Early proctocolitis is a routine sequel to pelvic irradiation; symptoms are cramping pain, diarrhea, and the passage of mucus and blood. This condition is self-limited and disappears soon after the completion of treatment. Late radiation colitis does not become apparent for months or years. Approximately one-half of colitis patients develop partial large bowel obstruction caused by radiation stricture. Nearly another one-half have cramping, pain, and diarrhea containing mucus and blood. In occasional patients, ulceration progresses to fistula formation or perforation.

Stercoral ulceration with perforation usually affects the sigmoid and rarely the cecum in patients with chronic constipation, ie, the institutionalized, the chronically ill, and those taking constipating drugs. Patients with scleroderma are especially susceptible.[133] These patients are frequently acutely ill, comatose, and have signs of peritonitis with a palpable fecal mass within the abdomen or rectum.[134]

Idiopathic perforation of a cecal ulcer accounts for about 8 percent of all cecal perforations.[135] These lesions occur most frequently in patients with cardiovascular disease, sepsis, and autoimmune disease, but young, previously healthy victims have been reported. The ulcers present with rectal bleeding or abdominal pain of acute onset and are often mistaken for acute appendicitis. When perforation occurs, the picture of peritonitis and sepsis develops quickly.

Diagnosis

Diagnostic features are similar for many ischemic disorders of the colon. Anemia is proportional to the amount of blood loss. Leukocytosis and left shift are usually moderate (10,000 to 20,000) but may be profound in the presence of gangrenous bowel. Conversely, leukopenia may reflect severe sepsis. Heikkinen et al [130] noted metabolic acidosis in patients with severe necrotizing colitis.

Colonoscopy is the ideal way to diagnose colonic ischemia, because the mucosal changes are the earliest. Because the rectum is involved in only 6 to 20 percent of patients, and the sigmoid colon in less than half,[128,129] proctosigmoidoscopy is frequently inadequate. The earliest visible changes are mucosal edema and pallor. A congested and bluish appearance accompanies submucosal bleeding. Blue nodules, the "thumbprints" seen on roentgenogram, may be seen. The mucosa then becomes friable, and ulceration occurs. The subsequent course of the ischemic process determines subsequent findings. The mucosa may become necrotic, and pseudomembranes may develop. The ulcers may coalesce, and one may see only a bed of granulation tissue as resolution occurs. Neither gross appearance nor biopsy may permit differentiation of ischemic colitis from inflammatory bowel disease or pseudomembranous colitis. Radiation colitis produces a rather pale, atrophic, granular mucosa. Radiation ulcers tend to be punched out with a shaggy yellow-gray base. Colon involved by radiation changes is often fixed and narrowed by fibrous stricture so that the endoscope cannot be safely passed. When bowel obstruction is present, a tumor, fecaloma, or other obstructing lesion may be seen. Endoscopy should be performed in all patients with possible ischemic colitis unless they are unstable from sepsis or shock or unless they have a frankly acute abdomen. After an ischemic area is found and the diagnosis made, undue effort should not be made to pass the instrument further because of the risk of perforating the bowel.

Contrast enema is the most useful study for diagnosing and following uncomplicated ischemic colitis; in the absence of signs of sepsis or peritonitis, barium enema should be performed within 48 hours of admission.[128] Usually, ischemic colitis is a segmental process. The splenic flexure and descending colon are most frequently involved (57 to 65 percent). The transverse colon is involved in 9 to 21 percent of patients, and the cecum and ascending colon in 4 to 8 percent. Involvement of more than one segment is seen in 12 to 39 percent.[128,129]

Thumbprinting is the classical (Fig. 39-8A), but transient, sign as ulceration soon occurs over the nodules of submucosal edema and hemorrhage. Subsequent changes include segmental spasm, ulcerations, and other changes noted in inflammatory colitis, as well as ischemic colitis. Evolution from the early findings to complete resolution within 2 weeks is essential to the diagnosis; barium enema must be repeated (Fig. 39-8B). Persistent early findings signify the presence of another disease. The late changes of segmental narrowing must be differentiated from other causes of narrowing.

Barium enemas should not be done when peritoneal signs are present. Findings on plain films may include free intraperitoneal air, intraperitoneal fluid, and distended small or large bowel. When the colon is distended, thumbprinting, thickening of the bowel wall, and ulceration may be apparent on plain films (Fig. 39-9). The presence of a distended colon or colonic segment on plain film may be of great diagnostic significance. When distension occurs secondary to obstruction, the dilated bowel retains haustral markings and appears otherwise normal. Distended ischemic colon is characterized by haustra that are thickened, blunted, or absent. Spontaneous distension of a segment of ischemic bowel indicates transmural involvement

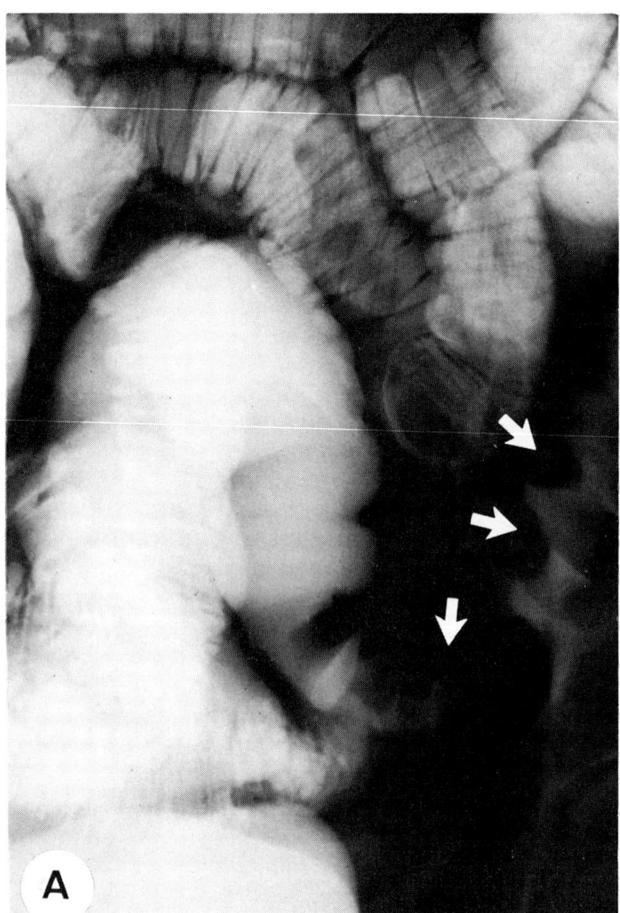

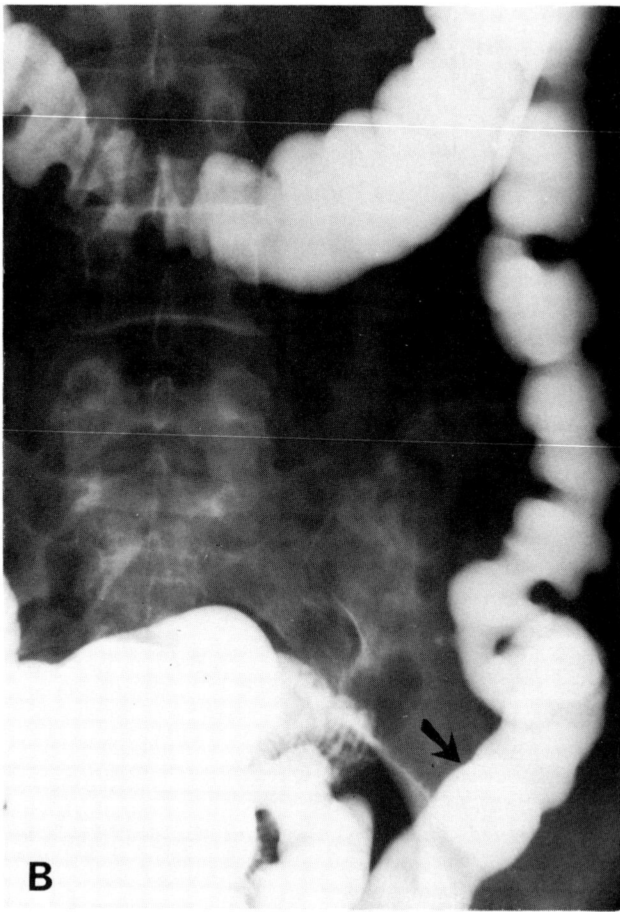

Fig. 39-8. **A. Ischemic colitis. Barium enema demonstrates narrowing of a sigmoid colon segment with "thumbprinting" (arrows).**

B. Ischemic colitis. Repeat barium enema performed 2 weeks later demonstrates resolution of the ischemic changes (arrow).

with impending or actual perforation.[125,130] Toxic dilatation of the colon may be seen in ischemic colitis.

Arteriography is relatively unproductive in ischemic bowel disease, because occlusion of large vessels (eg, the inferior mesenteric artery) occurs in only about 5 percent of patients.[129] However, the study should be performed in selected patients, since vascular reconstruction may be beneficial on occasion.

Treatment

Uncomplicated ischemic colitis does not require operation. Intravenous fluids, avoidance of oral intake, and nasogastric suction should prevent distension. Low molecular weight dextran is recommended by O'Connell et al.[126] Boley et al [128] feel the use of steroids is contraindicated. There are no reliable data on systemic or oral antibiotics.

Operation is indicated when the findings or clinical course suggest transmural involvement. Acute ischemic colitis that persists for more than 2 weeks results in irreversible bowel damage, for which operation is recommended. The operation of choice is resection of the entire segment of involved colon. Since the serosal surface of involved bowel may appear entirely normal, the extent of resection is determined by examining the margins of the removed segment of bowel. Primary colocolonic anastomosis is unwise when peritonitis is present, when bowel preparation has not been performed, and when resection is necessary during the acute phase of the disease.

When colitis is found proximal to an acutely obstructing lesion, the entire involved segment should be resected and colostomy performed. If a simple diverting colostomy is performed for distal obstruction, the patient must be observed closely for progression of the colitis.

When colon ischemia complicates an aortic operation, the management is the same. Ernst et al [132] stress several technical factors that prevent this complication: ligation of the inferior mesenteric artery flush with the aorta, restoration of hypogastric artery flow, avoidance of hypotension and trauma to the colon, preservation of a meandering mesenteric artery, and reimplantation of a patent inferior mesenteric artery if the collateral circulation appears inadequate.

Radiation colitis should be treated conservatively whenever possible. The symptoms of colitis usually respond to low-residue diet, stool softeners, local or systemic steroids, and Azulfidine. Operation is necessary for hemorrhage, complete obstruction, perforation, or fistula formation. The entire involved segment should be resected. End colostomy may be necessary, but anastomosis may be attempted if healthy bowel is present distally. If anastomosis is made to the rectum, a diverting colostomy is necessary. Rarely, colitis is severe enough to require a permanent

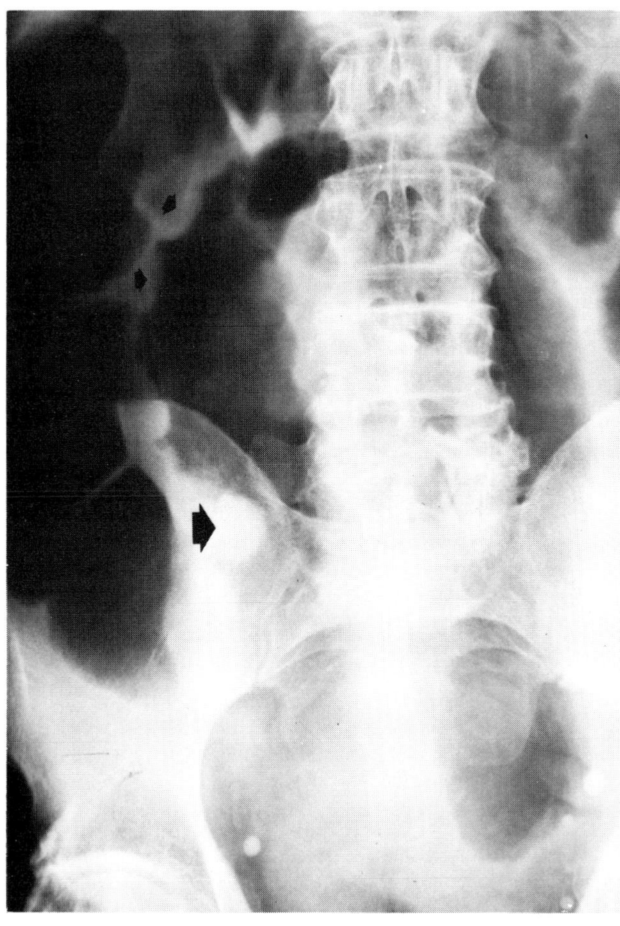

Fig. 39-9. **Transmural ischemic colitis. Plain abdominal film demonstrates dilation of the sigmoid colon with loss of haustra. Thickening of the bowel wall and "thumbprinting" (arrows) are apparent.**

diverting colostomy. Such a stoma must be made far enough proximally to avoid the irradiated bowel.

Fecal impaction causing stercoral ulceration must be removed rapidly but gently. Once the stool is evacuated, a nonperforated ulcer should heal as long as proper bowel management is maintained. If perforation has occurred, the defect must be exteriorized, resected, or closed and protected by a proximal stoma.

Spontaneous ulcers usually become apparent at the time of perforation. They should be managed by exteriorization or resection. Even though many of these occur in the cecum, primary colon anastomosis or closure is not recommended if peritonitis is present. Nonperforated cecal ulcers are usually detected during operations for suspected acute appendicitis. For these, excision with primary closure or imbrication is successful.

LARGE BOWEL FISTULAS

Although fistulas between the colon and many organs have been reported, most types are rare. The review of Webster and Carey [136] includes a comprehensive discussion of large bowel fistulas. A general discussion of intra-abdominal fistula abscesses and fistulas is given in Chapter 34.

Epidemiology and Pathogenesis

A listing of the anatomic types of large bowel fistula and the possible etiologic conditions for each type are presented in Table 39-3. Rectal fistulas are discussed in Chapter 41. Fistulas develop when a diseased organ comes into contact with other organs or when the space between organs is occupied by a mass, a focus of infection, or a foreign body. After the effects of pressure, nonspecific inflammation, and digestion by products of infection or digestive enzymes, the lumina of the organs communicate or the fistula opens onto the surface of skin.

Clinical Manifestations

Colocutaneous fistulas constitute 29 to 44 percent of all external gastrointestinal fistulas. Most colocutaneous fistulas (52 to 94 percent) occur as sequelae of surgical procedures, either as complications (eg, anastomotic leaks) or as persistent drainage or cecostomy tracts. Diverticular disease, carcinoma, and inflammatory bowel disease account for most spontaneous fistulas.

Spontaneous and complicating fistulas appear as a fluctuant, localized area of inflammation, which subsequently breaks down and drains pus or feces. After the removal of drains, feces continue to drain through persistent tracts. Under the best of circumstances, a colocutaneous fistula acts similar to a colostomy. All possible complications of fistula may occur, however, including intra-abdominal sepsis, fluid, electrolyte, and acid-base imbalance, malnutrition, hemorrhage, bowel obstruction, and skin breakdown. Since most large reported series come from referral centers, reported incidences of these complications in colocutaneous fistulas are probably not representative of the general situation.

Most gastrocolic fistulas result from carcinomas of the colon or stomach. Gastrojejunocolic fistulas were formerly occasional complications of retrocolic gastrojejunostomy performed for peptic ulcer disease.[136] Gastrocolic fistulas produce upper abdominal pain, diarrhea, and weight loss. Vomiting, occasionally feculent, frequently occurs.[136] A tumor mass may be palpated. Malabsorption is the most frequent complication. The colonization of the stomach and upper intestine with large numbers of fecal organisms alters digestion and absorption; undigested food and fluid may pass directly from stomach to colon.

Duodenocolic fistulas are also usually caused by malignancy, especially carcinoma of the right or transverse colon. Benign duodenocolic fistulas result from peptic ulcer disease or inflammatory bowel disease. The presentation is similar to that of gastrocolic fistula with pain, diarrhea, weight loss, malabsorption, and abdominal mass. Vomiting occurs less frequently than with gastrocolic fistula.

Intestinocolic and colocolic fistulas frequently result from septic complications of diverticular disease and inflammatory bowel disease. Systemic signs of infection are more prevalent than in gastric or duodenal fistulae. Otherwise, the symptoms are similar to those of the higher fistulas—abdominal pain, diarrhea, and weight loss. These symptoms may be minimal if the intestinal communication is located in distal small bowel. When cancer or abscess are present, abdominal or pelvic mass may be detected.

Biliary enteric fistulas occur in 0.4 to 2 percent of patients with biliary tract disease.[136-138] Of those patients

TABLE 39-3. LARGE BOWEL FISTULA: CLASSIFICATION AND ETIOLOGY

Anatomic Type	Etiology
Colocutaneous fistula	Iatrogenic (anastomotic leak, persistent cecostomy, postabscess drainage, intestinal injury), diverticulitis, carcinoma of large bowel, inflammatory bowel disease, trauma, ingested foreign body, tuberculosis, amebiasis, actinomycosis, strangulated hernia, appendicitis, ischemic perforation
Coloenteric fistula	
Gastrocolic and gastrojejunocolic fistula	Carcinoma of colon, carcinoma of stomach, peptic ulcer disease, gastric ulcer, inflammatory bowel disease, diverticulitis, carcinoma of pancreas or gallbladder, tuberculosis, syphilis, trauma, lymphoma, sarcoma, carcinoid, typhoid, pancreatic abscess, ingested foreign body, subphrenic abscess, iatrogenic (anastomotic leak, gastrostomy tube erosion, inadvertent gastrocolostomy, radiation therapy)
Duodenocolic fistula	Carcinoma of colon, carcinoma of gallbladder, carcinoma of duodenum, carcinoma of pancreas, lymphoma, peptic ulcer disease, duodenal diverticulitis, inflammatory bowel disease, biliary disease, pancreatitis, abdominal and subhepatic abscess, tuberculosis, typhoid, trauma, ingested foreign body, amebiasis
Intestinocolic fistula	Diverticulitis, inflammatory bowel disease, carcinoma of colon, ingested foreign body
Colocolic fistula	Sigmoid volvulus, diverticulitis
Appendicocolic fistula	Appendicitis
Cholecystocolic and cholecystoduodenocolic fistula	Chronic cholecystitis and cholelithiasis, carcinoma of colon, carcinoma of gallbladder, peptic ulcer disease, inflammatory bowel disease, diverticulitis coli, duodenal diverticulitis, lymphoma, trauma
Pancreaticocolic and pseudocystcolic fistula	Pancreatic abscess, pancreatic pseudocyst
Genitourinary-colon fistula	
Renocolic fistula	Renal disease—pyelonephritis, tuberculosis, echinococcosis, bilharziasis, renal calculus, renal tumor
Ureterocolic fistula	Renal disease—pyelonephritis, tuberculosis, renal and ureteral calculus, ureteral stricture, pregnancy, pelvic kidney, urinary tumor. Bowel disease—carcinoma of colon, diverticulitis, blunt and penetrating trauma, postileal conduit surgery
Vesicocolic fistula	Diverticulitis, carcinoma of colon, carcinoma of cervix, carcinoma of bladder, postradiation treatment, trauma, tuberculosis, amebiasis, syphilis, inflammatory bowel disease, other pelvic tumors
Colovaginal, colouterine, colocervical, tubocolic fistula	Diverticulitis, carcinoma of colon, pelvic cancer, operative trauma, radiation, tuberculosis, pelvic inflammatory disease, endometriosis
Intestinorespiratory fistula	Subphrenic abscess, rupture of the diaphragm, empyema, pyonephrosis
Vascular fistulas	
Aortocolic fistula	Ruptured aortic aneurysm, penetrating trauma
Inferior mesenteric artery-colic fistula	Arteriovenous malformation, arteriovenous fistula after bowel resection
Iliac artery-colic fistula	Foreign body perforation, iliac artery aneurysm, postvascular surgery

with fistulas, 8 to 24 percent have cholecystocolonic fistulas and another 2 to 8 percent have cholecystoduodenocolic fistulas.[136-138]

Because 80 to 90 percent of these fistulas are sequellae of chronic cholecystitis and cholelithiasis, many patients give a past history of right upper quadrant pain. The disappearance of right upper quadrant pain, particularly during an acute exacerbation, may herald the development of a fistula. Elderly cholecystitis patients with diabetes mellitus and atherosclerotic vascular disease are especially prone to fistula formation. Patients with biliary-enteric fistulas may develop gallstone ileus. The point of obstruction may be located in the terminal ileum if there is a cholecystoduodenocolic fistula or in sigmoid colon with a cholecystocolonic fistula.[138] Hematochezia, of moderate to severe degree, occurs if the cystic artery is involved in the fistula. Diarrhea and malabsorption occur if the duodenum is involved or if there is common bile duct obstruction with subsequent passage of all bile into the colon. Jaundice and cholangitis are more likely to occur when the duct is obstructed. Although the cholecystocolonic fistula is the most likely biliary-enteric fistula of all to cause cholangitis, the reported incidence ranges widely from 0 to 60 percent. Biliary colonic fistula may be asymptomatic, with only the roentgen finding of pneumobilia.

Complications involving the colon occur in about 1 percent of patients who are admitted with acute pancreatitis, and as many as one-half of these involve fistula formation. Pancreatocolonic fistulas occur spontaneously or as a sequel to operation in 10 to 18 percent of patients with pancreatic abscess,[139] and in 0.6 to 6 percent of patients with pseudocyst.[140] Most pancreatitis patients who develop colonic fistulas have a clinical course characterized by the presence of an abdominal mass, pain, and in the case of abscess, sepsis. Communication with the colon is heralded by the sudden passage of a brown or yellow watery diarrheal stool; pain and sepsis may be relieved. More than half of these patients subsequently develop severe hemorrhage. Passage of stool from a drain tract indicates the presence of a postoperative fistula.

Colourinary fistulas may originate from disease in either system. Fistulas that communicate with the upper urinary tract are more likely related to urinary disease,[136] whereas lower urinary tract fistulas arise as sequellae of bowel disease.[61] Colovesical fistulas are rare in females unless the woman has undergone hysterectomy.

Nearly all patients with urinary fistulas present with evidence of urinary sepsis—frequency, dysuria, and hematuria. Pneumaturia and fecaluria are noted in some, and if present, bowel disease may produce symptoms such as rectal bleeding, change in bowel habits, and lower abdominal pain. However, as many as half of patients with diverticulitis have no bowel symptoms. Other findings may include flank tenderness and pain, upper abdominal mass, presence of a psoas sign with upper tract disease, and lower abdominal or pelvic mass with bladder fistula. Urine may drain into the colon, causing watery diarrhea.

Colovaginal and colocervical fistulas occur in women who have had hysterectomy. These fistulas, along with colouterine fistula, occur secondary to diverticulitis or pelvic cancer. In women who have been treated for pelvic cancer, the development of a fistula frequently indicates tumor recurrence. Fistulas between the colon and the female reproductive organs usually present with the passage of pus, feces, and perhaps flatus per vagina.

Colorespiratory fistulas are rare. The most common cause is extension of a subphrenic abscess into both the colon and thorax. The presence of the fistula is indicated by mediastinitis, empyema, or recurrent pneumonitis.

Colovascular fistulas are unusual, relative to other vascular enteric fistulas. Aortocolic fistulas can result from a ruptured aortic aneurysm or penetrating tumor, but are more likely to occur at the distal suture line of an aortoiliac graft. Vascular fistulas present with rectal hemorrhage. The initial bleeding is usually minimal and of short duration; however, bleeding continues to occur and eventually reaches exsanguinating proportion.

Diagnosis

Most fistulas can be accompanied by sepsis, malnutrition, and fluid, electrolyte, and acid-base imbalance. Therefore, complete blood count, electrolyte, arterial blood pH, calcium, magnesium, and vitamin B levels are indicated in many patients. A complete nutritional assessment is frequently necessary. Cultures of blood and all drainage should be done when sepsis exists. The cause of the fistula should be determined.

The evaluation of a colocutaneous fistula must answer several questions: (1) what is the origin of the fistula? (2) is there continuity of the bowel? (3) is there distal obstruction of the bowel? (4) what is the nature of adjacent bowel? and (5) is there an undrained abscess? Plain abdominal roentgenogram series, abdominal ultrasound, and gallium scan may be used to investigate abdominal sepsis. However, the key studies are proctoscopy, barium enema, and injection of the fistula with contrast medium. An upper gastrointestinal series with small bowel follow-through and an intravenous pyelogram are sometimes helpful.

Gastrocolic, gastrojejunocolic, and colon intestinal fistulas are all best demonstrated by barium enema examination.[136] Upper gastrointestinal series and upper gastrointestinal endoscopy are less often successful, although both studies are indicated.[136,141,142] Neither proctoscopy nor colonoscopy demonstrate the fistula, but these studies may establish the diagnosis of specific colonic diseases that might account for fistulas.

Plain abdominal roentgenograms which show air in the biliary tree (Fig. 39-10A), or change in location of previously demonstrated biliary calculi, allow the diagnosis of biliary-colonic fistula. Communication with the colon is indicated by barium enema (Fig. 39-10B). An upper gastrointestinal series may demonstrate the presence of a cholecystoduodenocolic fistula.

Likewise, pancreatocolonic fistulas are usually visualized with barium enema examination. Concurrent gastric or duodenal involvement may be apparent on upper gastrointestinal series. Upper gastrointestinal roentgenograms, ultrasound, and computer tomography are indicated to determine the extent of the pancreatic disease process.

Urinarycolic fistulas are more difficult to demonstrate than are colenteric fistulas. Plain abdominal films may be of some help, since many of these patients harbor radioopaque calculi in the involved collecting system or in the

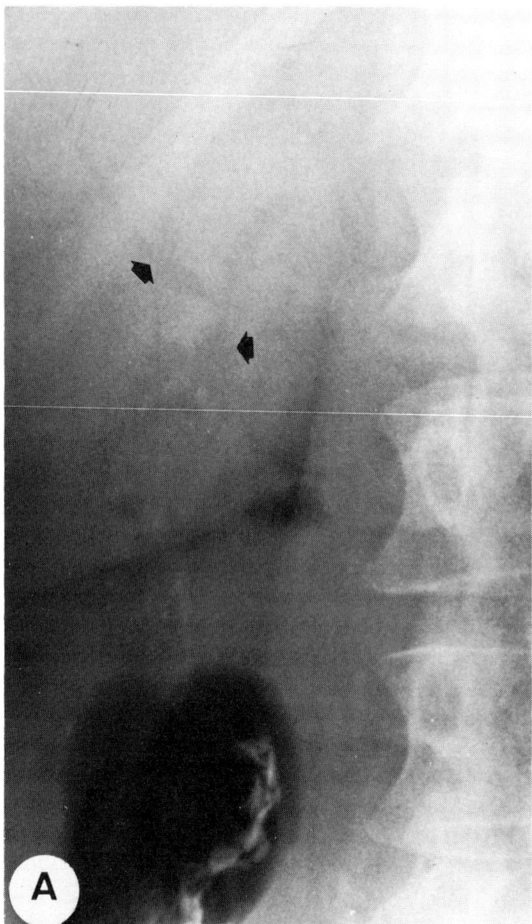

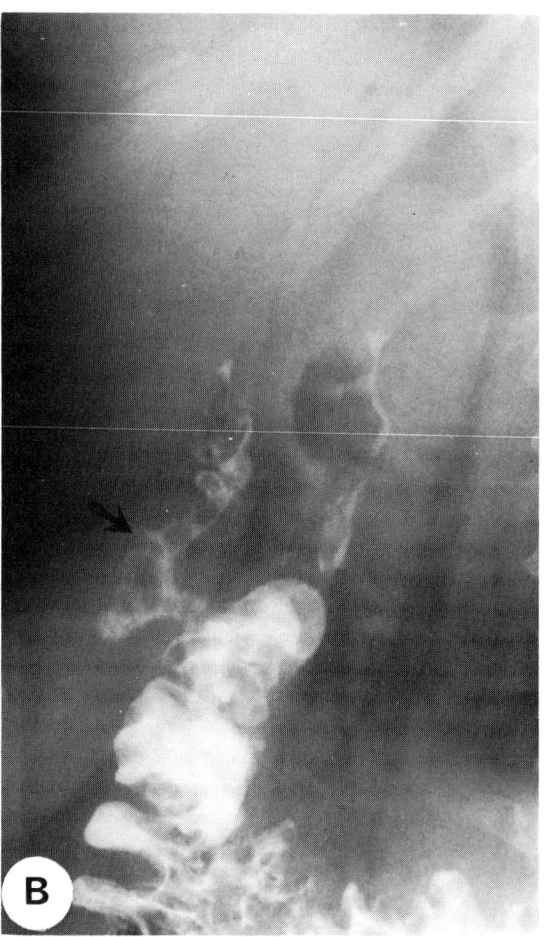

Fig. 39-10. **A. Cholecystocolonic fistula. Plain abdominal film demonstrates air in the biliary and hepatic ducts (arrows). B. Cholecystocolonic fistula. Barium enema demonstrates the fistula and the gallbladder containing calculi (arrow). Contrast from an intravenous pyelogram is seen in the pelvis of the right kidney.**

bladder. When renocolic or ureterocolic fistula is present, pneumonephrosis or air surrounding the renal shadow may be seen. Rarely, in upper or lower urinary tract fistulas an air fluid level may be seen in the bladder.

In contrast to coloenteric fistula, it is usually difficult to demonstrate colourinary fistulas by studying the bowel. In most instances, both endoscopy and barium enema reveal only the nature of the bowel disease (Fig. 39-3A). With renocolic or ureterocolic fistulas, the colon may be narrowed or inflamed at the site of the fistula. Methylene blue or indigo carmine injected intravenously or directly into the urinary tract will only rarely be seen emptying into the colon.

Urinalysis and urine culture nearly always prove urinary infection with enteric organisms. Intravenous pyelography and cystography almost never demonstrate the fistulas (Fig. 39-3B). However, in the event of upper tract fistula, the kidney may not be visualized on the involved side. Otherwise, hydronephrosis and hydroureter are seen. Likewise, although the fistula is not seen on the cystogram, a mass effect may be seen at areas of inflammation or tumor involvement. Retrograde ureterography is the examination most likely to demonstrate upper tract fistulas, whereas cystoscopy is the most useful examination in the evaluation of colovesical fistula. Cystitis, either diffuse or localized to the area of fistulization, is found in most patients. Tumor involvement of the bladder may be proved by biopsy. Fecal matter, pus, or air may be seen passing through the fistula or, in the case of upper tract fistula, from the ureteral orifice.

Fistula between the colon and the vagina, cervix, uterus, and fallopian tubes also is not frequently demonstrated on barium enema or large bowel endoscopy. Colon disease may be defined, however. Pelvic examination may demonstrate feces passing into the vagina or through the cervical os, but this is unusual. Hysterography and salpingography may demonstrate uterine and tubal fistulas.

Colorespiratory fistulas are usually demonstrated by barium enema.

Vascular fistulas are usually not diagnosed by either arteriography, barium enema, or large bowel endoscopy. However, arteriography may visualize contributing vascular malformations.

Treatment and Prognosis

Before definitive treatment of any fistula is undertaken, metabolic complications must be corrected. Fluid and electrolyte deficits must be replaced, and excessive losses must be controlled. Institution of complete bowel rest with nasogastric drainage and restriction of all oral intake may be necessary to control such losses. Nutritional requirements must be met to correct malnutrition and promote healing. For external colon fistulas, oral alimentation with low-residue nutritional supplements and elemental diets is usually adequate. However, if the volume of output is high (greater than 200 ml per day), if residue or digestive enzymes prevent healing, or if malnutrition is a sequella of an internal fistula, parenteral hyperalimentation must be used.

Failure to control sepsis is an ominous sign in patients with gastrointestinal fistulas; the mortality rate with uncontrolled sepsis is 85 percent. Appropriate antibiotics must be administered, and drainage of abscesses along the fistulous tracts must be performed. Diversion of enteric contents may be necessary to minimize drainage into the tissues from the fistula. Spontaneous closure of colocutaneous fistulas is expected in 30 to 70 percent of patients,[136] and recurrence is unusual after closure. When spontaneous closure does occur, it does so within 1 month of the control of sepsis in 91 percent of patients. Spontaneous closure is rare after more than 8 weeks of supportive care.[136]

Persistence is the result of a combination of factors: large size, large volume of output, a rigid wall of the fistula, presence of carcinoma, persistent foreign body, epithelialization of the tract, obstruction distal to the fistula, and separation of the ends of the bowel. Persistent sepsis or such infections as tuberculosis, actinomycosis, and amebiasis prevent spontaneous healing. Closure is relatively unlikely to occur when the fistula is secondary to diverticulitis, granulomatous colitis, and radiation colitis. Patients receiving steroids or chemotherapy heal poorly.

Unless drainage is minimal and acceptable, or the patient is a poor operative risk for medical reasons, external fistulas that persist for 8 weeks should be treated by operation. The most efficient treatment is excision of the fistula and the involved colon segment with end-to-end anastomosis. Simple turn-in repair leads to frequent recurrence. It may be necessary to achieve fistula closure in stages.[136]

Unless pressed by sepsis or hemorrhage, internal fistula can be treated by supportive measures until the patient is in optimum condition. Then, unless the patient is moribund due to the basic disease, surgical correction is indicated. Although operation may be necessary to treat sepsis, definitive repair of internal fistulas should not be attempted in the presence of uncontrolled infection.

Gastrocolic or gastrojejunocolic fistulas are tolerated poorly if untreated. Resection of the fistula and the involved stomach and bowel with primary anastomoses is recommended. When the fistula is due to recurrent peptic ulcer disease, the cause of recurrence must be treated.

Duodenocolic fistulas are lethal if not closed. The diseased colon, the fistula, and the involved portion of duodenum should be excised.[136,142] Duodenal closure may be a problem in these patients. Management options include: primary transverse closure, reinforcement of the closure with an omental patch or a jejunal serosal patch, anastomosis of the duodenal opening to either a loop or a Roux-en-Y limb of jejunum, or pancreaticoduodenectomy. Korelitz [141] suggests that duodenocolic fistula due to Crohn disease may be managed with a bypassing ileocolostomy or a diverting ileostomy with success equal to that of resection. When the lesion is resectable for cure, malignant duodenocolic fistula usually requires an extensive en bloc resection, often a colectomy and pancreatoduodenectomy. If the patient is not curable, a double bypass (gastrojejunostomy and ileocolostomy) provides the best palliation.[136,143]

Colointestinal and *colocolic* fistulas are treated by en bloc resection of the involved bowel and any focus of sepsis. The 5-year survival of colon cancer with fistula to small bowel is 43 percent.[136]

Elective operative treatment of cholecystocolonic fistula consists of cholecystectomy and closure or resection of the colon. Common duct exploration is performed if indicated. When the procedure is performed in the acute situation, the colon openings may be exteriorized as a colostomy to be closed secondarily. If gallstone ileus has occurred, one should try to milk the stone into the rectum for removal by proctoscopy. If this is unsuccessful, the stone may be removed through a colotomy, which is closed primarily and protected by a proximal colostomy. Opinion is divided as to whether the cholecystectomy should be performed at the same operation.[136,137] Patients who are poor operative risks, who have no complications, and who have no bile duct obstruction may be managed nonoperatively if carcinoma can be excluded.

Pancreatic fistulas to the colon require individualized management. The overall mortality is 33 percent—mostly due to sepsis and hemorrhage. When the fistula occurs secondary to a pancreatic abscess, radical debridement of the pancreas, and wide drainage of the pancreatic bed and retrocolic area are necessary procedures. In addition, the splenic flexure and left colon should be mobilized to assure complete drainage. Repair of the opening in the colon and proximal colostomy may suffice; however, resection of the involved colon segment with colostomy and mucous fistula are necessary in many cases.[136,139]

When a pseudocyst ruptures into the colon, spontaneous closure of the cyst and fistula is common; therefore, proximal colostomy alone is recommended in most instances.

If the fistula persists after 3 to 6 months of decompression, colon resection is necessary. Hemorrhage from the fistula carries a mortality of 50 percent.

Renocolic and ureterocolic fistulas usually require nephrectomy and ureterectomy with resection of the colon. Occasionally, the involved segment of the ureter may be excised and the remainder repaired. Nephrostomy drainage of the kidney may permit preservation of that kidney if any function persists.[136]

Definitive treatment of vesicocolic fistulas requires resection of the diseased colon segment, the fistula, and at least a small segment of involved bladder. This procedure may require one or more stages, depending on the presence of pelvic sepsis, bowel obstruction, inflamed bowel, and apposition of suture lines. When malignancy is the underlying problem, curative resection should be performed whenever possible. The 5-year survival is dependent on lymph node, rather than local, extension. In cases with massive tumor or involvement of the trigone, this may require pelvic exenteration with end colostomy and ileal conduit urinary diversion. If the disease is unresectable, diverting colostomy is indicated.[61]

Treatment of fistulas to the female reproductive organs involves resection of the involved colon segment and the cervix, uterus, or tubes as required. If recurrent carcinoma of the cervix is the cause of the fistula, pelvic exenteration is indicated if technically feasible and if there is no distant spread of tumor.[136]

After abscesses and other septic foci have been drained and controlled, *respiratory fistulas* are treated by resection of involved colon and irreversibly damaged pulmonary tissue.[136] Vascular fistulas require resection of aneurysms and involved grafts with closure of the colon. Extra-anatomic vascular reconstruction is the best method to avoid subsequent graft sepsis.[136]

BACTERIAL ENTEROCOLITIS WITH SURGICAL MANIFESTATIONS

Many bacterial diarrheas are caused by the effects of enterotoxins; diarrhea and dehydration are the usual complications of bacterial enterocolitis (Chapter 38). However, when the organism is capable of invading the bowel wall, surgical complications, such as hemorrhage or perforation, may occur. Such complications have been documented with *Shigella,*[144] *Salmonella,*[145] and *Yersinia*[146] infections. When perforation occurs, however, the resulting infection is caused by mixed fecal flora, in addition to the enteric invader.

Epidemiology

All three diseases are caused by ingestion of contaminated human fecal matter. Yersiniosis has been documented in man only in the past 20 years. Most cases have been reported in Western Europe and in North America, in colder rather than warmer climates. Cases appear in clusters,[146] many animals and birds probably serve as reservoirs for the organism.

Etiology and Pathogenesis

The etiologic agents of these diseases are discussed in Chapters 5, 7, and 38.

Shigella species causing human disease include *S. dysenteriae, S. flexneri, S. boydii,* and *S. sonnei.* All these organisms infect by penetrating the mucosa of the terminal ileum and colon. Both endotoxins and exotoxins result in superficial inflammation, coagulation necrosis, pseudomembrane formation, and ulceration. These ulcers may be deep, producing severe hemorrhage or perforation. Healing may be complete or may occur with stricture formation. Gram-negative bacilli are usually present on microscopic examination.

Salmonella gastroenteritis results from infection with *S. typhimurium, S. enteritidis,* and *S. cholerae suis.* Typhoid fever is caused by *S. typhi* and *S. paratyphi* A, B, and C. These organisms infect by penetrating the mucosa of the small bowel and invading lymphoid tissues. They gain access to the bloodstream by way of the lymphatics, and they are taken up by reticuloendothelial cells, where they proliferate. A second period of bacteremia occurs, and the bowel may be reinfected via the bloodstream or by passage of infected bile.

Reinfection of typhoid occurs in the bowel lymphoid tissues, especially the Peyer patches of the distal ileum. Hyperemia, hyperplasia, and mononuclear cell proliferation occur in these tissues. As the lymphoid aggregates undergo necrosis, ulcers develop in the distal small bowel and ascending colon, which may bleed or perforate. In the fourth week of infection, healing occurs with little or no scar formation. Bacteremia also produces metastatic infection resulting in lymphadenitis, splenomegaly, cholecystitis, pneumonitis, pyelonephritis, meningitis, osteomyelitis, thrombophlebitis, and soft tissue abscess.

Yersinia enterocolitica is responsible for yersiniosis. The pathogenesis of yersiniosis is similar to that of typhoid, with an initial enteritis and subsequent involvement of bowel and mesenteric lymphoid tissues. Bacteremia has occasionally been lethal. In addition, erythema nodosum and arthritis, apparently secondary to immune complex deposition, may occur.

Clinical Manifestations

The typical incubation period of shigellosis is 2 or 3 days (12 hours to 7 days). In severe acute diseases, the onset of fever (38 to 40C), headache, and malaise is abrupt. Abdominal cramping, vomiting, diarrhea, and severe tenesmus occur, and stool is converted to bloody mucus. Physical examination reveals abdominal guarding and tenderness, especially overlying the colon; peristalsis is hyperactive. Toxemia, dehydration, perforation, or bleeding may cause death. The disease lasts several days. Chronic disease with occasional episodes of diarrhea, flatulence, or rectal bleeding may occur. Asymptomatic patients may be carriers.

The incubation period of *Salmonella* gastroenteritis is short, usually less than 24 hours. Fever, nausea, vomiting, and diarrhea develop suddenly. The temperature usually ranges from 37.5 to 38.5C. The watery stools may contain blood or mucus. Colicky abdominal pain is common. The duration and severity of the disease vary, but surgical complications almost never occur.

The onset of typhoid fever is insidious. The patient may give a history of a mild, nonspecific respiratory infection or enteritis. Typhoid begins with malaise, headache, myalgia, and arthralgia; bronchitis, epistaxis, lethargy, anorexia, flatulence, and constipation often follow. During the first week, the temperature rises gradually. Fever is high and continuous during the second and third weeks and falls by lysis in the fourth week. Apathy, toxemia, delirium, and the typhoid rash (rose spots) accompany the high fever. Most surgical complications occur after the second week. Toxic dilation of the colon in a typhoid patient is reported. Death may result from septicemia, dehydration, or perforation and peritonitis (Chapter 38).

Yersinosis presents several clinical pictures. *Yersinia* gastroenteritis produces fever, headache, vomiting, diarrhea, and abdominal pain. Stools are usually watery and bilious. As many as a third of patients have an exudative pharyngitis.[146] In terminal ileocolitis and mesenteric adenitis, pain is localized to the right lower quadrant. A tender mass may be palpable, and it may be impossible to exclude the presence of acute appendicitis. Polyarthritis and erythema nodosum may be the only signs of disease. Rarely, especially in immunocompromised hosts, hepatosplenic abscesses and septicemia occur. In addition to pseudoappendicitis, surgical complications include hemorrhage from ileo-ascending colon ulcers,[93] bowel obstruction secondary to adhesions to inflamed nodes, and pseudocholecystitis. The duration is variable, but is in the range of weeks. Death is the usual result in untreated patients.

Diagnosis

In bacterial enterocolitis, radiologic examinations demonstrate nonspecific changes and are of no help in establishing a diagnosis. If a question of perforation exists, abdominal films are helpful. The rare toxic dilation of the colon is demonstrated on plain films.

If blood is lost, hematologic analysis reveals anemia in all these diseases; on the contrary, dehydration produces an apparent erythrocytosis. The leukocyte count may or may not be elevated; regardless, a left shift in the differential count is typical.

Serologic tests may be useful in the diagnosis of *Salmonella,* and to a lesser extent *Yersinia,* infections. For the tests to be meaningful, high titers of agglutinating antibody must be observed in repeated samples, and comparison with antibody levels in convalescent serum is worthwhile. In yersiniosis, the number of serotypes and false positives and negatives are problems.

With shigellosis, proctoscopy may show red, edematous mucosa, which subsequently develops dirty gray ulcers. Patches of granulation tissue may be present in patients with chronic disease. Proctoscopy is unlikely to reveal changes in salmonellosis and yersiniosis, since right colon involvement is most common.

Microscopic analysis of stool may be helpful. Leukocytes are present in the stained specimen in 69 percent of shigellosis patients. A positive stool analysis correlates with positive stool cultures and invasive disease. Only one-third of patients with salmonellosis have fecal leukocytosis; yersiniosis may produce similar findings.

Isolation of the organism on culture is the surest way to establish the diagnosis; stool specimens are productive in all three diseases. Blood cultures are useful in yersiniosis and typhoid and paratyphoid fever. When a normal appendix is found at appendectomy, culture of mesenteric nodes may be productive if the patient has yersiniosis. The microbiology laboratory must be alerted if *Yersinia* is suspected, because special culture methods are necessary to isolate these organisms.

Treatment

Since all three diseases are self-limiting, the essential task in treating bacterial enteritis is appropriate fluid and electrolyte support to prevent anemia, dehydration, and their complications.

It is often difficult to detect any effect of antibiotic treatment on the course of the disease. Presently, specific treatment is indicated in the following situations: (1) severe disease, (2) septicemia, (3) disease in children and the elderly, (4) disease in the immunocompromised patient, and (5) surgical complications, in which case antibiotics for the broad spectrum of fecal organisms should be selected.

If antibiotics are to be used, the choice should be dictated by in vitro sensitivity determinations, because drug resistance is a growing problem. Shigellosis usually responds to ampicillin, the sulfas, and tetracycline. The combination trimethoprim-sulfamethoxazole is highly successful against organisms resistant to ampicillin.[147] Although bacteriologic cure is usually achieved in 7 days, antibiotic treatment may prolong the carrier state.

Antibiotic treatment does not alter the duration of diarrhea or the carrier state in *Salmonella* enteritis. Treatment does decrease the degree of toxemia and prostration in septicemia and typhoid fever—several weeks' treatment is required. Ampicillin, chloramphenicol, and the tetracyclines are the first-line drugs. Trimethoprim-sulfamethoxazole is effective against resistant *Salmonella* as well.

Except for septicemia, the course of yersiniosis is not altered by antibiotic therapy. The antibiotics showing most effect are tetracycline, chloramphenicol, and the aminoglycosides, whereas ampicillin, trimethoprim-sulfamethoxazole, and cephalosporins are less effective.

Hemorrhage is treated the same as lower gastrointestinal bleeding from any other cause. Intraarterial vasopressor infusion and resection of the involved ileum and colon have been successful. Kim et al [145] have reported their experience in treating typhoid perforations of the ileum. Most patients were treated successfully by simple closure of the perforation; resection with anastomosis and bypass with ileostomy or ileotransverse colostomy also gave good results. Drainage alone was less successful, with a mortality rate of 10 to 32 percent. Most patients with toxic dilation of the colon respond well to nonoperative therapy.

Prognosis

Most patients who are supported adequately recover from *Shigella, Salmonella,* and *Yersinia* infection. Prompt treatment for complications yields successful results also. Repeated stool cultures are necessary until two to four successive test results, over a 3-week period, are negative. To prevent spread of the disease, fecal isolation precautions must be followed until the carrier state is cleared. Food handlers, especially, must not return to work until their stool results are negative.

PSEUDOMEMBRANOUS AND ANTIBIOTIC-ASSOCIATED COLITIS

Antibiotic treatment sometimes produces superinfection within the gastrointestinal tract. Antibiotic-associated colitis is one superinfection that often affects surgical patients.

Epidemiology

Diarrhea following the administration of antibiotics is common, but the true incidence depends on how one defines diarrhea. Friedman et al [148] found that lincomycin was the antibiotic most often associated with diarrhea (1.7 percent); next in order were clindamycin (0.65 percent), ampicillin (0.55 percent), erythromycin (0.28 percent), and tetracycline (0.17 percent). No pseudomembranous colitis was diagnosed. Although this study certainly underestimates the incidence of antibiotic-associated diarrhea, the relative risk of diarrhea for frequently used antibiotics is documented. In contrast, Tedesco's group [149] reported an incidence of diarrhea of 21 percent each in patients treated with ampicillin and clindamycin. During the study, pseudomembranous colitis did not occur in ampicillin-treated patients, but the incidence was 10 percent in the clindamycin-treated group. This incidence of clindamycin-associated colitis is the highest reported. Other studies [148] establish incidences of diarrhea in clindamycin-treated patients of 3.4 and 21 percent. No pseudomembranous colitis was noted in either study.

Although patients of all ages are at risk for antibiotic-associated colitis, white women of about 50 years of age are most frequently affected.

Many patients have severe underlying disease, such as cancer and leukemia, hepatic and renal failure, and diabetes.

Pathogenesis

A number of causes, among them the postoperative state, mucosal ischemia, heavy metal poisoning, and colon obstruction have been proposed. Although the disease was described in the preantibiotic era, attention has recently focused on the role of various antibiotics in changing the colonic flora.

Early in the antibiotic era, pseudomembranous colitis was seen mainly in patients having preoperative oral antibiotic bowel preparations. Such cases are now unusual. Slagle and Boggs [150] reviewed recent reports of antibiotic-associated colitis and identified cases related to the following drugs: clindamycin, lincomycin, tetracycline, ampicillin, erythromycin, penicillin, neomycin, cephalexin, and sulfamethoxazole-trimethoprim. During the 1970s, reports have most often implicated clindamycin.[151] Although cases of colitis after parenteral administration are reported, the majority follow oral intake. It has been suggested that these antibiotics may damage gastrointestinal epithelial cells, but no objective evidence has been produced to support this contention. Allergic reaction to the antibiotics has also been considered. Occurrence of antibiotic-associated pseudomembranous colitis in several members of one family has led to the suggestion that a genetic predisposition to this condition exists.

Overgrowth of the colon flora by toxin-producing bacteria has been discussed for three decades. In the first two decades, overgrowth with resistant *Staphylococcus* was emphasized.[152] Most recently, evidence supporting the etiologic role of *C. difficile* has been growing.[153] These organisms are resistant to clindamycin, and produce a toxin that can reproduce colitis in laboratory animals.

Clinical Manifestations

The clinical syndrome of antibiotic-associated pseudomembranous colitis is variable.[154] Symptoms occur anywhere from 1 day after the initial dose to 1 month following termination of antibiotic treatment. The cardinal features are fever (38 to 40C), diarrhea, and abdominal pain. The patient may have up to 20 mucoid or cloudy stools per day; occasionally, gross blood is noted. Steady or colicky abdominal pain occurs. On examination, tenderness overlying the colon is common, and rebound tenderness may be elicited. The abdomen may be distended. Findings suggestive of an acute abdomen are noted in 19 percent.[154]

A leukocytosis of 10,000–20,000 cells per mm^3 is common, and some counts as high as 32,000 per mm^3 have been reported. Microscopic stool analysis reveals abundant leukocytes with occasional red blood cells. Gram stain of the stool shows abundant gram-positive cocci if staphylococcal colitis is the problem. Stool culture using routine methods for demonstrating enteric pathogens detects no abnormal bacteria. Sophisticated anaerobic techniques allow isolation of *C. difficile*,[153] and a cytotoxic toxin can be demonstrated in tissue culture. The finding of the specific toxin is now considered diagnostic.

Barium enema is unwarranted but, when performed, shows thickened transverse folds, shallow ulcers, and flat plaques. Although not usually indicated, a gallium-67 scan may outline the colon.

The most useful diagnostic measure is proctoscopy or colonoscopy. Typically, cream to green colored plaques measuring 2–5 mm may be seen. In severe cases, the plaques may coalesce to form a pseudomembrane, which is adherent to a friable mucosa. It is necessary to carefully remove overlying mucus to see these features. Mucosal biopsy reveals a pseudomembrane of leukocytes, fibrin, and debris overlying an acutely inflamed mucosa. Defects in the epithelium are minimal. Mucus production is excessive. The submucosa is usually not involved except for edema and capillary engorgement. Absence of a pseudomembrane in the biopsy specimen does not rule out pseudomembranous colitis, since the membrane may be lost owing to technical factors. Colonscopy may be required to see lesions beyond 25 cm.

Treatment

Whenever diarrhea occurs in a patient who has recently received antibiotics, proctoscopy must be performed. The key to successful treatment is to discontinue the antibiotics immediately.[154] Intravenous fluids and electrolytes may be necessary to prevent dehydration. Tedesco [154] advocates the use of Lomotil to decrease the volume of diarrhea, although others feel this drug may exacerbate the colitis.[155] Use of local or systemic steroids has been suggested, but there are no controlled series to show whether this is helpful.

Cholestyramine will successfully control pseudomembranous colitis in about half the cases,[156] presumably because it binds the anionic *C. difficile* toxin.

Keighly et al [157] demonstrated rapid control of diarrhea in patients with pseudomembranous colitis using oral vancomycin. Almost 20 percent of patients will relapse, however, when this drug is stopped, and repeated treatment may be necessary.

In fulminant cases success has been achieved with diverting ileostomy and subtotal colectomy, but such measures should not often be necessary.

Prognosis

In the past, mortality rates in patients with pseudomembranous colitis have been high (50 to 75 percent); reports from the 1970s document mortality rates up to 25 percent. Tedesco[154] has shown that, with early diagnosis and cessation of antibiotic treatment, the mortality rate should approach zero. The disease may persist for as long as 4 to 8 weeks, but once it has subsided, the colon returns to normal. There may be an increased tendency to develop colitis following subsequent antibiotic treatment.

PNEUMATOSIS COLI

Pneumatosis coli is a manifestation of many diseases rather than a single disease itself. Table 39-4 lists conditions in which it has been described. Although pneumatosis may be associated with severe disease, it is more often a benign condition requiring no surgical treatment.

The gross appearance is that of multiple spherical and oblong cysts visible in the subserosa or submucosa of the small intestine or colon. The overlying mucosa may be normal or hemorrhagic.

Histologically, the cysts are located in the subserosa, submucosa, and occasionally the muscularis. There is no active inflammatory response or bacteria seen; multinucleated giant cells are often seen around the cysts.

TABLE 39-4. CONDITIONS ASSOCIATED WITH PNEUMATOSIS INTESTINALIS

Bowel ischemia
1. Circulatory
   a. Hypoperfusion
   b. Mesenteric vascular occlusion
2. Simple bowel obstruction (any cause)
3. Mechanical strangulation
   a. Volvulus
   b. Internal hernia
   c. Intussusception

Inflammatory
1. Neonatal necrotizing enterocolitis
2. Septic enterocolitis
3. Pseudomembranous enterocolitis
4. Toxic megacolon
5. Crohn disease
6. Inflammatory diarrhea of childhood

Pulmonary
1. Obstructive lung disease
2. Pneumothorax
3. Interstitial emphysema
4. Pneumomediastinum

Iatrogenic
1. Endoscopy
2. Umbilical vein catheter
3. Hydrogen peroxide enemas

Miscellaneous
1. Autoimmune diseases (especially scleroderma)
2. Whipple disease
3. Leukemia
4. Sprue
5. Peptic ulcer
6. Diverticulitis
7. Caustic injury
8. Trauma
9. Intestinal parasites

Adapted from Dodds WJ, Stewart ET, Goldberg HI: Pneumatosis intestinalis associated with hepatic portal venous gas. Am J Dis 21:992, 1976.

In 85 percent of patients, pneumatosis intestinalis is associated with other pathologic conditions. Pneumatosis of the distal colon more likely occurs in patients with no apparent underlying condition, whereas pneumatosis of the right colon is usually associated with small intestinal disease (Table 39-4).

Presently, two theories attempt to explain cyst formation. The most widely accepted theory is the mechanical theory: Gas reaches subserosa and submucosa in one of two ways: (1) intraluminal gas enters via a mucosal defect, or (2) air from ruptured pulmonary alveoli dissects down the mediastinum and out along mesenteric vessels. A large number of patients with chronic lung disease have asymptomatic pneumatosis, and the gas is mostly nitrogen and oxygen.

The other prevalent theory is that gas-producing bacteria gain access to the submucosa and cause cyst formation. This theory has not been accepted widely, because in adults bacteria are neither seen around nor cultured from the cysts. However, cyst cultures are positive in infants with necrotizing enterocolitis. Moreover, Yale et al [158] have reproduced pneumatosis in germ-free laboratory animals following monocontamination of the gut with *C. perfringens* and *C. tertium.*

The clinical features of the underlying disease predominate; [159] those patients with associated bowel disease are usually seriously ill. In asymptomatic patients, the discovery of pneumatosis on chest or abdominal roentgenograms is fortuitous. Pneumoperitoneum occurring in a patient without symptoms of abdominal disease suggests pneumatosis. Most asymptomatic patients have respiratory disorders.

Usually, the diagnosis may be made on plain abdominal films. The cysts are apparent as collections of air along the bowel (Fig. 39-11). Air may be located within the mesentery and may become confined under the diaphragm, regardless of the patient's position. Gastrointestinal contrast studies usually make visualization of the cysts easier. The appearance is that of polypoid or tumorlike lucent masses on the margin of the contrast column (Fig. 39-12).

Treatment

Treatment of underlying disease usually suffices to control secondary pneumatosis coli. It is unnecessary to treat asymptomatic pneumatosis; and for symptoms, oxygen therapy has been successful.[160]

TUBERCULOSIS OF THE LARGE BOWEL

Primary tuberculous enteritis is rare in countries in which pasteurization of milk is practiced, but recent reports document cases confined to the abdomen.[161]

In the prechemotherapy era, secondary bowel involvement was common, especially in patients with advanced pulmonary disease.

Tuberculous enterocolitis is a disease of young adults (third decade), and is more frequent in females.[162]

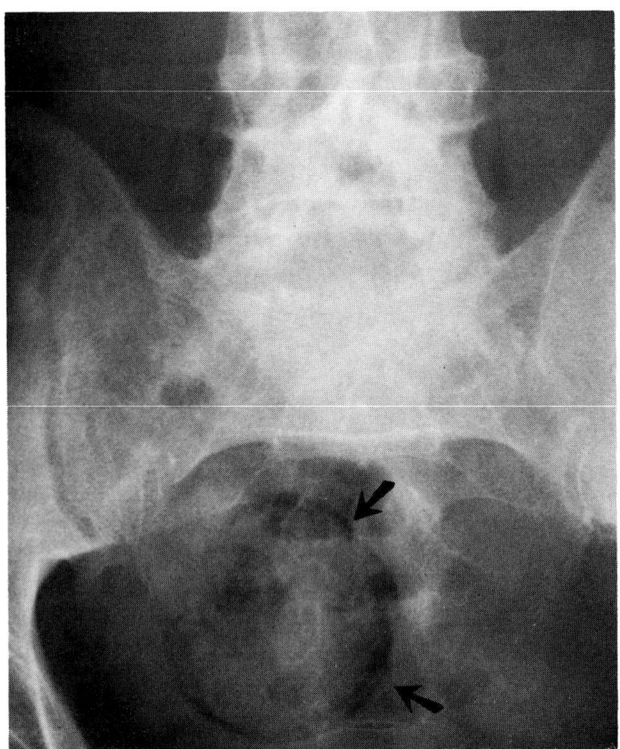

Fig. 39-11. **Pneumatosis coli indicative of infection. Plain abdominal film of a patient with peritonitis following a cardiac bypass procedure demonstrates intramural collections of air in an infarcted cecum (arrows).**

Pathogenesis

Intestinal tuberculosis can be caused by drinking milk contaminated with the bovine strain, but most recently cases have been caused by the human strains of the tubercle bacillus. The organisms are swallowed in infected sputum. Intestinal involvement may also result from hematogenous spread and perhaps direct spread from contiguous involved organs.[162]

The most frequently involved segments of the bowel are the ileocecal region, ileum, and the remaining large bowel, in that order,[163] although Paustian and Monto[162] indicate that disease of the ileum is being reported more frequently now. Anorectal disease, especially fistula, occurs, and is discussed in Chapter 41. The frequency of ileocecal involvement seems to be accounted for by the relative stasis of feces in this region, the abundance of lymphoid tissue, and the more digested state of the bowel contents. (Fig. 39-13)

The infection begins at the depths of the mucosal crypts. After invasion, phagocytes ingest and transport the bacteria to the submucosa, where lymphoid tissues become infected. Marked submucosal thickening occurs with edema, cellular infiltration, lymphoid hyperplasia, and tubercle formation. If the mucosal blood supply is impaired, ulceration occurs. As the process continues, the mesenteric lymph nodes become involved. Eventually, the process progresses to transmural involvement. Free perforation is unusual, because surrounding tissues adhere to the bowel before perforation. Healing of ulcers may be complicated by stricture formation.

Gross examination reveals inflamed bowel and edema of the mesentery and involved lymph nodes. Tubercles are often visible on the serosal surface. Ulcers are oriented in the transverse axis of the bowel and may become circumferential so that the strictures occupy only short segments of bowel.

Histologic analysis reveals a submucosal chronic inflammatory process with tubercles featuring epithelioid cells, giant cells, and central caseation necrosis. Fibrosis and hyalinization frequently surround the inflamed areas. Myobacteria may be seen with the acid-fast stain.

Clinical Manifestations

The clinical presentation of tuberculous enteritis, especially that involving the ileocecal region and the remaining colon, has been discussed in several articles.[161,162,164]

Prior to the chemotherapy era, tuberculous enterocolitis was usually detected in patients being treated for pul-

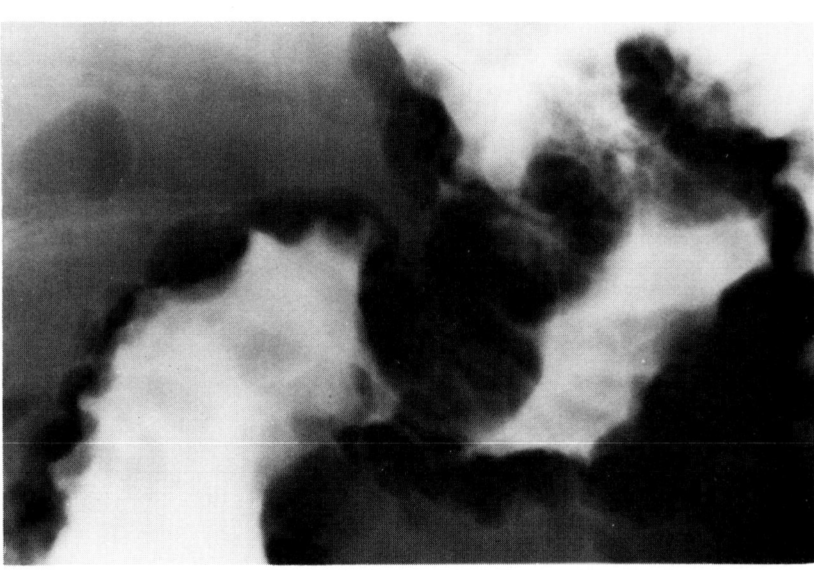

Fig. 39-12. **Pneumatosis coli—benign form. Barium enema of an asymptomatic patient demonstrates lucent masses surrounding the barium column.**

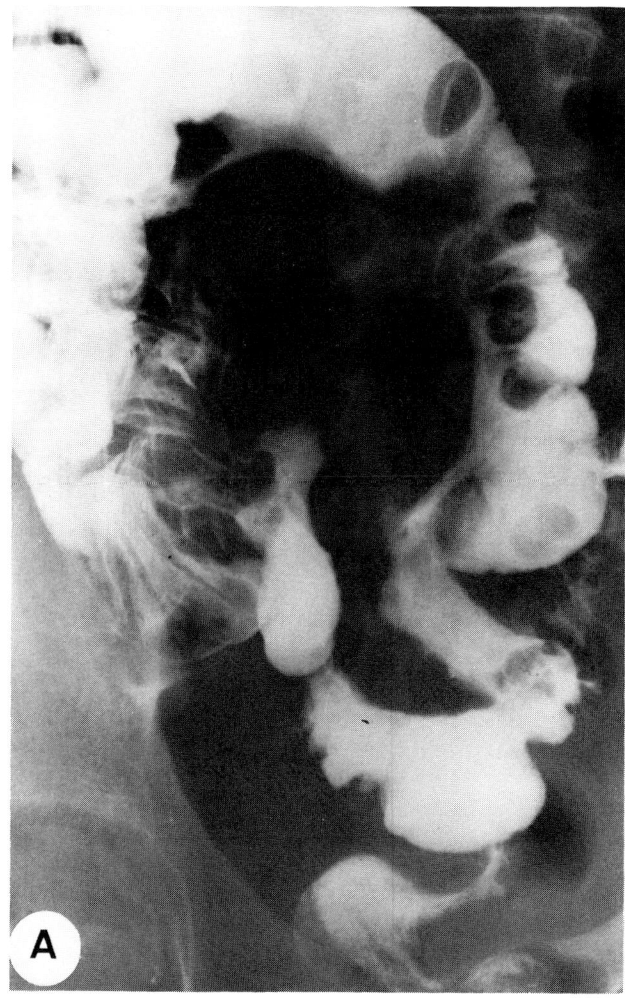

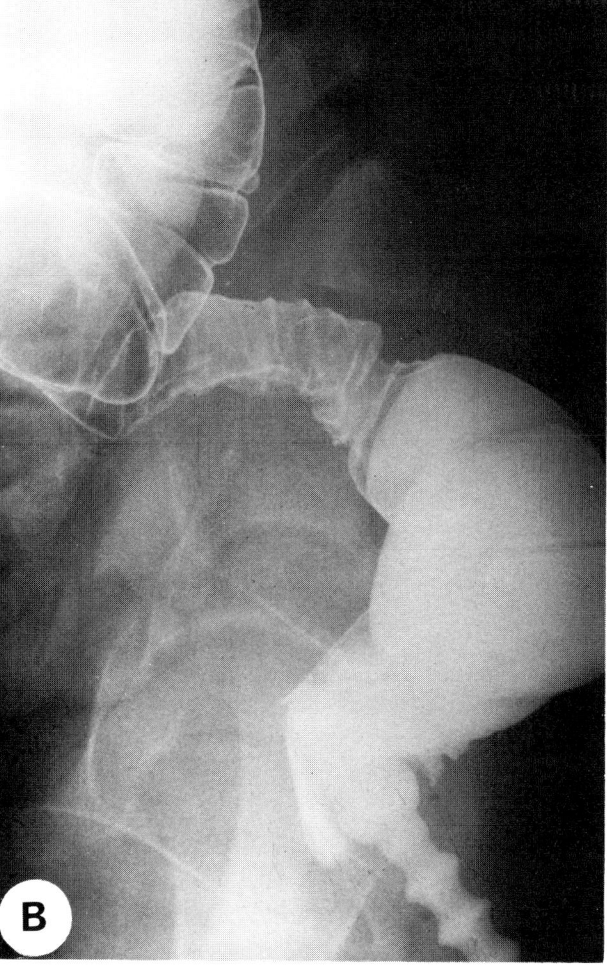

Fig. 39-13. **A. Tuberculosis. Barium enema with reflux into the terminal ileum demonstrates cecal distortion and filling defects, ileal narrowing with intervening dilated segments, and ileal inflammatory masses. B. Lateral rectal film demonstrates involvement of the first sacral vertebra and persistent narrowing of adjacent rectum.**

monary tuberculosis. The symptoms were protean and included fever, fatigability, nausea and vomiting, night sweats, weight loss, and dyspepsia. Abdominal pain and bowel changes were less common.

Currently, the most common surgical complications are obstruction and the presence of a mass, which cannot be differentiated from carcinoma, whereas bleeding, fistula formation, and perforation occur infrequently.

The symptoms and signs are those of chronic small bowel obstruction—colicky pain, distention, peristaltic activity, and right lower quadrant tenderness. Abdominal physical findings are those of small bowel obstruction. A palpable mass is present in up to two-thirds of patients.

Diagnosis

A positive skin test in a patient with abdominal symptoms is supportive, but not diagnostic, evidence of enteric tuberculosis. Conversely, a negative result, especially in a chronically or critically ill patient, does not rule out the possibility.

Roentgen signs on barium enema and small bowel follow-through examinations provide strong presumptive evidence of tuberculous enterocolitis, especially if the findings regress on appropriate antitubercular treatment. The following findings suggest tuberculous bowel disease: (1) motility disturbances, such as reduced transit time, hypersegmentation, stiffening, and thickening of mucosal folds, (2) lack of barium retention in the involved segment, (3) a short persistent narrow stream of barium in a small bowel segment, (4) delay of transit and dilation of short segments of small bowel, (5) cecal and colonic filling defects, with shortening of the ascending colon and cecal distortion, and (6) gapping of the ileocecal valve.[162]

Healing due to preoperative chemotherapy may cause difficulty in confirming the diagnosis of tuberculous enterocolitis. The only way to establish a definite diagnosis of tuberculous bowel disease is by culture and histologic analysis of resected tissue. The recovery of acid-fast bacilli from sputum or other sources is diagnostic of tuberculosis but is only strongly suggestive of bowel disease. After the bacilli are swallowed, they may be recovered from feces and fistula drainage in the absence of enteric infection.

Treatment

In active disease, antibiotic treatment is initiated with two or three drugs to which the organisms are sensitive (Chapter 18). The drugs presently used most frequently are isoniazid, ethambutol, and rifampin. Treatment is continued for at least 2 years. Antibiotic therapy of intestinal disease is effective within 1 or 2 weeks; however, Jordan and DeBakey [163] report perforation occurring in three patients with abnormal bowel involvement following the institution of antibiotics.

Operation is indicated to treat complications (obstruction, perforation with abscess or peritonitis, fistula, hemorrhage), to rule out carcinoma of the colon, and to remove disease that does not respond to systemic treatment. Since the diagnosis is frequently unclear, right hemicolectomy and resection of involved ileum is usually indicated.[164] Patients with tuberculosis and coexisting cecal carcinoma have been reported.

Free perforation usually occurs in the terminal ileum. Formerly, simple closure with drainage was performed; the mortality rate with this procedure was 50 percent. Thus, resection of the perforated segment is recommended by most surgeons. However, Porter et al [165] report a patient treated by drainage alone—a second stage became unnecessary when the resulting fistula healed with chemotherapy and nutritional support. Katariya et al [166] suggest that resection of all small bowel containing strictures is not necessary. They prefer to incise the bowel longitudinally through short strictures, closing the incision transversely. They reserve resection for segments with numerous strictures.

Adams and Miller [164] stressed the danger of operating on patients with uncontrolled pulmonary disease. In addition, they documented the danger of fistula formation and breakdown of anastomoses constructed in diseased bowel. Although this paper was written prior to the chemotherapy era, it points out two principles of surgical treatment of enteric tuberculosis. First, administer antibiotics for at least 2 weeks to patients with known disease in the lung or bowel before performing elective surgery. Second, it is unwise to attempt primary anastomosis in diseased bowel.

ACTINOMYCOSIS OF LARGE BOWEL

Abdominal actinomycosis is an uncommon disease, and the diagnosis is usually delayed. Since medical treatment is curative, surgeons should beware. The etiology and pathogenesis of abdominal actinomycosis is discussed in Chapters 6 and 34.

Most cases of abdominal actinomycosis occur in young adults, although patients of all ages are affected. There is no predilection to either sex.[167,168]

A. israelii is the species most often isolated from all forms of human disease. Most, if not all, infections occur following a break in the gut mucosa. Of 192 cases of abdominal actinomycosis,[168] 61 percent resulted from appendiceal perforation; large bowel perforation was associated in 14 percent. Association with perforating foreign bodies was frequent. The organism itself does not seem to be invasive. Actinomycotic infection in the abdomen never occurs without the involvement of other enteric bacteria.

Microscopically, an actinomycotic abscess consists of an outer zone of granulation tissue surrounding a central purulent loculation containing sulfur granules made up of numerous gram-positive bacilli. Necrosis in the abscess is unusual. The early actinomycotic abscess in the bowel wall spreads by direct extension and rarely disseminates. Eventually, fistulas characterized by the discharge of pus and sulfur granules develop.

Clinical Manifestations

Abdominal actinomycosis develops gradually; occasionally, the precipitating event goes unrecognized.[167] The initial symptoms are nonspecific, with malaise, night sweats, and fever. Abdominal pain suggests the source, and a mass may be noted. Frequently, one or more fistulous tracts discharge onto the abdominal wall or to the perineal region. Physical findings include abdominal tenderness, a palpable mass, and the fistulas. The diagnosis is rarely suspected, so that there is usually a history of chronicity with multiple failed attempts at treatment. Rarely, proctoscopy, barium enema, and intravenous pyelography may show evidence of a mass lesion. The differential diagnosis frequently includes carcinoma, Crohn disease, and other granulomatous infections such as tuberculosis and nocardiosis.

Diagnosis

Cultures from the fistula may yield only enteric organisms. Special attention must be paid to collection of material from deep within the fistula and to proper anaerobic methodology to successfully grow *Actinomyces.* The finding of sulfur granules may lead to the diagnosis, and histologic confirmation of actinomycotic granulomas in resected tissue is also diagnostic.

Treatment

Successful treatment of actinomycosis requires the appropriate combination of surgical and antibiotic therapy. Surgical measures may include only incision and drainage of abscesses and fistulas or resection of all affected tissues. Penicillin G must be administered in large doses for weeks or months. Alternative antibiotics include erythromycin, the tetracyclines, and clindamycin.[167] With antibiotics, the cure rate exceeds 90 percent,[167] and major operations are rarely indicated.

VIRAL INFECTIONS OF THE COLON

The only viral infections of surgical significance are ulcers that bleed or perforate. Although viruses have been implicated in the development of regional enteritis and ulcerative colitis (Chapter 10), the etiologic association has not been established.

Epidemiology

Viral ulcers of the colon are rarely clinically apparent. The most prevalent viral lesion is the sexually transmitted herpes simplex infection of the anus and rectum (Chapter 41). Of greater surgical significance are colonic ulcers due to cytomegalovirus. Many people have had subclinical infections with these viruses and carry latent viral genetic material within their body. The infections then become apparent under conditions of stress or impaired immune activity.

Etiology and Pathogenesis

The etiology of the herpesvirus infections, including cytomegalovirus, is discussed in Chapter 10. Most evidence suggests that the viruses infect the mucosal and endothelial cells to produce an ischemic vasculitis as part of an ischemic infection. Why the viruses become reactivated and produce clinical disease during stress, hyperthermia, neoplasm, and exposure to immunosuppressive and antineoplastic drugs is unknown. Why the colon, and especially the cecum, become infected is also unclear, but it may be related to local blood supply, colonic motility, or intralumenal bacteria. The ulcers become surgical problems when perforation or hemorrhage occur.[169]

Clinical Features

The clinical features of cytomegalovirus infections have been discussed in Chapters 10 and 47. The hemorrhage from cecal ulcers is usually profuse. The diagnosis can sometimes be made by angiography, but almost never by colonoscopy.

Diagnosis

The diagnosis depends on evidence of a fourfold rise in anticytomegalovirus titer or cultural isolation of the virus from blood. Histologic study of the ulcer reveals inclusion bodies at the base of the ulcer.

Treatment

Both successful and unsuccessful outcomes have followed resection, which is dangerous for the immunocompromised host. All efforts at conservative management should be tried, including intramesenteric pitressin infusion, reduction of immunosuppression, and maintenance of coagulation factors. There is no specific anticytomegalovirus agent available.

SURGICAL MANIFESTATIONS OF INFESTATION BY INTESTINAL PARASITES

Infestation with intestinal parasites is a problem of global significance because of population mobility. Colonic infestations of major significance include both amebiasis and schistosomiasis.

Amebiasis

Juniper[170] and Krogstad et al[171] have written recent reviews of amebiasis, and selected aspects are discussed in Chapters 11 and 36.

Epidemiology

The pathogenesis and epidemiology of amebiasis is discussed in Chapter 11. The infestation rate in the United States may be as high as 5 percent.[170,172]

Pathogenesis

Invasion by *Entameba histolytica* trophozoites occurs by release of lytic enzymes in contact with the intestinal mucosa. The trophozoite requires the anaerobic environment provided by the fecal flora for survival. Trophozoites appear in the stool of patients with dysentery. Ingestion of trophozoites does not result in infestation, since they are killed by gastric acid. Cysts, on the other hand, are found in the formed stool of asymptomatic carriers. Thus, spread of disease is accomplished via the asymptomatic carrier rather than the patient with dysentery.

Invasion results initially in the formation of minute ulcers located in the center of tiny nodules. A nodule is edematous mucosa with aggregations of chronic inflammatory cells. The process extends by undermining the mucosa, the flask-shaped abscess. If sufficient blood supply is compromised, ulcers enlarge. Occasionally, a proliferative granulomatous reaction occurs, the ameboma. The trophozoites are found at the junction of viable and necrotic tissue. Eventually, invasion of blood vessels allows dissemination of the trophozoites to other organs, particularly the liver.

Clinical Features

Nondysenteric colitis is the most frequent manifestation of amebiasis. Symptoms include anorexia, malaise, weight loss, cramping abdominal pain, mild diarrhea, and constipation.

Dysenteric colitis may occur at any time following infestation; dysentery is more likely to occur if host defenses are impaired by concurrent disease or use of immunosuppressive drugs (including chronic use of alcohol). Onset of dysentery may be gradual or rapid. The predominant symptom is diarrhea associated with abdominal cramps and lower abdominal pain. As many as 12 to 18 stools may be passed daily. The bowel movements are foul smelling, mushy or watery, and contain blood-streaked mucus. Dehydration is relatively uncommon, but severe weight loss, weakness, nausea, vomiting, and fever may occur. Abdominal examination reveals hyperperistalsis and tenderness, and the liver may be slightly enlarged and tender. Acute dysentery may last 1 to 4 weeks and often regresses without treatment. Recurrent episodes are typical.

Occasionally, localized amebiasis occurs. Localized ulcers may occur in the rectum or cecum. Rectal ulcers may be associated with passage of formed stools, but several discharges of bloody exudate are typical. Cecal ulcers produce right lower quadrant pain and massive hemorrhage, but little or no diarrhea.[173]

Ameboma may produce symptoms, usually pain without diarrhea. A tumor mass may be noted, usually in the cecum or rectosigmoid. Obstruction, intussusception, and volvulus may occur; carcinoma may be suggested.

Amebiasis becomes a surgical disease with the rare

occurrence of fulminating necrotizing amebic colitis, which is frequently complicated by perforation and peritonitis. Toxic dilation of the colon may occur. In these forms, amebic colitis may simulate ulcerative colitis.

Extraintestinal manifestations often are noted. Foremost among these is amebic liver abscess, which may exist along with fulminant colitis.

Endoscopy reveals punctate ulcers and tiny nodules, with normal intervening mucosa. More advanced changes are indistinguishable from those of ulcerative colitis. Tumor masses representing amebomas may be seen. Rectal biopsy usually reveals trophozoites.

Barium enema is usually unable to distinguish amebiasis from ulcerative colitis. However, with the localized type of disease, one may see a tumor mass or luminal narrowing; the cecum may fill incompletely (the cone-shaped cecum). These changes disappear more or less completely following antiameba therapy.

Diagnosis

Juniper [170] has written an extensive discussion of the diagnosis of amebiasis.

The diagnosis of colitis requires the finding of trophozoites on microscopic examination of fresh stool or colonic biopsy specimens, bloody mucus obtained at endoscopy or, best of all, scrapings taken from the ulcers themselves. It is most important to realize that feces are rendered unsatisfactory for diagnostic purposes for as long as 2 weeks following a number of otherwise routine maneuvers. These include administration of bismuth or kaolin containing antidiarrheals, nonabsorbable antacids, antimicrobials, barium, mineral oil, magnesium hydroxide, and enemas of tapwater, soap, or hypertonic solutions. Thus, fecal examination must be performed before any therapeutic or diagnostic maneuver; initial endoscopy must be performed without a preparation.

Even when other diagnostic maneuvers fail to demonstrate evidence of amebiasis, serologic tests are indicated to rule out the disease (see Table 11-1). The indirect hemaglutination test (IHA) is positive in 82 to 98 percent of patients with symptomatic amebiasis. Repeated assay may increase the yield. Serologic tests should be performed whenever amebiasis is considered, even if fecal and biopsy findings are negative.

Treatment

The treatment of amebiasis is discussed extensively in Chapter 11 (see especially Table 11-2). Metronidazole is the current drug of choice in the United States for extraintestinal amebiasis. Diiodohydroxyquin and diloxanide furoate are effective in asymptomatic patients, whereas diiodohydroxyquin and paromomycin used sequentially are effective in the dysenteric form of disease. Many investigators also administer broad-spectrum antibiotics, especially tetracycline, in addition to amebicides. When antiamebic therapy must be administered parenterally to a postoperative patient, parenteral metronidazole is now available.

Colon operations in the patient with unrecognized amebiasis often results in septic complications, and mortality is high. However, in acute fulminating colitis with perforation, toxic dilation, or some cases of ameboma, timely surgical treatment is necessary to avoid mortality rates approaching 100 percent. Latimer [172] lists the following indications for operation in acute fulminating amebic colitis: (1) impending or free intraperitoneal perforation, or perforation while receiving antiamebic chemotherapy, (2) failure of a localized perforation to respond to antiamebic therapy, (3) persistence or development of abdominal distension and tenderness while receiving treatment, (4) persistence of severe diarrhea following 5 days of chemotherapy, and (5) severe postamebic colitis symptoms with unremitting anemia and hypoproteinemia.

Indications for operation for ameboma include: (1) failure of the ameboma to regress after appropriate chemotherapy, (2) persistent ulceration, (3) intestinal obstruction, (4) stricture formation, (5) intussusception, (6) hemorrhage, (7) internal fistula formation, and (8) perforation. Most surgeons believe the procedure of choice is resection of all involved intra-abdominal colon; proctectomy is rarely necessary. Eggleston et al,[173] however, report better success with diversion and drainage procedures. Primary anastomosis should not be attempted in the presence of active amebiasis. Whenever possible, operative intervention should be postponed until antiamebic therapy has been administered for at least 24 hours.

Schistosomiasis

Schistosomiasis is the subject of several recent reviews,[174,175] and the etiology, epidemiology, and pathogenesis are discussed in Chapter 11.

The human phase is initiated when the individual is exposed to cercariae, second-stage larvae, which are released by the snail host into stagnant and slow-moving water. The cercariae penetrate skin or mucous membranes and become shistosomulae, which can migrate to the lungs and liver, where maturation to the adult worm occurs. The adult females lay their eggs in the venules of the colon, from which they may be carried back to the liver or deposited in intestinal tissues. Some of the eggs erode into the bowel lumen and are passed in the feces. The eggs that reach maturity provoke a granulomatous reaction within intestinal serosa, mesenteric and retroperitoneal tissues, and lymphatics. In the acute phase, involved rectum and colon become edematous and hyperemic, and many fine granulations, pinpoint hemorrhages, and small ulcerations result; in the chronic phase, granuloma formation predominates.

In severe bowel disease, pseudoneoplastic tumors, which may extend into the abdominal cavity or into the bowel lumen, develop. Polypoid lesions are found, especially in the rectosigmoid segment. Eventually, these lose their blood supply and slough, leaving behind an ulcer which may bleed. Rarely, severe stricture occurs.

Clinical Manifestations

The systemic clinical manifestations are discussed in Chapter 11. In the acute phase, diarrhea can be found. Chronic colonic disease is associated with a sporadic diarrhea, productive of bloody mucus, and constipation. Bowel polyps bleed, pseudoneoplastic tumors may compress or obstruct the bowel, and abdominal masses may be palpable.[175] Perforation through the ulcers may occur. Segmental ischemia of the colon due to vascular occlusion of small vessels has been reported.[176]

Endoscopy may reveal discrete or clustered punctate hemorrhages and erosions. Surrounding inflammation is absent. The mucous membrane is usually pale and edematous. Small excrescences and polypoid lesions may be noted.

The intestinal manifestations are important, but hepatic fibrosis, subsequent portal hypertension, and pulmonary hypertension are the more troublesome complications of this disease.

Diagnosis

Diagnosis of schistosomiasis depends on visualization of the eggs in feces or on rectal biopsy, which should be taken from an upper rectal valve. Serologic studies are sometimes helpful (Chapter 11).

Treatment

Effective drug therapy is outlined in Table 11-4. Surgical therapy is indicated to treat obstructive complications and to rule out neoplasm. Before proceeding to radical cancer procedures, it is imperative to have a tissue diagnosis of neoplasm.

INFECTIOUS COMPLICATIONS OF COLONIC OPERATIONS

ANASTOMOTIC LEAK

Anastomotic leak and its consequences constitute the major preventable complications of operations on the large bowel. The incidence of anastomotic leak in specific diseases and following specific procedures is noted in the other sections of this chapter. Other surgeons have noted clinically significant leaks in 3 to 23 percent of patients having colon resection.[177-181] One-third to one-half of patients with anastomotic leak die, and anastomotic leak accounts for one-quarter to one-half of the operative mortality of colon surgery.

Anastomotic Healing

Laboratory studies of anastomotic healing have focused on collagen metabolism at the anastomosis and in the adjacent colon. The amount, concentration, and structure of the collagen determine anastomotic strength, at least in part. Collagen lysis occurs at an increased rate at the anastomosis, and for several centimeters to each side, nearly immediately after operation. As a counterbalance to this, collagen synthesis increases in the same sites within 2 days. The balance of these factors is such that the total collagen content in the anastomosis and surrounding colon is decreased by about one-half on the third postoperative day, when the anastomosis is weakest. The collagen content then increases so that, at 1 week, the anastomosis is stronger than surrounding normal colon. Any factor that increases the rate of collagen lysis or retards its synthesis may contribute to anastomotic leak. Factors contributing to anastomotic leak are discussed by Schrock et al,[179] Morgenstern et al,[180] and Irvin and Goligher.[182]

The prime factor contributing to anastomotic leak is the presence at operation of peritonitis, abscess, or fistula. Sepsis causes both an increase of collagen lysis and a decrease in collagen synthesis. Any colonic anastomosis is subject to this effect—ileocolic as well as colocolic or colorectal. Debas and Thomson [181] found that because of leaks, right hemicolectomy in the presence of peritonitis was associated with a mortality rate of 23 percent, versus a rate of 3 percent for elective procedures.

An extraperitoneal anastomosis, eg, after a low anterior resection, is more likely to leak. Leak rates of 58 percent have been documented when routine contrast enemas have been used to detect early postoperative leaks.[177] The main reasons seem to be the presence of dead space around the anastomosis and the separation of the anastomosis from intraperitoneal defense and healing mechanisms. The dead space collects blood and serum, which easily become infected.[183] Otherwise, the segment of resected colon has no influence on leak rate.

Anything that decreases blood flow to the anastomosis results in increased leak rates. Hypoxia particularly retards collagen synthesis so that leaks are associated with a preoperative hematocrit of less than 35 percent, transfusion intraoperatively of more than two units of blood, or intraoperative hypotension. Colonic blood flow is particularly sensitive to hypovolemia. Blood flow to the colon decreased markedly when greater than 10 percent of the blood volume was lost; this decreased flow was only partially reversed by blood replacement. Other factors that increase leak rates, such as emergency operation, duration of operation of greater than 5 hours, or fixation of tumor to the pelvis probably relate to the degree of blood loss, too. Both trauma and hypovolemia have been shown to result in decreased collagen synthesis as well as decreased blood flow. Radiation injury of bowel leads to decreased protein synthesis, although no decrease in anastomotic strength results when anastomosis is made 8 to 23 days following radiotherapy.[184] Clinically, a history of prior radiotherapy is associated with an increased risk of leak. Chronic radiation damage is associated with decreased vascularity of tissue.

Nutritional factors should be important in anastomotic healing. Starvation (specifically protein depletion) is associated with decreased collagen synthesis and weaker anastomoses. Morgenstern et al [180] and Irvin and Goligher [182] identified malnutrition and hypoalbuminemia as factors associated with leak. In the paper of Schrock et al,[179] nutritional factors just missed being of statistical significance. Ascorbic acid, iron, and zinc, among other nutrients, are necessary for proper wound healing.

Drugs that impair collagen synthesis include dicumerol, chloramphenicol, and the cancer chemotherapeutic agents actinomycin D, nitrogen mustard, cyclophosphamide, 5-fluorouracil, and methotrexate. Steroids produce lysis of collagen as well as decreased synthesis. Morgenstern, et al [180] recognized an increase of leaks in patients dependent on steroids, but Schrock et al [179] could demonstrate no effect.

Other factors generally agreed on as influencing the leak rate are age greater than 60 years and cancer at the margin of resection. Schrock et al [179] found that neither the colon disease necessitating operation nor the presence of other illnesses was associated with increased leak rate. Morgenstern et al [180] found a positive correlation with obesity, coagulopathy, uremia, and diabetes mellitus.

Bowel preparations and use of systemic antibiotics are discussed in subsequent sections. In short, Schrock et al [179] found no effect of these factors or of degree of fecal loading on leak rate. Conversely, Morgenstern, et al [180] and Irvin and Goligher [182] found adequacy of mechanical preparation to be vital for proper healing.

Schrock et al [179] found that anastomotic leaks were not increased after operation for colon obstruction. Similarly, the experience of the surgeon and the need to resect other organs has no effect. Proximal diversion did not prevent leaks, but colostomy (not cecostomy) did prevent mortality due to leak. The use of neostigmine to reverse muscle relaxants is not associated with increased leak rate.[185]

Schrock et al [179] could find no technical factors that increased safety of colon anastomosis. A number of suture techniques have been tested. No significant difference between single-layer and two-layer anastomoses was demonstrable; [177] but, everting anastomoses were inferior to inverting anastomoses.[186]

Insertion of a rectal tube through the anastomosis to allow colon decompression and instillation of antibiotic solution has been associated with good results, but no prospective controlled studies have been reported.[187]

Many surgeons place drains in the vicinity of the anastomoses (particularly with low anastomoses) to establish a tract through which feces will drain if a leak occurs. Such drains increase the incidence of anastomotic leak.[188] Drainage was rarely used by Schrock's group,[179] so its effect was not analyzed. Fazio [183] reports good results using sump suction catheters with continuous irrigation in order to prevent the collection of a hematoma around a retroperitoneal rectal anastomoses. This practice has not been compared with alternative methods in a random trial.

Goldsmith [189] describes the use of a pedicle flap of omentum placed in the pelvis and wrapped around the low rectal anastomosis. The purposes of this maneuver are to fill the dead space and to utilize the protective properties of the omentum. This maneuver is helpful in experimental animals.[190]

In summary, the primary requirements for safe anastomosis are elementary—healthy bowel, good blood supply, absence of tension, and a watertight seal. We prefer an open, two-layer, inverting anastomosis using a running chromic catgut inner layer and an interrupted silk outer layer. No primary unprotected anastomosis should be constructed in any segment of colon in the presence of localized or general abdominal sepsis. A conservative attitude (ie, constructing a colostomy rather than performing a primary anastomosis) is indicated in any emergency.

Diagnosis of Anastomotic Leak

Debas and Thomson [181] stressed that the second most difficult problem with anastomotic leak is the usual delay in diagnosis and management. They classified anastomotic leaks into three types: minor separation, major separation, and gross necrosis of the bowel.

Minor separations occurred in 34 percent of patients with anastomotic leak. Patients with minor separation usually presented with a fecal fistula on about the seventh to tenth postoperative day. Fever and leukocytosis were minimal; sepsis was absent. These fistulas healed spontaneously with conservative management in all cases.

Major separations occurred in 56 percent. In these patients, fever and toxicity appeared in the early postoperative period. One-third presented findings of general peritonitis. Half the patients were treated conservatively for fecal fistula, and 31 percent died. The other half were treated by reoperation, with 11 percent mortality.

Gross necrosis of at least one segment of anastomosed colon occurred in 10 percent of patients. These patients demonstrated fever, disorientation, signs of peritonitis, and eventually septic shock within 36 hours. All patients passed blood per rectum or through a drain. All patients died.

Early diagnosis and treatment of major anastomotic leak is imperative. Postoperative examination of the anastomosis with water soluble contrast medium should be done in any patient who has unexplained signs of postoperative infection.

Treatment of Anastomotic Leak

The treatment of uncomplicated colocutaneous fistulas is described in a preceding section. Simple proximal diversion is sufficient treatment for some, but not all patients with major separations. The anastomosis itself should be explored (1) when the proximal segment is ileum, (2) when a fecal fistula presents with findings of peritonitis, and (3) when the patient deteriorates in the early postoperative period. One treatment option with major leaks is proximal diversion plus adequate drainage; in contrast, with a small leak, an attempt may be made to close the hole as well. When stool is present in proximal bowel, the defect is large, or necrosis has occurred, the anastomosis should be taken down and the ends exteriorized, or a Hartman procedure should be done. Reresection and anastomosis with proximal diversions is rarely indicated.

PREVENTION OF INFECTIOUS COMPLICATIONS OF COLONIC OPERATIONS

Preoperative Preparation of the Bowel

Preoperative bowel preparation has been the subject of considerable discussion for three decades. The ideal goals of bowel preparation are to empty the bowel of all bulk fecal matter (mechanical preparation) and to render the remaining bowel contents sterile (antimicrobial preparation). By accomplishing these goals, one should be able to reduce the rates of postoperative wound infection, anastomotic leak, intra-abdominal sepsis, and death.

There is little argument that adequate mechanical bowel preparation is important for successful bowel surgery. The standard method is restriction of diet to low-residue and liquid foods and purgation with laxatives and enemas for 3 to 5 days before operation. Our current regimen is listed in Table 39-5.

The standard method of mechanical bowel preparation has limitations. It does induce a state of dysentery. The nutritional status of patients who are already malnourished is made worse, and patients are depleted of water and electrolytes. In addition, most patients must be hospitalized for several days solely to accomplish proper preparation. For these reasons, alternative methods of mechanical preparation are being investigated.

Preoperative administration of an oral elemental diet (1800–2500 calories per day), plus laxatives has been tried.[191] These regimens are successful in producing a good to excellent mechanical preparation, but hospital time is not saved, and elemental diets currently available still taste terrible.

A new technique consists of the infusion of large quantities of warm (37C) saline solution through a nasogastric tube at the rate of 2–4 liters per hour.[192,193] The irrigation is continued until the fecal effluent is clear (2 to 6 hours). Whole-gut irrigation results in excellent mechanical preparation. The method requires a short time so that in most patients, mechanical and antibiotic preparation can be achieved in one day. Chung et al [193] noted an average weight gain of 1.6 kg following the procedure, but the excess water is excreted in the urine by morning.

Patient responses to whole-gut irrigation have been evaluated.[193] Abdominal cramps, epigastric fullness, nausea, and vomiting are frequent complaints.[193] Both the nasogastric tube and prolonged sitting on a hard commode seat was distressing to some. Nevertheless, it is rapid and tolerated well by most patients. Chung et al [193] and Hewitt et al [192] found that nearly all patients who had undergone both laxative and irrigation preparation preferred the latter. Because vomiting can be a problem, patients given irrigation must be alert and able to help themselves. The intelligent patient can control the rate of infusion to allow maximum comfort. Patients with obstructive bowel lesions and fluid retention states such as heart, kidney, and liver disease are not candidates for whole-gut irrigation.

Mechanical preparation of the bowel removes bulk fecal matter. In so doing, the total numbers of gut bacteria are reduced, and the chance for fecal spillage during operation is reduced. The most important factor determining the incidence of septic complications, however, is the concentration of colon bacteria, and the reduction of this concentration after mechanical preparation alone is modest at best.[192,194] In a recent prospective study,[195] none of three methods showed any significant differences from control or each other in bacterial concentrations. Thus, the use of antibiotic agents is necessary to produce a significant change in bacterial concentration in large bowel contents.

TABLE 39-5. MECHANICAL BOWEL PREPARATION REGIMEN

Preop day 3	Low-residue or clear liquid diet Bisacodyl, 1 capsule orally at 6:00 P.M.
Preop day 2	Low-residue or clear liquid diet Magnesium sulfate, 50% solution, 30 ml (15 gm) orally at 10:00 A.M., 2:00 P.M., and 6:00 P.M. Saline enemas at 7:00 P.M., 8:00 P.M., and hourly until no solid feces are returned
Preop day 1	Clear liquid diet Supplemental IV fluids as needed Magnesium sulfate, in dose above, at 10:00 A.M. and 2:00 P.M. No enemas
Operation day	Patient evacuates rectum at 6:30 A.M. No enemas. Operation at 8:00 A.M.

Poth [197] enumerated the ideal characteristics of a colonic antiseptic: (1) broad spectrum of effect, (2) low host toxicity, (3) chemical stability within the gastrointestinal tract, (4) low rate of stimulating bacterial resistance, (5) rapidity of action, (6) limited absorption from the gastrointestinal tract, (7) activity in presence of food, (8) capacity to aid bowel cleansing without causing dehydration, (9) lack of irritability to the gastrointestinal mucosa, (10) no interference with anastomotic healing, (11) low dosage requirement, (12) water solubility, (13) palatability, (14) inhibition of excessive fungal growth, and (15) limited clinical use. An additional characteristic has been stressed in subsequent discussions—efficacy against the pathogenic organisms. For over 30 years, investigators have been trying to find agents and regimens that fulfill these criteria; this experience has been reviewed.

Until the 1970s, the prominent role of anaerobic organisms in the septic complications of large bowel operations was not recognized. The target organisms were *E. coli*, other Enterobacteriaceae, and the aerobic streptococci and staphylococci. Special effort was made to avoid the pseudomembranous enterocolitis thought to be associated with staphylococcal overgrowth. The drugs and combinations that were used most widely were neomycin, neomycin and phthalylsulfathiazole, neomycin and tetracycline, neomycin and bacitracin, and kanamycin. Nystatin was added sometimes to prevent overgrowth of *Candida*. Many drugs were abandoned. Penicillin and the sulfonamides used alone did not have an adequate effect. Streptomycin, the first aminoglycoside antibiotic, was associated with rapid development of resistant organisms. The tetracyclines demonstrated a relatively poor spectrum of effect, and their use was associated with frequent overgrowth of staphylococci. Chloramphenicol was absorbed too rapidly from the intestine and was toxic. Use of erythromycin was discouraged to prevent staphylococcal resistance to this useful drug.

In 1971, Nichols and Condon [198] reviewed the status of antibacterial bowel preparation, and reached several important conclusions. First, in light of the frequency of *B. fragilis* in postoperative infections, the current regimens were inadequate. Second, nearly all prior clinical studies of the efficacy of antibacterial bowel preparation were retrospective and poorly controlled.

The effects of several commonly used regimens were evaluated for their effects on bowel flora,[199] using modern techniques of anaerobic microbiology. Kanamycin, neomycin, and neomycin-phthalylsulfathiazole preparations were effective against aerobic and facultative organisms. Kanamycin showed no effect on anaerobes. Neomycin alone or with phthalylsulfathiazole produced no effect on anaerobes in half the patients.

In the selection of agents to use for bowel preparation, it is reasonable to aim specifically against fecal organisms that most often cause postoperative sepsis. The most important aerobe is *E. coli,* and the most important anaerobe is *B. fragilis.* Drugs effective against these organisms are listed in Table 39-6.

Nichols et al [199] chose to test the combination of neomycin and erythromycin, drugs that best fit Poth's criteria. Neomycin and erythromycin produced nearly complete suppression of both aerobic and anaerobic organisms. Arabi et al [196] were able to produce equally remarkable reductions in bacterial counts using neomycin and metronidazole.

In the 1970s, a number of prospective randomized trials of preoperative antibacterial bowel preparation were conducted. These trials used drugs expected to have effect against anaerobes as well as aerobes. The results of these trials are tabulated in Table 39-7.

In all studies but two, the regimen combining an aminoglycoside with a drug active against anaerobes showed statistically significant reduction in infection rates. Nichols et al [200] had groups too small to prove significance. The control groups of Vargish et al [201] showed uncharacteristically low infection rates. Taylor et al [202] showed that the addition of metronidazole to phthalylsulfathiazole resulted in a significant improvement.

In all studies but one, the combination of neomycin and erythromycin produced wound infection rates of about 10 percent. Brass et al [203] had an infection rate of 25 percent with this combination—the combination of neomycin and metronidazole proved superior in their study. The administration schedule used by Brass et al varied from that of Nichols and Condon and may have resulted in an underdosage of erythromycin.

Studies that included microbiologic analysis [200,203] uniformly demonstrated suppression of aerobic and anaerobic organisms. There was no overgrowth of organisms resistant to aminoglycosides.

Thus, recent prospective, randomized, and often double-blind studies demonstrate a reduction in bacterial counts (aerobic and anaerobic) and a decrease in incidence of septic complications when appropriate antibiotic regimens are used. There were no instances of worse infection rates, overgrowth by resistant organisms, and no cases of pseudomembranous colitis. No impairment of anastomotic healing has been noted. These results speak to the arguments that some have against the use of preoperative oral antibiotic bowel preparation.[204] Preoperative antimicrobial bowel preparation may increase the risk of anastomotic recurrence of tumor,[205] a question not addressed in recent studies of bowel preparation.

There is a need for an instant preparation of the large bowel to increase the safety of primary repair and anastomosis during emergency colostomy. Jones et al [206] demonstrated that neomycin and erythromycin combined were unable to kill aerobic or anaerobic bacteria in a short time (20 minutes). On the other hand, povidone-iodine, 10 percent instilled into the colons of dogs [206] and humans,[207] reduced bacterial concentrations and was safe. Using povidone-iodine following colonic irrigation in the manner described by Gliedman et al [194] may allow increased use of one-stage operations in patients with large bowel emergencies.

TABLE 39-6. ANTIBIOTIC SENSITIVITIES OF FECAL BACTERIA

Aerobes *(E. coli)*	Anaerobes *(B. fragilis)*
Ampicillin	Clindamycin
Cephalosporins	Lincomycin
Chloramphenicol	Erythromycin (base)
Gentamycin	Chloramphenicol
Tobramycin	Tetracycline (one-half resistant)
Amikacin	Carbenicillin
Kanamycin	Metronidazole
Neomycin	Rifampin
Tetracycline (many resistant)	

Prophylactic Systemic Antibiotics

Another controversial practice is the prophylactic administration of systemic antibiotics to patients undergoing elective colon surgery and to patients undergoing emergency operations for possible perforation of the colon (Chapter 23). The difficulties encountered in the analysis of the literature, concerning the prophylactic use of antibiotics, are exemplified by the paper by Azar and Drapanas,[208] which concluded that the prophylactic use of antibiotics increased the incidence of wound infection after elective colon operations. However, this paper was a retrospective analysis and had a sizable discrepancy in numbers in each treatment group. The antibiotic regimens varied with individual surgeons, and systemic antibiotics were not administered until after the operation.

Laboratory experiments have shown that antimicrobial agents must be present in tissues before inoculation if maximum inhibition of infection is to be achieved [209-212] (Chapter 23). In order to determine how long prior to operation that antibiotics should be administered and by what route, antibiotic concentrations in tissues have been measured in several reports. Maximum tissue antibiotic levels are achieved within 1 to 2 hours when given intramuscularly; however, tissue levels were achieved faster by the intravenous route.[213] In the absence of tissue infection, there is no advantage to administration prior to the time required to achieve bactericidal tissue levels during operation.

Another question relating to the prophylactic use of systemic antibiotics concerns the postoperative duration of administration. In most prospective studies, these agents have been administered for 24 hours or less.[213-217] The longest duration was seven days. The only studies to examine this question specifically have shown no significant difference between groups who received antibiotics only during the perioperative period or for 5 to 7 days postoperatively.[218,219]

The results of prospective, randomized trials of prophylaxis with systemic antibiotics in colon surgery are listed in Table 39-8. Only those studies in which antibiotics were administered before or during operation are included.

In summary, we can endorse the principles of systemic antibiotic prophylaxis elucidated in Chapter 23. Antibiot-

TABLE 39-7. RESULTS OF TRIALS OF ANTIBACTERIAL BOWEL PREPARATION

Investigator	Number of Patients	Agents	Wound Infections (%)	Abdominal Infections (%)	All Infections (%)	Mortality (%)
Nichols et al, 1973 [200]	10	None	3 (30)	—	—	—
	10	Neomycin Erythromycin	0	—	—	—
Washington et al, 1974	63	Placebo	27 (43)	—	43 *	—
	68	Neomycin	28 (41)	—	34 *	—
	65	Neomycin Tetracycline	3 (5)	—	5 *	—
Farmer, 1975	23	None	—	—	8 (35)	—
	74	Neomycin Erythromycin	—	—	4 (5)	—
Clarke et al, 1977	60	Placebo	21 (35)	10 (17)	47 *	2 (4)
	56	Neomycin Erythromycin	5 (9)	2 (4)	10 *	0
Brass et al, 1978 [203]	40	Neomycin Erythromycin	10 (25)	—	—	—
	39	Neomycin Metronidazole	2 (4)	—	—	—
Vargish et al, 1978 [201]	32	Neomycin	4 (13)	—	—	—
	29	Neomycin Phthalylsulfathiazole	3 (10)	—	—	—
	30	Neomycin Erythromycin	3 (10)	—	—	—
Matheson et al, 1978	59	Placebo	25 (42)	10 (17)	36 (61)	7 (12)
	51	Neomycin Metronidazole	9 (18)	0	11 (22)	2 (4)
Wapnick et al, 1979	38	Kanamycin	18 (47)	—	—	—
	39	Kanamycin Erythromycin	5 (13)	—	—	—
Taylor et al, 1979 [202]	61	Phthalylsulfathiazole	29 (48)	—	—	—
	65	Phthalylsulfathiazole Metronidazole	8 (12)	—	—	—

* Cannot tell whether patients had more than one septic complication.

ics are useful in patients undergoing elective colectomy and in patients with possible perforation of the large bowel. Administration for periods longer than 24 hours postoperatively does not seem to improve results, although treatment of known intraperitoneal sepsis should certainly be more prolonged. Preoperative mechanical preparation with administration of oral antibiotics such as neomycin and erythromycin base seems to be more important in elective procedures than the use of systemic antibiotics.[214] It is not yet clear whether the combination of oral antibiotics with systemic antibiotics offers any advantage over either drug alone. Presently, a combination of an aminoglycoside and clindamycin seems to be most rational because of the variable results obtained when systemic prophylaxis has been directed against either aerobes or anaerobes alone.[204-224]

Drainage

Prophylactic drainage after operations of the large bowel is used by many. Although a widely accepted practice, drainage continues to be the subject of considerable debate.

No one argues against draining localized collections of infected body fluids (pus, blood, feces). The debate concerns prophylactic drainage. Suggested reasons for prophylactic drainage include: (1) prevention of generalized peritonitis, (2) prevention of fluid collection, and (3) obliteration of cavities.

Yates [225] confirmed earlier experiments by demonstrating that drains placed within the peritoneal cavity are sealed off from the cavity in less than 24 hours; this has been confirmed by Agrama, et al.[226] It is impossible to drain the peritoneal cavity adequately. Even if a large

TABLE 39-8. RESULTS OF TRIALS OF PROPHYLACTIC ANTIBIOTICS

Author	Indication for Surgery	Antibiotic Bowel Prep	Agents	Duration	Number	Wound Sepsis (%)	Intra-abdominal Sepsis (%)	Total Sepsis (%)
Altemeier et al, 1966 [204]	Elective colectomy	Neomycin and phthalylsulfathiazole	None	—	23	3 (13)	—	—
			Penicillin Tetracycline	3 days	19	1 (5)	—	—
Feltis and Hamit, 1967 [217]	Elective colectomy and emergency colostomy	None	None	—	77	—	—	7 (9)
			Penicillin, methicillin, chloramphenicol	1 day	38	—	—	0
Polk and Lopez-Mayor, 1969 [215]	Elective colectomy	None	Placebo	1 day	50	15 (30)	—	—
			Cephaloridine	1 day	54	4 (7)	—	—
Evans and Pollock, 1973	Elective colectomy, perforated appendix	None	None	—	46	20 (43)	—	—
			Cephaloridine	1 day	41	14 (34)	—	—
Stone et al, 1976 [213]	Elective colectomy	Neomycin Erythromycin	Placebo	1 day	43	7 (16)	3 (7)	—
			Postoperative cefazolin	1 day	46	7 (15)	3 (7)	—
			Preoperative cefazolin	1 day	101	6 (6)	2 (2)	—
Griffiths et al, 1976 [216]	Elective colectomy	None	None	—	6	3 (50)	—	—
			Tobramycin and clindamycin	1 dose	6	2 (33)	—	—
Kjellgren and Sellstrom, 1977 [220]	Elective colectomy	None	None	—	49	26 (53)	—	—
			Cephalothin	4 days	57	10 (18)	—	—
Burdon et al, 1977	Elective colectomy	Neomycin and sulfas in only 18 patients, all groups	Placebo	2 doses	47	24 (51)	—	—
			Cephalothin gram I	2 doses	18	5 (28)	—	—
			Cephalothin gram II	2 doses	28	13 (46)	—	—
Downing et al, 1977 [218]	Elective colectomy	None	None	—	29	11 (38)	3 (10)	13 (45)
			Lincomycin	1 day	31	5 (16)	1 (3)	7 (23)
			Lincomycin	5 days	33	4 (12)	1 (3)	6 (18)
Hojer and Wetterfors, 1978	Elective colectomy	None	Placebo	5 days	60	25 (42)	16 (27)	27 (45)
			Doxycycline	5 days	58	5 (9)	3 (5)	7 (12)
Slama et al, 1979 [221]	Elective colectomy	None	Cephalothin	2 days	16	3 (19)	2 (13)	5 (31)
			Cefamandole	2 days	18	4 (22)	2 (11)	6 (33)
Condon et al, 1979 [214]	Elective colectomy	None,	Cephalothin	1 day	67	20 (30)	19 (28)	26 (39)
		Neomycin and erythromycin	Placebo or Cephalothin	1 day	126	7 (6)	2 (2)	7 (6)
Barber et al, 1979	Elective colectomy	Neomycin and erythromycin	Placebo	2 doses	28	—	—	3 (11)
			gentamycin and clindamycin	2 doses	31	—	—	2 (7)
Stone et al, 1979 [219]	Elective colectomy	Not stated	Cephaloridine	3 doses	44	2 (5)	2 (5)	—
		Not stated	Cephamandol	3 doses	54	5 (9)	2 (4)	—
		Not stated	Cephamandol	5 days	47	5 (11)	1 (2)	—

amount of fluid remains within the abdominal cavity, the bowel or omentum usually adheres to the drain and isolates it from the peritoneal cavity.

While few suggest that it is beneficial to drain intraperitoneal anastomoses, many surgeons routinely drain low rectal anastomoses. It is reasoned that bloody fluid frequently collects in the sacral hollow, preventing apposition of the rectum to presacral tissues, and serves as a growth medium for bacteria—drainage is supposed to prevent this. The efficacy of such drainage has not been proved in controlled trials.

Another reason given for drainage is to provide a conduit through which pus will drain if an abscess develops. Stone [227] found that intraperitoneal abscesses, in patients whose wounds had already been drained, ultimately presented at the wound site three times more frequently than they did at the drain tract.

Drains are not innocuous. Yates [225] demonstrated that peritoneal resistance to infection was impaired by the presence of drains. Stone [227,228] documented in prospective and randomized studies that, following intraperitoneal contamination, prophylactic drainage increased the incidence of intraperitoneal sepsis and wound infections. Drains are two-way conduits, and surface bacteria quickly colonize the drain tract.[225] Even sump drains with bacterial filters allow drain tract infection when too much suction is used. Stone [228] showed that the combination of an intestinal stoma and drainage was associated with a higher incidence of sepsis than drainage alone. In addition, he showed that in "clean" cases, the infections that occurred in drained patients were caused by hospital pathogens more often than were infections in undrained patients.[227] Berliner et al [229] found that the presence of drains in the vicinity of an anastomosis resulted in impaired anastomotic healing and a higher leak rate.

When drainage is used, the type of drain must be carefully selected. Suction drains are superior to Penrose drains in almost all ways: (1) Penrose drainage by gravity is difficult and inefficient; (2) they are open to the environment, which facilitates secondary infections; (3) suction drains, as long as they remain patent, actively remove any liquid with which they come in contact; (4) the force of the suction assists obliteration of dead spaces; and (5) if low suction (15 cm H_2O) is used, sump drains allow only limited access of bacteria to the drain tract. Suction drainage of low rectal anastomoses results in a lower incidence of complications than does drainage using Penrose drains. Stone et al [227] suggest that if Penrose drains are used, they should be dressed with a sterile stoma appliance to prevent contamination from external sources. Duration of prophylactic drainage is easily determined. When nothing more comes from the drain, there is no reason to leave the drain in place.

Decompression of the Anastomosis By Colostomy or Cecostomy

Colon decompression is frequently performed as a preventive measure to direct the fecal stream and flatus from the anastomosis. Colostomy is indicated as a prophylactic procedure when it is unclear whether the ends of the resected bowel are healthy enough to support an anastomosis. Protective colostomy proximal to an anastomosis is, in addition, sometimes indicated when anastomotic healing is expected to be suboptimal, even after elective resection of a left colonic segment. Although there is some disagreement,[230,231] tube cecostomy is inadequate for protecting anastomoses because the fecal stream is not diverted.

There is still debate whether proximal decompression actually protects colon anastomoses. No prospective studies have been performed, and the documented experience suggests that proximal diversion does not prevent anastomotic leaks. Proximal decompression does seem, however, to reduce the morbidity and mortality associated with these leaks.[179]

The complications of large bowel decompression must be taken into consideration. The complications of cecostomy include the following: (1) leak of a protected anastomosis (0 to 4 percent), (2) intraperitoneal leakage from the cecostomy itself ($<$ 1 percent), (3) wound infection rate (7 percent), and (4) a persistent cecal fistula (1 to 77 percent).

Complications of prophylactic diverting colostomy include: (1) retraction (1 to 3 percent), (2) stoma necrosis (0.4 to 4 percent), (3) peritonitis secondary to stoma problems ($<$ 1 percent), (4) paracolostomy hernia (3 to 5 percent), (5) colostomy prolapse (3 to 14 percent), (6) paracolostomy abscess and colostomy fistulas (1 to 3 percent), and (7) wound infection [230-233] (2 to 11 percent). Some of these can be prevented by careful construction and placement, but all series report them. Stone and Hester [228] found that combined use of drains and colostomy in emergency colon operations led to an increased incidence of intra-abdominal sepsis.

Protective colostomies are constructed with the intention of subsequent closure. In practice, this is possible in only 27 to 55 percent of patients.[230,233] If elective protective colostomy is to be used, subsequent colostomy closure must be safe. The complications of colostomy closure have been reviewed in numerous publications [233-235] and include: (1) death (0 to 4 percent), (2) anastomotic leak and fecal fistula (0 to 18 percent), (3) intra-abdominal sepsis without leak (0 to 2 percent), (4) colon obstruction (0 to 7 percent), and (5) wound infection (2 to 43 percent, median 12 percent). Most surgeons report a greater incidence of complications when the colostomy is resected rather than closed without resection, and when the colostomy is closed within 6 to 12 weeks of construction. However, Todd et al [234] could document no significant effect of method of closure, timing of closure, or type of colostomy. Adeyemo et al [235] found that intraperitoneal closure was more successful than extraperitoneal closure.

We feel that protection of difficult anastomoses with a colostomy should be used liberally if an anastomosis is done at all. Since cecostomy does not divert the fecal stream, it provides inadequate protection when leak does occur. The complication rates of colostomy and colostomy closure are low enough to justify this procedure. We usually use a loop colostomy, which is completely diverting when proper attention is directed to the details of construction technique. When drains must be used, the drains and the stoma must be separated with occlusive sterile dressings.

BIBLIOGRAPHY

Abcarian H, Udezue N: Colonenteric fistulas. Dis Colon Rectum 21: 281, 1978.

Bartlett JG, Condon RE, Gorbach SL, Clarke JS, Nichols RL, Ochi S: Veterans Administration Cooperative Study on Bowel Preparation for Elective Colorectal Operations: Impact of Oral Antibiotic Regimen on Colonic Flora, Wound Irrigation Cultures and Bacteriology of Septic Complications. Ann Surg 188: 249, 1978.

Bull DM, Peppercorn MA, Glotzer DJ, Joffe N, Goldman H, Silen W: Crohn's disease of the colon. Gastroenterology 76: 607, 1979.

Condon RE, Anderson MJ: Diarrhea and colitis in clindamycin-treated surgical patients. Arch Surg 113: 794, 1978.

Finegold SM: Anaerobic Bacteria in Human Disease. New York, Academic, 1977.

Hinchey EJ, Schaal PGH, Richards GK: Treatment of perforated diverticular disease of the colon. In Rob C (ed): Adv Surg, Vol 12. Chicago, Year Book Medical Publishers, 1978, p 85.

Nahai F, Lamb JM, Harican RG, Stone HH: Factors involved in disruption of intestinal anastomoses. Am Surg 43: 45, 1977.

O'Connell TX, Kadell B, Tompkins RK: Ischemia of the colon. Surg Gynecol Obstet 142: 337, 1976.

Samhouri F, Grodinsky C, Fox T: The management of colonic and rectal injuries: A reappraisal. Dis Colon Rectum 21: 426, 1978.

Savage DC: Microbial ecology of the gastrointestinal tract. Annu Rev Microbiol 31: 107–133, 1977.

Schnaufer L: Hirschsprung's disease. Surg Clin North Am 56: 349, 1976.

Strauss RJ, Flint GW, Platt N, Levin L, Wise L: The surgical management of toxic dilation of the colon: A report of 28 cases and review of the literature. Ann Surg 184: 682, 1976.

REFERENCES

PATHOGENESIS

1. Finegold SM: Anaerobic Bacteria in Human Disease. New York, Academic, 1977.

COLONIC PERFORATIONS

2. Matolo NM, Cohen SE, Wolfman EF: Effects of antibiotics on prevention of infection in contaminated abdominal operations. Am Surg 42:123, 1976.
3. Altemeier WA, Culbertson WR, Fullen WD, Shook CD: Intra-abdominal abscesses. Am J Surg 125:70, 1973.
4. Lawrence PF, Tietjen GW, Gingrich S, King TC: *Bacteroides* bacteremia. Ann Surg 186:559, 1977.
5. Cochran DQ, Almond CH, Shucart WA: An experimental study of the effects of barium and intestinal contents on the peritoneal cavity. Am J Roentgenol 89:883, 1963.
6. Stone HH, Kolb LD, Geheber CE: Incidence and significance of intraperitoneal anaerobic bacteria. Ann Surg 181:705, 1975.
7. Anderson CB, Marr JJ, Ballinger WF: Anaerobic infections in surgery: clinical review. Surgery 79:313, 1976.
8. Polk HC, Shields CL: Remote organ failure: a valid sign of occult intra-abdominal infection. Surgery 81:310, 1977.
9. Norton L, Eule J, Burdick D: Accuracy of techniques to detect intraperitoneal abscess. Surgery 84:370, 1978.
10. Cruze K, Snyder WH: Acute perforation of the alimentary tract in infancy and childhood. Ann Surg 154:93, 1961.
11. Kosloske AM: Necrotizing enterocolitis in the neonate. Surg Gynecol Obstet 148:259, 1979.
12. O'Neill JA, Holcomb GW: Surgical experience with neonatal necrotizing enterocolitis. Ann Surg 189:612, 1979.
13. Barlow B, Santulli TV: Importance of multiple episodes of hypoxia or cold stress on the development of enterocolitis in an animal model. Surgery 77:687, 1975.
14. Book LS, Overall JC, Herbst JJ, Britt MR, Epstein B, Jung AL: Clustering of necrotizing enterocolitis: interruption by infection-control measures. N Engl J Med 287:984, 1977.
15. Howard FM, Flynn DM, Bradley JM, Noone P, Szawatkowski M: Outbreak of necrotizing enterocolitis caused by *Clostridium butyricum*. Lancet 2:1099, 1977.
16. Bell MJ, Feigin RD, Ternberg JL, Brotherton T: Evaluation of gastrointestinal microflora in necrotizing enterocolitis. J Pediatr 92:589, 1978.
17. Bell MJ, Ternberg JL, Feigin RD, Keating JP, Marshall R, Barton L, Brotherton T: Neonatal necrotizing enterocolitis: therapeutic decisions based upon clinical staging. Ann Surg 187:1, 1978.
18. Cohn I, Langford D, Rives JD: Antibiotic support of colon anastomoses. Surg Gynecol Obstet 104:1, 1957.
19. Kosloske AM, Papile L, Burstein J: Indications for operation in acute necrotizing enterocolitis of the neonate. Surgery 87:502, 1980.
20. Tonkin ILD, Bjelland JC, Hunter TB, Capp MP, Firor H, Ermocilla R: Spontaneous resolution of colonic strictures caused by necrotizing enterocolitis: therapeutic implications. Am J Roentgenol 130:1077, 1978.
21. Corkery JJ: Hirschsprung's disease. Clin Gastroenterol 4:531, 1975.
22. Sieber WK, Soave F: Hirschsprung's disease, with a note on the Soave operation. Curr Probl Surg 15:1, June 1978.
23. Bill AH, Chapman ND: The enterocolitis of Hirschsprung's disease: its natural history and treatment. Am J Surg 103:70, 1962.
24. Hung W: Experience with a modification of Duhamel-Grob-Martin operation for the treatment of Hirschsprung's disease. Surg 77:680, 1975.
25. Howell HS, Bartizal JF, Freeark RJ: Blunt trauma involving the colon and rectum. J Trauma 16:624, 1976.
26. Haas PA, Fox TA: Civilian injuries of the rectum and anus. Dis Colon Rectum 22:17, 1979.
27. Davis JJ, Cohn I, Nance FC: Diagnosis and management of blunt abdominal trauma. Ann Surg 183:672, 1976.
28. Flint LM, Voyles CR, Richardson JD, Fry DE: Missile tract infections after transcolonic gunshot wounds. Arch Surg 113:727, 1978.
29. Lorinc P, Brahme F: Perforation of the colon during examination by the double contrast method. Gastroenterology 37:770, 1959.
30. Burt CAV: Pneumatic rupture of the intestinal canal with experimental data showing the mechanism of perforation and the pressure required. Arch Surg 22:875, 1931.
31. Salvo AF, Leigh KE: Barium intravasation into portal venous system during barium enema examination. JAMA 235:749, 1976.
32. Schwesinger WH, Levine BA, Ramos R: Complications in colonscopy. Surg Gynecol Obstet 148:270, 1979.
33. Richman LS, Short WF, Cooper WM: Barium enema septicemia: occurrence in a patient with leukemia. JAMA 226:62, 1973.
34. Terranova O, Sandei F, Rebuffat C, Maruotti R, Bortolozzi E: Irrigation vs. natural evacuation of left colostomy: a comparative study of 340 patients. Dis Colon Rectum 22:31, 1979.
35. Gemer M, Feuchtwanger MM: Pneumatic rupture of the colon: sequential appearance of the symptoms. JAMA 233:355, 1975.

36. Sohn N, Weinstein MA, Gonchar J: Social injuries of the rectum. Am J Surg 134:611, 1977.
37. Christy JP: Complications of combat casualties with combined injuries of bone and bowel: personal experience with nineteen patients. Surgery 71:270, 1972.
38. Stone HH, Fabian TC: Management of perforating colon trauma. Ann Surg 190:430–436, 1979.
39. Roof WR, Morris GC, DeBakey ME: Management of perforating injuries to the colon in civilian practice. Am J Surg 99:641, 1960.
40. Vannix RS, Carter R, Hinshaw DB, Joergenson EJ: Surgical management of colon trauma in civilian practice. Am J Surg 106:364, 1963.
41. Beall AC, Bricker DL, Alessi FJ, Hartwell MD, Whisennand HH, DeBakey ME: Surgical considerations in the management of civilian colon injuries. Ann Surg 173:971, 1971.
42. McGown C, Khan MO, Rousufuddin M: Colon injuries in civilian practice. Am Surg 38:218, 1972.
43. Garfinkle SE, Cohen SE, Matolo NM, Getzen LC, Wolfman EF: Civilian colonic injuries: changing concepts of management. Arch Surg 109:402, 1974.
44. LoCicero J, Tajima T, Drapanas T: A half-century of experience in the management of colon injuries: changing concepts. J Trauma 15:575, 1975.
45. Chilimindris C, Boyd DR, Carlson LE, Folk FA, Baker RJ, Freeark RJ: A critical review of management of right colon injuries. J Trauma 11:651, 1971.
46. Quarantillo EP, Nemhauser GM: Survey of cecal and ascending colon injuries among Vietnam casualties in Japan (1967–1970). Am J Surg 125:607, 1973.
47. Bartizal JF, Boyd DR, Folk FA, Smith D, Lescher TC, Freeark RJ: A critical review of management of 392 colonic and rectal injuries. Dis Colon Rectum 17:313, 1974.

DIVERTICULAR DISEASE

48. Ochsner HC, Bargen JA: Diverticulosis of the large intestine: an evaluation of historical and personal observations. Ann Intern Med 9:282, 1935.
49. Willard JH, Bockus HL: Clinical and therapeutic status of cases of colonic diverticulosis seen in office practice. Am J Dig Dis Nutr 3:580, 1936.
50. Eusebio EB, Eisenberg MM: Natural history of diverticular disease of the colon in young patients. Am J Surg 125:308, 1973.
51. Morson CB: Pathology of diverticular disease of the colon. Clin Gastroenterol 4:37, 1975.
52. Marcus R, Watt J: The radiological appearances of diverticula in the anti-mesenteric intertaenia area of the pelvic colon. Clin Radiol 16:87, 1965.
53. Parks TG: Natural history of diverticular disease of the colon: a review of 521 cases. Br Med J 4:639, 1969.
54. Painter NS, Truelove SC: Potential dangers of morphine in acute diverticulitis of the colon. Br Med J 2:33, 1963.
55. Arfwidsson S: Pathogenesis of multiple diverticula of the sigmoid colon in diverticular disease. Acta Chir Scand (suppl) 342:47, 1964.
56. Painter NS, Burkitt DP: Diverticular disease of the colon, a 20th century problem. Clin Gastroenterology 4:3, 1975.
57. Wychulis AR, Beahrs OH, Judd ES: Surgical management of diverticulitis of the colon. Surg Clin North Am 47:961, 1967.
58. Ritchie JA: Rectosigmoidal mucosal puckering and diverticulosis. Dis Colon Rectum 18:221, 1975.
58a. Samuel E, Dean ACB: Investigative measures in diverticular disease: Radiology, colonoscopy. Clin Gastroenterol 4:71, 1975.
59. Morton DL, Goldman L: Differential diagnosis of diverticulitis and carcinoma of the sigmoid colon. Am J Surg 103:55, 1962.
60. Parks TG: Reappraisal of clinical features of diverticular disease of the colon. Br Med J 4:642, 1969.
61. Steele M, Deveney C, Burchell M: Diagnosis and management of colovesical fistulas. Dis Colon Rectum 22:27, 1979.
62. Wetstein L, Camera A, Trillo RA, Zamora BO: Giant sigmoidal diverticulum: report of a case and review of the literature. Dis Colon Rectum 21:110, 1978.
63. Eastwood MA: Medical and dietary management. Clin Gastroenterol 4:85, 1975.
64. Friedman G, Janowitz HD: Diverticular disease: the medical aspects. Contemporary Surg 11:29, 1977.
65. Painter NS, Almeida AZ, Colebourne KW: Unprocessed bran in treatment of diverticular disease of the colon. Br Med J 2:137, 1972.
66. Smithwick RH: Experiences with the surgical management of diverticulitis of the sigmoid. Ann Surg 115:969, 1942.
67. Boyden AM, Neilson RO: Reappraisal of the surgical treatment of diverticulitis of the sigmoid colon: with special reference to the choice of operative procedure. Am J Surg 100:206, 1960.
68. Smithwick RH: Surgical treatment of diverticulitis of the sigmoid. Am J Surg 99:192, 1960.
69. Madden JL, Tan PY: Primary resection and anastomosis in the treatment of perforated lesions of the colon, with abscess or diffusing peritonitis. Surg Gynecol Obstet 113:646, 1961.
70. Madden JL: Treatment of perforated lesions of the colon by primary resection and anastomosis. Dis Colon Rectum 9:413, 1966.
71. McSherry CK, Grafe WR Jr, Perry HS, Glenn F: Surgery of the large bowel for emergent conditions: staged vs. primary resection. Arch Surg 98:749, 1969.
72. Hinchey EJ, Schaal PGH, Richards GK: Treatment of perforated diverticular disease of the colon. In Rob C (ed.): Advances Surgery, Vol 12. Chicago, Year Book Medical Publishers, 1978, p 85.
73. Rodkey GV, Welch CE: Colonic diverticular disease with surgical treatment: a study of 338 cases. Surg Clin North Am 54:655, 1974.
74. Colcock BP: Diverticular disease: proven surgical management. Clin Gastroenterol 4:99, 1975.
75. Reilly M: Sigmoid myotomy. Part I: Development of the operation; its application and results. Clin Gastroenterol 4:121, 1975.
76. Smith AN: Sigmoid myotomy. Part II: Manometric and clinical results; comparison with resection and the effect of bran; transverse myotomy. Clin Gastroenterol 4:135, 1975.
77. Kettlewell W, Moloney GE: Combined horizontal and longitudinal colomyotomy for diverticular disease: preliminary report. Dis Colon Rectum 20:24, 1977.
78. Charnock ML, Rennie JR, Wellwood JM, Todd IP: Results of colectomy for diverticular disease of the colon. Br J Surg 64:417, 1977.

INFLAMMATORY BOWEL DISEASE

79. Kirsner JB: Inflammatory bowel disease: consideration of etiology and pathogenesis. Am J Gastroenterol 69:253, 1978.
80. Tompkins RK, Weinstein MH, Foroozan P, Marx FW, Barker WF: Reappraisal of rectum-retaining operations for ulcerative and granulomatous colitis. Am J Surg 125:159, 1973.
81. Brooke BN: The pathogenesis of ulcerative and granulomatous colitis: surgical implications. Surg Clin North Am 52:971, 1972.

82. Sloan WP, Bargen JA, Gage RP: Life histories of patients with chronic ulcerative colitis: a review of 2,000 cases. Gastroenterology 16:25, 1950.
83. Monteiro E, Fossey J, Shiner M, Drasar BS, Allison AC: Antibacterial antibodies in rectal and colonic mucosa in ulcerative colitis. Lancet 1:249, 1971.
84. Simonowitz D, Block GE, Riddell RH, Kraft SC, Kirsner JB: The production of an unusual tissue reaction in rabbit bowel injected with Crohn's disease homogenates. Surgery 82:211, 1977.
85. Hardin CA, Werder AA: Tissue culture of the sera in human ulcerative colitis. Am J Surg 130:20, 1975.
86. Sidi S, Graham JH, Razvi SA, Banks PA: Cytomegalovirus infection of the colon associated with ulcerative colitis. Arch Surg 114:857, 1979.
87. Nugent FW: Medical management of inflammatory disease of the colon. Surg Clin North Am 51:807, 1971.
88. Goligher JC: The outcome of excisional operations for primary and recurrent Crohn's disease of the large intestine. Surg Gynecol Obstet 148:1, 1979.
89. Turnbull RB, Hawk WA, Weakley FL: Surgical treatment of toxic megacolon: ileostomy and colostomy to prepare patients for colectomy. Am J Surg 122:325, 1971.
90. Watts JM, DeDombal FT, Watkinson G, Goligher JC: Long-term prognosis of ulcerative colitis. Br Med J 1:1447, 1966.
91. Korelitz, BI, Gribetz D, Kopel FB: Granulomatous colitis in children: a study of 25 cases and comparison with ulcerative colitis. Pediatrics 42:446, 1968.
92. Homan WP, Tang C, Thorbjarnarson B: Anal lesions complicating Crohn disease. Arch Surg 111:1333, 1976.
93. Binder SC, Miller HH, Deterling RA: Emergency and urgent operations for ulcerative colitis: the procedure of choice. Arch Surg 110:284, 1975.
94. Ritchie JK: Ulcerative colitis treated by ileostomy and excisional surgery: fifteen years' experience at St. Mark's Hospital. Br J Surg 59:345, 1972.
95. Lindner AE, Marshak RH, Wolf BS, Janowitz HD: Granulomatous colitis: a clinical study. N Engl J Med 269:379, 1963.
96. Sirinek KR, Tetirick CE, Thomford NR, Pace WG: Total proctocolectomy and ileostomy: procedure of choice for acute toxic megacolon. Arch Surg 112:518, 1977.
97. Meuwissen SGM, Pape KSSB, Agenant D, Oushorn HH, Tytgat GNJ: Crohn's disease of the colon: analysis of the diagnostic value of radiology, endoscopy, and histology. Am J Dig Dis 21:81, 1976.
98. Lennard-Jones JE, Powell-Tuck J: Drug treatment of inflammatory bowel disease. Clin Gastroenterol 8:187, 1979.
99. Summers RW, Switz DM, Sessions JT Jr, Becktel JM, Best WR, Kern F Jr, Singleton JW: National Cooperative Crohn's Disease Study: Results of Drug Treatment. Gastroenterology 77:847, 1979.
100. Singleton JW: National Cooperative Crohn's Disease Study (NCCDS): Results of Drug Treatment. Gastroenterology 72:A110, 1977.
101. Michener WM, Gage RP, Sauer WG, Stickler GB: The prognosis of chronic ulcerative colitis in children. N Engl J Med 265:1075, 1961.
102. De Dombal FT: Results of surgery for Crohn's disease. Clin Gastroenterol 2:493, 1972.
103. Homan WP, Dineen P: Comparison of the results of resection, bypass, and bypass with exclusion for ileocecal Crohn's disease. Ann Surg 187:530, 1978.
104. Jones JH, Lennard-Jones JE, Lockhart-Mummery HE: Experience in the treatment of Crohn's disease of the large intestine. Gut 7:448, 1966.
105. Fawaz KA, Glotzer DJ, Goldman H, Dickersin GR, Gross W, Patterson JF: Ulcerative colitis and Crohn's disease of the colon—a comparison of the long term postoperative courses. Gastroenterology 71:372, 1976.
106. Khubchandani IT, Trimpi HD, Sheets JA, Staski JJ, Kleckner FS: Ileorectal anastomosis for ulcerative and Crohn's colitis. Am J Surg 135:751, 1978.
107. Fry, PD, Atkinson KG: Current surgical approach to toxic megacolon. Surg Gynecol Obstet 143:26, 1976.
108. Block GE, Moossa AR, Simonowitz D, Hassan SZ: Emergency colectomy for inflammatory bowel disease. Surgery 82:531, 1977.

INFECTIOUS COMPLICATIONS OF CANCER

109. Welch JP, Donaldson GA: Perforative Carcinoma of Colon and Rectum. Ann Surg 180:734, 1974.
110. Peloquin AB: Factors influencing survival with complete obstruction and free perforation of colorectal cancers. Dis Colon Rectum 18:11, 1975.
111. Welch JP: Unusual abscesses in perforating colorectal cancer. Am J Surg 131:270, 1976.
112. Valerio D, Jones PF: Immediate resection in the treatment of large bowel emergencies. Br J Surg 65:712, 1978.
113. Welch JP, Donaldson GA: Management of severe obstruction of the large bowel due to malignant disease. Am J Surg 127:492, 1974.
114. Klein RS, Recco RA, Catalano MT, Edberg SC, Casey JI, Steigbigel NH: Association of *Streptococcus bovis* with carcinoma of the colon. N Engl J Med 297:800, 1977.

INFECTIONS RELATED TO LARGE BOWEL OBSTRUCTION

115. Greene WW: Bowel obstruction in the aged patient: a review of 300 cases. Am J Surg 118:541, 1969.
116. Byrne JJ: Large bowel obstruction. Am J Surg 99:168, 1960.
117. Greenlee HB, Pienkos EJ, Vanderbilt PC, Byrne MP, Mason JH, Banich FE, Freeark RJ: Acute large bowel obstruction: comparison of county, Veterans Administration, and community hospital populations. Arch Surg 108:470, 1974.
118. Michel ML, Tanner GR, Rohr ME: Obstructions of the colon. In Ballinger WF, Drapanas T (eds): Practice of Surgery—Current Review, Vol. II. St. Louis, Mosby, 1975, p 90.
119. Weilbaecher D, Bolin JA, Hearn D, Ogden W: Intussusception in adults: review of 160 cases. Am J Surg 121:531, 1971.
120. Smith GA, Perry JF, Yonehiro EG: Mechanical intestinal obstructions: a study of 1,252 cases. Surg Gynecol Obstet 100:651, 1955.
121. Payne RL, McAlpine RE: Obstruction of the colon: resection in two stages. Ann Surg 153:871, 1961.
122. Starling JR: Initial treatment of sigmoid volvulus by colonoscopy. Ann Surg 190:36, 1979.

COLONIC ISCHEMIA

123. Bernardino ME, Lawson TL: Discrete colonic ulcers associated with oral contraceptives. Am J Dig Dis 21:503, 1976.
124. Kistin MG, Kaplan MM, Harrington JT: Diffuse ischemic colitis associated with systemic lupus erythematosus—response to subtotal colectomy. Gastroenterology 75:1147, 1978.
125. Hagihara PF, Parker JC, Griffen WO: Spontaneous ischemic colitis. Dis Colon Rectum 20:236, 1977.
126. O'Connell TX, Kadell B, Tompkins RK: Ischemia of the colon. Surg Gynecol Obstet 142:337, 1976.
127. LeVeen EG, Falk G, Ip M, Mazzapica N, LeVeen HH: Urease

as a contributing factor in ulcerative lesions of the colon. Am J Surg 135:53, 1978.
128. Boley SJ, Brandt LJ, Veith FJ: Ischemic disorders of the intestines. Curr Probl Surg 15:1, April 1978.
129. Williams LF, Wittenberg J: Ischemic colitis: a useful clinical diagnosis, but is it ischemic? Ann Surg 182:439, 1975.
130. Heikkinen E, Larmi TKI, Huttunen R: Necrotizing colitis. Am J Surg 128:362, 1974.
131. Feldman PS: Ulcerative disease of the colon proximal to partially obstructive lesions: report of two cases and review of the literature. Dis Colon Rectum 18:601, 1975.
132. Ernst CB, Hagihara PF, Daugherty ME, Sachatello CR, Griffen WO: Ischemic colitis incidence following abdominal aortic reconstruction: a prospective study. Surgery 80:417, 1976.
133. Robinson JC, Teitelbaum SL: Stercoral ulceration and perforation of the sclerodermatous colon: report of two cases and review of the literature. Dis Colon Rectum 17:622, 1974.
134. Russell WL: Stercoraceous ulcer. Am Surg 42:416, 1976.
135. Albers JH, Smith LL, Carter R: Perforation of the cecum. Ann Surg 143:251, 1956.

LARGE BOWEL FISTULA

136. Webster MW, Carey LC: Fistulae of the intestinal tract. Curr Probl Surg 13:1, June 1976.
137. Haff RC, Wise L, Ballinger WF: Biliary-enteric fistulas. Surg Gynecol Obstet 133:84, 1971.
138. ReMine WH: Biliary-enteric fistulas: natural history and management. In Hardy JD, Zollinger RM (eds): Advances Surgery, Vol 7. Chicago, Year Book Medical Publishers, 1973, p 69.
139. Holden JL, Berne TV, Rosoff L: Pancreatic abscess following acute pancreatitis. Arch Surg 111:858, 1976.
140. Grace RR, Jordan PH: Unresolved problems of pancreatic pseudocysts. Ann Surg 184:16, 1976.
141. Korelitz BI: Colonic-duodenal fistula in Crohn's disease. Am J Dig Dis 22:1040, 1977.
142. Howat JMT, Schofield PF: Benign duodenocolic fistula. Br J Surg 65:513, 1978.
143. Ergin MA, Alfonso A, Auda SP, Waxman M: Primary carcinoma of the duodenum producing a malignant duodenocolic fistula. Dis Colon Rectum 21:408, 1978.

BACTERIAL ENTEROCOLITIS

144. Viranuvatti V: Infectious diarrheas, Part II. Cholera, salmonellosis and shigellosis. In Bockus H (ed): Gastroenterology. Philadelphia, Saunders, 1976, p 959.
145. Kim J, Oh S, Jarrett F: Management of ileal perforation due to typhoid fever. Ann Surg 181:88, 1975.
146. Gutman LT, Ottesen EA, Quan TJ, Noce PS, Katz SL: An inter-familial outbreak of *Yersinia enterocolitica* enteritis. N Engl J Med 288:1372, 1973.
147. Nelson JD, Kusmiesz H, Jackson LH, Woodman E: Trimethoprim-sulfamethoxazole therapy for shigellosis. JAMA 235: 1239, 1976.
148. Friedman GD., Gerard MJ, Ury HK: Clindamycin and Diarrhea. JAMA 236:2498, 1976.
149. Tedesco FJ: Ampicillin-associated diarrhea—a prospective study. Am J Dig Dis 20:295, 1975.
150. Slagle GW, Boggs HW: Drug-induced pseudomembranous enterocolitis: a new etiologic agent. Dis Colon Rectum 19:253, 1976.
151. Toffler RB, Pingoud EG, Burrell MI: Acute colitis related to penicillin and penicillin derivatives. Lancet 2:707, 1978.
152. Hummel RP, Altemeier WA, Hill EO: Iatrogenic staphyloccal enterocolitis. Ann Surg 160:551, 1964.
153. Bartlett JG, Chang TW, Gurwith M, Gorbach SL, Onderdonk AB: Antibiotic-associated pseudomembranous colitis due to toxin-producing clostridia. N Engl J Med 298:531, 1978.
154. Tedesco FJ: Clindamycin-associated colitis: review of the clinical spectrum of 47 cases. Am J Dig Dis 21:26, 1976.
155. Novak E, Lee JG, Seckman CE, Phillips JP, DiSanto AR: Unfavorable effect of atropine-diphenoxylate (Lomotil) therapy in lincomycin-caused diarrhea. JAMA 235:1451, 1976.
156. Kreutzer EW, Milligan FD: Treatment of antibiotic-associated pseudomembranous colitis with cholestyramine resin. Johns Hopkins Med J 143:67, 1978.
157. Keighly MRB, Arabi Y, Burdon DW, Alexander-Williams J, George RH: Randomized controlled trial of vancomycin for postoperative diarrhea and pseudomembranous colitis. Br J Surg 66:363, 1979.
158. Yale CE, Balish E: Pneumatosis cystoides intestinalis. Dis Colon Rectum 19:107–111, 1976.
159. Gruenberg JC, Grodsinsky C, Ponka JL: Pneumatosis intestinalis: a clinical classification. Dis Colon Rectum 22:5, 1979.
160. Gruenberg JC, Batra SK, Priest RJ: Treatment of pneumatosis cystoides intestinalis with oxygen. Arch Surg 112:62, 1977.

GRANULOMATOUS INFECTIONS

161. Shukla HS, Hughes LE: Abdominal tuberculosis in the 1970's: a continuing problem. Br J Surg 65:403, 1978.
162. Paustian FF, Monto GL: Tuberculosis of the intestines. In Bockus HL (ed): Gastroenterology. Philadelphia, Saunders, 1976, p 750.
163. Jordan GL, DeBakey ME: Complications of tuberculous enteritis occurring during antimicrobial therapy. Arch Surg 69:688, 1954.
164. Adams R, Miller WH: Surgical treatment of intestinal tuberculosis. Surg Clin North Am 26:656, 1946.
165. Porter JM, Snowe RJ, Silver D: Tuberculous enteritis with perforation and abscess formation in childhood. Surgery 71:254, 1972.
166. Katariya RN, Sood S, Rao PG, Rao PLNG: Stricture-plasty for tubercular strictures of the gastro-intestinal tract. Br J Surg 64:496, 1977.
167. Berardi RS: Abdominal actinomycosis. Surg Gynecol Obstet 149:257, 1979.
168. Cowgill R, Quan SH: Colonic actinomycosis mimicking carcinoma. Dis Colon Rectum 22:45, 1979.
169. Howard RJ, Balfour HH, Simmons RL: The surgical significance of viruses. Curr Probl Surg 14:1, 1977.
170. Juniper K: Amebiasis. Clin Gastroenterol 7:3, 1978.
171. Krogstad DJ, Spencer HC Jr, Healy GR: Amebiasis. N Engl J Med 298:262, 1978.
172. Latimer RG: Surgical intervention in intestinal amebiasis. Am Surg 41:385, 1975.
173. Eggleston FC, Verghese M, Handa AK: Amoebic perforation of the bowel: experiences with 26 cases. Br J Surg 65:748, 1978.
174. Warren KS: Schistosomiasis Japonica. Clin Gastroenterol 7:77, 1978.
175. Prata A: *Schistosomiasis mansoni*. Clin Gastroenterol 7:49, 1978.
176. Boley SJ, Schwartz S, Lash J, Sternhill V: Reversible vascular occlusion of the colon. Surg Gynecol Obstet 116:53, 1963.

INFECTIOUS COMPLICATIONS OF COLON OPERATIONS

177. Goligher JC, Lee PWG, Simpkins KC, Lintott DJ: A controlled comparison of one and two-layer techniques of suture

for high and low colorectal anastomoses. Br J Surg 64:609, 1977.
178. Jonsell G, Edelmann G: Single-layer anastomosis of the colon: a review of 165 cases. Am J Surg 135:630, 1978.
179. Schrock TR, Deveney CW, Dunphy JE: Factors contributing to leakage of colonic anastomoses. Ann Surg 177:513, 1973.
180. Morgenstern L, Yamakawa T, Ben-Shoshan M, Lippman H: Anastomotic leakage after low colonic anastomosis: clinical and experimental aspects. Am J Surg 123:104, 1972.
181. Debas HT, Thomson FB: A critical review of colectomy with anastomosis. Surg Gynecol Obstet 135:747, 1972.
182. Irvin TT, Goligher JC: Aetiology of disruption of intestinal anastomoses. Br J Surg 60:461, 1973.
183. Fazio VW: Sump suction and irrigation of the presacral space. Dis Colon Rectum 21:401, 1978.
184. Crowley LG, Anders CJ, Nelsen T, Bagshaw M: Effect of radiation on canine intestinal anastomoses. Arch Surg 96: 423, 1968.
185. Cofer TW, Ray JE, Gathright JB Jr: Does neostigmine cause disruption of large intestinal anastomoses? a negative answer. Dis Colon Rectum 17:235, 1974.
186. Goligher JC, Morris C, McAdam WAF, DeDombal FT, Johnston D: A controlled trial of inverting versus everting intestinal suture in clinical large-bowel surgery. Br J Surg 57:817, 1970.
187. Balz J, Samson RB, Stewart WRC: Rectal-tube decompression in left colectomy. Dis Colon Rectum 21:94, 1978.
188. Crowson WN, Wilson CS: An experimental study of the effects of drains on colon anastomoses. Am Surg 39:597, 1973.
189. Goldsmith HS: Protection of low rectal anastomosis with intact omentum. Surg Gynecol Obstet 144:584, 1977.
190. McLachlin, AD, Denton DW: Omental protection of intestinal anastomoses. Am J Surg 125:134, 1973.
191. Cooney DR, Wassner JD, Grossfeld JL, Jesseph JE: Are elemental diets useful in bowel preparation? Arch Surg 109:206, 1974.
192. Hewitt J, Rigby J, Reeve J, Cox AG: Whole-gut irrigation in preparation for large-bowel surgery. Lancet 2:337, 1973.
193. Chung RS, Gurll NJ, Berglund EM: A controlled clinical trial of whole gut lavage as a method of bowel preparation for colonic operations. Am J Surg 137:75, 1979.
194. Gliedman ML, Grant RN, Vestal BL, Karlson KE: Impromptu bowel cleansing and sterilization. Surgery 43:282, 1958.
195. Dickman MD, Chappelka AR, Schaedler RW: Evaluation of gut microflora during administration of an elemental diet in a patient with an ileoproctostomy. Am J Dig Dis 20:377, 1975.
196. Arabi Y, Dimock F, Burdon DW, Alexander-Williams J, Keighly MRB: Influence of bowel preparation and antimicrobials on colonic microflora. Br J Surg 65:555, 1978.
197. Poth EJ: Intestinal antisepsis in surgery. JAMA 153:1516, 1953.
198. Nichols RL, Condon RE: Preoperative preparation of the colon. Surg Gynecol Obstet 132:323, 1971.
199. Nichols RL, Condon RE, Gorbach SL, Nyhus LM: Efficacy of preoperative antimicrobial preparation of the bowel. Ann Surg 176:227, 1972.
200. Nichols RL, Broido P, Condon RE, Gorbach SL, Nyhus LM: Effect of preoperative neomycin-erythromycin intestinal preparation on the incidence of infectious complications following colon surgery. Ann Surg 178:453, 1973.
201. Vargish T, Crawford LC, Stallings RA, Wasilauskas BL, Myers RT: A randomized prospective evaluation of orally administered antibiotics in operations on the colon. Surg Gynecol Obstet 146:193, 1978.
202. Taylor SA, Cawdery HM, Smith J: The use of metronidazole in the preparation of the bowel for surgery. Br J Surg 66:191, 1979.
203. Brass C, Richards GK, Ruedy J, Prentis J, Hinchey EJ: The effect of metronidazole on the incidence of postoperative wound infection in elective colon surgery. Am J Surg 135:91, 1978.
204. Altemeier WA, Hummel RP, Hill EO: Prevention of infection in colon surgery. Arch Surg 93:226, 1966.
205. Herter FP, Slanetz CA: Preoperative intestinal preparation in relation to the subsequent development of cancer at the suture line. Surg Gynecol Obstet 127:49, 1968.
206. Jones FE, DeCosse JJ, Condon RE: Evaluation of "Instant" preparation of the colon with povidone-iodine. Ann Surg 184:74, 1976.
207. Arango A, Lester JL, Martinez OV, Malinin TI, Zeppa R: Bacteriologic and systemic effects of intraoperative segmental bowel preparation with povidone iodine. Arch Surg 114:154, 1979.
208. Azar H, Drapanas T: Relationship of antibiotics to wound infection and enterocolitis in colon surgery. Am J Surg 115:209, 1968.
209. Burke JF: The effective period of preventive antibiotic action in experimental incisions and dermal lesions. Surgery 50:161, 1961.
210. Miles AA, Miles EM, Burke J: The value and duration of defence reactions of the skin to the primary lodgement of bacteria. Br J Exp Pathol 38:79, 1957.
211. Polk HC, Miles AA: The decisive period in the primary infection of muscle by Eschericia coli. Br J Exp Pathol 54:99, 1973.
212. Fullen WD, Hunt J, Altemeier, WA: Prophylactic antibiotics in penetrating wounds of the abdomen. J Trauma 12:282, 1972.
213. Stone HH, Hooper CA, Kolb LD, Geheber CE, Dawkins EJ: Antibiotic prophylaxis in gastric biliary and colonic surgery. Ann Surg 184:443, 1976.
214. Condon RE, Bartlett, JG, Nichols RL, Schulte WJ, Gorbach SL, Ochi S: Preoperative prophylactic cephalothin fails to control septic complications of colorectal operations: results of controlled clinical trial. Am J Surg 137:68, 1979.
215. Polk HC, Lopez-Mayor JF: Postoperative wound infection: a prospective study of determinant factors and prevention. Surgery 66:97, 1969.
216. Griffiths DA, Shorey BA, Simpson RA, Speller DCE, Williams NB: Single-dose preoperative antibiotic prophylaxis in gastrointestinal surgery. Lancet 2:325, 1976.
217. Feltis JM, Hamit HF: Use of prophylactic antimicrobial drugs to prevent post-operative wound infections. Am J Surg 114:867, 1967.
218. Downing R, McLeish AR, Burdon, DW, Alexander-Williams J, Keighly MRB: Duration of systemic prophylactic antibiotic cover against anaerobic sepsis in intestinal surgery. Dis Colon Rectum 20:401, 1977.
219. Stone HH, Haney BB, Kolb LK, Geheber CE, Hooper CA: Prophylactic and preventive antibiotic therapy: timing, duration and economics. Ann Surg 189:691, 1979.
220. Kjellgren K, Sellstrom H: Effect of prophylactic systemic administration of cephalothin in colorectal surgery. Acta Chir Scand 143:473, 1977.
221. Slama TG, Carey LC, Fass RJ: Comparative efficacy of prophylactic cephalothin and cefamandole for elective colon surgery: results of a prospective, randomized, double-blind study. Am J Surg 137:593, 1979.
222. Thadepalli H, Gorbach SL, Broido PW, Norsen J, Nyhus L: Abdominal trauma, anaerobes and antibiotics. Surg Gynecol Obstet 137:270, 1973.

223. Barber MS, Hirschberg BC, Rice CL, Atkins CC: Parenteral antibiotics in elective colon surgery? A prospective, controlled clinical study. Surgery 86:23, 1979.
224. O'Donnell V, Mandal AK, Lou MA, Thadepalli H: Evaluation of carbenicillin and a comparison of clindamycin and gentamycin combined therapy in penetrating abdominal trauma. Surg Gynecol Obstet 147:525, 1978.
225. Yates JL: An experimental study of the local effects of peritoneal drainage. Reprinted in Am Surg 21:1048, 1955.
226. Agrama HM, Blackwood JM, Brown CS, Machiedo GW, Rush BF, Functional longevity of intraperitoneal drains: an experimental evaluation. Am J Surg 132:418, 1976.
227. Stone HH, Hooper CA, Millikan WJ: Abdominal drainage following appendectomy and cholecystectomy. Ann Surg 187:606, 1978.
228. Stone HH, Hester TR: Incisional and peritoneal infection after emergency celiotomy. Ann Surg 177:669, 1973.
229. Berliner SD, Burson LC, Lear PE: Use and abuse of intraperitoneal drains in colon surgery. Arch Surg 89:686, 1964.
230. Mirelman D, Corman ML, Veidenheimer MC, Coller JA: Colostomies-indications and contraindications: Lahey Clinic experience, 1963–1974. Dis Colon Rectum 21:172, 1978.
231. Chandler JG, Evans BP: Colostomy prolapse. Surgery 84:577, 1978.
232. Birnbaum W, Ferrier P: Complications of abdominal colostomy. Am J Surg 83:64, 1952.
233. Hines JR, Harris GD: Colostomy and colostomy closure. Surg Clin North Am 57:1379, 1977.
234. Todd, GJ, Kutcher LM, Markowitz AM: Factors influencing the complications of colostomy closure. Am J Surg 137:749, 1979.
235. Adeyemo A, Gaillard WE, Ali SD, Calhoun T, Kurtz LH: Colostomy: intraperitoneal or extraperitoneal closure? Am J Surg 130:273, 1975.

CHAPTER 40
Appendicitis

EDWARD H. STORER

The human vermiform appendix has had a checkered history during the past century. Until 1886, right lower quadrant suppuration was attributed to cecal disease and called "perityphlitis." In that year, Reginald Fitz [1] set the record straight with a landmark report. His term, "appendicitis," was quickly accepted, and appendectomy soon became the most common abdominal operation. Not all removed appendices were inflamed, but the prevailing attitude was that it was safer to remove some normal appendices than to allow an inflamed appendix to rupture during observation. In addition, the human appendix was considered an evolutionary vestige that served no useful function. By the mid-twentieth century, however, surgical tissue committees began to look critically at the removal of any normal tissue. Since then, the percentage of healthy appendices removed with a preoperative diagnosis of acute appendicitis has dropped from nearly 50 percent in the 1940s to around 15 percent in the 1970s.

Two events in the 1960s promised to change the status of the lowly, useless appendage. Retrospective studies [2,3] of necropsy data suggested that the incidence of previous appendectomy in patients who were dying of carcinoma of the colon was significantly higher than in comparable control groups. For a time, it appeared that the appendix would no longer be called a useless vestige if it might protect against cancer. The relationship could not be confirmed,[4,5] and Moertel et al [6] could find no evidence in a prospective study that appendectomy predisposed to cancer.

A second possible new role for the appendix was suggested by Good and his associates [7]—namely that the gut-associated lymphoid tissue (GALT), including the appendix, functions as a maturational organ for B lymphocytes. Other sites that serve this function have since been ascertained,[8] so the appendix presumably remains a useful, though not indispensable, immunologic organ.[9]

ANATOMY

The fetal appendix develops as the inferior tip of the funnel-shaped cecum, which is its configuration at birth.[10,11] In early childhood, bilateral sacculation of the cecum occurs, which sets off the cecum from the appendix. Further cecal growth is more rapid on the anterolateral aspects, so that the base of the now tubular appendix is rotated to its adult position on the posteromedial wall of the cecum, inferior to the ileocecal valve. The relationship of the base of the appendix to the cecum is fairly constant, but the free tip is found in a variety of locations—right lower quadrant, left lower quadrant, pelvic, or retrocecal. Arrest in rotation of the colon results in abnormal locations of the appendix and may confuse the diagnosis of acute appendicitis. The three taeniae coli join at the junction of the cecum with the appendix to form a continuous outer longitudinal muscle layer. The surgeon can always locate the elusive appendix by following the taeniae.

The adult human appendix is usually 9 ± 2 cm long but may vary from 1 to 27 cm.[11] Complete absence of the appendix has been reported in thalidomide children.[12] The diameter varies from 3 to 15 mm but is usually about 7 to 8 mm, with little tapering from base to tip. The capacity of the lumen of the entire organ is less than 0.5 ml—a fact that looms large in the pathogenesis of acute appendicitis.

HISTOLOGY

The appendix consists of several concentric tissue layers. From the outer layer inward, these are serosa, longitudinal muscularis propria, circular muscularis, submucosa, muscularis mucosae, lamina propria, and mucosa. In younger individuals, the lymphoid tissue in the epithelium, lamina propria, and submucosa occupies more than half of the cross-sectional area.

This lymphoid tissue is sparse at birth but gradually increases to a peak in the early teens. Thereafter, a more gradual reduction begins and continues until only a little lymphoid tissue remains in old age.[13] The appendiceal lymphoid tissue is predominantly a B cell pool but includes T cells as well.[8,14–16]

The epithelium of the appendix consists of simple tubular glands, the crypts of Lieberkühn, the ends of which are embedded in lymphoid tissue. Several types of cells—columnar epithelial, goblet, argentaffin, and Paneth—are present. The mucosal surface between the glands is flat, without villi, and composed principally of surface epithelial cells with striated borders, with occasional goblet cells. There are, however, discrete areas of morphologically distinct surface cells called follicle-associated epithelium,[17] or M cells (membranous epithelial [9] or microfold [18] cells), because they are found overlying the point of contact between lymphoid follicles and epithelium. These cells are characterized by the presence of irregular microvilli or microfolds and numerous micropinocytotic vesicles. Similar highly specialized epithelial cells have been previously described in the chicken bursa of Fabricius and in human Peyer patches.[17] These attenuated specialized epithelial cells allow the lymphoid cells to approach within 0.3 mm of the intestinal lumen while maintaining the integrity of the intestinal epithelium. It is thought that the biologic significance of follicle-associated epithelium is to provide a direct access for lumenal antigens into the dome of the follicle. Here the antigens stimulate clonal proliferation and seeding of B lymphocytes throughout the lamina propria of internal mucous surfaces.[19-23]

The appendix is not indispensable, even though it is an integral part of the GALT-mediated secretory globulin immune mechanism (Chapter 13). Appendectomy produces no detectable defect in the functioning of the immunoglobulin system. Conversely, selective s-IgA deficiency has no known effect on diseases of the appendix—it does not predispose to acute appendicitis.

ACUTE APPENDICITIS

Although the appendix is occasionally involved in inflammatory disease of the cecum or ileum such as tuberculosis, typhoid fever, actinomycosis, or inflammatory bowel disease, acute appendicitis is by far the most important disease of the appendix. Chronic appendicitis was a popular diagnosis in years past but probably does not exist. Recurrent acute appendicitis does occur.[24,25]

Incidence

The incidence of primary appendectomy in the United States (appendectomy done for a preoperative diagnosis of acute appendicitis as distinguished from appendectomy done as an incidental part of another abdominal operation) has fallen dramatically in the past 40 years. Most of the fall occurred in the first 15 years,[26] with a continued slower decline over the past 25 years. Similar declines have occurred in other developed countries.[27] The reasons for this decline are unknown, although part of it can be accounted for by better diagnosis. Other possibilities include the use of antibiotics and the increased roughage in the diets of North Americans. Burkitt [28] has attributed the remarkably low incidence of acute appendicitis in native Africans to their rough diet.

Acute appendicitis is rare in infants and uncommon in early childhood, presumably because of the configuration of the appendix, which makes lumenal obstruction unlikely. The peak incidence for both sexes is in the mid and late teens and continues at a high level through the third decade of life. The incidence is higher in males, but this distinction disappears at higher ages.

Etiology

The preponderance of the evidence is that acute appendicitis is not primarily an infection per se, but is caused by proximal obstruction of the appendix with resulting inflammation and secondary infection.

Aschoff, the nineteenth century pathologist, asserted that appendicitis is a specific bacterial disease (not unlike gonorrhea) caused by the enterococcus type B of Gundel.[29] This hypothesis is not true but still crops up periodically. Most recently, *Streptococcus milleri* [30] and *Yersinia enterocolitica* [31] have been reported to cause acute appendicitis. It is unlikely, however, that either agent is responsible for more than an occasional case.[32] The bacterial organisms that finally infect the obstructed and ischemic appendix are the mixed flora of the cecal lumen.

Jackson et al [33] have evaluated the hypothesis that an acute virus infection at the time of, or just before, appendicitis might lead to lymphoid hyperplasia in the appendix. This hyperplasia or subsequent healing and scarring might produce acute obstruction of the appendix. They found no difference in the viral recovery rate in children with appendicitis as compared to normal children.

Pathogenesis and Pathology

Zwalenberg proposed in 1905 [34] that obstruction is the basic pathophysiologic process in acute appendicitis. Wilkie demonstrated in 1930 [35] that acute appendicitis could, "with ease and certainty," be produced in the rabbit by milking fecal matter into the appendix from the cecum and then ligating the appendix at its cecal end, taking care not to interfere with its blood supply. The animal died within 24 hours from a perforated gangrenous appendix. Then Wangensteen and several associates [36-41] in the late 1930s and early 1940s extensively and systematically studied the comparative anatomy and pathophysiology of the appendix in many animal species. They concluded that acute appendicitis in the human is usually caused by proximal obstruction of the appendix.

For appendicitis to occur, the appendix must: (1) be susceptible to obstruction, ie, be tubular, and (2) continue to secrete in the face of increased pressure. Although a few animals (chimpanzee, gibbon, gorilla, orangutan, rabbit, and wombat) [42] have a tubular appendix, Wangensteen and associates found only three (man, chimpanzee, and rabbit) in which the obstructed appendix continued to secrete against a pressure gradient. Blackwood et al [42] have confirmed Wangensteen's observations. They concluded that the appendiceal epithelium of rabbit and man is a secreting intestinal epithelium without absorptive functions.

Wangensteen and Dennis's studies in patients are particularly illuminating.[36] They exteriorized the appendix in patients undergoing colon surgery, ligated the base without disturbing the blood supply, and inserted a small catheter connected to a manometer. Maximum pressures generated within the appendices ranged from 0 to 126 mm H_2O. The appendices were then removed and examined histologically. Appendices that had generated little pressure had little functioning mucosa, were mostly fibrotic, and showed little inflammation. On the other hand, the appendices that had generated high pressure demonstrated all the histologic criteria for acute appendicitis.

Obstruction is often caused by fecaliths, particularly in the more severe types of appendicitis. Fecaliths are found in about 40 percent of appendices with simple acute appendicitis, about 65 percent in gangrenous appendicitis without rupture, and about 90 percent in gangrenous appendicitis with rupture. Rare causes include cecal tumors,[43] appendiceal tumors,[44] vegetable and fruit seeds, inspissated barium,[45,46] foreign bodies,[47,48] and intestinal worms, particularly ascarids.[49] Hypertrophied lymphoid tissue is thought to be responsible for the remainder. The fact that the peak incidence of appendicitis coincides with the peak in the amount of lymphoid tissue in the appendix lends credence to this hypothesis. A fold of tissue in the cecum, called the valve of Gerlach, near the opening of the appendix has been proposed as a possible cause of appendiceal obstruction. Wangensteen [29] could find no evidence for this and feels that the valve of Gerlach may impede the entry of cecal content into the appendix, but that it does not impede egress of appendiceal content into the cecum.

Proximal obstruction of the appendiceal lumen from whatever cause creates a closed-loop obstruction. Continued secretion by the appendiceal mucosa rapidly builds pressure because of the miniscule capacity of the lumen. As pressure increases, normal lymphatic and venous pressures are sequentially exceeded producing edema, engorgement, and vascular congestion, because arteriolar inflow continues. The omnipresent bacteria multiply and soon invade the now compromised mucosa. Microscopic sections of appendicitis at this stage would be called catarrhal or acute focal appendicitis and would reveal submucosal edema, vascular congestion, beginning invasion of the organ by bacteria through mucosal microulcers, and some polymorphonuclear infiltrate.

Progression of the inflammatory process is probably not inevitable, because obstruction caused by lymphatic swelling or a soft fecal plug often relieves itself. Patients with acute appendicitis frequently have a history of similar attacks in the past that subsided spontaneously. These appendices are often thickened and scarred, suggesting previously healed inflammation.

If the obstruction is unrelenting, however, distention continues and all the appendiceal coats become involved in the combination of circulatory compromise, bacterial invasion, and the inflammatory response; thus *acute suppurative appendicitis.* When the intraluminal pressure approaches the arteriolar pressure, the blood supply to the antimesenteric border is cut off, and ellipsoidal infarcts appear; the result is *acute gangrenous appendicitis.* The infarcted areas now permit bacteria to reach adjacent peritoneal surfaces. Finally, perforation occurs, usually through one of the infarcted areas on the antimesenteric border, and *perforated* or *ruptured appendicitis* is present.

The sequelae of appendiceal rupture include confined perforation with phlegmon or abscess formation, unconfined perforation with spreading peritonitis, and secondary abscesses. Pylethrombophlebitis and intestinal obstruction may follow either confined or unconfined perforation.

Perforation of the appendix is nearly always distal to fecalith occlusion of the lumen. The presence of the fecalith will usually prevent retrograde spillage of cecal content through the perforation, but the occluding fecalith may be dislodged if the point of rupture of the appendiceal wall is at or near the site of the fecalith, permitting spillage of cecal content.

In the several hours between the onset of inflammation and appendiceal perforation, fibrinous adhesions usually form between adjacent peritoneal surfaces and confine the infection. This walling off is successful about 95 percent of the time but less often in the very young or very old. The periappendiceal phlegmon consists of inflamed matted omentum and adjacent intestinal loops, with little or no frank pus. This mass may slowly resolve spontaneously. Resolution can be hastened by removal of the necrotic appendix. In some patients, however, suppuration continues with the production of an expanding collection of pus—a periappendiceal abscess. The abscess may slowly resolve spontaneously or can be surgically drained. If it is neglected, further progression of the suppurative process may lead to the dreaded complication of secondary rupture of a periappendiceal abscess.

Spreading peritonitis results when the walling-off process is incomplete at the time of rupture. If the spread continues unchecked, diffuse generalized peritonitis is produced. The process may also be localized by the peritoneum's protective mechanisms with secondary abscess formation. Common sites are the pelvic cul-de-sac, which is seeded by gravity, the right subhepatic space by drainage up the right paracolic gutter, and between adjacent loops of intestine-interloop abscesses.

Clinical Manifestations

Symptoms. Abdominal pain is the principal symptom and is present in over 99 percent of patients. Early in the clinical course, the pain is diffuse (in the lower epigastric or periumbilical area), steady (sometimes with superimposed cramps), and only moderately severe. After 1 to 12 hours, but usually within 6 hours, the pain becomes localized to the right lower quadrant, where it becomes more severe and steady.

The early pain is characteristic of visceral pain, ie, dull, diffuse, midline pain, and is caused by distension of the appendix, which stimulates visceral afferent pain fibers. The later right lower quadrant pain is somatic in nature and is caused by involvement of segmental afferent nerves in the local parietal peritoneum.

There are many variations in the classical pain sequence. One of the more common variations is pain that begins and stays in the right lower quadrant; the visceral component is not perceived by the patient. The various locations of the appendix account for many of the variations in the location of the somatic pain component. A pelvic appendix may cause predominantly suprapubic pain; a retrocecal appendix, flank pain; and a retroileal appendix, testicular pain. Malrotation of the cecum may also produce puzzling pain patterns. The visceral pain component is felt in the usual midline location, but the somatic component is felt in that part of the abdomen where the cecum has been arrested during embryonic rotation.

Anorexia is an almost constant accompaniment to acute appendicitis and is often the first symptom. It is most likely the result of distension of the appendix because it is present before there is any infection or fever. Anorexia is so constant in appendicitis that the diagnosis must be questioned if the patient is hungry.

Nausea and vomiting occur sometime in the course of appendicitis in about 75 percent of patients. The vomiting is not prominent or prolonged and occurs after the onset of abdominal pain. If vomiting comes before pain, the diagnosis of appendicitis is in doubt.

Change in bowel habits is of little differential diagnostic value. Many patients complain of obstipation and state that a bowel movement would relieve the pain. Diarrhea occurs in about 15 percent, particularly in children.

The diagnosis usually becomes more obvious after perforation has occurred. The patient becomes obviously quite ill, toxic, and distended. The right lower quadrant pain increases in severity and spreads out over a larger area. The former teaching was that the pain of appendicitis lessens dramatically at the moment of perforation because of relief of distention of the appendix. This rarely occurs, probably because the gangrenous appendix contaminates the adjacent peritoneum before rupture with the production of the pain of localized peritonitis.

Physical Signs. Vital signs are scarcely altered early in appendicitis when appendiceal distention is present but before infection has supervened. With well-developed appendicitis, but before gangrene or perforation, the temperature is usually only about 38 to 38.5C; the pulse is modestly elevated. High fever and tachycardia indicate gangrene and perforation. Unstable blood pressure indicates peritonitis and septic shock.

Physical findings are determined by the stage of the disease when the patient is examined, as well as by the position of the inflamed organ. The classical physical signs are found with an unruptured appendix lying in an anterior position in the right lower quadrant. The point of maximal tenderness is often at or near McBurney's point, which he described as being "located exactly between an inch and a half and two inches from the anterior spinous process of the ileum on a straight line drawn from that process to the umbilicus." [50] Direct and referred rebound tenderness, indicating parietal peritoneal irritation, are also felt maximally in the right lower quadrant. Resistance of the abdominal wall muscles to palpation is roughly proportional to the extent of the inflammatory process. Early in the course, resistance consists mainly of voluntary guarding. As involvement of the parietal peritoneum increases, muscular spasm also increases and becomes largely involuntary, ie, true reflex spasm. Cutaneous hyperesthesia in the area of the T-10, 11, and 12 dermatomes on the right occurs frequently, and is often helpful to detect atypical, early appendicitis.

The position of the distal appendix often determines which physical signs will be found. Anterior abdominal signs may be completely absent if the inflamed appendix hangs into the pelvis, and the diagnosis may be missed unless a digital rectal examination is done. Pressure on the peritoneum in the cul-de-sac of Douglas produces pain both locally and in the hypogastric area. Similarly, abdominal signs are less striking with retrocecal positions of the appendix, and other signs must be relied on. A retrocecal appendix with the tip pointing cephalad often produces tenderness and spasm in the flank or back. Retrocecal appendices that point caudad often produce a positive psoas sign or obturator internus sign by virtue of local irritation of these muscles by the inflamed organ. The psoas sign is elicited by having the patient lie on his left side; the examiner then slowly extends the right thigh, thus stretching the iliopsoas muscle. The test is positive if extension produces pain. The obturator sign is elicited by passive internal rotation of the flexed right thigh with the patient supine. The test is positive if hypogastric pain is produced.

Physical findings become more definite after perforation of the appendix. If the perforation is confined to the right lower quadrant with the formation of a periappendiceal phlegmon or abscess, a tender boggy mass with ill-defined margins can be palpated. Tenderness that was confined to McBurney's point now extends to include most of the right lower quadrant. Muscular rigidity and rebound tenderness are also much more pronounced and conform to the area of localized peritonitis. As expected, the physical findings depend on the position of the diseased appendix. For example, abdominal examination may be entirely within normal limits with a confined rupture of a pelvic appendix—the only finding may be a boggy, tender mass on rectal examination.

If the perforation is not confined, the abdominal findings resemble generalized peritonitis, and tenderness is found over the extent of parietal peritoneal involvement. The greatest tenderness is usually over the site of the spillage but may be located over the advancing edge of the inflammatory process. Rebound tenderness, both direct and referred, is easily elicited. This is sometimes more accurate than palpation in locating the point of maximal tenderness as well as delineating the extent of peritoneal irritation.

Rigidity of the abdominal wall musculature overlying peritonitis usually results from both voluntary guarding and reflex muscular spasm. The rigidity in bacterial peritonitis is characteristically firm, but is not boardlike as in chemical peritonitis.

Early in the course of peritonitis, bowel sounds are often still present in the portions of the abdomen not yet involved. As the inflammation spreads, bowel activity ceases and the abdomen becomes silent. Extensive hyperresonance caused by gaseous intestinal distension can usually be demonstrated by percussion.

Laboratory Findings. Early in the course of acute obstructive appendicitis, laboratory values will be normal. After infection is present, the white blood cell count will range from 11,000–13,000 cells per mm^3, with a predominance of neutrophils with some young forms.[51,52] These findings do vary, but appendicitis is so consistently accompanied by a leukocytosis that white blood cell counts lower than 10,000 cells per mm^3 or a differential neutrophil count less than 75 percent should prompt review of the diagnosis.[53] Leukocytosis is more dramatic after perforation. A normal or depressed leukocyte count with a predominance of young forms can occur in overwhelming peritoneal sepsis, and is a grave sign.

Urinalysis may reveal white cells and occasional red blood cells, particularly if the inflammation is close to ureters or bladder. Significant bacilluria is not seen in appendicitis, however, and if present suggests urinary tract infection.

Blood chemistry determinations have no special diagnostic value but may be helpful in guiding intravenous therapy. Desalting water loss and metabolic acidosis are proportional to the extent of the inflammatory process. Massive fluid losses occur in generalized peritonitis and may require several hours of therapy before an operation should be done.

Roentgenography. Roentgenograms play little role in the diagnosis of straightforward acute appendicitis but are helpful in atypical presentations and in complicated appendicitis.[54]

Plain films of the abdomen in unruptured appendicitis usually have a dilated intestinal loop or two (the "sentinel loop") in the right lower quadrant. Although radio-opaque fecaliths are uncommon, when they are seen in association with right lower quadrant pain a gangrenous appendix is nearly always found.[55] Similarly a gas-filled appendix usually, but not invariably, indicates acute appendicitis with proximal appendiceal obstruction.

With unconfined perforated appendicitis and peritonitis, plain abdominal films reveal generalized adynamic ileus, with both small and large bowel loops visible. The space between adjacent gas-filled loops may be increased because of serosal inflammatory exudate and edema of the intestinal wall. Properitoneal fat lines and psoas shadows, particularly on the right, are usually obliterated. it is rare to find visible free air in appendicitis.[56]

Barium enema is proving to be a valuable diagnostic adjunct, particularly in children with an atypical presentation.[57,58] The procedure is done without preparation of the colon, with low pressure instillation of barium, and without external manipulation or pressure. Appendicitis is likely if the appendix does not fill or only fills for a short distance, if there is mass effect on the medial and inferior margins of the cecum, and mass effect and mucosal irregularities of the terminal ileum. Complete filling of the appendix and absence of mucosal irregularities and mass effects lessens the likelihood of appendicitis. An operation should be done nevertheless if the clinical picture is compelling, because there are about 5 percent false-negative results with barium enema.[59]

Appendicitis in the Young. The morbidity and mortality of acute appendicitis in infants and children is significantly higher than in adults, because the perforation rate is much higher. The diagnosis is more difficult to make in the young. Infants cannot describe their symptoms, the clinical picture is more often atypical with higher fevers and more vomiting, and physicians may not think of appendicitis, because it occurs much less frequently in the young.

Perforation, however, occurs in 30 to 50 percent of children [60] and up to 85 percent of infants.[61] After perforation, spreading peritonitis and intra-abdominal abscesses are more common than in adults because the inflammatory process proceeds more rapidly from onset to perforation and because the incompletely developed greater omentum cannot wall off the inflammation.

Even with perforation, a high mortality rate is not inevitable. Marchildon and Dudgeon [62] have reported a consecutive series of 89 children with perforated appendicitis, with a complication rate of 17 percent and no deaths.

It has been accepted practice in the past that it was better to remove an occasional normal appendix than to risk the rupture of an appendix in a child with an atypical presentation. Haller and his associates have reevaluated this practice.[63] Before their study, the perforation rate was 27 percent, and appendicitis was found during 80 percent of operations. By a policy of intensive in-hospital observation when the diagnosis of appendicitis was uncertain, appendicitis was found at operation in 94 percent while the perforation rate was unchanged. Leape and Ramenofsky[63a] have shown that the unnecessary appendectomy rate can be reduced to 1 percent with laparoscopy in children.

Appendicitis in the Elderly. Less than 10 percent of the operations for acute appendicitis take place in patients older than 60, but more than 50 percent of all deaths from appendicitis are in this age group. The composite mortality rate from seven recent large series is 6 percent.[64] The perforation rate of from 32 to 74 percent [64,65] (average 42 percent) is obviously responsible for the continuing high incidence of death and the high rate of septic complications which occur in one-half to two-thirds of this group.

There is a time-honored teaching that appendicitis in the elderly has a different clinical presentation that makes diagnosis much more difficult. Older patients are expected to have fewer symptoms, a less reliable duration of disease, a lower leukocyte count, and a lower temperature. This belief is only partially true—the symptoms and the signs are the same as in younger adults [65,66] but are less pronounced so that the findings are not proportional to the severity of the disease process.

The duration of the course of appendicitis in the elderly before operation correlates with the incidence of rupture and with increased morbidity and mortality. Delay in seeking medical attention is too frequent in this group—in one study [65] the mean duration was 58 hours. Also, more than 50 percent of these patients will have taken a cathartic, and about 40 percent will have serious concomitant disease.

Appendicitis During Pregnancy. Acute appendicitis is the most common surgical emergency occurring during pregnancy, with an incidence of about 1 in 2,000 deliveries. The incidence of appendicitis is not increased by pregnancy.[67]

Diagnosis is difficult. The symptoms of appendicitis (eg, abdominal pain and nausea) are common during pregnancy. Displacement of the appendix by the gravid uterus changes the location of the somatic component of abdominal pain and the point of maximal tenderness to a higher and more lateral position. At 5 months gestation, the appendix is at the level of the iliac crest and at 8 months about halfway between the iliac crest and lower ribs. Leukocytosis of pregnancy, where counts as high as 15,000 cells per mm^3 are normal, compromises the diagnostic

TABLE 40-1. CONDITIONS THAT MIMIC ACUTE APPENDICITIS

Acute mesenteric adenitis	Perforated peptic ulcer
Acute gastroenteritis	Diverticulitis coli, particularly cecal
Yersiniosis	Perforating carcinoma of the colon, particularly cecal
Urinary tract infection	Foreign body perforations of the bowel
Meckel diverticulitis	Closed-loop intestinal obstruction
Intussusception	Mesenteric vascular occlusion
Regional enteritis	Pleuritis of the right lower chest
Primary peritonitis	Acute cholecystitis
Henoch-Schönlein purpura	Acute pancreatitis
Gynecologic disorders	Right ureteral calculus
Pelvic inflammatory disease	Infarcted epiploic appendage
Ruptured graafian follicle	Hematoma of the abdominal wall
Ruptured ectopic pregnancy	
Diseases of the male	
Torsion of the testis	
Acute epididymitis	

Adapted from Storer EH: Appendix. In Schwartz SI, Shires GT, Spencer FC, Storer EH (eds): Principles of Surgery, 3d ed. New York, McGraw-Hill, 1979, p 1257.

value of this test.[68] Laparoscopy can be used in atypical cases and may make laparotomy unnecessary.

Maternal mortality from appendicitis is now about 0.2 percent and is nearly always associated with generalized peritonitis. Fetal mortality, overall, is about 8.5 percent but is about 35 percent when peritonitis develops.

Table 40-1 is a list of conditions that occasionally mimic the clinical findings of acute appendicitis. Detailed discussion is available in standard textbooks of surgery.[69]

Treatment

There is only one effective treatment for acute appendicitis—early removal of the diseased organ. Treating appendicitis with antibiotics ignores the obstructive etiology and is to be condemned. Nonoperative therapy may be elected only if symptoms of several days' duration are subsiding, and there is a discrete right lower quadrant mass when the patient is first seen. Antibiotic and supportive therapy are continued as long as the patient's clinical improvement continues. Interval appendectomy should be done 6 to 8 weeks after complete subsidence of the mass.

Prompt operation is essential, but the patient must be adequately prepared. Preparation requires very little time in acute unruptured appendicitis. The fluid and electrolyte shifts in ruptured appendicitis, particularly if extensive peritonitis is present, are of considerable magnitude, however, and should be corrected before anesthesia is induced. The temperature should be brought below 39C by the use of antipyretics and cooling blankets before induction of anesthesia. This is particularly critical in children.

Preoperative Antibiotics. There is still no unanimity of opinion concerning the role of antibiotics as part of preoperative preparation. Nearly everyone starts antibiotics in patients who might have perforated appendicitis. The difference of opinion concerns patients with acute but unruptured appendicitis. There are currently three different practices: (1) Antibiotics are started preoperatively in all patients with a diagnosis of acute appendicitis. If appendicitis of any stage is found, antibiotics are continued for 3 to 5 days. (2) Antibiotics are started preoperatively in all patients. If gangrenous or perforative appendicitis is found, antibiotics are continued, but if less advanced appendicitis is found, no further antibiotics are given. (3) Antibiotics are started preoperatively only if perforative appendicitis is thought to be present. I prefer opinion two.

Antibiotics, alone and in various combinations, that have been reported to be effective include ampicillin, kanamycin, gentamicin, cephalothin, cephaloridine, cefamandole,[69a] and clindamycin. The bacterial flora customarily found in acute appendicitis is a mixed colonic flora with both aerobic and anaerobic organisms. Because the most important pathogen in appendicitis-related infections is *Bacteroides fragilis*,[70] an agent effective against this species (such as clindamycin) should be part of the regimen. I prefer clindamycin plus an aminoglycoside.

The Operation. Most surgeons prefer a muscle-splitting incision for appendicitis, because the integrity of the layers is not entirely dependent on the sutures, and wound complications such as dehiscence and hernia occur less often. The incision may be placed obliquely in the right lower quadrant (McBurney) or transversely at a level just below the umbilicus (Rockey-Davis).[71] If the appendix is abnormally situated because of malrotation or pregnancy, the incision should be centered over the point of maximal tenderness. Some surgeons prefer a lower right paramedian incision if the diagnosis is in doubt, particularly in females. If generalized peritonitis is present, a midline incision is preferred.

On opening the peritoneum, any fluid should be aspirated into a syringe for Gram stain, aerobic and anaerobic cultures (Chapters 12 and 34). If a diseased appendix is found, it is removed and no exploration is done. On the other hand, if the preoperative diagnosis is incorrect, a systematic search for the cause of the symptoms is carried out. Most often another lesion, which does not require operative correction, such as mesenteric adenitis or pelvic inflammatory disease, will be found. Next in frequency is no identifiable intra-abdominal pathology, and finally another lesion requiring operative therapy such as Meckel diverticulitis or carcinoma of the cecum is found (Table 40-1).

There is still no unanimity of opinion concerning the management of the appendiceal stump. The traditional method of ligation and inversion gives secure hemostasis and covers the contaminated stump but inverts an infected stump into a closed cavity, which risks an intramural abscess of the cecum. Ligation with fine plain catgut minimizes this risk. Inversion without ligation avoids the risk of intramural abscess but risks bleeding from the intramural branch of the appendiceal artery. Ligation without inversion avoids burying a contaminated stump within the wall of the cecum and gives secure hemostasis, but is objectionable because it leaves a contaminated surface free in the peritoneal cavity. Contamination of the peritoneum can occur from the dirty stump, and there can be more massive contamination if the ligature slips off or the stump necroses.

A pursestring suture encompassing the base of the appendix is the time-honored method of inversion. Alternate methods include a "Z-stitch" [72] and an aseptic Parker-Kerr basting suture.[73]

If perforation of the appendix has occurred, and the inflammatory process is successfully confined, a phlegmon or abscess will be found. The phlegmon, consisting of a conglutinated mass of appendix, omentum, and adjacent viscera, but without a localized collection of pus, is much more common than is abscess per se. In the past, it was sometimes the practice to simply drain an abscess without trying to remove the appendix. Six weeks or more after subsidence of the acute episode, an elective "interval" appendectomy was done. This required two hospital stays for the patient, the first often prolonged, and was attended by an appreciable morbidity. Advances in patient care, antibiotics, and widely available well-trained surgeons have made this approach obsolete. In most patients, it is possible and advisable to remove the diseased appendix and any devitalized tissue surrounding it. Aspirates of the fluid or necrotic debris should be cultured for aerobic and anaerobic bacteria and antibiotic sensitivity studies performed.

If unconfined perforated appendicitis with spreading or generalized peritonitis is encountered, the appendix should surely be removed to prevent continued contamination of the peritoneum. After obtaining cultures, the peritoneal cavity is thoroughly cleansed by copious, repeated irrigations with 37C Ringer lactate or normal saline solution containing 0.1 percent povidone-iodine until the suctioned return is clear (Chapter 34).

Drains. The role of intraperitoneal drains in the therapy of appendicitis continues to be an area of controversy [52] and is extensively discussed in Chapter 34. Most surgeons do not use drains in simple acute appendicitis, whereas most do drain localized collections of pus. The difference of opinion concerns generalized peritonitis. Proponents of drainage assert that soft drains placed in sites of predilection for secondary abscess formation such as appendix fossa, pelvis, and colonic gutter provide an evacuation route for pus. Drainage is considered especially necessary in infants and children because they handle peritonitis poorly. Opponents of drainage point out that it is physically and physiologically impossible to drain the peritoneal cavity, that drains are walled off within 24 hours and so do not prevent abscess formation. They feel that drains not only do no good, they are potentially harmful because they enhance the formation of adhesions around the drain. And finally, drains act as a two-way street, also allowing bacteria ingress to the peritoneal cavity.

Prospective randomized studies [74,75] have not clearly settled the question. Magarey et al [74] felt that peritoneal drainage was of no benefit after appendectomy and actually increased the number of days of postoperative fever in patients who had turbid peritoneal fluid, but no local abscess, at operation. Haller et al [75] found that transperitoneal drainage did not decrease morbidity or mortality. They concluded that specific intensive antibiotic therapy and supportive treatment are the most effective for children with generalized peritonitis. They no longer use drains in this condition. I do not use drains in adults either.

Prevention of Wound Infection. The majority of complications of appendicitis and appendectomy are septic. By far the most common septic complication is wound infection. This occurs in at least 10 percent, but is proportional to the degree of appendiceal inflammation. In one large series,[76] the incidence of wound infection was 0.3 percent with normal appendices, 7.4 percent with acute suppurative appendicitis, 16.4 percent with perforation and localized abscess, and 35 percent with perforation and generalized peritonitis. Clark [77] has reported that if the incision is closed primarily, the incidence of wound infection is 50 percent with gangrenous appendicitis and 80 percent with perforated appendicitis. Several measures are effective in reducing the wound infection rate; systemic antibiotics, local irrigation and applications to the wound, wound drainage, and delayed or nonclosure of the superficial layers of the incision.

Many studies [69a,74,78-81] have been designed to evaluate the efficacy of systemic antibiotics in reducing the incidence of wound infections. Some studies were controlled, some had historic controls only, and some used no control groups. Many different antibiotics and many different dosage schedules have been used. Most researchers have concluded that systemic antibiotics *are* effective in reducing the wound infection rate. For this purpose, a single dose given immediately before operation appears to be as effective as longer, several day courses. Antibiotics are probably less beneficial if the appendix is not perforated.[74] Since there are other measures that are effective in reducing the wound infection rate, the use of antibiotics is probably not warranted solely for the purpose of avoiding wound infections. If antibiotics are indicated for perforation, however, reduction in wound infections is a welcome by-product.

Of the many local irrigants, two are emerging as clearly effective in reducing wound infections. These are povidone-iodine as a wound wash, spray,[82] or pack, and ampicillin powder dusted on the wound.[83-85] Both kanamycin [86] and an ammonium bromide antiseptic solution [85] are ineffective. Diluted povidone-iodine would seem to be the preferable agent because there are few contraindications to its use (iodine sensitivity). It is toxic to tissue, however (Chapters 22 and 34).

Everson and associates [79] studied the effect on the wound infection rate of extraperitoneal wound drainage and systemic antibiotics, separately and combined. They showed that drainage alone significantly reduced the incidence of postoperative wound infection in patients with gangrenous or perforative appendicitis. When drainage was combined with a 3-day course of cephaloridine, there was a further significant reduction. It would seem that if all layers of the wound are to be closed in patients with gangrenous or perforative appendicitis, a drain down to the peritoneum should be used. An increasing number of surgeons, however, do not close the superficial layers of the wound when gangrenous or perforative appendicitis is encountered.

Essentially all postappendectomy wound infections involve the subcutaneous fat layer, and more than 90 percent have anaerobic organisms as the predominant pathogens. It is therefore rational to leave the subcutaneous fat and skin layers open, to be closed later as a delayed primary closure or allowed to granulate. Grosfeld and Solit [87] found a wound infection rate of 34 percent in patients with perforated appendicitis and primary wound closure, versus a 2.3 percent incidence if delayed closure was carried out. Stuart [88] reported 100 consecutive appendectomies without a single wound infection. Delayed primary closure was used in those patients in whom the risk of infection was high.

I use the following regimen for minimizing the incidence of postappendectomy wound infections (adults).

Preoperative intravenous antibiotics: 600 mg of clindamycin and 2.0 mg per kg of gentamicin (with renal impairment or allergy, give 200 mg of doxycycline instead). If the appendix is gangrenous or perforated, antibiotics are continued. The incision is thoroughly irrigated layer by layer with 1 percent povidone-iodine solution (1:9 dilution of stock povidone-iodine aqueous solution with normal saline). If the appendix is not gangrenous or perforated, the incision is closed primarily, without drainage. If it is gangrenous or perforated, subcutaneous fat and skin are packed open with povidone-iodine soaked gauze. Tissue colony counts [89] are done daily starting on the fourth day postoperatively. When the count is less than 10^5 colonies per gram of tissue the skin is loosely approximated. If the count stays above 10^5, the wound is left open to granulate.

Septic Complications of Appendicitis

Peritonitis. Perforation of the inflamed appendix and, to a lesser extent, gangrene of the appendix contaminate the peritoneal cavity with a complex spectrum of aerobic and anaerobic bacteria. The anaerobic organisms, particularly *B. fragilis*,[70] are more important as pathogens, but symbiotic support must be furnished by their aerobic partners to create an anaerobic environment if they are to thrive and proliferate.[90]

Bacteriology of Peritonitis after Appendiceal Perforation. *B. fragilis* can be isolated in about 85 percent of intra-abdominal abscesses.[70,91] Other anaerobes include *B. melaninogenicus*, *Peptococcus*, *Peptostreptococcus*, *Fusobacterium*, *Eubacterium*, and *Clostridium*. *E. coli* is by far the most common aerobic isolate, followed by other coliforms, *Pseudomonas*, *Klebsiella*, and enterococci.

Peritoneal Toilet. Thorough mechanical cleansing of all peritoneal surfaces is mandatory when operating for appendicitis with spreading peritonitis. All devitalized tissue and discrete foreign matter are meticulously removed, and the contaminated surfaces are washed with warm Ringer lactate solution until the solution returns clear. The final wash should consist of a liter of 1 percent povidone-iodine solution in saline. This is sloshed around for a minute or so and then suctioned as completely as possible. Although antibiotic washes have had mixed results,[86,92] povidone-iodine has been shown to be effective. Sindelar and Mason [93] randomized patients with bacterially contaminated peritoneal cavities into either saline irrigation or povidone-iodine irrigation groups. All received appropriate systemic antibiotics. There were nine abscesses in 88 patients in the control group and one abscess in 80 patients in the povidone-iodine group ($p \leq 0.05$).

Antibiotics. The choice of antibiotics is critical in these mixed intra-abdominal infections and changes from time to time as new antibiotics are developed and as resistant strains of bacteria develop. The rationale for combination therapy directed against both aerobes and anaerobes in feculent peritonitis has been extensively discussed in Chapter 34. A combination of clindamycin and an aminoglycoside has been successful in clinical intra-abdominal infections. Bartlett et al [94] controlled intra-abdominal sepsis in 90 percent of their patients by using clindamycin and gentamicin. Swenson and Lorber [95] were successful in 80 percent of patients with intra-abdominal sepsis by using clindamycin plus either gentamicin or kanamycin. Clindamycin alone, which is active against over 97 percent of anaerobic isolates, has been effective in controlling both anaerobic and mixed aerobic-anaerobic infections,[96] suggesting that the anaerobic component is the more important.

Penicillin G is effective against most anaerobic bacteria found in intra-abdominal sepsis yet it is ineffective therapy. It is now known that penicillin G is inactivated within intra-abdominal abscesses by beta-lactamase, which is produced by some resistant strains of *B. fragilis*.[97]

Similarly, the tetracyclines were once effective agents against anaerobic intra-abdominal bacteria. More than 50 percent of these organisms are now resistant to tetracyclines.

Chloramphenicol has a broad spectrum of activity against anaerobes and has been an effective agent both alone and combined in the treatment of intra-abdominal sepsis. As with penicillin G and tetracyclines, chloramphenicol does not seem as effective as it once was, even though resistant organisms have not been clearly demonstrated. Animal experiments suggest that production of nitro-reductase by anaerobic organisms inactivates chloramphenicol.[98]

Metronidazole, which is used in the United States principally for the treatment of trichomoniasis and giardiasis, has been successfully used in England to control intra-abdominal sepsis.[99,100] It has been effective both alone and in combination with gentamicin or ampicillin. Metronidazole is now available in parenteral form in the United States.

Abscesses. The incidence of intra-abdominal abscesses secondary to peritoneal contamination from gangrenous or perforated appendicitis has decreased markedly since the introduction of potent antibiotics. The sites of predilection for abscesses are the appendiceal fossa, pouch of Douglas, subhepatic space, and between bowel loops which are usually multiple. Other sites are seldom involved.

The symptoms of an intra-abdominal abscess often come on insidiously. The patient who seemed to be recovering stops improving or regresses. Fever recurs, though it may be a daily spike initially, with normothermia between fever spikes. Later, high spikes, often with shaking chills, signal septicemia. Anorexia, vomiting, ileus, and abdominal distention are frequent.

The problems of diagnosis and localization of intraperitoneal abscesses are discussed in Chapter 34. Physical findings depend on the location of the abscess(es) and may be unrevealing. Abdominal pain and tenderness to palpation are present and related to the site of the abscess. With a pelvic abscess, abdominal signs can be entirely absent, but its presence will be easily revealed by a digital rectal examination, which should be done daily in patients at risk for abscess formation. Jaundice can accompany a subhepatic or subphrenic collection and is a grave sign.

The white blood cell count, which usually starts back toward normal after operation, reverses and starts back up as the abscess enlarges. The left shift in the differential count also becomes more pronounced, particularly if the abscess is seeding the bloodstream. Blood samples should be drawn for culture (before restarting antibiotics if they had been stopped), which will usually confirm bacteremia. Stopping antibiotics to obtain positive blood cultures is dangerous if intraperitoneal sepsis is suspected.

Plain films of the abdomen, in addition to confirming the paralytic ileus, may identify the focus of the abscess by the presence of an air-fluid level outside the bowel, or by a localized collection of gas bubbles. Barium contrast radiography is not particularly helpful except to show displacement of gastrointestinal organs by the abscess.

The newer diagnostic modalities of gallium-67 scanning, ultrasonography, and computed tomography are proving to be helpful at times in obscure cases.[101,102] Gallium-67 citrate, given intravenously, localizes in areas of inflammation and in some neoplasms as well as being excreted into the colon. Thus, the bowel must be evacuated to allow the radioactivity in the abscess wall to be "seen." Because of the ileus associated with intra-abdominal sepsis, it may be difficult to clean out the bowel well enough. The other problem with gallium-67 is its lack of specificity. In Taylor's series,[103] abscesses were present in only 43 percent of patients with gallium uptake. Indium-111 autologous leukocyte scanning may prove to be better.[103a]

Ultrasonography is safe, noninvasive, comparatively inexpensive, and does not involve radiation. It is highly sensitive to detection of fluid collections and is therefore well suited to search for fluid-containing abscesses. A relatively high degree of skill is necessary to perform the examination, produce the images, and interpret the resulting cross-sectional scans. This may limit its usefulness outside large teaching centers. Another limitation is the inability of ultrasound to penetrate a gas-tissue interface—gas is nearly always present in abundance in a patient with intra-abdominal sepsis. Obesity also degrades the image.

In areas impermeable to sound waves (the gas of adynamic ileus or the bony pelvis), computed tomography is clearly preferable. It also is better in obese patients. A major disadvantage is its high cost. The amount of radiation to the patient was considerable in the early machines but is now at or below the amount received in a barium enema examination.

Treatment. Pus must be evacuated. Once an abscess forms, failure to drain only produces a prolonged course of illness that nearly always culminates in death.

Antibiotic therapy may be successful in the treatment of a localized phlegmon without a discrete collection of pus, but is less often successful in the treatment of a true abscess. Antibiotics are an essential adjunct to drainage of abscesses to prevent bacteremia and metastatic abscesses. See Chapter 34 for a more complete discussion of intra-abdominal abscesses.

Pylephlebitis. Suppurative thrombosis of the portal vein has fortunately become rare since the advent of antibiotics. Pus gains access to portal tributaries, which cause multiple metastatic liver abscesses. The onset is heralded by high spiking fevers, shaking chills, and deepening jaundice. Blood cultures will nearly always be positive at the time of the chill. The liver becomes moderately enlarged and tender to palpation and percussion. Liver function tests become progressively deranged but without a particular pattern. Because the abscesses are small and multiple, liver scan will show only some enlargement and generalized decreased uptake of isotope. Similarly, attempts to aspirate an abscess are usually unsuccessful.

Treatment consists of high doses of antibiotics. If no culture results are available, ampicillin-clindamycin-gentamicin should be used empirically. As soon as the patient's condition permits, the septic focus responsible for seeding the portal vein must be eradicated.

Intestinal Obstruction. Many patients with peritoneal contamination from a ruptured appendix can be expected to have a problem with intestinal obstruction. Early on, all have adynamic ileus from the septic peritonitis. Fibrous adhesions often produce a component of mechanical obstruction as well. It is often difficult to differentiate ileus from mechanical obstruction, but this does not become important until after the first 2 postoperative weeks. Intestinal problems during the early period can nearly always be managed by the judicious use of gastric and intestinal tubes. After about 2 weeks, the adhesions become fibrous, and operative relief of the obstruction is usually required. Intestinal obstruction from persistent fibrous adhesive bands also occurs months or years later. The mechanism of the formation of adhesions has been elucidated in recent years and is discussed in Chapter 34.[102]

Prognosis

In 1941 in the United States, there were 10,789 deaths attributed to acute appendicitis—a rate of 8.1 per 100,000. In 1976, there were 752 deaths—a rate of 0.4 per 100,000. This is a 20-fold reduction in 35 years. Nearly all deaths now are in the very young or in the old with perforative appendicitis. The death rate from acute unruptured appendicitis in patients between the ages of 6 and 60 approaches the mortality from anesthesia alone and is about 0.1 percent. The only way to further lower mortality will be to get a larger proportion of patients with appendicitis to the operating table before perforation has occurred.

INCIDENTAL APPENDECTOMY

The prophylactic "incidental" removal of an easily accessible appendix during the performance of another abdominal procedure is a generally accepted practice,[104] which adds little if any to the morbidity of the procedure.[105-109] It should not be done, however, as a part of a procedure that introduces foreign material, such as a placement of a prosthetic arterial graft. Some surgeons do not do incidental appendectomy in elderly patients because the incidence of acute appendicitis is low in this group.[110] On the other hand, appendicitis is a much more serious disease in the elderly. Because of this, the appendix should be removed if it can be safely done. There is no convincing evidence that appendectomy causes any detectable deficit in secretory immunoglobulin function or loss of resistance to cancer.[6] It is concluded that unless and until new evidence is presented, incidental appendectomy should be done as a worthwhile prophylactic procedure.

BIBLIOGRAPHY

DeBoer HHM (ed): Intra-abdominal Sepsis. Utrecht, Bunge Scientific Publishers, 1979.

Mason JH, Byrne MP, Gau FC: Surgery of the vermiform appendix. Surg Clin North Am 57:1303, 1977.

Schwartz SI, Shires GT, Spencer FC, Storer EH (eds): Principles of Surgery, 3rd ed. New York, McGraw-Hill, 1979.

Ziegler MM, Bishop HC: Incidental appendectomy. JAMA 239: 295, 1978.

REFERENCES

1. Fitz RH: Perforating inflammation of the vermiform appendix with special reference to its early diagnosis and treatment. Trans Assoc Am Physicians 1:107, 1886.
2. McVay JR: The appendix in relation to neoplastic disease. Cancer 17:929, 1964.
3. Bierman HR: Human appendix and neoplasia. Cancer 21:109, 1968.
4. Howie JG, Timperly WR: Cancer and appendectomy. Cancer 19:1138, 1966.
5. Berndt H: Is appendectomy followed by increased cancer risk? Digestion 3:187, 1970.
6. Moertel CG, Nobrega FT, Elveback LR, Wentz JR: A prospective study of appendectomy and predisposition to cancer. Surg Gynecol 138:549, 1974.
7. Perry DY, Cooper MD, Good RA: The mammalian homologue of the avian bursa of Fabricius. Surgery 64:614, 1968.
8. Georgollon P: The normal human appendix: a light and electron microscopic study. J Anat 126:87, 1978.
9. Walker WA, Isselbacher KJ: Intestinal antibodies. N Engl J Med 297:767, 1977.
10. DeGaris CF: Topography and development of the cecum-appendix. Ann Surg 113:540, 1941.
11. Buschard K, Kjaeldgaard A: Investigation and analysis of the position, fixation, length and embryology of the vermiform appendix. Acta Chir Scand 139:293, 1973.
12. Smithells RW: Thalidomide, absent appendix, and sweating. Lancet 1:1042, 1978.
13. Hwang JMS, Krumbhaar EB: Amount of lymphoid tissue of human appendix and its weight at different age periods. Am J Med Sc 199:75, 1940.
14. Alexopoulos C, Papayannis AG, Gardikas C: Increased proportion of B lymphocytes in human tonsils and appendices. Acta Haematol (Basel) 55:95, 1976.
15. Mizumoto T: B and T cells in lymphoid tissues of human appendix. Int Arch Allergy Appl Immunol 51:80, 1976.
16. Toma VA, Retief FP: Human vermiform appendix. Immunocompetent cell topography and cell-to-cell interactions in situ. J Immunol Methods 20:333, 1978.
17. Backman DE, Cooper MD: Early lymphoepithelial relationships in human appendix. Gastroenterology 68:1160, 1975.
18. Owen RL, Jones AL: Epithelial cell specialization within human Peyer's patches: an ultrastructural study of intestinal lymphoid follicles. Gastroenterology 66:189, 1974.
19. Cebra JJ, Kamat R, Gearhart P, Robertson SM, Tseng J: The secretory IgA system of the gut. In Immunology of the Gut. Ciba Foundation Symposium 46 (new series). Amsterdam, Elsevier, 1977, pp 5–28.
20. Brown WR: Relationships between immunoglobulins and the intestinal epithelium. Gastroenterology 75:129, 1978.
21. Bienenstock J: The physiology of the local immune response and the gastrointestinal tract. Prog Immunol 4:197, 1974.
22. Katz AJ, Rosen FS: Gastrointestinal complications of immunodeficiency syndromes. In Immunology of the Gut. Ciba Foundation Symposium 46 (new series). Amsterdam, Elsevier, 1977, pp 243–261.
23. Kraft SC: The intestinal immune response in giardiasis. Gastroenterology 76:877, 1979.
24. Grossman EB Jr: Chronic appendicitis. Surg Gynecol Obstet 146:596, 1978.
25. Savrin RA, Clausen K, Martin EW Jr, Cooperman M: Chronic and recurrent appendicitis. Am J Surg 137:355, 1979.
26. Castleman KB, Puestow CB, Sauer D: Is appendicitis decreasing in frequency? Arch Surg 78:794, 1959.
27. Noer T: Decreasing incidence of acute appendicitis. Acta Chir Scand 141:431, 1975.
28. Burkitt DP: The aetiology of appendicitis. Br J Surg 58:695, 1971.
29. Wangensteen OH: The genesis of appendicitis in the light of the functional behavior of the vermiform appendix. Proc Inst Med Chicago 12:1, 1939.
30. Poole PM, Wilson G: *Streptococcus milleri* in the appendix. J Clin Pathol 30:937, 1977.
31. Jepsen OB, Korner B, Lauritsen KB, Hancke AB, Anderson L, Henrichsen S, Brenøe E, Christiansen PM, Johansen A: *Yersinia enterocolitica* infection in patients with acute surgical abdominal disease. Scand J Infect Dis 8:189, 1976.

32. Vilinskas J, Tilton RC, Kriz JJ: A new clinical entity: human infection with *Yersinia* presenting as an acute abdomen. Am Surg 37:568, 1971.
33. Jackson RH, Kennedy J, Gardner PS, McQuillan J: Viruses in the aetiology of acute appendicitis. Lancet 2:711, 1966.
34. Zwalenberg CV: The relation of mechanical distention to the etiology of appendicitis. Ann Surg 41:437, 1905.
35. Wilkie DPD: The etiology of acute appendicular disease. Can Med Assoc J 22:314, 1930.
36. Wangensteen OH, Dennis C: Experimental proof of the obstructive origin of appendicitis in man. Ann Surg 110:629, 1939.
37. Bowers WF: Appendicitis: with special reference to its pathogenesis, bacteriology, and healing. Arch Surg 39:362, 1939.
38. Dennis C, Burige RE, Wangensteen OH: An inquiry into the functional capacity of the cecal appendage in representative birds and mammals. Surgery 7:372, 1940.
39. Wangensteen OH, Dennis C: The production of experimental acute appendicitis (with rupture) in higher apes by luminal obstruction. Surg Gynecol Obstet 70:799, 1940.
40. Burige RE, Dennis C, Varco RL, Wangensteen OH: Histology of experimental appendiceal obstruction (rabbit, ape and man). Arch Pathol 30:481, 1940.
41. Dennis C, Burige RE, Varco RL, Wangensteen OH: Studies in the etiology of acute appendicitis. An inquiry into the factors involved in the development of acute appendicitis following experimental obstruction of the appendiceal lumen of the rabbit. Arch Surg 40:929, 1940.
42. Blackwood WD, Bolinger RA, Lifson N: Some characteristics of the rabbit vermiform appendix as a secreting organ. J Clin Invest 52:143, 1973.
43. Marshak RH, Kurzban JD, Maklansky D, Lindner AE: Carcinoma of the cecum producing appendicitis. Am J Gastroenterol 69:108, 1978.
44. Munk JF: Villous adenoma causing acute appendicitis. Br J Surg 64:593, 1977.
45. Sakover RP, Trotta PC: Barium appendicitis. Arch Surg 111:1168, 1976.
46. Merten DF, Lebowitz ME: Acute appendicitis in a child associated with prolonged appendiceal retention of barium (barium appendicitis). South Med J 71:81, 1978.
47. Balch CM, Silver D: Foreign bodies in the appendix. Arch Surg 102:14, 1971.
48. Carey LS: Lead shot appendicitis in northern native people. J Can Assoc Radiol 28:171, 1977.
49. Smedresman P: *Ascaris lumbricoides* as an unusual cause of appendicitis in an 8 year old girl. Clin Pediatr 16:197, 1977.
50. McBurney C: Experience with early operative interference in cases of diseases of the vermiform appendix. NY State Med J 50:676, 1889.
51. Doraiswamy NV: The neutrophil count in childhood acute appendicitis. Br J Surg 64:342, 1977.
52. Law D, Law R, Eiseman B: The continuing challenge of acute and perforated appendicitis. Am J Surg 131:533, 1976.
53. Raftery AT: The value of the leukocyte count in the diagnosis of acute appendicitis. Br J Surg 63:143, 1976.
54. Shimkin PM: Radiology of acute appendicitis. Am J Roentgenol 130:1001, 1978.
55. Gill B, Cudmore RE: Significance of faecaliths in the diagnosis of acute appendicitis. Br J Surg 62:535, 1975.
56. Saebo A: Pneumoperitoneum associated with perforated appendicitis. Acta Chir Scand 144:115, 1978.
57. Jona JZ, Belin RP, Selke AC: Barium enema as a diagnostic aid in children with abdominal pain. Surg Gynecol Obstet 144:351, 1977.
58. Rajagopalan AE, Mason JH, Kennedy M, Pawlikowski J: The value of the barium enema in the diagnosis of acute appendicitis. Arch Surg 112:531, 1977.
59. Fee HJ Jr, Jones PC, Kadell B, O'Connell TX: Radiologic diagnosis of appendicitis. Arch Surg 112:742, 1977.
60. Stone HH, Sanders SL, Martin JD Jr: Perforated appendicitis in children. Surgery 69:673, 1971.
61. Bartlett RH, Eraklis AJ, Wilkinson RH: Appendicitis in infancy. Surg Gynecol Obstet 130:99, 1970.
62. Marchildon MB, Dudgeon DL: Perforated appendicitis: current experience in a children's hospital. Ann Surg 185:84, 1977.
63. White JJ, Santillana M, Haller JA Jr: Intensive in-hospital observation: a safe way to decrease unnecessary appendectomy. Am Surg 41:793, 1975.
63a. Leape LL, Ramenofsky ML: Laparoscopy for questionable appendicitis: Can it reduce the negative appendectomy rate? Ann Surg 191:410, 1980.
64. Anderson A, Bergdahl L: Acute appendicitis in patients over sixty. Am Surg 44:445, 1978.
65. Owens BJ III, Hamit HF: Appendicitis in the elderly. Ann Surg 187:392, 1978.
66. Goldenberg IS: Acute appendicitis in the aged. Geriatrics 10:324, 1955.
67. Gomez A, Wood M: Acute appendicitis during pregnancy. Am J Surg 137:180, 1979.
68. Zaitoon MM, Mrazek RG: Acute appendicitis associated with pregnancy, labor, and the puerperium. Am Surg 43:395, 1977.
69. Storer EH: Appendix. In Schwartz SI, Shires GT, Spencer FC, Storer EH (eds): Principles of Surgery, 3d ed. New York, McGraw-Hill, 1979, p 1257.
69a. Busuttil RW, Davidson RK, Fine M, Tompkins RK: Effects of prophylactic antibiotics in acute nonperforated appendicitis: a prospective, randomized, double-blind clinical study. 101st Annual Meeting, Am Surg Assoc, April, 1981, p 73.
70. Gorbach SL: Treatment of intraabdominal sepsis. Ann Intern Med 83:377, 1975.
71. Meade RH: The evolution of surgery for appendicitis. Surgery 55:741, 1964.
72. Adams JT: Z-stitch for inversion of the appendiceal stump. Surg Gynecol Obstet 127:1320, 1968.
73. Sterling JA: Aseptic closure of appendiceal stump. Surg Gynecol Obstet 115:508, 1962.
74. Magarey CJ, Chant ADB, Rickford CRK, Magarey JR: Peritoneal drainage and systemic antibiotics after appendectomy. Lancet 2:179, 1971.
75. Haller JA Jr, Shaker IJ, Donahoo JS, Schnaufer L, White JJ: Peritoneal drainage versus non-drainage for generalized peritonitis from ruptured appendicitis in children. Ann Surg 177:595, 1973.
76. Kazarian KK, Roeder WJ, Mersheimer WL: Decreasing mortality and increasing morbidity from acute appendicitis. Am J Surg 119:681, 1970.
77. Clark AW: Management of appendicitis. Br Med J 2:881, 1976.
78. Fine M, Busuttil RW: Acute appendicitis: efficiency of prophylactic preoperative antibiotics in the reduction of septic morbidity. Am J Surg 135:210, 1978.
79. Everson NW, Fossard DP, Nash JR, MacDonald RC: Wound infection following appendectomy: the effect of extra peritoneal wound drainage and systemic antibiotic prophylaxis. Br J Surg 64:236, 1977.
80. Leigh DA, Pease R, Henderson H, Simmons K, Russ R: Prophylactic lincomycin in the prevention of wound infection following appendectomy: a double-blind study. Br J Surg 63:973, 1976.

81. Foster PD, O'Toole RD: Primary appendectomy. The effect of prophylactic cephaloridine on postoperative wound infection. JAMA 239:1411, 1978.
82. Gilmore OJA, Martin TDM: Aetiology and prevention of wound infection in appendectomy. Br J Surg 61:281, 1974.
83. Andersen B, Bendtsen A, Holbraad L, Schantz A: Wound infections after appendectomy. Acta Chir Scand 138:531, 1972.
84. Rickett JWS, Jackson BT: Topical ampicillin in the appendectomy wound: report of a double-blind trial. Br J Med 4:206, 1969.
85. Tanphiphat C, Sangsubhan C, Vongvaravipatr V, La-Ongthong B, Chodchoy V, Treesaranuvatana S, Ittipong P: Wound infection in emergency appendectomy: a prospective trial with topical ampicillin and antiseptic solution irrigation. Br J Surg 65:89, 1978.
86. Sherman JO, Luck SR, Borger JA: Irrigation of the peritoneal cavity for appendicitis in children: a double-blind study. J Pediatr Surg 11:371, 1976.
87. Grosfeld JL, Solit RW: Prevention of wound infection in perforated appendicitis: experience with delayed primary wound closure. Ann Surg 168:891, 1968.
88. Stuart M: The role of delayed primary wound closure in the prevention of wound sepsis after appendectomy. Med J Aust 2:421, 1976.
89. Robson MC, Krizek TJ, Heggers JP: Biology of surgical infections. In Current Problems in Surgery 10:3, 1973.
90. Stone HH: Bacterial flora of appendicitis in children. J Pediatr Surg 11:37, 1976.
91. Leigh DA, Simmons K, Norman E: Bacterial flora of the appendix fossa in appendicitis and post-operative wound infection. J Clin Pathol 27:997, 1974.
92. Stewart DJ, Matheson NA: Peritoneal lavage in appendicular peritonitis. Br J Surg 65:54, 1978.
93. Sindelar WF, Mason GR: Intraperitoneal irrigation with povidone-iodine solution for the prevention of intra-abdominal abscesses in the bacterially contaminated abdomen. Surg Gynec Obstet 148:409, 1979.
94. Bartlett JG, Miao PVW, Gorbach SL: Empiric treatment with clindamycin and gentamicin of suspected sepsis due to anaerobic and aerobic bacteria. J Infect Dis 135:580, 1977.
95. Swenson RM, Lorber B: Clindamycin and carbenicillin in treatment of patients with intra-abdominal and female genital tract infections. J Infect Dis 135:540, 1977.
96. Gorbach SL, Thadepalli H: Clindamycin in pure and mixed anaerobic infections. Arch Intern Med 134:87, 1974.
97. Joiner KA, Gorbach SL: Antimicrobial therapy of digestive diseases. In Clinics in Gastroenterology. 8:3, 1979.
98. Louie TJ, Bartlett JG, Onderdonk AB, Gorbach SL: Failure of chloramphenicol therapy of experimental intra-abdominal sepsis. 17th Interscience Conference on Antimicrobial Agents and Chemotherapy, New York, 1977.
99. Willis AT, Ferguson IR, Jones PH, Phillips KD, Tearle PV, Berry RB, Fiddian RV, Graham DF, Harland DHC, Innes DB, Mee WM, Rothwell-Jackson RL, Sutch I, Kilbey C, Edwards D: Metronidazole in prevention and treatment of *Bacteroides* infections after appendectomy. Br Med J 1:318, 1976.
100. Eykyn SH, Phillips I: Metronidazole and anaerobic sepsis. Br Med J 2:1418, 1976.
101. Korobkin M, Callen PW, Filly RA, Hoffer PB, Shimshak RR, Kressel HY: Comparison of computed tomography, ultrasonography, and gallium-67 scanning in the evaluation of suspected abdominal abscess. Radiology 129:89, 1978.
102. Hau T, Payne WD, Simmons RL: Fibrinolytic activity of the peritoneum during experimental peritonitis. Surg Gynecol Obstet 148:415, 1979.
103. Taylor KJW, Sullivan DC, Wasson JFM, Rosenfield AT: Ultrasound and gallium for the diagnosis of abdominal and pelvic abscesses. Gastrointest Radiol 3:281, 1978.
103a. Ascher NL, Forstrom L, Simmons RL: Radiolabeled autologous leukocyte scanning in abscess detection. World J Surg 4:392, 1980.
104. Hayes RJ: Incidental appendectomies. Current Teaching. JAMA 238:31, 1977.
105. Pollock AV, Evans M: Wound sepsis after cholecystectomy: effect of incidental appendicectomy. Br Med J 1:20, 1977.
106. Thal ER, Guzetta PC, Krupski WC, Jones RC: Morbidity of appendectomy in patients with acute salpingitis. Am Surg 43:403, 1977.
107. Pollack AV, Evans M: Wound sepsis: effect of incidental appendicectomy. Br Med J 2:124, 1977.
108. Waters EG: Elective appendectomy with abdominal and pelvic surgery. Obstet Gynecol 50:511, 1977.
109. Ziegler MM, Bishop HC: Incidental appendectomy. JAMA 239:295, 1978.
110. Nockerts SR, Detmer DE, Fryback DG: Incidental appendectomy in the elderly? No. Surgery 88:301, 1980.

CHAPTER 41
Anal and Perianal Infections

PATRICK F. HAGIHARA AND RICHARD J. HOWARD

Only a single layer of columnar epithelium in the rectum or multilayered squamous epithelium in the anus intervene between the feces (which contains 10^{11} bacteria per gram) and the perineal tissues. This barrier is so efficient that few infections result. Even if the barrier is interrupted by operation, the wounds most often heal without infection. No one knows whether the soft tissues of this region are intrinsically more resistant to infection than other areas.

Yet infections of the anorectal region can occur both with fecal bacteria and with exogenous microorganisms. If host defenses are compromised (ie, diabetes mellitus, immunosuppression, chemotherapy, leukemia, aplastic anemia), such infections can be florid and even fatal.

Treatment of anorectal infections requires a thorough knowledge of the regional anatomy and the proper preoperative localization of the infection to a given anatomic space or spaces. The relationship of the infection or fistulous tract to local muscular structures should also be defined preoperatively in order to choose the best surgical approach. Hasty attempts at treatment without adequate preoperative evaluation may result in inaccurate diagnosis or irretrievable damage to normal anorectal function.

SURGICAL ANATOMY OF THE ANORECTUM

The rectum extends from the rectosigmoid junction, which can be marked by a distinct flexure as the terminal sigmoid turns sharply downward in the curve of the sacrum. The anal canal is approximately 3 cm long, extending from the distal rectum to join the skin of the perineum. The anal canal is the part of the distal alimentary tract that is encompassed by the anal sphincters, and is below the sling of the levator ani muscle (Fig. 41-1).

The rectum and upper portion of the anus are lined by a mucosa, which is for the most part columnar epithelium. The cells take on a more cuboid and transitional appearance just above the dentate line. The distal 2 cm of the anal canal are lined by stratified squamous epithelium—modified skin devoid of hair, sebaceous, or sweat glands.

The junction of the upper mucosal and lower cutaneous portions of the anal canal is demarcated by a row of anal valves, referred to as the pectinate or dentate line because of the serrated appearance produced by the valves (Fig. 41-1). The dentate line is the junction of the embryologic hindgut and the proctodeum.

Above the dentate line, the mucosa is thrown into 8 to 14 folds known as the rectal columns or columns of Morgagni (Fig. 41-1). Two adjacent columns are joined by an anal valve at the dentate line. Each valve creates a small proximal pit called the anal crypt, anal sinus, or sinus of Morgagni. Foreign material may lodge in these crypts and initiate infection.

Anal glands or ducts extend from the mucosa through the wall of the anal canal (Fig. 41-1). Normally, four to eight such glands can be found. Each has a direct opening into an anal crypt, but not every anal crypt has a gland opening into it. The anal ducts ramify in the submucosa above and below the dentate line. Some of these glands extend into the internal anal sphincter and intersphincteric regions, so that infection can penetrate from the anal canal into the submucosal and intersphincteric spaces.

The relationships of the anorectum to the surrounding spaces and muscles are important, because infections can be confined to these spaces, and an appreciation of the normal anatomy (Fig. 41-2) will permit proper treatment without the risk of destroying normal anorectal function.

One-third to one-half of the rectum lies above the peritoneal reflection. The portion below the peritoneum is surrounded by the supralevator or pelvirectal space, a space filled with loose areolar tissue and fat (Fig. 41-2A). This space is confined by the peritoneum above, the pelvic wall laterally, and the levator ani muscles below. The ischiorectal space is bounded by the levator ani muscles superiorily, the external sphincter medially, the ischium laterally, and the perineal skin inferiorly (Fig. 41-2A).

The muscles of the anorectum hold the anus closed except during defecation, an act that requires the complex integration of sensory, cerebral, and muscular activities. The internal anal sphincter is a thickened continuation of the inner circular smooth muscle of the rectum (Fig. 41-1). The external anal sphincter, a striated muscle, extends below the internal sphincter and fuses with the puborectalis portion of the levator ani muscle at the upper end (Fig. 41-2B). Between the internal and external sphincter lies a thin layer of longitudinal muscle fibers. This layer of smooth muscle is a continuation of the outer longitudinal layer of the rectum, which is joined by some straited muscle fibers of the levator ani.

The levator ani muscle is a broad, thin muscle that attaches to the inner surface of the side of the pelvis and

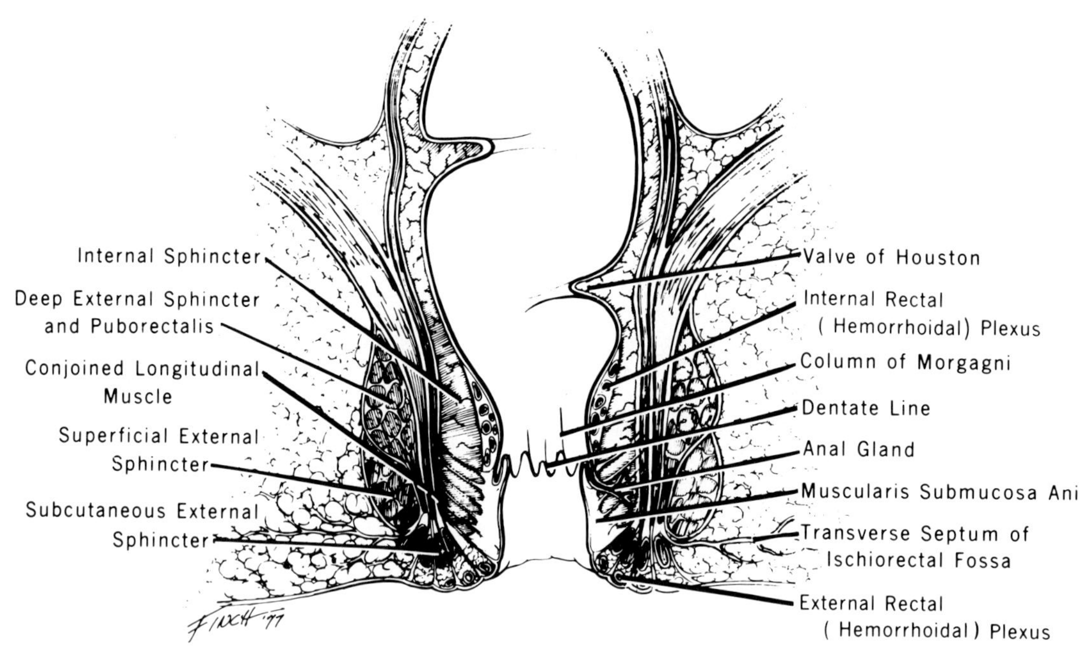

Fig. 41-1. **Coronal section of the rectum and anal canal, showing sphincter muscles and the lining of the anal canal. (Figures 41-1 to 41-8 from Storer EH, Goldberg SM, Nivatvongs S: Colon, rectum, and anus. In Schwartz SI, Shires GT, Spencer FC, Storer EH (eds): *Principles of Surgery* (3rd edition). New York: McGraw-Hill Book Company, 1979, p 1191.)**

medially unites with its fellow on the opposite side, thereby forming the greater part of the pelvic floor. The levator ani can be divided into three parts, depending on its pelvic site of origin. The iliococcygeus originates from the ischial spine and posterior part of the pelvic fascia covering the obturator internus, and inserts into the sacrum and anococcygeal raphe. The pubococcygeus originates from the back of the pubis and anterior part of the obturator fascia and fuses with its fellow on the opposite side posterior to the rectum to form a fibrous band, the anococcygeal raphe. Finally, the puborectalis originates from the back of the pubis and fuses with its contralateral pair to form a sling behind the rectum at the anorectal junction.

The anorectal ring is a functionally important ring of muscles, which surrounds the rectum and anal canal. This ring is composed of the upper borders of the internal and external sphincters, which completely encircle the anorectum and the medial aspects of the puborectalis sling. The puborectalis muscle does not contribute to the anorectal ring anteriorly. Appreciation of this ring is important in the treatment of fistulas and abscesses, because complete division invariably results in rectal incontinence.

ANORECTAL ABSCESS

Etiology and Pathogenesis

Most of the common anorectal abscesses originate as an infection of the anal ducts and glands, whether or not actual connection to the ducts is demonstrable.[1-3] Occlusion of the duct with feces or infective material initiates infection of the entire anal duct. By the time infection becomes clinically evident, most cases have developed frank suppuration. In a small number of cases, cryptitis, papillitis, or cellulitis may be present.

Because the termination of the anal gland lies between the internal sphincter and the longitudinal intersphincteric muscle fibers, an intersphincteric abscess forms (Fig. 41-3). The infection may then continue downward along the longitudinal muscle fibers and emerge subcutaneously at the anal orifice as a perianal abscess. If the pus migrates laterally through the longitudinal muscle and external sphincter, it enters the ischiorectal space and leads to an ischiorectal abscess. Upward extension in the intersphincteric space gives rise to a high intermuscular abscess. It may then break through the longitudinal muscle into the pelvirectal space to cause a supralevator or pelvirectal abscess (Fig. 41-3B).

If the theory of anal gland infection and intersphincteric abscess formation as the first step in the formation of most anorectal abscesses is correct, one would expect most anorectal abscesses to have an internal opening at the level of the anal valves and a definable intersphincteric abscess component. In many acute anorectal abscesses, an internal opening cannot be demonstrated, and external drainage leads to healing without development of a fistula into the anal canal.

The majority of anorectal abscesses involve the perianal and ischiorectal regions (Fig. 41-3B), and in the vast majority of cases, *S. aureus* or gram-negative enteric bacteria are the etiologic agents. Multiple organisms can usually be cultured. Dark yellow pus can be expressed from the abscess cavity. The surrounding tissues are edematous, and

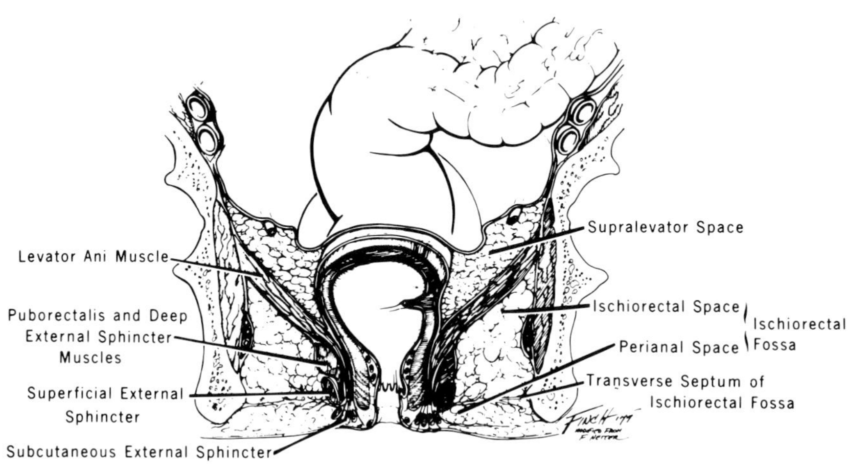

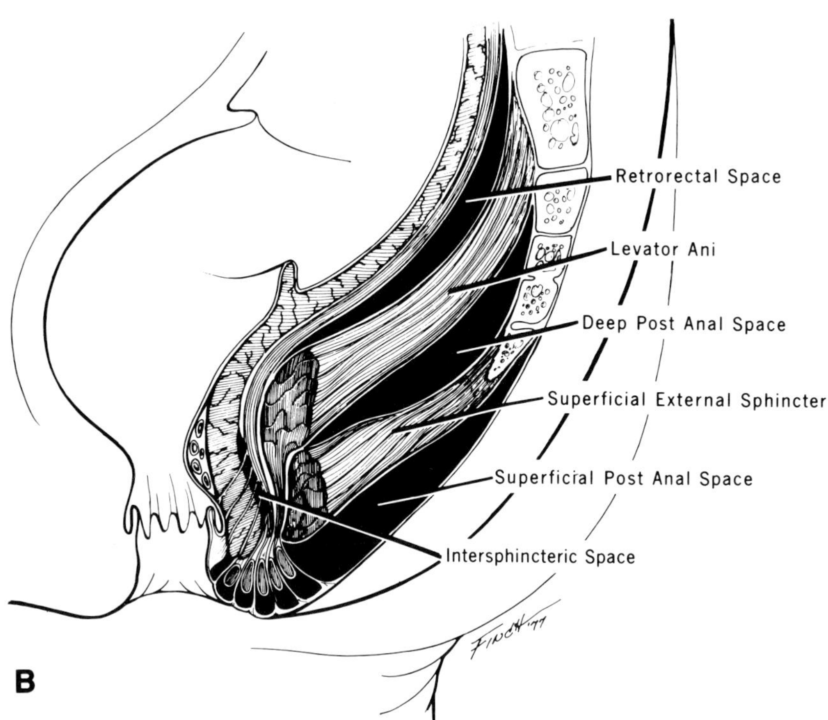

Fig. 41-2. **A. Coronal section of the perianal and perirectal spaces. B. Sagittal section of the perianal and perirectal spaces.**

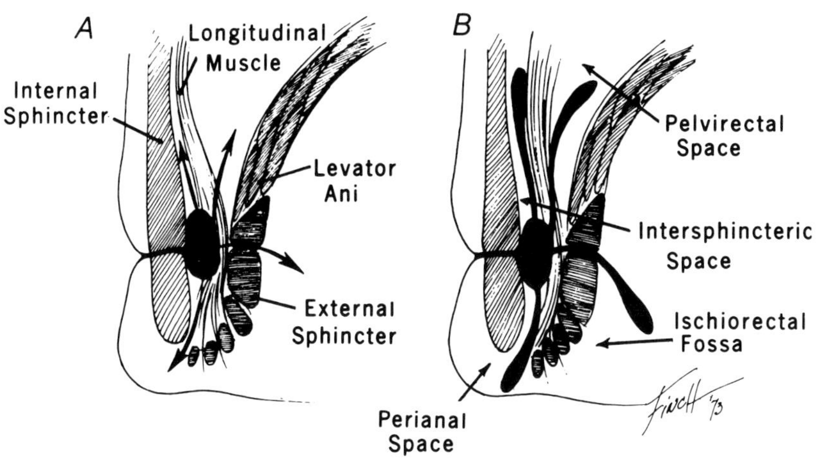

Fig. 41-3. **A. Pathways of infection from the intersphincteric space at the base of the anal duct. B. The intersphincteric abscess then spreads to form perianal, ischiorectal, or pelvirectal abscesses.**

the areolar tissue may be necrotic. In neglected cases, the muscles may also be destroyed.

While the majority of anorectal abscesses are thought to begin with infection of the anal glands, other conditions can also give rise to abscess formation—foreign bodies, anal fissure, gangrene of hemorrhoids, tuberculosis, Crohn disease, and ulcerative colitis.[4,5] In fact, any break in the lining of the anal canal will permit bacteria to penetrate the epithelial lining.[6] Supralevator (pelvirectal) abscesses can also be due to intra-abdominal disease such as acute appendicitis, acute salpingitis, and diverticulitis.

Clinical Manifestations

The initial symptom of most anorectal abscesses is severe acute pain in the anal region. The pain is usually throbbing and is aggravated by sitting, walking, and sudden increases in abdominal pressure, such as occur in sneezing and coughing. Defecation is also painful. Large abscesses may be accompanied by fever. Submucosal or high intermuscular abscesses usually do not cause severe anal pain; rather, the patient feels a dull aching in the rectum. The abscess may rupture spontaneously into the rectum, and the patient complains of passage of pus. A pelvirectal abscess by itself is not usually accompanied by rectal or anal pain—fever and constitutional symptoms may be the initial presentation.

Perianal Abscess. Examination of a perianal abscess shows an inflamed, tender, raised region adjacent to the anus. At a later stage, fluctuation occurs and the skin may become purple or necrotic, allowing pus to escape. The patient may not permit examination of the anal canal without anesthesia, but digital examination reveals no induration or bulging of the corresponding part of the anal canal.

Intersphincteric Abscess. Intersphincteric abscesses most frequently present posteriorly in the midline. The anal pain is somewhat higher than that due to a perianal abscess. Inability to perform a digital rectal examination because of the intense pain may suggest its presence. A posterior midline intersphincteric abscess frequently dissects into the postanal space and localizes there. Tenderness and swelling may be felt posteriorly in the midline by digital anal examination, and perianally posteriorly in the midline. Bidigital examination may allow further definition of this form of abscess. The abscess may extend laterally, into the perianal or ischiorectal space to become a horseshoe abscess. Under such circumstances, swelling, tenderness, and redness may be evident around the anus. If a horseshoe abscess exists, an abscess should be suspected posteriorly because an anterior intersphincteric abscess is only rarely the cause. Digital anal examination of a patient with a high intermuscular abscess or submucosal abscess reveals a highly localized, superficial tender swelling in the rectal wall.

Ischiorectal Abscess. An ischiorectal abscess causes a more diffuse swelling on one side of the anus. Digital examination reveals bulging into the rectum with induration on that side. Abscesses high in the ischiorectal space may produce no obvious external signs, and the only finding may be tenderness and induration on digital rectal examination.

Supralevator Abscess. A supralevator abscess is palpated as a high bulging mass outside of the rectum. It can be difficult to distinguish this form of abscess from a high ischiorectal abscess. Because a supralevator abscess is quite uncommon, one should consider intra-abdominal abscesses such as those originating from appendicitis, diverticulitis, or pelvic inflammatory disease before diagnosing a supralevator abscess. The lower abdomen may be somewhat tender on deep palpation. The concurrent or recent presence of more frequent forms of anorectal abscesses is a good clue to the diagnosis of supralevator abscess arising from anal duct infection.

Anorectal abscesses usually do not spontaneously subside. Infection continues until they are either drained or spontaneously burst through the rectum, perianal skin, anoderm, or anal canal.

Treatment

While cellulitis around the anus and rectum almost always proceeds to suppuration, occasionally some cases of cellulitis may respond to antibiotic therapy.

Perianal abscesses can be drained in the office with the aid of local anesthesia. Xylocaine can be injected into the overlying skin, or ethyl chloride spray can be used to freeze the overlying skin. Incision and drainage can then be accomplished. A sample of the purulent drainage should be sent for culture. The wound should be explored gently with the finger or a blunt instrument to divide septa and to bring secondary abscesses into communication with the main cavity. General, spinal, epidural, or caudal anesthesia facilitates examination and exploration of the wound.

An internal fistulous opening can also be sought with adequate anesthesia by attempting to pass a probe from the abscess into the anal canal. This procedure must be performed gently to avoid creating a false passage. In the majority of cases, no fistulous opening will be found. Most often, drainage only should be performed, and primary fistulotomy should be avoided. Primary fistulotomy can be successfully done only if the opening is low on the anal canal.[7] Most fistulotomies should be delayed until the inflammation from the abscess subsides. The patient is begun on sitz baths, at least twice a day, the day after operation. The anal pain subsides rapidly following operation.

General or regional anesthesia is necessary in other anorectal abscesses for proper localization and for determining the most appropriate site for drainage. Intersphincteric abscess may be unroofed by incising the anoderm and the mucosa and extending this incision through the internal anal sphincter. If the abscess is in the postanal space of Courtney, the space is opened in the perianal area, and the subcutaneous external anal sphincter is incised and the fibers of the superficial external anal sphincter are separated. The overlying internal anal sphincter is divided caudally. If extension into a horseshoe abscess is encountered, each limb should be drained.

High intermuscular abscesses should be unroofed by incising the overlying rectal mucosa and muscles, using an anal speculum. Occasionally, the abscess will already have drained into the rectum, and there may even be sloughing of the overlying mucosa. In these cases, the opening into the abscess cavity should be made larger to provide better drainage.

Ischiorectal abscesses may be drained with an incision in the perianal skin overlying the abscess. It is helpful to have a finger in the rectum in order to guide a clamp into the abscess once the skin incision has been made. Connection into the rectum should be avoided.

A supralevator abscess may be drained through the perianal skin. A scalpel or clamp can be pushed up through the supralevator muscle into the abscess (Fig. 41-4). A finger in the rectum may be useful to guide the instrument into the abscess. The abscess may also be drained into the rectum.

Drains are not usually necessary after evacuation of the pus. If abscesses are deep—as with a high ischiorectal or supralevator abscess—drains may be kept in for several days and then removed. The abscess cavity should not be packed. Packing may not allow the cavity to collapse and may encourage cellulitis.

Antibiotics are usually not required for perianal abscesses and for most other anorectal abscesses. Broad-spectrum antibiotics should be initiated prior to drainage if the patient is a compromised host (ie, receiving immunosuppressive therapy or chemotherapy), has a lymphoproliferative disorder, diabetes, or aplastic anemia, or has a foreign body elsewhere (ie, prosthetic valve). Antibiotic therapy should be continued for several days until the cavity wall is granulating. Antibiotics should also be added if the abscess is large or deep so that normal tissues have to be traversed to enter the abscess.

The empiric choice of antibiotic should reflect the fecal flora found in most cases—gram-negative enteric bacteria, enterococci, anaerobic gram-positive cocci, and anaerobic gram-negative bacilli (especially *B. fragilis*). For deep infections and infections in compromised hosts, hospitalization and intravenous treatment with an aminoglycoside plus clindamycin would seem rational. If enterococci are isolated, ampicillin may be added. Single agent regimens using chloramphenicol or cefoxitin should be effective empiric choices pending the return of culture and sensitivity results. In normal patients who are adequately drained, antibiotic therapy need not be continued for longer than the time necessary to control the cellulitis that surrounds the infection.

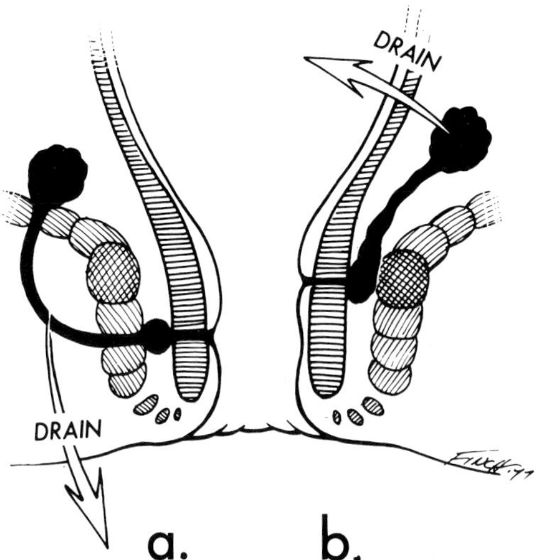

Fig. 41-4. **Two routes of drainage of supralevator abscesses. A. The usual perianal transcutanous route, useful even for abscesses that do not extend into the ischiorectal space, such as that shown in B, a transrectal drainage route, which is rarely used.**

Prognosis

In about half the patients, drainage alone is adequate treatment. In the other half, fistula-in-ano will develop. If drainage is properly done, fistulas are not complicated and are easily treated at a later time. Untreated anorectal abscesses lead to destruction of the surrounding normal structures. Necrotizing fasciitis may even develop in some cases (Chapter 25). Improper drainage may lead to recurrent abscess, complicated fistulas, or anal incontinence.

FISTULA-IN-ANO

A fistula is an unnatural connection between two epithelial lined surfaces. In fistula-in-ano, the two surfaces are the skin of the perianal region and the epithelium of the anal canal or rectum.

Etiology and Pathogenesis

Fistula-in-ano usually follows an acute anorectal abscess.[2] About 50 percent of all anorectal abscesses, which presumably originate in the anal duct gland, develop fistula-in-ano after proper surgical drainage. Experience indicates that when an anorectal abscess is allowed to drain spontaneously or is drained inadequately, the chances of its developing into a fistula-in-ano are even greater. A tract that has only one opening may still be called a fistula-in-ano if the tract is thought to originate in infection of the anal duct gland.

While most fistulas-in-ano appear without any specific predisposing cause, in some cases specific diseases or infections lead to anorectal abscess or fistula-in-ano. The most important of these causes is Crohn disease,[4,5] especially Crohn colitis.[4,5] Ulcerative colitis and malignant neoplasms of the anus and rectum (especially colloid carcinoma) also predispose to fistula-in-ano. *M. tuberculosis* may be a cause of anorectal abscess and fistula. Foreign bodies such as swallowed bone fragments and eggshells may lodge in the anus or lower rectum and act as a nidus of persistent infection. In some cases, congenital tract lined by transitional epithelium may be causes of repeated infection. Occasionally, diverticulitis, Crohn disease, and other intra-abdominal conditions can fistulize directly to the perineum from an intra-abdominal source.[8]

A part of the tract of fistula-in-ano is usually located in the intersphincteric zone between the internal anal sphincter and the external anal sphincter (Fig. 41-5A). The internal opening is usually found at an anal crypt and may be epithelial lined. The external opening is usually in the perianal area near the anal verge and is usually lined by granulation tissue. The tract may traverse through the external anal sphincter at various levels (Fig. 41-5B), in some cases quite cephalad (Fig. 41-5C). Fistulous tracts may be

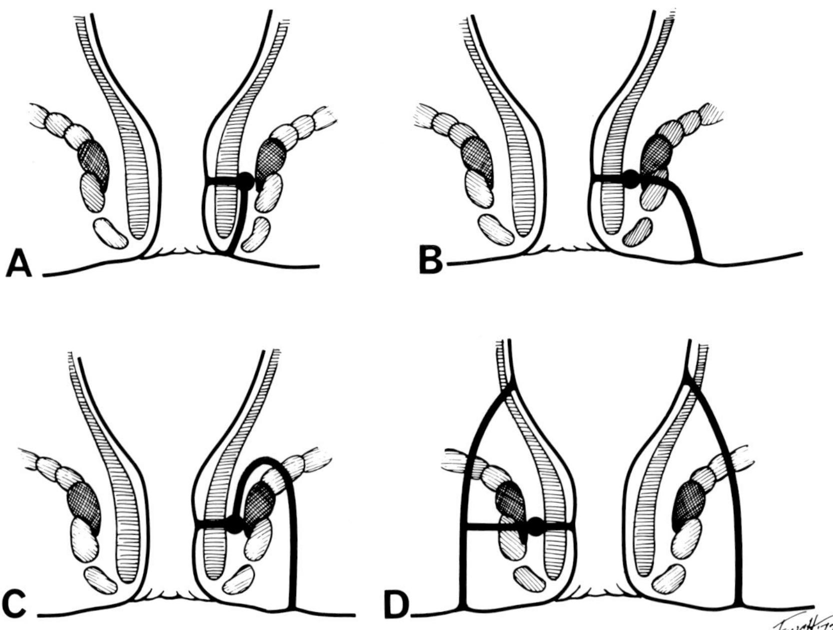

Fig. 41-5. **The four main anatomic types of fistula: A. intersphincteric (most common), B. trans-sphincteric (frequent), C. suprasphincteric (uncommon), D. extrasphincteric (rare).**

multiple, and more than one external opening may be found. It is less common to find more than one internal opening (Fig. 41-5D). A small internal opening may not allow passage of a probe, or it may be obliterated.

Classification

In order to apply proper treatment, some form of anatomic classification should be used. Accurate classification may be most difficult in just those cases where precise anatomic understanding is most crucial. In the classification of Milligan and Morgan,[9] the levels to which the cephalad end ascends are used to divide the fistulas-in-ano into low anal, high anal, and anorectal fistulas. Low anal fistulas have tracts that do not extend above the level of the anal crypts and usually open into the anal canal at this level. In a high anal fistula, the tract is above the level of the anal crypts but is below the anorectal ring. Anorectal fistulas have tracts above the level of the anorectal ring and thus lie opposite both the anal canal and the lower part of the rectum. With this classification, however, a fistula traversing the ischiorectal fossa, whose cephalad extension is at the inferior surface of the levator ani muscle, would be classified as an anorectal fistula, as would one that penetrates through the levator ani and into the rectum. Treatment is vastly different for these two types of fistula-in-ano. A fistulous tract that ascends in the intersphincteric zone to the rectum just deep to the circular muscle of the rectum is also an anorectal fistula by this definition, but its treatment is relatively simple.

Parks et al[10,11] have made a more useful classification—intersphincteric, transsphincteric, suprasphincteric, and extrasphincteric (Fig. 41-5). All, except the extrasphincteric fistula, pass through the internal anal sphincter. The tract of an intersphincteric fistula is deep to the internal anal sphincter or circular muscle of the rectum. The most common fistula-in-ano is an intersphincteric fistula, which dissects down into the anal verge or perianal area. If it dissects upward, it may be difficult to define by digital anal examination. Most of those labeled as high submucous or intermuscular are of this variety. Suprasphincteric fistulas dissect proximally between the internal and external anal sphincters from the level of anal crypt and pass cephalad over the puborectalis, then penetrate down into the ischiorectal fossa and then through the perianal skin (Fig. 41-5C). Extrasphincteric fistulas pass cephalad through the perianal skin outside of the external anal sphincter and puborectalis and penetrate through the levator ani (Fig. 41-5D). The internal opening may be in the rectum and may not be in the anus. The etiology of this type of fistula-in-ano may not be in the infection of the anal duct gland.

Fistulas-in-ano should also be viewed in a horizontal plane. Goodsall's rule states that if a line is drawn transversely across the center of the anus, a fistula with a cutaneous opening anterior to this line usually runs directly into the anal canal, whereas one with a cutaneous opening posterior to this line has a curved course, which terminates in the midline of the posterior wall of the anal canal (Fig. 41-6). There are many exceptions to Goodsall's rule, however.

High posterior fistulas, which are usually the result of ischiorectal abscesses that extend from the infection in the space of Courtney, are likely to follow a horseshoe pattern. The tract proceeds anteriorly through the ischiorectal space surrounding the anus so that there are two limbs, one on each side of the anus; in some, one limb may be incomplete. The infection of the space of Courtney usually follows an infection of the anal duct gland posteriorly in midline. The infection then dissects between the superficial and deep part of the external anal sphincter to reach the space of Courtney. Occasionally, dissection occurs between the puborectalis and the deep part of the

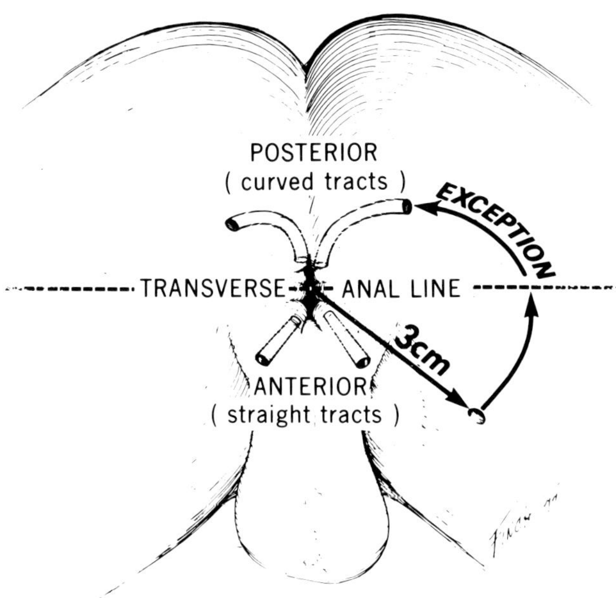

Fig. 41-6. **Goodsall's rule.**

external anal sphincter.[12] Thus, basically, a horseshoe fistula is a trans-sphincteric fistula-in-ano.

Clinical Manifestations

Usually, a history of anorectal abscess is present. Frequently, the preceding abscess had been surgically drained or had drained spontaneously with relief of symptoms. The opening persists to become the external opening of a fistula-in-ano. Purulent, and at times serosanguineous, drainage persists in small amounts. Pruritis ani or a sense of wetness may be present because of the persistent or intermittent drainage. Spontaneous healing of a well-established fistula-in-ano is rare, but intermittent breakdown is common. Some low-lying epithelial-lined fistulas are asymptomatic. A variety of malignant tumors have been found in long-standing fistulas—the most common is colloid carcinoma. It is more likely, however, that the colloid carcinoma was primary and fistulization occurred later. Although many fistulas-in-ano show stability over a long time, some may extend to become complex, rendering simple surgical solutions unsuccessful. It is always a potential source of sepsis, which is at times life-threatening.[13]

Inspection of the perianal area and anal verge, digital anal examination, and proctoscopy should be standard procedures. Further examination, including colonoscopy, tuberculin test, chest roentgenogram, and barium stool studies of the upper gastrointestinal tract and colon may be required, depending on the initial evaluation. The external opening of a fistula-in-ano is usually single but may be multiple. The opening may be found at the top of raised granulation tissue or in a slightly depressed area. If the opening is temporarily healed, it is marked by a raised, red papilla. Usually, a fibrous tract is palpable from the external opening leading to its internal opening. The internal opening of a fistula-in-ano may be identified as a depression at the dentate line on anoscopy and on digital anal examination. When the internal opening is located elsewhere, it may be surrounded by granulation tissue.

Injection of contrast material to define the tract may shed further light on complex, deep, or difficult fistulas-in-ano. This procedure should be done before operation.

Goodsall's rule is particularly helpful for complete and correct identification of a fistula-in-ano under anesthesia just before definitive surgical treatment. Under anesthesia, the tract can be probed in either direction. Through the external opening, the tip of the probe may be inserted, and with the guidance of the examiner's index finger in the anus, the tip may be passed through the internal opening. A prominent crypt may be probed with a hooked probe or bent malleable silver probe. At times, traction on the external opening with a clamp will cause dimpling of the internal opening, which is otherwise difficult to recognize. A malleable silver probe is versatile and should be available in any operation on fistula-in-ano. Gentleness in probing avoids creating a false passage.

Accurate and complete delineation of the tracts and openings is important to obtain a cure and minimize the consequence of anal incontinence from surgical division of the puborectalis or a major portion of the external anal sphincter. Correct anatomic classifications of the fistula (Fig. 41-5), according to its relationship to the muscles of the sphincter, is essential in planning the proper surgical treatment. Although more complete examination is possible under anesthesia at the time of operation, the relationship to the puborectalis may be more clearly defined on digital anal examination before operation. Anesthesia may so relax the puborectalis muscle that the relationship of the fistula to the muscle is obscured.

Differential Diagnosis

Other conditions whose treatment may differ from that of fistula-in-ano need to be delineated. Constant wet perianal soiling can be caused by fistula-in-ano, but it may be part of idiopathic pruritis ani or a variety of other conditions. An anterior fistula may be due to urethral fistula in the male or a Bartholin abscess in the female. Some of the diagnostic possibilities include tuberculosis, low-lying carcinoma in the rectum or anus with external fistulization, lymphogranuloma venereum, actinomycosis, fistulous tracts due to previous anorectal or obstetric operations, anal duct carcinoma, diverticulitis of the sigmoid colon with perineal fistulization, infected dermoid cysts, low lying pilonidal sinus, hydradenitis suppurativa, Crohn disease of the anus, leukemia, and agranulocytosis.

Treatment

Correct treatment of fistula-in-ano consists of eliminating the fistula while preventing anal incontinence. Since most fistulas are intersphincteric with well-defined external and internal openings, simple unroofing is adequate (Fig. 41-7). An intersphincteric fistula (Fig. 41-5A) that penetrates through the rectum may be completely unroofed. If the intersphincteric fistula proceeds cephalad into the pararectal tissue (Fig. 41-5C), it should be drained into the

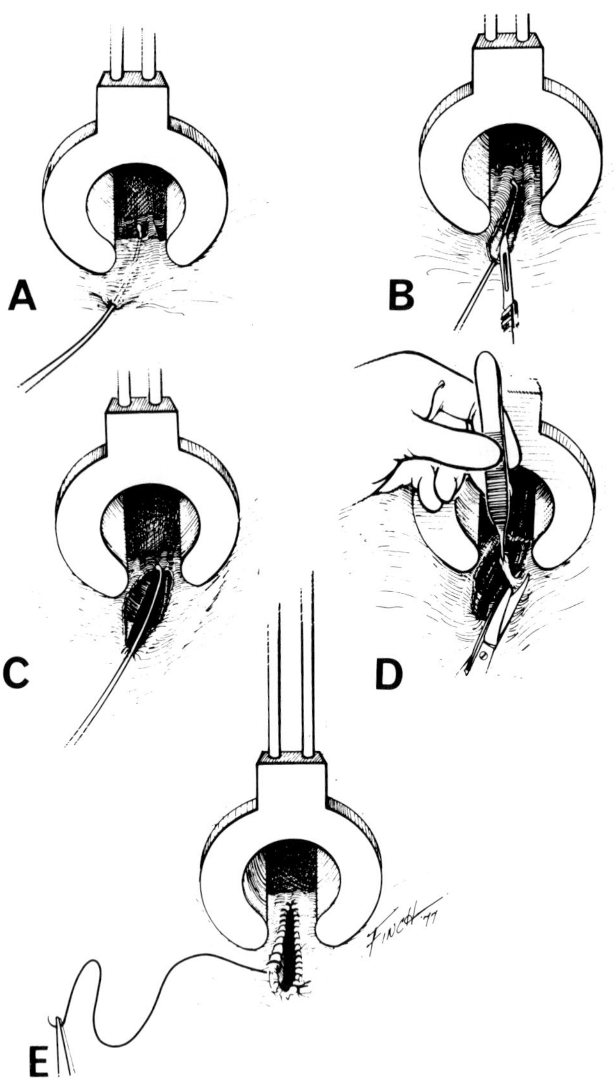

Fig. 41-7. **Fistulotomy. A. The probe is in the fistulous tract. B,C. Unroofing of the fistulous tract over the probe. D. Redundant skin is excised. E. The wound is marsupialized.**

rectum (Fig. 41-4B) following unroofing of the caudal part in the anus (Fig. 41-7). If caudal extension into the perianal or perineal area is lacking, the diseased anal duct gland in the internal anal sphincter around the internal opening should be curetted or excised, and the pararectal limb should be drained into the rectum at the site of the excision (Fig. 41-4B). It would be a grave error to drain it through the ischiorectal fossa, for such an attempt would convert the tract into a suprasphincteric variety. A fistula that traverses through the lower part of the external anal sphincter (Fig. 41-5B) can be similarly unroofed, transecting the internal anal sphincter and some of the external anal sphincter (Fig. 41-7).

A trans-sphincteric fistula-in-ano (Fig. 41-5C) that would require transection of a major portion of the external anal sphincter should not be unroofed primarily, for anal incontinence could result. Fortunately, such cases are relatively infrequent. The sphincteric muscle of the anterior wall of the anus is not as large as that of the posterior wall, which is buttressed cephalad by a large bundle of the puborectalis muscle. Unroofing of the external anal sphincter of the anterior wall is therefore relatively less well tolerated.

Several procedures are available as alternatives to the unroofing technique (Fig. 41-8). In a seton procedure, a thick thread, a rubber band, or a wire is threaded through the tract traversing the external anal sphincter and tied over the bundle of the sphincter to be transected some time later (Fig. 41-8). The bundle of the external anal sphincter to be transected later is isolated. The anoderm and internal anal sphincter overlying the bundle of the external anal sphincter are incised, and the inner surface of the external anal sphincter is exposed. The seton is then tied around the bundle of the external anal sphincter. In theory, the external anal sphincter to be divided gets fixed to the underlying fibrous tissue, so that transection of the external anal sphincter later as a second stage does not result in excessive parting of the muscle.

Another procedure, Park fistulectomy,[2] may be used if the fistula-in-ano traverses through the external anal sphincter quite cephalad. In this procedure, the mucosa, anoderm, and the internal anal sphincter in the vicinity of the internal opening are excised, exposing the inner surface of the external anal sphincter. The caudal part of the internal anal sphincter is excised in continuity. The diseased anal duct gland is thus removed. The tract that traverses the external anal sphincter is cored out to rid it of granulation and fibrous tissue. The internal opening on the exposed external anal sphincter is then closed with absorbable sutures. Thus, transection of the external anal sphincter is avoided.

A trans-sphincteric fistula-in-ano may not be simple. There may be a variable extension cephalad from the portion of the tract in the ischiorectal fossa. Some of the extensions may end in the inferior surface of the levator ani, whereas others may penetrate through it (Fig. 41-5D). In either case, complete unroofing, Park fistulectomy, or a seton procedure may be performed and the upward extension cored out. It is important to keep the perianal opening adequate until the cephalad extension heals. Drainage of the high infralevator or supralevator extension into the rectum would convert the trans-sphincteric fistula into an extrasphincteric one.

The suprasphincteric variety is rare (Fig. 41-5C). A suprasphincteric fistula ascends from the anal crypt area in the intersphincteric zone, curves over the puborectalis, and descends into the infralevator space, piercing through the levator ani and communicating with a perianal opening on the outside of the external anal sphincter. According to Parks,[11] this variety occurs as a horseshoe fistula-in-ano surrounding the lower rectum for about a half circumference, creating a ringlike fibrous band just above the puborectalis. This type of fistula usually occurs following anal duct infection posteriorly in midline. The puborectalis may be transected at this area, provided that such a fibrous reaction is present. Fibrous tissue prevents excessive parting of the puborectalis muscle on transection. Aside from

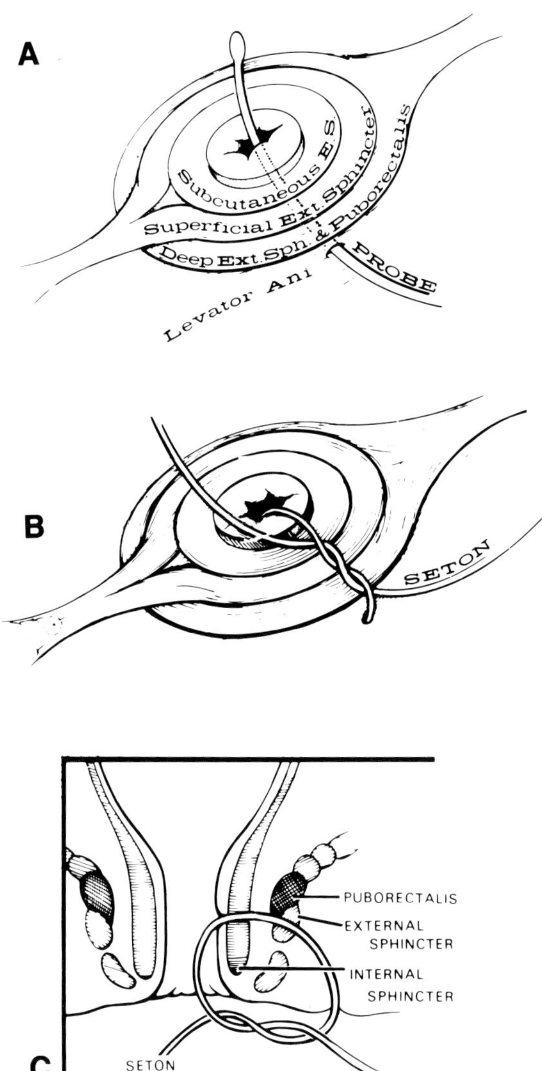

Fig. 41-8. Use of seton in high fistula. A. The probe is in the fistulous tract. B. A seton or suture is inserted into the fistulous tract and (C.) tied loosely over the sphincter to create fibrosis. The fistulous tract will be laid open in the second stage 6 to 8 weeks later.

the above special situation, division of the puborectalis muscle in suprasphincteric fistula is unsatisfactory. Some other procedure is warranted. The part of the tract medial to the external anal sphincter and the puborectalis may be unroofed, the transected tissue consisting of the anoderm, the rectal mucosa, and the internal anal sphincter and its cephalad circular muscle of the rectum. The portion of the tract that laterally penetrates through the levator ani on the outside of the puborectalis muscle downward into the ischiorectal fossa is cored out, and the cephalad end is closed from the rectal side. Colostomy is added to keep the intrarectal pressure low. A decision about to what extent, what portion, and when to transect the skeletal muscle seen during operation on a suprasphincteric fistulous tract requires considerable judgment and experience.

Extrasphincteric fistula may be of anal duct origin. As such, it may be a spontaneous or iatrogenic complication of either suprasphincteric fistula or trans-sphincteric fistula. The anal duct disease must be eradicated. The treatment would require staged operations. The extrasphincteric fistula is cored out, and the rectal entrance into the fistula is closed. Colostomy should accompany the operation.

Extrasphincteric fistula from intra-abdominal disease such as Crohn disease and diverticulitis requires removal of the diseased bowel causing the fistula. The internal opening in such a case is usually in the diseased bowel, and the fistulous tract usually traverses outside the rectum to the perianal area, although in some cases the tract runs immediately deep to the internal anal sphincter, simulating an intersphincteric fistula.

Operation is the only successful therapy for fistula-in-ano. Antibiotics are usually not necessary. If fistula-in-ano is associated with a large acute anorectal abscess or with cellulitis, antibiotics are indicated.

All wounds following operation should heal by granulation from the base of the wound. Twice daily sitz baths should be started 24 to 48 hours after operation in order to keep the base of the wound clean. The wound should be inspected regularly to make sure the skin does not heal over before the base of the wound does.

In the past, various sclerosing agents were injected into the fistulous tract in an attempt to close the fistula-in-ano. They were unsuccessful and are no longer used.

CROHN DISEASE OF THE ANORECTUM

Incidence

Crohn disease of the anorectum may occur by itself, but it is found more commonly in association with Crohn disease of the small or large bowel. Crohn disease has been described in Chapters 38 and 39. The National Cooperative Crohn's Disease Study found that 36 percent of 569 patients with Crohn disease had a history of perianal disease,[5] 46.7 percent with ileocolitis and 25.5 percent with disease confined to the small bowel. If the rectum is involved with Crohn disease, anal involvement is nearly 100 percent.[14]

Pathogenesis and Pathology

Crohn disease may not be an infection. Anal ulceration is the most common anal lesion, and its pathogenesis is unknown. In some cases, an infection may originate in the prominent lymphatic collections of the anal region. The surface anoderm overlying the infected lymphatics may ulcerate, and the ulcerated areas become the nidus for further extension of the disease. These ulcers frequently fail to heal. They are broad ulcers, with undermined edges, and may develop abundant granulation tissue and extensive fibrosis. They may extend deeply to involve the ischiorectal fat or sphincter muscles, sometimes with great destruction of tissue. Whether these ulcers can also extend into the duct system and lead to anal gland infection and anorectal abscess is not known.

Anorectal abscess and fistula-in-ano can also occur in

association with Crohn disease. Anorectal abscesses caused by Crohn disease may appear on superficial inspection to be like any other abscess. Histologic examination of granulation tissue in the wall of the abscess may reveal typical microscopic features. Fistulas that occur in patients with Crohn disease are likely to be extensive and complicated. Microscopically, the base of the fissure or ulcer, wall of the abscess, and tract of the fistula show fibrosis, acute and chronic granulation tissue, and occasionally granulomas.

Clinical Manifestations and Diagnosis

The clinical manifestations of anorectal Crohn disease do not differ substantially from those of fissure, ulcer, abscess, and fistula-in-ano in the absence of Crohn disease. Most patients have symptoms of intestinal Crohn disease, but occasionally Crohn disease affects the anus alone, and intestinal disease develops much later.

The diagnosis usually depends on determining Crohn disease of the intestine by typical symptoms and roentgenographic findings. Anal Crohn disease can be suspected, even in the absence of findings of intestinal Crohn disease, because the ulcers are located laterally or anteriorly and have a broad base. Crohn disease should be suspected, especially if the ulcer is 2 cm or larger and if the edges are undermined. Usual anal fissures are mere cracks located posteriorly in the midline. Unusually shaped or elongated anal skin tags may be present. Abundant granulation tissue and inflammatory edema are usually associated with Crohn disease of the anus.

The fistulas-in-ano associated with Crohn disease tend to be complicated with multiple cutaneous openings. In some cases, however, Crohn fissures and fistulas-in-ano look no different from the common varieties.

Treatment

Anal lesions may wax and wane with the intestinal disease, and they may heal only to recur as the intestinal disease recurs. Treating the anal manifestations of Crohn disease without treating the intestinal lesions is ineffective in most cases. On the other hand, with adequate treatment of intestinal lesions alone, anal fissures may heal with no further treatment. Perianal ulcers and fistulas are usually associated with Crohn disease of the rectum, and removal of the rectum may become necessary if they are extensive. Colostomy alone is usually not effective.

Acute anorectal abscesses must be drained. Fistula-in-ano should not be treated surgically until the intestinal disease has been treated, usually by excision. Then some of the fistula can be treated as discussed in the previous section on fistula-in-ano. Under most circumstances, the fistula should be left alone.

The National Cooperative Crohn's Disease Study reported that perianal abscesses responded to sulfasalazine and anal fissure to prednisone or azathioprine.[5] But the number of patients in each treatment group or control group was small (one to seven patients), and the response was as great in the placebo group. The natural waxing and waning of Crohn disease makes conclusions with such small groups unreliable. There is little evidence that drug therapy helps the anorectal manifestations of Crohn disease.

TUBERCULOSIS OF THE ANUS

Anorectal tuberculosis is almost always caused by *M. tuberculosis* and rarely by other mycobacteria.

In the past, when pulmonary tuberculosis was prevalent, the incidence of tuberculosis in fistula-in-ano was estimated as high as 16 percent.[15] However, other disease entities whose lesions characteristically show granulomatous changes with giant cells (Crohn disease) were probably included in the diagnosis. About 70 to 90 percent of fistulas-in-ano in patients with active pulmonary tuberculosis are complicated with tuberculous infection. Tuberculosis affects the anus less frequently than the ileocecal region, however.

Tubercle bacilli probably enter anorectal tissues via breaks in the mucocutaneous surface, ie, fistulas or fissures. The organisms may also enter the anal duct and induce tuberculous anorectal abscess; the abscess may then lead to fistulas or ulcers. Tuberculous fistulas are usually complex and multiple, and ulcers are usually undermined with thickened edges. The infection may start and remain as small nodules in the anal area without ulceration for a long time. In some cases, the most prominent gross feature of anal tuberculosis may be verrucous and papillary changes of the overlying anoderm without fistulization or ulceration. The tuberculous ulcers, fistulas, or abscesses produce thin watery-purulent discharge. If they are left untreated, anal function can be compromised and incontinence can result.

The lesion is a granulomatous process, sometimes with caseation. In the verrucous form, the overlying anoderm may demonstrate acanthosis and papillomatous hyperplasia. *M. tuberculosis* may be difficult to identify by the Zeil-Neilsen staining technique.

The diagnosis is suspected when fissures or ulcers reveal undermined edges or profuse watery discharge. Anal ulcers in combination with pulmonary changes suggestive of tuberculosis or with positive skin test to PPD are very suspicious. A biopsy showing caseation or acid-fast bacilli is confirmatory. Cultural isolation of *M. tuberculosis* from anal lesions is difficult.

Antituberculous therapy has been detailed in Chapters 7 and 18. Ulcerated anal lesions will heal, usually in 3 to 6 months. Fistula-in-ano will respond to operations for ordinary fistula-in-ano following appropriate antituberculous therapy. Abscesses require drainage. At times, complicated and extensive fistulas-in-ano may require fecal diversion. Anal incontinence may be given attention following complete healing of tuberculosis of the anus.

HIDRADENITIS SUPPURATIVA

Hidradenitis suppurativa is caused by infection of the apocrine sweat glands that results in abscesses and sinuses in the skin of axillary, inguinal, mammary, and perianal regions. Since apocrine glands do not become active until puberty, hidradenitis is not seen before that time (Chapter 25).

Perianal hidradenitis occurs in young adults. Subcutaneous nodules may appear in the early stages of the disease. These nodules usually coalesce to form an elevated cord or plaque, which gradually increases in size to form a large area of induration. Pustules may periodically open and drain small amounts of pus. Sinus tracts may develop, and ulceration of the perianal skin may occur. The pain is usually mild or moderate unless abscess occurs, in which case it can become severe. The patient more commonly complains of the bad odor from the constant drainage.

Proper treatment requires complete excision of the skin and underlying subcutaneous tissue down to the deep fascia. Large defects are thus produced, so that primary closure cannot be accomplished. Closure may require skin grafting, using a split-thickness graft or rotating a large flap of skin and subcutaneous tissue. This latter procedure is required if the disease involves the tissue overlying the ischial tuberosities, which bears weight when one sits. In extensive cases where removal of the diseased skin and underlying subcutaneous tissue leads to a large open wound, fistulas and sinuses may be unroofed, thoroughly curetted, and the overhanging skin edges excised; the intervening skin is left for adequate healing. Antibiotics are ineffective as the sole treatment of hidradenitis. They may be a useful adjuvant to operative therapy, especially if skin grafts or rotated flaps are used. Perianal plastic procedures may require a prior diverting colostomy.

PILONIDAL DISEASE

Pilonidal disease consists of a sinus or fistula located behind the anus or over the sacrum, usually containing hairs.

Etiology

Several theories have been elaborated to explain the cause of pilonidal disease. The theory that pilonidal disease is an acquired condition is favored by the occasional recurrence of pilonidal sinus after adequate excision. Patey and Scarff[16] proposed that hairs from the surrounding skin are somehow introduced into the tissues and cause the sinus. Pilonidal sinuses that occur in other places, the web of the fingers in barbers, amputation stumps, and the axilla, where no congenital sinuses occur, are almost certainly acquired by this mechanism. How these hairs penetrate the skin is uncertain. This theory fails to explain, however, why the hairs in the sinuses are longer and finer than those in the surrounding skin.

Congenital theories assert pilonidal disease is caused by some embryologic remnant such as an epithelial-lined sinus beneath the skin over the coccyx. The condition remains symptomless unless infection occurs leading to abscess formation and development of a sinus tract.

Pathology

A pilonidal sinus is a tract that is skin-lined at the orifice and extends subcutaneously for 2–5 cm. The tract often ends in a small cavity. Most of the length of the tract and cavity is lined with granulation tissue. Hairs are almost always found in the sinus tract, frequently projecting from the opening. Secondary openings are frequently present and are lined by granulation tissue. These openings may or may not be in the midline.

Clinical Manifestations

The first presentation of a pilonidal sinus is frequently an abscess over the coccyx, which drains spontaneously or is drained by the surgeon. The patient may remain well for several weeks or months, only to have the abscess recur. Alternatively, the patient often first complains of drainage from the sinus without a history of a previous abscess.

Examination reveals one or more openings at the base of the spine in the midline. If more than one opening is present, they communicate, so that a probe can usually be passed in one and out the other. The tract seldom extends far from the midline.

Treatment

A variety of operations have been used to treat pilonidal disease. Operations have generally involved complete excision of the sinus and the tract, a method favored by surgeons in the United States, or by simple incision of the sinus tract, a method popular with many British surgeons.

Complete excision of the sinus with a margin of normal tissue is most easily done with the patient in the prone position with the buttocks taped apart.

After excision, the wound can be dealt with in several ways. The wound can be left open to granulate. This method is associated with few complications and is favored by many surgeons for that reason. The patient is required to take sitz baths twice a day until granulation occurs, after which either sitz baths or showers can be used. In between, a single gauze pad can be used to keep the skin edges apart. Healing occurs in 4 to 10 weeks depending on the size of the wound. To facilitate healing and reduce the size of the wound, some surgeons suture the skin to the presacral fascia (marsupialization).

Primary suture of the wound is favored by some surgeons, but has several disadvantages. The wound infection rate is high (approximately 50 percent), and the wound ends up being treated open anyway.[16] To keep tension of the wound to a minimum, physical activity has to be greatly restricted, and prolonged hospitalization is required. Finally, the recurrence rate is high.

A variety of plastic procedures have been used to obtain primary closure without these defects. These have included relaxing incisions in the skin and fat of one buttock, rotational flaps, and muscle grafts of gluteus maximus. None of these procedures is easy to do, and if infection occurs, the patient is left with a much larger defect.

Simple incision of the sinus tracts is widely practiced in Britain. A probe is inserted in the sinus and out a second opening if it exists. The skin is then incised down to the tract, the tract and cavity are opened widely, hairs in the tract are removed, and the tract is curetted. This wound is not as deep as the one resulting from complete excision, but complete healing takes as long.

SEXUALLY TRANSMITTED DISEASES OF THE ANUS

All the diseases in this section are found predominantly in male homosexuals who perform anal intercourse. None require operative treatment, but they can be confused with anal diseases that do. For this reason, the differential diagnosis is critical.

ANORECTAL SYPHILIS

The etiology, pathogenesis, and serodiagnosis of syphilis are discussed in Chapter 7. Anorectal syphilis is reported with increasing frequency, especially among male homosexuals.

T. pallidum can penetrate directly through intact rectal mucosa or through a break in the anoderm or perianal skin. The incubation period ranges from 10 to 90 days, with an average of 21 days.

Primary anal syphilis begins with induration at the site of penetration, and there may be a break in the skin overlying the indurated area. The lesion then ulcerates to form an indurated, clean-based ulcer, the typical chancre.[17,18] The diagnosis may be difficult, however, since a wide ulcer with poorly defined, indurated margins is sometimes seen. If the chancre is at the anal margin or in the anal canal, it may be confused with an anal fissure. It is not confined to the posterior or anterior location as in an ordinary fissure-in-ano, and the lesions may be located in multiple areas. Some anal lesions develop into fistula-in-ano, and others may remain indurated without developing ulceration. Anal lesions may extend into the perianal region. The lesions usually heal in 3 to 12 weeks, but they may persist into the secondary stage of syphilis.

Soon after appearance of the primary lesion, inguinal adenopathy develops. The inguinal lymph nodes are enlarged and have a rubbery consistency. The enlarged lymph nodes are frequently described as being nontender, but secondary bacterial infection of the ulcerated syphilitic anal lesion may render them quite tender. Irritation, soreness, itching, and serous, purulent, or bloody discharge are common symptoms of anal syphilis.

Syphilitic proctitis is more often asymptomatic if it remains within the rectum, but it more frequently extends out to the anal region.[19-21] The lesion is a localized, thickened, edematous, granular area that bleeds easily when traumatized. Tenesmus, abdominal pain, and loose bowel movements have been noted. The affected area may be small or extensive. Circumferential extension may occur as a result of intramural lymphatic spread, and cephalad extension may occur by vascular spread. Rectal lesions can also present primarily as ulcers. When ulcerated lesions have raised margins, they can resemble adenocarcinoma of the rectum.[19]

Secondary syphilis appears 6 weeks to 6 months following the onset of the primary disease. Condyloma latum is the anal manifestation of secondary syphilis. It is a moist, raised, flat, wartlike lesion. It can occur as an isolated patch or in clusters. The appearance of condyloma latum is quite characteristic. Condyloma acuminatum is characterized by softer, drier, pedunculated lesions, and is usually easily differentiated from condyloma latum.

Dark-field examination of secretions or scrapings from ulcers or condyloma lata will show the motile spirochetes to the expert examiner. The lesion should first be rubbed with a dry sponge. Any initial exudate or blood should be discarded. Then the serous fluid that flows out or is squeezed out is mounted on a glass slide and is examined by dark-field microscopy. The spirochetes can also be seen in biopsy specimens stained with the Warthin-Starry silver stain. The serodiagnosis has been described in Chapter 7. Gonorrhea frequently coexists with syphilis, and cultures for *N. gonorrhoeae* should be obtained in all cases of anorectal syphilis.

The United States Public Health Service currently recommends benzathine penicillin G, 2.4 million units, intramuscularly at one time (Chapter 45). For patients who are allergic to penicillin, tetracycline, 500 mg orally four times a day for 15 days, can be used. Pregnant women who are allergic to penicillin should receive erythromycin, 500 mg orally four times a day for 15 days, because tetracycline can eventually stain the teeth of the child.

GONOCOCCAL PROCTITIS

Gonococcal proctitis, caused by *N. gonorrhoeae* (Chapter 4) is more common in male homosexuals than in females. *N. gonorrhoeae* can be recovered from the rectum of up to 65 percent of females with urogenital gonorrhea if they have proctoscopic examination. In women, proctitis probably occurs by direct extension when vaginal secretions flow over the anus and infect the rectal mucosa.

N. gonorrhoeae enters the rectal mucosa just above the dentate line. The infected rectal mucosa becomes erythematous and friable. Acute and chronic inflammatory cells—polymorphonuclear leukocytes, plasma cells, and lymphocytes—accumulate in the lamina propria. A light brown exudate is usually present over the mucosa, although it may become purulent. The anoderm and perianal skin may be erythematous. Obvious inflammatory changes may subside, and the proctitis may enter a chronic stage in which the disease may be transmissible, but changes in the rectal mucosa may not be clearly evident.

Most patients with gonococcal proctitis are completely asymptomatic, and the condition is detected only if it is specifically looked for. In symptomatic patients, it most commonly causes slight rectal discomfort with a rectal discharge and pruritis ani. Symptoms such as tenesmus, a burning sensation, and pain on defecation are rare. The organism can be identified by culturing the rectal exudate. Appropriate studies to rule out syphilis should also be performed.

Gonococcal proctitis in females usually responds to 4.8 million units procaine penicillin G administered intramuscularly, 2.4 million units into each buttock. Probenecid, 1 gm orally, can increase the effectiveness of penicillin by decreasing excretion in the urine. Because the failure rate for males with gonococcal proctitis is higher than that for females, 2.4 million units procaine penicillin G intramuscularly daily for 5 days may be required. Patients should observe strict sexual abstinence during the treatment period, and culture should be obtained 1 to 2 weeks after treatment.

Ampicillin may be given as a single oral dose of 3.5 gm together with 1 gm probenecid for urogenital gonorrhea. This regimen may not be satisfactory for rectal gonorrhea, and 2 gm ampicillin should be given orally daily for 5 days. Tetracycline, 1.5 gm orally followed by 500 mg four times a day for 5 days, can be used in patients who are allergic to penicillin. Spectinomycin, given as a single 4-gm intramuscular injection, is associated with the lowest failure rates in gonococcal proctitis, and a 100 percent cure rate has been claimed. Spectinomycin does not affect syphilis. Kanamycin, 2 gm intramuscularly, and trimethoprin-sulfamethoxazole, two tablets twice a day for 7 days, have also been used to treat gonococcal proctitis.

The failure rate for females with gonococcal proctitis is 2 to 7 percent. Failure rates may be somewhat higher for rectal gonorrhea in the male. No good large-scale studies on a standard antibiotic regimen are available. Recurrence or persistence of positive rectal cultures calls for antibiotic sensitivity testing. Some gonococcal strains produce penicillinase and are resistant to both penicillin and ampicillin. Such strains are also likely to be resistant to tetracycline.

GRANULOMA INGUINALE

The etiology, pathogenesis, and general features of granuloma inguinale *(Calymmatobacterium granulomatis)* are discussed in Chapters 7, 25, 44, and 45.

Granuloma inguinale is a disease of tropical regions, and fewer than 100 cases are reported per year in the United States.[22] Transmission occurs by sexual contact.[23] Usually, perianal lesions are an extension of genital lesions. An eroded papule appears first, and it gradually develops into a painless shallow ulcer. The ulcer has bright red granulation tissue in the base, with rolled serpiginous borders. Without treatment, the ulcer extends, usually along skin folds. Squamous cell carcinoma may develop in long-standing, neglected lesions. Elephantiasis of the local genital region can occur.

Granuloma inguinale should be suspected in any perianal ulcer associated with a genital ulcer. In the absence of inguinal adenopathy, a genital ulcer lasting more than several weeks should suggest the possibility of granuloma inguinale. Clusters of rod-shaped intracellular bacteria can be seen by examining small pieces of granulation tissue that have been crushed between two slides and stained with Giemsa or Wright stain.

Tetracycline, 2 gm daily for 2 weeks, is recommended for treatment. Some lesions may not heal with this regimen, in which case ampicillin or chloramphenicol may be used.

CHANCROID

The etiology, pathogenesis, and general features of chancroid have been discussed in Chapters 7, 25, 44, and 45. Chancroid has been noted particularly among military personnel from World War I to Vietnam.[24-26]

Two to 14 days after sexual contact, a pustule or papule develops over the genital area.[24] It rapidly becomes a nonindurated soft ulcer of variable size, with slightly undermined and irregular edges and a gray, purulent base. It is usually a singular, painful lesion, but multiple lesions may develop by contact. Large ulcers may result from confluence of the smaller lesions. Tender inguinal adenopathy develops in about one-half the individuals within 1 week after the genital lesion. Inguinal lymph nodes may develop fluctuance, and a sinus may form onto the skin surface. Fever, malaise, and anorexia may occur.

Perianal lesions are usually secondary to genital disease, and few cases of anal chancroid have been reported.

The diagnosis is frequently made on clinical impression, followed by a therapeutic trial. Cultures or smears of the exudate at the base of the ulcers are unreliable methods of diagnosis, but they should still be taken.[27] This entity is frequently confused with herpes genitalis. Chancroid ulcers are larger, deeper, and fewer in number than those of herpes. Moreover, chancroid lesions are not recurrent like herpes. Chancroid is less destructive than granuloma inguinale or lymphogranuloma venereum, and elephantiasis of the local genital area is not seen. The diseased inguinal nodes in chancroid usually develop simple and singular cutaneous sinusus, whereas the nodes in lymphogranuloma venereum may develop multiple complex sinuses and fistulas. Syphilitic lesions are indurated lesions and are usually painless. All other concurrent and confusing anogenital diagnoses should be excluded prior to treatment.

Sulfisoxazole, 4 gm per day for 2 to 3 weeks, is effective treatment for chancroid. The effectiveness may be enhanced by adding tetracycline, 2 gm per day. Either may be used alone. If the disease recurs, the course may be repeated. Other antibiotics used include chloramphenicol, chlorotetracycline, and streptomycin. If inguinal nodes are involved, the response may be poor and may require longer therapy.

LYMPHOGRANULOMA VENEREUM OF THE ANORECTAL REGION

The etiology *(Chlamydia trachomatis)*, pathogenesis, and general features of lymphogranuloma venereum are discussed in Chapters 7, 25, 44, and 45.

Clinically, lymphogranuloma venereum becomes manifest as inguinal, genital, or anorectal varieties.[28] In the inguinal variety, there is a transient sore, usually in the genital area. Lymphatic drainage to the inguinal nodes leads to lymphadenopathy. The nodes become fluctuant and develop cutaneous sinuses or fistulas. In the genital variety, there may be extensive edema due to lymphatic obstruction (Chapters 44, 45). In anorectal lymphogranuloma venereum, unlike the genital and inguinal forms, the findings are usually confined to the anorectal area. Inguinal adenopathy is absent.

Anorectal lymphogranuloma venereum in the male is probably acquired by direct implantation of the organism during anal intercourse.[29] In the female, vaginal discharge may enter into the anorectal area. Proctitis can gradually progress via submucosal fibrosis to contraction of the entire thickness of the rectum. There are two major theories on pathogenesis of rectal lymphogranuloma venereum in the female. One is that infection of the posterior vaginal wall leads to breakdown of the wall, and the disease spreads to the adjacent rectum by means of the lymphatics surrounding the rectum. In view of the usual lymphatic drainage and spread of cervical carcinoma, lymphatic permeation from the posterior vaginal wall and secondary rectal involvement appears a somewhat unlikely mechanism.

The second and probably more plausible theory is direct implantation of organisms into the rectum, as in the male. Experimental implantation of *Chlamydia* into the rectum of chimpanzees caused proctitis, which later developed into a stricture.

Local symptoms and signs of anorectal lymphogranuloma venereum may be predominantly anal or rectal.[30] Proctitis leads to bloody discharge with mucus or pus, diarrhea, tenesmus, and rectal pain. Blood loss may lead to anemia. Stricture may develop in a year, although many cases of proctitis may remain chronic without developing stricture. Strictures may be severe enough to produce partial obstruction with alternating diarrhea and constipation, colicky abdominal pain, abdominal distention, and ribbonlike stools. There may be left lower quadrant abdominal tenderness over the diseased distal left colon.

From the mucosal surface, proctitis may be seen extending for a variable distance beginning low in the rectum, most marked 5 cm from the anal verge.[30] The mucosal surface is hemorrhagic, granular, and friable, and may resemble ulcerative colitis. The rectum contains blood, pus, and mucus. In a long-standing proctitis, a ringlike stricture or stenosis over a long segment may be present in the rectum. Stricture is most frequently found 3–5 cm from the anal verge. In the female, the area is closely adherent to the posterior vaginal wall. At times, rectovaginal fistula is present at that level. Narrowing of the rectum may extend for a variable distance proximally. Stenosis or strictures may be present on the left side of the colon in skip areas. Active proctitis may not be evident in some of the patients with rectal stricture or stenosis. The overlying mucosal surface in such cases is pale, atrophic, and easily traumatized. A long segment of the left colon can become shortened, inelastic, and pipelike, losing normal haustral markings.

Complex or simple anorectal abscesses, ulcers, and fistulas may be seen in predominantly anal disease. They sometimes extend anteriorly to genital areas. Without specific antibiotic treatment, operations on these anal lesions are accompanied by repeated failures. Tuberculosis, Crohn disease, as well as a local malignant disease are appropriate differential diagnoses, and all other anorectal sexually transmitted diseases should be ruled out before treatment is instituted.

Rectal and anal samples are so frequently contaminated with other organisms that diagnosis based on cultural isolation is difficult. In addition, *C. trachomatis* requires special laboratory facilities for its culture. The serodiagnostic tests have been discussed in Chapter 7. The commonly used complement-fixation test is unreliable,[31] and a titer of 1:64 or greater should be taken as the lowest titer level for a firm diagnosis.[32] A titer of 1:16 is necessary to initiate treatment in clinically convincing cases.

The Frei skin test [33] may be negative in the early stage, and thus should be repeated in several weeks. Counterimmunoelectrophoresis using purified *C. trachomatis* protein antigen is highly specific for lymphogranuloma venereum.[34]

Tetracycline, 2 gm per day for 3 weeks, is standard therapy. The disease also responds to sulfasoxazole, 4 gm per day for 3 weeks after a 4-gm loading dose. Clinical response is usually rapid. If resolution does not occur, treatment may be repeated. Some cases are not responsive to medical treatment, particularly to sulfonamides; the lack of response may be due to strain characteristics.[35] In chronic cases, tetracycline or sulfasoxazole may not be effective.

The disease appears to respond more readily to ampicillin or minocycline.[35] Two gm of ampicillin are given daily for 3 weeks.[36] Minocycline is given as a 300-mg loading dose followed by 200 mg twice a day for 10 days.[37] In late cases, prednisone may be added in cases of proctitis to prevent progression of rectal stricture.

Other antibiotics such as chloramphenicol, erythromycin, and streptomycin may be used. They may be given for 2 to 3 weeks in a dosage of 2 gm per day.

Efficacy of treatment is reflected in resolution of systemic manifestations and local disease. Lowering of complement-fixation titers is also a measure of response to appropriate medical treatment. The Frei test does not become negative after treatment in most cases.

Medical therapy alone gives surprisingly good results in patients with stricture or stenosis. This may be due to resolution of active proctitis. In a soft stricture, gentle digital dilation may accompany antibiotic treatment. Hard fibrotic stricture does not respond to dilation. Overzealous attempts at dilation may result in rectal perforation. In others, colostomy may be necessary. In those free of disease in the anus and lower rectum, a sphincter-saving type of operation may be performed. The majority of those with advanced stricture, however, have extensive disease that precludes satisfactory function following sphinctersaving operation. In anal disease, one should give adequate medical therapy, and treatment of fistula-in-ano should follow ordinary surgical principles.

HERPES SIMPLEX INFECTION OF THE ANAL AND PERIANAL AREA

Herpes simplex infections are discussed in Chapters 10, 25, 44, and 45.

Herpes simplex virus-2 (HSV-2) is the usual etiologic agent in anal, genital, and cervical herpes.[38–40] Herpes simplex virus-1 (HSV-1) is being recovered from anal and perianal infections with increasing frequency.

The anal infection is acquired by anal intercourse [41] or as an extension of genital herpes infection in the female.

Primary and recurrent herpes have similar manifestations. Small vesicles, solitary or in clusters, surrounded by a red areola, are the first lesions to appear in the perianal area or the anal canal.[40] The vesicles soon rupture, leaving apthouslike shallow erosions, which may coalesce to become larger ulcers. If secondary bacterial infection sets in, the discharge may turn purulent.

In the anal canal, eroded areas have a grayish floor

bordered by edematous and erythematous mucosa. Almost all patients have local pain and itching, especially if the anal canal is involved.[42] The majority of patients have bilateral inguinal adenopathy. Constitutional symptoms of fever, chills, malaise, headache, and anorexia may be present. The herpetic lesions are usually self-limited and heal completely without residue in 2 to 3 weeks.

Laboratory tests can confirm the diagnosis.[43-46] The virus can be cultured from fluid aspirated from the vesicular lesions (Chapter 12). A more rapid diagnosis may be obtained by finding characteristic cytopathic changes in cells obtained from suspected lesions after staining scrapings from the base of lesions with Wright, crystal violet, or Giemsa stains. Immunofluorescence and immunoperoxidase staining techniques of lesion scrapings are the most rapid, reliable methods of identification.[43,44]

Concurrent venereal lesions must be ruled out.

Treatment of anal and perianal herpes infection is symptomatic—ie, wet packs soaked in Burow solution, local analgesic ointment such as 2 percent lidocaine, and sitz baths. At times, systemic analgesic or sedation may be necessary. Various antiviral agents have been tried for mucocutaneous lesions, particularly for genital lesions, but they have not been successful in treating genital lesions. A topical agent of 0.19 percent 2-deoxy-D-glucose in miconazole nitrate (2 percent) was found to be effective against genital herpes infection in shortening the primary as well as recurrent herpes infection and in lowering the incidence of subsequent recurrences.[47] Further studies with this agent are warranted. Acyclovir will probably be an effective antiherpetic agent when final license is given (Chapters 10, 18).

CONDYLOMA ACUMINATUM

Condyloma acuminatum is caused by a papovirus (common wart virus) [48-50] (Chapters 10, 25), but it is probably sexually transmitted. Anal intercourse is practiced by over 80 percent of both male and female patients. Males without homosexual history appear to have higher incidence of coexisting condylomatous lesions in the inguinal area and penis.

Condyloma acuminatum usually occurs in warm and moist areas of the body, including preputial sac of the penis, natal cleft, vulva, axilla, vagina, cervix, inguinal areas, anal and perianal area. It is a soft, friable, warty growth, pedunculated or sessile, which bleeds easily on contact. It may occur singly or in clusters. Condyloma acuminatum is usually white or pinkish, in contrast to brown or gray more common penile warts. Condyloma acuminatum occurring in the perianal and anal area is usually limited in cephalad extent by the dentate line. It may cover the entire anal verge like a cauliflower. Bleeding, pruritis ani, and pain on defecation are common symptoms. Some condylomatous lesions regress spontaneously.[51]

Under light microscopy, condyloma acuminatum differs from the common wart (verruca vulgaris) in that it shows little hyperkeratosis but more marked parakeratosis and extreme acanthosis. There is vacuolization of the upper prickle layer. Infrequently, condyloma acuminatum is associated with carcinoma in situ.[52] A rare so-called Buschke-Lowenstein tumor or giant condyloma, reported to occur more frequently in the male genital area than the perianal area, is a low-grade malignant lesion. It burrows through soft tissues forming fistulas and sinus tracts. The lesion may involve perineum and buttocks, and dip into the perirectal tissue and ischiorectal fossa.[53] Metastasis may occur to inguinal lymph nodes. Histologically, the lesion does not appear different from ordinary condyloma acuminatum.[53,54]

Diagnosis is made by clinical observation of the gross lesion, confirmed by biopsy. Patients may have the same lesions elsewhere on the body. Other veneral diseases may be present concomitantly. Condyloma latum is a major differential diagnosis. It is a whiter, flatter, and more moist papillary lesion. Condyloma latum and condyloma acuminatum may occur together, however. Some perianal papillary lesions are squamous cell carcinoma, which is usually easy to recognize. If in doubt, biopsies should be obtained.

Various local treatments are available. Podophyllin resin in mineral oil, tincture of benzoin, or glycerin may be applied over the lesions at weekly intervals. The normal skin and mucous membrane should be protected. Some lesions do not respond well to podophyllin. Large lesions, particularly extending cephalad into the anal canal, are difficult to treat with podophyllin or any other locally destructive solutions. Podophyllin occasionally causes polyneuritis. Since it has a teratogenic potential, it should not be used in pregnant women.[55] Severe local reaction may result from its use in patients with autoimmune disease, diabetes, and in those who are on corticosteroids. Bichloroacetic acid solution may also be used to locally destroy condylomatous lesions. The anal and perianal area should be dried, and the lesions may be touched with a swab or a small stick dipped in the acid. The lesions turn white, indicating the effect of the acid. If spillage occurs onto the normal skin or mucous membrane, the solution should be wiped off or sodium bicarbonate solution applied immediately. Other local agents used infrequently with some success for destruction of condyloma acuminatum are chloroquine, sulfa-cream, 5-fluorouracil, and Thiotepa.

For large circumferential condyloma acuminatum extending into the anal canal, electrocoagulation with curetting is probably most useful, accomplishing destruction of the lesion in one sitting. Care should be exercised to avoid excessive burn of the normal squamous cell layer between the individual condylomatous fronds. Local or regional anesthesia is needed for satisfactory exposure of the anal canal. Simple excision of large perianal and anal condyloma acuminatum in toto will entail removal of the normal intervening anoderm and skin, so that extensive scarring and anal stenosis would more likely result. Excision of the normal unaffected skin between the fronds can be minimized, however. Dilute adrenalin-saline solution may be injected subcutaneously under condyloma acuminatum. Fronds of the lesion separate to expose the intervening normal-appearing skin or anoderm, so that the fronds of condyloma acuminatum may be individually excised.[56]

Recurrence is reported to occur in as many as 70 percent of cases following various local treatments.[57] Anal stenosis and scarring can occur. Repeated injudicious procedures may even result in anal incontinence. Treatment failures may have several causes. Some virus may be in a latent phase when treatment is rendered. Lesions may be small and difficult to see, and thus not destroyed by local treatment. Reinfection and autoinoculation may occur.

More recently, immunotherapy using autologous vaccine has become a worthy alternative to other traditional treatment modalities. Abcarian and Sharon [57] obtained 83 percent complete disappearance in one course of immunotherapy. Powell et al [58] obtained similar results. A recurrence rate of 10 percent is far lower than the usual recurrence rates. No specific cellular or humoral immune reaction to the autovaccination has yet been demonstrated. It remains to be seen if this mode of therapy is lasting.

INFECTIONS THAT MANIFEST AS PRURITIS ANI

Pruritis ani is itching of the anal region, which may begin as a sensation of slight itching confined to one aspect of the anus. With time, it usually becomes more severe and involves the whole perianal skin. It may also extend onto the vulva and posterior aspect of the scrotum, but it is usually experienced along the anal verge and along the median raphe in front of and behind the anus. In many cases, the itching is felt only at night. At times, the itching can become nearly intolerable. Examination of the anal region shows a variety of appearances ranging from normal to red, raw, oozing skin around the anus.

Pruritis ani is a symptom not a disease, and as such can have a variety of causes—mental strain, overwork, strawberries, caffein, alcohol, shellfish, change in climate, lack of anal cleanliness, local anorectal lesions, sweating, chemicals passed in the feces, and infections. Of the infectious agents, parasites (scabies, pediculoses pubis, threadworms, pinworms, and cutaneous larva migrans), fungi (the tineas and *Candida*), and bacteria (especially *Corynebacterium minutissimum,* which causes erythrasma) can be responsible.[59] Most of these diseases are discussed in Chapter 25.

A thorough physical examination and culture or other laboratory and roentgenographic examinations where indicated are mandatory in an attempt to find a treatable cause of pruritis ani. Specific infections should be treated (Chapters 11, 18, and 25). Nonspecific therapies include anal hygiene, local medications designed to minimize itching, and sedatives. In very severe cases, injections of the perianal skin with alcohol or long-acting anesthetics or operations designed to denervate the perianal skin have been used.

GENERAL REFERENCE

Goldberg SM, Gordon PH, Nivatvongs S (eds): Essentials of Anorectal Surgery. Philadelphia, Lippincott, 1980.

REFERENCES

1. Granet E: Manual of Proctology. Chicago, Year Book Medical Publishers, 1954.
2. Parks AG: Pathogenesis and treatment of fistula-in-ano. Br Med J 1:463, 1961.
3. Kratzer GL: The anal ducts and their clinical significance. Am J Surg 79:32, 1950.
4. Homan WP, Tang CK, Thorbjarnarson B: Anal lesions complicating Crohn's disease. Arch Surg 111:1333, 1976.
5. Rankin GB, Watts HD, Melnyk CS, Kelley ML Jr: National cooperative Crohn's disease study: extraintestinal manifestations and perianal complications. Gastroenterology 77:914, 1979.
6. Goligher JC: Surgery of the Anus, Rectum, and Colon, 3rd ed. Springfield, Thomas, 1975.
7. McElwain JW, MacLean MD, Alexander RM, Hoexter B, Guthrie JF: Experience with primary fistulectomy for anorectal abscess: a report of 1000 cases. Dis Colon Rectum 18:646, 1975.
8. Parks AG, Gordon PH: Fistula-in-ano: perineal fistula of intra-abdominal or intrapelvic origin stimulating fistula-in-ano. Report of seven cases. Dis Colon Rectum 19:500, 1976.
9. Milligan ETC, Morgan CN: Surgical anatomy of the anal canal with special reference to anorectal fistulae. Lancet 2:1150, 1934.
10. Parks AG, Gordon PH, Hardcastle JD: A classification of fistula-in-ano. Br J Surg 63:1, 1976.
11. Parks AG: The classification of fistula-in-ano. In Hofenrichter J (ed): Progress in Proctology. New York, Springer-Verlag, 1969.
12. Hanley PH, Ray JE, Pennington EE, Grablowsky OM: Fistula-in-ano: a ten-year follow-up study of horseshoe-abscess fistula-in-ano. Dis Colon Rectum 19:507, 1976.
13. Marks G, Chase WV, Mervine TB: The fatal potential of fistula-in-ano with abscess: analysis of 11 deaths. Dis Colon Rectum 16:224, 1973.
14. Lockhart-Mummery HE: Anal lesions of Crohn's disease. Clin Gastroenterol 1:377, 1972.
15. Gabriel WB: Results of an experimental and histological investigation into seventy-five cases of rectal fistulae. Proc R Soc Med 14:156, 1921.
16. Patey DH, Scarff RW: Pathology of postanal pilonidal sinus: its bearing on treatment. Lancet 2:484, 1946.
17. Drusin LM: The diagnosis and treatment of infectious and latent syphilis. Med Clin North Am 56:1161, 1972.
18. Akdamar K, Martin RJ, Ichinose H: Syphilitic proctitis. Am J Dig Dis 22:701, 1977.
19. Marino AWM Jr: Proctologic lesions observed in male homosexuals. Dis Colon Rectum 7:121, 1964.
20. Gluckman JB, Kleinman MS, May AG: Primary syphilis of rectum. NY State J Med 74:2210, 1974.
21. Nazemi MM, Musher DM, Schell RF, Milo S: Syphilitic proctitis in a homosexual. JAMA 231:389, 1975.
22. Annual Summary 1978: (Section 1) Summary of notifiable diseases in the United States. MMWR 27 (No. 54):3, 1979.
23. Lal S, Nicholas C: Epidemiological and clinical features in 165 cases of granuloma inguinale. Br J Vener Dis 46:461, 1970.
24. Greenwald E: Chancroidal infection. Treatment and diagnosis. JAMA 121:9, 1943.
25. Asin J: Chancroid: a report of 1402 cases. Am J Syph Gonorrhea Vener Dis 36:483, 1952.
26. Kerber RE, Rowe CE, Gilbert KR: Treatment of chancroid: a comparison of tetracycline and sulfisoxazole. Arch Dermatol 100:604, 1969.

27. Hammond GW, Lian CJ, Wilt JC, Ronald AR: Comparison of specimen collection and laboratory techniques for isolation of *Haemophilus ducreyi*. J Clin Microbiol 7:39, 1978.
28. Schachter J, Smith DE, Dawson CR, Anderson WR, Deller JJ, Hoke AW, Smartt WH, Meyer KF: Lymphogranuloma venereum. I. Comparison of the Frei test, complement fixation test, and isolation of the agent. J Infect Dis 120:372, 1969.
29. Grace AW: Anorectal lymphogranuloma venereum. JAMA 122:74, 1943.
30. Annamunthodo H: Rectal lymphogranuloma venereum in Jamaica. Dis Colon Rectum 4:17, 1961.
31. Storz J: Chlamydia and Chlamydia-Induced Diseases. Springfield, Thomas, 1971.
32. Schachter J, Dawson CR: Lymphogranuloma venereum. JAMA 236:915, 1976.
33. Greaves AB: The frequency of lymphogranuloma venereum in persons with perirectal abscesses, fistula-in-ano, or both. With particular reference to the relationship between perirectal abscesses of lymphogranuloma origin in the male and inversion. Bull WHO 29:797, 1963.
34. Caldwell HD, Kuo CC: Serologic diagnosis of lymphogranuloma venereum by counterimmunoelectrophoresis with a *Chlamydia trachomatis* protein antigen. J Immunol 118:442, 1977.
35. Schachter J, Meyer KF: Lymphogranuloma venereum. II. Characterization of some recently isolated strains. J Bacteriol 99:636, 1969.
36. Shapiro SR, Breschi LC: Venereal disease in Vietnam: clinical experience at a major military hospital. Milit Med 139:374, 1974.
37. Sowmini CN, Gopalan KN, Rao GC: Minocycline in the treatment of lymphogranuloma venereum. J Am Vener Dis Assoc 2:19, 1976.
38. Nahmias AJ, Roizman B: Part I. Infection with herpes-simplex viruses 1 and 2. N Engl J Med 289:667, 1973.
39. Nahmias AJ, Naib ZM, Josey WE, Clepper AC: Herpes simplex infection of the female genital tract. Virologic and cytologic studies. Obstet Gynecol 29:395, 1967.
40. Centifanto YM, Drylie DM, Deardourff SL, Kaufman HE: Herpesvirus type 2 in the male genitourinary tract. Science 178:318, 1972.
41. Waugh MA: Anorectal herpesvirus hominis infection in men. J Am Vener Dis Assoc 3:68, 1976.
42. Jacobs E: Anal infections caused by herpes simplex virus. Dis Colon Rectum 19:151, 1976.
43. Benjamin DR: Use of immunoperoxidase for rapid diagnosis of mucocutaneous herpes simplex virus infection. J Clin Microbiol 6:571, 1977.
44. Brown ST, Jaffe HW, Zaidi A, Filker R, Hermann KL, Lylerla HC, Jove DF, Budell JW: Sensitivity and specificity of diagnostic tests for genital infection with herpesvirus hominis. Sex Transm Dis 6:10, 1979.
45. Hanna L, Keshishyan H, Jawetz E, Coleman VR: Diagnosis of herpesvirus hominis infections in a general hospital laboratory. J Clin Microbiol 1:318, 1975.
46. Nahmias AJ: The laboratory diagnosis of herpes simplex virus infection. Diagnostic Horizons 1:1, 1977.
47. Blough HA, Giuntoli RL: Successful treatment of human genital herpes infections with 2-deoxy-D-glucose. JAMA 241:2798, 1979.
48. Morgan HR, Balduzzi PC: Propagation of an intranuclear inclusion-forming agent from human condyloma acuminatum. Proc Nat Acad Sci 52:1561, 1964.
49. Shirodaria PV, Matthews RS: An immunofluorescence study of warts. Clin Exp Immunol 21:329, 1975.
50. Walter EL Jr, Walker DL, Cooper GA: Localization of specific antigen in human warts. Arch Pathol 79:419, 1965.
51. Oriel JD: Natural history of genital warts. Br J Vener Dis 47:1, 1971.
52. Oriel JD, Whimster IW: Carcinoma in situ associated with virus-containing anal warts. Br J Dermatol 84:71, 1971.
53. Dawson DF, Duckworth JK, Bernhardt H, Young JM: Giant condyloma and verrucous carcinoma of the genital area. Arch Pathol 79:225, 1965.
54. Dreyfuss W, Neville WE: Buschke-Loewenstein tumors (giant condylomata acuminata). Am J Surg 90:146, 1955.
55. Chamberlain MJ, Reynolds AL, Yeoman WB: Medical memoranda: toxic effect of podophyllun application in pregnancy. Br Med J 3:391, 1972.
56. Thompson JPS, Grace RH: The treatment of perianal and anal condylomata acuminata: a new operative technique. J R Soc Med 7:180, 1978.
57. Abcarian H, Sharon N: The effectiveness of immunotherapy in the treatment of anal condyloma acuminatum. J Surg Res 22:231, 1977.
58. Powell LC Jr, Pollard M, Jenkins JL Jr: Treatment of condyloma acuminata by autogenous vaccine. South Med J 63:202, 1970.
59. Boyer A, McColl I: The role of erythrasma in pruritis ani. Lancet 2:572, 1966.

CHAPTER 42
Infections of the Skeletal System

ROBERT H. FITZGERALD JR. AND PATRICK J. KELLY

WHEN a Cartilage therefore is inflamed, and soaked in purulent Matter, the transverse or connecting Fibres will the soonest give way, and the Cartilage becomes more or less red and soft. If the Disorder goes on a little longer, and Cartilage does not throw off a Slough, but separates from the Bone, where the Force of Cohesion is least, and where the Disease soon arrives, by reason of the Thinness of the Cartilage. . . . But if, unfortunately, the Patient labours under a bad Habit of Body, the Malignancy, having got Root in the Bone, will daily gain ground, the *Caries* will spread, and at last the unhappy Person must submit to Extirpation, a doubtful Remedy, or wear out a painful, though probably a short Life.

William Hunter, 1743 [1]

The introduction of antimicrobial drugs dramatically improved the treatment of a spectrum of serious infectious diseases. Although the results of treatment of acute hematogenous osteomyelitis have been improved, by the introduction of newer and more potent agents, over that described by William Hunter, chronic osteomyelitis and established septic arthritis remain recalcitrant.

Even though an extensive vascular network exists in osseous tissue, sequestration of devascularized areas of bone creates an environment that permits continued bacterial growth without interference by host defense mechanisms or antimicrobial agents. This basic response of infected osseous tissue isolated from the systemic circulation is fundamental in the development of chronic osseous infections.

Sepsis of the skeletal system can be divided into osteomyelitis, septic arthritis, and postoperative wound sepsis. The microbiologic findings and the medical and surgical treatment of septic arthritis and osteomyelitis differ with various causes, that is, hematogenous, posttraumatic, and postoperative.

OSTEOMYELITIS

Wilensky credits Nelaton with introducing the term "osteomyelitis" in 1834.[2] Nelaton distinguished inflammation of cortical bone, "osteite," from inflammation of the medulla, "osteomyelitie." Although osteomyelitis frequently begins in the medullary portion of tubular bones, the term is generally understood to signify an infection of either the cortical or the medullary portion of a bone. Pyogenic or bacterial osteomyelitis can be subdivided into hematogenous and secondary forms, which include osteomyelitis from a contiguous focus of infection, as well as posttraumatic and postoperative osteomyelitis.

PATHOBIOLOGY OF BONE INFECTIONS

Osteomyelitis is usually initiated by bacteremia lodging in a receptive bony site, usually the metaphysis in children and infants, and in the middle of the shaft of the long bone, pelvic bone, or body of a vertebra in adults.

The vascular supply of the metaphysis in a child older than 1 year seems to be critical for the localization of infection. In growing long bones, the blood supply to the metaphysis is separate from that of the epiphysis. The metaphyseal nutrient artery terminates in acutely looped capillaries beneath the cartilaginous growth plate that flow into venous sinusoids in which blood flow is sluggish. Septic emboli apparently lodge here and thrombose the terminal capillaries of the nutrient artery, which fosters spread of infection from the venous lakes. In the child, the cartilaginous growth plate is an effective barrier to communication between the blood supply of the shaft and that of the epiphysis. Thus, in a child older than 1 year, bacteremia that leads to metaphyseal osteomyelitis rarely involves the epiphysis. Septic arthritis is an unusual complication of metaphyseal or diaphyseal osteomyelitis in children.

In infancy, blood vessels from the metaphysis perforate the cartilaginous growth plates of the long bones and penetrate the epiphysis, forming venous lakes similar to those in the metaphysis. Because of these vascular communications through the growth plate, infection of the shaft and metaphysis via the nutrient artery can invade the epiphysis and extend secondarily into the joint to produce septic arthritis.

In adulthood, the growth plate has fused, and the old cartilage growth plate has been penetrated by metaphyseal vessels. Vascular communications are then reestablished between the metaphyseal and epiphyseal circulations so that osteomyelitis can once again extend beneath the articular cartilage and into the involved joint. For these reasons, infants have severe, often permanent epiphyseal damage and joint infection, a large involucrum, but only transient damage to the shaft and metaphysis. Children have extensive cortical damage with involucrum and, rarely, damage to the growth cartilage and to joints. Adults have cortical atrophy, chronic infection of the marrow cavity, and chronic discharging sinuses, often with extraperiosteal abscesses and joint involvement.

Infecting agents of low virulence may be inhibited and eradicated by host defense mechanisms. Alternately, host tissue may isolate and wall off the nidus of infection, forming a Brodie abscess (Fig. 42-1). When a Brodie abscess is formed, the remaining microorganisms are usually destroyed, resulting in serous fluid or fibrous tissues filling the cavity. When classic osteomyelitis occurs, necrosis and increased pressure result in the spread of the infection through paths of least resistance—the haversian and Volkmann canals—as well as the intramedullary space. A subperiosteal abscess occurs if the process continues unabated. When the endosteal and the periosteal blood supplies are occluded, sequestration or separation of the entire cortex can occur. Frequently, only a portion of the cortex is involved. The host attempts to isolate the infectious process with new periosteal and endosteal bone forming an involucrum about the necrotic bone (the sequestrum). An inflammatory reaction occurs in adjacent areas, which is the basis for the reactive synovitis so frequently seen in adjacent joints.

This sequence can be altered at any stage by host defense mechanisms or by the administration of antimicrobial agents. If significant necrosis has occurred, operative intervention is usually required to halt the progression of the disease.

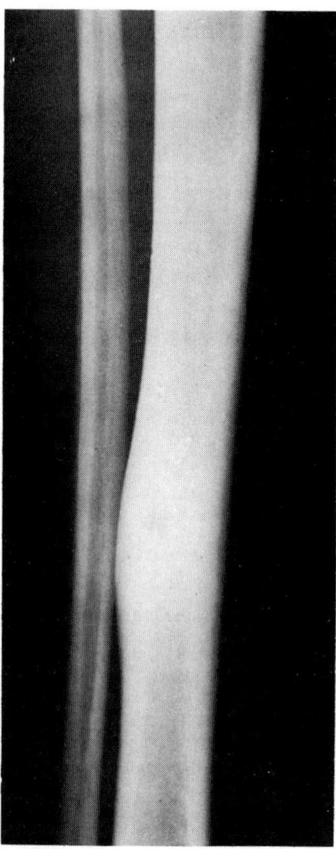

Fig. 42-1. **Brodie's abscess of tibial diaphysis. Lytic zone is surrounded by zone of sclerosis in middle third of tibia.**

Hematogenous Osteomyelitis in Infants and Children

Incidence

Acute hematogenous osteomyelitis is primarily a disease of children between the ages of 3 and 15 years [3] but has been noted in neonates. A predilection for the metaphyseal region of a long tubular bone is seen, so that the most frequent sites of involvement include the proximal tibial and distal femoral metaphysis. The humerus, fibula, radius, and ulna are involved less frequently. Spinal involvement in the pediatric patient is usually limited to the intervertebral disc (Table 42-1).

Most of the patients in whom the proximal femoral metaphysis is involved are infants, and most of these are associated with septic arthritis of the hip. In older children, the distal femur and proximal tibia are frequent sites of involvement. All three sites account for a large percentage of the growth of the extremity and can easily be damaged by uncontrolled infection.

Etiology

Staphylococcus aureus can be isolated from material obtained by aspiration or open biopsy in 80 to 90 percent of the patients. Most of the staphylococcal isolates will

TABLE 42-1. SITES OF INVOLVEMENT, BY AGE, IN CHILDREN WITH HEMATOGENOUS OSTEOMYELITIS *

	Age			
Site	2	3–8	9–16	Total
Femur (N = 50)				
Proximal	8	12	9	29
Middle	0	2	3	5
Distal	3	4	9	16
Tibia (N = 42)				
Proximal	3	3	12	18
Middle	1	1	2	4
Distal	2	7	11	20
Humerus	3	4	5	12
Fibula	1	3	4	8
Radius	1	1	1	3
Ulna	0	1	1	2
Pelvis	0	5	5	10
Total	22	43	62	127 †

* Three patients had multiple sites of involvement.

† Total does not reflect patients with involvement of cranium (2), talus (1), clavicle (2), calcaneus (3), tarsal navicular (1), scapula (1), and rib (1).

Adapted from Morrey BF, Peterson HA: Hematogenous pyogenic osteomyelitis in children. *Orthop Clin North Am* 6:935, 1975.

be resistant to penicillin. Streptococcal osteomyelitis is less frequent and is usually limited to patients who are 3 years of age or younger. In contrast to the adult patient with osteomyelitis, gram-negative bacilli are rarely isolated from infections in the pediatric patient (Table 42-2).

Clinical Manifestations

In Children. Clinically, acute hematogenous osteomyelitis is characterized by an abrupt onset of pain of increasing severity and pyrexia.[4] The patient may be lethargic, dehydrated, and irritable. Early in the infection, the lack of local signs of inflammation may be misleading. A limp or limited use of an involved extremity may be the only clinical finding. In the younger child, pseudoparalysis can be the earliest sign. Close scrutiny reveals that the adjacent joints are flexed and the regional muscles are in spasm. If examination is performed gently, passive motion can be demonstrated in adjacent joints, an important sign in differentiating osteomyelitis from septic arthritis. If an abscess has ruptured through the periosteum, a fluctuant mass can be palpated in the soft tissues. Leukocytosis with a definite shift to the left and an elevation of the erythrocyte sedimentation rate are characteristically present.

It is important to emphasize that roentgenographic examination initially will reveal only soft tissue changes. A technetium-99 scan can be helpful in making an early diagnosis and localizing the site of involvement. Not until 10 to 14 days after the onset of the infection will a localized destruction surrounded by a zone of decalcification in the metaphysis be visualized roentgenographically. Lacy periosteal new bone formation can be observed two to four weeks after onset. A moth-eaten appearance in the metaphysis appears if the infection continues without treatment (Fig. 42-2).

Inadequate administration of antimicrobial agents results in a subacute form of the disease characterized by persistence of regional physical findings and a lack of systemic symptoms. The erythrocyte sedimentation rate remains elevated in spite of a normal leukocyte count. Alteration of the osseous structures can be identified on roentgenographic examination.

Diagnosis

It is important to obtain a culture to identify the specific organism(s) and determine antibiotic sensitivities in all cases of osteomyelitis. Subperiosteal or intraosseous needle aspiration and aspiration of a contiguous joint are useful procedures when roentgenograms are unrevealing. If there is evidence, however, of a lytic lesion in a metaphysis, the area can be drained through a cortical window and tissue obtained for culture.

Osteomyelitis can be difficult to distinguish from Ewing sarcoma when roentgenographic changes have occurred in the subacute form. Urgent operative exploration, biopsy, and culture are mandatory.[4]

Treatment

When acute hematogenous osteomyelitis is diagnosed early, parenteral administration of an antimicrobial agent and splinting of the involved extremity will arrest the infection.[4] If, however, the infection has become established, debridement will be required. Usually, removal of a cortical window for the metaphyseal area permits decompression of intramedullary abscesses and excision of sequestrated osseous tissue. Closure can be accomplished over an irrigation–suction system a few days later.

Acute Osteomyelitis in Adults

Acute hematogenous osteomyelitis in adults is uncommon in diaphyseal long bones and usually is limited to the axial skeleton in debilitated patients who are in their fifth or sixth decade. The thoracolumbar segments of the spinal column are most frequently involved. *S. aureus* is the usual etiologic agent. Residual *S. aureus* infections from childhood osteomyelitis are sometimes seen in the long bones. When retrograde seeding of the vertebral body through the interconnecting plexus of valveless veins occurs from an antecedent infection of the pelvic organs or after instrumentation of the urogenital tract, gram-negative bacillary

TABLE 42-2. CULTURE RESULTS, BY AGE, IN CHILDREN WITH HEMATOGENOUS OSTEOMYELITIS

Culture	Age 2	Age 3–8	Age 9–16	Total
Staphylococci				
Penicillin-resistant	5	10	23	38
Penicillin-sensitive	0	6	5	11
Unclassified	2	7	11	20
Coagulase-negative	1	1	4	6
Streptococci	7	0	3	10
Gram-negative rods	1	1	0	2
Anaerobic	0	2	0	2
Culture negative	6	12	14	32
Not done	1	4	9	14
Total	23	43	69	135

Adapted from Morrey BF, Peterson HA: Hematogenous pyogenic osteomyelitis in children. *Orthop Clin North Am* 6:935, 1975.

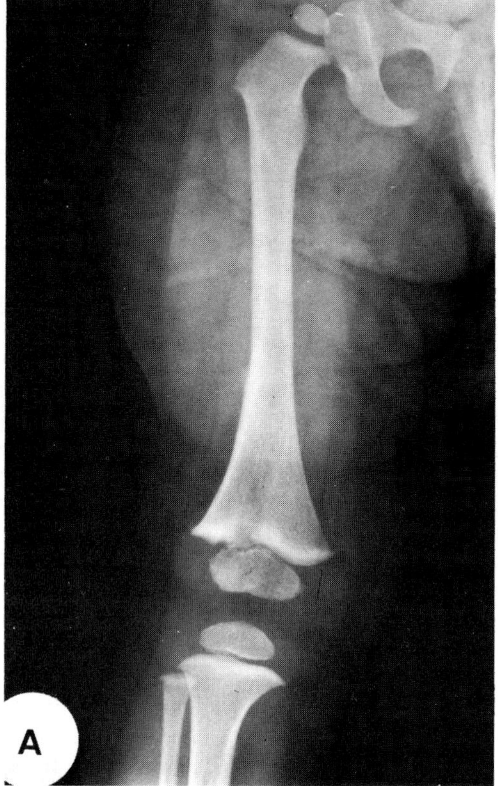

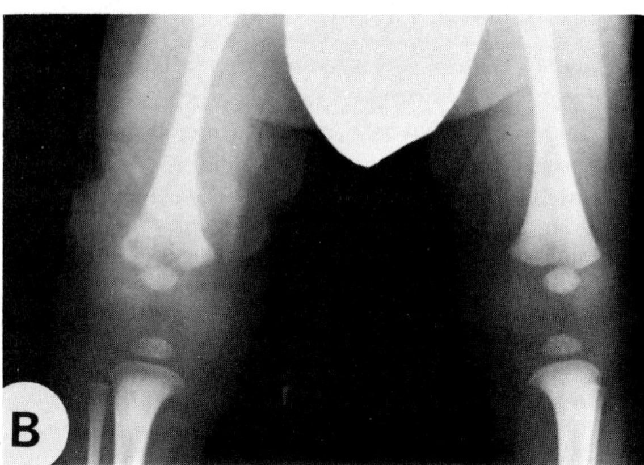

Fig. 42-2. A. **Newborn child with soft-tissue swelling and early lytic involvement of distal femoral epiphyseal plate. B. Three weeks later, further destruction of distal femoral epiphyseal plate and metaphysis has occurred despite parenteral antibiotic therapy. Surgical debridement was required to eradicate infection.**

organisms (most commonly *Pseudomonas aeruginosa, Proteus mirabilis, Enterobacter,* and *Escherichia coli*) are found.[5] Osteomyelitis caused by *Salmonella* is becoming more common, especially in immunocompromised patients and in the long tubular bones of patients with hemoglobinopathies. An increasing number of young adults, particularly drug addicts, have hematogenous vertebral or clavicular osteomyelitis.[6] Submission of tissue specimens to the microbiology laboratory before initiating antimicrobial therapy is important because unusual causative organisms, such as *P. aeruginosa* and *Candida albicans,* are frequently isolated.

Most adults with hematogenous osteomyelitis of the axial skeleton have fever symptoms and an elevated leukocyte count and sedimentation rate, and most can be treated with bed rest and specific antimicrobial therapy. After the initial symptoms subside, the spinal column should be protected with either a cast or a brace.

Contiguous Osteomyelitis

Osteomyelitis after incomplete antimicrobial therapy for exogenous contamination or an antecedent contiguous soft-tissue infection in children has been noted more frequently in recent years. Many of the children with this type of osteomyelitis have sustained puncture wounds of the foot. Their clinical course is altered by oral antimicrobial therapy prescribed in emergency rooms. A progressive limp indicates further medical consultation. The patient is usually afebrile. Examination reveals an exquisitely tender site with or without an inflammatory response near the previous plantar puncture wound. The erythrocyte sedimentation rate is elevated.

Previous antimicrobial therapy can make identification of the causal organism(s) difficult. Gram-negative bacillary rods predominate in patients with secondary forms of osteomyelitis.

P. aeruginosa has been isolated from tissue specimens in more than 90 percent of the patients who have sustained puncture wounds of the foot. Surgical debridement is invariably required for eradication of the infection. A retained foreign body frequently is identified at operation. When a foreign body is not located during debridement, the central nidus of the infection involves a cartilaginous surface—articular, epiphyseal, or apophyseal.

Chronic Osteomyelitis

Incidence and Etiology

Chronic osteomyelitis can be a sequela of trauma, postoperative sepsis, or acute hematogenous osteomyelitis. Chronic osteomyelitis after acute hematogenous osteomyelitis may be asymptomatic for many years before a persistent draining sinus tract appears. Chronic posttraumatic osteomyelitis occurs most often in the readily traumatized area of the tibia and femur, and less often, in the humerus and radius. Patients with concomitant nonunion account for almost one third of cases.[7]

Chronic osteomyelitis after elective musculoskeletal surgery accounts for only a small fraction of the patients with chronic osteomyelitis. The prognosis depends upon the area involved. In patients with spinal involvement, eradication of the septic process without sacrificing osseous stability or creating neural deficit can create formidable problems. If other areas are involved, a reasonably successful outcome can be anticipated, with removal of foreign bodies, saucerization, and sequestrectomy.

West and associates[7] report that the most frequent sites of involvement in chronic osteomyelitis include the tibia and femur. The upper extremity is less often involved.

However, when osteomyelitis occurs in the arm, the humerus, radius, and ulna are the most frequent sites. Osteomyelitis of the small bones of the hand is usually secondary to penetrating wounds. Involvement of the foot is frequently associated with occlusive vascular disease or diabetes mellitus. The prognosis obviously reflects the severity of the underlying problem, and when the appropriate vascular procedure is successful, a localized amputation will rectify the problem.

Etiology

Chronic osteomyelitis appearing as a late complication of the acute disease in childhood is most often due to a penicillin-sensitive *S. aureus.* Chronic posttraumatic osteomyelitis is usually polymicrobic, gram-negative organisms, especially *P. aeruginosa* and *P. mirabilis,* with or without *S. aureus.*

Anaerobes have been isolated infrequently from surgical specimens in patients with osteomyelitis. Actinomycosis of the mandible and other head and neck sites is an obvious exception. More recently, improved transportation vials and increased physician awareness have led to the isolation of increasing numbers of anaerobic organisms from tissue cultures in patients with osteomyelitis, especially after trauma. In a study of *Bacteroides* infections of the musculoskeletal system by Nettles and co-workers,[8] 4 of the 11 patients had chronic osteomyelitis. In a recent study of patients with osteomyelitis (posttraumatic osteomyelitis),[9] anaerobic organisms were isolated from 18 percent of the patients. A wide variety of gram-positive and gram-negative anaerobic isolates were recovered. In all but 1 patient, the anaerobes were isolated from a mixed culture consisting of both aerobic and anaerobic organisms.

In a recent series reported by Finegold,[10] 22 of 58 patients with osteomyelitis had anaerobes recovered. Only 3 of the 22 had only anaerobes. In the group of 22 patients, there were 92 aerobic or facultative isolates (14 *S. aureus,* 32 Enterobacteriaceae, 9 *P. aeruginosa,* 22 streptococci) and 98 anaerobic isolates (33 *Bacteroides,* 4 *Fusobacterium,* 29 *Peptococcus,* 8 *Peptostreptococcus,* 6 *Actinomyces*). In brief, the flora resembled that of long-standing soft tissue infections.

Diagnosis

The clinical and radiographic findings, including tomography results, should outline the diseased areas. Sinograms may be helpful in demonstrating the degree of soft tissue involvement. The microbiologic diagnosis is more complicated. Since various causal organisms are isolated from the different types of osteomyelitis, separate deep tissue specimens should be obtained from bone, muscle, and fascia. Swab cultures of sinus tract drainage are notoriously misleading. Most organisms isolated from sinus tract drainage will not be recovered from cultures of deep tissue. If *S. aureus* is isolated from the drainage, however, it will invariably be isolated from deep-tissue cultures. Furthermore, as treatment progresses the saucerized cavity should be recultured and susceptibility studies performed. If an irrigation–suction system is employed as an adjunct to delayed closure, culture of the egress fluid should be performed by the third or fourth day because gram-negative bacterial contamination and superinfection of the irrigation–suction system are common.

Treatment

The treatment of chronic osteomyelitis is prolonged, requiring at least four weeks of parenteral antimicrobial therapy and two operations. Surgical treatment of chronic osteomyelitis is based on four principles: (1) excision of dead bone, (2) removal of infected granulation tissue, (3) obliteration of dead space, and (4) obtaining union when nonunion exists.[11] Achieving union in an ununited and infected fracture may seem difficult, but many fractures unite without further operation after the infection has resolved. The recent introduction of external fixation devices has been invaluable in the management of the infected nonunion.

Chronic Hematogenous Osteomyelitis. Tomograms and bone scans are valuable in planning the operations. Exposure of cavities invaded by infected granulation tissue with unroofing procedures is essential. Because patients with chronic hematogenous osteomyelitis have bony stability, external splinting is unnecessary unless excessive bone has been excised, but pathologic fracture can occur when an extensive debridement and saucerization have been performed (Fig. 42-3).

Delayed closure over an irrigation–suction system often can be accomplished by the third to the fifth day after the initial debridement. If an irrigation–suction system is employed, it should be used to control the hematoma formation and should be removed within three to five days. An antimicrobial drug need not be administered in the irrigation–suction system.[12] If debridement is adequate, a sufficient blood supply should exist, permitting parenteral therapy to achieve bactericidal concentrations in the tissues. Prolonged use of an irrigation–suction system has a serious disadvantage—it permits the entry into the wound of ambient gram-negative bacilli, which in our experience invariably colonize the egress tubes by the twelfth to the fourteenth day.

Posttraumatic Chronic Osteomyelitis with Nonunion. Opinions differ on the management of chronic osteomyelitis and ununited fractures.[13] Traditionally, primary emphasis has been placed on controlling the infection. Once the infection is eradicated, those patients with a persistent nonunion are treated with autogenous bone grafts and stabilization. The alternate approach is based on the rationale that once union has been achieved, an adequate blood supply exists, permitting the host defense mechanisms to eradicate the infection. We believe that the latter approach, in which internal fixation devices were placed concurrently with wound debridement, has been followed too often by persistent sepsis. Thus, we continue to favor the traditional approach of controlling the infection first. However, if an intramedullary nail already provides stability when the infection appears, bone grafting procedures away from the site of the septic process can

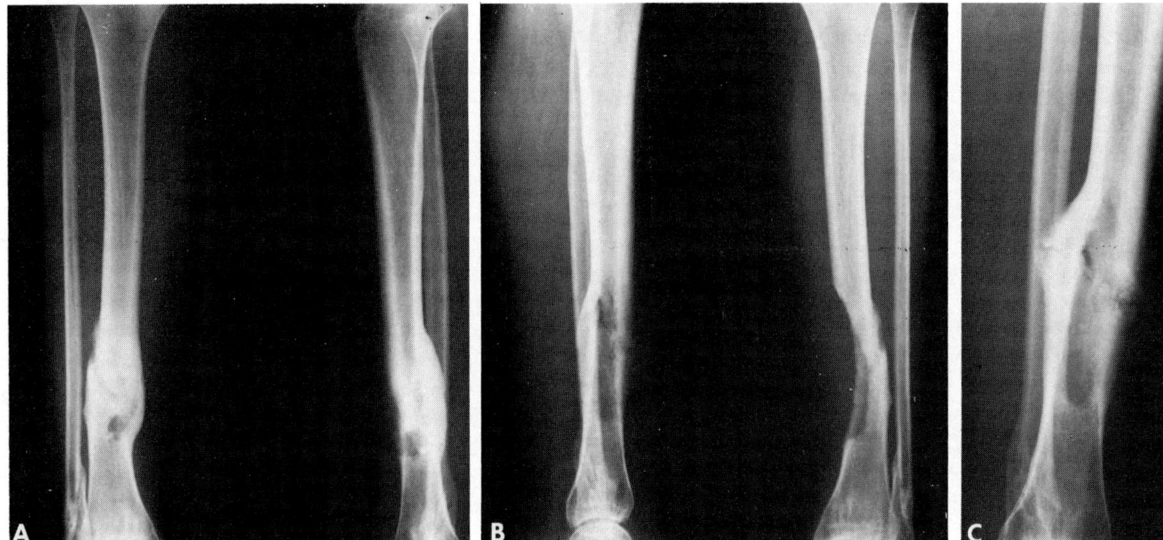

Fig. 42-3. **Pathologic fracture after saucerization of posttraumatic osteomyelitis of tibia. A. Posttraumatic osteomyelitis of tibia with a draining sinus one year after removal of foreign bodies (screws) used to achieve stabilization. Lytic destruction of proximal fracture fragment on anteroposterior view is noted. B. Tibia was saucerized, and local muscle flap placed in cavity. The degree of infected bone was greater than that appreciated on preoperative roentgenograms. Extensive unroofing procedure was required, leaving only posterior cortex intact. C. Healing fracture through saucerized cavity six months after surgical treatment.**

sometimes still achieve union, with eradication of the infection.

In our experience, 60 percent of patients with infected nonunions of the femur and tibia will obtain union of their fracture if the infection is eradicated, stability maintained, and early ambulation encouraged, especially if functional casts are used.

For the infected tibial nonunion, preservation of an intact fibula is important because removal of infected and dead bone may lead to diaphyseal discontinuities. After arrest of the infection, autogenous iliac grafts can be inserted posteriorly, above and below the nonunion, if the fibula is intact. Autogenous iliac crest bone is the material of choice.

In treating an infected nonunion of the femur, debridement and soft-tissue healing should be the first objective. After 6 to 12 weeks of freedom from clinical evidence of infection, long strips of autologous iliac bone are placed medially and posteriorly, with or without internal fixation, to effect bony union (Fig. 42-4).

For nonunion of the humerus, radius, or ulna, an iliac graft can be fashioned to fill in defects and maintain length. In these anatomic areas, plates are probably preferable to intramedullary rods for achieving stability, although the recently designed fluted rod for the humerus may offer another technique for achieving humeral fixation.

If primary stabilization is elected in the treatment of the infected nonunion, the newer devices that provide rigid internal fixation are probably necessary. Burri [13] proposed that rigid internal fixation and cancellous autogenous iliac bone grafts be used to achieve union of the fracture after thorough debridement. If soft-tissue closure is not possible, the wound is allowed to heal by granulation tissue and epithelialization. Utilizing these techniques in the treatment of 200 patients with posttraumatic osteomyelitis (102 patients had a united fracture), Burri arrested the osteomyelitic process in 180. Nine patients required amputation for persistent infection, and 11 patients developed recurrent sepsis.

In some infected nonunions of the femur, intramedullary fixation devices can be left in situ or, when loose, can be replaced to obtain stability at the time of debridement. These intramedullary rods will have to be removed later.

The advent of rigid external fixation has made the preceding debate academic because it permits concurrent stabilization and control of the infection without implanted foreign material traversing the nonunion. Currently, a complete debridement and saucerization can be done at the initial operation. When the secondary debridement is performed two to three days later, the application of either a Vidal-Hoffman device for infected nonunion of the tibia, humerus, radius, or ulna (Fig. 42-5) or a Wagner apparatus for infected nonunions of the femur (Fig. 42-6) will provide rigid external fixation.

Chronic Posttraumatic Osteomyelitis with Union. The treatment of posttraumatic osteomyelitis with a united fracture can be difficult. Repeated operation in an area of chronic infection causes extensive scars that make the anatomy obscure, dissection difficult, and healing poor. Excision of bone must be judicious if pathologic fracture is to be avoided, yet saucerization must be sufficient to permit the eradication of the infected granulation tissue and sequestra. Methylene blue can be used to identify avascular tissue and to follow the sinus tracts. If the dye

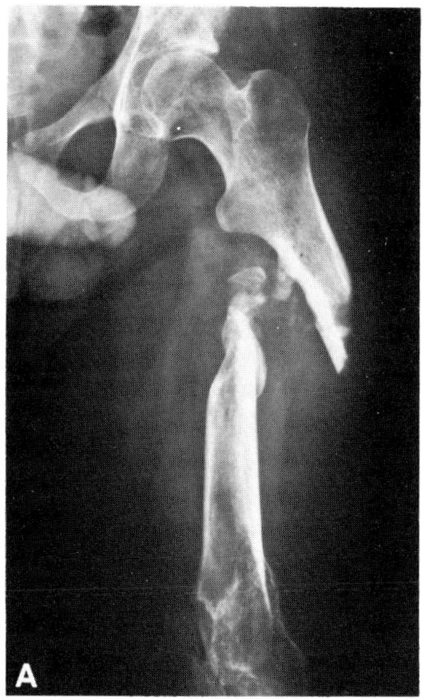

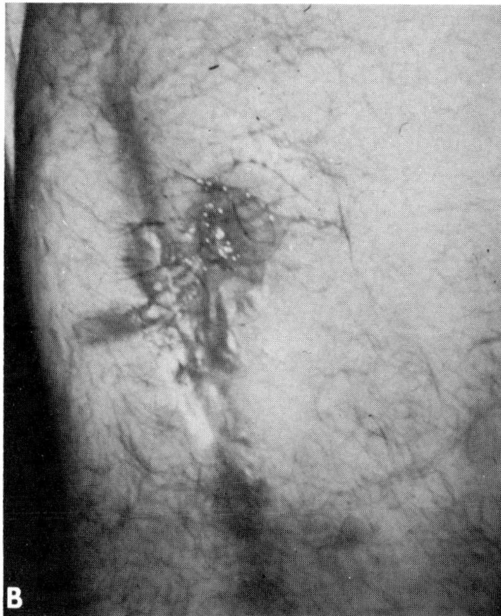

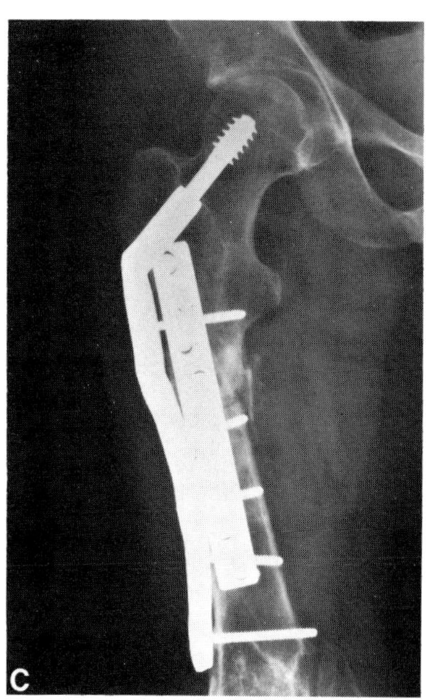

Fig. 42-4. **Infected nonunion of femur. A. Anteroposterior roentgenogram of femur demonstrating osteomyelitic changes with concomitant nonunion. B. Sinus tract located on lateral thigh. C. Anteroposterior roentgenogram one year after debridement and soft-tissue closure. Internal fixation and autogenous bone grafting were performed six months after debridement. Early roentgenographic union of femoral fracture is evident.**

is injected into the sinus tract with a soft catheter 12 hours before operation, all avascular tissues will be stained at the time of debridement.

Because bone is rigid and will not collapse and obliterate the dead space after saucerization, a variety of techniques are employed to close the dead space. The time-honored techniques include open packing of the wound, with healing from within, or, alternately, marsupialization of the osseous cavity, with subsequent application of a split-thickness skin graft directly to the granulating osseous cavity. The placement of cancellous bone grafts directly into the osseous bed was common two to three decades ago. In 1944, Mowlem [14] placed cancellous bone into mandibular defects, some of which communicated with the oral cavity. About the same time, Knight and Wood [15] and Robertson and Barron [16] initially applied a split-thickness skin graft to the saucerized cavity. When the infectious process was controlled, the skin graft was replaced by autogenous iliac bone graft. Coleman and co-workers [17] advocated a one-stage procedure consisting of saucerization, bone grafting, and closure. They noted that, although skin necrosis might occur, exposure of the bone grafts had no adverse effect. The exposed grafts were gradually covered by granulation tissue, which could be covered with a second split-thickness skin graft. Bickel and co-workers [18] reported a failure rate of 22 percent with this technique. Recently, this technique has been repopularized by Papineau,[19] who placed the cancellous grafts directly into the saucerized cavity. The grafts are slowly covered with granulation tissue. Secondary epithelialization or placement of split-thickness skin grafts can be used to achieve skin coverage.

In many anatomic locations, especially the tibia, a muscle flap can obliterate the dead space and provide a new blood supply to the saucerized osseous cavity.[20] Muscle tissue has excellent reconstructive properties,[21] rapidly attaches itself to the walls of the cavity, and introduces a new blood supply, which allows host defense mechanisms and parenterally administered antimicrobial agents to reach the wound. The muscle flap can be a pedicle graft or a local flap. Cross-leg pedicle grafts, utilized in the past, subject the opposite normal extremity to surgical trauma and expose it to infection.

Local flaps have been advocated recently by Ger [20] for the treatment of osteomyelitis. Although Uyama [22] and Popkirov [23] have each reported replacement of muscle fibers with fibrous tissue, newer techniques take both the blood supply and the innervation of the flap into consideration so that the muscle will remain viable and contractile. We have had gratifying results with this technique in those tibial and femoral lesions in which extensive scar tissue has replaced the soft-tissue envelope. Even in infected nonunions of the tibia, a local muscle flap and an external fixation device provide a new blood supply and rigid stabilization—prerequisites for healing (Fig. 42-7).

Specific parenteral antimicrobial therapy is as important as good surgical technique. Either modality alone results in a high incidence of recurrent sepsis. We have learned to give parenteral antimicrobial therapy for at least four weeks. Data on whether a shorter or longer course of parenteral antimicrobial therapy is better are not available. Recently, Nelson and co-workers [24] reported the successful management of pediatric osteomyelitis with oral agents if serum and tissue fluid levels were monitored frequently. The agent used must be selected on the basis of results of susceptibility studies, and some organisms,

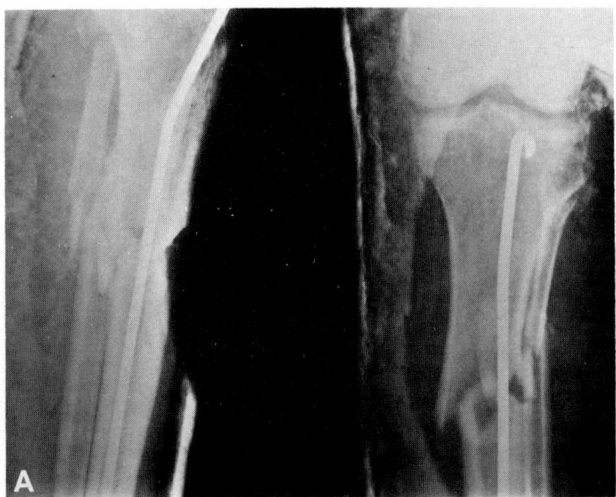

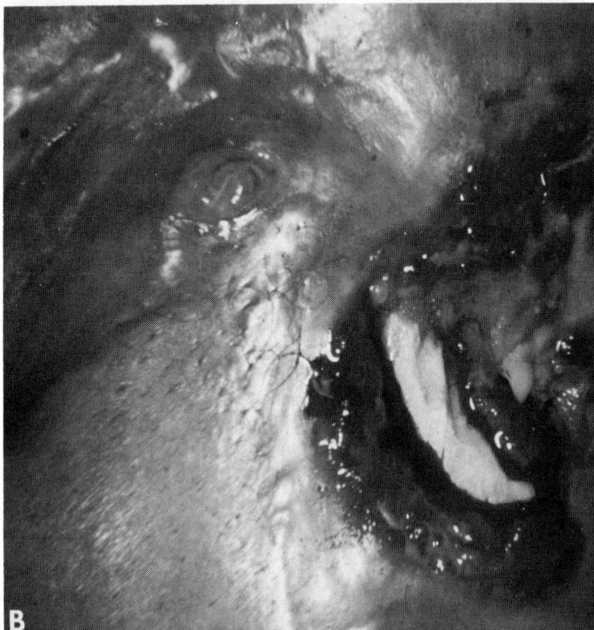

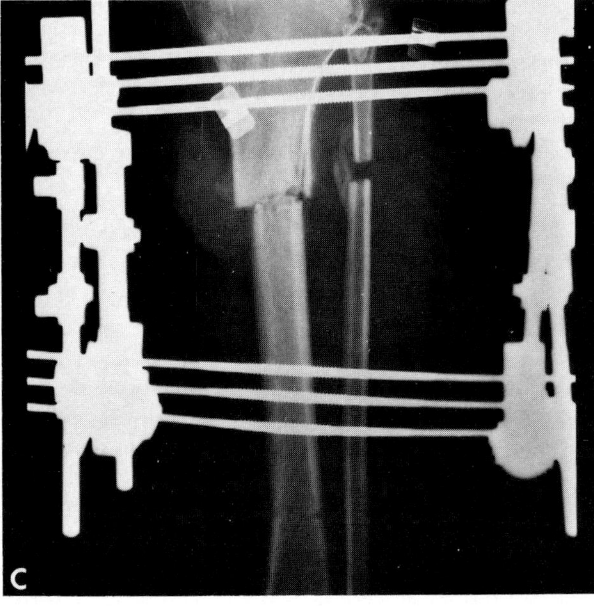

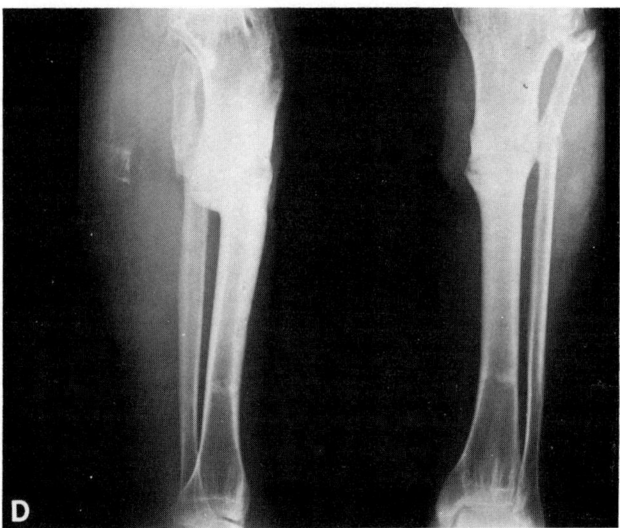

Fig. 42-5. Posttraumatic osteomyelitis of tibia with ununited fracture managed by external fixation. A. Compound fracture of tibia with extensive soft-tissue injury. Initial stabilization was attempted with a Rush rod. B. Five months later, patient was seen at the Mayo Clinic with exposed tibial diaphysis and a draining sinus. C. After excision of dead and infected tissue, stabilization was achieved with the Vidal-Hoffmann device. D. Sixteen months after surgical debridement and four weeks of parenteral antimicrobial therapy, there is no evidence of sepsis, and union has been achieved.

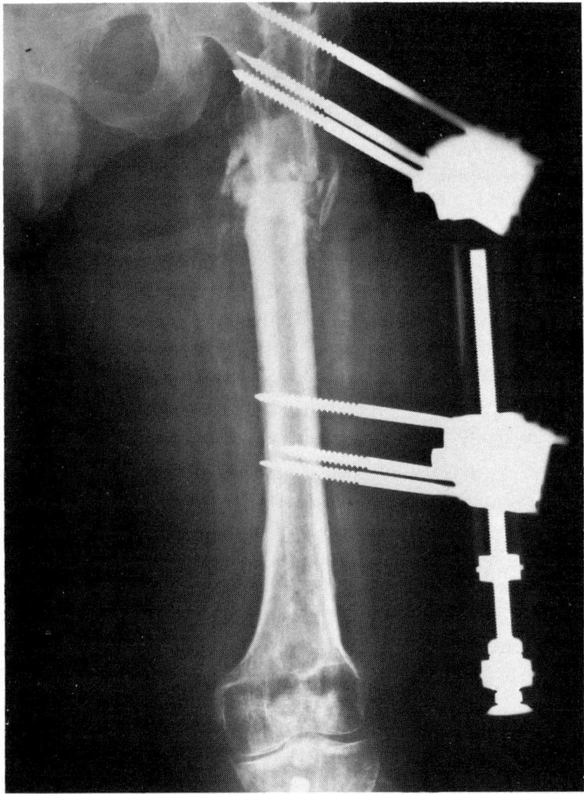

Fig. 42-6. Infected nonunion of femur after insertion of intramedullary nail. Intramedullary device was removed, wound debrided, and Wagner apparatus applied. Three months later, there was evidence of early union.

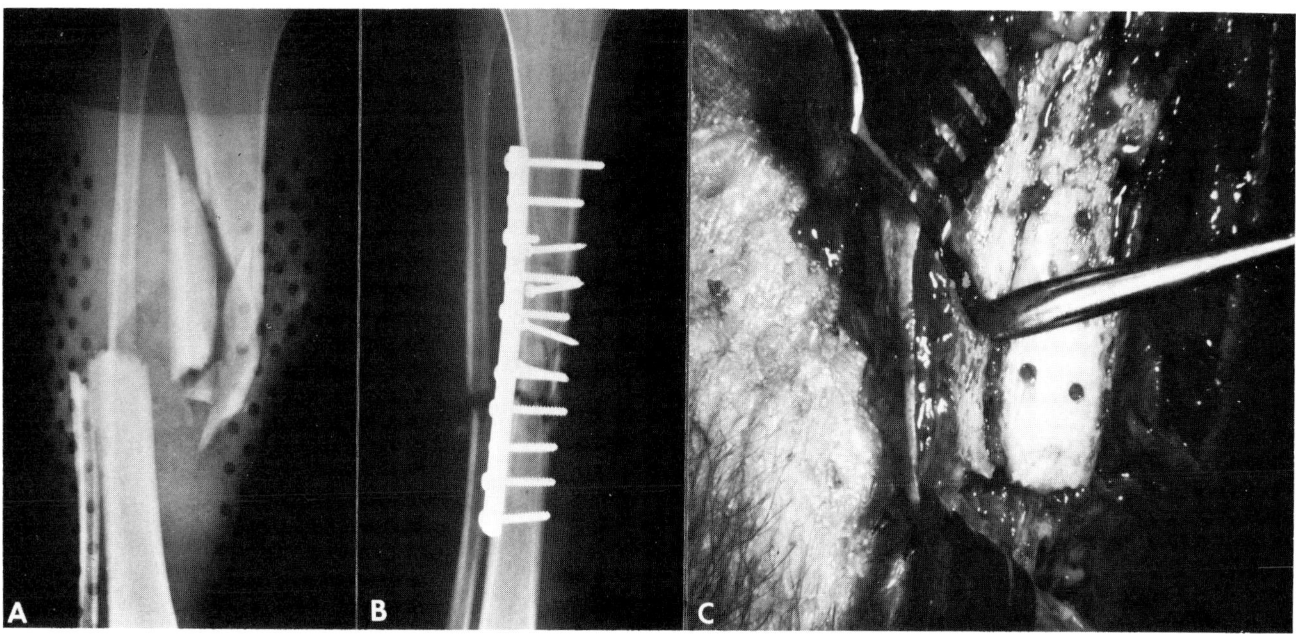

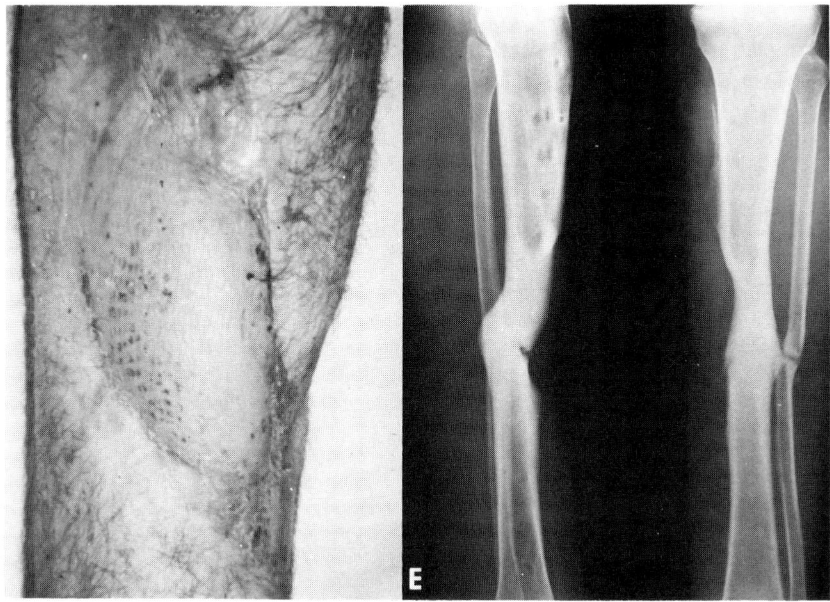

Fig. 42-7. Posttraumatic osteomyelitis of tibia with nonunion. A. Anteroposterior roentgenogram of compound fracture in tibia and fibula of 17-year-old boy. B. Drainage and resorption of osseous tissue at fracture line four months after open reduction and internal fixation. C. Multiple sequestra were excised at time of surgical debridement. Modified Vidal-Hoffmann external fixation device was utilized to stabilize nonunion. D. Localized gastrocnemius–soleus muscle flap was rotated into resulting saucerized cavity. Muscle flap was covered with split-thickness skin graft. Well-healed wound 10 months later. E. Ten months after surgical and antimicrobial treatment, union has occurred. Fracture line is almost obliterated on anteroposterior and lateral roentgenograms.

eg, *P. aeruginosa,* will still require synergistic parenteral treatment with an aminoglycoside and carbenicillin or ticarcillin. Because microorganisms can alter their susceptibility patterns, additional specimens for culture and susceptibility studies should be obtained at subsequent debridements. When the microbes are susceptible to an oral agent, we administer an oral agent for from four to six weeks after parenteral therapy.

Using the techniques described, we arrested the infectious process in 75 percent of the patients treated between 1967 and 1973. Our criteria for resolution of the osteomyelitic process included freedom from clinical signs and symptoms of the infection, a normal erythrocyte sedimentation rate, and resolution of the associated roentgenographic changes a minimum of two years after treatment.

SEPTIC ARTHRITIS

At the Mayo Clinic, only about 9 of the 250,000 adult patients seen yearly have septic arthritis. Almost any joint of the upper or lower extremity can be involved, but there is a predilection for the knee, hip, and glenohumeral joints (Table 42-3).

Etiology

Although a variety of bacteria have been isolated from synovial fluid, *S. aureus* is by far the most frequent. Table 42-4 lists those organisms found in patients with septic arthritis seen at the Mayo Clinic. Goldenberg et al [25] have noted a similar distribution. Gram-negative bacilli were isolated from 20 percent of patients with septic arthritis.

TABLE 42-3. BACTERIAL ARTHRITIS IN 161 PATIENTS

Joint Affected	Monarticular (Patients)	Polyarticular		Total Joints
		Patients	*Joints*	
Knee	64	10	11	75
Hip	29	5	5	34
Ankle	5	1	1	6
Sacroiliac	2	0	0	2
Subtalar	1	0	0	1
Glenohumeral	28	3	4	32
Elbow	5	4	5	10
Sternoclavicular	7	2	2	9
Wrist	4	2	2	6
Acromioclavicular	1	0	0	1
Second metacarpophalangeal	1	0	0	1
Total	147	14 *	30	177

* These 14 patients had two or more joints affected.

In recent years, many medical centers have noted a distinct increase in the incidence of gonococcal arthritis. Cultures of blood, skin lesions, endocervix, rectum, oropharynx, and urethra are frequently necessary for the isolation of the etiologic agent.

Hematogenous anaerobic septic arthritis is distinctly uncommon. Anaerobic septic arthritis in association with joint implants is increasingly being recognized. The gram-negative anaerobic bacilli predominate in patients with hematogenous anaerobic septic arthritis. These patients usually have a serious, debilitating, medical illness with gastrointestinal involvement. *Bacteroides fragilis* is the most frequently isolated organism.

Salmonella septic arthritis is rarely seen in adult patients. Goldenberg and associates [25] reported the isolation of *Salmonella choleraesuis* and *Salmonella typhimurium* from 2 of 13 patients with gram-negative septic arthritis. This type of septic arthritis often occurs in patients with sickle cell anemia and other types of hemoglobinopathies.

Although pneumococcal and streptococcal organisms were at one time frequently isolated from patients with septic arthritis, they are rare in the modern antibiotic era.

Predisposing Factors

The frequent association of bacterial arthritis with a systemic disease that alters host defenses is more than coincidental. Among the diseases most frequently associated with bacterial arthritis are diabetes mellitus, malignancy, and rheumatoid arthritis. The hypocomplementemic subgroup of patients with rheumatoid arthritis, described by Hunder and McDuffie,[26] appears to be predisposed to various infections, including bacterial arthritis. This group has peripheral manifestations of the rheumatoid process (increased IgM and decreased IgG levels) and depressed serum complement level.

Preexisting infection elsewhere in the body is frequently seen in patients with bacterial arthritis.

Many patients will report a history of corticosteroid use. Frequently, those who have received oral corticosteroids have rheumatoid arthritis or systemic lupus erythematosus. The frequent local injection of steroid preparations for tendinitis and bursitis has been associated with a precipitous increase in the incidence of septic arthritis, especially septic arthritis of the glenohumeral joint (Fig. 42-8). Prior to 1957, only one patient with septic arthritis of the glenohumeral joint had been seen at the Mayo Clinic. Since then it is as common as hip infection (Table 42-3).

In children, soft-tissue trauma has been implicated in the development of septic arthritis. Bacterial arthritis is a frequent complication of osteomyelitis—classically in infants and adults but also in children. In children, joints in which the metaphysis is located within synovial lining (the hip, shoulder, ankle, and radiohumeral joints) are typically involved.

Pathophysiology

In 1924, Phemister's investigation [27] of the destructive processes associated with septic arthritis demonstrated that articular cartilage does not have a purely passive role.

TABLE 42-4. BACTERIOLOGIC DATA FROM 161 PATIENTS WITH BACTERIAL ARTHRITIS

Organism	Number
Staphylococcus aureus	117
S. aureus with gram-negative bacilli	6
Gram-negative bacilli	
Pseudomonas	7
Proteus	1
Enterobacter and *Pseudomonas*	1
Bacteroides	2
Escherichia coli	9
Bacteroides and viridans streptococci	1
E. coli and β-hemolytic streptococci	1
Pseudomonas and *Proteus*	1
Citrobacter diversus	1
Streptococci	
S. pyogenes	2
Anaerobic streptococci	4
β-Hemolytic streptococci	3
S. pneumoniae	1
Viridans streptococci	1
Neisseria gonorrhoeae	1

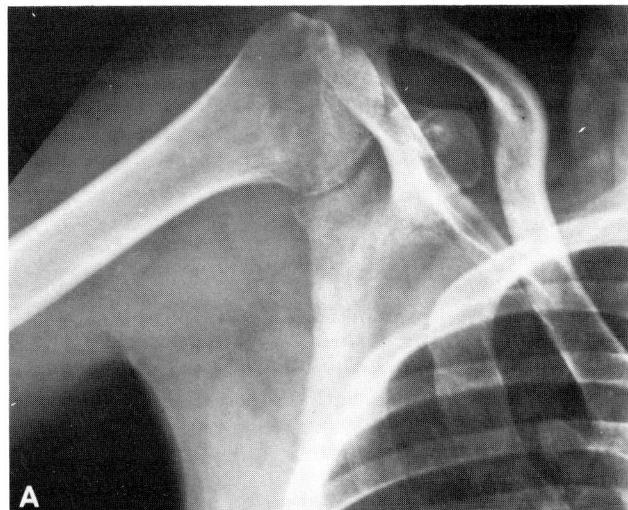

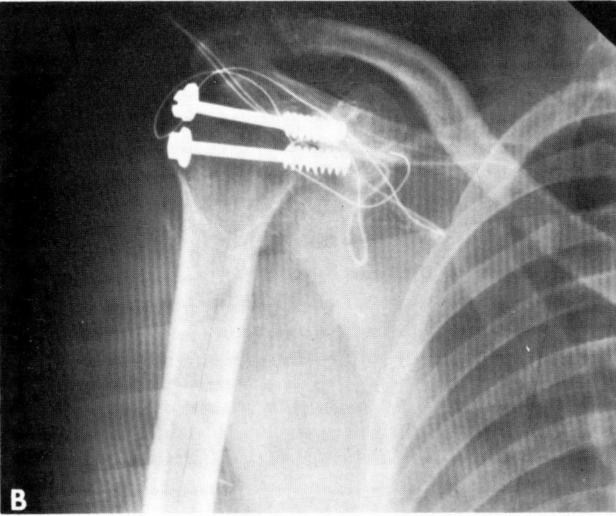

Fig. 42-8. **Septic arthritis of shoulder after local steroid injection. A. Destruction of articular surface of glenohumeral joint. B. Arthrodesis of shoulder at second-stage operation using lag screws after a primary debridement.**

Phemister incubated articular cartilage with a staphylococcal suspension, a purulent exudate, and saline at 55C. Because the bacterial action of staphylococci was inhibited at this temperature, he concluded that the resulting destruction of articular cartilage occurred through the action of proteolytic ferments present in the purulent exudate. He theorized that the ferments were released by polymorphonuclear leukocytes.

Curtiss and Klein [28] repeated these experiments in 1963. They noted that incubation of articular cartilage and a purulent exudate, with or without staphylococci, at 37C had no visible effect on the articular cartilage. However, incubation of articular cartilage and a purulent exudate at 55C resulted in destruction of the articular cartilage. By measuring the hydroxyproline content, these authors demonstrated that the dissolution of visible cartilage was directly related to the destruction of collagen. Thus, they concluded that Phemister's [27] observations were based on the action of proteolytic enzymes on the collagen of denatured cartilage. At the more physiologic temperature of 37C, they noted that various proteolytic enzymes, such as papain, trypsin, plasmin, streptococcal kinase, and leukocytic proteinase, had no deleterious effect on the collagen content of articular cartilage. In fact, at this temperature, only clostridial collagenase dissolved hyaline cartilage. Curtiss and Klein [29] demonstrated that the proteolytic enzymes had an adverse effect on the cartilage matrix, with a loss of chondroitin sulfate by articular cartilage.

Clinical Manifestations

In the past, bacterial arthritis was considered to be a disease of children. Although still prevalent in children and young adults, it is not exclusively a pediatric disease. In fact, at the Mayo Clinic, twice as many adult patients as children have been treated for bacterial arthritis during the past 25 years. Adult patients at greatest risk are those with remote infections, urinary tract or bowel disease, the elderly, the chronically ill, those with rheumatoid arthritis, and patients being treated for malignant disease with cytotoxic drugs or radiation. Bacterial arthritis begins as a painful, swollen joint, and the erythrocyte sedimentation rate and peripheral leukocyte count can be helpful in the diagnosis. An elevation of the sedimentation rate in a patient with hip joint or sacroiliac pain should alert the physician to the possibility of septic arthritis. Although roentgenographic changes are later findings, technetium or gallium scans can provide valuable information early in the disease.

Two clinical forms of gonococcal arthritis are seen. Patients with monarticular involvement, or less often polyarticular involvement, have asymptomatic bacteremia without fever and chills. The characteristic cutaneous manifestation of gonococcemia, that is, erythematous papules surmounted by a hemorrhagic vesiculopustular lesion, is uncommon. Usually, gonococci will be isolated from synovial specimens. The second group of patients with gonococcal arthritis have a septic course. A history of fever and chills, characteristic skin lesions, and polyarticular involvement are characteristic. Although blood and skin lesion cultures are frequently positive, the synovial fluid is usually sterile. In contrast to previous experience, gonococcal arthritis occurs more frequently in female patients.

Fever, chills, and a rash, found in patients with polyarticular involvement, can make differentiation from Reiter's syndrome difficult. Patients with Reiter's syndrome have histories of previous arthritis, persistent low-back pain, or previous urethritis. Patients with gonococcal arthritis experience a rapid clinical response to parenterally administered penicillin, whereas those with Reiter's syndrome respond more slowly to nonsteroidal anti-inflammatory agents. Reiter's syndrome tends to be associated with lower extremity involvement, as well as plantar fasciitis and tendonitis, whereas gonococcal arthritis occurs initially in the upper extremity and is associated with a fever and a positive culture from an orifice or synovial fluid.

More characteristic symptoms and physical findings occur in the pediatric patient with septic arthritis. Rheumatic fever and juvenile rheumatoid arthritis must be included in the differential diagnosis. A more difficult distinction to make is that between transient synovitis of the hip and septic arthritis. In bacterial infections of the hip, the patient tends to be febrile and younger. The erythrocyte sedimentation rate is elevated, and the synovial leukocyte counts are higher. Only the isolation of microorganisms from synovial fluid or blood can prove the final diagnosis.

Diagnosis

Salvage of a functional joint in septic arthritis requires early diagnosis, and tissue culture of synovial fluid obtained by aspiration (Table 42-5) or of synovial membrane obtained at arthrotomy should be done. Table 42-6 lists the differential diagnostic characteristics of joint fluid. The isolation and subsequent susceptibility studies of the infective agent are essential.

Treatment

Antimicrobial drugs cross the synovial membrane readily in health and disease.[30] If the etiologic diagnosis of septic arthritis is made promptly, antimicrobial therapy alone may result in eradication of the infection. The duration of parenteral antimicrobial therapy remains empiric. Four weeks of therapy can be considered a helpful, albeit arbitrary, guide.

The management of the infected synovial fluid precipitates considerable controversy. Animal experimentation suggests that infected synovial fluid interferes with hyaline cartilage metabolism. Daniel and co-workers[31] demonstrated that removal of the infected synovial fluid improved cartilage metabolism, with preservation of collagen content. Thus, most orthopedic surgeons favor removal of the synovial fluid. Arthrocentesis can be readily accomplished in superficially located joints (ie, knee, ankle, and shoulder). However, if thick purulent joint fluid is present or if the joint is not readily accessible, such as the hip or sacroiliac joints, open debridement and drainage are indicated. The use of an irrigation–suction system after joint debridement is common.[32] As mentioned in the treatment of osteomyelitis, such systems are not proper for the delivery of antimicrobial agents. If debridement has been thorough, the remaining tissue has an adequate blood supply that will allow bactericidal concentrations of parenterally administered antimicrobial agents within the tissues of the joint. The use of irrigation–suction beyond four or five days, however, may provide a route for colonization of the tissues with secondary invaders (usually gram-negative bacilli) and may precipitate superinfection.

The treatment becomes far more complex when the diagnosis of septic arthritis has been delayed. Frequently, delay in diagnosis and treatment precludes salvage of a functional joint. As William Hunter[1] pointed out two centuries ago, ". . . an ulcerated Cartilage is universally allowed to be a very troublesome Disease; . . . it admits of a Cure with more Difficulty than a curious Bone; and, . . . when destroyed, it is never recovered."

Even though it may be irregular and pitted, an attempt should be made to salvage a functional joint if some articular cartilage remains after debridement. Early functional rehabilitation after debridement may provide the patient with a stable and minimally painful joint. If, how-

TABLE 42-5. PROCEDURES FOR ASPIRATION OF JOINTS

Joint	Procedure
Knee	Medial approach with knee as fully extended as possible. Puncture site—anteromedial, 1 to 2 cm medial to inner border of patella in line with patellar midpoint. Needle tip directed laterally, slightly posteriorly, and distally. Needle slips between midpatella and femur.
Hip	Lateral approach. Use 19- or 20-gauge spinal needle. Puncture site—just anterior to greater trochanter with hip in extension. Needle directed medially and slightly cephalad; aim tip to point below middle of Poupart's ligament. Needle slips anterior to periosteum of femoral neck, follows bone into joint cavity.
Ankle (subtalar joint)	Anteromedial approach. Puncture site—medial to tendon of extensor hallucis longus, 2 cm in front of medial malleolus. Direct needle toward joint cavity.
Elbow (humero-ulnar joint)	Lateral approach with elbow at 90°. Puncture site—just distal to lateral epicondyle and just lateral to olecranon. Direct needle toward joint.
Shoulder	Anterior approach with arm at side and internally rotated, easily palpable. Puncture site—anterior into space between head of humerus and rim of glenoid. Needle directed posteriorly from point just below and lateral to coracoid process. Joint reached approximately 4–5 cm below skin.
Hands and feet (interphalangeal joints)	Dorsal approach with 23- or 24-gauge needle. Traction on finger or toe helps to widen joint. Direct needle at right angles into joint space.

From Pulaski EJ: In Pulaski EJ (ed): *Common Bacterial Infections,* 1964. (Courtesy of WB Saunders Co.)

TABLE 42-6. SYNOVIAL FLUID CHARACTERISTICS IN MAJOR JOINT DISEASES

Diagnosis	Appearance	Fibrin Clot	Mucin* Clot	WBC/mm³	PMN † (%)	Sugar (% of Blood Level)
Normal	Straw-colored, clear	None	Good	<200	<25	~100
Degenerative joint disease	Slightly turbid	Small	Good	<2,000	<25	~ 100
Traumatic arthritis	Straw-colored, bloody, or xanthochromic	Small	Good	2,000	<25	~100
Rheumatoid arthritis	Turbid	Large	Fair to poor	5,000–50,000	>65	75 ‡
Other types of inflammatory arthritis §	Turbid	Large	Fair to poor	5,000–50,000	>50	75
Acute gout or pseudo-gout	Turbid	Large	Fair to poor	5,000–50,000	>75	90
Septic arthritis	Very turbid or purulent	Large	Poor	50,000–200,000	>80	<50
Tuberculous arthritis	Turbid	Large	Poor	~25,000	Variable	<50

From Gilliland BC, Mannik M: Approach to disorders of the joints. In Thorn GW, Adams RD, Braunwald E, Isselbacher KJ, Petersdorf RG: *Harrison's Principles of Internal Medicine,* 1977, p 2048. (Courtesy of McGraw-Hill Book Company.)

* Correlates with viscosity.
† PMN, polymorphonuclear cells.
‡ May be less than 50 percent.
§ Includes Reiter's syndrome, psoriatic arthritis, ankylosing spondylitis (peripheral joints), arthritis associated with intestinal diseases.

ever, significant destruction of the articular surfaces with exposure or erosion (or both) of subchondral bone has occurred, a more definitive procedure is indicated. When the knee, ankle, elbow, wrist, interphalangeal, or subtalar joints are involved, compression arthrodesis with the Charnley or Hoffmann apparatus is indicated. Destruction of the articular surfaces of the hip can be treated by either arthrodesis or joint resection, depending upon the degree of involvement and the patient's occupation and level of activity. The acromioclavicular and sternoclavicular joints can be treated by joint resection, with remarkably good results (Fig. 42-9). The glenohumeral joint is amenable to treatment with debridement and protected motion or arthrodesis.

Septic arthritis of the hip in children is best treated by early debridement and drainage. Delay in diagnosis and treatment of septic arthritis in the hip in the child is catastrophic. Every effort should be made to salvage the involved joint. The child has an infinitely greater ability to attain a functional joint than does the adult patient. The presence of an open epiphyseal plate makes the salvage operation used in adult patients (which destroys the epiphyseal plate) far more difficult to use in children.

Prognosis

Death attributable to septic arthritis, even in this era of sophisticated antimicrobial therapy, has been noted in as many as 15 percent of afflicted patients. Joint instability and subluxation, when the capsule and associated ligaments are involved, necessitates external support, for example, cane, crutch, or braces. Prolonged immobilization can create stiff, immobile joints. If immobilization is inade-

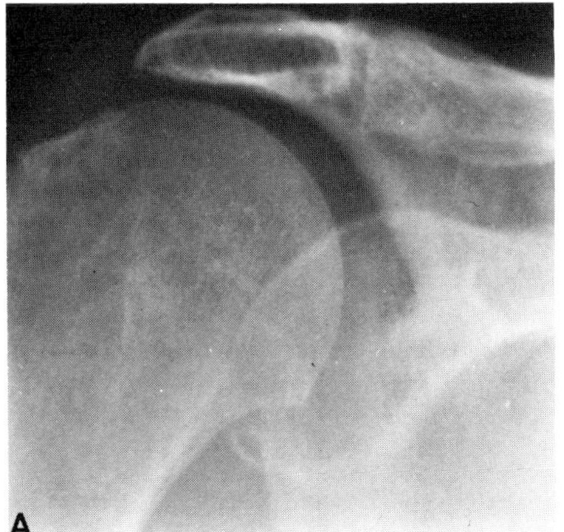

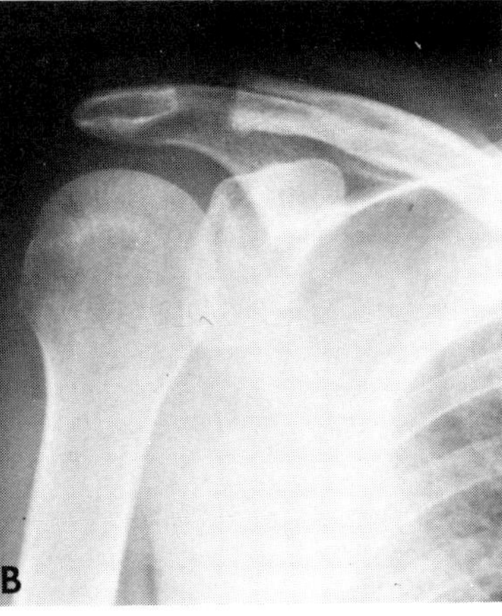

Fig. 42-9. Septic arthritis of acromioclavicular joint. A. Destruction of acromioclavicular joint with narrowing of joint space. Sinus tract communicates with joint. B. Sixteen months after resection of distal clavicle, the patient has full range of painless motion. No further drainage. Anteroposterior roentgenogram shows no evidence of infection.

quate, flexion contractures are common. Delay in diagnosis in children can result in functional impairment from discrepancy in leg length, persistent pain, limitation of motion, or soft-tissue contracture. Because the epiphysis is intra-articular in the glenohumeral and hip joints, septic arthritis can compromise the blood supply and result in osteonecrosis.

UNCOMMON SKELETAL INFECTIONS

MYCOBACTERIAL INFECTIONS

The various mycobacteria are discussed briefly in Chapter 7 and in many other chapters on regional infection. Although the incidence of tuberculosis has declined, tuberculosis of the spinal column and major joints is still seen. With the advent of total joint arthroplasty, many patients with joints destroyed by tuberculosis years before are now seeking reconstructive surgery. New cases can occur in patients of any age, but adults are more often affected. Since classic tuberculosis of bone appears to arise from a hematogenous source, primary tuberculosis, usually pulmonary, is said to be commonly present. In our experience, however, skeletal involvement with tuberculosis has seldom been associated with pulmonary tuberculosis, but disseminated disease can afflict both multiple bones and soft tissues simultaneously. The tubercle bacilli lodge in the metaphyseal region of long bones or in the anterior portions of vertebral bodies (Pott's disease). Tuberculous arthritis is probably secondary to tuberculous osteomyelitis.

The spinal column is the most frequent site of involvement with *Mycobacterium tuberculosis* and classically can lead to paraplegia. However, any bone or joint may be afflicted—the hip, knee, and tendons of the hand are the most frequent nonspinal sites. The usual clinical findings are insidious, with fever, malaise, and bone or joint pain. Rheumatoid arthritis is a common clinical impression in nonspinal disease.

Unfortunately, roentgenographic examination is not diagnostic. A range of radiographic alterations from soft-tissue swelling to joint destruction can be seen. Initially, soft tissue swelling and distention of a joint capsule may be seen. Cartilage destruction occurs. If bone destruction occurs, the lucent area is surrounded by sclerotic bone, and there may be subperiosteal new bone formation. When infection of the spinal column occurs, destruction of several contiguous vertebral bodies, narrowing of interpectoral spaces, and paraspinal abscess as indicated by anterior vertebral scalloping may be present. Kyphosis or scoliosis, or both, may be observed.

A positive skin test is helpful, but the diagnosis depends upon histopathologic demonstration of granulomas with caseous necrosis and Langerhans giant cells, acid-fast stain, and culture. Drug treatment for tuberculosis is essential regardless of the surgical treatment. Nondestructive bony lesions respond to prolonged chemotherapy and immobilization. Moderate joint involvement should probably be treated with synovectomy plus chemotherapy. Extensive joint disease responds best to debridement and arthrodesis. Spondylitis may be best treated with anterior spinal fusion and early drainage of any paraspinal abscess. Paraplegia demands operative decompression and responds remarkably well.[33]

There are four groups of atypical mycobacterial organisms (groups I, II, III, IV). Inoculation of the hand and fingers after minor trauma probably accounts for the frequent involvement of the tendon sheaths of the hand and wrist. Bone infections are rare, but synovial and bursal infections may be related to injections of anesthetics or steroids into these locations. Because these organisms do not respond to the standard antituberculosis drugs, bacteriologic culture, identification, and susceptibility studies are invaluable. Synovial biopsy is useful for culture. Surgical debridement of all of the involved synovial tissue is frequently required. Further discussion of laboratory diagnosis and treatment of mycobacterial infections appears in Chapters 7 and 18.

FUNGAL INFECTIONS

The more common but still rare fungal infections of bone include blastomycosis, cryptococcosis, coccidioidomycosis, and sporotrichosis.[33] The systemic character of these infections is discussed in Chapter 9. *Actinomyces* is an anaerobic bacterium that can grow like a fungus.

Blastomycosis

Blastomycosis *(Blastomyces dermatitidis)* is acquired by inhalation of the spores from soil, and bone lesions occur only with disseminated disease frequently in conjunction with cutaneous ulcers and subcutaneous sinuses.[34] Multicentric osseous lesions are common when the spinal column is infected, the most frequent sites being tubular bones (especially the tibia) and ribs.

Pathology and Pathogenesis

The metaphyses or epiphyses and subarticular regions are commonly involved. Joints become secondarily infected, and the synovium, ligaments, and surrounding soft tissues are destroyed with subluxation of the joints. Draining sinuses are common. Paravertebral dissection occurs after vertebral infection, and even skip areas occur as the infection dissects along the anterior longitudinal ligament.

Clinical Manifestations

Recent respiratory symptoms will have occurred in about half the patients who have skin involvement. The patient is acutely and chronically ill with fever, weight loss, night sweats, and cough. Skin ulcers and draining sinus tracts occur in association with bony involvement. The roentgenographic appearance of blastomycosis has been described by Gehweiler et al.[35] In spinal disease, several vertebral bodies are infected along with the adjacent ribs—an important differential point. Three forms of disease may be seen: a cystic or focal form, a diffuse form, and, in long bones, a circumscribed, soft, saucer-shape erosion of cortical bone. The differential diagnosis includes neoplasms, sarcoidosis, other fungal diseases, gout, and rheumatoid arthritis.

Diagnosis

Histopathologic examination with special stains may reveal the yeasts in tissue. Culture, however, is necessary for definitive diagnosis. Amphotericin B is the best treatment and is described in Chapter 9. Operative debridement of the extensive sinus tracts, drainage of the abscesses, sequestrectomy, or even amputation may be necessary.

Sporotrichosis

Sporotrichosis *(Sporothrix schenckii)* arthritis should be included in the differential diagnosis of chronic monarticular or polyarticular arthritis.[36] Bone and joint disease is most often the result of hematogenous spread in the rare systemic form of the disease, although direct extension from a local lesion or spread via lymphatic extension may occur. The unifocal form, in which joint infection is the sole manifestation of the disease, predominates. The roentgenographic findings are nonspecific, and the diagnosis depends on cultures of synovial tissue. Patients with destructive changes tend to have had symptoms for a longer time. Debridement with systemically administered amphotericin B is the treatment of choice. Treatment with potassium iodide will not suffice in this form of the disease.

Cryptococcosis

Osseous lesions in cryptococcosis *(Cryptococcus neoformans)* are rare and usually result from direct extension. For this reason, the cranium is the most commonly affected site, secondary to cryptococcal meningitis. The other osseous lesions are usually multiple because of hematogenous spread. Since cryptococcosis can be widespread without systemic or local signs of host response, sinuses and ulcers are unusual. Bone pain may be present. Radiolucent lesions without new periosteal bone formation are the characteristic radiographic alterations. The organisms can be demonstrated on clinical tissue specimens with the periodic acid-Schiff stain and can be grown on Sabouraud's medium. Cryptococcosis is rarely seen except in patients with debilitating disease. The patient frequently seeks medical attention for evaluation of a fever of unknown origin or dysfunction of the central nervous system. Amphotericin B and 5-fluorocytosine combinations are the treatment of choice. Surgical debridement is frequently necessary.[33]

Coccidioidomycosis

As noted in Chapter 9, primary infection with *Coccidioides immitis* can be accompanied by arthritis (desert rheumatism). Pain, tenderness, and swelling of a joint occur, but the condition is transient, as are most manifestations of the primary infection.

Some patients do not recover from the primary infection, and bone and joint complaints may be the initial signs of the chronic disease.[33] Pain, swelling, and draining abscesses may be the first findings.

Disseminated coccidioidomycosis will occasionally infect one or more joints or the vertebral column. The large joints—hip, knee, and shoulder—are most often afflicted. Coccidioidomycosis tends to involve the metaphysis of large tubular bones and bony prominences. When the vertebral bodies are infected, the disc is spared. The lesions are usually radiolucent and well demarcated without sclerosis or sequestra. As with the other fungal infections, diagnosis depends on the identification of spherules on histologic examination of biopsy material or on the isolation of the fungus on solid medium. (The serologic and skin tests interpretations are discussed in Chapter 9.) Systemic involvement requires parenteral administration of amphotericin B. Immobilization of joints and relief from weightbearing may be helpful. Synovectomy of extensively involved joints or saucerization of osseous lesions is occasionally necessary.[33]

UNUSUAL BACTERIAL INFECTIONS

Actinomycosis

Actinomycosis of bone occurs with the cervicofascial form and frequently invades the mandible after tooth extraction. Osseous infection at other sites is distinctly uncommon. Involvement of the second rib has been noted in the thoracic form of the disease. A mixed lytic and sclerotic appearance is seen radiographically, and the picture of cervical facial actinomycosis (Chapter 27) is easily recognized. This diagnosis depends on finding sulfur granules in the sinus drainage, gram-positive organisms in smear, and culture. Penicillin G in large doses of 10 to 20 million units per day should be given for an extended period. Surgical debridement can be helpful.[33]

Brucellosis

Brucellosis *(Brucella abortus)* in the United States is limited to farmers, veterinarians, and others working with infected cattle (Chapter 7). There are two forms of the disease: an acute form with systemic complaints and a chronic form with intermittent recurrent (undulant) fever. *Br. abortus* is isolated most frequently in the systemic form, and *Br. suis* in the localized form.

The spinal column, knees, and hip can be affected. However, invasion of phalanges, pelvis, and diaphyses has been reported. Brucellar spondylitis and prepatellar bursitis are the two most frequent types of skeletal involvement. An insidious onset of nonspecific symptoms is characteristic. Backache and joint pain are characteristic. Agglutination titers are elevated in the spondylitic form and may be normal in the localized form. Treatment of the patient with brucellosis includes debridement and the administration of tetracycline for three weeks.

POSTOPERATIVE WOUND SEPSIS

Even though postoperative skeletal sepsis is not associated with a high mortality rate, the increased morbidy and loss of function of the infected limb make it one of the most formidable complications of orthopedic surgery. The resultant loss of function and the reliance on crutches or canes frequently preclude the patient's return to his or her premorbid occupation. Although newer reconstructive procedures can restore function to a destroyed joint, they are contraindicated in the presence of sepsis. Even with eradication of the infection, the rate of failure of a total joint arthroplasty implanted into a previously infected joint is significantly increased. Thus, prevention of skeletal sepsis and early eradication when infection occurs are the primary goals of orthopedic surgeons.

Incidence and Etiology

The incidence of nosocomial wound infections of the skeletal system is unknown. In a prospective study of postoperative wound sepsis, by the National Academy of Sciences,[37] only 692 orthopedic procedures were included among the 15,613 operations studied. Septic complications occurred in 54 (7.8 percent) of the orthopedic procedures.

As expected, the regional anatomy and type of skeletal operation influence the incidence of deep sepsis. The rich vascular supply of the hand helps make postoperative infection uncommon. In contrast, Boyd et al [38] and Tengve and Kjellander [39] have noted wound sepsis in 4.8 and 16.9 percent, respectively, after internal fixation of fractured hips. Thus, in any evaluation of postoperative wound sepsis of the skeletal system, elective and traumatic operations should be considered separately. The variations in anatomy, dissection, and residual dead space necessitate subdivision of elective operations into adult, pediatric, and oncologic procedures. Traumatic procedures are subdivided into open and closed injuries.

In a prospective study, Miller and Counts [40] noted 22 (5.8 percent) wound infections after clean, elective skeletal procedures in 378 patients. In 12 (3.2 percent), the tissues deep to the fascia were infected. Patients treated for closed hip fractures had the highest incidence of deep infections (6 of 65 patients, 9.2 percent), whereas elective reconstructive hip procedures were associated with the lowest incidence (2 of 59 patients, 3.4 percent).

At the Mayo Clinic,[41] postoperative sepsis is defined as an inflamed wound that drains purulent material. Even wounds from which microorganisms cannot be isolated are included if many polymorphonuclear leukocytes can be seen. When purulent material extends beneath the fascia, the infection is classified as deep.

Elective Reconstruction. Deep sepsis after elective reconstructive procedures in adult patients occurs in 0.4 to 0.5 percent of our patients. The incidence has remained fairly constant.[41] Gram-positive isolates, staphylococci in particular, predominate. Gram-negative bacilli are isolated from 20 to 35 percent of the infected wounds. The anaerobic cocci, *Peptococcus* and *Peptostreptococcus,* have been noted with increasing frequency.

Total hip arthroplasty is a special procedure in which prophylactic antimicrobial therapy is frequently used because of the high incidence of early septic failures. Although the incidence of deep sepsis within the first two months after total joint arthroplasty has been similar to that observed after other types of elective reconstructive surgery, more than half of the clinical infections have been delayed two to five years after the procedure. The organisms isolated from infected total joints have varied. In 1974, only 17 percent of the isolates were gram-positive. In contrast, 57 and 81 percent of the organisms were gram-positive in 1975 and 1976 (Table 42-7).

Oncologic Procedures. The incidence of deep sepsis after orthopedic oncologic procedures is low (range, 0.7–1.4 percent) in spite of acquired immunologic defects in cancer patients and the magnitude of tissue dissection required to treat these diseases. Although gram-positive isolates predominate, gram-negative bacilli are noted after inguinal lymphadenectomies and hemipelvectomies.

Pediatric Orthopedics. Deep sepsis after elective orthopedic procedures in children tends to be associated with chronic urinary tract infections (patients with myelomeningoceles) and long operations requiring foreign body implantation (eg, scoliosis fusions with implantation of Harrington rods). Penicillin-resistant staphylococci are common isolates, and gram-negative bacilli are seen occasionally.

Trauma. In trauma surgery, the overall incidence of deep sepsis is low. However, when open fractures and dislocations are separated from closed injuries, a fourfold increase in the incidence of sepsis is seen. This difference reflects the contamination of devitalized tissue by soil and water organisms. The etiology of infections after operative treatment of closed fractures is similar to those seen after elective reconstruction. In contrast, after operations for open fractures and dislocations, gram-negative bacilli alone or in mixed cultures are found in most infections.

In a study of compound fractures, Gustilo and Anderson [42] noted deep sepsis in 2.5–9 percent of patients, proportional to the degree of soft-tissue injury. The surgical treatment of open fractures was accompanied by an

TABLE 42-7. MICROORGANISMS ISOLATED FROM INFECTED TOTAL JOINT ARTHROPLASTIES

	No. of Isolates		
Organism	**1974**	**1975**	**1976**
Staphylococcus aureus	2	4	7
Staphylococcus epidermidis	0	1	14
Group D streptococcus	1	0	3
β-Hemolytic streptococcus	0	2	0
Streptococcus pneumoniae	0	0	1
Streptococcus viridans	0	0	2
Corynebacterium	0	0	5
Peptococcus magnus	1	1	1
Clostridium perfringens, *Bacteroides fragilis*	0	1	1
Pseudomonas aeruginosa	2	1	3
Klebsiella	2	0	1
Escherichia coli	2	1	1
Veillonella	0	1	1
Proteus mirabilis	0	1	1
Proteus morganii	1	0	0
Proteus vulgaris	1	0	0
Enterobacter cloacae	1	0	1
Enterobacter aerogenes	0	0	1
Mycobacterium tuberculosis	0	1	0

infection rate of 13.9 percent in patients receiving no antimicrobial therapy.[42] A reduction of the incidence of deep sepsis to 2.3 percent occurred with the administration of cephalosporins. In that prospective study, *S. aureus* was the predominant organism in patients who received either no antimicrobial therapy or penicillin and streptomycin. Gram-negative bacilli were isolated in 11 of 14 infections occurring in patients who received cephalosporins.

Clinical Manifestations and Diagnosis

Elective Reconstructive Surgery. The clinical features of sepsis after skeletal operations vary with the procedure performed. Most infections occur within the first two weeks after elective reconstruction in adults if neither foreign body nor prophylactic antibiotics are used. Spiking temperatures (39–40C), increasing pain, progressive swelling, and an enlarging area of erythema are first seen. Frequently, there is either serous drainage or a draining hematoma. Because the leukocyte count and erythrocyte sedimentation rate are elevated after most major operations, they are of little value in the differential diagnosis. Similarly, routine roentgenograms and technetium-99 scans will reflect only postoperative changes. If sufficient time has elapsed for an abscess to form, a gallium-67 scan may be helpful. Most acute infections are diagnosed on clinical examination alone. At the time of debridement, fluid and tissue specimens should be submitted for aerobic and anaerobic cultures (Chapter 12). Susceptibility studies should be performed on all isolates to permit the selection of specific antimicrobial agent(s) for parenteral therapy.

Intervertebral Disc Operations. The clinical and laboratory expressions of postoperative wound infection after intervertebral diskectomy do not conform to the pattern described. The onset of symptoms varies from 1 to 10 weeks after operation. Excruciating pain, unrelieved by narcotics, is the most characteristic symptom. It is described as severe back spasms and extends into both flanks, the lower abdomen, and groin. Sciatic radiation is uncommon. Little fever is noted. Paraspinal spasm and resistance to all spinal motion are noted on physical examination. The erythrocyte sedimentation rate remains elevated for longer than the 6 to 8 weeks that are normally associated with this procedure. Roentgenographic examination during the first few weeks reveals only postoperative changes. Loss of the distinct margins of the usually sclerotic endplate of the cephalad and caudal vertebrae in the lateral projection is the first change. Subsequently, the disc space narrows. Eventually, the adjacent vertebrae fuse with new bone formation. The sedimentation rate remains elevated until bony fusion occurs.

Infected granulation tissue rather than gross purulence is noted if debridement is performed. Tissue specimens from the involved disc space obtained by either needle biopsy or at operation should be submitted for aerobic and anaerobic culture and susceptibility studies. Because *S. aureus* is generally cultured, intravenous antimicrobial therapy with a semisynthetic penicillinase-resistant penicillin or a cephalosporin should be administered until the results of the culture and susceptibility studies are available. The patient should be immobilized in a plaster jacket to control pain.

Elective Reconstructive Surgery with Foreign Body Implant. The use of prophylactic antimicroibial therapy during operations that require the implantation of plates, screws, or nail has altered the clinical manifestations of postoperative wound sepsis. The infection discloses itself late, three months or more after operation. Low-grade infection with commensal organisms, previously considered to be nonpathogenic, is partly responsible for this altered clinical course. The patient usually complains of pain but has little clinical evidence of sepsis. Fever is absent, and the wound appears normal but may be tender. Laboratory evaluation can reveal an elevated leukocyte count with a shift to the left, a moderate anemia, and, usually, an elevated erythrocyte sedimentation rate. Roentgenographic examination reveals various changes, but the roentgenographic alterations are usually subtle—lacy, periosteal new bone formation and cystic erosion around the screws or intramedullary nail.

Intra-articular Surgery. Septic arthritis after arthrotomy and intra-articular procedures can be difficult to differentiate from intra-articular hematoma. A swollen, painful joint occurs with both conditions. The febrile response associated with septic arthritis varies with the virulence of the bacteria. The peripheral leukocyte count and the erythrocyte sedimentation rate are elevated because of the operation itself. Needle aspiration of the involved joint can provide diagnostic information. If the infection seems superficial to the capsule, the subcutaneous or subfascial space (depending upon the joint) is aspirated without entering the joint. All material obtained is submitted for cell count, Gram stain, and culture. If few leukocytes are seen and no organisms are noted on Gram stain (or the process is definitely intra-articular), the intra-articular space can then be aspirated. If an infection is present, the aspirate will vary from turbid to purulent, and the viscosity will be decreased. Mucin clot, as measured by acid preparation, will be poor. An elevated total leukocyte count ranging from 15,000 to 200,000 per mm^3, with 90 percent polymorphonuclear leukocytes, is common. The synovial glucose level will be decreased, averaging 50 mg per dl less than the serum glucose level. Gram stain of the aspirate will identify microorganisms, allowing the physician to begin administering antimicrobial therapy. A portion of the specimen should be submitted for aerobic and anaerobic cultures. If a postoperative hematoma is present, the aspirate will be bloody with small clots. The viscosity and mucin clot test results are decreased and poor. The leukocyte count may be only slightly elevated, and the percentage of polymorphonuclear leukocytes is not elevated. No organisms will be seen on Gram stain.

Internal Fixation of Femoral Neck Fractures. When low-grade sepsis occurs after open reduction and internal fixation of femoral neck fractures, the patient experiences continuous pain. The erythrocyte sedimentation rate and total leukocyte count remain elevated. Roentgenographic examination reveals a series of characteristic changes, the first of which is the loss of height of the normal joint space. Subsequently, subluxation of the hip joint occurs (Fig. 42-10). With further progression of the infection, cystic erosion of the acetabulum and femoral head usually occurs.

Total Joint Arthroplasty. Deep sepsis after total joint arthroplasty can be subdivided into three stages based on the time of presentation and the clinical course: stage 1, an acute fulminating infection, which usually develops within the first four weeks after surgery, stage 2, delayed deep sepsis, which develops as creeping infection within the first two postoperative years, and stage 3, hematogenous infection, which develops in a previously asymptomatic patient, usually occurring two to five years after operation.

Because most patients who have an elective procedure in which a large foreign body is implanted receive prophylactic antimicrobial therapy, acute fulminating infections (stage 1) are uncommon. Most of these stage 1 infections are infected hematomas that drain postoperatively and can be diagnosed on examination (Fig. 42-11).

Stage 2 infections (delayed deep sepsis) can be difficult to diagnose because the usual clinical signs of wound infection—fever, drainage, and so forth—are rarely seen. The patient complains of pain about the joint, especially when using the extremity. The differential diagnosis includes mechanical loosening at the bone–cement interface and loosening secondary to low-grade infection. Although the leukocyte count is not generally abnormal, the erythrocyte sedimentation rate is frequently elevated—greater than 60 mm in 1 hour (Westergren) in females and greater than 40 mm in males. Roentgenographic examination reveals a lucent zone at the bone–cement interface about one or both components of the total joint arthroplasty. If cystic erosion or periosteal new bone formation is seen, an infection may be present (Fig. 42-12). An arthrogram of the joint frequently is helpful. Before the dye is injected, an aspirate should be sent for culture and susceptibility studies. Penetration of the dye into the bone–cement interface suggests loosening. Murray and Rodrigo,[43] however, have seen such penetration in the bone–cement interface of some asymptomatic patients who have had total hip arthroplasty. If lateral pocketing of the dye beyond the pseudocapsule is noted, an infectious cause is more likely (Fig. 42-13). A technetium-99 scan frequently reveals increased uptake with either mechanical or infectious loosening. Although a gallium-67 scan usually reveals increased uptake only if the cause is infectious, false-positive scan results have been encountered.

Frequently, the clinical and laboratory evaluations will not be diagnostic in the patient with low-grade *S. epidermidis* or anaerobic infections. Frozen-section histologic examination of tissue specimens obtained at operation has been diagnostic. If many polymorphonuclear leukocytes are seen in each high-power field, low-grade sepsis is present, and a complete debridement with removal of the prosthesis should be performed. However, if lymphocytes and histiocytes without polymorphonuclear leukocytes are seen on frozen-section study, mechanical

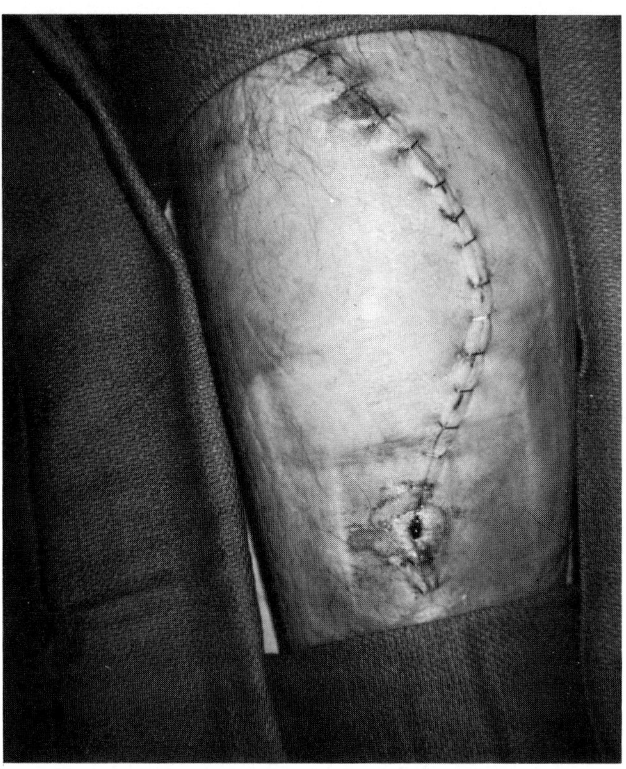

Fig. 42-11. **Draining hematoma from distal aspect of knee 12 days after total knee arthroplasty.**

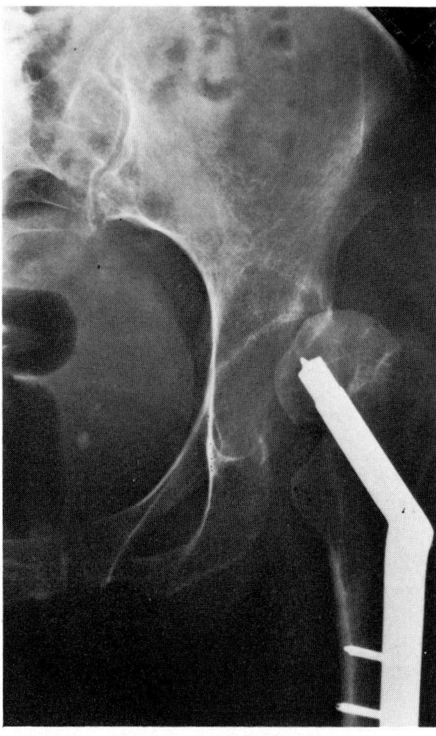

Fig. 42-10. Peptococcus **infection of hip after internal fixation of intracapsular femoral neck fracture. Subluxation of hip with erosion of acetabulum and cystic formation in femoral head.**

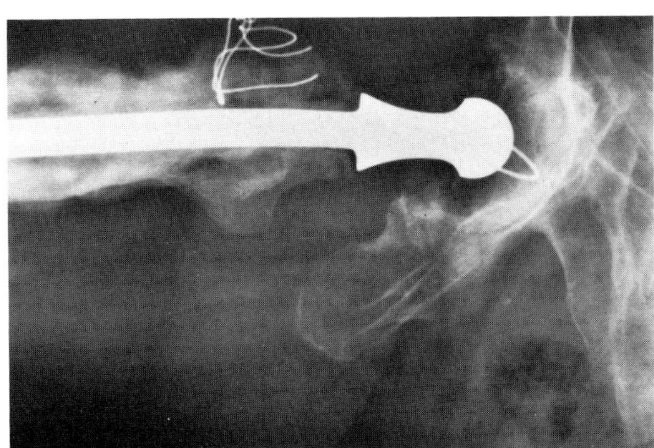

Fig. 42-12. **Lateral view of Charnley total hip arthroplasty. Periosteal new bone formation of anterior and posterior femoral cortices is well demonstrated. Erosion of bone–cement interface about femoral compartment. Lucent zone is present at bone–cement interface of entire circumference of acetabular component.**

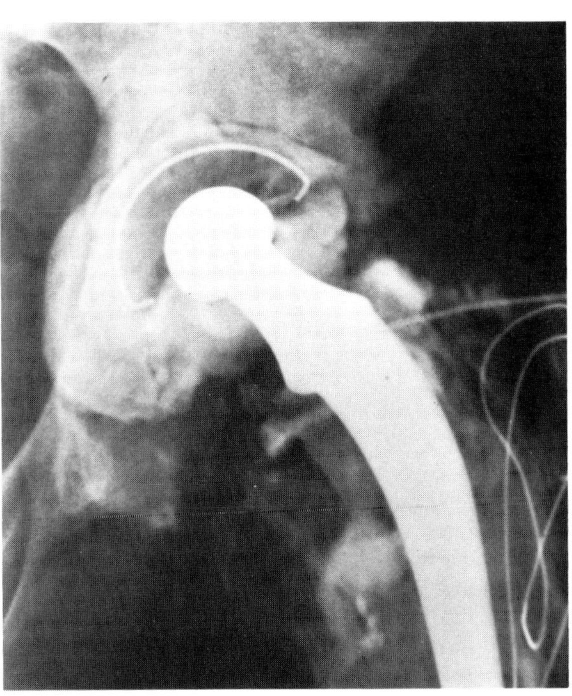

Fig. 42-13. **Arthrogram of hip reveals penetration of bone–cement interface of femoral components. Pocketing of dye inferomedially and superolaterally. Small pocket of dye indicating erosion of greater trochanter.**

loosening is the diagnosis, and revision arthroplasty is indicated.

In stage 3 infections (late hematogenous infections), the patient describes a previously asymptomatic arthroplasty with the acute onset of fever, chills, and pain around the involved joint. Unlike patients with stage 2 infection, who are never completely free of pain after operation, patients with stage 3 infection are asymptomatic until the acute episode. Frequently, the patient has a history of an antecedent infection at a remote site (eg, urinary tract infection, infected toenail). The leukocyte count is elevated, with a shift to the left, and the erythrocyte sedimentation rate is elevated. Roentgenographic examinations of the arthroplasty are normal. The acute nature of the infection usually precludes the use of bone scans. When debridement is performed early in the disease, purulent material is found rather than infected granulation tissue permeating the bone–cement interface, so characteristic of delayed deep sepsis (stage 2).

After Operation for Injury. Septic complications in the traumatized patient vary with the surgical techniques used in the initial management of the wound. Sepsis after debridement and open packing of the wound is usually associated with purulence within the depths of the wound. A progressive necrosis frequently can be the predominant clinical feature. Clostridial cellulitis or myonecrosis may occur when debridement, followed by primary closure, is the initial operative treatment. In fact, Brown and Kinman,[44] in a recent study of gas gangrene in 27 patients, stressed the association of clostridial myonecrosis and the premature closure of traumatic wounds.

Virulent microorganisms are associated with wound sepsis after the primary closure of traumatized wounds. Thus, most patients will have systemic signs and symptoms of sepsis. In addition to a spiking temperature, dehydration, and delirium, the patient will experience progressive localized pain. Occasionally, the organism will be one of the less virulent types, for example, *S. epidermidis*. In this group of patients, only local symptoms herald the presence of sepsis. Wound drainage is usually minimal. Roentgenographic examination reveals resorption of bone around internal-fixation devices, resulting in their loosening.

Treatment

The management of septic complications after skeletal operations usually requires aggressive intervention. To ignore a draining hematoma during the first few postoperative weeks in a patient with local or systemic signs of sepsis is an invitation to disaster. When there are no implanted foreign bodies in the wound, early debridement and specific parenteral antimicrobial therapy can frequently control, if no eradicate, the infection.

Although the factors influencing the incidence of postoperative sepsis are protean, careful evaluation of operative wound sepsis can identify changing trends in the microbiology of nosocomial infections and alteration in the susceptibility patterns. The information obtained can be invaluable to the physician in determining empiric therapeutic regimens for the patient with a postoperative septic complication while awaiting microbiologic identification and susceptibility studies.[5]

Debridement provides not only for excision of dead and infected tissue but also an opportunity to obtain deep-tissue specimens for aerobic and anaerobic cultures and susceptibility studies. While the results of the microbiologic studies are being awaited, empiric antimicrobial therapy should be initiated on the basis of the type of infection, the local anatomy, and Gram stain of the clinical material submitted to the laboratory. If necessary, the therapeutic agents can be altered after the organism is identified and the results of susceptibility studies become available.

Early aseptic debridement of hematomas that are about to drain or of those that begin to drain after suture removal can prevent deep sepsis. Foreign bodies that are providing stability to osseous structures (compression plates and intramedullary nails) should not be removed. Frequently, a thorough debridement, followed by fascial closure and secondary closure of the subcutaneous tissues and skin, will control the infection until first-stage osseous healing has occurred. When early bony union has been achieved, the internal fixation devices can be removed and cast-immobilization used until healing is complete.

In wounds without bone grafts or foreign bodies, debridement followed by open packing will control the sepsis. The wound can be closed in a delayed primary or secondary fashion. Alternately, the fascia alone can be closed, closure allowing the superficial tissues to heal by secondary intention.

Persistent sepsis after soft-tissue trauma is often associated with the presence of retained foreign bodies that are frequently radiolucent. Thus, roentgenograms are of little value in identifying their location (Fig. 42-14). Removal of the foreign body and debridement of infected and necrotic tissue, combined with specific antimicrobial therapy, usually will eradicate the infection.

The treatment of deep sepsis around an artificial joint varies with the stage of the infection. Stage 1 infected hematomas usually are amenable to debridement with retention of the artificial joint. In contrast, stage 1 fulminative infections require removal of the foreign bodies. Most stage 2 delayed deep infections require removal of the implant. Early operative debridement and parenteral antimicrobial therapy may permit retention of the arthroplasty in stage 3 hematogenous infections.

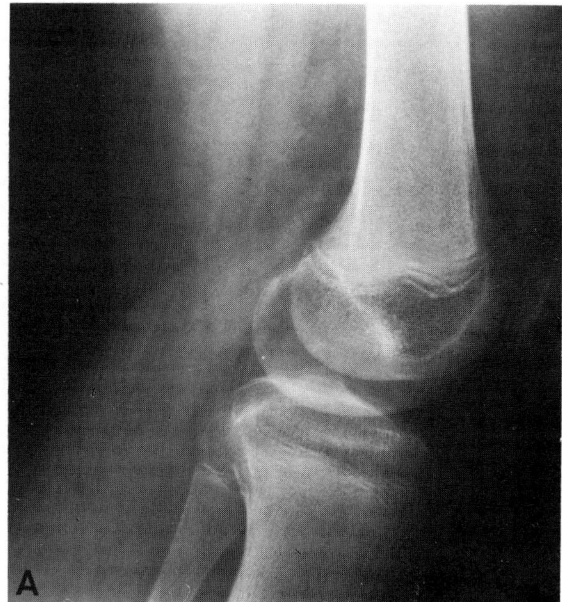

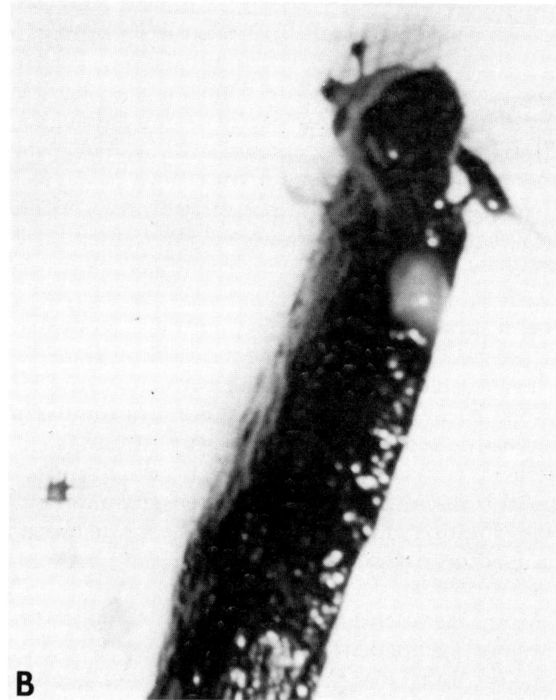

Fig. 42-14. **Persistent drainage about medial aspect of distal thigh, after two subsequent debridements, of 15-year-old boy one year after falling on tree branch. A. Lateral roentgenogram of knee. Soft-tissue swelling and effusion of knee are seen. B. Large (3 by 0.5 cm) twig found. Foreign body had eroded into suprapatellar pouch. Infection cleared after operation and specific antimicrobial therapy.**

Prevention

Quantitative microbiologic techniques have been useful in the management of open fractures and dislocations.[45] The technique, modified from Robson et al,[46] is described in Chapter 12. A 1 ml tissue specimen is weighed, homogenized, serially diluted, and stained, and bacteria are counted so that the result can be available to the surgeon within 30 minutes. Our experience suggests a high (98 percent) correlation between a positive quantitative Gram stain and a colony count of 10^5 per gram or greater. In our prospective study of open fractures and dislocation in 82 patients, a similar correlation was found between the results of quantitative microbiology techniques and the development of wound sepsis. For these reasons, positive quantitative Gram stains at the conclusion of the debridement are used as an indication for open packing of the wound and the parenteral administration of antibiotic drugs. A negative quantitative Gram stain allows the surgeon greater latitude in the management of the wound.

After Elective Reconstructive Surgery. Epidemiologic studies performed in response to the early high incidence of sepsis after total hip arthroplasty showed that many potential sources of bacterial contamination in the conventional operating room could be eliminated with a few modifications of operating room technique and strict discipline. For example, the older conventional operating rooms had low rates of room air exchange and high rates of infection compared with newer rooms with high rates of air exchange. A high rate of infection also followed procedures performed later in the day and in patients with previous hip operations.

Untraviolet light and unidirectional airflow facilities can reduce the level of airborne bacterial contamination in the operating room. Recent studies have implicated the poor barrier techniques provided by the mask and linens currently used for drapes and gowns as a source of airborne bacteria. Unidirectional airflow units with personnel isolator systems permit the use of more impermeable materials for gowns and eliminate contamination through the mask. Previously unattainable levels of postoperative wound sepsis after implant surgery (0.3–0.7 percent) have been reported in the early studies using unidirectional airflow systems (Table 42-8). The vertical airflow systems with a personnel isolater system appear to be more effective. Prospective studies of these techniques should provide more definitive answers to the questions raised by these environmental systems.

Preoperative and intraoperative prophylactic antimicrobial agents are effective in high-risk orthopedic procedures. Antimicrobial agents administered within three hours after an operation enter the hematoma and adjacent tissues in sufficient concentrations to lower the incidence of experimental infections.[47] Fogelberg and co-workers [47] noted a statistically significant reduction in the incidence of deep sepsis with the prophylactic administration of penicillin in a prospective randomized series of patients undergoing either mold arthroplasty of the hip or spinal fusion. Boyd and co-workers [38] also noted a significant reduction of wound sepsis in a randomized, prospective study with the prophylactic administration of nafcillin in patients undergoing operations for fracture of the hip. In a study with the randomized administration of cephaloridine to 1,591 patients undergoing elective orthopedic procedures, Pavel et al [48] noted a reduction in the incidence of deep sepsis from 5 percent in the placebo group to 2.8 percent in the treatment group ($P = 0.025$). A similar reduction in the incidence of deep sepsis was reported by Patzakis et al [49] with the use of cephalothin in adult patients who had open fractures. Thus, the prophylactic administration of antimicrobial agents reduces the incidence of deep sepsis in patients with open fractures, in those with extensive reconstructive procedures with the implantation of foreign bodies, or in those having procedures in which a large dead space remains. The choice of agent should be based not only on the expected contaminating flora but also on the distribution and excretion characteristics of the various drugs.[49a] Chapter 23 contains a comprehensive review on this subject.

Joint Reconstruction after Operative Wound Sepsis

Limited function and a painful joint occur frequently after alteration of the articular cartilage by the infection. In certain conditions, the residual pain can be alleviated by extra-articular reconstructive procedures. Pain after incomplete destruction of either the medial or the lateral compartment of knees can be relieved by transferring the weightbearing focus to the asymptomatic compartment with an upper tibial osteotomy (Fig. 42-15). More commonly, the partially destroyed joint will require that the articular surfaces be replaced by a total joint arthroplasty.

It is desirable to perform a second total joint arthroplasty after removal of the first and eradication of the infection. Few objective criteria are available, however, to determine whether the infection has been completely eliminated and whether a second implant will not be complicated by recurrent infection. Experience with reimplantation has been primarily limited to total hip arthroplasty.[50] Favorable results have been reported by Wilson et al [51] in the treatment of subacute sepsis of the hip with immediate total joint arthroplasty combined with large doses of parenteral antimicrobial drugs. Because many patients do not wish immediate reoperation, we believe that reimplantation generally should be delayed for one year after the treatment of the infection around the hip implant. Patients who have continued pain and difficulty in walking with a resection (Girdlestone) arthroplasty and have no evidence of sepsis are candidates for reimplantation. Recurrent deep sepsis is more common in pa-

TABLE 42-8. INCIDENCE OF DEEP SEPSIS AFTER TOTAL HIP ARTHROPLASTY

	No Previous Surgery			Previous Surgery			Total		
		With Sepsis			With Sepsis			With Sepsis	
Environment	*Total*	*No.*	*%*	*Total*	*No.*	*%*	*No.*	*No.*	*%*
Vertical unidirectional airflow	321	1	0.3	197	2	1.0	518	3	0.6
Horizontal unidirectional airflow	511	9	1.8	200	7	3.5	711	16	2.3
Vertical unidirectional airflow	1,187	5	0.4	234	2	0.9	1,500	7	0.5
Conventional operating room	2,224	19	0.9	991	23	2.3	3,215	42	1.3
Total	4,243	34	0.8	1,662	34	2.1	5,944	68	1.1

Modified from Fitzgerald RH, Bechtol CO, Eftekhar N, Nelson JP: Reduction of deep sepsis after total arthroplasty. Arch Surg 114:803, 1979.

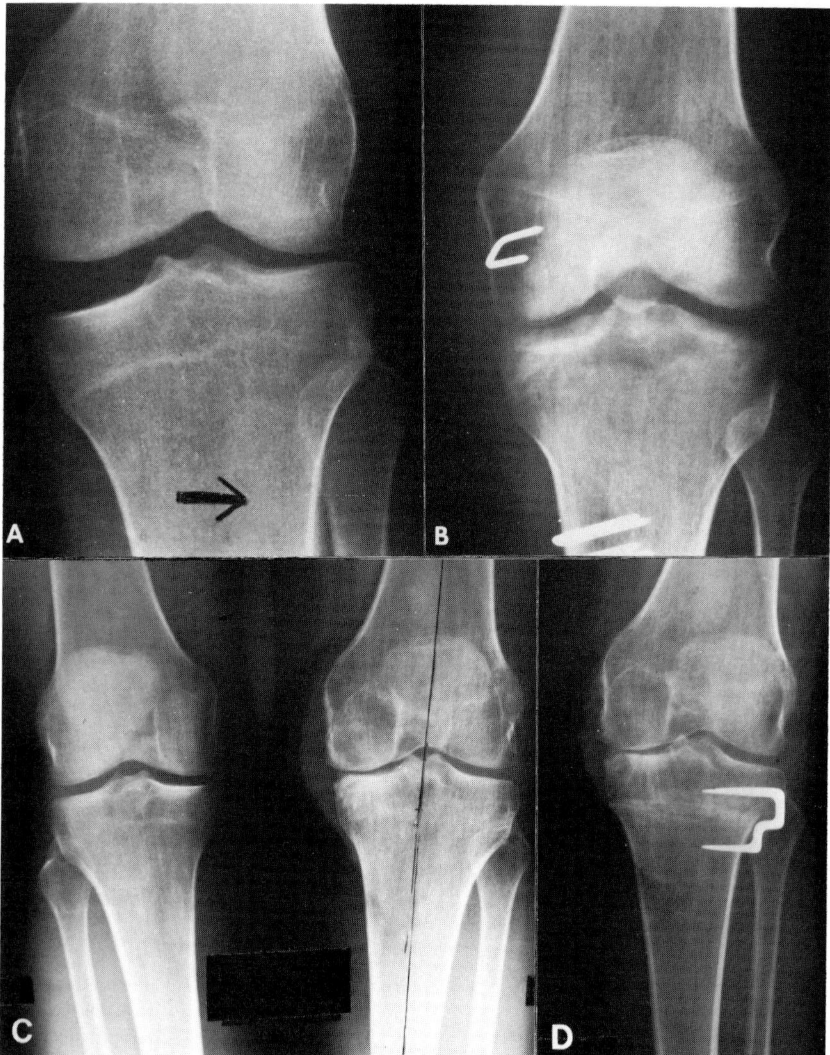

Fig. 42-15. Traumatic ligamentous disruption of medial collateral ligament repaired immediately. Postoperative wound sepsis, evident two weeks after operation, was treated by open debridement. Erosion of articular cartilage of medial compartment resulted in medial joint narrowing and early degenerative changes. A. Valgus stress view demonstrates medial joint opening (arrow) indicative of disruption of medial collateral ligament. B. Two months after repair, joint narrowing and subchondral reseparation are evident. C. Standing anteroposterior view of knees. Two years after injury, medial joint space degenerative changes have resulted in neutral anatomic position with loss of normal physiologic valgus. D. Standing anteroposterior view of left knee. Valgus upper tibial osteotomy has restored valgus alignment and shifted weightbearing forces to lateral compartment.

tients with previous gram-negative bacterial infections and those with early reimplantation (less than six months). In our experience, if organisms of low pathogenicity are isolated during the initial infection, reimplantation of a total joint is associated with a better prognosis.

Preliminary experience is promising with a similar technique in the treatment of the infected total knee arthroplasty. Reimplantation of the prosthetic components can be performed if, after three debridements, the bony and soft tissues are sterile.

Buchholz and Gartmann [52] used gentamicin-impregnated bone–cement in a single-stage treatment of the infected total hip arthroplasty. In contrast to the delayed reconstruction with total hip arthroplasty performed at the Mayo Clinic, their technique involved removal of the infected components, complete debridement of the bone and soft tissues, and immediate reimplantation of a new total hip with gentamicin-impregnated cement. Sixty-nine percent of their early results with this technique were successful. Further laboratory and clinical research into this technique is needed to clarify several points, such as the possible use of less toxic antimicrobial agents, the potential development of allergic reactions, and whether an allergy would require removal of the implant.

Complications of Chronic Skeletal Sepsis

Malignant degeneration and amyloidosis are occasionally seen in patients who have chronic infections of bones and joints.[9,13] Both carcinomas and sarcomas probably result from a long-standing reparative process. Squamous cell carcinoma appears in association with a draining sinus of long duration. Increased pain, drainage, hemorrhage, an enlarging mass, or a pathologic fracture suggests neoplastic degeneration. The sedimentation rate and leukocyte count are frequently normal. Roentgenograms usually demonstrate lytic and sclerotic changes indistinguishable from those of chronic osteomyelitis. However, a severely destructive lesion clearly different from the usual osteomyelitic process can be seen (Fig. 42-16). Biopsy of the sinus tract usually reveals bone invasion. Cure usually can be achieved with amputation

Sarcomatous change in chronic osteomyelitis is usually associated with a pathologic fracture or an enlarging mass. Biopsy delineates the histologic diagnosis.

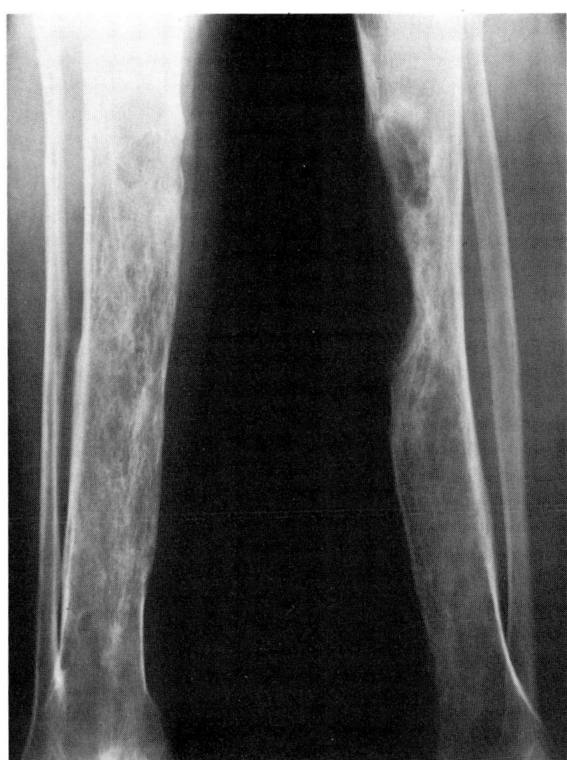

Fig. 42-16. **Squamous cell carcinoma in chronic osteomyelitis. Anteroposterior and lateral views demonstrating diffuse destruction of tibial diaphysis by lytic process, especially in distal third of tibia. Growing mass and sinus tract were located at junction of midthird and distal third of tibia.**

The association of amyloidosis with long-standing osteomyelitis and tuberculosis of the skeletal system was recognized years ago. Although secondary amyloidosis complicating chronic osteomyelitis has been seen occasionally in the patient who fails to receive treatment, modern drug therapy has significantly reduced this complication. Secondary amyloidosis is seen with equal frequency in patients who have chronic hematogenous and posttraumatic osteomyelitis. In general, chronic or recurring osteomyelitis will have been present for 20 years or more. Hepatosplenomegaly, a common finding in primary amyloidosis, is seldom noted. Laboratory evaluation of renal function reveals an elevation of the serum creatinine and blood urea nitrogen levels. Proteinuria is noted on routine urinalysis. Renal or rectal biopsies are necessary to confirm the diagnosis. A technetium-99 scan and a gallium-67 scan of the area reveal increased activity. An invasive type of subacute and chronic inflammatory granulation tissue is noted on tissue study.

BIBLIOGRAPHY

Fitzgerald RH Jr: The epidemiology of nosocomial infections of the musculoskeletal system. In Gröschel D (ed): Handbook on Hospital-associated Infections, Vol. 3. New York, Dekker, 1979, p 25.

Lobe G, Hierholzer: Posttraumatic Osteomyelitis. Berlin: Springer-Verlag, 1981.

REFERENCES

OSTEOMYELITIS

1. Hunter W: Of the structure and diseases of articulating cartilages. Philos Trans R Soc Lond 42:514, 1743.
2. Wilensky AO: Osteomyelitis: Its Pathogenesis, Symptomatology and Treatment. New York, Macmillan, 1934.
3. Dich VQ, Nelson JD, Haltalin KC: Osteomyelitis in infants and children: a review of 163 cases. Am J Dis Child 129:1273, 1975.
4. Morrey BF, Peterson HA: Hematogenous pyogenic osteomyelitis in children. Orthoped Clin North Am 6:935, 1975.
5. Waldvogel FA, Medoff G, Swartz MN: Osteomyelitis: a review of clinical features, therapeutic considerations and unusual aspects. N Engl J Med 282:198, 260, 317, 1970.
6. Lewis R, Gorbach S, Altner P: Spinal pseudomonas chondroosteomyelitis in heroin users. N Engl J Med 286:1303, 1972.
7. West WF, Kelly PJ, Martin WJ: Chronic osteomyelitis. I. Factors affecting the results of treatment in 186 patients. JAMA 213:1837, 1970.
8. Nettles JL, Kelly PJ, Martin WJ, Washington JA II: Musculoskeletal infections due to bacteroides: a study of eleven cases. J Bone Joint Surg [Am] 51:230, 1969.
9. Fitzgerald RH Jr, Kelly PJ: Recurrent sepsis, malignant change, and amyloidosis following posttraumatic osteomyelitis. In Lobe G, Hierholzer (eds): Posttraumatic Osteomyelitis. Berlin, Springer-Verlag, 1981.
10. Finegold SM: Anaerobic Bacteria in Human Disease. New York, Academic Press, 1977.
11. Kelly PJ: Infections of bones and joints in adult patients. Instructional Course Lectures. Am Acad Orthop Surg 26:3, 1977.
12. Weinstein AJ, McHenry MC, Gavan TL: Systemic absorption of neomycin irrigating solution. JAMA 238:152, 1977.
13. Burri C: Post-traumatic Osteomyelitis. Bern, Huber, 1975.
14. Mowlem R: Cancellous chip bone-grafts: report on 75 cases. Lancet 2:746, 1944.
15. Knight MP, Wood GO: Surgical obliteration of bone cavities following traumatic osteomyelitis. J Bone Joint Surg 27:547, 1945.
16. Robertson IM, Barron JN: A method of treatment of chronic infective osteitis. J Bone Joint Surg 28:19, 1946.
17. Coleman HM, Bateman JE, Dale GM, Starr DE: Cancellous bone grafts for infected bone defects: a single stage procedure. Surg Gynecol Obstet 83:392, 1946.
18. Bickel WH, Bateman JG, Johnson WE: Treatment of chronic hematogenous osteomyelitis by means of saucerization and bone grafting. Surg Gynecol Obstet 96:265, 1953.
19. Papineau LJ: L'excision-greffe avec fermeture retardée délibérée dans l'ostéomyélite chronique. Nouv Presse Med 2:2753, 1973.
20. Ger R: Muscle transposition for treatment and prevention of chronic posttraumatic osteomyelitis of the tibia. J Bone Joint Surg [Am] 59:784, 1977.
21. Prigge EK: The treatment of chronic osteomyelitis by the use of muscle transplant or iliac graft. J Bone Joint Surg 28:576, 1946.
22. Uyama S: Die Plombierung, von Knochenhöhlen durch Muskeltransplantation. Bruns Beitr Klin Chir 104:707, 1917.
23. Popkirov SG: Die Behandlung der hämatogenen und der traumatischen Osteomyelitis. Berlin, Volk und Gesundheit, 1971.
24. Nelson JD, Howard JB, Shelton S: Oral antibiotic therapy for skeletal infections in children. I. Antibiotic concentrations in suppurative synovial fluid. J Pediatr 92:131, 1978.

SEPTIC ARTHRITIS

25. Goldenberg DL, Brandt KD, Cathcart ES, Cohen AS: Acute arthritis caused by gram-negative bacilli: a clinical characterization. Medicine (Baltimore) 53:197, 1974.
26. Hunder GG, McDuffie FC: Hypocomplementemia in rheumatoid arthritis. Am J Med 54:461, 1973.
27. Phemister DB: The effect of pressure on articular surfaces in pyogenic and tuberculous arthritides and its bearing on treatment. Ann Surg 80:481, 1924.
28. Curtiss PH Jr, Klein L: Destruction of articular cartilage in septic arthritis. I. In vitro studies. J Bone Joint Surg [Am] 45:797, 1963.
29. Curtiss PH Jr, Klein L: Destruction of articular cartilage in septic arthritis. II. In vivo studies. J Bone Joint Surg [Am] 47:1595, 1965.
30. Marsh DC Jr, Matthew EB, Persellin RH: Transport of gentamicin into synovial fluid. JAMA 228:607, 1974.
31. Daniel D, Akeson W, Amiel D: The effect of joint lavage in preventing cartilage destruction in an experimentally produced *Staphylococcus aureus* joint infection (abstract). J Bone Joint Surg [Am] 57:583, 1975.
32. Anderson LD, Horn LG: Irrigation–suction technic in the treatment of acute hematogenous osteomyelitis, chronic osteomyelitis, and acute and chronic joint infections. South Med J 63:745, 1970.

GRANULOMATOUS INFECTIONS OF BONES AND JOINTS

33. Pritchard DJ: Granulomatous infections of bones and joints. Orthop Clin North Am 6:1029, 1975.
34. Bassett FH III, Tindall JP: Blastomycosis of bone. South Med J 65:547, 1972.
35. Gehweiler JA, Capp MP, Chick EW: Observations on the roentgen patterns and blastomycosis of bone. Am J Roentgenol Radium Ther Nucl Med 108:497, 1970.
36. Crout JE, Brewer, NS, Tompkins RB: Sporotrichosis arthritis: clinical features in seven patients. Ann Intern Med 86:294, 1977.

POSTOPERATIVE INFECTIONS

37. Ad Hoc Committee of the Committee on Trauma: Postoperative wound infections: the influence of ultraviolet irradiation of the operating room and of various other factors. Ann Surg 160[Suppl]:1, 1964.
38. Boyd RJ, Burke JF, Colton T: A double-blind clinical trial of prophylactic antibiotics in hip fractures. J Bone Joint Surg [Am] 55:1251, 1973.
39. Tengve B, Kjellander J: Antibiotic prophylaxis in operations on trochanteric femoral fractures. J Bone Joint Surg [Am] 60:97, 1978.
40. Miller WE, Counts GW: Orthopedic infections: a prospective study of 378 clean procedures. South Med J 68:386, 1975.
41. Fitzgerald RH Jr: The epidemiology of nosocomial infections of the musculoskeletal system. In Gröschel D (ed): Handbook on Hospital-associated Infections. Vol 3. New York, Dekker, 1979, pp 25–35.
42. Gustilo RB, Anderson JT: Prevention of infection in the treatment of one thousand and twenty-five open fractures of long bones: retrospective and prospective analyses. J Bone Joint Surg [Am] 58:453, 1976.
43. Murray WR, Rodrigo JJ: Arthrography for the assessment of pain after total hip replacement: a comparison of arthrographic findings in patients with and without pain. J Bone Joint Surg [Am] 57:1060, 1975.
44. Brown PW, Kinman PB: Gas gangrene in a metropolitan community. J Bone Joint Surg [Am] 56:1445, 1974.
45. Fitzgerald RH Jr, Cooney WP, Dobyns JH: Unpublished data.
46. Robson, MC, Lea CE, Dalton JB, Heggers JP: Quantitative bacteriology and delayed wound closure. Surg Forum 19:501, 1968.
47. Fogelberg EV, Zitzmann EK, Stinchfield FE: Prophylactic penicillin in orthopaedic surgery. J Bone Joint Surg [Am] 52:95, 1970.
48. Pavel A, Smith RL, Ballard A, Larson IJ: Prophylactic antibiotics in elective orthopedic surgery: a prospective study of 1,591 cases. South Med J 70[Suppl 1]:50, 1977.
49. Patzakis MJ, Harvey JP Jr, Ivler D: The role of antibiotics in the management of open fractures. J Bone Joint Surg [Am] 56:532, 1974.
49a. Hill C, Flamant R, Mazas F, Evrard J: Prophylactic cefazoline versus placebo in total hip replacement. Lancet 1:795, 1981.
50. Fremont-Smith P: Sepsis and total hip arthroplasty. Part I. Antibiotic management of septic total hip replacement: a therapeutic trial. Proc Sci Meet Hip Soc 2:301, 1974.
51. Wilson PD Jr, Aglietti P, Salvati EA: Subacute sepsis of the hip treated by antibiotics and cemented prosthesis. J Bone Joint Surg [Am] 56:879, 1974.
52. Buchholz HW, Gartmann HD: Infektionsprophylaxe und operative Behandlung der schleichenden tiefen Infektion bei der totalen Endoprosthese. Chirurg 43:446, 1972.

CHAPTER 43
Infections of the Hand

JOHN H. CRANDON

The studies of Kanavel [1] at the turn of the century revolutionized the concepts and treatment of infections of the hand. He demonstrated the various closed spaces of the fingers and hand, the significance of infections within them, and the importance of their early diagnosis and drainage for subsequent adequate restoration of function. Since the advent of antibiotics, both the incidence and the severity of infections have diminished, together with their crippling after-effects. Nevertheless, the principles of diagnosis and treatment have not changed. The use of local heat, particularly in the form of hot soaks, however, is less common. This chapter will focus on the anatomy and therapy of pyogenic hand infection. The more unusual infections of bone, joint, and soft tissue are discussed in Chapters 25 and 42.

ANATOMY

A requirement for the proper treatment of infections of the hand is knowledge of anatomy. This includes the course of neurovascular bundles, the location of flexor tendons and their sheaths, and their relationship to the closed spaces of the hand (Figs. 43-1 and 43-2).

Closed spaces of the hand, with the exception of the dorsal subaponeurotic space (which is rarely infected), occur on the volar aspect of the hand (Fig. 43-1). In the distal phalanx, the pulp space of the digit is a closed space bound anteriorly by the volar subcutaneous fascia, posteriorly by the bony phalanx periosteum, and proximally by the septum of Wilkinson, which separates it from the insertion of the flexor tendon (Fig. 43-1). In the middle phalanx, the space under the fascia is essentially a closed space and is bounded by the joint capsule and its ligaments and the tendon sheath at the distal and proximal interphalangeal joints.

Between the four fingers are three web spaces in the palm, which are bounded proximally by the ligaments between the metacarpal heads, anteriorly by the prolongations of the palmar fascia, and distally by the tendons of the lumbricals and interossei (Fig. 43-2). These spaces extend to the dorsum of the webs.

In the palm, the thenar space is a greatly enlarged web space between the thumb and the index finger (Fig. 43-2). Its floor is the adductor pollicis muscle, and its medial boundary is a septum running between the third metacarpal and the overlying flexor tendons to the middle finger.[2] This septum is also the lateral boundary of the midpalmar space. The floor of the midpalmar space is the interosseous septum between the fourth and fifth metacarpals. Its roof is the flexor tendons of the middle, ring, and little fingers, and its medial boundary is the hypothenar muscles.

The quadrilateral space (space of Perona) in the wrist lies between the flexor tendons and the fascia covering the pronator quadratus muscle. It is continuous with the radial and ulnar bursae in the proximal palm.

The flexor tendon sheaths terminate at the distal flexion crease of each finger. The proximal sheaths of the index, middle, and ring fingers begin proximal to the annular ligaments over the metacarpal heads (Fig. 43-1). The sheaths of the thumb and little finger also may be continuous with the radial and ulnar bursae respectively, which in turn may communicate with each other and with the space of Perona in the wrist. Tenosynovitis in the thumb can sometimes extend to the little finger and vice versa.

The dorsal subaponeurotic space is a potential space between the dorsal fascia and the extensor tendons. Swelling of the dorsum is common in many severe infections of the hand; however, infection in this space is rare.

The vital neurovascular bundles in the palm run between the flexor tendons; in the fingers, they run along the anterolateral aspect about 3 mm beneath the volar skin. A midlateral incision over the finger will avoid these structures (Fig. 43-3). A relatively superficial transverse incision across the entire volar aspect of the finger can divide both the neurovascular bundles, with resulting gangrene.

THE EPIDEMIOLOGY OF HAND INFECTIONS

Bell [3] reviewed the epidemiology of 400 consecutive pyogenic hand infections. Infections occurred in males twice as frequently as in females, and they occurred most commonly in manual and industrial workers, but also frequently in school children, housewives, and other types of workers (Table 43-1). Paronychial infections were most common, occurring in 202 of the 400 infections (Table 43-2). Other common infections were pulp infections (fel-

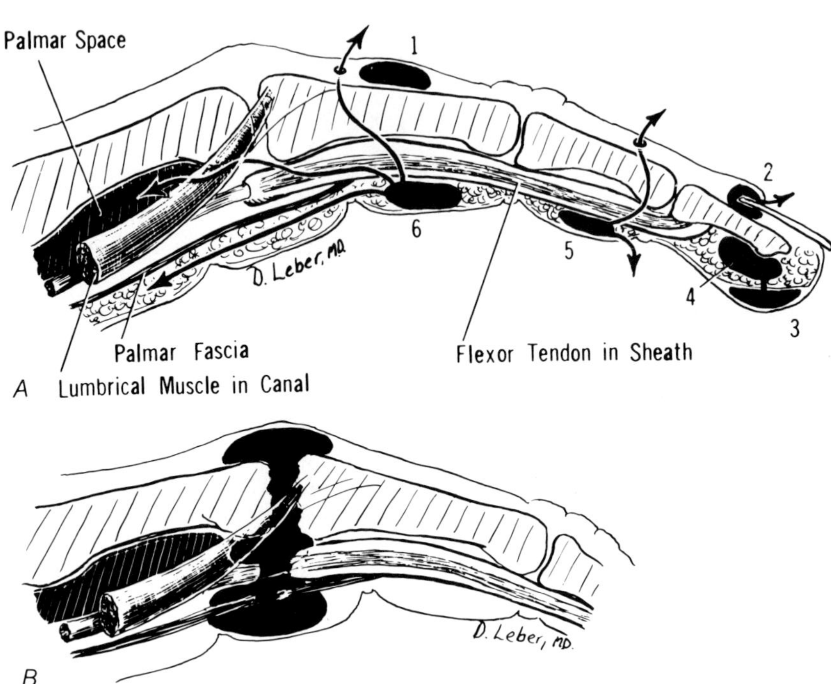

Fig. 43-1. **A. Diagram of the locations of common infections, showing spreading and pointing. 1. Dorsal subcutaneous abscess. 2. Paronychia. 3. A vesicle or pustule indicative of felon beneath. 4. Felon. 5. Abscess in volar fat pad; this can point in a palmar direction or track to the dorsum before pointing; the flexion creases frequently act as barriers to spread. 6. Abscess in palmar fat pad may spread by perforating dorsad, by passing the flexion crease barrier through bacterial action and going proximally to the subcutaneous tissue in the palm, or by spreading via the lumbrical canal to a palmar space. B. The collar button abscess. This advanced lesion, with abscess cavities on both the palmar and dorsal aspects, is common in the area of the metacarpophalangeal joint. It has the potential for spreading beneath the palmar fascia or into the dorsal compartment opposite the web space, or it may fill the web space and extend along the tendons into the midpalmar space or to the thenar space. (From Chase RA, Cramer LM: Hand. In Schwartz SI, Shires GT, Spencer FC, Storer EH (eds): *Principles of Surgery,* 3rd ed. New York, McGraw-Hill, 1979, p 2031.)**

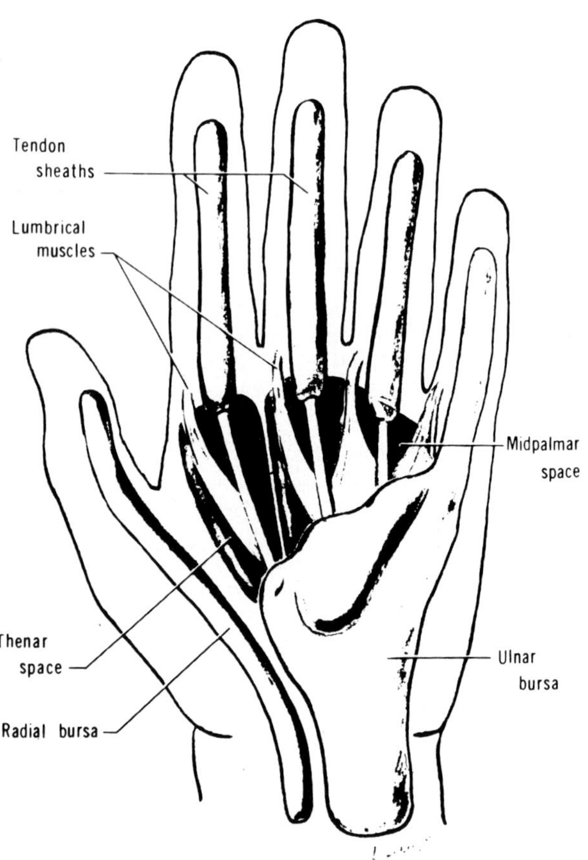

Fig. 43-2. **The anatomy of the synovial sheaths and deep spaces in the hand. (From Chase RA, Cramer LM: Hand. In Schwartz SI, Shires GT, Spencer FC, Storer EH (eds): *Principles of Surgery,* 3rd ed. New York, McGraw-Hill, 1979, p 2031.)**

ons), subcutaneous abscesses, and infected lacerations. *S. aureus* accounted for 61 percent of the infections, and an additional 20 percent were mixed infections (Table 43-3). Of the 400 hand infections, 306 required incision and drainage (Table 43-4).

PRINCIPLES OF TREATMENT OF HAND INFECTIONS

Elevation, immobilization, and heat have remained the most important features in the treatment of hand infections. Immobilization should always be maintained in the position of function. Heat should be applied in the form of hot wet packs changed every 2 to 4 hours. Hot soaks may be used for 20 minutes every 4 hours. Appropriate antibiotics may also aid in recovery, but they cannot replace elevation, immobilization, and heat.

Signs of a favorable response to treatment include decreasing discomfort, tenderness, swelling, and shininess of the overlying skin.

Abscesses and local collections of pus should be drained promptly. All drainage procedures should ensure adequate drainage and subsequent function of the hand. Adequate anesthesia should be provided, and a tourniquet should be used to provide a bloodless field so vital structures can be seen. In general, incisions for drainage should be placed on the volar aspect of the hand, and they should be transverse, as parallel to the flexion creases as possible (Fig. 43-4A–D). Care should be taken not to cut nerves or arteries. Vertical incisions can be made only over the midlateral aspects of the fingers, over the dorsum of the hand, and over the midulnar and midradial aspects of the wrist. When a long incision is required in the palm or

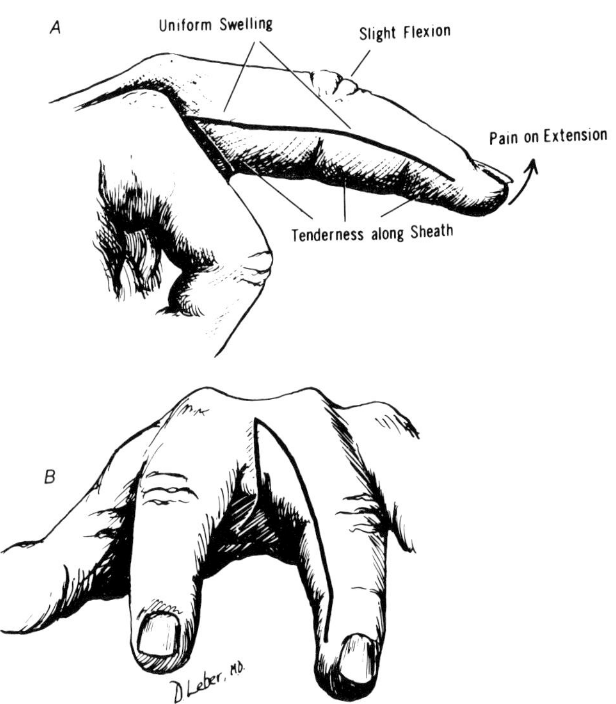

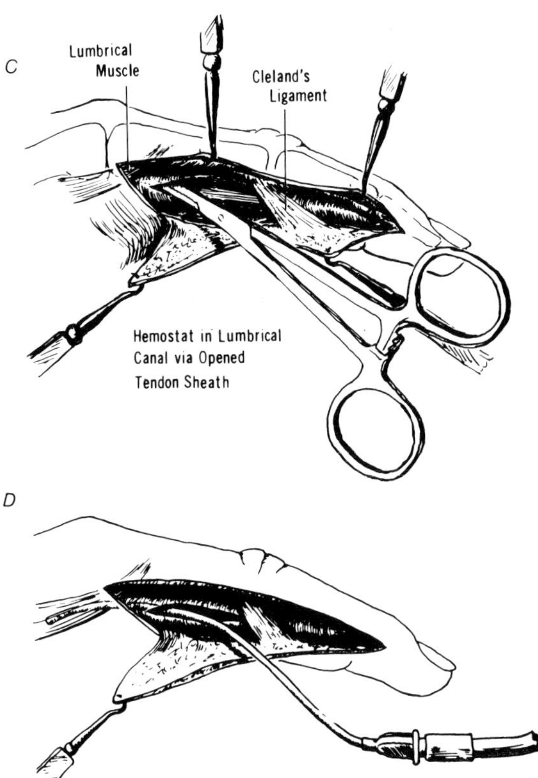

***Fig. 43-3.* Diagnosis and treatment of flexor tenosynovitis. A. The cardinal signs of inflammation related to flexor tenosynovitis. The entire digit will be swollen. The incision is placed on the neutral midlateral line. B. End-on view of the incision. If there is no suspicion of palmar spread, the incision should be placed on the ulnar side of the finger. If palmar spread is suspected, the incision should be placed on the radial side. The web extension of the incision is not always necessary for exposure. C. The fascial sheaths around the lumbrical muscles provide a point of least resistance and create a canal for spread of infection. Careful diagnosis in this region may allow effective drainage without opening the palm. D. Implantation of irrigating catheters and multiple postoperative instillations effectively control many infections. (From Chase RA, Cramer LM: Hand. In Schwartz SI, Shires GT, Spencer FC, Storer EH (eds): *Principles of Surgery,* 3rd ed. New York, McGraw-Hill, 1979, p 2031.)**

anterior wrist, it should be S-shaped parallel to flexion creases as much as possible, with gentle curves in between. Drains should be of inert nonporous materials like latex rubber or silastic—except in the case of a felon.

Goldner [4] has listed six do's and seven don't's that summarize treatment concepts in hand infections (Table 43-5).

CLINICAL MANIFESTATIONS

HISTORY AND PHYSICAL EXAMINATION

A complete history, in the case of an infected hand, should include the possible source of infection and the occupation of the patient—fish handler, garbage collector, stable boy, cook, hospital employee—whether or not the infection could have been acquired at work, the date of injury, and whether it is the dominant hand. The evaluation should also include any history of diabetes, gout, prior infections and allergies to antibiotics, as well as any recent treatment with these or other medicines.

Physical examination should include comparison of the finger or part involved with that of the opposite hand, with respect to both swelling and function. The arm should be carefully examined for evidence of lymphangitis, which may extend up the volar aspect of the forearm. The presence of tender enlarged epitrochlear or axillary lymph nodes should be noted. Particular attention should be paid to the involvement of the flexor tendon sheaths; failure to treat this infection is disastrous.

In many even moderately severe infections of the hand, there is associated severe swelling of the dorsum,

TABLE 43-1. OCCUPATION OF PATIENTS WITH HAND INFECTIONS

	Number
Under school age	21
Schoolchildren	72
Housewives	56
Manual and industrial workers	129
Other workers	90
Retired	13
Occupation unspecified	19

From Bell MS: The changing pattern of pyogenic infections of the hand. *Hand* 8:298,1976.

TABLE 43-2. SITES OF INFECTION

	Number
Pulp infection	64
Paronychia	202
Apical infection	11
Subcuticular abscess	2
Subcutaneous abscess	56
Infected laceration	43
Cellulitis	4
Web space infection	4
Thenar space infection	1
Middle palmar space infection	2
Tendon sheath infection	4
Carbuncle	1
Septic arthritis	1
Other infections	5

From Bell MS: The changing pattern of pyogenic infections of the hand. *Hand* 8:298, 1976.

since the lymphatics of the hand pass through this area. Frank abscess of this area, however, is extremely uncommon.

In all cases, cultures should be taken of infected material for Gram staining.

SPECIFIC INFECTIONS

Paronychia

The most common infection of the finger is the paronychia, which involves the soft tissue at the base of the nail, adjacent to the edge of the proximal portion of the fingernail. The offending organism, as in the majority of hand infections, is coagulase-positive *S. aureus,* but other etiologies are becoming more common. Paronychia may be divided into three types: superficial, deep, and chronic.

Superficial Paronychia

Superficial paronychia appears as a small area of cellulitis, with swelling at the base of paronychial tissue adjacent to the nail. On closer inspection, a small intracuticular or subcuticular abscess is seen arising in the sulcus at the nail border (Fig. 43-5). This type can be drained by passing the point of a bayonet-type knife blade into the sulcus at an oblique angle (Fig. 43-6). If a drop or two of pus is not obtained, the knife should be repositioned and a second, more liberal incision made. After drainage, warm sodium chloride solution soaks can be beneficial for promoting drainage from the wound. Intervening ointment dressings and splinting in the position of function should be used. Splinting of even so superficial an infection prevents changes in tissue tension produced by flexion of the finger, and thereby promotes healing. An antibiotic ointment such as Neosporin, if not topically active, at least keeps the affected tissue soft and adds to the patient's comfort.

TABLE 43-3. ORGANISMS CULTURED EXPRESSED AS PERCENTAGES OF TOTAL

	Percent
S. aureus, pencillin-sensitive	21
S. aureus, penicillin-resistant	40
β-hemolytic streptococci	7
Other streptococci	6
Coliforms	3
Proteus	1.5
P. pyocyaneus	1.5
Mixed infections	20

From Bell MS: The changing pattern of pyogenic infections of the hand. *Hand* 8:298, 1976.

TABLE 43-4. TREATMENT OF HAND INFECTIONS

	Number
Number of cases incised once	306
Number of cases incised more than once	9
Number of patients admitted	3
Average duration of disability in days	8
Number of patients given antibiotics	165

From Bell MS: The changing pattern of pyogenic infections of the hand. *Hand* 8:298, 1976.

Deep Paronychia

In deep paronychia, there is diffuse tender swelling and cellulitis of the entire proximal paronychial tissue, which frequently extends into the adjacent eponychia. There may be no evidence of underlying pus. Local heat, ointment dressings, splinting, and antibiotics may be helpful for 48 hours. Pus may localize or drain spontaneously from the sulcus. An incision like that used for superficial paronychia is usually appropriate to complete the drainage. Otherwise, an incision that extends proximally along the entire sulcus to the proximal corner of the nail is necessary to ascertain that there is neither early devitalization of the corner of the nail base nor pus under it. If either of these conditions exist, this portion of the nail must be removed (Figs. 43-7 and 43-8). Failure to recognize an early subungual abscess involving one corner of the nail base in conjunction with a deep paronychia is one of the most common errors in the treatment of hand infections and can lead to a protracted inflammation relieved only by removal of the entire nail.

Chronic Paronychia

Chronic paronychia is a low-grade inflammatory process that involves the paronychia. Generally, the eponychia, and occasionally the paronychia on the other side of the nail, are involved as well (Fig. 43-8). A complete history must be recorded. The normal cuticle in the involved area is absent. Instead, the tissue adjacent to the nail has a "rolled in" appearance. The most common cause is devitalized nail under the paronychial-eponychial junction (Fig. 43-9). Another common cause is mycotic infection. Smears, cultures, examination of the nail bed, and removal of the nail are necessary. A few patients have this infection on

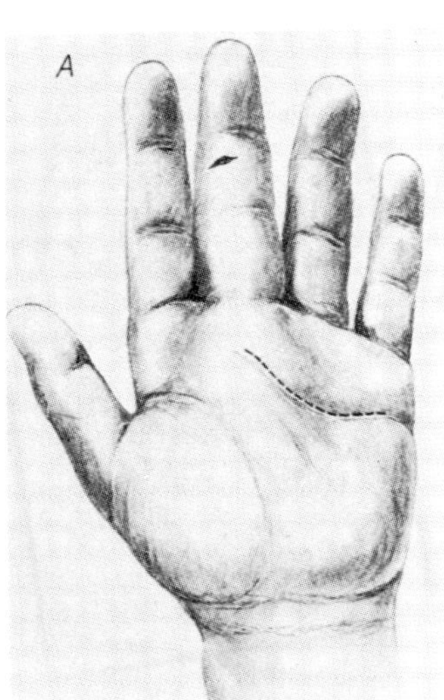

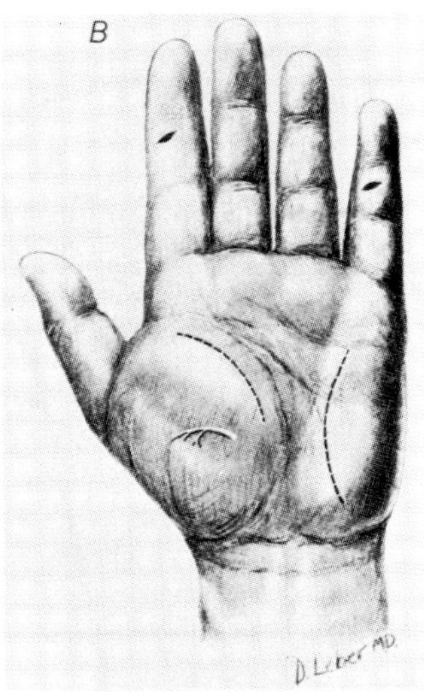

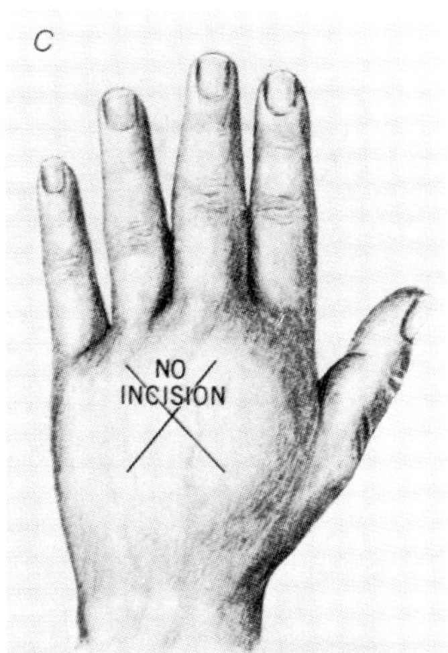

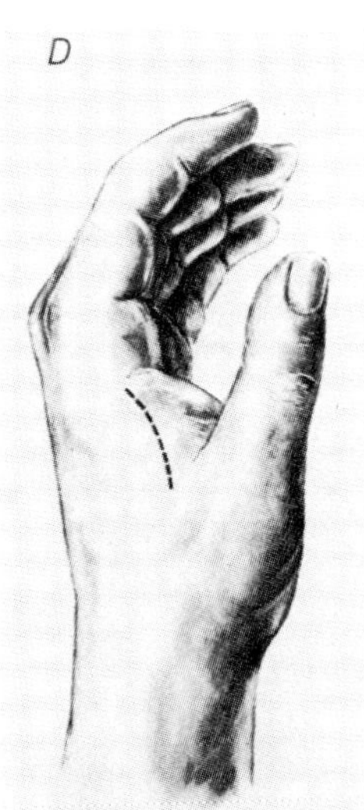

Fig. 43-4. **Spread of digital infection into the palm. A. Incision for drainage of the midpalmar space. B. Incisions for drainage of the radial bursa and the ulnar bursa. C. Palmar digital infections frequently create extremely swollen regions on the dorsum of the hand, because the lymphatic drainage runs from the palmar to the dorsal aspects. A common error is to expect to drain such a lesion at this lymphadenitis point. When there are dorsal infections, incision and drainage will be performed dorsally. D. The incision for drainage of the thenar space. (From Chase RA, Cramer LM: Hand. In Schwartz SI, Shires GT, Spencer FC, Storer EH (eds): *Principles of Surgery,* 3rd ed. New York, McGraw-Hill, 1979, p 2031.)**

several fingers. Squamous cell carcinoma of the nail bed should be considered [5] when infection of the nail bed of one finger persists.

Subungual Abscess

Subungual abscess is generally easy to recognize when suspected because pressure on the proximal nail will cause pain and give the impression that the nail is floating at its base. It is usually associated with and caused by a deep paronychia. Pus from the deep paronychia undermines the proximal nail and produces a devitalized foreign body (Fig. 43-10). The offending paronychia should be incised, the eponychia laid back, the nail removed, and a small vaseline gauze pack inserted under the eponychia and left for 48 hours, with concomitant administration of suitable antibiotics. Thereafter, hot soaks using a weak chlorine type of solution (0.5 percent sodium hypochlorite solution) with intervening ointment dressings and splinting should be used. Elevation of the hand is also helpful.

Felon (Whitlow)

A felon is a closed space infection in the pulp space of the terminal phalanx of a digit. Proper drainage is difficult, because the pulp space is made up of firm fat lobules tightly interspersed with multiple columellae of fascial strands.

Etiology and Pathogenesis

The felon most often results from a puncture wound of the volar aspect of the fat pad of the distal phalanx. Drainage through the puncture wound can often be seen. It can also develop from an infected blister on the volar surface of the fat pad, from a neglected deep paronychia or subungual abscess, and rarely from a severe contusion

TABLE 43-5. TREATMENT CONCEPTS IN HAND INFECTION

DO

1. Take a careful history; examine the entire extremity carefully, as well as the hand.
2. Think of conditions other than infections that might account for the condition.
3. Attempt a specific diagnosis before beginning therapy. There is a safe waiting period.
4. Wait for abscess localization in most instances except if the tendon sheath is involved; then early incision may be performed. Use immobilization, elevation, wet dressings, and antibiotics before and after drainage.
5. Use adequate anesthesia—either general or nerve block—for draining abscess. Use a tourniquet if a tendon is exposed.
6. Administer tetanus prophylaxis if there has been a puncture or laceration associated with the infection (Chapter 46).

DON'T

1. Incise every painful swollen digit.
2. Make incisions in the finger pads unless the infection has already localized to this area.
3. Injure digital nerves or motor branch of median or ulnar nerves in making incision for drainage.
4. Attempt to drain fingertip abscesses with a puncture-type incision.
5. Close human bites or puncture wounds.
6. Close puncture wounds or lacerations when the hand injury has occurred in dishwater, fishy water, sand, or dirt.
7. Forget to obtain adequate material for culture—give special instructions concerning organism suspected and type of injury, and ask for sensitivities.

From Goldner JL: The hand. In Sabiston DC Jr (ed): *Textbook of Surgery,* 11th ed. Philadelphia, Saunders, 1977, p 1609.

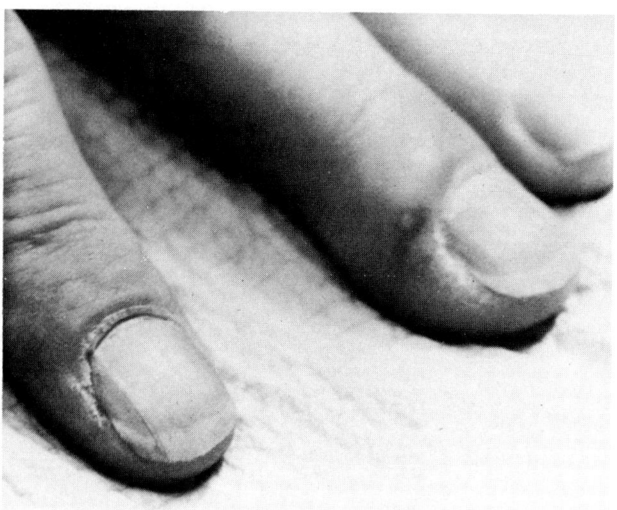

Fig. 43-5. **Superficial paronychia. The appearance suggests underlying localized pus.**

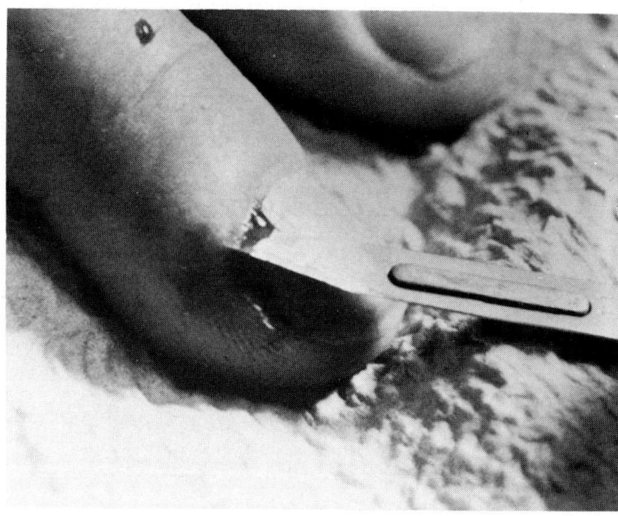

Fig. 43-6. **Incision and drainage of superficial paronychia. The knife blade should be almost parallel to the nail.**

of the pulp without obvious break in the skin. *S. aureus* is almost always cultured. A felonlike picture can also develop from herpesvirus (especially in dentists), in which case a history or presence of herpetic vesicles and possible exposure to such a virus can be helpful in the diagnosis.

Diagnosis

Early diagnosis is important, because progression of the process causes occlusion of the blood vessels which can result either in bony necrosis or slough of the volar fat pad (Figs. 43-11 and 43-12). The patient complains of constant severe pain until the infection is well advanced and the blood vessels become occluded, after which the digit may feel numb. The swelling of the digit may not be appreciated unless comparison is made with its contralateral member. Pressure over the volar aspect of the digit causes pain. Simultaneous transillumination of the affected digit and its counterpart on the other hand over a flashlight in a dark room will show increased opacity of the affected finger (Fig. 43-13).[5] When the felon is the result of extension from a deep paronychia, drainage of the paronychia in a bloodless field can reveal a sinus passing volarward into the pulp space. Pressure over the pulp can cause the pus to exude up through the sinus (Fig. 43-14). In all but the early cases, roentgenograms will help detect the presence of bony necrosis.

Treatment

Immediate drainage is indicated except when the lesion may have resulted from a severe contusion or from herpes.

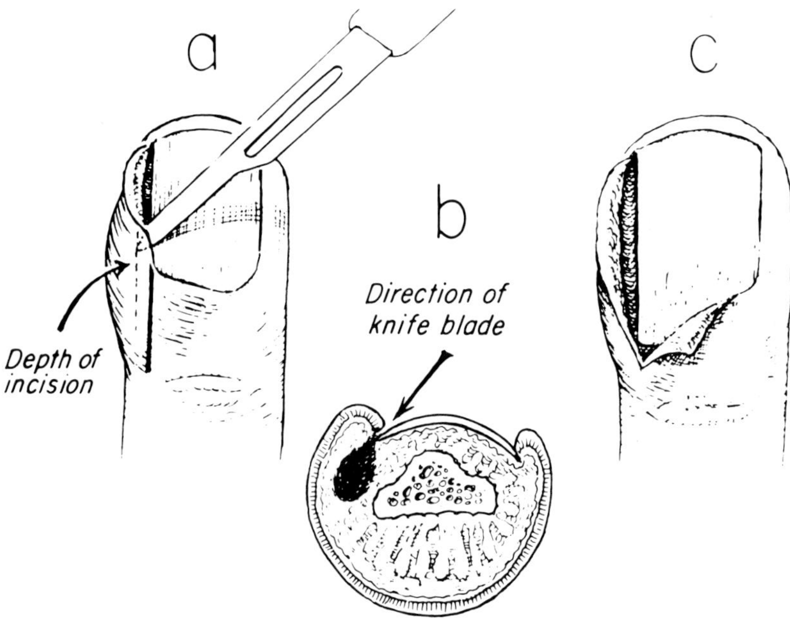

Fig. 43-7. **Incision and drainage of deep paronychia. The proximal corner of the nail must be exposed to ascertain early devitalization of subungual abscess. (From Flynn JE: *Hand Surgery.* Baltimore, William and Wilkins, 1975).**

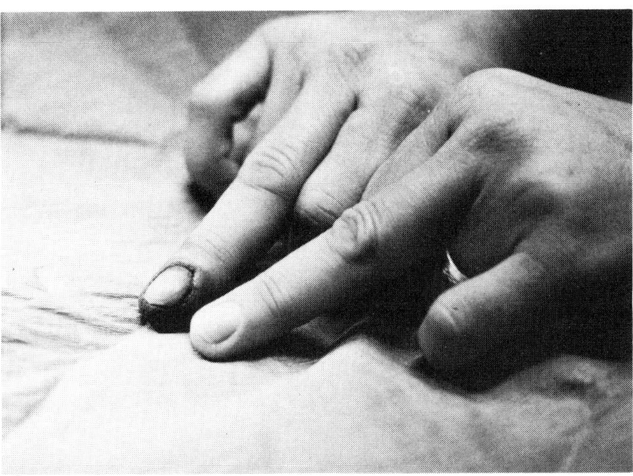

Fig. 43-8. **Chronic paronychia. The cuticle has disappeared. The proximal corner of the nail was devitalized. The nail was removed to stop the infection.**

A proper incision is of utmost importance and has been misrepresented in several texts. The incision should be hockey-stick in configuration, somewhat dorsal to the underlying lateral line, and made to come down directly onto the lateral aspect of the bony phalanx and curve around the tip of the finger down to the tip of the bony phalanx (Fig. 43-15). The tip of a small curved hemostat is forced under the volar aspect of the bony phalanx and opened to spread apart the underlying closed space (Fig. 43-16). A midlateral incision will not provide adequate drainage, and a fishmouth incision, extending around the entire tip of the finger to its other side, will frequently cause thrombosis of the digital vessels with resulting slough of the volar fat pad, a disastrous complication (Figs. 43-17 and 43-18). Following adequate breakdown of the trabeculae attached to the volar aspect of the bone, the space should be packed open for 24 to 48 hours (Fig. 43-19). A rather bulky dressing generally serves both to absorb the blood and to splint the finger. Antibiotics effective against *S. aureus* speed recovery. When the pack is removed after 48 hours (after a sterile soak), the wound cavity is frequently so clean that further soaks and repacking may be unnecessary. However, the cavity should be repacked if active infection still appears to be present, because reoperation is frequently necessary if premature closure is permitted.

When the felon is secondary to a deep paronychia or subungual abscess, the hockey stick incision should be made on the same side as the paronychia, and the fingernail should also be removed.

Roentgenographic evidence of osteomyelitis is not cause for great alarm. Adequate drainage will permit ultimate regeneration of the bone, providing that meddlesome curettage is not attempted. Any dead bone will be extruded or can be carefully picked out of the wound cavity during healing.

When the felon results from a puncture wound on the volar surface of the phalanx, or if the felon points or drains through the volar pad, the surgeon may be tempted

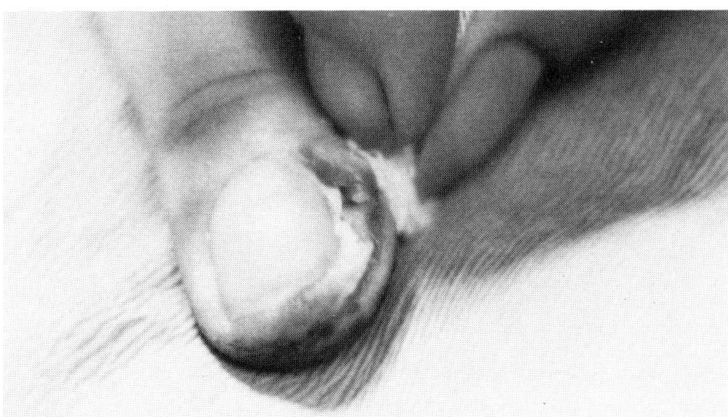

Fig. 43-9. **Devitalized nail. Deep paronychia progressed to felon, which was properly drained, but the nail was not removed—inflammation of paronychia continued.**

to drain the felon through a volar incision. This provides adequate drainage, but a permanently tender scar can result.

Prognosis

When adequate early drainage is carried out, the results are excellent. Delay or inadequate drainage can lead to osteomyelitis, slough of the volar fat pad, tenosynovitis, or deep fascial infection of the middle and proximal phalanges, all of which can occur by direct extension from the felon (Fig. 43-12).

Subfascial Infections of the Finger

Subfascial infections can occur in the volar aspects of the middle and proximal phalanges. These infections are usually the result of an infection or wound of the overlying volar skin. In the middle phalanx, subfascial infection involves a closed space which, if neglected, can extend into the underlying flexor tendon sheath or adjacent joint. In the proximal phalanx the process can extend into the lumbrical canal or web space. It is difficult to differentiate between a subfascial infection and tenosynovitis. In tenosynovitis, however, there is tenderness over the entire

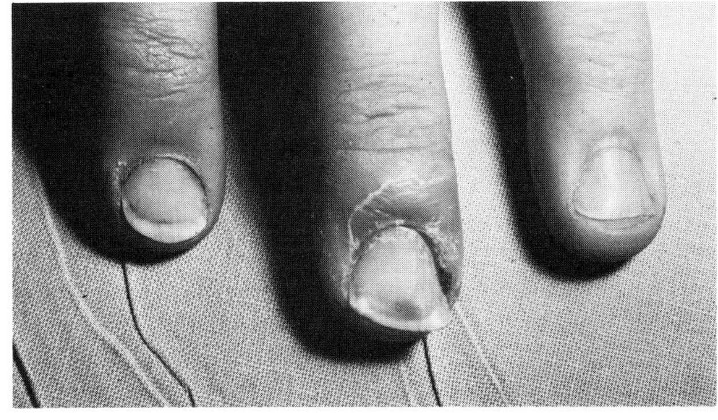

Fig. 43-10. **Subungual abscess. Pressure on the proximal nail causes pain, and the nail feels as though it were floating.**

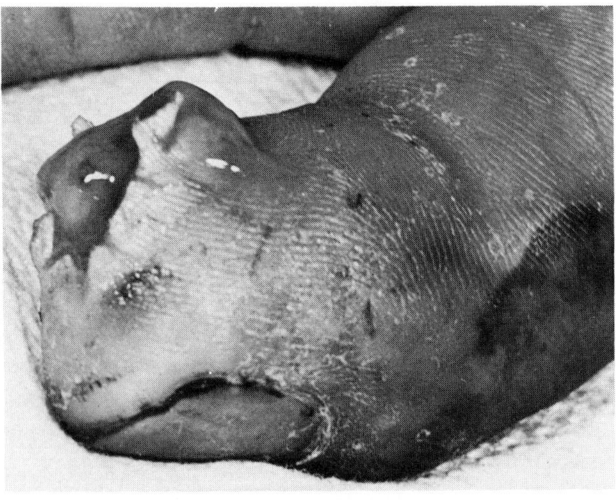

Fig. 43-11. Slough of volar fat pad, neglected felon.

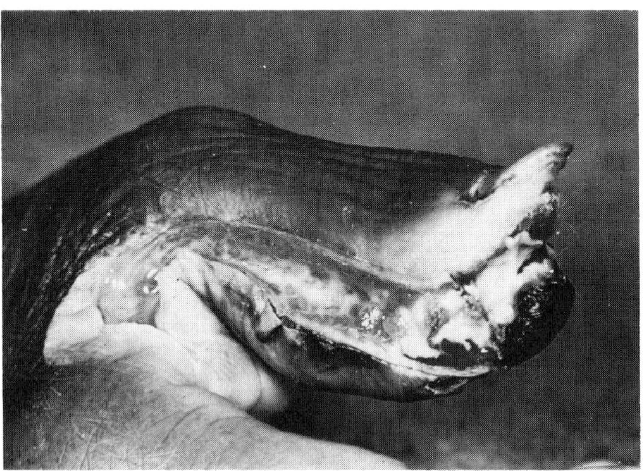

Fig. 43-12. The ultimate disaster of neglected felon—slough of fat pad, osteomyelitis, and tenosynovitis. The patient was a diabetic, and amputation of the ray was required.

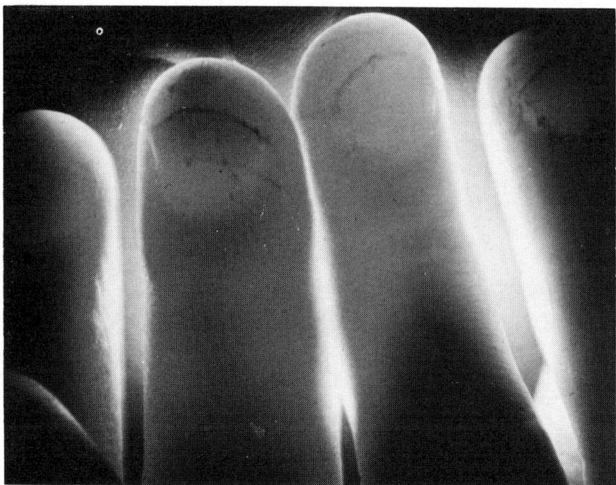

Fig. 43-13. Early diagnosis of felon by transillumination.

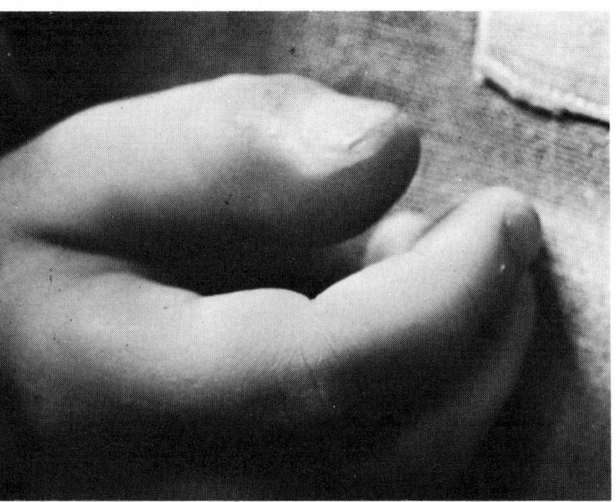

Fig. 43-14. Felon of undetermined cause, 1 week after first signs of infection.

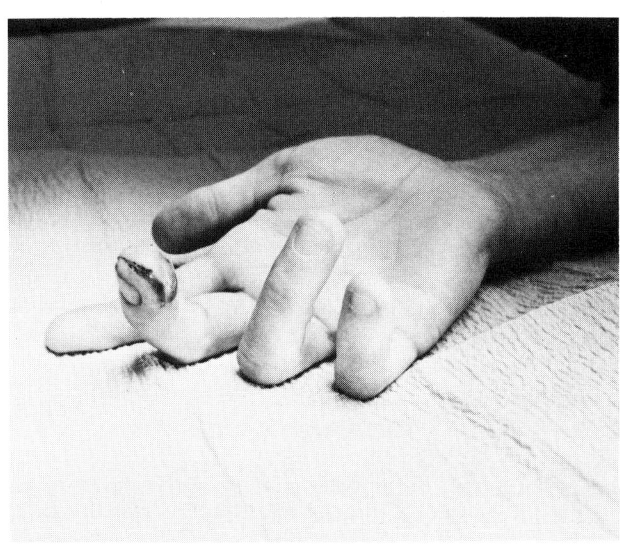

Fig. 43-15. Hockey-stick incision for felon, shown in a patient 5 days after incision and drainage and 3 days after removal of a pack.

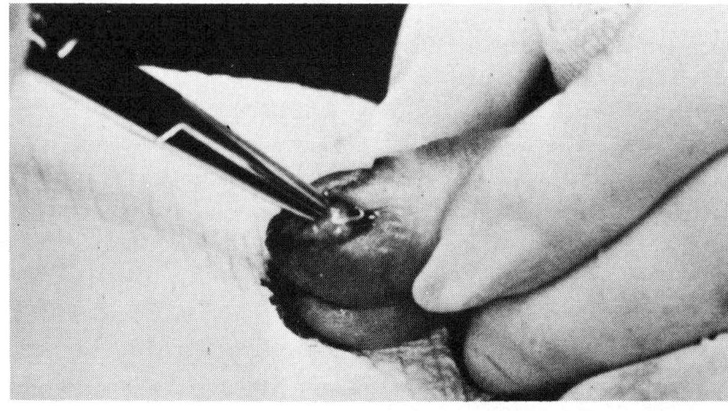

Fig. 43-16. The proper method of pushing the tip of a hemostat under the volar aspect of the bony phalanx and into pulp space. After the pulp space has been reached, the jaws of the hemostat are repeatedly opened to break down all the fibrous trabeculae in the space.

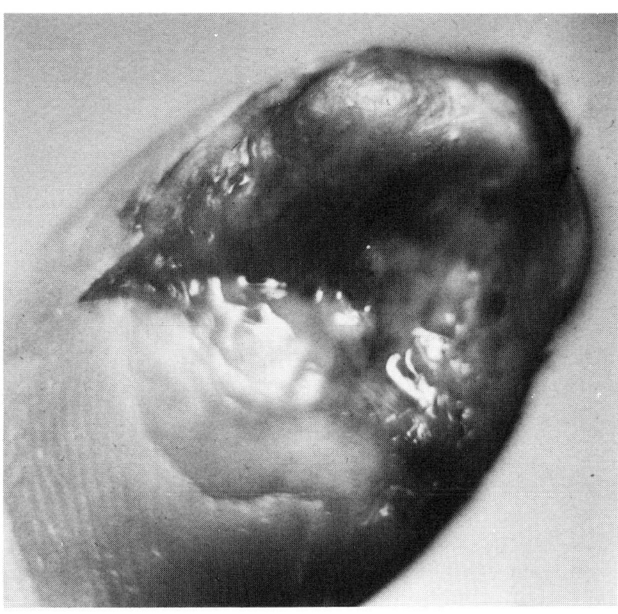

Fig. 43-17. **Felon. Fish mouth to shark mouth. The fish mouth incision may cause devitalization of the volar fat pad by interference with its blood supply from the volar digital vessels.**

length of the tendon sheath from middle phalanx to proximal extent in the distal flexion crease of the palm. In either case, approach is made through a midlateral incision, with exploration of the subfascial space deep to the neurovascular bundle before the tendon sheath is incised (Fig. 43-3A). Drainage should be promoted by placing small strips of rubber into the space and splinting the finger in a position of function.

Tenosynovitis

Bacterial tenosynovitis of the flexor tendon sheaths is the most dreaded and crippling infection of the hand. Much of the current thinking on this subject stems from the studies of Flynn.[6]

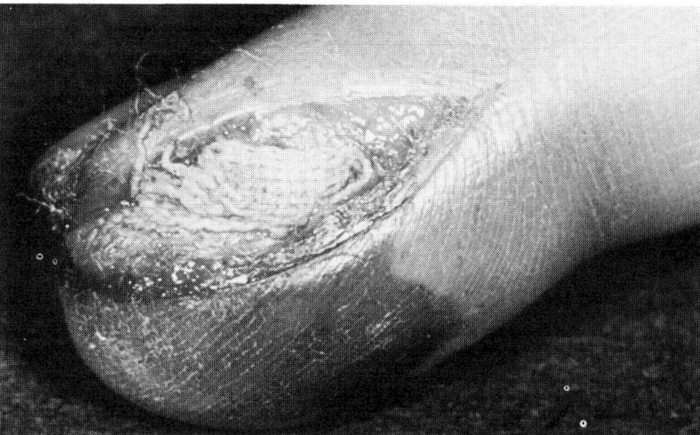

Fig. 43-19. **Proper packing of a felon; 3 days after incision and drainage.**

Pathology

In bacterial tenosynovitis, the flexor tendons and their blood supply are rapidly constricted by exudation and edema within the surrounding tendon sheath. Constriction is most marked at the level of the annular ligament and pulleys, which do not yield to tissue tension. It is therefore mandatory that the tendon sheath be laid open through midlateral incisions from one end to the other to avoid tendon necrosis (Fig. 43-3).

Clinical Manifestations

The cardinal signs of acute bacterial tenosynovitis of the flexor tendon sheath are: (1) diffuse swelling of the finger, (2) maintenance of the finger in a partially flexed position, (3) elicitation of pain by passively extending the finger from its partially flexed position, and (4) volar tenderness along the course of the tendon sheath where the infection has not extended beyond the confines of its sheath (Fig.

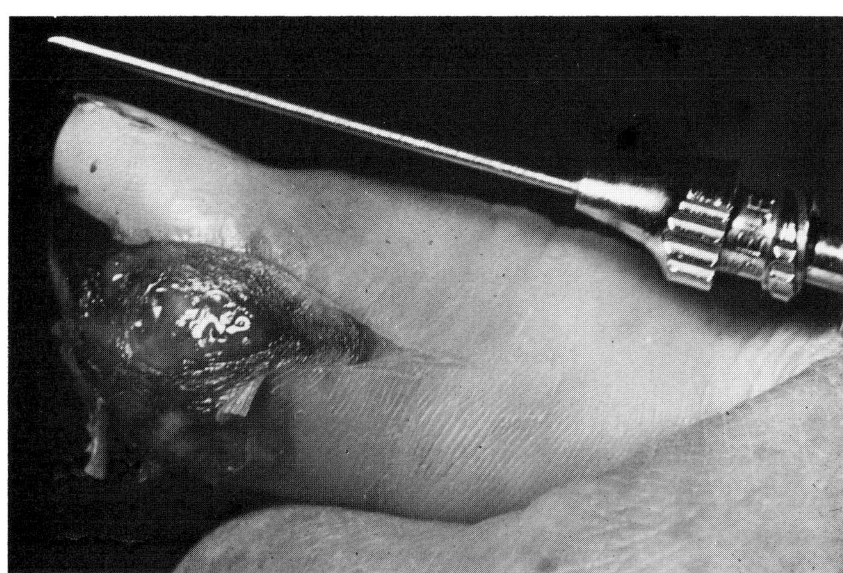

Fig. 43-18. **Felon. Fish mouth incision placed too anteriorly and injected with antibiotics.**

43-4C). Tenderness over the index, middle, and ring fingers will extend proximally only to the flexion crease in the palm. In the thumb and little fingers, however, where the infection can extend proximally into the radial or ulnar bursae, and even into the quadrilateral space deep to the tendons in the wrist, tenderness can extend along these pathways.

The main source of confusion in diagnosis is traumatic tenosynovitis, for which conservative treatment is indicated. In traumatic tenosynovitis, there is more gradual onset, no portal of entry, and a history of vigorous or traumatic use of the finger.

Treatment

Immediate drainage of the tendon sheath is mandatory (Fig. 43-4). The tendon and its blood supply are thereby released from the constricting force of its sheath. The blood supply to the tendon is poor, so that it is advisable to supplement the procedure with continuous or intermittent antibiotic irrigations of the tendon and its sheath (Fig. 43-4C). For this purpose, small plastic catheters can be threaded into the sheath or its adjacent tissue and tied in place for as long as necessary.[7] When the infection is in an advanced stage with thick pus present, most authorities agree that the tendon sheath should be laid open by a continuous midlateral incision from the distal to the proximal flexion crease of the finger. Another vertical incision should be made in the palm down to the proximal extremity of the sheath, avoiding the proximal flexion crease of the finger. In early cases of tenosynovitis, however, smaller incisions can be used—a midlateral incision over middle and proximal phalanges and a transverse incision in the palm over the distal flexion crease. By exposing the tendon sheath, pulley, and annular ligament through these incisions, the sheath can be opened with a knife through the annular ligament or pulley. The sheath can then be slit by using the slightly opened jaws of small scissors, the inner jaw of which acts as a guide within the sheath.

Complications

The most serious complication of bacterial tenosynovitis is necrosis of the tendon itself—destruction of the gliding surfaces of tendon and its sheath are early changes.

Extension into the deep spaces of the hands are a constant threat. Tenosynovitis of the thumb, index, and middle fingers can extend proximally into the thenar space. The tenosynovitis of the middle, ring, and little fingers can extend into the middle palmar space. Tenosynovitis of the thumb and little finger can extend into the quadrilateral space or space of Perona, which underlies the flexor tendons in the wrist. Incision of this latter space can best be made through a vertical medial incision directly down to the bony ulna in the wrist. A curved scissors can safely enter this space if it is pushed and spread with slight force over the anteromedial surface of the exposed bone (Fig. 43-20).

Infections of the Middle Palmar and Thenar Spaces

These spaces are separated by a septum running from the undersurface of the flexor tendons of the middle finger to its metacarpal bone.[2]

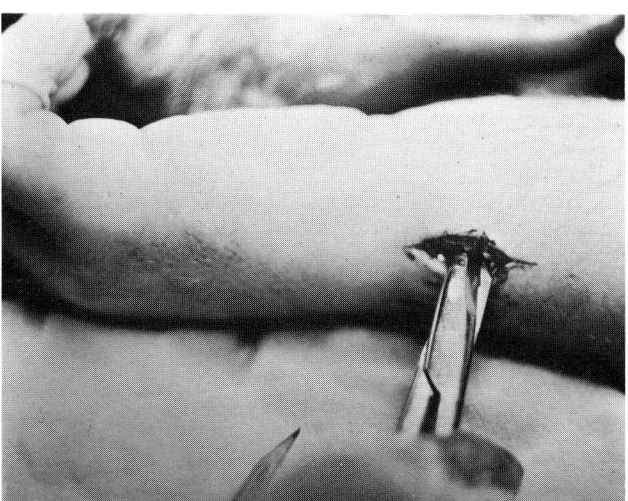

Fig. 43-20. **Abscess of the space of Perona (quadrilateral space). The incision is made down to bony ulna. Curved scissors can be slipped over the anterior aspect of bone and into space, avoiding the ulnar nerve. The bulge of the anterior wrist can be seen.**

Thenar Space Infections

Thenar space infection is more common and is easy to recognize by its associated tender, disabling swelling of the large web between thumb and index finger. The palmar portion of this web is involved before the dorsal aspect, which restricts adduction and opposition of the thumb. The proper incision for drainage of a thenar abscess is on the dorsum of the web, on a real or imaginary line from the proximal portion of the head of the second metacarpal to that of the first with the thumb fully extended (Fig. 43-21). When the space is entered, a hemostat can be pushed over the edge of the adductor muscle into the palm, and a transverse counterincision can be made over the nose of this instrument to establish through-and-through drainage (rubber drains only). Damage to the motor branch of the median nerve can be avoided by this maneuver.

Midpalmar Space Infection

The midpalmar space is best located by compression of the midpalm of the hand between thumb and middle finger of the other hand, thumb to palm and long finger to dorsum of hand. By pressing the fingertips into the interspace between the middle and ring fingers of the compressed palm, just proximal to its distal flexion crease, the midpalmar space can be located (Fig. 43-22). Infection of this space causes the natural concavity of the palm to be replaced by a tender bulge and is generally the result of infection in the third or fourth web spaces, overlying tenosynovitis, or penetrating injury of the underlying palm. A hockey-stick incision running transversely over the proximal palmar crease and curving over the vertical crease of the palm where the two creases intersect is the proper incision for drainage (Fig. 43-3A). After being carried through the palmar fascia, the direction of the incision should be vertical; the flexor tendons and intervening neurovascular bundles should be carefully identified if pus is not encountered before they are reached. Generally, pus will be encountered directly under the palmar fascia.

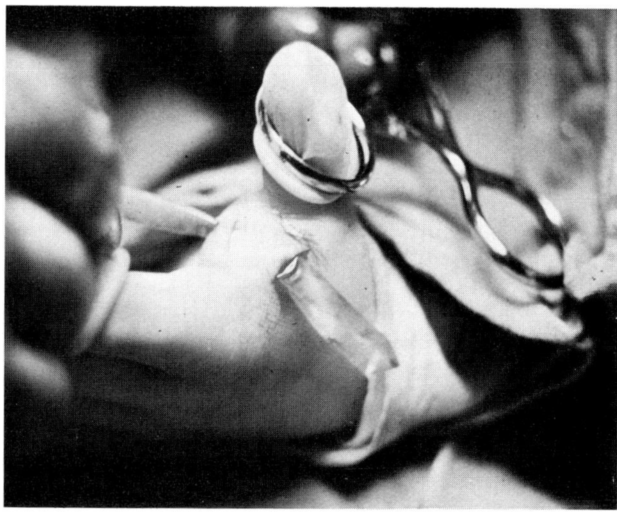

Fig. 43-21. **Thenar abscess. Incision is first made over dorsum of web in line between first and second metacarpal heads. Hemostat passed over edge of adductor muscle into palm. Counterincision made over nose of hemostat in palm, avoiding possible injury to motor nerve to thenar muscles.**

Web Space Infections

Web space infections arise most frequently from an abscess under a callus over an adjacent metacarpal head (collar button abscess). The fingers on either side of the web are characteristically held apart, and there is tenderness over the web both anteriorly and later posteriorly, with swelling extending over the entire dorsum of the hand (Figs. 43-23 and 43-24). If neglected, this infection can extend to the other two web spaces, rupture into the midpalmar space (medial two webs) or into the thenar space (web between the index and middle finger), extend into the adjacent flexor tendon sheath, and run up to the lumbrical canals, causing slough of the overlying tissues.

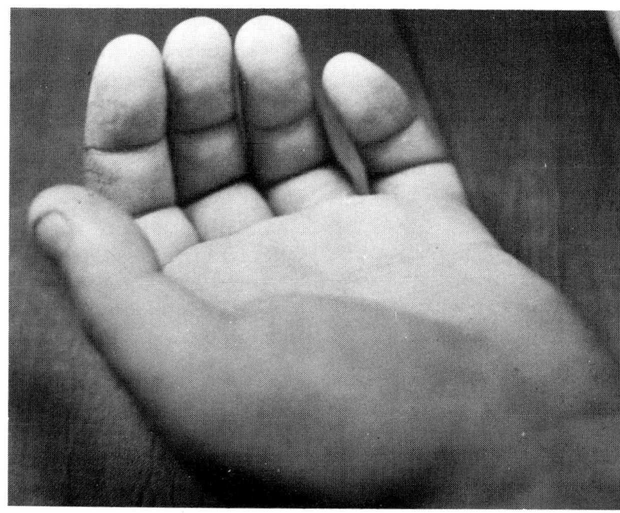

Fig. 43-23. **Web space infection is a common result of neglected collar button abscess or infection in distal palm. Involuntary separation of adjoining fingers with considerable swelling on the dorsum of the hand.**

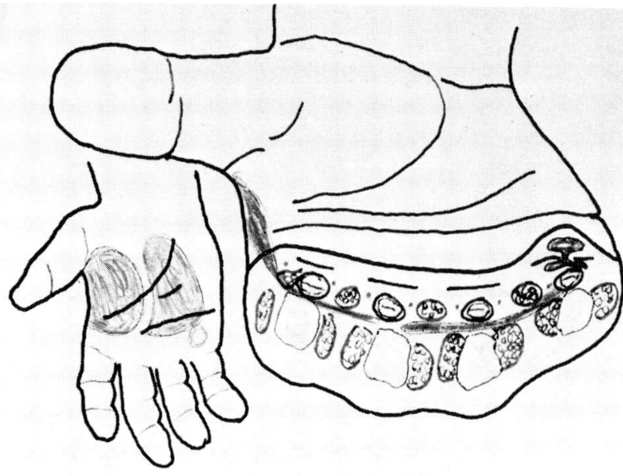

Fig. 43-22. **Thenar space, midpalmar space, and collar button abscess. Schematic presentation of configuration of collar button abscess, which most commonly occurs over metacarpal head #5, and rough outline of thenar and midpalmar spaces.**

For proper drainage, a through-and-through incision is made over the involved web, taking care not to incise the free edge of the web. A curving, semilunar incision is made in the distal palm, which follows what would be the line of the distal flexion crease of the palm if it extended to the base of the proximal phalanx. The incision is begun approximately 1 cm proximal to the edge of the web and gently curved medially to over the head of the next metacarpal. Care must be taken not to injure the underlying neurovascular bundle. After the space and the abscess have been reached, a hemostat can be passed through it to the dorsum of the web, where a vertical counterincision is made over its tip. A through-and-through rubber drain should be used.

Collar Button Abscess

A collar button abscess is common, frequently missed for some time, and frequently inadequately drained. These

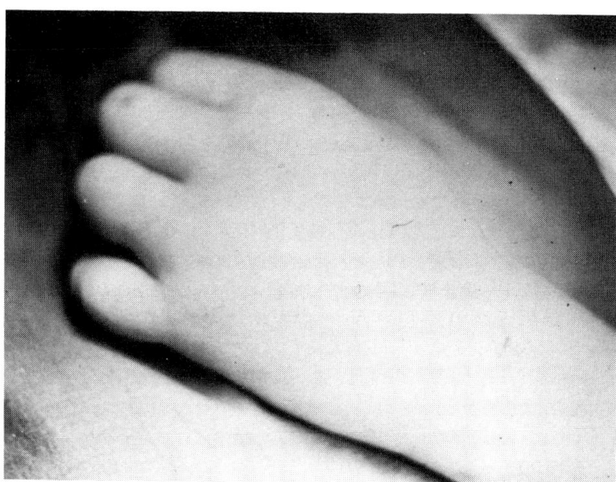

Fig. 43-24. **Web space infection, dorsal aspect.**

abscesses usually occur under a callus over a metacarpal head in the palms of people who do heavy work. The abscess cavity is shaped like a collar button, with one collection under the callus, which may hide it, and the other collection under the palmar fascia. The two collections are connected by a small opening in the intervening fascia (Fig. 43-22). If the superficial abscess is unroofed and evacuated in a bloodless field, pressure on the adjacent palm will generally cause pus from under the palmar fascia to well up through the connecting sinus, which can then be properly incised for adequate drainage.

Neglected collar button abscesses commonly enter the adjoining web space, but they can also rupture into the adjoining midpalmar or thenar spaces.

Dorsal Subaponeurotic Space Abscess

Abscess of this space is rare and is almost invariably the result of a penetrating wound. Swelling, tenderness, and occasionally fluctuations are present. The patient is reluctant to flex the metacarpophalangeal joints. Swelling over the back of the hand is common because of the lymphatic drainage to this area from an infected palm or finger. Sometimes, it is difficult to refrain from opening this space. Should drainage be performed, the lines of incision should run vertically rather than transversely.

Granuloma Pyogenicum

This raspberry-red protuberant tumor, generally on the finger, is associated with a history of protracted infection at the site. It is best treated by excision at its base, followed by electrodessication (Fig. 43-25). If the tumor is large (Fig. 43-26), a persistent bleeder in the base may require placement of a fine catgut suture for adequate control.

Furuncle and Carbuncle

Infections of the hair follicles can occur over the dorsum of the proximal phalanx. The follicles are aggravated by the frequent changes in tissue tension associated with flexion of the finger. It should be remembered that the carbuncle extends down to the fascia, so an incision should be carried down to this level. Splinting is mandatory for quick recovery (Chapter 25).

Human Bite

Human bite infections are usually the result of a misguided fist striking an opponent's front tooth, with resulting laceration of the dorsum of a metacarpophalangeal joint, generally the fourth or fifth. The history is frequently unreliable. The contaminating organisms are virulent and multiple, and a relatively small, innocuous-looking wound can hide a divided extensor tendon and a violated joint capsule. The wound should be cultured, debrided, drained, and splinted. Massive doses of penicillin should be administered.[8] A secondary, rather than primary, suture of a divided tendon is the safest procedure. Before the advent of antibiotics, infections in these wounds were among the most severe seen in the hand (Chapter 25).

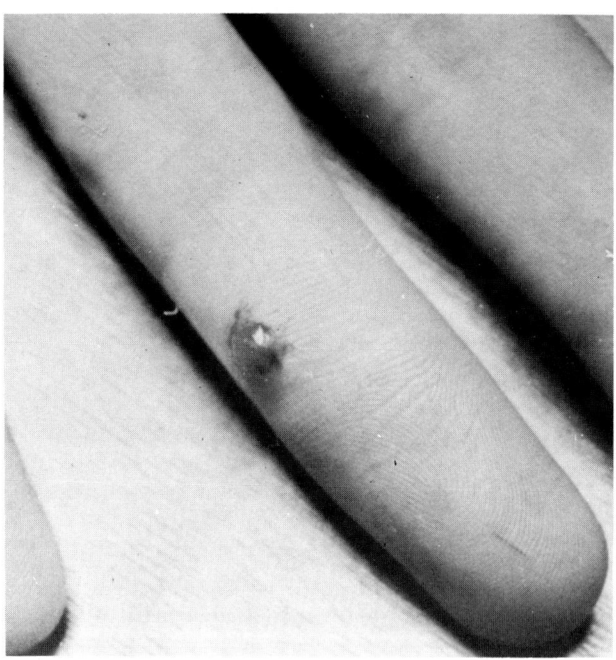

Fig. 43-25. **Granuloma pyogenicum (small).**

Cellulitis of the Hand

Occasionally, a hand will become beefy-red, with diffuse swelling but without an obvious source of infection. There can be a systemic reaction and lymphangitis. If an examination fails to demonstrate localized signs of infection, treatment should consist of bed rest, hot wet packs, elevation, and immobilization of the hand and arm. Roentgenograms should be taken to rule out the presence of foreign bodies or osteomyelitis. Systemic diseases such as gout should be considered. Antibiotics are frequently used, but resolution can take place without them in many cases.

POSTOPERATIVE INFECTIONS OF THE HAND

Postoperative infections of the hand after elective surgery are extremely rare. Low infection rates are the combined result of the generous blood supply to the hand, prophylactic antibiotics, and aseptic operative technique. The recent use of implants, such as artificial tendons, in reconstructive surgery has, however, been associated with a low but appreciable infection rate. If reconstructive or corrective surgery is planned following bacterial tenosynovitis, 6 weeks to 3 months should be allowed before the secondary operation is performed.

PREVENTION OF INFECTION AFTER TRAUMA

When an operation is indicated after injury, certain empirical rules must be followed to avoid complications. The type of wound and the duration of time between wounding and operation must be carefully considered.

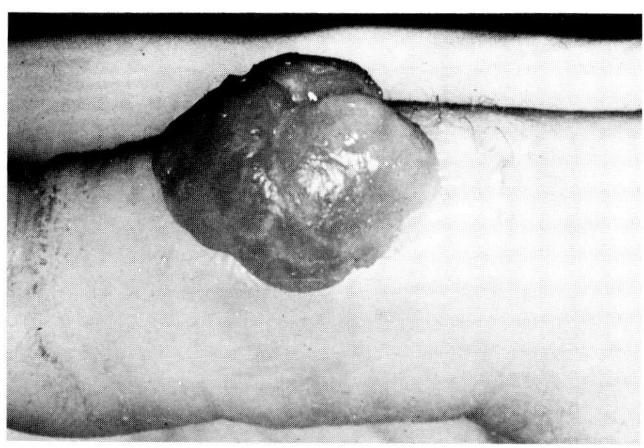

Fig. 43-26. **Granuloma pyogenicum (large). When a granuloma pyogenicum is shaved off at skin level (under local anesthesia), there is likely to be troublesome bleeding, which may require a suture or two in addition to the customary treatment of electrodessication. Generally, silver nitrate application is unsatisfactory in a lesion of this size.**

DIRTY WOUNDS

Extensive street wounds, wounds contaminated by feces, crushing wounds with extensive necrosis of tissue, and human bites are prone to infection. Fractures associated with severe crushing injuries (Fig. 43-27) should be aligned as well as possible with intramedullary or transversely running Kirschner wires. The wound should be debrided, extensively irrigated, and packed open with the use of antibiotics. Debridement in the hand should be extremely careful; better to leave a little dead tissue than to accidentally divide a vital neurovascular bundle. Smears should be made and cultures taken. The hand should generally be immobilized in a position of function. In all crushing injuries of the hand and fingers, traumatized arteries seemingly patent after wounding can thrombose up to 5 or more days later. Thrombosis results in delayed gangrene, which is better accepted by the patient if he or she has been forewarned of its possible occurrence.

OLD WOUNDS

If considerable time has elapsed between wounding and operation, particularly in the case of divided flexor tendons of the fingers, the "golden period" concept applies—after 6 hours have elapsed, bacterial growth within the wound increases rapidly. Therefore, flexor tenorrhaphy within a tendon sheath or primary repair of lacerated muscle bellies are contraindicated. Divided extensor tendons of the fingers, or of either flexor or extensor tendons within the wrist, can be repaired if the wound has been immediately treated properly.

REFERENCES

1. Kanavel AB: An anatomical, experimental, and clinical study of acute phlegmons of the hand. Surg Gynecol Obstet 1:221, 1905.
2. Flynn JE: Surgical significance of the middle palmar septum of the hand. Surgery 14:134, 1943.
3. Bell MS: The changing pattern of pyogenic infections of the hand. Hand 8:298, 1976.
4. Goldner JL: The hand. In Sabiston DC Jr (ed): Textbook of Surgery, 11th ed. Philadelphia, Saunders, 1977, p 1609.
5. Samuel EP: Transillumination of whitlows of terminal phalanx. Lancet 258(1):763, 1950.
6. Flynn JE: Modern considerations of major hand infections. N Engl J Med 252:605, 1955.
7. Flynn JE: Personal communication.
8. Farmer CB, Mann RJ: Human bite infections of the hand. South Med J 59:515, 1966.

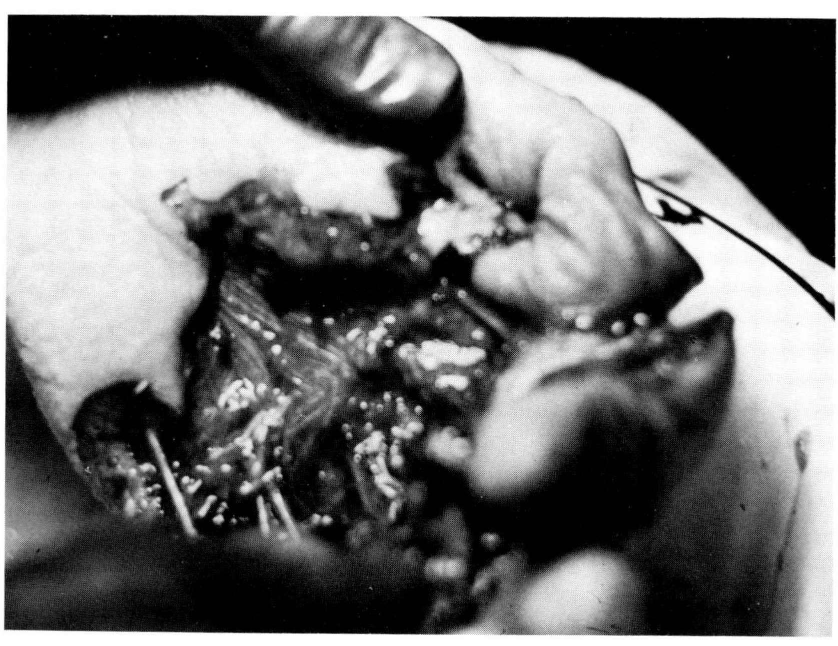

Fig. 43-27. **Severe crushing injury of a hand caught in the gears of a machine.**

CHAPTER 44
Infections of the Female Genital Tract

GORDON W. DOUGLAS AND RICHARD L. SIMMONS

Infections of the female genital tract have been the subject of renewed interest in the last decade, as new information on the microbiology of these infections has appeared and long-accepted concepts have been challenged and revised. The concept of a single microorganism producing a typical and predicted sequence of pathophysiologic events has been replaced by the recognition that many, if not most, serious upper tract infections are mixed infections caused by both aerobes and anaerobes.

These considerations have called for a reassessment of the surgical as well as the medical management of infection. Formerly, surgeons advocated prolonged preoperative palliative management in the hope of stabilizing infection, reducing technical difficulty, and minimizing complications. It is now clear that, when necessary, appropriate operations can be accomplished in an actively inflamed field and complications avoided with antibiotics. At one time, virtually all procedures for advanced pelvic infection resulted in a "pelvic cleanout." A more selective view is now taken, and it is often possible to salvage gonadal tissue.

Newer diagnostic techniques have also greatly improved management of pelvic infection. Pelvic sonography is a valuable means of assessing pelvic masses and can be repeated throughout management. Culdocentesis, long employed for the diagnosis of ruptured tubal pregnancy, is a valuable technique for the isolation of the pathogens responsible for pelvic infection.

THE VAGINAL FLORA AND CHOICE OF ANTIBIOTICS

The vagina should always be regarded as a contaminated surface. The normal vaginal flora are discussed in Chapter 3. Even after decontamination prior to vaginal hysterectomy, bacteria can be recovered from more than 95 percent of vaginal cultures. Most of the normal vaginal and endocervical bacteria are strict or facultative anaerobes.[1] Fecal organisms *(E. coli, Enterococcus, B. fragilis)* are commonly found. Although the menstrual cycle and pregnancy have some effect on the normal flora, the wide spectrum of flora remains essentially the same.[2-6] *Candida* species can be isolated from almost half of normal women.

The importance of the vagina as a portal of entry is therefore not restricted to sexually transmitted diseases, but is evident also whenever the upper genital tract is invaded, as in induced abortion, operative delivery, or the introduction of intrauterine devices. The vagina is also the source of contamination in all forms of pelvic operations, vaginal or abdominal, when the vagina is entered. Consequently, the organisms normally recovered from upper tract infections (eg, gonorrhea) are mixed. Even if a single pathogenic species initiates an infection, the normal mixed flora soon predominates.

The predominance of endogenous mixed aerobic and anaerobic flora in upper female genital tract infections is important in the selection of antibiotics. Monif[7] has devised a classification system in which each antibiotic is analyzed for its ability to cover the major bacteria involved in aerobic-anaerobic polymicrobial infection (the Gainsville Classification). Table 44-1 lists the four categories of bacteria that commonly compose the mixed flora in severe pelvic infections and some of the antibiotic combinations that have been used for treatment.[7] The gaps in certain combinations are noted. If infections fail to respond to certain combinations, an antibiotic can be selected to fill the gap in antimicrobial spectrum.

LOCAL HOST DEFENSES

The vagina itself is relatively resistant to invasive infection, and most vaginitis is superficial and caused by organisms not commonly found among the usual flora. Lacerations, however, make the soft tissue available for invasion.

The cervical canal contains deep clefts lined by mucus-secreting glandular epithelium. The secretion forms the mucus plug, which appears to seal off the canal effectively except at midmenstrual cycle, when the mucus becomes watery, or during menses, when the mucus may mix with defibrinated menstrual blood to form the clot described by some women. On the face of it, this does not seem to be an effective way of excluding microbes

TABLE 44-1. CRITICAL SPECTRUM IN UPPER GENITAL TRACT INFECTIONS (GAINESVILLE CLASSIFICATION)

Antibiotic	Gram-Positive Aerobes and Anaerobes*	Nonpenicillin-Sensitive Bacteroidaceae (Including B. fragilis)	Group D Streptococci (Enterococci)	Enterobacteriaceae†
Cephalosporin and gentamicin	+++	−	+ to ++	++++
Ampicillin and gentamicin	+++	−	++++	++++
Clindamycin and gentamicin	+++	+++ to ++++	+	++++
Ampicillin and clindamycin	+++	+++ to ++++	++++	++ to +++
Ampicillin and cefoxitin	+++	++ ½ to +++	+++	+++
Penicillin and doxycyline	++++	++ ½ to +++	++ to +++	++ to +++
Carbenicillin and gentamicin	+++	+++	+++ ½	++++
Carbenicillin	+++	++ ½ to +++	++ ½ to +++	+++
Penicillin, clindamycin, gentamicin	++++	+++ to ++++	+++ ½	++++

* As defined by their theoretical or demonstrated susceptibility to penicillin. Included are *Peptococcus, Peptostreptococcus,* penicillin-sensitive Bacteroidaceae, *Clostridium,* the majority of the *Fusobacterium,* etc.
† Included are *E. coli, K. pneumoniae, Enterobacter* species, indole-positive and indole-negative *Proteus* species.

Adapted from Monif GRG: *Ob/Gyn Infectious Diseases,* Gainesville, Infectious Disease Inc., 1979.

from the endometrial cavity, yet the fact is that normal midcycle endometrium is sterile and shows no trace of inflammatory reaction. Indeed, the endometrium is believed to be the site of only secondary inflammatory lesions, related to other processes.

When the endometrium has been traversed, however, the oviducts are prone to mucosal infection, and they lead directly to the pelvic peritoneal cavity. If the endometrium is disrupted, as after curettage or delivery, the myometrium itself can become infected. In pregnancy, the veins and lymphatics of the uterus are dilated, and infection within the uterine lumen can spread readily to the parametrial tissues to produce septic pelvic thrombophlebitis and septicemia.

THE FEMALE GENITAL TRACT AS A RESERVOIR FOR NEONATAL INFECTIONS

Surgeons seldom need to treat neonatal infections. All who deal with pregnant women, even occasionally, should be aware of the importance of the mother in the transmission of infections to the newborn. Table 44-2 lists diseases transmissible from mother to fetus and summarizes the methods of direction and prevention. The most feared infections are classified as TORCH (toxoplasmosis, other, rubella, cytomegalovirus, herpes) or STORCH (which includes syphilis)[9,10] syndrome. A few serious neonatal infections originate in the cervical or vaginal flora (gonorrhea, herpes simplex, cytomegalovirus, *Chlamydiae,* and most of the bacterial infections that cause neonatal septicemia, pneumonia, or meningitis). A detailed description of the important neonatal syndromes derived from the mother, their prevention, and treatment has been written by Charles.[8]

INFECTIONS OF THE LOWER FEMALE GENITAL TRACT

Many infections of the lower female genital tract can be classified among the sexually transmitted diseases—but many can also arise through different pathogenetic mechanisms. Thus, candidiasis, which can be transmitted by sexual intercourse, also occurs by other means of transmission or acquisition.

VULVOVAGINITIS

Monilial Vulvovaginitis (Candidiasis)

Etiology and Pathogenesis

C. albicans is a yeast that occurs in the mouth, vagina, or intestine of at least 50 percent of healthy individuals (Chapter 9). Proliferation in the region is enhanced by heat and moisture, and vulvovaginitis is more common in women who wear tight-fitting nylon clothing. Its growth is promoted by the use of broad-spectrum antibiotics (ie, for acne), which diminish competitive bacterial populations. *Candida* infections are more common in all situations associated with lowered resistance to infection—diabetes, steroid administration, chronic illness, cancer, malnutrition, overzealous dieting. *Candida* infections are also noted frequently in pregnancy (30 percent) and in women who take oral contraceptive pills.

Despite this multiplicity of predisposing conditions,

TABLE 44-2. NEONATAL INFECTIONS TRANSMITTED FROM MOTHER TO FETUS

Disease	Transmission to Fetus	Prevention in Neonate	Detection in Pregnancy	Management in Pregnancy
VIRAL				
Rubella	Intrauterine	Vaccination of all nonpregnant females	Prenatal antibody screening at time of registration. Positive antibody establishes immunity	Termination of pregnancy
Cytomegalovirus	Birth canal and intrauterine	None	Antibody surveillance for febrile illness	None available
Herpes simplex	Birth canal	If lesions are present at parturition, cesarean section	Clinical examination, viral isolation from lesions	None available
Influenza	Intrauterine	Suspected to cause birth defects but unproved in human beings.		
Coxsackie A	Intrauterine			
Coxsackie B	Intrauterine			
Echovirus	Intrauterine			
Hepatitis A	Intrauterine			
Hepatitis B	Intrauterine			
Lymphocytic choriomeningitis	Intrauterine			
Mumps	Intrauterine			
Rubeola	Intrauterine			
Poliomyelitis	Intrauterine			
BACTERIAL				
Syphilis	Intrauterine prior to 16th week of gestation	Treatment of pregnant patient with disease	Serologic screening and follow-up	24 million units penicillin G weekly for 3 wks
Gonorrhea	Birth canal	Treatment of pregnant patient with disease. Treatment of offspring of infected mother	Prenatal cervical cultures—screen at registration and 32–36 weeks	See Table 44-7
Chlamydial conjunctivitis and ophthalmia	Birth canal	Treatment of cervicitis in mother	Prenatal cervical cultures	Erythromycin
Group B streptococcus sepsis	Birth canal	None currently recommended	Normal flora in vagina	None
Haemophilus influenzae	Birth canal	None currently recommended	Occasionally in vaginal flora	None
Listeria monocytogenes	Birth canal	None currently recommended	Occasionally in vaginal flora	None
Salmonella typhi	Birth canal	None currently recommended	Occasionally in vaginal flora	None
Group A streptococcus	Birth canal	None currently recommended	Occasionally in vaginal flora	None
Vibrio fetus	Birth canal	None currently recommended	Occasionally in vaginal flora	None
Mycoplasma hominis	Birth canal	None currently recommended	Occasionally in vaginal flora	None
Ureaplasma urealyticum	Birth canal	None currently recommended	Occasionally in vaginal flora	None
PARASITIC				
Toxoplasma gondii	Intrauterine	Prenatal antibody screening for maternal infection. If mother positive, demonstrate specific IgM antibodies in neonatal serum. Screen again if febrile illness or lymphadenopathy occurs	Screen for antibody at registration	Pyrimethamine-sulfadiazine in first trimester. No treatment required in last two trimesters. Do not use sulfamanide last month of pregnancy

From Charles D[8] and Monif GRG[9]

little is known about the susceptibility of some individuals to candidiasis and the frequency of recurrence after apparently adequate treatment. Many clinicians have noted the difficulty of achieving cure by conventional methods in patients who are under chronic or recurrent emotional stress.

Clinical Manifestations

Vulvovaginal candidiasis is unusual in the prepubertal girl or the postmenopausal women, but is frequent in the menstruating or pregnant woman. The uniform complaint is of severe itching, usually associated with a scant discharge, which is not copious but thick and cottage cheese–like. Examination reveals varying degrees of erythema, edema, and excoriation. Most typical is a beefy-red, dry vagina with adherent patches of exudate.

Diagnosis

Since *Candida* is part of the normal vaginal flora, cultural isolation without the typical clinical signs is inconclusive evidence. Direct culture from swabs reveals typical brown-black cultures in 48 to 72 hours. An immediate presumptive diagnosis may be made by the identification of mycelia and budding cells in wet saline smear, or by addition of 10 percent KOH for identification of mycelia and budding cells. This is substantially less sensitive than cultures, and negative results do not exclude a candidal etiology. A Gram stain smear, however, will often demonstrate the organism. Simultaneous infection with other organisms should be considered in all cases.

Treatment

The treatment of choice for candidiasis is topical nystatin, administered in the form of vaginal suppositories of 100,000 units twice daily for 2 weeks. Nystatin cream is available for control of vulvar lesions. Clotrimazole or miconazole suppositories are equally effective and should be used nightly for at least 1 week. Any treatment should be continued without interruption through any intervening menstrual period. Male sex partners, if symptomatic, should be treated with nystatin or micronazole cream twice daily for 1 to 2 weeks. Recurrent *Candida* vulvovaginitis is common. Attempts should be made to remove presumptive predisposing conditions—avoid hot tight clothing, stop the use of antibiotics, change oral contraceptive regimens, rule out diabetes mellitus, and check for *Candida* balanitis in sex partners. Oral nystatin may be useful in eliminating a fecal reservoir.[11,12] Ketoconazole may be useful in resistant cases (Chapter 18).

Trichomoniasis

Etiology and Pathogenesis

T. vaginalis is a flagellate protozoan for which the human is the only known host. It is found in the vaginas of 12 to 15 percent of females, many of whom are asymptomatic. The organism seems to require glycogen-derived glucose, and a pH of 5.5 to 7.5 for growth; hence its predilection for younger women in their menstruating years. It usually infests the vagina, and may also be found in the endocervix, Bartholin and Skene glands, and in the bladder. Upper tract disease is rare. In men, trichomonas colonizes the lower urethra, but may also colonize the prostate, epididymis, and seminal vesicles. It is almost always spread by sexual transmission and produces a vaginitis with secondary vulvar irritation.

Clinical Manifestations

Women symptomatically infected with trichomonads uniformly complain of a vaginal discharge, usually watery, which may lead to vulvar irritation as well. Pruritus is a variable symptom, but often occurs. The discharge is typically gray or greenish, frothy, copious, and malodorous. Associated symptoms include dysuria, dyspareunia, and lower abdominal discomfort.

Diagnosis

The diagnosis is most readily made by immediate microscopic examination of a drop of vaginal secretions, diluted with saline. Prompt examination easily reveals the movement of trichomonads propelled by their whipping flagella. The diagnosis can also be made by culture in special media (Feinberg) or on Papanicolaou smear.

Treatment

Metronidazole is the treatment of choice. Treatment may consist of 250 mg given orally three times daily for 1 week, or 2 gm orally given once.[13] Abstinence from alcohol should be recommended during treatment. Simultaneous treatment of sexual partners is recommended to prevent reinfection. A second course of treatment is necessary in 10 percent of cases. No comparably effective treatment with vaginal medication is available.[14]

Hemophilus Vaginalis Vulvovaginitis

Etiology and Pathogenesis

Gardnerella vaginalis (H. vaginalis) can be isolated in nearly 15 percent of women of child-bearing age and may be the cause of what was formerly called nonspecific vaginitis.[15] There is growing evidence, however, to suggest that an anaerobe *(Bacteroides, Peptococcus)* may participate in the pathogenesis.[16,17]

Clinical Manifestations

Vaginitis due to this cause is often less dramatic, and 10 to 40 percent of women harboring this organism are asymptomatic. When symptoms occur, they typically consist of greyish-green watery discharge and mild itching. The vagina may appear to be only mildly irritated, and the discharge is not profuse. The pH of the vagina is usually 5 to 5.5, and there is no relationship to the menstrual cycle.

Diagnosis

A wet smear in these cases reveals the "clue cell," an epithelial cell with stippled appearance. A Gram stained smear is more dramatic evidence of the same phenomenon, a cornified cell studded with gram-negative pleomorphic coccobacilli.[11]

Treatment

The recommended treatment has long been 500 mg of ampicillin 4 times daily for 7 to 10 days. Metronidazole,

TABLE 44-3. CLINICAL AND LABORATORY FINDINGS IN SEXUALLY TRANSMITTED VAGINITIS

Category	Trichomoniasis	Candidiasis	*H. vaginalis* Vaginitis
Symptoms	Discharge: malodorous, thin to frothy, onset during or immediately after menstruation; pruritis; dysuria; dyspareunia	Intense pruritus; discharge: scanty, odorous; dysuria (rare); dyspareunia (occasionally)	Discharge: small amount, onset unrelated to menses; mild pruritus; dyspareunia (rare)
Clinical findings	Vulva: irritated, erythematous, edematous, excoriated; discharge: thin, frothy, malodorous; red-speckled ("strawberry") cervix and vagina; lower abdominal tenderness (rare)	Vulva: irritated, erythematous, edematous, excoriated; discharge: thick, white, curdy, adherent, or thin and watery; satellite lesions on external genitalia	Vulva: slightly irritated; discharge: homogenous in consistency ("flour paste"), thin, gray-white, adherent
pH range	5.5 to 6.5	4 to 5	5 to 5.5
Laboratory diagnosis, wet mount	Motile trichomonads	Hyphae, yeast cells	Granular, cornified, epithelial cells ("clue cells")
Gram stain (or other)	Trichomonads may be seen in Papanicolaou smear	Gram-positive budding yeast cells and hyphae	Epithelial cells studded with gram-negative pleomorphic coccobacilli
Culture	Feinberg medium	Sabouraud medium	Peptone-starch-dextrose medium

500 mg, twice daily for 7 days is more effective.[15] Treatment of the sexual partner is essential to prevent reinfection.[14]

DIFFERENTIAL DIAGNOSIS OF VULVOVAGINITIS

A summary of the clinical and laboratory findings of vulvovaginitis is included in Table 44-3.

Sometimes, the specific etiologic agent includes none of these agents. Vaginal infections with tuberculosis, *Salmonella,* enteric gram-negative bacteria, *Staphylococcus,* and *Actinomyocetes* are rare and are almost always associated with preexisting local or severely debilitating disease. Rapidly progressive fusospirochetal infections of preexisting lesions are sometimes found and respond to metronidazole.[18] Pinworms are an occasional cause of pruritis in children. Foreign bodies left in the vagina (tampon, diaphragm, condom) can be associated with foul discharge.

Noninfectious leukorrhea can be caused by genital neoplasms, atrophic vaginitis, allergic vulvitis, and normal responses to contraceptive medications.

INFECTIONS OF THE VULVA

Any disease of the soft tissues (Chapter 25) may affect the vulva. A list of the more commonly encountered infective vulvar lesions is presented in Table 44-4.[19,20]

Herpes Simplex Genitalis

Etiology

Herpes simplex virus infections of the female genital tract most commonly involve the cervix, but are far more painful when they infect the vagina and vulva. The etiologic agent is discussed in Chapter 10. In the genital area, HSV-2 infections are more common, although about 30 percent of patients under 25 years of age with HSV-1 infections will have associated genital lesions. Herpesvirus infections become latent after the primary infection, and during the latent period the HSV-2 virus appears to reside within the neurones of the sacral ganglia. Herpesvirus infections are transmitted by direct contact, and genital herpes is a sexually transmitted disease most commonly seen in the 15 to 30-year age group.

TABLE 44-4. COMMON INFECTIVE LESIONS OF THE EXTERNAL FEMALE GENITALIA

Ulcers
- Herpes genitalis
- Syphilis
- Chancroid
- Lymphogranuloma venereum
- Tularemia
- Donovanosis

Papules
- Venereal warts
- Scabies
- Molluscum contagiosum
- Syphilis
- Candidiasis

Vesicles
- H. genitalis

Crusts
- Scabies
- H. genitalis

Miscellaneous lesions
- Nits: crabs
- Hypertrophic: donovanosis
- Diffuse inflammation: Candidiasis
- Linear tracks: scabies

Modified from Rein MF: Skin and mucous membrane lesions. In Mandell GL, Douglas, RG Jr, Bennett JE (eds): *Principles and Practice of Infectious Diseases.* New York, Wiley, 1979, p 996.

Clinical Manifestations

The incubation period of primary HSV infection ranges from 2 to 12 days, but the clinical picture often represents reactivation of an earlier infection. A small cluster of vesicles appears, which ruptures early and becomes secondarily infected. The resulting shallow ulcers are painful out of proportion to their size and location, and regress slowly. Secondary infection is the rule, and inguinal adenopathy may occur. The lesions may involve any of the vulvar skin surfaces or the vagina, but are less symptomatic in the cervix.

Diagnosis

The diagnosis of genital herpes is usually clinical, because of the typical picture and painful nature of the lesion and the history of recurrence at the same site. Papanicolaou smears may show intranuclear inclusions, and typical multinucleate giant cells can be demonstrated on smears with Giemsa and Wright stains. The virus can also be cultured and antibody determinations done. These must be interpreted in the light of the fact that prior infection to herpesvirus may have occurred, and a reactivated lesion may appear without simultaneous rise in antibody titer.

Treatment

No completely safe or effective treatment is presently available, although much work on this problem continues. Therapeutic trials have been conducted using photodynamic dyes, smallpox vaccination, immune globulin, chloroform, ether, alcohol, deoxyuridine, and adenine arabinoside. Although many of these agents are lethal to the virus in vitro, none have been safe and effective in clinical use. At present, treatment is directed largely toward the secondary bacterial infection of herpetic ulcers, utilizing povidone-iodine or broad-spectrum antibiotics. The use of a condom or abstinence from sexual activity is strongly recommended when active lesions are present. The problem of herpesvirus infections in pregnancy is described in Table 44-2.

Vulvar Furunculosis

Vulvar furunculosis occurs when infections of the vulvar hair follicles spread and coalesce to create cellulitis, with resultant suppuration. The etiologic agent is nearly always *S. aureus.* The condition usually responds well to hot soaks, antibiotics, and appropriate incision and drainage (Chapter 25). In some patients, the condition tends to be chronic, with recurrences over a period of years. In such cases, an unusual etiology (foreign body, tuberculosis) or fistulous tracts should be suspected. Excision of the affected area, when feasible, may provide the only permanent relief.

Condyloma Acuminatum

Etiology and Pathogenesis

Condylomata acuminata are warts caused by the DNA virus called the papillomavirus (Chapters 10 and 25). Although the virus has not been cultured, its appearance on electron microscopy closely resembles the viruses of cutaneous and plantar warts.

Condylomata acuminata, or genital warts, are transmitted by sexual contact, and are rarely seen in children or the elderly. Following contact, the incubation period may range from 6 weeks to 8 months. Because the lesions are occasionally confused with condylomata lata, the lesion of secondary syphilis, it is strongly recommended that all cases have serologic tests for syphilis.

Clinical Manifestations

The typical lesions of condylomata acuminata are multiple, discrete, well-differentiated papillary growths, which may coalesce to form cauliflowerlike masses in the vulvar area, inner thighs, perineum, or perianal area. They are also seen in the vagina and on the cervix.

Growth of genital warts is often unpredictable. They tend to grow more rapidly during pregnancy and under moist conditions such as those created by severe leukorrhea. In some cases, they remain stationary for prolonged periods, and may even disappear. In pregnancy, the condylomatous mass can grow to block the introitus and necessitate cesarean section for delivery.

Diagnosis

The diagnosis is usually strongly suspected from the appearance of lesions on inspection, but it is important to differentiate condylomata acuminata from condylomata lata of syphilis, from granuloma inguinale, and from benign and malignant neoplasms. This requires serologic testing, a crushed tissue smear for Donovan bodies, and adequate biopsy. The biopsy is conclusive and reveals papillomatous folds of highly keratinized epithelium, with deep rete pegs, in an arborescent structure.

Treatment

The usual treatment consists of the application of a 25 percent solution of podophyllin in tincture of benzoin, applied carefully to the surface of the wart and allowed to dry. The patient is instructed to bathe 4 to 6 hours later, and the treatment is repeated once or twice weekly. Usually, several weeks are required. Podophyllin is teratogenic and is quite toxic if absorbed in any substantial quantity. Consequently, it is not recommended for use during pregnancy or for large or hemorrhagic lesions.

A number of modalities have been employed for destructive therapy. These include cryotherapy, which is effective with larger lesions. Unless stimulated by pregnancy, venereal warts tend to regress spontaneously.[14,20]

Syphilis

The etiology, pathogenesis, and systemic clinical manifestations of syphilis are discussed in Chapters 7, 25, and 45. In women, the lesions of early syphilis may escape discovery unless they involve the vulvar skin, and even then may not be noticed because they are relatively painless and tend to heal spontaneously. Consequently, successful detection requires that apparently innocuous sores in the vulvar or genital area be regarded with suspicion. The primary chancre is a genital sore, which develops 10 to 90 days (average, 21 days) after coitus. It may appear as an indurated, painless papule, or as a shallow ulcer with raised borders. It is usually single, and may be found on the surfaces of the labia, vagina, and cervix. The lesion heals spontaneously within 1 to 4 weeks.

Secondary syphilis develops 2 weeks to 6 months after the untreated primary infection has disappeared. This is a bilateral, symmetrical papulosquamous eruption with generalized distribution. On the vulva, secondary syphilis may appear as multiple raised but flat lesions of the cutaneous surface (condyloma latum), sometimes confused with condylomata acuminata. The lesions on mucous membranes have a gray surface and are known as mucous patches. Spontaneous healing of secondary syphilis skin lesions occurs in 2 to 6 weeks. If the disease is still untreated, one-third of patients develop tertiary syphilis.

Diagnosis

The diagnosis may be made by demonstration of *T. pallidum* on dark-field examination of material from fresh, untreated lesions. However, because this may not be available, diagnosis is often established by the serologic tests discussed in Chapter 7. These results become positive 1 to 4 weeks after the primary lesion become positive, when the secondary lesions are visible.

Treatment

Current recommendations for treatment of primary or secondary syphilis include, principally, benzathine penicillin G, 2.4 million units intramuscularly as a single injection. An alternative is aqueous penicillin G procaine, 600,000 units intramuscularly daily for 8 days (total dose, 4.8 million units). When a penicillin allergy is present, tetracycline 500 mg four times a day for 15 days, taken 1 hour before or 2 hours after meals, is recommended. Another alternative is erythromycin, 500 mg four times daily for 15 days. When syphilis is treated, serologic testing for a baseline value and then every 3 months for 1 year is advisable to detect any need for retreatment.[14]

Chancroid

Among the venereal lesions of the vulva, one of the more painful is chancroid, which is characteristically manifest as a painful, tender, shallow ulcer in the vulvar area, often at the fourchette. It is caused by a gram-negative bacillus, *H. ducreyi*, and is spread by sexual contact (Chapter 7).

The typical early lesion of chancroid is a ragged, saucer-shaped ulcer, which may occur on the vulvar skin, in the vagina, or on the cervix. It appears after an incubation period of 3 to 5 days, and is accompanied by a foul purulent discharge. The lesion is surrounded by cellular induration and is quite tender. Most cases develop a painful inguinal adenitis, which progresses to necrosis and spontaneous drainage if untreated. The lesion must be distinguished from syphilis, herpes, lymphogranuloma venereum, and granuloma inguinale.

Chancroid usually responds well to sulfisoxazole, 1 gm four times daily for 10 days, combined with vigorous local hygiene. Tetracycline, 500 mg four times daily for 10 to 14 days, may also be employed.[20,14]

Granuloma Inguinale

Granuloma inguinale is caused by *Calymmatobacterium granulomatis*, an organism that is encapsulated in mononuclear leukocytes and referred to in that form as the Donovan body (Chapter 7). It is a chronic, ulcerative disease process of the vulva and inguinal regions which produces extensive tissue destruction and scarring in advanced cases. Although rare, this vulvar disease remains an important clinical entity because it may coexist with vulvar carcinoma and because relapse after treatment occurs in at least 10 percent of patients.

The typical form of granuloma inguinale is one of an exuberant, hypertrophic granulating tissue growth coupled with scarring edema and tissue distortion. Secondary infection is the rule, so that the ulceration is associated with a malodorous discharge. Early lesions begin as papules, progressing to ulceration. These lesions develop a base of beefy-red granulation tissue with little tendency to heal. Lymphadenitis is not a prominent feature, unless node-bearing areas are directly involved.

The diagnosis is accomplished by a crushed tissue smear directly from an ulcerated area, and stained with Wright stain. This will reveal cytoplasmic inclusion of rod-shaped Donovan bodies in mononuclear leukocytes.

Tetracycline, 500 mg four times daily for 2 to 3 weeks, is the most effective treatment. Erythromycin in similar dosage, for a similar period, has been effective. Streptomycin is reported to be effective in high, nearly toxic, dosage (1 gm intramuscularly two to three times daily for a total of 21 gm).

As previously noted, the need to exclude vulvar carcinoma makes multiple biopsy samples mandatory in these cases. Moreover, in chronic cases the degree of tissue distortion may indicate a need for vulvectomy, following treatment with antimicrobials.[20,21]

Lymphogranuloma Venereum (LGV)

The recent discovery that lymphogranuloma venereum (LGV) and nongonococcal arthritis are caused by different serotypes of the same organism, *C. trachomatis*, has aroused new interest in LGV. The fact that this disease is not easily confirmed by readily available laboratory tests, and the low reported incidence (28 cases in New York City in 1977), suggest that the prevalence may be greater than is usually supposed.

LGV is a systemic, sexually transmitted disease, and of the 15 separate serotypes of *C. trachomatis*, three (L1, L2, L3) are known to cause LGV.[22] The disease is more common in the tropics than in temperate zones, and is more frequently reported in men than in women (Chapter 7).

The primary lesion of LGV develops at the site of contact with the infectious lesion of another individual, and is a painless vesicle or papule, which progresses to a small superficial ulcer. The lesions develops within 7 to 12 days after exposure in most cases, and heals rapidly. Like the primary lesion of syphilis, it may go untreated in women.

One to 4 weeks later, the secondary stage of the disease develops, which is usually the stage at which a diagnosis is made. When the primary lesion is on the anterior portion of the vulva, involving the upper labia or clitoris, ipsilateral inguinal adenopathy develops. The nodes, at first indurated and discrete, become matted together, suppurate, and drain with the persistent sinus tracts. Ulceration of tissues in the region of the labia and clitoris may persist. However, vulvar lesions of the posterior vulva or perianal area may drain to deeper nodes, skipping the inguinal and femoral chains entirely.

The tertiary stage of disease represents further progressive change of untreated secondary disease, with deep destructive ulcers, scar formation, elephantiasis, and lobular distortion of tissues. Enteric LGV also occurs to include the rectum and sigmoid, with production of annular strictures.[23]

The diagnosis is usually strongly suggested by the clinical appearance of the vulvar lesion, but other sexually transmitted diseases must be included in the differential diagnosis. The serodiagnosis is discussed in Chapter 7. Cultural isolation of the organism requires special techniques.

The Frei test, a skin test that uses antigen prepared from *C. trachomatis*, was in use until 1975 but has been abandoned because of numerous false-positive and false-negative results. A complement-fixation test to LGV is available, which also becomes positive with other chlamydial infections, but a titer of 1:64 or above strongly suggests LGV infection. Isolation of the organism by culture is not generally available as a diagnostic procedure.

For primary or secondary LGV, the treatment of choice is tetracycline, 500 mg four times daily for 3 weeks. Sulfisoxazole, 4 gm initially followed by 1 gm four times daily for 3 weeks, is also acceptable.

Surgical treatment should be conservative and undertaken in the knowledge that lymphatic obstruction is already present and may be aggravated by any operative procedure.[23]

Bartholinitis

The Bartholin gland is located on each side of the vagina near the base of the labia minora. It is drained by a 2-cm duct, which opens up at the junction of the posterior and middle thirds of each labia. Ductal obstruction can lead to a sterile cyst or infection of the blocked duct can result in a Bartholin gland abscess.

Etiology

Bartholin abscesses were once thought to be caused exclusively by the gonococci. In fact, gonococci can be recovered from a small minority of patients with Bartholin gland abscess,[24] and most patients from whom gonococci can be recovered are asymptomatic. Like most infections of the female genital tract, mixed infections of Bartholin glands are found, ie, *E. coli, P. mirabilis,* and multiple species of anaerobes including *Bacteroides* species are usually recovered.[10,24]

When the gland is palpable, gentle attempts to milk it and recover material for Gram stain and culture should be attempted. Sometimes, these lesions are too tender. When cellulitis and induration are present, hot soaks and oral antibiotics should be tried. Tetracyclines are frequently recommended, but ampicillin or amoxacillin, 500 mg orally four times daily, may be the best initial choice. Failure to respond or the development of an abscess pointing into the vulva requires simple drainage of the abscess. Excision of the gland is indicated when it is durated and chronically inflamed. Cyst formation is best treated by marsupialization of the cyst.

When gonorrhea is present, the usual treatment of gonorrhea (see below) is recommended.[11]

Skenitis

Skene glands empty into the urethra. Inflammation usually produces dysuria, and sometimes pus can be expressed. The gonococci produce some cases of skenitis, but the role of other pathogens has not been systematically studied.[11]

CERVICITIS

Cervicitis is a poorly defined clinical syndrome manifested by an increased amount of cervical discharge, which may be mucoid or purulent. The area immediately surrounding the cervical os may be intensely erythematous and may reveal ulcerations or frank necrosis. These findings may be present without accompanying vaginitis. The bacteria usually present in the endocervix mirror the normal vaginal flora.[2] Consequently, the etiologic diagnosis and even the presence of acute cervicitis cannot always be ascertained.

Acute Gonococcal Cervicitis

Gonococci are most frequently isolated from the endocervix in women with uncomplicated gonococcal infections. In the typical case, the cervical os is reddened and produces a purulent discharge.[25] Gram stain reveals typical gram-negative cell-associated diplococci in about half the women. For this reason, the negative results cannot rule out the diagnosis of gonorrhea and cultures must be taken. The endocervical culture is thought to be diagnostic in 90 percent of cases. Uncomplicated gonococcal cervicitis is asymptomatic in about two-thirds of women.[11]

Chlamydia Trachomatis Cervicitis

Sexual partners of men with chlamydial urethritis frequently develop *C. trachomatis* cervicitis. Most women are asymptomatic, and the cervix usually appears normal although vaginal discharge may be noted. The common association of chlamydia with gonococci makes the definition of a typical clinical picture impossible.[11,14] If chlamydial infection is present, tetracycline 500 mg by mouth four times per day for 10 days is curative. This regimen also cures gonococcal cervicitis.

Herpes Simplex Cervicitis

Herpetic cervicitis may be asymptomatic and have no clinical findings. On the other hand, it may progress to a severe necrotizing disease often associated with a clear vaginal discharge.[26] Herpetic cervicitis is the most important reservoir of the infection and may or may not be associated with lesions of the external genitalia. The diagnosis is made by observing multinucleatide giant cells with intranuclear inclusions in cervical smears. Cultural isolation of the virus may be essential, however, in necrotic cervicitis.[27]

Herpes cervicitis is important because of the possible transmission of the virus to the neonate during vaginal delivery.[28] Patients with active herpetic lesions at term should probably be delivered by cesarean section unless the fetal membranes have ruptured prematurely. Specific therapy is not currently available.

Herpetic cervicitis has also been linked to cancer of the cervix. The evidence is mostly circumstantial and relates to the high incidence of cancer in sexually active women, the fact that other herpes viruses are oncogenic, and that virus can occasionally be isolated from carcinoma of the cervix. Proof is as yet lacking.[11,29]

Other Causes of Cervicitis

Adenoviruses, type C viruses, mycoplasm, and *Enterobius vermicularis* have all been implicated as unusual causes of cervicitis.[11] Cervicitis should be treated with agents specific for the organism isolated.

PELVIC INFLAMMATORY DISEASE AND ITS COMPLICATIONS

ACUTE PELVIC INFLAMMATORY DISEASE

The term pelvic inflammatory disease (PID) refers to infections of the endometrium and the fallopian tubes with extension to the parametrial tissues and the pelvic peritoneum of the pelvis. Since community-acquired pelvic inflammatory disease differs so much in etiology and pathogenesis from similar diseases associated with pregnancy and parturition, the diseases will be discussed separately. Acute pelvic inflammatory disease is generally thought to be initiated in most cases by gonococci but can be caused by other organisms alone or as secondary invaders in combination with gonococci. Its importance rests not only with the acute infection itself but also with the residual damage to the tubes, which causes infertility.

Incidence and Epidemiology

Gonococcal pelvic inflammatory disease is the most serious gynecologic infectious disease. An estimate of more than 2,500,000 new cases of gonorrhea was made in the year ending June, 1973.[30] In 1974 Monif estimated that only 10 to 30 percent of the cases are actually reported and that approximately 65 million new cases occur worldwide each year.[10]

Gonorrhea is spread almost solely by sexual intercourse, because the organism requires implantation directly onto the susceptible mucosal surfaces—urethra, periurethral glands, and cervix. Its rising incidence is directly related to increased sexual activity of young adults and the relative decline in the use of condoms for contraception. Several additional factors encourage its spread: (1) therapy is frequently incomplete, (2) follow-up is often inadequate, (3) immunity is absent, (4) females are so often asymptomatic that they provide a community reservoir, and (5) the increasing resistance of the organism to penicillin is an important epidemiologic factor.[31]

Many, but not all, investigators report a higher incidence of pelvic inflammatory disease in patients who wear an intrauterine contraceptive device. The risk is relatively higher for nongonococcal pelvic inflammatory disease than for gonococcal disease.[31]

Etiology

N. gonorrhoeae has long been thought to be the major cause of acute pelvic inflammatory disease. It can be isolated from the cervix in approximately 60 percent of cases of acute pelvic inflammatory disease that present without preexisting pregnancy or operation. The growth characteristics and pathogenic characteristics of *N. gonorrhoeae* are discussed in Chapter 4.

Recent evidence suggest that the gonococcus is not alone in producing all the changes seen in this illness.[32,33] Chow et al [32] were the first to study the bacteriology of acute pelvic inflammatory disease by simultaneous cul-de-sac, cervical, and blood cultures with aerobic and fastidious anaerobic techniques. Cul-de-sac cultures were positive in almost all patients with pelvic inflammatory disease. Anaerobic bacteria were the most common isolates, and *N. gonorrhoeae* was rarely isolated from the cul-de-sac despite its presence in almost two-thirds of cervical specimens. There was poor correlation between the cul-de-sac and cervical culture results. Subsequent data obtained by others [34] (Table 44-5) confirmed these findings. Whereas two-thirds of cervical cultures reveal gonococci, only about one-third of cul-de-sac cultures do. Of the patients with positive gonococcal cervical cultures, two-thirds have positive cul-de-sac cultures, but half of these revealed mixed organisms. One third of cervical and cul-de-sac cultures reveal no gonococci at all. The data suggest that the gonococcus may be important in initiating acute pelvic inflammatory disease but that its primary function may be to facilitate secondary invaders from the normal vaginal flora to gain access to the upper genital tract. As the infection progresses, the gonococci are replaced by a mixed flora in which anaerobes predominate.[34-35]

This hypothesis would force reconsideration of the idea that there are two kinds of pelvic inflammatory disease—gonococcal and nongonococcal. It should be emphasized, however, that the two forms of disease are clinically indistinguishable and that treatment should be based on the clinical findings, the known high frequency of polymicrobial etiology, and the Gram stain of cervix and culdocentesis or laparoscopy specimens as modified by culture results.

Acute pelvic inflammatory disease can be initiated by many other organisms—*C. trachomatis*, group A. *S. pyogenes*, and *N. meningitidis*.[36] The clinical pictures are identical, and the latter two species are sensitive to penicillin. Therapeutic failure with penicillin is thought to be due to *C. trachomatis* or to superinfection with *Bacteroides* species (Table 44-5). There is some evidence to support the hypothesis that *Mycoplasma hominis* or *Ureaplasma urealyticum* may also be responsible for some cases.[37,38] *Actinomyces israelii* has been increasingly implicated in pelvic inflammatory disease associated with intrauterine devices.[39] A review of common and uncommon etiologic agents has been recently published.[39a]

Pathogenesis

The gonococcus has the capacity for intercellular penetration between the epithelial cells of the urethra, periurethral glands, Bartholin and Skene glands, and the cervix. It does not have the capacity to invade mature vaginal squamous epithelium. During pregnancy, the uterine route to the upper tract is blocked so that acute pelvic inflammatory disease rarely occurs in pregnancy. The infection seems to begin more often in the postmenstrual period, suggesting that the endocervix is a moderate barrier to the spread from cervix to endometrium. *C. trachomatis* shares many of the characteristic pathogenetic features of the gonococcus.[40,41]

The incubation period for gonorrhea ranges from 2 to 10 days (average of 5). The infection appears first to affect the urethra and to spread to the periurethral glands. The vagina provides a conduit to the upper genital tract and is rarely infected despite the appearance of inflammation under the purulent discharge. The gonococcus apparently shows a predilection for the columnar epithelium

TABLE 44-5. THE BACTERIOLOGIC SPECTRUM OF ISOLATES OBTAINED FROM THE CUL-DE-SAC OF 64 PATIENTS WITH ACUTE PELVIC INFLAMMATORY DISEASE

Category IA aerobes and facultative organisms		
Streptococci, not group D: A-hemolytic streptococci;		16
nonhemolytic streptococci		12
B-hemolytic streptococci, group B		4
Lactobacilli		2
Microaerophilic streptococci		8
Corynebacteria		12
Staphylococci: coagulase-negative;		8
coagulase-positive		3
Micrococci		1
Eikenella corrodens		1
N. gonorrhoeae		17
Category IB anaerobes		
Peptococci		
Peptococcus spp		5
P. morbillorum		2
P. prevoiii		11
P. asaccharolyticus		4
P. variabilis		1
	Total	23
Peptostreptococci		
Peptostreptococcus spp		17
P. anaerobius		9
P. productus		1
P. micros		2
	Total	29
Veillonella		6
Unidentified gram-negative		2
Bacteroides, species other than *fragilis*		
Bacteroides spp		11
B. corrodens		1
B. pneumonosintes		3
B. nodosus		1
B. melaninogenicus ss *intermedius*		2
B. capillosus		4
B. oralis		1
	Total	23
Fusobacterium spp		1
Unidentified gram-negative rods		3
Clostridia		
Clostridium spp		2
C. malenominatum		1
C. haemolyticum		1
	Total	4

TABLE 44-5. *(Continued)*

Gram-positive nonsporulating (GPNS)	
Eubacterium spp	2
E. lentum	2
E. tenue	1
E. aerofaciens	1
E. contortum	1
Propionibacterium acnes	1
P. avidum	1
Lactobacillus spp	1
L. salvarius	1
L. acidophilus	1
L. minutus	1
L. ferimentum	1
Bifidobacterium spp	1
B. infantis	3
B. longum	1
B. adolescentis	1
Unidentified GPNS rods	12
	Total: 32
	Total aerobes: 84
	Total anaerobes: 123
	Total category I: 207 (76.91%)
Category II *B. fragilis*	
ss *fragilis*	5
ss *ovatus*	1
ss *thetaiotaomicron*	2
ss *distasonis*	1
ss *vulgalus*	1
ss unknown ("no good fit")	12
H. influenzae	1
	Total 10
	Total category II: 24 (8.9%)
Category III group D streptococci (enterococci)	Total category III: 12 (4.5%)
Category IV	
Enterobacteriaceae	
E. coli	8
Serratia marcescens	2
P. mirabilis	1
Enterobacter cloacae	1
K. pneumoniae	3
Citrobacter diversus	1
	Total 16
Others	
H. vaginalis	9
	Total category IV: 25 (9.6%)
	Total isolates in all 4 therapy groups: 269

Grouped in accordance with the Gainesville classification.

From Monif GRG: Significance of polymicrobial bacterial superinfection in the therapy of gonococcal endometritis-salpingitis-peritonitis. *Obstet Gynecol* 55(S):154S, 1980.

of the endocervical glands. In the asymptomatic carrier, the cervix is the superior limit of the spread of the infection.

In the lower tract, two additional sites traditionally become infected—the periurethral glands of Skene and Bartholin glands. Bartholin abscesses, however, are not pathognomonic of gonococcal infection. Spread up the urethra to the bladder is relatively rare.

The endometrium is relatively resistant, and only a superficial endometritis results, with rare epithelial penetration. This is as much due to the periodic sloughing of the endometrium as to the intrinsic resistance of the endometrium to gonococcal invasion.

Acute pelvic inflammatory disease is essentially an infection of the fallopian tubes. The mucosa is initially involved with edema, hyperemia, leukocytic infiltration; the purulent exudate fills the tube and oozes out the fimbriated end, leading to pelvic peritonitis and tubo-ovarian abscesses. Obstruction of the fimbriated end leads to pyosalpinx. With treatment, the tube becomes scarred or, if fluid remains, develops into a hydrosalpinx or tubo-ovarian cyst. Serosal adhesions between the reproductive organs as well as other pelvic organs may also occur.

The infection can sometimes sterilize itself in part because of the fastidious nature of the gonococcus.[10]

By changing the microbiologic environment, the gonococcus permits superinfection by the normal vaginal flora.[34] These weakly pathogenic anaerobic organisms (Table 44-5) proliferate best in anaerobic environments established by preexisting infection. For this reason, chronic pelvic inflammatory disease is usually due to anaerobic infections.[42]

The mechanism for the high rate of pelvic inflammatory disease among intrauterine device users is probably a simple one: bacteria are probably introduced into the endometrium during insertion or migrate there along the fiber tails that pass through the cervical os. The IUD itself may help maintain colonization of the endometrial cavity or may erode or inflame it, thereby establishing conditions for better microbial growth.[35]

Clinical Manifestations

Acute gonorrhea is most often asymptomatic. Some women have symptoms of lower tract disease—dysuria, urinary frequency, and vaginal discharge—but gonorrhea is rarely the sole cause of vaginal discharge, and concurrent trichomoniasis should be suspected.

Infections of Bartholin glands may produce unilateral-bilateral erythema and tender swelling. Occasionally, pus can be expressed from the urethra or from the orifices of Skene glands.

Acute pelvic inflammatory disease (endometritis-salpingitis-peritonitis) has a classical presentation: fever, bilateral lower abdominal pain, a purulent cervical discharge, a tender cervix, bilateral adnexal tenderness, and adnexal induration or masses. The bilateral pelvic pain is aggravated by the Valsalva maneuver and made less by flexion of the thighs. Migration up the right pelvic gutter leads to a Fitz-Hugh-Curtis syndrome of perihepatitis. Occasionally, irregular bleeding occurs owing to the superficial endometritis, but this is rarely serious. The lower quadrants are both equally tender; rebound tenderness, percussion tenderness, and involuntary muscle guarding are present. There may be distension, tympany, and decreased or absent bowel sounds.

On pelvic examination, the cervix may appear acutely inflamed. Movement of the cervix causes exquisite pain. The adnexal regions are most tender, usually equally so, and may feel full or thickened on bimanual examination. The tubes are not normally palpable even in salpingitis, so that masses usually indicate a pyosalpinx or tubo-ovarian abscess.

The principal problem is to rule out other conditions in order to promptly institute treatment and avoid the complications of chronic pelvic pain, subsequent episodes of pelvic inflammatory disease, and infertility.

The reliability of the clinical diagnosis of acute PID has been studied by Jacobson and Westrom.[43] They found that laparoscopy could confirm the clinical diagnosis in only 65 percent of 814 women; 12 percent had other diagnoses, and 23 percent had grossly normal tubes and ovaries. The latter finding, of course, did not rule out endosalpingitis. Less than one-third of patients with salpingitis had a temperature elevation of 38C or greater. Less than 50 percent of cases had an elevated peripheral cell leukocyte count, and the erythrocyte sedimentation rate was normal in 25 percent of patients.[43] A high erythrocyte sedimentation rate suggested the diagnosis of tubular occlusion or a tubo-ovarian abscess.

Diagnosis

Confirmation of the clinical diagnosis depends on a positive smear for, or cultural isolation of, *N. gonorrhoeae* from the endocervix, or demonstration of this or other bacteria in the posterior cul-de-sac by culdocentesis or laparoscopy. Monif suggests the following sequence of diagnostic procedures: (1) a Gram stain of the endocervix, (2) culture of the endocervix on modified Thayer-Martin medium, and (3) culdocentesis. If fluid other than serous fluid is obtained with more than five white cells per high-powered field, the fluid should be stained and cultured using strict aerobic and anaerobic techniques.

The cervical Gram stain is helpful if gram-negative intracellular diplococci are demonstrated. False-positive results are sometimes due to saprophytic *Niesseria* or *Mimae* species.

The technique used to obtain cervical smears and culture is important— the instruments should not be lubricated with jelly. Cervical mucus is wiped away, and a sterile cotton-tip swab introduced into the cervical canal.[10] The swab is rotated or moved from side to side and allowed to remain long enough for absorption to occur. The swab is then rolled directly on Thayer-Martin medium at room temperature. Using either transport medium or cold media will reduce the incidence of positive results. Curettage of the endocervix probably improves the bacterial yield. The culture plate should be cross-streaked with a wire loop as soon as possible and promptly placed in a candle jar.

The anal canal culture is sometimes the only site from which the organism can be recovered.

Urethral and vaginal cultures are indicated only in molested children and posthysterectomy patients. The urethra should be stripped toward the meatus to express the exudate; the vaginal culture should be taken from the posterior fornix.

When *N. gonorrhoeae* is present in the endocervix, 35 to 55 percent of the cases will have positive cul-de-sac culture. When the gonococcus is neither demonstrated on Gram stain nor isolated from the endocervix, *N. gonorrhoeae* is rarely isolated from the cul-de-sac. A severely retroflexed uterus is a relative contraindication and a mass in the cul-de-sac an absolute contraindication to culdocentesis. Culdocentesis should otherwise be performed whenever there are peritoneal signs or a combination of marked cervical tenderness on motion and a positive finding by a jar test.[44] Culdocentesis is important because of the polymicrobial nature of the disease even when it has been initiated by *N. gonorrheae.* It is especially important in patients who wear intrauterine devices or have a history of prior pelvic infections that favor polymicrobial infection.[32,43]

Culdocentesis is helpful in other respects. Bloody culdocentesis fluid suggests a ruptured ectopic pregnancy, a ruptured corpus luteum cyst, or other cause of hemoperitoneum. Less often is it found as a sign of pelvic inflammatory disease. Cloudy fluid is found in abdominal or pelvic peritonitis, a ruptured appendix, or salpingitis. Purulent fluid is most often found in patients with pelvic or abdominal peritonitis, ruptured tubo-ovarian abscess, ruptured appendix, ruptured diverticular abscess, or pelvic inflammatory disease. In short, bloody, cloudy, or purulent fluid can be found on culdocentesis in pelvic inflammatory disease.

In the differential diagnosis, the results of the pregnancy test should be negative and the urinalysis of the midstream specimen normal.

Laparoscopy is not routinely performed unless there are serious doubts concerning the diagnosis.

Treatment

The full therapy of acute pelvic inflammatory disease is usually medical, although operation is occasionally indicated for specific reasons. Therapy should be predicated on: (1) Gram stain of the endocervix, (2) presence or absence of the intrauterine contraceptive device, (3) character and staining results of fluid obtained by culdocentesis, and (4) the presence or absence of cul-de-sac or adenexal mass.

Many of these infections can be cared for without hospital admission. Hospitalization is mandatory, however, if (1) the diagnosis is uncertain, (2) there are severe gastrointestinal symptoms, (3) the disease is recurrent, (4) the patient is unreliable, or (5) pus has been obtained on culdocentesis. Supportive treatment includes bed rest, analgesics, and intravenous fluid if oral intake is inadequate. The guidelines for the selection of antibiotics for acute pelvic inflammatory disease are listed on Table 44-6.[7] The approved treatment for uncomplicated gonorrhea is described in Table 44-7.[9]

Gonococcal Acute Pelvic Inflammatory Disease. Antibiotics are the crux of therapy (Table 44-6). In the uncomplicated case without cul-de-sac infection in which gram-negative intracellular diplococci are seen on endocervical Gram stain, single drug therapy with penicillin or doxycycline is adequate as listed in Table 44-7. Table 44-6 also lists some of the therapeutic considerations in selecting one effective agent over another.

Single-dose parenteral therapy is preferred in patients who are unreliable and in patients with anal, rectal, pharyngeal, or ectopic gonorrhea. Whatever treatment is selected, concurrent syphilis should be sought by serologic tests at the time of diagnosis and 6 weeks after treatment. Advanced syphilis will not be treated adequately by any of the brief regimens described. Incubating syphilis may be obliterated by penicillin and tetracycline, but spectinomycin will not even cure incubating syphilis. Men and women exposed to gonorrhea should be examined, cultured, and treated at once with one of the described regi-

TABLE 44-6. ADVOCATED GUIDELINES FOR THE SELECTION OF ANTIBIOTICS IN ENDOMETRITIS-SALPINGITIS (ES) AND ENDOMETRITIS-SALPINGITIS-PERITONITIS (ESP)

Endocervical Gram Stain	Presence or Absence of IUD	Character of Cul-de-sac Aspirate	Indicated Therapy*
Gram-negative intracellular diplococci (GNID)	None	Dry tap or serous fluid	Single-drug therapy with penicillin or doxycycline
GNID	None	Turbid or frankly purulent fluid (15 WBC/hpf)	Cefoxitin or chloramphenicol or ampicillin plus clindamycin
GNID	IUD	Dry tap or serous fluid	Attempt single-drug therapy with IUD in place. If significant response to therapy does not occur within 12 hours, pull IUD
GNID	IUD	Turbid or frankly purulent fluid	Cefoxitin or chloramphenicol or ampicillin plus clindamycin, and pull IUD after 2 hr
Mixed bacterial flora (MBF)	None	Dry tap or serous fluid	If endocervical Gram stain demonstrates a definite mixed flora, doxycycline. If endocervical Gram stain demonstrates heavy gram-positive cocci predominance, ampicillin
MBF	None	Turbid or frankly purulent fluid	Cefoxitin or chloramphenicol or ampicillin plus clindamycin
MBF	IUD	Immaterial	Pull IUD after 2 hours antibiotic coverage. Cefoxitin or chloramphenicol or ampicillin or clindamycin

* See text for alternative treatment.

Modified from Monif GRG: *Ob/Gyn Infectious Diseases.* Gainesville, Infectious Disease, Inc., 1979.

TABLE 44-7. GONORRHEA: CDC RECOMMENDED TREATMENT SCHEDULES, 1979

UNCOMPLICATED GONOCOCCAL INFECTIONS IN MEN AND WOMEN

Aqueous procaine penicillin G (APPG): 4.8 million units IM at 2 sites, with 1.0 gm of probenecid by mouth

or

Tetracycline hydrochloride: 0.5 gm by mouth 4 times a day for 5 days (total dosage 10 gm) (other tetracyclines are not more effective than tetracyline hydrochloride; all tetracyclines are ineffective as a single-dose therapy)

or

Ampicillin 3.5 gm, or amoxicillin 3.0 gm, with 1 gm probenecid by mouth (evidence shows that these regimens are slightly less effective than the other recommended regimens)

or

Spectinomycin hydrochloride 2.0 gm in one IM injection (for patients who cannot tolerate tetracycline or penicillin)

DISSEMINATED GONOCOCCAL INFECTION

Ampicillin 3.5 gm, or amoxicillin 3.0 gm by mouth with probenecid 1.0 gm, followed by ampicillin 0.5 gm, or amoxicillin 0.5 gm, 4 times a day orally for 7 days

or

Tetracycline 0.5 gm orally 4 times a day for 7 days

or

Spectinomycin 2.0 gm, IM twice a day for 3 days (treatment of choice for disseminated infections caused by penicillinase-producing *N. gonorrhoeae*)

or

Erythromycin 0.5 gm, orally 4 times a day for 7 days

or

Aqueous crystalline penicillin G, 10 million units IV per day until improvement occurs, followed by ampicillin, 0.5 gm 4 times a day to complete 7 days of antibiotic treatment

MENINGITIS AND ENDOCARDITIS

Highdose IV penicillin, chloramphenicol, may be used in penicillin-allergic patients with meningitis

Adapted from Monif GRG: *Ob/Gyn Infectious Diseases.* Gainesville, Infectious Disease, Inc., 1979.

mens. Follow-up culture samples should be obtained from the infected sites 3 to 7 days after completion of treatment, and cultures should be obtained from the anal canal of all women who have been treated for gonorrhea.

Infants born to mothers with active gonococcal infection should be treated with 50,000 units of aqueous penicillin G, with lesser amounts to low birth weight infants. Topical prophylaxis for neonatal ophthalmia is not adequate treatment for infants born to mothers with active gonococcal infection. Infants who develop clinical illness require additional penicillin treatment. For example, gonococcal ophthalmia in the neonate should be treated with aqueous crystalline penicillin G 50,000 units per kg per day in two doses intravenously for 7 days. In normal infants born of apparently healthy mothers, prophylaxis in neonatal gonococcal ophthalmia includes opthalmic ointment or drops containing tetracycline, erythromycin, or a 1 percent silver nitrate solution.[10]

Although the minimal treatments for uncomplicated gonococcal pelvic inflammatory disease are listed in Table 44-6, patients with peritoneal signs should probably be treated for a disseminated gonococcal infection, with high-dose intravenous penicillin within the hospital (Table 44-7).

Nongonococcal and Mixed Gonococcal–Nongonococcal PID. Because it is impossible to differentiate gonococcal from nongonococcal salpingo-oophoritis at the time of hospital admission, treatment of all pelvic inflammatory disease as gonococcal infection is sometimes unsuccessful. The strategy listed in Table 44-6 provides a guideline for therapy. Minimal treatment for nongonococcal salpingitis should include antibiotics that effectively deal with gonococcal salpingitis, and in addition deal with gram-positive aerobes, *S. viridans*, the enterococcus, gram-negative aerobes (particularly *E. coli*), and the anaerobes, including the anaerobic cocci and *Bacteroides fragilis* (Table 44-1). No single antibiotic will cure all such patients so that the choice of antibiotic regimen is controversial. Since the majority of patients will respond to penicillin, doxycycline, or a first-generation cephalosporin, many gynecologists initiate therapy with a single regimen and add antibiotics if a prompt (36-hour) clinical response is not obtained or if culture results indicate that one or another copathogen is untreated.[38] Culture results, especially of anaerobes, are so slow in being reported, however, that empiric therapy based on the criteria in Table 44-6 seems more rational.

The recommendations in Table 44-6 list only a few of the antibiotic choices available to cover the broad spectrum of organisms found. The others are listed in Table 44-1. The combinations of aminoglycoside plus clindamycin, penicillin plus chloramphenicol, ampicillin plus cefoxitin, carbenicillin (or ticarcillin) plus an aminoglycoside have all been tried to achieve therapeutic levels against both the gonococcal infection and the other organisms that frequently occur in complicated nongonococcal pelvic inflammatory disease.[45] A combination of ampicillin, aminoglycoside, and clindamycin, useful for the treatment of bacterial peritonitis caused by mixed enteric infections, may be indicated in serious pelvic inflammatory disease. No relative advantage of clindamycin or chloramphenicol for the treatment of the anaerobic component has been seen.[46]

There is considerable debate on whether the presence of an intrauterine device increases the incidence or severity of pelvic inflammatory disease.[44,47,48] Similarly, authorities differ on whether or not the device must be removed during the treatment of uncomplicated pelvic infection.[42,49] Most patients respond well despite the intrauterine device, but in infections complicated by cloudy culdocentesis fluid, the device is best removed (Table 44-6).[42,50,51]

Prognosis

Uncomplicated upper tract gonococcal infections respond readily to antibiotic therapy. Failure of the fever to lyse within 24 to 36 hours, particularly in association with persistent tachycardia, and failure to the physical findings of rebound tenderness and deep organ tenderness to abate within 36 to 48 hours, should lead to a reevaluation of the diagnosis and therapeutic course. Repeated pelvic and rectal examination should be performed in order to determine whether operation is indicated.

Fertility After Antibiotic Therapy. After a single episode of pelvic inflammatory disease, 13 percent of laparoscopies will reveal tubular occlusion. After two episodes of pelvic inflammatory disease, nearly 36 percent are occluded.[9] In addition, there may be increased wastage of pregnancy, caused by changes in the oviducts secondary to previous infections, and an increase in ectopic pregnancies.[42] Early antimicrobial therapy directed at the entire spectrum of polymicrobial flora might be expected to lessen the incidence of these complications, but that has not yet been demonstrated.

TUBO-OVARIAN ABSCESSES

Incidence

Tubo-ovarian abscesses are usually complications of acute pelvic infectious disease, although they may not become manifest for many years. Daly and Monif[52] suggest that approximately 3 percent of all patients with chronic pelvic inflammatory disease, who have structural alteration of the fallopian tube or ovary as a consequence, will have a concomitant tubo-ovarian abscess. Rupture of the abscess will occur in about 15 percent of these patients.

Ruptures generally occur on the left side, a fact that may be related to the propinquity of the descending colon and the possibility that the use of a laxative sometimes precedes the rupture. Although the rupture may occur at any place along the tube or the ovary, the ovarian abscess is apparently more prone to rupture.

Etiology

Although *N. gonorrhoeae* is important in the pathogenesis of most cases of pelvic inflammatory disease, cultures of ruptured tubo-ovarian abscess rarely yield gonococci. Instead, polymicrobial flora are usually found, especially *E. coli, S. aureus,* anaerobic streptococci, enterococci, and *B. fragilis.*[52] This would be expected considering the flora obtained from the cul-de-sac during acute uncomplicated pelvic inflammatory disease (Table 44-5) (see preceding discussion).

Clinical Manifestations

As a Complication of Acute Pelvic Inflammatory Disease. Most patients with acute pelvic inflammatory disease respond to antibiotics within 48 hours. Failure to respond should prompt reexamination and determination if a tubo-ovarian abscess is present. Routine repeated examination during the course of therapy and before hospital discharge should also suggest the possibility that tubo-ovarian abscess is present. Failure to respond adequately is frequently accompanied by rectal tenesmus, diarrhea, progressive tachycardia, prolonged fever, weight loss, and anemia.[44]

A pyosalpinx, peritubular abscess, tubo-ovarian abscess, or loculation of pus in the posterior cul-de-sac will all appear as a tender and sometimes fluctuant mass in the adnexal or postuterine regions. Most purulent collections are found in the posterior compartment. Both tubes are involved in 75 percent of cases, although one tube may be larger and more posterolateral.[53] Rectal examination may help to define these masses, since vaginal exam permits only the palpation of the anterior aspect of the mass.

In difficult cases in which masses cannot be palpated, ultrasound, computerized tomography, the gallium scan, and laparoscopy can provide diagnostic assistance. Ultrasound can demonstrate a fluid-filled mass, although it cannot differentiate abscess from cyst. The advantages and disadvantages of these techniques have been described in Chapter 34.

Ruptured Tubo-Ovarian Abscess. Sudden pain at the site of the rupture is the usual initial symptom. The pain localization is variable depending on the degree of peritonitis, but the left lower quadrant is more frequently affected with subsequent spreading pelvic and generalized peritonitis, so that upper abdominal signs may predominate by the time the patient is first examined. Pelvic pain and tenderness are almost always present, and diarrhea is a prominent symptom of pelvic abscess. Ileus, distension, nausea, and vomiting, as in many cases of peritonitis, are late signs. The degree of hypotension and dehydration correlates directly with the amount of inflammatory exudate liberated into the intraperitoneal cavity. Diaphragmatic pain referred to the shoulder is common in bedridden patients. Fever, tachycardia, and leukocytosis are usually present.

The diagnosis is made clinically rather than bacteriologically. If rupture of a tubo-ovarian abscess happens during an acute episode of pelvic inflammatory disease or acute exacerbation of chronic pelvic inflammatory disease, the diagnosis is obvious. Sometimes the tubo-ovarian abscess does not become apparent until pregnancy. This may be a result of preexisting pelvic inflammatory disease with abscess formation or abscess formation associated with intrauterine infections during pregnancy. Here the diagnosis is difficult—rupture usually occurs in the first few weeks of gestation making the differential diagnosis between ruptured tubo-ovarian abscess, appendicitis, ectopic pregnancy, or torsion-infarction of ovarian mass. Culdocentesis should reveal blood-tinged pus or seropurulent fluid. The presence of multiple forms on Gram stain or foul-smelling exudates suggests an anaerobic infection.

Treatment

Ruptured Tubo-Ovarian Abscess. The treatment is operation in addition to antibiotics, because an unoperated ruptured tubo-ovarian abscess carries a mortality rate of 65 to 96 percent.[54] The current death rate is directly proportional to the delay in operation—it should always be less than 12 hours.

The operation that is univerally recommended is hysterectomy and bilateral salpingo-oophorectomy.[55,56] Swartz and Tanaree[57] demonstrated that closed suction drainage via the vaginal cuff will prevent accumulation of purulent material in this deep pelvic space. In selected patients with unilateral disease, simple salpingo-oophorectomy will both cure the disease and preserve reproductive function. The pelvic veins should be carefully examined in all cases of tubo-ovarian abscess so that suppurative pelvic thrombophlebitis can be ruled out.[52] Prolonged antibiotic therapy against the polymicrobial aerobic and anaerobic flora commonly present is recommended [53]—ampicillin, an aminoglycoside, and clindamycin appear to be a good combination.

Unruptured Tubo-Ovarian Abscess. Before the advent of antibiotics, some abscesses that formed in the cul-de-sac of patients with acute pelvic inflammatory disease could be drained by a posterior colpotomy. Currently, with adequate antibiotic therapy, fluctuant masses rarely localize in this position, and posterior colpotomy is rarely indicated. If, however, a bulging fluctuant mass is found in the posterior fornix, it should certainly be drained. One should not expect, however, that drainage alone will totally cure the disease; the patient frequently requires subsequent laparotomy for removal of the infected pelvic organs. If the posterior colpotomy succeeds in draining the collection with total resolution of infection without residual tubo-ovarian abscess, no subsequent operation is necessary, and successful pregnancy can occur.[58] When an unruptured tubo-ovarian abscess remains after control of acute pelvic inflammatory disease, the standard therapy is hysterectomy and bilateral salpingo-oophorectomy. Agreement is not complete on the timing of the operation, however. Anderson and Bucklew [59] first suggested that a pelvic clean-out should be performed during the acute phase of resolution of pelvic inflammatory disease to prevent abscess rupture. Indeed, acute-phase operation with appropriate antibiotic coverage can be safely performed with little serious postoperative morbidity.[60,61] Such an operation is rarely required, however. Fewer than 10 percent of patients hospitalized for acute pelvic inflammatory disease fail to respond to systemic antibiotics, and intraperitoneal rupture of a tubo-ovarian abscess in such a hospitalized patient is rare. Ledger bases his own decision for acute-phase laparotomy on persistent fever and not on the presence of pelvic masses. Pelvic masses can be observed by clinical and ultrasonic examination and frequently disappear with resolution of the infection and are not per se indications for operation.[42]

Although unilateral abscesses are said to be uncommon after pelvic inflammatory disease, unilateral abscesses related to intrauterine devices are more frequently found.[62] When there is only unilateral disease present and reproductive function is desired in the future, unilateral salpingo-oophorectomy (and even simple drainage) can be performed on occasion without placing the patient at excessive risk. One should remember, however, that occasional reoperation will be necessary because of recurrence or unrecognized contralateral ovarian involvement.

RARE INFECTIONS OF THE UPPER FEMALE GENITAL TRACT

TUBERCULOSIS

Pelvic tuberculosis is now uncommon in the United States [63] but is much more common in the underdeveloped countries. Although the disease is spread to the pelvis by hematogenous dissemination, other foci may not be found even with careful investigation.

M. tuberculosis is discussed in Chapter 7. Pelvic tuberculosis is a disease of the oviducts which spreads to the endometrium. Discovery by endometrial biopsy during the investigation of the asymptomatic infertile woman is a frequent mode of diagnosis.[64] The most common subjective symptom, however, is chronic pelvic pain; some patients complain of menstrual irregularity or amenorrhea.

On examination, the cervix is rarely ulcerated. Adnexal masses are frequently palpable. Results of PPD skin test are positive, but pulmonary foci may not be found. Endometrial biopsy can suggest the diagnosis, and culture of the biopsy specimen should permit diagnosis when the uterus is involved. The diagnosis is often made inadvertently. A hysterosalpingogram may be suggestive, revealing tubal distortion, intrauterine adhesions, and pelvic nodal calcification.[65] Laparoscopy for pelvic pain or chronic pelvic inflammatory disease may reveal tubercles on the peritoneal surface; biopsy should establish the diagnosis. If pelvic tuberculosis is seriously suspected, however, laparoscopy is contraindicated because of the extensive adhesions usually present.

The treatment of pelvic tuberculosis is medical and is described in Chapters 7 and 18. The combination of rifampin, ethambutol, and isoniazid is commonly chosen. Long-term therapy and careful follow-up for recurrence are essential.[66,67] The only current indications for hysterectomy and salpingo-oophorectomy are clear failure of drugs to resolve the adnexal masses, relapse after cessation of chemotherapy, or persisting symptoms during drug therapy.[63] If extirpation of the pelvic organs is required, drug therapy should be continued for 12 to 24 months. Long-term infertility with a high incidence of spontaneous abortion and ectopic pregnancy is almost a universal consequence of pelvic tuberculosis, however successful the therapy.

ACTINOMYCOSIS

Actinomycosis is discussed in Chapters 6 and 25, and in other regional infection chapters. Pelvic actinomycosis was long considered to be a rare sequel to a ruptured appendix, and the right fallopian tube was almost always affected.[68] *A. israelii* is not a normal vaginal inhabitant, and the increasing incidence is related to prolonged wearing of intrauterine contraceptive devices. Users of copper-containing devices may be at higher risk.

Cases that come to clinical diagnosis are indistinguishable from chronic pelvic inflammatory disease. Patients have vaginal discharge, which sometimes contains sulfa granules. The disease can progress to involve the tubes, ovaries, and adjacent organs in adnexal masses, without severe symptoms. Vague pelvic pain, low-grade fever, and weight loss may go unnoticed. Pap smears will frequently reveal the diagnosis to alert cytologists, but technicians may ignore debris.[69] A Gram stain and anaerobic culture should confirm the diagnosis if suspected, but too often only cases with extensive pelvic abscesses are found.[70] Treatment is high-dose penicillin (10 to 20 million units intravenously) for 6 weeks. If the disease is confined to the uterus, removal of the intrauterine device plus oral penicillin for a month will suffice.[39] The diseased pelvic organs should be excised only if adnexal abscesses are present. Charles recommends operation after 6 weeks of treatment, with postoperative antibiotics for another 10 weeks. Long-term follow-up is important, because recurrence is frequent. If the etiologic agent is not recognized during operation for chronic pelvic inflammatory disease, short-term antibiotic therapy will be insufficient for cure and intra-abdominal infection will recur despite an adequate operation.[70]

COCCIDIOIDOMYCOSIS

Coccidioides immitis rarely causes pelvic inflammatory disease (Chapter 9), but it can result from hematogenous dissemination from a pulmonary focus that may have healed. The peritoneal cavity is usually diffusely involved with miliary granulomas as well as large tubo-ovarian abscesses. In this respect, it resembles tuberculous pelvic inflammatory disease. The symptoms and signs are those of chronic pelvic inflammatory disease—pelvic pain, menstrual disturbance, a history of infertility, vaginal discharge, and recurrent genital infections. The diagnosis is usually not made until laparoscopy or laparotomy, when a granulomatous histology with special stains or culture confirm the diagnosis. Amphotericin B is the only effective drug currently available and must be combined with hysterectomy and salpingo-oophorectomy in the treatment of pelvic abscesses.[71]

INFECTIONS ASSOCIATED WITH PREGNANCY

CHORIOAMNIONITIS

The intact fetal membranes and the cervical plug are strong barriers to ascending infection. After rupture of the membranes, however, the fetus is exposed to the vaginal flora. Neonatal infection is most commonly the result of premature rupture of the fetal membranes (Table 44-2). Within 24 hours of rupture, 75 percent of amniotic fluid cultures will be contaminated,[72] and 17 percent of neonates will have septicemia. Inflammation of the fetal membranes is suggestive evidence of disease, and umbilical vein vasculitis is indicative of fetal septicemia.

The maternal consequences of chorioamnionitis are a consequence of bacteremia or subsequent endometritis (see subsequent section on puerperal sepsis).

The diagnosis should be based on the finding of bacteria in amniotic fluid after amniocentesis, and should be suspected in any patient with ruptured membranes, because maternal fever and leukocytosis are late signs. Fetal tachycardia is a nonspecific sign, which should increase suspicion and prompt amniocentesis.

The only definitive therapy is evacuation of the uterus. Antibiotic therapy (ampicillin plus gentamicin) should be administered intravenously. After delivery, a neonatal gastric aspirate should be obtained for Gram stain and cultures. The placenta and cord should be sent to pathology for examination. In the absence of puerperal endometritis, antibiotics can be discontinued in 24 to 48 hours after the last fever.

PUERPERAL SEPSIS

Puerperal Endometritis and Its Complications

The gradual discovery by Pasteur, Holmes, and Semmelweis that puerperal fever was caused by a microbe was a landmark in clinical infectious disease. Clinical antiseptic precautions soon reduced its incidence and severity.

Charles [73] points out that postpartum endometritis is simply a wound infection. The wound is the large abraded area at the placental site, and the bacteria are either the endogenous bacteria of the vagina or those that contaminate the examining hand or the instrument of the obstetrician. Infection is aggravated by retained placental tissue or fetal membranes, blood clot, or traumatized tissue, which permit opportunistic microbes to replicate. Sweet and Ledger [74] reported a 3.8 percent incidence of puerperal endometritis. Spread to myometrial and parametrial tissues, pelvic peritoneum, and pelvic virus follows the course of other infections of the female upper genital tract (see sections on pelvic inflammatory disease and postabortal sepsis).

Etiology

Until the antibiotic era, Group A *S. pyogenes* caused most of the puerperal sepsis. Beta-hemolytic streptococcus still causes an occasional case of puerperal endometritis.[75]

Most microorganisms which cause postpartum endometritis after vaginal delivery are the endogenous vaginal bacteria. The vaginal and cervical flora of prenatal patients do not differ markedly from the flora of the normal vagina (Table 3-13).[77-79] Cervical cultures in healthy puerperal patients are virtually identical with endometrial cultures from patients with puerperal sepsis.[80] Occasionally, unusual microorganisms will be found. Table 44-8 differs from Table 44-5, however, because most cases of postpartum endometritis follow cesarean section. Skin bacteria, therefore, have come to play an important copathogenic role with the vaginal flora.

Pathogenesis

The number of clinical factors appears to increase the incidence of puerperal endometritis and its sequellae. These include prolonged (especially longer than 48 hours) rupture of the fetal membranes, chorioamnionitis, prolonged labor, genital tract trauma, retained placental tissue and devitalized tissue, preexisting anemia, and poor antepartum care and hygiene.

Increased incidence of infection is also said to be correlated with the use of scalp electrodes for fetal heart monitoring, but there is considerable difference of opinion in this regard. Short-term monitoring (less than 8 hours) apparently carries little danger.[81-83] Gassner and Ledger [84] noted an almost double incidence of postpartum endometritis in patients who had vaginal deliveries after continuous fetal heart rate recording during labor.[82] Bacteremia associated with the endometritis was also twice as common in monitored patients.[85] In all studies, however, fetal monitoring is most frequently performed in patients with desul-

TABLE 44-8. BACTERIA ISOLATED FROM ENDOMETRITIS

	Wayne County General Hospital	University of Michigan Medical Center	Total
AEROBIC GRAM-POSITIVE			
Coagulase-negative staphylococci	17	40	57
Viridans streptococci	28	26	54
Diphtheroids	4	27	31
S. faecalis	6	19	25
Gamma streptococci	14	6	20
Group B beta-hemolytic streptococci	11	6	17
Coagulase-positive staphylococci	6	4	10
Group A beta-hemolytic streptococci	6	2	8
S. lactis	0	3	3
AEROBIC GRAM-NEGATIVE			
E. coli	39	57	96
Proteus spp	13	5	18
H. vaginalis	8	9	17
Klebsiella spp	3	11	14
Enterobacter aerogenes	1	3	4
E. cloacae	—	3	3
Pseudomonas	1	—	1
MICROAEROPHILIC SPECIES			
N. gonorrhoeae	16	—	16
Microaerophilic streptococci	10	1	11
OBLIGATE ANAEROBES			
Bacteroides spp	31	10	41
Peptostreptococcus	32	5	37
Peptococcus	10	—	10
C. perfringens	5	4	9
Propionibacterium acnes	—	5	5

From Sweet RL, Ledger WJ: Puerperal infections morbidity: A two-year review. *Am J Obstet Gynecol* 117:1093, 1973.

tory labor or other potential obstetric complications, so that the effect of pure fetal monitoring cannot be determined.

Clearly, however, the most significant obstetric procedure contributing to puerperal infection is cesarean section. Cesarean section is now performed far more often than previously, and for a broader set of indications—high-risk pregnancies, whenever delivery per vagina seems difficult, for social reasons, and for the convenience of the obstetrician. Patients who undergo cesarean section have a higher incidence of puerperal morbidity and more severe pelvic infections. Endometritis after cesarean section is seven times as great than that following vaginal delivery,[74] and bacteremia is ten times as common. The combination of cesarean section with prolonged rupture of the membranes, prolonged labor, or anemia further increases the morbidity.

Clinical Manifestations

Puerperal endometritis is frequently an arbitrary diagnosis defined by the syndrome of fever, uterine subinvolution and tenderness, and increased lochea within 96 hours of parturition. The onset of fever within 24 hours may be associated with virulent infections due to group A streptococci. In these cases, the pelvic source may not be clear because both parametrial tenderness and purulent discharge are minimal. The clear cervical discharge is, however, loaded with cocci on Gram smear. Treatment is urgently required.

Most cases of postpartum endometritis are more insidious—low-grade fever, a mild increase in pulse rate, malaise, anorexia, and headache. A mild fever (38C) on the third or fourth postpartum day is typical. Uterine tenderness may not be elicited on abdominal examination, but the tenderness is characteristically present in the area of the broad ligament. The lochea may be foul or may be an odorless, serosanguinous discharge.

All postpartum fever must be considered to be due to endometritis until proved otherwise, but the differential diagnosis can be difficult—urinary tract infection, respiratory tract infections, retention of the lochea (possibly a precursor of endometritis), retained fetal membranes, and mastitis. Transcervical aspiration of the endometrium should be carried out to obtain samples for aerobic and anaerobic culture.

Chills, high fever, and lower abdominal pelvic pain are indicative of severe infection, pelvic cellulitis, peritonitis, and bacteremia. Ileus, distention, vomiting, constipation, and urinary retention are frequently noted, and septic thrombophlebitis of the pelvic veins must be suspect. Blood cultures are useful in febrile postpartum patients. About 1 percent of febrile postpartum patients have bacteremia, and almost 90 percent of these had endometritis.[85] After cesarean operations, a wound infection may present as puerperal fever and an abscess can even develop in the uterine incision.

Pelvic Thrombophlebitis. As noted in the preceding section, fever of unknown origin at the puerperal period can sometimes be attributed to septic thrombophlebitis. *Bacteroides* species, in particular, are associated with septic thrombophlebitis, and patients with persistent febrile courses despite treatment for anaerobic bacteria should be assumed to have thrombophlebitis and receive anticoagulation therapy. Clinically evident pulmonary emboli are uncommon, but direct tenderness of the parametrial tissues with guarding, rebound, and mild distension is common. The fever is more often hectic and spiking than sustained and low-grade. Brown and Munsick[86] describe a characteristic ropelike mass, lateral and superior to the uterine cornu, which they think is the palpable thrombosed ovarian vein. But most clinicians fail to detect a mass in patients with persistent fever in whom pelvic thrombophlebitis is suspect.[74] The diagnosis of pelvic thrombophlebitis is most often made when antibiotics effective against *Bacteroides* species (clindamycin, chloramphenicol, metronidazole) fail to control fever associated with a preexisting endometritis and parametritis. Positive lung scan is presumptive evidence of pelvic thrombophlebitis.

Prevention

Although puerperal infections of the upper genital tract are caused by microbes, good obstetric care is the most important factor in prevention. Although no reversal of the trend toward increased fetal monitoring or cesarean section is likely, prolonged labor (especially in the face of ruptured membranes), traumatic operations, and repeated internal examinations should be avoided. Retained placenta or fetal membranes must be removed to provide adequate uterine drainage.

Antimicrobial Prophylaxis. The incidence of puerperal sepsis in uncomplicated vaginal delivery is so low there is almost certainly no benefit, but real potential harm, in giving antibiotics to all patients in labor. Numerous studies have, however, shown that prophylactic antimicrobial agents directed against the major components of the vaginal flora will reduce the incidence and severity of puerperal sepsis after cesarean section. Most investigators administer the drug before operation, but some wait until the cord has been clamped. Direct comparisons between these two techniques have not been made. Ledger[76] speculates that myometrial antibiotic levels are so low that the apparent beneficial result depends on prolonged postpartum administration, rather than on intraoperative prevention. Most studies, however, have used short intraoperative and postoperative courses.

The following antibiotic combinations have been useful: penicillin G plus kanamycin,[87] ampicillin, methicillin, plus kanamycin,[80] ampicillin plus kanamycin,[88] and clindamycin plus gentamicin.[89] The aim of combination therapy is to encompass the sensitivities of most of the mixed vaginal flora. Larson et al[90] showed that cefoxitin is a highly effective single agent even if it is withheld until the cord has been clamped. Cefoxitin was given intravenously in three 2-gm doses, the first after the cord was clamped and the others at 4 and 8 hours. Cefoxitin was effective only in reducing the severe infections and had no significant effect on mild febrile illness. Harger and English[91] have confirmed these findings and further showed that cefoxitin prophylaxis reduced the incidence of incisional infection from 11 percent to 1 percent. Other randomized clinical trials have demonstrated the beneficial effect of prophylactic ticarcillin.[92] Unfortunately, it is impossible to compare the various drugs that have been used by various centers for prophylaxis, because the incidence of infection itself varies so much from place to place.

Treatment

The clinical spectrum of endometritis requires different therapeutic strategies. Fever that appears in the first 24 to 48 hours after delivery is suggestive of severe infections—group A streptococci or bacteremia due to enterococci, *E. coli*, *Bacteroides*, or anaerobic gram-positive cocci.[76] Triple antibiotic coverage—ampicillin, aminoglycoside and clindamycin—should be used.

In the usual case of fever that appears 48 to 96 hours after vaginal or cesarean delivery, retained products of gestation should be sought and removed. Antibiotic treatment of uncomplicated endometritis depends partially on the infecting organism. Obviously, total identification of the pathogen and determination of its sensitivity cannot be carried out before the institution of therapy. However, the physician must not only consider what organisms are involved but must also obtain a Gram stained smear as well as aerobic and anaerobic culture on the material obtained from the uterine cavity. Charles' recommendation[73] of penicillin G as a first treatment does not seem reasonable, since it will have little effect on enterococci, the Enterobacteriaceae, or *B. fragilis*. Cephalothin, also recommended by Charles, has similar limitations. A number of controlled and randomized studies found that a combination of penicillin and kanamycin or clindamycin and kanamycin were equally efficacious, but that *B. fragilis* escaped the first combination and enterococcus the second.[93] The combination of ampicillin, an aminoglycoside, and clindamycin would be expected to be effective against the entire spectrum, and the results of a recent controlled clinical trial[94] favored the inclusion of clindamycin in the original combination. Cunha et al[95] showed that mezlocillin, a semisynthetic ureidopenicillin with a wide antibacterial spectrum against gram-negative aerobes and anaerobes, was effective.

Sorrell et al[96] showed no difference between mezlocillin and ampicillin, both of which were effective treatment for puerperal endometritis. Patients who did not respond to either drug were treated successfully with clindamycin. Gall et al[97] found no difference in effectiveness between metronidazole in combination with tobramycin, when compared with clindamycin in combination with tobramycin.

Failure to respond to a combination of antibiotics that covers the entire spectrum of vaginal flora should prompt a reevaluation. If there is no evidence for abscess in the wound, uterine wall, or pelvis, a tentative diagnosis of septic thrombophlebitis is usually made and a continuous infusion of heparin started and used for 10 to 14 days. Inferior vena cava ligation and bilateral ovarian venous ligation is recommended only for patients who continue to throw pulmonary emboli despite adequate anticoagulation. At operation, any nidus of the infection should be sought and eliminated.

Abdominal exploration is rarely required [61] for puerperal sepsis, but if extensive myometritis and necrosis are present, hysterectomy is required. Extirpation of the uterus plus both tubes, broad ligaments, and ovaries is usually necessary because conservation of the gonads sometimes fails to control the pelvic infection. Closed-suction drainage of the pelvis through the vagina should be carried out; a T-tube suction drain is effective, but Penrose drains are not.

SOFT TISSUE INFECTION IN THE PUERPERAL PERIOD

Retroperitoneal Abscesses In the Postpartum Period

Perinephric, subphrenic, inguinal, femoral, and gluteal abscesses have been reported as complications of puerperal parametritis simply as extensions into the retroperitoneal space.[98] Subgluteal and retropsoas infections can also originate from the paracervical or paravaginal tissues following paracervical and pudendal block anesthesia.[99] Hibbard et al [99] showed how infections arising in the paravaginal or paracervical tissues can extend laterally into the space that underlies the gluteal muscles or upward into the lumbosacral nerve plexus beneath the psoas muscle. These patients present with pain in the hip, abdomen, and back, along with fever and malaise. Hip disease is frequently suspected and the pelvic source ignored.[100,101] Roentgenograms sometimes reveal interstitial gas. The organisms isolated are *E. coli*, anaerobic streptococci, *Proteus*, and *Bacteroides* species.

Necrotizing Fasciitis

Necrotizing fasciitis of the perineum, paravaginal tissues, and abdominal wall has been reported as an unusual cause of puerperal sepsis (Chapter 25). These infections are most often seen in patients with diabetes, and several have died.[102] Important predisposing soft tissue injuries include fourth-degree extension of a median episiotomy and vaginal laceration. The most common cause is a polymicrobial abdominal infection after cesarean section. Extensive debridement is required in addition to antibiotics directed against enterococci, Enterobacteriaceae, gram-positive and gram-negative anaerobes (Chapter 25).

SEPTIC ABORTION AND ITS COMPLICATIONS

Incidence

The incidence and morbidity of septic abortion have fallen inversely with the increase in the number of medically approved terminations of pregnancy. Burkman et al [103] report an incidence of endometritis after elective first trimester abortions of 1.1 percent, and after abortion in the second trimester of 3.2 percent. There now are basically two forms of septic abortion—that associated with abortions performed by appropriately trained physicians, and that which is acquired in the community by intrauterine chemical or mechanical manipulation. Most of the literature on septic abortion relates to the latter.

Etiology

As in other infections of the female genital tract, the etiology relates directly to organisms introduced into the body of the uterus during manipulation. For this reason, mixed infections with the normal vaginal and fecal flora are most common. Many older series state that *E. coli* and *Klebsiella* species predominate,[104] but the majority of careful microbiologic studies using aerobic and anaerobic techniques have revealed that mixed infections are most common. For example, Rotheram and Schick [105] found a total of 129 anaerobic isolates from 69 cervical cultures in postabortal sepsis; in only six cultures was there moderate or abundant growth of *E. coli* without anaerobes. One of the most commonly recovered anaerobes was *B. fragilis.* Anaerobic septicemia, especially *B. fragilis,* was frequent. Other investigators [42] found a low incidence of positive blood culture. Still others found that treatment with antibiotics directed against anaerobes is not always essential.

There are several organisms traditionally associated with a lethal outcome—*C. perfringens* and group A *S. pyogenes.* Neither infection is always serious, but occasional deaths will result.

Pathogenesis and Pathology

The factors predisposing to infection during or after the performance of abortion relate to the sterility of the instruments, the care taken in the preoperative decontamination of the cervix, vagina and perineal tissues, and the completeness of uterine evacuation. Hospital-associated infections are inversely proportional to physician experience, and directly related to gestational age.[106] Suction curettage has a lower rate of complications than sharp curettage that damages the uterine wall. Perforations of the uterus and retained products of conception increase the incidence of infection.

Both hysterotomy and the intra-amniotic injection of hypertonic solutions were associated with relatively high infection rates. Both have been discontinued as common modes of abortion. In 1974, several reports stressed the apparent high incidence of septic abortions associated with intrauterine contraceptive devices (IUD).[107] Mead et al [108] subsequently found that nine of ten patients admitted for septic abortion were wearing an IUD of a single type (Dalkon shield), and all abortions occurred in the midtrimester. No association of septic abortion with other type of IUD has been made, although PID has been associated with IUDs of all types.[108]

Community-acquired septic abortion results from the insertion of contaminated catheters, coat hangers, knitting needles, slippery elm stick, and other foreign bodies into the uterus. Additionally, irritating solutions such as lysol, soap, pine oil, turpentine, or hydrogen peroxide were once introduced directly into the uterine cavity. Parsons and

Sommers [109] point out that soap solutions are the most lethal since they produce extensive necrosis within the uterine cavity and thrombosis of the adjacent vessels. The soap bubbles embolize to the lung or kidney, leading to respiratory failure or producing renal tubular necrosis.

The primary sites of infection in septic abortion are the fetal membranes, placenta, and adjacent endometrium. In pregnancy, these tissues provide little resistance to the lymphatic or vascular invasion of bacteria through the myometrium along the thrombosed veins and distended lymphatics of the pelvis into the blood. Several diseases can result: (1) septic thrombophlebitis, (2) pelvic cellulitis, (3) salpingitis, and (4) pelvic peritonitis and abscess.

Clinical Manifestations

Illegal Abortions. Most patients present late in the first trimester, and few will admit to intrauterine manipulation. The patient usually complains of bloody vaginal discharge which may be foul or purulent, fever, chills, and lower abdominal pain.

The spectrum of severity of the infection is considerable: the uterus may be large or small, boggy or firm, but an open cervical os is fairly constant. Cramps suggest that the products of conception are still present. The uterus and pelvic floor may be tender. Parametrial masses may be palpable, depending whether the infection is confined to the body of the uterus or has spread to the parametrial and adnexal regions.[110] There may be localized or generalized peritonitis and ileus with distension and absent peristaltic sounds. An abdominal roentgenogram should always be obtained. If perforation has occurred, there may be air under the diaphragm. Note should be taken of the presence of intrauterine devices.

In patients with parametrial tenderness, septic thrombophlebitis should be presumed. Persistence of fever and septicemia following evacuation of the uterus is almost diagnostic of pelvic thrombophlebitis, which can lead to metastatic infection of the lungs, brain, liver, kidney, and heart valves. Postabortal sepsis was a common cause of hypotension and septic shock in the preantibiotic era.[111]

Although clostridia account for only a small percentage of postabortal infections, they are among the more dramatic and severe presentations. Infection of the closed uterus leads to fetal emphysema. This is a relatively benign process per se, but there is gaseous vaginal discharge, crepitance of the uterine wall, and roentgenographic evidence of intrauterine gas. When the infection spreads to the endometrium, vaginal discharge and uterine tenderness are present, with or without gas formation. At this stage, there is little toxemia, but when the infection spreads beyond the endometrium to the uterine muscle, the full-blown picture of myometrial gas gangrene appears. The gas in the uterine wall appears in layers (onion skin effect), and uterine perforation, peritonitis, and systemic sepsis follow. Such a patient is very toxic, with tachycardia out of proportion to the fever, uterine and abdominal pain, and foul gaseous vaginal discharge revealing numerous clostridia and disintegrated white cells on Gram stain.

With severe clostridial sepsis, a dramatic clinical picture consisting of hemolytic anemia, hemoglobinemia, hemoglobinurea, disseminated intravascular coagulation, bleeding tendency, bronze-colored skin, hyperbilirubinemia, hypotension, shock, and renal failure is present (Chapter 6). Hemoglobin may impart a peculiar bronze or magenta color to the skin (pink lady syndrome), and the urine is port wine colored.

Endometritis after Elective Abortion. This can be a vague syndrome with fever, abdominal pain, and pelvic tenderness indistinguishable from acute pelvic inflammatory disease. Endometrial culture results obtained during curettage are usually positive, most often for group A *S. pyogenes*, *Bacteroides* species, *E. coli*, and *S. aureus*.

In almost all types of postabortal sepsis, the leukocyte count parallels the severity of infection. Anemia is not severe. Positive blood culture results vary considerably from series to series. It is dangerous to base therapy only on the findings of blood culture, since mixed bacterial infections are frequently present.

Treatment

The principles of therapy for incomplete and septic abortion as well as in puerperal sepsis are the same—evacuation of the uterus and systemic antibiotics. If the infection has spread beyond the confines of the uterus, hysterectomy and bilateral salpingo-oophorectomy may be required, although simple drainage procedures sometimes suffice. If clostridial infection has spread into the myometrium or beyond, hysterectomy and bilateral salpingo-oophorectomy are required, but when the infection is confined to the products of conception, it can be treated by curettage and antibiotics.[112]

Most patients will have incomplete abortion confined to the uterus without parametrial tenderness or mass. Under these circumstances, the uterus should be evacuated by sharp curettage. A delay of approximately 8 to 12 hours is sufficient for antibiotic premedication and control of any parametrial cellulitis. If severe hemorrhage is present, no delay should be permitted. Antibiotics may not always be necessary in these cases,[113] but they should be started before the uterine curettage to minimize bacteremia.

A difficult area in patient management is the decision for abdominal exploration and the potential removal of pelvic organs. The indications are clear-cut when there is a history of a widespread pelvic infection as in the use of a soap intrauterine douche, myometrial gas, or evidence of massive pelvic infection with intraperitoneal gas. Operation should be considered if there are signs of intravascular hemolysis or clinical evidence of deterioration with spiking fevers, hypotension, or renal failure despite uterine evacuation and antibiotics. If laparotomy is required to treat infection of the myometrium, a total abdominal hysterectomy and bilateral salpingo-oophorectomy is likely necessary. Even when the adnexa appear grossly normal, small abscesses in the substance of the ovaries have been found from which clostridia grow.[42]

Antibiotic Therapy. Considerable controversy surrounds the choice of antibiotics in patients with septic abortion. Many studies have demonstrated that equivalent therapeutic results are obtained with a number of combinations—penicillin plus chloramphenicol, cephalothin plus kanamycin, penicillin plus kanamycin, or cephalothin alone.[42] These studies clearly demonstrate that antibiotics normally ineffective against *B. fragilis* are quite effective in the treatment of septic abortion despite the frequent isolation of *B. fragilis* from such infections. Nevertheless, an occasional patient fails to respond to a regimen such as penicillin and an aminoglycoside, and will require clindamycin or chloramphenicol therapy to adequately treat the mixed infection.

Clostridial infections should be treated with large doses of penicillin and clindamycin.

Supportive Measures. Careful attention to fluid electrolyte and hemodynamic considerations are important, as discussed in Chapter 16. In clostridial sepsis, hyperbaric oxygen has proved to be occasionally useful,[114] but the use of a polyvalent gas gangrene antitoxin is more controversial.

Treatment of Pelvic Thrombophlebitis. Any severe pelvic inflammatory disease, especially postabortal sepsis, may be associated with septic pelvic thrombophlebitis. This vascular extension of infection is particularly common after anaerobic pelvic inflammatory disease. The diagnosis should be suspected in patients who remain febrile despite apparently appropriate antibiotic therapy in whom no evidence of pelvic abscess can be found.

There is strong evidence that pelvic thrombophlebitis is a pathologic entity.[115] Ledger found suppurative thrombophlebitis at laparotomy in 25 women with infected incomplete abortion. On the other hand, it is uncommon following uncomplicated vaginal delivery.[106]

The therapy of pelvic thrombophlebitis is still controversial. Collins [115] originally proposed that patients have inferior venacaval and ovarian vein ligation. Such radical treatment is usually unnecessary, because this is essentially an infectious process—usually caused by anaerobic cocci or *B. fragilis.* Clindamycin or chloramphenicol should be utilized. If this fails to control the fever or if pulmonary emboli develop, intravenous heparin is indicated. Venous ligation should be reserved only for patients who develop pulmonary emboli despite adequate anticoagulants. Oral anticoagulation in such patients should be maintained for 3 to 6 months.[106]

Prevention

The prevention and treatment of hospital-acquired postabortal sepsis is worthy of consideration. Nontraumatic and complete evacuation of the uterus through a properly prepared field is most important. It is not clear that prophylactic antibiotics delay the onset or prevent the development of postabortion endometritis. In patients with a purulent discharge, fever, or tender uterus, penicillin and an aminoglycoside are a rational first choice to prevent parametrial spread.

Patients with a clearly traumatized uterus (eg, perforation at the time of curettage) should be maintained in the hospital without systemic antimicrobial agents and be observed for excessive bleeding and herniation of bowel into the vagina. If the bowel has been damaged, laparotomy should be carried out to repair the damage, in addition to administration of systemic antibiotics (ampicillin, an aminoglycoside, plus clindamycin) (Chapter 34).

WOUND INFECTIONS IN OBSTETRICS AND GYNECOLOGY

Abdominal wound infections are a frequent cause of fever following cesarean section. Preexisting infections can prolong labor, and multiple pelvic examinations seem to increase the risk of wound infection. Most appear on the fourth to seventh days of the puerperium. Obviously, such wounds should be treated as described in Chapters 20 and 25. Surgical drainage without antimicrobial therapy is adequate in the usual well-loculated infection. Infection of the anterior abdominal wall can extend into the uterine wound. This is more common after classical section than after lower uterine segment incision. The measures noted previously for the prevention of puerperal sepsis apply equally well to the prevention of wound infection. Prophylactic cefoxitin therapy is highly effective prophylaxis for wound, as well as endometrial, infections during the performance of cesarean section.[91]

Episiotomy wounds are seldom infected, unless extension into the rectum has occurred. In these cases, gangrenous wound infections can result. Charles [73] recommends that the second stage of labor should not exceed one half-hour in order to circumvent neonatal morbidity and reduce contusions of the maternal perineum with the consequent increase in local infections. He favors the early outlet forceps delivery with an adequate episiotomy. Most episiotomy wound infections can be avoided if the perineum is promptly closed carefully. However, infections sometimes extend to involve the pubococcygeal muscle and fascia. Induration, suppuration, and sinus tract formation may occur. These cases are frequently ignored for fear of disrupting the repair, but in fact the sutures must be removed to allow free drainage and prevent the extension to peracervical and peravaginal tissue. Secondary closure can then be carried out, after all evidence of infection has resolved and bacteriologic cultures demonstrate the absence of virulent organisms (less than 10^5 per gram).

In the prevention of these infections, all the principles noted in Chapter 22 must be observed to reduce the infection rate from very low to virtually nil.

WOUND INFECTIONS AFTER GYNECOLOGIC OPERATION

Wound infections following gynecologic procedures differ from other clean contaminated cases only in that the bacteria found derive from the endogenous vaginal flora (Chapter 3). The mixed bacterial infections they cause in the postpartum period are similar to those caused following cesarean section. The vagina is never sterile, and contamination with anaerobic gram-positive organisms and fecal organisms, especially *E. coli, Klebsiella,* and *Bacteroides* species, is common.

There are basically three kinds of infection in the wounds of patients undergoing hysterectomy or other gynecologic procedure: (1) vaginal cuff infection, (2) soft tissue wound infection, or (3) pelvic abscess (including the rare ovarian abscess).

Vaginal Cuff Infection

This complication is particularly common after vaginal hysterectomy and slightly less common after abdominal hysterectomy. Low-grade fever usually appears between the fifth and seventh postoperative days, and most such infections resolve without abscess formation or pelvic cellulitis when adequate drainage is instituted. Hot vaginal douches may be helpful, and the administration of broad-spectrum antibiotics is probably indicated.

Vaginal cuff abscess is associated with pelvic pain or pressure, especially in the rectovaginal septum, and results in painful defecation. Persistent fever necessitates pelvic examination and drainage. Antibiotics are necessary and helpful in the localization and shortening of the course.

Pelvic Abscess

Patients with pelvic abscess following gynecologic procedures present with persistent pyrexia, lower abdominal discomfort, adynamic ileus, distension, nausea, vomiting, and partial intestinal obstruction. Persistence of fever after evacuation of a vaginal cuff abscess may be suspicious, and failure to respond to antibiotics suggests that the pelvic cellulitis is not being successfully controlled by the antibiotics. Although the classical findings consist of tenderness, induration, and a mass, it may be difficult to palpate the mass through the vaginal cuff or rectum. The use of ultrasound, computerized axial tomography, gallium, or indium scans may be helpful.

In addition to antimicrobial agents directed against the usual vaginal flora, surgical drainage or extirpation of the residual infection should be carried out. These may require removal of pelvic organs left in place or simple drainage. Even after vaginal hysterectomy, the transabdominal drainage route is useful, because rupture of a tubo-ovarian abscess is associated with a high mortality. The major differential problem is septic pelvic thrombophlebitis, which may require prolonged antimicrobial therapy and/or anticoagulation.

The "fever index" of Ledger and Kriewall [116] has become popular in the evaluation of these infections. This is a quantitative indirect measure of infection indicating the number of hours the patient's temperature is above 99F when oral temperatures are recorded four or more times per day. Daily differential leukocyte counts and estimations of the erythrocyte sedimentation rate are also useful in assessing the patient's response to postoperative infections. Serial ultrasonic diagnostic studies can demonstrate regression of loculated infection under conservative therapy, but persistence of the erythrocyte sedimentation rate in excess of 100 mm per hour in the absence of anemia or malignancy indicates continued activity in the infectious process.

Ovarian Abscess

Ovarian abscess is a distinctive clinical entity, not to be confused with tubo-ovarian abscess. Whereas tubo-ovarian abscess is part of an ascending pelvic infection, an isolated bacterial ovarian abscess is almost always the result of an operation in which the ovarian capsule has been disrupted with accompanying bacterial contamination. Daly and Monif [52] speculate that suturing the ovarian pedicle to the angle of the vaginal cuff after hysterectomy is a common cause. Mixed vaginal flora, including *B. fragilis* and the anaerobic streptococci, are most commonly found. It is unlikely that spontaneous infection of ruptured ovarian cysts occurs without surgical operation.

In the characteristic case, the patient becomes febrile after operation, especially a vaginal hysterectomy, and responds initially to antibiotic therapy. The fever then recurs, and a mass can be discerned by bimanual rectal or vaginal examination. Once the diagnosis is made, an abscess that follows a vaginal hysterectomy can sometimes be drained through the vaginal vault. Most often, however, the adnexal mass has retracted into the pelvis and treatment requires transabdominal excision.

Wound Infections

Infections of the abdominal wall soft tissue are common following any gynecologic operation in which the vagina is entered, because it is impossible to sterilize the mucosal surface. Mixed vaginal flora predominate, but in all other ways these infections are similar to those discussed in Chapters 21 and 25. Necrotizing fasciitis and other gangrenous infections are fortunately rare. Treatment is identical to that discussed in Chapters 21 and 25.

Antibiotic Selection for Postoperative Wound Infections

The selection of antibiotics for infections caused by mixed vaginal flora in soft tissue, pelvis, or vaginal cuff are those which have been repeatedly discussed in this chapter (Table 44-6). The Gram stain of the smear may be of some assistance in the empiric selection, but in most cases drugs effective against *B. fragilis* will be required for optimum treatment. Antibiotics may not be necessary for well-confined minor wound infections, but pelvic infections can be fatal if not adequately treated.

Antibiotic Selection for Prophylaxis

Most evidence supports the perioperative and intraoperative administration of antibiotics whenever the vagina is to be entered during operation. Cephalosporin,[117] ampicillin, tetracycline,[118,119] and many other agents have proved useful. The principles of chemoprophylaxis discussed in Chapter 23 should be used. Coverage against vaginal aerobes and anaerobes appears most rational.

BIBLIOGRAPHY

Charles D: Infections in Obstetrics and Gynecology. Philadelphia, Saunders, 1980.

Ledger WJ: Infection in the Female. Philadelphia, Lea and Febiger, 1977.

Monif GRG: Infectious Diseases in Obstetrics and Gynecology. Hagerstown, Harper and Row, 1974.

St John RK, Brown ST (eds): International symposium on pelvic inflammatory disease. Am J Obstet Gynecol 138:845–1109, 1980.

REFERENCES

1. Levison ME, Corman LC, Carrington ER, Kaye D: Quantitative microflora of the vagina. Am J Obstet Gynecol 127:80, 1977.
2. Gorbach SL, Menda KB, Thadepalli H, Keith L: Anaerobic microflora of the cervix in healthy women. Am J Obstet Gynecol 117:1053, 1973.
3. Neary MP, Allen J, Okubadejo OA, Payne DJH: Preoperative vaginal bacteria and postoperative infections in gynecological patients. Lancet II:1291, 1973.
4. Onderdonk AB, Polk BF, Moon NE, Goren B, Bartlett JG: Methods for quantitative vaginal flora studies. Am J Obstet Gynecol 128:777, 1977.
5. Bartlett JC, Moon NE, Goldstein PR, Goren B, Onderdonk AB, Polk BF: Cervical and vaginal bacterial flora: ecologic niches in the female lower genital tract. Am J Obstet Gynecol 130:658, 1978.
6. Sparks RA, Purrier BGA, Watt PJ: The bacteriology of the cervix and uterus. Br J Obstet Gynecol 84:701, 1977.
7. Monif GRG: Part I. Antibiotics in Ob/Gyn. In Monif GRG: Ob/Gyn Infectious Diseases. Gainesville: Infectious Disease, Inc, 1979, pp 1–71.
8. Charles D: Infections in Obstetrics and Gynecology. Philadelphia, Saunders, 1980.
9. Monif GRG: Ob/Gyn Infectious Diseases, 2nd ed. Gainesville, Infectious Disease, Inc, 1979.
10. Monif GRG: Infectious Diseases in Obstetrics and Gynecology. Hagerstown, Harper and Row, 1974.

LOWER FEMALE GENITAL TRACT

11. Rein MF: Vulvovaginitis and cervicitis. In Mandell GL, Douglas RG Jr, Bennett JE: Principles and Practice of Infectious Diseases. New York, Wiley, 1979, p 985.
12. Charles D: Fungal infections. In Charles D: Infections in Obstetrics and Gynecology. Philadelphia, Saunders, 1980, p 51.
13. Fleury FJ, Van Bergen WS, Prentice RL, Russell JG, Singleton JA, Standard JV: Single dose of two grams of metronidazole for *Trichomonas vaginalis* infection. Am J Obstet Gynecol 128:320, 1977.
14. Charles D: Sexually transmitted disease. In Charles D: Infections in Obstetrics and Gynecology. Philadelphia, Saunders, 1980, p 9.
15. Pheifer TA, Forsyth PS, Durfee MA, Pollock HM, Holmes KK: Nonspecific vaginitis. Role of *Haemophilus vaginalis* and treatment with metronidazole. N Engl J Med 298:1429, 1978.
16. Kaufman RH: The origin and diagnosis of "nonspecific vaginitis." N Engl J Med 303:637, 1980.
17. Spiegel CA, Amsel R, Eschenbach D, Schoenknecht, F, Holmes, KK: Anaerobic bacteria in nonspecific vaginitis. N Engl J Med 303:601, 1980.
18. Finegold SM: Miscellaneous anaerobic infections. In Finegold SM: Anaerobic Bacteria in Human Disease. New York, Academic, 1977, p 463.
19. Finegold SM: Therapy and prognosis in anaerobic infections. In Finegold SM: Anaerobic Bacteria in Human Disease. New York, Academic, 1977, p 534.
20. Rein MF: Skin and mucous membrane lesions. In Mandell GL, Douglas RG Jr, Bennett JE (eds): Principles and Practice of Infectious Diseases. New York, Wiley, 1979, p 996.
21. Charles D: Granuloma inguinale. In Charles D: Infections in Obstetrics and Gynecology. Philadelphia, Saunders, 1980, p 37.
22. Grayston JT, Wang S: New knowledge of Chlamydiae and the diseases they cause. J Infect Dis 132:87, 1975.
23. Schachter J: Chlamydial infections (3 parts). N Engl J Med 298:428, 490, 540, 1978.
24. Lee YH, Rankin JS, Alpert S, Daly AR, McCormack WM: Microbiological investigation of Bartholin gland abscesses and cysts. Am J Obstet Gynecol 129:150, 1977.
25. Curran JW, Rendtorff RC, Chandler RW, Wiser WL, Robinson H: Female gonorrhea. Its relation to abnormal uterine bleeding, urinary tract symptoms, and cervicitis. Obstet Gynecol 45:195, 1975.
26. Willcox RR: Necrotic cervicitis due to primary infection with the virus of herpes simplex. Br Med J 1:610, 1968.
27. Morse AR, Coleman DV, Gardner SD: An evaluation of cytology in the diagnosis of herpes simplex virus infection and cytomegalovirus infection of the cervix uteri. J Obstet Gynecol Br Commonwealth 81:393, 1974.
28. Nahmias JA, Alford CA, Korones SB: Infection of the newborn with herpesvirus hominis. Advan Pediatr 17:185, 1970.
29. Charles D: Viral infections. In Charles D: Infections in Obstetrics and Gynecology. Philadelphia, Saunders, 1980, p 103.

PELVIC INFLAMMATORY DISEASE

30. Tyler CW, St John RK: Gonorrhea—diagnosis and therapy in the female. Am Coll Obstet Gynecol Tech Bull 28:1, 1974.
31. Eschenbach DA: Epidemiology and diagnosis of acute pelvic inflammatory disease. Obstet Gynecol 55(S):142S, 1980.
32. Chow AW, Malkasian KL, Marshall JR, Guze LB: The bacteriology of acute pelvic inflammatory disease. Value of cul-de-sac cultures and relative importance of gonococci and other aerobic or anaerobic bacteria. Am J Obstet Gynecol 122:876, 1975.
33. Falk V: Treatment of acute non-tuberculous salpingitis with antibiotics alone and in combination with glucocorticoids. A prospective double-blind controlled study of the clinical course and prognosis. Acta Obstet Gynecol Scand Suppl 44(Suppl 6):7, 1965.
34. Monif GRG: Significance of polymicrobial bacterial superinfection in the therapy of gonococcal endometritis-salpingitis-peritonitis. Obstet Gynecol 55(S):154S, 1980.
35. Eschenbach DA, Buchanan TM, Pollock HM, Forsyth PS, Alexander ER, Lin JS, Wang SP, Wentworth BB, McCormack WM, Holmes KK: Polymicrobial etiology of acute pelvic inflammatory disease. N Engl J Med 293:166, 1975.
36. Kappus SS: The bacterial pathogenesis of acute pelvic inflammatory disease. Obstet Gynecol 52:161, 1978.
37. Sweet RL, Mills J, Hadley KW, Blumenstock E, Schachter J, Robbie MO, Draper DL: Use of laparoscopy to determine the microbiologic etiology of acute salpingitis. Am J Obstet Gynecol 134:68, 1979.
38. Thompson SE III, Hager WD, Wong KH, Lopez B, Ramsey C, Allen SD, Stargel MD, Thornsberry G, Benigno BB, Thomson JD, Shulman JA: The microbiology and therapy of acute pelvic inflammatory disease in hospitalized patients. Am J Obstet Gynecol 136:179, 1980.
39. Hagar WD, Majmudar B: Pelvic actinomycosis in women using intrauterine contraceptive devices. Am J Obstet Gynecol 133:60, 1979.

39a. Mårdh P: An overview of infective agents of salpingitis, their biology and recent advances in methods of detection. Am J Obstet Gynecol 138:933, 1980.

40. Mårdh PA, Ripa T, Svensson L, Westrom L: *Chlamydia trachomatis* infection in patients with acute salpingitis. N Engl J Med 296:1377, 1977.
41. Muller-Schoop JW, Wang SP, Munzinger J, Schlapfer HU, Knoblauch M, Ammann RW: *Chlamydia trachomatis* as possible cause of peritonitis and perihepatitis in young women. Br Med J 1:1022, 1978.
42. Ledger WJ: Community-acquired gynecologic infections. In Ledger WJ: Infections in the Female. Philadelphia, Lea and Febiger, 1977, p 108.
43. Jacobson L, Westrom L: Objectivized diagnosis of acute pelvic inflammatory disease. Am J Obstet Gynecol 105:1088, 1969.
44. Monif GRG: Part II. The core infectious disease problems in Ob/Gyn. In Monif GRG: Ob/Gyn Infectious Diseases. Gainesville, Infectious Disease, Inc., 1979, p 74.
45. Louria DB, Sen P: Anaerobic infections of the pelvis. Obstet Gynecol 55(S):114S, 1980.
46. Ledger WJ, Moore DE, Lowensohn RI, Gee CL: A fever index evaluation of chloramphenicol or clindamycin in patients with serious pelvic infections. Obstet Gynecol 50:523, 1977.
47. Wright NH, Laemmle P: Acute pelvic inflammatory disease in an indigent population: an estimate of its incidence and relationship to methods of contraception. Am J Obstet Gynecol 101:979, 1968.
48. Golditch IM, Huston JE: Serious pelvic infections associated with intrauterine contraceptive device. Int J Fertil 18:156, 1973.
49. Willson JR, Ledger WJ, Bollinger CC, Andros GJ: The margulies intrauterine contraceptive device: experience with 623 women. Am J Obstet Gynecol 92:62, 1965.
50. Marshall BR, Hepler JK, Jinguji MS: Fatal *Streptococcus pyogenes* septicemia associated with an intrauterine device. Obstet Gynecol 41:83, 1973.
51. Scott RB: Critical illnesses and deaths associated with intrauterine devices. Obstet Gynecol 31:322, 1968.

TUBO-OVARIAN ABSCESS

52. Daly JW, Monif GRG: Tuboovarian and ovarian abscesses. In Monif GRG: Infectious Diseases in Obstetrics and Gynecology, Hagerstown, Harper and Row, 1974, p 396.
53. Charles D: Anaerobic infections. In Charles D: Infections in Obstetrics and Gynecology. Philadelphia, Saunders, 1980, p 198.
54. Black WT: Abscess of the ovary. Am J Obstet Gynecol 31:487, 1936.
55. Vermeeren J, TeLinde R: Intra-abdominal rupture of pelvic abscesses. Am J Obstet Gynecol 68:402, 1954.
56. Collins CG, Nix FG, Cerha HT: Ruptured tuboovarian abscess. Am J Obstet Gynecol 72:820, 1956.
57. Swartz WH, Tanaree P: T-tube suction drainage and/or prophylactic antibiotics. A randomized study of 451 hysterectomies. Obstet Gynecol 47:665, 1976.
58. Fraser AC: Surgical treatment of acute pelvic sepsis. J Obstet Gynecol Br Commonwealth 79:560, 1972.
59. Anderson GV, Bucklew WB: Abdominal surgery and tuboovarian abscesses. West J Surg Obstet Gynecol 70:67, 1962.
60. Kaplan AL, Jacobs WM, Ehresman JB: Aggressive management of pelvic abscess. Am J Obstet Gynecol 98:482, 1967.
61. Ledger WJ, Gassner CB, Gee C: Operative care of infections in obstetrics-gynecology. J Reprod Med 13:128, 1974.
62. Scott WC: Pelvic abscess in association with intrauterine contraceptive device. Am J Obstet Gynecol 131:149, 1978.

GRANULOMATOUS INFECTIONS OF THE UPPER GENITAL TRACT

63. Charles D: Tuberculosis. In Charles D: Infections in Obstetrics and Gynecology. Philadelphia, Saunders, 1980, p 234.
64. Schaefer G: Female genital tuberculosis. Clin Obstet Gynecol 19:223, 1976.
65. Klein TA, Richmond JA, Mishell DR Jr: Pelvic tuberculosis. Obstet Gynecol 48:99, 1976.
66. Sutherland AM: Twenty-five years experience of the drug treatment of tuberculosis of the female genital tract. Br J Obstet Gynecol 84:881, 1977.
67. Sutherland AM: Tuberculosis of the female genital tract. Br Med J 1:576, 1978.
68. MacCarthy J: Actinomycosis of the female pelvic organs with involvement of the endometrium. J Pathol Bacteriol 69:175, 1955.
69. Gupta PK, Hollander DH, Frost JK: Actinomycetes in cervico-vaginal smears: an association with IUD usage. Acta Cytol 20:295, 1976.
70. Lomax CW, Harbert GM Jr, Thornton WN Jr: Actinomycosis of the female genital tract. Obstet Gynecol 48:341, 1976.
71. Saw EC, Smale LE, Einstein H, Huntington RW Jr: Female genital coccidioidomycosis. Obstet Gynecol 45:199, 1975.

UPPER TRACT INFECTIONS ASSOCIATED WITH PREGNANCY

72. Pomerance W: Chorioamnionitis and maternal sepsis. In Monif GRG: Infectious Diseases in Obstetrics and Gynecology. Hagerstown, Harper and Row, 1974, p 292.
73. Charles D: Wound infections. In Charles D: Infections in Obstetrics and Gynecology, Philadelphia, Saunders, 1980, p 259.
74. Sweet RL, Ledger WJ: Puerperal infectious morbidity: two-year review. Am J Obstet Gynecol 117:1093, 1973.
75. Tancer ML, McManus JE, Bellotti G: Group A, type 33, β-hemolytic streptococcal outbreak on a maternity and newborn service. Am J Obstet Gynecol 103:1028, 1969.
76. Ledger WJ: Hospital-acquired obstetric infections. In Ledger WJ: Infections in the Female. Philadelphia, Lea and Febiger, 1977, p 201.
77. De Louvois J, Hurley R, Stanley VC, Jones JB, Foulkes JEB: Microbial ecology of the female lower genital tract during pregnancy. Postgrad Med J 51:156, 1975.
78. De Louvois J, Hurley R, Stanley VC: Microbial flora of the lower genital tract during pregnancy: relationship to morbidity. J Clin Pathol 28:731, 1975.
79. Goplerud CP, Ohm MJ, Galask RP: Aerobic and anaerobic flora of the cervix during pregnancy and the puerperium. Am J Obstet Gynecol 126:858, 1976.
80. Gibbs RS, DeCherney AH, Schwarz RH: Prophylactic antibiotics in cesarean section: a double-blind study. Am J Obstet Gynecol 114:1048, 1972.
81. Wiechetek WJ, Horiguchi T, Dillon TF: Puerperal morbidity and internal fetal monitoring. Am J Obstet Gynecol 119:230, 1974.
82. Larsen JW, Goldkrand JW, Hanson TM, Miller CR: Intrauterine infection of an obstetric service. Obstet Gynecol 43:838, 1974.
83. Hagen D: Maternal febrile morbidity associated with fetal monitoring and cesarean section. Obstet Gynecol 46:260, 1975.
84. Gassner CB, Ledger WJ: The relationship of hospital-acquired infection to invasive intrapartum monitoring techniques. Am J Obstet Gynecol 126:33, 1976.
85. Ledger WJ, Norman M, Gee C, Lewis W: Bacteremia on

an obstetric-gynecologic service. Am J Obstet Gynecol 121:205, 1975.
86. Brown TK, Munsick RA: Puerperal ovarian vein thrombophlebitis: a syndrome. Am J Obstet Gynecol 109:263, 1971.
87. Weisberg SM, Edwards NL, O'Leary JA: Prophylactic antibiotics in cesarean section. Obstet Gynecol 38:290, 1971.
88. Gibbs RS, Hunt JE, Schwarz RH: A follow-up study on prophylactic antibiotics in cesarean section. Am J Obstet Gynecol 117:419, 1973.
89. Gibbs RS, Weinstein AJ: Bacteriologic effects of prophylactic antibiotics in cesarean section. Am J Obstet Gynecol 126:226, 1976.
90. Larson P, Nelson KE, Ismail M, Geiseler PJ: Double-blind study of cefoxitin prophylaxis of post-cesarean section infection. In Nelson JD, Grassi C. (eds): Current Chemotherapy and Infectious Disease, Vol II. Washington, D.C., American Society for Microbiology, 1980, p 1212.
91. Hager J, English D: Perioperative cefoxitin prophylaxis in cesarean section at high risk for infection. 20th Interscience Conference on Antimicrobial Agents and Chemotherapy, 1980, Abstract #229.
92. Reyelt MC, Apuzzio J, Sen P, Louria DB: Randomized clinical trials of ticarcillin as prophylaxis of post-caesarean section endometritis and as a therapeutic agent for post-caesarean section endometritis. 20th Interscience Conference on Antimicrobial Agents and Chemotherapy, 1980, Abstract #229.
93. Ledger, WJ, Kriewall TJ, Sweet RL, Fekety FR Jr: The use of parenteral clindamycin in the treatment of obstetric-gynecologic patients with severe infections. A comparison of a clindamycin-kanamycin combination with penicillin-kanamycin. Obstet Gynecol 43:490, 1974.
94. Sen P, Apuzzio J Reyelt C, Kaminski T, Levy F, Kapila R, Middleton J, Louria D: Prospective evaluation of combinations of antimicrobial agents for endometritis after cesarean section. Surg Gynecol Obstet 151:89, 1980.
95. Cunha AC, Lima GR, Mello B, Miranda PR, Carvalho JA, Trabulsi LR: Postabortion and puerperal infections: treatment with mezlocillin. In Nelson JD, Grassi C (eds): Current Chemotherapy and Infectious Disease, Vol II. Washington, D.C., American Society for Microbiology, 1980, p 1221.
96. Sorrell TC, Yoshimori R, Marshall JR, Chow AW: Puerperal endomyometritis: prospective randomized comparison of mezlocillin and ampicillin. 20th Interscience Conference on Antimicrobial Agents and Chemotherapy, 1980, Abstract #226.
97. Gall SA, Ayers Q, Kohen F, Edmisten C, Addison A, Hill GB: Intravenous metronidazole in the therapy of anaerobic obstetrical and gynecological infections. In Nelson JD, Grassi C (eds): Current Chemotherapy and Infectious Disease, Vol II. Washington, D.C., American Society for Microbiology, 1980, p 1225.
98. Charles D, Klein TA: Postpartum infection. In Charles D, Finland M: Obstetric and Perinatal Infections. Philadelphia, Lea and Febiger, 1973, p 247.
99. Hibbard LT, Snyder EN, McVann RM: Subgluteal and retropsoal infection in obstetric practice. Obstet Gynecol 39:137, 1972.
100. Wenger DR, Gitchell RG: Severe infections following pudendal block anesthesia: need for orthopaedic awareness. J Bone Joint Surg 55:202, 1973.
101. Galask RP, Larsen B, Ohm MJ: Vaginal flora and its role in disease entities. Clin Obstet Gynecol 19:61, 1976.
102. Golde S, Ledger WJ: Necrotizing fasciitis in postpartum patients. A report of four cases. Obstet Gynecol 50:670, 1977.
103. Burkman RT, Atienza MF, King TM: Culture and treatment results in endometritis following elective abortion. Am J Obstet Gynecol 128:556, 1977.
104. Dahm CH Jr, Ostapowicz F, Cavanagh D: Use of cephalothin in septic abortion. Obstet Gynecol 41:693, 1973.
105. Rotheram EB Jr, Schick SF: Nonclostridial anaerobic bacteria in septic abortion. Am J Med 46:80, 1969.
106. Ledger WJ: Septic abortion and septic pelvic thrombophlebitis. In Monif GRG: Infectious Diseases in Obstetrics and Gynecology. Hagerstown, Harper and Row, 1974, p 275.
107. Christian CD: Maternal deaths associated with an intrauterine device. Am J Obstet Gynecol 119:441, 1974.
108. Mead PB, Beecham JB, Maeck JVS: Incidence of infections associated with the intrauterine contraceptive device in an isolated community. Am J Obstet Gynecol 125:79, 1976.
109. Parsons L, Sommers SC: Vol II. Gynecology 2nd ed. Philadelphia, Saunders, 1979.
110. Neuwirth RS, Friedman EA: Septic abortion. Changing concept of management. Am J Obstet Gynecol 85:24, 1963.
111. Studdiford WE, Douglas GW: Placental bacteremia: a significant finding in septic abortion accompanied by vascular collapse. Am J Obstet Gynecol 71:842, 1956.
112. O'Neill RT, Schwarz RH: Clostridial organisms in septic abortions. Report of 7 cases. Obstet Gynecol 35:458, 1970.
113. Barnes AB, Ulfelder H: Septic abortion. JAMA 189:919, 1964.
114. Perrin LE, Ostergard DR, Mishell DR Jr: The use of hyperbaric oxygen in the treatment of clostridial septicemia complicating septic abortion. Report of a case. Am J Obstet Gynecol 106:666, 1970.
115. Collins CG: Suppurative pelvic thrombophlebitis. A study of 202 cases in which the disease was treated by ligation of the vena cava and ovarian vein. Am J Obstet Gynecol 108:681, 1970.

POSTOPERATIVE INFECTIONS

116. Ledger WJ, Kriewall TJ: The fever index: a quantitative indirect measure of hospital-acquired infections in obstetrics and gynecology. Am J Obstet Gynecol 115:906, 1973.
117. Ledger WJ, Sweet RL, Headington JT: Prophylactic cephaloridine in the prevention of postoperative pelvic infections in premenopausal women undergoing vaginal hysterectomy. Am J Obstet Gyn 115:766, 1973.
118. Bolling DR Jr, Plunkett GD: Prophylactic antibiotics for vaginal hysterectomies. Obstet Gynecol 41:689, 1973.
119. Rosenhein GE: Prophylactic antibiotics in elective abdominal hysterectomy. Am J Obstet Gynecol 119:335, 1974.

CHAPTER 45
Infections of the Genitourinary Tract

RUSSELL K. LAWSON AND STEPHEN C. JACOBS

Urinary tract infections are ten times more common in women than in men. Approximately 10 to 20 percent of women will have a urinary tract infection some time in their lives, and the prevalence increases with age. Approximately 1 percent of school age girls have bacteriuria, 4 percent of young adult women have urinary tract infections, and 7 percent of women older than 50.[1] Although the early increased prevalence with age is related to the onset of sexual activity, the continued increase is unexplained.

Urinary tract infections seldom cause serious morbidity, and loss of renal function is rare. These infections are, however, accompanied by substantial physical discomfort and medical expense.

NORMAL BLADDER DEFENSE MECHANISMS

Although urine contains many nutrients that are suitable for bacterial growth, normally it is sterile.

Because the urethra (approximately 3.5 cm long in the female and 20 to 25 cm long in the male) is the first line of defense against infection, the long male urethra explains the lower rate of urinary infections in men.

Regular voiding flushes the bacteria from the bladder before they can proliferate sufficiently to produce a clinical infection.[2,3] This bacterial washout is important in both males and females; in fact, it is difficult to produce a lower urinary tract infection by direct instillation of organisms into the bladder, because voiding eliminates the bacteria faster than they can divide.[4] When complete washout does not occur with micturition, infection can become established in the residual urine. Boen and Sylvester [3] have established mathematical relationships among urinary frequency, bacterial growth, and residual urine in bladder infections. Pathologic conditions (eg, bladder diverticulum) give rise to residual urine, and elimination of this residual urine is the goal of operations for persistent bacteriuria.

Immunoglobulins, IgG, IgA, and IgM, are found in the urine.[4-6] These antibodies are believed to bind to bacterial surface antigens, so that microbial attachment to bladder epithelial cells is impaired. Bacterial adherence is the first step in invasive infection. IgG is found in higher concentrations in patients with bladder infections than in uninfected people. There is disagreement, however, whether IgG is secreted into the bladder or whether it is actually serum IgG that finds its way into the bladder through the inflamed bladder wall. Tuttle et al [7] found that vaginal IgA was lower in girls with recurrent urinary tract infections than in girls who had no infection. Vaginal IgA may reduce colonization of the vaginal introitis by pathogenic bacteria, thus eliminating the source for an ascending infection.

Parsons et al [8] have shown that the transitional epithelium of the bladder produces a mucopolysaccharide, which forms a thin layer that covers the epithelium and can prevent bacteria from adhering to the bladder epithelium. This bladder surface mucin provides an electrochemical coat on the bladder surface, making it a poor substrate for bacterial adherence and blocking receptor sites.[8]

Although the urine normally has a wide variation in pH—from 4.6 to 8.0 depending on the diet— it is usually acid. The acidity of urine inhibits bacterial growth and makes the electrochemical properties of the mucin more favorable for preventing bacterial adherence. An acid pH is so inhibitory to growth of some bacteria that in many cases *Proteus* and *Pseudomonas* urinary tract infections can be cleared by acidification of the urine alone. In addition, many antibiotics are effective only in an acid medium.

The previous suggestion [9] that an additional antibacterial factor was present in prostatic fluid has not been confirmed.

URINARY TRACT INFECTIONS

Etiology

The same pathogenic organisms are responsible for upper and lower urinary tract infections. Approximately 80 percent of the infections are caused by *E. coli.* Most of the remaining infections are caused by species of *Klebsiella, Enterobacter, Proteus, Pseudomonas,* and rarely, *Serratia.* Gram-positive organisms cause infection occasionally. *Streptococcus fecalis,* staphylococci, and other streptococci are relatively uncommon causes of urinary tract infection.

Pathogenesis

Stamey [10] has divided urinary tract infections into four categories: (1) first infections, (2) unresolved bacteriuria during therapy, (3) bacterial persistence, and (4) reinfections.

The causes for unresolved bacteriuria during therapy are usually selection of inappropriate antibiotic therapy, selection of resistant microbial mutants, and simultaneous infection with two bacterial species that have different antibiotic sensitivities; initial therapy reveals the presence of the second species. Less common causes for unresolved bacteriuria are reinfection with a resistant organism during therapy for the original bacteriuria, diminished renal function which precludes the kidney from excreting the antibiotics in concentrations sufficient to inhibit the organism, and renal calculi in which bacteria are lodged in the matrix of the stone, where the antibiotic cannot reach them.

Bacterial persistence and reinfections make up the group of recurrent urinary infections. Bacterial persistence—recurrence with the same organism from a site within the urinary tract after the urine has been sterile for 5 to 10 days—occurs in many circumstances: two examples are infection (struvite) stones and chronic bacterial prostatitis. Reinfection includes all other urinary tract infections. It is important to realize that the overwhelming majority of patients with urinary tract infections do not have stones or structural abnormalities.

Stamey [11] demonstrated in women with recurrent bacteriuria that the urethra, vagina, and vaginal vestibule are usually colonized by the same pathogenic organisms that caused the urinary tract infection. On the other hand, pathogenic bacteria could not be cultured from the urethra or introitus of most normal females.[12,13] It is clear from Stamey's studies [12,14] that colonization of the vaginal mucosa precedes the bacteriuria.

The urethral and vaginal mucosa are exposed to the same fecal bacteria in women with and without recurrent urinary tract infections, but pathogenic bacteria only colonize the urethra and vagina of women with recurrent bacteriuria. The same organisms that cause cystitis are present in the rectum, as determined by serotyping.[15-17] Urethral colonization and hence urinary tract infection are determined by vaginal bacteria. These findings suggest there is something different about the vagina and vaginal vestibule of women with recurrent bacterial infections that allows them to become colonized and thus leads to urinary tract infections. The difference may be susceptibility of the epithelium to bacterial adherence.[18]

Vaginal antibody (IgA) may play a role in determining colonization of the vaginal vestibule with enteric bacteria. Women who rarely have their vaginal vestibules colonized with enteric bacteria have specific antibody to their own *E. coli,* while women who are susceptible to urinary tract infections (ie, regularly colonized with enteric bacteria) do not.[19] Others, however, have not found any difference in urethral colonization between women with and without recurrent urinary tract infections.[20]

The short female urethra facilitates bladder contamination by urethral and vaginal organisms.[21,22] In addition, vaginal and urethral secretions are milked into the bladder by the penis during sexual intercourse. Hence, cystitis frequently follows sexual intercourse.

Incomplete bladder emptying is the underlying cause for urinary tract infections. Urine is not completely removed from the bladder: (1) when obstruction in present, (2) when there is pelvic relaxation with cystocele, (3) when bladder or urethral diverticula are present, and (4) with abnormal bladder muscle contraction (ie, neurogenic bladder).

Urinary obstruction is the underlying cause for many urinary tract infections. In the male, urethral strictures, benign prostate hyperplasia, carcinoma of the prostate, and bladder neck contractures are all common causes for lower urinary tract obstruction that can lead to infection. Urethral tumors, stones, diverticula, valves, and prostatic abscess are less common causes for obstruction, but all may present as lower urinary tract infection. Meatal stenosis, urethral stenosis, diverticula, and tumors may also be causes for urinary tract obstruction in the female.[23-25] Stones can cause upper and lower urinary tract infections in either sex.

With lower urinary tract obstruction, the bladder detrusor muscle hypertrophies, resulting in bladder wall trabeculation, which may lead to bladder cellule and diverticula formation. These bladder diverticula together with nonfunctioning duplications, and pericalyceal diverticula can cause persistent bacterial infections, because urine collects in these spaces and there is incomplete emptying of the upper and lower urinary tract. Stamey [12] has stressed that sterile residual urine per se does not predispose the patient to bacteriuria. Rather, patients with persistent bacteriuria may not be able to clear the already infected urine without surgical correction of these defects.

Other causes of bacterial persistence curable by operation include vesicoureteral reflux, infection, (struvite) stones, and unilateral pyelonephritic atrophy.[26]

Vesicoureteral reflux is a common cause for recurrent urinary tract infections, especially in children. In these patients, increased vesical pressure with voiding causes urine to reflux up the ureter to the kidney. The ureter gradually dilates, and a large amount of urine may be refluxed into the upper tract with voiding. When the intravesical pressure returns to normal after voiding, the urine drains back into the bladder. The effect of reflux, then, is residual urine.

Many children with recurrent urinary tract infections from vesicoureteral reflux can be managed by administration of long-term antibacterial therapy.[27-29] However, children and adults who break through the infection while on therapy or who show deterioration of renal function should have surgical correction of their reflux.

An interesting finding in both animals and man is that bladder infection may result in distortion of the ureterovesical junction by edema and can cause temporary reflux.[30,31] When the bladder infection subsides, the reflux disappears.

Reflux of infected urine does enable bacteria to reach the kidney. Hence, upper urinary tract infection can occur concomitantly with, or following, an episode of cystitis.

Thus, reflux can predispose to renal scarring and loss of renal function.

Several conditions that affect the ability of the bladder musculature to contract result in a flaccid, large-capacity, poorly emptying bladder. Neurogenic dysfunction of the bladder is a cause for incomplete emptying with voiding. Neurogenic dysfunction may manifest itself by inadequate detrusor contraction or by sphincter-detrusor dysynergia when the external sphincter contracts rather than relaxes with detrusor muscle contraction.

Patients with neurogenic bladder because of spinal cord injury, cerebrovascular accidents, and multiple sclerosis nearly all have persistent bacteriuria. Outlet obstruction by malfunction of the intact urinary sphincters (sphincter dysynergia) is a major cause of urinary retention and infections in these patients. Moreover, they develop problems such as ureterectasis, hydronephrosis, reflux, and renal calculi, which only compound the infection. Sphincterotomy, clean intermittent catheterization, and urinary diversion are all used to help control infection and damage to renal function. Fifty percent of spinal cord injury patients ultimately die from urinary tract complications.

Neurogenic and myogenic dysfunction of the bladder also occurs in patients with diabetes mellitus. After many years of infrequent voiding, the bladder capacity becomes huge, and the detrusor muscle stretches beyond the point where it can effectively contract and empty the bladder. By the time patients with diabetes mellitus develop a neurogenic bladder, they frequently have decreased renal function as well. The decreased renal function results in impaired antibiotic excretion, so the bladder infection is doubly difficult to cure. A similar type of problem is seen in some men who have had long-standing prostatic obstruction and have developed high-capacity, decompensated bladders that fail to empty properly when the obstruction is relieved.

There are several congenital disorders that result in a flaccid, large-capacity, poorly emptying bladder. Meningomyelocele can cause neurogenic dysfunction of the bladder with recurrent bouts of lower urinary tract infections. Congenital megacystis and megaureter are problems similar to Hirschsprung disease of the colon, which results in poor emptying of the bladder and susceptibility to recurrent urinary tract infections. A rare disorder of children called the prune-belly syndrome, characterized by poor development of abdominal wall musculature, results in poor bladder emptying and upper tract dilatation with a propensity to develop urinary tract infections.

Pelvic relaxation in the female, often related to childbirth, results in cystocele formation. Because of the cystocele, these women are unable to empty their bladder completely and are at greater risk for developing cystitis. A similar problem is seen in some men who have had abdominal-perineal resection of the colon, which results in a tipping back of the fundus of the bladder and inability to completely empty the bladder with voiding.[32] However, vesical dysfunction associated with abdominal perineal resection of the colon may also be due to a neurogenic bladder caused by nerve injury from the pelvic surgery.[33]

Catheter-induced infections of the lower urinary tract are very common in spinal cord–injured patients with neurogenic bladders and in other hospitalized patients. Bacteria gain entrance to the bladder through the lumen of the catheter via ascending infection from the collection bag. Microorganisms can also pass upward along the outside of the catheter to the bladder. This type of infection usually begins as a urethritis and then ascends to the bladder, causing cystitis. The catheter is a foreign body that diminishes the ability of the mucosa to eliminate the infection. The catheter therefore promotes infection by its irritative effect on the urethral and bladder mucosa and also serves as a route for bacteria to pass from the urethral meatus into the bladder. In the male, a urethral catheter not only causes urethritis, it may also lead to prostatitis and epididymitis.

Foreign bodies in the lower urinary tract other than catheters also tend to promote persistent infections. The two most common bladder foreign bodies are bladder stones and nonabsorbable suture material inadvertently placed into the bladder lumen by surgeons. Both of these foreign bodies make bladder infections impossible to cure unless they are removed. In the United States, the majority of bladder stones are a result of crystalization of salts from the urine on a chronic indwelling bladder catheter.

Foreign bodies and obstructions are also associated with infections of the upper urinary tract. Stones are the most common foreign bodies in the upper urinary tract. Calcium oxalate, calcium phosphate, and uric acid stones are not primarily associated with urinary tract infections, but they may cause obstruction and lead to infection.

Urea-splitting organisms such as *P. mirabilis*, *P. aeruginosa*, and some *E. coli* cause alkalinization of the urine, which favors precipitation of magnesium, ammonium, and phosphate in a crystal called struvite. Struvite stones may contain calcium deposits as a passive phenomenon and therefore show greater or lesser density on roentgenogram. Bacteria can persist inside these stones and can reinfect the urine even though it is initially sterilized. Such stones are soft and friable and adhere tightly to the mucosa of the renal pelvis, so that total removal is difficult and fragments are often left behind following nephrolithotomy. Small clusters of crystals collect under the mucosa of the renal papillae. These collections, called Randall plaques, may be the nidus for regrowth of stones in some patients.[34,35] Struvite stones can also lead to scarring of the renal parenchyma, which can harbor bacteria and may be resistant to antibiotic therapy because of the poor blood supply.

A second type of foreign body that may cause upper tract infection is a renal papilla that becomes necrotic and separates from the renal parenchyma. Papillary necrosis is seen in patients with diabetes mellitus and in patients with phenacetin abuse nephropathy. In both cases, the papilla often becomes infected when the tissue is devitalized and serves as a source of organisms for recurrent infection. The sloughed papilla may also drop into the ureter and cause obstruction and infection.

There are many causes for obstruction of the upper urinary tract. The more common congenital abnormalities of the kidney and ureter that cause obstruction and predispose to infection are ureteropelvic junction obstruction from external bands, blood vessels, or intrinsic stenosis, ureteral strictures, ectopic ureters, and congenital megaureter with an adynamic segment.

Secondary scarring in the kidney from chronic infection, particularly tuberculosis, can cause infundibular stenosis with obstruction of individual calices. Similarly, chronic infection with tuberculosis can cause ureteral strictures with obstruction of the upper tract. Prior operation on the ureter is a common cause for ureteral stricture and obstruction. Functional obstruction of the upper urinary tract accompanies infection because of poor ureteral peristalsis caused by the effect of bacterial toxins on the ureteral musculature.[36,37]

Pregnancy also predisposes to acute pyelonephritis. The ureters frequently become dilated and tortuous during pregnancy. The changes in the upper urinary tract are thought to be secondary to compression of the ureters in the pelvis by the uterus.

The mechanism for development of chronic pyelonephritis is unclear. Infection followed by scarring followed by poor blood supply to the scarred area with resultant low levels of antibacterial agents in the infected tissue has been thought by many to be the genesis of chronic infection that is resistant to therapy. There is some evidence that chronic pyelonephritis may be, in part, an immune disease with deposition and persistence of bacterial antigens in the tissue following an acute infection and a cellular immune response directed toward these antigens. In fact, killed bacteria injected into the rat kidney can produce a lesion that is histologically indistinguishable from chronic pyelonephritis.[38] There are also studies suggesting that the chronic scarring seen in patients with a long history of upper urinary tract infections results from multiple acute infections rather than a chronic smoldering infection.

Blood-borne bacteria can lead to pyelonephritis, renal abscess, and perinephric abscess. Hematogenous pyelonephritis is usually seen, however, only in patients with severe infections elsewhere who have septicemia. The renal infection occurs as the end stage of the primary infection.

Diseases of the colon and small bowel occasionally include the wall of the bladder, and vesicoenteric fistula can develop. Diverticulitis of the colon and colon cancer are the most common causes for fistula development. Often, these patients are first seen by the surgeon with the problem of a severe urinary tract infection that is resistant to treatment. Pneumaturia is usually present.

Pathology

With acute bacterial cystitis there is hypervascularity of the bladder mucosa with edema and infiltration of polymorphonuclear leukocytes into the submucosa. With progression of the inflammation, a friable hemorrhagic granular surface replaces the mucosa, and it may be covered with shallow focal ulcers. With persistent infection, chronic cystitis develops, mononuclear cells replace neutrophils in the submucosa, and the transitional epithelium may undergo squamous metaplasia. The elasticity of the bladder wall may be compromised by fibrous thickening. Epithelial cysts containing proteinaceous material can protrude into the bladder and can sometimes be seen radiographically, a condition called cystitis cystica. In another special type of chronic cystitis, cystitis follicularis, lymphoid follicles are found in the bladder mucosa and bladder wall.

In acute pyelonephritis, the kidney is enlarged and bulging owing to inflammation and edema. Histologically, there is extensive inflammation and edema in a focal distribution. Microabscesses can form in severe cases of pyelonephritis and cause destruction of surrounding tissue. Lymphocytes and plasma cells, characteristic of chronic pyelonephritis, can also be seen.

Diagnosis

Because urine is normally sterile, any degree of bacteriuria can be important. However, urine collected for culture is usually contaminated with bacteria washed from the introitus in the female and from the urethra of both sexes. Even when a catheter is passed into the bladder to obtain a specimen, urethral bacteria may cling to the catheter and contaminate the specimen. For this reason, the technique of quantitative urine culture was developed.[39-41] Kass[39,41] established that patients with three consecutive cultures with greater than 10^5 organisms per ml of urine have a 95 percent chance of having clinically significant bacteriuria rather than contamination. Kass based his data on a collection of the total voided specimen, however, not a midstream urine collection.

Several factors can affect the quantitative cultures. Frequent voiding from bladder irritation can reduce counts to less than 10,000 bacteria per ml of urine, because the bacteria are washed out at a rate similar to the rate at which they divide. The first voided specimen in the morning is likely to contain many more organisms than other specimens because of increased incubation time in the bladder. Recent or concurrent antibiotic therapy can also reduce the number of bacteria and lead to falsely low bacterial counts.

The technique of cleansing the introitus in the female and the penis in the male and of culturing urine specimens has been discussed in Chapter 12. The collection of urine specimens for culture is difficult because of the possibility of contamination by urethral flora, preputial flora, or vaginal secretions. The problem is more serious in females and children than in adult males. Urine passing through the urethral meatus is easily contaminated by introital bacteria. An alternative is a simple straight catheterization of the bladder following good preparation with antibacterials. The risk of causing an infection by a single catheterization in a female outpatient with a structurally normal urinary tract is less than 1 percent.[42] However, the risk of causing an infection by catheterization in a female outpatient rises sharply if a urinary tract abnormality is present or if the patient is hospitalized. Monzon and others have described the use of suprapubic needle aspiration of the bladder in both adult females and little children, and it is an excellent method for obtaining urine free from contamination.[43,44] Although little risk is associated with the procedure, it is painful and has poor patient acceptance when compared to the usual methods of urine collection. With a urine specimen obtained by suprapubic needle aspiration, 10^2 to 10^3 bacteria per ml should be considered significant of infection.

Microscopic examination of the urine is also useful. The specimen is centrifuged, and the sediment is examined under high dry power for white blood cells and bacteria. The sediment can be stained with methylene blue or Gram stain. In most patients, more than 3 to 5 polymorphonuclear cells per high power field is considered clinically significant. White blood cell casts are occasionally seen in patients with pyelonephritis and are helpful in establishing that diagnosis. There are a number of other causes for urinary tract inflammation that can cause pyuria with no associated infection. Red blood cells are also usually found with urinary tract infections.

The presence of bacteria in the sediment of catheter-collected urine in the female or midstream clean-catch urine in the male is highly suggestive of urinary tract infection. However, the absence of bacteria in the sediment has little diagnostic significance, because greater than 30,000 bacteria per ml of urine are required before they can be detected in a centrifuged specimen.[45]

Localization Techniques. Localization of infection to the upper or lower urinary tract or to one kidney or the other requires cystoscopy and bilateral ureteral catheterization by a method standardized by Stamey.[46] The validity of this technique depends on reducing the number of bacteria from the bladder that contaminate the ureteral catheters as they pass through the bladder into the ureteral orifices. Therefore, the bladder is thoroughly irrigated with sterile saline before the ureteral catheters are passed into the bladder. Multiple quantitative urine cultures are obtained before and after washout, and four serial cultures are obtained from each kidney individually through the ureteral catheters.[12,46]

Aspiration of urine through the renal parenchyma from a hydronephrotic kidney is also a useful technique to help localize infection in a patient with an obstructed upper urinary tract. Aspiration is best carried out using a 21-gauge spinal needle, which is passed into the kidney just below the 12th rib in the costovertebral angle.

Sequential urine specimens can be obtained in men to help localize the site of infection [47] After the penis is cleansed, the first 200 ml of urine is collected from the full bladder and a second culture tube is inserted into the stream for collection of the midstream specimen. The patient is told to stop voiding, and the physician massages the prostate. The few drops of prostatic fluid are collected in a separate container, the patient voids again, and the third specimen is collected. Quantitative urine cultures are then done. When the colony counts of the first (urethral) specimen significantly exceed the counts of the prostatic specimens, the diagnosis is urethral colonization or urethritis. When the colony counts of the prostatic specimens significantly exceed the urethral specimens, the diagnosis is prostatic infection. If the midstream specimen has significant colony counts, the site cannot be localized, because all specimens will show heavy growth.

Several investigators have described an immunofluorescence method to detect gammaglobulin (antibody) on the surface of bacteria as an indication of upper urinary tract infection.[48,49] Bacteria from the upper urinary tract are thought to be coated with gammaglobulin, whereas bacteria from the bladder are not coated. Despite its early promise, this technique is far less precise in localizing infection than are catheterization studies.

Indications for X-Ray Studies. The vast majority of urinary tract infections in women are not associated with underlying pathologic conditions of the upper or lower urinary tracts. Intravenous pyelograms should therefore be obtained only in women who have recurrent urinary tract infections. Intravenous pyelograms are of almost no value in the 99 percent of women with primary infections. In contrast, excretory urography should be obtained in men who have urinary tract infections because the likelihood of finding a significant structural abnormality (bladder stones, diverticula, urethral strictures, or upper tract abnormalities) is quite high.

Winberg [27] has outlined the indications for intravenous pyelography in children with apparent first infections (Table 45-1). Children of all ages and both sexes with a history of recurrent infections, who have not been examined earlier, should have intravenous pyelography and voiding cystourethography. The frequency of obstruction is higher in children than in adults—5 to 10 percent in boys and 1 to 2 percent in girls.

Clinical Manifestations

The clinical manifestations of urinary tract infection varies depending on whether it involves the upper or lower tract and whether the patient is an adult or a child.

Cystitis. Acute bacterial cystitis is usually accompanied by urinary frequency and urgency, dysuria, nocturia,

TABLE 45-1. INDICATIONS FOR RADIOLOGY IN APPARENT FIRST INFECTIONS IN CHILDREN

1. All infants and toddlers with symptomatic infections.
2. All boys with symptomatic infections, regardless of age.
3. All patients with screening bacteriuria.
4. When a mass is seen or palpated over the symphysis after micturition, indicating incomplete bladder emptying.
5. When a mass is palpated in the upper part of the abdomen, indicating hydronephrosis.
6. When blood urea nitrogen or serum creatinine is increased or concentrating capacity is persistently lowered.
7. When blood pressure is increased.
8. When an infection fails to resolve in spite of administration of an adequate antibiotic.
9. In all other patients, the experience of the doctor and the investigative facilities should be deciding factors.

From Winberg, J: Urinary tract infections in infants and children. In Harrison JH, Gittes RF, Perlmutter AD, Stamey TA, Walsh RC: *Urology,* 4th ed. Philadelphia, Saunders, 1978, Vol 1, p 485.

suprapubic discomfort, and low back pain. Gross hematuria occurs occasionally, but chills, fever, and flank pain are usually absent. With chronic bladder infections, the patient may be totally asymptomatic. If pneumaturia is present, a vesicovaginal or vesicoenteric fistula should be sought.

In children, the symptoms are influenced by age, sex, and presence of anatomic disorders of the urinary tract.[27] In the neonatal period, infections are manifested by weight loss, fever, feeding difficulties, and sluggishness. In older children frequency, dysuria, enuresis, urgency, abdominal discomfort, and flank pain can all be noted.

Pyelonephritis. The hallmarks of acute pyelonephritis are aching pain in the lumbar region, fever, and shaking chills. There may also be nausea, vomiting, and diarrhea. Dysuria, frequency, urgency, and malaise are also common. The most prominent sign on physical examination is tenderness on deep pressure over one or both costovertebral areas or on bimanual palpation of the kidney region. Occasionally, this sign is absent. Patients with acute pyelonephritis usually have a polymorphonuclear leukocytosis, whereas those with cystitis do not.

Patients with chronic pyelonephritis frequently come to the physician's attention because of renal failure or hypertension. Urography shows broad scars of the renal parenchyma with blunting of the corresponding calyx and papilla. Only in retrospect is there a history of bouts of pyelonephritis, and even this history is sometimes not obtained. The symptoms are frequently those of renal failure—fatigue and lassitude associated with anemia—rather than of bacterial infection.

Treatment

Treatment of bacterial cystitis is with an appropriate antibacterial, determined by microbiologic sensitivity testing. Pending results of sensitivity testing, a low-cost antibacterial drug, such as sulfisoxasole, that is effective against the commonly found enteric bacteria should be used. Sulfisoxasole should be given for about 10 days. The drug should be changed if the infecting bacteria are not sensitive to it. Pyridium, 100 mg twice a day, will help dysuria, but it should not be given for more than 3 days because of potential bone marrow toxicity. In addition to sulfonamides, other suitable first choice antibacterial agents are nitrofurantoin, nalidixic acid, and ampicillin. All should be used for approximately 10 days.

Chronic low-dose antibiotic prophylaxis in women with repeated bouts of lower urinary tract infections will diminish the frequency of infections and may help to prevent pyelonephritis. Appropriate antibacterials for suppression are sulfisoxasole, nitrofurantoin, and methenamine. More potent antibiotics should not be used for long-term prophylaxis, because they can cause emergence of resistant strains. Even the antibacterials can cause emergence of resistant fecal flora, because they are all taken orally and it is the fecal flora that is the source of the recurrent bacteriuria.

Patients with neurogenic bladder due to spinal cord injury, cerebrovascular accidents, multiple sclerosis, and diabetes mellitus may have indwelling urethral catheters for incontinence or to prevent urinary retention due to functional outlet obstruction caused by malfunction of the urinary sphincter. Clean intermittent catheterization four to six times daily to empty the bladder is a more effective method of preventing severe cystitis.[50] Bacteriuria is virtually unavoidable, however. Functional outlet obstruction due to malfunction of the internal sphincter can be remedied by internal sphincterotomy.

Operation can be effective in eliminating the cause for bacterial persistence. Infected stones can be removed from the urinary tract. Congenital and acquired abnormalities of the upper and lower urinary tract may be the cause for recurrent urinary tract infections and may require surgical correction. Causes of obstruction can be relieved: meatotomy for meatal stenosis, dilatation for urethral stricture, transurethral resection for prostatic hypertrophy, and transurethral resection of urethral valves.

Management of vesicoureteral reflux is still controversial. In children, there is a great tendency for reflux to disappear spontaneously.[51] Patients with recurrent infections should have long-term antibacterial prophylaxis. They should have the urine cultured periodically, and renal function should also be determined. Renal growth should be followed with isotope studies. So long as renal growth is normal and there is no breakthrough infection while the child is on antibacterial drugs, conservative management is appropriate. If renal growth is impaired or there is functional deterioration or the infection is not successfully controlled, operative repair should be performed. Loss of the intravesical urethral tunnel with a golf hole orifice and reflux to the kidney is an indication for corrective operation regardless of the bacteriologic status. Urologic surgeons generally agree that surgical correction should also be undertaken if there is progressive dilatation of the renal pelvis and minor calices.

INFECTIONS OF THE URETHRA

Urethritis in the male is a frequently encountered problem that requires surgical therapy only for its complications. *N. gonorrhoeae* causes a sexually transmitted disease that infects Cowper urethral glands and leads to acute urethritis with thick yellow purulent discharge from the urethra. It is surgically important for the complications it causes—urethral strictures. The microbiology of *N. gonorrhoeae* and gonorrhea in women have been discussed in Chapters 4 and 44. The most common sexually transmitted disease is now nongonococcal urethritis, also known as nonspecific urethritis.

GONORRHEA

Epidemiology and Incidence

There are now over 1 million cases per year in the United States (Fig. 45-1). In 1978, 598,000 cases of gonorrhea were reported in men and 416,000 cases occurred in women.[52]

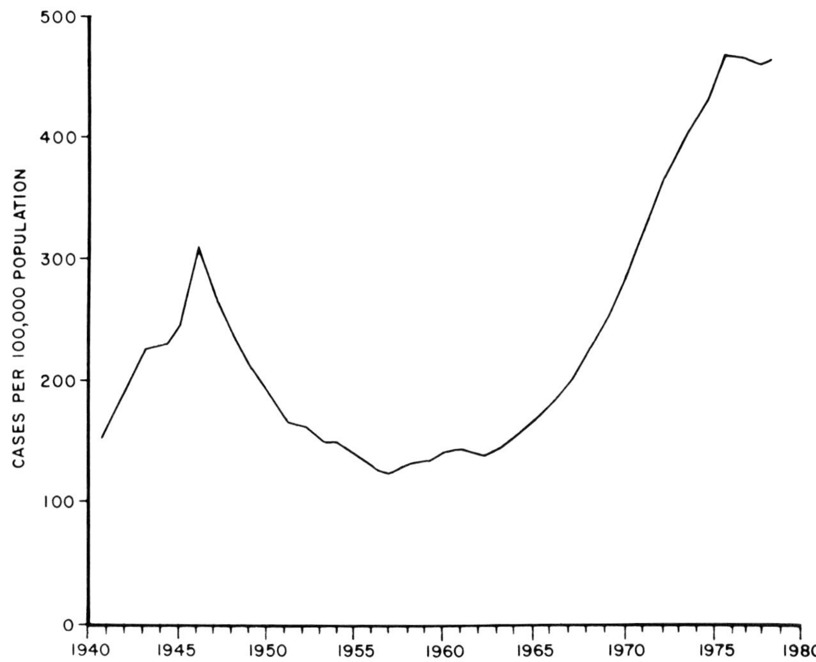

Fig. 45-1. **Reported cases of gonorrhea in the civilian population in the United States. (From *MMWR* 27:26, 1979.)**

In fact, the number of cases was probably a good deal greater, since many cases are not reported. The incidence of gonorrhea has increased markedly in the past 20 years. This increase is believed to be due to changing sexual mores and a decrease in the use of the condom, diaphragm, and vaginal spermicides, brought about in part by the widespread use of oral contraceptives. The incidence of gonorrhea in the United States is estimated to be three to ten times higher than in England because of the failure to trace and treat infected contacts. The highest incidence of gonorrhea occurs between 20 and 24 years of age.

Asymptomatic female carriers have long been known to be potential sources of spread. Handsfield et al [53] have now shown that men, too, can be asymptomatic carriers. The carrier rate is low, however, and more than 95 percent of men who become infected develop symptoms. Nevertheless, the males who remain asymptomatic or who ignore their symptoms become a reservoir of gonorrhea and can spread the infection to women. Handsfield et al [53] found that two thirds of the men with asymptomatic gonorrhea remained asymptomatic carriers for as long as 165 days if treatment was withheld.

Pathogenesis and Pathology

The gonococcus first adheres to the urethral epithelial cells by the pili on the bacterial cells. The bacteria then penetrate the interepithelial spaces to reach the subepithelial connective tissue. An intense inflammatory reaction develops, with extensive exudate and abundant polymorphonuclear leukocytes. The overlying epithelium may be destroyed. The inflammatory reaction gives rise to the characteristic purulent discharge.

The bacteria and neutrophils accumulate in the mucosal infoldings and in the periurethral glands of Littré. In these mucous glands, the detritis of the infection tends to plug the ducts, resulting in microabscesses. The infection may then extend to the corpus spongiosum. Lymphangitis and thrombophlebitis can result in extensive edema of the penis.

Gonococci can be demonstrated in prostatic secretions,[54] but infection of the prostate and seminal vesicles is rare. The infection can spread into the epididymus, however, through the vas deferens. Most infections are unilateral, but if both glands are involved the rate of infertility is high. The epididymus is involved in approximately 2 percent of cases of gonorrhea.[55]

Stricture of the urethra is due to periurethral inflammation deep to the urethral mucosa, which results in fibrosis in the corpus spongiosum and surrounding fascial sheaths. Infection of the periurethral glands of Littré leads to stricture, because of the cicatricial deformities that occur in the surrounding tissues in the natural course of healing.

In homosexual men, similar pathologic changes can also be seen in the pharynx and anal canal. Pharyngeal infection is found in 5 to 10 percent of cases in heterosexual men, however, probably the result of cunnilingus. Disseminated gonococcal infection occurs in approximately 1 percent of men with gonorrhea.[56]

Clinical Manifestations

The incubation period is 3 to 4 days, though it can be as long as 14 days. The patient usually has a purulent urethral discharge and symptoms of dysuria, urinary frequency, and meatal erythema. Because most symptomatic men seek prompt medical attention, the disease is usually promptly arrested. Men who do not develop symptoms and those who ignore their symptoms are at risk for developing complications. With the advent of effective chemotherapy, epididymitis, prostatitis, edema of the penis from dorsal lymphangitis or thrombophlebitis, inflammation of the corpus spongiosum, paraurethral abscess or fistula, infection of Cowper glands, and seminal vesiculitis are much less common.

Anorectal gonococcal infection causes rectal pain, tenesmus, mucopurulent rectal discharge, and rectal bleeding. Systemic gonococcal infection produces fever; arthralgia; petechial, pustular, and hemorrhagic skin lesions; and tenosynovitis. The infection may cause endocarditis, meningitis, myocarditis, and hepatitis.

Diagnosis

Goncoccal urethritis must be differentiated from nongonococcal urethritis because treatment, prognosis, and management of sex partners differs for various types of urethritis. The techniques for specimen collection, staining, and culture are discussed in Chapter 12.

Treatment

The preferred drugs for the treatment of gonococcal infection are penicillin G, ampicillin or amoxicillin, tetracycline, or spectinomycin. The preferred treatment is aqueous procaine penicillin G, 4.8 million units given in two equal portions intramuscularly in two sites at one visit. Probenecid, 1 gm orally, is also given as a single dose. This therapy is also adequate treatment for incubating syphilis. Spectinomycin, 2 gm intramuscularly as a single dose, or tetracycline, 30 mg per kg per day orally four times a day for 4 days, are alternate regimens if the patient is allergic to penicillin.

Postgonococcal Urethritis

One-fourth to two-thirds of men develop a mild form of urethritis, termed postgonococcal urethritis,[57] 1 to 3 weeks after treatment for gonorrhea. In about half the cases, *C. trachomatis* is responsible. The cause in the other half is unknown. Probably the gonorrhea and chlamydial infection were obtained together, but the incubation period for the *Chlamydia* is longer or antibiotic therapy may have eradicated the gonorrhea but only suppressed the chlamydiae.

URETHRAL STRICTURE AND ITS COMPLICATIONS

Urethral strictures can be a complication of gonococcal urethral infection as well as of trauma from indwelling catheters or urethral instrumentation. Dysuria, urgency, frequency, persistent urinary tract infections, alteration of the force, diameter, and appearance of the stream, and a split, narrowed, or dribbled flow of urine can all be due to urethral stricture. Strictures are occasionally discovered in asymptomatic patients when passage of a catheter is attempted. The diagnosis of stricture is established by cystoscopy, urethrography,[58] and calibration by bougie à boule.

Treatment depends on location, severity, age, and health of the patient. Strictures in nursing home patients, for instance, who require intermittent or continuous catheter drainage, are best managed by suprapubic cystostomy. In other patients, the initial treatment of strictures is dilatation. The stricture should be dilated without causing urethral tears, which in turn can lead to more scar formation and further narrowing. After the initial dilatation, progressive dilatation should be carried out within 3 to 5 days. Dilatation may then be performed weekly or biweekly until a 28 or 30 French sound may be passed easily. Dilatation can then be performed less frequently—once every 6 months. But dilatation may be required for life. If the stricture recurs or becomes resistant to dilatation, a number of surgical procedures can be performed: internal or external urethrotomy,[59,60] stricture excision with urethral reapproximation, patch-graft urethroplasty, and marsupialization with or without later reconstruction can all be performed.[59–64] If a stricture recurs quickly after dilatation, biopsy should be performed to rule out carcinoma. Chronic inflammation associated with urethral strictures can also lead to malignant degeneration and squamous cell carcinoma.

Urethral Diverticulum and Periurethral Abscess

Urethral diverticulum and periurethral abscess in the male are a complication of strictures and their treatment. Diverticula may be formed by infection behind the stricture or by traumatic urethral dilatations. Spinal cord injury patients develop diverticula and strictures as a result of applying condom catheters too tightly around the penis and causing compression and erosion of the penis and urethra. Urethral diverticula usually drain poorly and often become infected. Diagnosis is made by urethrography and cystoscopy. They should be resected and the associated urethral stricture repaired.[64]

Infected diverticula or infected periurethral glands may form periurethral abscesses. Infected urethral carcinoma may present as a periurethral abscess and should be looked for in any patient with the recent onset of stricture.

Periurethral abscesses present with fever and a fluctuant mass. They may rupture spontaneously or require incision and drainage. A urethrocutaneous fistula often forms after incision and drainage or spontaneous rupture. Adequate drainage and debridement are essential. Left undrained, the abscess may spread to involve the scrotum and lower abdominal wall. Frequently, suprapubic cystostomy will aid in local care by diverting urine from the wound. Extensive periurethral abscesses and urethrocutaneous fistulas in the bulbous urethra lead to the "watering pot perineum." Surgical repair of the causative strictures should be delayed until healing of the acute abscess has occurred.

Nongonococcal (Nonspecific) Urethritis

Etiology and Epidemiology

The most common sexually transmitted disease is now nongonococcal urethritis. Thirty to 50 percent of the cases are caused by *C. trachomatis*[65] (Chapter 7). Two genital mycoplasmas, *Ureaplasma urealyticum* and *Mycoplasma hominis*, may also cause nonspecific urethritis,[66,67] although their real importance as etiologic agents has been debated for years.

Nongonococcal urethritis occurs in the same age group as gonorrhea. Men with the disease are more likely to be Caucasian, in a higher socioeconomic group, better educated, and to have fewer sexual partners than men with gonorrhea.[68]

Clinical Manifestations and Diagnosis

The urethral discharge in nongonococcal urethritis is clear and watery, and the disease frequently causes only minor symptoms of mild dysuria, perineal ache, urinary frequency, premature ejaculation, and pain on ejaculation. Urethral stricture does not occur. The most serious sequela is Reiter syndrome, which consists of nongonococcal urethritis associated with ocular, arthritic, and dermatologic findings. Symptoms usually appear 1 to 4 weeks after onset of urethritis, but they occur in less than 1 percent of patients. The incubation period is approximately 14 days. The ocular manifestations vary from the usual mild transient conjunctivitis to anterior uveitis that may lead to blindness. The arthritis characteristically affects the large joints of the legs, achilles tendons, plantar fascia, and sacroiliac joints. The arthritis usually remits after several months, although permanent disability can occur. Recurrences are common. The skin lesions are distinctive; balanitis circinata, well-demarcated erythematous erosions surrounded by a light border, occur on the glans penis in up to 80 percent of cases. Hyperkeratotic lesions occur on the soles of the feet and occasionally on the hands. Small superficial ulcers may also occur on the palate, oral mucosa, and tongue.

Nongonococcal urethritis is important because of its frequency and the need to distinguish it from gonorrhea, prostatitis, and cystitis. The diagnosis is usually made by clinical features characteristic of the urethral discharge and failure to demonstrate gonococci by Gram stain or culture. *C. trachomatis* can be cultured if special techniques are used.[69]

Treatment

Tetracycline, 500 mg four times daily for 14 to 21 days, should be used for nongonococcal urethritis caused by *C. trachomatis*. Relapses are common: 17 percent of *Chlamydia*-positive and 47 percent of *Chlamydia*-negative patients recurred.[70] For patients who recur after tetracycline therapy, trimethoprim-sulfamethoxasole is the second-choice antimicrobial. Erythromycin, 500 mg four times daily for 7 days, is also active against *C. trachomatis* and is moderately active against *U. urealyticum*.

URETHRITIS ASSOCIATED WITH INDWELLING CATHETERS

A urethral catheter or urethral foreign body not only perpetuates infection by its irritative effect may also obstruct periurethral glands leading to periurethral infection. A thick yellow discharge from around a long-term indwelling urethral catheter is indicative of severe urethral infection. All urethral catheters left for more than a few days will have some associated mild urethritis. A thick yellow urethral discharge in the absence of a urethral catheter should make one think of gonorrhea, a foreign body, or a urethral cancer.

The patient with bacterial urethritis usually complains of urethral pain around the catheter. If the infection is not cleared quickly, the patient will likely develop a urethral stricture some time after the catheter is removed. Proper treatment is removal of the catheter to facilitate urethral drainage. Most often, bladder drainage will still be necessary, so a suprapubic catheter should be placed by either operative or percutaneous techniques. The urethral infections caused by catheters are usually mixed, with gram-negative organisms predominating, so that a broad-spectrum antibiotic should be given. Complications of urethral infections are stricture and periurethral abscess.

Catheter-induced urethritis can be reduced in incidence and severity by proper catheter care.[71] Cleansing around the meatus and removing the crusts or normal urethral secretions should be followed by application of an antibacterial ointment around the meatus. The choice of size and material of the urethral catheter will also bear on the frequency and severity of urethral infections.[71] Large-bore catheters obstruct free urethral drainage of secretions and should be avoided in routine use. There are advocates of cutting side holes in the urethral catheters to allow urethral secretion drainage.[48] Teflon-coated or silastic catheters cause less foreign body reaction than latex catheters.

INFECTIONS OF THE PROSTATE

ACUTE PROSTATITIS

Etiology and Pathology

Prostatic infections may be caused by almost any bacterial agent. The gram-negative organisms *E. coli*, *Proteus*, *Klebsiella*, *Enterobacter*, and *Pseudomonas* predominate in acute and chronic bacterial prostatic infection. The gram-positive organisms *S. epidermidis*, alpha-hemolytic *Streptococcus*, enterococci, and diphtheroids are often thought of as normal flora in the distal urethra but in fact can cause chronic prostatitis.[72] Infection of the prostate and urethra of young men by sexually transmitted *C. trachomatis*, *U. urealyticum*, or *M. hominis* is very common and has been discussed under infections of the urethra. Parasitic infections of the prostate do occur, but only *T. vaginalis* is a significant problem in the United States and Canada. Tuberculosis of the prostate occurs when mycobacteria invade the prostate from upper urinary tract infection. Rarely, tuberculosis prostatitis may occur as a sexually transmitted ascending infection.

Infections of the prostate are caused primarily by infectious agents ascending the urethra, entering the prostatic ducts, and proliferating within the prostatic acini, causing marked inflammation in part or all of the prostate gland.

Infection in the urine may also enter the prostatic ducts during voiding, particularly if there is urethral obstruction distal to the prostate causing high voiding pressures within the prostatic urethra. An intraurethral catheter provides an ingress for bacterial contamination and is also a foreign body that tends to promote inflammation and infection. Prostatic calculi and inspissated concretions may also act as foreign bodies to perpetuate infections.

Histologically, acute bacterial prostatitis shows polymorphonuclear leukocytes within and around prostatic acini and diffuse edema and hyperemia of the stroma. Small abscesses are common. Chronic infections are nonspecific with varying degrees of focal lymphocyte, plasma cell, and macrophage infiltration.

Clinical Manifestations

Acute bacterial prostatitis presents with sudden onset of moderate to high fever and chills. Symptoms are varied and nonspecific. Urinary symptoms include frequency, urgency, dysuria, decreased urinary flow rate, intermittency and spraying, a sensation of incomplete bladder emptying, and occasionally total urinary retention. Local prostatic tenderness such as pain at the end of voiding, pain on defecation or rectal examination, pain on ejaculation, and a perineal ache are also common. Pain is frequently referred to the tip of the penis and diffusely to the low back. Sexual dysfunction occurs with decreased turgidity of erections and premature ejaculation. Alterations in prostate secretions can lead to purulent discharge, initial or terminal hematuria, and hematospermia.

Rectal examination discloses a tender, edematous prostate that is indurated and warm to the touch. The expressed prostatic secretions contain numerous leukocytes, oval fat bodies, and bacteria. The prostate should not be examined too vigorously, because bacteremia may occur. Therefore, the prostate should not be massaged unless the patient is being treated with appropriate antibiotics. Bacterial endocarditis and brain abscess have occurred after bacteremia of prostatic origin. Manipulation or instrumentation can also cause retrograde movement of bacteria up the vasa deferentia, leading to epididymitis.

The laboratory assessment of acute bacterial prostatitis should include a white blood cell count, which is usually elevated. Urine specimens and expressed prostatic specimens should be cultured. Patients with acute bacterial prostatitis usually have ascending bacterial cystitis. Semen cultures may be even more accurate than expressed secretion cultures in establishing the diagnosis of bacterial prostatitis.[73] A saline mount of the prostatic fluid should be examined for *T. vaginalis.*

The irritative voiding symptoms caused by prostatic infection can be mimicked by carcinoma in situ of the bladder, a serious disease that can be cured if detected early. Patients should have urine cytologies performed for irritative voiding symptoms if infection is not present, and then undergo cystoscopy. Infections in the prostate, including tuberculosis, can lead to formation of a palpable nodule. Biopsy of these nodules is mandatory to rule out carcinoma of the prostate in patients over 40 years old.

Treatment

Treatment of acute bacterial prostatitis consists of hospitalization, bed rest, and antimicrobial therapy. The correct approach to therapy of prostatic infections depends more on physiology than on the infectious agents. Prostatic fluid has a pH of 7.3, and this fluid becomes more alkaline (pH 8.3) with infections.[74,75] This means that only a few antibiotics like trimethoprim-sulfamethoxazole and erythromycin are effective in prostatic fluid. Trimethoprim-sulfamethoxazole is the drug of choice for gram-negative infections, and erythromycin is useful for treating gram-positive infections. Antibiotics must also be lipid soluble to be effective in the prostate. The normal prostate appears to have a barrier to the diffusion of antibiotics similar to the blood-brain barrier. But as in meningitis, this barrier to antibiotics is broken down by the inflammatory response. If trimethoprim-sulfamethoxazole cannot be taken, aminoglycosides, cephalosporins, and ampicillin are all effective. After 1 week of parenteral antibiotics, oral antimicrobial therapy should be continued for an additional 3 weeks to guard against the development of chronic prostatitis.

Supportive measures such as hydration, analgesics, antipyretics, and stool softeners should also be used. Urethral catheters should be removed, and if the patient requires urinary drainage, a suprapubic catheter should be placed surgically or percutaneously.

CHRONIC PROSTATITIS

The clinical manifestations of chronic prostatitis vary widely. Although chronic prostatitis may follow acute prostatitis, most patients have no history of acute prostatitis.

Most patients have irritative voiding symptoms such as dysuria, urinary frequency and urgency, and nocturia. Low back pain, perineal discomfort, and painful ejaculation can also be found. Physical examination is frequently normal unless benign prostatic hyperplasia is also present.

Recurrent bacteriuria is the hallmark of chronic bacterial prostatitis. Antibacterial therapy frequently sterilizes the urine, but because most antimicrobial agents do not enter the prostatic fluid, the prostatitis continues and the bacteriuria recurs when therapy is stopped.

Chronic bacterial prostatitis is difficult to cure with antimicrobial agents, probably because they do not diffuse from the plasma to the prostatic tissue and fluid. The prostatitis can be kept under control with long-term suppressive antibacterial therapy. With this regimen, most patients remain relatively asymptomatic. Discontinuing the antibacterial therapy, even after months or years, may cause reinfection of the bladder urine and recurrence of symptoms.

Total prostatectomy offers the most definitive cure for patients with debilitating symptoms. Transurethral resection of the prostate can be curative if all infected tissue is removed. In a small series, Meares[47] cured only one-third of the patients. None of the patients who were not cured were made worse. In chronic prostatitis, however, transurethral resection of the prostate can make the patient's irritative voiding symptoms worse.

PROSTATIC ABSCESS

Occasionally, acute or chronic prostatitis may result in prostatic abscess. These abscesses are most often found in men 50 to 70 years old and in patients with diabetes mellitus. Transrectal needle biopsy of the prostate can also lead to abscess formation. Symptoms include acute urinary retention, frequency, dysuria, fever, epididymo-orchitis, and rectal discomfort. The gland is enlarged, tender, and fluctuant. The abscess may spontaneously rupture and drain intraurethrally, or it may require endoscopic transurethral incision or perineal incision for drainage. Appropriate antimicrobial therapy should also be given. Abscesses usually leave no sequelae and usually do not recur.

INFECTIONS OF THE SEMINAL VESICLES, VAS DEFERNS, AND SPERMATIC CORD

Infections of the seminal vesicles, vas deferens, and spermatic cord (funiculitis) rarely, if ever, occur alone; rather, they are almost always a part of infection elsewhere in the genital tract. Up to 80 percent of cases of prostatitis are accompanied by seminal vesiculitis.[76] Seminal vesiculitis without prostatitis is rare. Therapy is treatment of the primary disease.

EPIDIDYMITIS

Etiology and Pathogenesis

Epididymitis is a disease of adults and only rarely affects the prepubertal child. An indwelling urethral catheter is often the cause for urethritis and subsequent epididymitis.[77] It is usually caused by retrograde passage of bacteria from the prostatic urethra up the vas deferens. Many different organisms can cause epididymitis. In men under 35 years old, *C. trachomatis* is the most common organism.[78] In older men, enteric bacteria, staphylococci, and occasionally streptococci predominate. In patients with long-term indwelling urethral catheters, unusual bacteria such as *S. marcescens* may cause epididymitis under the influence of chronic antibiotic therapy. Epididymitis may also be due to syphilis, gonorrhea, tuberculosis, and trauma. Spinal cord injury patients and older disoriented men are occasionally found lying on their testes, which may cause epididymitis. Nursing staffs should be instructed in the proper protection of the testes in such patients.

Clinical Manifestations

The epididymis is enlarged and extremely tender. Severe infections present with fever and systemic symptoms of toxicity. With rapid progression, suppuration, abscess formation, and extension into the testicle may occur. Fluctuance is found with abscess formation. The prostate gland is also usually tender. Often, a reactive hydrocele will be present, making examination of the epididymis and testis difficult. Aspiration of the hydrocele may be of help in examining the patient. Infiltration of the spermatic cord with 1 percent xylocaine will reduce pain and allow better examination of the epididymis and testis. In chronic epididymitis, tenderness may be mild, and the epididymis may only be indurated and slightly enlarged.

Urine culture should be obtained before treatment to obtain a bacteriologic diagnosis. If there is doubt about the diagnosis or if epididymitis does not promptly resolve, inguinal exploration of the testis should be performed because of the possibility of testicular cancer. Torsion of the testis occurs in young males up to age 30. Here also, the distinction between epididymitis and torsion is difficult. Early exploration will resolve any diagnostic questions and save the testis.

Treatment

Treatment consists of systemic antibiotic therapy and scrotal support. Milder cases of epididymitis are treated by tetracycline or ampicillin until urine culture results are available. Aminoglycosides should be used in severe infections. In addition to antibiotic therapy, bed rest and scrotal elevation are very important in the treatment of acute epididymitis. The patient should be placed at bed rest and folded bath towels placed under the scrotum. Alternatively, a wide band of tape can be placed across the upper thigh to provide scrotal elevation. Anti-inflammatory agents like phenylbutazone may help if given early. Injection of the spermatic cord with 1 percent xylocaine yields immediate and frequent long-term pain relief. Walking while wearing a scrotal supporter is permissible after the pain and swelling have subsided, but lifting and manual labor should be avoided for 2 to 6 weeks. If an abscess forms, surgical drainage is required.

Chronic epididymitis is an annoying and painful condition. Patients with chronic epididymitis are liable to recurrent acute attacks, especially if there is infection of the prostate and seminal vesicles that cannot be eradicated. Epididymectomy is the procedure of choice. It results in sterility, but sterility is an almost inevitable consequence anyway.

INFECTIONS OF THE TESTIS (ORCHITIS)

Infections of the testis are rare and are usually caused by systemic viral infections, most notably mumps. The rich blood and lymphatic supply of the testis give it a high degree of resistance to bacteria.

The testis is covered with a thick, fibrous layer, the tunica albuginia, which is resistant to penetration by infection. Infections elsewhere in the body can spread via the bloodstream to the testicle, but most commonly infection occurs by direct extension from severe epididymitis to involve the testis producing epididymo-orchitis.

Etiology and Pathology

Any of the pyogenic or enteric organisms that cause epididymitis can cause orchitis: *Staphylococcus, Streptococcus, E. coli, K. pneumoniae, P. aeruginosa,* and so forth. In this form of orchitis, the testicle is swollen and tense and has many punctate hemorrhages on its surface. Multiple foci of necrosis may be found. Suppuration may progress to involve the entire gland.

Mumps orchitis is rare before puberty and occurs 4 to 6 days after mumps parotitis. Approximately 5 to 10 percent of adult males with mumps parotitis develop orchitis. The orchitis is unilateral in about 70 percent of cases and results in some degree of testicular atrophy.[79] The epididymis may also be involved, and sterility can result.

In rare instances, orchitis can occur with virtually any systemic infection including viral, fungal, rickettsial, bacterial, protozoal, and helminthic infections.

Clinical Manifestations

Acute pyogenic infection usually begins with chills and fever and sudden pain in the involved testicle. The pain radiates to the inguinal canal and is usually accompanied by nausea and vomiting. The involved testicle is swollen, tense, and extremely tender. There is usually acute hydrocele. If suppuration involves the entire gland, it becomes fluctuant. Testicular pain will often cause cremasteric contraction, drawing the testis high up in the scrotum where it is difficult to examine. The spermatic cord can be infiltrated with 1 percent xylocaine, which will reduce the pain and permit better examination of the testis.

Treatment

The patient is treated with bed rest, scrotal elevation, and antibacterial therapy. Bed rest, scrotal elevation, and warm or cold compresses provide symptomatic relief. Broad-spectrum antibiotic therapy should be initiated until the specific causative agent can be identified by Gram stain or culture of urine or aspirated material. With prompt institution of antibacterial therapy, there is less suppuration. Orchiectomy is usually required for testicular abscess. In any case, atrophy and fibrosis frequently cause sterility in orchitis from any cause.

Specific immunoglobulin or plasma can reduce the incidence of mumps orchitis 75 percent if given early after the onset of parotitis.[80,81] Steroids or ACTH have been reported to reduce testicular pain and swelling in men with mumps orchitis and reduce the incidence of orchitis if given prophylactically. Their efficacy has not been proved in controlled trials.[82]

INFECTIONS OF THE PENIS

Most acute inflammatory lesions on the surface of the penis are due to sexually transmitted diseases. These infections are usually self-limited and easily treated if prompt attention is sought. These diseases must be differentiated from other noninfectious diseases and malignant diseases.

SYPHILIS

Etiology and Epidemiology

The etiologic agent of syphilis, *T. pallidum* has been discussed in Chapter 7. Syphilis occurs most commonly in the sexually active years between 15 and 39 years of age, with the highest incidence in both men and women between 20 and 24. Between 25 and 73 percent of new cases occur in male homosexuals. In 1978, 21,656 cases of primary and secondary syphilis were reported in the United States.[52] Many more were probably unreported. The number of new cases reached a peak during World War II. The number of reported cases steadily declined until 1959 but increased dramatically between 1959 and 1965. There has been a slow, but steady increase since then. Surgeons are at risk from nicks and abrasions incurred during operations on patients with active syphilis. A VDRL test should be performed on all patients before operation and treatment instituted prior to operation if possible.

Pathogenesis and Pathology

T. pallidum enters the body through the intact mucous membranes, via tiny abrasions of the epithelium, and possibly through the unbroken skin by way of the hair follicles. The treponemal organisms replicate slowly after entry in the moist anaerobic conditions and cause a chancre to develop in 10 to 90 days (average 21 days). Microscopically, the primary chancre shows a dense infiltrate of mononuclear inflammatory cells, whereas secondary lesions show a sparser, nonspecific infiltrate, making histologic diagnosis more difficult. The most prominent feature is an endarteritis and periarteritis with endothelial cell swelling and proliferation and periadventitial cuffing of monocytes and plasma cells.

Clinical Manifestations of Primary Genital Syphilis

The chancre is classically painless, with a clean base and raised indurated borders (Fig. 45-2). It is usually single but may be multiple, and lymphadenopathy is usually present. The lesion usually disappears spontaneously in 1 to 5 weeks. Primary lesions of the oral cavity and perianal region are becoming more common (Fig. 45-3). In females, the chancre may go unnoticed altogether. In untreated cases, the lesions of secondary syphilis appear 6 to 12 weeks later.

Diagnosis

The only way to make an absolute diagnosis of primary syphilis is to find spirochetes in the exudate of the chancre by dark-field microscopy. Serologic tests are helpful in patients with dark-field–negative lesions and in patients in the secondary and later stages of syphilis. The Venereal Disease Research Laboratory test (VDRL) can be used as a screening test. This test is highly sensitive, but it is not specific. Patients with positive screening tests should be tested by the FTA-ABS (fluorescent treponemal antibody absorption) test, which is more specific but still has occasional false-positives (particularly in genital herpes, pregnancy, systemic lupus erythematosis, scleroderma, and alcoholic cirrhosis). A number of other serologic tests using cardiolipin-lecithin-cholesterol antigen (nontreponemal tests) or *T. pallidum* antigen (treponemal tests) are available, but the VDRL (nontreponemal) and FTA-ABS (treponemal) are standard tests used today.

Other genital skin lesions such as granuloma inguinale, chancroid, lymphogranuloma venereum, herpes simplex, Reiter syndrome, dry eruptions, fungus infections, and lichen planus should be excluded.

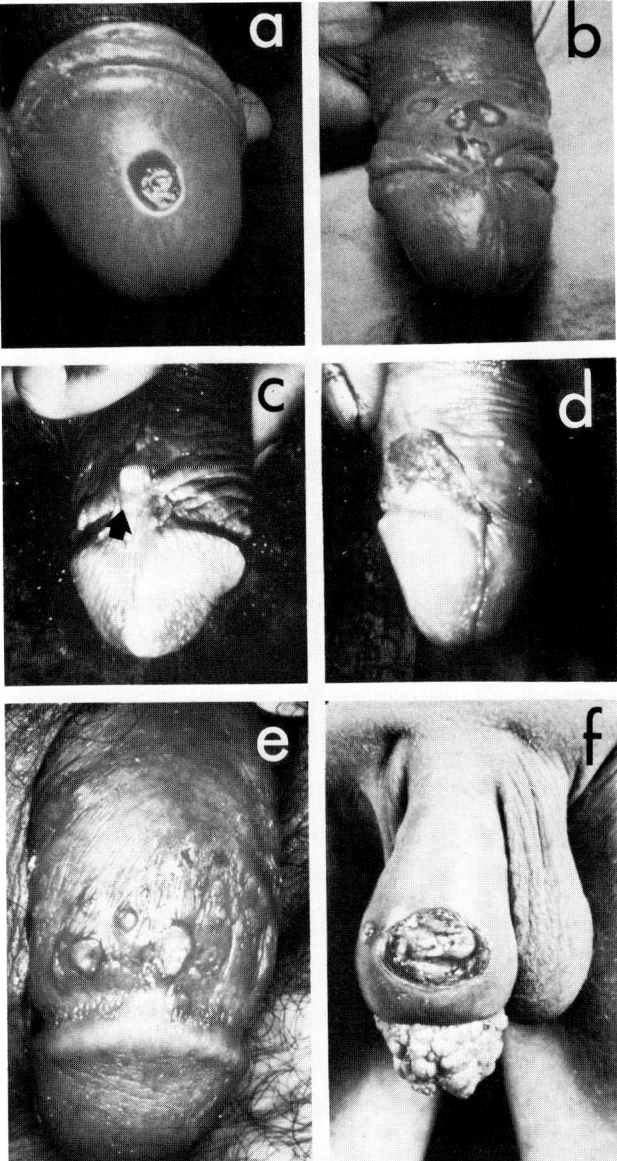

Fig. 45-2. A. Primary syphilis showing chancre of the glans. The surrounding borders are raised and firm. The base is clean, soft, and swarming with spirochetes. B. Chancroidal ulcers. The lesions are usually multiple, soft, tender erosions or ulcerations with a grayish base. Both the lesions and the associated adenopathy are often more pronounced on one side and are quite painful. Dark-field examination is negative. *H. ducreyi* can be demonstrated from the lesion by stained smear or culture. C. Lymphogranuloma venereum. The small soft ulcer (arrow) is usually missed. The patient shows unilateral, painful, inguinal adenopathy 10 to 30 days later. D. Granuloma inguinale. The lesion is soft, painless, raised, beefy red, smooth, and granulating. There is no significant adenopathy. Dark-field examination is negative. Donovan bodies *(Donovania granulomatis)* can be demonstrated in stained smears. E. Genital herpes begins as grouped vesicles, which ulcerate and heal without scarring. F. Condyloma acuminatum of foreskin and draining abscess of the shaft of the penis. (A–E. Courtesy U.S. Public Health Service, Centers for Disease Control, Atlanta, Georgia. F. Courtesy Dr. Birdwell Finlayson.)

Treatment

Treatment schedules for syphilis are published by the Center for Disease Control.[83,84] Early syphilis (less than 1 year) is treated with benzathine penicillin G, 2.4 million units intramuscularly once or aqueous procaine penicillin G 600,000 units intramuscularly daily, for 8 days. Late syphilis is treated by benzathine penicillin G, 2.4 million units intramuscularly weekly for 3 weeks, or aqueous procaine penicillin G, 600,000 units intramuscularly daily for 15 days. If penicillin allergy is present, oral tetracycline or erythromycin, 500 mg four times daily, can be used for 15 days for early syphilis and 30 days for late syphilis. Treatment is extremely effective in the early stages, with 97 percent of treated primary cases being serologically negative 2 to 10 years after therapy.

CHANCROID

Chancroid causes a painful ulcer of the corona, foreskin, or shaft of the penis (Fig. 45-2). The necrotic, suppurative ulcer bleeds easily and has less induration than the primary chancre of syphilis. Regional lymph nodes may also become suppurative. The gram-negative bacterium *Hemophilus ducreyi* causes this venereally transmitted infection, which is common in tropical and subtropical areas.

Three to 5 days after exposure to an asymptomatic female carrier, a penile papule appears, which quickly becomes ulcerated and necrotic. These painful ulcers are often multiple and may spread to other sites by autoinoculation. Extragenital lesions of the mouth and perianal area are common. At about 7 days, the inguinal nodes become involved, and half of these involved nodes will become fluctuant and spontaneously rupture. If superinfection occurs, rapid destruction of the penis and urethra may occur. The disease is usually self-limited, but most patients seek medical attention because of pain.

Biopsy of the ulcer will show a superficial zone of polymorphonuclear neutrophils and necrotic tissue, a middle zone of endothelial proliferation, and a deep zone of lymphocytes and plasma cells. The diagnosis can be made from the pathologic appearance, but biopsy is rarely required. Gram stain of the ulcer exudate or lymph node aspirate usually shows *H. ducreyi* as small clusters of gram-negative bacteria, often in chains, streaming along strands of mucus. Culture of the organism is difficult and not clinically useful. The diagnosis is usually made by the appearance of the ulcer, Gram stain of the exudate, and exclusion of syphilis, lymphogranuloma venereum, granuloma inguinale, infected human bites, and herpes simplex genitalis.

Sulfisoxazole, 1 gm, or tetracycline, 500 mg, four times daily for 14 days is effective treatment. If lymph node infection is not completely cleared in 14 days, the treatment should be continued longer.[85] Penicillin is ineffective.

As with syphilis, the disease poses a threat to medical personnel who come in contact with the lesion. With involvement of the foreskin, the resulting phimosis may make circumcision necessary. If at all possible, this should be delayed until after resolution of the acute ulcers.

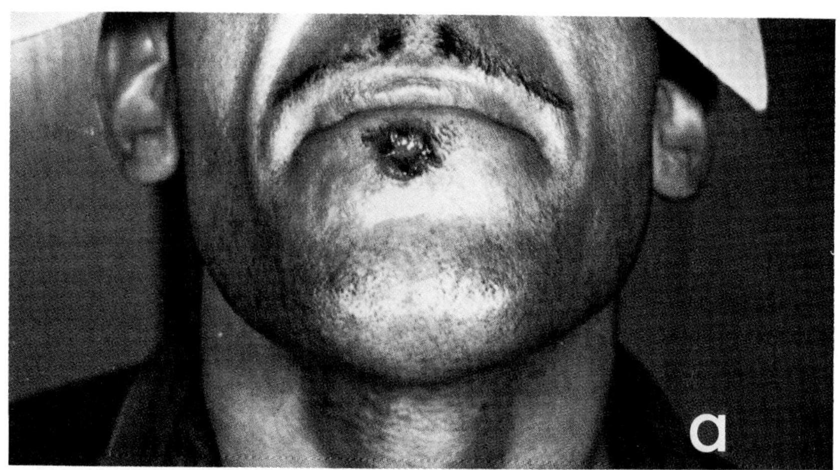

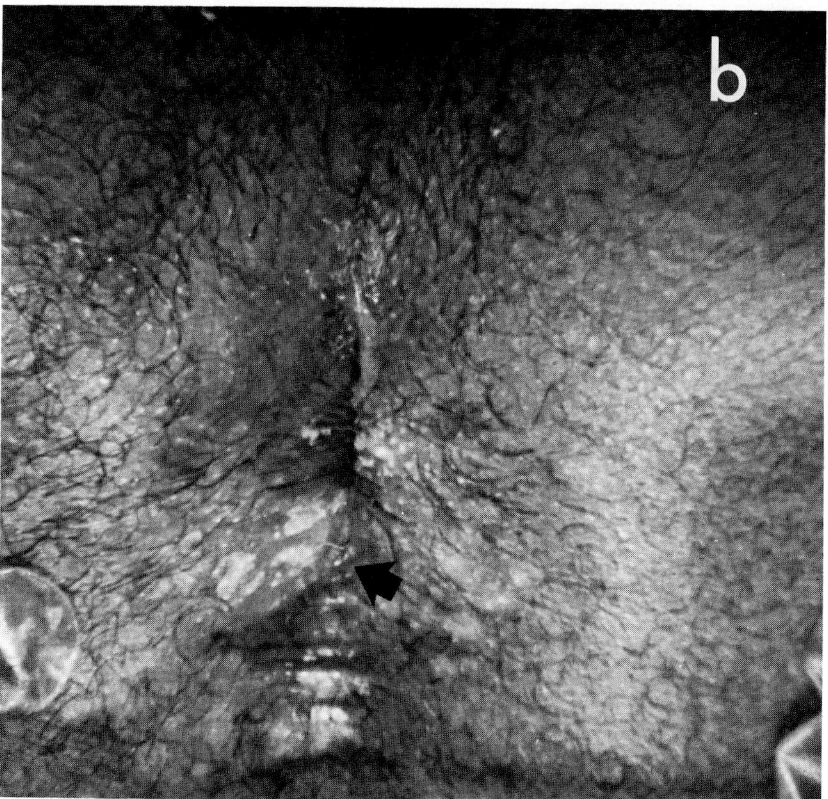

Fig. 45-3. **Extragenital syphilis. A. Chancre of the lower lip. B. Anal chancre (arrow) in a homosexual male. (Courtesy U.S. Public Health Service, Center for Disease Control, Atlanta, Georgia.)**

LYMPHOGRANULOMA VENEREUM

Lymphogranuloma venereum (LGV) is an uncommon sexually transmitted disease. It is caused by *C. trachomatis,* and is found primarily in the southeastern United States (Chapter 7). The primary lesion is a small soft painless erosion, which heals in a few days (Fig. 45-2). Inguinal adenopathy follows in 1 to 2 weeks and represents the major morbidity of the condition. Rupture of fluctuant nodes may lead to chronic draining inguinal sinuses, and lymphatic channel sclerosis may lead to genital lymphedema. The diagnosis is now made by a chlamydial group complement-fixation test titer of greater than 1:16. The Frei test is no longer performed. Treatment with sulfisoxazole, 1 gm four times daily, or tetracycline, 500 mg four times daily, for 3 weeks is effective. Fluctuant groin nodes are best managed by aspiration. Incision and drainage may lead to fistulas.

GRANULOMA INGUINALE

Just as with lymphogranuloma venereum, granuloma inguinale has a small primary penile lesion (papule or ulcer), but after an incubation period (2 to 12 weeks), papules and nodules appear by direct extension and quickly ulcerate (Fig. 45-2). The penile shaft, glans penis, and scrotum become involved with a spreading, ulcerated granulating surface. The disease is caused by a gram-negative rod, *Calymmatobacterium granulomatis* (Chapter 7). As the gross appearance mimics carcinoma, the diagnosis is made by biopsy, stained touch prep, and culture. Large mononuclear cells containing safety-pin-shaped gram-negative rods (Donovan bodies) are diagnostic. Superinfection can lead to serious genital tissue destruction and scarring, but early treatment with tetracycline, 500 mg four times a day for 4 weeks (or ampicillin, gentamycin, chloramphenicol, or streptomycin), is generally effective in curing the disease.

CONDYLOMA ACUMINATUM

Condylomata acuminata (venereal warts) are caused by an epidermotropic DNA virus, human papilloma virus. The exact incidence is unknown, but the lesions are common on the penis, scrotum, and perianal region. The infectivity rate by sexual intercourse is approximately 64 percent, though long latent periods may occur. The incidence in male homosexuals is high.

The painless small papillomata may be single or multiple and are raspberry- or cauliflower-shaped (Fig. 45-2). Microscopically, these are squamous papillomata with marked acanthosis and hyperplasia of the prickle cell layer of the dermis. The growth is upward toward the surface and not down into the tissue. A variant known as giant condylomata (Bushke-Lowenstein tumor) forms large cauliflowerlike warts with progressive extension, tissue destruction, and a tendency to become infected with bacteria. A number of authors believe that giant condylomata are malignant lesions.[86] Unless the urethra is involved, condylomata acuminata cause problems only by their unsightliness and tendency to bleed when traumatized. Recurrences after treatment are common, though few patients are seen with this problem after the age of 40. The warts flourish in immunosuppressed renal transplant patients. The diagnosis is made by gross appearance, with biopsy reserved only for suspicious lesions that raise the question of malignancy. There are no abnormal laboratory findings.

Initial therapy for condylomata of the external genitalia is topical. One percent podophyllin in benzoin can be repeatedly applied to the lesion on the penis and scrotum. Circumcision is usually required for recalcitrant lesions under the foreskin. Electrocautery and cryotherapy with liquid nitrogen are also effective. Surgical excision of external lesions is usually reserved for large or multiple lesions. Complete surgical excision is the treatment of choice for giant condylomata. Wearing a condom during intercourse will reduce the individual's propensity to acquire and spread the lesions.

Condylomata in the urethra may be a more difficult problem. These lesions may extend all the way to the bladder and cause symptoms of bleeding and urinary obstruction. Urethroscopy should be performed to determine the extent of the lesions; however, there is concern that instrumentation may seed lesions onto the normal urethral mucosa. Lesions at the meatus can be excised and fulgerated rather easily. Frequently, a meatotomy is required to provide exposure of the lesions or to help effect cure in recurrent lesions. For urethral lesions proximal to the fossa navicularis, electroresection can be performed using the Bugbee electrode at the base of the lesion. The most effective treatment for these more proximal lesions is intraurethral instillation of 5 percent 5-fluorouracil cream (Efudex).[87] The patient uses a urethral applicator to apply the cream into the urethra twice daily for 10 days. For the first few days, there may be slight dysuria. After each intraurethral application, the patient must take great care to cover the meatus with gauze. Any 5-flourouracil cream spilled on the scrotum will cause a severe burn. In extreme cases of extensive recurrent intraurethral condylomata, a first-stage Johanson urethroplasty may be required in order to resect and fulgurate all the lesions.

HERPES SIMPLEX VIRUS

Herpes simplex virus infections of the genitalia have become very common in recent years (Chapter 10). Either herpes simplex virus type 1 (3 percent) or herpes simplex virus type 2 (97 percent) may be isolated from the genital lesion. The virus is transmitted by direct contact, with an infectivity rate of about 75 percent. The incubation time is 5 days (range 3 to 14 days) before the prodrome of pain and tingling occurs. A vesicular eruption on an erythematous base is accompanied by severe pain; the lesions spontaneously subside (2 to 6 weeks) in all except the debilitated or immunosuppressed patient (Fig. 45-2). The virus is neurotropic and remains in sacral ganglia to cause reactivation and recurrence. Serum antibodies are ineffective in preventing reactivation or reinfection.

One of the complications of herpes progenitalis is urinary retention, probably caused by an acute lower motor neuron neurogenic bladder due to sacral root involvement[88] and not by voluntary retention as previously thought. Urinary retention is more common in females with acute herpes infection, but it also occurs in males.[89] Catheter drainage should be provided until resolution of the acute neurogenic bladder occurs (7 to 28 days). Reluctance to employ a urethral catheter will lead to bladder overdistention and may result in serious injury to the detrusor muscle.

BALANITIS AND BALANOPOSTHITIS

Bacterial infections of the glans penis usually occur in the uncircumcised male with poor hygiene. Initially, an acute viral infection may cause open sores, and superinfection with mixed organisms, often anaerobes, quickly follows in the warm, moist environment. Bacterial balanitis can be the initial presentation of other, more serious diseases or can be confused with these diseases such as Kaposi sarcoma, squamous cell carcinoma, and other premalignant conditions. Therefore, balanitis cannot be dismissed as a simple local inflammation. Other, dermatologic skin disorders can also present on the penis, such as drug eruptions, leukoplakia, psoriasis, neurodermatitis, eczematous eruptions, and so forth. Biopsy may be required to differentiate them from infections or neoplastic lesions.

Without treatment, the infection may progress to

cause gangrene and necrosis of the foreskin and glans penis. The organisms causing gangrenous balanitis are frequently oral anaerobes, the salivary contact occurring by fellatio. The first sign is erythema, which progresses to ulceration, induration, and swelling of the prepuce, which then turns black. Gangrene of the prepuce can be accompanied by necrosis of the glans and in some instances even of the entire shaft. The inguinal nodes become enlarged, and the patient may have systemic manifestations of infection such as malaise, chills, and fever.

Treatment consists in retraction of the foreskin, cleansing of the glans penis, application of topical antibiotics, and broad-spectrum systemic antibiotics. Exposure of the glans penis to the air is helpful in treating the infection, and often a dorsal slit of the foreskin under local anesthesia is required. After resolution of the infection, circumcision should be performed in sexually active males. Sexually inactive patients may be left with just a dorsal slit.

FULMINATING GANGRENE OF THE PENIS

Primary spontaneous fulminating gangrene of the penis is an entity distinct from the slowly progressive gangrenous conditions that may involve the penis secondary to other infections and other disease entities. Fulminating gangrene is commonly associated with gangrene of the scrotum (Fournier gangrene) and other types of perineal necrotizing infections (Chapter 25).

Alpha-hemolytic streptococci and staphylococci are commonly listed as the casual organisms, but *E. coli, C. perfringens,* and diphtheroids have also been implicated. Careful aerobic and anaerobic culture techniques will usually yield aerobic and anaerobic fecal flora. Thrombosed vessels are seen histologically at the periphery of the lesion.

The onset is sudden, with rapid progression to the gangrenous state. The infection may be confined to the penis, with only erythema noticeable on the adjacent scrotum. Within 24 hours, exudation and desquamation of the skin begins. Gangrene ensues and spreads rapidly to involve the entire penis. A line of demarcation spontaneously occurs, and the gangrenous portion sloughs down to the primary facial planes. The corpora and testicles are not involved. At times, the gangrene also involves the scrotum and even the entire pubic region. The sloughed region may bleed and soon begins to granulate and heal. Systemic symptoms occur such as chills, fever, and pain. The mortality rate has been estimated to be 17 to 27 percent.

Treatment consists of debridement of necrotic tissue, irrigation with antiseptic solutions, and systemic antibiotic therapy. Antibiotic therapy should initially be based on Gram stains of the tissue specimens and modified depending on the culture results. Penicillin should be instituted if clostridial species are suspected. An aminoglycoside and clindamycin are a good initial combination for polymicrobial perineal infections.

SCABIES

The itch mite, *Sarcoptes scabiei,* is usually contracted from a bed partner and produces pruritic inflammatory papules or nodules on the glans, shaft, and scrotum (Fig. 45-4). The lesions are often crusted. They can become secondarily infected. The mite or its eggs can be identified microscopically after a thin sliver of skin from a papule is digested with 10 percent potassium hydroxide.

Sulfur ointment is 97 to 100 percent effective in treating scabies, but it can produce dermatitis. Lindane, 1 percent in vanishing cream (Kwell lotion), and emulsions containing 20 to 25 percent benzyl benzoate are also effective treatments. Bed linens and clothing must be washed or dry cleaned. The penile and scrotal lesions can be slow to heal even though all parasites are dead.

GANGRENE OF THE SCROTUM

Etiology and Pathology

Gangrene of the scrotum is a rapidly progressive frequently mixed infection usually caused by microaerophilic streptococci, enteric organisms, and gas-forming anaerobes. It is probably similar to necrotizing, synergistic gangrene found in other sites (Chapter 25). Even *Entamoeba histolytica* and Rocky Mountain spotted fever (caused by *R. rickettsii*) have been associated with scrotal gangrene. Scrotal gangrene can on occasion also be due to arterial occlusive disease. Histologically, subcutaneous and dermal necrosis are seen together with an obliterative endarteritis caused by the microorganism.

The source of the infection is usually gastrointestinal organisms from such sources as an ischiorectal abscess or anal fissure.[90-92] But it can also occur after extravasation of urine, periurethritis, prostatitis, seminal vesiculitis, or epididymitis. The organisms may enter the scrotum through tiny defects in the skin caused by abrasions or scratching, or bacteria may be seeded into the scrotum from the blood. Another source is direct extension from an infection in neighboring tissue.

Clinical Manifestations

The onset is sudden. An otherwise healthy individual is suddenly stricken with pain. Scrotal edema and swelling soon appear. The scrotum becomes tense, red, glossy, and moist. The gangrene is usually limited to the scrotum, but it may involve the penis or extend onto the abdominal wall. Systemic manifestations of fever and chills, nausea, vomiting, and prostration are usually present. Left untreated, the infection progresses to rapid death from sepsis.

Treatment

Treatment is aimed at the scrotum gangrene and any underlying pathology. The necrotic tissue should be debrided aggressively and widely until uninfected tissues are exposed. Cultures of tissue and wound fluid should be incubated aerobically and anaerobically. Proper debridement will usually necessitate removal of most of the scrotum.

The testicles are not involved and can be left intact uncovered by skin or placed subcutaneously in the thigh. If clostridia are present, therapeutic hyperbaric oxygen should be considered. If the penis or abdominal wall is involved or if urine extravasation had a role in the etiology of the gangrene, a suprapubic catheter should be placed.

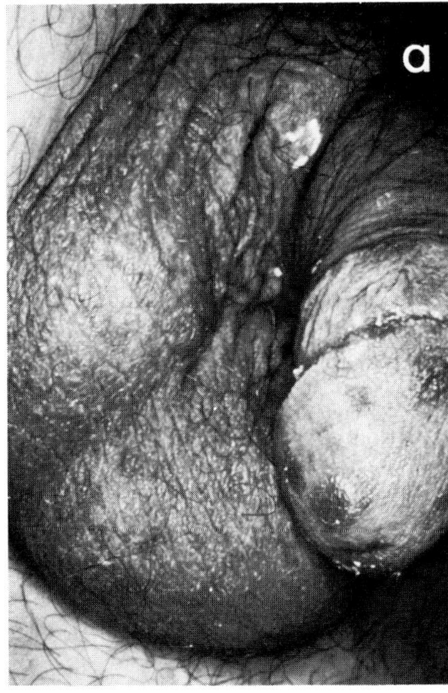

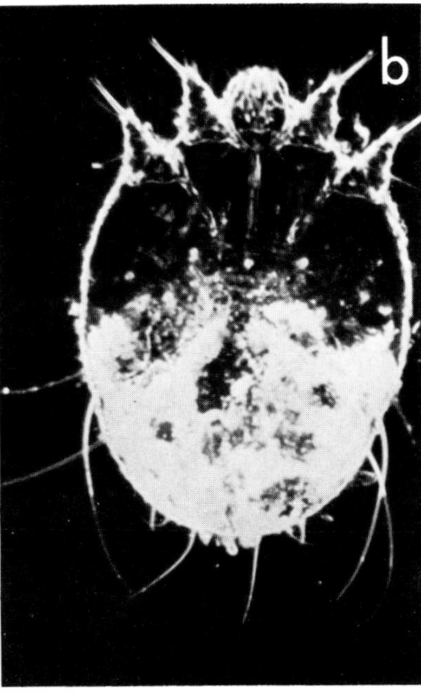

Fig. 45-4. **A. Scabies bites on the corona of the penis. B. The itch mite, *Sarcoptes scabiei.* (Courtesy U.S. Public Health Service, Center for Disease Control, Atlanta, Georgia.)**

Split thickness skin grafts can be placed on healthy granulation tissue when it appears over the exposed testicles. Ultimately, these grafts will assume the corrugated appearance of the normal scrotum.

Combination broad-spectrum antibiotics should be given because of the likelihood of a mixed infection. If crepitation is present, penicillin in high doses should also be administered. The antibiotic regimen should be adjusted on the basis of Gram stains of debrided tissue and the results of the cultures. Antibiotic therapy should never replace debridement. An underlying infection such as ischiorectal abscess, epididymitis, or prostatitis should also be sought and treated.

PERINEPHRIC ABSCESS

A perinephric abscess is a suppurative infection around the kidney that arises by direct extension from an infected kidney or by hematogenous spread, usually from sites of skin infection. The bacteria most frequently cultured are gram-negative enteric bacteria such as *E. coli, Proteus, Pseudomonas,* and *Klebsiella,* and gram-positive staphylococci and streptococci.

Clinical manifestations include chills and fever, dysuria, unilateral flank pain, tenderness, abdominal pain and tenderness, abdominal mass, and flank mass. Intravenous pyelography shows a mottled mass within the kidney or Gerota capsule and often reduced excretion of contrast agent on the affected side. Ultrasound is helpful in confirming the presence of a fluid-filled mass. However, computerized tomography scanning is now considered to be the best diagnostic study.

Pyelonephritis is a frequent misdiagnosis in patients with perinephric abscess resulting in delayed surgical drainage.

The treatment of perinephric abscess is surgical drainage through the flank. Relief of concomitant ureteral obstruction by ureteral catheterization or nephrostomy tube placement may be necessary. Definitive correction of renal abnormalities or nephrectomy should be avoided at the initial operative procedure. This is best done later, after the acute infection has subsided.

Initial antibiotic therapy should be broad-spectrum, because a variety of organisms can cause perinephric abscess. The antibacterial regimen can be more specific once a specimen has been obtained for Gram staining, and can be further altered by culture results.

GENITOURINARY TUBERCULOSIS

Genitourinary tuberculosis rarely, if ever, occurs as an isolated infection. Rather, it is a local manifestation of a generalized infection that is disseminated via the bloodstream to any part of the body. The etiologic agent, *M. tuberculosis,* was discussed in Chapter 7. Death from tuberculosis has been declining in the United States for the past 60 years, and the incidence of new cases of pulmonary and genitourinary tuberculosis is also decreasing.

Because tubercle bacilli reach the kidneys via the bloodstream, both kidneys should be assumed to be involved in patients with renal tuberculosis. From the kidney, the tubercle bacilli may migrate down the urinary tract to involve the ureter, bladder, prostate, seminal vesicle, and epididymis.

The kidneys in patients with renal tuberculosis can be destroyed by parenchymal involvement and destruction by *M. tuberculosis* or as a result of hydronephrosis due to ureteropelvic junction obstruction or ureteral stricture from tuberculous involvement of these sites.

The symptoms and signs of genitourinary tuberculosis vary markedly from one patient to another. In male patients, the earliest indication may be epididymitis.[93] Most other patients present with signs and symptoms of cystitis: urinary frequency, burning, and dysuria. However, patients may present in end-stage renal disease never having had any clinical findings of infection, or they may have fever, malaise, and cachexia from systemic tuberculosis.

Physical examination in females is frequently unrewarding. In males, the prostate may be shrunken and irregularly nodular from involvement of that organ. Epididymal involvement presents as a nontender spermatic cord mass that may be explored because of the suspicion of neoplasm. Rupture of an epididymal tuberculoma can lead to a chronic draining scrotal sinus tract.

The diagnosis is most commonly made by finding tubercle bacilli in the urine. Patients with pulmonary tuberculosis should have periodic urine cultures to rule out renal involvement. In patients suspected to have prostatic or epididymal involvement, the semen should be cultured as well. Culture and biopsy should also be performed on all nonhealing scrotal sinus tracts.

Antituberculous chemotherapy has been covered in Chapter 18. If surgical treatment should be required, at least 3 weeks, and preferably 3 months, of preoperative triple drug therapy is recommended. Because both kidneys are frequently involved, renal tissue should be preserved; heminephrectomy may be preferred to nephrectomy. Antituberculous chemotherapy should be continued for at least 1 year after nephrectomy.

BIBLIOGRAPHY

Andriole VT: Current concepts of urinary tract infections. In Weinstein L, Fields B (eds): Seminars in Infectious Disease, Vol. III, New York, Thieme-Stratton, 1980.

Buchsbaum HJ, Schmidt JD (eds): Gynecologic and Obstetric Urology. Philadelphia, Saunders, 1978.

Harrison JH, Gittes RF, Perlmutter AD, Stamey TA, Walsh PC: Urology. Philadelphia, Saunders, 1978.

Stamey TA: Pathogenesis and Treatment of Urinary Tract Infections. Baltimore, Williams and Wilkins, 1980.

REFERENCES

PATHOGENESIS

1. Stamey TA: The prevention of recurrent urinary infections. New York, Science and Medicine, 1973.
2. Hinman F Jr: Bacterial elimination. J Urol 99:811, 1968.
3. Boen JR, Sylvester DL: The mathematical relationship among urinary frequency, residual urine, and bacterial growth in bladder infections. Invest Urol 2:468, 1965.
4. Cox CE, Hinman F Jr: Experiments with induced bacteriuria, vesical emptying and bacterial growth on the mechanism of bladder defense to infection. J Urol 86:739, 1961.
5. Parsons CL, Greenspan C, Mulholland SG: The primary antibacterial defense mechanism of the bladder. Invest Urol 13:72, 1975.
6. Tomasi T: Secretory IG. N Engl J Med 287:500, 1972.
7. Tuttle JP Jr, Sarvas H, Jukka K: The role of vaginal immunoglobulin A in girls with recurrent urinary tract infections. J Urol 120:742, 1978.
8. Parsons CL, Shrom SH, Hanno PM, Mulholland SG: Bladder surface mucin. Examination of possible mechanisms for its antibacterial effect. Invest Urol 16:196, 1978.
9. Fair WR, Couch J, Wehner N: The purification and assay of the prostatic antibacterial factor (PAF). Biochem Med 8:329, 1973.

URINARY TRACT INFECTIONS

10. Stamey TA: A clinical classification of urinary tract infections based upon origin. South Med J 68:934, 1975.
11. Stamey TA, Sexton CC: The role of vaginal colonization with Enterobacteriaceae in recurrent urinary infections. J Urol 113:214, 1975.
12. Stamey TA: Urinary Infections. Baltimore, Williams and Wilkins, 1972.
13. Pfau A, Sacks T: The bacterial flora of the vaginal vestibule, urethra and vagina in the normal premenopausal woman. J Urol 118:292, 1977.
14. Stamey TA, Timothy M, Millar M, Mihara G: Recurrent urinary tract infections in adult women. The role of introital enterobacteria. Calif Med 115:1, 1971.
15. Turck M, Petersdorf RG: The epidemiology of non-enteric *Escherichia coli* infections: prevalence of serological groups. J Clin Invest 41:1760, 1962.
16. Vosti KL, Goldberg LM, Monto AS, Rantz LA: Host-parasite interaction in patients with infections due to *Escherichia coli.* I. the serogrouping of *E. coli* from intestinal and extraintestinal sources. J Clin Invest 43:2377, 1964.
17. Gruneburg RN, Leigh DA, Brumfitt W: *Escherichia coli* serotypes in urinary tract infection: studies in domiciliary, antenatal and hospital practice. In O'Grady F, Brumfitt W (eds): Urinary Tract Infections. London, Oxford Univ. Press, 1968, p 68.
18. Fowler JE Jr, Stamey TA: Studies of introital colonization in women with recurrent urinary infections. VII. The role of bacterial adherence. J Urol 117:472, 1977.
19. Stamey TA, Wehner N, Mihara G, Condy M: The immunologic basis of recurrent bacteriuria: role of cervicovaginal antibody in enterobacterial colonization at the introital mucosa. Medicine 57:47, 1978.
20. Kunin CM, Polyak F, Postel E: Periurethral bacterial flora in women: prolonged intermittent colonization with *Escherichia coli.* JAMA 243:134, 1980.
21. Alexander AR, Morrisseau PM, Leadbetter GW Jr: Urethral-hymenal adhesions and recurrent post-coital cystitis: treatment by hymenoplasty. J Urol 107:597, 1972.
22. Reed JF Jr: Urethral hymenal fusion: a cause of chronic adult female cystitis. J Urol 103:44.
23. Jacobo E: Diseases of the urethra. In Buchsbaum HJ, Schmidt JD (eds): Gynecologic and Obstetric Urology. Philadelphia, Saunders, 1978, p 325.
24. Leadbetter GW: Female urethral stenosis and valves. In Glenn JF (ed): Urologic Surgery. Hagerstown, Harper & Row, 1975, p 763.
25. Marshall FC, Uson AC, Melicow MD: Neoplasms and caruncles of the female urethra. Surg Gynecol Obstet 110:723, 1960.
26. Stamey TA: Urinary tract infections in women. In Harrison JH, Gittes RF, PerlmutterAD, Stamey TA, Walsh PC: Urology, Vol 1. Philadelphia, Saunders, 1978, p 451.
27. Winberg J: Urinary tract infections in infants and children. In Harrison JH, Gittes RF, Perlmutter AD, Stamey TA, Walsh PC: Urology, Vol 1. Philadelphia, Saunders, 1978, p 451.
28. Govan DG, Fair WR, Friedland GA, Frilly RA: Urinary tract infections in children. Part III. Treatment of ureterovesical reflux. West J Med 121:382, 1974.
29. Kendall AR, Karafin L: Urinary tract infections in children:

fact and fantasy. J Urol 107:1068, 1972.
30. Auer J, Seager LD: Experimental bladder edema causing urine reflux into ureter and kidney. J Exp Med 66:741, 1937.
31. King LR, Kazmi SO, Belman AB: Natural history of vesicoureteral reflux. Urol Clin NA 1:441, 1974.
32. Marshall VF, Pollack RS, Miller C: Observations on urinary dysfunction after excision of the rectum. J Urol 55:409, 1946.
33. Smith PH, Ballantyne B: The neuroanatomical basis for denervation of the urinary bladder following major pelvic surgery. Br J Surg 55:929, 1968.
34. Randall A: The origin and growth of renal calculi. Ann Surg 105:1009, 1937.
35. Nemoy NG, Stamey TA: Surgical, bacteriological and biochemical management of "infection stones." JAMA 215:1470, 1971.
36. Teague N, Boyarsky S: Further effects of coliform bacteria on ureteral peristalsis. J Urol 99:720, 1968.
37. Grana L, Kidd H, Idriss F, Swenson O: Effect of chronic urinary tract infection on ureteral peristalsis. J Urol 94:652, 1965.
38. Strong DW, Lawson RK, Hodges CV: Experimentally induced chronic pyelonephritis using bacterial antigen and its prevention with immunosuppression. Invest Urol 11:479, 1974.
39. Kass EH: The role of asymptomatic bacteriuria in the pathogenesis of pyelonephritis. In Biology of Pyelonephritis. Henry Ford Hospital International Symposium. Boston, Little, Brown, 1960, p 399.
40. Savage WE, Samir NH, Kass EH: Demographic and prognostic characteristics of bacteriuria in pregnancy. Medicine 46:385, 1967.
41. Kass EH: Asymptomatic infections of the urinary tract. Trans Am Phys 69:56, 1958.
42. Turck M, Goffe B, Petersdorf RG: The urethral catheter and urinary tract infection. J Urol 88:834, 1962.
43. Monzon OT, Ory EM, Dobson HL, Carter E, Yow EM: A comparison of bacterial counts of the urine obtained by needle aspiration of the bladder, catheterization and midstream voided methods. N Engl J Med 259:764, 1958.
44. Stamey TA, Pfau A: Some functional, pathologic, bacteriologic and chemotherapeutic characteristics of unilateral pyelonephritis in man. II. Bacteriologic and chemotherapeutic characteristics. Invest Urol 1:162, 1963.
45. Kunin CM: The quantitative significance of bacteria visualized in the unstained urinary sediment. N Engl J Med 265:589, 1961.
46. Stamey TA, Govan DE, Palmer JM: The localization and treatment of urinary tract infections: the role of bactericidal urine levels as opposed to serum levels. Medicine 44:1, 1965.
47. Meares EM Jr: Urinary tract infections in men. In Harrison JH, Gittes RF, Perlmutter AD, Stamey TA, Walsh PC: Urology, Vol 1. Philadelphia, Saunders, 1978, p 451.
48. Thomas V, Shelokov A, Forland M: Antibody-coated bacteria in the urine and site of urinary-tract infection. N Engl J Med 290:588, 1974.
49. Jones SR, Smith JW, Sanford JP: Localization of urinary-tract infections by detection of antibody-coated bacteria in urine sediment. N Engl J Med 290:591, 1974.
50. Lapides J: Neurogenic bladder. Principles of treatment. Urol Clin NA 1:81, 1974.
51. Smellie JM, Edwards D, Hunter N, Normand ICS, Prescod N: Vesicoureteric reflux and renal scarring. Kidney International 8:65, 1975.

URETHRAL INFECTIONS

52. Center for Disease Control MMWR: Morbidity and Mortality Weekly Report. Annual Summary, 1978. Vol 27, September 1979.
53. Handsfield HH, Lipman TO, Harnish JP, Tronca G, Holmes KK: Asymptomatic gonorrhea in men. Diagnosis, natural course, prevalence and significance. N Engl J Med 290:117, 1974.
54. Danielsson D, Mulin L: Demonstration of *Neisseria gonorrhoeae* in prostatic fluid after treatment of uncomplicated gonorrheal urethritis. Acta Derm Venereal 51:73, 1971.
55. Kraus SJ: Complications of gonococcal infections. Med Clin NA 56:1115, 1972.
56. Holmes KK, Beaty HN, Count GW: Disseminated gonococcal infection. Ann Intern Med 74:979, 1971.
57. Holmes KK, Johnson DW, Floyd TM, Kuale PA: Studies of veneral disease. II. Observations on the incidence, etiology and treatment of postgonococcal urethritis syndrome. JAMA 202:467, 1967.
58. Bissada NK, Cole HT, Fried FA, Rittenberg GM, Peterson DP, Biddle WS: Urethrography in the investigation of proximal urethral strictures. J Urol 110:299, 1973.
59. Kirchheim D, Tremann JA, Ansell JS: Transurethral urethrotomy under vision. J Urol 119:496, 1978.
60. Carlton FE, Scardino PL, Quattlebaum RB: Treatment of urethral strictures with internal urethrotomy and 6 weeks of silastic catheter drainage. J Urol 111:191, 1974.
61. Olsson CA, Krane RJ: The controversy of single versus multistaged urethroplasty. J Urol 120:414, 1978.
62. Devine PC, Fallon B, Devine CJ Jr: Free full thickness skin graft urethroplasty for urethral stricture disease. J Urol 118:392, 1977.
63. Wein AJ, Leoni JV, Sansone TC, Mulholland SG, Bogash M: Two-stage urethroplasty for urethral stricture disease. J Urol 118:392, 1977.
64. Devine CJ, Jr, Horton CE: Urethral diverticula. In Horton CE (ed): Plastic and Reconstructive Surgery of the Genital Area. Boston, Little, Brown, 1973, p 405.
65. Schachter J: Chlamydial infections (3 parts). N Engl J Med 298:428–435, 490–495, 539–549, 1978.
66. Bowie WR, Wang SP, Alexander ER, Holmes KK: Etiology of nongonoccal urethritis. In Hobson D, Holmes KK (eds): Nongonoccal Urethritis and Related Infections. Washington, D.C., American Society for Microbiology, 1977, p 19.
67. McCormack WM, Braun P, Lee YH, Klein J, Kars EH: The genital mycoplasmas. N Engl J Med 288:76, 1973.
68. Weisner PJ: Selected aspects of the epidemiology of nongonoccal urethritis. In Hobson D, Holmes KK (eds): Nongonoccal Urethritis and Related Infections. Washington, D.C., American Society for Microbiology, 1977, p 9.
69. Hobson D: Tissue culture procedures for the isolation of *Chlamydia trachomatis* from patients with nongonoccal genital infections. In Hobson D, Holmes KK (eds): Nongonoccal Urethritis and Related Infections. Washington, D.C., American Society for Microbiology, 1977, p 286.
70. Handsfield HH, Alexander ER, Wang SP, Pederser AHB, Holmes KK: Differences in the therapeutic response of chlamydia-positive and chlamydia-negative forms of nongonococcal urethritis. J Am Ven Dis Assoc 2:5, 1976.
71. Uehling DT: The normal caliber of the adult female urethra. J Urol 120:176, 1978.

INFECTIONS OF THE PROSTATE AND SEMINAL VESICLES

72. Drach GW: Prostatitis: man's hidden infection. Urol Clin NA 2:499, 1975.
73. Mobley DF: Semen cultures in the diagnosis of bacterial prostatitis. J Urol 114:83, 1975.
74. Fair WR, Cordonnier JJ: The pH of prostatic fluid: a reappraisal and therapeutic implication. J Urol 120:695, 1978.

75. Pfau A, Perlberg S, Shapira A: The pH of the prostatic fluid in health and disease: implications of treatment in chronic bacterial prostatitis. J Urol 110:384, 1978.
76. Alyea EP: Infections and inflammations of the prostate and seminal vesicles. In Campbell MF, Harrison JH (eds): Urology, 3rd ed. Philadelphia, Saunders, 1970, p 555.

EPIDIDYMITIS

77. Jacobs SC, Kaufman JM: Complications of indwelling urethral catheters in spinal cord injury patients. J Urol 119:740, 1978.
78. Berger RE, Alexander ER, Monda GD, Ansell J, McCormick G, Holmes KK: *Chlamydia trachomatis* as a cause of idiopathic epididymitis. N Engl J Med 298:301, 1978.

ORCHITIS

79. Gall EA: The histopathology of acute mumps orchitis. Am J Pathol 23:637, 1947.
80. Smith RG: Plasma treatment of mumps orchitis. US Navy Med Bull 44:159, 1945.
81. Burhans RA: Treatment of orchitis of mumps. J Urol 54:547, 1945.
82. Mongan ES: Treatment of mumps orchitis with prednisone. Am J Med Sci 237:749, 1959.

INFECTIONS OF THE EXTERNAL GENITALIA

83. Syphilis: CDC Recommended Treatment Schedules, 1976. Morbid Mortal Week Rep 25:101, 1976.
84. Idsoe O, Guthe T, Willcox RR: Penicillin in the treatment of syphilis. Bull WHO 47 (Suppl 1):1, 1972.
85. Marmar JL: Management of resistant chancroid in Vietnam. J Urol 107:807, 1972.
86. Hudson HC, Holcomb FL, Gates W: Giant condyloma acuminatum of the penis: case reports and review. J Urol 110:301, 1973.
87. Dretlet SP, Klein LA: The eradication of intraurethral condyloma acuminata with 5 percent 5-Flourouracil cream. J Urol 113:196, 1975.
88. Jacobs SC, Herbert LA, Piering WF, Lawson RK: Acute motor paralytic bladder in renal transplant patients with anogenital herpes infection. J Urol 123:426, 1980.
89. Oates JK, Greenhouse PRDH: Retention of urine in anogenital herpetic infection. Lancet 1:691, 1978.
90. Brown GS, Tremann JA: Fournier's syndrome: necrotizing subcutaneous infection of male genitalia. J Urol 122:279, 1979.
91. Burpee JF, Edwards P: Fournier's gangrene. J Urol 107:812, 1972.
92. Flanigan RC, Kursh ED, McDougal WS, Persky L: Synergistic gangrene of the scrotum and penis secondary to colorectal disease. J Urol 119:369, 1978.

TUBERCULOSIS

93. Wechsler H, Westfall M, Lattimer JK: The earliest signs and symptoms in 127 male patients with genitourinary tuberculosis. J Urol 83:801, 1960.

PART VIII: SPECIAL PROBLEMS IN SURGICAL INFECTIONS

CHAPTER 46
Tetanus

WESLEY FURSTE, IAN M. BAIRD, AND THOM E. LOBE

Tetanus (lockjaw) is a dreaded infectious complication of wounds, caused by the toxin-producing *Clostridium tetani.* This disease is characterized by tonic spasms of the voluntary muscles and by a tendency to episodes of respiratory arrest. Total prevention by immunization with tetanus toxoid is possible.

Tetanus has been recognized as a terrifying disease for 2,300 years. Hippocrates referred to a patient, the master of a large ship, who smashed the index finger of his right hand with the anchor: "Seven days later a somewhat foul discharge appeared; then trouble with his tongue . . . on the third day opisthotonos occurred with sweating . . . 6 days later he died."[1] In the second century, Aretaeus, the Cappadocian, called the disease an inhuman calamity, an unseemly sight, a spectacle painful even to the beholder.[2] He wrote, "The wish of the physician that the patient should expire, otherwise irreverent and objectionable, is, in this case well taken." (Fig. 46-1)

In spite of the many advances in medicine and surgery, tetanus, although completely preventable, still occurs and appears as it was described centuries ago. For example, in 1978 two cases of tetanus were reported. One patient was a 33-year-old housewife who had undergone rubber-band ligation of hemorrhoids,[3] and the other was a 77-year-old man who was stung by a bee.

At best, the results of the therapy of tetanus are not good. Tetanus can become a disease of only historical significance if physicians constantly consider and implement four basic principles: (1) administration of tetanus toxoid when indicated, (2) immediate, meticulous surgical care of all wounds, (3) administration of tetanus immune globulin (human) when indicated, and (4) use of emergency medical identification devices for all individuals (Fig. 46-2).

Incidence and Epidemiology

The clinical introduction of tetanus toxoid four decades ago was followed in many parts of the world by immunization of entire populations and contributed greatly to the control of tetanus. In developed countries, like the United States, the incidence of tetanus is less frequent (Fig. 46-3), but in other countries approximately one million deaths per year (900,000 caused by neonatal tetanus) may be caused by tetanus.[4] In 1973, 88 cases were reported in the United States, considerably less than 1 case per million population per year. Certain populations have a higher incidence; it is greatest in the Southeast—Louisiana and Alabama having the highest reported number of cases, with slightly lower incidences in adjacent states. Noncaucasians have a fivefold greater incidence, males are more frequently affected than females, and older adults who have not been immunized have the highest incidence. Most cases appear in the spring, summer, and early fall, when outdoor activity and exposure to the organism in the soil is the greatest. Heroin addicts are particularly susceptible, especially when quinine is injected, because this agent appears to produce locally anaerobic conditions.

Etiology

Microbiology. *C. tetani* is a large, gram-positive, actively motile bacillus, which in its spore-bearing form has a characteristic drumstick appearance. Spores may develop at either end of the bacillus, giving a dumbbell appearance. It is strictly anaerobic; spores will not germinate in the presence of even the smallest amount of oxygen. The spores of *C. tetani* are found worldwide in soils, dust, and the feces of man and beast. The spores resist killing by phenol and boiling, although autoclaving destroys them.

After germination, *C. tetani* produces two exotoxins, tetanospasmin and tetanolysin. Of these, tetanospasmin is the neurotoxin that produces the typical muscle spasms of tetanus. The organism itself apparently has almost no properties that permit it to invade tissue or elicit inflammatory responses.

Pathogenesis and Pathology

C. tetani is almost always acquired by implantation of the organism into tissues via breaks in mucosal or skin barriers. The routes of infection for a large number of cases of teta-

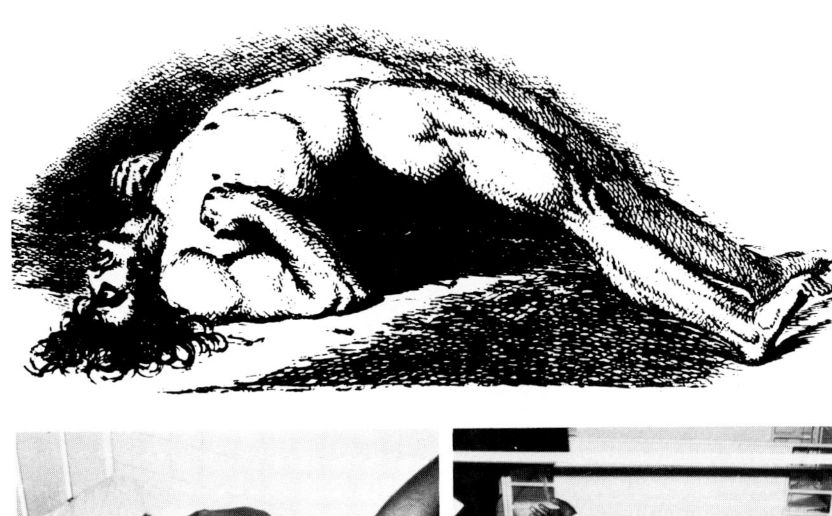

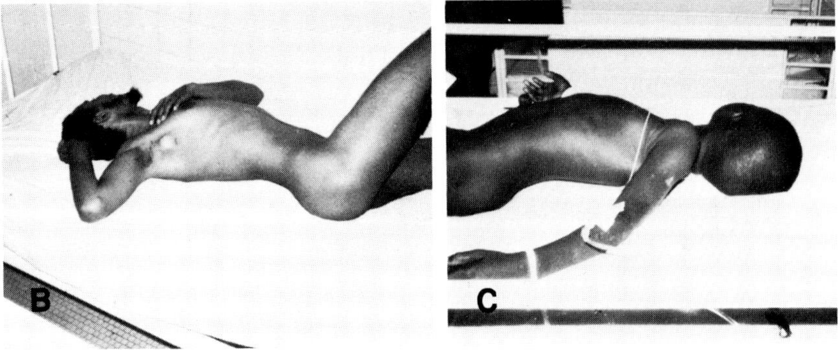

Fig. 46-1. **A. Tetanus as depicted by Sir Charles Bell during the nineteenth century, B. in a man and C. in a boy. (Courtesy of United States National Library of Medicine.)**

nus in India are listed in Table 46-1. Of particular interest is the absence of any apparent wounds in 14.2 percent, the high incidence of puerperal and umbilical tetanus (neonatal tetanus), and the high incidence associated with otorrhea.[5]

Table 46-2 lists the injuries associated with 285 American cases of tetanus.[6] The majority appeared after punctures, lacerations, and abrasions. Only a small number appeared in wounds classically associated with large amounts of anaerobic devitalized tissue. Many wounds appear to be healed (cryptogenic tetanus). No injury seems categorically unsuited for spore germination, especially if infection with facultatively anaerobic organisms further reduces redox potential. Spores may persist in healed wounds for years and will occasionally germinate later after reinjury or operation. Postoperative tetanus, however, usually results from breaks in sterile technique or wound contamination with intestinal contents.

The mere fact that *C. tetani* is present in a wound does not necessarily mean that the patient has tetanus or that it will develop. The organisms will proliferate only in the presence of an oxidation-reduction potential far lower than that existing in normal living tissue. As soon as *C. tetani* begins to grow, it produces tetanospasmin, which is transported to the central nervous system, where it becomes fixed and is responsible for the development of tetanus. Tetanospasmin is a protein of MW 67,000 with a potency equivalent to botulinus toxin; approximately 130 μg of purified tetanospasmin is lethal. There have been differences of opinion concerning the site of action of tetanospasmin and the route by which it spreads.[6] Apparently, wound toxin spreads centrally along the motor nerve trunks to the spinal cord and brain stem.[8] Tetanus will also follow the intravenous injection of toxin into animals, but the route by which toxin clears the blood-brain barrier and enters the central nervous system is not clear. Toxin injected intramuscularly apparently spreads both by passing centrally in nerves and by absorption into the blood.

The toxin becomes bound to central nervous system gangliosides. Early involvement of the lower cranial nerves is most frequent, but widespread central nervous system involvement is common when tetanus is fatal. The action of tetanospasmin mimics that of strychnine in suppressing the central inhibitory influences on motor neuron activity, leading to intensified reflex responses to afferent stimuli. Convulsions and spasticity result. The sympathetic, neurocirculatory, and neuroendocrine systems are also involved so that hypertension, tachycardia, peripheral vasoconstriction, and cardiac arrhythmias may be seen.

The causes of death in treated tetanus are complex. Pulmonary complications appear to be important in patients who survive more than 1 week. Degenerative changes in the respiratory muscles may play an important role, because such changes become more severe with increased survival time.[9]

Clinical Picture

In the largest American series, the median incubation period for fatal and nonfatal cases was 7 and 8 days respectively (range 1 to 54 days).[10] Tetanus almost always appears in a general form, but occasionally it may appear as local tetanus with increased muscle tone and spasms confined to muscles near a wound, without systemic signs. Neonatal tetanus is first recognized as a difficulty in sucking, beginning at 3 to 10 days of age, progressing to generalized

to put E.M.I. to work for you...

fill in both sides of this card. **For example,** under

Immunizations

The date is important. If you note immunization over three years old, ask your doctor about a booster immunization. For tetanus toxoid, note the date of your first immunization as well as your last.

Present Medical Problems

Epilepsy	Tracheotomy (neck breather)
Diabetes	Pneumothorax
Glaucoma	Pneumoperitoneum
Hemophilia	Colostomy
Chorea	

Dangerous Allergies

Drug allergies	Feathers (pillows)
Horse serum (as in tetanus antitoxin)	Common foods
	Penicillin sensitivity

Medicines Taken Regularly

Anticoagulants	When noting drugs, ask your doctor for the name to use that will be easy to identify in an emergency.
Cortisone or ACTH	
Heart drugs such as digitalis or nitrites	
Thyroid preparation	

Other Information

Scuba diver	Speak no English (note the language you speak)
Recurring unconsciousness	Wearing contact lenses
Hard of hearing	

Additional copies may be purchased from:
Order Department OP-2
American Medical Association
535 N. Dearborn St.
Chicago, Illinois 60611

YA 5025 907-N 25M 10/77

Medical Information

Last Immunization Date

diphtheria ______ mumps ______ tetanus toxoid ______

German measles ______ polio Sabin ______

measles ______ small pox ______ typhoid ______

Present Medical Problems ______

Medicine Taken Regularly ______

Dangerous Allergies ______

Other Information ______

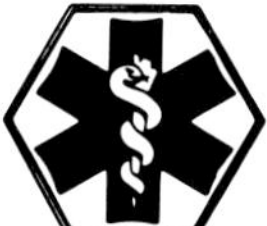

EMERGENCY MEDICAL IDENTIFICATION

American Medical Association
535 North Dearborn Street
Chicago, Illinois 60610

Why You Should Carry Emergency Medical Identification

An emergency medical identification card is your protection in an emergency. If you are not able to tell your medical story after an accident or sudden illness, the information entered on this card can save your life.

You may have health problems which can affect your recovery from an emergency. You may have a problem which is no emergency but often is treated as one, such as epilepsy. Even if you do not have a health problem, the information on this card can be of valuable assistance to the first aid attendant.

Why You Should Wear an Emergency Medical Signal Device

In an emergency, you may be separated from your pocket card. Possibly you are one who has a medical problem so critical that it must be immediately known to those who help you. If so, a signal device of durable material should be worn around your neck or wrist so that it can be present at all times, even while swimming.

The device should be fastened to the person wearing it with a strong nonelastic cord or chain so designed that it does not become an accident hazard in itself.

On this device there should be:

- The symbol of emergency medical identification
- The name of your major health problem
- For children and the aging, the name and address of a responsible relative and a telephone number, including area code.

Carry Your Card and Wear Your Signal Device at All Times!

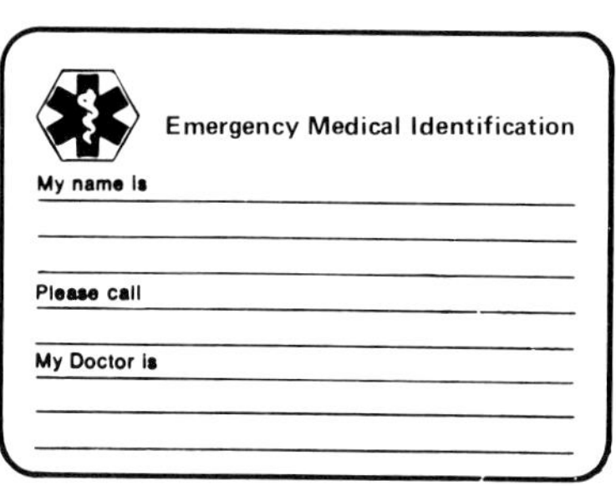

Emergency Medical Identification

My name is ______

Please call ______

My Doctor is ______

Fig. 46-2. Front and back sides of an effective emergency medical identification device. (Courtesy of American Medical Association.)

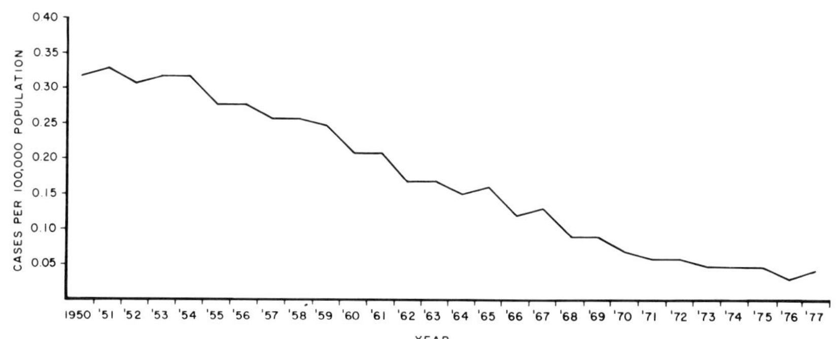

Fig. 46-3. Reported cases of tetanus per 100,000 population by year, United States, 1950–77. (Courtesy of Center for Disease Control, Public Health Service, U.S. Department of Health, Education, and Welfare. Annual Summary 1977, Morbidity and Mortality Weekly Report 26:69, 1978.)

tetanus. Cephalic tetanus follows injuries to the head or otitis. The incubation period is short and the mortality extremely high. In this form, cranial motor nerve palsies are common, but if the patient survives, total recovery ensues.

In general tetanus, some patients have prodromal symptoms of restlessness and headaches. In others, the first symptoms are those stemming from the developing muscle rigidity, with vague discomfort in the jaws, neck, or lumbar region. In an early stage, spasm of the muscles of mastication causes trismus and difficulty with chewing, ie, lockjaw. Sustained contraction of the facial muscles produces a distorted grin (risus sardonicus). Spasm of the pharyngeal muscles makes swallowing difficult; a stiff neck is among the early signs. Progressively, other muscle groups become involved. There is tightness of the chest and rigidity of the abdominal wall, the back, and the limbs, and orthotonos, opisthotonos, or emprosthotonos may de-

TABLE 46-1. ROUTE OF INFECTION OF *CLOSTRIDIUM TETANI* IN A LARGE SERIES OF TETANUS CASES AT THE KING EDWARD MEMORIAL HOSPITAL, BOMBAY, INDIA

Route	Total	Percent
Injury	892	44.5
Otorrhea	406	20.2
Umbilicus	292	14.5
Unknown	283	14.2
Puerperal	67	3.3
Injection	32	1.6
Vaccination	20	1.0
Operation	15	0.7

Adapted from Patel JD, Mehta BC: A study of 2,007 cases. *Indian J Med Sci* 17:791, 1963.

velop.[11] Generalized tonic convulsions are frequent, exhausting, and unpredictable. Any external stimulus (a breeze, sudden movement, noise, light) and many internal stimuli (cough, swallow, distended bladder) may trigger such generalized convulsions. In association with these convulsions, spasms may occur of the laryngeal and respiratory muscles, possibly with occasional fatal, acute asphyxia.

The patient is mentally alert throughout the course of the disease and suffers great pain from the muscle spasms. The pulse rate is elevated, and there is profuse perspiration. Fever may or may not be present. Neurologic examination discloses hyperactive tendon reflexes, often with sustained clonus. There are no sensory changes.

Cases have been classified as mild, moderate, and severe corresponding to the length of incubation, severity of paroxysms, and degree of autonomic dysfunction. In severe cases, patients may experience sudden changes in hemodynamic vital signs, either spontaneously or in response to external stimuli. Patients who survive more than 1 week gradually improve over 2 to 6 weeks, but total recovery may take months.

The diagnosis of tetanus must be based on the clinical picture, associated with no prior history of immunization, because laboratory examinations are of little assistance. The demonstration of *C. tetani* in a wound does not diagnose tetanus; the failure to demonstrate the bacillus in a wound does not eliminate the diagnosis. Fever is initially mild, leukocytosis moderate, and cerebrospinal fluid normal.

TABLE 46-2. TETANUS CASES BY TYPE OF ASSOCIATION INJURY IN THE UNITED STATES

Type of Wound	No. Cases	Proportion Total Cases (%)	Case-Fatality Ratio (%)
Puncture	105	36.8	51.5
Laceration	101	35.4	45.6
Abrasion	22	7.7	60.0
Crush	10	3.5	50.0
Surgical	9	3.2	62.5
Injection	2	0.7	100
Multiple injury	31	10.9	46.7
No injury	5	1.8	25.0
Total	285	100	49.4

From Smith A.[7]

Rarely has the surgical literature included notes on the progress of these patients. After giving the clinician's account of successful treatment of tetanus in a 20-year-old analytical chemist, Cole et al [12] included their patient's personal account of his illness.

> The first symptoms started approximately a week after I had cut my finger. They consisted in a sudden tightening around my throat causing extreme difficulty in breathing and making swallowing virtually impossible. During this spasm, coughing or expectoration added to the difficulty in obtaining air as my throat seemed to collapse when I tried to inspire.
>
> Spasms of the throat usually appeared at rest and lasted about ten minutes in the early stages. Later on, they were more prolonged. Two days after admission they seemed continuous, and about this time my voice became reduced to a whisper and my jaw felt stiff. The symptoms from then on are only snatches of memory. I felt like snarling, my upper lip involuntarily drawing back over the teeth, and a peculiar twitch was vaguely present in my limbs. . . .
>
> After several days I lost the fear of never being able to breathe when off the respirator, as it was always restored quickly. I only had one really scary time, when the tube fell out after replacement. I know it felt more secure when the tube from the ventilator was *screwed* into the tracheostomy socket and not just pushed in. Also, when the tube was taken off before the suction apparatus was made ready, the time taken was terrifyingly long. . . .

Diagnosis

The differential diagnosis may be difficult to make in early tetanus, but severe tetanus can be confused with a few other diseases, such as the following.

Heterologous serum sickness may be confused with early tetanus in patients who have received heterologous antisera in an effort to prevent the disease.

Hypocalcemic tetany is less severe than tetanus, and may follow operations on the thyroid or parathyroid glands when the latter are injured or removed. The upper extremities are primarily affected, the serum calcium is low, and calcium infusions provide easy control.

Meningitis and encephalitis usually provide enough signs to enable a physician to differentiate them from tetanus. In addition, the cerebrospinal fluid examination should be diagnostic.

Rabies is indicated early by an inability to swallow, drooling of saliva, and spasms of the muscles of deglutition. Trismus is rare, and spinal fluid pleocytosis is frequent. Animal bites may precede both tetanus and rabies, but the incubation period is much longer for rabies.

Strychnine poisoning may mimic tetanus closely, except that the muscles are relaxed between seizures in strychnine intoxication, whereas spasm tends to persist in tetanus.

Central nervous system cancer metastases can mimic the symptoms of tetanus.

Drug toxicity to penicillin, to haloperidol, to lead or

to phenothiazine tranquilizer drugs, may be differentiated from tetanus by an adequately taken history.

Acute hysteria and acute psychoses may be quite difficult to differentiate from early or mild tetanus until the patient has been evaluated for several days.

Spasms of a localized group of voluntary muscles that result from soft tissue or bone injuries may simulate local tetanus.

Trismus not caused by tetanus may occur with peritonsillar abscess, dental infections, and other local infections of the mouth and cervical regions, and with dentomandibular problems.

Meningitis, sepsis, hypocalcemic tetany, hypomagnesemia, metabolic alkalosis, and *intracranial hemorrhage* can be confused with neonatal tetanus. Newborns of drug-addicted mothers can have temporary tetanuslike symptoms.

Stiff-man syndrome, described by Moersch and Woltman in 1956,[13] can at first be confused with subacute tetanus, but the slow progression, for months or years, eventually differentiates it from tetanus.

Malingering, mimicking the signs of mild tetanus, may be used for monetary or other reasons. One unusual patient did so to remain near a ward nurse.[14]

The failure to demonstrate a wound does not eliminate a diagnosis of tetanus, for many cases have occurred without a demonstrable wound.

Prognosis

Even when treatment is adequate, the mortality rate may exceed 50 percent.[6] Patients who survive 10 days or more have a good chance of total recovery.[9] Many combinations of nonfatal complications may be responsible for death. Pulmonary atelectasis and aspiration can be followed by pneumonia. Traumatic glossitis is often seen. Compression fractures of the vertebrae may result from the convulsive seizures. Decubitus ulcers may occur. Constipation, fecal impaction, and urinary retention are often encountered. Cystitis and pyelonephritis may develop in patients who require catheterization. Foot drop and muscle contractures may follow prolonged unconsciousness. Asphyxia from respiratory or laryngeal muscle spasm or from aspiration of secretions, vomitus, or food can be the immediate cause of death. Coagulopathy can develop, as can fatal pulmonary emboli.

In long-term follow-up studies, irritability, insomnia, fits, myoclonus, decreased libido, postural hypotension, and electroencephalographic abnormalities have been recorded.

The professional liability law suit is an annoying complication for the physician, which can occur months or years after a case of tetanus, and for which well-documented records are most important.[9]

Prevention

Tetanus is of historical significance only due to worldwide implementation of the effective and inexpensive methods of tetanus prophylaxis that are available. Such methods are outlined in Table 46-3, which represents the combined thinking and recommendations of many [15-27]

Tetanus Toxoid

Active immunization with adsorbed tetanus toxoid is the best way to prevent tetanus. Unfortunately, many individuals, even in developed countries, are not adequately immunized (Fig. 46-4),[23,28] and primary immunization after wounding, though essential, will not provide protection from tetanus arising from this wound. In normal individuals, two injections of adsorbed toxoid 4 to 6 weeks apart provide the *initial series* and a third injection (the *reinforcing injection*) completes the primary *basic immunization.* Antibody (circulating antitoxin) develops soon after the second dose. Adsorbed toxoid should be used for primary immunization and for booster doses after injury, or routinely about every 10 years. In the previously immunized, booster injections will elicit protective levels of antitoxin in 4 to 7 days. Local reactions are unusual except in those who have received frequent booster injections. Most reactions are confined to local erythema and swelling. A few cases of tetanus have occurred with prior tetanus toxoid immunization (complete or incomplete).[29-33] One case has been reported with a circulating serum tetanus antitoxin titer greater than 0.01 units of antitoxin per ml of serum, which has been considered a protective level.[24,34]

The interval between wounding and the last previous tetanus toxoid booster should be a guide for the decision whether to administer a booster to wounded patients. Two hundred directors of emergency departments responded to a questionnaire in 1978. Sixty-five percent boost all patients with major wounds if a year or more has passed since the last booster. As many as 80 percent are observing a 5-year interval, or less, for minor wounds. In view of the few recent cases of tetanus in the United States, the use of these guidelines apparently are effective.

Surgical Wound Care

Operative prophylaxis consists of the removal of *C. tetani* and nonviable tissue from wounds and of the best possible reconstruction of aerobic wounds. Optimal prophylaxis includes the following steps.[9,35]

1. The wounds are treated at the earliest possible moment.
2. Aseptic technic must be observed, including the use of gloves, gowns, masks, sterile instruments, and proper antiseptic skin preparation.
3. During preparation of the skin, the wounds should be covered with gauze to prevent further contamination from surrounding contaminated tissue.
4. Proper lighting is needed to help identify and protect fine structures such as nerves and vessels.
5. Adequate instruments and assistance are needed for optimal exposure.
6. Hemostasis should be achieved with delicate instruments and with fine suture material to minimize the amount of necrotic tissue left in wounds.
7. Tissues should be handled gently to prevent more necrotic tissue.
8. Complete debridement with excision of necrotic tissue must be carried out so that no pabulum is left on which residual bacterium can propagate. If reevaluation of wounds indicates the development of more necrotic tissue, debridements must be repeated.
9. All foreign bodies must be excised.

10. The wound should be irrigated copiously with large amounts of physiologic salt solution.

11. If it might provide the anaerobic conditions for growth of tetanus bacillus and its lethal toxin, a wound should be left open and drainage instituted when necessary.

Antitoxin

Since 1966, the recommended prophylactic dose of tetanus immune globulin (human) (TIG[H]) in the United States has been 250 units. An increase to 500 units is recommended for severe, neglected, or old (more than 24 hours) tetanus-prone wounds.[24] During 1970 and 1971,

TABLE 46-3. A SUGGESTED OUTLINE FOR PROPHYLAXIS AGAINST TETANUS IN WOUND MANAGEMENT

A. GENERAL PRINCIPLES

1. Triple responsibility: physicians, public health officials, and patients are responsible for the prevention of tetanus.
2. Professional liability problems: to protect the medicolegal rights of the patient, of nonphysician personnel involved in the care of the patient, and of all physicians associated with the care of the patient, record the history and complete care of the patient, including all skin or other sensitivity tests performed and all injections on permanent and available records.
3. Basic immunization and nonwound booster immunization: Basic immunization for tetanus with adsorbed tetanus toxoid requires 3 injections, with the first 2 administered 4 to 6 weeks apart and the third given 6 to 12 months after the second injection. A booster of adsorbed tetanus toxoid is indicated 10 years after the third injection or 10 years after an intervening booster.

   All individuals, including pregnant women, should have basic immunization and booster injections when indicated. Neonatal tetanus is preventable by active immunization of the mother before or during the first 6 months of pregnancy. This immunization can be achieved by 2 intramuscular injections of adsorbed toxoid given 6 weeks apart. In the event that a neonate is borne by an immunized mother without adequate obstetric care, the infant should receive 250 units or more of TIG(H). Active and passive immunization for the mother should also be initiated.
4. Individualization of wounded patients: the attending physician must determine for each patient what is required for adequate prophylaxis against tetanus.
5. Surgical wound care: regardless of the status of the active immunization of the patient, immediately render optimal surgical care for all wounds, including removal of all devitalized tissue and foreign bodies.
6. Toxoid and antitoxin at the time of injury: whether or not to provide active immunization with tetanus toxoid and passive immunization with TIG(H) must be decided individually for each patient. The characteristics of the wound, conditions under which it was incurred, its treatment, its age, and the previous active immunization status of the patient must be considered. The patient's stating that he has had a significant reaction to tetanus toxoid may be a contraindication to the injection of toxoid, and requires investigation.
7. Emergency medical identification devices: to every wounded patient, give a written record of the immunization provided, instructing him to carry the record at all times, and if indicated, to complete active immunization. For precise tetanus prophylaxis, an accurate and immediately available history regarding previous active immunization against tetanus is required, or rapid laboratory titration to determine the patient's serum tetanus antitoxin level is necessary.
8. Antibiotics: the effectiveness of antibiotics for prophylaxis of tetanus remains unproved.

B. SPECIFIC MEASURES FOR PATIENTS WITH WOUNDS

1. Wounded individuals, who have received no previous injections or whose immunization history is unknown, are considered for the following:
   a. For non-tetanus-prone wounds (clean and/or minor) give 0.5 ml of toxoid * (initial immunizing dose) and instructions for completion of the basic series.
   b. For tetanus-prone wounds (severe, neglected, or more than 24 hours old), give 0.5 ml of toxoid * (initial immunizing dose), instructions for completion of the basic series, and 250 or more units of TIG(H).†
2. Wounded individuals, who have been given an indeterminate number of tetanus toxoid injections, are considered for the following:
   a. For non-tetanus-prone wounds, give a booster dose of toxoid * unless the patient has received his last dose during the previous 5 years.
   b. For tetanus-prone wounds, give a booster dose of toxoid * unless the patient has received his last dose within the previous year.
   c. For tetanus-prone wounds, give a booster dose of toxoid * and 250 or more units of TIG(H) † when the patient has received his last dose of toxoid more than 10 years previously.
3. Wounded individuals, who have received at least 4 unequivocally documented doses of tetanus toxoid, with the last given more than 10 years previously, are considered for the following:
   a. For non-tetanus-prone wounds, give 0.5 ml of toxoid.*
   b. For tetanus-prone wounds, give 0.5 ml of toxoid * and possibly 250 or more units of TIG(H).†
4. Wounded individuals, who have received at least 4 unequivocally documented doses of tetanus toxoid, with the last given within 10 years, are considered for the following:
   a. For non-tetanus-prone wounds, no booster dose is indicated.
   b. For tetanus-prone wounds, give 0.5 ml of toxoid * unless the patient has received a booster dose within the previous 5 years.

* With different preparations of adsorbed toxoid, the volume of a single booster dose should be modified as stated on the package label. The Public Health Service Advisory Committee on Immunization Practices recommended in 1977 DTP (diphtheria and tetanus toxoids combined with pertussis vaccine) for basic immunization in infants and children from 2 months through 6 years, and Td (combined tetanus and diphtheria toxoids: adult type) for basic immunization of those over 6 years. For the latter group, Td toxoid was recommended for routine or wound boosters; but if there is any reason to suspect hypersensitivity to the diphtheria component, tetanus toxoid (T) should be substituted for Td.

† Use different syringes, needles, and sites of injection for toxoid and TIG(H).

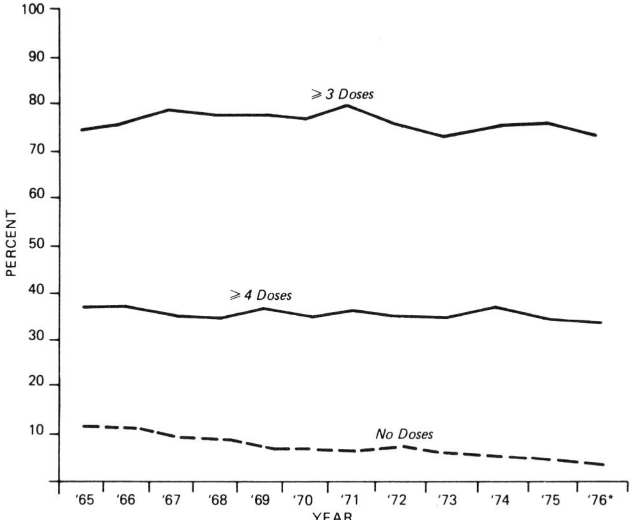

Fig. 46-4. **Diptheria-tetanus-pertussis immunization status of 1 to 4-year-old children, United States, 1965–76. (Courtesy of Center for Disease Control, Public Health Service, U.S. Department of Health, Education, and Welfare. United States Immunization Survey, 1976, HEW Publ No (CDC) 78–8221:9, 1977.)**

only five of 207 (2.4 percent) of the patients with tetanus in the United States, with information on prophylaxis, had received prophylactic antitoxin before the onset of tetanus; two of these received more than eight doses of tetanus immune globulin (more than 1,000 units). The two cases may represent therapy after the onset of tetanus that was incorrectly reported as prophylaxis.[36] Nevertheless, higher dosage of TIG(H) is indicated for major burns, septic abortions, retained foreign bodies, open fractures, inadequate debridement, or wounds contaminated with herbivore feces.[26,37] TIG(H) must not be given intravenously. Passive immunization with TIG(H) is no substitute for active immunization or adequate surgical care of a local wound.

Emergency Medical Identification Devices

In the United States, where more and more individuals are actively immunized for tetanus, emergency medical identification devices are becoming more important. Clinicians constantly ask these questions during the management of the wounded: (1) Has the patient been actively immunized for tetanus? (2) If actively immunized for tetanus, when? (3) Have there been severe—and hence significant—reactions to tetanus toxoid? (4) Should TIG(H) be given? Such questions can be answered immediately if every citizen carries an up-to-date emergency medical identification device (Fig. 46-2). Memory alone can be inadequate. Many who have thought they had received tetanous toxoid injections in the past are discovered to have received tetanus antitoxin, diphtheria toxoid, or perhaps typhoid vaccine instead. The possession of some type of emergency medical identification device could simplify and expedite history taking after injury before treatment is begun. Tetanus toxoid immunization could be performed accurately, and overdoses and unnecessary injections of tetanus toxoid could be avoided in the rare individual who is sensitive to toxoid (Table 46-4).

Antibiotics

The consensus reached at the Second International Conference on Tetanus in 1966 was that antibiotics, such as penicillin, are effective against vegetative tetanus bacilli, both in vitro and in experimental animals. Antibiotics have no effect against toxin and must not be relied on to the exclusion of active and passive immunization procedures. The effectiveness of antibiotics for prophylaxis remains unproved; if used, they should be given for at least 5 days.[38] Therefore, antibiotics should be used as a deterrent to the growth of tetanus organisms that cannot be surgically removed from wounds. Huge doses are generally recommended to penetrate into partially devitalized areas.

Treatment: Management of the Victim of Tetanus

The therapeutic recommendations that follow have been discussed in detail at the five International Conferences on Tetanus, most recently in June 1978.[26,36–40]

1. Establishment of a diagnosis of tetanus. Be as certain as possible of the diagnosis. Other diseases mimic tetanus.

2. Complete history and physical examination. This information forms a baseline for the recognition of complications.

3. Antitoxin: *Intramuscular Injection.* As soon as the diagnosis of tetanus is made, give intramuscular injections of 500–10,000 units of TIG(H). Intravenous administration of aggregated gammaglobulin may produce hypertension and is contraindicated. The exact, effective dosage of TIG(H) has not been established. A dose of only 500 units may be as effective as 3,000–10,000 units.[41] Patel and his associates [42] in Bombay, India, found no significant difference in mortality for doses ranging from 5,000 units (the lowest dose) to 60,000 units, and interpreted larger doses as being probably detrimental. In countries where there are adequate supplies of tetanus immune globulin (human), there are no indications for the administration of heterologous equine antitoxin. In countries in which it is not available, heterologous antitoxins are still being used.

Intrathecal Injection. Give an intrathecal injection of a mixture of prednisolone plus TIG(H), and TIG(H) intramuscularly. For neonatal tetanus, 250 units of TIG(H) and 12.5 mg of prednisolone are administered intrathecally by lumbar puncture and 250 units of TIG(H) is given intramuscularly. For adults, the dose of TIG(H) for the intrathecal route is increased to 1,000 units and for the intramuscular route to 1,000 units.[26,43,43a]

TABLE 46-4. USE OF THE EMERGENCY MEDICAL IDENTIFICATION DEVICE IN THE UNITED STATES

Period	No. of. Individuals	No. with E.M.I.D. (%)	No. with Tetanus Data on E.M.I.D. (%)
1970–72	428		22 (5.1)
1974–75	339	10 (2.9)	7 (2.1)
1978	122	16 (13)	8 (6.6)

These data were obtained by a survey of patients and their friends encountered in the practice of one of the authors (WF).

4. Laboratory tests. Our protocol for laboratory tests in the hospital is shown in Table 46-5.

5. Nursing care. Nursing care must be provided constantly in an intensive care unit. A respirator, oxygen, suction, and tracheostomy equipment must be immediately at hand.

6. Analgesics. The use of appropriate doses of codeine and meperidine (Demerol) will relieve the pain associated with the tonic contractions of tetanus, without causing excess respiratory depression.

7. Sedatives and muscle relaxants. The purpose of sedatives is to reduce the patient's threshold to external stimuli, with the hope of reducing the number and severity of seizures. The mildest cases of tetanus can be sedated adequately with phenobarbital or paraldehyde, but the more severe cases require thiopental sodium (Pentothal). Some physicians have been enthusiastic about the use of muscle relaxant drugs to control convulsive seizures. These drugs are difficult to administer because of the problems of overdosage or underdosage. Drugs more commonly suggested for use are diazepam (Valium), methocarbamol (Robaxin), D-Tubocurarine, succinylcholine (Anectine), and pancuronium (Pavilon).

8. Surgical wound care. Meticulous surgical care of wounds must be used, with removal of all necrotic tissue and foreign bodies, as outlined in the previous section on prevention.

9. Antibiotics. In vitro, penicillin and other antibiotics (Table 46-6) are effective against the tetanus bacillus. However, antibiotic therapy will be disappointing insofar as it is directed against the tetanus itself, because tetanus is a toxemia, not a bacteremia. In addition, the organism's lethal antibiotic concentrations within the wound may not be attained, because avascular conditions are frequently present. Nevertheless, penicillin may be a useful adjunct to surgical wound care.

On the other hand, antibiotics are part of the therapy plan. They are irreplaceable in the care of infectious complications of tetanus, especially in combating pneumonia or secondary invasive wound infections. Of course, the choice of most effective antibiotics for the infectious complications should be determined by prior experience and by culture and sensitivity tests.

10. Tracheostomy. If personnel and facilities, including adequate tracheostomy tubes and mechanical respiration units, are available to care adequately for it, perform a tracheostomy. Tracheostomy and controlled ventilation are not necessary for every patient, but patients with short incubation periods or those who manifest periods of respiratory arrest will require long-term respiratory control.

11. Iatrogenic problems. Be constantly on the alert to avoid iatrogenic problems. For example, rectal probes left in place for the constant recording of temperature must be checked to prevent trauma to the rectal mucosa and anorectal veins during convulsions.

12. Private, dark, quiet room. It is traditional to place the patient in a private, dark, quiet room, but with adequate sedation and muscle relaxation, this may no longer be necessary.

13. Proper environment for infants. Infants with tetanus must have a proper environment in which the oxygen partial pressure, temperature, and humidity can be monitored and maintained. An infant radiant warmer will maintain body temperature and allow for availability of nursing care.

TABLE 46-5. PROTOCOL FOR ADMISSION LABORATORY TESTS

Order the following:

1. Complete blood cell count with differential white blood cell count
2. Urinalysis
3. Prothrombin time and partial thromboplastin time
4. Blood chemistry test: urea nitrogen, creatinine, electrolytes, bilirubin, calcium, glucose
5. Arterial blood gases
6. Chest roentgenogram
7. Electrocardiogram
8. Electroencephalogram if it can be obtained so that—if necessary for later brain evaluation—serial electroencephalograms may be available from the time of initial care
9. Wound and—if the patient is febrile—both aerobic and anaerobic blood cultures and sensitivity tests
10. If necessary for diagnosis, cerebrospinal fluid for culture, Gram smear, cells, and chemistry tests
11. Diazepam levels of serum

14. Roentgenograms. Roentgenograms are useful for fractures associated with the initial injury, or with tonic muscle contractions, or for pulmonary complications.

15. Padded tongue depressor. A padded tongue depressor should be inserted to protect the tongue from being bitten during tonic contractions.

16. Oral hygeine. The lips, teeth, tongue, and oral cavity must be cleaned daily to lessen the possibility of growth of pathologic bacteria and viruses.

17. Nutrition. Central intravenous hyperalimentation is best during the convulsive phase of tetanus. Enteral alimentation via mouth, gastrostomy, or nasogastric tube is best deferred until convalescence so that aspiration is minimized.

18. Alimentary tract elimination. Provide for adequate gastrointestinal elimination by saline laxatives prophylactically, and enemas as required.

19. Urine elimination. When necessary, a Foley catheter can provide for elimination of urine. Remove the catheter as soon as possible to prevent urinary tract infections.

TABLE 46-6. ANTIBIOTICS WHICH MAY HAVE A POSSIBLE DETERRENT ACTION ON ANY *C. TETANI* THAT HAVE NOT BEEN OR CANNOT BE REMOVED SURGICALLY FROM A WOUND

Ampicillin
Cephalosporins
Chloramphenicol
Clindamycin
Erythromycin
Metronidazole
Penicillin *
Tetracyclines

* Penicillin is the most effective.

20. Intake and output records. Record the fluid and electrolyte balance. If facilities permit, weigh the patient daily.

21. Protection of the eyes. To prevent dessication, an ophthalmic ointment and moist gauze sponges should be used.

22. Prevention of decubitus ulcers. Decubitus ulcers can be prevented by appropriate cushions, pads, and skin hygiene.

23. Blood dyscrasias and bleeding problems. If there is a possibility of blood dyscrasias or bleeding problems, order frequent complete blood cell counts and promptly investigate the clotting mechanisms.

24. Prevention of pulmonary emboli. Some patients may require heparin to prevent or treat thromboembolic disease.

25. Prevention of cardiac exhaustion and circulatory disruption resulting from sympathetic overstimulation. Use propranolol to treat cardiac dysrhythmias, and add bethanidine for persistent hypertension.[44] When possible, if indicated, continuously monitor the heart rate and the arterial and central venous blood pressures.

26. Consideration of temporary endocardial pacemaker in cases with severe bradycardiac episodes. A temporary endocardial pacemaker may be indicated when severe, medically refractory bradycardia of unknown cause occurs.[45]

27. Prevention of muscle contractures. Prevent muscle contractures with resulting deformities, such as foot drop, by temporary splints. Physiotherapy should be started as soon as recovery permits.

28. Control of body temperature. Carry out necessary procedures to lower excessively high body temperatures.

29. Tetanus toxoid. One month after the diagnosis of tetanus is made, give 0.5 ml of adsorbed tetanus toxoid intramuscularly for active immunization, and instruct the patient to complete his basic immunization. Exposure to tetanospasmin does not provide immunity because the amount of tetanospasmin which causes tetanus is so very, very small. A complete course of active immunization is necessary.

30. Emergency medical identification device. At the time of discharge from the hospital, give the cured patient a completed emergency medical identification device (Fig. 46-2).

31. Hyperbaric oxygen. Hyperbaric oxygen is not recommended because it is ineffective and dangerous. Oxygen has no effect on the toxemia.

32. Recording of data. The possibility of professional liability problems require that complete and accurate records of the course of treatment of tetanus cases be kept.

Professional Liability Problems

Unfortunately, in the United States professional liability problems are greatly overemphasized (Table 46-7). In addition to the impressive dollar values involved, such problems encircle the physican with a girdle from which he or she cannot escape. Lawyers have been frequently consulted for professional liability problems involving tetanus prophylaxis or treatment.

TABLE 46-7. PROFESSIONAL LIABILITY ASPECTS OF A POSSIBLE CASE OF TETANUS

Tetanus (?); No Trial: 1978 *	
Responsible individual	$100,000
First care providers	231,000
Third care providers	100,000
Local government	19,800
SUBTOTAL	$450,800
Lawyers	?

* Estimate of $750,000 if trial.

Pretrial settlements, as indicated, were made because a much higher total settlement (possibly $750,000) might have resulted if the case had been evaluated by a judge and/or jury in court. The responsible individual (the defendant) was involved in an automobile accident with the plaintiff (Quinn, personal communication).

Progress in the United States

The tetanus prophylaxis record of the United States has steadily improved (Fig. 46-3). In 1978, only 82 cases of tetanus were reported to the Centers for Disease Control in Atlanta (Fig. 46-5).[46]

The United States armed forces has had an outstanding record of tetanus prophylaxis for many years (Table 46-8).

According to Vice Admiral W. P. Arentzen, surgeon general of the United States Navy, among the several million people who have served in the Navy and Marine Corps since World War II, none has had an injury while on active duty that was responsible for tetanus.[47] He noted that, during the summer of 1974, one man, who had never received a tetanus inoculation and was circumcised several

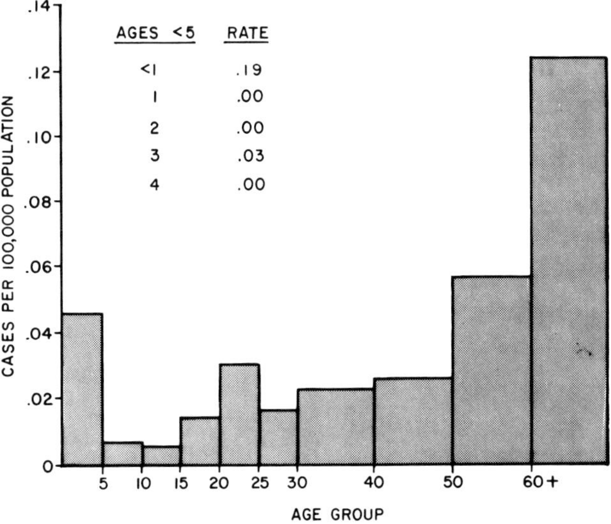

Fig. 46-5. **Reported cases of tetanus per 100,000 population by age group, United States, 1977. (Courtesy of Center for Disease Control, Public Health Service, U.S. Department of Health, Education, and Welfare. Annual Summary 1977, Morbidity and Mortality Weekly Report 26:69, 1978.)**

TABLE 46-8. CASES OF TETANUS IN THE UNITED STATES ARMED FORCES

Unit	U.S. Armed Forces Period	No. of Cases
Army	1956–77	0
Navy and Marine Corps	1946–77	1
Air Force	1958–77	2

days before enlisting in the Navy, developed tetanus several days after his induction. This case is obviously not a failure of the Navy tetanus prophylaxis program, but actually emphasizes how extremely effective the Navy program has been, and indicates that tetanus may occur even after operations.

Colonel Llewellyn J. Legters of the United States Army Medical Corps indicated for the surgeon general that there have been no confirmed cases of tetanus reported in Army personnel during the 20 years from 1956 through 1976.[48]

Lieutenant General George E. Schafer, surgeon general of the United States Air Force, stated that Air Force statistical data reveal two cases of tetanus in Air Force personnel since 1958.[49]

BIBLIOGRAPHY

Furste W, Wheeler W: Tetanus: A team disease. Curr Probl Surg, October, 1972.

Habermann E: Tetanus. In Vinken PJ, Bruyn GW (eds): Handbook of Clinical Neurology, Infections of the Nervous System (Vol 33), Amsterdam, North-Holland Publishing Company, 1978, p. 491.

Martin RR: Tetanus. In Mandell GL, Douglas RG Jr, Bennett JE (eds): Principles and Practice of Infectious Diseases. New York, Wiley, 1979.

REFERENCES

1. Hippocrates (with an English translation by WHS Jones), Vol 1. Cambridge, Harvard Univ. Press, 1923, p 165.
2. Aretaeus, the Cappadocian. On tetanus. In Adams F (ed): The Extant Works. London, 1856, pp 246–249, 400–404.
3. Murphy KJ: Tetanus after rubber-band ligation of haemorrhoids. Br Med J 1:1590, 1978.
4. Bytchenko B: Personal communication. June, 1978.
5. Patel J, Mehta B: Tetanus: a study of 2007 cases. Indian J Med Sci 17:791, 1963.
6. Center for Disease Control, Public Health Service, U.S. Department of Health, Education, and Welfare. Tetanus Surveillance. Report No 5, in press.
7. Smith A: Tetanus. In Beeson PB, McDermott W (eds): Cecil-Loeb Textbook of Medicine, 13th ed. Philadelphia, Saunders, 1971, p 566.
8. Kryzhanovsky G: Tetanus: a polysystemic disease. In Comptes rendus de la quatrieme conference internationale sur le tetanos (Proceedings of the fourth international conference on tetanus). Lyon (France), Lips, 1975, p 189.
9. Furste W, Wheeler W: Tetanus: a team disease. Curr Probl Surg, Oct 1972.
10. Communicable Disease Center, Public Health Service, U.S. Department of Health, Education, and Welfare: Tetanus Surveillance. Report No 1, February 1, 1968.
11. Glenn F: Tetanus—a preventable disease: including an experience with civilian casualties in the battle for Manila (1945). Ann Surg 124:1030, 1946.
12. Cole L, Youngman H, Gandy A: An attack of tetanus. Lancet 2:567, 1968.
13. Moersch F, Woltman H: Progressive fluctuating muscular rigidity and spasm (stiff-man syndrome). Proc Staff Meet Mayo Clin 31:421, 1956.
14. Wangensteen OH: Personal communication, November 20, 1972.
15. American Academy of Pediatrics: Report of the Committee on the Control of Infectious Diseases. Evanston, Illinois, The Academy, 1977, p 11.
16. Bennett J: Tetanus. In Hoeprich P (ed): Infectious Diseases, 2nd ed. Hagerstown, Harper and Row, 1977, p 954.
17. Center for Disease Control, Public Health Service, U.S. Department of Health, Education, and Welfare. Recommendation of the Public Health Service Advisory Committee on Immunization Practices. Morbidity and Mortality Weekly Report 26:401, 1977.
18. Committee on Control of Surgical Infections, American College of Surgeons: Manual on Control of Infection in Surgical Patients. Philadelphia, Lippincott, 1976, pp 180, 189.
19. Committee on Trauma, American College of Surgeons: A guide to prophylaxis against tetanus in wound management. 1979 revision. Bull Am Coll Surg, 64:19, 1979.
20. Department of the Army, the Navy, the Air Force, and Transportation. Immunization. AR 40–562, BUMEDINST 6230.1H, AFR 161–13, CG COMDINST 6230.4C. Washington, D.C., June 7, 1977.
21. Dull H: Active immunization for infectious diseases. In Conn H (ed): Current Therapy 1978. Philadelphia, Saunders, 1978, p 86.
22. Furste W, Aguirre A: Preventing tetanus. Am J Nursing 78:834, 1978.
23. Krugman S, Katz S: Childhood immunization procedures. JAMA 237:2228, 1977.
24. McComb J: The combined use of homologous tetanus immune globulin and toxoid in man. In Eckmann L (ed): Principles on Tetanus. Bern, Hans Huber, 1967, p 359.
25. Peebles T, Levine L, Eldred M, Edsall G: Tetanus toxoid emergency boosters. A reappraisal. N Engl J Med 280:575, 1969.
26. Proceedings of the Fifth International Conference on Tetanus. Ronneby, Sweden, June 1978, in press.
27. Sandusky W: Tetanus. In Conn H (ed): Current Therapy 1978. Philadelphia, Saunders, 1978, p 71.
28. Chase A: Immunization. Med Trib 19:11, 1978.
29. Long A: The Army Immunization Program. Vol III. Preventive Medicine in World War II, Medical Department, United States Army, Washington, D.C., United States GPO, 1955, p 287.
30. Long A, Sartwell P: Tetanus in the U.S. Army in World War II. Bull U.S. Army Med Dept 7:371, 1947.
31. Murphy K: Fatal tetanus with brainstem involvement and myocarditis in an ex-serviceman. Med J Aust 2:542, 1970.
32. Sakurai N, Hashizume S, Fujishiro K: Tetanus infection after immunization with tetanus toxoid. Part I. Human incidence. In Proc Fifth Internat Conf on Tetanus, 1978, in press.
33. Sakurai N, Ogonuki M, Niiro M, Takano S, Yamada S, Sugiura Y: Tetanus infection after immunization with tetanus toxoid. Part II. Cases in guinea-pigs in experiments and calves in

the farms. In Proc Fifth Internat Conf on Tetanus, 1978, in press.
34. Berger S, Cherubin C, Nelson S, Levine L: Tetanus despite pre-existing antitetanus antibody. JAMA 240:769, 1978.
35. Furste W: The role of surgical prophylaxis. In Eckmann L (ed): Principles on Tetanus. Bern, Hans Huber, 1967, p 369.
36. Center for Disease Control, Public Health Service, U.S. Department of Health, Education, and Welfare. Tetanus Surveillance. Report No 4, March 31, 1974, p 9.
37. Santangelo Y, Moreira I: Tetanus prophylaxis of wounds. Rev Brasileira de Med 33:257, 1976.
38. Eckmann L (ed): Principles on Tetanus. Bern, Hans Huber, 1967.
39. Furste W: The second international conference on tetanus. Int Med Dig 82:469, 1966.
40. Furste W, Editorial: The fourth international conference on tetanus, Dakar, Senegal, 1975. J Trauma 16:755, 1976.
41. Blake P, Feldman R, Buchanan T, Brooks G, Bennett J: Serologic therapy of tetanus in the United States, 1965–1971. JAMA 235:42, January 5, 1976.
42. Patel J, Mehta B, Nanavati B, Hazra A, Rao S, Swaminathan C: Role of serum therapy in tetanus. Lancet 1:740, 1963.
43. Ildirim I: Intrathecal treatment of tetanus with antitetanus serum and prednisolone mixture. Report at Third International Conference on Tetanus, Sao Paulo, Brazil, 1970.
43a. Editorial: Tetanus immune globulin: The intrathecal route. Lancet 2:464, 1980.
44. Prys-Roberts C, Corbett J, Kerr J, Spalding J, Crampton-Smith A: Treatment of sympathetic over-activity in tetanus. Lancet 1:542, 1969.
45. Pikelj F, Lazar M, Vidmar L: Treatment of asystole and bradycardia in tetanus with endocardial demand pacemaker. Proc Fifth Int Conf On Tetanus, in press.
46. Center for Disease Control, Public Health Service, U.S. Department of Health, Education, and Welfare. Morbidity and Mortality Weekly Report 27:538, 1979.
47. Arentzen WP: Personal communication, April 1977.
48. Legters LJ: Personal communication, April 1977.
49. Schafer GE: Personal communication, April 1977.

CHAPTER 47
Infection in the Immunocompromised Host

ROBERT H. RUBIN AND A. BENEDICT COSIMI

The major advances in immunosuppressive therapy have greatly increased the productive years of people who would formerly have succumbed quickly to uremia and malignant and autoimmune diseases. Such potential, however, may only be realized if life-threatening infections, which arise from the major host defense defects present in these patients, can be prevented or treated. Infection, not the primary illness, has become a major cause of both morbidity and mortality.

Physicians of every level of specialization must become familiar with both the unusual infectious diseases that occur in this population, and also the ways in which the underlying disease and its therapy can modify the clinical presentation and management of common conditions.

SPECIFIC AND NONSPECIFIC HOST DEFENSE DEFECTS AND THEIR INFECTIOUS COMPLICATIONS

NEUTROPHIL, B-LYMPHOCYTE, T-LYMPHOCYTE, AND COMPLEMENT FUNCTION

Host defenses have been discussed in Chapter 13. Both primary (inborn) and secondary (acquired) disorders of neutrophil, B-lymphocyte, T-lymphocyte, and complement function have been described,[1] and these disorders increase the host's susceptibility to infections. Each disorder gives rise to certain types of infections.[1] Thus, depressed neutrophil function increases susceptibility to bacterial infections. B-lymphocyte disorders increase the likelihood of infections with encapsulated bacteria and fungi, especially *Streptococcus pneumoniae, Haemophilus influenzae, Neisseria meningitidis* (the meningococcus), and group A streptococcus. Patients with depressed T-lymphocyte function have increased susceptibility to viruses, fungi, intracellular bacteria (*Salmonella* and *Listeria monocytogenes*), and some protozoans (*Pneumocystes carinii* and *Toxoplasma gondii*).

ADVERSE EFFECTS OF SPLENECTOMY

It has become apparent that the spleen is important to people who develop bacteremia with an organism to which they have little or no preexisting antibody. Although well-opsonized bacteria are removed primarily by the liver, the spleen is responsible for removing unopsonized bacteria from the bloodstream. The spleen also serves as a major site of synthesis of tuftsin, a basic tetrapeptide that coats polymorphonuclear leukocytes to promote phagocytosis, and the initiation of specific IgM antibody response to new antigens. The unique microcirculation of the spleen appears to be crucial to the survival of the nonimmune patient with pneumococcal or type B *H. influenzae* bacteremia. Even normal adults who are splenectomized after trauma exhibit an increased risk of catastrophic, overwhelming infection with these organisms. This phenomenon is particularly important in individuals who are asplenic after sickle cell anemia or as part of the management of hematologic malignancy. Children are clearly more susceptible than adults, especially during the first 6 to 12 months after splenectomy, although there have been several instances of late pneumococcal sepsis. Every effort should be made to protect the spleen from needless removal. Patients who have been splenectomized should receive the newly available pneumococcal vaccine. Although this vaccine is useful, the rate of seroconversion is inadequate in patients with malignant disease who are receiving combined radiation and chemotherapy. Therefore, all patients with functional or anatomic asplenia are susceptible to the development of overwhelming sepsis with the encapsulated organism, especially since the syndrome may follow otherwise trivial upper respiratory infections (Chapter 36).

MUCOCUTANEOUS ULCERATION AND NECROSIS

The mucocutaneous surfaces of the body serve as the primary barrier between the individual and the surrounding microbial world. Trauma and infection must be avoided at the two most susceptible mucosal sites, the mouth and the anorectal area, particularly in immunosuppressed patients.

MALNUTRITION

The interaction of inadequate nutrition and infectious agents is complex. The host defense defects produced by malnutrition predispose to infection, and the infection increases nutritional requirements. Increased nutrition is needed to avoid infection during malignant disease, major thermal injury, and conditions associated with major losses of protein from the body, such as the nephrotic syndrome, advanced cirrhosis, and malabsorption and gastrointestinal fistulas. Protein-calorie-vitamin malnutrition causes (1) atrophy of lymphoid tissue, particularly thymus and thymic-dependent areas of peripheral lymphoid tissues, (2) an associated decrease in the number and function of circulating T-lymphocytes, (3) normal or increased numbers of circulatory B-lymphocytes, with depressed primary antibody responses, (4) impaired intracellular killing of organisms by neutrophils, and (5) a decrease in both classic and alternate complement pathway components. It is little wonder that a major effort is now devoted to correcting and preventing nutritional abnormalities in all surgical patients but, most particularly, in those with other defects in host defense (Chapter 19).[2]

UREMIA

The metabolic abnormalities associated with uremia result in a number of abnormalities in host defense that lead to increased susceptibility to pneumonia, septicemia, and chronic viral hepatitis. Both specific and nonspecific components of host defense may be impaired. Although no single effect is sufficient to produce an increased propensity for infection by itself, the net result is a compromised patient. The most clearly demonstrable defect in host defense of the uremic patient is in cell-mediated immunity. Enhanced survival of skin, renal, and cardiac allografts, suppression of cutaneous delayed-type hypersensitivity reactions, defective lymphocyte blastogenesis in response to transplantation antigens and a variety of mitogenic agents, and, in some instances, lymphopenia and thymic atrophy have all been demonstrated in uremic patients and animals. An additional function of the T-lymphocyte, the production of interferon in response to viral infection, likewise seems to be significantly depressed in uremia. It is thought that these defects in cell-mediated immunity and interferon production are responsible for the uremic patient's frequent inability to eliminate hepatitis virus following acute exposure and the development of the prolonged carrier state.[3]

Less is known about the functioning of the B-lymphocyte system in uremia. Data suggest that the nature of the inciting antigen is important in predicting the antibody response. Although uremic patients appear to respond normally to the potent antigens of tetanus and diphtheria toxoids, other vaccines (most notably typhoid, influenza, and the new experimental cytomegaloviral vaccine), are less effective. Although the recently developed pneumococcal vaccine has been recommended for this population, there is no clinical proof of its effectiveness.[3]

Granulocyte function in uremia similarly may be impaired. Studies performed more than two decades ago show that the injection of noxious agents, such as sodium urate or bacteria, into the skin of uremic animals causes a diminished inflammatory response. More recent work in humans has shown that the generation of factors chemotactic for granulocytes, phagocytosis, and intraleukocytic killing of bacteria are relatively normal in the uremic patient. However, the ability of both polymorphonuclear and mononuclear leukocytes to respond to chemotactic factors may be depressed. This defect, which occurs in approximately 50 percent of nondialyzed uremic patients, is correctable by hemodialysis, although the cuprophane membrane used in hemodialysis may also create a more persistent defect in leukocyte function.[2,4]

There may be substances circulating in uremic serum that are inhibitory to the phagocytic function of both monocytes and macrophages—especially in the lung, where depressed alveolar macrophage function impairs bacterial clearance.[2,3] These uremic abnormalities are most likely caused by substances circulating in uremic plasma—the middle molecules, substances of 300 to 5,000 dalton molecular weight incompletely removed by hemodialysis. Bergstrom et al have isolated a single peptide from these middle molecules that is toxic for white cells. Newer dialysis techniques with better middle molecule clearance hold promise to partially repair host defense function.[5]

DIABETES

Diabetes mellitus is associated with an increased risk of infection, particularly mucocutaneous infections caused by *Staphylococcus aureus* and urinary tract infections. It is still unclear how much of the vulnerability is related to the patient's general debility, increased exposure to the hospital environment, and the vascular and neuropathic complications of the disease, as opposed to direct inhibitory effects of the molecular consequences of diabetes on host defenses. A recent review suggests that diabetics have an increased susceptibility only to (1) urinary tract infections in women, particularly a form of pyelonephritis complicated by renal papillary necrosis, (2) pulmonary tuberculosis, (3) vaginal candidiasis, (4) rhinocerebral mucormycosis, especially in association with ketoacidosis, and (5) malignant otitis externa caused by *Pseudomonas aeruginosa*. Other serious infections, for example staphylococcal and gram-negative bacteremias and viral influenza, may have a greater impact on the diabetic because of his or her general debility and metabolic complications. Individuals with impaired circulation secondary to diabetic vascular disease often develop osteomyelitis and chronic skin ulcerations of the feet, but the primary lesion is neuropathic and vascular.[6] Hyperglycemia may be a risk factor in predisposing organ transplant patients to infection. Finally, defects in neutrophil chemotactic responsiveness and phagocytosis can be demonstrated in patients with hyperglycemia.[7]

HEMOLYSIS

Blockade of the reticuloendothelial system renders the patient more susceptible to infection with intracellular parasites *(Salmonella, Listeria, Babesia).* Chronic hemolysis, malaria, relapsing fever, bartonellosis, and certain neoplastic conditions result in decreased monocyte–macrophage function.

EFFECTS OF TREATMENT REGIMENS ON HOST DEFENSE

There are many therapeutic programs that adversely affect a patient's ability to resist infection, particularly when more than one therapeutic agent is being used at a time—antimicrobial agents, hyperalimentation, radiation therapy, corticosteroids, and antineoplastic chemotherapeutic agents. Antimicrobial agents create selection pressures for colonization with antibiotic-resistant organisms. This is accomplished by both suppression of normal flora and increased availability of nutrients. All too often, the result is a treatment-resistant primary infection or superinfection, both of which are common in this patient population. Thus, antibiotic therapy should be as specific as possible and should not be used needlessly.

Intravenous hyperalimentation can be lifesaving in the repair of nutritional defects, but organisms can be infused in this way. Thus, staphylococcal and gram-negative bacteremias and, most importantly, *Candida* fungemias may occur. In the patient with underlying granulocytopenia or a defect in T-lymphocyte function, *Candida* introduced via this route is associated with at least a 50 percent rate of metastatic tissue invasion.[8]

Radiation therapy can cause a variety of dose-related systemic and local side effects that will impair the ability of the patient to resist infection. Factors influencing this impairment include the volume of irradiated marrow-bearing tissue, whether the bowel is included, and the extent of anatomic derangement caused by postirradiation fibrosis. The serious side effects caused by radiation therapy include (1) granulocytopenias and lymphopenia (especially T-cells), (2) decreased bactericidal function of monocytes and macrophages, (3) damage to mucocutaneous surfaces, providing a portal of entry for resident microbes, and (4) impaired circulation, providing a fertile soil for anaerobic infection.[9]

Corticosteroids have the most global immunosuppressive effects. They impair the mobilization, adherence, phagocytosis, and bactericidal activity of neutrophils, monocytes, and macrophages. They depress B- and T-lymphocyte activity, diminish production of interferon, and alter the gastrointestinal flora and local tissue integrity, resulting in easier invasion by endogenous flora. These effects are related to both the dose and the duration of therapy. Thus, high-dose steroids are usually well tolerated for one to two weeks, but after that the incidence of life-threatening infection is increased. Alternate-day steroids have less depressant effects on host defense and are associated with significantly fewer serious clinical infections than is daily therapy. When prolonged daily use is required, the dosage of prednisone should remain under 20 mg per day.[10-12]

Cytotoxic drugs also have broad-ranging immunosuppressive properties. The most common adverse effect is granulocytopenia. Patients myelosuppressed by cytotoxic drugs usually have both neutropenia and monocytopenia and, thus, may be at greater risk for infection than patients with chronic granulocytopenia of other etiologies. Other adverse effects include ablation or suppression of both antibody synthesis and cell-mediated immunity (although B cell function is usually depressed more than T cell function), suppression of the reticuloendothelial system, and damage to mucocutaneous surfaces. Since mucosal damage to the gut may predispose to gram-negative bacteremia, the stimulataneous reticuloendothelial depression may contribute to the high mortality rate from gram-negative sepsis observed in patients receiving cytotoxic therapy. Other defects of importance produced by some of these agents include decreased white cell mobilization, chemotaxis, phagocytosis, and bactericidal function (particularly by the *Vinca* alkaloids), and diminished opsonic activity by the cytotoxic agents, such as cyclophosphamide and nitrogen mustard compounds.

The cumulative effects of individual immunosuppressive agents may far exceed the effects of each alone. For example, splenectomized adult lymphoma patients are not at greater risk for overwhelming sepsis than are normal individuals undergoing posttraumatic splenectomies.[13] However, if one adds granulocytopenia, an age less than 12, or, most particularly, a history of combined radiation and chemotherapy, the risk is significantly increased. Patients with Hodgkin's disease subjected to this most intense of therapeutic regimens have lower circulating IgM levels and lower titers of antibody to *H. influenzae* type B and respond poorly to pneumococcal vaccine. Thus, the net effect of successful therapy of a T-lymphocyte disorder (Hodgkin's disease) has been the creation of a B cell disorder.[13,14]

APPROACH TO PATIENTS WITH POSSIBLE HOST DEFENSE DEFECT

The major clue to the presence of a significant host defense defect is an increased susceptibility to infection. This is usually manifested by increased frequency, severity, or duration of infection, the development of an unusual complication or manifestation of the primary infection, or the demonstration of invasive infection with organisms that are normally relatively avirulent. In children,[15] the clinical clues suggesting a primary immunodeficiency syndrome are as listed in Table 47-1.

The ideal test to screen for a possible immunodeficiency should be inexpensive, noninvasive, easy to perform, and reliable. Table 47-2 delineates the approach developed by Stiehm—initial screening tests followed by more specific evaluation of abnormalities.[15]

TABLE 47-1. PEDIATRIC PRIMARY IMMUNODEFICIENCY SYNDROME

Usually Present	Frequently Present	Occasionally Present
Recurrent respiratory infections	Draining ears	Mucocutaneous candidal infection
Severe infections	Irritability	
Pneumonia		Vaccinia gangrenosum
Bacteremia	Anemia	
Meningitis		*Pneumocystis carinii* pneumonia
	Chronic pneumonia	
Recurrent diarrhea		Skin rashes and alopecia
	Bronchiectasis	
Overall failure to thrive		Severe viral disease
	Pyoderma	
		Arthritis
	Chronic conjunctivitis	
	Malabsorption	Hepatosplenomegaly or lymphadenopathy
	A paucity of lymph nodes and tonsils	Hematologic abnormalities

INFECTION IN THE COMPROMISED HOST: EPIDEMIOLOGY AND PREVENTION

Epidemiologic aspects of infection in this population have, appropriately, been receiving increasing attention. Among hospitalized cancer and leukemia patients, careful studies have shown that although 86 percent of infections arise from the patient's endogenous flora, approximately half of these organisms were first acquired from the hospital environment (Chapter 24). The incidence of nosocomial infections among cancer patients is approximately four times that of the general population. Such infections are most frequently caused by Enterobacteriaceae, especially *Klebsiella* and *Enterobacter* species, *P. aeruginosa,* and *Candida.* Of particular importance is the fact that once colonization with *P. aeruginosa* occurs, 40–68 percent of patients will develop septicemia during periods of drug-induced severe neutropenia.[16] Goldschmidt and Bodey [17] have made the interesting observation that many of the cytotoxic agents employed for cancer chemotherapy have antibacterial activity for most of the intestinal flora, with the exception of *P. aeruginosa.*

Nosocomial infection appears to play an important role in pneumonia and septicemia in the immunosuppressed patient. We have observed a high rate of *P. aeruginosa* superinfection among kidney recipients temporarily housed on the same isolation floor as burn patients. Since the transplant patients have been moved to a different hospital site, apart from the burn patients who are heavily contaminated with *P. aeruginosa,* there has not been a single instance of *Pseudomonas* infection. However, colonization and superinfection with other relatively antibiotic-resistant gram-negative bacilli in the hospital environment (*Klebsiella, Serratia,* and *Acinetobacter*) remain a significant problem.[18]

Other microorganisms have caused epidemics of nosocomial pneumonia in the immunosuppressed patient. A probable outbreak of *P. carinii* infection has been identified on an oncology service, involving patients and staff alike.[19] Epidemic Legionnaires' disease has occurred on at least two renal transplant services due to probable nosocomial exposure,[20] but *Aspergillus* species have been the greatest nosocomial problem. Epidemic invasive aspergillosis has been documented in the following circumstances: (1) *Aspergillus fumigatus* spores were contaminating the air ducts leading to the rooms of immunosuppressed patients, (2) *A. fumigatus* was growing in pigeon excreta that was being sucked into the intake duct of ventilating systems leading to an operating room, and (3) three *Aspergillus* outbreaks were caused by spores present in fireproofing and/or insulating materials disturbed during renovation or used in the building of a new hospital facility.[18,21,22]

Constant surveillance of the immunosuppressed patient population is essential in order to identify an important infectious disease hazard before a major epidemic occurs. The compromised patient is like the old-fashioned sentinel chicken staked out in swamps to monitor the circulation of arboviruses between mosquitoes and birds.

Patients with neoplastic disease who have been rendered severely neutropenic by either the disease or its therapy are at greatest risk from infection. A great deal of attention has been devoted to attempts to prevent such infections. Observations in animals with and without tumors have shown that if the animals are rendered germ free, there is an increased tolerance of chemotherapy, and larger doses may be given with an enhanced tumoricidal effect and a greater chance for the induction of remission from the neoplastic condition. Germ-free animals can tolerate a greater degree and duration of myelosuppression without added risk. A great deal of effort has been expended to attempt to apply such a concept to the care of humans with neoplastic disease.

TABLE 47-2. LABORATORY EVALUATION OF POSSIBLE IMMUNODEFICIENCY

Type of Deficiency	Screening Test	Definitive Tests
Antibody deficiency	Immunoelectrophoresis Schick test Isoagglutinin titers	Quantitative immunoglobulin determination Enumeration of B-lymphocytes Secretory immunglobulins and antibodies Rectal or lymph node biopsy Lateral pharyngeal x-ray Preexistent antibodies to polio, tetanus, and so on Antibody response to injected antigens Immunoglobulin kinetics IgG subclass determination
Cell-mediated immunity deficiency	Lymphocyte count and morphology Thymic x-ray Skin tests with battery of skin test antigens (*Candida*, mumps, *Trichophyton*)	Enumeration of T-lymphocytes Dinitrochlorobenzene challenge Assay of lymphokine and blastogenic response in vitro Lymph node biopsy Skin homograft
Phagocytic deficiency	White blood cell count, differential, and morphology	Nitrobluetetrazolium assay Assays of chemotactic responsiveness, random migration, phagocytosis, bactericidal activity Antileukocyte antibodies Rebuck skin window Splenic scan
Complement and opsonic deficiency	Total hemolytic complement (CH_{50}) C3 level	Assay of specific complement components Generation of chemotactic factors Opsonic assay

Modified from Stiehm ER: Immunodeficiency disorders: General considerations. In Stiehm ER, Fulginiti VA (eds): *Immunologic Disorders in Infants and Children,* 1980, p 183. (Courtesy of W.B. Saunders Company.)

This hypothesis has been tested in man, using some form of protected environment (initially a self-contained patient isolation unit termed a "life island"), such as laminar air flow rooms employing filters, bowel and orificial decontamination, and sterile food and water. A 95 percent reduction in microbial colonization can be achieved at most body sites using the combination of oral gentamicin, vancomycin, and nystatin for bowel decontamination. The oropharynx, however, remains difficult to decontaminate, since *Candida albicans* is often impossible to eradicate with existing oral antifungal agents, and a period of up to three to four weeks is required to complete the task. Even then, certain organisms, particularly *P. aeruginosa* and *C. albicans,* are only suppressed and will reappear as soon as the program is relaxed. If the program is stopped while a patient is still severely granulocytopenic, these two organisms will rapidly repopulate the gut, with a 70 percent risk of septicemia. An additional problem is the increasing evidence that gentamicin-resistant gram-negative bacteria will emerge with this program.[23-25]

The drawbacks of these programs are major: increased cost (approximately $1,000 per day), patient intolerance of the taste of the oral antimicrobial agents, the associated abdominal cramps and diarrhea, and the profound psychologic effects of isolation. The benefits are minimal. When the total program of protected environment plus decontamination with antimicrobial agents is carried out, there appears to be a decrease in the incidence of life-threatening infection. Unfortunately, even with the maximal program, there has not been any clear-cut demonstration of increased patient survival, greater tolerance of increased doses of chemotherapeutic agents, or increased rate of remission. Such programs remain of research interest only.[26] Recently, several investigators have shown that bacterial decontamination can be achieved with oral trimethoprim-sulfamethoxazole prophylaxis, with a consequent lower rate of infection in neutropenic patients at reasonable cost.[27,27a]

SPECIAL CLINICAL PROBLEMS IN THE IMMUNOSUPPRESSED PATIENT

FEVER WITHOUT EVIDENT CAUSE

Perhaps the most common clinical infectious disease problem in the compromised host is fever without evidence of a localized infection. The compromised host defenses probably diminish the inflammatory response that is often used to guide diagnosis and therapy. For example, meningeal signs may be absent from patients with meningitis, or cough and sputum production may be impaired in patients with pneumonia.[28]

The differential diagnosis of fever in these patients is extensive. Figure 47-1 illustrates the evaluation procedures used at one transplant center when a kidney recipient develops a fever of unknown origin. Fever may be due to such noninfectious causes as malignancy, allograft rejection, graft-versus-host disease, thromboembolic disease, antilymphocyte serum, antimicrobial agents, anticonvulsants, and blood product transfusions. Over 50 percent of the fevers, however, are caused by infections.[28a]

Neutropenic patients, especially, can have life-threatening infection with few localizing findings. Gram-negative bacilli of gastrointestinal origin are particularly common and usually enter through minor defects in the gastrointestinal mucosa, particularly in the mouth and oropharynx and the anorectum. In addition to minimal lesions leading to serious bacteremias, large areas of cellulitis, phlegmon, and frank abscess formation may develop. The other major site of entry is the lungs, where even a minimal infiltrate can cause overwhelming bacteremia. Perhaps the best example of this phenomenon comes from the studies of children with leukemia who develop pneumonia. The incidence of bacteremia is directly related to the neutrophil count. Patients with neutrophil counts greater than 1,000 per mm^3 had no positive blood cultures, compared to an incidence of 64 percent in those with counts less than 1,000 per mm^3.[29]

Life-threatening sepsis may be present even though there is no fever. The more subtle signs of serious infection include unexplained tachypnea, hypotension, continuous volume requirement, and acidosis. Whatever the manifestation of infection, the critical consideration is speed, because these patients rapidly succumb unless antimicrobial therapy is instituted. When the initial physical examination, chest roentgenogram, Gram stain of the urine, and other immediate bedside evaluations are unrevealing, and cultures have been done, empiric therapy with broad-spectrum antibiotics directed against the hospital's own bacteria should be instituted. The first principle of antibiotic therapy in the neutropenic patient is speed, and the second is the use of synergistic therapy with bactericidal drugs whenever possible. Lau et al [30] evaluated the results of different types of antibiotic therapy used in neutropenic patients with bacteremia. If neither drug employed was effective in vitro, the mortality rate was 100 percent, if only one effective drug was used, the mortality rate was 71 percent, if two drugs that had an additive antimicrobial effect were used, the mortality was 44 percent, and if synergistic therapy was used, the mortality was 18 percent. Two-drug or three-drug combinations of a cephalosporin, carbenicillin (or ticarcillin), and an aminoglycoside (gentamicin, tobramycin, or amikacin) that are effective against over 95 percent of the gram-negative isolates at the particular hospital should be instituted as empiric therapy. These drugs have a potential for synergy. Particularly in elderly patients with preexisting renal disease, the combination of cephalothin and gentamicin is far more nephrotoxic than either of the drugs alone or the combination of penicillin and gentamicin. After a bacteriologic isolation is made and the antibiotic susceptibility pattern is known, a less toxic synergistic antibiotic combination should be chosen.

Transfusions of granulocytes are a useful adjunct to synergistic antibiotic therapy in patients with profound neutropenia plus proven gram-negative sepsis. It will keep patients alive long enough for the therapy aimed at their basic underlying condition to have an opportunity to work. It is unclear, thus far, whether such a prolongation can be translated into an increase in patient survival. There are several disadvantages of granulocyte transfusions, including cost, potential hazard to the donor who receives systemic anticoagulation and corticosteroids during leukophoresis, and possible damage to the white cells. Most important, there is the risk of transfusion reactions and life-threatening posttransfusion cytomegaloviral infection in the recipient. Despite these concerns, granulocyte infusion

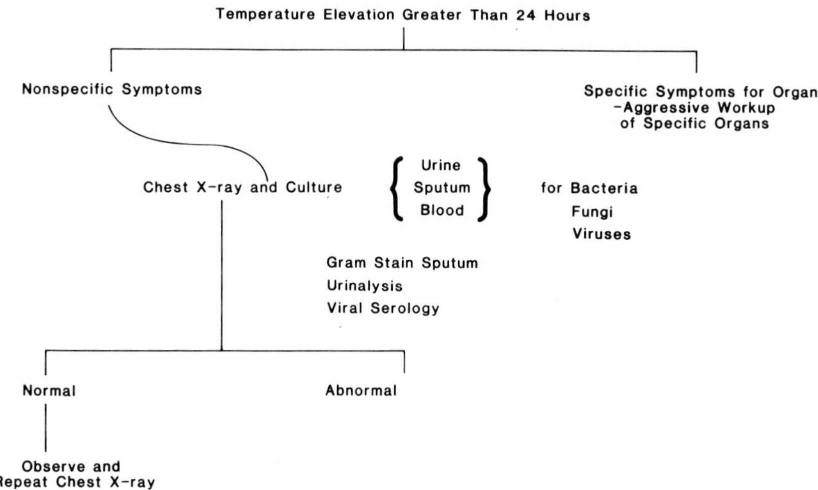

Fig. 47-1. **Flow diagram illustrating the evaluation of a transplant recipient with fever and nonlocalizing symptoms. (From Matas AS, Simmons RL, Najarian JS: In Hardy JD (ed): Critical Surgical Illness, 1980. Courtesy of W.B. Saunders Company.)**

provides a useful adjunct to the care of patients with sepsis and reversible neutropenia.[31,32a]

Several series show that early use of empiric antibiotics lowers mortality despite the fact that microbiologic proof of infection never emerges.[30,33,34] How, then, can therapy be terminated particularly because the risk of superinfection apparently goes up after seven days of broad-spectrum antimicrobial therapy? Empiric antibiotic treatment and clinical evaluation should be continued for five to seven days after antibiotics are initiated. If clinical infection has been documented or if a clinical response to therapy has been demonstrated, treatment should be continued for one to two weeks after evidence of the infection has disappeared. If no response and no bacteriologic isolation has been made, therapy should be stopped and the patient reevaluated. The most frequently missed infections in these patients include periodontal sepsis, perirectal abscess, pneumonia, and infections with fungi, protozoa, or viruses (particularly cytomegalovirus). In patients with esophagitis, prolonged diarrhea, history of exposure to broad-spectrum antibiotics for greater than 10 days, or positive surveillance cultures for fungi, and continuing unexplained fever, an empiric trial of parenteral antifungal therapy should be considered.

The same pressure for immediate empiric antimicrobial therapy is not present in patients with host defense defects who have normal levels of functioning neutrophils, and who have fever but no other local findings. Therefore, in the renal transplant patient or the lymphoma patient with a normal white count, a more leisurely diagnostic work-up can usually be undertaken. The indications for immediate initiation of antibiotics are usually related to where the patient is in his clinical course. For example, opportunistic infection with *Listeria, Nocardia,* and *Cryptococcus* are rare during the first two to four weeks after transplantation. Instead, the major diagnostic considerations are anatomic infections related to technical complications of the operation (eg, infected hematomas, or lymphoceles, infection associated with ureteral leaks), the usual forms of postoperative bacterial pneumonia, and acute allograft rejection. From one to three months posttransplant, cytomegaloviral infection is the most common cause of febrile illnesses, although allograft rejection, routine bacterial infection, and other opportunistic infections must be ruled out.[18,35,36] Urinary tract infection seems to be a particular problem on our transplant service. There is a 40 percent incidence of urinary tract infection in the first four months, and more than 80 percent of them are infections in the transplanted kidney. A prompt and prolonged course of therapy is indicated. Patients who develop their first urinary tract infection more than four months posttransplant predominantly have bladder infections that can be managed by more conventional methods.[37]

Patients with recently diagnosed lymphoma also appear to withstand infection relatively well. Zoster is their major infection and is especially common in the young, the female, and those recently irradiated. Early in the course, zoster is usually a relatively benign, well-localized disease. When it occurs a year or more after initial treatment, it is often a manifestation of tumor recurrence and may lead to encephalitis or pneumonia. Patients with progressive or recurrent lymphoma resemble renal transplant patients more than two or three months posttransplant. They develop high rates of disseminated cryptococcal infection, listeriosis, toxoplasmosis, and *Pneumocystis* and cytomegaloviral infections. As the disease progresses and the therapy is increased (with resulting granulocytopenia), the infections resemble those seen in acute leukemia—gastrointestinal tract-related bacteremias, pneumonia, esophagitis, pharyngitis. In addition, the tumor masses can cause tracheobronchial, urinary tract, biliary tract, and middle ear obstruction. Infections behind obstructions are difficult to eradicate—radiotherapy and surgery are necessary to relieve the obstruction.[38]

In patients treated with immunosuppressive agents, the kinds of infections observed are related not only to the drug, its dose, and the resulting level of immunosuppression but also to the time-related cumulative effect of the treatment. Therefore, the approach of the clinician to a patient with undiagnosed fever should be modified by the patient's underlying disease and course of therapy.

FEVER AND PNEUMONITIS

The differential diagnosis of fever and pneumonitis in an immunocompromised patient includes both noninfectious and infectious causes. The noninfectious causes include radiation pneumonitis, drug-induced pneumonitis (bleomycin, busulfan, methotrexate, and cyclophosphamide), parenchymal invasion of the lung by tumor (particularly lymphoma), leukoagglutinin reactions, pulmonary emboli, pulmonary hemorrhage, and atypical congestive heart failure.

True infection of the lung is the most common cause. Despite the occurrence of unusual opportunistic pathogens in these patients, the common bacterial pathogens predominate. Primary bacterial pneumonias occurring in outpatients are usually caused by gram-positive organisms (particularly, *S. pneumoniae*) and *H. influenzae.* Those that are nosocomially acquired are predominantly caused by enteric gram-negative bacilli. Bacterial pneumonia in the immunosuppressed population is similar to that in the general population. The onset is acute (within hours), the roentgenographic patterns are characteristic, and the response to therapy is prompt. The major difference lies in the risk of superinfection with antibiotic-resistant bacteria or fungi. In fact, superinfection is the major cause of death in immunosuppressed patients.[18,39,40] At autopsy, it is often impossible to find the original infecting pathogen, although several other agents are usually present (eg, herpes simplex virus, *Candida*). These organisms rarely cause primary pulmonary infection but are frequently part of a fatal polymicrobial superinfection.[18]

The major factor that predisposes to superinfection is a preexistent cytomegaloviral infection. This agent not only damages the lung and the alveolar macrophages but also is a potent inhibitor of systemic host defenses.[18,35,36,41]

Whatever the underlying factors, speed in establishing a diagnosis and initiating therapy is imperative. Important clues may be gained by using information concerning the pace of the illness, the history of the underlying disease, the therapy used to manage it, and the pattern of pulmonary infiltrate observed on chest roentgenogram. Thus, an illness that develops over a relatively few hours suggests acute bacterial infection, a pulmonary embolus, acute pulmonary edema, or pulmonary hemorrhage. A subacute onset (over a few days) suggests viral infection, *Pneumocystis, Aspergillus,* or *Nocardia.* A more chronic course (over several days to weeks) suggests fungal, nocardial, or tuberculosis infection or tumor-, drug-, or radiation-induced pneumonitis. The exemplary review of the subject by Williams and colleagues [22] points out that no radiologic pattern is specific for one particular pathogen, although certain patterns are more characteristic of some infectious agents than of others. Consolidation with air bronchograms suggests pneumococcal or *Klebsiella* infection, pulmonary hemorrhage, or other processes primarily affecting the distal air spaces. In contrast, an interstitial pattern suggests *Pneumocystis,* viral, leukoagglutinin, or drug-related disease. Cavitary lesions suggest fungal, nocardial, or tuberculosis infection. Thus, a series of clues will considerably narrow the diagnostic possibilities.

Even with these clues, an exact etiologic diagnosis must be aggressively sought so that specific therapy can be instituted quickly. Figure 47-2 shows the steps used at one center for evaluating a kidney transplant patient who has a fever and symptoms of pulmonary involvement. The classic approach to pneumonia has centered on the microscopic and cultural examination of expectorated sputum, but several factors make this approach unreliable in immunocompromised patients. (1) These patients often fail to produce sputum, even after the most aggressive induction methods.[28,42] (2) These patients have a high incidence of pharyngeal colonization by a variety of potentially invasive pathogens, particularly gram-negative bacilli, *S. aureus,* and fungi. Therefore, the distinction between colonizers and invaders is difficult. (3) Several of the pathogens that invade this population are not shed into the sputum (*Aspergillus, Pneumocystis,* Legionnaires' bacillus), so that false-negative results are to be expected.[22] (4) The noninfectious causes of the febrile pneumonitis syndrome in this population cannot be diagnosed in this fashion. Therefore, invasive techniques have been designed to obtain more accurate information—transtracheal aspiration, bronchial brushing, percutaneous aspiration and cutting needle biopsy, fiberoptic bronchoscopy with bronchial brushing and transbronchial biopsy, and open lung biopsy. Each technique carries its own advantages and complications.[43]

Transtracheal aspiration, in which a plastic catheter is introduced through the cricothyroid membrane into the trachea, collects pulmonary secretions uncontaminated by the pharyngeal flora. Bleeding, hemoptysis, and cervical cellulitis can be kept to a minimum (less than 1 percent) if the patients are cooperative and have no bleeding disorders. Thrombocytopenia is not a contraindication as long as platelet transfusions will sustain a platelet count of greater than 50,000 per mm^3 for at least six hours after the procedure.[43] Transtracheal aspiration reveals the diagnosis in 90 percent of conventional bacterial infections, 50 percent of nocardial infections, and 20 percent of *Aspergillus* and *Pneumocystis* infections. Any sputum obtained by this technique should be cultured broadly, undergo routine staining for acid-fast, fungal, and bacterial organisms, and be specially processed for methanamine silver staining for *Pneumocystis.*[22,42,43,44] Virtually every immunocompromised patient who develops pulmonary infection should undergo a transtracheal aspiration as part of the initial evaluation. This technique is the best for diagnosing bacterial infection because routine bronchial brushing and fiberoptic bronchoscopy will yield specimens

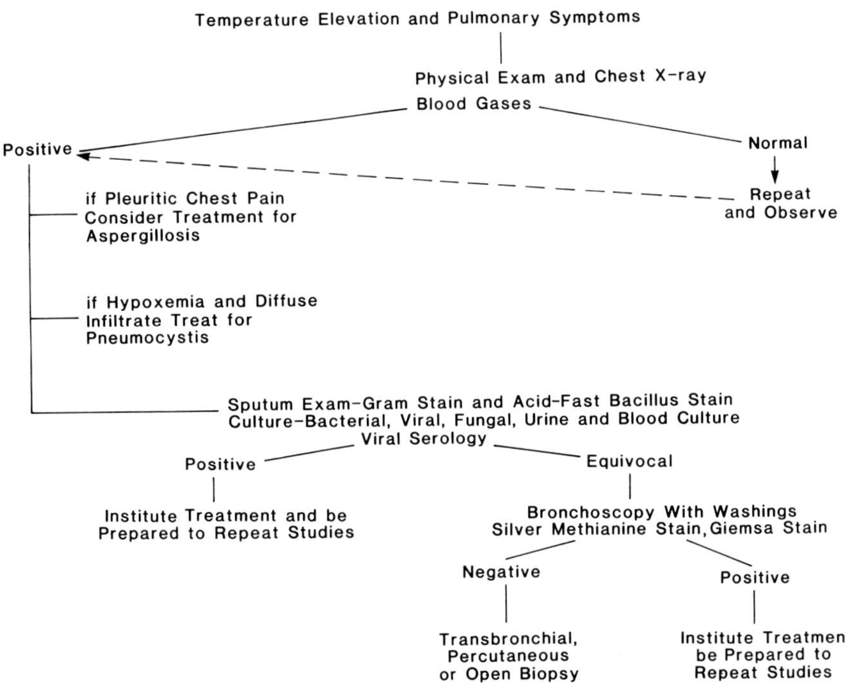

Fig. 47-2. **Flow diagram illustrating the evaluation of a transplant recipient with fever and pulmonary symptoms. (From Matas AS, Simmons RL, Najarian JS: In Hardy JD (ed): Critical Surgical Illness, 1980. Courtesy of W.B. Saunders Company.)**

contaminated by pharyngeal flora.[22,43]

If transtracheal aspiration fails, a more invasive procedure is needed. The choice, however, depends on the rapidity with which the patient is deteriorating, the expertise available at a particular hospital, and the type of roentgenographic abnormality. If the patient's pulmonary status is deteriorating rapidly, the most definitive diagnostic procedure, the open lung biopsy, should be done immediately. If the problem is more of a diagnostic dilemma, with a more desultory course, one may choose one of several less invasive diagnostic approaches, holding the open biopsy in reserve.[43]

Bronchial brushing, in which catheters are introduced through the nose or pharynx, is unreliable for the diagnosis of bacterial infection but is reliable in 75 percent of *Pneumocystis* infections and in 50 to 75 percent of fungal or nocardial infections. Major complications are rare. Major pneumothorax or hemorrhage occurs about 1 to 2 percent of the time.[22,43,45] Attempts by Aisner et al [42] to avoid oral contamination of the specimen by transtracheal bronchial brushing increased the diagnostic effectiveness, concurrently increasing the serious complication rate to 15 percent (severe neck cellulitis, major pneumothorax, and significant hemorrhage).

The percutaneous route, needle biopsy of the lung, yields excellent diagnostic specimens, but the turbine-powered trephine and the Vim-Silverman cutting needle carry high complication rates (hemorrhage, pneumothorax, air embolism).[22,43,46] In contrast, needle aspiration under fluoroscopic control, using a thin-walled, 18-gauge, noncutting needle, has yielded excellent results, particularly in patients with focal, peripherally located pulmonary lesions, especially when cavitation has been present. Major complications are unusual. This procedure has had its highest yield in patients with focal bacterial, fungal, and nocardial infections and is probably best when such infections are not diagnosed by the initial transtracheal aspiration. This technique is less useful in diagnosing diffuse lung disease, although it has been used successfully.[18,22,43,45-48]

Second to transtracheal aspiration, fiberoptic bronchoscopy combined with transbronchial biopsy and bronchial brushing is the best diagnostic technique for patients with diffuse lung diseases. The most common treatable cause of diffuse interstitial lung disease in the immunosuppressed host, caused by *P. carinii*, appears to be diagnosable in approximately 90 percent of patients. In addition, material sufficient for pathologic diagnosis of radiation-induced and drug-induced pneumonia may also be obtained in a comparable percent. Focal fungal or nocardial infection may also be identified, particularly when bronchial brushing as well as transtracheal biopsy are carried out through the fiberoptic bronchoscope. The complications associated with this procedure are pneumothorax (3 to 6 percent), hemorrhage (1 to 2 percent), and death (0.2 percent).[43,49,50] Life-threatening bacteremia and postbronchoscopy pneumonia have been reported in the neutropenic and debilitated patient. Appropriate safeguards should be taken to prevent these complications.[51,52]

A particular, unsolved problem is the etiology of diffuse pulmonary infiltrates in many patients who are immunosuppressed. Even after the most extensive work-up, up to and including open lung biopsy and autopsy examination, approximately half of these patients will remain undiagnosed. Some of these cases can represent instances of unusual drug-induced pneumonias, particularly that caused by bleomycin.[43,50]

SPECIFIC INFECTIONS IN THE COMPROMISED HOST

BACTERIAL INFECTIONS

Although unusual pathogens are important in this clinical setting, common bacteria are still the most frequent cause of serious infection. There are two groups of infections caused by aerobic gram-negative bacilli: those due to common endogenous organisms, *Escherichia coli, Klebsiella, Proteus,* and *Enterobacter,* and those acquired in the hospital environment, antibiotic-resistant *E. coli* and *Klebsiella, Pseudomonas, Serratia,* and *Acinetobacter.* In the past few years, there has been a resurgence in the incidence of infection with *S. aureus,* particularly in patients with skin breaks. Anaerobic infection, especially that with *Bacteroides* and *Clostridium,* is rare except in patients with solid tumors, particularly tumors involving the gastrointestinal or genitourinary tracts. In fact, unexplained bacteremias with one of these organisms can be a clue to the presence of such neoplasms.[53] Among the less common bacterial species, infections caused by *Salmonella, Listeria, Bacillus, Nocardia,* and *Mycobacterium tuberculosis* deserve comment.

Salmonella

Nontyphoidal *Salmonella* infections are more common and more severe in the immunocompromised patients (Chapter 5). Nosocomial transmission of the intracellular organism appears to be an important factor. The risk of bacteremia, metastatic infection, and a prolonged carrier state are significantly increased in renal transplant recipients and in patients with lymphoproliferative disorders, with defects in intracellular killing, with immunoglobulin disturbances, and with solid tumors that may actually get infected with these organisms. Prolonged therapy with bactericidal antibiotics is required.

Listeria Monocytogenes

L. monocytogenes is discussed in Chapter 7. Although listeriosis may occur among normal individuals, 50 to 75 percent of children above the age of 12 and adults who develop listerial infection have a significant predisposing disease. Underlying conditions associated with *Listeria* infection include lymphoproliferative disorders, prolonged corticosteroid or cytotoxic drug therapy, organ transplantation, and other diseases associated with impaired cell-mediated immunity, such as sarcoidosis and cirrhosis of the liver. Bacteremia without an obvious primary site or evidence of metastatic infection and central nervous system infection may lead to widespread metastatic infection, especially to the heart valves or bone.[54]

In the immunosuppressed patient population, listerial meningitis is a less dramatic infection and develops over days to even weeks, with absence of meningeal signs and, in some instances, no changes in mental status and minimal fever. Virtually all patients will have a headache, however (Fig. 47-3). Since the other major cause of meningitis in the compromised host, *Cryptococcus neoformans,* similarly may have minimal findings, the indication to perform a lumbar puncture is the presence of a sustained headache, particularly if a low-grade fever is present. The cerebrospinal fluid formula in listerial meningitis usually resembles that of other bacterial meningitis, with a polymorphonuclear leukocyte pleocytosis, low sugar, and high protein. An occasional patient, particularly one with a prolonged course, will have a lymphocytic predominance of cells on cerebrospinal fluid examination.[55] Occasionally *L. monocytogenes* may invade the brain, with or without simultaneous meningeal involvement, producing a bacterial encephalitis.

The treatment of listeriosis is discussed in Chapter 7. We use ampicillin (12–14 gm daily, intravenously in adults) or penicillin G (2,000,000 units intravenously every two hours in adults) with or without accompanying aminoglycoside therapy, which may be synergistic. High-dose intravenous tetracycline (1–2 gm per day in four divided doses), or erythromycin (4 gm per day in four divided doses) is satisfactory in allergic patients. Central nervous system infection with *Listeria* has a distinct tendency to relapse, so therapy should be continued for a minimum of 10–14 days after the patient has become afebrile, if treated with penicillin, and even longer if erythromycin or tetracycline has been used.

Bacillus

The saprophytic species of *Bacillus, Bacillus subtilis* and *Bacillus cereus,* particularly the latter, are capable of producing invasive pulmonary and disseminated bloodborne infections in the immunologically compromised host, comparable to that produced by *Bacillus anthracis* in the normal host (Chapter 7). In the lung, a hemorrhagic pneumonia, with evidence of blood vessel invasion, causing thrombosis, infarction, hemorrhage, and bacteremia, is commonly observed. Pulmonary infarction is the usual mistaken diagnosis. Although *B. subtilis,* like *B. anthracis,* is sensitive to penicillin, *B. cereus* requires therapy with gentamicin.[56]

Nocardia

The major focus of infection with *Nocardia* is the lungs, but there is a relatively high rate of disseminated disease, particularly to the brain, skeletal system, skin, and kidneys, sometimes without obvious preceding pulmonary disease (Chapter 7). Patients with chronic deficits of host defense (eg, lymphoma, organ transplant recipients) are most susceptible. Pulmonary nocardial infection is usually subacute or chronic, with fever, chills, cough productive of purulent (sometimes bloody) sputum, and pleurisy. Roentgenographic findings range from lobar consolidation to single or multiple nodules, all with a tendency to rapidly cavitate. Any pustular skin lesion, subcutaneous abscess, or superficial nodule may be the first clue to the presence of the systemic form of nocardial infection. Any patient with nocardial infection documented in the lungs or periphery should be examined for metastatic brain abscess.

Diagnosis of nocardial infection depends on the awareness of the clinical setting in which it occurs and the prompt and liberal use of biopsy wherever the lesion appears. Positive blood or sputum culture results are unusual, although nocardial colonization of the respiratory tract without disease has been noted. Treatment of nocardial infection in the immunosuppressed patient requires at least four to six months of therapy with high-dose sulfonamide or trimethoprim-sulfamethoxazole. Minocycline is an alternative agent.[22,57]

Tuberculosis

Tuberculosis in the immunosuppressed patient is unusual—so unusual that isoniazid prophylaxis is no longer recommended for tuberculin-positive patients undergoing transplantation. We only use prophylaxis in the patient with a grossly abnormal chest roentgenogram or a history of recent active infection.[18] When it occurs in transplant patients, musculoskeletal manifestations may predominate, but miliary tuberculosis has been reported. Tuberculosis is most common among patients with lung cancer (92 cases per 10,000) and Hodgkin's disease (96 cases per 10,000). Clinical tuberculosis is most severe in those patients receiving corticosteroid therapy or with an underlying lymphoproliferative disease.[58]

FUNGAL INFECTION

Fungal infections are the greatest concern in the compromised host. Aspergillosis, candidiasis, cryptococcosis, blastomycosis, coccidioidomycosis, histoplasmosis, and mucormycosis all occur in this population. These agents have been extensively discussed in Chapter 9. *Aspergillus* and *Candida* species require reemphasis here.

Invasive Aspergillosis

Two species, *Aspergillus fumigatus* and *Aspergillus flavus,* account for more than 90 percent of the invasive aspergillosis in compromised patients. The air supply in the hospital environment may serve as a source of epidemic infection in this patient population.[21] *Aspergillus* infection in the compromised host is invasive aspergillosis, a necrotizing bronchopneumonia and bronchitis featuring blood vessel invasion with hemorrhage, infarction, and dissemination to every conceivable organ. Brain abscesses are common and usually fatal.

The pneumonic form causes dyspnea, tachypnea, nonproductive cough, pleurisy, hemoptysis, fever, and chills. Twenty to thirty percent of these patients have these symptoms before the appearance of clear roentgenographic abnormalities, in which case lung scans can be useful in demonstrating perfusion defects and can suggest

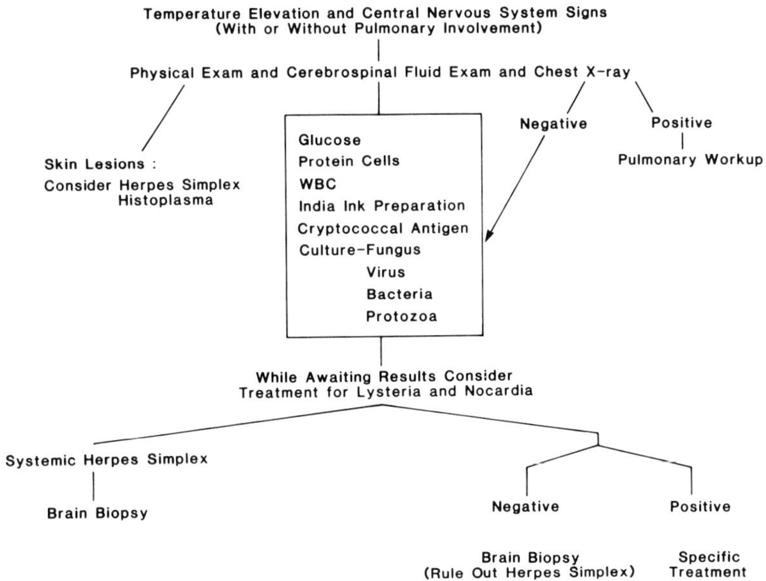

Fig. 47-3. **Flow diagram illustrating the evaluation of a transplant recipient with fever and neurologic symptoms. (From Matas AS, Simmons RL, Najarian JS: In Hardy (ed): Critical Surgical Illness, 1980. Courtesy of W.B. Saunders Company.)**

an etiologic diagnosis. The roentgenographic picture can be varied, with the most characteristic one showing single or multiple nodular lesions that progress rapidly to cavitation and frequently cross lung fissures. Less commonly, interstitial pneumonia, lobar consolidation, and miliary disease may be observed. Dual infections are common, with *Aspergillus* complicating primary cytomegaloviral or bacterial pneumonia or simultaneously presenting with *Nocardia* and *M. tuberculosis. Aspergillus* is by far the most lethal of the common superinfections afflicting this patient population.[22]

Aspergillus infections are difficult to diagnose. Positive sputum cultures appear in only 15 to 30 percent of cases. Nasal swabs may pick up a few more. Even then, the organism only grows transiently and in small numbers. Furthermore, *Aspergillus niger* is a major cause of laboratory contamination, and if speciation is not done, this saprophyte can confuse diagnosis. The isolation of *A. fumigatus* or *A. flavus* should be considered diagnostic of invasive aspergillosis in immunocompromised patients. Rarely are they laboratory contaminants.[59,60]

Even with careful culturing, the diagnosis will be missed in 75 percent of patients. Serologic techniques have not proved helpful. More promising are the immunologic techniques that measure the presence of circulating antigen as a measure of invasive infection.[61]

Invasive biopsy techniques are still the cornerstone of early diagnosis and therapy. The importance of early diagnosis is underscored by the results obtained in the treatment of this disease.[18,59] For example, Aisner et al [59] studied patients with acute nonlymphocytic leukemia. Of six patients diagnosed and treated within four days of onset, three were cured, and three showed a partial response. In contrast, all 11 patients in whom diagnosis was delayed for at least two weeks died with disseminated disease.

The best treatment for invasive aspergillosis is amphoterocin B (Chapter 9). Adjunctive treatment with granulocyte transfusions may benefit some neutropenic patients, although successful therapy of invasive aspergillosis has been reported in patients with hematologic malignancy and neutropenia without such transfusions.[22,43]

Candidiasis

Infection due to *Candida* in the immunocompromised host can range from the trivial to the life threatening (Chapter 9). The most virulent of the *Candida* species are *C. albicans* and *C. tropicalis*, which can maintain yeastlike and myceliumlike growth in human tissues. These pseudomycelia are quite resistant to phagocytosis. *Candida* produces two kinds of clinical disease, the most common being overgrowth at the mucocutaneous sites (oropharynx, vagina, and gastrointestinal tract) of normal colonization. Candidal growth is related to the amounts of glucose and glycogen present in mucosal secretions, and the organism grows well on macerated, intertriginous skin. Diabetes, pregnancy, and the administration of oral contraceptives or corticosteroids and broad-spectrum antibiotics all make more nutrients available. Thus, in the immunosuppressed patient population, the patient who is receiving concomitant steroid and antibiotic therapy is the best candidate for candidal overgrowth. Even with such overgrowth, however, candidal infection remains trivial unless the colonized mucocutaneous surfaces are penetrated. Tumor, trauma, operation, and immunosuppression encourage penetration into the bloodstream, with possible visceral dissemination. The most frequent means of penetration is provided by intravenous therapy, particularly hyperalimentation.[8]

In the normal human, even when *Candida* organisms penetrate beyond the primary mucocutaneous barriers into the bloodstream, infection is usually easily controlled by natural defense mechanisms. The host defenses that appear to be most important are adequate numbers of normally functioning neutrophils and normal T-lymphocyte–monocyte interactions. Patients with hematologic malignancy and those receiving corticosteroids are, therefore, particularly at risk for invasive candidal infection. A practical example of the difference in the nature of candidal infection in the normal and compromised patient is what happens after transient fungemia related to contaminated intravenous infusions. In the nonimmunosuppressed patient, transient fungemia results in serious disease in less than 5 percent of patients, as long as the source of the infection is removed promptly, and immediate institution of antifungal therapy is not necessary. In contrast, in the patient with leukemia or lymphoma or the patient on steroids, transient fungemia is associated with at least a 50 percent risk of visceral invasion, and antifungal therapy is indicated at the first sign of transient fungemia.[8,22,43]

In the compromised patient, overgrowth of *Candida* on mucosal surfaces may result in local discomfort and a risk of dissemination. In the oropharynx, raised, discrete, white patches on an erythematous base may appear. Such lesions are frequently painful but may be asymptomatic and, more important, may be associated with candidal overgrowth in the rest of the gastrointestinal tract. In the esophagus, the usual symptom complex is severe retrosternal pain and dysphagia, usually beginning in close association with a course of broad-spectrum antibiotic therapy. Although in the appropriate clinical setting a presumptive diagnosis can usually be made, diagnosis may be confirmed by esophagoscopy (the most sensitive technique) or barium swallow. On barium swallow, irregularities of the mucosal folds of the esophagus that resemble esophageal varices, atonicity, and impaired peristalsis are commonly seen. In a few patients, the esophageal lumen may be compromised, and similar findings may be observed in patients with severe herpetic esophagitis.

In the compromised host, *Candida* are by far the most commonly cultured fungal organisms recovered from sputum, bronchial secretions, or postmortem lung biopsies, although its clinical significance is often questionable. Most commonly, *Candida* are present as colonizers of the tracheobronchial tree but are not actually invading the pulmonary parenchyma. Even if the patient has concomitant pneumonia, the odds are overwhelming that the candidal isolates have more to do with the pathogenesis of an accompanying stomatitis or esophagitis than with the pneumonia. Although primary candidal pneumonia exists in the immunosuppressed host, it is rare, it cannot be reliably diagnosed by the examination of sputum or serologic testing, and it should be accepted as a diagnosis only when proved by lung biopsy. In contrast, *Candida* are frequently part of a multimicrobial superinfection. *Candida* may also invade the lung, producing miliary microabscesses as part of a generalized hematogenous dissemination of the organism.[18,22]

Disseminated candidal infection, with metastatic spread to one or more visceral organs, is common under the following circumstances: (1) intravenous catheter-related infections, (2) operative manipulations of sites of candidal overgrowth (particularly the gastrointestinal tract, and (3) spontaneous bloodstream invasion from gastrointestinal sites in patients who are severely neutropenic from their disease or its therapy and in patients with major defects in lymphocyte–monocyte interaction and function. All of these factors are exacerbated if concomitant steroid therapy is being given.[8]

The consequences of candidal dissemination are many. Perhaps the major site of metastatic seeding is to the kidneys. In fact, in a patient at risk for candidal invasion, the demonstration of candiduria indicates the presence of disseminated candidiasis and the need for systemic anticandidal therapy. The other easily diagnosed metastatic site of candidal infection is the eye—candidal endophthalmitis is a frequent complication of sustained candidemia. Repeated examination of the optic fundi should be carried out in any patient with suspected disseminated candidiasis or in any compromised patient who is on prolonged hyperalimentation. The classic funduscopic finding is one or more white, cottonball-like areas of chorioretinitis extending out into the vitreous.[8] Another site of metastatic infection that may be of diagnostic help is the skin. Hematogenous spread of *Candida* to the skin is usually associated with erythematous, macronodular, occasionally hemorrhagic, skin lesions that are 0.5–1.0 cm in size. Such lesions should be biopsied soon after they appear.[62,63] Less common sites of metastatic infection include the myocardium, the skeletal system, and the meninges.[8]

As with invasive aspergillosis, invasive candidiasis is difficult to diagnose. Routine blood cultures are usually negative (50 to 75 percent of the time), and even when positive, they may not be recognized for a long time. Serologic studies are useless in immunosuppressed patients.[64] It is little wonder that a premortem diagnosis of disseminated candidiasis was made in only 15 to 40 percent of patients. Even though newer techniques for demonstrating candidal antigen appear promising, aggressive biopsy techniques and empiric anticandidal therapy will have to be employed if mortality is to be reduced.[8]

There are two aspects to the therapy of candidal infection in the immunosuppressed host: (1) correction of the circumstances that lead to candidal overgrowth and invasion in the first place and (2) specific antifungal chemotherapy. The first step, then, is to remove urinary and intravenous catheters, discontinue broad-spectrum antibacterial therapy, control diabetes, and decrease, if possible, corticosteroid and other immunosuppressive therapy.

The antifungal therapy employed depends, in part, upon the type of candidal invasion observed. Even in immunosuppressed patients, mucocutaneous infection will often respond to correction of predisposing factors and topical therapy. Cutaneous and vaginal candidiasis are effectively treated with creams or lotions containing nystatin, clotrimazole, or miconazole. Frequent gargling and swallowing of suspensions of nystatin or amphotericin B will usually clear oropharyngeal and esophageal infection. Such therapy is more effective prophylactically, and, therefore, we place susceptible patients on prophylactic nystatin whenever antibacterial therapy is initiated. In individuals with severe mucosal disease, particularly of the esophagus, whose predisposing factors cannot be corrected, low-dose parenteral amphotericin B therapy (5–10 mg daily for 5–14 days) may be effective. Invasive candidiasis should be treated with a combination of intravenous amphotericin B and 5-fluorocytosine, as described in Chapter 9.

The new systemic antifungal agents, miconazole and ketoconazole, hold some promise as anticandidal agents. They lack significant renal, hepatic, and bone marrow toxicity (Chapter 18).[65,65a]

Cryptococcal Infection

C. neoformans is discussed in Chapter 9. Only a few points will be emphasized here. Approximately 50 percent of patients who develop cryptococcal infection have an easily recognizable defect in host defenses, usually caused by lymphoma, corticosteroid administration, or sarcoidosis. In fact, the diagnosis of cryptococcal infection indicates a disease state associated with defects in cell-mediated immunity. The major clinical impact of *C. neoformans* infection is on the lungs and central nervous system, although miliary disease occurs in patients with the most profound defects in host defense.[22]

Infection of the lung with *C. neoformans* produces a subacute, chronic illness. Despite the presence of rather extensive pulmonary infiltrates, the symptoms are often minimal, and at least one third of patients are asymptomatic. The most common symptoms are low-grade fever and nonproductive cough. The typical roentgenographic finding is a mass or a segmental consolidation, occasionally with some cavitation. Rarely, multiple nodules or diffuse disease, either in an interstitial or a miliary pattern, may also be seen. Hilar adenopathy is present in 10 percent of patients and pleural effusions in less than 5 percent.[18,22,66]

It is important to emphasize that the isolation of *C. neoformans* on sputum culture does not prove that a lesion seen radiographically is caused by this organism, since *Cryptococcus* may only be colonizing the tracheobronchial tree. There appears to be a particular association between cryptococcal colonization and lung cancer. A recent report from the Mayo Clinic[67] noted that 25 percent of their sputum isolates of *C. neoformans* were from patients with lung cancer without fungal pulmonary invasion. Relying on sputum cultures alone, particularly in patients with coin lesions, to rule out the presence of tumor and the need for thoracotomy could have disastrous consequences. Mixed infections with *Nocardia*, tuberculosis, and *Aspergillus* may be present. In the patient with depressed cell-mediated immunity, the diagnosis of pulmonary cryptococcal infection should lead to a search for disseminated disease, particularly of the meninges.

Cryptococcal meningitis is a chronic meningitis that follows a waxing and waning course over the months to years before death inevitably occurs. The clinical onset is usually insidious, and asymptomatic intervals may occur. The most common symptoms are fever and a persistent headache or headache alone, although headaches can be absent in 5 to 20 percent of patients. It is important to reemphasize that because of the benignity of the symptoms frequently associated with the onset of cryptococcal and listerial meningitis, the indications for a lumbar puncture in a compromised host include both unexplained fever and unexplained headache. Nausea, dizziness, impaired mentation, irritability, and ataxia are common. Seizures rarely occur early, but they occasionally develop as the disease progresses, as may decreased visual acuity, diplopia, and facial numbness and weakness. Papilledema is present in about one third of patients and cranial nerve palsies in about one fifth. Although patients commonly complain of neck stiffness, fully developed meningismus is rare. Focal neurologic lesions, except those due to the effects of the basilar meningitis on the cranial nerves, are rare. In patients who are severely immunosuppressed, meningitis can be associated with multiple sites of extraneural infection, particularly the skin, lungs, skeletal system, and urinary tract.[22]

Although cryptococci may be disseminated via the bloodstream to any organ in the body, the most commonly affected sites are the skin, skeletal system, and urinary tract. Any unexplained skin eruption in an immunosuppressed host merits biopsy to make an early diagnosis of disseminated opportunistic infection, whatever the cause. Cryptococcal skin lesions most commonly appear as erythematous papules or acneiform lesions at body sites atypical for acne. Cellulitis closely mimicking bacterial cellulitis and vesicular lesions resembling herpetic vesicles may also occur. Whatever the initial lesion, ulceration usually develops subsequently. Approximately 10–20 percent of patients with cryptococcal infection will have cutaneous involvement.[68]

Cryptococcal osteomyelitis and arthritis occur in approximately 10 percent of patients with cryptococcal infection and develop as slowly progressive osteolytic lesions without accompanying periosteal proliferation. In patients with long-standing bony infection, direct extension to the skin may occur. Particularly in patients with underlying malignancies, solitary bony lesions caused by *C. neoformans* may be mistaken, histologically, for Hodgkin's disease or osteogenic sarcoma unless special fungal stains are used.[69]

The diagnosis of cryptococcal infection depends on the isolation of the organism or the demonstration of cryptococcal antigen in the body fluid. These problems are discussed in Chapter 9, as is the appropriate therapy with amphotericin B and 5-fluorocytosine.

One final consideration is the need for antifungal therapy in patients who undergo operation for the removal of cryptococcal lesions. Campbell[66] has reported that 7 of 62 patients undergoing pulmonary resection for cryptococcal infection developed postoperative meningitis. Although amphotericin B is too toxic to justify its use as antifungal prophylaxis in this situation, we believe that the availability of the less toxic and more easily administered drugs, 5-fluorocytosine and miconazole, has obviated this problem and that a perioperative course of one of these drugs may safely prevent postoperative meningitis.

In immunosuppressed patients without evidence of extrapulmonary disease who undergo pulmonary resection of cryptococcal infection, we use a two-week course of full doses of 5-fluorocytosine or miconazole as a perioperative umbrella to prevent meningitis.

PROTOZOAN INFECTIONS

Although protozoan infections are discussed as a group in Chapter 11, the opportunistic protozoa are not considered there.

Pneumocystis carinii Infection

Pathogenesis

P. carinii causes a diffuse interstitial plasma cell pneumonia in patients who are immunosuppressed by a variety of diseases. Two epidemiologic patterns of disease have been noted. The first is an endemic infantile pattern found among the malnourished (war refugees). The second pattern of *Pneumocystis* infection is an acute to subacute interstitial pneumonia in patients immunosuppressed by malignancy or chemotherapy.[70]

Pneumocystis is probably acquired by airborne human-to-human transmission,[19,22] although there is considerable evidence that immunosuppression can reactivate a latent or asymptomatic infection.[22,70] The practical implications of such observations are that patients with active *Pneumocystis* pneumonia should be kept isolated from other immunosuppressed patients, and strict respirator precautions should be employed in their care.

Whatever the means by which *Pneumocystis* infection is acquired, clinical disease only occurs in combination with significant immunosuppression. Organ transplant recipients and cancer patients develop *Pneumocystis* infection only after exposure to corticosteroids and chemotherapy. Patients with hematologic malignancies that are themselves immunosuppressive, such as Hodgkin's disease, rarely develop *Pneumocystis* pneumonia unless immunosupressive therapy has been initiated. As far as steroids are concerned, the interesting observation has been made that, in many patients, *Pneumocystis* disease becomes clinically manifest only after the steroid dosage has been tapered. Nutritional status is clearly important, as shown by studies in which serum albumin levels and body weights were significantly lower in children with cancer who developed *Pneumocystis* infection than in children with cancer who did not. Likewise, normal B-lymphocyte function must be important in protecting against *Pneumocystis*, as shown by the many reports of *Pneumocystis* infection in patients with hypogammaglobulinemia, intact cellular immunity, and no history of steroid or cyclophosphamide exposure.

Pathology

Pneumocystis pulmonary infection is characterized by an interstitial pneumonia with thickening of the alveolar septa and the alveoli, hyperplasia of alveolar lining cells, and large numbers of infiltrating plasma cells in the septa. Foamy eosinophilic material fills the alveolar spaces. When Gomori methenamine silver stain is used, this material is shown to be filled with organisms. The diagnostic finding is a 4–6 μm cyst containing six to eight oval bodies, the merozoites. Rarely, *Pneumocystis* organisms have been found in draining hilar and thoracic lymph nodes, and a few instances of systemic dissemination have been reported.[22,70]

Clinical Manifestations

Pneumocystis pneumonia presents with fever, a hacking nonproductive cough, tachypnea, and progressive dyspnea without pleurisy over a few days to weeks. The patient is tachypneic and may be cyanotic but has normal breath sounds. A surprising degree of hypoxia is demonstrable on arterial blood gas determination. The differential diagnosis must include cytomegaloviral infection, which may coexist or predispose to *Pneumocystis* infection.[18,22,36,70]

The classical radiologic appearance of *P. carinii* pneumonia is a diffuse, bilateral, symmetric, interstitial and alveolar pattern with a predominantly perihilar distribution (Fig. 47-4A). Unilateral consolidations and nodular densities, however, have also been reported as being due to this organism, but about 80 percent of our patients have had the classic pattern. Pleural effusions, cavitation, and lymphoadenopathy on roentgenogram are quite unusual and, when present, should suggest the possibility of a concomitant process. There have been a number of reports of simultaneous infection by *Pneumocystis* and other opportunistic pathogens, such as *Nocardia* and *Aspergillus,* and an atypical chest roentgenogram or atypical clinical course or both should alert the clinician to that possibility.[18,22,49,50,70]

Diagnosis

The definitive means of diagnosing *Pneumocystis* infection is by demonstrating the organism. Sputum cytology will be diagnostic in less than 5 percent of patients.[71] Transtracheal aspiration will have a 15 to 20 percent yield,[44] and lung biopsy is necessary (Fig. 47-4B). Serologic studies may be useful in the endemic infantile form of the disease but useless in the immunosuppressed. More promising are recent reports that *P. carinii* antigen can be detected in sera of greater than 95 percent of infected patients by using the technique of counterimmunoelectrophoresis. No circulating antigen has been detected in normal individuals. However, 15 percent of cancer patients may have circulating antigen in the absence of overt *Pneumocystis* infection, an observation that suggests subclinical infection in this susceptible population. The technique of growing *P. carinii* organisms in tissue culture may yet prove to be useful for diagnostic purposes.[70]

Treatment

Pentamadine isethionate is an effective form of therapy, capable of decreasing the mortality rate from 100 to 25 percent. It must be obtained from the Parasitic Disease Drug Service of the Centers for Disease Control. The recommended course of therapy is 4 mg per kg per day administered as a single intramuscular dose for 14 days. In patients with clotting disorders, the drug may be given as a slow intravenous infusion, although anaphylaxis and hypotension may be more common when the intravenous route is used. Pentamadine therapy is frequently associated with major side affects (hypotension, tachycardia, nausea and vomiting, facial flushing, pleuritis, local irritation, hypoglycemia, azotemia, bone marrow toxicity, and sterile abscess formation at injection sites).[72] The combination of pyrimethamine and sulfadiazine also can be effective.[73] The treatment of choice, however, is trimethoprim-sulfamethoxazole administered over 14 days at a dosage of 20 mg of trimethoprim and 100 mg of sulfamethoxazole per kg per day in three to four divided doses.[74] The trimethoprim-sulfamethoxazole combination at the lesser dosage of 5 mg of trimethoprim and 20 mg of sulfamethoxazole per kg per day in two divided doses may be effective prophylaxis. In many centers, such prophylaxis is routinely used in populations at high risk for the development of *Pneumocystis* infection.

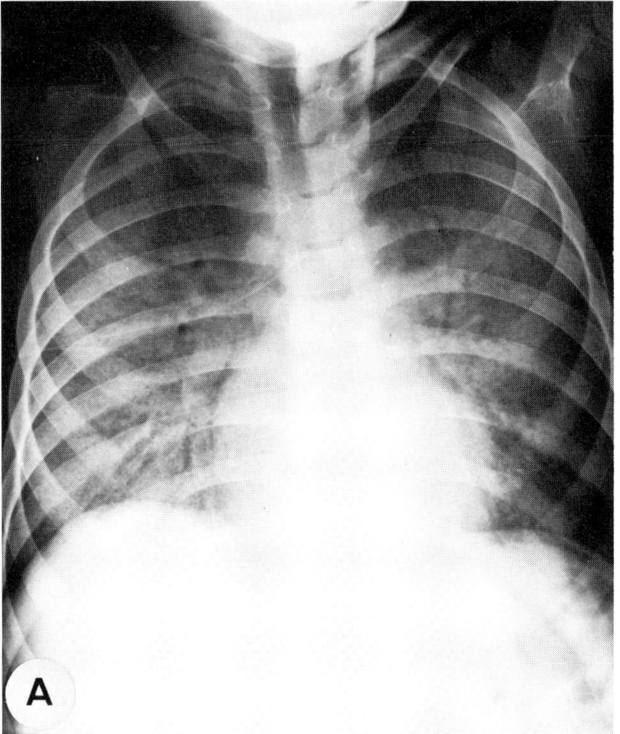

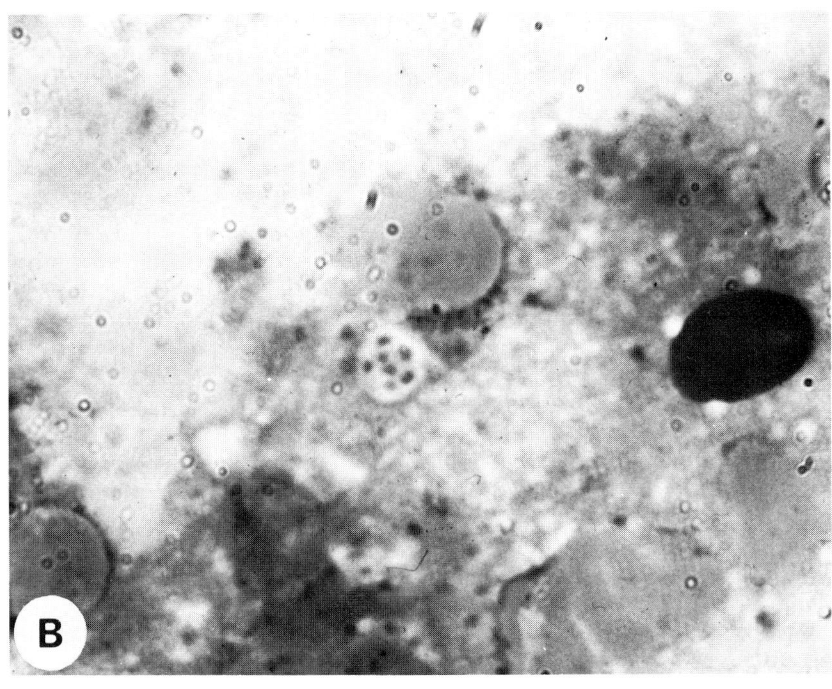

Fig. 47-4. A. The alveolar infiltrate that extends to the periphery of both lungs with an air bronchogram is characteristic of *P. carinii.* This patient, an 8-year-old boy, died three weeks after the disease was confirmed by open lung biopsy. B. Lung biopsy showing *P. carinii* with cysts (Giemsa stain). (Courtesy of B. Berke, MD. From Simmons RL, Kjellstrand CM, Najarian JS: In Hardy JD (ed): Critical Surgical Illness, 1971. Courtesy of W.B. Saunders Company.)

Toxoplasmosis

Toxoplasmosis, a systemic protozoan infection caused by *T. gondii,* is endemic the world over. It has a particular impact on the immunosuppressed patient, since life-threatening disease can develop following the acquisition of primary infection or the reactivation of previously acquired latent infection.[75] Primary infection with *T. gondii* may be acquired congenitally, when the mother develops primary infection during pregnancy, and postnatally, by ingestion (inadequately cooked meat,[76] oocysts in cat feces [77]) or by leukocyte transfusion.[78] Trophozoites of *T. gondii* eventually enter the bloodstream and metastasize to any body site. At these sites, the trophozoites proliferate, causing death of the invaded cells, with these foci of necrosis becoming surrounded by an intense inflammatory reaction. In the normal host, the chronic state of the disease develops. The tissue cyst survives in latent state for the life of the host.[75]

Pathogenesis and Pathology

The most common sites of tissue invasion and the subsequent formation of cysts are the brain, skeletal, and cardiac muscle, although all organs may be affected by this obligate intracellular parasite. Since intact cell-mediated immunity is most important in limiting the extent of toxoplasmosis, patients with Hodgkin's disease and those receiving immunosuppressive therapy are most commonly affected.[75]

Clinical Manifestations

In normal individuals, toxoplasmosis is often asymptomatic or is associated with silent lymphadenopathy. It is most frequently diagnosed when a full-blown infectious mononucleosislike syndrome occurs, with fever, myalgias, sore throat, headache, diffuse lymphadenopathy, hepatosplenomegaly, maculopapular rash, and atypical lymphocytosis. Rarely, acute acquired toxoplasmosis may develop, with carditis, hepatitis, encephalitis, polymyositis, pneumonitis, or choreoretinitis.

In the compromised host, the clinical manifestations are more serious—50 percent involve the central nervous system, with diffuse encephalopathy, meningoencephalitis, or a cerebral mass lesion. The heart and lungs are also affected in the compromised host. In patients with lymphoma, it is easy to misdiagnose a recurrence of lymphadenopathy as being due to the malignancy rather than to toxoplasmosis. Simultaneous infections with herpes group viruses, particularly cytomegalovirus, and *T. gondii* are quite common.[75,79,80]

Diagnosis

Ruskin and Remington [75] pointed out the difficulties in making a diagnosis of toxoplasmosis in this population by demonstrating the trophozoites themselves. Brain biopsy results appear to be most useful, particularly when electron microscopic examination is performed. Of more use is the fact that the lymph nodes exhibit pathognomonic changes in the absence of the parasite—reactive follicular hyperplasia associated with irregular groupings of epithelioid histiocytes in cortical and paracortical zones, as well as focal distention of subcapsular and trabecular sinuses by monocytoid cells.[75] Immunofluoroscent studies for *Toxoplasma* antigen and lymphangiograms are also useful.[75]

Serologic testing can be helpful. Greater than fourfold rises in titer by any serologic method and very high titers without a documented rise are diagnostic in a patient with a typical illness. Because some immunocompromised patients will not mount a characteristic serologic response, biopsy is required in a patient with a clinically compatible syndrome, particularly if this syndrome includes undiagnosed central nervous system disease.[75]

Pyrimethamine plus sulfadiazine is the treatment of choice. Trimethoprim–sulfamethoxazole is not adequate, however, because the trimethoprim component does not possess significant anti-*Toxoplasma* properties.[75] Pyrimethamine is given in an initial dose of 100–200 mg and 25 mg per day thereafter. The usual dose of sulfadiazine is 75–100 mg per kg per day in four divided doses after an initial loading dose of 50–75 mg per kg. Therapy should probably be continued for at least four to six weeks. To prevent pyrimethamine-induced bone marrow toxicity, folinic acid (calcium leucovorin) should be administered in dosages of 2–10 mg per day.[75]

VIRAL INFECTION

The most important viral infections to affect the compromised host are those caused by the four members of the human herpes group—herpes simplex virus, varicella-zoster virus, Epstein-Barr virus, and cytomegalovirus. Although the clinical impact of each of these may be different, they share a number of characteristics (Chapter 10).[81]

Herpesviruses are enveloped DNA viruses that range in size from 180–200 nm and characteristically produce intranuclear inclusion bodies in infected cells. Like other enveloped viruses, herpesviruses are relatively unstable at room temperature, and direct contact between susceptible cells and infected cell secretions is usually necessary for disease transmission. As soon as primary infection has occurred, latent infection develops, with the virus remaining dormant in one or more different cell types for months to decades, with poorly understood perturbations in host defenses resulting in viral reactivation and even dissemination. Although clearly recognized disease syndromes caused by these agents are commonly observed in the normal individual, the extent and impact of the illnesses are enhanced by immunosuppression. Antibody responses to each of these agents can be easily defined and are often useful for diagnosis. The role of antibody in preventing and limiting the extent of such infections remains undefined, with cell-mediated immunity apparently of greater importance. This is best shown by the clinical impact of these agents in patients with defects in cell-mediated immune function.

Herpes Simplex Virus Infection

Herpes simplex virus (HSV) is of two antigenic types. HSV-1, primarily transmitted by infected oral secretions, is the major cause of oral, encephalitic, and ocular infections in the adult. HSV-2 is venereally transmitted and is the major cause of genital and neonatal infection. Both primary and recurrent infections occur and are widespread.[81]

Pathogenesis

The pathogenesis of both primary and reactivation HSV infection requires the viral invasion of skin epithelium and mucous membranes. Viral replication kills the cell and elicits an inflammatory response, producing the typical vesicle on an erythematous base. Regional adenopathy may then occur, and systemic symptoms of viral infection, such as fever, myalgias, malaise, or anorexia, are common. After a primary infection, the virus travels centripetally via neuronal axons to reside in the sensory ganglia that correspond to the site of primary infection. The virus remains latent within these ganglia until reactivated by such factors as immunosuppression, fever, sunlight, trauma, operative manipulation of the nerve root, or a variety of circumstances, including menstruation. After reactivation, the virus travels centrifugally down the axon to reinfect the appropriate epithelial cells. This process may be repeated many times in the lifetime of a patient. In general, unless an acquired immunosuppressed state has developed, primary infection is more severe than recurrent infection, which is manifested by smaller lesions, fewer vesicles, less viral shedding, less adenopathy, fewer systemic symptoms, and a shorter time required for healing. Viremia has been documented in both normal and immunosuppressed individuals, but its importance is unclear, except in the few patients with disseminated visceral disease.[81]

Humoral antibodies to HSV are not protective. Recurrent and even fatal disease can occur with high titers. Humoral immunity may play a role in attenuating the severity of recurrent illness, making it less severe than primary infection. Such antibodies may act as blocking antibodies and contribute to the development of viral latency. Recent evidence suggests that an antibody-dependent cell-mediated cytotoxicity system is important in controlling HSV infection.[81]

Cell-mediated immunity appears to be more important than humoral immunity in protection. Prospective studies of organ transplant patients have correlated decreased lymphocyte transformation and interferon production in response to HSV antigen in the early posttransplant period with the peak incidence of both symptomatic and asymptomatic HSV excretion. The appearance of intravesicle interferon, in particular, appears to correlate with healing of the individual lesions.[81-83]

People at risk for severe HSV infection include all those with defects either in cellular immunity or in the mucocutaneous surfaces that are the primary sites of attachment, including organ transplant recipients, burn patients, and the debilitated, the malnourished, and the elderly.[81-84]

Clinical Manifestations

Chronic, large, ulcerated lesions (herpes phagedena) may persist at either oral or genital sites for weeks to months. Eczema herpeticum (Kaposi varicelliform eruption) is a diffuse vesicular eruption due to cutaneous dissemination of HSV at sites of previous skin damage (ie, burns, eczema). In addition to the cosmetic and physical discomfort associated with this condition, visceral dissemination may occur, with mortality rates of 10 to 50 percent.[81,84]

The prolonged presence of an endotracheal tube or a nasogastric tube can result in a superficial necrotizing mucositis, characterized grossly by multiple punched-out lesions. Coexistent candidal infection is often present. Primary infection of the lungs in the absence of endotracheal intubation or generalized visceral dissemination is rare.[18]

Widespread visceral dissemination of HSV may occur in the compromised host. This is often associated with disseminated intravascular coagulation. At present, treatment of this condition is ineffective, and mortality rates approach 100 percent.[81]

Treatment

Although adenine arabinoside is effective in the treatment of HSV encephalitis,[85] evidence of its efficacy in other syndromes does not exist. The major thrust of the therapeutic approach in these patients is to decrease their level of immunosuppression (by decreasing their steroid and cytotoxic drug therapy) and prevent superinfection. Acyclovir is an investigative agent with potent in vitro activity and little systemic toxicity (Chapter 18).

Varicella-Zoster Viral Infection

A single virus causes both varicella (chickenpox) and zoster (shingles).[81] Varicella-zoster virus (VZV) is presumably acquired through the lungs, with subsequent dissemination to skin and visceral organs, resulting in clinical varicella. It remains dormant within sensory ganglia until activated, then travels down the nerve root to the skin to produce zoster (Chapter 10).[81]

Pathogenesis

As with HSV infection, antibodies to VZV can be demonstrated during both varicella and zoster, with the pattern in zoster suggesting an anamnestic response. In transplant patients, serial antibody titers fluctuate, suggesting to Luby et al [86] that subclinical viral release and antigenic stimulation may be occurring. Humoral antibody must play some role in protection against this infection, as witnessed by the successful prophylactic use of zoster immune globulin or plasma when given early after exposure to immunosuppressed children at high risk for varicella, those with leukemia, lymphoma, and primary immunodeficiency syndromes.[87,88] In contrast, administration of antibody after the incubation period is ineffective.[87,88] Apparently, after this strongly cell-bound virus reaches cellular sites, circulating antibody has little effect on it, and cell-mediated immunity and the production of interferon become more important in limiting the extent of these infections. Patients with particular susceptibility to VZV, those on steroids or with lymphoma, have diminished lymphocyte responsiveness to this agent and delayed local interferon production, even with adequate antibody responsiveness.[81,89]

Disseminated visceral infection following varicella occurs in 20 to 35 percent of children with malignant disease who are receiving chemotherapy, with an associated mortality of 7 to 30 percent from varicella pneumonia or encephalitis.[87] Among adults, the risk of developing zoster is 13 to 15 percent for those with Hodgkin's disease, 7 to 9 percent for non-Hodgkin's lymphoma patients, and 1 to 3 percent for patients with solid tumors. Of the Hodgkin's patients, approximately 15 to 30 percent with zoster will develop disseminated disease.

Clinical Manifestations

Hirsch et al [81] recently pointed out that zoster develops more frequently at areas of regionalized tumor and localized radiation therapy. Its severity is proportional to the stage of cancer and the intensity of radiation and chemotherapy.

Seven to nine percent of organ transplant patients will develop localized zoster. Rarely, pain due to VZV without rash will be present. Although clinical zoster is usually well tolerated, primary varicella is often severe, with a high rate of visceral dissemination. Pediatric transplant recipients, in particular, should be carefully protected from exposure to VZV.[81,82] Fifty percent of bone marrow transplant recipients who survive longer than six months will develop either varicella or zoster, with an exceedingly high mortality rate. Similarly, children with primary immunodeficiency syndromes associated with impaired cell-mediated immunity have a high rate of disseminated VZV infection.[81]

Treatment

An attenuated live virus vaccine is being developed so that active prophylaxis of high-risk children may be possible.[90] In immunocompromised patients with zoster, trials of both adenine arabinoside [91] and exogenous interferon derived from human leukocytes [92] are encouraging, both in controlling dissemination and in preventing postherpetic neuralgia. Acyclovir is also effective against VZV in vitro (Chapter 18).

Epstein-Barr Viral Infection

Epstein-Barr virus (EBV) causes classic heterophil antibody-positive infectious mononucleosis (and some cases of heterophil-negative mononucleosis) and probably causes African Burkitt's lymphoma and certain forms of nasopharyngeal carcinoma. Here, too, cell-mediated immunity plays an important role in limiting the extent of the infection.[81]

The epidemiology of EBV infections in the compromised patient is unclear. It may be transmitted through blood transfusions. At least one epidemic of EBV infection occurred on a hemodialysis unit, related to blood contamination of an inadequately cleaned venous pressure monitor.[93] Reactivation of latent EBV with viral shedding from the oropharynx has been noted in 35 percent of patients receiving immunosuppressive therapy, 50 percent of patients with certain forms of malignancy, and 100 percent of seropositive patients seriously ill with leukemia.[94] The clinical impact of such reactivation infections is unclear, but some cases of unexplained fever and hepatitis are probably caused by EBV. An analogy to reactivation cytomegalovirus (CMV) infection (which may be present simultaneously in some of these patients, particularly transplant recipients) and the clinical disease caused by CMV would appear reasonable. In transplant patients, primary EBV infection has been associated with pneumonia [95] and an unusual lymphoproliferative disorder that may be caused by a polyclonal B-lymphocyte proliferation induced by the virus.[94] This latter condition bears some resemblance to an X-linked recessive immunodeficiency syndrome, in which EBV infection has appeared to cause both a B cell lymphoproliferative syndrome (eg, Burkitt's lymphoma, immunoblastic sarcoma, plasmacytoma) and an aproliferative syndrome (agammaglobulinemia, agranulocytosis, aplastic anemia).[81,94,96] Such observations have led to speculation that EBV, as well as cytomegalovirus, may play a role in the relatively high incidence of lymphoproliferative disorders among patients with defects in cell-mediated immunity, particularly transplant patients.[81,94,94a]

There is no treatment available for EBV infection. In patients with significant clinical manifestations, one should probably decrease the level of immunosuppression, whenever feasible.

Cytomegaloviral Infection

The viral infection with the greatest clinical impact on the compromised host is caused by cytomegalovirus (CMV). There are two patterns of CMV infection, primary and reactivation infection. Between the two, the virus remains latent within cells (probably leukocytes and epithelial cells) for the life of the individual. Reactivation occurs during pregnancy, immunosuppressive therapy, or immune reactions (graft rejection or graft-versus-host disease, for example). Approximately 80–90 percent of the normal population will be seropositive by the time they reach middle age. Close contact appears to be required for transmission of the virus. Because the virus is found in a variety of body fluids (saliva, cervical secretions, urine, semen, milk, and feces), it is likely that it can be acquired through multiple routes.[35,36,81,83,97]

Host defense against CMV, as with the other herpesviruses, appears to rely primarily on cell-mediated immunity, although some role for humoral immunity cannot be ruled out. Evidence of the importance of cell-mediated immunity comes from (1) the ability of immunosuppressive agents to reactivate latent virus in patients with rheumatic diseases, (2) the apparent increased severity of CMV infection in renal transplant patients receiving antithymocyte globulin in addition to routine immunosuppression, and (3) the abolition of measurable cell-mediated immunity to the virus in transplant patients during the time when CMV is clinically most manifest.[98,99]

Blood transfusion is an important means of acquiring primary CMV infection for both normal and immunosuppressed patients—from 2.7 to 12 percent of all blood donors may transmit CMV.[98,99] Since Kaariainen et al [100] first suggested that CMV was the major cause of the posttransfusion heterophil-negative mononucleosis syndrome, a number of attempts have been made to culture the virus from specific blood fractions. With few exceptions,[101] this has not been possible, and it would appear that in the majority of instances, CMV is not transmitted in an infectious form but in latent form within leukocytes. The blastogenic transformation that follows the transfusion of such leukocytes to another individual may activate latent virus and lead to viral replication and infection. Transfusion of blood products that are leukocyte-poor is associated with a lower risk of CMV transmission. Transfusion of a red cell preparation completely free of viable leukocytes is free of this risk.[102]

In the renal transplant population, both primary and reactivation infection may occur, and 60 to 90 percent of renal transplant patients demonstrate serologic evidence of infection with this agent one to four months posttransplant. Essentially 100 percent of patients seropositive pretransplant will reactivate CMV and excrete virus at some point. In addition, the virus may be passed from a seropositive donor via a latently infected kidney to a seronegative recipient. The site of latent virus within the kidney is currently unknown.[35,36,97,103-105a]

Within the transplant recipient, CMV can cause a syndrome of fever and leukopenia, sometimes accompanied by interstitial pneumonia, a mononucleosislike syndrome, and hepatitis. In addition, it suppresses host defenses, thus predisposing to potentially lethal superinfection. There is some suggestion that CMV has a role in producing kidney allograft rejection. One or more of these effects may be observed in patients with either primary or secondary disease. Approximately 70 percent of seronegative patients who receive kidneys from seropositive donors develop illness severe enough to require hospitalization posttransplant. Only about 20 to 25 percent of patients with reactivation disease require rehospitalization. Nevertheless, reactivation disease has at least an equal impact as primary disease on clinical transplantation, since most patients undergoing transplant are seropositive pretransplant.[35,36,104,105] Certain late complications of CMV infection (ie, progressive chorioretinitis and chronic active hepatitis) may also correlate with the existence of a chronic viremic state years after transplantation.[35,98,105b]

Cytomegaloviral infection appears to have a similar impact on cardiac transplantation, at least in terms of producing infectious disease syndromes and predisposing to severe superinfection.[105] In bone marrow transplant patients, CMV appears to play an integral role in the production of a highly lethal interstitial pneumonitis that frequently becomes superinfected. Such disease is closely intertwined with the occurrence of graft-versus-host disease in these patients, with half of all deaths being related to the development of this interstitial pneumonia syndrome.[81,106]

The primary concern of clinical management should be to decrease the level of immunosuppression in order to prevent serious superinfection. Viremia and leukopenia frequently precede superinfections.[36] Antiviral agents, in particular adenine arabinoside, have been both ineffective and possibly associated with major neurologic complications in the treatment of CMV. In contrast, the prophylactic use of human leukocyte interferon begun at the time of transplantation is promising. Trials of an attenuated live CMV vaccine in transplant patients are in progress.[107]

SURGICAL CONSIDERATIONS IN IMMUNOCOMPROMISED PATIENTS

With increasing frequency, surgical evaluation and therapy are required for patients with altered host defenses (malnutrition or advanced malignancy, steroid therapy, uremia, or diabetes, or patients who are immunosuppressed). Signs and symptoms of inflammation are frequently masked in immunologically compromised patients. Thus, peritonitis may be present in a patient receiving steroids, despite only modest abdominal pain, low-grade fever, and leukocytosis. Within hours, this same patient may be moribund, with gram-negative sepsis. For example, in several reports of colonic perforation in steroid-treated patients, the paucity of symptoms, signs, and laboratory evidence of visceral perforation led to frequent delays in treatment and to incorrect preoperative diagnosis in almost all cases.[108]

DIAGNOSTIC APPROACH

An aggressive diagnostic approach, therefore, must be undertaken. In patients with only mild abdominal pain, paracentesis and peritoneal lavage have been particularly helpful in diagnosis, often providing purulent fluid despite the absence of free air on plain roentgenograms. If the diagnosis remains in doubt, contrast roentgenographic studies of the gastrointestinal tract should not be delayed for fear of peritoneal soilage. In general, a water-soluble contrast agent is preferred.

In patients with occult fever but without evidence of peritonitis, the search of an intraperitoneal infection often requires the use of ultrasonography, computerized tomography, and radioactive isotope scanning. Negative results with any of these methods do not rule out active infection. Diagnostic laparotomy is probably indicated in any patient with steady, undiagnosed abdominal pain.

Previous, apparently healed incisions should also be regarded with suspicion in these patients with occult fever. Hidden infections may be demonstrated even years after apparent healing.[109] Needle aspiration of any area of tenderness, erythema, or questionable fluctuance is frequently helpful.

PREOPERATIVE PREPARATION

The degree to which preoperative preparation can be extended in an immunoincompetent patient is determined primarily by the nature and urgency of the operation. The usual preoperative resuscitative measures, including volume replacement, institution of antibiotic therapy, and correction of electrolyte imbalances should be followed. Certain conditions unique to these patients, however, must also be considered. For example, acute adrenal insufficiency must be avoided in patients receiving steroids. Adrenal crisis can be avoided by administering hydrocortisone, 300 mg the day of operation, 150 mg the following day, and 75 mg the third day. By this time, resumption of the preoperative maintenance dosage should be adequate, providing there is no continuing stress.

Uremia may necessitate preoperative dialysis or, at least, correction of hyperkalemia and fluid overload. Ketoacidosis should be corrected in diabetic patients. Given time, there may be some benefit in reducing immunosuppression or improving nutrition.

Selection of anesthetic techniques in these patients is limited primarily by precautions dictated by the underlying disease. In uremic patients, for example, agents eliminated almost exclusively via renal excretion should be avoided, or dosages should be appropriately decreased. The use of average doses of gallamine triethiodide in renal transplant recipients was found to result in prolonged paralysis in 20 percent of patients. We have observed a similar problem following administration of pancuronium bromide. This complication can be particularly serious because of the increased risk of pulmonary infection in immunosuppressed patients when prolonged endotracheal intubation is maintained. A primary goal of anesthesia management must, therefore, be to provide for return of adequate spontaneous respiratory activity and early postoperative extubation. Similar considerations should be observed when placing potentially contaminated percutaneous venous or arterial monitoring catheters. Recognition that any indwelling line in these patients can be the source of even fatal bacteremia should emphasize that their use should never be allowed for only marginal indications or convenience and that they should be removed as early as clinical conditions permit postoperatively.

INTRAOPERATIVE CONSIDERATIONS

Specific operative procedures often must also be modified in these patients. In urgent gastrointestinal tract operations, for example, stomas should be used in preference to anastomoses. Local drainage and proximal colonic diversion are inadequate therapy for sigmoid perforation. Despite the diversion of fecal stream, the inflammatory response is inadequate to provide local containment. Primary resection of the involved bowel and construction of a descending colostomy and distal mucous fistula must, therefore, be undertaken.

The technique of intraperitoneal toilet described in Chapter 34 should be followed in these patients.

Following abdominal surgery in the immunocompromised host, prolonged periods of bowel dysfunction will result. Some surgeons advocate gastric drainage via gastrostomy to avoid pulmonary and esophageal complications of nasogastric suction. Others object to unnecessary enterotomies that may leak. At the same time, consideration should be given to using the small bowel for resumption of nutritional support as soon as possible. In fact, it has been observed that most patients with a reasonable length of normal small intestine can be given full nutrition via jejunostomy in the early postoperative period.[110] Motility and absorption of the small intestine usually return within hours of abdominal exploration. Moreover, because the elemental diet is absorbed in the proximal intestine without the need for digestion, an early return to anabolism is achieved without the risks associated with prolonged hyperalimentation via central venous lines. Placement of a needle or tube catheter jejunostomy at the time of surgery for instillation of elemental diet postoperatively should be a regular consideration in these patients.

Wound complications and delayed healing should be expected. In transplant recipients, the incidence of wound infections may be as high as 39 percent,[111] but usually it is far less than 5 percent if the techniques described in Chapters 22 and 23 are used.

Specific Surgical Conditions

Certain surgical conditions are seen so regularly in the immunocompromised host that they deserve special emphasis. One of these is acute perforation of the colon in patients who are receiving steroids. Some authors suggest a direct adverse effect of steroids on normal colon. Certainly, inhibition of the normal inflammatory response, antifibroblastic activity, and atrophy of lymphoid elements of the bowel wall could interfere with normal barriers to invasive infection by intraluminal bacteria. Perforation could occur whether the colon wall was previously diseased or not and, indeed, has been documented in apparently normal areas of the bowel.[108]

Interestingly, appendicitis rarely occurs in most immunosuppressed hosts, except perhaps in children receiving chemotherapy for leukemia. In this group, abdominal pain and fever are often considered sufficient findings to justify immediate appendectomy. In renal transplant patients, on the other hand, appendicitis is seldom reported. Perhaps the lymphoid atrophy in the bowel wall makes obstruction and inflammation of the appendix unlikely.

Acute pancreatitis in immunosuppressed patients occurs with considerable frequency even in the absence of alcoholism or biliary tract disease. In one autopsy study of 54 patients who had received steroids, acute focal pancreatitis was found in 28.5 percent of the subjects, as compared with 3.7 percent of 54 matched but nonsteroid-treated autopsy subjects.[112] The mechanism whereby steroids could produce pancreatitis may be ductal ectasia and epithelial metaplasia, resulting in obstruction. Azathioprine is also suspect. Perhaps more important is the fact that many of these patients have coincident, severe, often viral infection. Cytomegaloviral inclusions have been found in the pancreas of many immunosuppressed patients. In a recent review of this condition in transplant patients,[113] the mortality was found to be 70 percent. The factors responsible for this high rate were the considerable delay in establishing the diagnosis and the unusually high incidence of postpancreatitis complications (pseudocyst and abscess).

BIBLIOGRAPHY

Allen JC (ed): Infection and the Compromised Host. Baltimore, Williams & Wilkins, 1976.

Aubertin J, Lacut JY, Hoerni B, Durand M: Opportunistic Infections in Cancer Patients (Armstrong D (tr)). New York, Masson Publishing USA, 1978.

Grieco MH (ed): Infections in the Abnormal Host. New York, Yorke Medical Books, 1980.

Matas AJ, Simmons RL, Najarian JS: Sepsis following kidney transplantation. In Hardy JD: Critical Surgical Illness. Philadelphia, Saunders, 1980, p 552.

Stiehm ER, Fulginiti VA (eds): Immunologic Disorders in Infants and Children, 2nd ed. Philadelphia, Saunders, 1980.

Verhoef J, Peterson PK, Quie PG (eds): Infections in the Immunocompromised Host—Pathogenesis, Prevention and Therapy. New York, Elsevier/North-Holland, 1980.

REFERENCES

PREDISPOSING CONDITIONS

1. Howard RJ: Host defense against infection. Curr Probl Surg 17:1, 1980.
2. Alexander JW, Good RA: Fundamentals of Clinical Immunology. Philadelphia, Saunders, 1977, p 311.
3. Tolkoff-Rubin NE, Rubin RH: Infection in patients with chronic renal failure. Infectious Disease Practice, 2(6,7):1, 1979.
4. Greene WH, Casann R, Mauer SM, Quie PG: The effect of hemodialysis on neutrophil chemotactic responsiveness. J Lab Clin Med 88:971, 1976.
5. Bergstrom J, Furst P: Uremic toxins. In Drukker W, Parson FM, Maher JF (eds): Replacement of Renal Function by Dialysis. The Hague, Martinus Nijhoff, 1978, p 334.
6. Weinstein L: Diabetes mellitus and infection. Infect Dis Pract 1:1, 1978.
7. Bagdade JD, Root RK, Bulger RJ: Impaired leukocyte function in patients with poorly controlled diabetes. Diabetes 23:9, 1974.
8. Edwards JE Jr, Lehrer RI, Stiehm ER, Fischer TJ, Young LS: Severe candidal infections: clinical perspective, immune defense mechanisms, and current concepts of therapy. Ann Intern Med 89:91, 1978.

9. Campbell AC, Hersey P, MacLennan ICM, Kay HEM, Pike MC, and Medical Research Council's Working Party on Leukaemia in Childhood: Immunosuppressive consequences of radiotherapy and chemotherapy in patients with acute lymphoblastic leukaemia. Br Med J 2:385, 1973.
10. Huber GL, LaForce FM, Mason RJ, Monaco AP: Impairment of pulmonary bacterial defense mechanisms by immunosuppressive agents. Surg Forum 21:285, 1970.
11. Dale DC, Petersdorf RG: Corticosteroids and infectious diseases. Med Clin North Am 57:1277, 1973.
12. Dale DC, Fauci AS, Wolff SM: Alternate-day prednisone: Leukocyte kinetics and susceptibility to infections. N Engl J Med 291:1154, 1974.
13. Donaldson SS, Moore MR, Rosenberg SA, Vosti KL: Characterization of postsplenectomy bacteremia among patients with and without lymphoma. N Engl J Med 287:69, 1972.
14. Weitzman SA, Aisenberg AC, Siber GR, Smith DH: Impaired humoral immunity in treated Hodgkin's disease. N Engl J Med 297:245, 1977.

DIAGNOSTIC APPROACHES

15. Stiehm ER: Immunodeficiency disorders: general considerations. In Stiehm ER, Fulginiti VA (eds): Immunologic Disorders in Infants and Children. Philadelphia, Saunders, 1980, p 183.

PREVENTION

16. Schimpff SC, Greene WH, Young VM, Wiernik PH: Significance of *Pseudomonas aeruginosa* in the patient with leukemia or lymphoma. J Infect Dis [Suppl] 130:S24, 1974.
17. Goldschmidt MC, Bodey GP: Effect of chemotherapeutic agents upon microorganisms isolated from cancer patients. Antimicrob Agents Chemother 1:348, 1972.
18. Ramsey PG, Rubin RH, Tolkoff-Rubin NE, Cosimi AB, Russell PS, Greene R: The renal transplant patient with fever and pulmonary infiltrates: etiology, clinical manifestations, and management. Medicine 59:206, 1980.
19. Singer C, Armstrong D, Rosen PP, Shottenfield D: *Pneumocystis carinii* pneumonia: A cluster of 11 cases. Am J Med 82:772, 1975.
20. Bock BV, Kirby BD, Edelstein PH, George WL, Snyder KM, Owens ML, Hatayama CM, Haley CE, Lewis RP, Meyer RD, Finegold SM: Legionnaires' disease in renal transplant recipients. Lancet 1:410, 1978.
21. Rose HD: Mechanical control of hospital ventilation and aspergillus infections. Am Rev Respir Dis 105:306, 1972.
22. Williams DM, Krick JA, Remington JS: Pulmonary infection in the compromised host. Am Rev Respir Dis 114:359, 593, 1976.
23. Levine AS, Siegel SE, Schreiber AD, Hauser J, Preisler H, Goldstein IM, Seidler F, Simon R, Perry S, Bennett JE, Henderson ES: Protected environments and prophylactic antibiotics. A prospective controlled study of their utility in the therapy of acute leukemia. N Engl J Med 288:477, 1973.
24. Schimpff SC, Greene WH, Young VM, Fortner CL, Jepsen L, Cusack N, Block JB, Wiernik PH: Infection prevention in acute nonlymphocytic leukemia. Laminar air flow room reverse isolation with oral, nonabsorbable antibiotic prophylaxis. Ann Intern Med 82:351, 1975.
25. Klastersky J, Debusscher L, Weerts D, Daneau D: Use of oral antibiotics in protected environment unit: Clinical effectiveness and role in the emergence of antiobitic-resistant strains. Pathol Biol 22:5, 1974.
26. Levine AS, Robinson RA, Hauser JM: Analysis of studies on protected environments and prophylactic antibiotics in adult acute leukemia. Eur J Cancer 11 [Suppl]: 57, 1975.
27. Gurwith MJ, Brunton JL, Lank BA, Harding GK, Ronald AR: A prospective controlled investigation of prophylactic trimethoprim/sulfamethoxazole in hospitalized granulocytopenic patients. Am J Med 66:248, 1979.
27a. Wade JC, Schimpff SC, Hargadon MT, Fortner CL, Young VM, Wiernik PH: A comparison of trimethoprim-sulfamethoxazole plus nystatin with gentamicin plus nystatin in the prevention of infections in acute leukemia. N Engl J Med 304:1057, 1981.

FEVER OF UNKNOWN ORIGIN

28. Sickles EA, Greene WH, Wiernik PH: Clinical presentation of infection in granulocytopenic patients. Arch Intern Med 135:715, 1975.
28a. Peterson PK, Balfour HH, Fryd, DS, Ferguson RM, Simmons RL: Fever in renal transplant recipients: Causes, prognostic significance and changing patterns at the University of Minnesota Hospital. Am J Med, in press, 1981.
29. Bodey GP: Microbiologic aspects in patients with leukemia. Hum Pathol 5:687, 1974.
30. Lau WK, Young LS, Black RE, Winston DJ, Linné SR, Weinstein RJ, Hewitt WL: Comparative efficacy and toxicity of amikacin-carbenicillin versus gentamicin/carbenicillin in leukopenic patients. A randomized prospective trial. Am J Med 62:959, 1977.
31. Herzig RH, Herzig GP, Graw RG Jr, Bull MI, Ray KK: Successful granulocyte transfusion therapy for gram-negative septicemia: a prospectively randomized controlled study. N Engl J Med 296:701, 1977.
32. Alavi JB, Root RK, Djerassi I, Evans AE, Gluckman SJ, MacGregor RR, Guerry D, Schreiber AD, Shaw JM, Koch P, Cooper RA: A randomized clinical trial of granulocyte transfusions for infection in acute leukemia. N Engl J Med 296:706, 1977.
32a. Newman KA, Schimpff SC, Wade JC: Antibiotic prophylaxis of infection for patients with granulocytopenia. In Verhoef J, Peterson PK, Quie PG (eds): Infections in the Immunocompromised Host—Pathogenesis, Prevention and Therapy. New York, Elsevier/North-Holland, 1980, p 187.
33. Bloomfield CD, Kennedy BJ: Cephalothin, carbenicillin and gentamicin therapy for febrile patients with acute non-lymphocytic leukemia. Cancer 34:431, 1974.
34. Pennington JE: Fever, neutropenia and malignancy: a clinical syndrome in evolution. Cancer 39:1345, 1977.
35. Fiala M, Payne JE, Berne TV, Moore TC, Henle W, Montgomerie JZ, Chatterjee SN, Guze LB: Epidemiology of cytomegalovirus infection after transplantation and immunosuppression. J Infect Dis 132:421, 1975.
36. Rubin RH, Cosimi AB, Tolkoff-Rubin NE, Russell PS, Hirsch MS: Infectious disease syndromes attributable to cytomegalovirus and their significance among renal transplant recipients. Transplantation 24:458, 1977.
37. Rubin RH, Fang LST, Cosimi AB, Herrin JT, Varga PA, Russell PS, Tolkoff-Rubin NE: Usefulness of the antibody-coated bacteria assay in the management of urinary tract infection in the renal transplant patient. Transplantation 27:18, 1979.
38. Schimpff SC: Diagnosis of infection in patients with cancer. Eur J Cancer 11 [Suppl]: 29, 1975.

FEVER AND PNEUMONITIS

39. Briggs WA, Merrill JP, O'Brien TF, Wilson RE, Birtch AG, Murray JE: Severe pneumonia in renal transplant patients. One year's experience. Ann Intern Med 75:887, 1971.
40. Simmons RL, Uranga VM, LaPlante ES, Buselmeier TJ, Kjellstrand CM, Najarian JS: Pulmonary complications in transplant recipients. Arch Surg 105:260, 1972.

41. Rand KH, Pollard RB, Merigan TC: Increased pulmonary superinfections in cardiac transplant patients undergoing primary cytomegalovirus infection. N Engl J Med 298:951, 1978.
42. Aisner J, Kvols LK, Sickles EA, Schimpff SC, Wiernik PH: Transtracheal selective bronchial brushing for pulmonary infiltrates in patients with cancer. Chest 69:367, 1976.
43. Rubin RH: The cancer patient with fever and pulmonary infiltrates: etiology and diagnostic approach. In Remington JS, Swartz MN (eds): Current Clinical Topics in Infectious Diseases (Vol I). New York, McGraw-Hill, 1980, p 288.
44. Lau WK, Young LS, Remington JS: *Pneumocystis carinii* pneumonia: diagnosis by examination of pulmonary secretions. JAMA 236:2399, 1976.
45. Finley R, Kieff E, Thomsen S, Fennessy J, Beem M, Lerner S, Morello J: Bronchial brushing in the diagnosis of pulmonary disease in patients at risk for opportunistic infection. Am Rev Respir Dis 109:379, 1974.
46. McCartney RL: Hemorrhage following percutaneous lung biopsy. Radiology 112:305, 1974.
47. Bandt PD, Blank N, Castellino RA: Needle diagnosis of pneumonitis. Value in high-risk patients. JAMA 220:1578, 1972.
48. Greenman RL, Goodall PT, King D: Lung biopsy in immunocompromised hosts. Am J Med 59:488, 1975.
49. Pennington JE, Feldman NT: Pulmonary infiltrates and fever in patients with hematologic malignancy: Assessment of transbronchial biopsy. Am J Med 62:110, 1979.
50. Singer C, Armstrong D, Rosen PP, Walzer PD, Yu B: Diffuse pulmonary infiltrates in immunosuppressed patients. Prospective study of 80 cases. Am J Med 66:110, 1979.
51. Beyt BE Jr, King DK, Glew RH: Fatal pneumonitis and septicemia after fiberoptic bronchoscopy. Chest 72:105, 1977.
52. Robbins H, Goldman AL: Failure of a "prophylactic" antimicrobial drug to prevent sepsis after fiberoptic bronchoscopy. Am Rev Respir Dis 116:325, 1977.

BACTERIAL INFECTIONS IN THE COMPROMISED HOST

53. Singer C, Kaplan MH, Armstrong D: Bacteremia and fungemia complicating neoplastic disease. Am J Med 62:731, 1977.
54. Louria DB, Hensle T, Armstrong D, Collins HS, Blevins A, Krugman D, Buse M: Listeriosis complicating malignant disease: a new association. Ann Intern Med 67:261, 1967.
55. Lavetter A, Leedom JM, Mathias AW Jr, Ivler D, Wehrle PF: Meningitis due to *Listeria monocytogenes:* a review of 25 cases. N Engl J Med 285:598, 1971.
56. Pennington JE, Gibbons ND, Strobeck JE, Simpson GL, Myerowitz RL: *Bacillus* species infection in patients with hematologic neoplasia. JAMA 235:1473, 1976.
57. Palmer DL, Harvey RL, Wheeler JK: Diagnostic and therapeutic considerations in *Nocardia asteroides* infection. Medicine 53:391, 1974.
58. Kaplan MH, Armstrong D, Rosen P: Tuberculosis complicating neoplastic disease. Cancer 33:850, 1974.

FUNGAL INFECTIONS

59. Aisner J, Schimpff SC, Wiernik PH: Treatment of invasive aspergillosis: relation of early diagnosis and treatment to response. Ann Intern Med 86:539, 1977.
60. Aisner J, Murillo J, Schimpff SC, Steere AC: Invasive aspergillosis in acute leukemia: correlation with nose cultures and antibiotic use. Ann Intern Med 90:4, 1979.
61. Shaffer PJ, Medoff G, Kobayashi GS: Demonstration of antigenemia by radioimmunoassay in rabbits experimentally infected with *Aspergillus.* J Infect Dis 139:313, 1979.
62. Bodey GP, Luna M: Skin lesions associated with disseminated candidiasis. JAMA 229:1466, 1974.
63. Kressel B, Szewczyk C, Tuazon CU: Early clinical recognition of disseminated candidiasis by muscle and skin biopsy. Arch Intern Med 138:429, 1978.
64. Filice G, Yu B, Armstrong D: Immunodiffusion and agglutination tests for candida in patients with neoplastic disease: Inconsistent correlation of results with invasive disease. J Infect Dis 135:349, 1977.
65. Stevens DA: Miconazole in the treatment of systemic fungal infections. Am Rev Respir Dis 116:801, 1977.
65a. Restrepo A, Stevens DA, Utz JP: First International Symposium on Ketoconazole. Rev Infect Dis 2:519–691, 1980.
66. Campbell GD: Primary pulmonary cryptococcosis. Am Rev Respir Dis 94:236, 1966.
67. Duperval R, Hermans PE, Brewer NS, Roberts GD: Cryptococcosis, with emphasis on the significance of isolation of *Cryptococcus neoformans* from the respiratory tract. Chest 72:13, 1977.
68. Schupbach CW, Wheeler CE Jr, Briggaman RA, Warner NA, Kanof EP: Cutaneous manifestations of disseminated cryptococcosis. Arch Dermatol 112:1734, 1976.
69. Burch KH, Fine G, Quinn EL, Eisses JF: *Cryptococcus neoformans* as a cause of lytic bone lesions. JAMA 231:1057, 1975.

PROTOZOAL INFECTIONS

70. Hughes WT: Current concepts: *Pneumocystis carinii* pneumonia. N Engl J Med 297:1381, 1977.
71. Walzer PD, Perl DP, Krogstad DJ, Rawson PG, Schultz MG: *Pneumocystis carinii* pneumonia in the United States: Epidemiologic, diagnostic, and clinical features. Ann Intern Med 80:83, 1974.
72. Western KA, Perera DR, Schultz MG: Pentamadine isethionate in the treatment of *Pneumocystis carinii* pneumonia. Ann Intern Med 73:695, 1970.
73. Young RC, DeVita VT Jr: Treatment of *Pneumocystis carinii* pneumonia: Current status of the regimens of pentamadine isethionate and pyrimethamine sulfadiazine. Symposium on *Pneumocystis carinii* infection. National Cancer Inst Monogr 43, p 193, 1976.
74. Hughes WT, Feldman S, Chandhary SC, Ossi MJ, Cox F, Sanyal SK: Comparison of pentamadine isethionate and trimethoprim-sulfamethoxazole in the treatment of *Pneumocystis carinii* pneumonia. J Pediatr 92:285, 1978.
75. Ruskin J, Remington JS: Toxoplasmosis in the compromised host. Ann Intern Med 84:193, 1976.
76. Kean BH, Kimball AC, Christenson WN: An epidemic of acute toxoplasmosis. JAMA 208:1002, 1969.
77. Teutsch SM, Juranek DD, Sulzer A, Dubey JP, Sikes RK: Epidemic toxoplasmosis associated with infected cats. N Engl J Med 300:695, 1979.
78. Siegel SE, Lunde MN, Gelderman AH, Halterman RH, Brown JA, Levine AS, Graw RG Jr: Transmission of toxoplasmosis by leukocyte transfusion. Blood 37:388, 1971.
79. Luna MA, Lichtiger B: Disseminated toxoplasmosis and cytomegalovirus infection complicating Hodgkin's disease. Am J Clin Pathol 55:499, 1971.
80. Gleason TH, Hamlin WB: Disseminated toxoplasmosis in the compromised host. Arch Intern Med 134:1059, 1974.

VIRAL INFECTIONS

81. Hirsch MS, Cheeseman SH, Hammer SM: Human herpesvirus infections: Pathogenesis and clinical implications. In Weinstein L, Fields BM (eds): Seminars in Infectious Disease (Vol 2). New York, Stratton Intercontinental, 1980.
82. Rand KH, Rasmussen LE, Pollard RB, Arvin A, Merigan TC: Cellular immunity and herpesvirus in cardiac-transplant patients. N Engl J Med 296:1372, 1977.
83. Pass RF, Long WK, Whitley RJ, Soong SJ, Diethelm AG, Reynolds DW, Alford CA Jr: Productive infection with cytomegalovirus and herpes simplex virus in renal transplant recipients: Role of source of kidney. J Infect Dis 137:556, 1978.
84. Foley FD, Greenawald KA, Nash G, Pruitt BA Jr: Herpesvirus infection in burned patients. N Engl J Med 282:652, 1970.
85. Whitley RJ, Soong S, Dolin R, Galasso GJ, Ch'ien LT, Alford CA, and Collaborative Study Group: National Institute of Allergy and Infectious Diseases Collaborative Antiviral study: Adenine arabinoside therapy of biopsy-proved herpes simplex encephalitis. N Engl J Med 297:289, 1977.
86. Luby JP, Ramirez-Ronda C, Rinner S, Hull A, Vergne-Marini P: A longitudinal study of varicella-zoster infections in renal transplant recipients. J Infect Dis 135:659, 1977.
87. Geiser CF, Bishop Y, Myers M, Jaffe N, Yankee R: Prophylaxis of varicella in children with neoplastic disease: Comparative results with zoster immune plasma and gamma globulin. Cancer 35:1027, 1975.
88. Winsnes R: Efficacy of zoster immunoglobulin on prophylaxis of varicella in high-risk patients. Acta Paediatr Scand 67:77, 1978.
89. Arvin AM, Pollard RB, Rasmussen LE, Merigan TC: Selective impairment of lymphocyte reactivity to varicella-zoster virus antigen among untreated patients with lymphoma. J Infect Dis 137:531, 1978.
90. Asano Y, Nakayama H, Yazaki T, Kato R, Hirose S, Tsuzuki K, Ito S, Isomura S, Takahashi M: Protection against varicella in family contacts by immediate inoculation with live varicella vaccine. Pediatrics 59:3, 1977.
91. NIAID Collaborative Antiviral Study: Adenine arabinoside therapy of herpes zoster in the immunosuppressed. N Engl J Med 294:1193, 1976.
92. Merigan TC, Rand KH, Pollard RB, Abdallah PS, Jordan GW, Fried RP: Human leukocyte interferon for the treatment of herpes zoster in patients with cancer. N Engl J Med 298:981, 1978.
93. Corey L, Stamm WE, Feorino PM, Bryan JA, Weseley S, Gregg MB, Solangi K: HBsAg-negative hepatitis in a hemodialysis unit: Relation to Epstein-Barr virus. N Engl J Med 293:1273, 1975.
94. Marker SC, Ascher NL, Kalis JM, Simmons RL, Najarian JS, Balfour HH Jr: Epstein-Barr virus antibody responses and clinical illness in renal transplant recipients. Surgery 85:433, 1979.
94a. Hanto DW, Frizzeria G, Gajl-Peczalska J, Purtilo DT, Klein G, Simmons RL, Najarian, JS: The Epstein-Barr virus (EBV) in the pathogenesis of posttransplant lymphoma. Transplant Proc 13:756, 1981.
95. Grose C, Henle W, Horwitz MS: Primary Epstein-Barr virus infection in renal transplant recipient. South Med J 70:1276, 1977.
96. Purtilo DT, Bhawan J, Hutt LM, DeNicola L, Szymanski I, Yang JPS, Boto W, Maier R, Thorley-Lawson D: Epstein-Barr virus infections in the X-linked recessive lymphoproliferative syndrome. Lancet 1:798, 1978.
97. Betts RF, Hanshaw JB: Cytomegalovirus in the compromised host(s). Annu Rev Med 28:103, 1977.
98. Pollard RB, Rand KH, Arvin AM, Merigan TC: Cell-mediated immunity to cytomegalovirus infection in normal subjects and cardiac transplant patients. J Infect Dis 137:541, 1978.
99. Rytel MW, Aguilar-Torres FG, Balay J, Heim LR: Assessment of the status of cell-mediated immunity in cytomegalovirus-infected renal allograft recipients. Cell Immunol 37:31, 1978.
100. Kaariainen L, Klemola E, Paloheimo J: Rise of cytomegalovirus antibodies in an infectious-mononucleosis-like syndrome after transfusion. Br Med J 1:1270, 1966.
101. Diosi P, Moldovan E, Tomescu N: Latent cytomegalovirus infection in blood donors. Br Med J 4:660, 1969.
102. Lang DJ: Cytomegalovirus infections in organ transplantation and posttransfusion: An hypothesis. Arch Gesamte Virusforsch 37:365, 1972.
103. Betts RF, Freeman RB, Douglas RG Jr, Talley TE, Rundell B: Transmission of cytomegalovirus infection with renal allograft. Kidney Int 8:385, 1975.
104. Ho M, Suwansirikul S, Dowling JN, Youngblood LA, Armstrong JA: The transplanted kidney as a source of cytomegalovirus infection. N Engl J Med 293:1109, 1975.
105. Balfour HH Jr, Slade MS, Lakis JM, Howard RJ, Simmons RL, Najarian JS: Viral infections in renal transplant donors and their recipients: A prospective study. Surgery 81:487, 1977.
105a. Peterson PK, Balfour HH, Marker SC, Fryd DS, Howard RJ, Simmons RL: Cytomegalovirus disease in renal allograft recipients: A prospective study of the clinical features, risk factors, and impact on renal transplantation. Medicine 59:283, 1980.
105b. Matas AJ, Simmons RL, Fryd DS, Najarian, JS: Persistent, recurrent, and late cytomegalovirus infections. Transplant Proc 13:291, 1981.
106. Meyers JD, Spencer HC Jr, Watts JC, Gregg MB, Stewart JA, Troupin RH, Thomas ED: Cytomegalovirus pneumonia after human marrow transplantation. Ann Intern Med 82:181, 1975.
107. Plotkin SA, Farquhar J, Hornberger E: Clinical trials of immunization with the Towne 125 strain of human cytomegalovirus. J Infect Dis 134:470, 1976.

SURGICAL CONSIDERATIONS

108. Warshaw AL, Welch JP, Ottinger LW: Acute perforation of the colon associated with chronic corticosteroid therapy. Am J Surg 131:442, 1976.
109. Moore TC, Hume DM: The period and nature of hazard in clinical renal transplantation. Ann Surg 170:1, 1969.
110. Page CP, Ryan JA, Haff RC: Continual catheter administration of an elemental diet. Surg Gynecol Obstet 142:184, 1976.
111. Schweizer RT, Kountz SL, Belzer FO: Wound complications in recipients of renal transplants. Ann Surg 177:58, 1973.
112. Carone FA, Liebow AA: Acute pancreatic lesions in patients treated with ACTH and adrenal corticoids. N Engl J Med 257:690, 1957.
113. Fernandez JA, Rosenberg JC: Post-transplantation pancreatitis. Surg Gynecol Obstet 143:795, 1976.

CHAPTER 48
Burns

P. WILLIAM CURRERI

Systemic sepsis, resulting from invasive infection of the wound or lungs, remains the leading cause of death of patients hospitalized with major thermal injury. During the past two decades, both clinical and basic investigation has resulted in improved understanding of the pathophysiology of burn wound infection, as well as recognition that burned patients have profoundly altered host defenses (Chapter 13). These perceptions have led to the development of new treatment methods that have been associated with reduction of the incidence of morbid complications associated with wound and pulmonary sepsis. Whereas death following burn injury exceeding 40 percent of the total body surface was almost universal in 1949,[1] modern burn centers today succeed in salvaging over half of the children and young adults with burns of 64 percent of the total body surface.[2]

PATHOPHYSIOLOGY OF INFECTIONS AFTER BURNS

ROUTES OF INFECTION

Burn Wound

One of the principal functions of intact skin is to act as a microbiologic barrier to bacteria, fungi, or viruses. Thermal injury breaks this barrier. Most burn wounds are initially free of major bacterial contamination, since the heat, which has destroyed the cutaneous elements, also kills surface microorganisms, with the exception of the gram-positive bacteria located at the depths of sweat glands or hair follicles. If topical antimicrobial agents are not used prophylactically to reduce the rate of bacterial proliferation, the wound may become colonized with up to 100 million gram-positive bacteria per gm of tissue within 48 hours. However, the rapid development of gram-positive bacterial overgrowth is rarely observed because potent topical chemotherapeutic agents are routinely used.

Nevertheless, complete wound sterilization is rarely achieved, even with the application of topical agents. Gram-negative bacteria often appear in the wound between 3 and 21 days, but topical chemotherapeutic agents inhibit gram-negative growth, and bacterial concentrations of less than 100 organisms per gm of tissue can be maintained.

If bacterial concentration is not controlled at levels below 10^5 organisms per gm of tissue, invasion of viable subcutaneous tissue usually occurs, with subsequent bloodstream dissemination.[3] This syndrome, *burn wound sepsis,* is characterized by early local deterioration of the wound and the late appearance of systemic sepsis.

The appearance of cellulitis in unburned skin surrounding the wound or of localized hemorrhagic necrosis within the burn wound (Fig. 48-1) should alert the physician to the possible development of burn wound sepsis. However, the diagnosis cannot be made unless histologic examination of full-thickness biopsies of the wound shows invasion of underlying viable subcutaneous fat and blood vessels by microbes.

Lungs

With improved methods of managing the burn wound, pulmonary infection with subsequent respiratory failure has now emerged as the most frequent cause of septic death in thermally injured patients. Prior to the utilization of local chemotherapeutic agents to control the proliferation of bacteria, about two thirds of pulmonary infections in burn patients represented hematogenous dissemination from wound to the lungs.[4] Hematogenous pneumonia is now relatively infrequent, and most pulmonary infections are bronchopneumonias secondary to the inhalation of organisms by an immunologically depressed host.

In addition, serious pulmonary compromise is often observed in patients with major burns secondary to the inhalation of the incomplete combustion products of smoke, resulting in severe chemical tracheobronchitis. The latter syndrome manifests itself by destruction of the lower respiratory epithelium, with loss of ciliary action, severe bronchospasm, and the development of mucous and cellular plugs within tertiary bronchi. All of these factors favor the proliferation of bacteria introduced into the lungs by inhaled air. Furthermore, if bacterial proliferation on the wound is not controlled, the patient is often exposed to a high concentration of aerosolized bacteria emanating from the wound during physical manipulation of the patient in bed.

Suppurative Thrombophlebitis

Suppurative thrombophlebitis represents the third most common infection observed in hospitalized burn patients. The diagnosis may be confirmed in approximately 5 per-

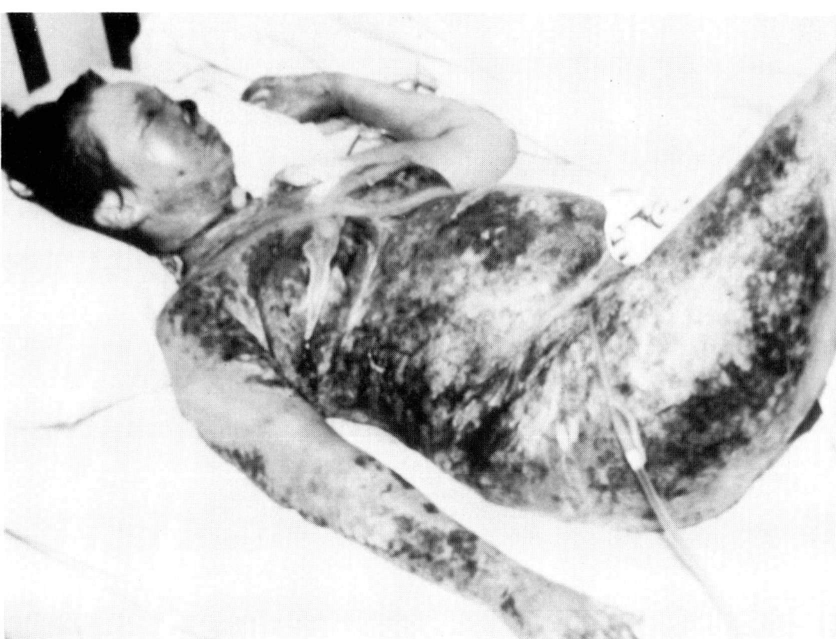

Fig. 48-1. **Burn wound sepsis. Note black hemorrhagic discoloration of the nose and flank secondary to ischemic necrosis induced by bacterial invasion of the microvasculature.**

cent of hospitalized patients with burns exceeding 20 percent total body surface area.[5] The complication is almost always associated with the peripheral insertion of synthetic catheters for venous infusion of fluids.

This disease is particularly insidious. The syndrome is rarely accompanied by any local or systemic signs prior to the development of bacteremia. Local tenderness over the involved vein, distal edema, or a positive Homan's sign are unusual. Late in the course of the disease, local abscesses may be noted surrounding the affected vein and involving the soft tissue. Suppuration within a thrombosed peripheral vein may occur as long as three weeks after the removal of an indwelling venous catheter, and, thus, the diagnosis may not be entertained unless careful records have been kept regarding the location of previously catheterized peripheral veins.

The diagnosis should be considered whenever systemic signs of sepsis are apparent or blood cultures are positive in the absence of obvious local infection. All peripheral veins used for prolonged intravenous infusions should be explored under local anesthesia. After a small venotomy is made, the vein should be milked by firm external pressure in a retrograde manner and the venotomy observed for the appearance of intraluminal pus. In addition, a small biopsy of a thrombosed vein should be examined histologically for the presence of bacteria within the intima of the vein. Either the presence of suppurative material within the vein or intimal colonization with bacteria confirms the diagnosis. Immediate operative excision (see subsequent section) is essential to prevent a progressive septic course.

Suppurative Chondritis

Because of the poor blood supply to cartilage, cartilaginous structures are particularly prone to becoming infected when they underlie a full-thickness burn wound. The cartilaginous support of the ear is at greatest risk, in part because it almost directly underlies the cutaneous tissue, with little subcutaneous insulation between the skin and the cartilage. Thus, not only is the cartilage frequently exposed to invading organisms from the overlying burn wound, but the cartilage itself is often damaged by the thermal insult. Cartilaginous coverings of the interphalangeal joints of the hands also are frequently affected because exposure of the joint often occurs during removal of the eschar. Full-thickness injury of the skin overlying the dorsum of the fingers is common because the skin is so thin there. Occasionally, chondritis of the costal chondral cartilage is observed following electrical injury when the entrance or exit wound of the current is directly over the sternum.

The diagnosis of suppurative chondritis of the ears is made by careful clinical examination. The patient will exhibit tenderness on movement of the earlobes and frequently has an increasing angle between the ear and the posterior scalp, resulting in obvious asymmetry when comparing both ears. During the late stages of suppurative chondritis, nonviable cartilage will often be extruded through the anterior surface of the auricle, and localized abscess formation may occur. If appropriate operative treatment (see subsequent section) is not performed, the infection may invade the mastoid bone, with later development of intracranial abscess.

Bacterial Endocarditis

Patients with major burns have frequent brief episodes of transient bacteremia (often associated with debridement of the burn wound) prior to definitive grafting. Patients with a prior history of valvular heart disease are particularly prone to develop either acute or subacute bacterial endocarditis and, therefore, must be monitored closely with frequent auscultatory examination. The incidence of bacterial endocarditis at autopsy has been reported to be as high as 0.6 percent.[6]

The diagnosis of bacterial endocarditis is essentially one of exclusion. In the absence of an obvious source of infection, the presence of positive blood cultures should be assumed to be bacterial endocarditis until proven otherwise. Patients with repetitive bacteremias or the development of a changing murmur should undergo echocardiography which may confirm the presence of valvular vegetations. The presence of either streptococcal or staphylococcal bacteremia in the absence of suppurative thrombophlebitis or burn wound sepsis should strongly suggest the presence of a complicating endocarditis.

Miscellaneous Infection

The Eye

Primary infection in other organs also occurs in burn patients. Patients with corneal burns (usually secondary to chemical injury) are at risk of secondary infection if corneal ulceration or corneal perforation occurs. Early examination of the eyes should be performed during the first few hours of fluid resuscitation because subsequent edema formation may prevent adequate exposure of the conjunctiva and cornea during the first several postburn days. In the presence of significant corneal damage, particular attention should be paid to the prevention of surface drying. The instillation of methyl cellulose and topical antibiotic ointments and early tarsorrhaphy should be considered. When severe ulceration or perforation of the cornea has occurred, immediate coverage of the defect is mandatory, using a conjunctival flap, a corneal transplant, or a protective soft lens.

The Urinary Tract

Patients with major burns require an indwelling Foley catheter to allow careful monitoring of renal function during fluid resuscitation. Periurethral and prostatic abscesses occasionally occur and may be diagnosed by rectal examination. When they are present, immediate incision and drainage are necessary to prevent systemic spread.

Intra-abdominal Infections

Intraperitoneal infection occurs in a small percentage of hospitalized patients. The diagnosis is frequently delayed because local peritoneal signs are masked by stress levels of circulating corticosteroids. Furthermore, the presence of burns on the surface of the abdomen may make physical examination difficult to interpret, since pressure on an area of second degree burn often elicits severe discomfort.

Most patients with major burns develop minor stress ulcerations during the first 24 hours following burn injury. However, progression to hemorrhage or perforation has become unusual during the past four years as a result of the prophylactic use of antacids, better control of burn wound bacterial proliferation, and better nutrition. The sudden appearance of paralytic ileus or abdominal distention should prompt the physician to obtain upright chest and abdominal roentgenographs to rule out the presence of free air.

Other infrequent causes of intra-abdominal sepsis include acalculous cholecystitis, appendicitis, and localized ischemic lesions of the colon. The presence of acalculous cholecystitis is suggested by fullness in the right upper quadrant or the presence of a palpable mass below the liver. It is often associated with prolonged periods of dehydration and nasogastric suction (Chapter 35). Confirmation is most easily obtained by abdominal sonogram.

Localized ischemic lesions of the colon with subsequent perforation are most often observed in the elderly and may follow prolonged hypotension due to an inappropriate fluid resuscitation in a patient with advanced atherosclerotic disease of the inferior mesenteric artery. It has also been observed in elderly patients when massive cecal dilation is unrecognized (Chapter 39).

ETIOLOGY

Gram-positive Bacteria

Prior to the availability of penicillin, *Streptococcus* was the most frequently isolated organism from burn wounds. The organism can proliferate rapidly and is often present in the hair follicles and sweat glands of the dermis and subcutaneous tissue. When streptococcal colonization of the burn wound occurs, the patient frequently exhibits fever, cellulitis of the unburned skin surrounding the wound, and later development of lymphangitis. Treatment with oral or systemic penicillin usually results in prompt resolution, within 24 to 48 hours. Failure to observe rapid improvement suggests a staphylococcal infection and dictates a change in antibiotic therapy. When topical chemotherapeutic agents are used, gram-positive bacterial colonization is often avoided, and initial colonization of the wound occurs with less pathogenic gram-negative bacteria.

Patients with burn injury must be considered to be at risk of clostridial infection and should be treated with appropriate prophylaxis. The incidence of colonization of the burn wound with anaerobic bacteria is extraordinarily low, however, unless significant associated soft tissue injury is also present. The potential for clostridial infection is greatest in patients with severe electrical injury or with major crush injuries associated with cutaneous burns (eg, wringer injuries or mangle injuries). Major ischemia of the muscular compartment is frequently observed after electrical injury, since current is primarily carried by nerves, blood vessels, and the well-vascularized muscular compartments. Thorough debridement of nonviable musculature is mandatory in such patients in order to prevent secondary bacterial infection with anaerobes or facultative aerobes.

Gram-negative Bacteria

The majority of burn wound infections are now caused by a single strain of gram-negative bacteria. Although *Pseudomonas aeruginosa* infections of these wounds were common in the early 1960s, the development of potent antibiotics and newer topical chemotherapeutic agents has reduced its incidence. A large number of other opportunistic gram-negative organisms have replaced *P. aeruginosa* in importance, but no single strain is responsible for a majority of burn would infections. However, almost all specialized burn facilities occasionally recognize local epidemics of burn wound infection with resistant opportunistic organisms. These miniepidemics arise secondary to persistent antibiotic pressure within a burn facility as a result of stereotyped prophylactic therapy.[7] The most troublesome gram-negative bacteria have included *Enterobacter cloacae*,[8] *Providencia stuartii*,[9] *Serratia marcescens*, and various strains of *Klebsiella*.

Regardless of the strain of gram-negative bacteria infecting the burn wound, rapid proliferation results in subcutaneous invasion and vascular dissemination. This process is associated with local ischemic necrosis within the burn wound, resulting in hemorrhagic discoloration of the subcutaneous tissue and granulation tissue. Frequently, small pitting lesions of the underlying viable tissue are visible.

Fungi and Viruses

Both fungal and viral burn wound infections have been described [10,11] but are extraordinarily rare. Invasive infection with fungi should be considered when a rapidly progressive change in the color and character of the burn wound is observed. The center of this rapidly expanding lesion usually appears infarcted and is surrounded by an area of inflammation characterized by purplish discoloration. The patient usually exhibits an unexplained and rapidly progressive toxemia. Diagnosis may be confirmed by biopsy of the lesion and the demonstration of invasive broad-based hyphae by light microscopy. Significant invasive infection, with subsequent dissemination, has been reported with *Aspergillus, Mucor, Candida,* and *Geotrichum* species.

Burn wound infections with viruses are usually only recognized in reepithelializing second degree burns. Such infections are most commonly caused by herpes simplex, although rare infections with cytomegalovirus have also been reported. Infection classically manifests itself with the appearance of small vesicles, followed by loss of superficial epithelium. Secondary infection with bacteria frequently occurs two to three days later, resulting in a hemorrhagic crusted lesion. Fortunately, most viral infections are self-limited and spontaneously disappear over 7 to 10 days. However, occasional invasion has been reported with subsequent viremia and spread to distant organs.[11] At autopsy, characteristic ulcerated lesions may be found in the tracheobronchial tree, esophagus, lung, liver, and adrenal glands. Viral infections are most easily diagnosed by scraping cutaneous lesions and examining the superficial cells under the light microscope. Characteristic intranuclear inclusion bodies are often observed (Fig. 48-2). Systemic dissemination is difficult to confirm. It should be suspected in patients with superficial lesions who also exhibit fever, disorientation, and pulmonary lesions that cannot be ascribed to bacterial infection. Tracheobronchial infection may be confirmed by cytologic examination of mucus obtained via bronchoscopy. Vital staining of recovered cells (Fig. 48-3) often reveals intranuclear inclusion bodies. Careful examination of the peritonsillar tissues and the undersurface of the tongue may also reveal secondary viral lesions.

ALTERATIONS OF HOST DEFENSE

Local Changes

A characteristic of full-thickness burn injury is a progressive development of local ischemia. The capillary supply to the epithelium is interrupted at the time of the injury due to thermal coagulation. Subsequent loss of the

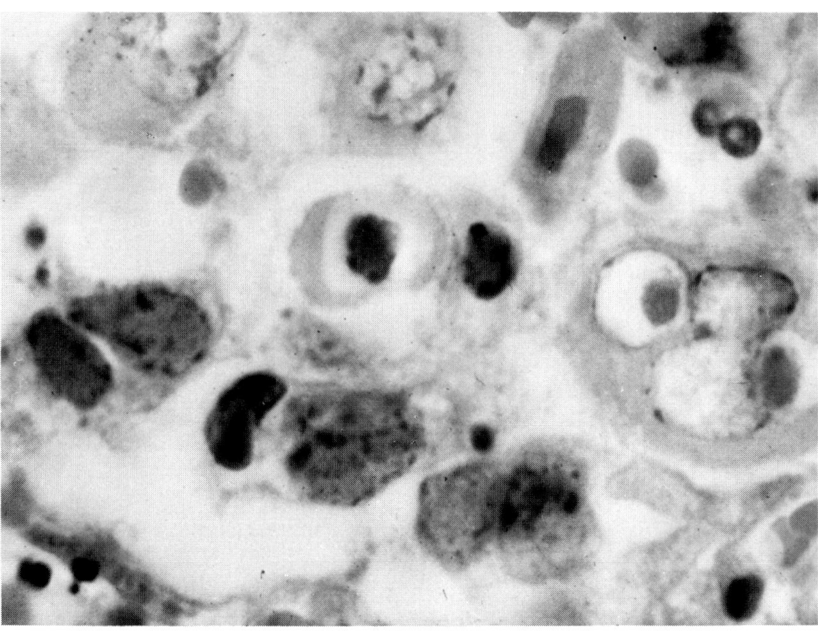

Fig. 48-2. **Cutaneous scrapings from vesicular lesion. The presence of intranuclear inclusion bodies confirms a viral etiology.**

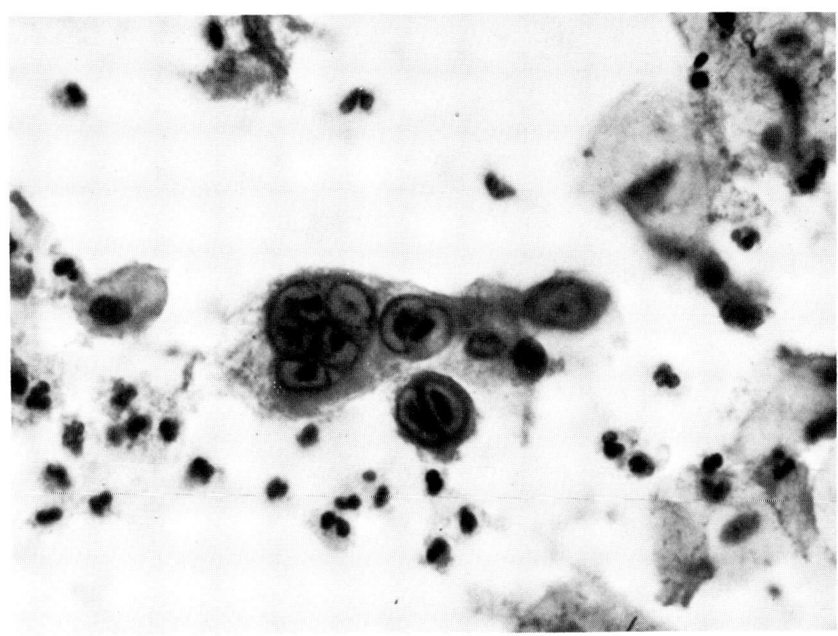

Fig. 48-3. **Cytologic examination of bronchial aspirate from a patient with pneumonic infiltrates and viral lesions of the skin. Intranuclear inclusion bodies are noted.**

vascular supply to the dermis and subcutaneous tissue results from progressive capillary thrombosis. By the fourth postburn day, the skin and superficial subcutaneous tissue are essentially avascular. New vascular ingrowth does not occur until the development of granulation tissue beneath the intact eschar. The development of granulation tissue may occur as early as two and a half weeks following the initial thermal insult but is often delayed until three and a half to four weeks in the elderly. Delayed fluid resuscitation may result in additional ischemic damage, since during hypovolemic states blood flow is normally diverted from the skin and subcutaneous tissue to maintain flow to vital organs.

Thus, full-thickness burn injury remains relatively avascular for approximately three weeks. Not only does the intact, nonviable tissue support bacterial growth, but the lack of vascular perfusion greatly impedes many of the host defense mechanisms. The delivery of phagocytes to the wound is delayed, and systemically administered antibiotics rarely reach the source of infection in sufficiently high concentrations to be effective as bactericidal agents.

Chemotaxis

There is a serious defect in leukocyte chemotaxis following burn injury. Utilizing modifications of the Boyden technique, leukocyte migration toward casein-serum, C5a, and bacterial chemotactic factor are all found to be seriously depressed. Warden et al [12,13] have shown that leukocyte chemotaxis is inversely correlated with clinical status and is predictive of ultimate survival. Those patients with recovery of leukocyte chemotaxis survive, whereas those in whom chemotactic recovery is not observed usually die of septic complications. Altman et al [14] described similar changes in chemotactic activity of monocytes recovered from burn plasma. Patients with burns involving less than 20 percent of the total body surface had normal monocyte chemotaxis, while monocytes from patients with burns over greater than 20 percent of the total body surface area had depressed activity. Patients with burns of greater than 40 percent of the total body surface showed an increasing depression of monocyte chemotaxis, reaching a nadir at approximately day 45. Thereafter, there was gradual return of chemotactic function in survivors.

Several defects have been identified that result in depressed chemotactic activity. Warden et al [13] and Fikrig et al [15] have confirmed intrinsic leukocytic abnormalities in cells recovered from the serum of burn patients. Warden has also demonstrated that two of the more commonly used topical chemotherapeutic agents, silver sulfadiazine and mafenide acetate, also suppress polymorphonuclear leukocyte chemotaxis. Significant serum concentrations of mafenide acetate and sulfadiazine are observed following the topical use of these agents, which presumably could contribute to the observed depression in chemotactic response. Altman et al [14] have identified a cell-directed chemotactic inhibitor that is present in the serum of patients with depressed monocyte chemotaxis. The inhibitor appears to be a protein (molecular weight 15,000–20,000). It has the capability of inhibiting the chemotactic function of normal monocytes from unburned individuals. Majeski et al [16] have shown that other antibiotics may alter serum chemotactic function. Tetracycline, ampicillin, and erythromycin inhibit the chemotactic responsiveness of neutrophils. On the other hand, high concentrations of chloramphenicol in the plasma showed a synergistic effect and appeared to enhance chemotactic responsiveness.

Phagocytosis

No consistent defect in neutrophil phagocytic activity has been noted following burn injury. Studies of granulocyte kinetics in the burned mouse [17] have suggested that tritiated thymidine uptake in bone marrow tissue is depressed by up to 50 percent during the first few hours after burn, but that the initial suppression of cellular synthesis is quickly overcome. Leukocytosis is observed during the first few days after burn and reflects a rapid release of marrow granulocyte reserves, resulting in temporary marrow exhaustion. The absolute number of granulocytic phagocytes is decreased from the third day to the seventh day postburn until cells are again available to the organism from the recovered bone marrow.

Phagocytic activity of the reticuloendothelial system appears to be depressed in animal models. DiMaio et al [18] showed depressed clearance of infused *Salmonella* in a 10 percent rat burn model. Depression of reticuloendothelial system function was evident 12 hours after burning and persisted until the second postburn day even though the burn model utilized was relatively nonstressful.

Neutrophil Function

Neutrophil bactericidal capacity is depressed after burn injury. Although phagocytosis is normal, intracellular killing is depressed. Cole et al [19] have suggested that there are defects in lysosomal enzyme levels (beta glucuronidase, lysozyme, and myeloperoxidase), and Curreri et al [20] have suggested that there are defects in the production of hydrogen peroxide and superoxide. In vitro oxygen consumption of neutrophils harvested from burn patients is significantly depressed when compared to cells harvested from unburned controls.[21] This observation is of particular interest because cells from other organs in the burned individual usually exhibit normal or increased oxygen consumption consistent with the hypermetabolic state of the thermally injured patient. However, no correlation has yet been shown between oxygen consumption and neutrophil bactericidal capability.

Alveolar Macrophages

Dressler et al [22] and Harmon et al [23] have emphasized the role of the pulmonary alveolar macrophage as a primary antibacterial defense of the lung. These investigators have documented increasing phagocytic ability of the alveolar macrophages for up to six days following a cutaneous burn. However, the activation of the alveolar macrophage did not occur in animals with infected burn wounds, and these animals exhibited little resistance to pulmonary infection when exposed to a standard bacterial aerosol challenge of *P. aeruginosa.* When parabiotic pairs of rats were studied and one of the rats was subjected to a 20 percent body surface burn, the number of alveolar macrophages, the percent of macrophage activation, and the phagocytic and intracellular killing capability of the macrophages were significantly increased in both the burned and unburned members of the parabiotic pairs. Alveolar macrophage function was unchanged when neither of the parabiotic members was burned or when one of the parabiotic members was sham-burned. These results suggested that there was a humoral or a cellular agent produced secondary to the cutaneous burn that activated alveolar macrophage function.

Immunoglobulin and Complement

Several reports have suggested that plasma immunoglobulin levels decrease following thermal injury as a result of extensive loss of plasma proteins into the burn wound. The concentration of immunoglobulin reaches its lowest level at two to five days following thermal injury. However, both burn patients and experimental animals retain the ability to produce antibodies following antigenic challenge.

The concentration of complement also decreases immediately after burn but returns to normal within a few days. The magnitude and length of depression appears related to the size of the burn. After two to three days, complement titer again rises and may remain elevated as long as five weeks. Although Bjornson et al [24,25] have demonstrated specific defects in a number of complement factors both prior to and during septic episodes in burn patients, in only one case could they demonstrate a decrease of opsonic capacity of the patient's own serum for the patient's infecting microorganism. These investigators have suggested that the classic complementary pathway is activated during septicemia in burn patients and that activation of this pathway occurs preferentially as a result of inhibition of the alternative pathway. Others have suggested that there is not a strong correlation between the incidence of sepsis and the level of serum complement.[26] However, there seems to be an inverse relationship between the severity of the burn trauma and the subsequent magnitude and rate of recovery of complement activity following the initial burn injury.

Lymphocyte Function

Many investigators have suggested that burn injury is associated with impairment of lymphocyte function, although the precise mechanisms are not completely understood. Delayed allograft rejection, altered rosette-forming ability, decreased delayed hypersensitivity, and diminished stimulative and responsive capacity of lymphocytes in mixed lymphocyte culture reactions have been reported in both thermally injured patients and in burned animal models.[27-30] No correlation has been repetitively demonstrated between the diminished lymphocyte function and total lymphocyte concentration, age of patients, nutritional state, number of operative procedures under general anesthesia, or cortisol levels. On the other hand, suppression of normal peripheral blood lymphocytes to phytohemagglutinin by serum from burned patients has been correlated with the magnitude of burn injury, as well as the presence of significant clinical sepsis.[31]

Although prolonged allograft survival in burned animals can be demonstrated up to three weeks following thermal injury, early excision of the burn wound with immediate application of isograft to the resulting defect does not restore cell-mediated immunity.[32] These observations suggest that the open wound is not solely responsible for toxic serum factors that alter lymphocyte function. A polypeptide subfraction (less than 10,000 daltons) with the ability to suppress the response of normal lymphocytes to phytohemagglutinin has been demonstrated in sera from burned patients.[33] The origin of these immunosuppressive peptides remains unknown.

Miller and Trunkey [34] have studied the effect of moderate burn injury (10 percent total body surface scald burn) on de novo antibody synthesis by lymphocytes in vitro. The number of antibody-forming cells generated by leukocytes from burned animals was reduced by 80 percent between the third and sixteenth postburn day when compared to leukocytes from normal mice. Addition of accessory cell (A) and T cell factors to the culture system restored antibody-forming cell capacity, suggesting that B cell integrity remains intact and that the burn-induced defect resides in either the T or the A leukocyte subpopulation.

One group of investigators has observed partial restoration of lymphocyte function following burn injury by the in vitro addition of thymosin.[35] Enhanced rosette-forming capacity and increased responsiveness to PPD, mumps antigen, streptokinase-streptodornase, and tetanus toxoid were noted following the addition of thymosin. However, both mixed lymphocyte culture response and stimulation remained significantly decreased whether or not thymosin was included in the in vitro assay.

ENVIRONMENTAL CONSIDERATIONS IN BURN WOUND SEPSIS

In general, surgical treatment of traumatic injury includes early debridement of nonviable tissue and immediate closure of the wound. Attempts to accomplish these goals in the severely burned patient have been frustrated in the past because of the massive amount of blood loss associated with early burn wound excision, a high perioperative mortality, and the inability to obtain wound closure when limited autologous skin donor sites are available. Therefore, most surgeons still attempt to control bacterial proliferation within the burn wound until spontaneous separation of eschar occurs, thereby allowing staged autografting of a granulating bed. Wounds treated in this manner eventually become colonized with a predominant strain of bacteria that liberates protease and collagenase, allowing separation of nonviable from viable tissue. However, when bacterial proliferation remains unchecked prior to the development of relatively resistant granulation tissue beneath the burn eschar, invasion of subcutaneous fat and capillaries may result in burn wound sepsis.

Equally important is the strain of colonizing bacteria, since particularly virulent strains of opportunistic organisms are occasionally identified in all burn specialty units. In addition, less virulent but antibiotic-resistant organisms may appear in any hospital environment following prolonged use of a single topical chemotherapeutic agent or repetitive use of a limited group of potent systemic antibiotics. Once an opportunistic organism appears, cross-contamination between patients becomes a hazard, since the organism is frequently harbored by patients with smaller burns (and therefore at little risk), preventing eradication of the bacterial strain from the unit.

Although it has been clearly demonstrated that most (70 to 90 percent) burn wounds are autocontaminated from the patient's own gastrointestinal or respiratory tract, Burke et al [36] have suggested that significant infection is present in only 39 percent of such wounds, as compared to 65 percent of wounds colonized by cross-contaminants.

Several investigators [37-39] have attempted to reduce the rate of cross-contamination by imposing physical barriers between patients. Patients can be isolated within a relatively sterile environment, either by means of bacterially controlled nursing units (eg, the life island) or laminar airflow systems. Advantages of such systems include the ability to better regulate environmental temperature and humidity. However, such physical barriers often also impose barriers to surveillance by medical personnel and increase psychologic distress for the patient as a result of isolation. Furthermore, the efficacy of these systems in the prevention of fatal burn sepsis has never been proved by randomized clinical trial. Because installation is extraordinarily expensive, the cost effectiveness of their routine use remains questionable. Similar survival results and rates of cross-contamination are reported from units utilizing careful isolation protocols that require the use of gloves, gowns, hats, and masks when attending patients, together with minimal opportunities for direct patient contact in central treatment facilities (such as in the hydrotherapy or physical therapy areas).

Jarrett et al [40-42] have reported delayed wound colonization, a decreased incidence of burn wound sepsis, and a diminished incidence of systemic infection when burned patients were given a prophylactic oral antibiotic regimen (neomycin-erythromycin-nystatin) and also treated within a laminar flow environment. Staphylococcal or fungal overgrowth of the gastrointestinal tract was not observed in this relatively small study of 20 patients. The use of a prophylactic oral antibiotic program in the absence of a laminar flow environment does not reduce the incidence of severe infections. In addition, the prophylactic administration of oral antibiotics has not yet been shown to result in improved survival.

MONITORING THE BURN WOUND

Clinical signs of burn wound sepsis usually appear late and often precede death by only a few days. Clinical symptoms usually occur too late to effect reversal of progressive sepsis. Marvin et al [43] were unable to show any correlation between the appearance of one or two clinical signs of sepsis and subsequent development of invasive burn wound infection. Only when three or more clinical signs of sepsis appeared simultaneously was a significant correlation with bacterial invasion of the burn wound documented. The most valuable clinical sign of burn wound sepsis is the sudden appearance of confusion or disorientation. Other clinical expressions of burn wound sepsis include tachycardia, tachypnea, hypothermia, paralytic ileus, thrombocytopenia, leukopenia, and hypotension.

Quantitative biopsy cultures of the burn wound, performed at 48-hour intervals, allow constant monitoring of the burn wound with regard to bacterial proliferation. Quantitation of bacterial concentration has proved to be the only reliable means of predicting incipient burn wound sepsis, allowing therapeutic intervention seven to nine days prior to systemic bacterial dissemination. Loebl et al [44,45] have described methods for performing quantitative burn wound biopsy cultures in detail. An even more rapid method is described in Chapter 22. In brief, surface bacteria, which are usually heterogeneous and reflect exposure to bacterial fallout from the immediate environment, are eliminated by local sterilization by the application of 70 percent alcohol. Full-thickness biopsies measuring 5 × 10 mm are then taken from representative areas of full-thickness injury. The tissue is weighed, homogenized, and then serially diluted prior to incubation on blood agar plates. At 24 hours, colony counts are performed, and concentrations of organisms can be calculated by multiplying the colony count by the number of serial dilutions and dividing the result by the weight of the tissue. Bacterial concentrations of 10^5 per gm of tissue or greater during the first three weeks postburn are indicative of incipient burn wound sepsis. Failure to intercede at this time with alternative therapy often is associated with progressive septicemia and the appearance of metastatic abscesses in multiple organs.

TREATMENT

PROPHYLAXIS AND TREATMENT OF BURN WOUND SEPSIS

Proliferation of microorganisms within the burn wound must be controlled if burn wound sepsis is to be avoided. Ideally, all nonviable tissue should be sharply excised within 48 hours of injury (after gaining hemodynamic stability but before wound colonization) and the wound closed by application of autograft or a synthetic skin substitute. However, until recently, such aggressive surgical approaches have been associated with an increased mortality and morbidity. Failure was attributed to massive intraoperative hemorrhage (often associated with cardiac arrhythmia or organ ischemia) as well as to the inability to achieve wound coverage because of limited donor sites and poor graft acceptance on recipient sites of subcutaneous fat. Furthermore, it became increasingly clear that *all* confluent burned areas had to be excised if secondary infection of grafts was to be avoided.

In the past several years, many investigators [46-49] have reexamined early excision as a mode for decreasing hospitalization time and minimizing the development of hypertrophic scar formation. Tangential excision of deep second degree burns allows salvage of viable deep dermis that may be immediately grafted, with greater expectation of complete graft survival. When full-thickness burn injury is present, excision of all the eschar and subcutaneous tissue to deep fascia also has been associated with improved graft acceptance. However, excisional therapy remains a stressful procedure that must be performed sequentially during the first postoperative week to gain any potential immediate advantage.

During this same period, the patient will exhibit profound hemodynamic, endocrinologic, metabolic, and respiratory alterations that often result in clinical instability. Therefore, early excisional therapy has been pursued primarily by major burn centers with a sufficiently large population of patients to justify a specialized burn intensive care facility. Major commitments are also required from anesthesiology, blood bank, respiratory therapy, and physical therapy departments to maximize patient perioperative survival and minimize postoperative morbidity. In addition, the availability of banked human skin (allograft) is required to achieve wound closure when insufficient donor sites are present. Although early excisional therapy has been associated with a decreased incidence of burn wound infection and postburn disability, there has been no convincing evidence that survival is greatly enhanced. Death from postoperative pulmonary infection still occurs.

Conventional therapy of the burn wound is directed at controlling the rate of bacterial proliferation in the burn until a sufficient bed of granulation tissue has developed beneath the eschar. The eschar is then debrided as it spontaneously separates, and split-thickness skin grafts are used to close the wound between the third and fifth postburn weeks. Partial-thickness burns are allowed to reepithelialize, a process which requires 10 to 30 days depending on the depth of injury.

Several topical chemotherapeutic agents are currently available that possess bacteriostatic properties and successfully retard rampant bacterial proliferation when used prophylactically. The successful use of these agents requires knowledge of their limitations and side effects. The four most commonly used preparations are described below.

Sodium mafenide (Sulfamyalon) cream exhibits bacteriostatic properties toward a wide spectrum of microorganisms.[50,51] It readily penetrates the eschar and, thus, is effective in treating wounds that are already colonized. The agent is applied twice a day and may be used without overlying dressings, which enhances the ability of therapists to maintain joint motion. The principal disadvantages of mafenide include cutaneous allergy (5 percent), pain on application (secondary to hypertonicity) [52] and profound inhibition of carbonic anhydrase activity. The last property often is associated with excessive urinary excretion of bicarbonate and compensatory hyperventilation. In the presence of pulmonary dysfunction, the rapid development of metabolic acidosis may be observed.

Silver nitrate solution (0.5 percent) is also effective against a wide spectrum of surface microorganisms. This agent is less favored because the active component, ie, the silver ion, does not penetrate the eschar readily so that the preparation is less effective after colonization has occurred. Its use, therefore, is limited to initial treatment of the wound, where it establishes a bacteriostatic barrier preventing bacterial access to the deep eschar. Significant side effects include hyponatremia, hypochloremia, and methemoglobinemia. Furthermore, the agent is applied within thick gauze dressings that must be kept saturated, thereby inhibiting efforts to maintain joint function. Increased numbers of nursing personnel are required to achieve dressing changes. Finally, although the preparation itself is relatively inexpensive, discoloration of linen, uniforms, and flooring requires frequent replacement and additional housekeeping, which significantly increases the total cost associated with its use.

Silver sulfadiazine (1 percent) (Silvadine) cream possesses most of the desirable features of sodium mafenide and few of the disadvantages.[53] It may be used without occlusive dressings, and the sulfadiazine readily penetrates the eschar. In contrast to mafenide, silver sulfadiazine is soothing on application. Between 3 percent and 5 percent of patients treated with silver sulfadiazine develop acute leukopenia, which spontaneously disappears if application of the cream is discontinued.[54,55] Cutaneous allergy is infrequently observed and may usually be alleviated by oral administration of antihistamines. Prolonged use occasionally is associated with the development of contact dermatitis.

Povidone-iodine (Betadine) foam exhibits bactericidal activity toward gram-positive bacteria, most gram-negative bacteria, and fungi. Its use does not require dressings. Excessive iodine absorption with the development of severe metabolic acidosis has been infrequently reported, and excessive drying of the wound is sometimes noted after application.[56,57]

Should bacterial concentration in the eschar increase by greater than 100-fold within 48 hours, or should the absolute concentration exceed 100,000 organisms per gm of tissue within the first 15 postburn days, it must be assumed that control of bacterial proliferation has been lost. A different topical chemotherapeutic agent should be selected. If systemic signs of septicemia are present, parenteral antibiotics should be administered to reduce the incidence of distant bloodborne infections. The half-lives of several antibiotics are considerably shortened in burned patients. Therefore, the dose of antibiotic may have to be increased to achieve effective serum concentrations.[58,59]

Low concentrations of antibiotics in eschar following parenteral administration are probably due to the relative avascularity of full-thickness burns.[60] Subeschar administration of appropriate antibiotics by clysis in patients with incipient burn wound sepsis ($>10^5$ organisms per gm of tissue) often reduces bacterial colonization to safer levels and has markedly reduced mortality even when administered to children with established burn wound sepsis.

Once eschar separation has occurred, further reduction of bacterial colonization within the granulation tissue may be accomplished by the temporary application of porcine xenograft or human allograft until definitive closure with autograft is performed. Similarly, bacterial colonization of partial-thickness burns may be prevented by immediate (first 24 hours) application of porcine xenograft or synthetic, bacteria-impervious polymers (such as the Hydron burn dressing), providing that firm adherence to the wound is obtained.

Treatment of Fungal and Viral Infections

Fungal infections within the burn wound are often multicentric in origin and rapidly spread along fascial planes.[61] After the fungus gains access to the bloodstream, distant metastases to the lung, brain, and kidneys are frequently observed. Because the lesion is characterized by avascular necrosis, systemic or topical antifungal agents do not, by themselves, eradicate the infection. Survival is dependent on aggressive wide excision of lesions on the trunk or head and proximal amputation of extremities that exhibit lesions extending to fascia. Reinspection of excisional sites at 48-hour intervals is mandatory, since repetitive excision may prove life saving if the lesion recurs at the margins.

Yeast infections, primarily *Candida albicans*, of the burn wound are not unusual in children and the elderly. They may be suspected on inspection of the wound whenever a layer of white necrotic tissue of cottage cheese consistency is identified beneath the eschar during debridement. The diagnosis is confirmed by Gram stain and conventional culture techniques. *Candida* is rarely invasive through the burn wound. Access to the bloodstream most frequently occurs via the lungs, the gastrointestinal tract, or along an intravenous catheter. Wound infections with *Candida* may be easily controlled by the addition of nystatin to one of the topical antibacterial creams.

Infections of the burn wound caused by viruses require no specific therapy, since they are usually self-limited. General nutritional support should be emphasized, and secondary bacterial infection of the cutaneous lesions may be treated with the topical chemotherapeutic agents discussed previously. If systemic infection is proved, parenteral administration of the newer antiviral agents should be considered (Chapter 18).

TREATMENT OF SUPPURATIVE THROMBOPHLEBITIS

When the diagnosis of suppurative thrombophlebitis within a peripheral vein is confirmed by venotomy, immediate operative excision of the vein is mandatory. Although only a small length of the vein may reveal macroscopic features of inflammation, the entire vein must be removed because skip areas, ie, normal appearing vessel between two infected portions of vein, occur. The resulting subcutaneous bed is left open and packed with one of the topical antibacterial chemotherapeutic agents. After three to five days, the wound may be covered with a porcine graft or allograft, followed by later application of autogenous skin graft, or the wound may be secondarily closed by loosely reapproximating skin edges with stainless steel wire sutures.

TREATMENT OF SUPPURATIVE CHONDRITIS

Infected cartilage must be aggressively excised to prevent local extension to underlying bone and subsequent introduction of bacteria into the bloodstream. Small areas of chondritis within the ear may be treated by partial chondrectomy. A small anterior window is made over the infected cartilage, which is then removed by sharp dissection or use of a curette. After the development of granulation tissue over the resulting defect, split-thickness skin may be applied to accomplish closure.

More extensive suppurative chondritis of the ear mandates complete excision of the cartilagenous substructure to prevent extension to the underlying mastoid. The ear is bivalved via an incision along the edge of the helix, and all of the infected cartilage between the anterior and posterior flaps is removed. The two flaps are then loosely approximated over a drain, and the ear is covered with a thick dressing, which avoids local pressure to the remaining skin flaps. Late reconstruction of the ear may be required when the deformed, unsupported external ear is not covered by hair.

Exposed cartilage of joints almost always becomes secondarily infected, and late destruction of the joint surface followed by spontaneous arthrodesis of the joint commonly occurs. Disability is dependent on the position of the opposing bones following arthrodesis. Therefore, when joint surfaces are exposed, timely operative excision of the infected cartilage, followed by fixation of the joint in the desired position, is indicated. Either Kirschner wires or Steinman pins may be used for fixation. In general, two wires should cross the obliterated joint space to prevent rotational deformity of the distal bone.

BIBLIOGRAPHY

Artz CP, Moncrief JA, Pruitt BA Jr (eds): Burns: A Team Approach. Philadelphia, Saunders, 1979.

REFERENCES

PATHOGENISIS

1. Bull JP, Squire JR: A study of mortality in a burn unit. Ann Surg 130:160,1949.
2. Curreri PW, Luterman A, Braun DW Jr, Shires GT: Burn injury: Analysis of survival and hospitalization time of 937 consecutive patients. Ann Surg, 192:472, 1980.
3. Lindberg RB, Moncrief JA, Mason AD Jr: Control of experimental and clinical burn wound sepsis by topical application of sulfamyalon compounds. Ann NY Acad Sci 150:950, 1968.
4. Pruitt BA Jr, DiVincenti FC, Mason AD Jr, Foley FD, Flemma RJ: The occurrence and significance of pneumonia and other pulmonary complications in burned patients: Comparison of conventional and topical treatments. J Trauma 10:519, 1970.
5. Stein JM, Pruitt BA Jr: Suppurative thrombophlebitis: A lethal iatrogenic disease. N Engl J Med 282:1452, 1970.
6. Baskin TW, Rosenthal A, Pruitt BA: Acute bacterial endocarditis: A silent source of sepsis in the burn patient. Ann Surg 184:618, 1976.
7. Overturf GD, Zawacki BE, Wilkins J: Emergence of resistance to amikacin during treatment of burn wounds: The role of antimicrobial susceptibility testing. Surgery 79:224, 1976.
8. Gayle WE Jr, Mayhall CG, Lamb VA, Apollo E, Haynes BW Jr: Resistant *Enterobacter cloacae* in a burn center: The ineffectiveness of silver sulfadiazine. J Trauma 18:317, 1978.
9. Curreri PW, Bruck HM, Lindberg RB, Mason AD Jr, Pruitt BA Jr: *Providencia stuartii* sepsis: A new challenge in the treatment of thermal injury. Ann Surg 177:133, 1973.
10. Bruck HM, Nash G, Foley D, Pruitt BA Jr: Opportunistic fungal infection of the burn wound with *Phycomycetes* and *Aspergillus*. Arch Surg 102:476, 1971.
11. Foley FD, Nash G: Herpesvirus infection in burned patients. N Engl J Med 282:652, 1970.
12. Warden GD, Mason AD Jr, Pruitt BA Jr: Evaluation of leukocyte chemotaxis in vitro in thermally injured patients. J Clin Invest 54:1001, 1974.
13. Warden GD, Mason AD Jr, Pruitt BA: Suppression of leukocyte chemotaxis in vitro by chemotherapeutic agents used in the management of thermal injuries. Ann Surg 181:363, 1975.
14. Altman LC, Klebanoff SJ, Curreri PW: Abnormalities of monocyte chemotaxis following thermal injury. J Surg Res 22:616, 1977.
15. Fikrig SM, Karl SC, Suntharalingam K: Neutrophil chemotaxis in patients with burns. Ann Surg 186:746, 1977.
16. Majeski JA, McClellan MA, Alexander JW: Evaluation of leukocyte chemotactic response in the presence of antibiotics. Surg Forum 26:83, 1975.
17. Asko-Seljavaara S: Granulocyte kinetics in burned mice: Inhibition of granulocyte growth studied in vivo and in vitro. Scand J Plast Reconstr Surg 8:185, 1974.
18. DiMaio A, DiMaio D, Jacques L: Phagocytosis in experimental burns. J Surg Res 21:437, 1976.
19. Cole WQ, Cook JJ, Grogan JB: In vitro neutrophil function and lysosomal enzyme levels in patients with sepsis. Surg Forum 26:79, 1975.
20. Curreri PW, Heck EL, Browne L, Baxter CR: Stimulated nitroblue tetrazolium test to assess neutrophil antibacterial function: Prediction of wound sepsis in burned patients. Surgery 74:6, 1973.
21. Heck EL, Browne L, Curreri PW, Baxter CR: Evaluation of leukocyte function in burned individuals by in vitro oxygen consumption. J Trauma 15:486, 1975.
22. Dressler DP, Skornik WA: Alveolar macrophage in the burned rat. J Trauma 14:1036, 1974.
23. Harmon JW, Skornik WA, McDonald J, Dressler DP: Pulmonary bacterial defense: Effect of burn wound on transfer of alveolar macrophage activation in rats by parabiosis. Am J Surg 131:447, 1976.
24. Bjornson AB, Altemeier WA, Bjornson HS, Tang T, Iserson ML: Host defense against opportunist microorganisms following trauma. I. Studies to determine the association between changes in humoral components of host defense and septicemia in burned patients. Ann Surg 188:93, 1978.
25. Bjornson AB, Alexander WJ: Opsonic activity of sera from patients after thermal injury. Surg Forum 24:44, 1973.
26. Dhennin C, Pinon G, Greco JM: Alterations of complement system following thermal injury: Use in estimation of vital prognosis. J Trauma 18:129, 1978.
27. Howard RJ, Simmons, RL: Acquired immunologic deficiencies after trauma and surgical procedures. Surg Gynecol Obstet 39:771, 1974.
28. Rapaport FT, Converse JM, Horn L, Ballantyne DL Jr, Mulholland JH: Altered reactivity to skin homografts in severe thermal injury. Ann Surg 159:390, 1964.
29. Chambler K, Batchelor JR: Influence of defined incompatabilities and area of burn on skin-homograft survival in burned subjects. Lancet 1:16, 1969.
30. Munster AM, Eurenius K, Katz RM, Canales L, Foley FD, Mortensen RF: Cell-mediated immunity after thermal injury. Ann Surg 177:139, 1973.
31. Neilan BA, Taddeini L, Strate RG: T-lymphocyte rosette formation after major burns. JAMA 238:493, 1977.
32. Fried DA, Munster AM: Does immunosuppression by thermal injury depend on the continued presence of the burn wound? J Trauma 15:483, 1975.
33. Constantian MB: Association of sepsis with an immunosuppressive polypeptide in the serum of burn patients. Ann Surg 188:209, 1978.
34. Miller CL, Trunkey DD: Thermal injury: Defects in immune response induction. J Surg Res 22:621, 1977.
35. Ishizawa S, Sakai H, Sarles HE, Larson DL, Daniels JC: Effect of thymosin on T-lymphocyte functions in patients with acute thermal burns. J Trauma 18:48, 1978.

36. Burke JF, Quinby WC, Bondoc CC, Sheehy EM, Moreno HC: The contribution of a bacterially isolated environment to the prevention of infection in seriously burned patients. Ann Surg 186:377, 1977.

PREVENTION AND TREATMENT

37. Nance FC: Absolute barrier isolation in the treatment of experimental burn wound sepsis. J Surg Res 10:33, 1970.
38. MacMillan BG, Edmonds P, Hummel RP, Maley MP: Epidemiology of *Pseudomonas* in a burn intensive care unit. J Trauma 13:627, 1973.
39. Demling RH, Perea A, Maly J, Moylan JA, Jarrett F, Balish E: The use of a laminar airflow isolation system for the treatment of major burns. Am J Surg 136:375, 1978.
40. Jarrett F, Chan CK, Balish E, Moylan JA: Antibiotic bowel preparation and burn wound colonization. Surg Forum 27:67, 1976.
41. Jarrett F, Balish E, Moylan JA: The use of oral antibiotic suppression for control of infections in patients with thermal injuries. J Surg Res 24:339, 1978.
42. Jarrett F, Balish E, Moylan J, Ellerbe S: Clinical experience with prophylactic antibiotic bowel suppression in burn patients. Surgery 83:523, 1978.
43. Marvin JA, Heck EL, Loebl EC, Curreri PW, Baxter CR: Usefulness of blood cultures in confirming septic complications in burn patients: Evaluation of a new culture method. J Trauma 15:657, 1975.
44. Loebl EC, Marvin JA, Heck EL, Curreri PW, Baxter CR: The use of quantitative biopsy cultures in bacteriologic monitoring of burn patients. J Surg Res 16:1, 1974.
45. Loebl EC, Marvin JA, Heck EL, Curreri PW, Baxter CR: The method of quantitative burn-wound biopsy cultures and its routine use in the care of the burned patient. Am J Clin Pathol 61:20, 1974.
46. Levine BA, Sirinek KR, Pruitt BA Jr: Wound excision to fascia in burn patients. Arch Surg 113:403, 1978.
47. Malfeyt GAM: Burns of the dorsum of the hand treated by tangential excision. Br J Plast Surg 29:78, 1976.
48. Burke JF, Quinby WC, Bondoc CC: Primary excision and prompt grafting as routine therapy for the treatment of thermal burns in children. Surg Clin North Am 56:477, 1976.
49. Levine NS, Salisbury RE, Mason AD Jr: The effect of early surgical excision and homografting on survival of burned rats and of intraperitoneally infected burned rats. Plast Reconstr Surg 56:423, 1975.
50. Moncrief JA: Topical therapy for control of bacteria in the burn wound. World J Surg 2:151, 1978.
51. Shuck JM, Thorne LW, Cooper CG: Mafenide acetate solution dressings: An adjunct in burn wound care. J Trauma 15:595, 1975.
52. Harrison HN, Shuck JM, Caldwell E: Studies of the pain produced by mafenide acetate preparations in burns. Arch Surg 110:1446, 1975.
53. Ballin JC: Evaluation of a new topical agent for burn therapy. JAMA 230:1184, 1974.
54. Kiker RG, Carvajal HF, Mlcak RP, Larson DL: A controlled study of the effects of silver sulfadiazine on white blood cell counts in burned children. J Trauma 17:835, 1977.
55. Chan CK, Jarrett F, Moylan JA: Acute leukopenia as an allergic reaction to silver sulfadiazine in burn patients. J Trauma 16:395, 1976.
56. Lavelle KJ, Doedens DJ, Kleit SA, Forney RB: Iodine absorption in burn patients treated topically with povidone-iodine. Clin Pharmacol Ther 17:355, 1975.
57. Pietsch J, Meakins JL: Complications of povidone-iodine absorption in topically treated burn patients. Lancet 2:207, 1976.
58. Glew RH, Moellering RC, Burke JF: Gentamicin dosage in children with extensive burns. J Trauma 16:819, 1976.
59. Zaske DE, Sawchuk RJ, Gerding DN, Strate RG: Increased dosage requirements of gentamicin in burn patients. J Trauma 16:824, 1976.
60. Curreri PW, Marvin JA: Advances in the clinical care of burned patients. West J Med 123:275, 1975.
61. Salisbury RE, Silverstein P, Goodwin MN: Upper extremity fungal invasions secondary to large burns. Plast Reconstr Surg 54:654, 1974.

Index